Conn's Current Therapy 1990

LATEST APPROVED METHODS OF TREATMENT
FOR THE PRACTICING PHYSICIAN

Edited by ROBERT E. RAKEL, M.D.

Chairman, Department of Family Medicine
Associate Dean for Academic and Clinical Affairs
Baylor College of Medicine, Houston, Texas

W.B. SAUNDERS COMPANY
Harcourt Brace Jovanovich, Inc.

Philadelphia
London   Toronto   Montreal   Sydney   Tokyo

Conn's **Current Therapy**

1990

W. B. SAUNDERS COMPANY
Harcourt Brace Jovanovich, Inc.

The Curtis Center
Independence Square West
Philadelphia, PA 19106

Library of Congress Cataloging-in-Publication Data

Current therapy; latest approved methods of treatment for the practicing physician. 1949–

v. 28 cm. annual.

Editors: 1949–   H. F. Conn and others.

1. Therapeutics.   2. Therapeutics, Surgical.
    3. Medicine—Practice.   I. Conn, Howard Franklin,
    1908–1982 ed.

RM101.C87   616.058   49–8328 rev*

ISBN 0–7216–2582–7

Editor: John Dyson
Developmental Editor: Kathleen McCullough
Designer: Ellen Bodner
Production Manager: Peter Faber
Manuscript Editor: Judith Gandy
Illustration Coordinator: Lisa Lambert
Indexer: Dennis Dolan
Cover Designer: Ellen Bodner

Conn's Current Therapy 1990   ISBN 0–7216–2582–7

Last digit is the print number: 9   8   7   6   5   4   3   2   1

Contributors

JAMES M. ADAMS, M.D.

Associate Professor of Clinical Pediatrics, Baylor College of Medicine; Director, Neonatal Intensive Care Unit and Transport, Texas Children's Hospital; Director, Neonatal Intensive Care Unit, Women's Hospital of Texas; Neonatologist, Methodist Hospital and Lyndon B. Johnson Hospital, Houston, Texas
Resuscitation and Stabilization of the Newborn

AUGUSTO AGUIRRE, M.D.

Clinical Assistant Professor of Pathology, Ohio State University College of Medicine; Senior Attending Staff, Department of Pathology, Riverside Methodist Hospitals, Columbus, Ohio
Tetanus

WILLIAM L. ALBRITTON, M.D., PH.D.

Professor and Head, Department of Microbiology, University of Saskatchewan; Medical Staff, University Hospital; Consulting Staff, St. Paul's Hospital and City Hospital, Saskatoon, Saskatchewan, Canada
Chancroid

JOAQUIN S. ALDRETE, M.D.

Professor and Vice Chairman, Department of Surgery, University of Alabama at Birmingham; Attending Surgeon, University of Alabama Hospital and Veterans Administration Hospital, Birmingham, Alabama
Acute Pancreatitis

JACK ANSELL, M.D.

Professor of Medicine and Pathology, University of Massachusetts Medical School; Attending Physician, University of Massachusetts Hospital, Worcester, Massachusetts
Platelet-Mediated Bleeding Disorders

ANN M. ARVIN, M.D.

Associate Professor of Pediatrics, Stanford University School of Medicine; Clinical Staff, Stanford University Medical Center and Children's Hospital at Stanford, Stanford, California
Chickenpox (Varicella)

DEAN G. ASSIMOS, M.D.

Assistant Professor of Surgery (Urology), Bowman Gray School of Medicine, Winston-Salem, North Carolina
Renal Calculi

ROBERT L. ATMAR, M.D.

Fellow, Section of Infectious Diseases, Department of Medicine, Baylor College of Medicine, Houston, Texas
Bacteremia

THEODORE M. BAILEY, M.D., M.P.H.

Associate Pathologist and Medical Director, Section of Microbiology, Maine Medical Center, Portland, Maine
Trichinellosis

FRANK J. BAKER, II, M.D., M.B.A.

Attending Physician, MacNeal Hospital and Medical Center, Berwyn, Illinois
Narcotic Poisoning

MARK BALLOW, M.D.

Professor of Pediatrics, State University of New York at Buffalo School of Medicine; Chief, Allergy-Immunology Division, Department of Pediatrics, Children's Hospital of Buffalo, Buffalo, New York
Anaphylaxis and Serum Sickness

DENNIS F. BANDYK, M.D.

Associate Professor of Surgery, Medical College of Wisconsin; Chief, Vascular Surgery Section, Veterans Administration Medical Center, Milwaukee, Wisconsin
Deep Vein Thrombosis and Thrombophlebitis

ROBERT BARAN, M.D.

Head, Dermatologic Unit, Centre Hospitalier, Cannes, France
Diseases of the Nails

ROBERT P. BAUGHMAN, M.D.

Associate Professor of Medicine, University of Cincinnati College of Medicine; Attending Physician, University Hospital, Cincinnati, Ohio
Sarcoidosis

CAROL A. BELL, M.D.

Clinical Professor of Pathology, University of California, Irvine, College of Medicine, Irvine. Clinical Professor of Pathology, University Southern California School of Medicine, Los Angeles; Director, Clinical Laboratory, Brotman Medical Center, Culver City, California
Adverse Reactions to Blood Transfusion

EDWARD J. BENZ, JR., M.D.

Professor of Internal Medicine and Human Genetics, Chief, Hematology Section, Associate Chairman, Department of Internal Medicine, Yale University School of Medicine; Attending Physician and Chief, Hematology Service, Yale—New Haven Hospital, New Haven, Connecticut
Thalassemia

DANIEL E. BERGSAGEL, M.D., D.PHIL.

Professor of Medicine, Faculty of Medicine, University of Toronto; Chief of Medicine, Princess Margaret Hospital, Toronto, Ontario, Canada
Multiple Myeloma

GERSON C. BERNHARD, M.D.

Clinical Professor of Medicine, Medical College of Wisconsin; Chairman, Division of Rheumatology, Columbia Hospital; Medical Director, Midwest Arthritis Treatment Center, Columbia Hospital, Milwaukee, Wisconsin
Osteoarthritis

ROBERT F. BETTS, M.D.

Professor of Medicine, Infectious Diseases Unit, University of Rochester School of Medicine and Dentistry; Associate Physician, Strong Memorial Hospital, Rochester, New York
Influenza

STEVEN D. BIGLER, M.D.

Chairman, Department of Obstetrics and Gynecology, Utah Valley Regional Medical Center, Provo, Utah
Antepartum Care

GARY BIRNBAUM, M.D.

Professor of Neurology, University of Minnesota School of Medicine; Attending Neurologist and Director, Multiple Sclerosis Research and Treatment Center, University Hospital, Minneapolis, Minnesota
Multiple Sclerosis

JOHN F. BOHNSACK, M.D.

Assistant Professor of Pediatrics and Director, Section of Pediatric Rheumatology, Division of Clinical Immunology and Allergy, University of Utah College of Medicine, Salt Lake City, Utah
Rheumatic Fever

JACQUES A. BOLLEKENS, M.D.

Hematology Fellow, Yale University School of Medicine; Fellow in Internal Medicine, Yale–New Haven Hospital, New Haven, Connecticut
Thalassemia

PHILIP BONOMI, M.D.

Associate Professor of Medicine, Associate Director, Section of Medical Oncology, and Senior Attending Physician, Rush–Presbyterian–St. Luke's Hospital, Chicago, Illinois
Primary Lung Cancer

HARISIOS BOUDOULAS, M.D.

Professor of Medicine and Pharmacy, Division of Cardiology, Ohio State University College of Medicine; House Staff, Ohio State University Hospital, Columbus, Ohio
Mitral Valve Prolapse and the Mitral Valve Prolapse Syndrome

ALAN BREIER, M.D.

Chief, Outpatient Department, Maryland Psychiatric Research Center, Baltimore, Maryland
Schizophrenic Disorders

JAMES B. BRIDENSTINE, M.D.

Board Examiner, American Board of Cosmetic Surgery; Clinical Staff, Montelepre Memorial Hospital, New Orleans, Louisiana. Clinical Staff, Lander Valley Regional Medical Center, Lander, Wyoming
Premalignant Lesions

DENISE M. BUNTIN, M.D.

Associate Professor of Medicine (Dermatology), University of Tennessee College of Medicine; Chief, Dermatology Section, Memphis Veterans Medical Center, Memphis, Tennessee
Urticaria and Angioedema

WALTER H. C. BURGDORF, M.D.

Professor and Chairman, Department of Dermatology, University of New Mexico School of Medicine, Albuquerque, New Mexico
Papulosquamous Eruptions

JOHN J. BYRNES, M.D.

Professor of Medicine and Chief, Division of Hematology, University of Miami School of Medicine; Professor of Medicine, University of Miami–Jackson Memorial Medical Center and Veterans Administration Hospital, Miami, Florida
Disseminated Intravascular Coagulation; Thrombotic Thrombocytopenic Purpura and the Hemolytic Uremic Syndrome

RIAD CACHECHO, M.D.

Assistant Professor of Surgery, Boston University School of Medicine; General Surgeon and Assistant Director, Surgical Intensive Care Unit, Boston University Hospital and Boston City Hospital, Boston, Massachusetts
Thrombophlebitis in Obstetrics and Gynecology

BLAKE CADY, M.D.

Associate Professor of Surgery, Harvard Medical School; Chief of Surgical Oncology, New England Deaconess Hospital, Boston, Massachusetts
Thyroid Cancer

THOMAS R. CARACCIO, Pharm.D., D.A.B.A.T.

Visiting Assistant Clinical Professor of Pharmacology and Toxicology, New York College of Osteopathic Medicine, Westbury. Affiliate Assistant Clinical Professor of Pharmacy, St. John's University College of Pharmacy, Jamaica; Assistant Director, Long Island Regional Poison Control Center. Clinical Pharmacist, Nassau County Medical Center, East Meadow, New York
Acute Poisonings

RALPH CARMEL, M.D.

Professor of Medicine and Pathology, University of Southern California School of Medicine; Physician Specialist, Los Angeles County–University of Southern California Medical Center. Consultant, Norris Cancer Center, Los Angeles, California
Pernicious Anemia and Other Megaloblastic Anemias

PAUL C. CARPENTER, M.D.

Assistant Professor of Medicine, Mayo Medical School, Rochester, Minnesota
Cushing's Syndrome

WILLIAM T. CARPENTER, Jr., M.D.

Director, Maryland Psychiatric Research Center, Baltimore, Maryland
Schizophrenic Disorders

THOMAS B. CASALE, M.D.

Associate Professor, Department of Internal Medicine, University of Iowa College of Medicine; Staff Physician, University of Iowa Hospitals and Clinics and Veterans Administration Medical Center, Iowa City, Iowa
Asthma in the Adolescent and the Adult

BAYARD D. CATHERWOOD, M.D.

Associate Professor of Medicine and Assistant Professor of Anatomy and Cell Biology, Emory University School of Medicine; Chief, Endocrinology-Metabolism Section, Veterans Administration Medical Center, Atlanta, Georgia
Hyperparathyroidism and Hypoparathyroidism

C. DAVID CAWOOD, M.D.

Clinical Associate Professor, Department of Urology, Baylor College of Medicine; Attending Physician and Associate Chief

of Urology, St. Luke's Episcopal Hospital; Associate Physician, Methodist Hospital, Houston, Texas
Bacterial Infections of the Urinary Tract in Women

ROBERTO CEDILLO-RIVERA, M.D., Ms.C.

Assistant Professor in Pediatrics, Medicine School, Universidad Nacional Autónoma de México; Clinical Staff, Department of Infectology, Hospital de Pediatría, Centro Médico Nacional, Instituto Mexicano del Seguro Social, Mexico City, Mexico
Typhoid Fever

DAVID A. CHAD, M.D.

Associate Professor of Neurology and Pathology (Neuropathology) and Attending Neurologist, University of Massachusetts Hospital, Worcester, Massachusetts
Peripheral Neuropathies

SUBHASH CHAUDHARY, M.D.

Associate Professor of Pediatrics, Southern Illinois University School of Medicine; Pediatric Infectious Diseases Consultant, St. John's Hospital and Memorial Medical Center, Springfield, Illinois
Measles (Rubeola)

CLARE L. CHERNEY, M.D.

Instructor in Medicine, St. Francis Medical Center, Trenton, New Jersey; formerly Instructor in Medicine, Medical College of Pennsylvania, Philadelphia, Pennsylvania
Salmonellosis

ANTHONY W. CHOW, M.D.

Professor of Medicine and Head, Division of Infectious Disease, University of British Columbia; Head, Division of Infectious Disease, Vancouver General Hospital, Vancouver, British Columbia, Canada
Toxic Shock Syndrome

NICHOLAS P. CHRISTY, M.D.

Senior Lecturer in Medicine, Columbia University College of Physicians and Surgeons; Attending Physician, Department of Medicine, Presbyterian Hospital, New York, New York
Hyperprolactinemia

ARNOLD C. CINMAN, M.D.

Assistant Clinical Professor of Urology, University of California, Los Angeles, School of Medicine; Attending Urologist, Cedars-Sinai Medical Center, Los Angeles, California
Genitourinary Tuberculosis

DAVID P. CLARK, M.D.

Assistant Professor of Dermatology, University of Missouri School of Medicine; Attending Physician, University of Missouri Hospital and Clinics, Columbia, Missouri
Verruca Vulgaris (Warts)

KEITH F. CLARK, M.D.

Associate Professor, Department of Otorhinolaryngology, University of Oklahoma Health Sciences Center; Active Staff, Oklahoma Memorial Hospital, Children's Hospital of Oklahoma, Veterans Administration Medical Center, O'Donoghue Rehabilitation Institute, and Central State Hospital; Courtesy Staff, Presbyterian Hospital, Oklahoma City, Oklahoma
Hoarseness and Laryngitis

STEVEN L. CLARK, M.D.

Director, Maternal-Fetal Medicine, Utah Valley Regional Medical Center, Provo, Utah
Antepartum Care

HARRIS R. CLEARFIELD, M.D.

Professor of Medicine, Hahnemann Medical College; Director, Division of Gastroenterology, and Attending Physician, Hahnemann University Hospital, Philadelphia, Pennsylvania
Diverticula of the Alimentary Tract

THOMAS G. CLEARY, M.D.

Associate Professor of Pediatrics, University of Texas Health Science Center at Houston Medical School, Houston, Texas
Cholera

FRANKLIN R. COCKERILL, III, M.D.

Assistant Professor of Medicine, Mayo Medical School; Consultant in Infectious Diseases and Internal Medicine, Mayo Clinic, Rochester, Minnesota
Blastomycosis

LAWRENCE H. COHN, M.D.

Professor of Surgery, Harvard Medical School; Chief, Division of Cardiac Surgery, Brigham and Women's Hospital, Boston, Massachusetts
Acquired Diseases of the Aorta

CAROL COLA, M.D.

Hematology/Oncology Fellow, University of Massachusetts Medical Center, Worcester, Massachusetts
Platelet-Mediated Bleeding Disorders

REX B. CONN, M.D.

Professor of Pathology, Jefferson Medical College of Thomas Jefferson University; Director, Clinical Laboratories, Thomas Jefferson University Hospital, Philadelphia, Pennsylvania
Laboratory Values of Clinical Importance

DAVID S. COOPER, M.D.

Associate Professor of Medicine, Johns Hopkins University School of Medicine; Director, Division of Endocrinology, Sinai Hospital of Baltimore; Attending Physician, Johns Hopkins Hospital and Sinai Hospital of Baltimore, Baltimore, Maryland
Simple Goiter

JOSEPH N. CORRIERE, Jr., M.D.

Professor of Surgery (Urology) and Director of Urology, University of Texas Medical School at Houston, Texas Medical Center; Chief of Urology, Hermann Hospital; Academic Staff, St. Joseph Hospital; Consultant, Shriners Hospital for Crippled Children, Houston, Texas
Trauma to the Genitourinary Tract

JOHN H. CRANDON, M.D.

Associate Clinical Professor of Surgery, Tufts University Medical School, Boston, Massachusetts
Scurvy and Vitamin C

JAMES P. CROWLEY, M.D.

Associate Professor of Medicine, Brown University; Acting Director, Division of Clinical Hematology, Rhode Island Hospital, Providence, Rhode Island
Therapeutic Use of Blood Components

KENNETH B. CUMMINGS, M.D.

Professor and Chief of Urology, Robert Wood Johnson Medical School; Chief of Urologic Surgery, Robert Wood Johnson University Hospital, New Brunswick, New Jersey
Malignant Tumors of the Urogenital Tract

NANCY P. CUMMINGS, M.D.

Assistant Clinical Professor, Stanford University School of Medicine; Clinical Faculty, Stanford University Hospital, Stanford, California
Asthma in Children

RICHARD O. CUMMINS, M.D., M.Sc., M.P.H.

Associate Professor of Medicine, University of Washington School of Medicine; Associate Director, Emergency Medical Services, University of Washington Medical Center, Seattle, Washington
Sudden Cardiac Arrest

GREGORY D. CURFMAN, M.D.

Assistant Professor of Medicine, Harvard Medical School; Assistant in Medicine, Massachusetts General Hospital, Boston, Massachusetts
Acute Myocardial Infarction

DAVID C. DALE, M.D.

Professor, Department of Medicine, University of Washington School of Medicine, Seattle, Washington
Neutropenia

KIRON M. DAS, M.D., Ph.D.

Professor of Medicine, Robert Wood Johnson Medical School; Clinical Staff, Robert Wood Johnson University Hospital, New Brunswick, New Jersey
Ulcerative Colitis

RICHARD J. DAVEY, M.D.

Clinical Associate Professor of Medicine, Georgetown University Hospital, Washington, D.C.; Deputy Chief, Department of Transfusion Medicine, National Institutes of Health, Bethesda, Maryland
Autoimmune Hemolytic Anemia

RICHARD A. DAVIDSON, M.D., M.P.H.

Associate Professor, Department of Medicine, University of Florida College of Medicine; Clinical Staff, Shands Hospital and Veterans Administration Medical Center, Gainesville, Florida
Amebiasis

G. WILLIAM DEC, M.D.

Assistant Professor of Medicine, Harvard Medical School; Assistant Physician (Medicine), Medical Director, Cardiac Transplantation Program, and Director, Bigelow Intensive Care Unit–Coronary Care Unit, Massachusetts General Hospital, Boston, Massachusetts
Acute Myocardial Infarction

VINCENT A. DELEO, M.D.

Assistant Professor, Department of Dermatology, Columbia University College of Physicians and Surgeons; Florence Irving Assistant Professor of Dermatology, Columbia-Presbyterian Medical Center, New York, New York
Sunburn and Photosensitivity

CHARLES L. DERUS, M.D.

Rheumatologist, Dreyer Medical Clinic, Copley and Mercy Hospitals, Aurora, Illinois
Fibrositis, Bursitis, and Tendinitis

RICHARD D. DeSHAZO, M.D.

Professor of Medicine and Pediatrics and Chairman, Department of Medicine, Division of Allergy and Immunology, University of South Alabama College of Medicine, Mobile, Alabama
Anaphylaxis and Serum Sickness

JEAN DESLAURIERS, M.D.

Associate Professor of Surgery, Laval University Faculty of Medicine; Chief Thoracic Surgeon, Hôpital Laval, Ste-Foy, Quebec, Canada
Atelectasis

PIETER P. DEVRIESE, Ph.D., M.D.

Staff, University of Amsterdam; Clinical Staff, Department of Facial Medicine, Academic Medical Centre, Amsterdam, The Netherlands
Acute Peripheral Facial Paralysis (Bell's Palsy)

DAVID A. DIAMOND, M.D.

Associate Professor of Urology and Pediatrics, University of Massachusetts Medical Center; Consultant Pediatric Urologist, Worcester Memorial Hospital, Worcester Hahnemann Hospital, and St. Vincent Hospital, Worcester, Massachusetts
Bacterial Infections of the Urinary Tract in Girls

KRISTINE C. DONEY, M.D.

Associate Professor of Medicine, University of Washington School of Medicine; Associate Member, Fred Hutchinson Cancer Research Center, Seattle, Washington
Aplastic Anemia

JOSÉ ERNESTO DOS SANTOS, M.D.

Associate Professor, Faculdade de Medicina, Universidade de São Paulo, São Paulo, Brazil
Pellagra

MARGARET C. DOUGLASS, M.D.

Staff Dermatologist, Henry Ford Hospital, Detroit, Michigan.
Granuloma Inguinale (Donovanosis); Lymphogranuloma Venereum

BERNARD J. DREILING, M.D.

Professor of Medicine, University of Mississippi School of Medicine; Staff Hematologist, Veterans Administration Medical Center, Jackson, Mississippi
Iron Deficiency Anemia

DAVID J. DRISCOLL, M.D.

Professor of Pediatrics, Mayo Medical School; Head, Section of Pediatric Cardiology, Mayo Clinic, Rochester, Minnesota
Congenital Heart Disease

HOWARD M. DRUCE, M.D.

Assistant Professor of Medicine and Director, Nasal and Paranasal Sinus Physiology Laboratory, St. Louis University School of Medicine; Attending Physician, St. Louis University Medical Center, Cardinal Glennon Children's Hospital, and John Cochran Veterans Administration Medical Center, St. Louis, Missouri
Allergic Rhinitis Caused by Inhalant Factors

DAVID L. DUNNER, M.D.

Professor, Department of Psychiatry and Behavioral Sciences, University of Washington School of Medicine; Chief of Psychiatry, Harborview Medical Center, Seattle, Washington
Affective Disorders

CORWIN Q. EDWARDS, M.D.

Associate Professor of Medicine, University of Utah College of Medicine; Medical Director, LDS Hospital Outpatient Clinic, Salt Lake City, Utah
Hemochromatosis and Hemosiderosis

MORVEN S. EDWARDS, M.D.

Associate Professor of Pediatrics, Baylor College of Medicine; Active Staff, Texas Children's Hospital, Ben Taub General Hospital, and Jefferson Davis Hospital, Houston, Texas
Rubella and Congenital Rubella

HANS E. EINSTEIN, M.D.

Professor of Clinical Medicine, University of Southern California School of Medicine Los Angeles; Medical Director, Bakersfield Memorial Hospital, Bakersfield, California
Coccidioidomycosis

EDWARD EISENBERG, M.D.

Assistant Professor of Medicine, Albert Einstein College of Medicine, Bronx, New York; Clinical Staff, Mountainside Hospital, Montclair Community Hospital, and St. Barnabas Hospital, Montclair, New Jersey
Rat-Bite Fever

JERRY J. ELLER, M.D.

Clinical Professor of Pediatrics and Community Medicine, College of Community Health Sciences, University of Alabama; Associate Physician, Lloyd Noland Foundation Hospital, Fairfield, Alabama
Diphtheria

CHARLES N. ELLIS, M.D.

Associate Professor of Dermatology, University of Michigan Medical Center; Consultant Dermatologist, Veterans Administration Medical Center, Ann Arbor; Consultant Dermatologist, Chelsea Community Hospital, Chelsea, Michigan
Acne Vulgaris and Rosacea

STANLEY FAHN, M.D.

H. Houston Merritt Professor of Neurology, Columbia-Presbyterian Medical Center, New York, New York
Parkinsonism

WILLIAM E. FANN, M.D.

Professor of Psychiatry and Associate Professor of Pharmacology, Baylor College of Medicine; Chief of Psychiatry, Veterans Administration Medical Center, Houston, Texas
Anxiety Disorders

NADIR R. FARID, M.D.

Professor of Medicine, Department of Medicine, and Professor of Immunology, Division of Basic Sciences, Memorial University of Newfoundland Faculty of Medicine; Chief, Division of Endocrinology and Metabolism, and Consultant, Health Sciences Center, St. John's, Newfoundland, Canada
Thyroiditis

PETER F. FEDULLO, M.D.

Assistant Professor, Department of Medicine, Pulmonary–Critical Care Division, University of California, San Diego, Medical Center; Assistant Professor, Department of Medicine, Pulmonary–Critical Care Division, Veterans Administration Medical Center, San Diego, California
Pulmonary Embolism

NEIL A. FENSKE, M.D.

Professor and Director, Division of Dermatology, Department of Internal Medicine, and Professor of Pathology, Department of Pathology, University of South Florida College of Medicine; Chief, Dermatology Section, James A. Haley Veterans Hospital; Chief, Section of Dermatology, Medical Service, H. Lee Moffitt Cancer Center and Research Institute, Tampa, Florida
Parasitic Infestations

LAWRENCE J. FENTON, M.D.

Professor and Chairman, University of South Dakota School of Medicine; Attending Staff, Sioux Valley Hospital, Sioux Falls, South Dakota
Care of the High-Risk Neonate

DOUGLAS P. FINE, M.D.

Professor of Medicine and Chief, Infectious Diseases Service, University of Oklahoma Health Sciences Center; Staff Physician, Oklahoma Memorial Hospital; Chief, Infectious Diseases Service, Veterans Administration Medical Center, Oklahoma City, Oklahoma
Rocky Mountain Spotted Fever

SYDNEY M. FINEGOLD, M.D.

Professor of Medicine, University of California, Los Angeles, School of Medicine; Staff Physician and Associate Chief of Staff for Research and Development, Wadsworth Veterans Administration Medical Center, Los Angeles, California
Brain Abscess

FAITH T. FITZGERALD, M.D.

Professor of Medicine and Vice-Chairman, Department of Internal Medicine, University of California, Davis, School of Medicine, Davis, California
Disturbances Caused by Cold

NICHOLAS J. FIUMARA, M.D., M.P.H.

Belmont, Massachusetts
Syphilis

BARRY S. FOGEL, M.D.

Associate Professor of Psychiatry and Human Behavior and Associate Director, Center for Gerontology and Health Care Research, Brown University, Providence, Rhode Island
Delirium

KENNETH A. FOON, M.D.

Professor, Department of Medicine, State University of New York at Buffalo School of Medicine; Chief, Division of Clinical Immunology, Roswell Park Memorial Institute, Buffalo, New York
The Chronic Leukemias

STEPHEN J. FORMAN, M.D.

Clinical Professor of Medicine, University of Southern California School of Medicine, Los Angeles; Director, Department of Hematology and Bone Marrow Transplantation, City of Hope National Medical Center, Duarte, California.
Malignant Lymphoma (Non-Hodgkin's Lymphomas)

JACKSON E. FOWLER, Jr., M.D.

Professor of Urology, University of Illinois College of Medicine; Chief of Urology, University of Illinois Hospital, Chicago, Illinois
Nongonococcal Urethritis

GARY S. FRANCIS, M.D.

Professor of Medicine, University of Minnesota Medical School; Director of Cardiovascular Research, Veterans Administration Medical Center, Minneapolis, Minnesota
Congestive Heart Failure

ANDREW G. FRANTZ, M.D.

Professor of Medicine, Columbia University College of Physicians and Surgeons; Attending Physician, Presbyterian Hospital, New York, New York
Hypopituitarism

ARNOLD I. FREEMAN
Children's Mercy Hospital, Kansas City, Missouri
Acute Leukemia in Childhood

WESLEY FURSTE, M.D.
Clinical Professor of Surgery Emeritus, Ohio State University College of Medicine; Active Staff, Department of Surgery, Mt. Carmel Medical Center; Senior Attending Staff, Department of Surgery, Riverside Methodist Hospitals, Columbus, Ohio
Anaerobic and Necrotizing Infections Including Gas Gangrene; Tetanus

ROBERT PETER GALE, M.D., Ph.D.
Associate Professor of Medicine, University of California, Los Angeles, School of Medicine, Los Angeles, California
The Chronic Leukemias

PHILLIP C. GALLE, M.D.
Associate Professor, Southern Illinois University School of Medicine; Attending Staff, Memorial Medical Center and St. John's Hospital, Springfield, Illinois
Ectopic Pregnancy

NELSON M. GANTZ, M.D.
Professor of Medicine, Microbiology, and Molecular Genetics, University of Massachusetts Medical School; Clinical Director of Infectious Diseases and Hospital Epidemiologist, University of Massachusetts Medical Center, Worcester, Massachusetts
Streptococcal Pharyngitis

GALE GARDNER, M.D.
Clinical Professor, Department of Otolaryngology, University of Tennessee College of Medicine; Attending Physician, Baptist Memorial Hospital, Memphis, Tennessee
Meniere's Disease

DOUGLAS GENTLEMAN, M.B., Ch.B.
Honorary Clinical Teacher in Neurosurgery, University of Glasgow; Senior Registrar in Neurosurgery, Institute of Neurological Sciences, Southern General Hospital, Glasgow, Scotland, United Kingdom
Acute Head Injuries in Adults

LAWRENCE D. GERMAN, M.D.
Attending Physician, St. Thomas Hospital, Nashville, Tennessee.
Heart Block

DAVID F. GIANSIRACUSA, M.D.
Associate Professor of Medicine and Director, Division of Rheumatology and Immunology, University of Massachusetts Medical Center, Worcester, Massachusetts
Hyperuricemia and Gout

HARRIET S. GILBERT, M.D.
Professor of Medicine, Albert Einstein College of Medicine, Bronx; Lecturer, Mount Sinai School of Medicine, New York; Attending in Medicine, Montefiore Medical Center and Bronx Municipal Hospital Center, Bronx; Attending in Medicine, Mount Sinai Hospital, New York, New York
Polycythemia Vera and Other Polycythemic Conditions

W. PAUL GLEZEN, M.D.
Professor of Microbiology and Pediatrics, Baylor College of Medicine; Adjunct Professor of Epidemiology, University of Texas School of Public Health, University of Texas Health Science Center at Houston; Attending Pediatrician, Harris County Hospital District; Courtesy Staff, Infectious Diseases, Texas Children's Hospital, Houston, Texas
Viral and Mycoplasmal Pneumonias

ALVIN F. GOLDFARB, M.D.
Professor of Obstetrics and Gynecology, Jefferson Medical College of Thomas Jefferson University, Philadelphia, Pennsylvania
Dysmenorrhea

MICHAEL T. GOLDFARB, M.D.
Lecturer, University of Michigan Medical School; Attending Physician, University Hospital, Ann Arbor, Michigan
Acne Vulgaris and Rosacea

JONATHAN C. GOLDSMITH, M.D.
Associate Professor and Director, Hematology Program, Viral Syndrome Clinic, and Nebraska Regional Hemophilia Center, University of Nebraska Medical Center, Omaha, Nebraska
Vitamin K Deficiency

JOSEPH GOODGOLD, M.D.
Professor of Rehabilitation Medicine, New York University Medical Center; Attending Physician, University Hospital and Rusk Institute for Rehabilitation Medicine; Consultant, Bellevue Hospital, Manhattan Veterans Administration Hospital and St. Claire's Hospital, New York, New York
Rehabilitation of the Patient with Hemiplegia

ALAN N. GORDON, M.D.
Assistant Professor, Department of Obstetrics and Gynecology, Vanderbilt University School of Medicine; Attending Physician, Vanderbilt University Hospital and Metropolitan Nashville General Hospital, Nashville, Tennessee
Neoplasms of the Vulva

DANIEL M. GORDON, M.D.
Clinical Staff, Infectious Disease Service, Walter Reed Army Medical Center, Washington, D.C.
Leishmaniasis

JACK M. GORMAN, M.D.
Associate Professor of Clinical Psychiatry, Columbia University College of Physicians and Surgeons; Associate Attending Psychiatrist, Presbyterian Hospital; Director, Biological Studies Unit, and Chief, Department of Clinical Psychobiology, New York State Psychiatric Institute, New York, New York
Panic Disorder and Agoraphobia

JUDITH REID GRAVES, R.N., E.M.T.-P.
Research Associate, Center for Evaluation of Emergency Medical Services, Seattle–King County Department of Public Health, Seattle, Washington
Sudden Cardiac Arrest

J. THOMAS GRAYSTON, M.D.
Professor of Epidemiology and Pathobiology, School of Public Health and Community Medicine, University of Washington, Seattle, Washington
Psittacosis (Ornithosis)

RICHARD N. GREENBERG, M.D.
Assistant Professor of Medicine and Microbiology, St. Louis University Medical School; Attending Physician, St. Louis University Hospital, St. Louis, Missouri
Osteomyelitis

JOSEPH GREENSHER, M.D.
Professor of Clinical Pediatrics, State University of New York at Stony Brook; Medical Director and Associate Chairman, Department of Pediatrics, Winthrop-University Hospital, Mineola; Associate Director, Poison Control Center, Nassau County Medical Center, East Meadow, New York
Acute Poisonings

GERALD C. GROGGEL, M.D.
Assistant Professor of Medicine, Division of Nephrology, University of Utah School of Medicine; Clinical Staff, Division of Nephrology, Department of Medicine, University of Utah Health Sciences Center, Salt Lake City, Utah
Glomerular Disorders

JOHN H. GROSSMAN, III, M.D., PH.D.
Director, Division of Maternal-Fetal Medicine, Department of Obstetrics and Gynecology, George Washington University School of Medicine and Health Sciences; Professor of Obstetrics, Gynecology, and Microbiology, George Washington University Hospital, Washington, D.C.
Chlamydia Trachomatis

STEVEN GRUNBERG, M.D.
Associate Professor of Medicine, University of Southern California School of Medicine; Attending Physician, Los Angeles County–University of Southern California Medical Center, Kenneth Norris Jr. Cancer Hospital, Barlow Hospital, and Hospital of the Good Samaritan, Los Angeles, California
Nausea and Vomiting

SHARON GRUNDFEST-BRONIATOWSKI, M.D.
Staff, Department of General Surgery, Cleveland Clinic Foundation, Cleveland, Ohio
Diseases of the Breast

HÉCTOR GUISCAFRÉ GALLARDO, M.D.
Professor of Infectology and Epidemiology, Faculty of Medicine, Universidad Nacional Autónoma de México; Associate Researcher, Clinical Investigation of Infectious and Parasitic Diseases Unit, Hospital de Pediatría, Centro Médico Nacional, Instituto Mexicano del Seguro Social, Mexico City, Mexico
Whooping Cough (Pertussis)

ARNOLD W. GUREVITCH, M.D.
Professor of Clinical Medicine (Dermatology), University of California, Los Angeles, School of Medicine, Los Angeles; Chief, Division of Dermatology, Harbor–University of California, Los Angeles, Medical Center, Torrance, California
Bacterial Diseases of the Skin

GARY R. GUTCHER, M.D.
Professor of Pediatrics, Medical College of Virginia, Richmond, Virginia
Hemolytic Disease of the Newborn

BRIAN C. HALPERN, M.D.
Clinical Staff, Riverview Hospital, Princeton Medical Center, Princeton, New Jersey
Common Sports Injuries

HUNTER A. HAMMILL, M.D.
Assistant Professor, Baylor College of Medicine; Attending Physician, St. Luke's Episcopal Hospital, Methodist Hospital, and Harris County Hospital District, Houston, Texas
Vulvovaginitis

STEPHEN C. HAMMILL, M.D.
Division of Cardiovascular Diseases, Mayo Clinic, Rochester, Minnesota
Tachycardia

WILLIAM P. HAMMOND, M.D.
Associate Professor, Department of Medicine, Division of Hematology, University of Washington School of Medicine, Seattle, Washington
Neutropenia

LEWIS H. HAMNER, III, M.D.
Assistant Professor of Gynecology and Obstetrics, Emory University School of Medicine; Assistant Professor, Department of Gynecology and Obstetrics, Grady Memorial Hospital; Director of Obstetrical Ultrasound, Crawford Long Hospital of Emory University, Atlanta, Georgia
Chlamydia Trachomatis

E. WILLIAM HANCOCK, M.D.
Professor of Medicine (Cardiology), Stanford University School of Medicine; Active Staff and Medical Director, GCG Laboratory, Stanford University Hospital, Stanford, California
Pericarditis

PHILIP M. HANNO, M.D.
Associate Professor of Urology, University of Pennsylvania School of Medicine; Chief of Urology, Veterans Administration Medical Center, Philadelphia, Pennsylvania
Bacterial Infections of the Urinary Tract in Men

JOHN T. HARRINGTON, M.D.
Professor of Medicine, Tufts University School of Medicine, Boston; Chief of Medicine, Newton-Wellesley Hospital, Newton, Massachusetts
Acute Renal Failure

T. MICHAEL HARRINGTON, M.D.
Associate Professor, Vice Chairman and Medical Director, Department of Family Medicine, University of Alabama at Birmingham; Attending Physician, Children's Hospital of Alabama and University of Alabama Hospital, Birmingham, Alabama
Disturbances Caused by Heat

RICHARD L. HARRIS, M.D.
Assistant Professor of Medicine, Baylor College of Medicine; Medical Epidemiologist, Methodist Hospital, Houston, Texas
Bacteremia

CHISTOPHER J. HARRISON, M.D.
Assistant Professor of Pediatrics, University of Cincinnati College of Medicine; Attending Physician, Children's Hospital Medical Center, Cincinnati, Ohio
Mumps (Epidemic Parotitis)

WILLIAM S. HAUBRICH, M.D.
Clinical Professor of Medicine, University of California, San Diego, School of Medicine, San Diego; Senior Consultant Emeritus, Division of Gastroenterology, Scripps Clinic and Research Foundation, La Jolla, California
Gastritis

FREDERICK W. HENDERSON, M.D.
Professor of Pediatrics, University of North Carolina School of Medicine; Attending in Pediatrics, North Carolina Memorial Hospital, Chapel Hill, North Carolina
Viral Respiratory Infections

ROBERT E. HERMANN, M.D.

Clinical Professor of Surgery, Case Western Reserve School of Medicine; Chairman, Department of General Surgery, Cleveland Clinic Foundation, Cleveland, Ohio
Diseases of the Breast

CHRISTIAN HERRMANN, Jr., M.D.

Professor Emeritus of Neurology, University of California, Los Angeles, School of Medicine; Honorary Consultant, Neuropsychiatric Institute and Hospitals, University of California, Los Angeles, California
Myasthenia Gravis

HARRY R. HILL, M.D.

Professor of Pediatrics and Pathology and Head, Division of Clinical Immunology and Allergy, University of Utah School of Medicine, Salt Lake City, Utah
Rheumatic Fever

RICHARD T. HOPPE, M.D.

Professor, Department of Radiation Oncology, Stanford University School of Medicine, Stanford, California
Mycosis Fungoides

JOHN W. HOUSE, M.D.

Assistant Clinical Professor, Department of Otolaryngology–Head and Neck Surgery, University of Southern California School of Medicine; Attending Physician, St. Vincent's Medical Center, Hospital of the Good Samaritan, Children's Hospital of Los Angeles, Los Angeles County–University of Southern California Medical Center, Los Angeles, California
Tinnitus

HARRY F. HULL, M.D.

Assistant Clinical Professor of Pediatrics, University of New Mexico School of Medicine, Santa Fe, New Mexico
Plague

VINCENT C. HUNG, M.D.

Assistant Professor of Clinical Medicine, Section of Dermatology, and Director of Mohs Micrographic Surgery Service, University of Southern California School of Medicine, Los Angeles, California
Moles and Melanoma

JOHN L. HUNT, M.D.

Professor of Surgery, University of Texas Southwestern Medical Center, Dallas, Texas
Burns

DUANE G. HUTSON, M.D.

Professor of Surgery, University of Miami School of Medicine; Attending Surgeon, Jackson Memorial Hospital; Staff Surgeon, Veterans Administration Hospital, Miami, Florida
Bleeding Esophageal Varices

J. THOMAS HUTTON, M.D., Ph.D.

Professor, Department of Medical and Surgical Neurology, and Director, Alzheimer's Disease Institute, Texas Tech Health Sciences Center, Lubbock, Texas
Alzheimer's Disease

FRANK L. IBER, M.D.

Professor of Medicine, Loyola University of Chicago Stritch School of Medicine, Maywood; Chief of Gastroenterology, Edw. Hines Jr. Veterans Administration Hospital, Hines, Illinois
Cirrhosis

MAUREEN A. JARRELL, M.D.

Assistant Professor, Department of Obstetrics and Gynecology, University of Vermont College of Medicine; Staff, Gynecologic Oncology, Medical Center Hospital of Vermont, Burlington, Vermont
Carcinoma of the Uterine Cervix

SUZANNE R. JENKINS, V.M.D., M.P.H.

Staff, Department of Public Health, Richmond, Virginia
Rabies

CYNDA ANN JOHNSON, M.D.

Associate Professor, University of Kansas Medical Center, Kansas City, Kansas
Contraception

J. MICHAEL JORDAN, M.D.

Fellow in Pulmonary Disease, University of Texas Health Science Center at San Antonio, San Antonio; Attending Physician, Baylor University Medical Center, Houston, Texas
Acute Respiratory Failure

JOSEPH L. JORIZZO, M.D.

Professor and Chairman, Department of Dermatology, Bowman Gray School of Medicine, Wake Forest University; Attending Physician, North Carolina Baptist Hospital and Veterans Administration Clinic, Winston-Salem, North Carolina
Connective Tissue Disorders: Lupus Erythematosus, Dermatomyositis, and Scleroderma

DIANE K. JORKASKY, M.D.

Assistant Clinical Professor of Medicine, University of Pennsylvania School of Medicine; Attending Nephrologist, Presbyterian Medical Center; Director of Clinical Research, Smith Kline & French Laboratories, Philadelphia, Pennsylvania
Diabetes Insipidus

MARILYN KACICA, M.D.

Fellow and Clinical Instructor, Children's Hospital Medical Center, Cincinnati, Ohio
Mumps (Epidemic Parotitis)

DONALD P. KADUNCE, M.D.

Research Fellow in Dermatology, University of Utah Health Science Center, Salt Lake City, Utah
Bullous Diseases

NERI M. KANDAWALLA, M.D.

Clinical Assistant Professor of Pathology, Ohio State University College of Medicine; Senior Attending Staff, Department of Pathology, Riverside Methodist Hospital, Columbus, Ohio
Anaerobic and Necrotizing Infections Including Gas Gangrene

K. SHASHI KANT, M.D.

Professor of Clinical Medicine, University of Cincinnati College of Medicine; Director, Dialysis Programs, University of Cincinnati Hospital, Cincinnati, Ohio
Chronic Renal Failure

MICHAEL M. KAPLAN, M.D.

Southfield, Michigan
Hypothyroidism

CARLOS S. KASE, M.D.

Professor of Neurology, Boston University School of Medicine; Attending Neurologist, University Hospital, Boston, Massachusetts
Intracerebral Hemorrhage

SOL KATZ, M.D.

Professor of Medicine, Georgetown University School of Medicine, Washington, D.C.
Primary Lung Abscess

JAMES R. KEANE, M.D.

Professor of Neurology, University of Southern California School of Medicine; Attending Physician, Los Angeles County Hospital, Los Angeles, California
Optic Neuritis

DAVID W. KENNEDY, M.D.

Associate Professor, Department of Otolaryngology–Head and Neck Surgery, Johns Hopkins University School of Medicine; Attending Physician, Johns Hopkins Hospital, Baltimore, Maryland
Sinusitis

ROBERT M. KENNEY, M.D.

Assistant Professor, Brown University; Director, Transfusion Service, Rhode Island Hospital, Providence, Rhode Island
Therapeutic Use of Blood Components

M. YOUSUF KHAN, M.D.

Director, Infectious Diseases, and Assistant Professor of Medicine, University of Minnesota Medical School, Minneapolis, Minnesota; Head, Division of Infectious Diseases, King Fahad Hospital, Riyadh, Saudi Arabia
Brucellosis

OK DONG KIM, M.D.

Fellow in Gastroenterology, University of Illinois at Chicago Medical Center, Chicago, Illinois
Constipation

CRAIG S. KITCHENS, M.D.

Professor and Vice-Chairman, Department of Medicine, University of Florida College of Medicine; Chief, Medical Service, Veterans Administration Medical Center, Gainesville, Florida
Hemophilia and von Willebrand's Disease

VICTOR R. KLEIN, M.D.

Assistant Professor of Obstetrics and Gynecology, Cornell University Medical College; Attending Physician, North Shore University Hospital, New York, New York
Vaginal Bleeding in Late Pregnancy

J. B. KOPSTEIN, M.D.

Consultant in Dermatology, Hotel Dieu Hospital, Grace Hospital, Windsor Western Hospital, and Metropolitan Hospital, Windsor, Ontario, Canada
Atopic Dermatitis

JOYCE A. KORVICK, M.D.

Assistant Professor, University of Kentucky Medical School; Infectious Disease Specialist, Albert Chandler Medical Center; Staff Physician, Veterans Administration Medical Center, Lexington, Kentucky
Legionellosis (Pontiac Fever and Legionnaires' Disease)

MARY KORYTOWSKI, M.D.

Instructor, Johns Hopkins University School of Medicine; Attending Physician, Francis Scott Key Medical Center, Baltimore, Maryland
Simple Goiter

JAMES P. KUSHNER, M.D.

Professor of Medicine, and Head, Division of Hematology-Oncology, University of Utah College of Medicine, Salt Lake City, Utah
Hemochromatosis and Hemosiderosis

SAMUEL B. LABOW, M.D.

Clinical Assistant Professor of Surgery, Cornell University Medical College; Attending Physician, North Shore University Hospital, New York, New York
Hemorrhoids, Anal Fissure, and Anal Fistula and Abscess

PEARON G. LANG, JR., M.D.

Associate Professor of Dermatology, Medical University of South Carolina; Staff, Medical University Hospital; Consultant, Charleston Memorial Hospital; Consultant, Veterans Administration Hospital, Charleston, South Carolina
Cutaneous Vasculitis

RENEE LANTNER, M.D.

Clinical Assistant Instructor, Department of Pediatrics, State University of New York at Buffalo School of Medicine; Attending Physician, Division of Allergy-Immunology, Children's Hospital of Buffalo, Buffalo, New York
Anaphylaxis and Serum Sickness

ALAN E. LASSER, M.D.

Associate Professor of Clinical Dermatology, Northwestern University Medical School; Senior Attending Physician, Evanston Hospital; Consultant, Rush North Shore Medical Center and Children's Memorial Hospital, Chicago, Illinois
Erythemas

GUY W. LEADBETTER, JR., M.D.

Chairman and Professor, Department of Urology, University of Vermont College of Medicine; Attending Physician, Medical Center Hospital of Vermont, Burlington, Vermont
Urethral Stricture

EUGENE LEIBSOHN, M.D.

Attending Staff, St. Joseph Hospital, Phoenix, Arizona
Pruritus Ani and Vulvae

MYRON J. LEVIN, M.D.

Professor of Pediatrics (Infectious Diseases) and Medicine, University of Colorado School of Medicine, Denver, Colorado
Viral Meningoencephalitis

MATTHEW E. LEVISON, M.D.

Professor of Medicine and Chief, Division of Infectious Diseases, Medical College of Pennsylvania, Philadelphia, Pennsylvania
Salmonellosis

JAMES H. LEWIS, M.D.

Associate Professor of Medicine, Division of Gastroenterology, Georgetown University School of Medicine; Attending Physician, Georgetown University Hospital, Washington, D.C.; Consulting Physician, National Institutes of Health, Bethesda, Maryland
Peptic Ulcer

CLAUDIA R. LIBERTIN, M.D.

Assistant Professor of Medicine and Pathology, Loyola, University of Chicago Stritch School of Medicine; Attending Physician, Loyola University Medical Center, Marywood, Illinois
Infective Endocarditis

MARTA M. LITTLE, M.D.

Associate Physician, University of Iowa College of Medicine; Staff Physician, University of Iowa Hospitals and Clinics, Iowa City, Iowa
Asthma in the Adolescent and the Adult

CHARLES H. LIVENGOOD, III, M.D.

Assistant Professor, Division of Gynecology, Department of Obstetrics and Gynecology, Duke University Medical Center, Durham, North Carolina
Leiomyomas of the Uterus

SIMON K. LO, M.D.

Assistant Clinical Professor of Medicine, University of California, Los Angeles, School of Medicine; Attending Physician, Division of Gastroenterology, Harbor–UCLA Medical Center, Los Angeles, California
Irritable Bowel Syndrome

GEORGE M. LORDI, M.D.

Associate Professor of Medicine, University of Medicine and Dentistry of New Jersey, New Jersey Medical School; Attending Physician, Pulmonary Disease, University Hospital, Newark, New Jersey
Tuberculosis and Other Mycobacterial Diseases

RODNEY A. LORENZ, M.D.

Associate Professor of Pediatrics, Vanderbilt University School of Medicine; Attending Physician, Vanderbilt University Hospital, Nashville, Tennessee
Diabetes Mellitus in Children and Adolescents

CHRISTY A. LORTON, M.D.

Clinical Instructor of Dermatology, University of Cincinnati College of Medicine; Attending Physician, University Hospital, Cincinnati, Ohio
Pigmentary Disorders

LINDA M. LUXON, B.Sc.

Consultant Physician in Neuro-otology, National Hospital for Nervous Diseases, London, England
Episodic Vertigo

DAVID R. MacDONALD, M.D.

Assistant Professor (Neurology), Departments of Clinical Neurological Sciences and Oncology, University of Western Ontario; Attending Neurologist, London Regional Cancer Centre and Victoria Hospital; Consulting Neurologist, University Hospital and St. Joseph's Hospital, London, Ontario, Canada
Brain Tumors

D. W. MacPHERSON, M.D.

Assistant Professor, Department of Pathology, McMaster University; Attending Physician, Infectious Disease and Tropical Medicine Clinic, Chedoke-McMaster Hospitals, and Regional Parasitology Laboratory, St. Joseph's Hospital, Hamilton, Ontario, Canada
Intestinal Parasites

JOHN H. MALFETANO, M.D.

Associate Professor, Department of Obstetrics and Gynecology, and Director, Division of Gynecologic Oncology, Albany Medical Center; Staff, St. Peter's Hospital, Albany; Consulting Staff, Mercy Community Hospital, Port Jervis; Mary McClellan Hospital, Cambridge; Veterans Administration Hospital, Albany; and Nathan Littauer Hospital, Gloverville; Assistant Attending Physician, Children's Hospital, Albany, New York
Cancer of the Endometrium

JOHN A. MANNICK, M.D.

Brigham and Women's Hospital, Boston, Massachusetts
Acquired Diseases of the Aorta

CHARLES M. MANSBACH, II, M.D.

Professor of Medicine and Physiology and Chief, Division of Gastroenterology, University of Tennessee College of Medicine; Staff Physician, Veterans Administration Medical Center and Baptist Memorial Hospital, Memphis, Tennessee
Malabsorption Syndromes

COLIN D. MARCHANT, M.D.

Associate Professor of Pediatrics, Tufts University School of Medicine; Assistant Pediatrician, Division of Infectious Diseases, Floating Hospital for Infants and Children, New England Medical Center, Boston, Massachusetts
Otitis Media

JAY MARION, M.D.

Assistant Professor of Clinical Medicine, Washington University School of Medicine; Attending Physician, Barnes Hospital and Missouri Baptist Medical Center, St. Louis, Missouri
Hodgkin's Disease: Chemotherapy

THOMAS MARRIE, M.D.

Professor of Medicine and Head, Division of Infectious Disease, Dalhousie University Faculty of Medicine; Chief, Infectious Disease Service, Victoria General Hospital, Halifax, Nova Scotia, Canada
Q Fever

EDWARD L. MARUT, M.D.

Assistant Professor of Obstetrics and Gynecology, University of Chicago College of Medicine; Director, Division of Reproductive Endocrinology and Director, Program for Assisted Reproductive Technology, Michael Reese Hospital and Medical Center, Chicago, Illinois
Amenorrhea

D. MATHERS, M.B., B.S.

Fellow in Rheumatology, University of Alberta Faculty of Medicine, Edmonton, Alberta, Canada
Ankylosing Spondylitis

MICHAEL E. MAYO, M.B.

Professor of Urology, University of Washington School of Medicine; Attending Physician, University of Washington Medical Center, Children's Hospital and Medical Center, and Veterans Administration Hospital, Seattle, Washington
Benign Prostatic Hyperplasia

RICHARD B. McELVEIN, M.D.

Professor, Division of Cardiothoracic Surgery, Department of Surgery, University of Alabama at Birmingham; Assistant Chief of Staff, University of Alabama at Birmingham; Chief, Thoracic Surgery, Veterans Administration Hospital, Birmingham, Alabama
Pleural Effusion and Empyema Thoracis

EDWARD J. McGUIRE, M.D.

Professor and Head, Section of Urology, University of Michigan Medical Center, Ann Arbor, Michigan
Urinary Incontinence

EDWIN M. MEARES, JR., M.D.

Charles M. Whitney Professor and Chairman, Division of Urology, Tufts University School of Medicine; Chairman, Department of Urology, New England Medical Center Hospitals, Boston, Massachusetts
Prostatitis

DAVID R. MELDRUM, M.D.

Clinical Professor, Department of Obstetrics and Gynecology, University of California, Los Angeles, School of Medicine, Los Angeles; Director, Female Infertility Services, AMI–South Bay Hospital, Redondo Beach, California
Endometriosis

NANCY PRICE MENDENHALL, M.D.

Associate Professor, University of Florida, College of Medicine, Gainesville, Florida
Hodgkin's Disease: Radiation Therapy

LEO C. MERCER, M.D.

Assistant Professor, Department of Surgery, Texas Tech University School of Medicine; Attending Staff, R.E. Thomason General Hospital, El Paso, Texas
Cholecystitis and Cholelithiasis

RUSSELL J. MERRITT, M.D., PH.D.

Associate Professor of Pediatrics, University of Southern California School of Medicine; Director, Nutrition Support Team, Children's Hospital of Los Angeles, Los Angeles, California
Normal Infant Feeding

RODNEY A. MICHAEL, M.D.

Assistant Professor of Medicine, F. Edward Hebert School of Medicine, Bethesda, Maryland; Chief, Infectious Disease Service, Madigan Army Medical Center, Tacoma, Washington
Bacterial Meningitis

J. PARKER MICKLE, M.D.

Professor, University of Florida College of Medicine; Chief, Pediatric Neurosurgery, Shands Hospital at the University of Florida, Gainesville, Florida
Acute Head Injuries in Children

KENNETH B. MILLER, M.D.

Assistant Professor of Medicine, Tufts University School of Medicine; Director, Leukemia Service, New England Medical Center, Boston, Massachusetts
Acute Leukemia in Adults

RODNEY R. MILLION, M.D.

Professor, University of Florida College of Medicine; Chairman, Department of Radiation Oncology, University of Florida J. Hillis Miller Health Center, Gainesville, Florida
Hodgkin's Disease: Radiation Therapy

DANIEL R. MISHELL, JR., M.D.

Professor and Chairman, Department of Obstetrics and Gynecology, University of Southern California School of Medicine; Chief of Professional Services, Women's Hospital, Los Angeles County/USC Medical Center, Los Angeles, California
Menopause

JAMES E. MITCHELL, M.D.

Associate Professor, Department of Psychiatry, University of Minnesota Medical School; Staff Psychiatrist, University of Minnesota Hospital, Minneapolis, Minnesota
Bulimia Nervosa

SOHRAB MOBARHAN, M.D.

Associate Professor of Medicine and Nutrition and Assistant Chief of Gastroenterology, University of Illinois at Chicago Medical Center, Chicago, Illinois
Constipation

HOWARD C. MOFENSON, M.D.

Professor of Clinical Pediatrics, State University of New York at Stony Brook; Professor of Pharmacology and Toxicology, New York College of Osteopathy, Old Westbury; Professor of Clinical Pharmacy, St. John's University College of Pharmacy, Jamaica; Director, Long Island Regional Poison Control Center, Nassau County Medical Center; Staff, Winthrop University Hospital, Mineola, New York
Acute Poisonings

KENNETH J. MOISE, JR., M.D.

Assistant Professor, Department of Obstetrics and Gynecology, Division of Maternal-Fetal Medicine, Baylor College of Medicine; Attending Physician, St. Luke's Episcopal Hospital, Methodist Hospital, and Harris County Hospital District, Texas
Postpartum Care

MARK E. MOLITCH, M.D.

Associate Professor of Medicine, Northwestern University Medical School; Attending Physician, Northwestern Memorial Hospital, Chicago, Ilinois
Diabetes Mellitus in Adults

WILLIAM J. MORAN, D.M.D., M.D.

Assistant Professor of Head and Neck Surgery, Pritzker School of Medicine, University of Chicago; Attending Staff, University of Chicago Hospitals and Clinics, Chicago, Illinois
Diseases of the Mouth

AUAYPORN P. NADEMANEE, M.D.

Staff Physician, Department of Hematology and Bone Marrow Transplantation, City of Hope National Medical Center, Duarte, California
Malignant Lymphoma (Non-Hodgkin's Lymphomas)

MARK S. NANES, M.D., PH.D.

Assistant Professor of Medicine, Emory University School of Medicine; Staff Physician, Veterans Administration Medical Center, Decatur, and Grady Memorial Hospital, Atlanta, Georgia
Hyperparathyroidism and Hypoparathyroidism

ROBERT S. NELSON, M.D.

Professor of Medicine, University of Texas Health Science Center at Houston Medical School; Professor of Medicine, Baylor College of Medicine; Attending Physician, M.D. Anderson Hospital and Tumor Institute, Houston, Texas
Tumors of the Stomach

JACK NEWMAN, M.D.

Assistant Professor, University of Toronto Faculty of Medicine; Acting Chief, Division of Emergency Pediatrics, and Director, Breastfeeding Clinic, Hospital for Sick Children, Toronto, Ontario, Canada
Fever

JAMES C. NIEDERMAN, M.D.

Clinical Professor of Medicine and Epidemiology, Yale University School of Medicine; Medical Staff Member, Yale–New Haven Medical Center, New Haven, Connecticut
Infectious Mononucleosis

PETER T. NIEH, M.D.

Associate Professor (Urology), University of Connecticut Health Center, Farmington, Connecticut; Senior Staff Urologist, Lahey Clinic Medical Center, Burlington, Massachusetts
Epididymitis

JAMES J. NORDLUND, M.D.

Professor and Chairman, Department of Dermatology, University of Cincinnati College of Medicine; Attending Physician, University Hospital, Cincinnati, Ohio
Pigmentary Disorders

JOHN W. NORRIS, M.D.

Professor of Neurology, University of Toronto Faculty of Medicine; Staff Neurologist, Sunnybrook Hospital, Toronto, Ontario, Canada
Ischemic Cerebrovascular Disease

G. ROBERT NUGENT, M.D.

Professor of Neurosurgery, West Virginia University Medical Center, Morgantown, West Virginia
Trigeminal Neuralgia

PATRICK T. O'GARA, M.D.

Instructor in Medicine, Harvard Medical School; Medical Director, Phillips House Coronary Care Unit and Baker Medical Intensive Care Unit, Massachusetts General Hospital, Boston, Massachusetts
Acute Myocardial Infarction

JEFFREY P. OKESON, D.M.D.

Director and Professor, Orofacial Pain Center, University of Kentucky College of Dentistry, Lexington, Kentucky
Temporomandibular Disorders

ANGELA M. O'NEAL, M.D.

Stroke Fellow, Boston University Hospital, Boston, Massachusetts
Intracerebral Hemorrhage

STEVEN M. OPAL, M.D.

Assistant Professor of Medicine, Brown University Program in Medicine, Providence; Infectious Disease Physician, Memorial Hospital of Rhode Island, Pawtucket, Rhode Island
Pyelonephritis

MIGUEL L. O'RYAN, M.D.

Fellow in Pediatrics, University of Texas Health Science Center at Houston Medical School, Houston, Texas
Cholera

P. J. OSMUNDSON, M.D.

Associate Professor of Medicine, Mayo Medical School; Attending Physician, St. Marys Hospital and Rochester Methodist Hospital, Rochester, Minnesota
Venous Stasis Ulcers

DENNIS R. OWNBY, M.D.

Clinical Associate Professor of Pediatrics and Communicable Diseases, University of Michigan Medical School; Director, Pediatric Allergy Immunology Research Laboratory, Henry Ford Hospital, Detroit, Michigan
Adverse Reactions to Drugs

J. CAMILO PALACIO, M.D.

Fellow in Surgical Metabolism and Nutrition, Harrison Department of Surgical Research, University of Pennsylvania School of Medicine; Metabolic and Nutrition Support Service, Department of Surgery, Hospital of the University of Pennsylvania, Philadelphia, Pennsylvania
Parenteral Nutrition in Adults

THOMAS D. PALELLA, M.D.

Associate Professor of Internal Medicine, Chief, Division of Rheumatology, and Director, Rackham Arthritis Research Unit, University of Michigan Medical School, Ann Arbor, Michigan
Rheumatoid Arthritis

NORMAN M. PANITCH, M.D.

Assistant Clinical Professor of Medicine, University of California, Los Angeles, School of Medicine, Los Angeles; Director, Endoscopy and Special Procedures, Torrance Memorial Hospital Medical Center; Consultant and Attending Staff, Harbor General Hospital–University of California, Los Angeles, Medical Center, Torrance, California
Gaseousness and Indigestion

LASZLO A. PAPP, M.D.

Assistant Professor of Clinical Psychiatry, Columbia University College of Physicians and Surgeons; Assistant Attending Physician, Presbyterian Hospital; Attending Psychiatrist, Hillside Hospital and Gracie Square Hospital; Director, Phobia, Anxiety and Stress Disorders Clinic, Hillside Hospital, New York, New York
Panic Disorder and Agoraphobia

ELDRYD H. O. PARRY, M.D.

Visiting Professor, London School of Hygiene and Tropical Medicine, University of London, London, England
Relapsing Fevers

JAMES N. PARSONS, M.D.

Clinical Assistant Professor of Internal Medicine, Ohio State University College of Medicine; Active Staff, Department of Medicine, Mt. Carmel Medical Center, Columbus, Ohio
Anaerobic and Necrotizing Infections Including Gas Gangrene

RICHARD D. PEARSON, M.D.

Associate Professor of Medicine and Pathology, University of Virginia School of Medicine; Attending Physician, University of Virginia Health Sciences Center and University of Virginia Hospitals, Charlottesville, Virginia
Toxoplasmosis

JAY I. PETERS, M.D.

Associate Professor of Medicine and Program Director, University of Texas Health Science Center Hospitals at San Antonio, San Antonio, Texas
Acute Respiratory Failure

JOHN M. PETTIFOR, M.B., PH.D.(MED.)

Professor of Paediatric Mineral Metabolism, Department of Paediatrics, University of the Witwatersrand Medical School, Johannesburg; Consultant Paediatrician and Director, MRC/University Mineral Metabolism Research Unit, Baragwanath Hospital, Bertsham, South Africa
Rickets and Osteomalacia

BRENT G. PETTY, M.D.

Associate Professor of Medicine, Johns Hopkins University School of Medicine; Active Staff, Johns Hopkins Hospital, Baltimore, Maryland
Viral Diseases of the Skin

BARBARA PHILLIPS, M.D.

Associate Professor, University of Kentucky College of Medicine; Active Teaching Staff, Albert B. Chandler Medical Center; Consultant, Veterans Administration Medical Center, Lexington, Kentucky
Chronic Obstructive Pulmonary Disease

WILLIAM REVELLE PHIPPS, M.D.

Assistant Professor, Department of Obstetrics and Gynecology, University of Minnesota Medical School; Staff Physician, University of Minnesota Hospital and Clinic, Minneapolis, Minnesota
Dysfunctional Uterine Bleeding

CLAUS A. PIERACH, M.D.

Associate Professor of Medicine, University of Minnesota Medical School; Attending Physician, Abbott Northwestern Hospital, Minneapolis, Minnesota
Porphyria

HAROLD PLOTNICK, M.D.

Clinical Professor of Dermatology, Wayne State University School of Medicine; Vice-Chief, Department of Dermatology, Harper-Grace Hospitals, Detroit Medical Center, Detroit, Michigan
Occupational Dermatitis

ROGER J. PORTER, M.D.

Clinical Professor of Neurology and Adjunct Professor of Pharmacology, Uniformed Services University of the Health Sciences; Staff, Clinical Center, National Institutes of Health; Staff, National Naval Medical Center, Bethesda, Maryland
Epilepsy in Adolescents and Adults

WILLIAM A. PRIMACK, M.D.

Associate Professor of Pediatrics, University of Massachusetts Medical School; Active Staff, University of Massachusetts Hospital and St. Vincent Hospital, Worcester, Massachusetts
Parenteral Fluid Therapy in Infants and Children

THOMAS J. PULLIAM, M.D.

Assistant Chief, Department of Medicine, Bowman Gray School of Medicine; Attending Physician, North Carolina Baptist Hospital, Winston-Salem, North Carolina
Dysphagia and Esophageal Obstruction

GARY F. PURDUE, M.D.

Associate Professor, University of Texas Southwestern Medical Center, Dallas, Texas
Burns

THOMAS REA, M.D.

Professor and Chairman, Section of Dermatology, University of Southern California School of Medicine, Los Angeles, California
Moles and Melanoma

LAWRENCE D. RECHT, M.D.

Assistant Professor of Neurology, University of Massachusetts Medical School; Attending Neurologist, University of Massachusetts Medical Center, Worcester, Massachusetts
Peripheral Neuropathies

LEE B. REICHMAN, M.D., M.P.H.

Professor of Medicine, University of Medicine and Dentistry of New Jersey; Director, Pulmonary Division, University Hospital, Newark, New Jersey
Tuberculosis and Other Mycobacterial Diseases

HERBERT Y. REYNOLDS, M.D.

Professor of Internal Medicine and Chairman, Department of Medicine, Milton S. Hershey Medical Center, Pennsylvania State University; Attending Physician, University Hospital, Hershey, Pennsylvania
Hypersensitivity Pneumonitis

HOBART K. RICHEY, M.D.

Resident in Dermatology, Division of Dermatology, Department of Internal Medicine, University of South Florida College of Medicine, Tampa, Florida
Parasitic Infestations

JOEL E. RICHTER, M.D.

Associate Professor of Medicine, Gastroenterology Section, Bowman Gray School of Medicine; Attending Physician, North Carolina Baptist Hospital, Winston-Salem, North Carolina
Dysphagia and Esophageal Obstruction

MICHEL E. RIVLIN, M.D.

Associate Professor, Department of Obstetrics and Gynecology, University of Mississippi Medical School; Director, Ambulatory Ob/Gyn, University of Mississippi Medical Center, Jackson, Mississippi
Pelvic Inflammatory Disease

O. G. RODMAN, M.D.

Dermatology Department, Henry Ford Hospital, Detroit, Michigan
Keloids

BLAKE J. ROESSLER, M.D.

Postdoctoral Fellow, University of Michigan, Ann Arbor, Michigan
Rheumatoid Arthritis

JOHN L. ROMBEAU, M.D.

Associate Professor, School of Medicine, Hospital of University of Pennsylvania; Staff, Hospital of University of Pennsylvania, Philadelphia, Pennsylvania
Parenteral Nutrition in Adults

E. WILLIAM ROSENBERG, M.D.

Professor, Departments of Medicine (Dermatology) and Community Medicine, University of Tennessee College of Medicine; Consultant, Veterans Administration Medical Center, St. Jude Children's Research Center, Regional Medical Center at Memphis, and William F. Bould Hospital, Memphis, Tennessee
Hair Disorders

HOWARD L. ROSNER, M.D.

Assistant Professor, Department of Anesthesiology, Columbia University College of Physicians and Surgeons; Assistant Attending Anesthesiologist and Co-director, Pain Treatment Service, Presbyterian Hospital, New York, New York
Pain

HARLEY A. ROTBART, M.D.

Assistant Professor of Pediatrics (Infectious Diseases) and Microbiology-Immunology, University of Colorado School of Medicine, Denver, Colorado
Viral Meningoencephalitis

H. GIL RUSHTON, M.D.

Assistant Professor of Urology and Pediatrics, George Washington University School of Medicine; Vice Chairman, Department of Pediatric Urology, Children's Hospital National Medical Center, Washington, D.C.
Childhood Enuresis

A. S. RUSSELL, M.B., B.CHIR.

Professor of Medicine, University of Alberta Faculty of Medicine; Consultant, University of Alberta Hospitals, Edmonton, Alberta, Canada
Ankylosing Spondylitis

JULIUS SAGEL, M.D.

Professor of Medicine, Division of Endocrinology-Metabolism-Nutrition, Medical University of South Carolina; Chief, Medical Service, Veterans Administration Medical Center, Charleston, South Carolina
Adrenocortical Insufficiency

EDWARD C. SALTZSTEIN, M.D.

Professor and Associate Chairman, Department of Surgery, Texas Tech University School of Medicine; Director of Surgical Services, R.E. Thomason General Hospital, El Paso, Texas
Cholecystitis and Cholelithiasis

JOEL R. SAPER, M.D.

Clinical Associate Professor of Medicine, Michigan Headache and Neurological Institute, Michigan State University; Attending Physician, St. Joseph Mercy Hospital, Ann Arbor, Michigan
Headaches

GEORGE A. SAROSI, M.D.

Professor of Medicine, University of Texas Health Science Center at Houston; Attending Physician, Hermann Hospital, Lyndon B. Johnson General Hospital, and M. D. Anderson Hospital, Houston, Texas
Bacterial Pneumonia

MICHAEL G. SARR, M.D.

Assistant Professor of Surgery, Mayo Medical School; Consultant in Surgery, St. Mary's Hospital and Mayo Clinic, Rochester, Minnesota
Chronic Pancreatitis

WILLIAM D. SAWYER, M.D.

China Medical Board, New York, New York
Typhus Fevers

ERNST J. SCHAEFER, M.D.

Associate Professor of Medicine, Tufts University School of Medicine; Associate Professor of Medicine, New England Medical Center, Boston, Massachusetts
Hyperlipoproteinemia

PETER M. SCHANTZ, V.M.D., PH.D.

Epidemiologist, Parasitic Diseases Branch, Centers for Infectious Diseases, Centers for Disease Control, Atlanta, Georgia
Trichinellosis

ARTHUR B. SCHNEIDER, M.D., PH.D.

Professor of Medicine, University of Chicago Pritzker School of Medicine; Head, Section of Endocrinology and Metabolism, Michael Reese Hospital and Medical Center, Chicago, Illinois
Hyperthyroidism

ROBERT T. SCHOEN, M.D.

Assistant Clinical Professor and Co-director, Lyme Disease Program, Yale University School of Medicine; Attending Physician, Yale–New Haven Hospital; Assistant Attending Physician, Hospital of St. Raphael, New Haven, Connecticut
Lyme Disease

HOWARD J. SCHWARTZ, M.D.

Clinical Professor of Medicine, Case Western Reserve University School of Medicine; Associate Physician and Chief, Adult Allergy Clinic, University Hospitals of Cleveland, Cleveland, Ohio
Allergic Reactions to Insect Stings

WAYNE H. SCHWESINGER, M.D.

Professor of Surgery, University of Texas Health Science Center at San Antonio; Attending Physician, Audie Murphy Memorial Veterans Medical Center and Medical Center Hospital, San Antonio, Texas
Cancer of the Large Bowel

DOUGLAS SEATON, M.D.

Consultant Physician in Respiratory and Internal Medicine, Department of Respiratory Medicine, Ipswich Hospital, Suffolk, England
Silicosis

RICHARD B. SEWELL, M.D.

Senior Lecturer, University of Melbourne; Deputy Director of Gastroenterology, Austin Hospital, Melbourne, Australia
Acute and Chronic Viral Hepatitis

HEIDI SHALE, M.D.

Junior Assistant Attending Physician, St. Lukes–Roosevelt Hospital; Associate in Clinical Neurology, Columbia-Presbyterian Medical Center, New York, New York
Parkinsonism

JAMES C. SHEININ, M.D.

Clinical Associate Professor of Medicine, University of Chicago Pritzker School of Medicine; Attending Physician, Division of Endocrinology and Metabolism, Michael Reese Hospital and Medical Center, Chicago, Illinois
Hyperthyroidism

PHILIP D. SHENEFELT, M.D.

Assistant Professor of Medicine, Division of Dermatology, Department of Internal Medicine, University of South Florida College of Medicine; Assistant Chief, Dermatology Section, James A. Haley Veterans Hospital, Tampa; Chief, Dermatology Section, Bay Pines Veterans Administration Medical Center, St. Petersburg, Florida
Parasitic Infestations

SHELDON G. SHEPS, M.D.

Professor of Medicine, Mayo Medical School, Rochester, Minnesota
Pheochromocytoma

ALAIN H. SHIKHANI, M.D.

Senior Resident, Department of Otolaryngology–Head and Neck Surgery, Johns Hopkins Hospital, Baltimore, Maryland
Sinusitis

CLARENCE SHUB, M.D.

Associate Professor of Medicine, Mayo Medical School; Consultant, Cardiovascular Diseases, Mayo Clinic, Rochester, Minnesota
Angina Pectoris

FREDERICK P. SIEGAL, M.D.

Professor of Medicine, State University of New York at Stony Brook, Stony Brook; Attending Physician, Department of Medicine, and Head, Hematology Research Division of Hematology-Oncology, Long Island Jewish Medical Center, New Hyde Park, New York
Management of HIV Infections

GARY L. SIMON, M.D., PH.D.

Professor of Medicine and Associate Chairman, Department of Medicine, George Washington University School of Medicine, Washington, D.C.
Tularemia

ROBERT B. SKINNER, Jr., M.D.

Associate Professor of Medicine (Dermatology), Regional Medical Center at Memphis; Attending Physician, Veterans Administration Medical Center, William F. Bowld Hospital, Baptist Memorial Hospital, Lebohneur Children's Medical Center, and St. Jude's Children's Research Hospital, Memphis, Tennessee
Hair Disorders; Urticaria and Angioedema

EDWIN A. SMITH, M.D.

Assistant Professor of Medicine, Medical University of South Carolina; Attending Physician, Medical University Hospital, Charleston Memorial Hospital, and Veterans Administration Medical Center, Charleston, South Carolina
Polymyalgia Rheumatica and Giant Cell Arteritis

WILLIAM J. SNAPE, Jr., M.D.

Professor of Medicine and Director, Inflammatory Bowel Disease Center, University of California, Los Angeles, School of Medicine, Los Angeles; Chief, Gastroenterology Section, Harbor–University of California, Los Angeles, Medical Center, Torrance, California
Irritable Bowel Syndrome

CONSTANTIN R. SOLDATOS, M.D.

Associate Professor, Department of Psychiatry, University of Athens; Director, Sleep Disorders Unit, Eginition Hospital, Athens, Greece.
Insomnia

HUMBERTO A. SORIANO, M.D.

Associate Professor of Pediatrics, School of Medicine, Catholic University of Chile; Attending Pediatrician, Pediatric Unit, Clinical Hospital, Catholic University of Chile, Santiago, Chile
Acute Infectious Diarrhea

MAREK A. STAWISKI, M.D.

Clinical Associate Professor of Internal Medicine, Michigan State Medical School; Chief, Dermatology Section, Saint Mary's Hospital; Member, Department of Internal Medicine, Butterworth Hospital, Grand Rapids, Michigan
Pruritus (Itching)

MARTIN H. STEINBERG, M.D.

Professor of Medicine, University of Mississippi School of Medicine; Associate Chief of Staff for Research, Veterans Administration Medical Center, Jackson, Mississippi
Iron Deficiency Anemia

ROBERT A. SWERLICK, M.D.

Assistant Professor, Department of Dermatology, Emory University School of Medicine; Staff Physician, Emory University Hospital and Grady Memorial Hospital, Atlanta, Georgia
Skin Diseases of Pregnancy

RONALD W. SWINFARD, M.D.

Assistant Professor, Dermatology Division, University of Missouri–Columbia School of Medicine; Attending Physician, University of Missouri Medical Center and Harry S. Truman Veterans Administration Hospital, Columbia, Missouri
Spider Bites and Scorpion Stings

CHRISTINE L. TERRELL, M.D.

Instructor of Medicine, Mayo Medical School; Consultant in Infectious Diseases and Internal Medicine, Mayo Clinic, Rochester, Minnesota
Blastomycosis

DAVID H. THOM, M.D., M.P.H.

Senior Fellow, Department of Epidemiology, School of Public Health and Community Medicine, University of Washington, Seattle, Washington
Psittacosis (Ornithosis)

SUMNER E. THOMPSON, III, M.D., M.P.H.

Director, Infectious Disease Clinic, and Associate Professor of Medicine, Grady Memorial Hospital, Atlanta, Georgia
Gonorrhea

IAN H. THORNEYCROFT, Ph.D., M.D.

John Rock Professor and Vice-Chairman and Chief, Section of Reproductive Endocrinology and Infertility, Department of Obstetrics and Gynecology, and Adjunct Professor of Physiology, Tulane University School of Medicine; Staff Physician, Tulane Medical Center Hospital, Touro Infirmary, and Baptist Hospital, New Orleans, Louisiana
Osteoporosis

CHARLES P. TIFFT, M.D.

Associate Professor of Medicine, Boston University School of Medicine; Attending Physician, Cardiovascular Institute, University Hospital, and Boston City Hospital, Boston, Massachusetts
Hypertension

DORIS A. TRAUNER, M.D.

Professor of Neurosciences and Pediatrics, University of California, San Diego, School of Medicine, La Jolla; Chief, Pediatric Neurology, University of California, San Diego, Medical Center, San Diego, California
Reye's Syndrome

JOHN R. TRAUTMAN, M.D.

Director, International Programs, Gillis W. Long Hansen's Disease Center, Carville, Louisiana
Leprosy (Hansen's Disease)

WILLIAM J. TREMAINE, M.D.

Assistant Professor of Medicine, Mayo Graduate School of Medicine, Mayo Clinic; Consultant in Gastroenterology and Internal Medicine, Rochester Methodist Hospital and St. Mary's Hospital, Rochester, Minnesota
Crohn's Disease

JAIME A. TSCHEN, M.D.

Associate Professor, Department of Pathology and Dermatology, and Director of Dermatopathology, Baylor College of Medicine; Attending Physician, Methodist Hospital and Veterans Administration Medical Center, Houston, Texas
Cancer of the Skin

WILLIAM N. VALENTINE, M.D.

Professor Emeritus, Department of Medicine, University of California Center for Health Sciences, Los Angeles, California
Nonimmune Hemolytic Anemia

JON A. van HEERDEN, M.D.

Professor of Surgery, Mayo Medical School; Consultant in Surgery, St. Marys Hospital, Rochester, Minnesota
Chronic Pancreatitis

L. GEORGE VEASY, M.D.

Professor and Associate Chairman, Department of Pediatrics, University of Utah School of Medicine; Physician in Chief, Primary Children's Hospital Medical Center, Salt Lake City, Utah
Rheumatic Fever

GREGORY RAY VEST, M.D.

Attending Surgical Staff, Valley Baptist Medical Center, Harlingen, Texas
Tetanus

JAMES P. VIGLIANCO, M.D.

Surgical Resident, Mt. Carmel Medical Center, Columbus, Ohio
Tetanus

RICHARD W. VILTER, M.D.

Professor Emeritus of Medicine, University of Cincinnati College of Medicine; Attending Physician, University Hospital, Cincinnati College of Medicine; Consultant, Christ Hospital, Jewish Hospital of Cincinnati, Deaconess Hospital, and Good Samaritan Hospital, Cincinnati, Ohio
Beriberi (Thiamine Deficiency)

EILEEN P. G. VINING, M.D.

Associate Professor of Neurology and Pediatrics, Johns Hopkins University School of Medicine; Active Staff, Department of Neurology and Department of Pediatrics, Johns Hopkins Hospital, Baltimore, Maryland
Epilepsy in Infants and Children

MARSHA L. WAKEFIELD, M.D.

Assistant Professor of Anesthesiology, Medical College of Georgia; Attending Physician, Medical College of Georgia Hospital and Veterans Administration Medical Center, Augusta, Georgia
Obstetric Anesthesia

WILLIAM D. WALDEN, M.D.

Clinical Associate Professor of Obstetrics and Gynecology, Cornell University Medical College; Associate Attending Obstetrician and Gynecologist, New York Hospital, New York, New York
Abortion

STANLEY WALLACH, M.D.

Professor and Associate Chairman, Department of Internal Medicine, University of South Florida College of Medicine, Tampa; Chief, Medical Service, Veterans Administration Medical Center, Bay Pines, Florida
Paget's Disease of Bone

ROBERT W. WARREN, M.D., PH.D.

Head, Section of Rheumatology, Department of Pediatrics, Baylor College of Medicine; Attending Physician, Harris County Texas Children's Hospital, Houston, Texas
Juvenile Rheumatoid Arthritis

CODY WASNER, M.D.

Assistant Professor of Rheumatology, Oregon Health Sciences University; Attending Physician, Sacred Hospital, Eugene, Oregon
Connective Tissue Disorders: Lupus Erythematosus, Dermatomyositis, and Scleroderma

W. DOUGLAS WEAVER, M.D.

Associate Professor of Medicine and Director, Cardiovascular Critical Care, University Hospital, Seattle, Washington
Rehabilitation After Myocardial Infarction

SUZANNE K. WEDEL, M.D.

Assistant Professor of Surgery and Medicine, Boston University School of Medicine; Associate Director, Surgery Intensive Care Unit, Boston City Hospital and University Hospital, Boston, Massachusetts
Thrombophlebitis in Obstetrics and Gynecology

CARL P. WEINER, M.D.

Associate Professor, University of Iowa College of Medicine, Iowa City, Iowa
Hypertensive Disorders of Pregnancy

ROBERT N. WEINREB, M.D.

Professor and Vice Chairman, Department of Ophthalmology, University of California, San Diego, School of Medicine, San Diego, California
Glaucoma

ROLAND L. WEINSIER, M.D., DR.P.H.

Professor and Chairman, Department of Nutrition Sciences, and Professor, Department of Medicine, University of Alabama at Birmingham School of Medicine, Birmingham, Alabama
Obesity

KATHARINE D. WENSTROM, M.D.

Fellow Associate, University of Iowa Medical School and University of Iowa Hospitals and Clinics, Iowa City, Iowa
Hypertensive Disorders of Pregnancy

L. JOSEPH WHEAT, M.D.

Professor of Medicine, Indiana University School of Medicine; Attending Physician, Wishard Memorial Hospital, Indiana University Hospital, and Richard L. Roudebush Veterans Administration Hospital, Indianapolis, Indiana.
Histoplasmosis

JOHN L. WHITING, M.D.

Formerly Fellow in Division of Infectious Diseases, Department of Medicine, University of British Columbia, Vancouver, British Columbia, Canada; Practicing Internist and Infectious Diseases Consultant, Brisbane, Queensland, Australia
Toxic Shock Syndrome

BERNHARD L. WIEDERMANN, M.D.

Assistant Professor of Pediatrics, George Washington University School of Medicine and Health Sciences; Director, Infectious Diseases Clinic, and Attending in Infectious Diseases, Children's Hospital National Medical Center, Washington, D.C.
Food-Borne Illness

SAMUEL E. WILSON, M.D.

Professor of Surgery, University of California, Los Angeles, School of Medicine, Los Angeles; Chairman, Department of Surgery, Harbor–University of Caifornia, Los Angeles, Medical Center, Torrance, California
Bacterial Diseases of the Skin

WILLIS A. WINGERT, M.D.

Professor of Pediatrics, Emergency Medicine and Public Health, University of Southern California School of Medicine; Director, Venom Laboratory, Los Angeles County–University of Southern California Medical Center, Los Angeles, California
Snakebite

A. WODAK, M.D., M.B.

Honorary Lecturer, School of Medicine, University of New South Wales; Director, Alcohol and Drug Service, St. Vincent's Hospital, Darlinghurst, New South Wales, Australia
Alcoholism

JOHN E. WOLF, JR., M.D.

Professor and Chairman, Department of Dermatology, Baylor College of Medicine; Chief of Service, Methodist Hospital, Texas Children's Hospital, and Ben Taub General Hospital; Consultant, Veterans Administration Medical Center; Acting Staff, St. Luke's Episcopal Hospital, Houston, Texas
Contact Dermatitis

MARTIN S. WOLFE, M.D.

Clinical Professor of Medicine and Clinical Associate Professor of Medicine, Georgetown University Medical School; Attending Physician, George Washington University Hospital and Georgetown University Hospital, Washington, D.C.
Malaria

DOUGLAS L. WOOD, M.D.

Assistant Professor of Medicine and Consultant in Cardiovascular Disease, Mayo Medical School, Mayo Foundation, Rochester, Minneosta
Tachycardia

GERALD M. WOODS, M.D.

Associate Professor of Pediatrics, University of Missouri–Kansas City Medical School; Staff Pediatric Hematologist-Oncologist, Children's Mercy Hospital, Kansas City, Missouri
Acute Leukemia in Childhood

CHARLES F. WOOLEY, M.D.

Professor of Medicine, Division of Cardiology, Ohio State University; House Staff, Ohio State University Hospitals, Columbus, Ohio
Mitral Valve Prolapse and the Mitral Valve Prolapse Syndrome

GEORGE C. XAKELLIS, M.D.

Assistant Professor, Department of Family Practice, University of Iowa College of Medicine; Staff Physician, Mercy Hospital and Iowa City Care Center, Iowa City, Iowa
Decubitus Ulcers

JAMES S. T. YAO, M.D., PH.D.

Magerstadt Professor of Surgery and Chief, Division of Vascular Surgery, Northwestern University Medical School; Attending Vascular Surgeon and Director, Blood Flow Laboratory, Northwestern Memorial Hospital, Chicago, Illinois
Peripheral Arterial Disease

JAMES D. YATES, M.D.

Clinical Associate Professor, Department of Internal Medicine, University of Tennessee College of Medicine, Memphis; Clinical Associate Professor, Department of Internal Medicine, University of Tennessee Memorial Hospital, Knoxville, Tennessee
Artrial Fibrillation

JOHN A. YEUNG-LAI-WAH, M.B., CH.B.

Assistant Professor of Medicine, Division of Cardiology, and Staff Cardiologist, University Hospital, Vancouver, British Columbia, Canada
Premature Beats

WILLIAM F. YOUNG, JR., M.D.

Assistant Professor of Medicine, Mayo Graduate School of Medicine; Consultant in Endocrinology, Hypertension, and Internal Medicine, Mayo Clinic and Mayo Foundation, St. Mary's Hospital, and Rochester Methodist Hospital, Rochester, Minnesota
Acromegaly

NARDO ZAIAS, M.D.

Director, Residency Program, Mt. Sinai Medical Center, Miami Beach, Florida
Fungal Diseases of the Skin

ROBERT ZANE, M.D.

Resident, Department of Surgery, Harbor–University of California at Los Angeles Medical Center, Torrance, California
Bacterial Diseases of the Skin

HAROLD ZARKOWSKY, M.D.

Associate Professor, Washington University School of Medicine; Associate Pediatrician, St. Louis Children's Hospital, St. Louis, Missouri
Sickle Cell Disease

IRWIN ZIMENT, M.D.

Professor of Medicine, University of California, Los Angeles, School of Medicine, Los Angeles; Chief of Medicine, Olive View Medical Center, Sylman, California
Cough

JOHN J. ZONE, M.D.

Chief, Division of Dermatology, University of Utah Health Science Center, and Veterans Administration Medical Center, Salt Lake City, Utah
Bullous Diseases

Preface

The practicing physician is under constant pressure to remain current with medical advances. It is a struggle to keep up with the enormous volume of articles published and to find pearls that can be used in practice. This book seeks to ease that struggle in that it

1. Offers annually new and useful information on the management of common problems in a format that is concise and easy to reference

2. Selects authorities in the field who see the problem frequently and are on the leading edge of new developments

3. Provides thorough editorial review by physicians, editors, and pharmacists to ensure accuracy

In this edition, 347 international authorities give their methods for managing 284 clinical problems. The article on management of HIV infections has been expanded greatly compared with previous editions to address more adequately the challenge of caring for patients with this complex and devastating disease. The Acute Poisoning Section also has undergone major revision, and we have added glaucoma as a new topic.

In all, more than 75 per cent of the articles in this edition are entirely new (written by new authors); the remainder have been thoroughly revised and updated. Where appropriate, important diagnostic features are discussed in addition to therapy.

The goal of *Current Therapy* today is the same as that conceived by the late Howard Conn more than 40 years ago and first published in 1949: to provide the practicing physician with a concise, practical reference that includes the most recent advances in therapy. In view of the information explosion that physicians confront, this is no small task.

Many people have shared in our efforts to realize this goal. I want to express my thanks to all the contributors who agreed to share their preferred treatment methods with other physicians. My special thanks also to John Dyson and the editorial staff at W. B. Saunders; Roxy Cuddy, my editorial assistant; Lucinda Miller, Pharm.D., and Barry Carter, Pharm.D., who reviewed all drug uses and dosages; and most especially my wife Peggy, who tolerates my penchant for writing and editing.

ROBERT E. RAKEL, M.D.

Table of Contents

SECTION 3. THE RESPIRATORY SYSTEM

SECTION 4. THE CARDIOVASCULAR SYSTEM

SECTION 5. THE BLOOD AND SPLEEN

SECTION 6. THE DIGESTIVE SYSTEM

SECTION 7. METABOLIC DISORDERS

SECTION 8. THE ENDOCRINE SYSTEM

SECTION 9. THE UROGENITAL TRACT

SECTION 10. THE SEXUALLY TRANSMITTED DISEASES

SECTION 11. DISEASES OF ALLERGY

SECTION 12. DISEASES OF THE SKIN

SECTION 13. THE NERVOUS SYSTEM

SECTION 14. THE LOCOMOTOR SYSTEM

SECTION 15. OBSTETRICS AND GYNECOLOGY

SECTION 16. PSYCHIATRIC DISORDERS

SECTION 17. PHYSICAL AND CHEMICAL INJURIES

SECTION 18. APPENDICES AND INDEX

Section 1

Symptomatic Care Pending Diagnosis

PAIN

method of
HOWARD L. ROSNER, M.D.

*Columbia University College of Physicians
 and Surgeons*
Columbia-Presbyterian Medical Center
New York, New York

Pain is a universal condition whose sequelae are often incapacitating. By all definitions and tests available, pain is a subjective phenomenon. Unfortunately, there are as yet no readily available, reliable objective criteria to measure and quantitate pain. Emphasizing the subjective nature of pain, the International Society for the Study of Pain has defined pain as "an unpleasant sensory and emotional experience associated with actual or potential tissue damage, or described in terms of such damage." The assessment of pain cannot be made through purely objective criteria; rather, the patient's subjective report is essential for diagnosis and management. Social and cultural factors have a major role in the self-assessment of pain. Behavioral patterning learned in early childhood influences the patient's pain experience. It is not that there are cultural differences in the experience of sensation; rather, the *report* of pain from a given sensation can differ greatly from patient to patient.

Pain is classified most commonly on the basis of the duration of symptoms. Table 1 describes five categories based on this temporal classification: acute, subacute, ongoing acute, recurrent acute, and chronic benign. The etiology and treatment of these entities differ. Acute pain is self-limited and easier to manage. Chronic benign pain, especially with poor coping mechanisms, has been termed "chronic intractable benign pain syndrome" or "chronic pain syndrome" and is extremely difficult to treat. Although acute pain can be managed by a single physician, chronic intractable benign pain requires a multimodal approach that must include psychologic evaluation and treatment in addition to any physical modalities.

Basic scientists have elucidated much of the pain transmission system. From peripheral nociceptors (pain receptors) to the cortex, many of the neurotransmitters, modulators, and receptors have been identified. Medications are available that can interfere with or augment aspects of this transmission and modula-

tion system to diminish the input of pain impulses into the cortex. These medications include conventional narcotic analgesics, nonsteroidal anti-inflammatory drugs (NSAIDs), and neuroactive and psychoactive agents. Each has its place in the pharmacologic management of one or more of the pain syndromes. Alternative or adjuvant modalities to medications include transcutaneous electrical nerve stimulation, hypnosis and biofeedback, nerve blocks, and physical therapy. These alternative treatments are beyond the scope of general office practice but are widely used by specialists in pain management.

MANAGEMENT

The management of pain syndromes should begin with an attempt to identify and treat the underlying cause of the pain. Sometimes this task is easy; however, often the underlying cause is obscure or cannot be treated. This does not preempt the management of pain; it makes the focus of treatment the pain itself rather than its cause. The objective of any treatment is threefold: to reduce pain, to decrease anxiety, and to return to function. There are no easy recipes or formulas to treat all of these problems. Treatment must be individualized because each problem is unique and each patient responds differently from his or her peers.

Medications

The majority of pain complaints arise from acute and subacute causes, when the underlying problem is most commonly tissue injury, either intrinsic or extrinsic. For acute and subacute pain, the major step in management is to provide analgesic support while the body has time to heal itself. The causes of ongoing and recurrent acute pain are rarely self-limited. On the basis of objective signs and subjective reports, pain is subdivided into three classes: mild, moderate, and severe. An analgesic regimen can be constructed that is related to the severity of pain. For such a regimen, three classes of medications are available: (1) non-narcotic analgesics, (2) narcotic an-

TABLE 1. **Pain Classification by Duration of Symptoms**

Category	Characteristics
Acute	Duration of 0–7 days
	Mild to severe
	Etiology known or unknown; usually a single, "fixable" event
	Input from nociceptors (peripheral pain receptors)
	Treatment of causes and reduction of pain: often an emergency
	Analgesics: narcotic and non-narcotic
	Mild psychologic contribution
Subacute	Duration of 7 days–6 mo
	Mild to severe
	Etiology as in acute pain
	Input from nociceptors
	Treatment of causes and reduction of pain: usually not an emergency
	Mild psychologic contribution
Ongoing acute	Any duration
	Usually severe
	Etiology related to ongoing tissue damage from neoplasms
	Input from nociceptors
	Treatment of causes and reduction of pain
	Analgesics: narcotic and non-narcotic
	Depression and anxiety common
Recurrent acute	Any duration
	Mild to severe
	Etiology related to chronic organic non-malignant pathology
	Input from nociceptors
	Treatment of causes and reduction of pain
	Analgesics: non-narcotic and coanalgesics as first treatment; narcotics sometimes indicated
	Depression and anxiety common
Chronic benign	Duration of more than 6 mo
	Mild to severe
	Etiology unknown
	No known nociceptive input
	Treatment aimed at reduction of pain
	Analgesics: non-narcotic and coanalgesics; usually no indication for narcotics
	Psychologic factors very important; psychotherapy indicated
	Patient may or may not have adequate coping mechanisms

algesics, and (3) coanalgesics. As a simple rule of thumb, the more severe the pain, the more potent the medications used in its management.

Non-narcotic analgesics consist of acetaminophen, aspirin, and the NSAIDs. These drugs are the mainstay of management of mild pain and can be part of the overall management of moderate to severe pain. NSAIDs exert a peripheral action by reducing prostaglandin synthesis (prostaglandins are major activators of nociceptors after tissue injury); they relieve mild to moderate inflammation and have an antipyretic action. Aspirin, because of its long history of safety and effectiveness, has been the standard against which all NSAIDs have been judged. Table 2 presents the most commonly used NSAIDs together with dosage schedules, maximum daily doses, and side effects. These agents have a ceiling effect (a dose above which there is no additional benefit) and have no potential for tolerance or addiction. These drugs all tend to have the same activity when given in equipotent doses. The major limiting factors are adverse reactions and convenience of dosage schedules.

Acetaminophen (which has many trade names) is not an NSAID. Although it is an antipyretic agent, it has no peripheral anti-inflammatory or prostaglandin inhibitory activity. It does, however, have analgesic properties, probably from central activity. The usual dose is 650 to 1000 mg every 4 to 6 hours by mouth or per rectum, with a maximum daily dosage of 6 to 8 grams (however, chronic daily ingestion of 5 to 8 grams over several weeks or 3 to 4 grams per day per year can result in liver damage). It can be given in conjunction with NSAIDs as well as with narcotic analgesics (whose activity it can potentiate).

Narcotic analgesics are rarely used for mild pain; however, they are frequently used for moderate to severe pain. Pharmacologically, they are placed in one of two classes: (1) pure opiate receptor agonists or (2) mixed agonist-antagonists, which have some properties of naloxone (an opiate receptor antagonist) plus properties of a direct agonist. The model of a pure receptor agonist is morphine, although there are many drugs of this class available. The mixed agonist-antagonist analgesics have been slow to achieve much popularity because of several factors, including a ceiling effect for analgesia, reversal of analgesia for patients taking pure agonists, and (with the exception of pentazocine) the unavailability of oral preparations. Medications in this group include buprenorphine, nalbuphine, and butorphanol. Tables 3 and 4 describe many commonly used narcotic analgesics that are used for mild to moderate pain and for severe pain, respectively. In outpatient situations, the most convenient route of administration is via the gastrointestinal tract (oral or rectal). This route has the added benefit of preventing abrupt swings in serum levels by providing a slow onset and decline of drug levels. Care must be taken when prescribing parenteral narcotics that adequate time is given for gastrointestinal absorption (which can take up to 90 minutes), and repeated doses should be given before levels in blood are reduced. The ideal way to use narcotics is to titrate them to a desired level of efficacy for each individual case. Unlike the NSAIDs, narcotics

TABLE 2. **Non-Steroidal Anti-Inflammatory Drugs***

Generic (Trade) Name	Usual Dosage and Route	Maximum Dose Per Day	Major Side Effects†
Aspirin (many)	650–1000 mg orally or rectally q 4 hr	4 grams	Tinnitus
Choline magnesium trisalicylate (Trilisate)	500–1000 mg orally, up to 3 times daily	3 grams	Tinnitus
Diclofenac (Voltaren)	25–75 mg orally, 2 or 3 times daily	150 mg	Headache, edema, dizziness, tinnitus
Diflunisal (Dolobid)	500 mg orally, 2 or 3 times daily	1.5 grams	Headache, rash, fatigue, dizziness
Fenoprofen (Nalfon)	200–600 mg orally, 4 times daily	3.2 grams	Dizziness, headache
Flurbiprofen (Ansaid)	50–100 mg orally, 2 or 3 times daily	300 mg	Headache, central nervous system stimulation or inhibition
Ibuprofen (Advil, Nuprin, Rufen, Motrin)	200–800 mg orally, 3 or 4 times daily	3.2 grams	Dizziness, rash
Indomethacin (Indocin)	25–75 orally q 8–12 hr, or 50 mg rectally q 6–12 hr	200 mg	Confusion, headache
Ketoprofen (Orudis)	50–100 mg orally, 3 times daily	300 mg	Headache, dizziness, drowsiness
Meclofenamate (Meclomen)	50–100 mg orally, 4 times daily	400 mg	Diarrhea, rash
Naproxen (Naprosyn)	250, 375, or 500 mg orally, 2 or 3 times daily	1.25 grams	Dizziness, rash, tinnitus, edema
Piroxicam (Feldene)	10 mg twice daily or 20 mg once daily orally	20 mg	Malaise, dizziness
Salsalate (Disalcid)	500–750 mg orally, 3 or 4 times daily	3 grams	Tinnitus, dizziness, headache, confusion
Sulindac (Clinoril)	150–200 mg orally, twice daily	400 mg	Headache, edema, dizziness, rash
Tolmetin (Tolectin)	400 mg orally, 3 times daily	2 grams	

*Phenylbutazone has not been included here because of the severity of its side effects.
†Common side effects include gastritis, platelet suppression, bowel disturbances, and mild renal suppression.

usually have no peak doses (with the exception of meperidine, propoxyphene, and pentazocine). The major limiting factor in increasing doses of narcotics is the escalation of undesirable side effects such as constipation, sedation, respiratory suppression, and confusion. When narcotics are used for treatment of pain, habituation is unlikely, and the specter of addiction should *not* be a consideration in the use of these analgesics if they are deemed to be necessary for the management of pain.

The goal for any analgesic regimen should be to ensure a serum level sufficiently high for pain relief in the resting state, with additional medication available to provide analgesia for breakthrough pain (pain that "breaks through" the baseline analgesia). Doses should be well within the established serum half-life of the medication

TABLE 3. **Narcotic Analgesics for Mild to Moderate Pain**

Generic (Trade) Name	Starting Dose and Route	Duration of Action (hr)	Comments and Side Effects*
Codeine† (many)	30–60 mg orally q 4–6 hr	4–6	See comment‡
Hydrocodone† (Vicodin)	5–10 mg orally q 4–6 hr	4–6	Dysphoria
Oxycodone† (Percodan, Percocet, Tylox)	2.25–4.5 mg orally q 3–6 hr	3–6	Dysphoria, shorter acting
Pentazocine (Talwin NX)	25–50 mg orally q 3–4 hr; can be given by injection for more severe pain	3–6	Dysphoria, agonist-antagonist type, sometimes mixed with naloxone; may cause withdrawal; peak dose per day 600 mg orally, 360 mg injected
Propoxyphene HCl†	32–65 mg orally	4–6	Dysphoria, hepatic dysfunction, convulsions with overdose
Propoxyphene napsylate (Darvon, Darvon-N, Darvocet-N)	50–100 mg orally q 4–6 hr	4–6	

*Common side effects include respiratory suppression, constipation, somnolence, nausea and vomiting, tolerance with continued use, urinary retention, and pruritus.
†These narcotics are commonly compounded with aspirin or acetaminophen and are known by various trade names.
‡In compounds the dose of codeine is noted by a numeral from 1 to 4; 1 indicates a dose of 7.5 mg, 2 a dose of 15 mg, 3 a dose of 30 mg, and 4 a dose of 60 mg. Other constituents of these compounds may include caffeine, barbiturates, and sympathomimetics.

TABLE 4. **Narcotic Analgesics for Severe Pain**

Generic (Trade) Name	Route and Starting Dose	Peak Duration of Action (hr)	Equianalgesic Dose* (mg)	Comments†
Hydromorphone (Dilaudid)	Oral: 4–6 mg q 3–4 hr	1–2	7.5	Good gastrointestinal (GI) uptake
	Intramuscular: 1–2 mg q 3–4 hr	½–1	1.5	
	Rectal: 3–6 mg q 4–8 hr	1–2	6	
Levorphanol (Levo-Dromoran)	Oral: 2–4 mg q 6–8 hr	1–2	4	Can accumulate during 2–3 days; long plasma half-life; good GI uptake
	Intramuscular: 2 mg q 4–6 hr	½–1	2	
Meperidine (Demerol)	Oral: 50–200 mg q 2–4 hr	1–4	150–200	Poor GI uptake; normeperidine (toxic metabolite) can accumulate; central nervous system excitation; avoid in anyone receiving monoamine oxidase inhibitor
	Intramuscular: 50–100 mg q 2–4 hr	½–3	100	
Methadone (Dolophine)	Oral: 5–10 mg q 6–12 hr	1–2	15–20	Good GI uptake; can accumulate with chronic use yielding half-life up to 2 days
	Intramuscular: 5–10 mg q 4–6 hr	½–1	10	
Morphine Immediate-release (Roxanol)	Oral: 20–60 mg q 3–4 hr	1–2	20–60	Poor GI uptake, improves with use, from 6:1 ratio to 2–3:1 ratio of oral to intramuscular dosing
	Intramuscular: 5–10 mg q 3–4 hr	½–1	10	
Controlled-release (Roxanol SR)	Oral: 20–60 mg q 6–12 hr	2–4	20–60	
Oxymorphone (Numorphan)	Intramuscular: 1 mg q 4 hr	½–1	1	No oral preparation
	Rectal: 5–10 mg q 4–6 hr	1–3	5–10	

*Equianalgesic doses are stated in comparison to 10 mg of intramuscular morphine.

†Common side effects include respiratory suppression, constipation, somnolence, nausea and vomiting, pruritus, urinary retention, tolerance with continued use, dysphoria, and euphoria. Caution should be used in patients at risk of carbon dioxide retention or increased intracranial pressure.

to maintain stable serum levels. This process is easily accomplished by providing medication on a *fixed schedule* for the background analgesia, and rapid-onset medication should be available for breakthrough pain on an as needed basis. The longer-acting narcotic analgesics have the advantage of providing extremely stable serum narcotic levels with only a few doses per day. The shorter-acting narcotics can do the same thing but require frequent dosing. The shorter-acting narcotics do, however, provide good coverage for breakthrough pain.

Coanalgesics are drugs that are used for various medical problems other than pain states. These medications are usually not considered by themselves to be analgesic, but they potentiate the activity of a narcotic or non-narcotic analgesic. For some pain states, these medications are the drugs of choice. For other syndromes, they act to enhance the analgesic regimen. Table 5 gives information for commonly used coanalgesics, including antidepressants, anticonvulsants, antipsychotics, analeptics, and others.

Adjuvant Therapies

Physical modalities available for treatment of pain include conventional physical therapy, transcutaneous electrical nerve stimulation, hypnosis, and biofeedback. Also, several nonconventional therapies can sometimes be helpful in the management of pain patients: chiropractic manipulation, Shiatsu and other massage techniques, acupuncture and acupressure, Alexander's technique, and numerous others. These therapies are aimed at stress reduction and myofascial release. The advantages of these treatments are their lack of invasiveness and low risk to the patients. Disadvantages are their often low rates of efficacy and lack of credibility. However, correct application of these treatments offers choices and alternatives above and beyond conventional medicine and surgery with some success.

Work-up and Treatment

The work-up for a patient presenting with a pain complaint is similar to that for any other patient (Table 6). A detailed history should be taken including a complete pain history, other present and past medical problems, current medications, allergies, social factors, and a detailed review of systems. The severity of the pain should be scored on a consistent scale. The visual analog

TABLE 5. **Coanalgesic Medications***

Drug Class	Indications for Use	Suggested Generic (Trade) Drugs	Starting Total Daily Dose† (mg)	No. of Doses Per Day	Usual Total Daily Dose (mg)	Comments
Analeptic	Reversal of narcotic-induced sedation, euphoria	Dextroamphetamine (Dexedrine)	5	2	Up to 40	Possess analgesic effects
		Methylphenidate (Ritalin)	5	2	Up to 40	
Anticonvulsant	Intermittent, lancinating neuropathic pain	Carbamazepine (Tegretol)	200	3–4	600–800	
		Clonazepam (Klonopin)	0.5	3–4	1.5–8	
		Phenytoin (Dilantin)	100	Up to 3	300 mg	
		Valproic acid (Depakene)	500	3	750–1500	
Antidepressant	Continuous pain of neuropathic origin, depression, or insomnia	Amitriptyline (Elavil)	10–25	1	50–150	Sedating dose at bedtime
		Doxepin (Sinequan)	10–25	1	50–150	
		Imipramine (Tofranil)	10–25	1	50–150	
		Nortriptyline (Pamelor)	10–25	1	25–75	
Antihistamine	Anxiety of nausea with pain	Diphenhydramine (Benadryl)	50	Up to 4	100–200	Needs very high doses for analgesia
		Hydroxyzine pamoate (Vistaril)	50	Up to 4	100–200	
Neuroleptic	Nausea, delirium, refractory neuropathic pain	Chlorpromazine (Thorazine)	10	3–4	200	Complicated by tardive dyskinesia; not first line drugs
		Fluphenazine (Prolixin)	2	1–2	4	
		Haloperidol (Haldol)	2	2–3	Up to 10	

*There are other medications currently under investigation and anecdotal reports of their success, particularly in the management of neuropathic pain. This group includes mexiletine, tocanide, baclofen, cannabinoids, L-tryptophan, and L-dopa.

†These medications are administered orally, and all dosages and schedules are based on oral administration. With the exception of analeptic agents (which are stimulants), all these medications are sedating. Care must be exercised in their use.

scale is a common tool for measuring pain and consists of a line of a given length on which the patient is asked to indicate the level of pain if the left side represents no pain and the right side, the worst possible pain. The pain score is then the distance from the left origin to this pain level divided by the total length of the line. An alternative is to ask the patient to score the pain on a numerical scale such as 0 to 9, with 0 being no pain and 9 being the worst possible pain. This quantitates the pain so that each visit can be compared with the previous visit and the extent of success of the treatment can be measured. During an examination of the patient who complains of pain, palpation and manipulation are vital. Soft tissue injury and muscle spasm are common causes of pain and are readily diagnosed from palpation. Low-back pain requires a detailed neurologic examination, as do cervical and arm pain and headache. Direct examination of the painful area is mandatory.

On the basis of the history and physical examination, the pain problem can be quantitated as mild, moderate, or severe and can be temporally categorized as acute, subacute, ongoing acute, recurrent acute, or chronic benign. Management should progress in a stepwise fashion. Table 7, an example of the decision tree approach, delineates the steps that should be taken to manage pain.

A patient suffering from acute, subacute, ongoing acute, or recurrent acute pain can usually be managed by pharmacologic means. It is not that these patients would not benefit by psychologic support or adjuvant therapies. However, for most patients whose pain complaints are shorter

TABLE 6. **Work-up of Patient Presenting with Pain**

1. Location and radiation of pain
2. Date of onset of symptoms
3. Progression of symptoms
4. Accompanying factors
5. What worsens or improves the problem
6. Effects on
   a. Sleeping
   b. Sexual function
   c. Social function
   d. Employment
   e. Appetite
7. Scale severity of pain
8. Previous treatments
9. Involvement of litigation in pain problem
10. Accompanying psychologic features and overtones
11. Medications taken for pain
12. Patient's expectations

TABLE 7. **Stepwise Management of Pain**

1. Determine if pain is acute, subacute, ongoing acute, recurrent acute, or chronic benign.
2. Separate and refer patients with chronic benign pain, which often requires a multimodal, multispecialty center for optimal management.
3. Determine if pain is mild, moderate, or severe.
4. For mild to moderate pain of all categories, treat with a non-narcotic analgesic combined with a coanalgesic if there is a specific indication for one of these medications.
5. For patients with more severe pain, or if treatment fails with non-narcotic or coanalgesic medications alone, an oral narcotic analgesic for mild to moderate pain should be added to the regimen started in No. 4. For continuous pain, narcotics should be administered on a fixed schedule, not on an as needed basis.
6. Patients who have insufficient analgesia with mild to moderate narcotic analgesics should be switched to a more potent agent used to treat more severe pain. Again, medication should be administered on a fixed schedule if the pain is constant.
7. For patients who cannot take medications by mouth, alternative delivery routes for analgesics are indicated, such as the intramuscular, subcutaneous, sublingual, intranasal, rectal, transdermal, and spinal routes.

than 6 months, simple office management with medication is enough. Even pain from cancer that has continued for months or pain from rheumatoid arthritis that has been ongoing for years produces many of the signs and symptoms of true acute pain and can be managed in the stepwise method presented in Table 7. Recently, there has been much attention in the literature on the treatment of recurrent acute pain. This chronic pain disorder is due to ongoing nonmalignant pathology, and narcotic analgesics have usually been avoided in these patients. However, this practice is now being questioned. Many pain therapists currently advocate the use of narcotic analgesics for the treatment of these chronic pain disorders. Certainly the use of narcotic analgesics is not questioned when treating patients with ongoing acute pain, the pain from chronic cancer. In fact, for these patients, narcotics become the mainstay of management.

Chronic benign pain, on the other hand, often requires intense simultaneous involvement of a number of different specialties, including physical therapy, psychotherapy, and rehabilitation medicine, for successful treatment. For many patients afflicted with this syndrome, particularly those with chronic intractable benign pain syndrome, the goal of treatment is a return to function, not an ablation of pain. The cost to society from this small number of patients is great, in both lost productivity and expenses of health care. These patients do not do well if they are ignored or if their discomfort is minimized because they suffer as much as patients with acute pain. However, narcotic analgesics should not be primary in management of their pain. A nonpharmacologic, structured, integrated approach is usually in their best interest.

SUGGESTED READING

An excellent monograph, entitled *Principles of Analgesic Use in the Treatment of Acute Pain and Chronic Cancer Pain, a Concise Guide to Medical Practice,* is available at cost from the American Pain Society, 1615 L St., N.W., Suite 925, Washington, D.C., 20036, 202–296–9200.

NAUSEA AND VOMITING

method of
STEVEN GRUNBERG, M.D.
*Los Angeles County–University of Southern
   California Medical Center
Los Angeles, California*

Vomiting is basically a protective reflex for the expulsion of noxious materials from the gastrointestinal tract. Nevertheless, the sensation of nausea and the experience of vomiting may be extremely distressing to the patient. Nausea and vomiting have been identified as the two most feared complications experienced by patients who receive cytotoxic chemotherapy and may lead patients to discontinue even curative therapy. However, one must remember that nausea and vomiting may be the presenting signs of numerous diverse physiologic and anatomic disorders. Identification of the etiology and control of the symptoms of nausea and vomiting therefore become significant concerns to the physician.

THE NAUSEA AND VOMITING REFLEX ARC

Nausea and vomiting are controlled by an anatomic system that is analogous to a reflex arc. The midpoint of this arc is the vomiting center, which is located in the brain stem near the nucleus of the tractus solitarius. The vomiting center is the beginning of the final common pathway that carries efferent impulses to the thoraco-abdominal musculature to initiate the actual act of vomiting. The nausea and vomiting reflex arc can be triggered by at least four different afferent pathways that may be activated simultaneously through the same stimuli, simultaneously through different stimuli, or independently. The humoral pathway is activated by various drugs, metabolites, or intermediary substances that travel through the blood stream and cerebrospinal fluid to the chemoreceptor trigger zone (CTZ). The CTZ consists of two small portions of the area postrema that abut the fourth ventricle. Activation of the CTZ leads to transmission of neural messages to the nearby vomiting center. The classic activator of this pathway is apomorphine. The peripheral pathway involves activation of peripheral nerve endings in the gastrointestinal tract, with transmission of afferent neural impulses to the vomiting center mainly by way of the vagus nerve. Activators of this pathway, such as copper sulfate taken orally, may trigger peripheral nerve endings even without significant systemic absorption. The cerebral pathway is the afferent limb that is activated by nonchemical stimuli such as unpleasant sights, unpleasant odors, or seemingly innocuous memories that recall an unpleasant experience. Both reactive vomiting when an unpleasant event is witnessed and anticipatory nausea and vomiting when a memory or other stimulus causes vomiting before exposure to the chemical emetogenic stimulus are mediated through the cerebral pathway. The fourth afferent limb is the vestibular pathway by which the vestibular apparatus of the inner ear can generate afferent impulses to activate the vomiting center. Repetitive unpleasant motions (which may cause air sickness, car sickness, or seasickness), conditions that prevent normal vestibular function (which may cause air sickness or space sickness experienced by pilots and astronauts under conditions of low or no gravity), and Meniere's disease can activate this pathway.

ETIOLOGIES OF NAUSEA AND VOMITING

Antiemetic agents suppress the nausea and vomiting reflex arc and therefore should be considered symptomatic rather than etiologic interventions. Proper management of a patient presenting with nausea and vomiting should begin with a thorough evaluation to identify, if possible, the etiology of the problem (Table 1). Direct treatment of the etiology is more effective than symptomatic suppression. Identification and treatment of the underlying condition may also prevent further complications or worsening of the condition

TABLE 1. **Common Etiologies of Nausea and Vomiting**

Gastrointestinal dysfunction
   Obstruction
   Ileus
   Volvulus
   Pyloric stenosis
Intracranial pressure
   Brain tumor
   Hydrocephalus
   Cerebral edema
Cerebral cortical reaction
   Anticipatory
   Reactive
Vestibular dysfunction
   Motion sickness
   Meniere's disease
Metabolic and endocrine abnormalities
   Uremia
   Hepatic insufficiency
   Adrenal insufficiency
   Hypercalcemia
Pregnancy (morning sickness)
Exogenous toxins
   Chemotherapy
   Other medications
   Postoperative vomiting
   Radiation therapy
   Heavy metal poisoning
   Food poisoning

itself. Treatment with antiemetic agents as a sole modality should be reserved for situations in which nausea and vomiting are unavoidable complications of a necessary treatment, situations in which the underlying etiology has been established and symptomatic control is desirable while the cause is being corrected, and situations in which etiologies requiring immediate intervention have been excluded and symptomatic control is the primary goal.

Nausea and vomiting may be triggered from any location within the reflex arc. Abnormalities of the gastrointestinal tract itself are an immediate consideration, and an abdominal film series (kidney, ureter, and bladder films and films taken with the patient in the upright position) may be an extremely valuable tool. Vomiting may result from obstruction of the gastrointestinal tract from either malignant disease (gastrointestinal neoplasm) or benign causes (peptic ulcer disease, volvulus, impaction). In infants, congenital abnormalities such as pyloric stenosis are also a consideration. Decompression of the gastrointestinal tract through nasogastric suction may provide extremely effective palliation. Early surgical consultation is advisable in most cases of gastrointestinal obstruction because immediate surgical intervention may be necessary, or the condition (e.g., intermittent small bowel obstruction), which may be initially amenable to nasogastric suction alone, may progress to the point of requiring surgical intervention. Abnormal gastrointestinal motility (ileus and gastric atony) may also cause nausea and vomiting. The finding of gastric atony or ileus may indicate an underlying condition, such as diabetes or pancreatitis, or may result from a recent therapeutic intervention, such as abdominal surgery or administration of the antineoplastic vinca alkaloids. Gastrointestinal decompression is again the primary modality for relief of the nausea and vomiting associated with these conditions.

The humoral pathway may be activated by metabolic abnormalities or by the introduction of extraneous chemical substances. Uremia and hepatitis may lead to nausea and vomiting. Patients with metabolic abnormalities (e.g., hypercalcemia) may present with vomiting and dehydration. Treatment should be aimed at correction of the underlying metabolic abnormality as well as suppression of the symptoms. The presence of renal or hepatic insufficiency must be appreciated early in the clinical course because adjustments of doses of therapeutic agents may be necessary. Illicit drugs or approved pharmacologic agents—from opiates to antibiotics to chemotherapeutic agents—may cause nausea and vomiting. In some cases nausea and vomiting may be delayed or operate through a secondary mechanism (e.g., vinblastine-induced ileus). A careful history of drug use for not only the hours but also the days before onset of nausea and vomiting is an essential part of the initial work-up.

Elevated intracranial pressure may lead directly to activation of the vomiting pathway. Steroids, particularly dexamethasone (Decadron) or methylprednisolone (Solu-Medrol), may reduce edema around an intracranial mass lesion sufficiently to improve or relieve nausea and vomiting. If increased intracranial pressure poses an immediate risk of herniation, mannitol diuresis, induction of alkalosis, or neurosurgical intervention and decompression may be necessary. Vomiting caused by increased intracranial pressure can present as projectile vomiting without nausea and should be considered in the evaluation of any cancer patient who has unexplained vomiting.

COMPLICATIONS OF NAUSEA AND VOMITING

Fluid and electrolyte imbalances are the major complications of extended or severe nausea and vomiting. However, these abnormalities themselves may further aggravate precipitating causes such as hypercalcemia or uremia. Carefully monitored intravenous hydration and electrolyte replacement are important parts of the symptomatic management of severe nausea and vomiting. Although gastrointestinal hemorrhage may lead to vomiting (as in peptic ulcer disease), severe vomiting itself may cause gastrointestinal hemorrhage through mechanisms such as esophageal tearing (Mallory-Weiss syndrome). New onset of hemorrhage during the management of a patient with vomiting must suggest further evaluation for an additional cause. Aspiration of gastric contents with resultant pneumonitis is not generally a major problem in patients who are alert and awake. However, this possibility must be considered in patients who are sedated or in those who have abnormalities of intracranial or oropharyngeal structures.

TREATMENT

Pharmacologic Classification of Antiemetics

Antiemetic agents may be classified either by the neurotransmitter involved or by the site of action (Table 2). Because specific neurotransmitter neurons tend to be concentrated in specific anatomic areas, these classifications are often interchangeable. Dopaminergic neurons are found in the CTZ and the periphery (gastrointestinal tract). Because the CTZ and the periphery are the two major afferent portals to the vomiting center, the antiemetic properties of antidopaminergic agents have long been recognized. The phenothiazines were one of the first families of antidopaminergic compounds to be used as antiemetics. Most phenothiazines have some antiemetic activity. Use of these compounds is dictated by the frequency of toxicities. Chlorpromazine (Thorazine), for example, causes more sedation than other members of the family. Prochlorperazine (Compazine), thiethylperazine (Torecan), and perphenazine (Trilafon) have therefore gained wider use as antiemetics. The butyrophenones, including haloperidol (Haldol) and droperidol (Inapsine), are another family of antidopaminergic agents with significant antiemetic activity. Metoclopramide (Reglan), particularly in high doses, is a potent antiemetic that has been classified with the antidopaminergics. Metoclopramide in low doses (10 mg orally three times daily) significantly increases peristaltic activity and may be of value when nausea and vomiting are due to gastric atony or decreased gastrointestinal motility. However, because of the increase in peristalsis, metoclopramide is contraindicated in cases of bowel obstruction, thereby emphasizing the importance of determining the etiology of nausea and vomiting before the institution of therapy. Antidopaminergic antiemetic agents may also cause antidopaminergic toxicities, including extrapyramidal syndromes, oculorgyric crisis, pseudoparkinsonism, akathisia, and anxiety reactions. Younger patients are more prone to experience extrapyramidal reactions. Metoclopramide by the oral route is also more likely to cause extrapyramidal reactions than an equal dose administered by the intravenous route.

Histaminergic and cholinergic neurons are found in the vomiting center and in the vestibular area. Antihistamines have only low-level antiemetic activity and cause sedation at higher doses. However, antihistamines decrease the incidence and severity of extrapyramidal syndromes associated with the antidopaminergic agents and are commonly used in combination antiemetic therapy. Anticholinergic agents, including scopolamine (Transderm Scōp), dimenhydrinate (Dramamine), hydroxyzine (Atarax, Vistaril), and meclizine (Bonine, Antivert), are particularly effective in the prevention of nausea and vomiting of vestibular origin (motion sickness).

Two families of agents act directly on receptors at the cerebral cortex. Benzodiazepines do not have major intrinsic antiemetic activity. However, their anxiolytic properties can be extremely important in preventing or ameliorating anticipatory nausea and vomiting. Lorazepam (Ati-

TABLE 2. **Site of Action (and Mechanism) of Common Antiemetic Agents**

Site (Mechanism)	Agents
Chemoreceptor trigger zone/periphery (antidopaminergic)	Prochlorperazine (Compazine)
	Thiethylperazine (Torecan)
	Perphenazine (Trilafon)
	Haloperidol (Haldol)
	Droperidol (Inapsine)
	Metoclopramide (Reglan)
	Trimethobenzamide (Tigan)
Vestibular apparatus/ vomiting center (anticholinergic/ antihistaminergic)	Scopolamine (Transderm Scōp)
	Dimenhydrinate (Dramamine)
	Meclizine (Antivert, Bonine)
	Hydroxyzine (Atarax, Vistaril)
Cerebral cortex (benzodiazepine/ cannabinoid)	Lorazepam (Ativan)
	Diazepam (Valium)
	Dronabinol (Marinol)
Unknown	Dexamethasone (Decadron)
	Methylprednisolone (Solu-Medrol)

van), the most commonly used of the benzodiazepines, acts as an anxiolytic, a hypnotic/sedative, and an inducer of retrograde amnesia, thereby providing the patient with needed rest and at times erasing the memory of chemotherapy itself. Diazepam (Valium) has also been used in the prevention of anticipatory nausea and vomiting and may be particularly useful when extreme sedation is not desired (e.g., in patients who develop anticipatory nausea and vomiting several days before scheduled administration of chemotherapy). The cannabinoid dronabinol (Marinol) has definite antiemetic activity, although it is not as potent as the high-dose antidopaminergics. Significant toxicities associated with dronabinol include euphoria, dysphoria, drowsiness, hallucinations, dry mouth, hypertension, and paresthesia. Dysphoria may be the most disturbing of these toxicities and may negate the benefit achieved by antiemetic protection. Addition of a low-dose phenothiazine can prevent dysphoria while maintaining the antiemetic activity of the cannabinoid agent.

Steroids, including methylprednisolone (Solu-Medrol) and dexamethasone (Decadron), have shown significant antiemetic activity. In cases of intracerebral mass with surrounding edema, steroids may act through reduction of the edema. However, even in the absence of intracranial pathology steroids may be potent antiemetics. The mechanism of action of steroids in this setting is unknown.

A new family of antiemetics of particular interest is the antiserotoninergic agents, which appear to act by specifically blocking 5-hydroxytryptamine receptors. These receptors are found in the gastrointestinal tract and recently in various sections of the brain. Metoclopramide is considered to have antidopaminergic activity at low doses but also to gain antiserotoninergic activity when administered at high doses, which perhaps explains the marked increase in antiemetic activity seen at these higher doses. The newer antiserotoninergic agents tend to be analogues of either metoclopramide or serotonin. Although investigational, these agents have shown excellent antiemetic activity without the toxicity of antidopaminergic agents and may soon be commercially available.

Chemotherapy

Nausea and vomiting are considered to be the worst toxicities of chemotherapy. However, the emetogenic potentials and patterns of different chemotherapeutic agents actually vary greatly. Certain agents, such as cisplatin, dacarbazine, nitrogen mustard, and high-dose cyclophosphamide, are extremely emetogenic and produce vomiting in almost all patients who do not receive antiemetics. Bleomycin (Blenoxane) and vincristine (Oncovin), on the other hand, have extremely low emetogenic potential and may often be given without antiemetics. Emetogenicity of combination chemotherapy regimens can be estimated based on the emetogenic potential of the individual agents. Patterns of emetogenicity of chemotherapeutic agents are also quite variable. The greatest emetogenic potential of most agents begins several hours after chemotherapy and ends within 24 hours. However, the toxicity of cyclophosphamide may have a delayed onset, with nausea and vomiting beginning up to 18 hours after administration of the agent. The major emetic risk for cisplatin occurs from 6 to 24 hours after administration, but nausea or vomiting may persist for 2 to 7 days in approximately 50 per cent of patients and may require continued treatment with low-dose oral antiemetics.

Because most chemotherapeutic agents act through the CTZ or the peripheral pathway, the antidopaminergic agents have been the mainstay of chemotherapeutic antiemetic therapy. The phenothiazines were demonstrated to decrease the incidence of 5-fluorouracil-induced nausea and vomiting 25 years ago and were for many years the standard major antiemetic agents. Introduction of highly emetogenic agents such as cisplatin in the mid-1970s revealed the inadequacy of standard-dose phenothiazines for antiemetic protection. Metoclopramide, which has little activity against cisplatin-induced nausea and vomiting when given at standard oral doses (10 mg orally three times a day), has excellent antiemetic activity when administered at much higher doses (2 mg per kg intravenously every 2 hours for five doses) and is now the mainstay of many major antiemetic regimens. Both haloperidol and prochlorperazine also have increased antiemetic activity when administered at intravenous doses higher than those normally used.

Combination antiemetic therapy is often used to gain an increased antiemetic effect. The goal of combination therapy should be an increased spectrum and potency of activity, with agents being combined that act on different afferent pathways of the vomiting reflex arc so that more complete coverage is obtained. When added to high-dose metoclopramide, dexamethasone increases the frequency of complete protection from nausea and vomiting in patients receiving cisplatin. A benzodiazepine such as lorazepam may also be added to block cerebral pathways and provide sedation. Finally, an antihistamine such as diphenhydramine (Benadryl) may be used to decrease the incidence of antidopaminergic toxicity. Recent studies with the new antiserotoninergic agents have demonstrated efficacy against cisplatin- and cyclophosphamide-induced nausea and vomiting that is similar to that of high-dose metoclopramide. These agents may prove to be extremely useful as members of antiemetic combinations.

Radiation Therapy

Radiation therapy may also induce nausea and vomiting. Although abdominal radiation is most often associated with this phenomenon, nausea and vomiting may also appear after either cranial or thoracic radiation therapy. Radiation therapy appears to act through the CTZ because ablation of this area prevents the onset of radiation-induced emesis. Haloperidol is effective in the treatment of radiation-induced nausea and vomiting.

Anticipatory Nausea and Vomiting

Anticipatory nausea and vomiting are learned responses in which various stimuli can be associated with the experience of chemotherapy and therefore produce nausea and vomiting. In patients who receive repeated courses of chemotherapy, the frequency of development of anticipatory nausea and vomiting is related directly to the intensity and duration of the emetic experience during early courses of chemotherapy. The best method of preventing anticipatory nausea and vomiting is therefore aggressive antiemetic therapy during early courses of chemotherapy. Once this anticipatory response has developed, therapeutic strategies are aimed at blunting the cerebral pathways that serve as the afferent limb of this particular reflex arc. Benzodiazepines have been effective because of their anxiolytic and amnesic properties. Use of antiadrenergic agents has been suggested. Behavioral therapy, relaxation therapy, and hypnosis may also be used to decrease and ameliorate this phenomenon.

A variant of anticipatory nausea and vomiting that may appear during chemotherapy is learned taste aversion. Studies with both animals and humans have demonstrated that pairing of a strongly flavored pleasant food stimulus with chemotherapy-induced nausea and vomiting results in future avoidance of that particular food stimulus. Although one might be tempted to encourage a patient to eat favorite foods at the time of chemotherapy in the hope of maintaining adequate nutrition, such activity may actually lead to later avoidance of these foods and a decrease in overall nutritional status. A better strategy would encourage small meals or bland meals at the time of chemotherapy so that more strongly flavored favorite foods would be available to supplement oral nutrition later.

Motion Sickness

Motion sickness results from alteration of vestibular function and may be ameliorated by numerous agents that block the cholinergic pathways from the vestibular apparatus to the vomiting center. Both antihistamines and anticholinergic agents, including dimenhydrinate, meclizine, and cyclizine (Marezine), can prevent motion sickness when taken before exposure to the emetogenic stimulus. A particularly useful method of drug delivery for such an agent has been the development of patches containing scopolamine for transdermal application. Maximal drug levels are not achieved until 4 to 8 hours after application of the patch, but a single patch may continue to be effective for up to 72 hours, which allows continuous protection during extended travel. Because the vestibular pathway appears to be a minor pathway for the induction of chemotherapy-induced nausea and vomiting, these agents have had little direct use in the prevention of chemotherapy-induced emesis. Although single-agent transdermal scopolamine is not effective in the prevention of cisplatin-induced vomiting, efficacy in the prevention of methotrexate-induced nausea and vomiting has been suggested and may warrant further study.

Anesthesia-Related Vomiting

Postanesthesia vomiting is seen particularly after the use of inhalation anesthetics or spinal anesthesia. Nasogastric suction and administration of phenothiazine antiemetics may be useful. Nausea and vomiting may also be seen after first administration of opiate analgesics, particularly meperidine (Demerol). Use of a different analgesic, reduction of the dose to a minimal effective level, or administration of antiemetic phenothiazines may be necessary.

Morning Sickness

Nausea and vomiting (morning sickness) are commonly seen in the early stages of pregnancy but generally subside by the end of the first trimester. Although comfort of the mother is important, an over-riding concern has been the possibility of pharmacologically induced damage to the fetus. The mixture of doxylamine succinate, dicyclomine hydrochloride, and pyridoxine hydrochloride (Bendectin) had often been used for nausea and vomiting of pregnancy. However, suggestion of an association between use of this drug and some congenital abnormalities led to its removal from the market. Meclizine and dimenhydrinate have been proposed as alternative antiemetics because their teratogenicity has not been proved. Avoidance of all drugs by pregnant patients unless their use is absolutely necessary is still the best strategy. Patients may be encouraged to take frequent light meals and to rest when possible.

Poisoning

Food poisoning may present as nausea and vomiting with or without accompanying diarrhea. Sudden onset without other precipitating causes or a series of cases with a common food exposure are highly suggestive of food poisoning. Many different organisms, including *Staphylococcus, Salmonella,* and *Clostridium,* may be associated with food poisoning. In general, rest and rehydration are sufficient therapy. However, phenothiazine antiemetics may be used in particularly severe cases. The physician must also carefully observe the patient for the appearance of additional symptoms, such as the neurologic depression of botulism, which may require more aggressive support of vital functions.

Vomiting may be one of the manifestations of numerous forms of acute poisoning caused by heavy metals, including antimony, arsenic, gold, mercury, silver, and thallium. Supportive care and hydration are the mainstays of therapy for this type of poisoning. However, gastric lavage or intravenous therapy with a chelating agent may be valuable in certain cases.

GASEOUSNESS AND INDIGESTION

method of
NORMAN M. PANITCH, M.D.
University of California, Los Angeles
Los Angeles, California

Patients who complain of gas and indigestion can, at times, be harboring life-threatening disease, but the vast majority, after an appropriate work-up, are usually found to have a functional disorder. When taking the initial history and performing a physical examination on these patients, precise questioning is essential, for "gas" and "indigestion" mean different things to different people. The passage of excess flatus with urgency, for example, is a common complaint of patients harboring a painless, partially obstructing rectal carcinoma. For the purpose of this discussion, "indigestion" means a burning, gnawing, unpleasant sensation felt in the epigastrium, at times radiating into the mid-chest, and "gaseousness" refers to the unpleas-

ant sensation of abdominal fullness, distention, and bloating, associated, at times, with excessive belching, flatus, and borborygmi.

GASEOUSNESS

Gaseousness can be subdivided into (1) excessive belching, (2) abdominal bloating, fullness, and distention, and (3) excessive passage of flatus.

Most patients who belch excessively are aerophagic. Excessive air swallowing occurs during jogging, gum chewing, cigarette smoking, talking while eating, and using straws, and during emotional crises, either perceived or real. Excessive belching can become a difficult habit to break. A minor tranquilizer given before meals for a short time is occasionally helpful in the refractory patient.

Abdominal bloating and distention are the most common functional complaints encountered by gastroenterologists in consultative practice. These symptoms are usually expressed as part of the symptom complex known as the "irritable bowel syndrome." Bloating, which can be incapacitating, may be seen alone or associated with alternating diarrhea, constipation, or both. Bloating is attributed by these patients to excessive gas, but studies reveal that they have no more than the normal amount of intestinal gas (100 to 200 ml). These patients seem to be trapping, moving, and reacting to intestinal gas in an abnormal fashion. Intestinal motility and psychologic studies in these patients have not been consistent or reproducible. The treatment of bloating is also difficult. Anticholinergics, the mainstay of treatment for years, with or without tranquilizers, have variable results. These medications should be used in increasing doses for an adequate period—for example, dicyclomine (Bentyl), 10 to 30 mg 1 hour before meals and before sleep. Promotility medications such as metoclopramide, 5 to 10 mg before meals, appears to be more effective than anticholinergics and tranquilizers in these patients. Dietary manipulation can be extremely helpful. Patients with bloating should attempt to avoid (1) milk and milk products (except for yogurt); (2) gas-producing foods such as legumes, Brussels sprouts, peas, raw onions, and pectin-containing fruits such as pears, peaches, melons, and apples; and (3) carbonated and diet beverages and chewing gum, especially those containing Sorbitol.

A complaint of excessive flatulence is treated similarly to abdominal bloating. Most gas passed rectally consists of carbon dioxide, hydrogen, and methane produced by colonic bacterial metabolism of carbohydrates that were either not digested or malabsorbed in the proximal small intestine. Ingestion of beans containing raffinose and stachyose may result in a tenfold increase in flatus volume. Antibiotics are not helpful in these patients unless certain conditions are present, such as blind or stagnant loop syndrome or small intestinal dysmotility disorders as seen in severe diabetes or scleroderma. Bulking agents such as psyllium seed (Metamucil), 1 to 2 heaping tablespoons in juice or water, along with unprocessed bran in flake or tablet form (Fibercon), are sometimes helpful in achieving improved bowel evacuation and symptomatic relief of excessive flatus in a patient with the irritable bowel syndrome. Charcoal (Charcocaps), one capsule four times daily, is occasionally helpful. Products containing simethicone (Mylicon-125) and pancreatic and "digestive" enzymes have not been consistently of value in these patients. These compounds are relatively harmless and therefore can be given for 3 to 4 weeks to the refractory patient. A rare individual will show a dramatic response.

INDIGESTION

Most patients who complain of indigestion have symptoms related to injury to the esophagus, stomach, and/or duodenum caused by acid. Acid bathing of the lower esophagus results from reflux of gastric acid through an incompetent lower esophageal sphincter (LES). Symptoms are usually postprandial and positional. Occasional, sporadic "heartburn," or acid reflux associated with dietary indiscretion, is treated with 15 to 30 ml of liquid antacid, taken immediately and 1 or 2 hours later. The sodium, magnesium, and aluminum contents of the different antacids vary. Antacid tablets are less effective than liquid antacids. Persistent, recurrent, and/or nocturnal reflux symptoms should be treated with any one of the H_2 histamine receptor antagonists on a twice daily schedule, that is, ranitidine (Zantac), 150 mg every 12 hours; cimetidine (Tagamet), 400 mg twice daily; or famotidine (Pepcid), 20 mg twice daily. Endoscopy is recommended in these patients to ascertain whether silent Barrett's transformation of the esophagus (a premalignant disorder) has developed. None of the treatment regimens (either medical or surgical) have been proved to reverse Barrett's transformation. Other measures that are symptomatically helpful in these patients include cessation of cigarette smoking, elevation of the head of the bed with 6-inch blocks of wood or brick (extra pillows do not help), and the avoidance of coffee and food high in fat content. Such foods, especially ice cream and chocolate, further weaken the LES, leading to intense postprandial reflux symptoms. Metoclopramide (Reglan), 5 to 10 mg

given 1 hour before meals and at night, has been shown to tighten the LES and enhance gastric emptying.

Indigestion perceived in the epigastrium usually denotes acid-peptic injury to the stomach, duodenum, or both. A 3-week trial of full doses of an H_2 histamine antagonist, given once or twice daily, or a cytoprotective medication such as sucralfate (Carafate), 1 gram orally four times daily before initiating an in-depth diagnostic work-up, has been advocated. Patients who do not respond completely within this time period are candidates for endoscopy. Gastric and duodenal ulcers take about 6 to 8 weeks to heal completely. There are, however, two conditions that are, at times, clinically indistinguishable from acid-peptic disorders and that require specific therapy: giardiasis of the upper small intestine and duodenum and *Campylobacter pylori* infection of the distal stomach and duodenal bulb. Endoscopic biopsy, aspiration, and culture can sometimes identify these organisms in patients unresponsive to standard ulcer regimens. *Campylobacter* infection responds to bismuth subsalicylate, penicillin, cephalosporins, and the quinolones. Giardiasis is treated with either quinacrine (Atabrine) or metronidazole (Flagyl).

Indigestion is sometimes related to delayed or disorganized gastric emptying. This disorder is commonly described in young women. Mild anorexia and postprandial nausea are associated symptoms. A fairly firm diagnosis can be made by using the radioactive isotope gastric emptying study. Promotility drugs such as metoclopramide, 5 to 10 mg 15 to 30 minutes before meals, can be effective in these patients. Many patients have the false impression that gallbladder disease causes indigestion, gaseousness, or both. Biliary colic is, however, extremely painful and episodic. It can usually be diagnosed by a careful history and confirmed by ultrasound.

ACUTE INFECTIOUS DIARRHEA

method of
HUMBERTO A. SORIANO, M.D.
Catholic University of Chile
Santiago, Chile

Almost 70 per cent of acute diarrheal diseases (ADDs) are infectious. They affect billions and kill millions of people each year throughout the world. In the developing nations, morbidity rates from ADDs are tens times higher and mortality rates are hundreds to thousands times higher than those in developed countries. In less developed countries, ADDs are responsible for 40 to 60 per cent of all deaths in children younger than 5 years of age. In the developed world, ADDs cause less than 5 per cent of all deaths at that age.

Fecal contamination of hands, water, or food, with rapid growth of bacterial enteropathogens because of hot and sometimes humid weather, is usually involved in summer epidemics.

ADDs are by far the most common disease among travelers leaving developed areas and going to less developed and tropical areas (there is a 30 per cent chance for a traveler to have a diarrheal episode).

Most ADD episodes do not require diagnostic laboratory tests or drugs for treatment. Adequate hydration and diet therapy suffice. However, severe secretory-type diarrhea of the summer, enterocolitis, and patients with systemic clinical signs of toxicity benefit from early and complete diagnostic studies and aggressive treatment.

ETIOPATHOGENESIS

ADDs are caused by enteropathogenic microorganisms in about 60 to 80 per cent of cases. Etiologic agents of ADDs are the same throughout the world. Their relative importance varies significantly with the geographic, socioeconomic, and sanitary conditions of the populations affected (Table 1), as well as with the yearly epidemic trend.

Rotavirus is by far the most common cause (50 to 80 per cent) of ADDs in winter epidemics in children 6 to 24 months of age in developed countries. Norwalk and adenoviruses are common causes of vomiting and/or epidemics of diarrhea in school-age children and adults during the winter. In developing countries, rotavirus maintains a fairly steady yearly frequency of 10 to 30 per cent of ADD cases in children younger than 3 years. The frequency of rotavirus diarrhea is surpassed by "summer" epidemics of disease caused by enteropathogenic bacteria, mainly enteropathogenic *Escherichia coli* (EPEC) or enterotoxigenic *E. coli* (ETEC), *Campylobacter jejuni*, and *Shigella* species. ETEC causes one-half to two-thirds of traveler's diarrhea (TD) cases.

Enteropathogenic microorganisms cause morphologic or functional intestinal damage that leads to diarrhea by one or more of the following direct or indirect mechanisms (Table 1): (1) direct penetration of the intestinal epithelium; (2) damage to microvilli, villi, and/or crypts secondary to adherence, to cytotoxin production, or to yet unknown mechanisms; (3) enterotoxins causing hypersecretion without primary morphologic abnormalities; (4) disaccharidase deficiency secondary to brush border damage leading to osmotic diarrhea because of accumulation of nonabsorbed disaccharides in the lumen; (5) abnormal bile acid metabolism in the intestine secondary to overgrowth of small intestine bacteria, which causes lipid malabsorption and direct villous damage by the action of abnormal bile acids present in the lumen; and (6) abnormal motility, either propulsive hyperperistalsis with accelerated intestinal transit time (e.g., *Shigella*) or decreased propulsive peristalsis with delayed intestinal transit time (e.g., EPEC).

CLINICAL SYNDROMES, INITIAL STUDY, AND THERAPY

Several clinical syndromes can be recognized by the practicing physician according to the way an episode of acute diarrhea begins. This recognition helps the physician to establish a presumptive etiologic diagnosis, to decide what laboratory tests to perform, and to initiate appropriate supportive and drug therapy.

Nonspecific Diarrhea. Nonspecific diarrhea (NSD) is the most common clinical acute diarrheal syndrome at any age, in any season, or in any geographic region. It presents with little or no nausea and/or vomiting; loose or watery (not high-volume) stools; an abnormal number of bowel movements per day for that person, usually three to five; scant or no mucus, no blood, and no distinct odor in stools; little or no fever; moderate malaise; few and not intense abdominal cramps; and no tenesmus.

No initial laboratory procedures are necessary. In cases with borderline enterocolitis or with the secretory type of summer diarrhea (SD), fecal leukocyte assays may help to initiate therapy with trimethoprim-sulfamethoxazole (TMP-SMX) (Bactrim, Septra) if the tests are positive and with bismuth subsalicylate or nonabsorbable antibiotics if the tests are negative. If there is any epidemiologic support, time may be saved by taking a sample for stool culture and/or initiating stool collection from each intestinal evacuation, for protozoan cysts and/or trophozoites (up to six samples). These samples may be discarded if clinical evolution makes them unnecessary.

TREATMENT. Most cases of NSD are mild and do not need hydration or drug treatment (see later supportive therapy discussion).

Enterocolitis Syndrome. This syndrome implies bloody diarrhea by definition. The classic clinical picture is represented by *Shigella* infection: mucous or mucopurulent bloody diarrhea with polymorphonuclear leukocytes always present, and frequent, small evacuations ("rectal sputum") accompanied by intestinal cramps and tenesmus. There is usually a high fever with moderate signs of toxicity (sometimes neurotoxic signs, even with convulsions, in small children).

Almost identical initial clinical manifestations may be caused by enteroinvasive *E. coli* (EIEC) and non-*typhi Salmonella* (Table 1). The following initial laboratory tests are helpful in diagnosing this clinical syndrome: (1) fecal leukocytes (Table 2); (2) search for occult blood in stool if it is not macroscopically evident; (3) Gram's stain for *C. jejuni;* (4) special stain for *Cryptosporidium;* (5) direct search for ameba trophozoites or cysts in fresh stools; (6) ova and parasites in stools collected in preservative media from each evac-

TABLE 1. **Acute Diarrheal Diseases: Etiology, Pathogenesis, Clinical Syndromes, Frequency**

Etiology and Agent	Pathogenic Mechanisms	Clinical Syndromes	Frequency		
			Developed World	*Traveler's Diarrhea*	*Third World*
I. Infectious					
A. Bacteria					
1. *Vibrio cholerae*	T, HS	SD	VR	VR	Ep Asia Africa
2. *Escherichia coli*			UC	MC	MC, Ep
Enteropathogenic (EPEC)	U, ED, HS	NS	UC	C	C
Enteroadherent-aggregant (EAEC)	ED, HS	NS, SD	UC	C	C
Enterotoxigenic (ETEC)	T, HS	NS, SD	UC	MC	C
Enteroinvasive (EIEC)	I, ED	EC	R	R	R
Enterohemorrhagic (EHEC)	C, ED	EC	R	R	R
3. *Shigella (dysenteriae, flexneri, boydii, sonnei)*	I, C, T, HS, ED	ED, SD, NS	UC, Ep. C	UC	C, Ep
4. *Salmonella (typhi, enteritidis, choleraesuis)*	I, C, T, HS, ED	FP, EC, NS	C, food borne	UC	UC
5. *Campylobacter jejuni*	I, C	EC	UC	UC	UC
6. *Yersinia enterocolitica*	I, ED, T	EC	R, VR	R	R, VR
7. *Aeromonas hydrophila*	T, HS, C, ED	SD, EC, NS	VR	VR	VR
8. *Clostridium difficile*	C, ED, HS	I	VR	—	VR
9. *Staphylococcus aureus*	T, I, ED	I, FP	VR	VR	VR
10. *Pseudomonas aeruginosa*	T, I, ED	I	VR	—	VR
11. *Clostridium perfringens*	T, HS	SD	VR	VR	VR
12. *Vibrio parahaemolyticus*	T, HS, I, ED	FP, SD	VR	VR	VR
13. *Bacillus cereus*	T, HS	SD	VR	VR	VR
14. Overgrowth of small intestinal fecal bacteria	HS, O, BA, ED	NS	VR	Unknown	C ?
15. Others (e.g., *Legionella, Edwardsiella*)	Variable	Variable	VR	VR	VR
B. Virus			MX, Ep	VR	C
1. Rotavirus	ED, HS	VTD, SD, NS	MC, Ep (6–24 mo)	VR	C
2. Small round viruses (e.g., Norwalk, Astrovirus Wollan)	ED, HS	VTD, SD, NS	R, Ep	VR	VR
3. Enteric adenoviruses	ED, HS	VTD, SD, NS	VR, Ep	VR	VR, Ep
4. Coronaviruses	ED, HS	VTD, SD, NS	VR, Ep	VR	VR
5. Enteroviruses (ECHO, coxsackie viruses D and B)	ED, HS	VTD, SD, NS	VR, Ep	VR	VR
C. Parasites			R, Ep	UC	UC, En, Ep
1. Protozoa					
a. *Entamoeba histolytica*	I, T	EC, NS	R	R	UC
b. *Giardia lamblia*	U, O, I	NS	R	R, Ep	UC
c. *Cryptosporidium*	U	NS	VR	VR	VR
d. *Balantidium coli*	I	EC, NS	VR	VR	VR
e. *Isospora hominis*	U	SD, NS	VR	VR	VR
2. Nematodes			VR	VR	VR, En
a. *Strongyloides stercoralis*	I	EC	VR	VR	VR, En
b. *Trichuris trichiura*	I	EC	VR	VR	VR, En
D. Fungi			VR	VR	VR
1. *Candida* species	U, I	NS	VR	—	VR
2. *Mucor* species	U, I	NS	VR	—	VR
II. Noninfectious			R	R	R
A. Carbohydrate intolerance	O	NS	R	R	UC
B. Food allergy (especially milk)	Immune	FP, EC	UC	—	VR
C. Nonbacterial food poisoning (mushrooms, solanine, seafood, green fruit)	T	FP	VR	VR	VR
D. Celiac disease	Immune, ED	NS	VR	—	VR
E. Cystic fibrosis	EPI	NS	VR	—	VR
F. Neoplasms	HS	SD	VR	—	VR
G. Laxatives	O, HS	Variable	VR	VR	VR
H. Drugs	Variable	Variable	VR	VR	VR

Abbreviations: Pathogenic mechanisms: T = toxigenic; C = cytotoxic; HS = hypersecretory; I = invasive; ED = epithelial damage; O = osmotic; BA = abnormal bile acid metabolism in intestine; U = unknown; EPI = exocrine pancreatic insufficiency. Clinical syndromes: SD = secretory diarrhea; EC = enterocolitis; VTD = viral-type diarrhea; TD = traveler's diarrhea; FP = food poisoning; NS = nonspecific. O = osmotic. Frequency: MC = most common (≥30% of ADD cases); C = common (15–30%); UC = uncommon (10–15%); R = rare (5–10%); VR = very rare (<5%); Ep = epidemic; En = endemic.

TABLE 2. **Acute Infectious Diarrhea: Stool Leukocytes**

Cause	Leukocytes	
	Type	Frequency (%)
Shigella, Salmonella (not typhi), Campylobacter jejuni, Clostridium difficile	Polymorphonuclear	90–100
Yersinia enterocolitica, Vibrio parahaemolyticus	Polymorphonuclear	Variable
Salmonella typhi	Mononuclear	100
Amebic dysentery	Mononuclear	100
Ulcerative colitis	Eosinophilic	100
Viruses, Vibrio cholerae, ETEC, EPEC, Giardia	Polymorphonuclear	0–10
EHEC	None	None

uation, up to three to six samples in each container; (7) stool culture, including special culture methods for C. jejuni and Yersinia enterocolitica, plus detection of EIEC when regional epidemiologic data suggest it.

TREATMENT. Initial therapy with TMP-SMX should be started in a patient who has enterocolitis syndrome with polymorphonuclear leukocytes in the stool if there is no other clinical or epidemiologic evidence suggesting a specific etiology that would require another drug or no treatment. If bacteriologic surveillance in the area detects frequent TMP-SMX-resistant strains of Shigella, proper antibiotic therapy based on that surveillance should be started (e.g., ampicillin or nalidixic acid) (Table 3).

If no leukocytes are present, evidence of enterohemorrhagic E. coli (EHEC) must be sought. Careful supervision is necessary after results of stool culture for EHEC are known and on appearance of oliguria (hemolytic-uremic syndrome) or blood diseases (thrombotic thrombocytopenic purpura). If mononuclear leukocytes are present in stool of a dysenteric patient, sigmoidoscopy and examination for ameba are indicated. If there has been previous antibiotic treatment, a search for Clostridium difficile toxins (or/and culture) is also justified. If pseudomembranous colitis is present or C. difficile toxins or positive culture results are found, metronidazole or vancomycin treatment should be initiated.

If seafood ingestion precedes the enterocolitis, culture media for Vibrio parahaemolyticus must be used.

Secretory Diarrheal Clinical Syndrome. This syndrome is best represented by cholera diarrhea and by the "summer" epidemic E. coli diarrhea in infants in less developed countries. Little or no vomiting, mild or moderate intestinal cramping, low-grade fever, and profuse watery diarrhea containing no pus or blood and scant or no mucus are present, as is a sui generis "coli" or "cholera" odor. There is a rapid tendency to dehydration.

Routine stool cultures at the beginning of the epidemic are highly advisable in countries where E. coli SD is prevalent (EPEC and ETEC being the most frequent). This culture identifies the dominant enteropathogenic strain and the antimicrobial susceptibility for that epidemic.

TREATMENT. Initial therapy must include hydration, feeding, and symptomatic treatment (see later). Useful drugs include (1) tetracyclines or other drugs (Table 3) in cholera epidemics or in endemic areas; and (2) bismuth subsalicylate or nonabsorbed antimicrobial agents or TMP-SMX (Table 3) in summer noncholera epidemics.

Viral Type of Diarrhea. The old term "winter vomiting disease" is the best clinical summary description for viral type of diarrhea (VTD). It marks the season in which VTD epidemics occur in developed countries and the main and almost invariable initial symptom, which is vomiting. Vomiting usually precedes diarrhea by hours and up to 2 days. Most of the cases are accompanied by mild respiratory common cold–type symptoms. The diarrhea is usually variable in amount and consistency, with scant or no mucus, no blood, and no fecal leukocytes.

TREATMENT. Rehydration is the mainstay of ambulatory treatment. Bismuth subsalicylate used early may decrease the duration of the disease (Table 3).

Traveler's Diarrhea. Each year, more than 1 million American travelers develop diarrhea. Although ETEC is responsible for two-thirds of all cases, Shigella accounts for 5 to 20 per cent, and several other enteropathogens may be present. Nevertheless, in 25 to 30 per cent of cases, no pathogen is found. Most of the time, the clinical syndrome is similar to that of secretory diarrhea.

TREATMENT. Bismuth subsalicylate or antimicrobial agents (Table 3) are indicated early in moderate or severe cases. Mild cases are alleviated by proper hydration, feeding, and symptomatic treatment (see later).

Food Poisoning. Food poisoning is caused by food contaminated with bacteria, such as Salmonella, or their products, such as staphylococcal toxin, or by naturally occurring food toxins. Symptoms are noted in one or more persons who have ingested

TABLE 3. **Anti-Infective Drug Therapy for Acute Infectious Diarrheal Diseases**

Drugs	Doses and Duration of Therapy		Clinical Syndrome or Etiology Where Indicated[1]
	Adults	*Children*	
Tetracycline HCl (Achromycin)	250–500 mg, PO, q 6 hr, × 2–5 days	20–40 mg/kg/day, PO, q 6 hr, × 2–5 days (only for > 7 yr)[2]	Cholera,[3] TD, *Yersinia, Campylobacter, Aeromonas*
Demeclocycline HCl (Declomycin)	150–300 mg, PO, q 8 hr, × 2–5 days	7–15 mg/kg/day, PO, q 8 hr, × 2–5 days (only for > 7 yr)	Same as for tetracycline
Doxycycline hyclate (Vibramycin)	100 mg, PO, q 12 hr, × 2–5 days	4–6 mg/kg/day, PO, q 12 hr, × 2–5 days (only for > 7 yr)	Same as for tetracycline; TD[3]
Bismuth subsalicylate (Pepto-Bismol)	524 mg (30 ml or two tablets), PO, q 30–60 min, 8 doses/day × 2 days	100 mg/kg/day, PO, q 4 hr, × 5 days	EPEC,[3] ETEC,[3] EAEC,[3] TD,[3] rotavirus,[3] Norwalk virus,[3] NS[3]
Ampicillin (Omnipen, Penbritin)	500–1000 mg, PO, q 6 hr, × 5 days	25 mg/kg/day, PO, IM, IV, q 6 hr, × 5 days	*Shigella,* EIEC, *Salmonella*
TMP-SMX (Bactrim, Septra)	160–800 mg, PO, q 12 hr, × 3–5 days	8–10/40–50 mg/kg/day, PO, q 12 hr × 5 days	*Shigella,*[3] EIEC,[3] TD,[3] *Yersinia, Salmonella,* ETEC, EPEC, EAEC, EHEC, NS, SD, *Aeromonas,* cholera
Erythromycin (Pantomycin, Mercine)	500 mg, PO, q 6 hr, × 5–7 days	40–50 mg/kg/day, PO, q 6 hr, × 5 days	*Campylobacter*[3] (early treatment)
Neomycin (Mycifradin)	—	50–60 mg/kg/day, PO, q 6–8 hr, × 5 days	EPEC-ETEC ?, NS, SD
Colistin (Polymyxin E, Colymycin-S)	—	5–15 mg/kg/day, PO, q 6 hr, × 5 days	EPEC-ETEC ?, NS, SD
Polymyxin B sulfate (Aerosporin)	750,000 U, PO, q 8 hr, × 5 days	250,000–500,000 U, PO, q 8 hr, × 5 days	EPEC-ETEC ?, NS, SD
Furazolidone (Furoxone)	100 mg, PO, q 6 hr, × 3–7 days (max 400 mg/day)	6–10 mg/kg/day, PO, q 6 hr, × 5–10 days	EPEC-ETEC ?, NS, SD, giardiasis, *Cryptosporidium,* cholera
Nifuroxazide[4] (Ercefuryl)	200 mg, PO, q 6–8 hr, × 3–5 days	10–30 mg/kg/day, PO, q 6–8 hr, × 5 days	EPEC-ETEC ?, NS, SD
Norfloxacin	400 mg, PO, q 12 hr, × 5 days	—	TD, *Shigella*
Ciprofloxacin (Cipro)	500 mg, PO, q 12 hr, × 5 days	Not recommended for children	TD, *Shigella*
Nalidixic Acid (NegGram)	15 mg/kg/day, PO, q 6 hr, × 5 days	Not recommended for children	*Shigella*
Chloramphenicol (Chloromycetin)	12.5–50 mg/kg/day, PO or IV, q 6–8 hr, × 5–14 days	25–75 mg/kg/day, PO or IV, q 6–8 hr, × 5–14 days	Septic salmonellosis,[3] *Shigella, Campylobacter, Yersinia,* cholera
Vancomycin (Vancocin)	10–40 mg/kg/day, PO, q 6 hr, × 7–10 days	20–50 mg/kg/day, PO, q 6 hr, × 7 days	*Clostridium difficile*[3]
Gentamicin (Garamycin)	1.7 mg/kg/day, IM, IV, q 8 hr, × 7–10 days	3–7.5 mg/kg/day, IM or IV, q 8 hr, × 7–10 days	Septic or persistent yersiniosis,[3] EPEC
Cefotaxime (Claforan)	—	25–33 mg/kg, IV, q 4–6 hr, × 7–10 days	Septic salmonellosis under 1 yr of age[3]
Ceftriaxone (Rocephin)	—	25–50 mg/kg/day, IM or IV, q 12 hr, × 7–10 days	Same as for cefotaxime
Metronidazole (Flagyl)[5]	250–500 mg, PO, q 6–8 hr, × 7–10 days	15–30 mg/kg/day, PO, q 8 hr, × 7–10 days (max 750 mg/day)	*Clostridium difficile, Giardia lamblia,*[3] intestinal amebiasis,[3] *Balantidium*
Tinidazole[4, 5] (Fasigyn)	2 grams, PO, 1 dose 2 grams/day, PO, × 3 days	60 mg/kg, PO, 1 dose 60 mg/kg/day, PO, × 3 days	*Giardia lamblia,*[3] intestinal amebiasis[3]
Quinacrine HCl (Atabrine)[6]	100 mg, PO, q 8 hr, × 7 days	6 mg/kg/day, PO, q 8 hr, × 7 days	*Giardia lamblia*

TABLE 3. **Anti-Infective Drug Therapy for Acute Infectious Diarrheal Diseases** *Continued*

| Drugs | Doses and Duration of Therapy | | Clinical Syndrome or Etiology Where Indicated[1] |
	Adults	*Children*	
Dehydroemetine[5, 7, 8] (Mebadin)	1 mg/kg/day, IM, q 12 hr, × 5 days (max 90 mg)	0.5 mg/kg/day, IM, q 12 hr, × 5 days	Intestinal amebiasis
Diloxanide[8] (Furamide [2-furoate])	500 mg/day, PO, × 10 days	20 mg/kg/day, PO, q 8 hr, × 10 days	Asymptomatic amebic cyst excretor
Diiodohydroxyquin (Diodoquin, Yodoxin)[9]	650 mg/day, PO, × 20 days, 2–3 times daily	15 mg/kg/day, PO, × 10 days (usual dose, 40 mg/kg/day)	Asymptomatic amebic cyst excretor
Paromomycin (Humatin)	10–20 mg/kg/day, PO, q 8 hr, × 7 days	30 mg/kg/day, PO, q 8 hr, × 7 days	Asymptomatic amebic cyst excretor

[1]See text. See Table 1 for abbreviations.
[2]Tetracyclines are not recommended for use in patients younger than 12 yr old.
[3]The drug is the first choice from among others for the disease.
[4]Not commercially available in the United States.
[5]Should be accompanied by a luminal amebicide.
[6]More than 20 per cent of patients have side effects: bitter taste, yellow discoloration of skin and sclerae, nausea, vomiting, toxic psychosis, exfoliative dermatitis, exacerbation of psoriasis.
[7]Cumulative toxic effect upon myocardium. Careful control of cardiac rhythm and frequency, blood pressure, ECG.
[8]Available through the Centers for Disease Control.
[9]Prolonged use may cause optic neuritis, optic atrophy, and peripheral neuropathy.

the same food. The diarrhea starts a few hours after ingestion with abdominal cramping and pain, followed by nausea and vomiting and later by loose stools.

TREATMENT. Only close clinical supervision and supportive treatment are needed (see later). Symptoms disappear in 1 or 2 days.

SUPPORTIVE THERAPY

Most ADD episodes resolve spontaneously 2 or 3 days after initiating treatment and are cured by days 5 to 7. Adequate hydration is the only essential therapeutic measure. Proper feeding in ADD is particularly important in small children to avoid the nutritional cost of diarrhea.

Hydration

Regardless of the clinical diarrheal syndrome, any patient with severe dehydration, signs of cardiovascular collapse or uncompensated acidosis, or signs of toxicity (intense pallor or pale-gray skin color, hyperthermia or hypothermia, prostration, decreased alertness or excitation) should be immediately placed under intensive care, including administration of intravenous fluids, separate urine and stool collection, cardiorespiratory monitoring, kidney function surveillance, and sepsis work-up. In children with vomiting and diarrhea, there may be potentially fatal diseases or complications (e.g., sepsis, meningitis, pneumonia, pyelonephritis, acute organic kidney failure). Also regardless of the clinical syndrome, any patient with moderate or severe diarrhea and/or vomiting or with mild to moderate dehy-

dration should be given appropriate carbohydrate-electrolyte oral fluids.

If the patient has a mild to moderate dehydration, the oral rehydration solution (ORS) from the World Health Organization, or a similar solution (Table 4), must be used for 2 to 6 hours. It should be offered as rapidly as the patient will accept it, in an amount at least equivalent to the estimated deficit. In infants, 50 to 100 ml per kg body weight in 2 to 6 hours can be given. This amount must be fractionated every 5 to 15 minutes. Gastroclysis should be tried if the patient does not accept or tolerate oral ingestion. The goal is proper diuresis and progressive disappearance of clinical signs of dehydration. If this goal is not achieved within 6 hours, or if dehydration worsens, intravenous fluids should be started.

If the patient is not dehydrated (<3 per cent of weight loss, no sunken eyes, humid mucous membranes), any of the maintenance oral fluid solutions shown in Table 4 (sodium, 30 to 50 mEq per liter) may be offered without other liquids, or the ORS or similar solution (Table 4) (sodium, 60 to 90 mEq per liter) may be used alternating with electrolyte-free fluids. The fluids must be given frequently, as much as the patient is willing to take each time, fractionating the volume but offering some every 5 to 15 minutes if there is a tendency to persistent vomiting.

The recommended World Health Organization formula for ORS can be prepared easily and cheaply at home by mixing ¾ teaspoon of table salt, 1 teaspoon of baking soda, 1 cup of orange juice, and 4 tablespoons of sugar to a liter (1.05 quart) of clean water.

TABLE 4. **Composition of Oral Electrolyte-Carbohydrate Solutions**

Solution	Electrolytes (mEq/liter)					% Carbohydrate (Glucose)
	Na	*K*	*Cl*	*Citrate*	*Bicarbonate*	
REHYDRATION						
ORS (WHO)	90	20	80	30	(−)	2.0
Gastrolyte	90	20	80	30	(−)	2.0
Rehydralyte	75	20	65	30	(−)	2.5
Pedialyte RS	75	20	65	30	(−)	2.5
Hydralate	84	10	59	(−)	15	2.5
Winhydran "90"	90	20	80	(−)	30	2.0
MAINTENANCE						
Pedialyte	45	20	35	30	(−)	2.5
Lytren	50	25	45	30	(−)	2.0
Infalyte	50	20	40	(−)	30	2.0
Resol	50	20	50	34	(−)	2.0
Winhydran "60"	60	20	50	30	(−)	2.0

Most cases of ADD, specially in adults, are mild enough not to need any particular hydration solution. Uncontaminated fluids are all the hydration necessary in these cases: pure boiled water, weak tea, or herbal infusions with about 3 per cent carbohydrate added, either sugar or starch refined from cereals (rice, corn, potato, wheat), suffice.

Feeding

ADD patients who previously received a full, normal diet will spontaneously select, on free demand and according to appetite, what is recommended traditionally: no residue (e.g., no peels, no seeds), no fiber (no raw fibrous vegetables: e.g., green beans, lettuce, celery), no spices (e.g., garlic, onion, pepper), low fat (not fried, no animal grease), and soft foods. These patients will eat smaller portions than usual to avoid postprandial discomfort, nausea, and vomiting. Fluids should be given ad libitum (see earlier). Three to 5 days of this diet, at the most, are usually needed to restore normal intestinal habit. Children 6 to 24 months of age should have their own regular nonmilk diet modified in the same way as adults. Children previously taking cow milk or modified milk formulas should have them diluted to one-half or three-quarters of the usual dilution to avoid lactose overload. Rice or other starch may be added to keep the calorie content and consistency to which the baby is accustomed. Normal bottle feeding can be restarted in 3 to 5 days. Lactose-free formulas may be used instead of the already mentioned modifications to bottle-feeding, but in most cases this adjustment is not necessary and is expensive. By contrast, the use of lactose-free formulas for 10 to 15 days is mandatory when the diarrhea affecting an infant is severe, or if the infant does not recuperate after the third day and has a fresh stool pH less than 6 and/or reducing substances are present in the stool.

Breast-fed children should be fed for less time (one-half or two-thirds) and more frequently (up to twice as often) than usual until diarrhea stops.

If vomiting is prominent in the clinical picture, only hydration measures are important, and feeding may be stopped for a few hours (usually 4 to 8). Care must be taken to extend this period in small infants and malnourished children. Care must also be taken not to restart feeding too soon in a patient with signs of "third space" in the abdomen: distention, intestinal "splash" (sounds on quickly and lightly shaking the abdominal wall), high-pitched intestinal sounds, persistent nausea, anorexia, and no or scant diarrheal stools passed in several hours. These patients tolerate oral refeeding poorly until intestinal propulsive motility has been restored.

Coadjuvant Therapy

If vomiting is persistent and there is no doubt about acute gastroenteritis being the only diagnosis or there are difficulties in providing intravenous administration of fluids, one dose of an antiemetic drug may be used: chlorpromazine (Thorazine) intramuscularly, adults 25 to 50 mg, children 0.5 mg per kg.

Antiperistaltic agents are contraindicated in cases of enterocolitis because they may prolong the illness and because the reduced stool output that they produce may reflect enteropooling rather than reduced body fluid losses. In addition, several diseases requiring surgical treatment may present initially as ADD, particularly in children, for example, acute appendicitis, intestinal intussusception, and intestinal subocclusion. These reasons make antiperistaltic drugs almost always contraindicated in children and rarely advisable in adults. Loperamide (Imodium), an initial dose of 4 mg followed by 2 mg taken as needed to a maximum of 16 mg per day, may be of benefit in reducing cramping and meeting social or professional obligations during a course of mild to moderate nonenterocolic adult ADD.

Antisecretory drugs like aspirin, indomethacin, chlorpromazine, and nicotinic acid have been tried without any significant or consistent result in secretory diarrheas. Recently, berberine, an alkaloid from a plant used for centuries in India and China as antidiarrheal in the sulfate form, has been shown to reduce stool volume significantly in patients with ETEC infection, although it has no effect on cholera diarrhea, in one dose of 400 mg, orally.

Absorbants like kaolin, pectin, activated charcoal, and cholestyramine have shown no benefit in ADD.

Bismuth subsalicylate has proved its efficacy and safety in ADD in adults, mainly in TD and in children, especially in *E. coli* and rotavirus diarrheas (see Table 3 for doses). Although the mechanisms of action of bismuth subsalicylate are not well understood, direct antimicrobial, intestinal mucosal protective, and antisecretory effects seem to operate together.

CONSTIPATION

method of
OK DONG KIM, M.D., and
SOHRAB MOBARHAN, M.D.
*University of Illinois College of Medicine at
    Chicago and Veterans Administration
    West Side Medical Center
Chicago, Illinois*

Constipation is a common problem, especially in the elderly, about one-third of whom use laxatives at least once a week. The discomfort to each individual from constipation may be attributed to infrequent bowel movements, hard stools, small stools, the necessity for excessive straining, or the sense of incomplete evacuation. Patients often have a combination of these symptoms. It is important to identify what "constipation" means to each patient because this definition often helps in diagnosing an underlying problem. There are several ways to define constipation, such as fewer than three bowel movements a week, excessive straining more than 25 per cent of the time, or stool weight less than 35 grams a day. The frequency of bowel movements is used most often. However, the exact definition may not be important because in most patients, mild to moderate constipation can be dealt with in a rather simple way by treating underlying diseases, removing offending medications, modifying dietary habits or lifestyle, and using laxatives. Young women have a greater predisposition to constipation than young men, particularly during the luteal phase of their menstrual cycles, which reflects the influence of progesterone on intestinal motility.

EVALUATION

The most common causes of constipation are presented in Table 1. A complete medical history and thorough physical examination, as well as appropriate laboratory tests, are required to rule out organic causes of constipation. A careful examination of the anorectal area cannot be overemphasized to rule out anorectal disorders. Barium enema or colonoscopy should be done if there is any clinical suspicion of a colorectal tumor. Anorectal manometry is useful to diagnose Hirschsprung's disease, which rarely manifests itself in adulthood. It is equally important to obtain a complete history of drug intake. Any potential offending agents should be discontinued or changed if possible. The physician should keep in mind that a patient complaining of constipation may actually be a laxative abuser.

A good, detailed account of dietary habits is important because low intake of fiber secondary to other medical problems such as poor dentition is a frequent cause of constipation in the elderly population. In some parts of the world, constipation is called a "summer disease" and is usually traceable to inadequate intake of fluid. Physical inactivity is another important factor in the etiology of constipation. Indeed, one study has shown prolonged colonic transit time of up to 3 weeks in bedridden patients as opposed to 5 days in healthy people. Repeated voluntary suppression of the urge to move the bowels may cause constipation, as it may make the fecal mass hard because of prolonged absorption of fluid in the colon, and the fecal mass may become so large that it is difficult to expel. Squatting or leaning forward on a low pedestal is so important to some people that they cannot defecate if they are unable to flex their hips. Ineffective Valsalva's maneuver related to cardiopulmonary diseases or a large abdominal hernia is sometimes responsible for constipation.

Colonic transit time can be measured easily by using radio-opaque materials to confirm delayed intestinal transit when the symptom is severe and does not improve with treatment. There is a rare subset of patients with severe idiopathic constipation whose life is disabled by progressive disease that does not respond to conventional measures. Surgical specimens of the colons of these patients have shown abnormalities of the myenteric plexus; however, the etiology of this illness is not totally clear. These patients are usually young females, and they frequently have associated gynecologic problems, including irregular and painful menstruation, difficulty starting a pregnancy, painful breasts, and increased incidence of hysterectomy or ovarian cyst removal. In some of these patients, constipation dates back to a previous childbirth or gynecologic operation. They may need to be referred to specialists for further evaluation with such tests as anorectal manometry, cinedefecogram, balloon proctogram, balloon expulsion test, or electrophysiologic studies of the puborectalis or anal sphincters.

TREATMENT

The initial therapy is aimed at treating the underlying diseases, side effects of medications,

TABLE 1. **Diseases and Drugs That May Cause Constipation**

Diseases		Drugs
Metabolic and Endocrine	*Neurogenic*	Opiates and analgesics
Diabetes	Intestinal pseudo-obstruction	Antacids containing calcium or aluminum
Porphyria	Chagas's disease	Anticholinergics
Amyloidosis	Autonomic neuropathy	Antidepressants
Hypercalcemia	Cauda equina tumor	Antiparkinsonian agents
Hypokalemia	Meningocele	Barium sulfate
Hypothyroidism	Trauma to lumbosacral cord	Diuretics
Pregnancy	Paraplegia	Iron
Uremia	Tabes dorsalis	Antihypertensive agents
Pheochromocytoma	Multiple sclerosis	Psychotherapeutic agents
Colonic	Parkinson's disease	Contraceptive pills
Tumors	Cerebral tumors	Laxatives
Volvulus	Cerebrovascular accident	
Hernias	Shy-Drager syndrome	
Intussusception and prolapse	*Anorectal*	
Inflammatory strictures	Rectocele	
Ulcerative proctitis	Anal stenosis	
Diverticular disease	Anal fissure	
Irritable bowel syndrome	Perianal abscess	
Dystrophia myotonica	Anterior mucosal prolapse	
Systemic sclerosis	Hemorrhoids	
Dermatomyositis		

and various predisposing factors in dietary habit or lifestyle. Daily intake of 30 grams or more of fiber, as well as 1.5 to 2 liters of fluid, is recommended to provide an adequate stool bulk. Routine daily exercise should be emphasized. The patient should also be instructed to be sensitive to the bowel function and answer the urge for a bowel movement promptly. It is better to avoid straining because it may cause unnecessary irritation and may aggravate hemorrhoids. There is also some evidence that excessive straining for many years may damage the pudendal nerves, thereby leading to incontinence. The patient needs to be aware of the concept of bowel training. Sitting on the toilet at the same time every day, whether or not the urge to defecate exists, may help to regulate bowel movement. This is best done after a meal to take advantage of the gastrocolic reflex. Some physicians use various laxatives for a few weeks to start this defecation habit and then taper them gradually.

The mainstay of laxative treatment is the bulk-forming agent. Included in this group are methylcellulose (Citrucel, Cologel), malt soup extract, polycarbophil, psyllium (Metamucil, Naturacil), and plant gums. They have the common property of forming a gel, thereby increasing total softness and bulk of the stool. They induce proliferation of intestinal bacteria, which adds to the laxative effect. The importance of stool bulk was confirmed by a study that demonstrated an inverse relationship between the minimum intra-abdominal pressure required to expel a sphere and the size of a sphere up to 2.5 cm. Several studies have clearly shown that a high-fiber diet shortens intestinal transit time. The bulk-forming agent should be taken with enough fluid, and it should not be used if there is a stenotic lesion in the gastrointestinal tract because it may hasten intestinal obstruction. Some patients may develop abdominal bloating and discomfort because of excessive gas production by intestinal bacteria, but this problem can be avoided if the amount of agent taken is increased slowly. Compounds such as methylcellulose are relatively resistant to bacterial degradation and therefore less likely to produce these side effects.

One particular concern has been the use of a bulking agent in bedridden patients because it may aggravate the "terminal reservoir" syndrome by adding to the fecal residue in the colon. Enemas or other laxatives have been suggested for these patients to treat constipation. Recent experience questions these ideas and supports the use of bulking agents in bedridden patients. The traditional recommendation was to continue use of a high-fiber diet and bulk-forming laxatives for 1 month to see the full effect. A recent study with wheat fiber reported that a shorter equilibration time of 1 week is necessary to demonstrate the maximum increase in fecal output. Bulk supplements are available in several forms, such as powder, granules, tablets, biscuits, candies, and cookies. Some patients prefer one of these products, and the time spent explaining these modalities is worthwhile.

Stool softeners such as docusate sodium (Colace) or docusate potassium (Dialose) act as secretagogues and dispersing agents. They are used mainly in the short-term treatment of patients with painful anorectal conditions such as anal fissure, hemorrhoids, or recent anorectal surgeries. They are often prescribed for patients with acute myocardial infarction to keep the stool soft. A study has suggested that soft and deformable stool is more easily expelled from the rectum. In this regard, stool softeners may well be prescribed in the first place for those patients who complain mainly of hard stool but who have adequate stool bulk and normal frequency of bowel movement. However, chronic use of stool softeners is not recommended.

Lubricants are mineral oil products. They are used occasionally for patients with fecal impaction as a retention enema before digital disimpaction. Otherwise, their use is not generally recommended. When ingested at night, a small amount remaining in the pharynx may be aspirated and cause lipoid pneumonia. They may be absorbed from the intestine and cause a foreign body reaction in lymph nodes. Chronic use has been reported to decrease absorption of fat-soluble vitamins.

Stimulant laxatives are often, unfortunately, agents of substance abuse. Included in this category are bisacodyl (Dulcolax), cascara, castor oil, casanthranol, danthron, phenolphthalein (Ex-Lax), and senna (Senokot). These agents are thought to work by stimulating peristalsis, although some may work by altering fluid and electrolyte transport. Bisacodyl stimulates the myenteric plexus of the colon, and it was used to test the functional integrity of myenteric plexus by some investigators. The abuse of these laxatives may damage the myenteric plexus and cause significant dilation of the colon leading to cathartic colon syndrome. Long-term use of these laxatives may also lead to melanosis coli, which is a reversible pigmentation of the colonic mucosa. We ask our patients to take these medications only under supervised situations because of their potential for dependency and long-term sequelae. It should be mentioned that prolonged use of any laxative can lead to dehydration and electrolyte depletion.

Agents that are believed to act primarily by their osmotic properties are saline laxatives, glycerine, and lactulose. Polyethylene glycol–electrolyte solutions (Colyte, GoLYTELY) were recently added to this category, and their main use now is in preparation for barium enema, colonoscopy, and bowel surgery. Owing to the large volume of oral fluid intake within 2 to 3 hours, there is a potential risk of vomiting from acute gastric distention with subsequent aspiration.

Saline laxatives include magnesium citrate, magnesium hydroxide (Milk of Magnesia), magnesium sulfate, and sodium phosphates (Fleet Enema, Phospho-Soda). Like polyethylene glycol–electrolyte solutions, they are used mainly for specific situations, including preparation of the bowel for radiologic and endoscopic studies, cleansing of the bowel after barium studies, purging of ingested toxins, or preparation of patients for bowel surgery. They are used either orally or as an enema. When used as an enema, they may irritate the rectal mucosa and alter its proctoscopic appearance. The problem of sodium and magnesium overload should be considered in patients with renal failure. There have been case reports of severe hypocalcemia after the use of a sodium phosphate preparation because of absorption of phosphate ion.

Glycerine is used only rectally because it is absorbed when ingested orally. It is used often for children as a suppository. Lactulose is another effective laxative; however, its high cost prevents its widespread use. It is valuable in the treatment of hepatic encephalopathy as well.

Idiopathic constipation may be so severe that some patients require surgical procedures. Ileostomy or total abdominal colectomy with ileorectal anastomosis is occasionally done as a last resort. Partial resection or division of the puborectalis and anorectal myectomy have been investigated as possible treatments. Although they are less extensive and more acceptable procedures, the results have been variable. Anorectal myectomy is a fairly simple procedure and is effective for some cases of short-segment Hirschsprung's disease. These patients, however, are best referred to a center that has experience with severe refractory constipation.

FEVER

method of
JACK NEWMAN, M.D.
Hospital for Sick Children
Toronto, Ontario, Canada

Myths about fever have abounded in all societies and at all times. In our Hollywood-influenced culture, movies show the frontier child who appears to be dying of fever, shivering in a tub of ice-cold water, and surrounded by anxious friends and relatives. The next scene shows the dozing father, suddenly awakened by the joyous mother who informs him that "the fever has broken." Of course, all is well.

PATHOPHYSIOLOGY

Fever is the body's response to viruses, bacteria, fungi, and immune complexes. These agents interact with macrophages to produce interleukin-1 (endogenous pyrogen), which then acts on the hypothalamus to reset the body's "thermostat" (thermoregulatory center), usually set at about 37° C. It was previously thought that neutrophils were a necessary part of the system, but this theory could not explain how the neutropenic patient developed fever. In response to the order to raise body temperature, several physiologic changes occur, including vasoconstriction of the skin vasculature (producing pallor or mottling as well as cold extremities) and shivering. Voluntary behavior to raise body temperature, such as covering with blankets, also occurs. Body temperature then rises until the new setting is reached. When the body has received the order to reduce the temperature (either naturally or as a result of medication), the skin vasculature dilates (causing the person to be hot, flushed, and sweaty) and the person tries to become cool by removing blankets or clothes. Acetaminophen, aspirin, and nonsteroidal anti-inflammatory agents block the resetting of the body's thermostat by interfering with the production of the prostaglandins by which interleukin-1 acts. External cooling (such as sponging the body with tepid water) may accelerate heat loss when the temperature is dropping but is unlikely to have much effect when the peripheral vasculature is already constricted. Furthermore, external cooling does not affect the thermoregulatory center of the hypothalamus. Therefore, even if the temperature is lowered by external cooling, the thermostat continues to try to maintain the body's temperature and produces more shivering and discomfort.

It should be remembered that an elevated temperature is not necessarily fever. Adults doing heavy exercise may increase body temperature to above 39° C. Body temperature may also rise to above normal if the ambient temperature is high. This is particularly true in the very young baby (younger than 4 weeks old) or the premature baby whose temperature control mechanisms are not yet mature. In these situations the thermoregulatory center has not been reset at a higher level. The athlete's temperature begins to decrease as soon as exercise stops; the baby's temperature drops if heavy clothing is removed.

SHOULD FEVER BE TREATED?

Whether or not to treat fever—like any other symptom or sign—depends on the relative benefits and disadvantages of the treatment. Reducing the temperature with an antipyretic agent does not eliminate the cause of the fever; a child with meningitis still has meningitis even if the temperature is returned to normal.

Is fever harmful in itself? This question immediately suggests the problem of febrile convulsions. However, there is no evidence that treating the fever prevents febrile convulsions. Furthermore, although febrile convulsions are extremely frightening for the child's caretakers, the convulsion has little or no consequence for the child. The convulsion itself does not mean that the cause of the fever is serious, and because of its usually short duration (almost always less than 20 minutes and usually much less), the convulsion does not cause brain damage or epilepsy.

Fever *does* cause discomfort for some children, especially if they are older than 3 years of age. Headache, muscle and joint pains, and occasionally delirium and hallucinations may occur, but they tend to resolve if the temperature is lowered. Many doctors perceive that children younger than 3 years of age also are bothered by fever, but the special circumstances of the office or emergency room may make a small child irritable when, if left alone with a parent, the child would merely put his or her head on the parent's shoulder and fall asleep.

Is fever beneficial? There is evidence from both studies of animals and in vitro studies from the laboratory that fever helps the host fight off the invading organism. Fever occurs in all mammals, and there is a suggestion that it occurs in reptiles as well (reptiles that are ill seek the sun to get warm). The cost to the organism of developing fever is not negligible. In the human, a temperature of 40° C increases the metabolic rate by approximately 36 per cent. It seems likely that this cost would be repaid to the host in some way, probably as an increased chance of survival. Would such a reaction be maintained over hundreds of millions of years if there were no survival benefit? This question should be considered in light of the fact that for most of history, humans have not lived in a state of excess energy reserve.

In normal children with an infectious disease, it appears that the body temperature does not rise higher than 41.6° C, and that this temperature, although dramatic, is not dangerous in itself. Children with severe brain damage, children with syndromes that interfere with temperature regulation (e.g., Riley-Day syndrome), and children taking medication that interferes with sweating (e.g., anticholinergic agents) may develop very high temperatures, above 41.6° C.

It would seem reasonable to lower the temperature of the child who is uncomfortable with fever. Some children seem to vomit when they are febrile, and lowering the temperature may alleviate this problem. It is obvious, however, that a febrile child may vomit for reasons other than the fever itself. Finally, the decision to seek medical advice should depend on deterioration or change in the child's condition. When the parents are unsure if there has been a significant change, lowering the temperature may help them decide what to do. If the child's temperature is reduced and the child seems to be livelier, they could continue observation; however, if the temperature is reduced and the child remains unwell, they should seek immediate medical attention.

When fever is chronic, such as that occurring with rheumatoid arthritis or other collagen vascular diseases, the metabolic cost of the fever may become debilitating. In such a situation, treating the etiology of the fever, if it can be determined, is obviously the best strategy; however, lowering the temperature may result in a subjective amelioration of the child's condition.

TREATMENT OF FEVER

Lowering the temperature, if it is thought to be necessary, should be done with acetaminophen. The usual dose is 10 to 15 mg per kg of body weight every 4 to 6 hours. In the usual therapeutic doses, acetaminophen is extremely safe and causes very few side effects. Overdose may be serious because irreversible hepatic failure may occur. Aspirin, because of its association with Reye's syndrome, should not be used. Nonsteroidal anti-inflammatory agents have potentially serious side effects similar to those of aspirin (gastric irritation and platelet function disturbances). Although use of these agents has not been associated with Reye's syndrome, it should be remembered that aspirin was in common use for almost 100 years before Reye's syndrome was recognized. Sponging the body with tepid water, because it does not deal with the fever at the level of the hypothalamus and because most children find it uncomfortable, should not be used except under special circumstances (e.g., for a child whose sweating mechanism is not operating properly).

Many health professionals suggest that fever should be treated to "give the parents something to do." However, concentrating on lowering the temperature takes the parents' attention away from their real task—watching the general condition of their child. The well child who is rushed to an emergency room because of a high temperature is a common phenomenon, as is the ill child who is kept home because the temperature is well controlled. Some parents, in their anxiety to lower the temperature, have given antipyretic agents in toxic amounts, which resulted in a "cure" that was much worse than the disease.

COUGH

method of
IRWIN ZIMENT, M.D.
Olive View Medical Center
Sylmar, California

Numerous agents have been used in the treatment of cough, although only a select minority are available in the United States. Because acute coughs, particularly those accompanying viral respiratory illnesses, are usually self-limited to within 2 to 3 weeks, most cough medications appear to be useful even if they are only serving as placebos. Thus, the management of cough is frequently carried out with apparent success by simple agents of unproven value. More serious etiologies, such as lung cancer, may demand the use of highly effective narcotic antitussives. It is therefore reasonable to approach cough management with respect to the apparent severity of the cough, and to advance if necessary from simple measures to the prescription of potentially hazardous drugs. Special cases of cough will be discussed. Underlying all treatment approaches is the requirement to evaluate the cause of the cough and to treat this directly if possible. It is of course well known that smoking and its complications are major causes of cough.

SIMPLE TREATMENT MEASURES

Airway irritation or inflammation may be palliated by inhaling warm moist air or steam with or without the addition of aromatic inhalants such as friar's balsam (compound tincture of benzoin). Oral medications, including the popular over-the-counter cough candies and throat lozenges, may also help. Simple syrups may provide a soothing cover to irritated oropharyngeal receptor sites that initiate reflex coughing. Hot drinks of teas, soups, or other beverages may be used. Applying an embrocation or aromatic lubricant externally to the skin, neck, or lips is favored by many people, who have thus enabled proprietary products such as Vicks Vaporub and Tiger Balm to achieve worldwide reputations that have not been supported by controlled studies.

Many proprietary cold remedies are also advertized to be effective for treating coughs. Alleviation of nasal inflammation and reduction of postnasal drip can undoubtedly result in an improvement in the cough that accompanies a common cold. Thus, mucosal vasoconstrictors and antihistamines can be effective in the management of cough, but the specific antitussive value of most of these drugs has not been demonstrated. Diphenhydramine and to a lesser extent tripelennamine have been reported to be more effective than other antihistamines, although the evidence for this is minimal. Antihistamines may be of further help in treating allergic coughs that are sometimes more of a problem than rhinitis in patients with allergy to pollen and other airborne antigens. Chlorpheniramine may be equally as effective as other antihistamines for allergic coughs, but a sedating agent is of added value at night.

DRUGS FOR SEVERE COUGH

A severe cough can be considered to be both persistent and subjectively distressing to the patient or to those who have to live or work with the patient; it could also be one that threatens the patient's life or daily activities. An effective cough suppressant is mandatory for patients undergoing eye surgery or those with fractured ribs.

For severe, nonproductive distressing or involuntary coughs that need to be suppressed, a narcotic medication is usually reliable (Table 1). In subjects with terminal diseases, such as cancer

TABLE 1. **Major Antitussive Products**

Drug	Marketed Products	Adult Dosage Range (mg)	Relative Effects Antitussive	Relative Effects Narcotic
Morphine	MSIR, Roxanol	2–8	+ + +	+ + +
Hydromorphone (dihydromorphinone)	Dilaudid	0.5–2	+ + +	+ + +
Methadone	Dolophine	2.5–10	+ +	+ +
Codeine	Bromarest-DC,* Dimetane-DC,* Medi-Tuss AC,* Medi-Tuss DAC,* Penntuss, Robitussin A-C,* Robitussin-DAC,* Ryna-C,* Ryna-CX*	5–20	+ +	+
Hydrocodone (dihydrocodeinone)	Hycodan,* Hycomine,* Tussend,* Tussionex*	5–20	+ +	+
Pholcodine	Not available in United States		+ +	+
Noscapine (narcotine)	Conar,† Tusscapine†	15–60	+ +	–
Dextromethorphan (dormethan)	Benylin DM,* Delsym, Hold, Robitussin-CF,* Robitussin-DM*	15–60	+ +	–
Benzonatate	Tessalon	100–400	+ +	–
Caramiphen edisylate	Tuss-Ornade*	10–30	+	–
Carbetapentane (pentoxyverine)	Rynatuss,* Tussar*	15–45	+	–
Levopropoxyphene	Novrad†	50–150	+	–

*Combination preparation.
†No longer marketed.

of the lung, morphine, hydromorphone (Dilaudid), or methadone may be appropriate, but for individuals in whom the risk of narcotic addiction must be avoided, hydrocodone (dihydrocodeinone) and codeine are safer. In other countries, heroin, dihydrocodeine, morpholinylethylmorphine, normethadone, and pholcodine are sometimes preferred. Occasionally, analgesics such as hydrocodone, oxycodone, and meperidine are indicated to suppress pain as well as cough. In practice, morphine and hydrocodone may be the most suitable agents for a severe distressing cough, but codeine, which is less effective, has the advantage of being virtually nonaddictive. It may be necessary to use larger doses than are usually recommended in persistent nonproductive coughs, and in the case of codeine, as much as 40 to 60 mg every 4 to 6 hours may be prescribed in adults if side effects are not a problem.

As an alternative to narcotics, several non-narcotic agents can be used. The most popular is dextromethorphan, which is usually given to adults in doses of 15 to 30 mg every 4 to 8 hours. This agent is generally well tolerated, and the dosage can be doubled to control a stubborn cough. An alternative drug is benzonatate (Tessalon); it is a local anesthetic that apparently acts on cough receptors in the lung. This agent can be particularly useful in coughs caused by interstitial lung diseases in which stretching of the damaged lung readily stimulates coughing. Lidocaine (Xylocaine), in contrast, is not used in similar circumstances, although it is a valuable local anesthetic for preventing cough during bronchoscopy. The drug has also been given intravenously to suppress a severe cough. Cocaine and other topical anesthetics may be effective but are rarely suitable for use in clinical situations.

A surprising number of additional antitussive agents are known, most of which are not available in the United States. The drugs that have been marketed in the United States include caramiphen edisylate, carbetapentane, chlophedianol, levopropoxyphene, and noscapine; of these, only noscapine appeared to be as effective as dextromethorphan. For economic reasons, caramiphen, chlophedianol, noscapine, and levopropoxyphene have been withdrawn from the market in recent years. In other countries, the numerous available antitussives include alloclamide, aminothiazoline, benzobutamine, bibenzonium, brospasmin, butamyrate, cloperastine, dibunate derivatives, dimenorfan, dimethoxanate, drotebanol, ethyl orthoformate, fedrilate, fominoben, glaucine, hydrocotarnine, isoaminile, morclofone, oxeladin, oxolamine, picoperine, pipazethate, piperidione, prenoxdiazin, viminol, and zipeprol. There is no evidence to suggest that any of these agents offers any advantages over codeine, dextromethorphan, or benzonatate. Similarly, the many Oriental and Western folk medicine cough medications have not been shown to be superior to established antitussives. Oriental medications that are readily available include Fritillary and Loquat Mixture, Ma-huang (ephedrine), Lo-han-kuo (mangasteen), and rhododendron extract.

Popular Western folk medications include colts-foot (which has the Linnaean name *Tussilago farfara*), horehound, eucalyptus, and extract of wild cherry.

SPECIAL THERAPEUTIC CONCERNS

It is important to try to tailor therapy to the particular characteristics of a cough. The nonspecific measures just discussed may not be suitable in the following situations.

Pulmonary Infection. A new or persistent cough with or without sputum may result from bacterial infection, in which case the use of one or more specific antibiotics is required. Bronchitis may respond to almost any antibiotic, whereas cystic fibrosis usually requires antistaphylococcal or antipseudomonal therapy. Bronchiectasis in exacerbation may present as a mixed infection, and broad-spectrum coverage is needed, as is the case with lung abscess or severe aspiration pneumonia in a compromised host. Legionnaires' disease and *Pneumocystis carinii* may present with a cough, and every effort must be made to diagnose and treat these conditions appropriately. Tuberculosis is becoming more common, and a persistent cough with an abnormal chest radiograph may be caused by typical or atypical mycobacterial infection, for which treatment with several drugs (e.g., isoniazid, rifampin, pyrazinamide) is required.

Abnormal Sputum. Persistent hyperviscous sputum in cystic fibrosis, the immotile cilia syndrome, or Young's syndrome may require postural drainage and chest percussion to alleviate the associated cough. Expectorants and other mucus-loosening drugs may help, with acetylcysteine (Mucomyst) being the best mucolytic agent, and the saturated solution of potassium iodide being the most favored general mucokinetic agent. Occasionally, bronchoscopy and pulmonary lavage are required to remove inspissated secretions.

Asthma. Some patients with latent asthma present with a chronic cough. Routine examination and pulmonary function tests may not conclusively demonstrate bronchospasm, and an inhalation challenge test may be needed for diagnosis. However, in suspicious cases it may be reasonable to give an empiric trial of bronchodilator therapy with an adrenergic aerosol or oral theophylline. If there is evidence of bronchitis, a course of ipratropium (Atrovent) inhalation should be initiated.

Allergy. In some patients, airborne allergens cause an annoying cough rather than rhinitis or conjunctivitis. The diagnosis may be suggested by the presence of an atopic history or the finding of eosinophilia, increased serum IgE level, a positive radioallergosorbent test, or a positive inhalation challenge test. The cough may respond best to a combination of codeine and chlorpheniramine in a slow-release preparation (Penntuss). A course of cromolyn (Intal) inhalation may be effective in selected patients, particularly in younger subjects with clear evidence of allergy or with coughing induced by cold air or exercise.

Nasal Disease. A large proportion of persistent coughs results from nasal disorders, the most important being postnasal drip. The presence of allergic rhinitis, sinus infection, or nasal polyps may explain the cough, and treatment with vasoconstrictors, antihistamines, topical steroids, or intranasal cromolyn should improve the nasal condition and alleviate the cough.

Heart Failure. Heart failure can present as a cough, which may respond to diuretic and specific cardiac therapy. It is of interest that the angiotensin-converting enzyme inhibitors captopril, enalapril, and lisinopril, which may be useful in heart failure, can cause an annoying cough in a small minority of patients. It is thought that these inhibitors allow the accumulation of bradykinin by inhibiting its metabolism; this peptide is believed to induce the cough.

Other Causes. Psychologic causes or habit can account for some coughs, including the hacking or throat clearing that may not be accompanied by sputum production. Many of these cases originate with a physical cause, but the cough may persist once the cause has been eliminated. Reassurance can usually be given without the need for an extensive work-up, but in more dubious cases it should be recognized that auditory, laryngeal, diaphragmatic, pericardial, chest wall, or gastric irritation can account for reflex coughing. In all cases, the physician should demonstrate that a thorough physical examination, chest radiographs, evaluation of sputum, and pulmonary function tests are normal before concluding that a persistent cough is of psychologic origin.

HOARSENESS AND LARYNGITIS

method of
KEITH F. CLARK, M.D.
University of Oklahoma Health Sciences Center
Oklahoma City, Oklahoma

Hoarseness is a nonspecific symptom that can result from various disease processes ranging from a short-lived viral laryngitis to a progressive and potentially life-threatening disease such as squamous cell carcinoma of the larynx. Furthermore, hoarseness can be a manifestation of systemic disease (e.g., hypothyroidism or rheumatoid arthritis) that may affect the larynx. A thorough history and physical examination of the patient complaining of hoarseness are required, in addition to a proper visual inspection of the larynx. Recall the old adage that "any patient with hoarseness of 2 weeks or longer duration must undergo a visualization of the vocal cords."

HOARSENESS IN CHILDREN

The most important consideration in the evaluation of children with hoarseness is whether there is airway compromise. Parents may confuse hoarseness with stridor, which is a wheezing sound produced by the flow of air through a partially obstructed airway during inspiration, expiration, or both. By using topical nasal anesthesia and the fiberoptic scope, the larynx can be examined with little trauma in children of all ages. Congenital cysts, laryngeal stenosis, recurrent respiratory papillomatosis, and laryngeal hemangiomas are examples of lesions that may present with hoarseness that progresses to airway obstruction. Children, in contrast to adults, can experience airway distress with unilateral vocal cord paralysis. A foreign body in the larynx or in the esophagus may produce hoarseness with concomitant airway obstruction. Many times the parents are not aware of a foreign body ingestion, but the physician must always think of this possibility in a child with airway compromise.

Screamer's Nodes

Probably the most common causes of hoarseness in children is vocal nodules or "screamer's nodes." These nodules are caused by vocal abuse and do not produce airway compromise. Speech therapy with behavior modification may be the only treatment needed. Surgical removal is not recommended unless the nodules are extremely large or persist despite adequate behavior modification.

Recurrent Respiratory Papillomatosis

Recurrent respiratory papillomatosis (RRP) is a potentially life-threatening disease that is characterized by the relentless growth of wart-like masses on the vocal cords. Although RRP is rare, it is the most common tumor of the larynx in children. Hoarseness is usually the initial symptom. Within several weeks or months the airway may become obstructed as these warty masses grow to fill the larynx completely. About 15 per cent of children with RRP continue to experience the disease well into adulthood. RRP can occur primarily in adults, but it usually has a less aggressive course.

Treatment

Treatment consists of laser removal of the papillomas. Because they have a marked propensity for recurrence, it is not unusual for a child to require monthly excisions of the papillomas to keep the airway open and to avoid tracheotomy. Spread to the trachea and lungs occurs more commonly in patients in whom a tracheotomy is performed. Adjuvant therapy with interferon has been successful in many patients but is still experimental. Vaccines, vitamins, antibiotics, and antimetabolites are not helpful. Radiation therapy is to be condemned because radiation is thought to cause malignant degeneration of the papillomas.

HOARSENESS AND LARYNGITIS IN ADULTS

Acute Laryngitis

Acute laryngitis is an inflammation of the mucosa of the larynx that usually occurs in association with an upper respiratory tract infection and is characterized by laryngeal and throat pain, hoarseness, and occasionally aphonia. Examination of the larynx reveals erythema and edema of the vocal cords. The infectious agent may be bacterial or viral. Acute laryngitis is usually self-limited; however, to assure the patient that there is no serious problem, the physician must perform a fiberoptic or indirect laryngoscopy.

Treatment

Symptomatic treatment with humidity, fluids, rest, and vocal care is helpful. Antibiotics should be given only in severe cases associated with fever and cervical lymphadenopathy.

Chronic Laryngitis

Chronic inflammation of the vocal cords can be caused by several factors, including allergy, chronic rhinitis, chronic sinusitis, voice abuse, reflux of gastric contents, and tobacco and alcohol abuse. Patients with chronic laryngitis usually do not have throat pain but simply complain of a long-standing abnormal voice that fatigues easily. The patient's occupation and personality are important etiologic considerations. An energetic, aggressive salesperson may be prone to voice abuse, whereas a janitor who breathes cleaning fluid fumes could experience a chemical or allergic laryngitis. Mild cases of chronic laryngitis may be caused by postnasal drainage from allergies, chronic rhinitis, or sinusitis, and treatment of these upper airway conditions improves the laryngitis. Patients with hoarseness related to gastroesophageal reflux may have posterior laryngeal inflammation visible on laryngoscopy. These patients may respond to antireflux management. However, in a significant number of patients with reflux there are no cervical symptoms and barium swallow, esophagoscopy, and esophageal biopsy are normal. Acid reflux may be documented in these patients by 24-hour esophageal pH monitoring.

The appearance of the vocal cords in chronic laryngitis varies from mild erythema and edema to thick, red, and boggy with patches of leukoplakia. Leukoplakia is a descriptive term for white patches on the mucosal surfaces of the larynx and is considered to be a precancerous lesion that requires biopsy. In the more severe forms of chronic laryngitis, polyps can be seen focally or spread over the entire surface of the vocal cords.

Treatment

The offending agent or habit must be eliminated to produce a long-term cure. Abstinence from smoking is a particularly important goal but a difficult one to achieve for most patients. Symptomatic treatment with humidity is helpful and is accomplished by increasing fluid intake and by the use of a bedside humidifier. Voice therapy may also play a useful role. Antibiotics and steroids may relieve inflammation, but often the benefits are only temporary.

Vocal cord stripping of hyperplastic mucosa and areas of leukoplakia is effective as a means of biopsy and may produce a more normal-appearing vocal cord with an improved voice.

Contact Ulcers and Vocal Process Granulomas

Another form of chronic laryngitis is caused by trauma produced either by an endotracheal tube lying between the posterior portion of the vocal cords or by prolonged abuse of the vocal cords presumably related to repeated throat clearing. Damage and breakdown of the mucosa covering the vocal process of the arytenoid cartilage results in ulceration with ensuing infection of the perichondrium and sometimes of the cartilage itself. Occasionally a large granuloma grows out of the initial ulcer. These entities can produce throat pain or discomfort and sometimes cause referred pain in the ears. The quality of the voice is not primarily affected because the vocal process portion of the vocal cords is not involved in phonation. However, voice changes can be caused by thickened tissue around a contact ulcer or by the mass of a granuloma itself, both of which can prevent proper closure of the vocal cords.

Treatment

Large granulomas should be removed surgically. Both granulomas and contact ulcers can be treated with antibiotics and steroids along with speech therapy. The course of treatment requires months and sometimes more than 1 year, with slow resolution. Serial laryngoscopy in the office will confirm the response to therapy. Biopsy should be considered to rule out a neoplasm, especially if there is a history of tobacco abuse.

Laryngeal Stenosis

Serious laryngeal and tracheal scarring can be caused by endotracheal tubes that are left in place for long periods. The cricoid cartilage lies below the vocal cords and is the only circumferential skeletal structure in the laryngeal and tracheal passage. Necrosis of the thin mucosal lining of the cricoid cartilage occurs rapidly when the endotracheal tube compresses this lining against the rigid cartilage. Subsequent scarring may result in mild stenosis or complete closure of the airway. Laryngeal stenosis can be prevented by the use of small endotracheal tubes and early conversion to a tracheostomy tube. The advent of large-volume, low-pressure cuffs has greatly reduced the incidence of tracheal stenosis. Because after only 48 hours of intubation significant inflammation and ulceration can be seen in the larynx, a tracheotomy should be considered early. In the adult patient, if intubation is anticipated to last longer than 1 week, tracheotomy is indicated. Neonates can tolerate long-term intubation (i.e., 4 to 6 weeks) with a lower incidence of cicatricial complications, probably because of the elasticity of the cricoid cartilage at this age.

Treatment

Treatment of laryngeal stenosis is often difficult and requires multiple surgical procedures. Mild cases may be treated with later excision and laryngeal dilation. Severe laryngeal stenosis may require laryngotracheal reconstruction with tracheotomy, cartilage implants, and internal stenting. The best form of treatment for laryngeal stenosis is prevention.

Vocal Nodules or Singer's Nodes

Vocal nodules do not cause airway obstruction or interfere with cord closure enough to cause aspiration. They are a form of chronic laryngitis caused by voice abuse and are a dreaded occupational hazard for singers. Acute nodules form during screaming when hemorrhage occurs beneath the mucosa of the free edge of the vocal cord. If this hemorrhagic injury organizes and becomes fibrotic, a chronic submucosal nodule results. Nodules can be quite small and almost invisible or so large that the vocal cords cannot close. They occur at the junction of the anterior and middle third of the vocal cords and seem to grow much like a callus, especially with continued heavy vocal abuse.

Treatment

Speech therapy, including behavior modification techniques, is frequently successful in curing vocal cord nodules. Surgical removal is not indicated unless the nodules are large or persistent despite adequate behavior modification. If behavior modification is not successful and poor vocal habits are not corrected, the nodules will recur after surgical excision.

Laryngeal Trauma

Improper or difficult intubation can occasionally cause an anterior dislocation of the arytenoid cartilage with resulting hoarseness but usually no airway distress. If the arytenoid cartilage is not returned to its proper position within several days, the dislocation may become a permanent complication with an immobile vocal cord.

Foreign bodies lodged between the vocal cords, such as a piece of glass or denture plate aspirated during an automobile accident, produce hoarseness and airway distress.

Injury to the larynx during motor vehicle accidents is common and is usually caused by compression of the larynx between the steering wheel or dashboard and the spine. Fractures of the cartilages of the larynx can greatly disturb laryngeal function. Hoarseness from laryngeal trauma can be minor when there is only submucosal hematoma. More serious laryngeal fractures can be recognized because of subcutaneous emphysema in the neck, point tenderness of the larynx on palpation, ecchymosis over or within the larynx, palpable deformity or crepitance of the laryngeal cartilages, voice change, and airway compromise. Computed tomography is helpful for the recognition of these fractures.

Treatment

Early treatment prevents the subsequent stenosis and hoarseness that occur when treatment is delayed. Open reduction and fixation of the fractures, repair of mucosal lacerations, and short-term internal stenting are required for satisfactory outcome in severe cases.

Laryngeal Carcinoma

All smokers with hoarseness need a careful laryngeal examination to rule out carcinoma because the vast majority of patients with laryngeal carcinoma have a history of tobacco abuse. Hoarseness caused by a carcinoma of the vocal cords is constant and slowly progressive. As the tumor enlarges, it may invade deeper structures to cause vocal cord paralysis or metastatic lesions in the neck. Throat pain is unusual in the early stages.

Treatment

When identified early and treated properly, laryngeal carcinoma can be cured with a success rate of over 90 per cent. Moderate-sized tumors may be treated successfully with conservative laryngeal surgery, laser surgery, or radiation therapy without total laryngectomy. Larger lesions, however, may require laryngectomy combined with radiation therapy for cure. Fortunately, many techniques are available for the rehabilitation of a patient's speech after total laryngectomy.

Vocal Cord Paralysis

Injury of the recurrent laryngeal nerve during surgery of the thyroid gland and the aortic arch is the most common cause of vocal cord paralysis. In patients in whom no apparent cause is found, a viral neuritis is thought to be the etiology. Neoplasms of the mediastinum, lungs, thyroid gland, base of skull, and vagus nerve can produce vocal cord paralysis. The patient with unilateral vocal cord paralysis presents with a breathy voice and may experience aspiration. The diagnostic work-up should consist of a thorough examination of the head and neck, a chest x-ray to identify a neoplasm of the lungs or mediastinum that may be affecting the left recurrent nerve as it loops under the arch of the aorta, and a barium swallow. Suspicious cases of neoplasia need computed tomography of the base of skull, neck, and/or mediastinum.

Treatment

Idiopathic vocal cord paralysis usually resolves within 6 to 12 months after onset. Patients whose paralysis does not resolve may learn to compensate with the mobile cord and achieve good vocal cord closure despite a complete lack of motion of the involved vocal cord. Gelfoam can be injected lateral to the paralyzed vocal cord to displace it medially. This technique allows the patient a good voice during the recovery period and is temporary because the Gelfoam is absorbed in several months. Gelfoam is used when it is critical to maintain voice or laryngeal competence while waiting for vocal cord movement to recover.

Patients who have a vocal cord paralysis that persists for a year after onset, without sufficient compensation by the mobile cord, are candidates for Teflon injection. This is a method of permanent vocal cord medialization that is successful, is painless, and can be performed in an outpatient setting. More than one injection may be necessary to achieve optimal results.

Bilateral Vocal Cord Paralysis

Bilateral vocal cord paralysis is unusual. It may be caused by thyroid surgery, amyotrophic lateral sclerosis (ALS), traumatic laryngotracheal separation, and Shy-Drager syndrome. Paralysis of both vocal cords produces airway obstruction. An immediate tracheotomy and eventually a vocal cord lateralization procedure may be needed to establish the airway.

Neurologic Diseases

Cerebrovascular accident (CVA), ALS, multiple sclerosis (MS), and myasthenia gravis are some of the neurologic disorders that can cause hoarseness.

Cerebrovascular Accident

Patients with a lateral brain stem CVA and a paralyzed vocal cord can be devastated by the resulting effects on communication and deglutition. Patients may literally drown in their own secretions, and tube feedings are often required to prevent aspiration and pneumonia. A Gelfoam or Teflon injection may be all that is needed to alleviate the aspiration and restore the voice. The addition of cricopharyngeal myotomy should be considered if a cine-esophagram demonstrates delayed passage of barium through the cricopharyngeus muscle.

Amyotrophic Lateral Sclerosis

Patients with ALS present with progressive weakness of cranial nerves. They have a prominent bilateral fasciculation of the tongue, which is almost pathognomonic. At first, the voice becomes weak. With progression, ALS patients may become aphonic and unable to swallow owing to hypopharyngeal muscle and tongue weakness, nasal regurgitation, and aspiration. Teflon injection is not an option for ALS patients: progressive airway obstruction is the rule because of their inability to abduct the vocal cords. Cricopharyngeal myotomy may help in the early stages because it may improve swallowing and decrease aspiration temporarily.

Myasthenia Gravis

Myasthenia gravis is a readily treatable cause of hoarseness. As the problem lies with neurochemical transmission, improvement after the patient receives 1 mg of edrophonium (Tensilon) may be diagnostic. Ptosis and dysphagia also suggest the diagnosis of myasthenia gravis.

Spastic Dysphonia

Spastic dysphonia is a neurologic disorder that is characterized by a choked, strangled speech pattern, with only a few words escaping before the sentence is ended prematurely by the involuntary spasm of the cords. At one time, patients with spastic dysphonia were labeled as malingerers or neurotics. The disorder is now thought to be due to a focal demyelinating process of the recurrent laryngeal nerve.

Treatment

Unfortunately, there is no successful medical or behavioral therapy for this debilitating disease. Unilateral recurrent nerve section may improve the voice in spastic dysphonia for several years, but reports of recurrence are common between 3 and 5 years after nerve section. The effectiveness of nerve section can be tested preoperatively by inducing a temporary recurrent laryngeal nerve paralysis with local anesthetic injection.

Systemic Disease

Myxedematous changes occur in the laryngeal mucosa in patients with hypothyroidism. The vocal cords become edematous and thickened with a corresponding drop in pitch. Thyroid replacement therapy results in a normal voice.

Rheumatoid arthritis may affect the cricoarytenoid joint, a true synovial joint. Pain is often quite severe. Hoarseness is caused by inflammation surrounding the joint and by limitation of cord motion. Corticosteroid treatment is helpful: the drug is given systemically or, in severe cases, may be injected into the joint.

INSOMNIA

method of
CONSTANTIN R. SOLDATOS, M.D.
University of Athens
Athens, Greece

The term "insomnia" applies to the condition of unsatisfactory quantity and/or quality of sleep. Insomniacs complain of difficulty in falling asleep, difficulty in staying asleep, awakening in early morning, or any combination of these symptoms. Not infrequently, however, patients suffer from poor quality of sleep, and the amount of their sleep may be judged subjectively and/or objectively to be within normal limits.

Insomnia is a prevalent condition both in the general population and in patient populations; surveys of the general public show a 20 to 30 per cent prevalence of insomnia, and physicians report that about 20 per cent of their adult patients have had sleep problems. The prevalence of insomnia tends to be higher among women, older individuals, and psychologically disturbed and socioeconomically disadvantaged persons.

Chronic insomniacs report that at bedtime they feel tense, anxious, worried, or depressed and as if their thoughts were racing. They also report rumination about getting enough sleep, personal problems, health status, and death. Further, they often attempt to reduce tension by taking medication and drinking alcohol. In the morning, they typically feel physically and mentally tired, and during the day they report being depressed, worried, tense, irritable, and overly preoccupied.

ETIOLOGIC CONSIDERATIONS

Insomnia is often a symptom of various psychiatric or medical conditions. It may also be a result of drug use. Amphetamines, energizing antidepressants, steroids, bronchodilators, and beta blockers are notorious for their sleep-disturbing effects. Rapidly eliminated benzodiazepine hypnotics such as triazolam often cause sleeplessness during the last few hours of nights during therapy (early morning insomnia) or intense sleep difficulty after their discontinuation (rebound insomnia). Substances other than drugs may lead to the development of insomnia: coffee and colas, as well as cigarette smoking, are associated with sleep disruption, particularly difficulty in falling asleep; use and abuse of alcohol are usually related to difficulty in staying asleep. Other common causes of insomnia include various environmental disturbances, stressful life events, and the process of aging. It should be emphasized that in most cases, multiple factors are involved in the etiology of insomnia.

Although insomnia is most often a secondary condition, when it is chronic and severe it becomes the focus of the patient's distress and is in fact perceived as a disorder itself. The most common cause of chronic insomnia is psychopathology. Extensive psychologic and psychiatric research has shown that chronic insomniacs tend to cope with stress and conflicts by internalizing their emotions, which leads to increased emotional arousal. This arousal causes physiologic activation, as indicated by the high levels of autonomic activity before sleep. In turn, this state of hyperarousal leads to difficulty in initiating sleep either at the beginning of the night or later on returning to sleep after a nocturnal awakening. Fear of sleeplessness further increases emotional arousal, thus perpetuating insomnia.

DIAGNOSTIC ISSUES

An adequate assessment of insomnia can be accomplished in the physician's office. The cornerstone of this assessment is the sleep history, as outlined in Table 1. Through the sleep history, relevant clinical information that accurately describes the patient's sleep problem and its important correlates can be collected. In addition, a thorough medical work-up, a careful psychiatric assessment, and a complete drug history should be obtained.

For the diagnosis of chronic insomnia to be established, the following criteria are required: (1) the complaint of sleep disturbance is either difficulty in falling asleep or maintaining sleep or poor quality of sleep; (2) the complaint has occurred at least three times per week for at least 1 month; (3) the patient is preoccupied with sleeplessness and is excessively concerned about its consequences; and (4) the unsatisfactory quantity or quality of sleep either causes marked distress or interferes with social and occupational functioning.

THERAPEUTIC PRINCIPLES

Insomniacs are so preoccupied with sleeplessness itself and invested in the secondary gain they receive that they are resistant to a systematic therapeutic approach. Thus, a major task of the physician is to overcome resistance and engage the patient in a comprehensive treatment plan. Such a plan should be multidimensional and should combine the following modalities: general measures for the improvement of sleep hygiene and the patient's lifestyle; psychotherapeutic techniques, selectively or in combination; and pharmacotherapy, only when indicated, as an adjunct.

General Measures and Psychotherapies

A number of general measures for improving the patient's sleep hygiene and overall lifestyle are relatively easy to implement (Table 2). These measures are often quite beneficial, especially when combined with other treatment modalities. The patient should be instructed to schedule times for hobbies and other interesting daytime activities. Particular emphasis should be given to increased exercise levels, although exercise close to bedtime should be avoided because of its arousing effect. Similarly, stressful situations

TABLE 1. **Steps in Taking the Sleep History***

Delineation of the specific sleep difficulty
Description of the condition's clinical course
Differentiation among various sleep disorders
Reassessment of previous diagnoses
Evaluation of sleep-wakefulness patterns on a 24-hr basis
Interview of bed partner
Evaluation for presence of other sleep disorders
Assessment of a family history of sleep disorders
Evaluation of the impact of the sleep disorder

*From Kales A, Soldatos CR, and Kales JD: Taking a sleep history. Am Fam Physician 22:101–107, 1980, published by the American Academy of Family Physicians.

TABLE 2. **General Measures for Treating Insomnia***

Regular exercise, but not close to bedtime
Avoidance of stress and tension
Restricted use of sleep-disturbing substances
Flexible, but not irregular, schedule for retiring and arising
Optimization of sleep duration
Improvement in sleep environment

*Derived from Kales A and Kales JD: Evaluation and Treatment of Insomnia. New York, Oxford University Press, 1984, p. 195. Used by permission.

and the use of coffee, colas, cigarette smoking, and other stimulating substances should be avoided close to bedtime.

It is important for the patient to observe a regular schedule for going to bed at night and arising in the morning; however, such a schedule must be reasonably flexible and take into account the fact that sleep cannot be forced on oneself. The patient can be taught that 7 to 8 hours of sleep per 24 hours is usually adequate and that any naps should be added up when the total duration of sleep is estimated. Special attention should be given to minimization of sleep-disrupting environmental stimuli, such as noise, light, and temperature extremes; uncomfortable beds should be corrected.

Any psychotherapeutic approach to treating insomnia should be tailored to meet the individual's needs. Most insomniacs require reassurance to alleviate their fear of sleeplessness; a full explanation should be offered of how anxiety becomes part of the vicious circle that exacerbates and perpetuates insomnia. Patients also need to be taught to reduce stress through effective management of emotions and appropriate expression of feelings. On an interpersonal level, they often need to become adequately assertive. From a technical standpoint, supportive, insight-oriented, and behavioral elements are usually combined for psychotherapy of insomnia. Although supportive psychotherapy can be performed successfully by almost any physician, appropriate referral is indicated for the application of highly specialized psychotherapeutic techniques.

Pharmacotherapy

A hypnotic drug may be used only as an adjunct to the multidimensional treatment of insomnia. Before prescribing a hypnotic, the physician must thoroughly assess the various factors involved in the etiology of the patient's insomnia and address them appropriately. A hypnotic can be quite beneficial in alleviating sleeplessness, thus providing the patient with a most needed sense of mastery. This beneficial effect, however, can be properly achieved only when certain principles are taken into account, as outlined in Table 3.

Because of their efficacy and safety, benzodiazepines have replaced other classes of hypnotics in the adjunctive treatment of insomnia. Benzodiazepines used as hypnotics in the U.S. market include flurazepam (Dalmane), temazepam (Restoril), and triazolam (Halcion). Because of their pharmacokinetics, these three drugs have different effects and side effects. Flurazepam and triazolam are absorbed rapidly and therefore are quite effective in inducing sleep; temazepam, a slowly absorbed formulation, has little efficacy for sleep induction. The long elimination half-life of flurazepam makes it possible for this drug to be effective during a 4-week period of nightly administration, whereas tolerance develops rather rapidly with triazolam and temazepam, both drugs having relatively shorter elimination half-lives.

Administration of slowly eliminated benzodiazepines, such as flurazepam, is often associated with higher degrees of daytime sedation. This side effect, however, is less of a problem with the 15-mg dose of flurazepam. Tolerance to daytime sedation develops much earlier than tolerance to the hypnotic effect of the drug. In contrast, rapidly eliminated benzodiazepines, such as triazolam, are practically devoid of this side effect, but they are more likely to cause rebound phenomena both during their administration (early morning insomnia, daytime anxiety) and after their withdrawal (rebound insomnia, rebound anxiety). Administration of triazolam has also been associated with episodes of amnesia, depersonalization, hallucinations, and other behavioral side effects.

Nonbenzodiazepine hypnotics are somewhat effective initially, but they lose most of their efficacy within about 2 weeks of nightly use. Thus, an escalation of their dosage often takes place, and a severe abstinence syndrome may occur with their abrupt withdrawal. Over-the-counter sedatives have been proved to be ineffective, and in high doses they may cause unwanted effects, such as confusional states, because of their atropine-like action. In the small subgroup of chronic

TABLE 3. **Considerations During Use of Hypnotic Medication for Treatment of Insomnia***

Thorough evaluation of the patient should be done before treatment
Hypnotics should be used only as adjuncts
Limited amounts should be prescribed
Initial and continued efficacy should be considered
The patient has to be cognizant of side effects
Withdrawal problems need to be addressed
Drug interactions should be avoided

*Derived from Kales A and Kales JD: Evaluation and Treatment of Insomnia. New York, Oxford University Press, 1984, p. 267. Used by permission.

insomniacs who are endogenously depressed, the use of tricyclic antidepressants is indicated. For psychiatric patients with the symptom of insomnia, neuroleptics with sedative effects should be prescribed.

TREATING THE ELDERLY

Before any treatment, the elderly insomniac should be assessed for the presence of medical and psychiatric disorders. If conditions such as organic brain syndrome or depression are present, the treatment plan must be adjusted accordingly. For example, haloperidol (Haldol) should be prescribed to the organically impaired elderly insomniac with nocturnal agitation and confusion.

Monosymptomatic elderly insomniacs should be educated about the extent of age-related sleep changes. Special emphasis should be placed on the effects of daytime naps on nocturnal sleep. These naps should be generally discouraged. Instead, the elderly insomniac is advised to increase daytime activities and to try to be engaged in stimulating social contacts.

The use of hypnotic drugs should generally be avoided in the elderly because the age-related impairment of renal function may lead to retention of the drug, which is often associated with increased likelihood of daytime sedation, amnesia, and other side effects. If a hypnotic is needed, one that is lastingly effective may be preferable. All hypnotic drugs should be administered in about one-half the dosage intended for young adults.

PRURITUS
(Itching)

method of
MAREK A. STAWISKI, M.D.
St. Mary's Hospital
Grand Rapids, Michigan

Pruritus is a common chronic problem that is often severe and unrelenting. Itching is an unpleasant sensation perceived in the skin that provokes an urge to scratch. Pruritus can prevent sleep and interfere with concentration. Anxiety, boredom, and mental distraction influence the perception of pruritus. The perception of the itching sensation is conducted from the unmyelinated fibers in the skin through the myelinated fibers, the dorsal root ganglia, the opposite spinothalamic tracts, and the thalamus to the cortex. Endopeptidases, trypsin, pepsin, prostaglandins, epidermal proteases, kallikrein, and histamine are some

TABLE 1. Skin Problems, Chemical Agents, and Skin Infestations Associated with Pruritus

Atopic eczema
Contact dermatitis
Seborrhea of scalp
Dermatitis herpetiformis
Scabies
Lice
Urticaria
Mastocytosis
Lichen planus
Psoriasis
Irritant chemicals
Miliaria rubra (heat rash)
Insect bites

chemicals that produce itching when applied or injected into the skin.

Generalized pruritus is caused by systemic disease in about 20 per cent of patients (Table 1). Primary cutaneous diseases such as eczema, contact dermatitis, scabies, pediculosis, dermatitis herpetiformis, and others are found in about one-third of patients with pruritus (Table 2). Pruritus can occur as a condition without a specific cutaneous or systemic cause. In many of these patients, dry skin (xerosis) and psychologic factors can exacerbate the symptoms of itching.

A careful history taken by the physician is mandatory in every patient with generalized pruritus. Physical examination can reveal cutaneous and systemic causes of pruritus. Laboratory investigation includes a

TABLE 2. Systemic Conditions Associated with Generalized Pruritus

Pregnancy
Obstructive hepatic disease
    Intrahepatic cholestasis
    Extrahepatic cholestasis
    Drug-induced disease
Chronic renal failure
Lymphoma
    Hodgkin's lymphoma
    Non-Hodgkin's lymphoma
    Mycosis fungoides
Leukemia
Multiple myeloma
Polycythemia rubra vera
Carcinoid tumors
Acquired immunodeficiency syndrome
Endocrine conditions
    Diabetes
    Hyperthyroidism
    Hypothyroidism
    Hypoparathyroidism
    Secondary hyperparathyroidism
Parasitic infections
Drug reactions
    Opiates
    Isoniazid
    Hydralazine
    Chlorpromazine
    Antimalarial agents
Multiple sclerosis
Sjögren's syndrome
Iron deficiency anemia
Psychiatric disorders

TABLE 3. **Treatment of Special Pruritic Conditions**

Condition	Treatment	Relative Success of Treatment
Hemodialysis in chronic renal failure	Ultraviolet B therapy in suberythema doses every other day for 15–20 treatments	Sometimes effective
Dermatographism	Hydroxyzine (Atarax, Vistaril), 10–25 mg 2–4 times daily	Sometimes effective
Dermatitis herpetiformis	Diaminodiphenylsulfone (Dapsone), 50–100 mg daily; gluten-free diet	Always effective
Obstructive biliary disease	Cholestyramine (Questran), 4 grams 2–3 times daily	Usually effective
Neurotic excoriations	Imipramine (Tofranil), 10–25 mg at bedtime, or chlorpromazine (Thorazine), 10–25 mg 3 times daily	Sometimes effective

complete blood count, urinalysis, liver function tests, renal function tests, stool examination for occult blood and parasites, and basic thyroid function tests. Patients with pruritus of more than 1 month's duration might require a radiologic examination of the chest and a barium enema. Pregnant women should not receive a radiologic examination. When all the test results are negative, a psychiatric evaluation might be needed.

Dermatologic conditions are usually apparent from a careful history and examination of the skin. However, skin scrapings to demonstrate scabies, KOH examination for fungal hyphae, and skin biopsy for diagnosis of dermatitis herpetiformis are some of the laboratory tests used to establish the causes of pruritus.

Localized pruritus is usually restricted to the anal area, the vulva, or the scalp. A physical examination is needed to rule out local malignancy as a cause of pruritus ani and vulvae. Candidiasis and dermatitis/eczema are frequent causes of pruritus ani and vulvae. Seborrheic dermatitis, psoriasis, and lice are frequent causes of pruritus of the scalp. Cosmetics, sprays, dyes, Benzamycin, neomycin, and balsam of Peru can initiate pruritus of the vulva, anus, or scalp. Psychologic factors such as depression and anxiety can aggravate these localized forms of pruritus.

TREATMENT

General Measures

The patient's skin must be kept moist and cool. The fingernails should be trimmed. Relaxation and rest can alleviate the psychologic component of pruritus. Because coffee and alcohol can exacerbate pruritus, they should be avoided. Patients should be instructed not to wear wool or tight-fitting clothing. Daily or alternate-day lukewarm showers or baths are recommended. A bath oil (Alpha-Keri) or baking soda may be added to bath water. Mild soaps (Basis, Neutrogena, Dove) are recommended. Moisturizing lotions (Moisturel, Cetaphil, Lubriderm, Eucerin, Complex 15) or humectants (LactiCare, Aquacare Lotion 2 per cent) should be applied to damp skin immediately after bathing.

Topical Treatment

Soothing cool or lukewarm water compresses applied for 1 hour a few times daily sometimes increase the effectiveness of antipruritic medications. Bland ointments and creams free of sensitizers (Eucerin cream and lotion) are important in treating xerosis. Mild antipruritic agents such as 0.5 per cent phenol or menthol can be added to an emollient base such as Eucerin. A lotion with phenol added (Sarna) has a cooling, antipruritic effect on the skin. Scalp pruritus secondary to seborrhea or psoriasis can be treated with tar shampoos (T/Gel) or zinc shampoos (Zincon). Only mild topical corticosteroids (1 per cent hydrocortisone cream or lotion) should be used if there is evidence of cutaneous dermatosis because of the risk of cutaneous atrophy or adrenal suppression from prolonged application of potent fluorinated corticosteroids. Antipruritic agents such as 0.5 per cent methol or phenol may be added to 1 per cent hydrocortisone mixed with Eucerin. Crotamiton 10 per cent (Eurax) is an antipruritic agent that is effective against scabies.

Systemic Therapy

Treatment of pruritus is often ineffective, especially in patients who have no associated cutaneous dermatoses or systemic disease. Oral H_1 histamine blockers are the mainstay of systemic therapy for pruritus. They may be beneficial partly because of their sedative effect on the central nervous system, although they are ineffective in some patients. Because of this sedative effect, antihistamines are frequently used at bedtime. Patients should be warned about the hazards of driving or operating machinery after ingestion of these medications. Hydroxyzine (Atarax, Vistaril), 10 to 25 mg, or diphenhydramine (Benadryl), 25 to 50 mg, or cyproheptadine (Periactin), 4 mg, is used twice or three times daily. Other oral H_1 receptor histamine blockers that can be used include chlorpheniramine (Chlor-Trimeton), 4 mg, or trimeprazine (Temaril), 2.5 mg. Terfenadine (Seldane), 60 mg given twice a day, has fewer sedative effects than hydroxyzine but is usually less effective. An H$_2$ histamine receptor blocker such as cimetidine (Tagamet), 300 mg three times daily with meals, can be added to these medications but is not always effective.

The tricyclic antidepressant doxepin (Sinequan), 25 to 50 mg daily, can be useful in the treatment of pruritus secondary to urticaria.

Corticosteroids such as prednisone can have a beneficial effect on severe, intractable pruritus. Prednisone is administered in doses of 20 to 30 mg daily and is rapidly tapered during a 2-week period. The drug should be used only for acute, intense pruritus in healthy patients who are free of diabetes mellitus, high blood pressure, and peptic ulcers.

Therapy of Special Pruritic Conditions

Special pruritic conditions include pruritus secondary to hemodialysis in renal patients, dermatographism, dermatitis herpetiformis, obstructive biliary disease, and neurotic excoriations. The treatment of pruritus secondary to these conditions and the relative success of these therapies are summarized in Table 3.

TINNITUS

method of
JOHN W. HOUSE, M.D.
Otologic Medical Group and House Ear Institute
Los Angeles, California

As has been often stated, tinnitus is a symptom and not a disease. Therefore, when patients complain of noise in their ears or head, an evaluation is necessary to establish the etiology of their tinnitus. All patients complaining of tinnitus require an audiogram, including air conduction, bone conduction, and speech, to evaluate the nature of any hearing loss if in fact there is such a loss. Approximately 10 per cent of our patients who have a primary complaint of tinnitus have normal hearing. In addition to routine audiometric studies, a history is taken, and an otologic examination is performed by the otologist.

A unilateral sensorineural hearing loss, unilateral symptoms, or an asymmetric hearing loss may indicate serious pathology. In these cases a neuro-otologic evaluation is necessary. An auditory brain stem response (ABR) is performed as a screening test. If this result is positive, we proceed to magnetic resonance imaging (MRI), initially without gadolinium; if the MRI result is equivocal, intravenous gadolinium may be intro-

duced. When we are strongly suspicious of a retrocochlear lesion, we proceed directly to MRI without performing the ABR test. On the other hand, if the ABR result is negative, we rarely proceed to MRI.

In patients who describe the tinnitus as pulsatile, auscultation of the ear is performed by using Toynbee's tube. The neck and mastoid are auscultated by using a stethoscope. This objective type of tinnitus can be associated with arterial plaques, arteriovenous malformations, enlarged jugular bulb, or vascular tumors (e.g., glomus tympanicum or jugulare). In such cases, we obtain a high-resolution computed tomography scan with a bone program to look at the bony details of the jugular bulb, carotid artery, and middle-ear structures. If these studies are normal, we do not usually proceed to angiography. In rare cases we obtain vascular studies such as an arteriogram, jugular venogram, Doppler, or ultrasound studies.

TREATMENT

Eighty-six per cent of patients with an ear disorder have associated tinnitus. Approximately 95 per cent of these patients are not particularly concerned about the tinnitus and are satisfied with an evaluation, an explanation, and any treatment of the underlying cause. A small number of patients are driven to distraction by the tinnitus and tend to focus on their complaints. Many of these patients complain of lack of sleep caused by the tinnitus. They also complain of difficulty in concentrating; in some cases they find everyday tasks difficult. We have evaluated the personality of these patients and have found that depression is a significant factor in their symptoms. We therefore recommend antidepressants as a first line treatment for these patients.

If the tinnitus is associated with a conductive hearing loss, correcting the hearing loss may be of benefit. Seventy-five per cent of patients with otosclerosis report resolution of the tinnitus after successful surgery. On the other hand, 5 per cent of patients report that the tinnitus is worse after surgery. Our experience with translabyrinthine removal of acoustic neuromas has shown that about one-half of the patients report improvement of the tinnitus, whereas the other half report that the tinnitus is worse. For this reason we do not recommend a cochlear nerve section for the treatment of tinnitus.

Because most tinnitus is associated with a sensorineural hearing loss, hearing aids can be helpful. We have found that most patients with a hearing loss and associated tinnitus report an improvement in the tinnitus while they wear hearing aids. The hearing aids act to improve the patients' performance and allow for environmental sounds to enter the ear, thus masking the tinnitus. We use tinnitus maskers on rare occasions. We have found that a small number of patients find the tinnitus masker to be helpful because they believe that it gives them some control of the tinnitus.

For many years we have been using biofeedback training as a treatment of tinnitus. Our experience has indicated that patients who are depressed or have anxiety attacks do well with biofeedback. Approximately 80 per cent of these patients report some relief or control of the tinnitus. Patients who are more severely disturbed tend to do poorly with biofeedback training. We believe that biofeedback training is successful in helping patients because the tinnitus is exacerbated by muscle tension around the neck and head and by constriction of the peripheral circulation. When patients learn to relax the muscles and to increase the peripheral circulation, the tinnitus tends to decrease. In addition the patients gain insight into the causes of the tinnitus and how it is exacerbated by tension and stress.

All patients complaining of tinnitus deserve an evaluation that should include at least routine audiometric studies. If any of these results are positive, further neuro-otologic or vascular studies are necessary. The general treatment is aimed at the underlying cause of the problem. A complete explanation of the situation is beneficial, and hearing aids, tinnitus maskers, biofeedback, and antidepressants may be helpful.

Section 2

The Infectious Diseases

MANAGEMENT OF HIV INFECTIONS

method of
FREDERICK P. SIEGAL, M.D.
Long Island Jewish Medical Center
New Hyde Park, New York

Infection with human immunodeficiency virus (HIV), a lentivirus transmitted by intimate (usually sexual or parenteral) contact among people, leads gradually to a state of immunodeficiency and mental deterioration known as acquired immunodeficiency syndrome (AIDS). The process by which this syndrome ultimately develops is gradual, with a mean incubation period after the infecting event estimated to be approximately 7.5 years. During much of this period, the infected individual may be unaware of the presence of the virus. Management of HIV infection depends on the stage of the illness when the patient first visits the physician, and it involves major psychosocial concerns as well as medical considerations. Optimal care in this complex situation should be pre-emptive, anticipatory, and preventive rather than reactive. The last 2 to 3 years have seen a revolution in management that promises ultimate conversion of this disorder from invariably fatal to chronic but amenable to prolonged life under close clinical observation.

Unfortunately, HIV infection has become prevalent since the virus was first introduced into the United States in the middle to late 1970s. Although its geographic distribution is variable, there are few locales in this country in which physicians will not have to address this problem. As of April 1989, more than 91,000 cases of frank AIDS had been seen nationwide, and estimates of numbers of persons infected range from 500,000 to 3 million Americans.

CLINICAL STAGING OF HIV INFECTION

Care of patients with HIV infection is guided by recognition of the presence of the virus and definition of the patient's immune competence. The presence of HIV infection is usually established serologically, through the use of screening immunoassays, and is confirmed by tests, such as the Western blot, that are highly specific because they measure antibodies to unique viral proteins. People with confirmed positive serologic tests for HIV almost certainly will harbor and be capable of transmitting the virus to some degree for the remainder of their lives; most patients will have gradually progressive immunologic dysfunction.

The level of immune function, which relates to prog-nosis and stage, is ascertained most directly by determination of the helper T cell (T4, CD4) count. CD4 lymphocyte counts are widely available through commercial laboratories and should be obtained for both initial staging and subsequent monitoring. Declining CD4 counts correlate well with increasing susceptibility to infection and to clinically important HIV-related encephalopathy and neuropathy. However, counts can be very variable: single determinations that do not fit with the patient's clinical status should be regarded with suspicion and repeated. A good practice is to repeat the initial CD4 count within 1 to 2 months, to confirm the original determination, and subsequently to monitor this value at an interval dependent on how far these two determinations are above the critical level of 250 cells per mm³. This level, associated with the development of opportunistic infections (OI), should prompt the institution of preventive therapies in all patients regardless of whether they appear to be clinically ill (see later section on symptomatic phase). It is not unusual to have patients with virtually no symptoms present with severe immunodeficiency; intervention should be immediate, as described later. A useful clinical staging system, which is summarized in Table 1, corresponds roughly to other staging systems but relates closely to the CD4 count and to prognosis.

MANAGEMENT BY STAGE

Early Infection

Initial infection is usually inapparent; however, some individuals have an acute illness resembling infectious mononucleosis around the time of seroconversion; management of this relatively unusual (or usually unrecognized) acute retroviral syndrome is supportive. Most persons who visit the physician at this stage do so because of a history of contact with a patient with AIDS, after birth of an infected infant, or after a serologic finding during blood donation, a physical examination required for insurance, or military screening tests. These patients feel well, have no clinical findings related to HIV infection, and usually have CD4 counts well in excess of the lower limit of the reference range for the laboratory.

The initial evaluation (of all HIV-infected people; Table 2) should include serologic tests for syphilis, cytomegalovirus (CMV), and toxoplasma and tests for tuberculin delayed-type hypersen-

TABLE 1. **Staging System for HIV Infection**

Stage	Clinical Findings	Usual CD4 Cell Count (Cells/mm^3)	Intervention
Early infection	No findings (rare acute illness)	>500	Psychosocial counseling; monitor q 3–6 mo.
Lymphadenopathy syndrome (PGL)	Axillary and inguinal adenopathy, splenomegaly, "hairy" leukoplakia	>250	Consider lymph node biopsy for unusual site or prominence; monitor q 3–4 mo.
Symptomatic (ARC)	Weight loss,* diarrhea, oral thrush, zoster, intermittent fever, nocturnal diaphoresis, malaise, reactivation pulmonary tuberculosis,† hairy leukoplakia, headache, bacterial pneumonia, pericarditis	<250	Search for OI, treat specific illnesses; begin zidovudine, prophylaxis for *Pneumocystis carinii* pneumonia (? and other OI); monitor q 1–2 mo.
Kaposi's sarcoma*	Dermal, oral, nodal, or visceral lesions	Any	Depends on immune status and extent of disease.
Lymphoma*	Prominent lymph nodes, extranodal (retroperitoneal, gastrointestinal, central nervous system involvement)	<300	Usually requires chemotherapy or radiotherapy.
AIDS-dementia complex*	Slow mentation, gait disturbance, peripheral neuropathy, urinary retention or incontinence	<250	Assess central nervous system; begin zidovudine, prophylaxis for *P. carinii* pneumonia.
AIDS/OI*	Case-defined OI	<250	Treat specific OI; search for other OI; start zidovudine when feasible.

*These conditions must be reported to local health departments as meeting the AIDS surveillance definition; loss of more than 10% of normal body weight in an HIV-seropositive individual meets this case definition.

†Pulmonary tuberculosis should be reported to local health departments.

Abbreviations: OI, case-defining opportunistic infections; PGL, progressive generalized lymphadenopathy; ARC, AIDS-related complex.

sitivity, along with a panel of skin test antigens to assess the patient's ability to respond. (Skin test anergy does not appear to be related to prognosis or even directly to stage of immune decline.) We find the Multitest-CMI (Merieux, Miami, Fl.) to be convenient for this purpose, but we confirm positive tuberculin reactors with a 5-TU intradermal test. These data provide information that may be useful later when progressive immunodeficiency develops. The eventual use of prophylactic isoniazid for the known tuberculin reactor, the use of cytomegalovirus-screened blood products for the previously uninfected per-

TABLE 2. **Initial Evaluation for HIV Infection**

Complete medical history and physical examination, with special attention to skin, mucous membranes, lymphoid organs, and central nervous system.

Confirmation of HIV seropositivity by enzyme-linked immunosorbent assay and Western blot

Complete blood count with differential, platelet count, and reticulocyte count

Erythrocyte sedimentation rate

Chemical assessment of hepatic and renal function: lactate dehydrogenese, creatine phosphokinase, uric acid, and electrolytes

Serologic tests for pre-existing infection with *Treponema pallidum, Toxoplasma gondii,* and cytomegalovirus

Skin tests for tuberculosis and competence to respond by delayed-type hypersensitivity (anergy panel)

T cell subset ratio and calculation of circulating helper (CD4, T4) lymphocyte count

son, and the recognition or exclusion of central nervous system (CNS) toxoplasmosis may hinge on these early determinations. A positive test for syphilis should be evaluated carefully; re-treatment for latent neurosyphilis may be justified. The clinician should remember that lumbar puncture in HIV-infected persons frequently yields abnormal results that cannot easily be distinguished from results of latent neurosyphilis.

Such individuals should be counseled extensively on the use of safe sexual practices (Table 3) and avoidance of situations in which parenteral transmission to others is likely to occur, such as sharing needles during intravenous drug abuse or allowing the HIV carrier's blood to come into contact with the skin of another person. Areas of remaining uncertainty (e.g., the role of intimate kissing in HIV transmission) should be explained to the patient.

TABLE 3. **Safe Sexual Practices**

Avoidance of
  Unprotected intercourse with exchange of semen or vaginal secretions with the infected partner
  Exposure of abraded or nonintact skin to semen or vaginal secretions of infected partner
  Prolonged intimate kissing (highly controversial)
Use of condoms supplemented with contraceptive creams or gels containing the spermicide (and virucide) nonoxynol 9
Finding satisfying alternatives to sexual practices likely to transmit HIV

HIV carriers should be warned not to divulge their status to persons other than those with a true need to know because of the stigma of this disorder in society today, but they should be urged to share the information with spouses, sexual or needle partners, and health care personnel with whom they come into contact. In certain states, the physician may be legally obligated, or at least permitted, to divulge this information to a known sexual partner of the patient as part of the "duty to warn." In some localities, reporting of HIV-seropositive patients to health authorities is mandatory. The physician's role, however, usually is to protect the patient's confidentiality to the greatest extent possible.

Symptom-free seropositive individuals with CD4 counts higher than 500 per mm³ may be monitored with follow-up visits every 3 to 6 months, during which an interim history, complete physical examination, complete blood and CD4 counts, routine urinalysis, and chemistry assays should be done. HIV-infected women should have a Pap smear for cervical cytology every 6 months because of an apparent increase in the frequency of cervical carcinoma.

Lymphadenopathy Syndrome

This stage of HIV infection may persist for years; the pattern of lymphadenopathy usually associated with early HIV infection involves variable, usually painless enlargement of axillary and inguinal/femoral node groups. Modest cervical adenopathy also is seen. Nodes can appear in clusters and be as large as 3 to 4 cm. People at this stage lack the systemic, "B" symptoms that characterize more advanced disease. Discrimination of lymphoma, nodal Kaposi's sarcoma (KS), and coincidental adenopathic disorders is the principal problem. Splenomegaly, usually nontender and modest in degree, is common. The presence of retroperitoneal, intrathoracic, epitrochlear, or very tender, extremely prominent, or rapidly enlarging nodes should prompt the physician to do a biopsy. However, even impressive, more or less symmetric adenopathy involving the usual sites seen in HIV-seropositive patients may often be observed without biopsy. Progressive decreases in adenopathy usually herald progressive immune depletion and retroviral activity.

Management of patients presenting at this stage involves the same considerations described for early infection (see earlier section). An appropriate interval of follow-up and monitoring CD4 counts in this stage is every 3 or 4 months.

Intercurrent illness during this stage of rela-

tively preserved immunity should be treated promptly. Even in the presence of CD4 counts higher than 300 per mm³, acyclovir given orally (800 mg five times daily with ample fluids) may be appropriate for a dermatomal zoster. Occasionally, a worrisome manifestation (e.g., oral "hairy" leukoplakia) can appear transiently, sometimes at a lower CD4 count, without ominous prognostic significance. Such occurrences should prompt closer follow-up and reassurance of the usually anxious patient.

Early Symptomatic Phase (AIDS-Related Complex)

Patients with HIV infection at this stage most often become symptomatic as the immunodeficiency worsens, presumably via the emergence of some opportunistic agent, which may not ever be specifically recognized. Because certain organisms—such as *Mycobacterium tuberculosis*, varicella-zoster virus, or *Candida albicans* (oral thrush)—are sufficiently pathogenic to cause disease in the nonimmunocompromised host, they may cause disease earlier than the generally nonpathogenic true opportunists that emerge only in very late stages and define AIDS/OI (see later section). Most people with the symptoms given in Table 1 are in the process of shifting into a more rapid loss of CD4 cells and should be considered to be immunocompromised regardless of the measured count. Some individuals remain in this metastable condition for months or (unusually) years. Occasionally, an acute illness that appears to be severe may occur despite CD4 counts considerably higher than 300 per mm³, may be coincidental to the HIV infection, and should not prompt the diagnosis of AIDS-related complex (ARC). On the other hand, some severely immunodeficient persons have minimal or no clinical symptoms because of the sporadic and unpredictable nature of complicating illnesses; they should be managed preventively once the CD4 count is established to be low.

The patient who has CD4 counts of 250 per mm³ has reached a critical point in his or her HIV infection. Counts lower than 250 per mm³ are increasingly associated with the development of severe OI and AIDS-dementia complex (ADC). Rarely, opportunistic complications can occur with higher numbers of circulating CD4 cells. Consequently, we begin prophylaxis against *Pneumocystis carinii* infection (Table 4) at this point, while confirming the lymphocyte determinations with monthly CD4 counts. Exploration of the patient's tolerance for trimethoprim-sulfamethoxazole (TMP-SMZ) (Septra, Bactrim) (one double-strength tablet on alternate days) is a reasonable precaution, with the realization that

TABLE 4. **Prophylactic Regimens for *P. carinii* Infections**

Drug	Dose	Efficacy	Comment
Trimethoprim-sulfamethoxazole	1 double-strength tablet, bid, qod, or tiw	Close to 100%	Rash and fever are common; may not be truly allergic; lower-frequency dosing appears equally effective and minimizes leukopenia.
Fansidar (pyrimethamine-sulfa-doxine)	1 weekly	Close to 100%	Stevens-Johnson syndrome can occur, but drug is convenient for many patients.
Dapsone	50–100 mg daily	Close to 100%	Leukopenia, anemia, and pancytopenia; bullous and other skin reactions; hemolysis can be associated with glucose-6-phosphate dehydrogenase deficiency.
Pentamidine	100 mg* via aerosol, weekly for 2–4 doses, then every other week	80–90%	Dose of aerosolized drug is not yet established; particle size delivered by nebulizer may be critical; wheezing may require prior use of aerosolized bronchodilator; extrapulmonary *P. carinii* infections are not prevented; drug is incompatible with saline solution and sterile water should be used for administration.

*Generally higher doses are recommended (up to 600 mg).

the CD4 counts of some patients improve significantly under close observation and obviate the need for further prophylaxis.

Prophylaxis against *P. carinii* infection is a life-prolonging mainstay of management; it usually avoids hospitalization and invasive diagnostic procedures for this otherwise debilitating complication. Systemic administration of TMP-SMZ may prevent reactivation toxoplasmosis as well as pneumocystosis; we have not observed the former complication in patients who are seropositive for *Toxoplasma gondii* who have been successfully maintained with TMP-SMZ. The alternative regimens (Table 4) may be tried if TMP-SMZ is not tolerated because of reactions (fever or severe skin eruption), or when pre-existing leukopenia is likely to limit the concurrent use of TMP-SMZ and zidovudine. With the low-dose alternate-day regimen recommended, however, TMP-SMZ does not usually produce appreciable leukopenia. Current investigations may eventually indicate the utility of chemoprophylaxis against other OI (e.g., mycobacterial disease), but the potential for adverse drug interaction through the inevitable introduction of additional drugs must be defined before any drug can be recommended.

Also at this stage of immune decline, institution of specific antiretroviral therapy should be seriously considered. Current labeling of zidovudine (Retrovir, AZT) gives CD4 counts below 200 per mm³ or the appearance of *P. carinii* pneumonia (PCP) as approved indications. However, we begin administration of this drug once the symptomatic phase has become established even if the CD4 count has not yet fallen to 200 per mm³ or below. The decision to begin use of zidovudine is not simple at this stage and depends on careful consideration of the entire situation. As statistical data from current clinical trials become available, the point in immunologic decline at which the drug is recommended will probably change; however, it is not clear now that early institution prevents progression of immunodeficiency. The use of zidovudine is discussed in greater detail later.

Specific illnesses at this stage require prompt recognition (by isolation of the organism, if possible) and treatment; usually, therapy can be that offered to the immunocompetent host. Such therapy often needs to be prolonged, perhaps "forever"; the tuberculous patient, for example, should probably never have chemotherapy stopped entirely because the underlying process (immunodeficiency) is likely to worsen rather than to improve during therapy of its complication (tuberculosis). Treatment of these complications is discussed in more detail in the later section on AIDS/OI. Occasionally, febrile illness with or without diaphoresis may represent true B symptoms of an emerging lymphoproliferative disease.

Kaposi's Sarcoma

This complication of HIV infection can occur at almost any time in the course of the decline of the immune system. It occurs almost exclusively among homosexual and bisexual males; a few gay men with KS have been reported to be HIV seronegative, thus fitting the surveillance definition of the Centers for Disease Control without actually having AIDS. Although KS usually presents with skin involvement, it often involves oral or intestinal mucous membranes and lymph nodes and later affects visceral organs and the lungs.

Management of KS depends on the extent of disease and the state of the immune system. Follow-up intervals and the point of institution of prophylactic antimicrobial drugs and zidovudine should be determined by placing the patient in the appropriate stage of HIV-related manifestations (Table 1) and by considering issues other than the presence of KS.

The specific care of KS (Table 5) is complicated by the fact that the patients who would respond best to therapy are those who probably do not require any. In general, the best results of intervention with chemotherapy or interferon-alpha have been reported for patients with minimal disease and better immune function. Inappropriately aggressive management can precipitate worsening immunodeficiency, severe neutropenia, and a rapidly fatal outcome. Management should involve consultation with a clinical oncologist unless minimal or intermediate disease responds (as it may after 1 to 3 months) to the institution of zidovudine alone. Active chemotherapeutic agents include etoposide (VP-16, VePesid), doxorubicin (Adriamycin), bleomycin (Blenoxane), vinblastine (Velban), vincristine (Oncovin), and others. The results from therapy with single agents are unpredictable in individual patients, and initial failure to respond to one does not preclude success with others. Multiple-agent regimens should be used with extreme caution in the severely immunocompromised patient but may be justified under certain circumstances. Recombinant interferon-alpha (Roferon-A, Intron A) is now approved by the U.S. Food and Drug Administration (FDA) for use in patients with KS.

Close observation and patient education for self-monitoring of new skin and oral lesions are essential in planning a stepwise, rational response to this disease.

Lymphoma

Non-Hodgkin's lymphomas, usually of B cell but sometimes of mature T cell origin, have been observed among the HIV-immunocompromised population. Hodgkin's disease has also been observed frequently, but whether there is a true statistical association between this disorder and HIV infection is not yet defined.

The emergence of lymphoproliferative diseases, like that of KS, is not as closely tied to immune competence as is the development of OI. Consequently, some patients may present with lymphomas, often in extranodal sites including the CNS, when their immune and bone marrow dysfunction may not be profound. Such persons may respond well to appropriate multidrug chemotherapy. Others, particularly patients with histologically high-grade lymphomas, may prove to be highly resistant to therapy.

There is no standard approach to the therapy of this complication, but the same considerations limiting the therapy of KS (see earlier section on KS) should be applied. Prevention of *P. carinii* infection and the provision of zidovudine as tolerated should be components of care. Patients

TABLE 5. **Management of Patients with Kaposi's Sarcoma**

Stage of Disease	Clinical Findings	Treatment
Early	Few (less than 10) skin lesions, little progression under close observation, normal chest film, CD4 count > 300/mm³	Observation, excision, or local radiotherapy for cosmetic effect; may consider zidovudine as monotherapy.
Intermediate	Multiple lesions at presentation; involvement of oral mucous membranes; lymphadenopathy; CD4 count > 250/mm³	Institute zidovudine; observe closely for progression of disease (1–2 mo); consider therapy* with interferon-alpha, vinca alkaloids, etoposide, doxorubicin, or bleomycin in consultation with clinical oncologist; use radiotherapy for locally troubling lesions.
Advanced	Multiple skin, oral, and nodal involvement; lymphedema; visceral or pulmonary disease at presentation; CD4 count 0–300/mm³	Institute zidovudine as tolerated in conjunction with systemic therapy as above; use prophylaxis for PCP; observe closely.

*Drug dosage is variable and depends on leukocyte and platelet counts, hepatic and renal function, presence of pre-existing peripheral neuropathy, lung disease, and patient tolerance for systemic side effects (e.g., flu-like syndrome with interferon-alpha) and extent of KS.

with lymphoma limited to the CNS may benefit from the use of whole-brain radiation and corticosteroids (dexamethasone [Decadron] in standard doses), but the hazards of daily steroid therapy in the severely immunodeficient patient should be recognized. The management of lymphoproliferative disease in the setting of HIV infection, although essentially that of the individual lymphoma, is highly complex and should be carried out by specialists in hematology/oncology in centers committed to the management of AIDS patients. Facilities for the support of patients with severe neutropenia and thrombocytopenia are essential; the role of bone marrow transplantation is under investigation.

AIDS-Dementia Complex and Other Neuropsychiatric Manifestations of HIV Infection

HIV, like its cousins the caprine and ovine lentiviruses, is a neurotropic retrovirus. The virus enters the CNS early in infection, which accounts for the sometimes abnormal cerebrospinal fluid findings seen in those stages of disease. Acute aseptic meningitis and Bell's palsy have been associated with recent primary HIV infection. Clinically, neurologic complications are generally seen when the immune system is profoundly compromised, but unusual cases have been reported of dementia or other neurologic disease appearing even in the absence of significant CD4 cell depletion.

The late neurologic expression of HIV infection involves progressive difficulty in concentrating, loss of memory for recent events, apparent depression, apathy, inattention to the environment, bradyphrenia, frank dementia, seizures, and, ultimately, coma. A myelopathy with gait disturbance and leg weakness, and peripheral neuropathy, can also be seen and are frequently associated with urinary retention or incontinence, and, later, with fecal incontinence.

Neurologic signs and symptoms of HIV infection must be discriminated from those of an OI involving the CNS (toxoplasmosis, tuberculosis, cryptococcal disease, and progressive multifocal leukoencephalopathy) and from those of lymphoproliferative disease (CNS, epidural, or retroperitoneal lymphoma). Computed tomography, magnetic resonance imaging, lumbar puncture, prior serologic tests for toxoplasma, and the mode of clinical presentation and of response to empiric antimicrobial drugs in selected cases usually permit a diagnosis. In certain situations brain biopsy may be justified.

HIV-mediated neurologic disease, defined by exclusion, is sometimes remarkably responsive to therapy with zidovudine. Because of limitations in access to the CNS, zidovudine should be given at the highest dose tolerated by the patient. Addition of acyclovir (Zovirax) at 200 to 800 mg orally every 4 hours may be a useful adjunct (see later). General supportive care (avoidance of pulmonary embolism, decubitus ulceration, oversedation, and urinary tract infection) is an essential component of management.

The patient presenting with neurologic complications should be evaluated for level of immunocompetence and should be managed on the basis of these findings and the presence of coexisting complications according to principles delineated in other sections.

AIDS/OI

Expression of systemic or CNS OI in patients with HIV infection marks the last stage of the disease. It often coexists with varying degrees of neurologic dysfunction (see earlier section on ADC). Patients presenting at this stage have lost the opportunity to benefit fully from earlier institution of zidovudine and prophylactic antimicrobial drugs, but they may nevertheless do well for a significant period if their disease is addressed aggressively. Containment of the complicating presenting illness usually must take precedence over the institution of preventive approaches, so as to avoid drug interaction that can further complicate therapy. For example, we do not start zidovudine at the time of initial therapy for PCP because an early neutropenia may compromise the use of high-dose TMP-SMZ and force the use of pentamidine, often a more toxic alternative (which can also contribute to leukopenia).

Diagnosis and management of OI in AIDS are summarized in Table 6.

Patients at this stage need close monitoring to detect early manifestations of OI. The follow-up interval should probably not exceed 1 month even when the situation appears to be stable. At the onset of zidovudine therapy (see later), close observation is essential. Attempts to define the cause of any symptoms should include blood cultures (with the Dupont Isolator, which enhances the detection of intracellular pathogens) for mycobacteria, assay for serum cryptococcal antigen, repeated chest radiography, bone marrow aspiration (primarily for culture for mycobacteria), and biopsy (which must always be stained for acid-fast organisms, even in the absence of granulomas). A gallium scan sometimes points to an unexpected localized inflammatory or lymphomatous process. Paranasal sinusitis, otitis media, mastoiditis, bacterial peritonitis, and pericarditis (usually viral), as well as the possible emergence

TABLE 6. **Diagnosis and Management of Opportunistic Infections in HIV Infection***

| Organism/Disease | Diagnostic Procedure | Therapy | | Comments |
		First Choice	Alternatives	
P. carinii: pneumonia, otitis, systemic dissemination (rare)	Bronchoalveolar lavage, transbronchial biopsy, induced sputum (Gomori methenamine silver, Giemsa), gallium scan, pulmonary function test with DL_{CO}; chest film	TMP-SMZ, 15–20 mg/kg TMP daily IV in 3 or 4 doses or as double-strength tablets, dose as for IV	Pentamidine, 4 mg/kg/day IV or via aerosol, 300–600 mg daily Trimetrexate with leukovorin obtained on compassionate use protocol from National Institutes of Health Trimethoprim, 5 mg/kg qid, with dapsone, 100 mg/day (oral regimen) Difluoromethylornithine (see text)	Early treatment and close daily monitoring essential (see text); corticosteroids used concurrently for brief course only (see text)
Cytomegalovirus: retinitis, colitis, pneumonitis	Funduscopic examination, colonoscopic or transbronchial biopsy	Gancyclovir on protocol (from Syntex; call 301–497–9888)	Foscarnet on protocol	Toxicities may preclude use of zidovudine; limited use; utility in pneumonitis uncertain (see text)
Toxoplasma gondii: CNS mass lesion, cerebritis	Computed tomographic scan with and without contrast, magnetic resonance imaging scan, brain biopsy, therapeutic trial	Pyrimethamine 100 mg, then 25 mg PO daily with sulfadiazine, 4–6 grams daily	Clindamycin 900 mg tid to replace sulfadiazine	Folinic acid supplement possibly useful; chronic suppression essential
Cryptococcus neoformans: meningitis, pneumonia, fungemia	Lumbar puncture with cryptococcal antigen, India ink preparation, serum antigen, blood culture	Amphotericin B, 0.5 mg/kg IV daily after test dose or 0.3 mg/kg daily with flucytosine, 150 mg/kg PO daily	Fluconazole, a promising experimental oral agent	Chronic suppressive maintenance essential
Mycobacterium avium complex: disseminated disease, pulmonary disease, scrofula	Blood culture, bone marrow biopsy with acid-fast stain and culture, buffy coat smear for acid-fast bacilli; node biopsy; bronchoscopy	Ansamycin, 150–450 mg with clofazimine, 300 mg initially, then 100 mg PO daily	Isoniazid, 300 mg, rifampin, 600 mg, ethambutal, 25 mg/kg PO daily	Continued suppressive therapy indefinitely at reduced doses of some agents

*TMP-SMZ = trimethoprim—sulfamethoxazole.

of a lymphoproliferative disease, must not be forgotten. Empiric antibiotic trials may be fully justified once proper studies have been obtained. Therapeutic trials should be based on the restrictions of the situation, not to obscure meaningful clinical responses or to increase the likelihood of inducing microbial resistance; for example, a clinical trial of antimicrobial drugs without activity against mycobacteria should probably precede a trial including rifampin or quinolones.

Two OI constitute true emergencies in HIV infection, and patients should be made aware of them by the physician because early specific treatment tends to mitigate their severity. These are the exceedingly common (at least 65 per cent of patients at risk without intervention) PCP and the relatively uncommon CMV retinitis.

Pneumocystis carinii *Pneumonia*

PCP is far more likely to have a fatal outcome if it is recognized or treated only late in its course. Patients known to be at risk because of low CD4 counts, especially those unable to tolerate or unwilling to follow the most effective prophylactic regimens, should be warned to report minimal but progressive dyspnea on exertion, fever, and productive or nonproductive cough. Careful history-taking usually excludes patients with stable dyspnea. If the chest film, done immediately, is negative, we obtain a measure of carbon monoxide diffusion capacity (DL_{CO}) and a flow-volume loop with a trial of bronchodilators. A DL_{CO} value at or below 65 per cent of predicted in the absence of pulmonary infiltrate or physical findings in the chest usually prompts the start of therapy, while confirmatory cytologic or histologic evaluation is arranged. Exposure of the patient to a few days of oral or intravenous TMP-SMZ, intravenous or high-dose aerosolized pentamidine (see Table 6 for doses) while the situation is clarified is far preferable to waiting for confirmation; treatment does not affect the results of diagnostic tests done within a reasonable time.

Interstitial pneumonitis in the AIDS patient is most often attributable to *P. carinii* but can result from a number of other opportunistic processes that need to be excluded and that sometimes occur simultaneously with PCP. Induction of sputum with a heated aerosol of 3 to 10 per cent saline sometimes yields a positive smear when stained with Gomori's methenamine silver or Giemsa's stain and may obviate the need for bronchoalveolar lavage. However, in AIDS, bronchoscopy with bronchoalveolar lavage has been the most reliable diagnostic approach to confirmation of the typical case. The washings obtained can be submitted for routine bacteriologic studies with Gram's stain, with direct fluorescent antibody for both *Legionella* species and CMV (the latter still of somewhat dubious significance), with acid-fast stain (which may reveal *Legionella* as well as some *Nocardia* species and mycobacteria), and for cryptococci. If pulmonary CMV or other processes (e.g., lymphocytic interstitial pneumonitis) are suspected, or if initial lavage has not provided a diagnosis, transbronchial biopsy may be done in addition to bronchoalveolar lavage. However, the diagnostic yield of transbronchial biopsy for pulmonary KS is relatively low, and the biopsy carries a significant risk of pneumothorax. Interstitial pneumonitis and fibrosis of unknown cause have been observed.

Determination of serum cryptococcal antigen may be useful for rapid diagnosis of disseminated cryptococcosis, which can clinically resemble PCP, even in the absence of manifestations of meningitis. We have not used gallium scan for pulmonary disease because of delayed results and relative nonspecificity. However, a positive scan in the absence of findings on chest films suggests the likelihood of a diffuse pneumonitis.

We usually discontinue use of zidovudine when beginning high-dose TMP-SMZ therapy for PCP unless the leukocyte count is well above 3000 per mm³. This maneuver may minimize the tendency toward progressive leukopenia, which is frequent with the latter drug and also occurs with pentamidine.

Clinical responses to these drugs are often delayed up to 3 to 5 days after starting therapy; high fever and a moderate erythroderma may not reflect a drug reaction, and even late skin eruptions, if mild and not involving the mucous membranes, may not warrant discontinuation of TMP-SMZ in favor of pentamidine. There is no evidence favoring either drug in terms of efficacy, but we prefer TMP-SMZ to pentamidine as generally being less toxic. (TMP-SMZ, unlike pentamidine, also covers *Haemophilus influenzae* and *Streptococcus pneumoniae,* which may co-infect patients with PCP.) A switch from one drug to the other because of adverse drug reactions does not usually signify a worsened prognosis; a change in drug because of apparent treatment failure, however, often bodes ill for the patient. If during intravenous pentamidine use the clinician is confronted with improvement in pulmonary function but severe problems with hypo- or hyperglycemia, electrolyte disturbances, or renal dysfunction, the clinician may switch to the aerosol route, 300 to 600 mg per day. Yet another regimen consists of oral dapsone, 100 mg per day, and trimethoprim, 20 mg per kg per day in divided doses. Dapsone may cause severe hemolysis in cases of glucose-6-phosphate dehydrogenase deficiency. Patients who are unable to tolerate either first line agent or who have progressive disease unresponsive to either drug may be eligible for clinical trials with trimetrexate with leukovorin rescue (for information, call National Institute of Allergy and Infectious Diseases, National Institutes of Health, Bethesda, Md.), or for trials with difluoromethylornithine eflornithine (available through Merrell Dow). Brief, high-dose use of corticosteroids for PCP that is rapidly progressive or far advanced at presentation may be justified, but the efficacy of such an approach has not been established.

Intubation and ventilatory support, when necessary because of respiratory failure in advanced

PCP, only occasionally result in a favorable outcome. Some patients cannot be weaned from support and remain tied to the ventilator for the remainder of their lives. Thus the decision to intubate is a difficult one, and probably should be anticipated so that the wishes of the patient and family members can be appropriately ascertained.

Drug treatment of confirmed PCP probably should continue for 21 days; shorter courses have led to relapse. Although some patients with uncomplicated illness may have chemotherapy continued at home, most drug-related toxicity develops relatively late in the course of treatment. Adequate, close monitoring of blood cell counts (for both TMP-SMZ and pentamidine), blood glucose level, renal function, and blood pressure (for pentamidine) should be available. Once a full course of therapy has been completed, there is generally a "honeymoon" period during which PCP prophylaxis may be omitted; it should generally be resumed within a few weeks.

Cytomegalovirus Retinitis

CMV retinitis, the other AIDS emergency, occurs in only a small proportion (probably less than 5 per cent) of patients at risk. It may be asymptomatic; careful routine funduscopy should reveal its presence, which should be distinguished from the rather common finding of cotton wool spots in advanced HIV disease. This variety of CMV retinitis, especially if uniocular, may be observed closely by an ophthalmologist familiar with the problem because unless vision is threatened, specific antiviral therapy is probably not indicated. Patients with advanced immunodeficiency (fewer than 250 CD4 cells per mm³) should be advised to check their vision daily by first closing one eye and then the other, and to report any abnormalities. Uniocular CMV retinitis that threatens vision may be treated under experimental drug protocols with gancyclovir (DHPG, available through Syntex Corporation) and, possibly, foscarnet. Bilateral CMV retinitis may rapidly and unpredictably result in blindness and should be treated under an existing compassionate use protocol for gancyclovir. Unfortunately, this drug cannot reverse permanent vascular damage once it has occurred; in addition, it must be given intravenously, sometimes as chronic maintenance. Its principal side effect is leukopenia, which usually precludes the simultaneous administration of zidovudine. Thus the clinician and the patient must decide whether preservation of vision justifies the reduction or elimination of zidovudine from the regimen (see later).

Oral and Esophageal Manifestations

Candidal infections of the oral cavity and esophagus (frequently associated with odynopha-gia) are often, but not invariably, concurrent. Esophageal involvement can be confirmed by barium swallow, but only endoscopy (or a therapeutic drug trial) can discriminate between candidiasis and other ulcerative processes (see later). Oral thrush alone usually responds to clotrimazole (Mycelex) troches, which should be allowed to slowly dissolve in the mouth, with the resulting saliva swallowed one to four times daily; some patients need only an occasional troche to suppress this organism effectively. Less tasty alternatives include nystatin (Mycostatin) solution, as "swish and swallow," or nystatin vaginal tablets dissolved orally, both three to five times daily. Esophageal candidiasis and more severe degrees of oral candidiasis generally respond to addition of ketoconazole (Nizoral), 200 to 400 mg daily, orally; only rarely is low-dose amphotericin B (0.3 mg per kg daily for 5 to 10 days) required.

AIDS and ARC are associated with other troubling oral and esophageal manifestations. Aphthous-like ulceration is common and sometimes intractable. True mucosal herpes simplex ulcers occasionally develop at these sites and generally respond promptly to use of acyclovir (Zovirax), orally 200 mg five times a day, or intravenously (5 mg per kg every 8 hours). Nonherpetic aphthae may respond to use of topical or intralesional corticosteroids in small doses or to application of pediatric oral suspension of tetracycline (125 mg per 5 ml, given three to five times daily). Oral penicillin may have a positive effect if anaerobes in the mouth are involved. For symptomatic relief, a "magic mouthwash," consisting of Kaopectate, 150 ml; viscous lidocaine (Xylocaine) 2 per cent, 100 ml; and diphenhydramine HCl (Benadryl), 12.5 mg/ml, 30 ml, appears to be comforting when applied locally as needed.

Diarrhea

Diarrhea, which is often severely debilitating, may be idiopathic, but specific causes should be identified and treated if possible. Conventional enteric pathogens, including salmonella, shigella, Clostridium difficile, enteropathogenic Escherichia coli, and campylobacter, may be detected by stool culture or by analysis for enterotoxin. Trichomoniasis, amebiasis (rarely, if ever, an opportunistic agent), and giardiasis may be identified in fresh specimens submitted for analysis of ova and parasites, but cryptosporidiosis requires special identification by using modified acid-fast stains of concentrated fresh stool and will not be found on routine examination. Detection of acid-fast bacteria—in contrast to that of cryptosporidia—in stool does not conclusively define their pathogenic role. Flexible sigmoidoscopy with biopsy often leads to a diagnosis via dem-

onstration of invasive mucosal disease by mycobacteria, CMV, herpes simplex virus (typical inclusions), or cryptosporidia, or reveals other
intraluminal or mucosal processes.

Treatment of diarrhea in the patient with AIDS
or ARC should be directed at the causative organism if possible; if CMV, a trial of gancyclovir
is justified (see earlier section on retinitis). Sometimes the modest increment in cellular immunity
that results from the institution of zidovudine
may be beneficial when there is no specific treatment. Cryptosporidiosis, in particular, is usually
intractable and has no well-defined effective therapy. The experimental drug spiramycin, available from Rhone-Pouleuc Pharmaceuticals, may
be tried. Occasionally cryptosporidiosis resolves
spontaneously. Replacement of fluid and electrolyte losses, if necessary, can be based on the
analysis of stool electrolytes, as in therapy of
cholera. Narcotics (tincture of opium, 5 to 10
drops in water given after every loose stool up to
five times daily, or paregoric) or loperamide HCl
(Imodium), one or two capsules or 2 to 4 teaspoons
of liquid after each unformed movement, may be
helpful in some cases but should probably be
avoided in acute, febrile diarrheal states until
the diagnosis is established. In secretory diarrhea, trials of indomethacin and of more arcane
agents may be attempted with the assistance of
a gastroenterologist.

Mycobacterial Infections

Mycobacterial infections, as noted earlier, may
present both early in the course of HIV-induced
immunodeficiency, when the organism is usually
M. tuberculosis hominis, and late, when atypical
organisms, usually of the *Mycobacterium avium-
intracellulare* complex (MAC), are more common.
Treatment of the former includes use of conventional chemotherapy but must be prolonged indefinitely and should probably be initiated with
at least three drugs (e.g., isoniazid, 300 mg daily;
rifampin, 600 mg daily; and ethambutal, 25 mg
per kg daily for 2 months, then 15 mg per kg per
day, with the usual precautions and observation
for drug toxicity). The third drug may be discontinued once a clinical response has been seen for
a few months and drug susceptibility results are
known. Therapy of MAC disease has been controversial, in part because of uncertainty about what
constitutes disease and in part because of an (in
our experience) unwarranted therapeutic nihilism among many specialists in infectious disease.
Recovery of MAC from sputum or stool may have
no significance (where these organisms may be
commensal) but should be regarded with extreme
suspicion in the immunodeficient host and should
prompt a search for tissue disease via biopsy. A

positive blood or bone marrow culture or histologic evidence of invasive disease in the marrow,
gastrointestinal tract, or lung indicates that
treatment is required because MAC infection can
be severely debilitating.

Clinicians must realize the limitations of such
therapy; once established, MAC infection resembles lepromatous leprosy in the enormous tissue
load of organisms that can be present, particularly intracellularly in macrophages. Optimal
treatment cannot be accomplished without patience on the part of both physician and patient.
MAC sometimes responds surprisingly well to
conventional antituberculosis drug combinations.
In the clinically typical MAC disease (with fever,
sweating, and evidence of disseminated infection
with or without apparent pulmonary disease),
however, we generally start therapy with ansamycin (Rifabutin), 150 to 300 mg daily, and
clofazimine (Lamprene, recently approved by the
FDA for the treatment of leprosy), 300 mg per
day, reduced to 100 mg daily after a response has
been established or skin pigmentation is noticeable. By tradition, isoniazid is often added to this
regimen, but the organisms are usually resistant
in vitro and the combination may only produce
additional drug toxicity. Ansamycin and clofazimine both produce pigmentation of skin, urine,
and other tissue sites and body fluids. The toxicities of ansamycin are essentially those of rifampin. Splenic infarction, gastrointestinal obstruction, bleeding and severe abdominal pain,
in addition to the more usual types of gastrointestinal intolerance, have been reported with clofazimine, which is also associated with various
less common adverse reactions. Therapy for mycobacterial disease may be needed indefinitely.

Other Opportunistic Infections

Treatment of the other OI associated with advanced HIV infection is summarized in Table 6;
detailed discussions of specific management of
these infections are found elsewhere in this volume. Special problems associated with AIDS need
to be recognized. A chief problem is the persistence of both microorganisms and underlying immunodeficiency after apparent remission. Thus
for both cryptococcal disease and CNS toxoplasmosis, chronic suppressive treatment is needed
after clinical response is achieved. Another problem, like those with neoplasms, is the limitation
of the bone marrow reserve.

Reactivation toxoplasmosis generally presents
with CNS manifestations and is most often recognizable on computed tomographic scan of the
brain. The diagnosis is best confirmed by brain
biopsy, but circumstances frequently dictate a
therapeutic drug trial. Management is usually

initiated with pyrimethamine (Daraprim), 100 mg initially and then 25 mg daily, and sulfadiazine, a 4-gram oral loading dose, thereafter 1 gram orally, four times daily, given with ample fluids. Folinic acid (leukovorin factor [Wellcovorin]), 5 to 15 mg daily, may protect bone marrow function but is quite expensive. Patients intolerant of sulfonamides may be given clindamycin (Cleocin), at a dose of 900 mg every 8 hours instead. If a clinical response is not apparent within 2 weeks, a brain biopsy should be undertaken. Duration of therapy is not defined, but we generally employ a chronic suppressive drug regimen (e.g., oral sulfadiazine, 1 gram daily, and pyrimethamine, 25 mg daily) after complete resolution of abnormalities noted by computed tomography. Discontinuation of all medications generally leads to relapse.

Cryptococcosis probably requires protracted maintenance therapy after initial remission induction with high-dose amphotericin B (Fungizone). We have had satisfactory results with that agent alone, at intravenous doses of 0.5 mg per kg daily. Once an adequate clinical response has occurred, reduction of the dose to 0.3 mg per kg three times weekly may be sufficient to maintain remission. Current clinical trials of a new oral agent, fluconazole, may provide a reasonable and less toxic alternative, for both induction and maintenance, because the chronic intravenous therapy needed for amphotericin B often requires the introduction of permanent intravenous catheters (Hickman, Infusaport). The use of oral flucytosine (Ancobon), 150 mg per kg daily in divided doses, with a lower dose of amphotericin B (0.3 mg per kg) is an alternative induction regimen. The severe systemic reactions (rigors, fever, myalgias) often associated with amphotericin use may be mitigated by premedication with intravenous diphenhydramine (Benadryl), meperidine (Demerol), or small doses of corticosteroids. We have occasionally avoided these reactions, which seemed to be exacerbated by intermittent infusion that was used for maintenance, by continuous (24-hour) intravenous administration via a portable infusion pump, which can be used by patients at home.

THERAPY OF HIV INFECTION

Management of HIV infection has been substantially affected by the recent availability of drugs that inhibit the replication of the virus itself, which provide the clinician with the means to treat the underlying disease. As of this writing, the only such drug to be licensed is zidovudine (AZT, Retrovir); other drugs of the same class (dideoxynucleosides), such as dideoxycytidine and dideoxyadenine, are under study. These agents inhibit the reverse transcriptase of HIV, an enzyme unique to retroviruses and, therefore, the most obvious target for chemotherapy.

Indications for Initiating Zidovudine

Zidovudine is best started when the clinician believes, on the basis of available data, that the patient's immune status is in progressive decline and nearing dangerous levels of dysfunction (Table 7). These considerations are also discussed earlier. If information from current clinical trials indicates that earlier initiation of treatment leads to hematologic and immunologic stabilization, it may become appropriate to begin well above the now critical level of approximately 200 to 250 CD4 cells per mm^3. However, the somewhat unpredictable hematologic toxicity of zidovudine may preclude its early use. In addition, although large studies indicate that on average, CD4 cell counts tend to fall in a predictably progressive manner, the natural history of HIV infection is highly variable. The use of very-low-dose zidovudine early in HIV infection to prevent disease progression, as advocated by some physicians, may promote the emergence of viral strains resistant to this drug.

Recent studies (August 1989) appear to indicate that the early use of zidovudine in asymptomatic HIV-infected patients retards the development of ARC symptoms or AIDS in patients with CD4 counts less than 500 per mm^3. Doses of 500 mg daily were as effective as 1000 mg daily. It is not yet clear whether early use of the drug in patients who have CD4 counts between 250 and 500 per mm^3 will prolong life. The clinician should follow developments in this field closely.

Although their utility has still to be defined, certain markers of disease progression other than the CD4 cell count may aid the physician in making the decision to initiate zidovudine therapy. These markers include levels of antiviral antibody (anti-p24, anti-p17), viral antigenemia (p24 antigen capture assay), and immune cell activation or destruction (serum levels of beta$_2$-microglobulin, neopterin, and interferon-alpha). We have found anemia, leukopenia, and elevated erythrocyte sedimentation rates, as well as the presence of certain early clinical manifestions (oral hairy leukoplakia and thrush; hair loss), to be useful components of the equation leading to the decision to begin zidovudine. Certain HIV-infected individuals with comparatively competent immune function (CD4 counts higher than 300 per mm^3) who develop idiopathic thrombocytopenic purpura or moderate KS benefit from zidovudine therapy with resolution of either man-

TABLE 7. **Indications for Institution
of Zidovudine Therapy**

HIV-infected persons with
Progressive reductions in CD4 counts to 250–200/mm³ (confirmed on repeat assay, if on initial visit)

and

Development of *persistent* symptoms
  Oral thrush
  Oral hairy leukoplakia
  Aphthous stomatitis
  Other manifestations of early symptomatic phase of HIV
   infection (see Table 1)

**and/or these possibly useful markers of progression to
AIDS**

  Rising erythrocyte sedimentation rate, falling hemoglobin
   level or leukocyte count
  Loss of antibody to viral core proteins (p24, p17)
  Appearance of viral antigenemia (p24)
  Rising serum neopterin level
  Rising serum interferon-alpha activity
  Rising serum beta$_2$-microglobulin level

or

CD4 count reduction to or below 200 (± 30)/mm³ (confirmed
  on repeat assay, if on initial visit) *without* symptoms

or

Development of a case-defining systemic OI

or

Development of *late** neurologic manifestations of HIV infection (requires careful exclusion of specifically treatable OI
in CNS)

or, possibly, with the appearance of

KS except for minimal (fewer than five skin lesions) disease
Idiopathic thrombocytopenic purpura associated with HIV infection
**Uninfected persons with very recent, single exposures to
HIV**
Health care workers with significant inoculation of blood or
  other body fluids from a known or likely carrier of HIV
  may be candidates for 6-wk course, 200 mg q4 hr (see text)

*There is no information supporting the use of zidovudine in
therapy for aseptic meningitis or other neurologic events occurring early in HIV infection.

ifestation. People presenting with more advanced disease should be started on the drug without much delay.

Many potential drug recipients are frightened by the bad press accorded this drug, especially by grassroots organizations interested in alternative, "nontoxic" approaches to HIV infection. The clinician must be prepared to overcome such objections. The patient must be educated to expect some difficulties, such as headache and nausea in the initial days or weeks of therapy, with the knowledge that these will pass with persistence or adjustment of dose. The patient must also be told that anemia or leukopenia, or both, may eventually develop. However, he or she can also be reassured that very few people are unable to tolerate at least moderate doses of the drug. In addition, persistent dosing may be essential: We have encountered patients whose physicians permitted, or who themselves insisted on, prolonged "AZT holidays"; such individuals had progressive HIV-mediated neurologic disease, whereas most patients with consistent, even low-level, dosing appeared to be better able to avoid these complications. It is our strong impression that consistent zidovudine use retards the development of many of the CNS complications of HIV infection.

Zidovudine is safely begun at the recommended dose (200 mg orally every 4 hours around the clock) in most adults of average height and weight, but many patients in whom the drug is indicated are particularly small or have pre-existing hepatic disease, anemia, leukopenia, or polypharmacy that suggests or demands a lower starting dose, which can be raised as tolerance is assessed. Under such circumstances, we usually begin at 100 mg five times daily. The optimal dose and dosing schedule of zidovudine have not been determined. We currently use this agent at the maximal dose tolerated (up to 1200 mg daily), on the basis of the cancer chemotherapy model. However, consistent use of lower doses, particularly if there is evidence of poor marrow reserve, may prolong the period of utility of the drug for that individual.

The drug is titrated continuously to the leukocyte count, which is limiting; if the neutrophil count declines progressively, we first eliminate the nighttime dose, to avoid disturbing sleep, and then use 100 mg five times daily, after which capsules are spaced further apart. Patients with advanced AIDS appear to tolerate leukocyte counts higher than 1200 cells per mm³ and neutrophil counts higher than 500 cells per mm³ without developing severe bacterial infections, but the margin for error is comparatively small; when the leukocyte count is less than 2000 per mm³, close monitoring (weekly or on alternate weeks) is appropriate. Because the hematologic suppression associated with zidovudine use usually begins only after a few weeks or months, we do complete blood counts weekly, starting with the second or third week of therapy, and we gradually increase the interval as tolerance is assessed; once the hematologic measures are stable, monthly observation is appropriate. Patients should be alerted to report symptoms that suggest leukopenia (mouth sores, fever, chills) or anemia (dyspnea, pallor). Because these problems would indicate closer observation of patients with advanced immunodeficiency even without zidovudine therapy, the well-educated patient should already be primed to report to the physician. Anemia, commonly normocytic, also prompts reductions of dose, which depend on the patient's tolerance for support with packed erythrocyte transfusions. Most individuals who tolerate the drug well develop a macrocytosis but often have minimal or no anemia. In the absence of either anemia or macrocytosis, questions of compliance should arise. The object is to keep the patient continuously taking some dose of the drug, even if quite small. Sometimes, a period of discontinuing the drug may be beneficial, but it should be brief.

The use of multiple drugs is generally unavoidable during zidovudine therapy; the cardinal management principle is concomitant use of effective prophylactic regimens against PCP (discussed earlier). Drug interactions are being explored; official labeling indicates that acetaminophen (Tylenol) should be avoided because of its potential to compete for the glucuronidation pathways by which zidovudine is metabolized and excreted. Other drugs eliminated via the same pathways should also be avoided (e.g., nonsteroidal antiinflammatory agents). Serum levels of zidovudine and glucuronidated zidovudine (gAZT) can be measured with some difficulty, but titration to tolerance presumably avoids difficulty.

Unfortunately, zidovudine when used alone appears to have a limited, if currently undefined, period of utility. Ultimately, drug toxicity, viral evolution, or incomplete inhibition of HIV activity leads to "the dwindles" in a significant proportion of patients, or an untreatable complication supervenes. It is hoped that combinations of agents may enhance or prolong the utility of zidovudine.

Experimental Approaches to HIV Infection

Clinicians caring for HIV-infected patients should be aware that the field is changing rapidly. A number of new agents are under investigation as antiretroviral drugs that may become available to the practitioner as early as 1990. In addition to the other dideoxynucleosides, which have toxicity profiles somewhat different from that of zidovudine, a number of other experimental agents may be found to be useful as part of multidrug regimens. These include castanospermine, which affects glycosylation of retroviruses; interferons, which interfere with assembly of viruses; dextran sulfate, which inhibits viral attachment to cells; and the antimycobacterial ansamycin (Rifabutin), which, like zidovudine, inhibits the viral reverse transcriptase. Because

the CD4 molecule that marks helper T cells appears to be a preferential binding site for HIV, there is interest in using recombinant soluble or erythrocyte-bound CD4 molecules to inhibit viral binding to target lymphocytes. Recombinant colony-stimulating factors (granulocyte colony-stimulating factor; granulocyte-monocyte colony-stimulating factor) may improve dose-limiting leukocyte counts, and recombinant erythropoietin may be useful for some drug-induced or HIV-induced anemic patients.

Certain combinations are already being evaluated in clinical trials: acyclovir provides some in vitro synergy to zidovudine. The combination of acyclovir at 200 to 800 mg orally every 4 hours with zidovudine at a standard or reduced dose is used by some practitioners, but it is not clear that the added expense is justified by any detectable clinical benefit. Interferon-alpha also has in vitro synergy, whereas ribavirin appears to antagonize the activity of zidovudine.

Health Care Workers, HIV Exposure, and Zidovudine

Infection challenge experiments with cats and mice indicate that zidovudine can prevent the establishment of retroviruses other than HIV. The drug must be given promptly (within approximately 1 hour) after viral challenge to be most effective, but a residual preventive effect is evident when the drug is given up to 1 week after inoculation of virus. These experiments suggest that humans inadvertently inoculated or otherwise exposed to HIV could avoid infection by taking the drug. Although no data are available to substantiate this idea, and the long-term side effects of a course of the drug in healthy people are unknown, a national study is under way for needle stick recipients. A telephone hot line has been established, 1–800–HIV-STIK, to provide information and entry. For minor needle stick exposures, the risk of infection is comparatively small, around 1 per 200 events, but for more extensive blood or tissue inocula, there is a more serious risk of infection. Such incidents must be evaluated individually. Some institutions in high-prevalence areas have established a policy of offering the drug to personnel who have been exposed to blood or other infectious body fluids. Specific body fluids include blood, serous effusions, semen, vaginal secretions, and other tissue fluids that contain leukocytes and exclude nonbloody urine, stool, saliva, and tears. The exposures that are considered to be significant are inoculation through intact skin by a sharp object (needle or scalpel), splash onto mucosal surfaces, or prolonged exposure to nonintact skin. Guidance is available in case of such an exposure through the Centers for Disease Control (Atlanta, Ga.), but the clinician's response to such injury should be as rapid as possible because of the possibility of instituting zidovudine therapy.

Additional Issues for HIV Infection

Use of Steroids

We try to avoid use of systemic corticosteroid therapy in patients with HIV infection, particularly patients with CD4 cell counts in decline. Injudicious use of these agents has apparently precipitated the onset of OI earlier than would have been expected. However, under certain circumstances, patient tolerance has been remarkable, particularly in patients with idiopathic thrombocytopenic purpura associated with middle-level HIV infection. Limited use of topical steroids for skin eruptions or intralesional injection into large oral aphthae may be justified at times. Administration of systemic steroids in large doses (60 to 100 mg prednisone equivalent daily) for brief periods also may have a role in the management of severe interstitial pulmonary disease, particularly if appropriate antimicrobial agents are administered simultaneously. Reduction of cerebral edema during therapy for CNS lymphoma or toxoplasmosis may also dictate the use of dexamethasone (Decadron). If their disease manifestation permits, immunodeficient individuals requiring systemic steroids may be less likely to develop severe infectious complications if prednisone is used at the lowest dose possible, given as a single morning dose on alternate days.

Use of Blood Components in AIDS

The transfusion of viable lymphoid cells from unrelated donors into severely immunodeficient people has been reported to result in graft-versus-host disease. Most blood components, particularly packed red blood cells and platelets, contain such lymphoid elements. However, graft-versus-host disease has not been noted in AIDS patients, possibly because HIV interferes with its development. If this is so, the use of effective antiviral agents may increase the likelihood of graft-versus-host reactions. We generally avoid this issue via routine irradiation (1200 to 2000 rad) of all blood products given to AIDS patients. However, no evidence mandates this procedure, which is simple only if the requisite equipment is available.

Idiopathic Thrombocytopenic Purpura

This occasional complication, which occurs often during relatively early-stage HIV infection, can be more frightening to the clinician than dangerous to the patient, and the clinician should beware of overaggressive therapy that may place the patient at later risk. Platelet counts done by automated techniques may be misleading and should always be confirmed by blood smears with Wright's or Giemsa's stain. Platelet counts higher than 20,000 per mm^3 in patients educated to avoid trauma-inducing circumstances seem to be well tolerated and are not generally associated with clinically significant bleeding. Specific therapy other than close observation is probably not necessary for counts higher than 50,000 per mm^3. If therapy is thought to be necessary, we use a trial of corticosteroids (usually prednisone, 60 to 80 mg orally each morning) in patients with CD4 counts in excess of 300 per mm^3. This schedule is tapered by halving the alternate day's dose every week or two and then discontinuing it entirely. The remaining alternate day's dose is then similarly tapered as tolerated, to maintain platelet counts higher than 20,000 to 30,000 per mm^3. A good alternative, or a potentially steroid-sparing approach, appears to be the institution of full-dose zidovudine. This often leads to significant improvement but seems to work less rapidly than high-dose steroids. Zidovudine alone is the approach of choice in patients with CD4 counts less than 300 per mm^3. We have not found it necessary to use splenectomy, cytostatic agents, or vincristine, which are alternative approaches to idiopathic thrombocytopenic purpura in more conventional situations. Splenectomy, in particular, may be ill advised in the long run because many of these patients become progressively deficient in antibody production and are thus at increased risk from complications of bacteremia with encapsulated pathogens. High-dose intravenous immunoglobulins (Sandoglobulin, Gammagard, Gamimune-N) at 400 mg per kg daily for 4 days, or 1000 mg per kg in a single infusion, may be used to raise the platelet count in an emergency situation (significant bleeding or preoperatively); this approach is expensive and, like others, does not always work. Some patients may continue to respond to periodic booster doses of gamma globulin, but even full-dose zidovudine therapy pales before chronic use of these immunoglobulins in terms of cost.

Coagulopathies

Derangements in blood coagulation are common among patients with HIV infection. In particular, the clinician should be familiar with the association of AIDS with circulating anticoagulants that prolong activated partial thromboplastin time, particularly in patients with PCP. The prothrombin time is not usually prolonged, and the problem comes to the attention of the physician during routine preoperative coagulation screening. Use of an inhibitor screen, or "mixing studies," will clarify this annoying but seldom clinically significant laboratory phenomenon, which is usually the result of antibodies directed against the phospholipids that are used to activate clotting in the performance of the test. In general, a trained hematologist should be consulted if major surgery is contemplated in this situation.

Pregnancy and AIDS

With the rising prevalence of HIV infection among heterosexual people (intravenous drug abusers, bisexual men, hemophiliacs, and their sexual partners), pregnancy has become more of a problem for the clinician. Approximately 35 per cent (in some studies, the percentage is higher) of pregnancies from HIV-infected women result in an infected infant. Pregnancy by itself does not appear to worsen the prognosis in an HIV-infected woman. Pregnancy in the sexual partner of a known HIV-positive male should raise the issue of therapeutic abortion, if the woman is infected. Because serologic testing may yield false-negative results, particularly in a woman who has recently become infected, the reliability of the tests may be improved by using additional and possibly more sensitive, but still experimental, tests for viral infection. Available through consultation with research centers, they include determination of circulating viral p24 antigen, direct culture for retroviruses, and use of the polymerase chain reaction to amplify and thus detect specific retroviral nucleic acid sequences in blood cells.

The safety of zidovudine in pregnancy has not yet been determined.

AMEBIASIS

method of
RICHARD A. DAVIDSON, M.D., M.P.H.
University of Florida
Gainesville, Florida

Worldwide, it is estimated that 480 million persons are infected with *Entamoeba histolytica* each year. Although only a small percentage of these persons (probably less than 10 per cent) have mild clinical illness and a much smaller percentage have dysentery or extraintestinal infection, approximately 40,000 deaths annually can be attributed to the infection. In the developed world, however, serious infection seems to be decreasing. Most new cases of amebic infection are found in immigrants or travelers from endemic areas. A new problem is the dramatic increase in infected homosexual men. The infection is transmitted

through contaminated food or water or through person-to-person contact. Although treatment decisions are clear-cut in patients with invasive or symptomatic amebiasis, opinions differ as to the benefits of treating asymptomatic carriers.

Infection is divided into two categories: intestinal and extraintestinal. The diagnosis of intestinal disease requires demonstration of either cysts or trophozoites in the stool, but accurate recognition is difficult, even in experienced laboratories. Extraintestinal disease is most frequently diagnosed by serologic tests, such as the amebic indirect hemagglutination titer, which is positive in more than 90 per cent of extraintestinal infections.

INTESTINAL INFECTION

Amebic Dysentery

Amebic trophozoites burrow into the intestinal mucosa where they secrete lytic enzymes that form the characteristic flask-shaped ulcers. These ulcers may become contiguous, especially when organisms reach the submucosa, resulting in undermining and necrosis of the mucosa. Sloughing of various amounts of mucosa results in bloody diarrhea. Tenesmus, prostration, and dehydration are common. If appropriate therapy is not undertaken promptly, progression to fulminant disease with fever, megacolon, and possible colonic rupture may occur. The characteristic trophozoites should be rapidly sought in fresh diarrheal stools.

Treatment

The mainstay of treatment in invasive colonic amebiasis is metronidazole (Flagyl), given either orally or intravenously, in a dosage of 750 mg three times daily for 10 days. (Pediatric dosages for all drugs are given in Table 1.) Metronidazole is a tissue amebicide, with good absorption; it also has some intraluminal activity. Major side effects are few, but include nausea and metallic taste. Patients taking metronidazole may have a disulfiram (Antabuse)-like reaction if they ingest alcohol, causing abdominal pain, nausea, and vomiting. Concern about carcinogenicity and mutagenicity of the drug exists, and it should not be given chronically or to pregnant women.

Alternatives to metronidazole include emetine and dehydroemetine; both are potent drugs that can cause cardiac toxicity, including arrhythmias and possibly ischemia. Patients given either drug should be monitored electrocardiographically and kept at bed rest throughout therapy. Both drugs are contraindicated in pregnancy. Emetine is given intramuscularly or subcutaneously in a dosage of 1 mg per kg per day (maximum 60 mg per day) for up to 5 days. Dehydroemetine, which may be less toxic, is also given subcutaneously

TABLE 1. **Pediatric Dosages of Amebicidal Drugs**

Drug	Dose
Tissue Amebicides	
Metronidazole (Flagyl)	30–50 mg/kg/day for 10 days*
Emetine	1 mg/kg/day (maximum 60 mg/day) IM for 5 days† ‡
Dehydroemetine‡	1–1.5 mg/kg/day (maximum 90 mg/day) IM for 5 days†
Luminal Amebicides	
Iodoquinol (Yodoxin)	30–40 mg/kg/day for 20 days*
Diloxanide furoate (Furamide)§	20 mg/kg/day for 10 days*
Paromomycin (Humatin)	25–30 mg/kg/day for 7 days*
Hepatic Amebicide	
Chloroquine (Aralen)	15 mg/kg/day (maximum 480 mg/day) for 14 days

*Give in three divided daily doses.
†Give in two divided daily doses.
‡In children younger than 8 yr, do not exceed 10 mg/day; in children older than 8 yr, do not exceed 20 mg/day.
§Available only from the Centers for Disease Control: telephone 404–639–3670; nights and weekends, 404–639–2888.

or intramuscularly for 5 days. Doses of 1 to 1.5 mg per kg per day are used, with a maximum dose of 90 mg per day. Dehydroemetine is available only through the Centers for Disease Control (telephone 404–639–3670).

The tissue amebicides are effective against invasive trophozoites but may not eradicate all luminal organisms. Therefore, a luminal amebicide that is poorly absorbed is usually given after the dysentery resolves. The most effective drug is diiodohydroxyquin (Yodoxin), also known as iodoquinol. It is given for 20 days in a dosage of 650 mg three times daily. This dosage should not be exceeded because the drug may cause optic neuritis. A less toxic alternative, diloxanide furoate (Furamide), 500 mg given three times daily for 10 days, would be preferable; however, the drug is available only from the Centers for Disease Control.

Additional supportive care, including antibiotics, fluid and electrolyte management, hyperalimentation, and surgery, may be necessary in severe amebic colitis.

Mild Intestinal Infection

Patients may present with mild diarrheal symptoms or with symptoms and x-ray findings mimicking colonic carcinoma caused by amebic granulomas (amebomas). Metronidazole is the drug of choice, in the same dosage as that used for serious infections. Use of a luminal amebicide such as iodoquinol should be considered. An alternative approach, which has been studied recently, is the use of the nonabsorbable aminogly-coside paromomycin (Humatin) in a dosage of 25 to 30 mg per kg per day in three divided doses for a total of 7 days. The most frequent side effects include minor gastrointestinal complaints and change in stool frequency or consistency. This drug should not be used alone in cases of ameboma, which require multiple drug therapy.

Asymptomatic Carriers

Not all strains of *E. histolytica* are pathogenic, and there are no morphologic differences between pathogenic and nonpathogenic strains. Analysis of isoenzyme patterns, known as zymodemes, has suggested that there are differences between pathogenic and nonpathogenic strains when categorized by zymodeme. The permanence of these classifications, however, is unknown. There are suggestions that isolates may change their zymodemes (and their pathogenicity) on exposure to certain bacteria or viruses or on transmission to a different host. This question is becoming increasingly important because of the dramatic increase in infected homosexuals.

Screening of male homosexuals has revealed that 15 to 40 per cent have asymptomatic infections with *E. histolytica;* a variety of the protozoans and helminths have also been found in increased frequency. The overwhelming majority of these individuals have few, if any, symptoms, and isolates from their stools have been found to be among the nonpathogenic zymodemes. Some authorities have recommended not treating these individuals because they frequently become reinfected, and most of the therapeutic alternatives should not be used chronically. Nonetheless, the possibility of zymodeme alteration represents a potential public health risk if such patients are not treated. An unproven theoretical reason for treating such patients is that chronic infection may decrease the latency period of the human immunodeficiency virus by mitogenic stimulation of infected T lymphocytes. Last, as many as 50 per cent of persons in whom extraintestinal infection develops have no history of intestinal symptoms, which suggests that these individuals were asymptomatic carriers. Long-term prospective studies are needed to demonstrate the true benign nature of chronic asymptomatic infection. A reasonable course of action is to treat asymptomatic carriers with nonabsorbed drugs such as paromomycin or drugs with low toxicity such as diloxanide furoate. Limiting sexual contacts and treating regular sexual partners may be useful.

EXTRAINTESTINAL DISEASE

The overwhelming majority of extraintestinal infections involve the liver; erosion into portal venules in the gut wall results in the migration of the trophozoites to the liver. Three-fourths of hepatic abscesses are solitary, right lobe lesions that are easily localized by computed tomography. One-half of all abscesses involve the diaphragm and may rupture into the lung by direct extension. Other sites of infection include the skin, genitalia, brain, adrenals, kidney, bladder, and pericardium. Serologic tests, such as the indirect hemagglutination titer and the gel diffusion precipitin, are usually positive in extraintestinal disease. In general, aspiration of hepatic abscesses is not necessary for the diagnosis. Symptoms of infection depend on the site involved. In hepatic abscess, right upper quadrant pain, fever, and leukocytosis may make differentiation from bacterial abscess difficult; in this setting, serologic tests are most useful.

Treatment

Patients with extraintestinal infection should be treated with metronidazole, either orally or intravenously, in a dosage of 750 mg three times daily for 10 days. Alternative tissue amebicides include emetine and dehydroemetine. An additional drug that is effective against hepatic amebiasis is chloroquine, given as a 1-gram loading dose per day for 2 days followed by 500 mg per day for 14 days. Chloroquine is used only in combination with other tissue amebicides and is effective only in hepatic disease. Eradication of intestinal infection is usually recommended with a course of a luminal drug after specific tissue treatment.

Surgical intervention in hepatic amebiasis should generally be avoided. In cases of rupture or threatened rupture, lack of therapeutic response in a reasonable period, or a large, slowly responding abscess, surgery may be performed. Drug therapy should be given for at least 48 to 72 hours before surgery if at all possible.

BACTEREMIA

method of
ROBERT L. ATMAR, M.D., and
RICHARD L. HARRIS, M.D.
Baylor College of Medicine
Houston, Texas

Bacteremia is a surprisingly common event and occurs in association with such activities as toothbrushing and during certain diagnostic and therapeutic procedures. It becomes important in patients when it causes clinically significant disease such as sepsis or prosthetic infection because of the considerable morbidity and mortality associated with these infections.

The best approach to the management of bacteremia is prevention, but when this is not possible, prompt recognition of clinically significant bacteremia to allow appropriate diagnostic and therapeutic maneuvers is of the utmost importance.

Bacteremia is defined as bacteria in the blood stream. Sepsis is defined as the physiologic changes and the clinical consequences of microorganisms in the blood or tissues. There are numerous different manifestations of sepsis (Table 1). It is not difficult to suspect sepsis in a febrile, hypotensive patient with rigors; however, signs of sepsis may be more subtle. Alteration of mental status may be the initial sign of sepsis in the elderly patient. Fever is usually present, but it may be absent in the elderly patient or in the patient with chronic liver or renal disease. Respiratory alkalosis, metabolic acidosis (lactic acidosis), or worsening renal function may be the first clue to sepsis in the intensive care unit. Septic shock is an advanced manifestation of sepsis in which there is circulatory failure resulting in inadequate tissue oxygenation and cell death. Because recognition of sepsis may be difficult, it is necessary for the clinician to maintain a high index of suspicion for its presence.

Once sepsis is suspected, a careful search for an underlying focus should be instituted. Identification of a focus of infection is helpful for selection of a therapeutic regimen before culture results become available. The most useful tool in identifying a source of infection is a careful history and physical examination. For example, a history of cough, sputum production, and pleuritic chest pain suggests a pulmonary focus, whereas recent passage of a kidney stone may suggest a urinary tract focus. The history and physical examination findings may also lead the physician to do certain supplemental investigations (such as x-rays or sonograms), which will identify a focus of infection. It is important to obtain blood and other indicated cul-

TABLE 1. **Manifestations of Sepsis***

Common Manifestations	Less Common Manifestations or Those Seen Only in Severe Sepsis
Fever, rigors, myalgias	Hypothermia
Tachycardia	(Shock (see Table 3)
Tachypnea (respiratory alkalosis)	Lactic acidosis
Hypoxemia	Adult respiratory distress syndrome
Proteinuria	Azotemia, oliguria
Leukocytosis (left shift, toxic granules, Döhle's bodies)	Leukopenia, leukemoid reaction
Eosinopenia	Thrombocytopenia
Hypoferremia	Disseminated intravascular coagulation
Irritability, lethargy	Anemia
Mild liver function abnormalities	Stupor, coma
Hyperglycemia in diabetics	Overt upper gastrointestinal tract bleeding
	Cutaneous lesions
	Hypoglycemia

*From Harris RL, Musher DM, Bloom K, et al: Manifestations of sepsis. Arch Intern Med 1987, *147*:1895–1906. Copyright 1987, American Medical Association.

tures in all patients suspected of having sepsis so that antibiotic therapy may be adjusted for organism-specific treatment. Identification of a pathogen by blood culture may also suggest a focus in a patient who does not otherwise have a readily identifiable site of infection, for example, *Bacteroides fragilis* bacteremia suggesting an intra-abdominal focus.

ADJUNCTIVE THERAPY

Because antibiotic therapy alone is frequently not sufficient for the treatment of sepsis, several other measures should be carried out while antibiotic therapy is being instituted. One of the most important additional steps in the treatment of bacteremia is the removal or drainage of septic foci. Potentially infected intravascular lines should be removed. Intra-abdominal abscesses, empyema, and most other abscesses require surgical drainage; infected or gangrenous tissue may need debridement; obstructions of the urinary and biliary tracts must be relieved; and infected prosthetic devices generally need to be removed.

Several of the manifestations of sepsis require additional therapy (Table 2). Hypoxemia is treated with supplemental oxygenation, whereas respiratory failure and adult respiratory distress

TABLE 2. **Manifestations of Sepsis That May Benefit from or Require Specific Therapy*,†**

Manifestations	Therapy
Fever, rigors, myalgias	Antipyretics, cooling blanket
Hypotension	Volume replacement, dopamine (naloxone)
Hypoxemia	Supplemental oxygen administration
Respiratory failure, ARDS	Mechanical ventilation (PEEP)
Lactic acidosis	Bicarbonate administration
Azotemia, oliguria	Fluid and electrolyte management, reduction of renally cleared drugs
Thrombocytopenia	Platelet and/or RBC transfusions if active bleeding
DIC	Fresh frozen plasma, platelet, and/or RBC transfusions if active bleeding (heparin)
Altered mentation	Monitoring or restraint of patient to prevent self-harm
GI tract bleeding	Nasogastric lavage or suction, RBC transfusions as needed (antacids, H₂ receptor antagonists
Hyperglycemia	Insulin administration
Hypoglycemia	Constant 10% dextrose infusion

*From Harris RL, Musher DM, Bloom K, et al: Manifestations of sepsis. Arch Intern Med 1987, *147*:1895–1906. Copyright 1987, American Medical Association.

†Therapeutic maneuvers that may be effective are given in parentheses.

Abbreviations: ARDS = adult respiratory distress syndrome; PEEP = positive end-expiratory pressure; RBC = red blood cell; DIC = disseminated intravascular coagulation; GI = gastrointestinal; and H_2 = histamine₂.

TABLE 3. **Hemodynamics of Sepsis***

	Preshock	Early Shock	Late Shock
Blood pressure	→↓	↓	↓↓†
Systemic vascular resistance	↓	↓↓	→↑
Cardiac output	↑↑	↑	↓
Volume responsive	++	+	—
Acid-base status	RA	RA, MA	MA

*From Harris RL, Musher DM, Bloom K, et al: Manifestations of sepsis. Arch Intern Med 1987, *147*:1895–1906. Copyright 1987, American Medical Association.

†Often pressor dependent.

Abbreviations: RA = respiratory alkalosis; MA = metabolic acidosis.

syndrome require mechanical ventilation with or without positive end-expiratory pressure. Hemorrhagic disorders are treated with factor replacement and blood components (fresh frozen plasma, packed red blood cells, and platelets) to control bleeding. Hyperglycemia is treated with insulin administration; hypoglycemia is treated by infusion of a 10 per cent dextrose solution.

Septic Shock. Septic shock requires immediate recognition and therapeutic intervention. It is characterized by a range of hemodynamic findings, from a preshock state to a late shock state (Table 3). The preshock state is characterized by a decrease in the systemic vascular resistance and an increase in the cardiac output. The blood pressure is normal or slightly depressed. The acid-base status is usually a respiratory alkalosis caused by primary hyperventilation. As the preshock state advances to early shock and then late shock, the cardiac output declines and hypotension and metabolic acidosis develop. Persistence of hypotension and metabolic acidosis may result in multisystem organ failure and death.

Septic shock is characterized by hypotension. Septic patients are usually relatively volume depleted secondary to increased venous capacitance, increased vascular permeability, increased insensible fluid loss, or decreased fluid intake. A fluid challenge with either crystalloid or colloid is generally appropriate, and a pulmonary artery catheter may be useful in monitoring fluid therapy. The goal of fluid replacement is to restore adequate circulatory perfusion, which can be determined by organ function (mentation or urinary output) and which generally occurs at a systolic blood pressure of 90 to 100 mmHg. If a pulmonary artery catheter is used, a pulmonary capillary wedge pressure of 12 to 14 mmHg is recommended for guidance of fluid replacement therapy.

If volume replacement does not restore the perfusion pressure, vasopressor therapy should be initiated. Dopamine HCl as a constant infusion

TABLE 4. **Initial Antibiotic Selection Based on Likely Focus of Infection**

Site or Type of Infection	Organisms	Antibiotics
Urinary tract	GNR	Aminoglycosides, ceftazidime
	GDS	Ampicillin, vancomycin
Pneumonia*		
Community-acquired	Pneumococcus, aspiration	Pencillin G
	Haemophilus influenzae	Ampicillin
	Legionella, atypical pneumonias	Erythromycin
Nosocomial	GNR†	Piperacillin, ceftazidime
	Staphylococcus aureus	Nafcillin, vancomycin
	Legionella	Erythromycin
Endocarditis, native valve		
Non-IVDA	Alpha streptococci, *S. aureus*	Penicillin, nafcillin
IVDA	*S. aureus*	Nafcillin, vancomycin
	GNR†	Ticarcillin or ceftazidime and aminoglycosides
Meningitis		
Adult	Pneumococci, meningococci	Penicillin, chloramphenicol
Postneurosurgery, immunosuppressed	*S. aureus, Staphylococcus epidermidis*	Nafcillin, vancomycin
	GNR†	Ceftazidime
Gastrointestinal and genital tracts	GNR	Ceftazidime, aminoglycoside
	GDS	Ampicillin, vancomycin
	Anaerobes	Clindamycin, piperacillin, metronidazole, chloramphenicol
Wound infection	*S. aureus*	Nafcillin, vancomycin
	GNR	Ceftazidime, aminoglycoside
Line sepsis	*S. aureus, S. epidermidis*	Vancomycin
	GNR	Ceftazidime, aminoglycoside
Other Risk Factors		
Neutropenia	GNR	Ceftazidime or ticarcillin and aminoglycoside
	S. aureus, S. epidermidis	Vancomycin
Postsplenectomy	Pneumococcus, *H. influenzae,* meningococcus	Penicillin, ampicillin
Raw shellfish consumption	*Vibrio*	Tetracycline and aminoglycoside
	Listeria	Penicillin, ampicillin
	Salmonella	Chloramphenicol, ampicillin
Empiric	*S. aureus,* streptococci	Vancomycin
	GNR	Ceftazidime, aminoglycoside

*Gram's stain of sputum may help initial therapy.
†Combination therapy with a penicillin or cephalosporin and an aminoglycoside should be given.
Abbreviations: GNR = gram-negative rod; GDS = group D streptococci; IVDA = intravenous drug abuse.

is the most commonly used pressor agent and should be titrated to maintain adequate perfusion. A low dose (1 to 2 micrograms per kg per minute) results in increased renal blood flow. At 5 to 10 micrograms per kg per minute, there is increased beta-adrenergic stimulation, which results in increased cardiac output while urinary sodium levels and volume excretion are maintained. At doses higher than 15 to 20 micrograms per kg per minute, alpha-adrenergic stimulation predominates and results in peripheral vasoconstriction and maintenance of blood pressure, usually at the expense of renal perfusion.

Steroids have been used for treatment of septic shock in the past, but there are now several well-designed, placebo-controlled trials showing that there is no long-term benefit from their use and that they may cause potential harm. In the absence of specific indications (e.g., Addison's disease), steroids should not be given.

Other therapies that must be considered investigational at this time include the use of the opioid antagonist naloxone in the treatment of septic shock and the use of monoclonal antibodies against gram-negative endotoxemia.

SELECTION OF ANTIBIOTIC THERAPY

Selection of an appropriate antibiotic regimen requires knowledge of the organisms most likely to be responsible for the infection. Information that may be available to the clinician includes the following: (1) previous culture data, for example, a urine culture obtained several days earlier; (2) Gram's stain of specimens of body fluids; (3) expected flora (Table 4) of a site, such as enterococcus and gram-negative bacilli in the urinary tract; and (4) hospital-specific resistance patterns in nosocomially acquired infections. At times, a clinical situation allows specific therapy

TABLE 5. **Dosage of Selected Antibiotics in Adult Patients with Normal Renal Function**

Antibiotic	Dose	Usual Dosing Interval (hr)
Beta-lactamase susceptible, non-antipseudomonal penicillins		
Penicillin G	1–2 million U	4
Ampicillin	1–2 grams	4–6
Beta-lactamase susceptible, antipseudomonal penicillins		
Ticarcillin	3 grams	4
Piperacillin	3–4 grams	4–6
Beta-lactamase resistant penicillins		
Nafcillin	1–2 grams	4–6
Methicillin	1–2 grams	4–6
Penicillins with beta-lactamase inhibitor		
Ampicillin with sulbactam	1.5–3 grams	6
Ticarcillin with clavulanate	3.1 grams	4
First-generation cephalosporin		
Cefazolin	1–1.5 grams	8
Second-generation cephalosporin		
Cefotetan	1–2 grams	12
Third-generation cephalosporins		
Ceftazidime	1–2 grams	8–12
Cefotaxime	1–2 grams	4–8
Carbapenem		
Imipenem with cilastatin	0.5–1 gram	6–8
Monobactam		
Aztreonam	1–2 grams	6–8
Aminoglycosides		
Gentamicin	1 mg/kg	8
Tobramycin	1 mg/kg	8
Amikacin	7.5 mg/kg	12
Others		
Vancomycin	15 mg/kg	12
Clindamycin	300–600 mg	8
Erythromycin	500–1000 mg	6
Doxycycline	50–100 mg	12
Metronidazole	7.5 mg/kg	6
Chloramphenicol	25 mg/kg	6
Ciprofloxacin*	250–750 mg	12

*Not yet available in the intravenous form.

from the outset, for example, penicillin in pneumococcal pneumonia or meningococcal meningitis, but more than one antibiotic is usually necessary to provide comprehensive antibacterial therapy until culture data become available.

When the physician selects the antibiotic regimen, the following should be considered.

(1) Initial treatment with two antibiotics is generally superior to treatment with one antibiotic because (a) the spectrum of antibacterial coverage is broadened with two antibiotics, (b) there may be synergy between the antibiotics for certain infections (e.g., enterococcal infections treated with ampicillin and an aminoglycoside), (c) development of resistance to the antibiotics may be prevented, and (d) the pharmacokinetics of the antibiotics may allow more continuous antibacterial coverage (i.e., when serum concentration of one antibiotic falls below the minimum inhibitory concentration of the bacteria being treated, the serum concentration of the other antibiotic may still be in the therapeutic range).

(2) Bactericidal agents (penicillins, cephalosporins, aminoglycosides) are preferred in the initial treatment of endocarditis, meningitis, and neutropenia. However, except for cefuroxime, first- and second-generation cephalosporins do not cross the blood-brain barrier and should not be used in the treatment of meningitis.

(3) Intravenous therapy should be instituted initially. This ensures that the antibiotics achieve adequate serum levels when dosed appropriately. Orally administered medications may not be absorbed because of an ileus, and medications given intramuscularly may have undependable absorption because of hypoperfusion during shock.

(4) Once culture data are available, the antibiotic regimen should be changed to the least toxic regimen that allows appropriate treatment.

(5) The appropriate length of therapy for most patients with bacteremia is not well defined but has generally been 10 to 14 days. Factors that may cause a change in the duration of treatment include the following: (a) organism, (b) host, (c) site of infection, and (d) clinical response of the patient. In some patients a switch from parenteral to oral therapy may be made to complete a course of treatment if a good clinical response has been achieved and an appropriate site is infected (e.g., in pyelonephritis).

Dosages of selected antibiotics are shown in Table 5.

Empiric Therapy. If a careful search for a site of infection fails to reveal a likely source, the physician must make an empiric decision about the initial antibiotic regimen. Gram-negative bacilli and *Staphylococcus aureus* are the most common pathogens in this situation, and therapy should be directed to them. Ceftazidime or an aminoglycoside provides good coverage of gram-negative bacilli, and vancomycin is a good antistaphylococcal drug.

Monitoring Therapy. Once therapy is initiated, it is important to monitor the patient for adequacy of therapy and for signs and symptoms of antibiotic toxicity. If there is no clinical response after 1 to 3 days of antibiotic therapy, blood cultures should be repeated to evaluate the adequacy of therapy in eradicating the bacteremia; persistently positive blood cultures may be secondary to inadequate antibiotic therapy or to an undrained focus of infection.

All antibiotics have side effects for which patients should be monitored. Peak and trough levels of aminoglycosides and vancomycin should be checked and adjusted to the therapeutic range. Impaired hearing and tinnitus may occur during the administration of aminoglycosides and may be due to elevated serum levels. Rash is another common side effect of therapy with most antibiotics; it is usually mild and self-limited after treatment stops, but occasionally it can be severe. Diarrhea is another common, generally self-limited, side effect of virtually any oral or parenteral antibiotic; it resolves after discontinuation of the antibiotic. If the diarrhea persists, the patient should be evaluated for colitis caused by *Clostridium difficile*.

Laboratory tests may be useful in the monitoring of patients for antibiotic toxicity. Leukopenia may be seen during the administration of beta-lactams or vancomycin; it usually resolves and is of little clinical significance if the antibiotic therapy is discontinued. Renal function may deteriorate during antibiotic therapy; aminoglycosides may cause renal tubular damage and beta-lactams or sulfonamides may cause interstitial nephritis. Early recognition of toxicity and adjustment of antibiotic therapy may prevent more serious complications.

BRUCELLOSIS

method of
M. YOUSUF KHAN, M.D.
King Fahad Hospital
Riyadh, Saudi Arabia

Brucellosis is a microbial infection of domestic animals that is transmissible to humans. This infection is caused by gram-negative bacteria belonging to the genus *Brucella*. *Brucella* species commonly involved in human infections are *B. melitensis* (goats, sheep), *B. suis* (hogs), *B. abortus* (cattle), and *B. canis* (dogs). Human infection most frequently results from ingestion of unpasteurized milk or milk products, or by direct contact with infected animal tissues. Workers in certain occupations, especially those working in meat-packing plants or on dairy farms or performing veterinary surgery or laboratory bacteriologic tests, can be at risk of brucellosis. This infection is frequently reported from the Middle East, Africa, Russia, India, Europe (Spain, France, and Italy), South America, and Mexico. In the United States, the number of cases of brucellosis has decreased from a peak of 6000 in 1947 to approximately 200 annually in recent years.

In humans, the acute infection is manifested by fever, chills, weakness, sweats, malaise, headache, backache, and arthralgia. Acute arthritis, especially of the sacroiliac and hip joints, is a common finding.

Various complications may occur in 5 to 10 per cent of patients with brucellosis. These complications include osteomyelitis of the spine, epididymo-orchitis, granulomatous hepatitis, meningoencephalitis, and infective endocarditis. This infection, because of its varied manifestations, can be easily misdiagnosed.

Brucellosis should be suspected in patients with a febrile illness, arthralgia or arthritis, and a history of exposure. Routine laboratory tests are not diagnostic. Diagnosis depends on serologic test results, with or without culture of *Brucella* from body fluids. Cultures are not always positive and even if they are, results may be available in 7 to 21 days; therefore, serologic tests are most helpful for early diagnosis. Nearly all cases of acute brucellosis show an agglutinin titer of 1:160 or higher. Cultures of body fluids should be attempted before antimicrobial therapy is begun. Blood cultures are most useful in acute disease and may be positive in 50 to 75 per cent of patients. Cultures of infected tissues and biopsies of bone marrow and abscesses may also be helpful. Bone marrow cultures may be positive even when blood cultures are negative and may remain positive after antibiotic therapy.

TREATMENT

Most patients with acute brucellosis require a few days of hospitalization for bed rest, rehydration, and nutritional support. Patients may be treated in an outpatient setting provided that they are not very ill. A combination of tetracycline and streptomycin is the current treatment of choice and results in the lowest relapse rates. The adult dose of tetracycline is 0.5 gram orally, four times daily for 6 weeks. Streptomycin is given at a dose of 1 gram intramuscularly once daily for 2 weeks. Doxycycline (Vibramycin), 100 mg orally twice daily, may be substituted for tetracycline. Although doxycycline is expensive, it is easier to administer and results in better patient compliance. Rifampin is generally active against *B. melitensis* but not always against *B. abortus*. To avoid emergence of resistant strains, rifampin should not be used as a single agent. It has been effective as a companion to tetracycline or doxycycline. Rifampin is used at a single daily dose of 900 mg orally. The combination of doxycycline and rifampin has shown satisfactory results and is suitable for outpatient use.

Relapses are rarely caused by resistant *Brucella* strains. They are due mainly to the intracellular nature of the infection because organisms may remain protected from antibodies and certain antimicrobial agents for long periods. Relapses can be treated successfully with a second course of treatment.

Brucellosis commonly causes abortion in the first and second trimesters of pregnancy. Early treatment may prevent this complication. Tetracycline should not be used in pregnant women because of the dangers of staining the developing teeth of the fetus and inducing skeletal deformities. Streptomycin is also considered to be unsafe in pregnancy. We have treated pregnant women with trimethoprim-sulfamethoxazole (co-trimoxazole). The treatment course consists of one double-strength tablet (160 mg trimethoprim plus 800 mg sulfamethoxazole) given twice daily by mouth for 6 weeks. This treatment prevents abortion when given early in the course of illness in pregnant women. In areas where prevalence of strains resistant to trimethoprim-sulfamethoxazole is high, rifampin may be used in combination with trimethoprim-sulfamethoxazole. We have used this regimen in a few patients with a satisfactory outcome of pregnancy.

Children younger than 8 years of age should not be treated with tetracycline. Treatment consisting of trimethoprim-sulfamethoxazole and rifampin has been successful in eradicating infection in children. The dose of trimethoprim is 10 mg per kg per day and that of sulfamethoxazole, 50 mg per kg per day orally as two equal portions, 12 hourly. The dose of rifampin is 10 mg per kg per day once daily orally. In complicated cases, streptomycin, 15 mg per kg as a single intramuscular injection, may be added to this combination for the first 3 weeks of the total course of 6 weeks.

Neurobrucellosis is difficult to diagnose and treat. A regimen combining tetracycline, rifampin, and trimethoprim-sulfamethoxazole has generally been found to be effective. A longer course of therapy from 2 to 4 months is required in these patients. The actual duration of therapy depends on clinical improvement and favorable response of pleocytosis in the cerebrospinal fluid. Streptomycin may have to be added to this regimen in patients who are quite ill. Streptomycin given intramuscularly and trimethoprim-sulfamethoxazole given intravenously should be used, together with rifampin and tetracycline by nasogastric tube, in unconscious patients who cannot take medications orally. Streptomycin use is limited to 2 to 4 weeks, to avoid toxicity.

Brucella osteomyelitis (spondylitis) also requires a longer course of therapy. A combination of doxycycline or tetracycline with rifampin for 6 to 9 months gives satisfactory results. *Brucella* spondylitis can mimic tuberculous spondylitis. If tuberculosis cannot be excluded, isoniazid, 300 mg per day orally, should be added to this combination. If possible, abscesses should be drained surgically. Abscesses of the spleen or of one kidney are cured by the removal of the organ.

Infective endocarditis is the most serious complication of brucellosis. Once established, *Brucella* endocarditis is difficult to treat and may result in death. Surgical replacement of the damaged valve with a prosthetic valve, together with treatment with bactericidal drugs, may be curative. We used ceftriaxone (Rocephin), 1.0 gram intravenously twice daily, together with tetracycline and rifampin orally, with an excellent clinical response and sterilization of blood cultures. However, surgical replacement of the diseased aortic valve (with ring abscess) was necessary because of relapse of bacteremia 1 year later. New antimicrobial agents such as third-generation cephalosporins (e.g., ceftriaxone) and quinolones have shown in vitro activity against *Brucella* species. In the past, cephalosporins have been ineffective in brucellosis. Results of clinical trials with these new agents are not yet available.

CHICKENPOX
(Varicella)

method of
ANN M. ARVIN, M.D.
Stanford University
Stanford, California

Varicella is a generalized vesicular exanthem caused by varicella-zoster virus, a DNA virus that belongs to the herpesvirus group. The scattered cutaneous lesions of the primary infection with the virus result from a viremia that is associated with peripheral blood mononuclear cells. After primary infection, the virus produces latent infection of neuronal cells in the dorsal root ganglia that may reactivate to cause herpes zoster (shingles).

EPIDEMIOLOGY

Varicella is transmitted to a susceptible individual by contact with another person who has varicella or herpes zoster. Airborne transmission occurs via respiratory droplets from patients with varicella but not from those with herpes zoster; transmission from individuals with herpes zoster requires direct contact with the lesions. The incubation period of varicella is 10 to 21 days, and transmission can occur from patients 24 to 48 hours before the appearance of the exanthem. Varicella should be considered contagious until no new lesions have appeared for 24 to 48 hours and crusting of old lesions is noted. Children with varicella need not be isolated from other healthy children. However, exposure of adults and pregnant women who are susceptible and of immunocompromised patients should be avoided. More than 90 per cent of adults who are natives of the United States have had varicella, but only about 50 per cent have a clinical history of past infection; the percentage of immune adults is significantly lower among individuals from tropical areas.

DIAGNOSIS AND MANAGEMENT IN THE NORMAL HOST

The diagnosis of varicella is usually made based on the characteristic vesicular exanthem and does not require laboratory documentation. The management of varicella in healthy individuals is supportive. Discomfort caused by the rash can be decreased by application of calamine lotions or cool compresses and by bathing. Daily bathing is indicated to minimize risk of secondary bacterial infection of the lesions; use of medicated soaps is not necessary. The initial lesions appear on the face, scalp, and trunk and are followed by new lesions for up to 7 days; in most cases, new lesions appear for 3 to 5 days. Mucous membrane lesions are common. Later lesions usually appear on the extremities and may be maculopapular rather than vesicular. Oral antihistamines may be helpful during the first few days if pruritus is severe and interferes with sleep, but care should be taken that their administration does not mask neurologic symptoms. Fever and malaise can be treated with acetaminophen; salicylates are contraindicated because of the association with Reye's syndrome. Discomfort of urethritis and vaginitis can be eased by bathing. Activity should be allowed as tolerated. Scabbed lesions may take several weeks to resolve. Areas of increased or decreased skin pigmentation may be prominent but gradually resolve. A few of the larger lesions may produce scarring, but these scars become less obvious with time.

COMPLICATIONS OF VARICELLA IN THE NORMAL HOST

The most common problem in normal individuals with varicella is secondary bacterial infection of the skin lesions; however, significant pyoderma or cellulitis occurs in fewer than 5 per cent of patients. The usual organisms causing secondary infections are *Staphylococcus aureus* and group A beta-hemolytic streptococci. Manifestations include rapidly progressive enlargement of skin lesions, impetigo, and cellulitis surrounding involved lesions; rarely, staphylococcal scalded skin syndrome or scarlet fever may develop. Bacteremia is rare, even in patients with infected skin lesions. After the lesions have been cultured, erythromycin or a semisynthetic penicillin (cloxacillin, dicloxacillin) should be given. If the organism is a streptococcus or penicillin-sensitive *S. aureus,* penicillin may be used.

Vesicular lesions of the conjunctivae can occur. These lesions usually resolve without residua, but if ocular infection is extensive ophthalmologic evaluation for keratitis and possible topical antiviral therapy is indicated.

The most common neurologic complications of varicella are cerebellar ataxia and encephalitis. Cerebellar ataxia is a self-limited syndrome that may occur in the acute phase of the illness or within 2 or 3 weeks after the exanthem appears. It resolves without treatment in 1 to 3 weeks and leaves no sequelae. Encephalitis in the normal host usually begins with symptoms of personality change: confusion, drowsiness, irritability, or seizures 5 to 7 days after the appearance of the rash. Symptoms may progress rapidly to obtundation and coma. Encephalitis is estimated to occur in 1 per 1000 cases of varicella. Lumbar puncture is indicated to rule out bacterial infection; the cerebrospinal fluid usually shows a moderate increase in white blood cells, predominantly lymphocytes, with a normal glucose level and normal or moderately elevated protein level. Lumbar puncture should be done only after careful assessment for signs of increased intracranial pressure. Management of these patients requires intensive supportive care with attention to maintaining the airway, fluid restriction, and monitoring vital signs. Seizures are treated with anticonvulsants. Patients who have increased intracranial pressure should be treated with dexamethasone, 1.5 mg per kg initially, with a maintenance dose of 1.5 mg per kg per day divided every 4 to 6 hours. Mannitol, 20 per cent solution, can be given at a dose of 0.25 gram per kg by intravenous push and increased to 1 gram per kg per dose if necessary. Mannitol should not be given if the serum osmolality is above 320 mOsm per liter. Steroid therapy for increased intracranial pressure should be tapered as soon as the problem has resolved. Symptoms of varicella encephalitis reverse rapidly after 24 to 48 hours, and sequelae are unusual. The fatalities that occur, estimated at 10 per cent, are attributed to increased intracranial pressure. The pathogenesis in healthy children is considered to be demyelination rather than viral infection of brain tissue. Antiviral therapy is not indicated unless encephalitis appears to be associated with visceral dissemination of the virus, as may occur in immunocompromised children.

Other neurologic manifestations that have been associated with varicella include Guillain-Barré syndrome, cranial nerve palsies, optic neuritis with transient blindness, and transverse myelitis. Reye's syndrome may follow varicella infection. Children with persistent vomiting should be evaluated for this complication because repeated vomiting is unusual with varicella.

Varicella pneumonia is estimated to occur in about 15 per cent of healthy adults who acquire varicella. Its severity may range from asymptomatic pulmonary infiltrates on chest films to life-threatening pneumonia. Respiratory symptoms develop within 2 to 5 days after the onset of the rash and are usually accompanied by continued formation of new skin lesions. Tachypnea is the initial sign; other findings on physical examination may be minimal. The chest film shows diffuse infiltrates with multiple modular densities, often in the hilar and perihilar regions. This pattern is quite distinct from pneumonia caused by secondary bacterial infection, which produces a unilateral lobar infiltrate with effusion in most cases. Arterial Po_2 should be measured in patients with extensive pneumonia demonstrated by chest film, even if respiratory symptoms appear mild. In severe cases, there is rapid progression with increased dyspnea, cyanosis, pleuritic pain, and tachycardia. Assisted high-pressure ventilation with 100 per cent oxygen may be required. Steroids are of no known benefit in this complication of varicella. Antiviral therapy is indicated because varicella pneumonia is caused by replication of the virus in lung tissue. Intravenous acyclovir (10 mg per kg per dose, given every 8 hours*) should be given. Clinical recovery generally parallels the cessation of formation of new skin lesions. Antibiotics are not indicated unless there is evidence of secondary bacterial infection.

Although the virus appears to infect the liver (normal children with varicella have moderately abnormal liver function tests), severe hepatitis with varicella is rare.

Thrombocytopenia may occur during acute varicella as part of a generalized intravascular coagulopathy associated with purpura fulminans and hemorrhage into the skin lesions. Patients with these symptoms should be treated with broad-spectrum antibiotics until bacterial sepsis can be ruled out. Intensive supportive care is required, including platelet and blood transfusions. Some patients who develop transient thrombocytopenic purpura may actually have a postinfectious complication of varicella. These patients may require platelet support and steroid therapy. Henoch-Schönlein (anaphylactoid) purpura can occur after varicella; patients with this sequela should be observed for abnormalities of renal function and gastrointestinal symptoms.

Varicella can cause arthritis during or immediately after the acute infection. Patients with bone or joint symptoms should be evaluated carefully because osteomyelitis caused by *S. aureus* may follow varicella. Varicella arthritis is self-limited and does not require surgical management other than aspiration if necessary.

Other rare but important complications of varicella include glomerulonephritis, which may be caused by the virus or by intercurrent group A streptococcal infection, and myocarditis.

*Usual dose is 5 mg per kg every 8 hours.

DIAGNOSIS AND MANAGEMENT IN SPECIAL RISK POPULATIONS

Pregnant Women and Infants

Varicella during pregnancy is unusual because most women of childbearing age are immune. Varicella is more likely to cause pneumonia in pregnant women, but whether the risk is age related or associated with pregnancy is uncertain. Varicella-zoster virus can cause embryopathy, but the risk is estimated to be less than 5 per cent even after maternal varicella during the first trimester. Clinical findings reported with intrauterine varicella include microcephaly, cerebral atrophy, mental retardation, seizures, chorioretinitis, limb atrophy, and cicatricial skin scars. Spontaneous abortion may also occur. If an exposed pregnant woman is proved to be susceptible by a sensitive serologic assay for antibodies to varicella-zoster virus, such as enzyme immunoassay or the fluorescent antibody membrane antigen method, varicella-zoster immune globulin (VZIG) prophylaxis should be given to modify the severity of varicella. However, there is no evidence that its administration prevents infection of the fetus or decreases the risk of sequelae. VZIG is available through the American Red Cross Blood Services.

If the mother develops varicella within 4 days before to 2 days after delivery, the infant is at risk for severe disseminated varicella, which may be fatal. These infants should be given VZIG as soon as possible after delivery. Infants who receive VZIG may develop varicella and should be treated with acyclovir if progression occurs. If varicella occurs in an infant born under these circumstances who was not given VZIG, antiviral therapy should be given. Varicella in infants born to mothers who develop the rash more than 4 days before delivery will be modified by transplacentally acquired antibody. Some of these infants have skin lesions at birth, but their prognosis for uncomplicated infection is good. In general, infants who are exposed to siblings or other contacts with varicella are usually protected from severe disease by transplacentally acquired maternal antibody. Although there is no definite evidence that varicella is more severe during the first few months of life, if an infant under 2 months of age whose mother is not immune to varicella has a close exposure it seems prudent to give prophylaxis.

Immunocompromised Children

Risk of visceral dissemination of varicella is increased in patients with congenital immunodeficiency, such as Wiskott-Aldrich syndrome and thymic dysplasia, or immunodeficiency related to treatment with immunosuppressive agents. Children with human immunodeficiency virus infection are also at risk because severe varicella is associated with impaired cellular immunity. Corticosteroids, cytotoxic chemotherapy, antithymocyte globulin, and radiation diminish the immune response to varicella. Children who are receiving prednisone therapy for asthma, idiopathic thrombocytopenic purpura, juvenile rheumatoid arthritis, nephrotic syndrome, or other diseases at doses less than or equal 0.25 mg per kg per day are not at significantly increased risk. Severe varicella may develop in children who are receiving more than 2 mg per kg per day of prednisone. Children with malignancies who are most likely to have life-threatening varicella are those whose absolute lymphocyte count is 500 cells per mm^3 or less and whose disease is in relapse. Bone marrow and organ transplant recipients are likely to develop progressive varicella.

Parents of high-risk children should immediately report any exposure to varicella or herpes zoster. Prophylaxis with VZIG should be given for household contact or other close indoor exposure. Modification of varicella is optimal if passive antibody prophylaxis is administered within 3 days after the exposure and is not likely to modify the disease if given after 4 to 5 days. Parents should also be educated to recognize possible varicella lesions. The diagnosis of suspicious lesions should be pursued by scraping cells from the base of the lesion and staining with immunofluorescent reagents that detect varicella-zoster virus–infected cells. If possible, children who are receiving high-dose steroids or chemotherapy should have the steroid dose decreased and chemotherapy interrupted for the duration of the incubation period. Although varicella is modified in most children who receive prophylaxis shortly after exposure, some children develop severe varicella despite its administration and may require intravenous acyclovir therapy.

Immunocompromised children who develop varicella may have fulminant infection with pneumonia, hepatic failure, and disseminated intravascular coagulation during the first few days of the illness. However, most children appear to do well initially but develop progressive varicella with new lesion formation for more than 5 to 6 days after the appearance of the exanthem. Progressive cutaneous infection may be accompanied by pneumonia, hepatitis, thrombocytopenia, encephalitis, and glomerulonephritis with severe hypertension. Severe abdominal or back pain is an ominous prognostic sign. Bacterial sepsis may also occur. To be effective, antiviral therapy should be initiated early in the clinical course, preferably within 3 days after the appearance of the rash. Acyclovir is preferred to vidarabine because it is more effective than vidarabine in high-risk patients with herpes zoster. Acyclovir is given at 500 mg per M^2 per dose, every 8 hours.* The drug must be given as a 1-hour infusion, and the patient should be kept well hydrated. The dose must be decreased in patients with impaired renal function if the creatinine clearance rate is less than one-half of normal. Some children develop severe varicella despite antiviral therapy, and intensive support is essential for the management of these patients. There is no evidence that passive antibody administration after the appearance of clinically apparent varicella modifies the severity of the disease. Immunosuppressive therapy can be resumed 1 week after skin lesions have crusted.

A live attenuated varicella vaccine is being evaluated for safety and efficacy in healthy children and adults and in selected immunocompromised children, but its use is investigational.

NOSOCOMIAL TRANSMISSION OF VARICELLA

Nosocomial varicella can be a serious problem in pediatric wards. All patients being admitted to the hospital should be questioned about recent exposures to varicella and herpes zoster; if an exposure has occurred, elective admissions should be delayed. If hospital exposure occurs, high-risk susceptible patients with close exposure should be given prophylaxis. Susceptible patients should be discharged during the incubation period if possible, and those who must remain in the hospital should be placed in strict isolation at the end of the incubation period. Hospital personnel who are susceptible to varicella should not care for these children. Isolation rooms for children with varicella should have negative airflow relative to the corridor and should be vented to the outside. In implementing these measures, it is helpful to screen high-risk susceptible patients for antibody to varicella at the time the underlying disease is diagnosed.

Infants with nosocomial exposure to varicella or herpes zoster are rarely at risk because most infants have maternally acquired antibodies to varicella. The maternal history should be determined; if there is doubt about the mother's immunity, the maternal varicella antibody titer should be measured. Infants with close exposure whose mothers have no antibodies to varicella should receive VZIG.

---

*Manufacturer's recommended dose is 250 mg per M^2, every 8 hours (750 mg per M^2 per day).

CHOLERA

method of
MIGUEL L. O'RYAN, M.D., and
THOMAS G. CLEARY, M.D.
*The University of Texas Medical School
at Houston
Houston, Texas*

Cholera is an extremely severe acute diarrheal disease characterized by abrupt onset of vomiting and watery diarrhea, with stool loss of up to 1 liter per hour in adults and 350 ml per kg per day in children. The disease is caused by *Vibrio cholerae,* a gram-negative, highly motile, curved bacillus that can be rapidly detected by dark-field microscopy of fresh feces and cultured on selective media. A large inoculum (10^8 to 10^{10} bacteria) is necessary for bacteria to survive the gastric acid barrier and colonize the small intestine. Any defect in gastric acid production enhances colonization. In the small intestine, *V. cholerae* adheres to the microvilli by surface pili and secretes a polypeptide toxin. The holotoxin, of about 84 kilodaltons (kDa), is composed of a catalytically active 27-kDa A subunit and five or six 12-kDa B subunits that bind to the intestinal receptor, ganglioside GM_1. After binding, the A subunit is cleaved and penetrates the cell membrane by an incompletely understood mechanism. In the cell, it catalyzes the adenosine diphosphate ribosylation of the stimulatory G component of adenylate cyclase, resulting in an increase in intracellular cyclic adenosine monophosphate. The net result is inhibition of sodium chloride absorption across the intestinal brush border of villous cells and active chloride secretion in the crypt cells; the result of these events is loss of chloride, sodium, and water.

Two main serogroups, defined by their somatic O antigen as 01 and non-01, have been identified. The first group has been associated with typical cholera. The 01 *V. cholerae* organisms are further subdivided into serotypes based on hemagglutination properties and biotypes based on specific biochemical reactions. There are two serotypes (Ogawa and Inaba) and two biotypes (classic and El Tor). El Tor biotype epidemics have been associated with a less severe course, a higher frequency of asymptomatic infections, and prolonged carriage.

The major sources of *V. cholerae* are thought to be contaminated water, particularly estuarine environments, or contaminated aquatic animals, especially in endemic areas. Even though person-to-person fecal-oral transmission is less important, it probably plays a key role in epidemic outbreaks.

Endemic and epidemic areas of cholera are located mainly in southern and southeastern Asia. Since 1961, cholera caused by the El Tor biotype has been epidemic throughout much of Asia, the Middle East, Africa, and certain parts of Europe. In the United States, endemic regions have been detected in the Gulf Coast areas of Texas and Louisiana, where shrimp and crab have been found to be contaminated with *V. cholerae* serotype Inaba, biotype El Tor.

TREATMENT

Because the immediate effects of cholera toxin are mild to massive loss of water, chloride, sodium, potassium, and bicarbonate, the patient is at risk of developing dehydration (sometimes with shock), hyponatremia, hypokalemia, metabolic acidosis, and acute renal failure. Children may also develop hypoglycemia, probably related to decreased intake of carbohydrates and diminished reserves.

Rehydration

A correct assessment of the severity of dehydration is crucial in the initial evaluation of a person with cholera (Table 1). Oral fluid therapy plays a key role in the management of these patients. Table 2 shows the composition of the most commonly recommended oral solution compared with the stool loss in cholera patients. Therapy is initiated according to the estimated severity of fluid loss. Comparing the patient's current weight with the previous weight may be helpful.

Mild Dehydration. Oral rehydration therapy (ORT) with appropriate formula is sufficient in most mild cases (Table 3).

Moderate Dehydration. Initiate treatment with ORT and evaluate serum electrolyte levels and acid-base status. Intravenous therapy is required if the patient is hemodynamically unstable, has acute renal failure, has an ileus related to electrolyte abnormalities, has vomiting sufficient to interfere with replacement, is too lethargic, or refuses to take fluids orally. Once oral therapy is initiated, the patient should be closely followed (vomiting, stool loss, urine output and specific gravity, weight, and fluid intake) to ensure that losses are being replaced adequately. If dehydration progresses, intravenous therapy should be initiated.

Severe Dehydration. The severely dehydrated patient always requires parenteral fluid therapy (Table 3). If the patient is in shock (e.g., with tachycardia, tachypnea, feeble pulse, delayed capillary refill, compromised consciousness, oligoanuria, and/or low blood pressure), rapid infusion of isotonic fluids is critical (Table 3). Assessment and correction of abnormalities of serum electrolytes, bicarbonate, urea nitrogen, and creatinine levels are mandatory. After the patient has improved, oral rehydration can be added to the regimen. During the next 24 to 72 hours, oral fluids can be increased progressively and parenteral fluids tapered rapidly according to clinical judgment and laboratory evaluation.

TABLE 1. **Clinical Assessment of Dehydration**

Signs	Mild Dehydration	Moderate Dehydration	Severe Dehydration
General appearance	Alert, restless, thirsty	Restless or moderately drowsy; irritable to touch; very thirsty	Drowsy; little or no reaction to touch or extremely irritable
Radial pulse	Normal	Rapid	Rapid; may be weak
Respiration	Normal	Deep, varying according to severity of acidosis	Deep and rapid
Systolic blood pressure	Normal	Normal or low	Low
Skin	Retracts immediately on being pinched*	Retracts slowly on being pinched	Retracts very slowly (>2 sec) on being pinched
Eyes	Normal, cry with tears	Sunken, absence of tears	Grossly sunken
Urine flow	Normal	Reduced for several hours	Absent for several hours†
Percentage of body weight loss	<5%	6–10%	>10%
Estimated fluid deficit	<50 ml/kg	60–100 ml/kg	>100 ml/kg

*Perform preferably on anterior thorax; severe malnourishment may result in abnormal retraction.
†If absent for more than 12 hours, acute renal failure should be suspected.

Correction of Electrolyte and Acid-Base Imbalance

Electrolyte and bicarbonate losses can be managed with ORT in most cases. Severe, symptomatic hyponatremia requires parenteral therapy. The severe loss of sodium, chloride, and bicarbonate in cholera stools (Table 2) requires the use of formulas with an adequate electrolyte concentration (World Health Organization [WHO]) or an analogue. Although WHO ORT was designed for cholera, it has been used for other dehydrating diarrheal syndromes with equal efficacy. The supplement of free water in these cases, administered either ad libitum or two parts ORT to one part water, is recommended to avoid hypernatremia. Formulas with a lower electrolyte content have been used extensively for noncholera diarrheas with good results (e.g., Infalyte, Pedialyte, Lytren, Resol). Rice-based formulas that substitute glucose for rice flour (50 to 80 grams per liter) are currently being evaluated; such formulas may

TABLE 2. **Cholera Stool Content and World Health Organization (WHO) Rehydration Formula Composition**

Component	Cholera Stool Content (mEq/ liter)	WHO ORT Formula* Composition (mEq/liter)
Sodium	133 ± 21	90
Potassium	20 ± 8	20
Chloride	100 ± 7	80
Bicarbonate	41 ± 9	30
Glucose	0	111

*Premeasured packets containing NaCl 3.5 grams, KCl 2.5 grams, NaHCO$_3$ 1.5 grams, and glucose 20 grams are diluted in 1 liter of water. Home preparation of a nearly equivalent solution involves use of ½ tsp of NaCl, ¼ tsp of KCl, ½ tsp of NaHCO$_3$ and 2 tbsp of sucrose per quart of water. Obviously, it is critical that the caretaker of the child understand that this formula must be rigidly adhered to so that the risk of hypernatremia and other electrolyte abnormalities is minimized.

further decrease fluid losses by reducing the osmotic load of glucose-based solutions.

Refeeding

Cholera often strikes the malnourished. Because of the severe impact of delayed refeeding in patients whose nutritional status is already compromised, fasting should be minimized to the interval necessary to stabilize the patient's fluid and electrolyte status. Generally, this is 6 to 18 hours after initiation of oral rehydration therapy. Because carbohydrate absorption is not typically impaired, dilution of milk formulas is not usually necessary in cholera patients. It is reasonable to offer frequent, small volumes initially, alternating with ORT, and to increase these progressively as tolerated. Breast-feeding should not be stopped in small infants.

Antibiotic Therapy

Antibiotic therapy reduces the amount of stool loss, the duration of disease, and the shedding of vibrio organisms in stools. The most effective antibiotic is tetracycline, 50 mg per kg per day, given every 6 hours orally in children and 2 grams per day every 6 hours orally in adults. Because tetracycline stains the teeth in children less than 7 years of age, other antibiotics are appropriate for the younger child. Furazolidone (Furoxone), 5 to 6 mg per kg per day given every 6 hours; trimethroprim-sulfamethoxazole (TMP-SMX), 8 mg TMP plus 40 mg SMX per kg per day given twice daily; and chloramphenicol, 50 mg per kg per day every 6 hours, have been used. Treatment is usually given for 3 days. Physicians should be aware that multiple antibiotic-resistant strains of *V. cholerae* are emerging. Other drugs, including chlorpromazine, berberine, sali-

TABLE 3. **Rehydration Therapy**

	Oral Fluids	Parenteral Fluids
Situation	Mild to moderate dehydration; cooperative patient	Severe dehydration Contraindication to ORT (see text) Failure of ORT
Fluids	WHO ORT (as described in Table 2)	Isotonic saline Ringer's lactate Hartmann's solution (DTS)* Dhaka's or other solutions†
Fluid therapy	Initial: ad libitum in small volumes as tolerated. As a guideline, give 50–100 ml/kg in first 4 hr in children and 2–3.5 liters in adults, depending on stool loss. First 24 hr: consider fluid deficit (percentage dehydration) plus ongoing stool losses plus daily fluid requirements (age related). As a guideline, 150–300 ml/kg or more is needed in children and at least 5–6 liters in adults. Continued monitoring is essential to treat these patients adequately. Subsequent days: progressive decline in oral fluids as parameters improve. To avoid hypernatremia, alternate use of formula and water as stool improves.	Shock: isotonic fluid, 20–30 ml/kg in 30 min (may be repeated) in children and 50–100 ml/min until pulse and blood pressure return toward normal in adults. Calculate volume needed, as in ORT. Administer one-half of the volume in 8 hr and one half of the volume in following 16 hr. Add K+ and bicarbonate according to estimated deficit and ongoing losses. Introduce oral fluids as soon as possible. Progressively increase ORT and decrease IV fluids. In 12–48 hr, IV therapy may be discontinued if the patient has adequate oral intake. Adequate monitoring is essential.

*DTS (diarrhea treatment solution): contains, in 1 liter, NaCl 4 grams, sodium acetate 6.5 grams, KCl 1 gram, glucose 10 grams.

†Such solutions approximate cholera stool losses. Example: Dhaka's solution: Na^+ 133 mEq/liter, K^+ 13 mEq/liter, Cl^- 98 mEq/liter, HCO_3^- 48 mEq/liter.

cylic acid, opiates, absorbents, and anticholera toxin antibodies, have not proved to be clinically useful.

PREVENTION

The main measures to control cholera epidemics are adequate isolation and treatment of symptomatic cases, adequate disposal of stools, emphasis on handwashing, and proper food and water handling. Control of endemic cholera depends on education and on improvements in sanitation. Vaccination is of limited benefit. In field trials conducted in areas with endemic cholera, vaccines have been only about 50 per cent effective in reducing the incidence of clinical illness for 3 to 6 months. Vaccines do not prevent transmission and infection. WHO no longer recommends cholera vaccination for travel to or from cholera-infected areas, nor does the U.S. Public Health Service require it for travelers coming to the United States from endemic areas.

DIPHTHERIA

method of
JERRY J. ELLER, M.D.
Lloyd Noland Foundation Hospital
Fairfield, Alabama

Diphtheria is an acute infectious disease caused by a pleomorphic gram-positive bacillus, *Corynebacterium*

diphtheriae. The organism usually colonizes mucous membranes of the upper respiratory tract, less commonly colonizes the skin, and produces a powerful exotoxin. The exotoxin causes local cellular necrosis and then diffuses into the circulation and may result in serious damage to the heart or to nerves, which causes myocarditis or polyneuritis. Death may occur early from respiratory obstruction or from overwhelming toxemia and circulatory collapse, or somewhat later from cardiac damage. Patients usually survive neurotoxic injury if they are medically attended and given supportive care. The hallmark of the disease is the presence of a diphtheritic pseudomembrane that is produced by exotoxin and that is composed of necrotic epithelium plus exuding fibrin, red and white blood cells, and colonizing bacteria. The clinical course of diphtheria depends on (1) the location and extent of the membrane, (2) the amount of toxin produced and absorbed, (3) early institution of treatment with antitoxin, and (4) the patient's age and immune status.

Corynebacterium organisms are gram-positive rods that possess irregular swellings at one end, which gives them a club-shaped appearance. The rods contain irregularly dispersed, deeply staining metachromatic granules when smears are made with Albert's stain. Individual bacteria tend to lie parallel or at acute angles to each other in stained smears. They form acid, but not gas, in certain carbohydrates. Members of *Corynebacterium* form part of the normal flora of the respiratory tract, conjunctivae, intestinal tract, vagina, and skin. *C. diphtheriae* must be distinguished from other *Corynebacterium* species that normally colonize the respiratory tract and conjunctivae, which are called diphtheroids.

Three biotypes of *C. diphtheriae*—*gravis, intermedius,* and *mitis*—may be identified. All toxigenic strains can produce the same exotoxin. Mitis strains have produced less severe clinical disease than the other strains.

Transmission of *C. diphtheriae* is by intimate contact with infected droplets, nasopharyngeal secretions, or skin exudates. Less often, transmission is by fomites, milk, or animals. A carrier state develops when a person with toxigenic immunity harbors the organism in the nasopharynx or on the skin and remains free of symptoms. Such a carrier must be identified by appropriate cultures. A convalescent carrier state after clinical disease also develops. These carriers comprise the reservoir of infection from which susceptible persons contract the disease. The incubation period is 2 to 6 days.

Cutaneous and wound diphtheria is characterized by ulcerative skin lesions with membrane formation and only slight absorption of toxin. Often skin disease is more common than respiratory tract disease in tropical and subtropical areas. In temperate climates, skin lesions caused by *C. diphtheriae* may occur in fully immunized children during late summer and early fall and be mistaken for common impetigo or pyoderma. These lesions may be of major importance in the transfer of *C. diphtheriae* organisms from one person to another, in whom they eventually reach the respiratory tract and cause recognizable disease.

During recent years, outbreaks of diphtheria have occurred in urban areas of the United States when immunity in the population has dropped to critical levels. Disease then occurs predominantly in parts of the city occupied by economically and socially deprived families. In the 1960s and 1970s, attack rates in the United States were highest among Mexican-American and black persons who were 5 to 14 years old. Morbidity may be appreciable in many age groups regardless of immune status. Since 1980, the proportion of cases in adults has been increasing in the United States. Fourteen of 18 cases have occurred in persons older than 15 years of age. Recent Scandinavian outbreaks have occurred in adult alcohol and drug abusers who lacked protective antitoxin serum levels. We can anticipate that this trend will continue in the United States provided that "herd immunity" among children remains high and that virulent, toxigenic strains are introduced into segments of our population. The case fatality rate has continued to be in the range of 5 to 10 per cent. However, the potential exists for increased mortality among elderly and immunocompromised individuals.

PREVENTION

Diphtheria is a preventable disease. Everyone must be immunized. Induction of active immunity is successful in preventing diphtheria. The following recommended schedules for active immunization, as found in the 1988 report of the Committee of Infectious Diseases of the American Academy of Pediatrics, are endorsed. A normal infant should receive 0.5 ml of diphtheria and tetanus toxoid combined with pertussis vaccine (DTP) at 2, 4, and 6 months, with a booster at 1½ years of age. A booster is also given at age 4 to 6 years. At age 14 to 16 years, an adult-type combined tetanus and diphtheria toxoid (Td) injection is given; thereafter it is given every 10 years. For a child younger than 7 years of age, a DTP injection is given at the first visit and then boosters are given 2 and 4 months later. A repeat injection is given 6 to 12 months later or in school. For children 7 years of age and older and for adults, on the first visit a Td injection is given, with a repeat injection 2 months later, which is followed by a booster 6 to 12 months later. A Td injection should be given every 10 years. A serum antitoxin level of 0.01 IU per ml or higher is protective. Primary care physicians should maintain protective levels by responsibly giving Td boosters to adult patients.

DIAGNOSIS

Diagnosis is a clinical judgment (Table 1). In general, direct smears are unreliable. Methylene blue staining of a throat smear only suggests the diagnosis. Although this procedure can be done quickly, its usefulness is limited because diphtheroids usually found in the throat are indistinguishable from *C. diphtheriae*. The organisms responsible for Vincent's angina also resemble *C. diphtheriae,* and some patients have Vincent's angina associated with diphtheria. Albert's stain of a smear is more reliable if it is carried out and interpreted by an experienced technologist. Identification by the fluorescent antibody technique is reliable only when done by experienced personnel. The complete blood count often shows only a mild leukocytosis.

The first procedure is to obtain material from the nose and throat and from skin lesions, if present, for culture. It is best to carry the material by hand to the laboratory and tell the technologist that the patient is suspected of having diphtheria. Swabs are usually streaked on Löffler's blood agar, tellurite, or fresh Pai's or Tinsdale's media. From 16 to 48 hours of incubation is required before *C. diphtheriae* colonies can be identified. A toxigenicity test must then be carried out, preferably by using the modified Elek's diffusion technique. A positive reaction consists of a white streak, which usually appears at 16 to 24 hours.

TREATMENT

Specific Management

Antitoxin

Every effort must be made to administer diphtheria antitoxin as soon as possible after the

TABLE 1. **Clinical Diagnosis of Diphtheria**

Category of Evidence	Characteristics
Clinical	Yellow to gray-green membrane on tonsils that 1. Bleeds if dislodged with swab 2. Crosses anatomic barriers
Laboratory	Smears usually unreliable Culture of nose, throat, or skin that grows on Löffler's and other media in 16–48 hr; then positive toxigenicity test (Elek's diffusion technique) in 16–24 hr

disease is suspected (Table 2). Delay beyond 48 hours must be avoided because the administration of even very large doses of antitoxin after this time may have little effect in altering the incidence or severity of complications. A syringe containing 1 ml of epinephrine chloride (1:1000) solution should always be available when antitoxin is being injected. The dose is 0.01 ml per kg of a 1:1000 aqueous solution, with a maximum dose of 0.5 ml.

Preliminary sensitivity testing—both a skin test and an eye test—of the patient to horse serum should always be done before antitoxin is administered. For the skin test, 0.1 ml of a 1:1000 dilution in isotonic saline of antitoxin should be injected intradermally. A positive skin test consists of the appearance of a significant wheal and flare at the injection site after 15 to 20 minutes. For the eye test, 1 drop of a 1:10 dilution in isotonic saline of antitoxin is instilled into the conjunctival sac. A positive reaction consists of conjunctivitis occurring 15 to 20 minutes after instillation. If either of these tests is positive, the patient is considered to be sensitive to horse serum, and desensitization should be accomplished. Before desensitization, the patient should be given diphenhydramine hydrochloride (Benadryl) as indicated: 2 to 5 years of age, 25 mg intramuscularly; 6 to 14 years of age, 50 mg intramuscularly; adults, 50 to 100 mg intramuscularly. Serial injections of diluted antitoxin as indicated in Table 3 may be given at intervals of 15 minutes if no reaction occurs. If a reaction occurs after an injection, the physician should wait 1 hour and then repeat the last dose that failed to cause a reaction.

The intravenous route is preferable in all cases. A single dose should suffice; re-treatment should never be necessary because of the serious risk of

TABLE 2. Treatment of Diphtheria

1. Preliminary sensitivity testing to horse serum—skin test and eye test

   If either test result is positive, use rapid desensitization before IV antitoxin; if both results are negative, then give

2. IV antitoxin, then start

3. Antibiotics
   If patient *is not* allergic to penicillin, and
   a. Can swallow: penicillin V, 250 mg PO tid × 10 days
   b. Cannot swallow: procaine penicillin G, 600,000 U IM q 12 hr × 10 days*

   If patient *is* allergic to penicillin, and
   a. Can swallow: erythromycin, 25 to 50 mg/kg/day PO qid × 10 days
   b. Cannot swallow: clindamycin, 25 to 40 mg/kg/day IV q 6 hr × 10 days*

*Or until able to swallow.

TABLE 3. Desensitization of Persons Allergic to Horse Serum

Serial Doses Given Every 15 Min Provided No Reaction Occurs

1. SC, 0.05 ml of 1:30 dilution of antitoxin
2. SC, 0.05 ml of 1:10 dilution of antitoxin
3. SC, 0.1 ml of undiluted antitoxin
4. SC, 0.2 ml of undiluted antitoxin
5. IM, 0.5 ml of undiluted antitoxin
6. IV, 0.1 ml of undiluted antitoxin
7. Then a therapeutic dose, given slowly IV, in 200 ml isotonic saline during 30 min

increasing sensitization to horse serum. Diphtheria antitoxin is administered on the basis of the following schedule (Table 4): mild pharyngeal diphtheria or when careful examination indicates that the membrane is small or confined to the anterior nares or tonsils, 40,000 units; moderate pharyngeal diphtheria, 80,000 units; severe pharyngeal or laryngeal diphtheria, combined types, or late cases, 120,000 units. Diphtheria antitoxin in 200 ml of isotonic saline is infused during a 30-minute period.

Immediate allergic reactions to antitoxin occur with an overall incidence of about 15 per cent. Such early reactions bear no relation to subsequent development of serum sickness. In children older than 10 years of age and in adults, the incidence of serum sickness has been 20 to 30 per cent. Clinical manifestations have occurred between the seventh and sixteenth days after antitoxin administration and have lasted from 2 to 6 days. The prophylactic use of antagonists of vasoactive amines seems to be worthwhile for the prevention of serum sickness when the agents are orally administered during the period of significant risk after the infusion of horse serum products. Either one of two drugs, cyproheptadine or hydroxyzine, has been found to be efficacious.

Antibiotics

Antibiotics eliminate the organism from the respiratory tract and skin, terminate the carrier state, stop exotoxin production, and eliminate secondary bacterial infections, particularly those caused by beta-hemolytic streptococci.

Penicillin is the drug of choice. If the patient

TABLE 4. Dosage of Diphtheria Antitoxin

Type of Disease	Dosage (U)
Nasal, tonsillar, mild pharyngeal diphtheria	40,000
Moderate pharyngeal diphtheria	80,000
Severe pharyngeal or laryngeal diphtheria, combined types, late cases	120,000

In 200 ml isotonic saline, infused during 30 min

can swallow, 250 mg of phenoxymethyl penicillin is given by mouth three times a day. Patients unable to swallow may receive intramuscular procaine penicillin G, 600,000 units twice daily. The duration of therapy is 10 to 14 days. For patients who are allergic to penicillin, erythromycin is given, 25 to 50 mg per kg per day, preferably by the oral route, for 10 to 14 days. In vitro sensitivity testing must confirm that the strain is sensitive to erythromycin since the occurrence of resistant strains is increasing. Clindamycin (Cleocin), 150 mg by mouth every 6 hours for 10 days, has also been used successfully. For patients who are allergic to penicillin and unable to swallow, intravenous erythromycin produces an unacceptable incidence of thrombophlebitis. Instead, clindamycin, 25 to 40 mg per kg per day intravenously, divided into four doses every 6 hours, is efficacious until the patient can take oral medications.

Myocarditis

Patients developing electrocardiographic changes during the course of diphtheria should have continuous cardiac monitoring to watch for serious arrhythmias and heart block. Monitoring is usually done in special intensive care or cardiac care units. Strict bed rest is enforced. Pharmacologic agents such as lidocaine and procainamide are used to suppress or control specific arrhythmias when indicated. Ventricular tachycardia or fibrillation is treated according to published recommendations by the American Heart Association for Advanced Cardiac Life Support. Transvenous or transthoracic pacing electrodes may need to be inserted for emergency treatment of heart block. Congestive heart failure is usually treated by careful monitoring of fluids and restriction of salt intake. Use of digitalis with congestive heart failure related to diphtheritic myocarditis has been controversial. However, short-acting digitalis preparations are recommended for severe congestive heart failure. Circulatory collapse and shock are managed according to guidelines for treatment of gram-negative sepsis and shock. The value of adrenocorticosteroid therapy is difficult to assess. However, prednisone in the usual doses may be given for approximately 2 weeks to lessen the severity of myocarditis. Bed rest is continued for at least 1 month, with gradually increasing activity as tolerated.

Laryngeal and Bronchial Diphtheria

Bronchoscopy may be used to remove dislodged membrane from larger bronchi, where it may cause death by asphyxia. Tracheostomy may be required early for severely ill patients. Secondary bronchopneumonia caused by hospital-acquired gram-negative bacilli should be watched for. Corticosteroids may be of use in acute laryngeal diphtheria. Hydrocortisone sodium succinate (Solu-Cortef), 5 mg per kg per day intramuscularly or intravenously, is given in three divided doses for 1 or 2 days or longer. An equivalent dose of prednisone is then given orally when possible and gradually reduced over 5 to 8 days.

Neurologic Complications

Palatal paralysis, the most common and often the only paralysis, usually appears early during the course of diphtheria. Intravenous therapy or nasogastric feeding may be required. Paralysis of respiratory muscles usually appears from 6 to 8 weeks after the onset of pharyngitis. Assisted or controlled ventilation by mechanical means is indicated until the patient can resume spontaneous respiration with satisfactory alveolar ventilation.

General Management

Bed rest in the hospital for 10 to 14 days is usually required. No special food restrictions or additions are needed. Food of a consistency that can be swallowed comfortably and a diet adequate in all the nutritional elements are sufficient. Parenteral therapy is indicated only for patients who cannot swallow, generally because of dysphagia, palatal paralysis, or airway obstruction. Patients may have considerable pharyngeal discomfort during the first few days of illness, and irrigation of the pharynx with warm isotonic saline solution may be helpful. Occasionally, codeine phosphate, 3 mg per kg per day divided into six doses, may be helpful; it is given either orally or subcutaneously.

Isolation

All patients must be isolated from other people until antibiotic treatment has rendered the respiratory secretions noninfectious. A private room is preferable. Because antibiotic administration is effective in eliminating the carrier state, many patients may be free of organisms early in the course of the disease (1 to 7 days). Isolation may usually be discontinued after 5 days of specific antibiotics. The staff should wear gowns and masks and should wash their hands thoroughly after attending patients with diphtheria.

Prophylaxis of Contacts

Any patient with a clinical diagnosis of diphtheria who requires antitoxin treatment should be reported to the local health department. Laboratory confirmation of the diagnosis should be communicated in a follow-up telephone report. Household members and close contacts of the patient are cultured and observed at home until culture results are available. Contacts whose immunizations have lapsed and the contacts who are not immunized are given diphtheria toxoid. Carriers are always treated, usually with erythromycin or clindamycin.

Diphtheria is a serious infectious disease with mortality associated with respiratory tract obstruction and toxemia leading to myocarditis and circulatory collapse. Diagnosis is a clinical judgment that is confirmed by isolation of the organism and demonstration of toxin production. Treatment with antitoxin must be instituted early to save lives.

FOOD-BORNE ILLNESS

method of
BERNHARD L. WIEDERMANN, M.D.
*Children's Hospital National Medical Center
and George Washington University
Washington, D.C.*

Illness can be caused by ingestion of foods contaminated by pathogenic microorganisms, microbial toxins, or chemicals. In the last situation, substances may have been added to the food or may be an inherently toxic component of the food itself. Most of the symptoms associated with food-borne illnesses include gastrointestinal or neurologic elements. Although most illness related to foods requires only nonspecific supportive therapy, some situations require specific therapeutic interventions. Also, a proper diagnosis may aid in prevention or termination of an outbreak of food-related disease. Therefore, it is important to be aware of important clues to the differential diagnosis of food-related illnesses.

The medical history is probably the most valuable clue to diagnosis of food-borne illness. It is important to take a detailed dietary history in cases of suspected food poisoning and to include not only the type of foods but also methods of food preparation and storage and the origins of foods. If a specific food or meal is suspected to be the source of the illness, a consideration of incubation periods for the various syndromes can be helpful in leading to an accurate diagnosis. For example, if several members of a group become ill with vomiting, diaphoresis, and severe abdominal cramps 6 hours after a picnic, exposure to *Bacillus cereus* toxin or *Staphylococcus aureus* enterotoxin can be entertained and supportive therapy provided. If, however, the clinical scenario involves severe bloody diarrhea

with cramping beginning the day after the picnic, *Shigella* enteritis could be considered, and appropriate cultures and specific antimicrobial therapy may be indicated.

TREATMENT

Treatment of food-related illness involves restoration and maintenance of adequate fluid balance, amelioration of other symptoms, and removal of the specific inciting agent. In most cases of food poisoning, dehydration from vomiting and/or diarrhea is not severe, and fluid status can be maintained with oral solutions. For infants, a commercially available oral rehydration solution, such as Pedialyte, allows discontinuation of formula or other dairy products while providing adequate fluid and electrolyte replacement. For these infants, it is important not to continue these solutions for more than 1 to 2 days without clinical reassessment because nutritional support can become further impaired with prolonged use of rehydrating solutions. For older children and adults, clear liquids such as juices or soups are better accepted for short-term hydration.

For more severe dehydration, particularly if oral feeding is not tolerated, it may be necessary to provide intravenous fluids temporarily. An estimation of fluid deficit can be made clinically, and the rate of fluid infusion can be calculated to restore the deficit while providing maintenance fluids. This calculation can be made most easily by using a system based on body surface area, which is applicable to both adults and children. Maintenance fluid requirements are between 1600 and 2000 ml per M^2 of body surface area per day. Additional allowances for ongoing losses (such as stool or gastric) and deficit can be added to this total and permit correction of imbalances during a 24-hour period. It is particularly important for infants requiring intravenous fluids that an electrolyte determination be done, primarily to identify hypernatremic dehydration (serum sodium level higher than 150 mEq per dl). These individuals are at risk for cerebral edema if the serum sodium level is reduced too rapidly, which will occur with standard rehydration techniques. In hypernatremic dehydration, correction of fluid deficit should be done during a 48-hour period, with no rapid rehydration unless shock is present. The overall goal is to lower the serum sodium level by no more than 10 mEq per day, and serial determinations of serum electrolyte levels are required during the rehydration period.

It is usually best to avoid administration of antiemetic or antimotility medications in cases of food poisoning because the episodes are generally self-limited and potential side effects of the drugs may outweigh any benefits. In general, none of these medications should be used for treatment of gastrointestinal symptoms in children younger than 2 years of age. Also, certain agents may actually worsen the course of some enteroinvasive gastrointestinal infections, such as *Salmonella*- or *Shigella*-associated enteritides, and therefore should be avoided in patients with bloody diarrhea or diarrhea associated with fever or fecal leukocytes. If an antiemetic drug is needed, a phenothiazine such as prochlorperazine (Compazine) can be given rectally (2.5 mg per dose in children or 25 mg per dose in adults) or intramuscularly (0.06 mg per pound in children or 5 to 10 mg per pound in adults). Repeated doses should not be given to children. For adults with moderate to severe diarrheal symptoms without the above-mentioned signs of enterinvasive bacterial infection, loperamide (Imodium) can be given orally as an initial dose of 4 mg, followed by 2 mg after each loose stool to a maximum of 16 mg per day. Antimotility therapy should not be continued beyond 48 hours in treatment of presumed food-borne illness, and it is preferable to withhold this therapy entirely in children who are otherwise healthy because potential side effects outweigh the minimal benefit obtained from these agents.

Over-the-counter agents containing kaolin and pectin, such as Kaopectate, have no proven efficacy for relief of diarrheal symptoms, but bismuth subsalicylate (Pepto-Bismol) can decrease the symptoms of traveler's diarrhea. The usual dose for adults is 2 tablespoons of liquid or two tablets orally every 30 to 60 minutes for eight doses. Individuals with aspirin sensitivity, renal failure, or gout should not receive Pepto-Bismol, and individuals receiving warfarin compounds, oral hypoglycemic agents, and high-dose aspirin therapy should also avoid its use.

Removal of the inciting agent, either by induction of emesis or with the use of activated charcoal or cathartics, is occasionally indicated in treatment of food-borne illness. Patients with altered sensorium should first have an adequate airway ensured before gastric lavage or emesis is attempted. Emesis is achieved with syrup of ipecac (15 ml orally) or apomorphine (subcutaneously, 1 to 2 mg in children, 6 mg in adults). Cathartics such as magnesium citrate may help to accelerate elimination of chemicals or toxins. However, some of these preparations contain sorbital, which can be absorbed and cause hyperosmolality in some individuals, particularly children.

The remainder of this chapter provides a brief discussion of the different food-borne illness syndromes, arranged by broad clinical manifestations.

ACUTE FOOD POISONING SYNDROMES

Acute food-poisoning syndromes can be characterized by the presence of gastrointestinal and other, varied symptoms that have an acute, sudden onset and a relatively rapid resolution. The classic representatives of this group include syndromes seen with ingestion of bacterial toxins from *S. aureus, B. cereus,* and *Clostridium perfringens. S. aureus* can produce at least five distinct enterotoxins (A to E), which typically produce severe vomiting, abdominal pain and cramping, and nausea approximately 1 to 6 hours after ingestion of a tainted meal. Fever and diarrhea are not common. Foods often associated with staphylococcal food poisoning are high-protein foods such as ham, poultry, egg salad, and pastries with cream filling. Episodes occur more frequently in the summer when foods are left unrefrigerated. *B. cereus* food poisoning produces two clinically distinct illnesses. A short (1 to 6 hour) incubation period precedes a syndrome characterized by vomiting and, in about one-third of cases, diarrhea that persists for a few days. Diarrhea is the predominant symptom in the disease with the longer (6- to 14-hour) incubation period, which generally resolves in 1 or 2 days. Fried rice, creams, and meats are the most common sources of *B. cereus* intoxications. In *C. perfringens* food poisoning, a slightly longer incubation period of 8 to 12 hours precedes a diarrheal illness, which generally resolves quickly. Fever and vomiting are rare. Beef, poultry, gravy, and Mexican foods are common sources of this illness.

The so-called Chinese restaurant syndrome represents a different type of acute food poisoning. Approximately 30 minutes after ingestion of monosodium glutamate, which is a common additive in Chinese foods, certain individuals can develop symptoms of flushing, nausea, headache, and facial paresthesias. Symptoms resolve gradually over several hours, and no specific therapy is needed. A flushing-type syndrome can also be seen with coprine ingestion, such as that occurring with the mushroom *Coprinus atramentarius.* Three to 48 hours after a mushroom-containing meal, coprine, acting as a disulfiram-like compound, produces flushing, vomiting, nausea, headache, tachycardia, hypertension, and a metallic taste sensation when alcohol is ingested. The response gradually subsides afer a few hours.

A third entity in the differential diagnosis of flushing with food poisoning is scombroid fish poisoning. Here, the clinical manifestations are most suggestive of massive histamine release, with flushing, nausea, headache, cramping abdominal pain, diarrhea, bronchospasm, and urticaria. Dark-meat fish such as tuna, mackerel, bonito, amberjack, mahi-mahi, and bluefish are primarily implicated in scombroid poisoning, although even aged cheeses have caused a similar clinical picture. Histamine or toxins such as scombrotoxin or saurine present in the fish are the likely cause of the symptoms, which usually resolve in a few hours. Sometimes, antihistamines such as diphenhydramine (Benadryl, others) or bronchodilators are needed. Recently, anecdotal reports of successful therapy of scombroid poisoning by use of intravenous cimetidine (Tagamet) have been published, but experience with this approach is too limited to recommend it for routine use. It should be noted that individuals receiving the antituberculous drug isoniazid can be at increased risk for illness with scombroid poisoning because isoniazid blocks activity of diamine oxidase, an enzyme that is required to oxidize histamine.

Two other forms of mushroom poisoning deserve mention here because initial symptoms are predominantly gastrointestinal and may mimic some of the other entities discussed earlier. Ingestion of improperly prepared mushrooms of the genus *Gyromitra,* such as *G. esculenta,* is followed 6 to 8 hours later by nausea, abdominal discomfort, headache, fatigue, and dizziness. These symptoms can be followed by severe hemolysis, methemoglobinemia, hepatic failure, metabolic acidosis, seizures, and coma. The monomethylhydrazine metabolite from the toxin of these mushrooms is a competitive inhibitor of pyridoxal phosphate, and specific therapy with pyridoxine hydrochloride, 25 mg intravenously, is indicated in severe intoxications with neurologic symptoms. Mortalities of 40 per cent have been recorded for this particular poisoning.

Finally, some mushrooms of the genus *Amanita (A. phalloides, A. ocreata, A. verna, A. virosa, A. suballiacea,* and *A. bisporigera)* and the genus *Galerina (G. autumnalis, G. marginata,* and *G. venenata)* produce a syndrome accounting for most of the fatal mushroom-related poisonings in North America. After a latent period of 10 to 12 hours after ingestion, clinical symptoms begin with vomiting, diarrhea, and abdominal pain. These symptoms resolve within a day and are followed by 1 to 2 days of well-being, after which the second phase of the illness begins. This second phase is characterized by renal and hepatic failure with a fulminant course. Treatment consists of supportive therapy, with particular attention to fluid and electrolyte balance and prevention of hypoglycemia. Oral or nasogastric charcoal lavage and charcoal hemoperfusion may help to remove circulating toxin early in the course before hepatic necrosis has developed. Although thioctic acid, penicillin G, and corticosteroids have all been advocated for therapy, most authorities do not use these compounds. It is advisable to check with local or regional poison control centers for all cases of suspected *Amanita* or *Galerina* ingestions.

INFECTIOUS DIARRHEA SYNDROMES

Ingestion of contaminated food or water is a frequent cause of infectious diarrheal illness, particularly in travelers. Incubation periods are usually longer than those for the food-poisoning syndromes and last 1 to 7 days. Fever is relatively common, and two distinct types of clinical illness can be identified. In inflammatory or invasive diarrhea, stools often contain blood and mucus, and fecal leukocytes can be observed on methylene blue–stained smears of stool samples. Complications such as bacteremia, septic arthritis, or bowel perforation can occur. These syndromes contrast with the noninflammatory, or secretory, diarrheas, in which profuse, watery stools are the chief clinical hallmark. Gradual resolution of symptoms without specific therapy is the rule for all of these entities, but young infants, elderly persons, and immunocompromised individuals are at risk for complications.

Salmonella species are the most common cause of food-borne inflammatory diarrhea; poultry, eggs, and some meats are often implicated. Illness generally resolves spontaneously in a few days, and treatment may actually increase the rate of symptomatic relapse and prolong fecal carriage of the organism. Therefore, treatment of *Salmonella* enteritis should be avoided except in cases of enteric fever (caused by *S. typhi* and the paratyphoid strains) or in situations where metastatic foci of infection, such as meningitis, have appeared. Some authorities also believe that all cases of febrile *Salmonella* enteritis in infants younger than 3 months of age should be treated to prevent complications of bacteremia. Most cases of *Salmonella* bacteremia in normal hosts are transient and do not require therapy. However, all bacteremic children younger than 12 months of age and all individuals with bacteremia caused by *Salmonella choleraesuis* should receive therapy because they appear to be at greater risk for progressive disease. Ampicillin (intravenously or orally) and amoxicillin (orally) are appropriate therapeutic choices, but drug resistance is common, particularly in *Salmonella* infections that are acquired abroad. Chloramphenicol has been commonly used in therapy of typhoid fever, and recent data suggest that intravenous ceftriaxone (Rocephin, 75 mg per kg in children and 3 to 4 grams in adults once daily) is also effective for this illness.

Shigella and *Campylobater* organisms also produce an inflammatory diarrhea, which is usually self-limited. The choice of antibiotic for treatment of persistent or severe cases of *Shigella* enteritis depends on susceptibility testing, but oral trimethoprim-sulfamethoxazole (Bactrim, Septra), 160 mg/800 mg or 10 mg per kg/50 mg per kg twice daily for 5 days, is usually effective. *Campylobacter* species are susceptible to erythromycin, but treatment may not alter the clinical course. Enteroinvasive strains of *Escherichia coli* produce a similar clinical illness, particularly in travelers, and can also be treated with trimethoprim-sulfamethoxazole if desired. Verotoxin-producing strains of *E. coli*, such as serotype 0157:H7, can cause a hemorrhagic colitis that is usually self-limited but has been associated with the hemolytic-uremic syndrome and thrombotic thrombocytopenic purpura. *Yersinia enterocolitica* can also cause inflammatory diarrhea, but treatment is not usually necessary.

Although not common in North America, the prototype food-borne secretory diarrhea is cholera, which is caused by *Vibrio cholerae*, and is characterized by profuse, watery diarrhea resolving over the course of 4 to 7 days. The mainstay of therapy for secretory diarrheas is aggressive fluid replacement, which can usually be done orally. Antibiotic treatment with tetracycline, 250 mg every 6 hours for 5 days, or trimethoprim-sulfamethoxazole, may shorten the clinical course. Strains of *E. coli* that produce heat-stable or heat-labile toxins can produce a similar, less severe illness, and Norwalk and other 27-nm viruses, *Vibrio vulnificus*, and *Vibrio parahaemolyticus* are increasingly implicated in diarrheal outbreaks related to seafood ingestion. The illnesses are self-limited in otherwise healthy hosts.

Two other causes of infectious diarrhea deserve comment. *Listeria monocytogenes* infection can be acquired via milk products or raw vegetables and can cause disseminated disease in otherwise healthy hosts as well as in immunocompromised individuals. For serious illness, ampicillin is the drug of choice. Finally, a chronic diarrhea syndrome has been reported in some areas after consumption of raw milk. No specific etiology has been identified, and the syndrome does not appear to be altered by treatment with various antibiotics. Dietary history is the key to diagnosis of this syndrome.

NEUROTOXIC SYNDROMES

In this group of food-borne illnesses, neurologic symptoms are the most prominent clinical features. Botulism is a relatively uncommon intoxication that occurs in two forms. In adults, a syndrome develops several hours to days after ingestion of preformed *Clostridium botulinum* toxin in food, usually from spores contaminating canned goods. Early symptoms of nausea, vomiting, dry mouth, and weakness are followed by signs of peripheral nerve weakness, usually involving ocular function. Weakness of extremities and respiratory compromise can develop. In infants, a similar syndrome develops not from ingestion of preformed toxin but rather from generation of toxin within the gastrointestinal tract, presumably from ingestion of *C. botulinum* spores contained in honey or from other environmental sources. Symptoms are similar to those in adults, with constipation being an early finding. Support of respiratory function is the most important therapy. Removal of existing toxin by cathartics (in infants and adults) and by emesis or lavage (in adults) may be useful. Use of antimicrobial therapy is controversial, and some authorities believe that release of toxin could be increased with penicillin therapy in infant botulism. Therapy with trivalent equine *C. botulinum* antitoxin is indicated for adult botulism but has no role for treatment of infants. Antitoxin can be obtained from the Centers for Disease Control (telephone 404–639–3753 weekdays and 404–639–3311 at other times).

Ingestion of certain varieties of mushrooms can produce various neurologic syndromes. Certain species of *Inocybe* and *Clitocybe* mushrooms contain muscarine and within minutes after ingestion can produce a parasympathetic syndrome of sweating, salivation, miosis, blurred vision, lacrimation, rhinorrhea, and abdominal cramps. Treatment is usually not necessary, although atropine can be of benefit. Consumption of members of the psilocybin group of mushrooms produces a state of emtional lability, incoherent speech, and visual disturbances or hallucinations, whereas *Amanita muscaria* and *Amanita pantherina* produce a state of alternating drowsiness and elation with delirium. Onset of symptoms is also rapid. Children may react unpredictably or more severely to these intoxications. Only symptomatic treatment and reassurance are needed for management.

Ingestion of contaminated seafood can also result in predominantly neurologic syndromes. Ciguatera poisoning is the most common of these syndromes and is caused by a toxin produced by the dinoflagellate *Gambierdiscus toxicus*. This organism is passed up the marine food chain to large predatory fish, such as the amberjack, red snapper, barracuda, grouper, sea bass, king mackerel, and many others. Risk of ciguatera intoxication is highest from reef-feeding fish in areas where the dinoflagellate has proliferated. Common sources of North American cases are Hawaii, south Florida, and the Caribbean, but reports have also originated from the north Atlantic coast. Symptoms usually begin 3 to 5 hours after ingestion, although this time is highly variable. Patients initially experience minor gastrointestinal symptoms followed by paresthesias, pruritus, and cholinergic or anticholinesterase-like manifestations. Later, cold-to-hot sensory reversal can occur and provide a clue to the diagnosis. Ciguatoxin is toxic to sodium channels of cells and may be the pathophysiologic mechanism of this disease. Many different types of therapies have been attempted, with no conclusive benefits yet demonstrated. Recently, treatment with intravenous mannitol in 24 patients and oral tocainide (Tonocard) in 3 patients resulted in improvement, but experience with these modalities is still minimal.

Paralytic shellfish poisoning results from ingestion of bivalve and gastropod mollusks such as clams, oysters, mussels, and scallops that have ingested the dinoflaggelates *Protogonyaulax catenella* or *P. tamarensis* and, in North America, is most common along the Pacific coast. Symptoms usually begin within 30 minutes and include circumoral paresthesia, cranial nerve and cerebellar dysfunction, and paralysis. Treatment is supportive, although removal of toxin by lavage, hemodialysis, and charcoal hemoperfusion has been reported. Patients usually recover if respiratory failure does not supervene. Neurotoxic shellfish poisoning is associated with ingestion of clams and oysters carrying a toxin from the dinoflagellate *Ptychodiscus brevis*. In the United States, cases have been reported from the west coast of Florida. Symptoms appear rapidly and again involve circumoral paresthesia, which progresses to other areas of the body. Cerebellar dysfunction and seizures may also be prominent. Therapy is supportive, and recovery is the rule.

Puffer fish poisoning is being seen more in the United States because of the increasing popularity of this risky culinary experience. Puffer fish is considered to be a delicacy in Japan and other areas, but skilled preparation is required to remove large amounts of a tetrodotoxin that is present in the liver and roe. Symptoms of dysesthesias, paralysis, and respiratory failure are seen, although mortality may be higher than that for paralytic shellfish poisoning. Treatment is supportive.

ANAEROBIC AND NECROTIZING INFECTIONS INCLUDING GAS GANGRENE

method of
WESLEY FURSTE, M.D.,
NERI M. KANDAWALLA, M.D., and
JAMES N. PARSONS, M.D.
Ohio State University
Columbus, Ohio

PROPHYLAXIS

Prophylaxis of anerobic and necrotizing infections (Tables 1 and 2) requires optimal, meticulous surgical technique and the indicated use of antibiotics. Table 1 consists of diagnoses that have been reported in the literature or that have been used in clinical practice. Closely related diagnoses are grouped together. Table 1 is more for retrospective than prospective use, inasmuch as the most important considerations in these infections are (1) determination, by surgical exploration, of the extent of necrotic tissue, (2) removal of this tissue, (3) production of an aerobic environment, and (4) supportive and adjunctive therapy.

Surgical Wound Care. The most effective prevention of the precipitating anaerobic conditions continues to be early and adequate wound care. Such surgical care includes wide incision, thorough debridement of all devitalized and potentially devitalized tissues, removal of contaminating dirt and all foreign bodies, and effective drainage. Adequate débridement is especially important in irregular deep wounds in which there are loculations and recesses that favor growth of anaerobic bacteria. Dead and devitalized tissues and foreign bodies must be removed at the time of the initial operation. In war wounds and in wounds for which treatment has been inordinately delayed, thorough débridement should be coupled with delayed surgical closure of the wound. The wound should be left open from 4 to 7 days after the débridement, and then delayed surgical closure should be accomplished if the wound has remained clean and shows no evidence of infection.

These surgical principles should be observed when elective surgery is performed for lesions of any of the body cavities or of the extremities.

Antibiotics. Antibiotic therapy is of prophylactic value when combined with proper surgical procedures. Experimental and clinical experience affirms this principle but indicates that antibiotic therapy alone cannot be relied on to prevent the

TABLE 1. **Diagnoses of Anaerobic and Necrotizing Infections, Including Gas Gangrene**

A. Deep infections with muscle involvement and with or without abscess
  1. Gas gangrene
      a. Gas gangrene resulting from soft tissue trauma; clostridial myositis; clostridial myonecrosis
      b. Abdominal wall gas gangrene; postoperative clostridial sepsis of the abdominal wall; clostridial myonecrosis of the abdominal wall
      c. Metastatic gas gangrene; gas gangrene without a visible wound; nontraumatic gas gangrene
      d. Uterine clostridial infections
      e. Gas gangrene of the heart
      f. Gas gangrene of the brain
  2. Streptococcal myositis; anaerobic streptococcal myonecrosis; anaerobic streptococcal myositis
  3. Infected vascular gas gangrene; nonclostridial gas gangrene; nonclostridial myositis
  4. Synergistic necrotizing sepsis; synergistic necrotizing cellulitis*
B. Superficial infections with or without abscess
  1. Hemolytic streptococcal gangrene
  2. Acute, infectious, staphylococcal gangrene
  3. Anaerobic cellulitis; crepitant phlegmon; clostridial cellulitis
  4. Necrotizing fasciitis*; synergistic gangrene; nonclostridial anaerobic cellulitis; anaerobic cutaneous gangrene; Fournier's gangrene†
  5. Panophthalmitis
C. Simple clostridial contamination of wounds
D. Infiltration or injection or aspiration of gas into wounds
  1. Wounds with gas not produced by bacteria
  2. Injection of gas into wounds
      a. Therapy (H₂O₂)
      b. Pranksters' jokes
      c. Malingerers
      d. Psychiatric problems
  3. Aspiration and dissemination of air into wounds by muscular activity
E. Gas in tissues after industrial accidents
  1. Magnesiogenous pneumagranuloma
F. Gas in tissues after injections of chemicals
  1. Injection of drugs
  2. Accidental injection of a foreign agent
      a. Benzene

*These are similar infections but are in different locations.
†If there is extension to the tissues of the abdominal wall below the deep fascia, such as the anterior sheath of the rectus muscle, Fournier's gangrene is a synergistic necrotizing sepsis rather than just a necrotizing fasciitis.

occurrence of clostridial myositis. Penicillin G, clindamycin, metronidazole, chloramphenicol, and the cephalosporins are effective against most strains of *Clostridium perfringens* (Table 3).

Penicillin G administered intravenously in doses of 1 to 2 million units every 4 hours is the antibiotic of choice, to be used in conjunction with adequate surgical intervention for the prevention of gas gangrene. Massive doses of penicillin can prolong the period during which surgical intervention short of amputation can be effective.

Antitoxins. Gas gangrene antitoxins have no place in the prophylaxis of gas gangrene.

There may be multiple species of clostridia involved, each requiring a specific antitoxin for neutralization of its exotoxin. Moreover, the antitoxin cannot be distributed to neutralize the exotoxin being produced in the nonviable, avascular tissue involved. In addition, there are often significant reactions to the large amounts of antitoxin that have been recommended. Large series of cases have not unequivocally proved the desirability of prophylactic gas gangrene antitoxin.

Even more important than such considerations, however, are studies of the hemolytic action of *C. perfringens* alpha-toxin. It has been shown that the amount of hemolysis has a high correlation with the phospholipase C activity of the toxin. In addition, the influence of such factors as enzyme concentration and concentration of red blood cells has been studied. The problem with the previous data was that the analyses were performed on only a qualitative basis. Ikezawa, however, used enzyme kinetics to study the mechanism of hemolysis by *C. perfringens* alpha-toxin. His work was of special interest with regard to the role of antitoxin.

As a summary of Ikezawa's work, it may be stated that (1) when antitoxin is added before the EMS complex is formed, the result is complete inhibition of lysis, (2) only partial inhibition is observed when antitoxin is added after the EMS complex is formed, and (3) the calcium ion is essential for the hemolytic reaction.

Hyperbaric Oxygen Therapy. Hyperbaric oxygen therapy remains experimental and unproved as a prophylactic therapeutic measure in gas gangrene. Experimental evidence indicates that it has little value without adequate surgical debridement.

THERAPY

For proper treatment, there must be an accurate diagnosis with respect to which tissues are involved and the types of bacteria and their drug sensitivities. Deep and spreading infections may require mutilating operations; superficial and localized infections may require only multiple incisions; and pure gas infiltrations and contaminations may require only diagnostic incisions. The extent and depth of a gas-forming infection are easily and—relatively safely—determined by longitudinal incisions of the skin, superficial fascia, and deep fascia.

An immediate Gram's stain provides a rapid determination of the type of bacteria, and subsequent culture and sensitivity tests can yield a more definitive bacterial identification for decisions about subsequent antibiotic therapy.

The major goals of treatment in a soft tissue

TABLE 2. **Microorganisms Reported to Produce Gas in Human Tissues**

Gram's Stain Result	Aerobes	Anaerobes

Gram-positive		Cocci
		   Peptostreptococcus (anaerobic *Streptococcus*)
		     (usually with group A *Streptococcus*
		     [*Streptococcus pyogenes*, beta-hemolytic
		     Streptococcus] or *Staphylococcus aureus*)
		Bacilli
		   Clostridium perfringens and other clostridia

Gram-negative	Bacilli
	   Escherichia coli
	   Klebsiella pneumoniae
	   Enterobacter species
	   Proteus species
	   (all usually in mixed infections)
		Bacilli
		   Bacteroides fragilis (usually with other anaerobic gram-negative bacilli)

infection include (1) complete removal of necrotic tissue, (2) limitation of the spread of infection, (3) control of bacteremia, (4) correction of deficits of fluid and electrolytes, and (5) prevention of organ failure (e.g., renal and cardiac).

Radical Surgical Wound Care. Treatment should be initiated as soon as a clinical diagnosis is established. Optimally, treatment consists of multiple incisions for decompression and drainage of the fascial compartments, excision of the involved muscles, or open amputation when necessary, followed by immobilization of the affected part. *Early and meticulous operation is the primary and most effective means of treating clostridial myositis.* If the diagnosis is made early, while the gangrene is relatively localized, radical

TABLE 3. **Antibiotic Treatment of Anaerobic and Necrotizing Infections Based on Gram's Stain Results, Cultures, and Sensitivity Tests**

Gram's Stain Result	Presumptive Microorganism	Antibiotics
Gram-positive cocci	Anaerobic *Streptococcus*	Penicillin G Clindamycin Metronidazole Chloramphenicol Cephalosporins
Gram-positive bacilli	*Clostridium* species	Penicillin G Clindamycin Metronidazole Chloramphenicol Cephalosporins
Gram-negative bacilli	*Bacteroides* species	Clindamycin Metronidazole Cefoxitin Chloramphenicol Ticarcillin Mezlocillin
	Coliforms	Gentamicin Tobramycin Amikacin Cephalosporins Ampicillin Ticarcillin Mezlocillin Chloramphenicol

decompression of the involved fascial compartments by extensive longitudinal incisions and excision of infected muscle usually arrests the progress of infection and eliminates the need for amputation. If the diagnosis is delayed and made when the process is extensive and has caused irreversible gangrenous changes, open amputation of the guillotine type becomes necessary.

Gas gangrene of the abdominal wall or perineum presents special problems, but the same surgical principles apply. *Multiple incisions, fasciotomy,* and *extirpation of* as much *involved tissue* as is technically feasible should be undertaken.

Marlex, Mersilene, and Prolene mesh may be used for temporary and permanent containment of abdominal viscera after extensive clostridial myonecrosis of the abdominal wall. Débridement is carried out through parallel incisions with maximum preservation of skin and subcutaneous tissues. Mesh is used temporarily until the infection is completely controlled. The mesh is then removed, and the skin and subcutaneous tissues are reapproximated. Such a procedure gives excellent wound coverage and markedly shortens the hospital stay.

On occasion, a postabortal infection may be caused by *C. perfringens*. Women infected with this organism may be critically ill with bacteremia, shock, and renal failure. Parenteral antibiotic therapy and heroic measures, such as peritoneal dialysis or hemodialysis, may be necessary. Hysterectomy is also often indicated.

In contrast to deep and anaerobic infections, treatment of superficial infections may require only debridement of the wound. Devitalized tissues must be excised. When the infection extends along fascial planes beyond the traumatized area of the wound, long incisions must be made to open these areas and to excise the necrotic fascia. After débridement, the wounds should be copiously irrigated with antibiotic isotonic solutions, such as 0.1 per cent cefazolin in normal saline solution, before a dressing is loosely applied. Such wounds are obviously not closed primarily.

Antibiotics. These drugs add much to the successful care of patients with gas-forming infections. The selection of optimal antibiotic therapy depends on identification of the pathogens involved.

Major considerations in anaerobic bacteriology include proper specimen collection, immediate transport to the laboratory, and prompt inoculation and placement of the specimen under aerobic and anaerobic conditions. Special collection and transport methods to ensure the survival of even the most fastidious anaerobic organisms should be instituted, such as the following:

1. The syringe technique can be effective in the case of abscess. The skin is decontaminated, and pus is removed with a needle and syringe. All air is eliminated, the needle is inserted into a cork or rubber stopper, and the specimen is carried promptly to the laboratory, where it must be processed immediately.

2. Specimens can be collected in rubber-stoppered tubes that have been gassed with CO_2 or N_2.

3. Transport systems containing reducing agents that help to maintain a low oxidation-reduction potential are commercially available.

It is important to remember in the interpretation of the smear and the culture that the presence of gram-positive rods or other organisms in either smear or culture does *not necessarily* indicate that *infection* is present. Colonization of uninfected wounds by microorganisms is not uncommon. The clinical picture should be considered before the institution of unwarranted antimicrobial therapy. Although an infection occasionally develops in these contaminated lesions, in most cases thorough cleaning and débridement will suffice.

Antimicrobial drugs are useful in the management of patients with soft tissue infections. These drugs limit the spread of infection within the tissues and are critical in the treatment of bacteremia. Note, however, that antibiotics used without adequate surgical measures often cannot control these infections, and their use must be coupled with the other modalities outlined.

Major considerations in the selection of antimicrobial agents include a knowledge of the bacterial pathogens involved and their antibiotic susceptibilities, the patient's sensitivity to antibiotics (e.g., penicillin allergy), and factors such as hepatic or renal insufficiency, which may affect drug metabolism and excretion.

The initial choice of an antibiotic should be based on the findings of the gram-stained smear of wound exudate, with therapy later modified as indicated by the results of the culture and sensitivity tests. Because these infections are often mixed and contain both aerobic and anaerobic organisms, more than one antibiotic is frequently necessary. Antibiotics are given intravenously and in high doses.

Table 3 gives the antibiotics commonly used in the management of necrotizing soft tissue infections but does not include all available antibiotics. By using Gram's stain as a guide, patients with a large number of gram-positive bacilli or gram-positive cocci in chains can be treated with penicillin G, 3 to 4 million units intravenously every 4 hours. *C. perfringens* is often isolated from these lesions. Patients who are allergic to penicillin may be given intravenous therapy with clindamycin, 600 mg every 6 hours, chloramphenicol, 12.5 mg per kg every 6 hours, or metronidazole, 500 mg every 6 hours.

For patients from whom a gram-stained smear of exudate shows pleomorphic gram-negative bacilli or pale gram-negative rods with tapered ends, clindamycin, chloramphenicol, or metronidazole may be selected. *Bacteroides* species and fusobacteria are often cultured in these cases.

When multiple morphologic forms are seen by Gram's stain—as in many cases—a combination of penicillin and chloramphenicol or a combination of clindamycin and an aminoglycoside is often effective.

Aminoglycosides that are used include gentamicin, tobramycin, and amikacin. The intravenous dose of gentamicin and tobramycin is 1.5 to 1.7 mg per kg every 8 hours, and that for amikacin is 7.5 mg per kg every 12 hours. Aminoglycoside serum levels should be monitored to ensure adequate therapy and reduce toxicity, particularly in patients with impaired or changing renal function.

If gentamicin-resistant strains of *Pseudomonas* are present, tobramycin, 1.5 to 1.7 mg per kg every 8 hours intravenously, or amikacin, 7.5 mg per kg every 12 hours intravenously, may be used.

These recommendations are guidelines. Other agents with broad activity against aerobic and anaerobic bacteria are also available. These agents include broad-spectrum penicillins and first-, second-, and third-generation cephalosporins. Because of some gaps in coverage, these drugs should be reserved for use against isolates with known antibiotic susceptibility. In addition, the aminoglycosides and metronidazole have no activity against anaerobic or aerobic bacteria, respectively, and must be used together with another agent in mixed aerobic-anaerobic infections.

Because the degree of activity of antibiotics is not always predictable, it is important to collect specimens for culture before starting antibiotic therapy. Such information may be used later to choose the most appropriate antibiotic. The selection and dose of an antibiotic depend on the clinical setting, the isolated pathogen or pathogens, and specific host features that may modify response and toxicity. Final therapy will be determined largely by these factors and especially by the culture and sensitivity results.

Antitoxin. Antitoxin therapy is not recommended for the reasons already given in the section on prophylaxis.

Hyperbaric Oxygen. The administration of hyperbaric oxygen is controversial. Good results have been reported in certain medical centers. The following factors, however, must be considered: (1) oxygen penetrates poorly into necrotic tissue; (2) there are certain associated hazards, such as oxygen toxicity with disorientation and convulsions; (3) seriously ill patients are difficult to manage in a hyperbaric oxygen chamber; and (4) the apparatus is frequently not available. When this treatment is used, 100 per cent oxygen at 3 atmospheres pressure for 1 to 2 hours at 8-hour intervals is recommended. One salient advantage of hyperbaric oxygen is that the involved tissues quickly become demarcated so that the extent of resection is readily apparent. Hyperbaric oxygen treatment may be worthwhile for a patient with gas gangrene before radical excisional surgery, *provided the apparatus is reasonably convenient and provided there is no delay in the indicated and necessary surgical intervention.*

Tetanus Prophylaxis. For all wounds, the best possible tetanus prophylaxis—including, when indicated, the administration of adsorbed tetanus toxoid and/or tetanus immune globulin—is to be effected. *Although gas gangrene is a complication primarily of severe wounds, tetanus may occur after wounds of any size and even in individuals in whom no wound can be demonstrated.*

Adequate Supportive Therapy. The general supportive measures of value in the management of gas gangrene include maintenance of satisfactory hematocrit levels, monitoring of the fluid and electrolyte balance, adequate immobilization of the infected and injured parts, respiratory and ventilatory therapy, and relief of pain. Blood or blood product transfusions may be necessary to correct the profound anemia with which this condition is frequently associated; such transfusions are one of the mainstays of postoperative management. Plasma is usually reserved for the correction of coagulation factor deficiencies seen with disseminated intravascular coagulation. Platelet transfusions may also be necessary.

Exchange Transfusions. Exchange transfusion is another technique advocated for cases with hemolysis caused by the toxemia. This approach has been used in uterine and abdominal wall gas gangrene. It is a measure of desperation, which has not been proved to be effective in controlled trials.

Control of Renal Failure. Hemodialysis or peritoneal dialysis may be needed to control renal insufficiency related to septic shock or rhabdomyolysis, the latter being characterized by elevation of serum creatine kinase levels.

Secondary Operative Procedures. Secondary operative procedures to facilitate healing of the wound and normal function of the extremity should be performed as indicated. These procedures should obviously be postponed until after the infection has been brought completely under control.

INFLUENZA

method of
ROBERT F. BETTS, M.D.
*University of Rochester School of Medicine
and Dentistry
Rochester, New York*

Influenza is caused by two types of influenza virus, Type A and Type B. The former occurs almost every year, whereas the latter occurs every 4 to 6 years. Influenza A has hemagglutinin and neuraminidase antigens on its surface. Three major hemagglutinins (H1, H2, and H3) and two major neuraminidase types are recognized. Combinations of these make up separate viruses. During the last few years, H1N1 and H3N2 subtypes have been recognized to circulate either in the same year together or separately in different years, often interspersed with Type B or concomitantly with Type B.

Three pieces of evidence make the diagnosis highly likely. Influenza almost always strikes in seasonal outbreaks, and the first type of evidence is virologic proof through laboratory means indicating that influenza is in the community. The second is epidemiologic evidence that influenza is present, that is, excess absenteeism from work and school. The third is the presence of specific symptoms and signs in the patient, with myalgia, cough, and headache predominating.

PREVENTION

Prevention of influenza is the major means of control. The currently available vaccines, which should be administered in the fall, are safe and effective, and their widespread use for high-risk individuals can provide important protection.

Vaccines provide benefit as soon as 10 days after administration. Vaccines should also be given to health care workers because nosocomial influenza is an important cause of increased mortality, and patients acquire infection from nurses and doctors who have not been immunized.

However, the use of vaccines falls short of the mark for control of influenza, for at least three reasons. First, and by far the most important, the majority of high-risk subjects either do not seek out or do not accept vaccine that is available. Second, not all subjects develop protective immunity after vaccine administration. This is especially true when the circulating strain drifts away from the antigen that is contained in the vaccine. Third, in the years when a completely new surface antigen type (antigenic shift) appears, vaccine for the old type of virus is ineffective, and vaccine for the new type cannot be produced with sufficient speed to be available. Examples of this occurred in 1957 when H2N2 first appeared, and in 1968 when H3N2 appeared.

One other method of control of influenza is the use of daily prophylactic amantadine hydrochloride (Symmetrel) or the soon to be marketed rimantadine hydrochloride (Flumadine). One potential benefit of the use of these drugs is the prevention of acute influenza. Prophylaxis may be useful in two settings: first, for the family members of a patient with clinical influenza, preventive drug treatment could be used for the 5 to 7 days after onset of the index case; second, for the high-risk subject who is vaccinated when it is likely that influenza has already appeared locally and before protective immunity develops. In both of these instances, duration of prophylaxis and therefore duration of risk can be shortened (Table 1). However, under most circumstances, to prevent influenza, a drug must be taken each day during the duration of the influenza season, usually a period of 4 to 6 weeks. It has been assumed that because amantadine is effective in young people prophylactically, it will be useful in the high-risk elderly. There are no available data to confirm or deny this conclusion; the frequency of side effects in young subjects is similar to the maximum influenza attack rate that has been described in the vaccinated elderly. Perhaps rimantadine, with its virtual absence of side effects in young subjects, will offer a lower risk/benefit ratio in the elderly. Carefully conducted studies of each of these compounds in the target population will be necessary to define their role.

TREATMENT

Although most of the studies showing the benefit of therapy have been conducted in young adults, the evidence that the duration of the influenza syndrome can be shortened by treatment is commanding. There is also evidence that dysfunction of small airways, which occurs and progresses during 2 weeks in untreated influenza, can be blocked or at least shortened by such therapy. There is reason to believe that similar results would be achievable in high-risk populations. It is important to recognize that with appropriate clinical symptoms and influenza in the community, the clinician need not and should not wait for virologic proof in each patient to initiate therapy. Treatment is most beneficial if it is started early, so to wait for confirmation would render treatment much less effective.

Amantadine hydrochloride is the only approved specific anti-influenza agent, although rimantadine hydrochloride will soon be available. These drugs probably impart their antiviral effect by blocking uncoating of the virus. Concentrations that are achievable in serum will, if used in vitro, inhibit synthesis of virus in tissue culture. Although the evidence is limited, it appears that 100 mg per day of either rimantadine or amantadine has less antiviral effect than 200 mg per day, but the meaning of this from a clinical standpoint is unknown. Dosage recommendations for treatment with either of these drugs can be made (Table 1) on the basis of the knowledge that both drugs are cleared by renal excretion and that therapy is necessary for only a few (5 to 7) days. If a young child is being treated, 6.6 mg per kg up to 200 mg per day is used (Table 1) (150 mg per day should not be exceeded in children 9 years old or younger).

There is also limited but convincing evidence that fever is reduced within 10 to 12 hours of initiation of antipyretic therapy, compared with 24 hours if antiviral medication is used alone. Despite the more rapid defervescence shown with aspirin and presumably acetaminophen, the overall feeling of well-being is improved more rapidly with antiviral than with antipyretic therapy.

TABLE 1. **Dosage Schedule for Antivirals in Patients by Age, Weight, and Renal Function**

Parameter	Dose (mg)	
	Days 1–2	Days 3–7*
Age ≥ 70 yr	200	100
Age < 70 yr	200	200
Weight < 50 kg	200	100
Creatinine		
≤1.4†	200	200
1.5–3.0	200	100 on even days (4, 6)
≥3.1	200 on day 1	100 on days 3, 6, 9,* 12*

*Dosage schedule can be continued until day 14 for high-risk subjects after vaccination.

†Age or weight takes precedence.

Pulmonary function is not improved by antipyretics. Therefore, logic dictates that acetaminophen in an appropriate dose be taken along with the antiviral medication at the onset of symptoms. Thereafter, the antipyretic should be taken twice at 4-hour intervals and then discontinued while use of the antiviral is maintained. In addition, fluid intake should be increased appropriately to replace losses caused by fever. Bed rest should be prescribed as needed. Prophylactic antibiotics should not be used because there is no evidence that they prevent secondary bacterial infection.

COMPLICATIONS

Most cases of pneumonia after influenza virus infection are caused by bacteria as a secondary process. Some patients, however, have pure viral pneumonia. The bacteriology of pneumonia after influenza is somewhat different from that of most cases of community-acquired pneumonia. Experience has demonstrated that in addition to pneumococcal disease, pneumonia caused by *Staphylococcus aureus, Haemophilus influenzae,* and Enterobacteriaceae can follow influenza. Often these infections can be controlled only by parenteral antibiotic therapy, and hospitalization is required.

The spectrum of empiric therapy for secondary bacterial pneumonia after influenza should include all of these possible bacteria. A drug such as cefotaxime (Claforan), with appropriate spectrum to match the possible causes, should be considered. Otherwise, a combination of antibiotics is necessary. If the pneumonia has the characteristics of primary viral pneumonia, an antiviral should be used as well, although proof of its efficacy in this setting is lacking. Once sputum cultures are mature, the antibiotic regimen should be narrowed to the specific agent that has been identified. The severe consequences of the infection, including fever and hypoxia, which may aggravate cardiac disease and produce heart failure and arrhythmias, probably contribute in a major way to the excess mortality seen in those individuals with heart or lung disease during influenza outbreaks. Administration of oxygen and control of the heart failure and arrhythmias are essential in these cases.

In young children the major complication of influenza is Reye's syndrome, which occurs more commonly after influenza B than after influenza A. To reduce the incidence of Reye's syndrome, use of acetaminophen rather than aspirin is recommended.

LEISHMANIASIS

method of
DANIEL M. GORDON, M.D.
Walter Reed Army Institute of Research
Washington, D.C.

The term "leishmaniasis" refers to a group of zoonotic diseases caused by protozoan parasites of the genus *Leishmania.* There are two major clinical syndromes caused by these protozoa: visceral leishmaniasis and cutaneous leishmaniasis. Cutaneous leishmaniasis has traditionally been further divided into two additional syndromes, Old World cutaneous leishmaniasis and New World cutaneous leishmaniasis, on the basis of geographic, parasitologic, and clinical aspects.

Leishmania organisms are transmitted to humans by the bite of sandflies. As the fly obtains a blood meal, the motile, flagellated promastigote is introduced into the vertebrate host. Once inside the host, the promastigotes invade reticuloendothelial (RE) cells, where they transform into the nonflagellated amastigote form. Amastigotes multiply by binary fission, eventually rupturing the host's RE cell, which releases varying numbers of daughter amastigotes that then invade other RE cells. Reinvasion may occur locally or amastigotes may be distributed by the blood stream to regional or systemic components of the RE system. Sandflies feeding on infected individuals ingest parasitized RE cells. Ingested amastigotes transform into the flagellated promastigote form, which reproduces by binary fission and eventually migrates to the anterior portion of the midgut, the esophagus, and the head of the insect host, thus completing the cycle.

CLINICAL SYNDROMES

Visceral leishmaniasis, also known as kala-azar, which is Hindi meaning black fever, is a chronic infection of the spleen, liver, and bone marrow that is caused by *Leishmania donovani.* It occurs in the Mediterranean Basin, India, Pakistan, China, southern Russia, Central and South America, northeastern Brazil, and Africa, primarily in a band between the Tropic of Cancer and the equator. Various species of sandflies serve as vectors, with humans, dogs, foxes, and perhaps rodents serving as reservoir hosts depending on the subspecies of *Leishmania* and the vector involved. Visceral leishmaniasis typically has a long incubation period, generally from 2 to 6 months after the primary skin lesion, which is usually just a small papule and is often not remembered. During the incubation period, patients may notice the gradual onset of low-grade intermittent fevers, malaise, and vague abdominal discomfort associated with an enlarging liver and spleen. Initially, patients may maintain a good appetite, but eventually weighted loss ensues. By the time the infection has become well established, hepatosplenomegaly, lymphadenopathy, fevers, cachexia, and pancytopenia are often found. Frequently, especially in light-skinned people, one finds a darkening of the skin (hence the name kala-azar). One may also find peripheral edema, trophic changes of the hair, ecchymoses, epistaxis, and diarrhea. The major pathologic findings in this disease reflect the multiplication of parasites in cells of the RE system. Hepatosplenomegaly and lymphadenopathy are caused by marked hyperplasia of the RE cells, which are filled with amastigotes. The bone marrow is another site where parasitized RE cells are found relatively easily. Parasites have also been reported in the RE cells in the gastrointestinal tract. In severe infections, parasitized histiocytes may be seen in almost any organ. One of the most common laboratory abnormalities noted with visceral leishmaniasis is anemia, which is attributed to bone marrow depression, at times coexisting iron deficiency, and decreased erythrocyte survival related to hypersplenism. Other hematologic abnormalities include thrombocytopenia and leukopenia, primarily related to neurotropenia, with relative lymphocytosis. Eosinophilia is not seen with visceral leishmaniasis; in fact, eosinophils are almost completely absent. Mild elevations in serum transaminase levels with normal bilirubin levels are common, as are moderate prolongations of the prothrombin time and decreases in the serum albumin levels. It is not unusual to find a polyclonal hypergammaglobulinemia.

The differential diagnosis of visceral leishmaniasis varies somewhat with the stage of the disease and may include malaria, African trypanosomiasis, schistosomiasis, brucellosis, typhoid fever, histoplasmosis, tuberculosis, and bacterial endocarditis, as well as other noninfectious diseases such as chronic myelocytic leukemia, lymphomas (including Hodgkin's disease), multiple myeloma, Waldenström's macroglobulinemia, sarcoidosis, and cirrhosis. Although complement fixation tests with either *L. donovani* or *Mycobacterium phlei* (because of its cross-reacting antigens) have been used in the past to suggest the diagnosis of visceral leishmaniasis, these tests have largely been replaced by the indirect fluorescent antibody test with promastigotes as the test antigen, or an enzyme-linked immunosorbent assay with soluble promastigote antigens. These tests, however, find their primary usefulness in epidemiologic studies of leishmaniasis because definitive diagnosis of cutaneous leishmaniasis rests on the demonstration of parasites in appropriate tissue samples. Splenic aspiration is considered to be the diagnostic procedure of choice. In one study involving more than 700 splenic aspirations, parasites were demonstrated in 98 per cent of cases, with only two significant complications (intra-abdominal bleeding in two individuals, both of whom recovered without surgery). Other diagnostic procedures are less sensitive, including bone marrow, liver, or lymph node biopsy or aspirations, and buffy coat smears of whole blood.

Old World cutaneous leishmaniasis, which is also known as Oriental sore, Aleppo button, Jericho boil, Delhi boil, or bouton de Biskra, presents as nodular or ulcerative skin lesions and is caused by members of the *Leishmania tropica* complex (*L. major, L. tropica,* and *L. aethiopica*). Zoonotic infections with these parasites occur in areas of the Middle East, the Mediterranean Basin, Saudi Arabia, Russia, India, and sub-Saharan Africa. The incubation period for Old World cutaneous leishmaniasis is 2 to 8 weeks, although occasionally incubation periods as long as 3 years have been noted. The lesions vary somewhat in appearance on the basis of the infecting parasite and the immune status of the infected individual. Lesions caused by *L. major* tend to be multiple and are associated with a more pronounced inflammatory reaction, although they generally heal within a few months, often with significant scarring. Lymphatic spread may occur and may present as a linear array of subcutaneous nodules associated with regional lymphadenopathy that mimicks sporotrichosis. *L. tropica* lesions, on the other hand, tend to be single, but may last for 12 months or more before completely healing. *L. aethiopica* lesions elicit the least pronounced inflammatory response and are typically more chronic, often persisting several years before healing occurs. In rare cases of *L. aethiopica* infection, a form of disease known as diffuse cutaneous leishmaniasis (DCL) may develop. DCL begins as a single nodular lesion and eventually progresses to the development of multiple nodular lesions that involve predominantly the face, extremities, and trunk. The lesions are nonulcerating. DCL appears to be associated with a specific defect in the host's cell-mediated immune response to leishmanial antigens.

New World cutaneous leishmaniasis, or American leishmaniasis, is known by various regional names, such as espundia, uta, chiclero ulcer, úlcera de Baurú, or forest yaws, and is caused by members of the *L. mexicana* complex (*L. mexicana mexicana* and *L. mexicana amazonensis*) and the *L. braziliensis* complex (*L. braziliensis braziliensis, L. braziliensis panamensis, L. braziliensis guyanensis,* and *L. peruviana*). The primary host varies from rodents, sloths, and dogs to primates, depending on the species of *Leishmania,* with the prevalence in humans directly related to exposure to and the biting habits of the principal insect vector. For example, forest rodents are the principal vertebrate hosts for *L. braziliensis braziliensis.* The principal vector, *Lutzomyia wellcomei,* readily bites both humans and rodents and feeds during the day, unlike most species of sandflies. As a result, *L. braziliensis braziliensis* is a fairly common human pathogen. *L. mexicana amazonensis* also causes disease primarily of forest rodents. However, because its principal vector, *Lutzomyia flaviscutellata,* is nocturnal, inhabits swampy areas of the Amazon forests, and is not very anthropophilic, human infection is relatively uncommon. The incidence of *L. mexicana amazonensis* in humans may increase as an increasing number of settlers move into the Amazon forest areas to establish logging and farming communities.

The incubation period in American leishmaniasis ranges from weeks to months. The lesion typically begins as an erythematous, pruritic papule that gradually enlarges and then ulcerates. The ulcer has a raised, indurated margin and is typically painless unless it is secondarily infected. Satellite lesions may be seen, as can subcutaneous nodules, which are similar to those seen with *L. major* infection and can be confused with sporotrichosis. A significant complication of *L. braziliensis braziliensis* infection and rarely of *L. braziliensis panamensis* infection is the development of mucosal disease, mucocutaneous leishmaniasis. Nasal, pharyngeal, or buccal mucosal involvement, which may develop years after resolution of the primary cutaneous lesion, can result in severe disfigurement and, at times, death. DCL similar to that seen with *L. aethiopica* has also been reported with *L. mexicana amazonensis*. The differential diagnosis of cutaneous leishmaniasis in general includes tropical ulcer, syphilis, yaws, lupus vulgaris, blastomycosis, histoplasmosis, coccidioidomycosis, leprosy, sporotrichosis, mycobacterial infections, and malignancy.

Definitive diagnosis of cutaneous leishmaniasis again depends on identification of parasites in appropriate tissue samples. At our institution, evaluation of suspected skin lesions involves both fine-needle aspiration and a 4-mm punch biopsy. Fluid obtained from the aspirations is used for inoculation into Schneider's medium and Novy, MacNeal, and Nicolle's medium for culture. Tissue obtained by biopsy is trisected: one-third for pathologic evaluation (routine hematoxylin and eosin, periodic acid–Schiff, and silver stains), one-third for leishmanial culture, and one-third for fungal and mycobacterial culture. Because some strains of *L. braziliensis* are difficult to isolate in culture and to identify in histologic sections, we are also investigating the use of species-specific monoclonal antibodies for the identification of leishmania amastigotes in biopsy tissue as well as in cells obtained by fine-needle aspiration. Work is also being done to evaluate the utility of DNA hybridization techniques for the diagnosis of leishmaniasis.

TREATMENT

The therapeutic agents that have been studied in the treatment of both visceral and cutaneous leishmaniasis and that have been shown to be efficacious at acceptable levels of toxicity are the pentavalent antimonials sodium stibogluconate, which is available from the Wellcome Foundation, United Kingdom, as Pentostam, and meglumine antimonate, which is available from Rhone Poulenc, France, as Glucantime. The only pentavalent antimonial currently available in the United States is Pentostam (through the Centers for Disease Control [CDC] in Atlanta, Ga.; telephone number 404–639–3670). Because leishmaniasis is relatively rare in the United States, the manufacturer has never applied to the U.S. Food and Drug Administration to license this drug. As a result, this drug is available only under investigational new drug status. On the basis of efficacy and toxicity data collected during Pentostam therapy of patients with kala-azar in Kenya and elsewhere, the World Health Organization and the CDC have recommended that kala-azar be treated with 20 mg of antimony (Sb) per kg of body weight per day, with a maximum total daily dose of 850 mg of Sb, for at least 20 days, or for 2 weeks after parasitologic cure. The dose for cutaneous leishmaniasis is less well established. We completed a randomized, double-

blind trial of Pentostam administered intravenously in a single daily dose of either 10 or 20 mg of Sb per kg of body weight per day (with no upper limit of Sb) for 20 days in adult Americans with cutaneous leishmaniasis that had been acquired in Panama. In this study, 21 patients received the 10-mg dose, and 19 patients received the 20-mg dose. There was no significant increase in toxicity noted between the two groups. However, all 19 patients receiving the 20-mg dose were cured 6 weeks after completion of therapy, whereas only 16 of 21 patients (76 per cent) receiving the 10-mg dose were cured (p = 0.03). Currently at our institution, all patients with confirmed cutaneous leishmaniasis undergo a complete history and physical examination and baseline laboratory evaluation including routine serum chemistry profile, complete blood cell count with differential and platelet counts, urinalysis, and electrocardiogram. If no significant cardiac, hepatic, or renal abnormalities are discovered, patients are offered therapy with Pentostam at a dose of 20 mg per kg of body weight per day for 20 days infused via a 21-gauge butterfly needle over 15 minutes. Side effects associated with the use of the pentavalent antimonials include cardiotoxicity, as manifested by T wave flattening and/or inversion, prolongation of the QT interval, and, rarely, premature ventricular contractions. The cardiac toxicities appear to correlate with the cumulative dose of Sb administered but appear to be transient and resolve within 6 weeks after completion of therapy. Patients may complain of arthralgias, which are usually controllable with aspirin or other nonsteroidal anti-inflammatory agents.

Although Pentostam is the drug of choice for the treatment of leishmaniasis in the United States, the cost of the drug as well as the inconvenience of administration hinders extensive use in countries where leishmaniasis is more prevalent. As a result, various other treatment modalities are under investigation by several groups. Pentamidine has been reported to be useful in the treatment of kala-azar in East Africa and India. However, significant side effects that are associated with administration of the drug, such as hypotension immediately after the injection, sterile abscess formation at the site of injection, and the potential for nephrotoxicity, limit its use to cases that are unresponsive to antimonials. Limited experience with amphotericin B in the treatment of visceral leishmaniasis suggests that this drug may be useful, but here again its use will be limited by the need for parenteral administration, as well as its toxicity. Incorporation of antimony or amphotericin B into liposomes (artificial lipid particles that are predominantly phagocytosed by macrophages) appears to abrogate some of the toxicity of the drug and may offer the added benefit of targeting the drug to the primary site of infection; these preparations, however, are just now undergoing initial safety and tolerance trials in humans.

Clinical trials of oral agents for leishmaniasis are also under way. Ketoconazole, in doses ranging from 200 mg once a day to 400 mg twice a day for between 4 and 12 weeks, has been used to treat both New World and Old World cutaneous leishmaniasis. Various degrees of success have been reported and may reflect not only differences in the treatment regimen used but also differences among parasites from different areas of the world. As a result, no definitive treatment regimen for ketoconazole in cutaneous leishmaniasis has been established. Itraconazole, a related compound being evaluated for use in the treatment of New World cutaneous leishmaniasis, also has the advantage of oral administration but does not depress testosterone levels at pharmacologic doses as has been reported for ketoconazole. At present, there are no licensed oral agents that are active in visceral leishmaniasis.

Local therapy of cutaneous disease should also be mentioned, although no study has definitively demonstrated the utility of any such treatment modality. Obviously, to be considered for local therapy, the patient must have no evidence of disseminated disease. Local and regional lymphadenopathy excludes a significant number of patients from local treatment because parasites can often be isolated from these nodes. Various agents have been applied topically, ranging from caustic chemicals such as battery acid and local plant preparations to various antibiotics. Heat (either by way of a knife heated in a campfire or a more modern battery-operated heating unit that can deliver defined temperatures to a well-defined surface area and depth) and cryotherapy (with either carbon dioxide or liquid nitrogen) have also been used. Local administration of antileishmanial drugs has also been attempted. The evaluation of the various treatment modalities currently in use and the establishment of a clearly superior therapeutic modality have been severely hampered by the inherent difficulties in conducting randomized trials, which must include sufficiently large numbers of individuals and appropriate control groups, with adequate follow-up periods for the demonstration of treatment efficacy in a disease process in which there is a variable incidence of self-cure and relapse. Future progress in the treatment of leishmaniasis will depend on the diligence of investigators to conduct these difficult studies.

LEPROSY
(Hansen's Disease)

method of
JOHN R. TRAUTMAN, M.D.
Gillis W. Long Hansen's Disease Center
Carville, Louisiana

The term "Hansen's disease" (HD) is used here instead of leprosy because of a previous commitment to patients and because it is recognized by the U.S. Public Health Service.

This disease is one of the most serious infectious diseases in the world, being of major import in India, Southeast Asia, Central Africa, and South America, especially Brazil. A moderate problem exists in Mexico. There may be 12 to 15 million cases worldwide. Some 6000 cases are known in the United States, and of about 300 new cases per year more than 90 per cent are contracted in a foreign country.

Methods used to diagnose HD have changed little in recent years. Important is a family history of the disease or of citizenship in a country in which the disease is known to be endemic. Clinically, HD can imitate various cutaneous and neurologic problems. The physical examination should include a skin biopsy stained for acid-fast bacilli *(Mycobacterium leprae)*, but this may not be feasible everywhere. Attention should be paid not only to the physical characteristics of lesions but also to the presence or absence of anesthesia or hypesthesia in individual lesions or in other areas of the skin, and to any enlargement of nerves such as the great auricular, ulnar, median, radial, and posterior tibial nerves. The examination should be carried out in a setting with as much natural light as possible. In testing for cutaneous sensation, a wisp of cotton or a nylon filament may be used.

Skin smears (skin scrapings), although not as reliable for diagnosis as a skin biopsy, can provide much information. These are best performed by someone trained in the technique. The presence of acid-fast bacilli in a smear, combined with skin lesions and some degree of sensory loss, is tantamount to a diagnosis of HD; however, the absence of bacilli does not rule out the disease. The classification of HD depends in large part on the characteristics of the lesions and the number of bacilli present. Internationally popular terms are "multibacillary," which refers to HD in which one or more acid-fast bacilli can be visualized microscopically on skin smears, and "paucibacillary," which refers to HD in which no bacilli are seen on skin smears. In the latter instance, the diagnosis must be made entirely on clinical grounds. In the United States, both skin smears and biopsies are usually taken. The bacilli are counted by using a semilogarithmic scale ranging from 0 to 6+, as per the Ridley-Jopling method. In the United States, a diagnosis of HD (or leprosy) is usually confirmed by skin biopsy.

TYPES OF HANSEN'S DISEASE

The treatment regimen used depends, in large part, on the type of disease present. There are four generally recognized types:

1. *Intermediate:* Lesions are variable and often insignificant in appearance. There may be no sensory loss. It is important for the examiner to have a high index of suspicion. Skin smears are of little or no value. Biopsy reveals a somewhat nonspecific tissue response with perineural or perivascular infiltration by small, round cells and a few histiocytes. A similar infiltration may surround various skin appendages. Bacilli may be difficult to locate even on extensive searching. The finding of even one bacillus, however, is of considerable aid in making a diagnosis.

2. *Tuberculoid:* Lesions tend to be single or few and relatively large (usually 3 cm or more in diameter). Anesthesia or hypesthesia of lesions is characteristic. Biopsy reveals a granulomatous process composed primarily of lymphocytes, epitheloid cells, and occasional Langhans-type giant cells. Examination of cutaneous nerve twigs may reveal mononuclear infiltration with an occasional acid-fast bacillus; these findings are essentially diagnostic.

3. *Lepromatous:* This most disseminated type of the disease is characterized by smaller, frequently multiple, skin lesions, with anesthesia found more often in the distal extremities. There is also a diffuse type without visible discrete lesions. On biopsy, lepra cells (foam cells or Virchow's cells) filled with *M. leprae* organisms are seen. Globi, which are coalesced lepra cells, may be common.

4. *Borderline:* Formerly known as dimorphous, this type of HD is, for practical purposes, a combination of tuberculoid and lepromatous HD. The spectrum is wide, ranging from almost pure tuberculoid to almost pure lepromatous; thus are derived terms such as BT (borderline tuberculoid), BB (borderline), and BL (borderline lepromatous). Skin lesions are quite variable as is the sensory pattern. Microscopically, the findings are those of tuberculoid and lepromatous disease in various degrees.

TREATMENT

In the 1940s, treatment with chaulmoogra oil gave way to sulfone therapy. Intravenous promin (glucosulfone) was supplanted permanently by an oral sulfone called dapsone (4,4'-diaminodiphenylsulfone; Avlosulfon; DDS). In the 1960s, other drugs became available, including clofazimine (B663; Lamprene), which is a riminophenazine dye; rifampin (Rimactane; Rifadin); ethionamide (Trecator-SC); and thalidomide, which was found to be effective for a specific complication of HD. Because resistance to dapsone by *M. leprae* was a steadily increasing problem, and for logistic and economic reasons, the World Health Organization (WHO) recommended a multidrug therapy regimen for HD. In countries with the largest problems, it had proved difficult, if not impossible, to treat patients for the many years required of earlier treatment regimens. The WHO regimen is presented here first, followed by the treatment regimen recommended in the United States.

WHO Regimen

The WHO regimen for *lepromatous and borderline lepromatous HD* (multibacillary) is dapsone, 100 mg daily, and clofazimine, 50 mg daily (unsupervised), with clofazimine, 300 mg monthly, and rifampin, 600 mg monthly (supervised). Therapy is continued for at least 2 years, preferably until skin smears are negative (5 or more years). However, some leprologists use only the minimal regimen. For patients who refuse clofazimine (usually because of skin pigmentation), ethionamide, 250 to 375 mg daily, can be substituted. Caution is indicated, however, when using ethionamide because of its hepatotoxicity, especially when combined with rifampin.

The WHO regimen for *tuberculoid, borderline tuberculoid, and indeterminate HD* (paucibacillary) is dapsone, 100 mg daily (unsupervised), and rifampin, 600 mg monthly (supervised) for 6 months.

Regimen Used in the United States

In the United States and in other areas where the relatively expensive mouse footpad drug sensitivity studies are available to determine the existence of drug resistance, the recommended treatment is as follows: borderline and lepromatous HD (multibacillary): dapsone, 100 mg daily indefinitely, and rifampin, 600 mg daily for 3 years. Borderline HD (paucibacillary): dapsone, 100 mg daily for 5 years, and rifampin, 600 mg daily for 6 months. Indeterminate and tuberculoid HD (paucibacillary): dapsone, 100 mg daily for 3 years, and rifampin, 100 mg daily for 6 months.

Primary dapsone resistance is not sufficiently common to warrant triple chemotherapy in all areas of the world, although as of this writing, studies of short-term double and triple chemotherapy are planned for the United States. Mouse footpad studies require 7 to 9 months. If they indicate dapsone resistance, rifampin alone should suffice for that period, after which clofazimine, 50 mg daily, can be added and continued for the same duration as dapsone would have been prescribed. If a patient's bacilli have become resistant to both dapsone and rifampin, clofazimine plus ethionamide can be given for 3 years followed by clofazimine monotherapy.

That treatment is having a beneficial effect can be determined during the early weeks with serial skin smears. Although the bacterial index, which is the number of bacilli present using the Ridley-Jopling technique, may not change appreciably until months or years after effective chemotherapy has been initiated, the morphologic index, which represents the percentage of solid-staining or viable *M. leprae* organisms, is reduced, often within 1 to 4 weeks. If there is no improvement in the morphologic index, the physician should suspect either that the patient is not taking the medication or that the bacilli may be resistant to the drugs in use—it is assumed that the person performing the laboratory studies is trained, proficient, and consistent in his or her readings.

Other Drugs. The ansomycins (which include rifampin) all appear to have similar activities. Thiacetazone (amithiazone) is not available in the United States and thiambutosine (CIBA 1906) is no longer manufactured. Streptomycin, 1 gram three times weekly, can be of benefit, but resistance to the drug usually develops within 2 years. Otherwise, side effects and the need for it to be injected limit its use.

REACTIONS

Reactive episodes in Hansen's disease can be troublesome, from both diagnostic and therapeutic standpoints. There are two common types of reactions and an uncommon one.

Reversal Reactions. These Type 1 reactions occur in borderline HD. They are delayed hypersensitivity reactions and are thought to be cell-mediated immune responses with a shift of the disease toward the tuberculoid end of the spectrum. They may be seen occasionally in what appears clinically to be tuberculoid HD. In this reaction, existing lesions become erythematous and often edematous. The onset may be rapid and may be associated with acute peripheral neuritis, which can lead to permanent paralysis and contractures.

Erythema Nodosum Leprosum. These Type 2 reactions represent a phenomenon initiated by antigens of *M. leprae* combining with antibodies to form immune complexes with complement. Their resultant precipitation in tissue causes a reaction. The process is thought to be a humoral antibody response. Erythema nodosum leprosum (ENL) is characterized by painful erythematous nodules (but many other types of erythematous lesions may occur) with associated fever, neuritis, and often one or more other entities such as iridocyclitis, arthritis, orchitis, and glomerulonephritis. Reactive episodes probably occur to some degree in 50 per cent or more of patients with lepromatous or borderline HD.

Lucio Phenomenon. This uncommon but serious complication occurs in diffuse lepromatous HD in patients usually of Mexican ancestry. It is characterized by the development of deep cutaneous ulcers. The ulcers may coalesce and eventually involve much of the skin, leading occasionally to death.

Treatment of Reactions

As soon as possible after the diagnosis is made, the patient should be told to expect what appear to be setbacks during the treatment program. Explanations should cover the possibility of a reaction's occurring, what the patient should expect, and the fact that a reactive episode usually means that treatment is effective.

Reversal Reactions. If mild erythema and some swelling of existing lesions occur, and there is no evidence of impending ulceration or of neurologic involvement, symptomatic treatment with an analgesic is all that may be needed. Whenever rapidly developing erythema, edema, and nerve involvement appear, with or without ulceration, swift action is needed in the form of corticosteroid therapy. Prednisone, 60 to 80 mg per day, should prove to be beneficial within 1 week, after which the dose can be reduced gradually over a period of a month or so, maintained if possible at 20 to 30 mg per day for approximately 2 months (longer if clinically indicated), and then slowly withdrawn. Reactive episodes that appear to be particularly severe can be treated during the first 2 days with intramuscular corticosteroid therapy such as prednisolone (Hydeltrasol), 60 to 80 mg per day or more. Prednisone can then be substituted. Rapid therapeutic action is sometimes necessary to prevent paralysis, which can develop within hours. If there are subsequent reactions, corticosteroid therapy can again be prescribed using the lowest dosage sufficient to control the episodes.

Erythema Nodosum Leprosum. Many anti-inflammatory agents have been used in an attempt to treat ENL. Mild reactions can be treated symptomatically. At times nothing specific is required. More severe reactions can be treated for 2 to 3 weeks with prednisone, 40 to 60 mg a day for up to 1 week, after which the dose can be gradually reduced and possibly withdrawn within several weeks. Long-term corticosteroid therapy is not recommended for persistent ENL. Thalidomide* is the drug of choice for moderate to severe ENL, except in a fertile woman. Thalidomide is given in a dose of 100 mg four times daily orally for 3 days, after which the dose can be reduced to 50 to 100 mg daily at bedtime. In 3 to 10 weeks, treatment can be stopped but should be restarted at maintenance levels should the reaction recur. Repeated reactions can at times be managed each time with short courses of thalidomide. More

---

*Investigational drug in the United States.

refractory reactions may have to be treated for months or years. Severe, protracted ENL may require treatment with both corticosteroids and thalidomide. Clofazimine may also be effective for the management of chronic ENL in a dose of 200 to 300 mg per day* for 3 to 4 weeks, followed by a maintenance dose of 100 mg per day. It is not useful for control of the acute reaction.

Lucio's Phenomenon. There is no known effective therapy for this serious reaction. Treatment is similar to that given for third-degree burns. High doses of a corticosteroid may be of limited benefit but may also be a negative factor in the face of secondary infection. In severe cases the prognosis is grave.

TREATMENT OF THE EYE

A large number of problems can occur in HD that involve the eye. Most of these problems should be treated by an ophthalmologist when possible, but if none is available many patients will still require care. Diminished tearing, often coupled with diminished corneal sensitivity, can be alleviated with artificial tears (Liquifilm drops), and a bland eye ointment at night. Lepromatous iridocyclitis reactions usually require treatment with a topical mydriatic such as 1 or 2 per cent atropine and corticosteroid drops such as cortisone acetate (1.5 per cent), prednisolone (1 per cent), or dexamethasone (0.1 per cent). If the pupil is already wide open, atropine should not be used because of the possibility of coexisting primary glaucoma. The drops may need to be administered as often as hourly during the first day. Other ocular reactions such as episcleritis and scleritis should also benefit from use of topical corticosteroids. Many other ocular area problems can occur, such as lagophthalmos, entropion, and ectropion.

SIDE EFFECTS OF PRINCIPAL HD DRUGS

Dapsone. This drug, which is bacteristatic toward *M. leprae,* should not be prescribed before the presence of glucose-6-phosphate dehydrogenase deficiency has been ruled out. In areas of the world where the test is not available, dapsone should be stopped if there is any sign of significant hemolysis. Dapsone otherwise not infrequently causes a mild hemolytic anemia. Agranulocytosis is uncommon but serious. True allergy to dapsone has been reported, and the severe allergic syndrome can be fatal. At the center in Carville, however, this problem has not been

seen. Gastric intolerance is occasionally troublesome. Overall, the drug is well tolerated and safe to use, including during pregnancy.

Rifampin. Effectively and rapidly bactericidal against *M. leprae,* the drug is known to be hepatoxic and care should be exercised in its use, especially in patients with pre-existing liver disease. It has not been shown to be contraindicated during pregnancy in women, but animal studies have shown fetal abnormalities. The wisest course would be to avoid its use during pregnancy if feasible. Avoiding pregnancy is the other option. Rifampin may reduce the effectiveness of oral contraceptives and can discolor urine, sweat, and sputum.

Ethionamide. This drug appears to be bactericidal against *M. leprae,* but it can be hepatotoxic, especially when given with rifampin. Gastrointestinal tract distress may limit its use, and its safety during pregnancy has not been proved. Concomitant administration of pyridoxine is recommended to prevent neuropathy.

Clofazimine. This agent appears to be as bactericidal for *M. leprae* as dapsone, and it also has an anti-inflammatory effect that is sometimes useful for the treatment of ENL. It can cause upper and lower gastrointestinal tract distress, especially in doses higher than 50 mg per day. It produces dark pink to bluish-black skin pigmentation, especially in existing lesions, which may cause patients to refuse to use the drug. It can also cause pinkish discoloration of urine, sweat, sputum, and stools. The pigmentation and discoloration usually disappear within 1 year after treatment is stopped. Although it can cause some skin pigmentation in newborns, it is considered to be safe to use during pregnancy.

Thalidomide. Because of its proven severe teratogenic effects, its use is prohibited during pregnancy, and in fact it should never be given to a fertile woman on an outpatient basis unless she is sterilized voluntarily. In practice, the wisest course is to seek alternative therapy.

In the United States, thalidomide is obtainable only from the Gillis W. Long Hansen's Disease Center in Carville, either directly or through the medical director in charge of one of the Regional Hansen's Disease Centers that are under contract to the Carville facility. The investigational license for the drug is currently limited to these centers.

Outside the United States, thalidomide may be obtainable on an experimental basis from Chemie Gruenthal, Stothbert, Germany, or from Champion Farmacenteria, LTDA, São Paulo, Brazil.

Rehabilitation and Follow-Up

With prevention of permanent disability in mind, care of the patient after the disease is

---

*Doses above 200 mg per day are not recommended by the manufacturers.

inactivated may be just as important as the drug treatment itself. No matter how effective chemotherapy may be, many patients are often left with permanent anesthesia of hands, feet, or corneas. Close attention to activities of daily living that prevent injury to these areas are of vast importance during and after drug treatment. Special devices to prevent burning of hands while cooking or handling other hot objects, special footwear to prevent ulcerations and amputations, and periodic examination of the eyes by an ophthalmologist are all essential and provide the opportunity for patients to lead productive lives. Surgical procedures exist to help correct certain disabilities such as claw hand or drop foot.

Prophylaxis

Family contacts of patients should be examined at least once yearly for 5 years. Prophylatic sulfone therapy or vaccination with bacille Calmette-Guérin is not recommended. Vaccines are being studied in various parts of the world, but trial results will not be known until well into the 1990s.

Isolation of patients is not indicated, either at home or in the hospital. Most patients should be able to continue to work, provided their physical condition permits this activity. Information about all aspects of HD control for medically orientated personnel and patients can be obtained from the Gillis W. Long Hansen's Disease Center, Carville, La. 70721, 1–800–642–2477. Information is also available about the location and contacts at regional Hansen's Disease Centers located in the United States that are sponsored by the U.S. Public Health Service.

MALARIA

method of
MARTIN S. WOLFE, M.D.
George Washington University Medical School
Washington, D.C.

Malaria occurs worldwide, particularly in tropical areas, and is a serious potential threat to those living in or traveling to these areas. Malaria must be suspected in anyone living in or returning from a malaria endemic location who has fever, chills, and headache. It must be considered even if the patient claims to have taken malaria prophylactic drugs because with the widespread occurrence of chloroquine-resistant *Plasmodium falciparum* (CRPF) malaria, no presently available chemoprophylactic regimen can be assuredly protective. Even where *P. falciparum* remains sensitive to chloroquine, malaria can occur unless adequate suppressive medication is taken for at least 4 weeks after leaving the malaria endemic area. Less commonly, *Plasmodium vivax* and

Plasmodium ovale malaria may occur for up to 3 years after the last exposure, unless primaquine is taken to eradicate the exoerythrocytic (liver) stage of these species.

SYMPTOMS

The typical malaria paroxysm consists of shaking chills, high fever, and headache, followed by severe sweating. Attacks may recur at 48-hour intervals (or every 72 hours in *Plasmodium malariae* infection). Often, however, such periodicity is lacking, or typical paroxysms do not occur at all, especially in *P. falciparum* malaria, which characteristically causes an intermittent fever. Malaria mimics other infections and may cause malaise, myalgias, arthralgias, cough, or diarrhea, among other signs and symptoms. The liver and spleen are often enlarged. When severe, *P. falciparum* infections may cause cerebral malaria, renal failure, pulmonary edema, or hemolytic anemia, which can lead to a fatal outcome.

DIAGNOSIS

In any febrile patient who may have been exposed to malaria, both thick and thin blood smears should be stained and examined promptly; freshly prepared Giemsa's solution is the preferred stain, but a Wright's stain may be used. A single negative result from a thin smear cannot rule out malaria; sometimes, thick and thin smears must be repeated every 6 hours to make the diagnosis. Malaria infection can also be partially suppressed or masked by subtherapeutic doses of antimalarial or certain antibiotic drugs. A technician experienced in diagnosing malaria should examine all smears. Once malaria is diagnosed, the species must be identified and the patient's travel history reviewed to determine if CRPF malaria is likely.

TREATMENT (Table 1)

Uncomplicated Chloroquine-Sensitive *Plasmodium falciparum* Infection

P. falciparum remains sensitive to chloroquine in Central America, Haiti and the Dominican Republic, northwest tropical Africa, and the Middle East. Malaria developing in someone while in or coming from these areas almost invariably occurs in persons who are not taking appropriate chloroquine or other drug prophylaxis. Sporadic chloroquine resistance occurs in South Asia, and if malaria develops in someone in or from this area who is being given appropriate chloroquine suppression, treatment should be with other drugs used for CRPF malaria. Treatment with chloroquine in an uncomplicated case with low parasitemia (less than 3 per cent of red blood cells parasitized) is usually adequate. This is given with 25 mg per kg chloroquine base over a 48-hour period. Chloroquine comes as chloroquine phosphate, generically in 250-mg salt (equal to 150-mg base) tablets, or as Aralen in 500-mg salt (equal to 300-mg base) tablets. An initial dose of 10 mg base per kg (600 mg for adults) is followed at 6, 24, and 48 hours later with 5 mg base per kg (300 mg for adults). Chloroquine is

TABLE 1. **Treatment Regimens for Malaria**

Form	Drug	Dosage	
		Adults	*Children*
P. falciparum Acquired where chloroquine resistance does not occur and	Chloroquine phosphate* (Aralen)	600 mg base PO stat; then 300 mg at 6 hr; then 300 mg daily for next 2 days (total of 1500 mg base)	10 mg base/kg PO stat, then 5 mg/kg as per adult doses
P. malariae	Chloroquine hydrochloride IM	If patient is vomiting, give 200 mg IM q 6 hr until oral ingestion possible (maximum 800 mg/day)	IM chloroquine not recommended
P. falciparum Acquired in areas with chloroquine-resistant strains	Quinine sulfate (salt) plus Pyrimethamine-sulfadoxine (Fansidar)	650 mg tid for 3 days Single 3-tablet dose	25 mg/kg/day in 3 doses for 3 days See Table 3—same doses
P. falciparum—alternative; or where resistance occurs to pyrimethamine-sulfadoxine	Quinine sulfate (salt) plus Tetracycline or Mefloquine	650 mg tid for 3 days 250 mg qid for 7 days 1250 mg single oral dose	25 mg/kg/day in 3 doses for 3 days 5 mg/kg qid for 7 days <45 kg: 25 mg/kg single dose >45 kg: same as adult
Severe or complicated (usually *P. falciparum*)	Quinine dihydrochloride‡ (salt IV) (see text) or Quinidine gluconate IV	10 mg/kg in 300 ml normal saline IV over 2–4 hr; repeat every 8 hr until oral therapy can be started (maximum 1800 mg/day) See text	25 mg/kg/day; give ⅓ of daily dose in normal saline or 5% dextrose over 2 to 4 hr; repeat every 8 hr until oral therapy can be started (maximum 1800 mg/day) See text
P. vivax and *P. ovale* (relapsing forms)	Chloroquine phosphate followed by Primaquine phosphate (base)†	As above—PO 15 mg base daily for 14 days	As above—PO 0.3 mg/kg base daily for 14 days

*A 500-mg salt tablet contains 300 mg base; a 250-mg salt tablet contains 150 mg base.
†Screen for glucose-6-phosphate dehydrogenase deficiency before administration.
‡Available through the Centers for Disease Control, 400–639–2888 (24-hr emergency).

generally well tolerated, but side effects in some patients may include headache, dizziness, blurred vision, gastrointestinal upset, or pruritus. Pruritus may be particularly severe in natives of Africa. Patients must be closely monitored during treatment with at least daily blood smears to ensure that the drug is adequately absorbed and that possible CRPF is not present. If severe vomiting or diarrhea is present, parenteral chloroquine hydrochloride may be administered intramuscularly as 200 mg base every 6 hours until oral therapy can be taken. Caution must be exerted to avoid rapid intravenous infusion or excessively high doses, particularly in infants and young children. With adequate treatment of a chloroquine-susceptible, uncomplicated *P. falciparum* malaria episode, the patient should improve and parasitemia should clear in about 48 hours. Persistence of typical sausage-shaped *P. falciparum* gametocytes (sexual forms) after clinical improvement and clearance of asexual blood schizont forms does not indicate treatment failure or drug resistance. Gametocytes do not cause disease, and they will clear spontaneously in due course.

Uncomplicated Chloroquine-Resistant *Plasmodium falciparum* Infection

CRPF malaria presently occurs in most of tropical Africa, Southeast Asia, Papua New Guinea and other malarious areas in the Southwest Pacific (Oceania), and the Para-Amazon region of South America (Table 2). As indicated earlier, CRPF occurs sporadically in South Asia (India, Pakistan, Sri Lanka), but most cases appear to be with sensitive strains of *P. falciparum*. Many patients who have acquired CRPF have been taking recommended chloroquine prophylaxis alone; some may have taken no or irregular chloroquine prophylaxis. Thus, initial treatment of suspected CRPF must be with a drug other than chloroquine.

In areas where resistance has not developed to it, pyrimethamine-sulfadoxine (Fansidar) can be given in a single three-tablet dose for those weighing more than 45 kg. Possible disadvantages of Fansidar alone are that it acts more slowly than quinine and that Fansidar resistance is becoming more prevalent. Some experts therefore recommend that initial treatment be with oral quinine sulfate in an adult dose of 650 mg three times daily for 3 days, along with or followed by a three-tablet dose of Fansidar. Children's doses are given in Tables 1 and 3. Fansidar cannot be given to those allergic to sulfa. Although Fansidar carries a significant risk of death from hypersensitivity reactions in weekly prophylactic doses, no deaths have as yet been reported in those taking a single dose. Fansidar resistance is widespread in Southeast Asia and Oceania, and it

TABLE 2. **Areas with Reported CRPF***

Africa[†]		South America	Asia
Angola	Madagascar	Bolivia	Burma
Benin	Malawi	Brazil[‡]	China (Hainan Island and
Burkina Faso	Mali	Colombia	southern provinces)
Burundi	Mauritania	Ecuador§	Indonesia‖
Cameroon	Mozambique	French Guiana	Kampuchea[†]
Central African Republic	Namibia	Guyana	Laos¶
Comoros	Niger	Panama (east of Canal Zone,	Malaysia
Congo	Nigeria	including San Blas Islands)	Philippines (Luzon, Basilan,
Djihanti	Rwanda	Peru (northern provinces)	Mindoro, Palawan,
Equatorial Guinea	Senegal	Surinam	and Mindano Islands;
Ethiopia	Sierra Leone	Venezuela	Sulu Archipelago)
Gabon	Somalia		Thailand
Gambia	Sudan		Vietnam
Ghana	Swaziland	**Indian Subcontinent**[†]	
Guinea	Tanzania	Bangladesh (north and east)	**Oceania**[†]
Guinea Bissau	Togo	Indian (isolated areas)	Papua New Guinea
Ivory Coast	Uganda	Pakistan (isolated areas)	Solomon Islands
Kenya	Zaire	Sri Lanka (central)	Vanuatu
Liberia	Zambia		
	Zimbabwe		

*Note: There is no malaria risk in urban areas unless otherwise indicated. Reports of CRPF as of June 1989.
†Malaria risk exists in most urban areas.
‡Malaria risk exists in urban areas of interior Amazon River region.
§Malaria risk exists in urban areas of Esmeraldes, Manabi, El Oro, and Buayas provinces (including city of Guayaquil).
‖Malaria risk exists in urban areas of Timor and Kalimantan provinces. Irian Jaya should be considered as Oceania.
¶Malaria risk exists in all urban areas except Vientiane.

is not recommended for either treatment or prophylaxis in these areas. Reports of Fansidar resistance have also come from East Africa and South America.

Where Fansidar resistance occurs, or as an alternative in other CRPF areas, quinine plus a tetracycline can be used. For adults, quinine, 650 mg of salt, is given orally three times daily for 3 days, although some experts extend this to 7 to 10 days. These longer courses have not been proved to be more effective but are more likely to cause side effects. Tetracycline, 250 mg four times daily, is given along with or after the quinine and continued for 7 days. The use of this drug in children less than age 8 is controversial. It can be argued that the benefit of a virtually assured cure of a potentially life-threatening infection is worth any teeth staining that might occur. However, some experts treat these children with quinine alone and monitor for recurrence of malaria, or substitute clindamycin for tetracycline.

Optimal treatment for all CRPF is with mefloquine (Lariam), where available. Mefloquine was approved by the FDA in May 1989 but is not expected to be commercially available in the United States until late 1989. It is available in some European and African countries. Treatment of mild to moderate infection with *P. falciparum* strains resistant to other antimalarial agents in adults is five tablets (1250 mg) as a single oral dose. Children's doses are given in Table 1. The drug should not be taken on an empty stomach and should be given with at least 8 oz of water. Mefloquine should not ordinarily be used concomitantly with quinine or quinidine. If these drugs are used in the initial treatment of severe malaria, mefloquine administration should be delayed at least 12 hours after the last dose.

Halofantrine (Halfan) has been used for treatment of multi–drug-resistant *P. falciparum* malaria in France and some African countries. It is not approved or available in the United States. Firm dosages to cure all nonimmune caucasian patients have not yet been established. Currently, 500 mg every 4 hours for three doses (total 1500 mg) is being used.

Complicated *Plasmodium falciparum* Infection

Severe or complicated infection can occur with both chloroquine-sensitive *P. falciparum* and CRPF strains. Patients with more than 3 per cent of their erythrocytes parasitized generally have more severe problems. Higher parasitemias are usually related to cases not readily recognized as malaria and in which diagnosis and initiation of treatment are delayed. An abnormal level of consciousness, shock, hemolytic anemia, hepatic dysfunction, renal insufficiency or failure, pulmonary or cardiac dysfunction, vomiting, and diarrhea are indications of severe malaria.

Patients with severe or complicated malaria should be managed with intensive care, immediate intravenous antimalarial drug treatment, and necessary supportive management. The initial therapy for these patients is intravenous quinine dihydrochloride not commercially available in the United States; for civilian use it can be obtained only through the CDC in Atlanta (24-hour emergency telephone number: 404–639–2888). If this product is not readily available, or until it can be obtained, intravenous quinidine gluconate should be used.

Some experts initiate intravenous quinine treatment with a loading dose of 20 mg salt per kg, followed by doses of 10 mg salt per kg every 8 hours. Others, particularly in Africa, do not use the loading dose but begin with a dose of 10 mg salt per kg. Administration is in 300 ml normal saline or 5 per cent dextrose infused over 4 hours. Intravenous treatment is given at 8-hour intervals until parasitemia is considerably decreased and the patient is definitely improved. A 3- to 7-day total course of quinine can then be completed with oral quinine sulfate.

Where intravenous quinine is unavailable or in the presence of *P. falciparum* resistance to quinine, intravenous quinidine gluconate can be given. Two different regimens have been used. Studies in Thailand have been with an initial dose of 24 mg per kg of the salt (15 mg per kg of base) infused over 4 hours in 300 ml of normal saline or 5 per cent dextrose. Additional doses of 12 mg per kg of salt (7.5 mg per kg of base) were similarly infused at 8-hour intervals. More limited investigations in the United States on adults and children have been with an initial loading dose of 10 mg per kg of salt (6.2 mg per kg of base) given over 1 hour, followed by a continuous infusion of 0.02 mg per kg of salt (0.0125 mg per kg of base) per minute. With both regimens, oral quinidine sulfate was substituted when patients could swallow and retain oral medications. Oral quinidine doses are as with intravenous quinidine at 8-hour intervals, using quinidine sulfate capsules, 300 mg of salt (248 mg of base). Quinidine treatment should continue for 72 hours. Results were similar to those achieved with intravenous quinine. Quinidine has also been effective in Thailand in the face of resistance to quinine. During intravenous quinidine use, infusion speed must be carefully monitored and the blood pressure and ECG should be followed closely for evidence of toxicity. After the quinidine or quinine course, oral tetracycline, 250 mg four times daily for 7 days, should be taken to ensure total cure.

The role of mefloquine and halofantrine, presently available only in oral dose form, in the treatment of severe and complicated malaria remains to be determined.

In patients with parasitemia higher than 10 per cent and/or marked deterioration of neurologic, renal, or hematologic function, or other grave prognostic signs, exchange transfusion may be lifesaving. Advantages include much more rapid removal of parasites than with antimalarial drugs and the potential restoration of platelets and clotting factors from fresh whole blood. The reduction of parasitemia to a desired 1 per cent or less often occurs after 8 to 10 units of exchange. Studies also suggest a continuous infusion of quinidine gluconate be combined with exchange transfusion.

Plasmodium malariae, Plasmodium vivax, and Plasmodium ovale Infections

These species give lower parasitemias than does *P. falciparum,* and pure infection with them is rarely severe. Treatment is with chloroquine, 25 mg base per kg over 3 days, as with uncomplicated chloroquine-sensitive *P. falciparum* infection. These three parasites have not developed resistance to chloroquine. Mefloquine, in doses used for *P. falciparum,* has also been effective against *P. vivax.* Chloroquine alone is sufficient for *P. malariae.* However, *P. vivax* and *P. ovale* have persistent exoerythrocytic liver-stage parasites that can be eliminated only with primaquine. After initial chloroquine or mefloquine treatment, primaquine, 15 mg base daily for 14 days, is given. Primaquine comes only in hard tablet form that cannot be put into solution. Young children should receive 0.3 mg base per kg daily for 14 days, which requires breaking the 15-mg-base (equal to 26.3 mg of primaquine phosphate salt) tablet into the approximate dose portion. Some strains of *P. vivax* from Southeast Asia and the Southwest Pacific (so-called Chesson strains) are relatively resistant to the usual dose of primaquine; these usually respond to 30 mg base primaquine daily for 14 days. Primaquine can cause hemolysis in persons with glucose-6-phosphate dehydrogenase (G6PD) deficiency. All persons receiving primaquine should be first tested to ensure absence of G6PD deficiency. In those with the mild (African) deficiency, primaquine can be tolerated in a weekly dose of 45 mg base for 8 weeks. In other varities of G6PD deficiency, in which hemolysis can be so severe as to be life-threatening, primaquine must be avoided. If relapses occur, they can be treated with chloroquine.

General Supportive Care

Patients with pure *P. malariae, P. vivax,* and *P. ovale* infections rarely have heavy parasitemias or severe illness or complications. They can generally be treated as outpatients. Those infected with *P. falciparum* always have the potential for rapidly developing severe illness or complications and are best treated in the hospital. Chloroquine-sensitive *P. falciparum* infection recognized early should quickly respond to chloroquine. Patients with heavier *P. falciparum* infections or those with CRPF infection (some of whom may already have been unsuccessfully treated with chloroquine) are more likely to develop complications and may require parenteral therapy, which must be closely monitored, and other intensive care. Treatment with analgesics, antiemetics, and antipyretics may be necessary. Thrombocytopenia, sometimes quite marked, often occurs with all forms of acute malaria, but this condition quickly reverts to normal with appropriate antimalarial chemotherapy.

Management of Complications

Cerebral malaria must be differentiated from other causes of coma; the airway must be carefully maintained. Adjuvant treatments, e.g., corticosteroids, high-molecular-weight dextran, mannitol, heparin, and epinephrine, have not been useful and may be harmful; these should be avoided.

Hyperpyrexia should be controlled with sponging, cooling blankets, and antipyretics.

Seizures are not uncommon, particularly with cerebral malaria, and should be treated with standard anticonvulsants. Status epilepticus may require diazepam therapy.

Severe anemia (hematocrit 20 ml/dl or less) should be treated with whole blood or packed red blood cell transfusions.

Hypoglycemia may occur with severe malaria and is especially common in pregnant women and in patients with hyperparasitemia. Blood glucose levels must be carefully monitored. Treatment initially is with 50 per cent dextrose injection followed by a 10 per cent dextrose infusion.

Pulmonary edema can be a fatal complication of severe *P. falciparum* infection and can develop after clearance of blood parasitemia and apparent clinical improvement. It presents as adult respiratory distress syndrome (ARDS). Prevention is by careful attention to fluid intake monitored by central venous pressure. Treatment is with diuretics, fluid restriction, and other methods used for pulmonary edema and ARDS.

Renal failure is related to decreased renal capillary blood flow, most frequently due to underhydration but also associated with hyperparasitemia and intravascular hemolysis. In the absence of fluid overload and with a low central venous pressure and high urine specific gravity, the patient should be challenged with a normal saline infusion. If this is unsuccessful, a diuretic or vasopressor is given. Persistent oliguria may require renal dialysis.

Disseminated intravascular coagulation with bleeding is rarely a clinically important occurrence in the absence of hyperparasitemia or multiorgan failure. Treatment is with fresh whole blood transfusions. Heparin has not been useful and is not recommended.

PROPHYLAXIS

In choosing an appropriate chemoprophylactic regimen before travel, various factors must be considered (Table 3). The full itinerary should be carefully reviewed to determine whether the person will be in specific areas where malaria actually occurs in a recognized malarious country. For example, most major cities of Asia and South America do not have endemic malaria; if only these cities are visited, chemoprophylaxis is not necessary. In tropical Africa, however, risk of acquiring malaria occurs in many cities as well as in rural areas. If travel to rural areas where malaria occurs is only during daytime hours, prophylaxis may not be required. It should also be determined if the area to be visited is one with CRPF. Any previous allergic or other reaction to the antimalarials chosen should be determined. Duration of travel and availability of adequate medical care must also be weighed in the decision.

The continuing spread of CRPF malaria has created serious problems in protecting against infection. There is no available drug or drug combination with proven efficacy or safety to prevent all malaria infections. Various recommendations for different countries have resulted, leading to confusion. The following recommendations are now believed to be most appropriate as offering the best combination of safety and relative effectiveness.

For areas with chloroquine-sensitive malaria species, or where only low-level or focal CRPF has been reported (South Asia), the drug of choice is chloroquine. This is taken in an adult dose of 300 mg base (equal to 500 mg salt) once weekly, beginning 2 weeks before arrival to ensure tolerance and adequate blood levels, while in the malarious area, and for at least 4 weeks after leaving. Chloroquine suspension is available for young children. Those unable to tolerate chloroquine should take proguanil (Paludrine), 200 mg daily for the same times.

For those going to Africa where CRPF is endemic (see Table 2), weekly chloroquine (as above) is recommended. Proguanil 200 mg daily should also be taken. This latter drug is not yet approved in the United States by the FDA, but is available in England, France, and Kenya and many other places in Africa. Limited data suggest that it is effective in Africa, but not in Thailand or Papua New Guinea. Proguanil has not been evaluated in other CRPF areas. A three-tablet treatment dose of Fansidar can also be carried by longer-term travelers or residents. They should be advised to take the Fansidar promptly in the event of a febrile illness while abroad, but only when professional medical care is not readily available; this measure is only temporary, and prompt medical evaluation is imperative. Fansidar is no longer recommended for routine prophylaxis.

In some malarious areas, particularly in Southeast Asia, Papua New Guinea, and the Amazon basin, multidrug resistance by *P. falciparum* parasites occurs. Doxycycline alone, 100 mg daily, can be considered in these areas for short-term travel, but users should be cautioned about side effects (see later). Doxycycline should be continued daily for 4 weeks after leaving the malarious area.

When mefloquine is commercially available in the United States and more definite recommendations for its use have been made, this drug will

TABLE 3. **Drug Prophylaxis for Malaria**

Condition	Drug	Dosage	
		Adults	*Children*
Areas with chloroquine-sensitive strains	Chloroquine phosphate* (Aralen)	300 mg base (500 mg salt) weekly; take for at least 4 wk after leaving malaria area	5 mg base kg weekly; same as for adults
Areas with chloroquine-resistant strains	Chloroquine plus	As above	As above
	Proguanil† (Paludrine)	200 mg daily during and for 4 wk after exposure	4–9 kg: 25 mg daily 10–14 kg: 50 mg daily 15–29 kg: 100 mg daily 30–50 kg: 150 mg daily >50 kg: 200 mg daily
	plus		
	Pyrimethamine-sulfadoxine (Fanisdar)	Carry a single (3 tablets) self-treatment dose	5–10 kg: ¼ tablet 11–20 kg: ½ tablet 21–30 kg: 1 tablet 31–45 kg: 2 tablets >45 kg: 3 tablets
	or		
	Mefloquine (Lariam)	250 mg salt orally once/wk for 4 doses. Subsequent doses at 2-wk intervals	15–19 kg: ¼ tablet 20–30 kg: ½ tablet 31–45 kg: ¾ tablet >45 kg: 1 tablet
	or		
	Doxycycline	100 mg daily during and for 4 wk after exposure	Contraindicated in children younger than 8 years >8 years: 2 mg/kg daily, up to 100 mg daily
Possibility of later relapsing malaria	Primaquine	15 mg base daily for 14 days; do not give to patients with deficiency of glucose-6-phosphate dehydrogenase	0.3 mg base/kg/day for 14 days

*Provided in 500- or 250-mg salt tablets, which equal 300 mg and 150 mg base, respectively.
†Not available in the United States.

likely become the prophylactic drug of choice in all CRPF areas. It is currently available in some countries. Where available, it may be considered for use by travelers to areas where there is risk of CRPF infection and particularly by travelers to areas where multidrug resistance to *P. falciparum* occurs. The adult prophylactic dose is 250 mg weekly for the first 4 weeks, and then once every other week until three doses have been taken after return to a malaria-free area.

Amodiaquine and Maloprim (a combination of pyrimethamine and dapsone) are recommended by some experts. Neither is commercially available in the United States. Both have been associated with bone marrow problems and are not recommended.

Primaquine has no role in prophylaxis for individuals who are in malarious areas. However, because persisting liver forms of *P. vivax* and *P. ovale* occur in most malarious areas (Haiti being a major exception), returnees from malarious areas run some risk of acquiring later relapsing malaria. This is more likely in persons having prolonged exposure in malaria-endemic areas. As long as G6PD status is normal, primaquine is considered to be safe and the only effective way of protecting against this risk. The optimal adult dose is 15 mg base daily (pediatric dose of 0.3 mg/kg base daily) for 14 days, and it is best taken after completing the terminal 4-week prophylaxis with chloroquine and/or other drugs.

PERSONAL PROTECTION MEASURES

Malaria transmission by mosquitos occurs primarily between dusk and dawn. During those hours, measures to reduce contact with mosquitos are most critical and include (1) remaining in well-screened areas, (2) using mosquito nets, (3) wearing clothes that cover most of the body, (4) using insect repellents containing DEET (*N,N*-diethyl-*m*-toluamide) on exposed parts of the body, and (5) using a pyrethrum-containing flying insect spray in living areas.

The most effective repellents contain DEET in an approximately 32 per cent concentration lotion. Higher concentrations of DEET in some repellents may cause a severe rash, and if absorbed in significant amounts through the skin, can produce seizures and neurologic damage in children. High concentrations of DEET should be used sparingly, if at all, on infants and children.

CONTRAINDICATIONS AND SIDE EFFECTS OF ANTIMALARIAL DRUGS

Chloroquine. This drug exacerbates psoriasis and should not be taken by persons with this condition.

Chloroquine in higher doses used for rheumatoid arthritis or lupus, or in the 600 mg base per week used in some French-speaking areas of Africa, has been associated with irreversible retinopathy and blindness. This is virtually unheard of in persons taking the recommended 300 mg base weekly dose. However, some experts consider it prudent to recommend periodic ophthalmologic examinations for those using chloroquine for more than 6 years of cummulative weekly prophylaxis. Temporary, minor side effects (usually adequately tolerated) include headache, blurred vision, gastrointestinal disturbances, and rashes. Uncomfortable side effects may be alleviated by taking chloroquine with meals or in divided, twice weekly doses.

Proguanil. This drug has been considered perhaps the best tolerated of all antimalarial drugs. With the 200-mg daily dose, mouth ulcers have been rarely reported and there have been some minor gastrointestinal problems. There are no contraindications.

Fansidar. The long-acting sulfa component, sulfadoxine, has been associated with fatal cutaneous reactions with weekly Fansidar use. In Americans, the incidence of fatal reactions ranges from 1 in 11,000 to 1 in 25,000 users. These reactions have not yet been recognized with a three-tablet treatment dose. Fansidar has also caused serum sickness reactions and hepatitis. Fansidar is no longer recommended for weekly prophylaxis. Fansidar is contraindicated in persons who are allergic to sulfa and in infants younger than age 2 months.

Quinine. Cinchonism (tinnitus, headache, nausea, abdominal pain, visual disturbance) is common. Drug-related fever rarely occurs.

Tetracyclines. Tetracyclines are contraindicated in children less than age 8 years. Doxycycline may produce photosensitivity, usually manifested as an exaggerated sunburn reaction, in those using it in tropical climates; users should avoid direct and prolonged sun exposure or use a high SPF sunscreen when prolonged sun exposure is anticipated. Tetracyclines may also lead to *Candida* vaginitis or gastrointestinal candidiasis or to gastrointestinal upset.

Mefloquine. Minor side effects have been reported rather frequently, including dizziness and gastrointestinal disturbances. Mefloquine has occasionally been associated with asymptomatic sinus bradycardia and prolonged QT interval, and it should not be used by those receiving calcium channel antagonists or beta blockers. If mefloquine is to be used for more than 1 year, periodic evaluations including liver function tests and ophthalmic examinations are recommended.

Primaquine. Severe hemolysis may occur in G6PD-deficient individuals, and it is generally contraindicated in this condition. Gastrointestinal symptoms rarely occur.

Malaria in Pregnant and Breast-Feeding Women. Malaria poses a serious threat to pregnant women and may cause abortion, premature labor, maternal anemia, and congenital infection. A pregnant woman should *never* go to a malarious area without taking appropriate malaria chemoprophylaxis. Chloroquine is considered safe for both prophylaxis and treatment. Proguanil has been safe in pregnancy. The safety of Fansidar in pregnancy has not been completely established. The safety of mefloquine is questionable and it should not be used during the first 3 months of pregnancy. Women with childbearing potential who are taking mefloquine should be warned against becoming pregnant. Tetracyclines and primaquine are contraindicated in pregnancy. When radical cure or prophylaxis with primaquine is indicated, chloroquine should be taken weekly until delivery, after which primaquine may be taken.

In treating severe CRPF malaria in pregnant women, any concern about side effects must necessarily be secondary to the potential lifesaving value of quinine along with either tetracycline or Fansidar.

The small amounts of antimalarial drugs secreted in the breast milk of lactating women are not considered to be harmful to the nursing infant. Insufficient amounts of these drugs are transferred in breast milk to protect infants, who require dosages recommended in Table 3.

BACTERIAL MENINGITIS

method of
RODNEY A. MICHAEL, M.D.*
Madigan Army Medical Center
Tacoma, Washington

Bacterial meningitis is a life-threatening medical emergency with high morbidity and mortality despite advances in both diagnosis and management. Approximately 5 to 10 cases per 100,000 population occur annually in the United States and account for more than 2000 deaths.

INITIAL TREATMENT

Reduction of morbidity and mortality depends principally on rapid, aggressive initiation of appropriate antibiotic therapy. Adherence to several key principles of management underlies the successful treatment of this potentially devastating infection:

1. *Rapid diagnostic assessment.* Blood and cerebrospinal fluid for analysis, Gram's stain, and culture need to be obtained rapidly. The initial

---

*The views of the author do not necessarily reflect the position of the Department of the Army or the Department of Defense.

Gram's stain of cerebrospinal fluid helps to direct early therapy in approximately 80 per cent of patients. The presence or absence of other cerebrospinal fluid abnormalities, including depressed glucose level, elevated protein level, bacterial antigens, and neutrophilic pleocytosis, assists in assessment and management.

2. *Do not delay therapy.* Treatment should not be delayed until diagnostic studies are complete. Empiric antibiotics should be initiated within 30 to 60 minutes of presentation. Therapy must be initiated if lumbar puncture is to be delayed for any reason. Available literature suggests that cerebrospinal fluid culture results and Gram's stain, as well as other laboratory features of acute bacterial meningitis, are affected minimally when preceded by antibiotic therapy given for only 1 or 2 hours. Antibiotics can be discontinued if cerebrospinal fluid analysis done within 1 to 2 hours of their initiation does not support the presumptive diagnosis of meningitis.

3. *Use bactericidal antibiotics.* The central nervous system has poor resources for the destruction of invading bacteria. Immunoglobulin and complement levels, numbers of polymorphonuclear cells, and phagocytic activity are all decreased in cerebrospinal fluid. The bactericidal activity of the chosen antibiotic is of paramount importance.

4. *Antibiotic penetration of the central nervous system.* The chosen antibiotic must penetrate the central nervous system. Not all antibiotics do this equally well, and several factors may inter-act to affect antimicrobial penetration. Of the agents that are active against usual central nervous system pathogens, beta-lactam drugs and chloramphenicol penetrate most predictably.

5. *Use adequate doses of antibiotic.* Even the best antibiotics have failed when insufficient levels in the cerebrospinal fluid are obtained. Several studies have demonstrated that optimal therapeutic outcomes are associated with cerebrospinal fluid levels of antibiotic that exceed the minimum bactericidal concentration of the pathogen by a factor of 10 or more.

ANTIBIOTIC SELECTION AND USE

Antibiotic Selection Based on Results of Gram's Stain. Gram's stain of the cerebrospinal fluid, when organisms are seen, allows early, more specific therapy. Table 1 correlates these findings with likely pathogens and recommendations for therapy.

Empiric Antibiotics Based on Patient's Age or Setting. In the absence of Gram's stain or other microbiologic information, empiric antibiotics can generally be selected accurately by using knowledge of age-associated pathogens or correlation with clinical setting (Tables 2 and 3). The initial regimen can be modified as more complete information (e.g., culture, Gram's stain, counter-immunoelectrophoresis, latex agglutination) is received.

Modification of Original Antibiotic Regimen. When the pathogen has been identified, usually within

TABLE 1. **Gram's Stain Findings and Antibiotic Selection**

Appearance of Gram's Stain	Possible Pathogens	Treatment of Choice	Alternative Therapy
Gram-positive cocci in short chains and pairs	*Streptococcus pneumoniae*	Penicillin G	Chloramphenicol or third-generation cephalosporin*
Gram-positive "large" cocci in clusters	*Staphylococcus*	Nafcillin	Vancomycin
Gram-positive bacilli, "Chinese characters"	*Listeria monocytogenes*	Ampicillin ± gentamicin	Trimethoprim-sulfamethoxazole
Gram-negative kidney bean–shaped cocci, in pairs or singles	*Neisseria meningitidis*	Penicillin G	Chloramphenicol or third-generation cephalosporin*
Gram-negative coccobacilli	*Haemophilus influenzae*	Third-generation cephalosporin*	Ampicillin + chloramphenicol
Gram-negative bacilli	Enterobacteriaceae	Third-generation cephalosporin* ± gentamicin†	Aztreonam‡ or ceftazidime ± gentamicin†
	Pseudomonas aeruginosa	Ceftazidime + gentamicin†	Antipseudomonal penicillin§ or aztreonam‡ + gentamicin†

*Ceftriaxone, cefotaxime, or ceftizoxime.

†Tobramycin, netilmicin, or amikacin may be substituted depending on local susceptibility patterns. Aminoglycosides should be used at least systemically until antibiotic susceptibilities are available. If *Pseudomonas aeruginosa* is suspected or if the patient is especially toxic, intrathecal or intraventricular use should be considered.

‡Clinical experience with aztreonam is small, but studies with animals and humans suggest a role for aztreonam in the treatment of some types of gram-negative meningitis. Infectious disease consultation should be considered when use of this drug is contemplated.

§Piperacillin, mezlocillin, azlocillin, or ticarcillin.

TABLE 2. **Age-Associated Pathogens in Bacterial Meningitis**

Age	Usual Pathogens	Treatment of Choice	Alternative Therapy
Neonates 0–2 mo	Group B *Streptococcus* Enterobacteriaceae *Listeria monocytogenes*	Cefotaxime + ampicillin	Gentamicin* + ampicillin
Infants 2 mo to 10 yr	*Haemophilus influenzae* *Streptococcus pneumoniae* *Neisseria meningitidis*	Third-generation cephalo-sporin†	Chloramphenicol + ampicil-lin
Adults 10–60 yr	*Streptococcus pneumoniae* *Neisseria meningitidis*	Penicillin G	Chloramphenicol or third-generation cephalosporin†
Adults older than 60 yr	*Streptococcus pneumoniae* Enterobacteriaceae *Listeria monocytogenes*	Third-generation cephalo-sporin† + ampicillin	Gentamicin* + ampicillin

*Tobramycin, netilmicin, or amikacin may be substituted depending on local susceptibility patterns.
†Ceftriaxone, cefotaxime, or ceftizoxime.

24 to 72 hours of specimen submission, empiric therapy can be modified to use of more specific antibiotics if appropriate. Antibiotic selection should be guided (in descending order of importance) by activity against identified or suspected pathogens (Table 1); central nervous system penetration; potential toxicity; and cost.

Special Considerations in Selecting Antibiotics. Some antibiotics may be appropriately selected despite poor central nervous system penetration. This is particularly true for aminoglycoside antibiotics that, because of a narrow therapeutic window, achieve inadequate cerebrospinal fluid levels when administered systemically. Aminoglycoside antibiotics continue to be indicated for meningitis caused by certain gram-negative bacilli, especially *Pseudomonas aeruginosa*. In such circumstances, direct instillation of the aminoglycoside into the central nervous system may be indicated, in combination with systemic aminoglycoside and beta-lactam administration. In this difficult situation, serious consideration should be given to infectious disease consultation.

Antibiotic Dosing and Duration of Therapy. Appropriate dosing may at times involve doses larger or more frequent than those recommended by the manufacturer for other severe infections (Table

4). In general, antibiotics must be given as intravenous solutions to achieve adequate systemic and cerebrospinal fluid levels, with the single exception of chloramphenicol (Chloromycetin), which may be used successfully as an oral agent. Duration of therapy depends somewhat on the organism cultured. *Haemophilus influenzae* infection may be successfully treated in 7 to 10 days; *Neisseria meningitidis* infection in 7 days; and *Streptococcus pneumoniae* infection in 14 days. Infections with other pathogens should usually be treated a minimum of 3 weeks or more.

ADJUNCTIVE MANAGEMENT

Isolation. Patients with suspected or proved meningococcal meningitis should be placed in respiratory isolation for the first 24 hours of hospitalization to minimize transmission to other patients or staff. Isolation is not necessary for infections caused by other central nervous system bacterial pathogens.

Radiologic Studies. X-rays of the chest, sinuses, and mastoids should be performed routinely to rule out primary foci of infection. Computed tomography of the brain should be considered when the history or physical examination suggests fo-

TABLE 3. **Clinical Settings and Bacterial Pathogens Causing Meningitis**

Clinical Setting	Likely Pathogens	Empiric Therapy
Skull fracture, especially basilar	*Streptococcus pneumoniae*	Penicillin G
After neurosurgical procedure or open head trauma	*Staphylococcus aureus* Gram-negative bacilli	Nafcillin + ceftazidime + gentami-cin*
Ventricular shunts	Staphylococcal species Gram-negative bacilli	Vancomycin + third-generation ceph-alosporin†
Neutropenic host or intensive chemo-therapy	Gram-negative bacilli including *Pseu-domonas aeruginosa* and staphylo-coccal species	Ceftazidime + gentamicin* + nafcil-lin
Transplant patient	*Listeria monocytogenes*	Ampicillin ± gentamicin
Asplenism	*Streptococcus pneumoniae* *Haemophilus influenzae* *Neisseria meningitidis*	Third-generation cephalosporin†

*Tobramycin, netilmicin, or amikacin may be substituted depending on local susceptibility patterns.
†Ceftriaxone, cefotaxime, or ceftizoxime.

TABLE 4. **Antibiotic Dosing in Bacterial Meningitis**

Antibiotic	Daily Adult Dose	Daily Pediatric Dose*	Dosing Interval† (hr)
Aqueous penicillin G	18–24 million U	300,000 U/kg	2–4
Ampicillin	8–12 grams	200–300 mg/kg	4–6
Nafcillin	12 grams	200 mg/kg	4
Piperacillin	18 grams	300 mg/kg	4
Cefotaxime	12 grams	200 mg/kg	4
Ceftriaxone	4 grams	100 mg/kg	12
Ceftazidime	6 grams	100 mg/kg	8
Aztreonam	6 grams	NA	8
Vancomycin	2 grams	50 mg/kg	6
Chloramphenicol	4 grams	100 mg/kg	6
Gentamicin	6 mg/kg	6 mg/kg	8
Tobramycin	6 mg/kg	6 mg/kg	8
Amikacin	15 mg/kg	15 mg/kg	8
Intrathecal or intraventricular gentamicin	5 mg	2.5 mg	24

*Daily neonatal dose may be different. Check manufacturer's recommendations.
†Dosing intervals for neonates and infants may vary from those shown. Check manufacturer's recommendations.
Abbreviation: NA = not available.

cal, intracranial suppuration (abscess). Computed tomography should also be considered to rule out focal suppuration when the patient shows a poor response to appropriate therapy.

Increased Intracranial Pressure. Brain edema with markedly elevated cerebrospinal fluid pressures occasionally complicates bacterial meningitis. Such edema probably accounts in part for neurologic sequelae, and when it occurs it requires rapid pharmacologic management to prevent herniation of brain substance. Mannitol, 100 grams in 500 ml, may be used acutely to reduce swelling. Dexamethasone, 10 mg intravenously initially and then 4 mg every 6 hours, may then be used until edema resolves.

Other Indications for Use of Corticosteroids. Recent literature suggests that high-dose dexamethasone may ameliorate or prevent neurologic sequelae, especially hearing loss, in children. However, the toxicity of high-dose dexamethasone is not clearly defined, and its use may be associated with increased risk of gastrointestinal hemorrhage or neuronal ischemia. I would continue to reserve its use for those patients who are seriously ill at presentation with either severe cerebral edema or coma.

Seizures. Generalized seizures occur commonly with bacterial meningitis and require aggressive management with anticonvulsants. In addition, high-dose penicillin may exacerbate the potential for seizures, especially if there is renal dysfunction. Attention should also be given to the potential for aspiration and pneumonia in patients with recurrent seizures.

Fluid and Electrolyte Management. Careful attention is required for management of fluid and electrolyte status, especially in patients with cer-

ebral edema. In addition, the syndrome of inappropriate antidiuretic hormone secretion may accompany meningeal inflammation with resulting hyponatremia. The use of high-dose potassium salt of penicillin G instead of the sodium salt may result in hyperkalemia, especially in the presence of pre-existent renal failure.

Repeat Lumbar Puncture. Repeated examination of the cerebrospinal fluid is probably indicated only when the patient fails to respond to therapy, generally within 72 to 96 hours. Routine cerebrospinal fluid examination after clinically successful therapy is not recommended and most often serves only to cause confusion for the clinician.

RECURRENT MENINGITIS

Recurrent episodes of bacterial meningitis most often represent anatomic defects in the dura, which serve as portals for re-entry of pathogens into the central nervous system. Such defects may be congenital or traumatic and may occur at any location in the central nervous system. Another cause of recurrent meningitis is incompletely treated or undrained parameningeal infection such as sinusitis, mastoiditis, or osteomyelitis. Sinuses and mastoids should be included in the initial evaluation of any patient presenting with bacterial meningitis. Also, immunologic defects including immunoglobulin deficiency, asplenia, and terminal complement deficiency may be associated with recurrent central nervous system infection. Data suggest that any patient with a disseminated infection with a *Neisseria* species, including meningococcal meningitis, should be evaluated for deficiency of terminal complement factors by measurement of total hemolytic complement (CH_{50}).

PROPHYLAXIS

Neisseria meningitidis. *N. meningitidis* is the only central nervous system bacterial pathogen that is associated with epidemic meningitis. Chemoprophylaxis is indicated for the index case before discharge from the hospital; for close personal contacts, including other household members; for day care contacts; and for recruit populations. Health care workers without close personal contact (e.g., mouth-to-mouth resuscitation) are not at increased risk for infection. Prophylaxis consists of rifampin, 600 mg given every 12 hours for 2 days. Polyvalent meningococcal polysaccharide vaccine may enhance the effectiveness of prophylaxis.

Haemophilus influenzae. Infection of close household contacts and day care contacts may occur but at a much lower frequency than that for meningococcal infection. However, data suggest that rifampin may be effective prophylaxis for such contacts. Prophylaxis, when elected, should be administered to the index case before discharge from the hospital and to contacts, 20 mg per kg per day for 4 days. Immunization for *H. influenzae* may improve success with prophylaxis. Either the recently released polysaccharide-diphtheria toxoid conjugate vaccine or the polysaccharide vaccine may be used. The former is more immunogenic and is preferred in infants younger than 24 months of age.

INFECTIOUS MONONUCLEOSIS

method of
JAMES C. NIEDERMAN, M.D.
Yale University School of Medicine
New Haven, Connecticut

Infectious mononucleosis (IM) is an acute lymphoproliferative disease caused by the Epstein-Barr virus (EBV). Primary EBV infection in the first few years of life is usually subclinical; however, infection in older children and in young adults is associated with symptoms of IM in 50 per cent of cases. Characteristic clinical features include (1) fever, pharyngitis, and lymphadenopathy; (2) an absolute lymphocytosis of 50 per cent or more, of which 10 per cent or more are atypical lymphocytes; (3) appearance of transient heterophil antibody responses; (4) development of persistent antibodies against EBV; and (5) abnormal liver function tests.

EBV infections and IM occur regularly in humans throughout the world. The disease is well recognized in areas of advanced sociohygienic standards where EBV exposure and infection are delayed until adolescence or early adulthood. Conversely, IM is rare in crowded, densely populated regions with lower standards of hygiene, where most EBV infections occur early in life and are subclinical.

An incubation period of 30 to 50 days in the adult has been suggested on the basis of studies of contact infections. In the usual case of IM, the sequence of events to control EBV infection of B lymphocytes induces self-limited immunologic lymphoid responses, which are associated with characteristic clinical features.

EBV is present in saliva of IM patients, and excretion of virus continues for long periods after acute infection and then intermittently for life; surveys of previously infected subjects have indicated that at any one time, at least 25 per cent shed infectious virus in the oropharynx. In preschool children and young adults in whom salivary exchange is high, EBV transmissibility is high; it is low where this exchange of saliva is uncommon.

Because the agent is present in cell-free form in saliva and has been recovered in secretions from parotid gland orifices and ducts, the salivary glands appear to be productive sites of EBV. There is increasing evidence suggesting that EBV replicates in pharyngeal epithelium and not in B lymphocytes. EBV DNA has been detected in parotid duct epithelium and exfoliated buccal mucosal cells; cell-free virus has also been demonstrated in the uterine cervix of several women with recent infection; and epithelial cells in cervical washings have been found to contain EBV DNA.

TREATMENT

Acute Illness

Most cases of IM are mild or moderate in severity. During a prodromal period lasting 4 to 5 days, malaise, headache, myalgia, and fatigue are frequent symptoms. Frank clinical features include sore throat, fever, and cervical adenopathy. Enlargement of both anterior and posterior cervical nodes usually occurs and axillary as well as other lymph nodes may be palpable; such lymphadenopathy persists for several weeks to months. Irregular fever is present for 1 to 2 weeks, and subjective symptoms of malaise and fatigue often continue for an additional 2 to 3 weeks. In the acute febrile phase of disease, rest in bed is advisable; limited activity is recommended as long as sore throat, headache, and malaise persist. During acute illness there is no need for isolation of patients.

Fever is usually controlled by salicylates, and both headache and pharyngeal discomfort are relieved by aspirin therapy, 1 grain or 60 mg per dose per year of age up to 10 grains (0.6 gram) every 4 hours. Codeine may be occasionally necessary for the relief of pharyngeal symptoms. In patients in a toxic state who develop severe pharyngotonsillitis and oropharyngeal edema and in whom potential airway obstruction may ensue, a short course of steroids should be instituted and a tracheostomy set should be made available for emergency use. Prednisone or its equivalent in other steroid preparations may be used; an initial dose of 10 to 15 mg four times daily is given for 24 to 48 hours. The dose is then decreased by 5 mg each day so that steroid treatment is terminated in approximately 10 days. Pharmacologic doses of steroids should also be used in the treatment of other severe complications of this infection, such as neurologic sequelae, thrombocytopenic purpura, hemolytic anemia, myocarditis, and pericarditis. However, steroid therapy is not recommended for treatment of the usual uncomplicated case.

Antibiotics have no effect on the course of EBV infection, and use of gamma globulin does not prevent or modify the illness. However, approximately 20 per cent of patients with IM have concurrent beta-hemolytic streptococcal tonsillitis and should receive appropriate antibiotic therapy for this. A 10-day course of oral penicillin, 125 to 250 mg (250 mg = 400,000 units) four times daily, or an equivalent amount of erythromycin or parenteral penicillin should be administered. Administration of ampicillin should be avoided because of the high frequency of generalized hypersensitivity rashes associated with use of this drug in patients with IM.

Treatment with acyclovir has no significant effect on clinical symptoms or on humoral and cellular immune responses in uncomplicated IM; EBV oropharyngeal shedding is inhibited, however.

Complications

Splenomegaly is present in approximately 50 per cent of patients with acute disease and is usually maximal during the second and third weeks after the onset of symptoms. Such patients should avoid vigorous athletics, heavy lifting, and any abdominal trauma until splenic enlargement has subsided. Splenic rupture is a rare but potentially fatal complication of the disease; severe abdominal pain in IM is unusual except in the presence of splenic rupture, a development necessitating immediate splenectomy.

Although hepatic enlargement is detectable in only 10 to 15 per cent of cases, liver function tests, especially measures of transaminase values, are abnormal for several weeks in almost all patients. Transient, mild jaundice is present in about 5 per cent of patients and requires only bed rest until the serum bilirubin level returns to normal.

Hematologic changes including mild anemia, granulocytopenia, and slight to moderate thrombocytopenia occur transiently in approximately half of patients with IM. Autoimmune hemolysis

is a rare complication and usually subsides within 4 to 6 weeks.

Less than 1 per cent of patients, usually adults, develop central nervous system complications including aseptic meningitis, Bell's palsy, Guillain-Barré syndrome, acute cerebellar ataxia, meningoencephalitis, and transverse myelitis. Recovery is usually complete, although fatal cases associated with encephalitis have been reported.

IM may be complicated by interstitial pneumonitis, pleuritis, and pleural effusion. In childhood pneumonia, EBV may be a primary, co-primary, or secondary pathogen; pulmonary complications usually result from superinfection with bacterial pathogens or *Mycoplasma pneumoniae*.

Fatal EBV infections have been reported in patients with cellular immunodeficiencies, who are unable to restrict EBV-induced B cell proliferation. Polyclonal or monoclonal B cell lymphoproliferative disorders may develop in recipients of organ transplants and in patients with acquired immunodeficiency syndrome. Rarely, complications such as agammaglobulinemia and aplastic anemia result from excessive suppressor T cell responses initiated by EBV infection of B cells.

Convalescence

After acute symptoms subside, most patients with IM recover uneventfully and gradually resume normal activities in 4 to 6 weeks. Rarely, symptoms persist for several months or more and laboratory abnormalities resolve slowly; during this period, supportive and symptomatic therapy is indicated. Medical knowledge is still incomplete on the events that follow primary EBV infection, such as the anatomic sites of virus latency and the factors that regulate virus production and excretion in seropositive persons.

MUMPS
(Epidemic Parotitis)

method of
MARILYN KACICA, M.D., and
CHRISTOPHER J. HARRISON, M.D.
Children's Hospital Medical Center
Cincinnati, Ohio

Mumps virus causes a contagious self-limited disease, has only one serotype, and is worldwide in distribution. Licensure of live mumps vaccine produced a 90 per cent decline in the occurrence of mumps in developed countries. The age of highest incidence also shifted from 5- to 9-year-olds to 10- to 14-year-olds, and the incidence in 15- to 19-year-olds is now nearly that of 5- to 9-year-olds. This is due to a relatively larger pool of unvaccinated older children rather than to vaccine failures. Mumps is transmitted by direct contact with infected secretions, respiratory droplets, or fomites. It is contagious 1 week before and up to 14 days after the onset of parotitis.

CLINICAL MANIFESTATIONS

The mean incubation period is 17 days (range 2 to 3 weeks). Mumps infection is subclinical in 25 to 40 per cent of cases, but it usually produces a nonspecific prodrome (anorexia, low-grade fever, malaise, and headache) and occasionally pain referred to the ear. Parotid size and tenderness increase during the first 2 to 3 days, obscure the mandibular angle, and displace the ear upward and outward. During the first 3 days of parotitis, a temperature up to 40° C, trismus, and increased pain with ingestion of citrus fruits or juices may occur. The parotid swelling peaks on the fifth to the tenth day and usually resolves during the next week. If parotid swelling persists for longer than 10 days, ultrasonography or computed tomography can rule out obstruction that might lead to sialectasia. Mumps parotitis is unilateral in about 25 per cent of cases. Although parotitis is most common, the submandibular and sublingual glands may be involved about 10 per cent of the time. However, nonparotid involvement is rarely the sole presenting feature. Presternal edema also occurs in 5 to 10 per cent of mumps cases and presents as tender and mildly erythematous swelling over the upper sternum. This may be confused with cellulitis, but it resolves spontaneously in 3 to 5 days. Mastitis, myocarditis (ST changes in up to 13 per cent of adults), optic neuritis, thyroiditis (usually in adults), bartholinitis, and oophoritis (in 5 per cent of postpubertal women) may occur.

Meningitis/Encephalitis

Clinical meningitis occurs concomitantly with parotitis in 1 to 10 per cent of patients; it appears approximately 4 days after clinical parotitis is noted. Pleocytosis in the cerebrospinal fluid (10 to 2000 white blood cells per mm³) occurs in 50 per cent of patients undergoing lumbar puncture, usually with a predominance of lymphocytes, although polymorphonuclear leukocytes may predominate. The level of glucose in cerebrospinal fluid is less than 50 per cent of the level of glucose in serum in 6 to 30 per cent of cases. Mumps meningitis usually resolves without sequelae; 1 per cent of aseptic meningitis is currently attributed to mumps. Encephalitis is rare and more serious, with the usual onset 10 to 14 days after salivary gland enlargement. The patient may become severely ill and obtunded or develop seizures.

Epididymo-orchitis

In postpubertal men, epididymo-orchitis is the most common extrasalivary gland manifestation. It occurs in 20 to 30 per cent of cases and is bilateral in 2 to 6 per cent. The onset of orchitis in 75 per cent of cases is during the first week of parotitis, but orchitis may occur without parotitis. A concomitant epididymitis is present in 85 per cent of cases. With defervescence, testicular pain and swelling resolve rapidly.

Pancreatitis

Severe pancreatitis is rare and presents with vomiting, epigastric pain, and an increase in the level of amylase in serum. Therapy is supportive: intravenous fluids, no oral intake, and nasogastric drainage are used. Spontaneous resolution usually occurs during 1 to 3 weeks. Subclinical pancreatitis may be more common than is thought.

Arthritis

Mumps-associated arthritis is rare, is usually polyarticular, and occurs mostly in young adult males. It may involve large and small joints; it begins 10 to 14 days after the onset of parotitis and lasts 2 days to 6 months before spontaneous resolution without residual damage. The duration of arthritis is unaltered by salicylates. Two-week courses of nonsteroidal anti-inflammatory agents may reduce symptoms of high fever and arthritis; an additional 2-week course should be given if symptoms recur.

Mumps During Pregnancy

Spontaneous abortions are possible when mumps occurs in the first trimester. A prospective study by Siegel in 1973 reported abortion in 27 per cent of women with mumps compared with 13 per cent in controls. The incidence of mumps during pregnancy is estimated at 0.8 to 10 cases per 10,000 population. There is a controversial association of intrauterine mumps infection with endocardial fibroelastosis.

DIAGNOSIS

The diagnosis of mumps is easily made in patients with a history of exposure, parotid swelling and tenderness, and mild to moderate systemic symptoms. Laboratory confirmation by either serologic tests or virus isolation may be necessary if the course is atypical or if extrasalivary gland manifestations are severe. A fourfold rise between acute and convalescent sera 3 to 5 weeks apart by complement fixing, hemagglutination-inhibition, or neutralization antibodies confirms the diagnosis. Complement-fixing antibodies to the soluble antigen (nucleoprotein) are detectable often at the onset of clinical disease and decline during 8 to 9 months; anti-V antibody (against a surface antigen) rises more slowly, peaking at 2 to 4 weeks, and persists for years. Mumps virus may be isolated from saliva from 6 days before to 9 days after the onset of symptoms, from cerebrospinal fluid during the first 3 days of meningeal symptoms, from urine for 2 weeks, and from blood during the first 2 days. Virus has been found in breast milk.

DIFFERENTIAL DIAGNOSIS

Parainfluenza virus type 3, coxsackievirus, influenza virus type A, lymphocytic choriomeningitis virus, and human immunodeficiency virus can also present with parotitis. Suppurative parotitis caused predominantly by group A *Streptococcus* or *Staphylococcus aureus* presents as a unilateral warm, hard, tender gland with purulent drainage from Stensen's duct, often accompanied by systemic symptoms of fever, lethargy, and headache. Drugs (phenylbutazone, thiouracil, nifedipine, iodides, and phenothiazines) can produce nontender bilateral parotitis, as can diabetes mellitus, malnutrition, cirrhosis, sarcoidosis, and renal failure. Patients with Sjögren's syndrome can also have parotitis.

TREATMENT

No specific antiviral therapy is currently available; thus therapy is supportive and symptomatic and involves antipyretic medications, cold packs to areas of painful swelling, and perhaps nonsteroidal anti-inflammatory agents. Hyperimmune globulin or pooled IgG does not prevent infection, lessen the severity of illness, or decrease the incidence or severity of orchitis. Adequate hydration is recommended to prevent sludging of inflammatory material and damaging obstruction of the salivary gland duct. Therapy of orchitis is also symptomatic with bed rest and perhaps narcotic analgesics. Support of the inflamed testes and ice packs may help. Regional anesthetic nerve block in the spermatic cord with 1 per cent procaine hydrochloride can relieve severe pain.

PREVENTATIVE MEASURES

Live attenuated mumps vaccine (licensed in December 1967) produces 95 to 100 per cent serologic conversion. Immunization is recommended using the measles, mumps, rubella vaccine at 15 months of age, but good serologic response occurs as early as 12 months of age. Immunization is recommended for older children, adolescents, and adults with no history of natural infection or previous immunization. Antibody levels, although lower than after natural infection, persist at least 15 years. Infectious virus cannot be recovered from persons who have been vaccinated. Side effects other than local tenderness are rare and include mild transient parotitis several weeks after immunization, rash, and pruritus. Mumps immunization during the incubation of mumps neither ameliorates nor prevents disease, but there are no ill effects of such vaccine administration, and these patients given vaccine acquire protection if clinical disease fails to develop.

Mumps vaccine should not be administered to pregnant women; to patients allergic to neomycin, eggs, chickens, or chicken feathers; or to severely immunocompromised patients (patients with malignancies or T cell or B cell defects, or patients receiving immunotherapy), although the Centers for Disease Control recommends immunization of pediatric patients with acquired immunodeficiency syndrome. Patients who receive whole blood, plasma, or gamma globulin in the 8 weeks before vaccine administration may not seroconvert.

SEQUELAE

In patients with orchitis, some degree of testicular atrophy occurs in 50 per cent, some degree of infertility occurs in 13 per cent, and sterility occurs in 2 per cent. Transient high-frequency deafness has been reported in approximately 4 per cent of cases. Permanent unilateral deafness occurs rarely (1 per 15,000 cases), but mumps is considered to be the leading cause of unilateral sensorineural deafness. Sialectasia, from damage to the salivary gland duct, may lead to recurrent sialadenitis.

PLAGUE

method of
HARRY F. HULL, M.D.
Lovelace Medical Center
Santa Fe, New Mexico

Plague is a rare, zoonotic disease of humans that is caused by the bacterium *Yersinia pestis*. In the United States, the disease is propagated in rodents and fleas in rural environments in an area bounded by the Mexican and Canadian borders, the Pacific Ocean, and a line stretching from the Texas panhandle to western North Dakota. The only major urban areas where plague-infected rodents have been identified since 1980 are Los Angeles, California and Albuquerque, New Mexico. Ten to 40 human cases occur each year in the United States, two-thirds of which are seen in New Mexico. Although cases may occur at any time during the year, most occur during the summer. Native Americans have an attack rate that is much higher than that of other ethnic groups. More than one-half of all patients are younger than 20 years old; the sex ratio is nearly 1:1.

There are three major forms of human plague: bubonic, septicemic, and pneumonic. Bubonic plague is the most common form and affects 75 to 90 per cent of patients. Within 1 week of exposure, but usually within several days, the patient will have fever, malaise, and discrete lymph node pain. These symptoms are followed rapidly by regional lymphadenopathy. The nodes (buboes) are exquisitely painful, and an overlying, brawny edema is typical. The inguinal and femoral nodes are most commonly affected (70 per cent), followed by the axillary nodes (20 per cent) and cervical and occipital nodes (10 per cent). Headache, chills, nausea, vomiting, and diarrhea are common. Septicemic plague occurs in about 20 per cent of patients. Presentation is indistinguishable from that of other forms of gram-negative sepsis. Symptoms include fever, chills, malaise, headache, nausea, vomiting, and diarrhea. Abdominal pain occurs in about one-half of cases. Tachypnea, tachycardia, and hypotension are common. The elderly, infants, and persons with immune deficiency or other underlying disease appear to be at increased risk of contracting this form of plague. Secondary pneumonic plague is a late complication in 10 per cent of cases. Primary pneumonic plague may result from airborne spread of bacilli from another patient with pneumonic plague. The pneumonia has no characteristic features except for the preterminal production of bloody sputum. Less common manifestations of plague include meningitis, endophthalmitis, and cutaneous and pharyngeal infections.

DIAGNOSIS

Because of the high mortality associated with plague and the potential for person-to-person spread of pneumonic plague, prompt diagnosis and treatment of persons with plague are imperative. Physicians who practice in New Mexico or on Native American reservations of the Southwest need to maintain a high index of suspicion, especially during the summer. Patients who have fever with or without buboes who reside or have a history of outdoor activity in plague-endemic rural areas should undergo an aggressive diagnostic work-up and be considered for presumptive treatment. A complete blood count with differential count and blood cultures should be obtained for patients with suspected plague. Leukocytosis with a shift to the left is characteristic of plague. If a bubo is present, it should be aspirated for microscopic examination and culture. (Precaution: masks should be worn during this procedure.) A rapid presumptive diagnosis can be made with fluorescent antibody testing of bubo aspirates. Fluorescent antibody testing can be arranged through state health department laboratories. The presence of gram-negative rods in a bubo aspirate strongly suggests plague. These rods have a bipolar appearance when stained with Wayson's, Geimsa's, or Wright's stain. Plague bacilli may occasionally be observed in the peripheral blood smear or a stained smear of the buffy coat. Definitive diagnosis depends on the isolation of Y. pestis from cultures, which usually requires 3 to 5 days. Patients with plague should have a chest film to rule out pneumonia. Serum should be saved for serologic testing, but this study is useful only for retrospective diagnosis when cultures are negative.

TREATMENT

Three antibiotics are accepted as effective against plague: streptomycin, tetracycline, and chloramphenicol. Gentamicin and trimethoprim-sulfamethoxazole are probably effective as well. Penicillins are clearly not effective. Likewise, cephalosporins are probably not effective and should not be used. The optimal antibiotic regimen depends on the form and severity of the illness, as well as the patient's age. Intramuscular streptomycin is the mainstay of therapy. The dosage for streptomycin is 30 mg per kg per day in two to four divided doses for adults and 20 to 30 mg per kg per day in two to four doses for children. Concern about ototoxicity and the discomfort of repeated intramuscular injections may limit the course of therapy with streptomycin to 5 days. In this case, oral tetracycline should be given to complete a 10-day course of therapy. Herxheimer's reactions have been described for streptomycin therapy of plague. Intramuscular streptomycin should not be used for patients with septic shock. Tetracycline may be given intravenously or by mouth to persons older than 8 years. An oral loading dose of 15 mg per kg (not to exceed 1 gram) should be given, followed by 30 mg per kg per day for a total of 10 days. The dosage for intravenous tetracycline is 12 to 20 mg per kg per day until the patient can be started on oral therapy. Chloramphenicol is useful in children and for the treatment of plague meningitis or endophthalmitis. The dosage is 50 to 75 mg per kg per day either orally or intravenously in four divided doses. Patients receiving chloramphenicol should be observed for bone marrow toxicity. Because of its apparent efficacy in plague, gentamicin (Garamycin) is recommended for the treatment of sepsis of unknown etiology in plague-endemic areas.

Plague responds quickly to appropriate antibiotic therapy. Fever disappears within 3 to 5 days. Buboes usually regress during several weeks without local therapy, but occasionally incision and drainage are required. Patients with plague should be placed in respiratory isolation for the first 24 to 48 hours until it is certain that no pneumonia is present. Respiratory isolation of patients with pneumonic plague should continue until at least 72 hours of effective antibiotic therapy have been completed. Wound and secretion precautions should be used for patients with draining buboes or ulcers.

Complications of plague may include overwhelming sepsis and shock, adult respiratory distress syndrome, and disseminated intravascular coagulation. Patients who remain febrile after 5 days of appropriate antibiotic therapy should be examined for metastatic foci of infection, particularly meningitis.

PREVENTION

Persons who have face-to-face contact with a patient who has pneumonic plague should receive prophylactic antibiotics. Persons who are exposed to the same source of plague infection as the patient may also be given prophylactic treatment. Tetracycline, 250 to 500 mg orally four times a day for 5 to 7 days, is the drug of choice for most adults. Therapeutic doses of trimethoprim-sulfamethoxazole (Bactrim, Septra) are used for children older than 2 months of age. Contacts for whom antibiotics are contraindicated (e.g., a pregnant woman) should be observed and treated with antibiotics if fever develops. Plague vaccine plays no role in the management of plague contacts.

Reporting of plague is mandatory. Because plague can generate a considerable fear among both the average person and medical personnel, the state or local health department should be involved in establishing both isolation procedures in the hospital and criteria for prophylactic treatment of contacts. The health department should also assist in identifying and locating contacts outside of the hospital.

PSITTACOSIS
(Ornithosis)

method of
DAVID H. THOM, M.D., M.P.H., and
J. THOMAS GRAYSTON, M.D.
University of Washington
Seattle, Washington

Human psittacosis (also called ornithosis) is caused by *Chlamydia psittaci,* an obligate intracellular bacterium. The infection is typically manifested by fever, pneumonitis, and systemic symptoms, although subclinical infections are known to occur as well. Birds that are infected with *C. psittaci* have been implicated as the source of human psittacosis since 1879. Virtually all common pet birds and many species of wild birds can carry the organism and often remain healthy while shedding organisms in their excreta and secretions. Human exposure occurs through inhalation of aerosolized particles containing *C. psittaci* or by direct contact with infected birds. Even brief exposure to birds or their excreta can cause infection. Turkey processing in the United States and duck processing in Europe account for the bulk of occupational psittacosis. Exposure to pet birds, including parakeets, parrots, and pigeons, accounts for most of the 150 to 200 cases of psittacosis reported annually in the United States.

Recently, a *Chlamydia* organism, *C. pneumoniae* strain TWAR, which is related to but distinct from *C. psittaci,* has been linked by culture and serology to human respiratory infections. No avian source of *C. pneumoniae* has been identified, which suggests that it is transmitted by human-to-human contact. Epidemics of *C. pneumoniae* strain TWAR in military and other populations have been documented. Several studies have found *C. pneumoniae* to be responsible for 6 to 12 per cent of community-acquired pneumonias and for a smaller percentage of bronchitis and pharyngitis, which makes *C. pneumoniae* infections more common than infections with *C. psittaci.* In addition, it is likely that some of the sporadic cases and past outbreaks of respiratory disease that were diagnosed as psittacosis by complement fixation serology were actually *C. pneumoniae* infections.

DIAGNOSIS

The clinical presentation of *C. psittaci* infection can range from mild symptoms in the upper respiratory tract to respiratory failure. Severe psittacosis typically presents with a moderate to high fever, headache, prominent cough, and relative paucity of pulmonary findings on physical examination. The suspicion of psittacosis is usually raised only when a history of exposure to birds is obtained. Infections with *C. pneumoniae* tend to be milder than diagnosed *C. psittaci* infections but can also range from a mild upper respiratory tract infection to severe pneumonia. Patients with *C. pneumoniae* infections may have a biphasic illness, with pharyngitis and upper respiratory tract symptoms followed in 1 to 3 weeks by pneumonia or bronchitis, or they may have a gradual onset of symptoms with an increasingly severe cough. Hoarseness was reported by 25 per cent of patients in one study. Neither leukocytosis nor fever is common.

In a patient with pneumonia, a history of recent exposure to a new pet bird or to a bird that sickens and dies makes psittacosis a likely diagnosis. However, no features of the clinical presentation, common laboratory tests, or chest radiograph are diagnostic of either *C. psittaci* or *C. pneumoniae* infections. *C. psittaci* is rarely isolated from the patient, and laboratory diagnosis depends on a fourfold rise in the *Chlamydia* complement fixation antibody titer between acute and convalescent serum samples taken 2 to 4 weeks apart. Early treatment with tetracycline may blunt or prevent the antibody response to *C. psittaci* infections. The complement fixation test that is usually used to diagnose psittacosis does not distinguish between *C. psittaci* and other systemic chlamydial infections, including *C. pneumoniae.* Isolation techniques and *C. pneumoniae*–specific antibody tests are available only in specialized laboratories.

TREATMENT

General treatment measures depend on clinical status. Patients with dyspnea, hypoxia, confusion, or other signs of severe disease should be hospitalized. Case fatality rates are usually less than 1 percent with treatment but can be higher in the elderly. Case fatality rates up to 40 per cent have been reported in untreated cases. To prevent transmission to humans, respiratory isolation is recommended. Patients should be observed for the rare nonrespiratory complications of psittacosis, which include endocarditis, pericarditis, myocarditis, encephalitis, meningitis, renal failure, spontaneous abortion, and reactive arthralgias. Health department authorities should be notified immediately.

The only widely accepted antibiotic therapy for psittacosis is tetracycline, 2 to 3 grams per day, which usually results in a clinical response within 24 to 48 hours, although delayed responses have been reported. Alternatives have been less well studied. Doxycycline (Vibramycin), an oxytetracycline derivative, has been used successfully to treat *C. psittaci* endocarditis in doses of 200 mg per day. Rifampin (Rifadin, Rimactane) and erythromycin have in vitro activity against *C. psittaci* and have been used alone or in combination in doses of 600 to 1200 mg per day for rifampin and 2 to 4 grams per day for erythromycin. Beta-lactam antibiotics such as penicillin are generally not recommended. If tetracycline or erythromycin is used, treatment with 2 grams per day should be continued for 14 days after defervescence, or for a total of 14 to 21 days, to prevent relapses.

Future immunity should not be assumed because reinfections have been reported. A prolonged convalescence after successful treatment is not uncommon. *C. pneumoniae* infections should be treated by using the same guidelines.

PREVENTION

There is no vaccine for psittacosis. The disease still occurs in turkeys, inadequately treated pet birds, and some wild birds. Appropriate surveillance of poultry flocks and pet shops and prompt investigation of outbreaks of psittacosis are needed to determine and eradicate sources of exposure. Limited information is now available on *C. pneumoniae,* and no method of prevention has been found.

Q FEVER

method of
THOMAS MARRIE, M.D.
Dalhousie University
Halifax, Nova Scotia, Canada

Q fever is the illness that results from infection by the rickettsial organism *Coxiella burnetii*. This zoonosis is widely distributed in nature, but the main reservoirs for transmission of this organism to humans are infected cattle, sheep, and goats. The placenta of these animals is heavily infected, and the organism is excreted in large amounts into the environment at the time of parturition. Humans become infected after inhaling the microorganism. The incubation period ranges from 4 to 30 days and is usually 2 weeks.

The most common manifestations of this infection are a self-limited febrile illness; atypical pneumonia, which ranges from mild to severe and rapidly progressive; hepatitis; and chronic Q fever, manifested mainly as endocarditis.

SUPPORTIVE TREATMENT

The severe headache that is part of Q fever often requires analgesics. Fever may persist for up to 10 days, although usually it lasts for only 3 to 4 days. During this period, antipyretics are useful. In some individuals, parenteral fluid therapy is necessary to correct dehydration.

SPECIFIC THERAPY

In 1962 it was demonstrated that the administration of tetracycline during the first 3 days of the illness reduced the duration of fever by 50 per cent. In spite of this observation, tetracycline has no activity against *C. burnetii* in infected L 7929 cells. In this situation, rifampin, difloxacin, oxolinic acid, and ciprofloxacin are most effective.

Our approach is to treat patients with severe, atypical pneumonia (in whom Q fever is considered likely) with both erythromycin and rifampin. Erythromycin is useless against *C. burnetii,* but rifampin is effective. For adults we use 600 mg of rifampin (Rifadin, Rimactane) every 12 hours* for the first 72 hours and then 300 mg every 12 hours to complete a 10-day course of treatment. This approach also allows us to treat the other causes of atypical pneumonia, such as *Mycoplasma pneumoniae* and *Legionella pneumophila.* For patients who cannot tolerate rifampin, tetracycline, 500 mg every 6 hours, or doxycycline, 100 mg every 12 hours, is used. Trimethoprim-sulfamethoxazole (Bactrim, Septra) may also be used in a dose of one double-strength tablet every 12 hours.

Patients with endocarditis (chronic Q fever) present with the features of culture-negative endocarditis and have Phase I titers that are severalfold higher than the Phase II titers, a situation that we have never found in acute Q fever. Controversy exists as to the proper treatment for Q fever endocarditis. We start therapy with tetracycline, 500 mg every 6 hours, and trimethoprim-sulfamethoxazole, one double-strength tab-

---

*This dose may exceed the manufacturer's recommended dose.

let every 12 hours. These medications are continued for at least 2 years. During this period, the Phase I and Phase II antibody titers should be monitored every 3 months. We discontinue therapy when the Phase I titer has declined to 1:512 by the indirect fluorescent antibody technique. (Some authorities recommend continuing therapy indefinitely.) If tetracycline cannot be tolerated, rifampin, 600 mg every 12 hours,* may be used in combination with trimethoprim-sulfamethoxazole. Although the quinolones have been shown to be active against *C. burnetii* in vitro, there are too few data to allow us to make a recommendation regarding their use in the treatment of Q fever endocarditis. Patients with Q fever endocarditis need careful follow-up, and valve replacement is frequently necessary for hemodynamic reasons.

PREVENTION

All cattle, sheep, and goats used in research laboratories should be serologically tested for *C. burnetii* before being admitted. Several outbreaks of Q fever have occurred when infected animals have been brought into research institutions.

VACCINATION

A Phase I vaccine has proved to be effective in Australia. When available, this vaccine should be offered to individuals at high risk for infection, such as veterinarians, abattoir workers, livestock dealers and transporters, auctioneers, bulk milk transporters, and meat inspectors.

---

*This dose may exceed the manufacturer's recommended dose.

RABIES

method of
SUZANNE R. JENKINS, V.M.D., M.P.H.
Virginia Department of Health
Richmond, Virginia

Although rabies in humans is extremely rare in the United States (an average of two cases per year), animal bites are very common (more than 1 million per year). Thus the clinician is more likely to be faced with a decision about the management of a potential rabies exposure than with the diagnosis and treatment of the actual disease. Rabies in animals, particularly in wild animals, is not uncommon in this country. In 1987, only 12 per cent of the 4729 rabid animals reported were domestic animals.

Rabies is caused by a rhabdovirus that can infect any warm-blooded animal but tends to predominate in a particular species in a specific geographic area. Although the predominant species may be involved in more than 85 per cent of the animal rabies cases in an area, spillover to any other mammal, including humans, is possible. In addition to the predominant species associated with the endemic rabies areas of North America (mid-Atlantic and southeastern raccoon, midwestern and California skunk, and northeastern fox), the potential for isolated cases of rabies exists in bats or other species bitten by rabid bats.

Recent research with panels of monoclonal antibodies has been used to define various rabies virus ecotypes and to help identify the source of some human cases. Humans whose rabies infection was acquired in the United States and for whom virus characterization was done have been found to be infected with the same virus type that circulates in the local wildlife.

POSTEXPOSURE DECISION-MAKING

Although the rabies biologics presently available in the United States are relatively safe, the decision to administer rabies postexposure prophylaxis should not be undertaken lightly because of the potential for reactions and the high cost. Each case needs to be evaluated separately to decide the most appropriate action (Figure 1). Consultation with local or state public health officials who are familiar with the epidemiology of rabies and the availability of biologics in that area should be sought.

The first part of the decision-making process is to ascertain whether an exposure actually took place. In rabid animals, rabies virus is present in concentrations that are considered to be infectious in the saliva, salivary glands, brain, and, less often, the spinal cord or large peripheral nerves of livestock. The virus usually enters the body through broken skin; it rarely enters through intact mucous membranes. Thus the most likely route of entry is via the bite of a rabid animal or contamination of a fresh open wound by saliva. Aerosol transmission of rabies has occurred only under special circumstances: two laboratory researchers acquired rabies while working with high concentrations of virus used for vaccine production, and two cases were reported in persons who spent time in bat caves that contained unusually high numbers of bats. There have also been cases that resulted from corneal transplants.

If it is established that a true exposure has taken place, the next step is to evaluate the possibility of rabies in that animal. Dogs and cats account for less than 11 per cent of the rabid animals in the United States but are responsible for the majority of postexposure prophylaxis given in this country. In dogs and cats, signs of rabies usually accompany the shedding of virus in saliva. Rarely, the onset of signs can be delayed for up to 5 days. If a dog or cat that bites someone is considered to be normal by a veterinarian, animal control officer, or public health official, it should be placed under confinement and observation for 10 days. As long as no signs of illness or behavioral changes indicative of rabies occur, rabies postexposure treatment of the exposed person is not necessary. Dogs

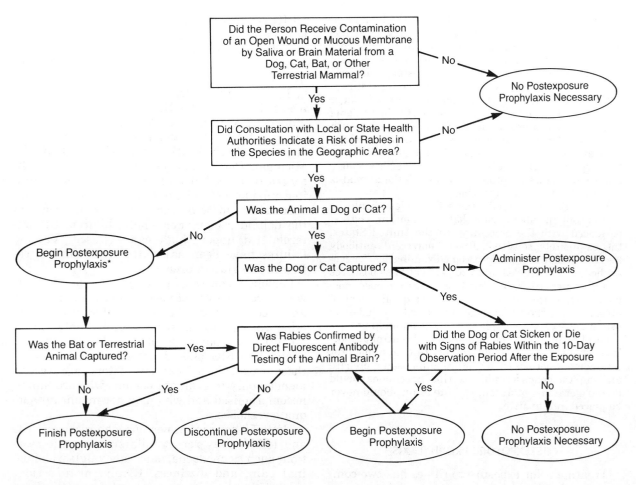

Figure 1. Algorithm for human rabies postexposure prophylaxis. *In exposures of low risk, when the animal brain is available for testing, the decision to administer postexposure prophylaxis is sometimes delayed for up to 2 days after the exposure pending the results of fluorescent antibody testing of the animal brain. (Modified from Fishbein DB. *In* Fishbein DB, Sawyer LA, and Winkler WT (eds): Rabies Concepts for Medical Professionals, 2nd ed. Miami, Merieux Institute, 1986, p. 56. Used by permission.)

and cats that show signs at the time of the bite or develop them during the period of confinement should be killed immediately and the head should be shipped to an appropriate laboratory for testing. The 10-day confinement applies to both vaccinated and unvaccinated animals. Although the risk of rabies in a vaccinated dog or cat is extremely low, vaccine failures do occur.

If exposure is from a dog or cat that is not available for observation or testing (i.e., a stray animal that cannot be located or a pet that disappears), the decision on postexposure prophylaxis should be based on the presence of animal rabies in the area and the circumstances of the biting incident, that is, whether the animal was behaving normally and whether the bite was provoked. The expertise of local or state public health officials should always be sought in these cases.

Although exposures from other domestic animals such as livestock have the potential for rabies, the risk of acquiring the disease from these species is extremely low, and treatment of the person is not indicated unless

the animal is symptomatic and its brain is found to be positive in the test for rabies. Because the period of shedding of rabies virus in wild and exotic animals is not known, even those that are kept as pets cannot be managed in the same way as domestic animals. Pet skunks, foxes, raccoons, and the increasingly popular European ferrets (a member of the skunk family) that bite a person should, under almost all circumstances, be killed and tested for rabies.

The major wildlife reservoirs of rabies in this country are skunks, raccoons, foxes, coyotes, bobcats, and bats, and exposure from these animals carries a high risk for rabies. Unless the animal's brain can be tested for rabies, postexposure prophylaxis should always be instituted when a person has been bitten by one of these species.

Animals that are unlikely to be rabid and for which exposure rarely requires postexposure prophylaxis include hooved mammals (such as deer, moose, and antelope), small rodents (such as mice, rats, gerbils, hamsters, guinea pigs, squirrels, and chipmunks), and lagomorphs (rabbits and hares). Despite the high number of rodent bites that occur in this country, there has never been a human rabies case resulting from such a bite. Abnormal, aggressive behavior by any of these animals might indicate the need for postexposure prophylaxis if the animal were not available for testing.

Woodchucks (ground hogs) and beavers are large rodents that account for the majority of rabid rodents in the United States, particularly in association with the mid-Atlantic raccoon outbreak. The potential for transmission via these animals is unknown. Bites by these species in areas where wildlife rabies is endemic require postexposure prophylaxis unless the animal is found to be negative on testing.

The testing of animal brains for rabies should be carried out in laboratories that are familiar and experienced with the procedure. In the United States, the exquisitely sensitive direct fluorescent antibody test has replaced the microscopic examination for Negri bodies that yielded up to 20 per cent false positives and false negatives. In some laboratories, mouse inoculation tests are still done as part of a quality control program, but the 21-day waiting period precludes its use in postexposure prophylaxis decision-making.

Local health department and animal control authorities should be contacted to institute and monitor confinement periods or to capture animals and prepare and ship the heads for rabies testing. Specimens should be refrigerated, not frozen, and the brain should never be placed in a fixative.

POSTEXPOSURE PROPHYLAXIS

Treatment for exposure to rabies has two components, local wound treatment and immunization. The risk of acquiring rabies can be reduced markedly if the wound is immediately and thoroughly washed with soap and water. In animal studies, the use of water or saline alone was not as effective as soap and water. Two products are used for immunization of persons who have had no prior experience with rabies biologics. Human rabies immune globulin (HRIG) is administered on the first day of treatment (designated day 0) to confer passive immunity until the body mounts a defense in response to the rabies vaccine (approximately 7 to 10 days after the initial vaccination). The dose of HRIG is 20 IU per kg body weight. If anatomically possible, up to one-half of the HRIG dose should be infiltrated around the wound; the remainder should be given deep in the gluteal area. Under no circumstances should the HRIG be given in the same site as the vaccine, where it might compromise vaccine activity. HRIG is supplied in 2-ml (300-IU) and 10-ml (1500-IU) vials, which are standardized to contain 150 IU per ml. Rabies immune globulin made from horse serum is available but carries a high risk (>40 per cent) of serum sickness and should be used only if HRIG is not available. If HRIG is inadvertently not given on day 0, it can be administered up to the eighth day after the first dose of vaccine.

Rabies vaccine is administered in a series of five 1-ml injections during a 28-day period (days 0, 3, 7, 14, and 28). Of the two vaccines currently licensed for use in the United States, only human diploid cell vaccine (HDCV; manufactured by the Merieux Institute) is widely available. The rabies vaccine, adsorbed (RVA; manufactured by the Michigan Department of Public Health) was licensed in 1988, but its availability remains limited outside of Michigan. Administration of either vaccine should be by the intramuscular route in the deltoid region. For small children, the anterolateral upper thigh can be used. Vaccine failures have been associated with administration in the gluteal area.

Persons requiring postexposure prophylaxis who have a history of vaccination with HDCV or an adequate postvaccination titer from some other rabies vaccine should receive only two 1-ml intramuscular doses of HDCV given on days 0 and 3. HRIG should not be administered in these cases. Post-treatment titers are recommended only to evaluate persons who are immunocompromised and who may not mount an adequate response.

Up to 50 per cent of persons who receive HRIG and HDCV may report mild symptomatic reactions such as headache, nausea, myalgias, abdominal pain, and dizziness. Rarely, more serious side effects have been reported, but none have been life-threatening. Two cases of Guillain-Barré syndrome after the administration of HDCV have been reported with no permanent sequelae. Immune complex–like illness has been reported in about 6 per cent of persons who have a history of HDCV vaccination and then receive a booster of the same vaccine. Pregnancy, existing illness, and previous allergy to rabies vaccine are not contraindications for postexposure prophylaxis if the person has been exposed to rabies. Patients with a history of allergic reactions should be closely monitored during postexposure prophylaxis. If a different brand of vaccine is available, its use may avert a reaction. Otherwise, allergic reactions can be controlled with antihistamines, epinephrine, or corticosteroids. The latter should be used as a last resort because corticosteroids may interfere with the production of rabies antibodies.

PRE-EXPOSURE PROPHYLAXIS

Rabies vaccines can be used for pre-exposure immunization in persons who are likely to experience an inapparent exposure, such as wildlife workers, veterinarians and their staff members, animal control officers, laboratory workers conducting research on rabies, spelunkers, and others having direct contact with animals at high risk for having rabies. Travelers to foreign countries who will be spending more than 30 days in areas with endemic rabies should also receive rabies pre-exposure immunization. This immunization may offer protection if there are delays in receiving postexposure treatment or if rabies immune globulin is not available. A history of pre-exposure immunization does not eliminate the need for postexposure treatment after a known exposure. However, the need for HRIG is eliminated and only two doses of vaccine are required, one on day 0 and one on day 3. Pre-exposure immunization consists of three 1-ml intramuscular doses of HDCV or RVA given on days 0, 7, and 28. HDCV (for intradermal use: Imovax Rabies I.D. Vaccine) may also be given in three 0.1-ml intradermal doses in the deltoid region by using the same schedule as that for the 1-ml intramuscular doses. Travelers should either receive the 1-ml intramuscular series or complete the 0.1-ml intradermal series at least 30 days before departure. Those receiving chloroquine for malaria chemoprophylaxis, which may interfere with the immune response to HDCV, should be administered only the 1-ml intramuscular regimen. Postvaccination serologic testing is not recommended unless the vaccinated person is immunocompromised. For persons who have a continuing potential for exposure, a booster dose should be considered every 2 years. Because of the risk of immune complex–like illness from boosters, a titer should be assayed and a booster administered only if the titer is inadequate. Either HDCV or RVA, 1-ml intramuscularly, or HDCV, 0.1-ml intradermally, can be administered as a booster.

CLINICAL DISEASE IN HUMANS

Although rabies in humans is extremely rare in the United States, it should be included in any differential diagnosis of a person with a rapidly progressive encephalitis even if there is no history of an exposure to an infected animal. Of the 11 cases of rabies in humans reported to the Centers for Disease Control since 1980, 5 had no known animal exposure. In many cases, the patient's condition precluded obtaining an accurate history. Two cases involved children who had emigrated from areas with endemic rabies 4 and 7 years previously, which raised the possibility of extended incubation periods in humans.

Fortunately, humans are not very susceptible to rabies. The risk of developing clinical disease depends on the amount of virus that is inoculated, the location of the inoculation, and host factors such as the number of nerve endings at the inoculation site, environmental stress, administration of corticosteroids, and administration of postexposure prophylaxis treatment. The probability of developing rabies from an animal with confirmed rabies varies from less than 1 per cent for contamination of minor wounds to more than 80 per cent for severe bites by wolves. Unfortunately, once symptoms develop there is little likelihood of recovery. Only two recoveries have been documented in the United States, one complete and the other with permanent sequelae; both patients had received some form of either pre- or postexposure prophylaxis.

Although some symptoms of rabies may be considered to be pathognomonic, such as hydrophobia and aerophobia, most symptoms are nonspecific and so varied that the diagnosis of rabies is rarely entertained until late in the disease. Clinical rabies in humans is classically divided into five stages: incubation period, prodrome, acute neurologic phase, coma, and recovery or death. The usual incubation period is between 20 and 90 days, although it can be as short as 9 days and up to several years long. A bite on the head results in a shorter incubation period.

The initial symptoms experienced during the 2- to 10-day prodrome are the most nonspecific and may include malaise, fatigue, headache, anorexia, and fever, and less often, mild respiratory or gastrointestinal signs. Approximately 50 per cent of patients report pain or paraesthesia at the site of the exposure. Neurologic involvement may be suggested by apprehension, anxiety, agitation, irritability, nervousness, insomnia, or depression. The first objective signs of neurologic involvement may include hyperactivity, disorientation, hallucinations, seizures, bizarre behavior, nuchal rigidity, or paralysis. In most cases, hyperactive episodes either occur spontaneously or are precipitated by various stimuli. It is during this time that attempts to drink may produce severe spasms of the pharynx or larynx. Fever (temperature $> 100°$ F) occurs in almost all patients. As the disease progresses (unless respiratory or cardiac arrest causes the patient's death), paralysis develops and mental status deteriorates from confusion to disorientation, stupor, and finally coma. Throughout the acute neurologic period, the mental status alternates between severe obtundation and relative normalcy. Coma occurs 4 to 10 days after onset of symptoms. In the absence of intensive supportive care, death can occur as early as 7 days after the first appearance of symptoms. With care, most patients survive for another week.

Rabies can be diagnosed by such laboratory procedures as detection of antigen in direct immunofluorescent antibody–stained impressions of corneal epithelium or neck skin biopsies, isolation of virus from saliva, and demonstration of significant titer to rabies virus in cerebrospinal fluid or serum (in the absence of a history of passive or active immunization). If these tests are positive, it is usually not until late in the course of illness.

If rabies is suspected in a patient, state public health authorities should be notified. These authorities can contact the Centers for Disease Control to assist in evaluating the patient, provide information on proper hospital isolation procedures, and facilitate the rapid processing of laboratory tests for rabies.

RAT-BITE FEVER

method of
EDWARD EISENBERG, M.D.
Montclair, New Jersey

Rat-bite fever is an acute febrile illness that is usually acquired by means of the bite or scratch of a rat, mouse, or other rodent. In some instances mere contact with a rodent or with another animal that recently killed a rodent has preceded human infection. The term rat-bite fever refers to two similar yet distinct disease syndromes caused by two different organisms that are part of the normal oral flora of the rat. *Streptobacillus moniliformis* is a pleomorphic gram-negative bacillus that grows poorly in routine blood culture bottles. It is best isolated in liquid media supplemented by serum, in which it forms characteristic puffball colonies. It is the major cause of rat-bite fever in North America and can be isolated from the oropharynx of 50 to 100 per cent of rats, including laboratory rats. *Spirillum minus* is a gram-negative, short, thick, tightly coiled spiral organism that does not grow on standard culture media. It can be identified by dark-field microscopic examination of infected material from patients or after injection of infected material into animals.

CLINICAL MANIFESTATIONS

Both illnesses are characterized by the acute onset of fever, malaise, chills, and rash. If the illnesses are untreated, relapse may occur for months or, rarely, for years. Distinguishing features of the illnesses are summarized in Table 1. Both illnesses may occur simultaneously. Occasionally, the chronic complications of arthritis, endocarditis, and abscess may occur. Although joint fluid is usually sterile, *S. moniliformis* has been cultured from the fluid. *S. moniliformis,* but not *S. minus,* may also cause epidemic disease by ingestion of raw milk contaminated by rat excrement.

TABLE 1. **Distinguishing Features of Rat-Bite Fevers**

	S. moniliformis	*S. minus*
Mode of transmission	Rat bite or ingestion	Rat bite
Incubation period to fever	A few days	More than 1 wk
Bite wound	Heals promptly	Heals, then ulcerates
Lymphadenopathy	Uncommon, mild	Prominent, usually regional
Arthritis	Common	Rare
Rash appearing days after fever onset	Morbilliform-purpuric	Maculopapular
False-positive syphilis serology	25%	50%

Such outbreaks of Haverhill's fever are characterized by rash, arthritis, upper respiratory symptoms, and vomiting.

DIAGNOSIS

The initial diagnosis of rat-bite fever is based on clinical suspicion in a patient with exposure to the animals. Routine laboratory tests are of little value, and in many cases blood and body fluid cultures do not reveal *S. moniliformis*. Dark-field microscopic examination of infected material from patients or intraperitoneal injection of such material into animals may establish the diagnosis of rat-bite fever caused by *S. minus*. Gas-liquid chromatography remains an experimental means of diagnosing disease caused by *S. moniliformis*. The differential diagnosis of the acute illness includes viral exanthems, rickettsial diseases, leptospirosis, Lyme disease, syphilis, infective endocarditis, and collagen vascular diseases.

THERAPY

The treatment of any bite begins with meticulous local wound care. Many authorities recommend prophylaxis with an oral antibiotic.

The drug of choice for rat-bite fever caused by either pathogen is penicillin. Procaine penicillin, 600,000 units intramuscularly twice daily, and aqueous penicillin G, 400,000 to 600,000 units intravenously every 4 to 6 hours, have been used with success. After clinical improvement of the patient, penicillin V, 500 mg every 6 hours, may be administered for a total course of 10 to 14 days. Septic complications may require drainage. Endocarditis should be treated with 12 to 24 million units of penicillin G intravenously for 4 weeks. In the penicillin-allergic patient, tetracycline or erythromycin, each at 2 grams per day, has been efficacious. Streptomycin, 500 mg intramuscularly every 12 hours, has also been used, either alone or with one of the previously mentioned regimens.

RELAPSING FEVERS

method of
ELDRYD H. O. PARRY, M.D.

The Wellcome Tropical Institute
London, England

Tick-borne relapsing fever (TBRF) is a zoonosis caused by several species of *Borrelia* spirochetes. It is transmitted from small mammals (e.g., squirrels and chipmunks) to humans by bites of soft (argasid) ticks. It occurs in most parts of the world except Australasia and the Pacific. It is endemic in the western United States, but it may be seen in persons who have traveled outside the endemic area before the disease became manifest. Outbreaks have been associated with summer camping in log cabins in the Rocky Mountains (Colorado and Washington) and the Grand Canyon.

In louse-borne relapsing fever (LBRF), human head and body lice transmit *Borrelia recurrentis* spirochetes when the louse is crushed against broken skin or an open wound, and the spirochetes then enter the blood stream of the patient. The human-to-human transmission depends thus on the body louse. LBRF is found chiefly in the Horn of Africa—Ethiopia, Djibouti, Somalia, and Sudan—but is also found in Rwanda and Burundi.

CLINICAL FEATURES

These illnesses are acute fevers that, if untreated, resolve by crisis in about 5 days. A series of relapses follow with afebrile intervals of 5 to 9 days. Symptoms include sudden high fever with rigors, headaches, and pains in the back, muscles, and joints; upper abdominal pain; vomiting and diarrhea; cough; and nosebleeds. Physical signs include jaundice, petechial hemorrhages, spontaneous bleeding, enlarged and tender liver and spleen; conjunctivitis; meningism; and impaired consciousness.

DIAGNOSIS

LBRF is easily confirmed by finding spirochetes in blood smears (dark-field or Giemsa's, Wright's, or fluorescent acridine orange stains). TBRF is more difficult to detect. Mouse inoculation may reveal the infection. Other laboratory abnormalities include thrombocytopenia, hyperbilirubinemia, elevated serum enzyme levels, false-positive Weil-Felix and syphilis reactions, and a lymphocyte pleocytosis.

TREATMENT

Antimicrobial Treatment

Table 1 presents the antimicrobial therapy for relapsing fevers. In adults, tetracycline is the drug of choice for both LBRF and TBRF. For children younger than 8 years old and for pregnant women, erythromycin is the best substitute.

TBRF is milder than LBRF but is more difficult to eradicate because spirochetes persist in the central nervous system. Treatment of TBRF should be continued for 10 days, but in LBRF a single dose is curative. Benzathine penicillin and long-acting penicillins, alone, clear spirochetemia too slowly and do not always prevent relapses. Doxycycline in a single dose of 100 mg is effective for mixed infections of LBRF and louse-borne typhus (which occur in the highlands of East Africa).

In an epidemic, a dose of procaine penicillin, 300,000 units on day 1 followed on day 2 by a single dose of doxycycline, 100 mg, has proved to be excellent. But health teams may have to manage with whatever is available—penicillin, tetracycline, or chloramphenicol—and must ensure that patients lie down for at least 24 hours after treatment to avert hypotension (see later).

Jarisch-Herxheimer Reaction

The problem in treatment is to balance the harmful effects of continuing spirochetemia against the known dangerous phases of the inevitable Jarisch-Herxheimer reaction (J-H R). Mortality is now less than 5 per cent in LBRF and is rare in TBRF. It was 30 to 70 per cent before antimicrobial agents were used. The spirochete is rapidly eliminated by tetracycline and other antimicrobial drugs, but the resulting J-H R can be fatal. The reaction is maximal about 1 hour after administration of intravenous tetracycline, with severe rigors and a dramatic and rapid rise in temperature and respiratory and pulse rates. The patient is confused or delirious and has autonomic and gastrointestinal symptoms, cough, and muscle pains. The temperature can reach 41° to 42° C, but it then falls precipitously in the flush phase with sweating, vasodilation, and a steady fall of blood pressure. Death is due to hyperthermia, irremediable hypotension, and, more rarely, myocarditis causing pulmonary edema.

The infection is more severe in women in the last trimester of pregnancy, and fetal loss is possible.

To avoid a severe J-H R, current practice in Ethiopia is procaine penicillin, 400,000 units by intramuscular injections, on day 1, with tetracycline, 500 mg every 6 hours, on days 2 and 3.

Pretreatment with high-dose corticosteroids does not prevent the reaction, but hydrocortisone, 20 mg per kg, and acetaminophen reduce peak temperatures, hasten the fall in temperature, and lessen the fall in blood pressure during the flush phase. Meptazinol,* an opioid antagonist with

---

*Investigational drug in the United States.

TABLE 1. **Antimicrobial Treatment of Relapsing Fevers**

Drug	LBFR (Single Adult Dose)	TBRF (Daily for 10 days)
Oral		
Tetracycline*,†	500 mg	25–50 mg/kg 6 hourly
Erythromycin	500 mg (8 mg/kg)	8 mg/kg 6 hourly
Intravenous		
Tetracycline	250 mg	10 mg/kg 8 hourly
Erythromycin lactobionate	500 mg (8 mg/kg)	8 mg/kg 6 hourly
Chloramphenicol‡	500 mg (8 mg/kg)	8 mg/kg 6 hourly

*Not for children or pregnant women.
†Single-dose doxycycline (100 mg), chloramphenicol (500 mg), and ampicillin (500 mg) are also effective (adult doses).
‡Not for infants.

agonist properties, diminishes the reaction when given in a dose (adults) of 100 mg by intravenous injection. Collapse from postural hypotension is prevented by keeping patients in bed for at least 24 hours after treatment. Hypotension during the J-H R should be prevented by infusion of isotonic saline which is controlled by monitoring of central venous pressure.

COMPLICATIONS

Hyperpyrexia must be prevented by fanning, tepid sponging, cooling blanket, or antipyretic drugs such as acetaminophen, 10 to 15 mg per kg given by mouth, by suppository, or via nasogastric tube.

Acute myocardial failure with pulmonary edema is signaled by a rise in central venous pressure. Furosemide, 40 mg, and digoxin, 1 mg (adult loading dose), should be given by intravenous injection during 5 to 10 minutes; oxygen should be given by mask.

Spontaneous bleeding and disseminated intravascular coagulation are not controlled by heparin. Vitamin K_1, 10 mg (adult dose), should be given by intravenous injection, and severe bleeding should be treated by cautious transfusion of fresh whole blood, fresh-frozen plasma, cryoprecipitate, or platelet-rich concentrate.

Complicating Infections

In Africa, LBRF may be associated with typhus, typhoid fever, malaria, or tuberculosis.

Splenic Rupture

In very ill patients, an unexplained fall of blood pressure and restlessness may be the only early signs. Be alert if the patient develops sudden abdominal pain.

Loss of Fetus

Abortion, uterine bleeding, and other obstetric complications must be anticipated. Maternal temperature should be controlled, and uterine contractions and fetal heart rate should be monitored for evidence of fetal distress. The outlook for the fetus in LBRF is poor, and the prognosis for a mother who is jaundiced and bleeding is poor.

CONTROL AND PREVENTION

Patients with LBRF remain infectious until they have been deloused by washing with soap or 1 per cent Lysol solution or by dusting with 10 per cent DDT or 1 per cent lindane. Clothes are disinfected by use of heat. In TBRF, ticks are rarely found. Cabins known to be the source of TBRF should be sprayed with insecticides such as 2 per cent benzene hexachloride or 0.5 per cent malathion, and attempts should be made to exclude or control local rodent populations.

RHEUMATIC FEVER

method of
JOHN F. BOHNSACK, M.D.,
L. GEORGE VEASY, M.D., and
HARRY R. HILL, M.D.
University of Utah School of Medicine
Salt Lake City, Utah

Acute rheumatic fever is a nonsuppurative sequela of group A streptococcal pharyngitis that can affect the heart, joints, integument, and central nervous system. The most important site is the heart, with effects resulting mainly from long-term damage to valvular structures from the initial attack and, even more so, from recurrent rheumatic fever. Although the number of cases of acute rheumatic fever has definitely declined in the United States and other developed countries, the incidence remains high in developing countries, in which rheumatic fever is a major public health problem. Furthermore, recent outbreaks of rheumatic fever in several areas of the United States demonstrate that it continues to constitute a problem that has not completely disappeared even in developed countries.

Acute rheumatic fever occurs from early childhood through adult life but has its peak incidence at 5 to 15 years of age. Strict diagnosis of rheumatic fever relies on the use of the revised Jones criteria (Table 1). The presence of two major or of one major and two minor manifestations indicates a high probability of acute rheumatic fever, *if* there is evidence of a recent streptococcal infection. Particular attention should be paid to establishing or ruling out the presence of *carditis* because carditis is the only life-threatening manifestation of acute rheumatic fever and because damage to the heart is the only significant cause of residual morbidity. In children and young adults, carditis is manifested predominantly by mitral regurgitation, although pancarditis can involve all portions of the heart. Aortic regurgitation may also be present, but it is usually associated with mitral valve involvement. Thus, confirmation of carditis in children depends on hearing a new murmur of mitral regurgitation, which is a high-frequency systolic murmur heard at the apex with transmission to the axilla. If the physician is unsure of the physical findings, regurgitant flow can be confirmed by echocardiography. In the young patient with moderate to marked mitral regurgitation, echocardiography often demonstrates mitral valve prolapse, which is due to chordal elongation. In the older (more than 30 years of age) individual, the predominant hemodynamic alterations and clinical manifestations are due to mitral stenosis. This different clinical picture of rheumatic heart disease in the older patient may be best explained by repeated attacks of rheumatic fever, or by a continued low-grade inflammatory reaction that results in the contraction and fusion of the chordae and deformity and fusion of the mitral leaflets. Therefore, a change in the murmur or the appearance of a new murmur is necessary to establish the diagnosis in the adult. These changes can be subtle and may be recognized only by a skilled cardiologist. Thus, when carditis is suspected or confirmed at any age, it is advisable to have the patient examined by an experienced cardiologist.

Arthritis has always been considered to be the Achilles' heel of the Jones criteria. Because there is a virtually unending list of diseases that can present with arthritic symptoms, there must be strong evidence of a preceding streptococcal infection to support the diagnosis of rheumatic fever. Recent experience suggests that pulsed Doppler ultrasound may demonstrate mitral regurgitation when the regurgitation cannot be heard and thus can help to establish the diagnosis in patients with polyarthritis. If Doppler ultrasound is used, strict criteria must be followed to avoid overdiagnosis. Specifically, regurgitant flow must be detected at least 1 cm above the mitral annulus and should be holosystolic. Until we have gained more experience with this new modality, a positive Doppler examination should perhaps be considered as another minor, not a major, manifestation.

The latent period for presentation of Sydenham's *chorea* is characteristically longer, that is, 6 weeks to several months after the preceding streptococcal infection. It is often more difficult, therefore, to establish a preceding streptococcal infection. Doppler echocardiography may be useful in "pure" chorea as in isolated arthritis.

In our experience, the skin manifestations of acute rheumatic fever, although strongly diagnostic, are characteristically seen only with another manifestation, that is, *erythema marginatum* with arthritis or carditis, and *subcutaneous nodules* only with carditis.

Much evidence indicates that rheumatic fever is a result of a preceding streptococcal pharyngitis. Thus, it is imperative to establish the diagnosis of a recent streptococcal infection in an individual who is suspected of having acute rheumatic fever. A throat culture for beta-hemolytic streptococci should be obtained, and evidence should be sought for a serologic response to group A streptococci. Throat cultures are frequently negative at the time of the initial presentation and should not be the sole test to determine streptococcal infection. Use of several serologic tests, for example, the antistreptolysin O, antihyaluronidase, and antideoxyribonuclease (anti-DNase) B titers, enhances the sensitivity of serologic diagnosis. Repeated determinations during 2 to 4 weeks can document a rise in serologic titer and establish the diagnosis of preceding streptococcal infection. The anti-DNase B test, which remains positive for 2 to 3 months after the acute streptococcal infection, is often useful in cases of isolated chorea.

TABLE 1. **Jones Criteria (Revised)***

Major Manifestations	Minor Manifestations
Carditis	Fever
Polyarthritis	Arthralgia
Chorea	Previous rheumatic fever
Erythema marginatum	Elevated erythrocyte sedimentation rate or positive C-reactive protein test or leukocytosis
Subcutaneous nodules	Prolonged PR interval

plus

Supporting evidence of preceding streptococcal infection: history of recent scarlet fever; positive throat culture for group A *Streptococcus;* increased antistreptolysin O titer or other streptococcal antibodies.

*From Jones criteria (revised) for guidance in the diagnosis of rheumatic fever. Circulation *69*:204A, 1984, by permission of the American Heart Association, Inc.

TREATMENT

Acute rheumatic fever varies in its presentation and severity. The following dosage and time schedules should serve as guidelines to be adapted for the treatment of the specific patient's particular manifestations. Eradication of residual streptococci and prophylaxis of recurrent attacks, however, are an indispensable part of every patient's management because further cardiac damage results from recurrences of acute rheumatic fever.

Bed Rest

In the past, patients with rheumatic fever were prescribed prolonged bed rest, but the value of this therapy was probably overestimated. On the other hand, no one denies that the patient with acute rheumatic fever improves both symptomatically and objectively with this treatment. The physician should restrict the patient's activity severely and carefully observe the patient during the first 2 weeks of illness because carditis characteristically appears during this time. If the patient improves and there is no evidence of carditis, normal activity can be rapidly restored. If the patient has moderate to severe carditis, activity should be resumed slowly and cautiously with frequent, thorough clinical assessment. Return to full activity is permitted after signs and symptoms have resolved and the acute phase reactants have returned to normal.

Eradication of Streptococci

Antibiotic therapy to eradicate residual streptococci is instituted as soon as the diagnosis of acute rheumatic fever is established, even when the throat culture is negative. A single intramuscular injection of benzathine penicillin G (600,000 units intramuscularly for children under 60 pounds, and 1.2 million units for heavier patients) is recommended. Alternatively, oral penicillin V (125 to 250 mg four times a day for 10 days) can be used. In the penicillin-allergic patient, erythromycin estolate 20 mg per kg per day in three divided doses may be substituted if erythromycin-resistant group A streptococci are not prevalent in the geographic area. Clindamycin is an alternative drug for the penicillin-allergic patient, but sulfa drugs should not be used in an attempt to eradicate streptococci. Prophylaxis of recurrent infections should begin immediately after the eradicating regimen (see later).

Anti-Inflammatory Agents

Aspirin

Aspirin is extremely effective in the control of arthritis and is used to suppress carditis when there is no associated cardiomegaly and no evidence of congestive heart failure. Aspirin is generally started at an oral dose of 100 mg per kg per day given in four equal doses. The dose is usually decreased to 70 mg per kg per day after 2 to 3 days. This lower dose is usually adequate to maintain a therapeutic serum level of 20 to 25 mg per dl. Because absorption can be quite variable, it is probably wise to check a serum salicylate level 5 to 7 days after starting treatment. A salicylate level should also be checked if the patient continues to complain of pain because aspirin consistently provides relief at therapeutic

levels. Aspirin should be continued until the erythrocyte sedimentation rate returns to normal. Because of the risk of Reye's syndrome, aspirin should be discontinued if the patient develops influenza or varicella.

Corticosteroids

The use of corticosteroids is recommended in the presence of moderate or severe carditis. Although symptomatic relief is often dramatic with these medications, there is no consensus that corticosteroids reduce the amount of residual cardiac disease. Prednisone, 2 mg per kg per day, is given orally in four divided doses and continued at this level until all clinical evidence of inflammatory activity has disappeared and the erythrocyte sedimentation rate has returned to normal. At this dosage, the patient almost always develops undesirable side effects, including moon facies, acne, and hirsutism. The patient should be monitored for the development of hypertension, and oral antacids may be given to prevent peptic ulcer. All side effects should disappear gradually after the medication is discontinued. Prednisone should not be discontinued abruptly but rather tapered during a 2- to 3-week period. To avoid rebound inflammation, aspirin should be started during the initiation of the taper and should be continued for 2 to 3 weeks after steroids have been totally discontinued.

In general, therapy to suppress inflammation should not be instituted before the diagnosis of rheumatic fever is established because the symptoms may improve dramatically or may disappear in response to salicyclates or steroids.

Congestive Heart Failure

Congestive heart failure should be managed in a conventional manner with the use of oxygen, diuretics, and digoxin. Rapid digitalization should probably be avoided because of possible sensitivity in the presence of myocarditis. It is also important that the patient be at rest to reduce demands for increased cardiac output.

Sydenham's Chorea

Sydenham's chorea generally resolves after several months but can last for more than 1 year. Management of chorea varies with its severity. When chorea is mild, patients need only to be mildly sedated and placed in a more tranquil environment, usually by keeping them out of school for a limited period. Hospitalization may be required for patients with chorea so severe that it does not permit them to feed or dress themselves. Recently, the anticonvulsants val-

TABLE 2. **Prophylaxis Against Bacterial Endocarditis***

Dental Procedures and Surgery of the Upper Respiratory Tract

1. Standard regimen: for dental procedures that cause gingival bleeding, and oral and respiratory tract surgery	Oral: penicillin V, 2 grams 1 hr before then 1 gram 6 hr later Parenteral: 2 million units of penicillin G IV or IM 30–60 min before a procedure and 1 million units 6 hr later
2. Penicillin-allergic patient	Oral: erythromycin, 1 gram 1 hr before, then 500 mg 6 hr later Parenteral: vancomycin, 1 gram IV slowly during 1 hr starting 1 hr before; no repeat dose necessary
3. Parenteral regimen for high-risk patients, e.g., with prosthetic valves	Ampicillin, 1–2 grams IV or IM, *plus* gentamicin, 1.5 mg/kg IV or IM 30 min before procedure, followed by 1 gram penicillin orally 6 hr later; alternatively, repeat parenteral regimen once 8 hr later

Gastrointestinal and Genitourinary Procedures

1. Standard regimen	Ampicillin, 2 grams IM or IV *plus* gentamicin, 1.5 mg/kg IM or IV, given 30 min to 1 hr before procedure; one follow-up dose may be given 8 hr later
2. Penicillin-allergic patient	Vancomycin, 1 gram IV slowly during 1 hr, *plus* gentamicin, 1.5 mg/kg IM or IV, given 1 hr before the procedure; may be repeated once 8–12 hr later
3. Oral regimens for minor or repetitive procedures in low-risk patients	Amoxicillin, 3 grams orally 1 hr before procedure and 1.5 grams 6 hr later

NOTE: Pediatric Doses: ampicillin, 50 mg/kg per dose, erythromycin, 20 mg/kg for first dose, then 10 mg/kg; gentamicin, 2.0 mg/kg/dose; penicillin V, full adult dose if more than 60 lb (27 kg), one-half adult dose if less than 60 lb (27 kg); aqueous penicillin G, 50,000 units/kg (25,000 units/kg for follow-up); vancomycin, 20 mg/kg/dose. The intervals between doses are the same as those for adults. Total doses should not exceed adult doses. *Renal Failure:* It may be necessary to omit or modify the second dose in patients who have compromised renal function.

*Adapted from Shulman ST, Amren DP, Bisno AL, et al: Prevention of bacterial endocarditis. Circulation *70*:1123A, 1984, by permission of the American Heart Association, Inc.

proate sodium and carbamazepine have been used with some success. We have used prednisone in the same dosage as that used for carditis with encouraging results. Haloperidol has been successfully used, but toxicity can be a problem. Therefore, haloperidol should be used only in the hospitalized patient who is observed carefully.

Prevention of Primary and Recurrent Rheumatic Fever

As the incidence of rheumatic fever declined, sentiment grew among physicians that vigorous diagnosis and treatment of streptococcal pharyngitis in the United States were not warranted. The recent outbreaks of rheumatic fever in this country indicate, however, that the medical community should not have this degree of complacency about this disease, particularly in areas where rheumatic fever is endemic. The treatment of streptococcal pharyngitis is outlined in another chapter in this volume.

Estimates of the incidence of recurrent rheumatic fever after a new episode of untreated streptococcal pharyngitis range from 5 to 50 per cent per infection. Excellent evidence exists that the prophylaxis of streptococcal infection with antimicrobial agents prevents the recurrence of rheumatic fever. All patients who are diagnosed as having rheumatic fever, including those without apparent carditis, should receive antibiotic prophylaxis. The best regimen is benzathine pen-

icillin, 1.2 million units intramuscularly every 4 weeks. In developing countries, many physicians prefer to give the same dose every 3 weeks. Oral penicillin V, 250 mg twice a day, is an alternative to intramuscular injections, but compliance is easier to ensure with intramuscular injections. The penicillin-allergic patient may be treated with sulfadiazine (0.5 to 1.0 gram daily) or erythromycin (250 mg twice a day). The physician should consider the possibility of erythromycin-resistant streptococci in the geographic area before using erythromycin.

Although the incidence of recurrent rheumatic fever decreases as the interval from the primary attack increases, it is prudent to administer antibiotic prophylaxis for the life of the patient. Compliance with regimens may require considerable effort and education on the part of the physician. The physician should particularly attempt to ensure prophylaxis of patients in high-risk situations: childhood and adolescence; crowded living situations such as military camps, prisons, or schools; teachers and others whose occupations bring them into contact with children; persons living in or visiting areas in which rheumatic fever is endemic or areas experiencing rheumatic fever outbreaks; and patients with residual cardiac abnormalities.

PROPHYLAXIS AGAINST BACTERIAL ENDOCARDITIS

Patients with cardiac valvular abnormalities secondary to rheumatic fever are at increased risk of developing infective endocarditis during episodes of transient bacteremia, such as might occur during dental work or during genitourinary or gastrointestinal surgery or instrumentation. This risk of endocarditis emphasizes the need to search carefully for evidence of valvular disease in patients with suspected rheumatic fever, by echocardiography if necessary. Table 2 details recommendations (developed by a committee of the Council on Cardiovascular Disease in the Young of the American Heart Association) for antibiotic prophylaxis for such bacterial endocarditis. The physician should stress equally the value of good dental hygiene in preventing endocarditis in the patient with rheumatic heart disease.

Routine follow-up of patients with acute rheumatic fever should include at least yearly examinations to document the presence and extent of residual or developing cardiac disease. In addition to monitoring disease activity, such examinations give the physician the opportunity to re-emphasize and re-educate the patient about prevention of recurrent rheumatic fever and prophylaxis against bacterial endocarditis.

LYME DISEASE

method of
ROBERT T. SCHOEN, M.D.
Yale University School of Medicine
New Haven, Connecticut

Lyme disease is a complex, multisystem disorder recognized in 1975 in patients living near Lyme, Connecticut. Erythema chronicum migrans (ECM), a characteristic rash seen in 30 to 60 per cent of individuals with Lyme disease, was described in Sweden in 1909. Lyme disease has been reported in 33 states and all continents except Antarctica. In the United States, the number of new cases approximately doubles each year. Lyme disease is a spirochetal infection caused by a newly recognized organism, *Borrelia burgdorferi,* and is transmitted primarily by ticks of the *Ixodes ricinus* complex, including *Ixodes dammini.* Lyme disease is now the most commonly reported tick-transmitted illness in the United States.

DIAGNOSIS

As many as 50 per cent of individuals who acquire Lyme disease remain asymptomatic in spite of serologic evidence of recent infection. Like other spirochetal infections, the illness can be divided into three stages or grouped into early and late manifestations. Also as in other spirochetal infections, antibiotic therapy is most effective early in the illness and cure becomes less certain in patients with chronic disease.

The greatest challenge in the care of patients with Lyme disease is to recognize and treat the illness as early as possible. The diagnosis of Lyme disease depends on (1) a history of potential exposure to ticks in an endemic area, particularly during the spring and summer; (2) recognition of characteristic clinical features; and (3) the use of Lyme disease–specific serologic testing.

The early diagnosis and treatment of Lyme disease are often made difficult by several factors.

1. Not all patients are symptomatic early in the illness. For example, patients may present with arthritis (Stage 3) but even in retrospect have no history to suggest earlier stages of Lyme disease.

2. Currently available serologic testing for Lyme disease by enzyme-linked immunosorbent assay (ELISA) detects diagnostic antibody titers (IgG and IgM) in most patients with established disease (Stages 2 and 3). Only 40 to 65 per cent of individuals with Stage 1 disease, however, have disease-specific IgM or IgG antibody titers even when acute and convalescent sera are obtained.

3. ECM, the characteristic rash in Lyme disease, is not always present or may have an uncharacteristic appearance.

4. Diagnosis of Lyme disease is suggested by travel or residence in an endemic area, but the disease is now recognized over an expanding geographic range. Nonetheless, in the United States most cases continue to occur in the northeastern coastal New England and Mid-Atlantic states, in Minnesota and Wisconsin, and in Northern California and surrounding states. It should be remembered that later stages of the illness can begin throughout the year, but Stage 1 disease is most likely from April to July when nymphal ixodid ticks are active and is unlikely to occur during the winter.

5. Increasing information about Lyme disease has led to an expanding clinical spectrum of disease manifestations. For example, uveitis and progressive dementia have recently been attributed to Lyme disease. In most patients, however, the disease has characteristic, well-described disease manifestations.

6. The Centers for Disease Control has reported that 5 of 19 pregnancies in women who acquired Lyme disease during pregnancy were associated with adverse fetal outcomes in spite of antibiotic therapy; this has added uncertainty as to how this disease should be treated during pregnancy.

7. Although *B. burgdorferi* has been cultured from the blood, cerebrospinal fluid, skin, and synovial fluid of patients with Lyme disease and has been visualized in patient specimens, direct identification of the organism requires specialized techniques that are not routinely used by the clinician.

STAGE 1 (EARLY DISEASE)

Erythema Chronicum Migrans. Approximately 30 per cent of individuals remember a tick bite several days to 1 month before they develop Lyme disease. A red macule or papule (ECM) may develop at the site of the bite; when present in its typical form, it is diagnostic of Lyme disease. The rash begins as a red macule or papule and then expands during several days, often to larger than 10 cm in diameter. The advancing ECM rash has a distinct outer border. There may be clearing, bluish discoloration, vesicle formation, or necrosis of the center of the rash. If untreated, the rash usually fades within 1 to 4 weeks, although occasionally it persists for months. During this early period, when Lyme disease is most successfully treated, the organism is thought to disseminate hematogenously; this may explain the presence in some patients of secondary annular skin lesions. These resemble the primary ECM lesion but are usually smaller, lack indurated centers, and wax and wane over short periods independent of the initial ECM lesion. These lesions also occasionally recur during later stages of the illness—for example, with the onset of arthritis.

Constitutional Symptoms. Hematogenous dissemination of *B. burgdorferi* may also explain the constitutional symptoms, which are sometimes, but not always, seen during this stage. Fatigue, malaise, fever, and migratory arthralgias suggest a flu-like illness. Headache and stiff neck may suggest aseptic meningitis. The presence, severity, and duration of these symptoms are highly variable.

STAGES 2 AND 3 (LATE DISEASE)

Neurologic Manifestations. Weeks to months after the tick bite, about 15 per cent of patients develop neurologic abnormalities. These include meningitis (associated with a lymphocytic pleocytosis), encephalitis, cranial neuropathy (Bell's palsy may be the only manifestation of Lyme disease), peripheral radiculoneuropathies, or myelitis. These manifestations may occur alone or in combination. In untreated patients, neurologic abnormalities usually resolve completely within months, although chronic neurologic disease is increasingly recognized. Patients with late neurologic illness have been reported to have neuropsychiatric symptoms, focal disease of the central nervous system, or a fatigue syndrome. Brain imaging by nuclear magnetic resonance scanning has shown demyelinative plaques in some patients.

Cardiac Involvement. About 5 per cent of patients develop cardiac involvement within several weeks after the onset of Lyme disease. In one series, 18 of 20 patients with cardiac disease had fluctuating degrees of atrioventricular block; 8 of these patients developed complete heart block that was more likely to occur when the PR interval was longer than 0.30 second; 13 had acute myopericarditis. These patients did not have valvular heart disease. The duration of Lyme carditis is usually brief (several days to several weeks), but recurrences are possible. Patients usually recover completely, although a cardiac death from Lyme disease has been reported.

Arthritis. Within several days to weeks after disease onset, about 20 per cent of patients develop arthralgias. Typically these are brief episodes of migratory joint, periarticular, and musculoskeletal pain; however, patients may continue to have attacks of arthralgias for up to 6 years without developing objective joint abnormalities. In addition to arthralgias, within days to years after untreated ECM, about 50 per cent of patients develop frank arthritis occurring as single or intermittent attacks of joint swelling lasting from several days up to 1 year. In most patients, asymmetric involvement of large joints, particularly the knee, is seen; involvement of more than 5 joints is unusual. About 10 per cent of patients with Lyme disease develop chronic arthritis, which can be associated with permanent joint destruction.

Acrodermatitis chronica atrophicans is a late skin manifestation of Lyme disease reported frequently in Europe; however, perhaps because of strain heterogeneity of *B. burgdorferi,* it is an unusual skin skin manifestation in North America.

TREATMENT

Stage 1 (Early Disease)

The goals of antibiotic therapy at the onset of Lyme disease are to shorten the duration of ECM and associated symptoms and to prevent the development of later stages of illness. During Stage 1, the disease can be cured in approximately 90 per cent of patients.

The drug of choice for adults (except pregnant women) and for children with permanent dentition is an oral tetracycline—either tetracycline, 250 to 500 mg four times daily, or doxycycline (Vibramycin), 50 to 100 mg twice daily, given for 14 to 21 days. The range of dosages and duration of treatment reflects the variability of severity of symptoms at disease onset. Severe disease at onset correlates with a greater likelihood of late complications such as arthritis than does mild disease at onset. In general, because antibiotic therapy is most effective early in the illness, it is appropriate to treat most patients with more than mild illness at onset for a full 3-week course of antibiotic therapy.

Phenoxymethyl penicillin (penicillin V), 250 to 500 mg four times daily, or amoxicillin, 250 to 500 mg three times daily, given for 14 to 21 days is also effective therapy for Stage 1 Lyme disease. Phenoxymethyl penicillin is the drug of choice for pregnant and lactating women and for children with deciduous dentition. Because an association between the onset of this infection during pregnancy and fetal malformations has been suggested and because transplacental infection is postulated to occur soon after disease onset, it is probably appropriate to treat pregnant women in whom Lyme disease is suspected with a lower threshold than other individuals. There may also be a role for intravenous penicillin in Stage 1 Lyme disease in some pregnant women with relatively severe symptoms, although this is unproved. Children with deciduous teeth should receive phenoxymethyl penicillin, 50 mg per kg per day (not less than 1 gram or more than 2 grams per day).

For adults who are allergic to tetracyclines or penicillins, erythromycin, 250 to 500 mg four times daily for 14 to 21 days, is a slightly less effective alternative. In children who are allergic to penicillin, erythromycin, 30 mg per kg per day in divided doses for 14 to 21 days, can be used.

Stages 2 and 3 (Late Disease)

Neurologic Manifestations. In patients with mild disease (for example, Bell's palsy alone), tetracycline, 250 to 500 mg four times daily for 14 to 31 days, is effective. For individuals with frank meningitis, cerebrospinal fluid pleocytosis, and cranial or peripheral neuropathies, intravenous penicillin G, 20 million units daily in divided doses for 10 to 14 days, is usually effective. Ceftriaxone, 2 grams daily for 14 days, is an alternative. In one patient, chloramphenicol at a dose of 1 gram intravenously after every 6 hours for 10 days was effective after unsuccessful intravenous penicillin therapy. Patients with Stage 3 neurologic complications of Lyme disease, including neuropsychiatric disease, focal central nervous system disease, and fatigue syndromes, have been treated with variable success with intravenous penicillin G in the regimens suggested for serious Stage 2 neurologic disease.

Cardiac Involvement. Patients with Lyme carditis should probably receive, in addition to antibiotic therapy, aspirin, six to twelve 325-mg tablets daily, or an equivalent nonsteroidal anti-inflammatory drug (NSAID) in therapeutic dosage. In patients with minor cardiac involvement (first-degree atrioventricular [AV] block, with PR interval less than 0.30 second) and no other significant symptoms, therapy with tetracycline as described for Stage 1 disease is effective. Such patients should restrict their activity, however, and should be monitored closely. Patients with more severe manifestastions of Lyme carditis (including first-degree AV block with PR interval more than 0.30 second) should be hospitalized and have cardiac monitoring and should be treated with intravenous penicillin or ceftriaxone as described for serious neurologic manifestations. Some of these patients have complete heart block requiring temporary transvenous cardiac pacemaker insertion, usually for less than 1 week. Persistent conduction system abnormalities requiring permanent pacemaker insertion are unusual but have occurred.

Arthritis

Several oral regimens are successful in treating Lyme arthritis in approximately 50 per cent of patients and avoid the morbidity and expense of intravenous antibiotic therapy. In adults these regimens include doxycycline, 100 mg twice daily given for 31 days; and amoxicillin, 500 mg three times daily, with probenecid, 500 mg three times daily, for 31 days.

Children should receive phenoxymethyl penicillin, 50 mg per kg per day (not less than 1 gram or more than 2 grams per day) in four doses for 31 days.

Penicillin G, 20 million units intravenously daily in divided doses for 14 to 21 days, or ceftriaxone, 1 to 2 grams intravenously daily for 14 to 21 days, is effective in approximately 75 per cent of patients with established Lyme arthritis. Children should receive penicillin G, 250,000 units per kg per day intravenously in divided doses every 4 hours for 14 to 21 days.

In some adults who do not respond to antibiotic therapy, especially individuals with chronic knee arthritis, arthroscopic synovectomy has been successful. Other patients require management with NSAID therapy or intra-articular corticosteroid injection. In some patients with arthritis, retreatment with an alternative antibiotic regimen results in an improved outcome. Ultimately, in most patients, Lyme arthritis can be arrested without significant joint destruction.

ROCKY MOUNTAIN SPOTTED FEVER

method of
DOUGLAS P. FINE, M.D.
University of Oklahoma Health Sciences Center
Oklahoma City, Oklahoma

Rocky Mountain spotted fever, an acute systemic febrile illness with a prominent exanthem, is caused by infection with *Rickettsia rickettsii*. Despite the name of the disease, most cases now occur in the mid-Atlantic Coast states and upper South, extending west to Oklahoma, which in some recent years has had the highest per capita incidence in the country. Because of its rapid clinical evolution and potential lethality, this is a disease for which physicians should maintain a high index of suspicion and that should be treated presumptively if it is considered to be at all likely.

R. rickettsii is maintained in a tick reservoir: *Dermacentor andersoni* (the wood tick) in the western United States and *Dermacentor variabilis* (the dog tick) in the eastern parts of the country. Most patients give a history of potential tick exposure (work or recreation in an outdoor setting or close contact with dogs) and a sizable proportion recall a tick bite. Thus, questioning about tick exposure is useful, but the absence of such a history should not preclude the diagnosis. Rocky Mountain spotted fever tends to be a disease of spring and summer, when ticks are most active, but it may occur at other times of the year, particularly in warmer climates.

CLINICAL MANIFESTATIONS

The clinical presentation of Rocky Mountain spotted fever reflects the diffuse vasculitic pathophysiology. A typical case begins with fairly abrupt onset of fever and headache, which is often severe. Rash follows in the majority of cases within a few days, usually beginning as erythematous maculopapular lesions on the wrists and ankles, spreading centripetally, and often becoming petechial or even purpuric. "Typical" involvement of palms and soles may not be obvious early, and the rash may be hard to detect in black patients. However, only about two-thirds of patients have the triad of fever, headache, and rash, and presentation may be highly varied and subtle. Therefore, Rocky Mountain spotted fever must be strongly considered in any febrile patient in an area in which the illness is endemic.

Most patients have multiple symptoms and signs reflecting the multisystem nature of the infection. Neurologic symptoms in addition to headache are common and include depression or confusion, lethargy, dizziness, and irritability. Approximately one-third of patients may have stiff neck; focal neurologic signs or coma can be seen in about 10 per cent of hospitalized patients. Seizure disorders or focal paresis may be long-term sequelae. Gastrointestinal symptoms and signs are common but nonspecific: nausea, vomiting, abdominal pain or tenderness (at times presenting as an acute abdomen), anorexia, diarrhea or constipation, and hepatomegaly. Myalgias and arthralgias are frequently noted. About 15 per cent of patients report a nonproductive cough. The vasculitis may be severe enough to result in necrosis of skin, particularly on distal appendages, but this complication is fortunately rare.

The mortality of Rocky Mountain spotted fever treated promptly is thought to be less than 5 to 10 per cent. This can be contrasted with a 25 per cent or higher death rate before the introduction of effective chemotherapy.

DIAGNOSIS

Presumptive diagnosis is based on the acute febrile presentation, especially if neurologic and cutaneous manifestations are present, in an area of endemic illness, particularly if there is history of tick contact. Thrombocytopenia is a suggestive laboratory finding; other hematologic changes are not specific or useful. Cerebrospinal fluid pleocytosis and an elevated protein level are the rule; hypoglycorrhachia is rare.

If the test is available, direct immunofluorescent antirickettsial antibody staining of organisms in tissue biopsy is useful for rapid diagnosis of Rocky Mountain spotted fever. Rash must be present to guide the biopsy; thus, this test is not helpful in patients who have not yet developed rash.

Serologic tests are useful only for retrospective confirmation of the diagnosis. Therapy should not be delayed pending these tests if Rocky Mountain spotted fever is suspected. Proteus OX-19 (Weil-Felix) agglutination and complement fixation tests are nonspecific and insensitive; microagglutination and indirect fluorescent antibody assays are more useful. Paired serum samples should be obtained approximately 2 weeks apart.

THERAPY

Tetracyclines are the primary therapeutic agents for Rocky Mountain spotted fever. Patients who are not severely ill and can tolerate oral medications can be treated with tetracycline, 500 mg orally every 6 hours (10 mg per kg orally every 6 hours for children older than 9 years) or doxycycline (Vibramycin), 200 mg orally as a single loading dose, followed by 100 mg orally every 12 hours (2 to 2.5 mg per kg orally every 12 hours for children). Tetracyclines should not be ingested at the same time as milk, milk products, antacids containing aluminum or magnesium, or iron because these agents interfere with absorption; however, tetracyclines can be administered with meals to minimize gastrointestinal toxicity.

Tetracycline and doxycycline can also be administered intravenously if needed for severe illness (nausea, vomiting, or excessive gastrointestinal toxicity precludes oral administration): tetracycline 0.5 to 1.0 gram every 12 hours (10 mg per kg every 12 hours in children) or doxycycline 200 mg loading dose and 100 mg every 12 hours (4.4 mg per kg as a loading dose and 2.2 mg per kg every 12 hours in children).

The principal toxicity of tetracyclines is gastrointestinal, primarily nausea, vomiting, and cramping abdominal pain. Children younger than 9 years old may develop yellow staining of teeth from tetracyclines and generally should not receive this therapy. Tetracyclines may also cause severe hepatic disease in pregnant women and retard fetal bone growth. Photosensitization is an infrequent complication of tetracycline therapy and is unlikely to be a concern. Tetracycline should not be used in patients with renal failure, but doxycycline can be used, at a slightly lower dosage (100 mg every 24 hours).

The alternative drug to tetracyclines is chloramphenicol. Usual dosage is 500 to 750 mg orally every 6 hours (20 mg per kg orally every 6 hours in children) or 20 mg per kg intravenously every 6 hours (adults and children); the usual maximum is 4 grams daily. Oral therapy is preferred if possible because of more predictable blood levels. Chloramphenicol is usually preferred for children younger than 9 years old, for pregnant women, and for patients unable to tolerate tetracyclines. The principal toxicity of chloramphenicol is a rare but fatal idiosyncratic bone marrow aplasia. Young infants or children with underlying liver disease should have chloramphenicol blood levels monitored to ensure that these are within therapeutic and nontoxic range.

Antimicrobial therapy should be continued at least until the patient has been afebrile for 48 to 72 hours and probably for a minimum total of 7 to 10 days. Adjunctive therapy is symptomatic and depends on manifestations of the disease (e.g., fluids, pressor agents, oxygen, diuretics). No data suggest that anticoagulation or corticosteroid therapy is beneficial.

PREVENTION

Rickettsial vaccines are experimental at this time but have shown some promise. Prevention is primarily a matter of taking appropriate precautions to minimize chances of tick bites in an area of endemic disease; occlusive clothing and insect repellants are helpful. When ticks are removed from animals, care should be taken to avoid direct human contact with the tick, its secretions, or its blood. Each day after being in an outdoor environment or around tick-infested dogs, one should inspect all areas of the body, particularly legs and groin areas, external genitalia, and belt lines, for adherent ticks, which should then be removed carefully to avoid further direct contact. The duration of tick attachment appears to be a factor in the severity of the disease episode. Postexposure antimicrobial prophylaxis cannot be recommended.

RUBELLA AND CONGENITAL RUBELLA

method of
MORVEN S. EDWARDS, M.D.
Baylor College of Medicine
Houston, Texas

POSTNATALLY ACQUIRED RUBELLA

Postnatally acquired rubella is usually a mild disease. During the 1 to 5 days preceding the exanthem, prodromal symptoms (which occur more frequently in adults than children), such as eye pain, fever, headache, malaise, sore throat, or mild coryza, may be observed. After an incubation period of 16 to 18 days (range 14 to 21 days), the maculopapular rash of rubella begins on the face and spreads downward and centrifugally. The pink-red lesions may coalesce on the trunk but remain discrete on the extremities. The rash clears from the face on the second day of illness and from the extremities by the end of the third day. Neither the rash nor the lymphadenopathy involving suboccipital, postauricular, and cervical nodes is sufficiently distinctive to be pathognomonic for rubella. It may be difficult clinically to distinguish rubella from infections such as erythema infectiosum, enteroviral illness, or infectious mononucleosis.

Postnatally acquired rubella generally is diagnosed serologically. Hemagglutination inhibition (HAI) is the most commonly used technique. Because HAI antibody is detectable by the third day of rash, reaches a peak by 1 month, and persists indefinitely, a single titer may not suffice for diagnosis of acute infection. A fourfold or greater increase in antibody titer *or* demonstration of rubella-specific IgM by an adaptation of the HAI is diagnostic of recent infection. Rubella-specific IgM tests are advantageous in that a diagnosis may be established from a single serum specimen; conversely, the extraction methods used to separate IgM from IgG reduce the sensitivity of these assays. A number of tests equal to or exceeding the HAI in sensitivity, including the latex agglutination and enzyme immunoassay methods, are gradually replacing the HAI. Sera must be treated to prevent false-positive results when rheumatoid factor is present, but the newer methods are rapid and easy to perform.

Treatment

No specific therapy is required or indicated for uncomplicated postnatally acquired rubella.

Complications

The most common complications of rubella are arthralgias or arthritis. Arthritis is most common in adults, affecting up to 30 per cent of women with rubella, has its onset during recovery and may persist for weeks to months. The treatment of choice, which usually results in dramatic improvement, is aspirin, 60 mg per kg per day for children and 2 grams daily for adults, given in four equal doses. Corticosteroids are not required and are contraindicated because synovial fluid may contain live virus. Treatment of the infrequently observed complications of encephalitis (1 per 5000 cases) and the hemorrhagic consequences of immune-mediated thrombocytopenia or vascular damage (1 per 3000 cases) is primarily supportive, although blood replacement may occasionally be required for the latter.

Management of Pregnant Contacts

Ideally, the rubella immune status of women should be determined early in pregnancy. An HAI antibody titer of 1:8 or higher or the presence of antibody by another properly performed test before or at the time of exposure indicates that the individual is immune and is not at risk. If antibody is not detectable, a second specimen should be obtained 2 weeks later. Infection can be assumed if seroconversion is documented. If the second specimen is negative, the test should be repeated 6 weeks after exposure; if it remains negative, infection did not occur. To document infection, detection of rubella-specific IgM or isolation of virus from the throat also can be useful.

The relative risk of congenital malformations as a consequence of maternal rubella during the first 4 weeks of gestation is 30 to 60 per cent. The risk declines to 25 per cent during the fifth to eighth weeks of gestation and to 8 per cent during the ninth to twelfth weeks. Occasionally, fetal damage occurs if rubella occurs up to the twentieth week of gestation. By the fifth month of gestation, some centers are able to obtain and process fetal blood for rubella-specific IgM to document the presence or absence of transmission to the fetus.

The relative risks to the fetus should be discussed in detail with the patient, and a decision should be made regarding potential pregnancy termination if infection is documented. If termination of pregnancy is not an option, administration of immune globulin (IG) for postexposure prophylaxis should be considered. Although not uniformly efficacious, IG administered within 72 hours of exposure at a dosage of 0.55 ml per kg may prevent or modify infection in an exposed susceptible patient.

CONGENITAL RUBELLA

The classic manifestations of the congenital rubella syndrome include intrauterine growth retardation, microcephaly, cataracts and microphthalmos, congenital heart disease, and developmental retardation. Deafness, usually severe and bilateral, occurs frequently and may be the only manifestation of congenital rubella. As the result of intense investigation surrounding the epidemic of 1964, the later effects of congenital rubella syndrome have been elucidated. These include endocrinopathies (particularly diabetes), progressive hearing loss, and progressive rubella panencephalitis related to persistent and extending rubella infection of the brain.

The best method for the definitive diagnosis of congenital rubella syndrome is isolation of the virus. Specimens for viral culture should be obtained from the nasopharynx, throat, urine, and cerebrospinal fluid. The virus persists for many months in the urine and nasopharynx. An alternative method for establishing the diagnosis is documentation in serum of rubella-specific IgM.

For questionable cases, declining levels of maternally acquired IgG antibody may be a helpful adjunct for excluding the diagnosis.

Treatment

No drugs are available to curtail viral shedding or to prevent progressive symptoms. Multidisciplinary supportive care should be provided.

Isolation Procedures

Patients with postnatal rubella are most contagious when the rash is erupting. Viremia peaks just before the onset of exanthem and resolves shortly after the appearance of rash. Viral shedding in the nasopharynx occurs for approximately 1 week before and 1 week after the onset of rash. Patients should be isolated from susceptible pregnant contacts during this interval. Children with postnatal rubella should be excluded from school for 7 days after the onset of rash. In the hospital setting, contact isolation is required for 7 days after the onset of rash.

Infants with congenital rubella remain chronically infected for many months. The hospitalized patient and those in day care should be considered to be contagious for the first year of life, unless nasopharyngeal and urine cultures obtained after 3 months of age are negative for rubella virus. Contact isolation should be used in the hospital setting. Severely affected infants may shed virus beyond the first year of life. Virus may persist in the eye for many years. Susceptible pregnant caretakers should be made aware of the potential hazard of exposure to these infants.

Prevention

Major rubella epidemics occurred at 6- to 9-year intervals before licensure of live attenuated rubella vaccine in 1969. Since then, more than 125 million doses of vaccine have been administered, and the incidence of congenital rubella syndrome has declined by 97 per cent. However, 10 to 20 per cent of women in the childbearing years are susceptible to rubella. The low incidence of congenital rubella syndrome is attributed to reduced exposure of susceptible adults to acutely infected school-age children.

The only rubella vaccine currently available in the United States is the RA 27/3 strain of virus grown in human diploid cell cultures. Serum antibody is induced in more than 95 per cent of recipients. Although antibody titers after vaccine administration are somewhat lower than those elicited from natural infection, they persist for at least 15 years after immunization and are probably lifelong. The vaccine is administered as a single subcutaneous dose of 0.5 ml, alone or in a preparation containing mumps and/or measles components.

In children, rubella vaccine is efficacious at or after 12 months of age. Currently, vaccine administration is recommended at 15 months of age in combination with measles and mumps vaccine. The vaccine may be given simultaneously at a different site from that of diphtheria-tetanus-pertussis vaccine and oral polio vaccine without reducing efficacy. Immunization is also indicated for susceptible prepubertal girls, day care personnel, college students, and military and health care personnel. Postpubertal seronegative women should be immunized if they are not pregnant and agree to avoid pregnancy for 3 months after receiving the vaccine.

The most common adverse reaction to rubella vaccine is arthralgia or arthritis. Involvement of joints tends to occur most often (10 to 20 per cent) in postpubertal females. Symptoms usually begin within 3 weeks after immunization and may persist for weeks or months. Less common reactions to vaccine include rash, lymphadenopathy, low-grade fever, or upper respiratory tract symptoms.

There are several specific contraindications to administration of rubella vaccine. It should be avoided in patients with primary or acquired immunodeficiency, such as leukemia; those with other malignancy; and those receiving steroid or cancer chemotherapy. After considering reports of severe measles (rubeola) in symptomatic children infected with human immunodeficiency virus (HIV) and in the absence of reports of serious or unusual adverse effects of measles, mumps, and rubella (MMR) vaccination, the Immunization Practices Advisory Committee suggested that administration of MMR vaccine should be considered for children with symptomatic HIV infection. The Immunization Practices Advisory Committee also recommended that children and young adults infected with HIV who have no overt clinical manifestations of immunosuppression may receive rubella vaccine. These patients should be monitored for possible adverse reactions, and it should be noted that immunization may be less effective in these individuals than in uninfected persons.

Pregnant women should not be given rubella vaccine. Although congenital rubella syndrome resulting from rubella vaccination in pregnancy has not been observed, the theoretical maximal risk for its occurrence may be as high as 1.7 per cent. This estimate is based on the outcome of pregnancy in a cohort of 254 susceptible women reported to the Centers for Disease Control who receive vaccine either 3 months before or 3 months after the estimated date of conception.

All of the 212 living infants delivered to women susceptible to rubella were free of defects compatible with congenital rubella. Virus was isolated from the products of conception in 1 of 35 women who underwent abortion.

Rubella vaccine should be deferred for 3 months after the administration of blood transfusion or IG. It may be given to postpartum women who require blood products or Rho (D) IG, but in that circumstance serum should be tested at 6 to 8 weeks after immunization to document seroconversion. Finally, vaccine administration should be deferred until resolution of acute febrile illnesses.

Because rubella vaccine virus is not transmitted from vaccinated individuals to others, there is no contraindication to immunization of susceptible children whose mothers are pregnant or to a child residing in the household of a patient with acquired immunodeficiency syndrome. Breast-feeding does not constitute a contraindication to immunization in the immediate postpartum period.

MEASLES
(Rubeola)

method of
SUBHASH CHAUDHARY, M.D.
Southern Illinois University School of Medicine
Springfield, Illinois

Measles virus is a single-stranded RNA virus with one antigenic type. Humans are the natural host, although other primates are susceptible to naturally transmitted measles infection. Measles occurs in all parts of the world. Measles is uncommon in the first 6 months of life because of the protection conferred by passively acquired maternal antibody. Beyond that period, the age at infection depends largely on contact with a contagious person. The incidence of measles in the United States is now less than 1 per cent of what it was before the introduction of vaccine. In developing countries, measles is still a serious problem.

The disease has an incubation period of 10 to 12 days. Measles virus is transmitted by direct contact with respiratory secretions from an infected person and by exposure to aerosols created by coughing and sneezing from as early as 3 days before onset of symptoms until the rash desquamates. Infectivity is maximal during prodrome and drops rapidly after the onset of rash. Measles virus, like human immunodeficiency virus (HIV), infects T4 lymphocytes, and T4/T8 ratios may be reversed during acute illness.

TREATMENT OF ACTIVE DISEASE
Uncomplicated Measles

In most patients, measles is associated with moderately severe symptoms and signs, like fever, coryza, brassy cough, conjunctivitis, abdominal pain, diarrhea, adenopathy, and the typical exanthem (confluent maculopapular erythematous rash) accompanied by a pathognomonic enanthem (Koplik's spots). Photophobia and headache occur regularly. Treatment, mainly symptomatic, includes bed rest, judicious use of acetaminophen for fever and headache, cough suppressants if the cough does not let the patient sleep, attention to humidity and to fluid intake, and a darkened room for photophobia. The conjunctivitis is self-limited. Isolation because of respiratory symptoms is recommended for 4 days after the onset of rash.

Ribavirin, a synthetic nucleoside analogue with broad-spectrum antiviral activity, has been used orally in studies of children with measles in Mexico, Brazil, and India. Severity and duration of measles were reduced, especially when the drug was given in the pre-eruptive phase of illness.

Complicated Measles in Normal Host

Respiratory Complications. Otitis media and bacterial pneumonia are frequent complications and should be treated with appropriate antibiotics. Tuberculosis may be exacerbated by measles. In addition, measles virus can cause croup, bronchiolitis, and giant cell pneumonia.

Encephalitis. Transient electroencephalographic abnormalities occur in approximately 50 per cent of patients, but encephalitis complicates 1 per 1000 cases of measles. Ten to 15 per cent of measles encephalitis cases are fatal and 25 per cent of survivors may have permanent sequelae.

Subacute Sclerosing Panencephalitis. This type of encephalitis is a rare (incidence of 1 in 1 million) delayed complication of measles. It has been treated by numerous therapeutic procedures, antiviral drugs, and biologic agents, but none have effectively altered the course of the disease. Recent uncontrolled trials suggest that inosiplex (Isoprinosine) and interferon given intraventricularly may be of some benefit. Use of ribavirin is being investigated.

Miscellaneous. Myocarditis, thrombocytopenic purpura, and appendicitis are rare complications.

Measles in the Altered Host

Immunosuppressed Host. Measles in patients with T cell abnormalities may be clinically aberrant, prolonged, and fatal. Death is frequently due to giant cell pneumonia; however, fatal measles encephalitis has also been reported. In many of these patients, rash may be absent. Six children with HIV infection have acquired measles

in the United States; two died of measles. Three of four patients with measles pneumonia were treated with aerosolized ribavirin, and two of these patients survived. Because of prolonged shedding of virus, isolation should be continued for the duration of the hospital stay.

Malnourished Children. Measles causes more severe disease in children who are malnourished, and there is a higher likelihood of poor outcome in these children. Measles accounts for a large number of cases of childhood blindness in Africa. Vitamin A supplementation has been shown to reduce mortality, particularly in children younger than 2 years old and for cases complicated by croup. Ribavirin may reduce the severity and duration of illness, particularly when administered in the pre-eruptive phase of illness.

PREVENTION AND CONTROL

Postexposure Prophylaxis. Unimmunized individuals who have been exposed to measles for more than 72 hours but less than 6 days should receive immune globulin (IG). IG is particularly useful for contacts younger than 12 months of age because of the higher risk of complications. The dose of IG is 0.25 ml per kg intramuscularly for a healthy host and 0.5 ml per kg (up to 15 ml) for immunocompromised patients. Individuals who have been exposed to measles for less than 72 hours can be protected with measles vaccine.

Active Immunization. Live attenuated measles vaccine should be used for protection against measles. The measles vaccine available in the United States is prepared in chick embryo cell culture, and it does not contain penicillin. The vaccine must be protected from heat and light during storage. Measles vaccine in association with mumps and rubella vaccines (MMR) is the vaccine of choice for routine immunization of children. A single subcutaneous injection at 15 months of age or older provides rapid and long-lasting protection with a seroconversion rate of 95 per cent. Evidence now extending through 23 years indicates that booster doses of vaccine are not indicated. In areas with recurrent measles transmission, a routine two-dose vaccination schedule, with the first dose at 9 months of age followed by MMR at 15 months of age, should be followed. When an outbreak of measles occurs, infants as young as 6 months old may be vaccinated. Revaccination should be carried out in children who were previously given (1) live measles vaccine before 12 months of age; (2) killed measles vaccine; or (3) live measles vaccine simultaneously or within 3 months after receiving IG. Revaccination should also be done if there is a doubt about the details of measles immunization history.

HIV-infected children, regardless of symptoms, should be given MMR vaccine at age 15 months. This recommendation is given because of recent reports of severe measles in symptomatic HIV-infected children, and the lack of reported serious or unusual reactions to immunization with MMR vaccine.

Contraindications. Vaccination should be deferred for 3 months in a child who has received IG, plasma, or whole blood. It is contraindicated in any child with compromised immunity except HIV infection. Measles vaccine is also contraindicated during active untreated tuberculosis or during a febrile illness. Live measles vaccine should not be given to women who are pregnant or who are considering pregnancy within 3 months of immunization. Persons with a history of anaphylactic reaction to neomycin should not receive measles vaccine, and those with a history of anaphylactic reaction after ingestion of eggs should be vaccinated with extreme caution. The presence of an immunosuppressed host in a family is not a contraindication for measles immunization of children.

Adverse Reactions. The vaccine can cause a mild subclinical infection that is not contagious. Fever and mild toxicity may develop 5 to 12 days postvaccination in 5 to 15 per cent of persons who are vaccinated. A transient faint rash may be seen in approximately 5 per cent of persons. Postvaccination central nervous system complications are rare (approximately 1 in 1 million doses); a causal relationship between these complications and the vaccine is unproved.

TETANUS

method of
WESLEY FURSTE, M.D.
Ohio State University,
Columbus, Ohio,

GREGORY RAY VEST, M.D.
Valley Baptist Medical Center
Harlingen, Texas,

JAMES P. VIGLIANCO, M.D.
Mt. Carmel Medical Center,
Columbus, Ohio,

and

AUGUSTO AGUIRRE, M.D.
Riverside Methodist Hospitals
Columbus, Ohio

Tetanus (lockjaw) is a severe and dreaded infectious complication of wounds and is caused by the toxin-producing *Clostridium tetani*. This disease is characterized by tonic spasms of the voluntary muscles, by a tendency toward episodes of respiratory arrest, and, over the entire world, by a mortality rate of approximately 50 per cent.

PROPHYLAXIS

Adequate tetanus prophylaxis is based on (1) proper use of tetanus toxoid, (2) immediate surgical care of all wounds of violence, (3) proper use of antitoxin (heterologous equine antitoxin, and more recently tetanus immune globulin, and (4) proper use of emergency medical identification devices.

Tetanus can be prevented by proper immunization. For healthy infants and children younger than age 7 years, tetanus toxoid is administered along with diphtheria and pertussis vaccines using DTP (diphtheria and tetanus toxoids and pertussis vaccine adsorbed). Primary vaccination is given at age 2 months or older; the second dose, 2 months after the first dose; the third dose, 2 months after the second dose; and the fourth dose, approximately 15 months after the third dose. A DTP booster is given at 4 to 6 years of age, before the child enters school. Additional boosters using Td (tetanus and diphtheria toxoids adsorbed) are given every 10 years after the last dose. For persons 7 years or older who have not had a complete immunization series for tetanus, this can be accomplished by using Td in the following sequence: primary vaccination, first visit; second dose, 1 to 2 months after the first dose; third dose, 6 to 12 months after the second; and subsequent Td boosters, every 10 years.

Prophylaxis against tetanus in wound management requires an adequate history and careful wound evaluation in accordance with the principles outlined in Tables 1, 2, and 3.

TREATMENT

The following recommendations for management are given in order of chronologic priority.

Complete History and Physical Examination

A complete medical and surgical history of the patient should be obtained and a complete physical examination performed. In particular, the information obtained should include the date of injury, the circumstances of injury, the depth of the injury below the skin, and allergies. Such information forms a baseline for the recognition of such complications as atelectasis, pneumonia, traumatic glossitis, muscle injuries, fractures of the vertebrae, decubital ulcers, and fecal impaction.

TABLE 1. General Principles for Tetanus Prophylaxis*

1. Active immunization against tetanus with tetanus toxoid plays a major role in markedly reducing the incidence of cases of this disease, and the resulting deaths.

2. Recommendations for tetanus prophylaxis are based on (a) the condition of the wound, especially as related to its susceptibility to tetanus, and (b) the patient's immunization history.

3. Regardless of the active immunization status of the patient, all wounds should receive immediate surgical treatment, with meticulous aseptic technique, to remove all devitalized tissue and foreign bodies. Such care is an essential part of prophylaxis against tetanus. (See *A Guide to Initial Therapy of Soft-Tissue Wounds,* American College of Surgeons.)

4. Warning: The only contraindication to tetanus and diphtheria toxoids for the wounded patient is a history of neurologic or severe hypersensitivity reaction to a previous dose. Local side effects alone do not preclude continued use. If a systemic reaction is suspected to represent allergic hypersensitivity, postpone immunization until appropriate skin testing is performed later. If a contraindication to a tetanus toxoid–containing preparation exists, consider passive immunization against tetanus for a tetanus-prone wound.

Contraindications to pertussis vaccination in infants and children younger than 7 years old include a previous adverse reaction after diphtheria and tetanus toxoids and pertussis vaccine adsorbed (for pediatric use) (DTP), or single antigen pertussis vaccination; and/or the presence of a neurologic condition characterized by changing developmental or neurologic findings. If such a contraindication to using pertussis vaccine adsorbed (P) exists, diphtheria and tetanus toxoids adsorbed (for pediatric use) (DT) are recommended. Neither a static neurologic condition, such as cerebral palsy, nor a family history of convulsions or other central nervous system disorders is a contraindication to giving vaccines containing the pertussis antigen.

Disposition: Give each patient an appropriate written record describing treatment rendered and providing instructions for follow-up that outline wound care, drug therapy, immunization status, and potential complications. Arrange for completion of active immunization.

Give every wounded patient a wallet-sized card documenting immunization dosage and date received.

*From American College of Surgeons, Committee on Trauma: Prophylaxis Against Tetanus in Wound Management. Chicago, American College of Surgeons, 1987.

Antitoxin

Intramuscular Injection

As soon as the diagnosis of tetanus is made, deep intramuscular injection of 500 to 10,000 units of tetanus immune globulin (TIG) should be given. Five hundred units may be as effective as the dose of 3000 to 10,000 units that has been recommended in the past.

Because TIG causes no hypersensitivity phenomena when injected intramuscularly and because it appears to be at least equal in efficacy to equine antitoxin, TIG should be given instead of the heterologous tetanus antitoxin (equine).

TIG is to be given intramuscularly in the proximal portion of the extremity in which the wound

TABLE 2. Wound Classification*

Clinical Features	Tetanus-Prone Wounds	Non–Tetanus-Prone Wounds
Age of wound	>6 hr	≤6 hr
Configuration	Stellate wound, avulsion, abrasion	Linear wound
Depth	>1 cm	≤1 cm
Mechanism of injury	Missile, crush, burn, frostbite	Sharp surface (e.g., knife, glass)
Signs of infection	Present	Absent
Devitalized tissue	Present	Absent
Contaminants (e.g., dirt, feces, soil, saliva)	Present	Absent
Denervated and/or ischemic tissue	Present	Absent

*From American College of Surgeons, Committee on Trauma: Prophylaxis Against Tetanus in Wound Management. Chicago, American College of Surgeons, 1987.

occurred, or in the gluteal muscles when the wound is not in an extremity or when the causative wound cannot be found.

In the United States, where there are now adequate supplies of TIG, there are no indications for the administration of heterologous tetanus antitoxin (equine), which has been responsible for serum sickness, myocardial infarctions, peripheral neuritis, and anaphylactic shock with death. Moreover, in the human being, the life span of the heterologous antitoxin cannot be predicted with certainty.

In countries in which TIG is not available, heterologous tetanus antitoxin (equine) is still being used. A dosage of 10,000 units is considered adequate. No significant lowering of the mortality rate has been found for doses ranging from 5000 to 60,000 units of equine antitoxin in adults. Fifteen hundred units of heterologous tetanus

TABLE 3. Immunization Schedule*

History of Adsorbed Tetanus Toxoid (Doses)	Tetanus-Prone Wounds		Non–Tetanus-Prone Wounds	
	Td†	TIG	Td†	TIG
Unknown or fewer than 3	Yes	Yes	Yes	No
3 or more‡	No§	No	No‖	No

*From American College of Surgeons, Committee on Trauma: Prophylaxis Against Tetanus in Wound Management. Chicago, American College of Surgeons, 1987.

†For children younger than 7 years old: DTP (DT, if pertussis vaccine is contraindicated) is preferable to tetanus toxoid alone. For persons 7 years old and older, Td is preferable to tetanus toxoid alone.

‡If only three doses of fluid toxoid have been received, a fourth dose of toxoid, preferably an adsorbed toxoid, should be given.

§Yes, if more than 5 years since last dose. (More frequent boosters are not needed and can accentuate side effects.)

‖Yes, if more than 10 years since last dose.

antitoxin (equine) appears to be as effective as a larger dose in neonates.

Intrathecal Injection of a Mixture of Antitoxin and Prednisolone

Serious consideration should be given to simultaneous single injections of TIG and prednisolone intrathecally and of TIG intramuscularly. For neonatal tetanus, 250 units of TIG and 12.5 mg of prednisolone are administered intrathecally, and 250 units of TIG is given intramuscularly. For adults, the dose of TIG for the intrathecal route is increased to 1000 units and for the intramuscular route to 1000 units. Complications of intrathecal administration are believed to be due to the preservatives rather than to the antitoxin itself.

Laboratory Tests

The following tests are recommended:
1. Complete blood cell count with differential white blood cell count
2. Urinalysis
3. Serologic test for syphilis
4. Prothrombin time and partial thromboplastin time
5. Blood chemistry tests: urea nitrogen, creatinine, electrolytes, serum protein electrophoresis, bilirubin, calcium, glucose
6. Arterial blood gases
7. Chest roentgenogram
8. Electrocardiogram
9. Electroencephalogram
10. Wound and, if the patient is febrile, blood cultures
11. If necessary for diagnosis, cerebrospinal fluid for culture, smear, cells, and chemistry tests
12. Serum diazepam levels
13. Serum tetanus antitoxin levels if the diagnosis is questionable

Nursing Care

Provide 24-hour constant nursing care. Having a resident or intern immediately available to treat complications, particularly respiratory problems such as respiratory arrest, greatly increases the patient's chance for recovery from tetanus.

Analgesics

Analgesics should be administered that relieve the pain associated with the tonic contractions of tetanus but do not cause respiratory depression. Codeine, meperidine (Demerol), meperidine with promethazine (Phenergan), and morphine are acceptable analgesic drugs.

Sedatives and Muscle Relaxants

Sedatives and muscle relaxants must be used correctly. A most important consideration is that the physician know how to use safely the sedatives and muscle relaxants that are ordered for the patient with tetanus and that drugs are used that give the best results.

Patients with the mildest cases of tetanus can be sedated adequately with phenobarbital, pentobarbital, secobarbital, paraldehyde, diazepam (Valium), and midazolam (Versed).

In the more severe cases, thiopental sodium (Pentothal) may be administered intravenously in a dilute solution (0.5 to 1 gram per 1000 ml) at a rate of 20 to 25 drops per minute in an effort to lower the patient's threshold of irritability to external stimuli and to reduce the number and severity of seizures and respiratory arrests. Care is taken to avoid overdosage. The optimal level of continuous sedation is obtained when the patient remains sleepy but can still be aroused by moderate external stimuli sufficiently to obey commands. Objectively, the best indication of this level is that the rectus muscles of the abdomen lose their hypertonic states and have only a normal degree of resistance to palpation. When a severe convulsive seizure occurs, with respiratory arrest, 2 to 8 ml of a 2.5 per cent solution of thiopental sodium is injected intravenously immediately and as necessary. This usually produces muscle relaxation within 30 to 45 seconds and permits spontaneous re-establishment of the respiratory cycle.

Some centers have been enthusiastic about the use of muscle-relaxant drugs to control convulsive seizures. Such drugs are difficult to manage and have not prevented death from respiratory arrest. Drugs more commonly suggested for such use are d-tubocurarine, succinylcholine (Anectine), pancuronium (Pavulon), atracurium (Tracrium), and vecuronium (Norcuron). The margin of safety with these drugs is narrow; they seem to be best designed for patients who are excessively difficult to manage—and then only under careful observation of an experienced anesthesiologist and with endotracheal intubation.

Surgical Wound Care

Optimal surgical care of wounds should be carried out in accordance with the following concepts:
1. The wounds cared for at the earliest possible moment.

2. Aseptic technique is observed, with the use of gloves, gowns, masks, and sterile instruments and the application of proper solutions to prepare the skin before the necessary operative procedures at the injured site.

3. During skin preparation, the wound should be covered with gauze to prevent further contamination.

4. Proper lighting is provided so that the surgeon can exactly identify and protect vital structures such as nerves and vessels.

5. Adequate instruments and adequate help should be available so that there is the best and gentlest possible retraction of structures in wounds.

6. Hemostasis is effected with delicate instruments and with fine suture material so that there is a minimum of necrotic tissue left in wounds.

7. Tissues are handled gently at all times so that necrotic tissue is not produced.

8. Complete débridement is carried out with scalpel excision of necrotic tissue and with removal of foreign bodies so that no pabulum is left on which any unremoved bacteria can propagate.

9. The wound is irrigated copiously with large amounts of physiologic salt solution to wash out minute avascular fragments of tissue and to eliminate foreign bodies.

10. If there is any doubt concerning a wound providing anaerobic conditions so that the tetanus bacillus can grow and produce its lethal toxin in it, the wound is left open. Drainage is instituted when necessary.

Antibiotics

Antibiotics may be administered for the treatment of the infectious complications of tetanus.

In vitro, penicillin is effective against the tetanus bacillus. It is not surprising, however, that antibiotic therapy is clinically disappointing when it is directed against the tetanus disease itself. Tetanus is not a bacteremia, for the bacillus remains at the place of its entry. By the time antibiotic therapy is begun, the wound often has been excised, and the toxins often are already spread in the circulation. When the site of infection is not known and the antibiotic effect would be particularly desired, there is little probability that the bacteria are reached by parenteral administration of an antibiotic owing to avascular conditions in a concealed, closed puncture wound. Despite the in vitro effects of penicillin, a noticeable, specific therapeutic reaction cannot be expected.

On the other hand, the antibiotics given according to sensitivity tests do play their part in the therapy plan. They are irreplaceable in the care of infectious complications of tetanus, especially in combating pneumonia or secondary, invasive wound infections. A combination of clindamycin phosphate injection, 600 mg every 6 hours, and gentamicin sulfate injection, 80 mg every 8 hours, may be given intravenously. A broad-spectrum antibiotic, such as a cephalosporin, may be administered intravenously.

The possible complications that may develop with antibiotic therapy must be given particular attention in the case of tetanus patients. Especially in the more severe cases, in which nourishment is accomplished through less than ideal methods, there is a tendency toward gastrointestinal disturbances.

Tracheostomy

Tracheostomy is performed when indicated if personnel and facilities are available to care adequately for the tracheostomy.

If the incubation period has been only a few days so that the patient may have severe tetanus, a tracheostomy probably will be necessary and can be performed with general anesthesia when extensive wound debridement is necessary, with local anesthesia, or with a combination of local and general anesthesia.

Tetanus patients in whom a tracheostomy is necessary will also need, in most cases, continuous artificial respiration. Such respiration is facilitated by attaching, with a gas-tight adapter, a tracheostomy tube with double inflatable cuffs to a volume-controlled respiration unit.

Nursing care of the seriously ill tracheostomy patient is not easy. Inspired air must be moist. If the patient can breathe spontaneously, moisturizing apparatus is set up in the patient's hospital room; if, however, the patient is being given artificial respiration, the respirator used must be one that continuously moistens the gas mixture. Dehydration of the respiratory tract can lead to severe hemorrhagic tracheobronchitis, which can be fatal. Even with absolutely correct conditioning of the inspired air, secretions can collect in the airway. A suction machine must always be at the patient's bedside. Patients with paralyzed respiratory muscles must be suctioned every hour. Also of extreme importance is the cleanliness of the tracheostomy tube; dehydrated secretions, pseudomembranes, and crusts can form on the inner margin of the cannula and may lead to narrowing of the respiratory airway. The tracheostomy tube should be changed whenever it cannot be made to function correctly by cleaning and manipulation.

A tracheostomy that is improperly cared for may be worse than none.

Tracheostomy may be poorly tolerated in the newborn infant, and decannulation may be quite difficult. In infants, particularly those with neonatal tetanus, endotracheal intubation by insertion of an endotracheal tube through the nose, or, less preferably, through the mouth, should be considered before tracheostomy.

Iatrogenic Problems

Constant alertness is required to avoid iatrogenic problems. For example, if rectal probes are left in place for constant recording of temperature, they must be checked carefully to prevent trauma to the rectal mucosa and anorectal veins during convulsions.

Private, Dark, Quiet Room

The patient should be placed in a private, dark, quiet room. Efforts should be made to reduce all external stimuli as much as possible. Visitors should be limited to the absolute minimum number. It should be pointed out that, with adequate sedation and muscle relaxation, some patients no longer require the dark, quiet room. Conversations with patients who have recovered from tetanus indicate that the constant attention to them 24 hours a day is most unpleasant and annoying for them.

Proper Environment for Infants

Place infants with neonatal tetanus in an incubator in which the oxygen partial pressure, the environmental temperature, and a nebulized atmosphere of distilled water can be monitored and maintained.

Roentgenograms

Roentgenograms may be indicated for (1) fractures associated with the initial injury, (2) determination of pulmonary problems such as atelectasis and pneumonia, (3) fractures or avulsions of muscle insertions produced by the tonic muscle contractions of tetanus, and (4) evaluation of resulting osteoarthropathies. Compression fractures of the vertebrae may be the result of the intense paroxysms that characterize the disease, and their diagnosis may be easily missed without roentgenograms.

Padded Tongue Depressor

Insertion of a padded tongue depressor can protect the tongue from being bitten during tonic contractions.

Oral Hygiene

The lips, teeth, tongue, and oral cavity should be cleaned daily to lessen the possibility of growth of pathologic bacteria and viruses. Remove all loose debris from the oral and nasal cavities.

Nutrition

Correct amounts of nourishment should be given by oral, nasogastric tube, gastrostomy tube, or intravenous routes. The relaxed patient is totally dependent on artificial nourishment. Initially, tube feedings through a soft nasogastric or nasojejunal tube are indicated. Aspiration pneumonia is a common complication of such feedings, and care must be taken that the stomach empties. Frequent, *small* feedings are indicated. If difficulties are encountered with the tube feedings, it may be necessary to resort to intravenous supplements. Central venous pressure systems that use the subclavian vein provide an excellent route for feeding, including hyperalimentation. Transfusions of blood, plasma, and human albumin can be supplemented with electrolyte solutions of glucose, alcohol, fructose, and protein hydrolysates. The infusions can be further supplemented with high doses of vitamins C and B complex. Serum protein and electrolyte levels should be checked repeatedly. Nothing is given by mouth until improvement begins. In choosing a diet, the fact that the patient on occasion may feel pain when eating and when trying to open his or her mouth should be considered.

Alimentary Tract Elimination

Adequate gastrointestinal elimination must be maintained. Spontaneous defecation usually is absent. Defecation can be controlled by saline laxatives given orally or into the nasogastric tube and by enemas as required.

Elimination of Urine

When necessary, elimination of urine can be facilitated by the insertion of Foley's catheter into the bladder. The catheter should be removed as soon as possible to reduce the possibility of urinary tract infections.

Intake and Output Records

Record intake and total output and alter intake as indicated.

Protection of the Eyes

In protecting the eyes, particular attention must be given to incomplete closure of the eyelids.

Without prophylactic measures, exsiccation, keratitis, and corneal ulcer can develop. An ophthalmic ointment may be covered with a moist gauze sponge.

Prevention of Decubital Ulcers

Keeping the patient's skin dry and cushioning pressure points can reduce the chance that the patient will develop decubital ulcers.

Blood Dyscrasias and Bleeding Problems

If there is a possibility of blood problems, complete blood cell counts should be obtained, clotting mechanisms promptly investigated, and any indicated treatment promptly rendered.

Prevention of Pulmonary Emboli

Indicated procedures, including ordering of heparin, must be carried out to avoid the risk of pulmonary embolization.

Prevention of Cardiac Exhaustion and Circulatory Disruption

Advances during the past decade have indicated the importance of proper use of alpha and beta blockers for sympathetic overactivity, which may be manifested by tachyarrhythmias and hemodynamic instability.

Temporary Endocardial Pacemaker

A temporary endocardial pacemaker may be indicated in cases with severe, medically refractory bradycardia of unknown cause.

Prevention of Muscle Contractures

As the patient improves, muscle contractures with resulting deformities, such as foot drop, must be prevented. Use of foam rubber padding, pillows, sandbags, and splints may be indicated. When necessary for muscle imbalance, physiotherapy should be instituted as soon as possible.

Electroencephalograms

Electroencephalograms should be ordered when it is technically possible to obtain them and when the procedure will not interfere with the patient's recovery. Such records may be of considerable importance in the long-range evaluation and care of the patient, particularly with regard to the possibility of brain damage.

Steroid Therapy

Steroid therapy should be considered if there is a possibility of adrenal gland exhaustion. Although not used routinely, steroid therapy has been used in a few severe cases of tetanus in which the prolonged course of the disease was throught to exhaust the adrenal glands. Before administration of corticosteroids for adrenal insufficiency, cortisol levels should be checked and an adrenocorticotropic hormone stimulation test should be performed to assess the need for supplemental steroids.

Tetanus Toxoid

At the end of the hospital treatment of tetanus, 0.5 ml of adsorbed tetanus toxoid intramuscularly should be given for active immunization, 1 month later another dose, and then 6 months later one more dose to complete the basic active immunization. Then, routine tetanus topxoid boosters are given every 10 years. Such immunization is necessary because *an attack of tetanus does not produce antibodies to prevent another attack.*

Emergency Medical Identification Devices

At the time of discharge from the hospital, the cured patient should be given a completed emergency medical identification device and should be instructed to complete the course of active immunization with tetanus toxoid to prevent recurrent tetanus.

Hyperbaric Oxygen

Hyperbaric oxygen is not recommended in view of its minimal good effects, if any, and the complications of such treatment. Tetanus is a toxemic state and is not due to bacteria that are spreading throughout the body and that might be acted on by oxygen in the circulating blood.

Control of Body Temperature

Necessary procedures to lower excessively high body temperatures should be carried out. Tetanus per se does not cause fever, but the complications of tetanus cause fever. Hence, tetanus and its complications should be treated, not the fever itself.

Recording of Data

In view of professional liability problems, the progress and treatment, and especially significant reasons for giving or not giving drugs, should be recorded completely and accurately.

TOXOPLASMOSIS

method of
RICHARD D. PEARSON, M.D.
University of Virginia School of Medicine
Charlottesville, Virginia

Toxoplasmosis is one of the most common parasitic infections of humans. Depending on the area, 20 to 70 per cent of adults in the United States have serologic evidence of infection with *Toxoplasma gondii*. The parasite has three morphologic forms: tachyzoite (trophozoite), tissue cyst, and oocyst. The cat is the definitive host of *T. gondii*. Humans become infected by ingestion of oocysts in food or water that has been contaminated with cat feces, by ingestion of tissue cysts contained in inadequately cooked meat, or by transplacental transmission. The early stage of infection is characterized by multiplication of tachyzoites and hematogenous dissemination to virtually every organ. Tissue cysts appear as immune responses of the host develop. The cysts persist for life and are the cause of recrudescent disease.

Most people infected with *T. gondii* are asymptomatic, but a wide spectrum of disease can occur. It is helpful to divide the clinical manifestations of toxoplasmosis into five categories (Table 1). The decision to treat and, to some degree, the selection of drugs depend on the location and extent of infection, the age and immunocompetence of the patient, and whether or not a woman with acute toxoplasmosis is pregnant.

TREATMENT

Treatment regimens for toxoplasmosis are based largely on clinical experience. Well-controlled, comparative therapeutic trials have not been conducted in humans. Pyrimethamine, a diaminopyrimidine, in combination with a sulfonamide has been the most widely used regimen. These drugs act synergistically against *T. gondii* tachyzoites, but they do not affect tissue cysts. They block sequential sites in the folic acid met-abolic pathway and thereby inhibit the synthesis of purines, pyrimidines, and certain amino acids.

Pyrimethamine (Daraprim) inhibits the dihydrofolate reductase of *T. gondii*. It is lipid soluble, readily absorbed from the gastrointestinal tract, and capable of entry into body compartments, including cerebrospinal fluid, which is of obvious importance for the treatment of toxoplasmic encephalitis. Trimethoprim, another dihydrofolate reductase inhibitor, is not as active as pyrimethamine against toxoplasma dihydrofolate reductase, and it should not be used for the treatment of toxoplasmosis.

The usual adult dose of pyrimethamine is 25 mg per day. In patients with toxoplasmosis and significant organ involvement, a loading dose of pyrimethamine 2 mg per kg (maximum dose 100 mg per day for adults) can be given daily in two divided doses for the first 2 days. When sulfonamides cannot be given concurrently or patients fail to respond, the dose of pyrimethamine is occasionally increased to 50 mg per day in adults.

Pyrimethamine can produce dose-related bone marrow suppression. Thrombocytopenia, neutropenia, and, less commonly, anemia may develop. Complete blood and platelet counts should be obtained at least once a week. The toxic effects of pyrimethamine on the bone marrow can be reduced, without altering the lethal effects against *T. gondii,* by administering folinic acid (leucovorin), 2 to 10 mg per day orally. Folic acid interferes with the action of pyrimethamine and should not be used. Pyrimethamine may also cause gastrointestinal side effects, but they are usually mild. Pyrimethamine is teratogenic in animals and is contraindicated during the first 14 to 16 weeks of pregnancy in humans.

Sulfonamides act synergistically with pyrimethamine against *T. gondii*. Sulfadiazine or trisulfapyrimidines are the most active and are given in conjunction with pyrimethamine. The dose of sulfonamides for adults is 75 to 100 mg per kg per day (maximum 6 grams per day) given in four divided doses. The loading dose is 75 mg per kg up to 4 grams. Other sulfonamides such as sulfisoxazole and sulfamethoxazole are less active and should not be used. The potential toxicities of sulfonamides are well known: crystalluria; hypersensitivity reactions, including rash and fever; blood dyscrasias; and gastrointestinal effects such as nausea, vomiting, and diarrhea. Crystalluria can be avoided by adequate hydration; a fluid intake in adults of at least 1 to 2 liters per day is recommended. Rash, fever, or neutropenia occurs in approximately 60 per cent of persons with acquired immunodeficiency syndrome (AIDS) who are treated with sulfonamides for toxoplasmic encephalitis. These toxic effects

TABLE 1. **Syndromes Associated with Toxoplasmosis**

1. Acute acquired toxoplasma infection in immunocompetent persons who are not pregnant
   a. Asymptomatic
   b. Self-resolving mild disease: adenopathy, malaise, and/or fever
   c. Symptomatic involvement of central nervous system, heart, or other organs (rare)
2. Acute acquired toxoplasma infection during pregnancy
3. Congenital toxoplasma infection
4. Ocular toxoplasmosis, usually caused by reactivation of congenital or acquired infection
5. Toxoplasmosis in immunodeficient patients, usually reactivation of disease
   a. Central nervous system infection
   b. Disseminated infection (e.g., heart, lungs)

not infrequently necessitate discontinuation of sulfonamide therapy.

Other drugs that have a potential role in the treatment of toxoplasmosis include spiramycin (Rovamycine) and clindamycin (Cleocin). Spiramycin, a macrolide antibiotic, is given at 50 to 100 mg per kg per day (2 to 4 grams per day for adults) in three or four doses. Spiramycin has been widely used in France for the treatment of toxoplasmosis acquired during pregnancy and for congenital toxoplasma infection. It is available in the United States only by special request from the U.S. Food and Drug Administration. Spiramycin has not been associated with teratogenicity. Its toxicities include gastrointestinal side effects such as nausea, vomiting and abdominal pain, and, less commonly, rash. Spiramycin is often administered in alternating courses with the combination of pyrimethamine and a sulfonamide.

Clindamycin has been reported to be effective when used with prednisone for the treatment of ocular toxoplasmosis and with pyrimethamine for the treatment of toxoplasmic encephalitis in persons with AIDS who could not tolerate sulfonamides. It should be noted that clindamycin is not lethal for *T. gondii* in vitro and the concentrations reached in brain tissue are low. Gastrointestinal side effects including diarrhea and pseudomembranous colitis are important potential toxicities of clindamycin treatment.

The recent increase in the number of cases of toxoplasmic encephalitis in persons with AIDS has stimulated the search for more effective, less toxic antitoxoplasmic drugs. Several new compounds including dihydrofolate reductase inhibitors and macrolides have been studied. One, trimetrexate, a low-molecular-weight, lipid-soluble dihydrofolate reductase inhibitor, has been shown to have excellent activity against *T. gondii*, but additional studies are needed to determine whether it or other new compounds are superior to currently available drugs.

The optimal duration of therapy for toxoplasmosis has never been carefully studied, but it clearly varies with the clinical syndrome. In immunocompetent adults and children with acquired toxoplasmosis who are treated with pyrimethamine and a sulfonamide, 4 to 6 weeks is usually adequate. Patients with AIDS and toxoplasmic encephalitis require long-term therapy, probably for the remainder of their lives.

Acquired Toxoplasmosis. Immunocompetent children or adults who acquire *T. gondii* are usually asymptomatic or experience a mild, self-limited disease characterized by lymphadenopathy, fever, or malaise. Chemotherapy is rarely indicated except for the unusual person in whom disease is severe or persistent or in whom there is symptomatic involvement of the central nervous system, heart, or lungs. However, infection acquired through a laboratory accident or blood transfusion should be treated. Pyrimethamine plus sulfadiazine along with folinic acid is administered for 4 to 6 weeks in immunocompetent persons who require therapy.

Infection During Pregnancy. Congenital infection is a feared complication in women who acquire toxoplasmosis during pregnancy. The likelihood of fetal infection has been reported to be 14 per cent in women infected in the first trimester, 29 per cent in the second trimester, and 59 per cent in the third trimester. The severity of infection is greatest when infection is acquired early in pregnancy. Treatment of women who become infected with *T. gondii* during pregnancy can decrease the incidence of congenital infection. Several regimens have been proposed. In a recent French series, acutely infeted women were given 3 grams of spiramycin per day in divided doses once maternal infection was diagnosed or suspected. Spiramycin was continued throughout pregnancy. Amniocentesis, fetal blood monitoring, and fetal ultrasonography were used to assess infection in the fetus. If fetal toxoplasmosis was diagnosed and the pregnancy was continued, pyrimethamine and a sulfonamide were administered to the mother. The most commonly used regimen was pyrimethamine, 50 mg, with sulfadiazine, 3 grams daily for 3 weeks, alternating with 3 weeks of daily spiramycin. This approach resulted in a lower frequency of congenital infection and less severe disease than expected based on previous experience. However, the number of women with infected fetuses was small. Establishing the efficacy of treating toxoplasma infection in the fetus by giving the mother pyrimethamine and sulfadiazine will require larger numbers of patients. Finally, because of potential teratogenicity, pyrimethamine should not be used during the first 14 to 16 weeks of pregnancy, and the efficacy of sulfonamides used alone has not been documented.

Congenital Toxoplasmosis. It is estimated that 0.1 to 1 per 1000 children born each year in the United States has congenital toxoplasmosis. It is not known how effective postnatal treatment is for ameliorating or preventing development of sequelae, but all infected neonates should be treated. Even neonates who appear to be normal at birth may later demonstrate serious sequelae. Twenty-one-day courses of pyrimethamine plus sulfadiazine are often alternated with 4- to 6-week courses of spiramycin. Pyrimethamine, 1 mg per kg (maximum dose 25 mg) every 2 days, plus sulfadiazine or trisulfapyrimidines, 75 to 100 mg per kg per day divided into two doses, plus folinic acid, 5 mg every other day, is used for 21 days. Twice the daily dose of pyrimethamine can be given on the initial 2 days of therapy in seriously infected infants. A complete blood count and platelet count should be obtained twice a week. Corticosteroids (1 mg per kg per day) are added in patients with active macular involvement. Initial therapy with pyrimethamine and sulfadiazine is followed by spiramycin, 100 mg per kg per day in two or three doses, for 4 to 6 weeks. Alternating cycles of therapy are given for a minimum of 6 months in asymptomatic children, and for 1 year or longer in symptomatic children. In healthy-appearing neonates whose mothers are known to have acquired toxoplasmosis during pregnancy, pyrimethamine plus sulfadiazine for 3 weeks followed by spiramycin or sulfadiazine alone is given until laboratory confirmation of congenital infection is obtained.

Ocular Toxoplasmosis. Local reactivation of infection is usually responsible for ocular toxoplasmosis. An aggressive immune response contributes to the observed retinochoroiditis. Corticosteroids along with antitoxoplasma chemotherapy are indicated when vision-threatening lesions involve the macula, optic nerve head, or papillomacular bundle. Prednisone is given at a daily dose of 1 to 2 mg per kg (total of 60 to 100 mg in adults). Equivalent doses of other steroids can be used. Pyrimethamine and sulfadiazine are administered along with folinic acid for 4 to 6 weeks. Small peripheral retinal lesions may subside spontaneously with time, and corticosteroids are not necessary for them. When prednisone is administered, it is usually tapered after retinal lesions demarcate and pigmentation begins. Some ophthalmologists use clindamycin (1200 mg per day in four divided doses) in place of pyrimethamine and sulfonamides for ocular toxoplasmosis, but controlled, double-blind studies comparing the efficacy of pyrimethamine and sulfonamides with clindamycin have not been reported.

Toxoplasmosis in Immunocompromised Patients. *T. gondii* has evolved as an important cause of encephalitis in patients with AIDS and occasionally in other persons who are immunocompromised by Hodgkin's disease or by use of immunosuppressive drugs for neoplasms, connective tissue diseases, or transplantation. It has been estimated that as many as 10 per cent of persons with AIDS develop this complication. Although most immunocompromised patients who develop toxoplasmosis present with encephalitis, some have cardiac or pulmonary involvement. Treatment with pyrimethamine plus sulfadiazine and folinic acid is the regimen of choice. In many instances, therapy is begun empirically in persons who have clinical findings consistent with toxoplasmic encephalitis and ring-enhancing central nervous system lesions on computed tomographic (CT) scan. A rapid response to therapy suggests that the patient has *T. gondii*. Patients who fail to respond within 2 weeks should be evaluated for other causes of central nervous system disease. Relapses have been the rule in patients with AIDS in whom therapy has been stopped, so treatment is usually continued at full or reduced doses until death occurs from other causes.

Rash, fever, neutropenia, or thrombocytopenia occurs in approximately 60 per cent of patients with AIDS who receive sulfonamides and pyrimethamine for toxoplasmic encephalitis. These side effects not infrequently necessitate discontinuation of sulfonamides. In that instance, both successes and failures have been reported with the combination of pyrimethamine (25 mg per day) and clindamycin (1800 to 2400 mg per day given in three or four divided doses). Alternatively, pyrimethamine can be used alone; the dose can be increased to 50 mg per day, particularly if there is evidence of progression of disease. More effective, less toxic drugs are needed for the treatment of toxoplasmosis, and the increasing number of cases of toxoplasmic encephalitis in persons with AIDS is stimulating research in this important area.

TRICHINELLOSIS

method of
THEODORE M. BAILEY, M.D., M.P.H.,
and PETER M. SCHANTZ, V.M.D., Ph.D.
Division of Parasitic Diseases, Centers for Disease Control
Atlanta, Georgia

Trichinellosis is caused by eating meat that is infected with larval cysts of the parasitic worm *Trichinella spiralis*. The larvae excyst in the stomach and the adult worms establish themselves in the small bowel. Within 1 week the adults produce larvae that invade the mucosa, enter the blood stream, and migrate through skeletal muscle and other internal organs, including the heart, brain, and lungs. Only larvae that encyst in skeletal muscle mature. In the United States, clinical trichinellosis has declined markedly in the past 30 years. From 1982 to 1986, the mean annual number of cases reported to the Centers for Disease Control was 57.

T. spiralis larvae are found in different kinds of meat, and a history of eating raw or poorly cooked pork, homemade pork sausage, or wild boar, bear, walrus, or other carnivorous game within 30 days of the onset of symptoms should suggest the diagnosis. The severity of signs and symptoms parallels the number of larvae ingested. In classic trichinellosis, patients have muscle soreness and pain, periorbital edema, fever, and eosinophilia.

Migrating and encysting larvae damage skeletal muscle fibers and increase levels of creatine phosphokinase. However, in most cases the diagnosis is difficult to make because in the enteric or the migratory phase of the parasite, patients either are asymptomatic or have nonspecific symptoms (gastrointestinal complaints, weakness, chills, or headache) lasting only a few days. Although a positive serologic test helps to establish the diagnosis, a negative test does not eliminate it because serologic tests do not become positive for 3 to 6 weeks after infection. Some tests may not become positive even after documented exposure. A positive muscle biopsy establishes the presence of the parasite and indicates the intensity of infection, but it must be performed no earlier than 14 days after eating the infective meat product to allow migrating larvae to encyst in skeletal muscle. Complications of infection depend on the intensity of larval migration through major organ systems.

TREATMENT

A patient who is seen within 6 weeks of ingesting the implicated meat product should be treated with mebendazole (Vermox)* (5 mg per kg orally three times a day for 13 days†; children, regardless of age, should take a minimum of 200 mg for 13 days). This treatment eliminates the intestinal phase of the adult *Trichinella* worm, stops the production of larvae, and kills migrating and encysted larvae. During the first trimester of pregnancy, mebendazole should be used with extreme caution because of its possible embryotoxic and teratogenic effects.

Because mebendazole acts on the larval tissue phase of trichinellosis, the treatment may cause systemic hypersensitivity reactions depending on the number of migrating and encysted larvae in the body. Hypersensitivity reactions should be treated with corticosteroids.

Persons who are asymptomatic or have mild symptoms (myalgias and low-grade fever) should be treated with mebendazole, antipyretics, and analgesics. Patients with more pronounced symptoms (fever, myalgias, leukocytosis, and eosinophilia) may need corticosteroids (20 to 40 mg of prednisone per day until symptoms disappear) in addition to mebendazole.

Symptoms of severe trichinellosis include fever, myalgias, generalized weakness, conjunctival

---

*This use of this agent is not listed in the manufacturer's official directive.

†Usual adult dose for trichinellosis is 200 to 400 mg three times daily for 3 days followed by 400 to 500 mg three times daily for 10 days.

hemorrhages, periorbital edema, and high eosinophilia. Corticosteroids (40 to 60 mg prednisone per day or higher) must be given in addition to mebendazole until fever and other allergic signs disappear. The intensity of infection increases the potential for complications. Bed rest and close medical supervision are required because patients may need treatment directed toward circulatory, respiratory, or neurologic complications caused by the large number of larvae migrating through vital organs. Myocardial failure and death can occur.

Thiabendazole, long used to treat trichinellosis, kills adult *Trichinella* worms but not migrating or encysted larvae and frequently causes side effects.

TULAREMIA

method of
GARY L. SIMON, M.D., Ph.D.
*The George Washington University School
of Medicine*
Washington, D.C.

Tularemia is caused by a small gram-negative coccobacillus, *Franciscella tularensis*. This organism is widely distributed throughout the Western hemisphere and has been isolated from more than 100 different mammals, fish, amphibians, and insects. The major reservoirs for human infection in the United States are rabbits, hares, and ticks. Infection in humans follows exposure to tissues or body fluids from an infected animal or through the bite of an infected insect. The organism is virulent, and infection may also follow inhalation of an infectious aerosol or ingestion of inadequately cooked meat.

The clinical features of tularemia are quite variable. The incubation period ranges from hours to 3 weeks. Systemic symptoms include fever, chills, headache, malaise, myalgias, and fatigue. Ulceroglandular tularemia is the most frequently encountered clinical syndrome and accounts for more than 75 per cent of all cases. In this form of the disease, there is a cutaneous lesion at the site of entry of the organism and associated regional lymphadenopathy. The disease may also present as a nonspecific febrile illness (typhoidal) or as pneumonia. Purulent conjunctivitis or exudative pharyngotonsillitis may be seen in the oculoglandular and oropharyngeal forms of the disease. The disease is usually sporadic, but clusters and small epidemics have been observed among populations at risk.

The diagnosis of tularemia requires a high index of suspicion and is confirmed by serologic studies. A fourfold rise in the level of serum agglutinins establishes the diagnosis. A single titer of 1:160 or higher suggests acute disease. The organism can be grown on cysteine-enriched media, but laboratory accidents are common and isolation should not be attempted in the routine clinical microbiology laboratory.

MANAGEMENT

General Measures

Hospitalization is indicated for all patients with pulmonary involvement and/or systemic symptoms. Stringent isolation procedures are not necessary because person-to-person transmission has not been reported, but routine precautions dictate that draining lesions should be covered by sterile dressings. Buboes should be treated conservatively because aspiration drainage may result in a draining sinus. If rupture appears imminent or the bubo becomes fluctuant, it may be necessary to aspirate the lesion.

Antibiotics

Streptomycin is the drug of choice for the treatment of all forms of tularemia. The drug should be given intramuscularly in a dose of 0.5 gram twice daily for 7 to 10 days. In children the dose is 7 to 10 mg per kg twice daily. For patients with more severe infections, especially those with pulmonary involvement or the typhoidal form of the disease, it may be prudent to give 1 gram (30 mg per kg per day) twice daily for the first 2 to 3 days. Treatment should not be withheld pending the results of serologic tests but rather should be initiated in response to clinical suspicion because early treatment reduces complications and mortality.

Gentamicin, 1.7 mg per kg every 8 hours, is a useful alternative agent and also provides coverage against other gram-negative organisms when the diagnosis is uncertain. The aminoglycoside antibiotics are potentially nephrotoxic and ototoxic. Serum concentrations should be monitored to ensure adequate therapeutic levels and to minimize the risk of toxicity. In patients who develop renal insufficiency, the dose must be adjusted accordingly. Development of vestibular or auditory toxicity may necessitate discontinuation of the drug.

Tetracycline or chloramphenicol, 500 mg four times daily, can be used to treat tularemia in patients who are not severely ill. The appropriate dose in children is 30 mg per kg per day. These drugs may be given orally and are continued for 14 days. Tetracycline should not be used in pregnant or lactating women, children younger than 8 years of age, or patients with renal or hepatic insufficiency. Side effects include nausea, vomiting, diarrhea, and photosensitivity. The hematologic toxicities of chloramphenicol are well known, and its use should be avoided when equally efficacious alternatives are available.

Tetracycline and chloramphenicol are bacteriostatic, and relapse may occur in up to 30 per cent of patients who are treated with these drugs, especially when the drugs are given for less than 14 days. Relapse is characterized by the recurrence of fever, usually within the first few weeks after therapy. Relapses are not due to resistant organisms, and re-treatment with the same drug is usually curative. The aminoglycoside antibiotics are bactericidal, and relapse does not occur after their use.

The mortality related to tularemia before the use of antibiotics ranged from 5 to 30 per cent. With the use of appropriate antibiotics, mortality has been reduced to less than 1 per cent. Individuals with pulmonary involvement or typhoidal disease have the highest mortality. Immunity after an episode of clinical tularemia appears to be lifelong, although a few well-documented reinfections have occurred in laboratory workers.

Prevention

The risk of infection can be reduced by avoiding exposure to potentially contaminated animals. Persons who handle such animals should wear thick rubber gloves. Rabbit meat should not be eaten unless it is thoroughly cooked. In tick-infested areas, insect repellants may be of value and clothing should fit tightly at the wrists and ankles.

A live, attenuated vaccine is available for administration to laboratory workers and other individuals whose occupation or avocation makes it likely that they will be frequently exposed to *F. tularensis*. This vaccine does not provide complete protection; however, the severity of the illness is modified in persons who develop overt disease. This vaccine is available from the Centers for Disease Control in Atlanta, Ga.

SALMONELLOSIS

method of
CLARE L. CHERNEY, M.D., and
MATTHEW E. LEVISON, M.D.
The Medical College of Pennsylvania
Philadelphia, Pennsylvania

Salmonellosis refers to a group of diseases caused by *Salmonella*. These organisms are motile, non–spore-forming, non–lactose-fermenting gram-negative rods of the family Enterobacteriaceae. *Salmonella* has three primary species, *S. typhi*, *S. choleraesuis*, and *S. enteritidis*, the last of which contains more than 2000 serotypes. The most common serotype isolated at the Centers for Disease Control is *S. enteritidis*, serotype *typhimurium*. Although humans are the only known reservoir for *S. typhi*, the non-*typhi Salmonella* colonize the majority of the animal kingdom, including humans. Humans become infected by ingesting large numbers of salmonellae in contaminated food or water. *Salmonella* is the most common etiologic agent identified in outbreaks of food-borne illness. Improperly cooked poultry (chicken, turkey, and duck) and poultry products (eggs) have been implicated as the source of non-*typhi Salmonella* in most investigated outbreaks, although beef, pork, dairy products, frozen pasta, water, marijuana, biologic extracts, and pet turtles are also known vectors. Direct human-to-human transmission can occur, but usually only in impaired hosts, such as infants or the old and debilitated.

Host characteristics play an important role in susceptibility to salmonellosis. Altered humoral or cellular immunity increases the risk of infection. Patients with human immunodeficiency virus (HIV) infection, diabetes mellitus, malignancy, splenectomy, or malnutrition, as well as infants and patients receiving immunosuppressive drugs (e.g., organ transplant recipients or those receiving steroids), are known to have an increased risk of salmonellosis. Impaired gastric acidity, whether surgically or medically induced, also enhances the risk of salmonellosis. This enhancement is probably a result of diminished killing of these acid-sensitive organisms in the gastric lumen, which allows for a low inoculum of ingested salmonellae to colonize the bowel. Patients with hemolysis (e.g., related to malaria, sickle cell disease, or bartonellosis) also are at increased risk of infection because of an impaired ability to clear salmonellae from the blood. Areas of anatomic abnormalities such as infarcted tissue, tumors, atherosclerotic plaques, and renal or biliary stones are especially prone to focal infection after *Salmonella* bacteremia.

ENTEROCOLITIS (GASTROENTERITIS)

Acute enterocolitis is the most common form of salmonellosis and accounts for 70 per cent of documented clinical disease. *S. typhimurium* is the usual pathogen in the United States. The majority of patients have an acute, self-limited illness consisting of fever, myalgia, headache, nausea, abdominal cramping, and diarrhea, which occurs 6 to 48 hours after the ingestion of contaminated food or water. Diarrhea may be either watery and profuse or dysenteric (containing blood and mucus). White blood cells are often seen on Wright's stain of stool samples. Fever may last 2 to 3 days and diarrhea may last 7 to 10 days. Early in the course of *Salmonella* enterocolitis, transient bacteremia has been estimated to occur in fewer than 5 per cent of adults, in 8 to 15 per cent of children, and in up to 40 per cent of infants (less than 3 months of age). Complications, such as intravascular infection or a localized extraintestinal infection, should be suspected if the patient has persistently positive blood cultures or a prolonged febrile illness.

Most episodes of *Salmonella* enterocolitis can be managed conservatively with attention to hydration and electrolyte replacement. Intravenous fluids may be necessary, especially in the infant or young child, when adequate intravascular volume cannot be maintained orally. Drugs that slow intestinal motility (e.g., diphenoxylate hydrochloride with atropine sulfate [Lomotil] or loperamide hydrochloride [Imodium]) are not recommended because they may decrease clearance of salmonellae or bacterial toxic products from the bowel.

Antimicrobial therapy is not indicated for this self-limited disease because it neither shortens the length of illness nor decreases the time of stool carriage of the organism, and it may select for resistant organisms. Antimicrobial therapy has been recommended in patients with sickle cell disease, infants younger than 3 months of age, and patients older than 50 years of age, and perhaps HIV-positive patients as well, because these groups have been shown to be at increased risk of developing complications from bacteremia; however, there is no evidence to support the hypothesis that antimicrobial therapy for *Salmonella* enterocolitis in these groups can actually prevent these complications. In one study of *Salmonella* enterocolitis in children, the occurrence of bacteremia was unpredictable and did not worsen the prognosis.

ENTERIC (TYPHOID) FEVER

Enteric fever is a prolonged, febrile illness caused by any serotype of *Salmonella*, although the usual pathogen is *S. typhi*. Enteric fever begins insidiously with progressively worsening systemic symptoms that include fever, headache, anorexia, myalgia, and generalized weakness. Nausea, vomiting, and diarrhea are not strikingly characteristic of this disease. In fact, constipation, cough, sore throat, and/or abnormal mentation may dominate the clinical picture at the time of presentation. A pulse that is slower than expected for the height of the body temperature, rose spots on the lower chest and upper abdomen, hepatosplenomegaly, and rales may be noted on physical examination. Blood and stool cultures are positive in the majority of cases. If untreated, enteric fever may last 3 to 4 weeks and may have a 1 to 30 per cent mortality.

Complications, including intestinal hemorrhage, bowel perforation, localized infections, and relapse, occur in up to 10 to 20 per cent of patients, even among treated individuals. Therapeutic measures important in the care of patients with enteric fever include antibiotics, rehydration, and nutritional supplementation. In the severely ill patient, a short course of high-dose corticosteroids (e.g., prednisone, 60 mg orally per day for 3 days, or dexamethasone, 1 to 3 mg intravenously every 6 hours for 3 days) has been shown to decrease morbidity and mortality. Steroids, as well as nonsteroidal anti-inflammatory drugs, should be given with extreme caution because they can lead to a precipitous fall in temperature and blood pressure.

Chloramphenicol (Chloromycetin) has traditionally been the antimicrobial drug of choice for enteric fever since its first documented success in 1948. There are well-known problems with this drug, including idiosyncratic aplastic anemia and dose-related marrow suppression, but it can generally be used safely. Resistance to chloramphenicol has been documented in Mexico, Great Britain, Vietnam, India, and parts of the United States, although the frequency is low (less than 1 per cent).

Ampicillin is a therapeutic alternative for enteric fever if the organism is sensitive to this drug. Ampicillin resistance is common among non-*typhi Salmonella* in this country, although most strains of *S. typhi* are susceptible. Ampicillin should not be used alone as first line therapy for enteric fever, when the pathogen or its sensitivities are not as yet known. Trimethoprim-sulfamethoxazole (Bactrim, Septra) can also be used as alternative treatment for enteric fever, especially when strains are resistant to both ampicillin and chloramphenicol, but in one study this agent was associated with an unacceptably high failure rate.

There is a growing, albeit small, amount of literature attesting to the efficacy of ciprofloxacin (Cipro) in the treatment of enteric fever. This drug has not been recommended for children less than 18 years of age (because of cartilage malformations reported in certain animals) or pregnant women (because of reported teratogenicity). Advantages include no known resistance, excellent intracellular penetration, and rapid bactericidal action.

Table 1 lists dosages of the aforementioned drugs.

BACTEREMIA

Patients with *Salmonella* bacteremia present with spiking fever, sometimes persisting for weeks, and no localizing signs of infection. Gastrointestinal symptoms usually do not occur. Blood cultures are positive, but stool cultures are usually negative. *S. choleraesuis* is the most common species that causes this disease. Complications include focal suppurative infections and a high relapse rate, especially in the immunocompromised patient.

It has recently become evident that patients with HIV infection are at increased risk for *Salmonella* bacteremia and, in fact, that this may commonly be their first manifestation of the acquired immunodeficiency syndrome (AIDS). These patients appear to have a high rate of relapse, and some experts have advocated chronic suppressive therapy in this group.

Treatment of *Salmonella* bacteremia is similar to that of enteric fever. Chloramphenicol and extended-spectrum cephalosporins, as outlined in Table 1, are alternative agents. In the nonpregnant adult with adequate oral absorption, ciprofloxacin is efficacious. Duration of therapy is 14 days unless a complication requiring more prolonged therapy is discovered. Because more than 40 per cent of non-*typhi Salmonella* strains are ampicillin-resistant, ampicillin should be used only if the in vitro sensitivity to this antibiotic is confirmed.

Hepatosplenic schistosomiasis is known to predispose patients to persistent *Salmonella* bacteremia and to relapse after therapy. Treatment of the salmonellosis may be facilitated in these patients by treatment of schistosomiasis.

CHRONIC CARRIER STATE

Most patients continue to carry salmonellae in their stools for up to 8 weeks after enterocolitis

TABLE 1. **Therapeutic Alternatives for Enteric Fever and *Salmonella* Bacteremia**

Drugs	Dosage*	Comments
Chloramphenicol (Chloromycetin)	12.5 mg/kg IV or PO q 6 hr for 14 days	Still considered drug of choice; do not use alone as initial therapy when resistance suspected; attention to side effects
Ciprofloxacin (Cipro)	500–750 mg PO q 12 hr for 14 days	To be used only in the nonpregnant adult; must have adequate oral absorption
Ampicillin	25 mg/kg IV or PO q 6 hr for 14 days	Use alone only if sensitivity confirmed
Ceftriaxone (Rocephin)	25–50 mg/kg IV or IM q 12 hr (up to 2 grams daily for children and 4 grams daily for adults)	Largest clinical experience for the cephalosporins
Trimethoprim-sulfamethoxazole (Bactrim, Septra)	4 mg/kg of trimethoprim component IV or PO q 12 hr	An alternative agent, but may have significant hematologic, hepatic, and dermal toxicity, especially in HIV-positive patients

*In older children and adults with normal renal function.

TABLE 2. **Therapeutic Alternatives for Chronic Carriage of *Salmonella***

Therapy	Dosage*	Comments
Ampicillin plus probenecid	1.5 grams ampicillin PO q 6 with 500 mg probenecid PO q 6 hr for 6 wk	May need to repeat 2 or 3 times but often is ineffective in patients with gallbladder disease
Ciprofloxacin (Cipro)	500–750 mg PO q 12 hr for 3–6 wk	Only in the nonpregnant adult
Trimethoprim-sulfamethoxazole (Bactrim, Septra) plus rifampin (Rifadin)	1 double-strength tablet (160 mg trimethoprim/400 mg sulfamethoxazole) q 12 hr with 600 mg rifampin PO daily	For 3 mo
Cholecystectomy	—	Consider only if: 1. Cholelithiasis is present 2. Eradication of the carrier state is mandatory 3. Benefits outweight risks 4. Multiple medical trials have failed

*In adults with normal renal function.

or enteric fever. Patients who continue to excrete salmonellae for more than 1 year are considered to be chronic carriers. In adults, chronic stool carriage after infection with *S. typhi* occurs in 1 to 3 per cent of patients. Chronic carriage after infection with non-*typhi Salmonella* is rare in the adult and probably occurs in fewer than 1 per cent of patients.

It is difficult to eradicate the chronic carrier state, especially when cholelithiasis is present. Chronic carriers should be counseled as to the practice of strict personal hygiene. If eradication is thought to be necessary, prolonged courses of ampicillin or trimethoprim-sulfamethoxazole may be tried (Table 2). Some studies have noted success with trimethoprim-sulfamethoxazole along with rifampin (Rifadin) when gallbladder disease is present. A preliminary report suggests that ciprofloxacin may also be effective. In only the unusual chronic carrier who is unresponsive to medical therapy and in whom eradication of the carrier state is mandatory should cholecystectomy be considered. However, the chronic carrier state may persist even after cholecystectomy in some patients.

LOCALIZED INFECTION

Focal suppurative infections caused by *Salmonella* can occur anywhere, especially at sites of previously damaged tissue. Abnormalities such as atherosclerotic plaques, scars, infarcts, tumors, or stones are often predisposing lesions. Clinical manifestations include those of osteomyelitis, infected arterial aneurysms, endocarditis, pericarditis, meningitis, pyelonephritis, pneumonia, empyema, abscesses in the liver or spleen, and soft tissue infections. Most of these complications require prolonged antimicrobial therapy and consideration of surgical drainage. Individualized

therapeutic regimens are obviously needed but are beyond the scope of this review.

TYPHOID FEVER

method of
ROBERTO CEDILLO-RIVERA, M.D., Ms.C.
*Instituto Mexicano del Seguro Social
Mexico City, Mexico*

Typhoid fever is an acute, systemic infection caused by *Salmonella typhi*, found exclusively in humans. It is found worldwide and affects mainly developing countries. The infection is acquired through ingestion of water or food contaminated by feces of patients or carriers. Bacteria penetrate the intestinal mucosa, are disseminated in the blood stream, and infect primarily the reticuloendothelial system. The disease is characterized by fever, malaise, headache, diffuse abdominal pain, and leukopenia. The diagnosis is confirmed by isolation of *S. typhi* from blood or bone marrow. Serologic tests may be of use for diagnosis when they are performed after 1 week of evolution of the illness. Early recognition and prompt antibiotic therapy are necessary to prevent complications and death. Lethality of untreated or inadequately treated disease is up to 15 per cent as a result of complications such as septic shock, hemorrhage, and intestinal perforation.

THERAPY

Antimicrobial Agents

Since the introdution of chloramphenicol in 1948, mortality from typhoid fever has decreased from 10 to 15 per cent to 1 to 3 per cent and the duration of illness from 5 weeks to 1 week; however, the appearance of bacterial strains that are resistant to chloramphenicol has obliged physicians to search for alternative drugs.

Chloramphenicol. Most strains that cause endemic typhoid fever are sensitive to chloramphenicol and the therapeutic results with this drug are superior to those obtained with other antibiotics; hence, chloramphenicol is the drug of choice. The recommended dosage in adults is 3 grams per day, and that in children is 100 mg per kg per day, divided in four doses. Treatment must be maintained for 10 to 12 days, and a reduction of fever generally occurs within 3 to 5 days; lower doses of chloramphenicol delay fever control until the seventh day. The total dose regimen should not exceed 30 grams. The route of choice is oral; when this route is not possible, the intravenous route is used until the switch to oral medication can be made. Chloramphenicol should not given intramuscularly because this route is painful and low and variable drug serum levels are achieved.

Chloramphenicol does not change the rate of occurrence of carriers, and it is ineffective for the treatment of these patients. Relapses occur in 5 per cent of patients, and case fatality rates range from 1 to 3 per cent. The major side effect of chloramphenicol is its hematologic toxicity and generally corresponds to reversible hematopoietic depression, which is dose related. Irreversible aplastic anemia occurs in approximately 1 in 40,000 to 50,000 recipients and is not dose related.

Since 1972, chloramphenicol-resistant strains of S. typhi have been reported during epidemics in Mexico, Southeast Asia, and India. In this situation alternative drugs should be used.

Furazolidone. As a result of experience in India and Mexico, we consider furazolidone (Furoxone) as the drug of second choice. We recommend a high dosage: 800 mg per day in adults and 10 to 15 mg per kg per day in children, divided in four doses, for 10 to 12 days.* Control of fever is obtained after 5 to 7 days of treatment. One disadvantage of the use of this drug is that it can be administered only by the oral route, but it has the advantage of being less expensive than other drugs. Side effects are gastrointestinal discomfort and headache. S. typhi is sensitive to furazolidone in vitro.

Amoxicillin. Amoxicillin (Amoxil) is a cogener of ampicillin but with superior intestinal absorption and thus higher serum levels than the latter. The recommended dosage in adults is 4 grams per day divided in four doses and in children is 100 mg per kg per day. Treatment should be continued for 14 days. The clinical response to this drug is slower than that with chloramphenicol; fever disappears after 7 days of treatment.

---

*These doses exceed the manufacturer's recommended dosages.

Certain chloramphenicol-resistant strains of S. typhi that have appeared since 1972 may also carry plasmid-mediated resistance to ampicillin and amoxicillin. The resistance of endemic strains of these antibiotics is higher than that for chloramphenicol and furazolidone. Rashes and gastrointestinal upsets occur with amoxicillin use, as with ampicillin.

Trimethoprim-Sulfamethoxazole. Trimethoprim-sulfamethoxazole (Bactrim) is less effective than those drugs mentioned earlier, and therapeutic failures have been reported in 8 to 10 per cent of infections with sensitive strains of bacteria. As with amoxicillin and ampicillin, the resistance of endemic strains to this drug combination is higher than that for chloramphenicol and furazolidone. However, it is considered to be an acceptable choice for treatment of cases resistant to the above-mentioned drugs. The recommended dosage is 160 mg of trimethoprim and 800 mg of sulfamethoxazole orally every 12 hours in adults and 8 mg of trimethoprim and 40 mg of sulfamethoxazole per kg per day in children, divided in two doses, for 12 to 14 days. Fever disappears after 5 to 7 days of treatment. The most frequent side effects are nausea, vomiting, and rash.

Cephalosporins and Quinolones. Third-generation cephalosporins, such as cefotaxime (Claforan), ceftriaxone (Rocephin), and cefoperazone (Cefobid), and new quinolones, such as norfloxacin (Noroxin) and ciprofloxacin (Cipro), have good activity in vitro against S. typhi. The clinical studies performed thus far indicate that these new classes of antimicrobial agents offer significant potential improvement for the treatment of typhoid fever; however, they must now be considered as alternative treatments for resistant strains of S. typhi.

Supportive Measures

In addition to antimicrobial therapy, the following measures must be taken: bed rest during the febrile period; normal low-residue diet, even enriched in calories; physical measures to control fever (the use of antipyretics should be avoided because they may cause hypothermia and hypotension). Intravenous fluids must be given as necessary to those patients who are unable to maintain hydration orally. Corticosteroids have been used in some patients with severe toxicity, but in our experience this measure is not useful and increases the risk of gastrointestinal bleeding, intestinal perforation, and superinfections.

Management of Complications

Intestinal Complications. Hemorrhage occurs in 10 per cent of patients. It appears more frequently during the second week of the illness, and its major clinical sign is melena; hypovolemic shock related to acute anemia can develop. Treatment involves blood transfusions and management of the shock.

Intestinal perforation occurs in 3 to 5 per cent of patients and is more common during the second and third weeks of disease. It is manifested by severe abdominal pain with signs of peritoneal irritation, perforation of hollow viscera, and septic shock. Treatment is based on (1) correction of shock; (2) administration of additional antimicrobial agents to treat peritoneal infection caused by aerobic and anaerobic bacteria by using amikacin together with metronidazole or cefoxitin; and (3) surgical correction, which may vary from the single closure of the perforation with drainage to intestinal resection with ileostomy.

Septic Extraintestinal Complications. Hepatitis, myocarditis, pneumonia, osteoarthritis, meningitis, typhoidic status, parotitis, and nephritis usually respond to basic antimicrobial treatment but in some cases may require drainage or surgery.

Septic Shock and Intravascular Coagulation. Special measures in addition to antimicrobial treatment are required for these complications (see specific chapters).

Relapses. Relapses occur despite adequate antimicrobial therapy in about 5 per cent of patients. Symptoms are usually less severe than those of the initial episode and occur 10 to 20 days after the cure. Treatment is the same as that given initially unless chloramphenicol was used at the maximal dose, in which case an alternative drug is preferred.

Carrier State. Approximately 10 per cent of patients continue to eliminate the bacillus for weeks or months. This is a self-limited condition and these *convalescent carriers* do not need treatment. It is only necessary to insist on strict hygienic measures and to prevent these persons from working as food handlers. If after a year *S. typhi* organisms are still being eliminated in the stool, these subjects are considered to be *chronic carriers* (about 1 per cent). Women and older adults are at increased risk of becoming typhoid carriers. The gallbladder is the common site of infection. Many of these patients have gallstones and gallbladder dysfunction, which make management difficult. Treatment involves a medical or combined medical-surgical approach: cholecystectomy accompanied by 4 weeks of amoxicillin, 2 grams three times a day, can cure the carrier state in about 90 per cent of cases. If only medical treatment is indicated, there have been therapeutic successes with 4 to 6 weeks of amoxicillin, 6 grams per day. Early reports indicate that third-generation cefalosporins and new quinolones, cited earlier, are also useful in the treatment of chronic carriers.

Prevention

The rational prevention of typhoid fever is based on hygienic education, environmental sanitation, and improvement of the quality of life. However, during epidemics and in subjects who travel from nonendemic areas to epidemic areas, vaccination is in order. One of the most effective vaccines available is prepared by acetone extraction, which preserves the Vi antigen and confers protection for up to 3 years in 90 per cent of the subjects immunized. The vaccine is administered parenterally in two doses of 0.5 ml at 1-month intervals. Side effects are fever, malaise, and adverse local reactions.

A new live oral vaccine has been developed by using a mutant strain of *S. typhi* (Ty21a). It has been tested in a field trial in Egypt with good results (95 per cent of protection for at least 3 years); however, in Chile the vaccine provided protection in only 67 per cent of those immunized. The advantage of this vaccine is the lack of notable adverse reactions, and it will probably be a good alternative for prevention of typhoid fever.

TYPHUS FEVERS

method of
WILLIAM D. SAWYER, M.D.
China Medical Board of New York, Inc.
New York, New York

Two species of *Rickettsia* are responsible for the diseases of the typhus fever group. These are *Rickettsia prowazekii,* the cause of epidemic (louse-borne) typhus and recrudescent typhus (Brill-Zinsser disease), and *Rickettsia typhi,* the cause of murine (endemic) typhus. The three diseases present similarly but differ in severity and in epidemiology.

Certain other rickettsial diseases are sometimes known as a form of typhus. Scrub typhus, caused by *Rickettsia tsutsugamushi,* differs clinically and epidemiologically from the typhus fevers. The spotted fever group of diseases, sometimes called tick typhus, results from infection by different rickettsial species in different parts of the world. The most severe form, Rocky Mountain spotted fever, which is caused by *Rickettsia rickettsii,* is found in the United States.

Although they are not called typhus and are quite different clinically, two other rickettsial infections are considered here because they respond to the same therapy: Q fever, caused by *Coxiella burnetti,* and rickettsial pox, caused by *Rickettsia akari.*

The *Rickettsia* species are widely distributed in nature, are transmitted primarily by arthropod vectors, and have various mammalian reservoirs. Except for epidemic typhus and Brill-Zinsser disease, human infection is incidental to the perpetuation of the organisms in nature. The global distribution of the rickettsial diseases depends on the ecology of the arthropod vectors and the mammalian reservoirs. Epidemic typhus, for example, is transmitted primarily from human to human by lice. Conditions such as war and disaster promote such transmission and can lead to major outbreaks of disease.

The common rickettsial diseases in the United States are Rocky Mountain spotted fever, endemic typhus, and Q fever. Epidemic typhus, Brill-Zinsser disease, and rickettsial pox occur only rarely. Rocky Mountain spotted fever, transmitted by ticks, occurs throughout the country, but most often in the south Atlantic and Gulf states. The reservoir is ticks and a variety of wild mammals. The peak period of the disease is in the spring and summer when ticks are most active. The incidence is highest in rural and suburban areas where humans are exposed to ticks. Endemic typhus is an infection of rats and other rodents that is transmitted to humans by fleas. Rickettsialpox is an infection of the house mouse and other rodents that is transmitted to humans by mites. Cases of both diseases occur when there is interaction of the requisite species. Q fever is an infection of small mammals, cattle, sheep, and goats that is transmitted both by ticks and by inhalation of dried infected material from mammals with the disease.

In humans the rickettsiae may multiply locally at the site of inoculation and, in some instances, produce a local lesion. The organisms spread throughout the body and multiply within and injure the endothelial cells of the small blood vessels. The injury and inflammation lead to leakage and extravasation of blood elements into the tissues and also lead to thrombosis with resultant damage to tissues. The specific manifestations of each disease relate to the location of the dominant organ involved and the consequences of the angiitis.

The key features of the diseases are an acute, febrile illness that develops after an incubation period of a few days to 3 weeks, a rash (except for Q fever), and the consequences of the angiitis such as decreased effective circulating blood volume, azotemia, electrolyte imbalance, delirium, stupor, coma, myocarditis, hepatitis, a consumptive coagulopathy, and shock. The clinical manifestations and epidemiologic setting are the basis of initial diagnosis. Specific serologic tests provide confirmation. The nonspecific Weil-Felix reaction may help during the second week of illness. Rocky Mountain spotted fever is the most severe rickettsial disease. It may be fulminant and fatal before the results of serologic tests can be obtained. Antirickettsial therapy must not be delayed in cases of clinically suspected Rocky Mountain spotted fever until a diagnosis is made.

THERAPY

Prompt antirickettsial therapy is the principal concern in the treatment of rickettsial diseases.

Patients who are cooperative and mildly ill can be treated as outpatients. Those who may be unreliable or who are moderately or severely ill should be hospitalized to ensure proper antimicrobial treatment and to attend to complications that tend to occur in the second week of untreated disease.

Supportive care is vital for the severely ill patient and must be directed to the complications, for example, azotemia, hypovolemia, and hypoproteinemia. Corticosteroids in large doses for up to 3 days may be tried in severely toxic patients.

General therapeutic measures include provision of a nutritious diet, protection of the agitated patient from injury, and skin and mouth care. The severe headache that is common in these diseases is most often intractable and not eased by the usual drugs.

Specific Therapy

Both tetracycline (or an equivalent congener) and chloramphenicol are highly effective in the treatment of the typhus group of infections and the other rickettsial diseases. Other common antibiotics are ineffective. Chloramphenicol is preferred in cases in which typhoid fever is included among the possible causes of illness and in children younger than the age of 8 years. Clinical response begins quickly. Fever remits and dramatic overall improvement typically occurs in the first 2 days of antimicrobial therapy. In Rocky Mountain spotted fever, the vascular lesions may be so extensive that permanent tissue damage occurs despite effective antibiotic treatment.

Patients who can tolerate oral medication should receive one of the following drugs:
1. Tetracycline
   a. Initial dose: 25 mg per kg
   b. Daily dose: 25 mg per kg per day in four equal doses every 6 hours
2. Chloramphenicol
   a. Initial dose: 50 mg per kg
   b. Daily dose: 50 mg per kg per day in four equal doses every 6 hours

Intravenous preparations should be administered to patients who are unable to tolerate oral treatment. Warnings on package inserts should be observed. Oral therapy should replace intravenous administration as soon as possible. Adults and children should receive one of the following drugs:
1. Tetracycline
   a. Initial dose: 15 mg per kg infused in 30 to 45 minutes
   b. Daily dose: 25 mg per kg per day infused in equal doses every 6 hours
2. Chloramphenicol sodium succinate

a. Initial dose: 20 mg per kg infused in 30 to 45 minutes

b. Daily dose: 50 mg per kg per day infused in equal doses every 6 hours

Treatment should continue until the patient is improved and has been afebrile for 24 to 48 hours. Treatment with these drugs stops the proliferation of organisms and hence treats the disease. The antibiotics do not, however, eradicate the organisms. Eradication depends on the host's immune response, which is relatively slow to develop. A relapse may follow cessation of therapy, especially if the treatment was instituted early in the course of the disease and was short. Such a relapse responds quickly to a new course of the same antibiotic.

Doxycycline is a long-acting derivative of tetracycline. A single oral dose is effective in the treatment of typhus and is both convenient and safe. This is probably the treatment of choice for the typhus fever group, especially in situations such as refugee camps or disasters when medical service is limited. A single dose of doxycycline is not, however, reliable therapy for Rocky Mountain spotted fever. For this disease, doxycycline should be continued until the patient has improved and been afebrile for 24 to 48 hours. Doxycycline should be given as follows:

1. Doxycycline
   a. Single dose: 100 or 200 mg

PREVENTION

Prevention of rickettsial disease relies primarily on reducing human contact with the arthropod vectors, for example, delousing and using insect repellants, and on reducing the number of reservoir hosts and vectors. A commercial vaccine for epidemic typhus is available. It consists of killed rickettsiae prepared as a formalin-treated suspension of infected yolk sac. The vaccine prevents or ameliorates the disease.

Local health authorities should be informed of the occurrence of a case of rickettsial disease.

WHOOPING COUGH
(Pertussis)

method of
HÉCTOR GUISCAFRÉ GALLARDO, M.D.
Instituto Mexicano del Seguro Social
Mexico City, Mexico

Pertussis is a highly contagious infectious disease of the respiratory tract that is seen mainly in children of preschool and early school age. However, recently it has been seen with greater frequency in infants younger than 6 months of age, in older children, and in adults. In preschool children and those of early school age, the cough is manifested by recurrent severe paroxysms that end in a musical, stridulous inspiratory gasp or whooping sound—hence, the name whooping cough. In infants younger than 6 months of age, the whoop may not be present, and they may have only severe paroxysms of cough ending with cyanosis and apnea. In older children and in adults, there may be only a chronic severe cough.

Classic pertussis presents in three clinical stages: (1) the catarrhal stage, which may be indistinguishable from a simple cold (1 to 2 weeks); (2) the paroxysmal stage (2 to 4 weeks); and (3) the convalescent stage (3 to 4 weeks), which is manifested only by chronic cough. If the patient has a viral infection in this stage, the paroxysmal cough may occur again.

The disease is caused by *Bordetella pertussis,* a small and fastidious gram-negative coccobacillus, that can be cultured from material taken by nasopharyngeal swab from individuals during the catarrhal stage or early paroxysmal stage, by using Bordet-Gengou agar. However, in these stages the isolation rate is less than 40 per cent. Hence, the diagnosis is made mainly on the basis of clinical characteristics, epidemiologic aspects, and the presence of leukocytosis higher than 15,000 cells per mm^3, with lymphocytosis (in 70 per cent of cases).

The mortality caused by pertussis is lower than 10 per cent, but in infants younger than 6 months of age it may be 30 or 40 per cent. Death is caused mainly by severe complications: early pneumonia caused by *B. pertussis* (first 3 weeks); later pneumonia caused by secondary bacterial infection (after 3 weeks of disease); and encephalopathy caused by hypoxemia and cerebral microhemorrhages.

THERAPY

Antimicrobial Treatment. Antibiotics do not alter the clinical course of the disease when the paroxysmal stage is already present. Antibiotics can modify the disease if they are administrated during the catarrhal stage. However, in clinical practice, whooping cough is not diagnosed at this stage. *B. pertussis* is eradicated in 3 or 4 days in patients who are treated with erythromycin, which shortens the contagious period. Some studies have shown a failure of erythromycin to erradicate pertussis organisms from patients with whooping cough, but these patients were treated with a low dose of antibiotic or with a preparation of erythromycin (ethylsuccinate or stearate) that is known to produce significantly reduced serum and respiratory secretion levels. For these reasons, the antimicrobial treatment recommended is the estolate ester of erythromycin (Ilosone), at a dosage of 50 mg per kg per day (maximum 1.5 grams) for 14 days; shorter courses of 5, 7, or even 10 days are associated with a 10 per cent bacteriologic relapse. (Note: the estolate salt has been associated with hepatotoxicity.)

Other antibiotics such as ampicillin, co-trimoxazole, chloramphenicol, or tetracycline have in vitro activity against *B. pertussis,* but they do not inhibit the growth of the organism at concentrations that are judged as achievable in vivo in respiratory secretions.

The scheme of antimicrobial treatment that we use depends on the clinical condition of the patient and the stage of the disease and is shown in Table 1.

Symptomatic Treatment. Cough supressants, expectorants, mucolytic agents, and sedatives have not been shown to be of benefit. The value of corticosteroids has not been properly evaluated; we do not use them.

Although preliminary results have shown that beta$_2$-adrenergic stimulants such as salbutamol (albuterol [Ventolin]) were of benefit, we have not observed a favorable effect and do not recommend them.

Unfortunately, there is no treatment to lessen the frequency or intensity of the paroxysms of cough.

Supportive Care. Patients with pneumonia or encephalopathy or patients with hypoxemia must be hospitalized. Continuous humidified oxygen is

TABLE 1. **Antimicrobial Treatment of Whooping Cough**

Clinical Condition	Treatment
Without pneumonia	
Early paroxysmal stage (<2 wk)	Estolate ester of erythromycin, 50 mg/kg/day q 8 hr
Later paroxysmal stage (>2 wk)	None
With pneumonia	
Early pneumonia (<3 wk of the disease)	Ampicillin, 50–100 mg/kg/day, q 6 hr for 10 days
Later pneumonia (>3 wk of the disease)	Penicillin G, 100,000 U/kg q 4 or 6 hr parenterally for 7 days

indicated for patients who show evidence of hypoxemia. Nasopharyngeal suctioning of secretions is frequently required, particularly in young, weak, and exhausted infants. Patients with severe hypoxemia must receive ventilation assistance in a timely fashion. Parenteral fluid administration and electrolyte and nutritional supplementation are frequently required in patients with severe and protracted disease. Patients with encephalopathy related to whooping cough must be treated for cerebral edema.

PREVENTION

Strict respiratory isolation of infected patients is essential during the contagious period (until the third week of the paroxysmal stage). Passive immunization with pertussis hyperimmune globulin has been shown to have no benefit, nor is active immunization after exposure useful.

Susceptible children (children younger than 2 months or unvaccinated children) who are exposed to an infected person during the contagious period must receive erythromycin. The effectiveness of this measure is not fully demonstrated, but most authors agree that it is beneficial.

The best way to prevent pertussis is active immunization at 2, 4, and 6 months of age (with booster doses at 2 and 4 years) with the whole cell vaccine. Efficacy is estimated to be approximately 80 per cent. Pertussis vaccine given as diphtheria-tetanus-pertussis vaccine has many transient side effects that are not serious (local pain in 50 per cent and fever in 30 per cent of patients). However, in some cases this combination vaccine may produce seizures (0.6 per cent) or encephalopathy (1 in 180,000 applications).

Given the efficacy and the side effects of the whole cell vaccine, the development of an acellular vaccine is exciting. The experience of Japanese physicians is favorable, and this new vaccine provides a hope for the future.

Section 3

The Respiratory System

ACUTE RESPIRATORY FAILURE

method of
JAY I. PETERS, M.D., and
J. MICHAEL JORDAN, M.D.
The University of Texas
San Antonio, Texas

The term "respiratory failure" implies the inability to maintain the normal delivery of oxygen to the tissues or removal of carbon dioxide from the tissues. Thus, three processes are actually involved: transfer of oxygen across the alveolus, transport to the tissues (by cardiac output), and removal of carbon dioxide from the blood into the alveolus with exhalation into the environment. Failure of any part of this system can lead to respiratory failure or can worsen pre-existing respiratory failure. Clinically, most physicians define "respiratory failure" by analysis of arterial blood gases. Although levels of Pa_{O_2} and Pa_{CO_2} that are said to constitute respiratory failure are obviously somewhat arbitrary, an arterial P_{O_2} of less than 60 mmHg or a P_{CO_2} of more than 45 mmHg generally indicates serious respiratory compromise.

CLASSIFICATION

Respiratory failure may be usefully classified by distinguishing between "ventilatory failure" and "oxygenation failure."

Ventilatory Failure

Ventilatory failure is diagnosed when the Pa_{CO_2} exceeds 45 mmHg and may be due to defective respiratory control mechanisms, impaired function of the respiratory muscles, or mechanical abnormalities of the lungs or chest wall. Thus, ventilatory failure may occur in patients with normal lungs, although mechanical impairment of the lungs—usually caused by chronic airway obstruction—is the most frequent cause. In addition to an elevated Pa_{CO_2}, ventilatory failure is always associated with hypoxemia if the patient is breathing room air because of the effect of an increased Pa_{CO_2} on the alveolar oxygen tension. This effect is defined by the alveolar air equation, which relates alveolar oxygen tension (PA_{O_2}) to Pa_{CO_2}:

$$PA_{O_2} = FI_{O_2} \times (PB - PH_2O) - Pa_{CO_2}/RQ$$

where PB is barometric pressure, PH_2O is water vapor pressure at 37° C (usually assumed to be 47 mmHg), and RQ is the respiratory quotient (generally taken to be 0.8). From this equation, it can be seen that at a constant FI_{O_2} (fraction of oxygen in inspired air) and PB, PA_{O_2} (and thus Pa_{O_2}) decreases as Pa_{CO_2} rises. As a general rule, the Pa_{O_2} decreases by 5 mmHg for every increase of P_{CO_2} of 3. Thus, in hypoventilation states reflected by an elevated PA_{CO_2}, ventilatory failure leads to oxygenation failure as well.

Oxygenation Failure

In addition to alveolar hypoventilation, failure of oxygenation may be caused by shunting, $\dot{V}/\dot{Q}$ (ventilation perfusion ratio) mismatching, and impaired diffusion. Of these, impaired diffusion is a rare cause of arterial hypoxemia, except during exercise in patients with interstitial lung disease or at extreme altitude. To distinguish the remaining three causes, the magnitude of the difference between alveolar and arterial oxygen tensions, $P(A - a)_{O_2}$, is useful.

The measured arterial P_{O_2} is always somewhat lower than the ideal alveolar oxygen tension calculated by the alveolar air equation, owing to the presence of $\dot{V}/\dot{Q}$ mismatching and normal anatomic shunts. The normal $P(A - a)_{O_2}$ is about 10 mmHg in young persons but increases with age to about 30 mmHg in healthy people by age 70 years. Oxygenation failure related to shunting and $\dot{V}/\dot{Q}$ mismatching causes increases in $P(A - a)_{O_2}$ above normal, whereas alveolar hypoventilation causes hypoxemia with a normal $P(A - a)_{O_2}$ gradient.

Physiologic shunting is defined as the persistence of an increased $P(A - a)_{O_2}$ during oxygen breathing and is due to anatomic right-to-left shunts or to continued perfusion of lung units that receive no ventilation ($\dot{V}/\dot{Q} = 0$). The latter abnormality is usually associated with alveolar filling processes such as pneumonia, atelectasis, or severe pulmonary edema, which are readily apparent on radiographs of the chest. Hypoxemia that is not relieved by breathing oxygen in the presence of clear lung fields radiographically suggests the presence of an intracardiac shunt, pulmonary arteriovenous fistula, or microatelectasis (most often seen in postoperative patients). Arterial hypoxemia related to shunting is worsened by conditions that reduce the oxygen content of the mixed venous blood, such as a low cardiac output.

$\dot{V}/\dot{Q}$ mismatching is the most common cause of arterial hypoxemia in hypoxemic patients. Lung units that have low $\dot{V}/\dot{Q}$ ratios contribute to arterial hypoxemia in a fashion similar to shunt units; this effect is termed "venous admixture." However, in contrast to true shunts, the effect of low $\dot{V}/\dot{Q}$ units is eliminated by oxygen breathing. Hypoxemia related to $\dot{V}/\dot{Q}$ mismatching is thus improved by small increases in FI_{O_2}, whereas hypoxemia related to shunting requires a high FI_{O_2}, and often other measures as well.

Respiratory failure caused by pure hypoventilation (as seen most commonly after strokes, head trauma, central nervous system [CNS] infections, or ingestion of CNS-depressant drugs) is characterized by carbon dioxide retention as well as by hypoxemia. The degree of hypoxemia is directly related to the rise in Pa_{CO_2}, resulting in a normal $P(A - a)_{O_2}$. Calculation of the $P(A - a)_{O_2}$ can thus distinguish hypoventilation from other causes of oxygenation failure.

TREATMENT

When approaching the patient in acute respiratory failure, whatever the underlying cause, the physician must remember the ABC's of resuscitation: airway, breathing, and circulation. A patent airway is the first priority. Upper airway obstruction may be manifested by stridor in awake patients or by inability to elevate the chest with inspiratory efforts applied at the nose or mouth in unconscious patients (via mouth-to-mouth resuscitation or face mask and self-inflating bag). Obstruction must be dealt with rapidly by manually clearing the obstruction or instrumenting the airway. Important information may be gained by a quick assessment of the presence or absence, as well as the apparent adequacy, of the patient's spontaneous breathing, as well as its rate, pattern, and laboredness. Similarly, rapid assessment of the patient's circulatory status—pulse, jugular venous pressure, and blood pressure—provides useful clues to the patient's overall status. Once these initial observations are made and any necessary emergency support measures are instituted, decisions regarding specific therapies may be made on the basis of arterial blood gas determinations.

Oxygen Therapy

Two primary considerations are involved in deciding on the method of oxygen administration for a hypoxemic patient: How much oxygen will be required? Is it important to know the FI_{O_2}? For many patients, "some" oxygen is sufficient, whereas for others each of these considerations is an important issue.

Administration of oxygen via nasal cannulas at flow rates of 1 to 5 liters per minute provides some augmentation of the FI_{O_2} and is the best tolerated means of O_2 therapy. However, the magnitude of increase in FI_{O_2} is unknown, being determined primarily by the patient's ventilatory pattern. On average, provision of low-flow oxygen

increases FI_{O_2} by 3 per cent per liter per minute of oxygen flow, but the increase is greater in patients with low minute ventilation and smaller in patients with large minute ventilation. In general, low-flow nasal oxygen provides adequate oxygen supplementation for patients whose hypoxemia is due to $\dot{V}/\dot{Q}$ mismatching (in contrast to shunting), who are not excessively tachypneic, and whose oxygen requirement is not great. These criteria would include patients with airway obstruction, mild heart failure, mild pneumonias, or pulmonary embolism, for example, but would not include patients with extensive pneumonias, severe pulmonary edema, or any of these problems associated with cardiogenic shock.

In the latter conditions, provision of a known, high concentration of oxygen is often necessary to correct hypoxemia. High-flow oxygen devices generally incorporate a dilution apparatus that reduces the final concentration of oxygen by entraining and adding air to the stream of oxygen, usually using Venturi's principle. Because of entrainment characteristics, fixed oxygen concentration devices can provide oxygen-enriched gas at flow rates that are likely to exceed the patient's inspired flow at low oxygen concentrations ($FI_{O_2} \leq 0.40$). However, delivery of high oxygen concentrations requires less air entrainment and results in lower flow rates. Patients often "overbreathe" these systems, resulting in lowering of the effective FI_{O_2}. This may explain why in some tachypneic patients, increasing the FI_{O_2} fails to improve the patient's oxygenation. To provide high FI_{O_2} levels, tight-fitting masks with reservoir bags and unidirectional valves must be used; with these devices, FI_{O_2} in the range of 0.8 to 0.95 is achievable.

Mechanical Ventilation

Absolute indications for initiation of mechanical ventilation include apnea and the need for administration of paralyzing agents. Mechanical ventilation is also usually required in patients who exhibit ineffectual respiratory efforts, inspiratory muscle fatigue, refractory hypoxemia, or progressive hypercapnea with acidosis. More specific indications are advocated by some physicians, and these include a vital capacity less than 15 ml per kg, FEV_1 less than 10 ml per kg, Pa_{O_2} less than 60 mmHg on supplemental oxygen, and PCO_2 more than 55 mmHg.

Although a number of types of ventilators exist, volume-cycled ventilators (i.e., ventilators that deliver a preset tidal volume) are by far the most common. When mechanical ventilation is instituted with such a ventilator, tidal volumes in the range of 10 to 15 ml per kg are reasonable. Tidal volumes of this size minimize atelectasis but at the upper end of this range may generate high peak airway pressures. In general, if peak pressures exceed 40 cmHg at higher tidal volumes, the tidal volume should be lowered to the range of 10 to 12 ml per kg to minimize the risk of barotrauma.

When the respiratory rate of a patient who is being mechanically ventilated is to be determined, a crucial decision concerns which ventilator "mode" is most appropriate. In the assist-control mode, the ventilator delivers a full preset tidal volume each time the patient initiates an inspiration. This mode is preferred by most conscious patients and should be used in patients with cardiogenic or other forms of shock. This method decreases the blood flow to the diaphragm and allows blood to be diverted to more critical organs. In addition, patients with diffuse lung disease and metabolic acidosis should be placed on assist-control to allow them to reduce their level of carbon dioxide to compensate for the acidosis. However, problems may arise with patients who "fight the ventilator" and with patients with hyperventilation. The former situation arises when the patient perceives that the ventilator settings as determined by the physician are inadequate and breathes out of synchronization with the ventilator. This problem can be corrected by changing the settings, by sedating the patient, or by switching to another mode. Hyperventilation results when the patient's drive to breathe is not diminished by correction of hypoxemia or the provision of large tidal volumes, as often occurs with diffuse pulmonary processes and in patients with altered sensorium and increased central drive. This condition can most readily be corrected by changing modes to intermittent mandatory ventilation (IMV).

IMV is a mode of ventilation in which the patient draws spontaneous tidal volumes from a reservoir and receives intermittent breaths from the ventilator at mandatory intervals. Thus, IMV combines assisted and unassisted ventilation. IMV should always be used in patients who are intubated for chronic carbon dioxide retention. Rapid reduction of carbon dioxide leads to CNS alkalosis and results in seizures. IMV may be useful in patients with central hyperventilation by avoiding the delivery of large tidal volumes each time the patient inspires. Also, IMV may be useful in weaning patients from mechanical ventilation because it provides a method for gradually reducing the amount of mechanical assistance to ventilation. IMV is obviously not well suited to the patient with respiratory muscle fatigue in whom rest is required; indeed, if the spontaneous circuit is not properly adjusted, the work of breathing with IMV may be substantially greater than with unassisted breathing.

One other newer mode is available on some ventilators, namely "pressure support." A preset inspiratory pressure is maintained throughout inspiration, whereas tidal volume depends on patient effort. This mode helps to overcome the systemic resistance during spontaneous ventilation, thereby decreasing the work of breathing. Pressure support may prove to be helpful in weaning patients from the ventilator.

To select the initial FI_{O_2} when instituting mechanical ventilation, there are two reasonable approaches. With many patients, previous blood gas determinations will be of help in knowing what oxygen concentrations were previously inadequate, and a somewhat higher FI_{O_2} should be selected initially. With other patients, a level around 0.80 is a good place to start. If an acceptable Pa_{O_2} (approximately 60 mmHg) is not obtained with an FI_{O_2} of more than 0.6, positive end-expiratory pressure (PEEP) should be instituted and invasive hemodynamic monitoring considered.

The principal value of PEEP is that it often allows a reduction in the FI_{O_2} required to achieve adequate oxygenation of the arterial blood, and it should be used in most patients who require an FI_{O_2} of 0.6 or more without it. The beneficial effects of PEEP derive from a number of factors, including improved lung compliance, increased functional residual capacity, and diminished shunting. The use of PEEP may be associated with deleterious effects as well. The incidence of barotrauma is greater among patients ventilated with PEEP than without, although it is uncommon when less than 15 cmH_2O PEEP is used. Because PEEP tends to decrease cardiac output, the usual increase in Pa_{O_2} and arterial oxygen content with PEEP may be offset, resulting in an actual reduction in oxygen delivery (the product of cardiac output and oxygen content).

Weaning from Mechanical Ventilation

Minimal criteria for discontinuing mechanical ventilation include (1) awake and cooperative mental status; (2) FI_{O_2} of 0.40 or less; (3) ventilatory capacity sufficient to support unassisted breathing for 30 to 60 minutes while intubated; and (4) ability to control secretions through spontaneous coughing. More objective measures of ventilatory capacity have been suggested: Successful weaning is unlikely if FVC is less than 15 mg per kg, maximal inspiratory pressure is less than −25 cmH_2O, or maximal voluntary ventilation is less than twice the patient's minute ventilation while being assisted. Weaning in most patients may be accomplished by "T tube trials," which involve connecting the endotracheal tube to a high-flow gas source delivered via tubing that connects at a right angle to the endotracheal tube. The critical determinations are based on clinical observation rather than blood gas analysis. If heart rate, respiratory rate, and blood pressure remain stable for 30 to 60 minutes on the T tube, blood gases should then be checked. If the patient becomes obviously dyspneic or tachycardic, blood gas analyses are not necessary to confirm failure. Patients who fail an extended T tube trial may be weaned by progressive tube trials, gradually increasing the length of time that the T tube is used until it is clear that the patient no longer requires ventilatory support. Alternatively, IMV may be used in weaning by gradually reducing the mandatory rate until the patient is essentially breathing without assistance. This latter technique is especially useful in chronically ventilated or debilitated patients and in those with severe lung disease. Finally, some patients with severe underlying lung disease may fail weaning attempts because the added resistance of an endotracheal tube precludes adequate spontaneous ventilation. In these patients, it may be necessary to proceed with a trial extubation once all reversible components of the patient's disease have been corrected, with the knowledge that reintubation may be necessary.

Chronic Obstructive Pulmonary Disease

The hallmark of respiratory failure in patients with chronic obstructive pulmonary disease (COPD) is worsening dyspnea. Most often, respiratory failure is precipitated by infection. Sputum becomes discolored, yellow or green, and is more difficult to raise than usual. The pattern of breathing may have important prognostic implications. A slow respiratory pattern, with expiratory flow rates controlled by pursed-lip breathing, is a favorable sign, whereas rapid panting respirations are usually ineffectual and signify rapid deterioration. Asking the patient to cough is a useful test; ineffectual efforts indicate that intubation may be required. Heart rates in excess of 130 beats per minute and pulsus paradoxus of 15 mmHg or more correlate with severe obstruction.

Relief of hypoxemia is the first goal in the treatment of respiratory failure. Hypoxemia in COPD patients is due principally to $\dot{V}/\dot{Q}$ mismatching, and thus only a small increment in $F_{I_{O_2}}$ is usually required. This may be accomplished by either low-flow oxygen by nasal cannulas or high-flow oxygen delivering fixed oxygen concentrations by face mask. On average, the Pa_{O_2} increases by 10 mmHg in acutely ill COPD

patients when the $F_{I_{O_2}}$ is increased from 0.21 (air) to 0.24, equal to about 1 to 2 liters per minute by nasal prongs, and by 20 mmHg when the $F_{I_{O_2}}$ is increased to 0.28. In about 10 per cent of acutely ill COPD patients, relief of severe hypoxemia is followed by respiratory depression, respiratory acidosis, and mental obtundation. In general, such patients cannot be accurately identified beforehand, although they are more likely to have a high Pa_{CO_2} and to be acidemic on presentation. In managing such patients, if the initial $F_{I_{O_2}}$ was high (>0.30) and the Pa_{O_2} exceeds 60 mmHg, it may be reasonable to attempt to lower the $F_{I_{O_2}}$. However, it must be remembered that the patient may become profoundly hypoxemic at the lower $F_{I_{O_2}}$ because of the time required to "blow off" the accumulated stores of carbon dioxide. Prompt intubation is often required. This problem can best be avoided by starting with a low $F_{I_{O_2}}$ and increasing it incrementally until an acceptable Pa_{O_2} is reached.

Pharmacologic management of respiratory failure in COPD is important. Intravenous aminophylline is usually given. The loading dose for a patient who has not taken a theophylline preparation in the last 24 hours is 5 to 6 mg per kg given over 20 minutes; this dose is reduced by 50 per cent if the patient is taking oral theophylline. After this, an infusion of aminophylline is maintained at a rate of 0.5 to 0.6 mg per kg per hour. Inhaled beta agonists such as isoetharine or metaproterenol are administered by hand-held nebulizer. Epinephrine should be avoided in COPD patients because of its cardiac effects and because it may induce bronchospasm in patients being given beta blockers. Intravenous corticosteroids in doses of 4 mg per kg of hydrocortisone or 0.5 mg per kg of methylprednisolone should be given every 6 hours initially to most COPD patients with severe respiratory failure. Antimicrobial agents have not been clearly shown to have a role in management of acute respiratory failure in COPD and should be reserved for patients whose sputum shows a single predominant organism by Gram's stain or for those with concomitant pneumonia.

Adult Respiratory Distress Syndrome

Patients who present with respiratory failure requiring high $F_{I_{O_2}}$ in the presence of diffuse radiographic infiltrates may be divided into two categories based on results of Swan-Ganz catheterization: those with high wedge pressure are defined in terms of cardiac failure, and those with a normal or low wedge pressure are said to have adult respiratory distress syndrome (ARDS). In ARDS, hypoxemia is the patient's major threat to life. This hypoxemia is due mainly to shunting and thus responds poorly to increments in $F_{I_{O_2}}$. These patients almost always require intubation and mechanical ventilation, although high-flow oxygen delivery by mask may be attempted initially. Frequently, patients remain hypoxemic even after intubation despite increasing $F_{I_{O_2}}$. PEEP is usually initiated at 5 to 10 cmH$_2$O when $F_{I_{O_2}}$ requirements reach the 0.60 to 0.80 range, in an effort to increase Pa_{O_2} while minimizing the toxic effects of high oxygen concentrations. With the initiation of PEEP, most patients should undergo Swan-Ganz catheterization to ensure rapid identification of untoward hemodynamic effects. It should be remembered that although PEEP increases Pa_{O_2}, it also tends to decrease cardiac output; it is the amount of oxygen delivered to tissues that is the important end point in ARDS, and oxygen delivery (the product of oxygen content and cardiac output) may actually decrease with increasing PEEP. This situation can be rapidly identified with a Swan-Ganz catheter in place. Daily chest x-ray films should be obtained of patients with ARDS who require mechanical ventilation and PEEP as a result of the increased incidence of barotrauma (tension pneumothorax, pneumomediastinum). In all patients with ARDS, vigorous measures should be undertaken to maintain the lowest possible wedge pressure without inducing hypotension; this minimizes the transudation of fluid from the vasculature into the alveoli, thus minimizing shunt.

Neuromuscular Diseases

Patients with neuromuscular disorders affecting the respiratory system characteristically breathe with rapid, shallow tidal volumes. They often complain of dyspnea before deterioration of arterial blood gas levels is evident. Tachypnea usually maintains normal blood gas levels until respiratory reserve is markedly diminished. The onset of frank respiratory failure is often initiated by the development of a complication, such as aspiration, atelectasis, or a minor respiratory infection.

In acute neuropathies, such as Guillain-Barré syndrome, serial measurements of respiratory muscle function are useful in determining the timing of intervention with ventilatory support. In previously normal patients, a reduction of FVC to less than 40 per cent of predicted, or a maximum inspiratory pressure of less than -20 cmH$_2$O, identifies a high-risk patient who is likely to require intubation in the near future. When mechanical ventilation is required, most patients are best managed in an assist mode,

which allows the patient to set the ventilator rate. Weaning of patients with neuromuscular diseases from ventilatory support is more difficult if the respiratory muscles are "loaded" by breathing through the added resistance of an endotracheal tube, and early tracheostomy may allow for earlier weaning.

The question of whether to provide long-term ventilation support for patients with progressive neuromuscular disease is difficult to answer. If the nature of the disease is known beforehand, the prognosis and likely outcome should be discussed with the patient and the family. Faced with the prospect of relentless loss of body function plus the limitations imposed by continuous ventilatory support, many patients decide that intubation should not be performed. Alternatively, the physician may decide that the patient's sudden deterioration is due to a reversible process, such as pneumonia, and that only short-term ventilatory support will be required.

ATELECTASIS

method of
JEAN DESLAURIERS, M.D.
Unité de Recherche, Centre de Pneumologie
 Hôpital Laval
Sainte-Foy, Québec, Canada

Atelectasis is usually an acquired disorder that is characterized by the collapse of a lung, a lobe, a segment, or an acinar unit from any cause. The loss of volume reflects the resorption of air from distal lung units, a situation that occurs when normal communication between air passages (central or peripheral) and alveoli is interrupted (resorption atelectasis).

The clinical relevance of atelectasis is threefold: (1) It may be the only indication of an occult thoracic pathology such as an endobronchial obstructing neoplasm. (2) It can predispose the lung to bacterial pneumonia not only because retained mucus is an ideal medium for bacterial growth but also because decreased blood flow impairs local defense mechanisms. Indeed, it has been shown that atelectasis affects the antibacterial function of alveolar macrophages and decreases mucociliary clearance. (3) Perfusion of underventilated areas of the lung may result in significant shunting of blood, with resultant hypoxemia.

Proper management of atelectasis depends on a clear understanding of its mechanisms and on the presence and the severity of secondary complications.

TREATMENT

Segmental or Lobar Atelectasis in Nonoperative Patients

Segmental or lobar atelectasis in nonoperative patients is mainly due to airway obstruction by a neoplasm, a foreign body, or an inflammation. The diagnosis can sometimes be suspected from a review of previous chest radiographs, but bronchoscopic examination is mandatory to determine the cause, the site, and the degree of obstruction. Biopsies of intraluminal masses can readily be performed. If the obstruction is in the distal bronchial tree and cannot be seen by the endoscopist, or if it is extrinsic, bronchial brushings or transbronchial biopsies can be obtained for histopathologic examination.

In all of these situations, management should be that of the primary lesion.

Atelectasis in the Postoperative or Critically Ill Patient

Atelectasis in postoperative or critically ill patients is mainly the cumulative result of decreased tidal volume, absence of sigh mechanism, and ineffective cough. It can present as "plate" atelectasis in lung bases or as lobar atelectasis when secretions are retained and mucous plugging occurs. Atelectasis is a common problem after thoracic or upper abdominal operations and often causes significant venoarterial shunting.

The incidence of postoperative atelectasis can be decreased substantially by proper prophylactic measures. In all patients, medical operability must be carefully assessed with reference to age, weight loss, coexisting diseases, and cardiopulmonary function. Patients should be prepared preoperatively by physiotherapy training, and the nature of the surgery and its possible complications should be properly explained. Bronchodilators or antibiotics should be given preoperatively when indicated. The surgery itself should be performed rapidly and with minimal tissue trauma. The anesthetist must be familiar with modern techniques of intubation, one-lung anesthesia, and perioperative monitoring. The anesthetist must make sure that residual anesthetic effects are minimized. Postoperatively, active chest physiotherapy must be started early, and modern analgesia methods should be routinely used. Most important, imminent atelectasis must be recognized and treated vigorously.

Once atelectasis has developed, active respiratory therapy is the mainstay of treatment. This therapy includes chest physiotherapy with deep breathing and cough exercises, frequent changing of body positions, early ambulation, and postural drainage with percussion maneuvers. To facilitate vigorous coughing and deep breathing, control of pain must be optimal. The use of intercostal block therapy, cryotherapy, or spinal narcotics (epidural analgesia) is preferred to systemic analgesia. When these conservative measures fail to initiate proper cough and/or to reverse atelectasis, therapeutic bronchoscopy is indicated.

In most circumstances, bedside flexible bronchoscopy under local anesthesia suffices. Large mucous plugs are first aspirated from major bronchi. The bronchoscope is then advanced into lobar or segmental bronchi where any inspissated mucus is carefully suctioned. Individual segments of the lung are then lavaged with a sterile saline solution. In some cases, selective lobar re-expansion can be achieved with a balloon-cuffed bronchoscope. Unstable or hypoxic patients may require endotracheal intubation to enable a safe bronchoscopy through the endotracheal tube.

Because the primary objective in preventing atelectasis is to maintain the best possible tidal volumes and functional residual capacities, any maneuver that emphasizes inflation is likely to be useful. Acceptable techniques include incentive spirometry and continuous positive airway pressure (CPAP). The current belief is that intermittent positive pressure breathing is of little use and that medications such as albuterol (Ventolin), which may be useful in relieving bronchospasm and/or potentiating clearing of secretions, are best given by nebulization.

Incentive spirometer devices are designed to ensure a large inspired volume. They stress a sustained inspiratory effort and are recommended by most investigators. CPAP techniques are similarly effective, but their use requires trained personnel and more cooperative patients.

Compression Atelectasis

Compression or passive atelectasis is defined as a reduction in lung volume secondary to a contiguous pulmonary abnormality or to a space-occupying lesion within the chest wall or pleural space. Primary therapy should be aimed at removing the underlying cause.

Accumulation of fluid or gas in the pleural space can readily be treated by needle aspiration or tube thoracostomy. When the disease process is more chronic, the lung may have to be surgically decorticated. In most of these cases, proper anatomic expansion of the lung can be achieved, although pulmonary function does not always return to normal.

Decreased Ventilation

Several disorders can be associated with alveolar hypoventilation and secondary atelectasis. In these cases, atelectasis is secondary to the loss of surface tension within the alveoli, or decreased distending pressure and alveolar size, or the failure to generate an adequate negative inspiratory pleural pressure. The physiologic consequences depend on the amount of lung involved.

Decreased ventilation results from either a decreased central drive or faulty chest wall or lung mechanics. Although central origins include various rare brain disorders, decreased ventilation is more commonly associated with improper use of narcotic analgesia. In patients with trauma or in postoperative patients, for example, intercostal block therapy (bupivacaine [Marcaine] every 8 to 12 hours) can be effective while avoiding the central depression that is associated with intramuscular administration of analgesics. As noted earlier, spinal analgesia, particularly with morphine, can also be useful.

Decreased ventilation may also occur in patients in whom there is interference with chest wall mechanics or respiratory muscle function. One example of this problem is seen in patients with flail chests, when pain and instability of the chest wall can lead to hypoventilation, atelectasis, and ultimately respiratory failure. Prevention of atelectasis in these patients may be achieved through adequate pain control, aggressive respiratory therapy, and, on occasion, open stabilization of the chest wall. In the post-thoracotomy patient, the function of intercostal and diaphragmatic muscles can be severely perturbed. Because both of these muscles are important for normal respiration, this malfunction can lead to significant hypoventilation and atelectasis. Therapy should be primarily aimed at preventing surgical damage to the phrenic nerve, relieving pain, and/or encouraging deep breathing exercises.

CHRONIC OBSTRUCTIVE PULMONARY DISEASE

method of
BARBARA PHILLIPS, M.D.
University of Kentucky College of Medicine
Lexington, Kentucky

DEFINITIONS

The term chronic obstructive pulmonary disease (COPD) encompasses bronchitis, emphysema, bronchiectasis, and, perhaps, asthma. Although these entities have different definitions and manifestations, they have one thing in common: retardation of expiratory airflow. A reduced ratio of forced expired volume in 1 second (FEV_1) to forced vital capacity (FVC) is the manifestation of this airflow obstruction, which can be measured in the pulmonary function laboratory. An FEV_1/FVC of less than 70 to 75 per cent is diagnostic of airflow obstruction.

Chronic bronchitis is defined as cough and production of sputum on most days for 3 months or more for 2 consecutive years. Thus, the diagnosis is a clinical one based solely on the patient's history. It is possible to have chronic bronchitis without abnormal pulmonary function tests. Emphysema is defined as permanent, abnormal enlargement of any part or all of the respiratory acinus, which is accompanied by destruction of respiratory tissue (alveolar capillary bed). Although emphysema is defined and diagnosed histologically in the strictest sense, the diagnosis is often made on clinical grounds in the "pink puffer," the patient who has dyspnea, a barrel chest, decreased breath sounds, and hyperlucent lung fields on chest radiographs. Most older patients who have chronic bronchitis also have some degree of emphysema (and vice versa) because the etiologies of the two illnesses are the same. Bronchiectasis is defined as irreversible dilatation of a part of a bronchial tree. It is diagnosed by bronchography or by computed tomography of the chest. We suspect the diagnosis in patients who have cough with large amounts of purulent sputum, clubbing noted at the physical examination, and increased lung markings on chest radiographs. Asthma is defined simply as reversible bronchospasm with hyper-reactivity of the airways. It is diagnosed clinically in patients who have wheezing or airflow obstruction that disappears spontaneously or with treatment.

Because the manifestations of these disorders coexist and overlap within individuals, the term chronic obstructive pulmonary disease, although it is somewhat imprecise, is widely used.

TREATMENT

General Measures

Smoking Cessation

A treatment protocol for COPD that does not include emphasis on smoking cessation is inadequate. Physicians who treat patients with bronchitis and emphysema must be knowledgeable about smoking cessation techniques and about the physician's role in encouraging smoking cessation. Table 1 lists seven steps recommended by the National Institutes of Health to prevent relapse from tobacco abstinence. It is also important to remember that nicotine is highly addictive (causing the release of both endorphins and catecholamines as it enters the blood stream). For this reason, heavy smokers may benefit from the addition of nicotine replacement therapy (nicotine polacrilex [Nicorette]) to the regimen of advice and close follow-up. Detailed verbal advice about how to use the nicotine medication should accompany the prescription. Most patients who ultimately quit make several attempts before succeeding. Personalized smoking cessation advice by a physician is a highly effective and inexpensive form of treatment for nicotine dependence.

TABLE 1. **Nicotine Addiction:
Seven Steps to Prevent Relapse**

1. Remind patients at each office visit of the clinical consequences of smoking.
2. Provide positive reinforcement and emphasize the benefits of quitting.
3. Provide take-home materials that encourage maintenance of cessation.
4. Refer patients to community maintenance programs or ex-smokers' hot lines.
5. Emphasize that repeated cessation attempts are often necessary for success.
6. Prepare patients for the short-term results of cessation: possible withdrawal symptoms and immediate benefits (e.g., better-smelling breath, better ability to taste).
7. Follow up patients between office visits by telephone or by mail.

Immunizations

Patients with chronic airflow obstruction should receive the pneumococcal vaccine once in their lifetime and the influenza vaccine yearly. The best time to administer the influenza vaccine is in November so that antibody levels will be highest during flu season. The pneumococcal and influenza immunizations can be given simultaneously, but at different sites.

Medical Therapy

Beta-Adrenergic Agents

Beta-adrenergic agents are the cornerstone of treatment for patients with chronic airflow obstruction. A large number of these agents are available (Table 2). If they are used in adequate doses, these agents are essentially equipotent, although there are slight variations in side effects and half-lives. If at all possible, beta-adrenergic agents should be given by inhalation because they act more quickly, require lower doses, have fewer side effects, and are much less expensive when administered by this route. Unfortunately, many patients with COPD are unable to master the metered-dose inhaler (MDI) technique. For

these patients, use of a spacer (reservoir device) may be helpful. Spacers have been shown to increase the amount of drug that reaches the distal airways and to increase the bronchodilator response in patients who have poor MDI technique. Administration of beta-adrenergic agents by spacer is probably as efficacious in nonemergent patients as administration by nebulizer. Table 3 provides information about commercially available spacers.

Although the manufacturers' recommended dosages for beta-adrenergic agents by MDI are typically two or three actuations four times a day, a higher dosage often results in greater bronchodilatation with a minimal increase in side effects. This is especially true in patients with marginal MDI technique who waste a great deal of their medication. Patients should be instructed to take four to six puffs of the beta-adrenergic agents at regular intervals. The two main adverse consequences of increased doses of these agents are more rapid development of tolerance (a downgrading of beta-adrenergic receptors, which results in a lessened bronchodilator response with subsequent doses) and more severe side effects. Most commonly used beta-adrenergic agents are sufficiently $beta_2$ selective that the major consequence of higher doses is tremor (a $beta_2$ side effect). This issue may be put into perspective by the realization that one of the reasons that patients perceive nebulizer treatments to be more effective than MDI treatments is that nebulizer treatments may contain as much as *10 times* the dose delivered by two puffs of an MDI (Table 2).

Anticholinergic Agents

Ipratropium bromide has been available for clinical use in the United States since 1987. It is available only as an MDI, and the recommended dose is two puffs four times a day (although, as with the beta-adrenergic agents, this is almost certainly an underdose). Ipratropium bromide

TABLE 2. **Sympathomimetic Agents**

| Drug | Recommended Dosage Per Treatment | | | | Duration of Action (hr) |
	Subcutaneous (ml)	Metered-Dose Inhaler (mg)	Nebulizer* (mg)	Oral (mg)	
Epinephrine (1:1000 solution)	0.1–0.5	0.32–0.9	2.5–22	—	1–2
Isoproterenol	—	0.16–0.39	0.63–3.8	—	1–2
Isoetharine	—	0.68–1.02	1.25–5	—	2–3
Metaproterenol	—	1.3–1.95	10–15	5–20	3–4
Albuterol	—	0.18–0.27	—	1–4	4–6
Terbutaline	0.25–0.5	0.4–0.6	—	1.25–5	4–6
Bitolterol	—	0.37–1.11	—	—	4–6
Pirbuterol	—	0.2–0.6	—	—	4–6

*Dosages vary widely. These are typical treatment doses, usually given at intervals of 3–6 hr.

TABLE 3. **Characteristics of Spacer Devices**

Device	Description	Requires Synchronization of Actuation and Inhalation	Aerosol Deposition in Oropharynx	Adapts to Different MDIs	Regulates Inspiratory Flow
Brethancer	Straight tube spacer	Yes	Moderately reduced	Adapts to terbutaline	No
Azmacort	Straight tube spacer	Yes	Moderately reduced	Adapts only to triamcinolone	No
Inhal-Aid	700-ml rigid plastic reservoir with one-way valves (designed for children)	No	Markedly reduced	Adapts to all available MDIs	Yes (visual feedback)
Inspirease	700-ml collapsible plastic reservoir bag	No	Markedly reduced	Adapts to many but not all MDIs	Yes
Aerochamber	145-ml rigid holding chamber with one-way valve	No	Markedly reduced	Adapts to all MDIs	No

(Atrovent) is a quaternary derivative of atropine. Because it is not absorbed from the tracheobronchial tree, its only side effect is the possibility of increased cough. Considerable data indicate that ipratropium is at least as effective a bronchodilator in patients with bronchitis and emphysema as are the beta-adrenergic agents. It is also a useful agent for the treatment of asthma, but it is probably not as effective in the treatment of asthma as are the beta-adrenergic agents. However, there is no U.S. Food and Drug Administration approval for the use of ipratropium for treatment of asthma at this time. Because of its lack of toxicity and its remarkable efficacy, ipratropium has supplanted theophylline as the second line treatment for patients with COPD. Indeed, the National Institutes of Health uses ipratropium as its only agent for the treatment of patients with early airflow obstruction in the Lung Health Study.

When ipratropium and beta-adrenergic drugs are given in combination, the ipratropium should probably be administered first. Unlike the beta-adrenergic drugs, which have an onset of action in 5 minutes and a peak action within 30 minutes, ipratropium does not reach its peak effect for 45 minutes to 1½ hours. Patients are more likely to be compliant with its use if they are advised of its delayed onset of action.

Also unlike beta-adrenergic agents, ipratropium does not seem to induce tolerance; that is, the drug is just as efficacious after months of use as it is with the initial inhalation. It has a slightly longer half-life than those of the beta-adrenergic drugs, and it probably exerts significant effects for 4 to 6 hours after use.

Theophylline

Theophylline has many effects in addition to bronchodilatation. It enhances mucociliary clearance; it is an inotrope, a chronotope, a diuretic, and a respiratory stimulant; and it may enhance mental alertness. It also increases the strength of diaphragmatic contraction and reduces diaphragmatic fatigue. Like caffeine, it is a xanthine and has similar side effects: nausea, dyspepsia, diarrhea, insomnia, tremor, nervousness, and cardiac ectopy. Unfortunately, many of the gastrointestinal side effects are manifested in the so-called therapeutic range (10 to 20 micrograms per ml) of theophylline. This is particularly true in elderly patients. Further, there is a long and growing list of drugs and conditions that interfere with theophylline metabolism, which results in an increased risk of toxicity with this agent. The toxicity of theophylline, coupled with its relatively weak bronchodilator effect when compared with beta-adrenergic and anticholinergic drugs, has resulted in theophylline's recent decline in importance for the treatment of COPD.

Nevertheless, theophylline does have many potential beneficial effects for patients who have COPD, and its use often results in symptomatic or subjective improvement in the absence of significant objective evidence. For this reason and because it can be taken orally and is inexpensive, theophylline is still commonly used. The tendency is to use more sparing doses, both because of its multiple drug interactions that push levels upward and because of its toxicity at higher drug levels; we consider a level of 5 to 15 micrograms per ml to be adequate and rarely use levels above 15 micrograms per ml in patients who have COPD.

When outpatient treatment with oral theophylline is started, initial doses usually should not exceed 400 mg in nonsmoking adults or 600 mg in smokers. Various agents are available. Plain aminophylline (salt of theophylline) is not often used because it has a short half-life and requires

TABLE 4. **Maintenance Dosages of Aminophylline***

Patient Group	Calculated Dosage (mg/kg/hr)
Nonsmokers	0.5–0.6
Young smokers	0.8
Cimetidine users	0.3–0.4
Patients with cor pulmonale	0.25–0.3
Patients with hepatic insufficiency	0.2–0.25

*Recommended loading doses of aminophylline for patients who have not been given maintenance oral therapy: 5–7 mg/kg, delivered during 20–30 min.

dosing four times a day. Sustained-release preparations reduce dose frequency, result in more stable blood levels, and probably improve compliance and control of symptoms. Although the manufacturers recommend that these medications (e.g., Theo-Dur and Slo-bid) should be taken twice daily, they may need to be taken three times a day by patients with a high clearance rate, such as young adult smokers. Two theophylline preparations are now available for use once daily: Uniphyl and Theo-24. Despite their increased cost and the possibility of "dose dumping" (with the entire dose acutely absorbed and resultant toxicity), these preparations may be useful for selected patients, particularly those with nocturnal asthma who have symptoms in the early morning.

The U.S. Food and Drug Administration's guidelines for the intravenous administration of aminophylline are given in Table 4. It is prudent to underdose rather than to overdose if there is a question, and to check a theophylline blood level within 12 to 24 hours of initiating the drip. In patients who have been taking theophylline before initiation of intravenous therapy, one-half of the usual initial loading dose should be given, followed by the usual maintenance dose. Obese patients should receive a dose according to ideal body weight, although this dose will probably result in levels that will be slightly lower than predicted.

Corticosteroids

Intravenous corticosteroids are of benefit for acute exacerbations of COPD. Recommended (although somewhat arbitrary) doses of the three most commonly used agents are given in Table 5. Certain caveats are in order. Beta-adrenergic agents, diuretics, and corticosteroids with mineralocorticoid activity promote hypokalemia. Potassium losses can be a significant problem in patients who are undergoing intense in-hospital treatment for COPD exacerbation. It is important to anticipate this possibility and to check potassium levels frequently. In patients who have marked hypokalemia, dexamethasone may result in less potassium wasting than methylprednisolone or hydrocortisone. It is also reasonable to remember that patients with liver disease may respond better to methylprednisolone than to the other preparations. Patients usually receive maintenance therapy with intravenous corticosteroids until their clinical condition stabilizes; they are then given oral corticosteroids (typically, prednisone), at 40 to 60 mg per day, and are tapered rapidly. In patients who have not previously demonstrated steroid dependence, corticosteroid therapy can be abruptly terminated within 2 weeks of initiation of treatment. Patients who tend to have problems whenever their corticosteroid treatment is tapered may benefit from a more gradual taper and the addition of inhaled corticosteroids. Most patients who develop trouble during the tapering do well until the dose reaches 20 mg of prednisone per day or below. Thus, it is reasonable to start inhaled corticosteroids at this point. Attempts can then be made to further taper the oral prednisone.

A subset of patients with stable COPD may benefit from chronic oral corticosteroid use. It is difficult to tell without a trial of steroid therapy who these patients are. A therapeutic trial consists of measuring baseline spirometry when the patient is given an optimum regimen of standard bronchodilators and then administering the equivalent of 32 mg of methylprednisolone (40 to 60 mg prednisone) orally for approximately 2 weeks. Spirometry is then repeated. If there is no significant improvement (i.e., an increase of 15 per cent or more) in FVC, FEV_1, or peak flow, the steroids should be discontinued. If there is a positive response, the steroid dose is tapered to a maintenance dose. The optimal chronic steroid dose for patients with COPD is the lowest possible dose that results in symptomatic relief, prevents or reduces exacerbations, and causes objective improvement in pulmonary function. In some cases this optimum can be accomplished by using

TABLE 5. **Intravenous Corticosteroids**

Generic Name	Trade Name	Route of Administration	Dose
Hydrocortisone	Solu-Cortef	IV	100–200 mg q 4–6 hr
Dexamethasone	Decadron	IV	4–6 mg q 4–6 hr
Methylprednisolone	Solu-Medrol	IV	60–125 mg q 4–6 hr

alternate-day steroid therapy combined with inhaled corticosteroids. Although there is more myth than data concerning the use of inhaled steroid therapy in COPD, this type of treatment may reduce the need for oral corticosteroids. Table 6 provides information about inhaled corticosteroids. Because of the hazards of long-term corticosteroid therapy, patients should be well educated about the risks of such treatment before the trial is undertaken, and the risks and benefits of long-term corticosteroid therapy should be weighed carefully. When a corticosteroid trial and long-term steroid therapy are being contemplated, the patient should undergo purified protein derivative (PPD) testing, preferably before corticosteroids are started, because long-term corticosteroid use is an indication for isoniazid treatment in a person who has a positive test result.

Antibiotics

Antibiotics are used routinely in patients admitted to the hospital with exacerbation of chronic airflow obstruction, even though bacteria usually play no role in these exacerbations. Many physicians treat outpatients with COPD with a 5-day to 2-week course of oral antibiotics when there is change in the quantity or type of sputum production. Although antibiotic treatment of COPD exacerbations and sputum changes is fairly standard practice, it has not been convincingly shown to confer added benefit to other standard care.

Oxygen Therapy

Chronic Use of Oxygen

Supplemental oxygen has prolonged life of patients who have stable arterial oxygen tension (Pa_{O_2}) values of less than 55 mmHg or Pa_{O_2} values of less than 59 mmHg in combination with pulmonary hypertension (by physical examination, chest radiograph, or electrocardiogram), congestive right-sided heart failure, or hematocrit of greater than 55 per cent. In addition to prolonging life, oxygen treatment can improve cognitive function, lower pulmonary artery pressure, reduce hematocrit, and improve stroke volume index. To be beneficial, oxygen must be used for at least 12 to 15 hours per day; maximum benefit is conferred by round-the-clock use. Arterial blood gas determinations are required to document hypoxemia so that oxygen therapy will be reimbursable. Blood gas determinations should be made when the patient's condition is stable and the patient is receiving maximum bronchodilator therapy. The usual dose is 1 to 2 liters per minute nasal oxygen; the adequacy of therapy should be documented by repeat arterial blood gas testing. Therapy should raise the resting Pa_{O_2} value to 65 to 80 mmHg. Oxygen therapy is indicated and appropriate for two other groups of patients with COPD who do not meet the above-mentioned criteria:

1. Patients with nocturnal hypoxemia. COPD patients who have a Pa_{O_2} value of greater than or equal to 60 mmHg and who are obese or who have carbon dioxide retention, polycythemia, or evidence of right-sided heart failure probably should undergo sleep studies with continuous measurements of arterial oxygen saturation. If such patients meet the regular criteria noted earlier or if they demonstrate a significant fall in oxygen levels (as evidenced by a decrease in Pa_{O_2} of more than 10 mmHg or in oxygen saturation of more than 5 per cent), nocturnal treatment with oxygen is warranted.

2. Patients who complain of dyspnea on exertion and who meet the criteria outlined earlier with exercise should be provided with oxygen for use during exercise.

In both of these two conditions, it is reasonable to attempt to maintain a Pa_{O_2} value higher than 60 mmHg (Sa_{O_2} higher than 88 per cent).

In all patients who receive oxygen therapy, at least yearly reassessment of the adequacy and need for treatment, either by a measurement of arterial oxygen saturation or arterial blood gases, should be undertaken. Portable oxygen can be prescribed for use during exercise in patients with exercise-induced hypoxemia or for complementing a stationary system. Documentation of the need for portable oxygen (e.g., to permit exercise in muscle reconditioning, to extend ambulation, to reduce the risk of thrombophlebitis) should accompany the prescription. Prescriptions for home oxygen therapy should include the flow rate, frequency, and duration of use (e.g., nasal oxygen, 2 liters per minute, 24 hours per day).

TABLE 6. **Relative Cost and Dose of Inhaled Steroids***

Generic Name	Trade Name	Interval Dose	Actuations/MDI	Cost/Inhaler	Cost/Day
Beclomethasone dipropionate	Beclovent	2 puffs qid or tid	200	$18.51	56¢
Beclomethasone dipropionate	Vanceril	2 puffs qid or tid	200	$18.60	56¢
Flunisolide	Aerobid	2 puffs bid	100	$18.52	74¢
Triamcinolone	Azmacort	2 puffs qid or tid	200	$15.34	38¢

*As of December 1985, average of 10 retail pharmacy costs in Lexington, Kentucky.

Oxygen can probably be safely started on an outpatient basis in patients who do not retain carbon dioxide. However, in patients who retain carbon dioxide or who are severely hypoxemic (Pa_{O_2} value less than 45 mmHg), hospitalization for initiation of oxygen is probably appropriate.

Two new forms of oxygen delivery are now available. Oxygen-conserving devices deliver oxygen only during inspiration, thus avoiding the waste of oxygen that occurs during the expiratory phase of breathing. These devices have been shown to be equivalent to continuous flow devices in short-term studies, but there is not much economic benefit to their use as yet because the devices themselves are so expensive.

Transtracheal oxygen administration not only facilitates oxygen delivery, but also enhances cosmetic improvement. This method of oxygen delivery may be particularly useful for patients who require unusually high flow rates because of severe hypoxemia.

Acute Use of Oxygen

In COPD patients with acute exacerbations and hypoxemia, oxygen should be given in sufficient doses to raise the arterial PO_2 to 60 mmHg. It is difficult to predict which patients will retain carbon dioxide when they receive supplemental oxygen. However, severe hypoxemia causes death, whereas severe carbon dioxide retention usually does not. Thus, the first goal of oxygen therapy should be adequate oxygenation even if the need for mechanical ventilation arises. It is usually not worthwhile to increase the Pa_{O_2} value above 80 mmHg, because increases in Pa_{O_2} beyond 65 to 70 mmHg result in only minor additional increases in arterial oxygen content but often require relatively huge increases in oxygen flow rates. Although each liter of supplemental oxygen will increase the FI_{O_2} of a normal individual who has a normal respiratory pattern by 2 to 4 per cent, patients with COPD exacerbations have abnormal breathing patterns and usually have much greater minute ventilations than do normal people. Thus they dilute the supplemental oxygen in a larger volume of inspired air, and the increase in FI_{O_2} is difficult to predict. For this reason, venturi masks are sometimes preferable because the FI_{O_2} is more precise, but there can still be considerable variation, particularly at higher FI_{O_2} values. It is imperative to sample arterial blood gases after starting oxygen therapy, both to assess the adequacy of treatment and to detect the possibility of carbon dioxide retention and impending narcosis. In patients with severe COPD, 20 to 30 minutes may be necessary for a steady state to result after addition of supplemental oxygen, so arterial blood gas determinations should not be done at intervals much shorter than that.

PULMONARY REHABILITATION PROGRAMS

Several different types of programs are available for patients with COPD. The general aim of these programs is to improve the quality of life. Specific programs vary and often are individualized for patients. The components of a pulmonary rehabilitation program are given in Table 7. Some of the potential benefits of pulmonary rehabilitation include reduced respiratory symptoms, less severe anxiety and depression, enhanced ability to carry out activities of daily life, improved exercise tolerance, reduced hospital days required, and prolonged life in selected patients.

The American Lung Association's Better Breathers Club is available through local chapters of the American Lung Association in many cities and towns. Although it is not an extensive pulmonary rehabilitation program, it is an education and support group that is free of charge to COPD patients.

PROGNOSIS

The most important determinants of survival in patients who have COPD are the patient's age

TABLE 7. **Components of a Pulmonary Rehabilitation Program**

1. *General*
   Patient and family education
   Proper nutrition including weight control
   Avoidance of smoking and other inhaled irritants
   Avoidance of infection (e.g., by immunization)
   Adequate hydration
2. *Medications*
   Bronchodilators
   Expectorants
   Antimicrobial agents
   Corticosteroids
   Cromolyn sodium
   Digitalis
   Diuretics
   Psychopharmacologic agents
3. *Respiratory Therapy*
   Aerosol therapy
   Oxygen therapy
   Home use of ventilators
4. *Physical Therapy Modalities*
   Relaxation therapy
   Breathing retraining
   Chest percussion and postural drainage
   Deliberate coughing and expectoration
5. *Exercise Conditioning*
6. *Occupational Therapy*
   Evaluate activities of daily living
   Outline energy conserving maneuvers
7. *Psychosocial Rehabilitation*
8. *Vocational Rehabilitation*

and postbronchodilator FEV_1 value. Although extrapolation to individual patients is difficult, population studies have shown that patients who have a postbronchodilator FEV_1 value of less than 30 per cent predicted have a reduced life expectancy with a 3-year survival rate of 50 to 70 percent. Untreated hypoxemia also has a negative impact on anticipated survival.

Although physicians may be reluctant to discuss the patients' prognosis and treatment options in general terms, most patients with COPD welcome the opportunity to do so. It is tragic for everyone when patients with end-stage COPD receive mechanical ventilation against their wishes in the face of no reversible or treatable conditions. A brief discussion of mechanical ventilation, cardiopulmonary resuscitation, and the patient's concerns and feelings about them in the outpatient clinic during a routine visit may enable the patient to prepare for the possibility of mechanical ventilation and to participate more effectively in making the decision about whether this type of treatment is appropriate.

PRIMARY LUNG CANCER

method of
PHILIP BONOMI, M.D.
Rush Medical College
Chicago, Illinois

The incidence of lung cancer in the United States is increasing annually. It has been the leading cause of cancer-related death in men for decades. Within the last several years, it has become the leading cause of cancer-related death in women and has surpassed colon and breast cancer as causes of cancer-related death. In 1989, 155,000 new cases of lung cancer will be diagnosed, and approximately 142,000 deaths will occur because of lung cancer. It is encouraging to see that the percentage of U.S. adults who smoke is decreasing. Unfortunately, the reduction in the smoking rate has not been apparent in all population subsets. In particular, the smoking rate remains high among men of lower socioeconomic background and among young women from all backgrounds. Preventing the onset of smoking is extremely important because of the difficulty of breaking this habit and because it takes 8 to 15 years after cessation of smoking for a smoker's risk of acquiring lung cancer to return to that of a nonsmoker.

The number of persons with lung cancer mandates continuing efforts to educate the population about the risks of smoking. Greater physician involvement in these educational efforts is essential.

NON–SMALL CELL LUNG CANCER

The four major histologic subtypes of lung cancer include small cell carcinoma, squamous cell carcinoma, adenocarcinoma, and large cell carcinoma, with the latter three histologic categories collectively referred to as non–small cell lung cancer (NSCLC). Seventy-five per cent of lung cancer patients have non–small cell tumors, and within this group of patients (120,000 cases in 1988), approximately one-third will be surgical candidates, one-third will not be surgical candidates because of locally advanced disease, and one-third will not be surgical candidates because of distant metastases. Although there are biologic differences among the NSCLC subtypes, the primary therapy is resection when feasible. There are no significant survival differences among the different histologies when survival durations for patients within a given stage are compared.

SMALL CELL LUNG CANCER

Unlike NSCLC, the primary treatment for small cell lung cancer (SCLC) is combination chemotherapy rather than pulmonary resection. Early studies of local therapy showed that distant metastases appeared rapidly after surgery or thoracic radiation in virtually all patients. High rates of tumor regression were observed in subsequent trials of combination chemotherapy; more important, there was a three- to fourfold improvement in median survival duration in patients receiving systemic therapy versus those treated with local therapy or supportive care only.

There are subcategories within small cell carcinomas, including oat cell or lymphocyte-like type, intermediate type, variant form (a combination of large cell and small cell), and mixed histology (small cell carcinoma plus adenocarcinoma or squamous cell carcinoma). In general, combination chemotherapy remains the primary therapy for each category, and the natural history for each subtype is similar. One exception is the patient whose tumor contains mixed histologies (SCLC plus NSCLC). In these patients, pulmonary resection should be considered when the tumor is technically resectable and there is no evidence of distant metastases. These patients should also receive combination chemotherapy.

LUNG CANCER STAGING

Staging of any type of cancer is designed to group similar patients for selection of treatment and interpretation of the results of treatment. The staging systems of the American Joint Committee on Cancer, the tumor, node, metastases (TNM) system, is used by most physicians who are involved in treating lung cancer patients. This system has been revised recently (Tables 1 and 2).

For staging SCLC, the TNM system is not usually used. In its place, patients are categorized as having limited or extensive disease. For the purposes of most studies, limited disease is defined as gross tumor that is encompassable within a radiation field that would include the primary intrathoracic tumor, ipsilateral hilar and/or mediastinal nodal metastases, and ipsilateral supraclavicular nodal metastases. Patients who have evidence of gross disease beyond these areas, including hematogenous pulmonary metastases and

TABLE 1. **International TNM Staging for Lung Cancer***

Tumor size (T)

TX   =   Occult carcinoma (cytologically positive; bronchoscopically and radiographically nondetectable)
T1   =   Tumor 3 cm or less surrounded by lung or visceral pleura
T2   =   Tumor more than 3 cm
T3   =   Tumor of any size with direct extension into chest wall, or with 2 cm of the carina, or associated with atelectasis or obstructive pneumonia of the entire lung
T4   =   Tumor of any size invading the mediastinal structures or vertebral body, presence of malignant pleural effusion

Nodal Status (N)

N0   =   No hilar or mediastinal nodal involvement
N1   =   Ipsilateral hilar nodal involvement
N2   =   Ipsilateral mediastinal nodal or subcarinal nodal involvement
N3   =   Contralateral hilar or mediastinal nodal involvement, supraclavicular nodal involvement (ipsilateral or contralateral)

Metastases (M)

M0   =   No distant metastases
M1   =   Distant visceral metastases present

Stage

Occult carcinoma	TX, N0, M0
Stage I	T1–2, N0, M0
Stage II	T1–2, N1, M0
Stage IIIA	T3, N0–1, M0
	T1–3, N2, M0
Stage IIIB	T4, N1–3, M0
	T1–3, N3, M0
Stage IV	Any T, any N, M1

*Adapted from Mountain CF: A new international staging system for lung cancer. Chest 89(Suppl):2255, 1986.

metastases to contralateral supraclavicular areas, bone, liver, brain, adrenal, or other distant sites, are classified as having extensive disease.

In addition to histologic subtype and stage, other factors must be considered when selecting treatment. Overall performance (ambulatory versus nonambulatory), recent changes in body weight, and cardiopulmonary status are important prognostic factors that should be considered when recommending therapy. Poor performance status, recent weight loss, and a history of non–cancer-related cardiopulmonary disease are associated with worse survival and can be associ-

TABLE 2. **Five-Year Disease-Free Survival Rates for Surgical Resection in Patients with Non–Small Cell Lung Cancer**

	Stage	5 Yr Disease-Free (%)
I	T1, N0, M0	70–85
	T2, N0, M0	55–65
II	T1, N1, M0	30–50
	T1, N2, M0	25–30
IIIA	T3, N0, M0	25–35
	T3, N1, M0	15–20
	T1–2N2, M0	9–24
	T3, N2	0–5

ated with increased incidence and severity of treatment-related complications.

TREATMENT

Non–Small Cell Lung Cancer

Surgery

Most patients with NSCLC present with unresectable disease because early lesions are frequently not associated with symptoms. In addition, there is no clearly effective means of screening for lung cancer in high-risk individuals. In general, patients with Stage I and Stage II disease and some patients with Stage IIIA disease are candidates for pulmonary resection. Before thoracotomy, pulmonary function should be assessed. Virtually all patients who have a predicted forced expiratory vital capacity at 1 second (FEV_1) of less than 1 liter after pulmonary resection will have respiratory insufficiency after surgery. Similarly, patients who have a history of congestive heart failure or who have suffered a recent myocardial infarction (within 3 months) have an increased risk of surgical mortality.

Patients with T1 or T2 lesions that have not metastasized to regional lymph nodes have a 60 to 80 per cent chance of being cured by surgical excision. In contrast, the 5-year survival rate decreases to 20 to 25 per cent in patients who have T2 tumors that have metastasized to hilar lymph nodes (N1).

Although the cure rate for all clinical Stage IIIA cases is approximately 5 per cent, it is important to identify subsets of patients who have considerably higher 5-year survival rates and for whom surgery by an experienced thoracic surgeon should be considered. Patients who have T3 tumors by virtue of chest wall invasion and who have no mediastinal lymph node metastases have a 30 to 40 per cent 5-year survival rate. Also, a subset of patients with metastases to ipsilateral mediastinal lymph nodes (N2), which are discovered at the time of thoracotomy, have been reported to have 5-year survival rates of 15 to 30 per cent. Patients who have clinical evidence of N2 disease (evident on chest film), tumor extending beyond the lymph node capsule, or metastases in the highest mediastinal nodes or in multiple levels of mediastinal nodes are excluded from the subset of patients who have relatively a good prognosis. For this group with poor prognosis, surgery is unlikely to result in long-term survival.

Surgery provides no benefit for metastastic Stage IIIB patients who have contralateral mediastinal or supraclavicular lymph nodes or for patients who have distant metastases (M1, Stage

IV). However, surgery may provide long-term survival for some Stage IIIB patients who have tumor invading the lower trachea.

Postoperative Adjuvant Treatment

Postoperative thoracic radiation therapy has not improved survival in patients with regional lymph node metastases, despite the fact that local recurrence is reduced by this adjunctive therapy. Many radiation therapists recommend postoperative radiation therapy because it reduces local recurrence.

Most lung cancer patients develop distant metastases, and thus various systemic therapies have been used as surgical adjuvants in lung cancer. Immunotherapy has not improved survival in lung cancer patients. Recent randomized trials have shown that postoperative chemotherapy with cyclophosphamide (Cytoxan), doxorubicin (Adriamycin), and cisplatin (Platinol) has resulted in prolongation of the median survival, but does not appear to improve long-term survival. At this point, adjuvant therapy in lung cancer patients must be considered to be experimental.

Radiotherapy

Palliation of symptoms including cough, dyspnea, hemoptysis, and chest pain is frequently achieved with thoracic radiation. In addition, control of local disease can be achieved with this modality and, in a small percentage of cases, long-term survival results. However, progressive distant disease, local disease, or both occur in most patients. Approximately 20 per cent of patients who received thoracic irradiation with curative intent survive for 2 years. Although there is not a great amount of data comparing supportive care only to radiation therapy, and although some physicians recommend reserving radiation therapy until significant symptoms appear, the standard care for Stage IIIB and most Stage IIIA NSCLC patients in the United States is primary thoracic irradiation.

Randomized trials have demonstrated that higher doses of irradiation produce greater reduction of local disease. In addition, giving uninterrupted as opposed to split-course irradiation appears to yield better results. The suboptimal results observed with split-course irradiation are probably related to tumor regrowth, which occurs between treatments as a result of repair of sublethal irradiation injury. Recent radiation biology studies suggest that multiple daily treatments result in greater cell kill. An ongoing clinical trial comparing irradiation given as a single daily fraction versus twice daily fractions is testing this concept.

Chemotherapy

The use of combination chemotherapy for Stage IV NSCLC patients has created considerable controversy. Opinions have ranged from therapeutic nihilism to considerable enthusiasm in favor of treating this group of patients with combination chemotherapy regimens. Initial reports for a variety of cisplatin-containing regimens have shown response rates of 40 to 50 per cent. In subsequent larger studies, the same regimens have produced response rates of 25 per cent, with responding patients living twice as long as the nonresponders. Critics argue that "responders" may have had a longer survival because of pretreatment prognostic factors rather than chemotherapy treatment. This issue has been at least partially resolved by a recently reported prospective, randomized study in which supportive care alone was compared with two cisplatin regimens. Although the differences were modest, patients receiving chemotherapy survived longer than those receiving supportive care only. On the basis of these results, it is reasonable to treat Stage IV NSCLC patients who have good performance status (ambulatory) with combination chemotherapy. However, in patients who have lost 5 per cent or more of their usual body weight or who are not ambulatory, treatment-related toxicity is frequently severe, and this group of patients should not usually be treated with combination chemotherapy. Also, the results with systemic therapy are clearly suboptimal. The major objective in these patients is identification of more effective systemic therapy, based on clinical trials and lung cancer biology.

Combined Modality Treatment in Stage III NSCLC

The same regimens that produce a 25 per cent response rate in Stage IV NSCLC patients have been shown to produce a 50 per cent response rate in Stage III patients. These reports have resulted in considerable interest in using combination chemotherapy before radiation therapy or surgery in Stage III patients. This approach, in which systemic therapy is administered before local therapy in patients who have locally advanced disease, has been termed "neoadjuvant" therapy or "protochemotherapy."

Recent neoadjuvant studies have confirmed the earlier reports of a relatively high response (50 per cent) in Stage III patients, and in a randomized trial comparing vinblastine plus cisplatin followed by no radiation therapy to radiation therapy alone, a modest improvement in median survival was observed in patients who received both treatment modalities. Despite these encouraging results, neoadjuvant treatment remains investigational. Accordingly, Stage III patients should be considered for entry into randomized trials of the neoadjuvant approach or of other combined modality approaches, such as the simultaneous use of chemotherapy and thoracic irradiation, because long-term survival in this group of patients treated with irradiation alone is poor.

Small Cell Lung Cancer

For several decades, it has been recognized that SCLC is a distinct clinical entity because this neoplasm has high propensity for rapid appearance of distant metastases. More recently, it has become apparent that this tumor is also a distinct pathologic entity and exhibits neuroendocrine differentiation, which is manifested by the presence of neurosecretory granules and neural filaments seen by electron microscopy. These cells can synthesize various polypeptide hormones, including adrenocorticotropic hormone and antidiuretic hormone, as well as autocrine growth factors, such as bombesin. Ongoing research is aimed at autocrine growth factors to determine whether interference with the action of these growth factors will result in regression of SCLC.

At presentation, two-thirds of SCLC patients have metastases to distant sites including liver, bone, brain, adrenal glands, bone marrow, and remote lymph nodes. The remaining one-third of patients have disease that is apparently limited to one hemithorax and 10 to 15 per cent of them have "very limited" disease (3 to 5 per cent of all SCLC patients) that is potentially resectable.

Surgery

Although response rates for patients with limited SCLC who are treated with chemotherapy and/or thoracic irradiation are high (70 to 90 per cent), most patients experience recurrent disease, and approximately 50 per cent of all limited SCLC patients have recurrence at the primary site. This observation, together with reports of long-term survival in small groups of patients whose primary SCLC was resected, has resulted in renewed interest for surgery plus chemotherapy in SCLC. At present, this approach is still investigational. However, for tumors that contain mixed histologies (i.e., small cell carcinoma plus adrenocarcinoma) or that are pure SCLC Stage I, resection is appropriate as long as these patients also receive combination chemotherapy.

Radiation Therapy

SCLC is the most radiosensitive of the different histologic subtypes of lung cancer. This treatment modality can palliate symptomatic central nervous system metastases (brain and spinal cord), painful osseous metastases, and symptomatic intrathoracic disease such as lesions causing post-obstruction pneumonitis, cough, respiratory insufficiency, chest wall pain, superior vena cava syndrome, and esophageal compression.

Although studies have shown conflicting results, there is increasing evidence that combining thoracic irradiation with chemotherapy produces a modest improvement in median survival duration and a trend for a higher 2-year survival rate. The optimum dose and schedule for thoracic irradiation and for chemotherapy have not been determined. However, it appears that radiation doses of 4500 to 6000 cGy, which are given without interruption, are superior to lower doses or to split-course irradiation. Also, there is preliminary evidence suggesting that concurrent use of thoracic irradiation and chemotherapy, particularly the combination of cisplatin plus etoposide (Platinol plus VePesid), is more effective than using chemotherapy and radiotherapy sequentially.

A high percentage of SCLC patients develop brain metastases. For patients who are long-term survivors, the percentage with brain metastases may reach 50 to 60 per cent. Currently available chemotherapy regimens do not appear to reduce the frequency of brain metastases, a phenomenon that is probably related to the inability of these drugs to cross the blood-brain barrier in appreciable amounts. Prophylactic cranial irradiation in doses ranging from 2500 to 3000 cGy has been shown to reduce the incidence of brain metastases but has not improved overall survival. The failure to improve survival is because most relapsing patients develop metastases at multiple extracranial sites, and these areas of disease become refractory to all types of available chemotherapeutic agents.

Subsequent dementia and dystaxia have been reported in patients who have received prophylactic cranial irradiation. Some physicians have recommended that prophylactic cranial irradiation not be used because of these neurologic problems, which may be treatment related. Despite these concerns, it seems reasonable to give prophylactic cranial irradiation to patients who have limited disease that has responded to chemotherapy and/or thoracic irradiation because in a high percentage of patients brain metastases will develop and tumor-related neurologic deficits may not be reversible even when cranial irradiation produces intracranial tumor regression.

Chemotherapy

Some of the most commonly used regimens include (1) cyclophosphamide, doxorubicin, and vincristine; (2) cyclophosphamide, doxorubicin, and etoposide; (3) cisplatin plus etoposide. Since the advent of combination chemotherapy, there has been a four- to fivefold increase in median survival in SCLC, and long-term survival is observed in a small percentage of patients with limited disease. Initially, most SCLC patients respond to various combination chemotherapy regimens. Although the response rate to initial chemotherapy is high, virtually all patients with extensive disease and most patients with limited disease experience widespread tumor recurrence with disease that is refractory to all currently available agents.

Various treatment strategies have attempted to overcome drug resistance. One approach has involved the use of extremely high doses of chemotherapy with subsequent bone marrow transplantation. So far, this strategy does not seem to have improved the results that can be achieved with conventional doses of chemotherapy. These results with a single course of high-dose chemotherapy do not suggest that dose is unimportant. Currently, there is considerable interest in testing multiple courses of relatively high-dose chemotherapy in the hope that repeated administration of substantial amounts of drugs given during a relatively short time may produce superior results. The concept of drug dose delivered per unit time is called dose intensity. The recent discovery of granulocyte colony-stimulating factors may improve our ability to use chemotherapy regimens with a high dose intensity.

Another attempt to overcome drug resistance has involved alternating different chemotherapy regimens, for example, the cyclophosphamide, doxorubicin, and vincristine regimen alternating with the cisplatin plus etoposide regimen. Although this strategy has been associated with longer survival, its effect has been minimal, and there does not appear to be an increased percentage of long-term survivors.

Clearly, more effective systemic therapy is needed for SCLC. The identification of new cytotoxic agents may be facilitated by testing new antineoplastic drugs in cultures of cell lines established from human small cell lung carcinomas. The identification of growth factors in small cell lung carcinomas and the development of methods that block these cells from stimulating their own growth offer the promise of developing a completely new type of systemic therapy. Similarly, the identification of cancer genes (oncogenes) within small cell lung carcinomas and the identification of oncogene-related proteins, some of which may not be growth factors, may lead to another type of systemic therapy.

COCCIDIOIDOMYCOSIS

method of
HANS E. EINSTEIN, M.D.
Bakersfield Memorial Hospital
University of Southern California
School of Medicine
Los Angeles, California

Coccidioidomycosis is one of the so-called endemic mycoses and is, after histoplasmosis, the most common mycosis in the United States. The causative agent, *Coccidioides immitis*, is a dimorphic fungus living in well-defined areas of the southwestern United States and contiguous parts of Mexico. Localized endemic areas exist in parts of Central and South America. Arthroconidia (spores) are inhaled by susceptible human or animal hosts, and a localized pneumonitis, which is characterized by granuloma formation, results.

More than one-half of the primary infections are subclinical. When there are symptoms, there are cough, chest pain, and fever; x-ray films show an infiltrate with ipsilateral hilar adenopathy. Pleural effusion is seen in 8 per cent of cases. Hypersensitivity syndromes such as erythema nodosum or erythema multiforme, arthralgia with arthritis, and joint effusions frequently accompany the primary infection, which is then referred to as the valley fever syndrome.

The lesions just described usually clear but leave a cavity, coccidioidal lung abscess, or a nodule (coccidioidoma) in 5 per cent of cases. The nodules need to be distinguished from neoplasms, whereas the cavities can progress to significant hemoptysis, an occasional rupture with pneumothorax, and empyema formation.

Fewer than 1 in 1000 infections progress to metapulmonary dissemination. Risk factors include race or ethnicity (Filipinos, black persons [Afro-Americans], Native Americans, Orientals, and Hispanics are the most susceptible), immunosuppression (such as that found with corticosteroid use), malignant diseases, cytotoxic chemotherapy, pregnancy, and diabetes. The most commonly involved sites are skin, bones and joints, liver, serous membranes, lymph nodes, and meninges.

DIAGNOSIS

The mature sporangium (spherule) can be demonstrated in body secretions or pus by potassium hydroxide wet mount and cytologic stain. Cultures should be done from sputum, pus, urine, and cerebrospinal fluid. Biopsy is a useful procedure for the lung, liver, bone, and skin.

Immunologic tests are specific, sensitive, and generally available. Skin reactivity to coccidioidin or spherulin indicates past infection and is useful diagnostically only when a conversion is witnessed. Tube precipitin tests detect the IgM response that occurs early in the disease; standard complement fixation or immunodiffusion tests demonstrate IgG antibodies.

The latter can be quantitated and correlated with the extent and progress of the disease.

THERAPY

The primary infection is self-limited and usually requires only symptomatic and supportive care. Occasionally, ketoconazole, an orally active agent, is given to hasten recovery or to prevent dissemination. No data exist to substantiate this practice. There is general agreement that chemotherapy should be considered under the following circumstances:

1. Any type of coccidioidal disease in infants
2. Progressive primary pneumonia (persistent hilar or paratracheal adenopathy, accompanied by rising antibody titer)
3. Significant pneumonia with high antibody titer in susceptible racial and ethnic groups
4. Coexisting congenital or acquired immunodeficiency, diabetes, or pregnancy
5. Surgical coverage if disease is extensive, active, or disseminated, or if surgery is being repeated
6. All forms of metapulmonary spread, combined whenever possible with local amphotericin B therapy

Amphotericin B (Fungizone)

This agent, a water-insoluble polyene, remains the drug of first choice after more than three decades of use, despite multiple toxicities and difficulty of administration. The initial dose, 5 to 10 mg, is suspended as a 10 per cent solution in dextrose and water and is infused slowly for the first 1 mg as a test dose; the remainder is infused in 1 to 4 hours, with most patients tolerating the more rapid infusion better. The dose is increased daily by 10 to 15 mg until the maximum tolerated dose, or 1 mg per kg, is reached. In severely ill patients, this process can be shortened to 3 days. The drug has a half-life of 24 hours, which makes therapy given every other day feasible.

Nausea, vomiting, chills, and fever are almost universal. Premedication with aspirin and antiemetics is helpful, as is meperidine (Demerol), which terminates severe, shaking chills. If reactions persist, corticosteroids can be effective. It is not necessary to add heparin to the infusion or to protect it from light.

Systemic manifestations of amphotericin B toxicity include self-limited anemia, hypokalemia, and hypomagnesemia, which respond well to replacement therapy. Renal function impairment, the most significant side effect, is dose related. Creatinine levels or creatinine clearance should be measured to monitor renal function. The dose

of amphotericin B should be decreased or the interval between infusions lengthened if the creatinine level is raised to above 2.5 or 3 mg per dl. Renal function usually returns to normal if the total dose of drug remains below 3 grams.

The amount of drug required for a given lesion is determined empirically. A predetermined amount is delivered and the patient is then carefully monitored for effect; there is a delay before radiographic, serologic, or even clinical changes become manifest. Between 1 and 2 grams is usually sufficient for progressive primary disease, simple meningitis, skin lesions, and isolated bone lesions; more widespread disease requires longer treatment.

Amphotericin B is active locally and thus is useful in the management of coccidioidal osteomyelitis and synovitis. A 10 per cent suspension of drug is infused into surgically exposed areas. In meningitis, intrathecal administration is invariably required because the agent does not cross the blood-brain barrier. The intracisternal route has been the safest and therapeutically most successful approach. Initially, 0.05 mg is given, gradually increasing to 0.25 mg and then to 0.5 mg or even 1 mg if tolerated daily initially, then decreasing to 3 times weekly. As pleocytosis normalizes and cerebrospinal fluid antibody titers decrease, the interval between intrathecal injections can be lengthened. Two months after all parameters, including protein and glucose levels, have become normal, treatment can gradually be discontinued.

Miconazole (Monistat)

This azole must be given intravenously, and it is quite toxic (causing phlebitis, thrombocytosis, hyperlipidemia, severe pruritus, fever, chills, nausea, vomiting, and electrolyte disturbances). Because of its short half-life, the drug is started at 200 mg every 8 hours, gradually increasing to a daily dose of 1200 to 2400 mg for 1 to 3 months. The use of miconazole has remained limited for these reasons.

Ketoconazole (Nizoral)

This orally active azole has moderate activity against *C. immitis*. It is usually given at 400 mg once daily in the morning, after fasting. Absorption is impaired by food, H_2 antagonists, and antacids. Larger doses, up to 1800 mg, have been given in disseminated disease, including meningitis, when tolerated. Although results early in the disease appear to be satisfactory, relapses occur often (in 35 to 40 per cent of patients), even after long initial courses of therapy (at least 6 months).

The drug is generally well tolerated. Nausea, drug-induced hepatitis (1 in 10,000), and marked suppression of testosterone and cortisol production are the chief metabolic side effects, which at times result in reversible impotence, hypospermia, gynecomastia, and decreased libido. Replacement therapy with androgens is helpful. Clinical hypoadrenalism is extremely rare.

Other azoles, specifically the triazoles fluconazole and itraconazole, are currently under investigation and will probably be superior to ketoconazole because of better tissue penetration, less toxicity, and longer half-lives. Relapses appear to be a problem with these drugs also.

Surgery

Excisional surgery of residual cavities is mandatory in severe hemoptysis and manifest or threatened rupture. Cavities should be removed electively should they persist with intermittent bleeding, enlargement, and development of air fluid levels, which indicates coccidioidal or bacterial abscess formation. Nodules (coccidioidoma) need a tissue diagnosis unless their origin can be definitely established as being from proven previous coccidioidal pneumonitis.

HISTOPLASMOSIS

method of
L. JOSEPH WHEAT, M.D.
Indiana University School of Medicine
Indianapolis, Indiana

Histoplasmosis is the most common systemic mycosis in the United States. Histoplasmosis is endemic in the Ohio and Mississippi River valleys, but cases have been reported from most states. *Histoplasma capsulatum* is not evenly distributed in the environment but is rather localized to microfoci contaminated by bird or bat droppings. These foci include bird roosts, caves, buildings inhabited by birds or bats, chicken coops, wood piles, and farms. Although some individuals may recall exposure to such microfoci, in most cases the exact source of exposure cannot be determined. These individuals presumably have been exposed during their daily activities to wind-borne infectious microconidia from microfoci that have been disturbed during construction, demolition, or excavation.

Microconidia convert into yeast phase organisms within the lungs and produce a self-limited pulmonary infection. The outcome of this infection is influenced by the magnitude of the exposure and the immune status of the patient. Infection is usually asymptomatic in the normal host after low-level exposure. Symptomatic patients with primary, self-limited histoplasmosis usually present with flu-like pulmonary illness, arthritis or arthralgia accompanied by erythema nodosum or erythema multiforme, or pericarditis. Chronic pulmonary histoplasmosis develops predominantly in patients with underlying emphysema. In addition to underlying lung disease, heightened cellular hypersensitivity to *H. capsulatum* resulting from prior unrecognized histoplasmosis may affect the course and pathologic response observed in chronic pulmonary histoplasmosis. Disseminated histoplasmosis is characterized by widespread involvement of the reticuloendothelial system and progresses ultimately to a fatal outcome without treatment. Development of cellular immunity to *H. capsulatum* is required for recovery from histoplasmosis. Disseminated infection occurs primarily in individuals with impaired cellular immunity. Rarely, patients may develop late fibrotic complications of histoplamosis, including mediastinal fibrosis and constrictive pericarditis. A sarcoidosis-like illness may also develop in some individuals.

Diagnosis of histoplasmosis is based on serologic tests, special stains of tissue sections, and cultures. Histoplasmin skin testing is not useful for diagnostic purposes; rather, it complicates interpretation of serologic tests because of a booster phenomenon that follows a positive skin test. The immunodiffusion test for H and M precipitins is highly specific but may be falsely negative in up to 20 per cent of cases. The complement fixation test is more sensitive but less specific, particularly at low titers of 1:8 or 1:16. Serologic tests may be falsely negative during the first month after exposure and thus should be repeated in appropriate clinical settings. Serologic tests are also falsely negative in approximately one-quarter of immunocompromised patients with disseminated infection. Cultures provide the basis for diagnosis in 90 per cent of cases of disseminated infection, 60 per cent of cases of chronic pulmonary disease, but in only about 10 per cent of self-limited disease syndromes. Delays of 2 to 6 weeks are required to identify *H. capsulatum* in positive cultures. A rapid diagnosis may be established by histopathologic visualization of yeast phase organisms in the blood or tissues of patients. Detection of a polysaccharide antigen in the urine, blood, cerebrospinal fluid, or bronchoalveolar lavage fluid has proved to be a valuable new method for rapid diagnosis of histoplasmosis.

TREATMENT

Acute Self-Limited Disease

As the title implies, patients with acute pulmonary, rheumatologic, or pericardial manifestations of histoplasmosis recover without treatment. Restriction of activity and symptomatic treatment with antipyretics are recommended. The effectiveness of antifungal treatment in modifying the course of self-limited histoplasmosis has not been investigated. A trial of ketoconazole

(Nizoral) therapy may be warranted in patients with more severe or prolonged (≥3 weeks) illness or with obstructive symptoms caused by mediastinal or paratracheal lymphadenopathy.

Occasional patients develop diffuse pulmonary infiltrates with respiratory insufficiency after exposure to a heavy inoculum. Treatment with amphotericin B (Fungizone) intravenously at a dose of approximately 0.7 mg per kg per day for 10 days, in conjunction with 40 to 60 mg per day of prednisone, is appropriate in these individuals. Clinical manifestations are caused in part by the inflammatory response to *H. capsulatum,* which justifies corticosteroid treatment. Ketoconazole should not be used in these cases because the response to it is slower than the response to amphotericin B.

Disseminated Disease

Without treatment, nearly all patients with disseminated disease experience progressive and eventually fatal outcomes. Treatment with amphotericin B results in cure of at least 75 per cent of such cases. In patients receiving at least 30 mg per kg of amphotericin B given over 6 to 10 weeks, relapse is uncommon, occurring in fewer than 25 per cent of cases. Relapse is more common in patients with underlying immunosuppression, endocarditis, infection of vascular grafts or mycotic aneurysms, meningitis, and adrenal insufficiency. About one-half of patients with meningitis have a relapse despite prolonged courses of amphotericin B. Relapse occurs predictably in patients with acquired immunodeficiency syndrome (AIDS) and histoplasmosis. Treatment with ketoconazole has produced response rates of 70 to 100 per cent in nonimmunocompromised patients with disseminated histoplasmosis, but the response to ketoconazole is slower than the response to amphotericin B, which reduces its usefulness for severely ill patients. Ketoconazole should be given for 6 to 12 months. Individuals should be followed carefully for at least 5 years to identify relapsing infection. Relapse probably occurs more frequently in patients treated with ketoconazole than in those treated with amphotericin B, because ketoconazole is fungistatic, whereas amphotericin B is fungicidal. The usual adult dose of ketoconazole is 400 mg daily, administered with a meal. Antacids and H_2 blockers impair absorption of ketoconazole and should be avoided. Patients who must receive antacids or H_2 blockers should not take these drugs within 4 hours of administration of ketoconazole.

Absorption of these drugs is impaired in patients with AIDS and bone marrow allograft recipients because of high gastric pH in these patients. Rifampin (Rifadin) and isoniazid accelerate the metabolism of ketoconazole and have caused treatment failure. If absorption is questioned or if patients are receiving antituberculous therapy, blood levels of ketoconazole should be determined to ensure proper therapy. Higher doses* (600 to 800 mg per day) of ketoconazole or alternative therapies are appropriate for patients with inadequate blood levels (<5 micrograms per ml).

Ketoconazole causes few significant adverse effects. Nausea and vomiting have been the most frequent symptoms and may compromise patient compliance. Mild elevation of hepatic enzyme levels occurs fairly often, but severe hepatitis is rare. Ketoconazole also inhibits synthesis of sterol hormones and causes adrenal insufficiency, gynecomastia, loss of libido, loss of sexual potency, oligospermia, and menstrual irregularity. Patients receiving ketoconazole should be followed clinically for side effects, and liver function tests should be done frequently, perhaps monthly.

Patients with AIDS respond appropriately to amphotericin B but relapse when treatment is stopped. Thus, the goal of therapy should be suppression of infection rather than cure. An induction phase of 1 to 2 grams of amphotericin B is usually sufficient to induce remission of infection, and chronic maintenance treatment is required to prevent relapse. Treatment with amphotericin B administered twice weekly, weekly, or biweekly may be more effective maintenance therapy (90 per cent) than treatment with ketoconazole (50 per cent).

Chronic Pulmonary Histoplasmosis

Although some patients may improve without treatment, most experience a chronic, slowly progressive course with gradual loss of pulmonary function; some patients (5 per cent) develop disseminated infection. Treatment with amphotericin B halts progression of the pulmonary disease. Relapse occurs in fewer than one-quarter of patients receiving at least 35 mg per kg of amphotericin B. Although a response rate of 80 per cent has been observed with ketoconazole, additional follow-up is required to determine the long-term relapse rate. Ketoconazole, 400 mg per day, is the appropriate initial treatment in patients who are not severely ill with mild or moderate respiratory insufficiency. Amphotericin B, 35 mg per kg given during 10 to 16 weeks, should be administered to patients who are severely ill or have severe respiratory insufficiency and to pa-

---

*Exceed manufacturer's recommended dose.

tients who fail ketoconazole treatment. Patients treated with ketoconazole should be followed for 5 to 10 years to identify relapse.

Antifungal treatment is not indicated for fibrous mediastinitis. These clinical syndromes are not caused by the infection per se but by an exaggerated scarring response to a past infection. Limited experience suggests that antifungal treatment is not effective in these cases, nor does treatment with anti-inflamatory agents appear to be helpful. Surgical resection of fibrotic mediastinal tissue is often complicated by hemorrhage or damage to pulmonary structures that are embedded in the scar, and it rarely alleviates the obstruction. Some patients with symptomatic superior vena cava obstruction have benefited from construction of a venous bypass around the obstruction.

Investigational treatments include liposomal amphotericin B, which appears to be better tolerated than amphotericin B; itraconazole, which is better absorbed, better tolerated, and more active than ketoconazole; and fluconazole, which crosses the blood-brain barrier well and provides a potential alternative to amphotericin B for treatment of meningitis.

BLASTOMYCOSIS

method of
FRANKLIN R. COCKERILL, III, M.D., and
CHRISTINE L. TERRELL, M.D.
Mayo Clinic
Rochester, Minnesota

Blastomyces dermatitidis is a dimorphic fungus that causes a pyogranulomatous infection in humans and some animals, especially dogs. The organism exists as a spore-forming mycelium in nature and as a yeast in the infected host. A regional distribution of the organism occurs in North America including the south central United States and the valleys of the Mississippi, Ohio, and St. Lawrence rivers.

Spores are inhaled by hosts who inadvertently disturb soil and decomposed vegetation that under certain environmental conditions supports growth of the organism. Rarely, transmission to humans has been by animal bite. After spores are inhaled, the organism may cause pneumonitis; if the infection is unchecked, it spreads to extrapulmonary sites, including the skin, bones, genitourinary system, reticuloendothelial organs, and central nervous system (CNS). Although blastomycosis is seen primarily in immunocompetent patients, severe disseminated disease may occur in immunocompromised patients.

Clinical manifestations depend on the organ system involved. Some patients may be asymptomatic despite an abnormal chest x-ray film. Fever, headache, myalgias, pleuritic chest pain, and nonproductive cough may occur with pulmonary blastomycosis. The chest film may show localized infiltrates, which may be consolidated or nodular densities indistinguishable from bronchogenic carcinoma.

Extrapulmonary disease may be elusive with a paucity of early signs and symptoms. *B. dermatitidis* skin lesions mimic pyoderma gangrenosum (papulopustular) or squamous cell carcinoma (verrucoid, ulcerative); subcutaneous nodules are also seen. Bone infection is usually manifested by osteolytic lesions. Genitourinary infection presents as chronic "aseptic" prostatitis, prostatic nodules, prostatic abscess, or acute epididymitis. *B. dermatitidis* infection in the reticuloendothelial system or CNS may present as "sterile" abscesses. Chronic meningitis also occurs. Stains and cultures for *B. dermatitidis* should be performed when a pyogranulomatous (polymorphonuclear leukocytes with or without noncaseating granulomata) tissue reaction is observed and conventional aerobic and anaerobic bacterial cultures are negative.

DIAGNOSIS

A presumptive diagnosis of *B. dermatitidis* infection is achieved by demonstrating the yeast form on direct examination of samples of spontaneous or induced sputum, bronchoalveolar lavage fluid, or normally sterile body fluids (e.g., joint or pleural fluid), or in histopatholgic sections of infected tissues. Methods of direct examination include potassium hydroxide preparations (viewed by using phase contrast microscopy), cytologic preparations (Papanicolaou's smear), or silver stains. Silver stains are used most often for histopathologic sections; *B. dermatitidis* may also be seen with routine hematoxylin and eosin stains. The organism characteristically is large (8 to 15 micrometers in diameter) and has a double-thick refractile wall and flat broad-based connecting buds to parent cells. A definitive diagnosis is achieved by culture isolation of the organism (usually within 5 days). Standard serologic methods for diagnosis (complement fixation and immunodiffusion) are of little use because of low sensitivity in both acute and chronic infections. An enzyme-linked immunoassay has recently been developed that in preliminary studies appears to be more sensitive than the conventional serologic methods. Skin tests have been of little diagnostic use and are no longer available.

TREATMENT

The following comments summarize the methods generally followed at our institution for treating blastomycosis.

1. With the introduction of ketoconazole, an oral agent with fewer side effects than amphotericin B, some clinicians would treat all patients with symptomatic pulmonary blastomycosis. However, certain asymptomatic or mildly symptomatic immunocompetent patients with nonprogressive pulmonary disease can be observed with-

out treatment because spontaneous resolution is common.

2. If the radiographic appearance of a chest lesion is worrisome for malignancy or progresses despite antifungal therapy, surgical treatment should be strongly considered.

3. In general, ketoconazole is the drug of choice in mild to moderately ill immunocompetent patients with nonmeningeal blastomycosis. All severely ill patients should be treated with amphotericin B.

4. Ketoconazole should not be administered to patients with CNS disease because it penetrates the blood-brain barrier poorly.

5. Ketoconazole has cured genitourinary blastomycosis but is not as reliably effective as amphotericin B because of poor penetration into the genitourinary system. For this reason, many physicians consider amphotericin B to be the drug of choice in genitourinary blastomycosis. If ketoconazole is used, 600 to 800 mg per day* should be administered and the patient should be followed closely.

6. Amphotericin B is preferred in all forms of blastomycosis in immunocompromised patients, except in the mildest cases.

7. Ketoconazole should be administered at a minimal dosage of 400 mg per day for at least 6 months. Higher doses of 600 to 800 mg per day* or a more extended duration of therapy, or both, may be necessary depending on the severity of illness and the clinical response. Side effects are more common with the higher dose of ketoconazole. Amphotericin B should be used if *B. dermatitidis* infection persists or worsens when ketoconazole is given.

8. The exact dose for a full course of amphotericin B is unknown, although most clinicians familiar with treating the disease recommend a total cumulative dose of 1.5 to 2.5 grams. In certain clinical circumstances, lesser amounts of amphotericin B can be given if ketoconazole is subsequently administered.

9. Chronic suppressive therapy using either ketoconazole or amphotericin B after initial treatment may be necessary in immunocompromised patients, especially those with infection with human immunodeficiency virus. Use of immunosuppressive agents (e.g., corticosteroids) should be reduced or eliminated if possible.

10. 2-Hydroxystilbamidine, an effective although toxic antifungal agent, was occasionally used to treat *B. dermatitidis* infections before the availability of amphotericin B and ketoconazole. It has no use in current clinical practice.

---

*May exceed manufacturer's recommended dose.

AMPHOTERICIN B

Amphotericin B (Fungizone) is a naturally occurring polyene antibiotic that binds to fungal membrane sterols, increases permeability of the membrane, and produces cell lysis. The drug is complexed with a bile salt (desoxycholate), which increases bioavailability. It is insoluble in many solutions and should be diluted in 5 per cent dextrose and water. After intravenous infusion, the drug binds to beta-lipoproteins and probably to sterols in human cells. Most of the drug is metabolized slowly in vivo; little is excreted in the urine, bile, or feces. Concentrations of the drug in infected tissues (pleura or peritoneal, joint, or vitreous fluid) are essentially two-thirds of trough serum levels.

It is our institution's practice to deliver a 1.0-mg test dose during 1 to 2 hours in adult patients (anaphylaxis rarely occurs), followed by 5 mg in 6 to 12 hours and 10 mg after an additional 6 to 12 hours if the drug is tolerated. Alternatively, 15 mg may be given as the second dose. Daily increments of 5 to 10 mg are provided until 0.5 to 0.7 mg per kg of body weight is achieved. A more rapid increase of the dose of amphotericin B is occasionally necessary in severely ill patients. Some clinicians favor alternate-day amphotericin therapy (i.e., 50 mg every other day).

Adverse physical side effects of amphotericin B include fever, chills, myalgias, headaches, nausea, vomiting, and hypotension. It is our policy to premedicate patients with acetaminophen (Tylenol), 650 mg, and/or diphenhydramine hydrocholoride (Benadryl), 25 to 50 mg orally or parenterally, 30 to 60 minutes before the infusion is begun. If side effects are not alleviated, decreasing the rate of infusion or adding 10 to 20 mg of hydrocortisone sodium succinate to the infusate are further options. In most cases, the above-mentioned side effects resolve spontaneously with continued daily infusions. Some clinicians advocate the addition of heparin, 1000 to 2000 units, to the infusion to prevent phlebitis, especially if peripheral veins are used.

Azotemia occurs universally during a therapeutic course, and a permanent reduction in glomerular filtration rate can result, especially if the total amphotericin dose exceeds 3 grams. Most physicians continue amphotericin B treatment until the serum creatinine level reaches 3.0 mg per dl. The drug can be reinstituted once the creatinine level falls to 2.5 mg per dl. Renal toxicity may be enhanced with the use of other nephrotoxic drugs such as cyclosporin.

Hypokalemia and normocytic and normochromic anemia occur frequently. Renal tubular acidosis, hypomagnesemia, hepatic dysfunction, leukopenia, and thrombocytopenia are less common. Recently, pulmonary toxicity related to aggregation of leukocytes in lungs was reported when leukocyte transfusions followed amphotericin infusions. Appropriate serial laboratory studies should be obtained to monitor for these toxicities. When administering amphotericin to pregnant women and to children, the clinician should consult specialists who have experience in its use.

KETOCONAZOLE

Ketoconazole (Nizoral) is an imidazole that interferes with the formation of fungal membrane sterols. Unlike amphotericin B, the drug can be given orally and has fewer and less severe side effects. Because oral absorption is decreased by an alkaline gastric pH, the concomitant use of oral hydrochloric acid (dissolve each 200-mg tablet in 4 ml aqueous solution of 0.2 N HCl) is necessary in patients with achlorhydria. Antacids and H_2-blocking agents also interfere with the absorption of ketoconazole. Rifampin and isoniazid given in conjunction with ketoconazole may reduce the blood levels of the latter. Furthermore, ketoconazole may increase levels of cyclosporin, potentiate the action of warfarin, and have an insulin-sparing effect. Once absorbed, ketoconazole is highly protein bound; degradation occurs in the liver with inactivated drug excreted in the bile and to a lesser extent in the urine. Penetration of active drug into the cerebrospinal fluid and genitourinary system is poor. Dosage recommendations were presented earlier.

Side effects that occur with ketoconazole use, especially with higher doses (800 mg per day), include nausea and vomiting (which is minimized if the drug is taken with food), elevated transaminase level (which is often transient; rarely, fatal hepatoxicity has occurred), and depression of serum testosterone level leading to decreased libido, impotence, and gynecomastia. Ketoconazole also dampens the cortisol response to adrenocorticotropic hormone. Periodic clinical laboratory studies should be conducted to monitor these potential toxicities.

PLEURAL EFFUSION AND EMPYEMA THORACIS

method of
RICHARD B. McELVEIN, M.D.
The University of Alabama at Birmingham
Birmingham, Alabama

PLEURAL EFFUSION

Pathophysiology

In healthy persons, there is a small amount of fluid in the pleural space, which has its origin in the capillaries of the parietal pleura. Fluid is transferred into the pleural space where it is absorbed by the visceral pleural capillaries (80 per cent) and pleural lymphatics (20 per cent). The estimated flow across the pleural membrane is 5 to 10 liters a day. Any abnormality that results in an increased production of fluid, decreased absorption, or loss of oncotic pressure with increased capillary permeability leads to the development of an effusion.

Accumulation of pleural fluid generally produces pain followed by dyspnea, cough, and fever. Other symptoms related to the causative disease may be present.

Etiology

A pleural effusion may be the result of increased capillary permeability and decreased lymphatic flow, such as in primary or metastatic malignancy or tuberculosis. Increased capillary permeability also leads to pleural effusion, such as with pulmonary embolus or in pneumonia, uremia, and subdiaphragmatic infection. When there is a reduced lymphatic flow such as in sarcoidosis, an effusion may develop and can be chylous. Various drugs may produce pleural effusion, including nitrogen mustard (Alkeran), quinacrine (Atabrine), nitrofurantoin (Furadantin), methysergide (Sansert), and amiodarone (Cordarone). When increased hydrostatic pressure and decreased oncotic pressure occur, such as in congestive heart failure, cirrhosis, nephrotic syndrome, myxedema, and superior vena cava syndrome, a transudate pleural effusion may result. Despite all diagnostic efforts, there are a small number of patients in whom a definitive etiology is never established.

Diagnosis

Clinical assessment of a patient with an effusion demonstrates diminished respiratory excursion on the affected side, diminished vocal and tactile fremitus, dullness to percussion, decreased breath sounds, and, on occasion, a friction rub. Posteroanterior and lateral x-ray films of the thorax are generally all that is required to establish a diagnosis of pleural effusion. Lateral decubitus films of the chest are of no value unless there is a suspected subpulmonic effusion. Rarely is a computed tomographic scan of the thorax required. Echopleurography and magnetic resonance imaging examinations are superfluous.

Treatment

The management of a patient with pleural effusion involves treatment of the underlying disease while remembering that an effusion is not an entity itself but is instead a manifestation of disease. However, if the patient has a symptomatic pleural effusion or if the diagnosis is not known, removal of the fluid by thoracentesis is indicated.

The patient is informed of the reason for thoracentesis and of the technique to be used. Morphine, 4 to 6 mg 30 minutes before the procedure, is used for premedication. The patient is placed in the sitting position, leans forward on a pillow-covered table, and is made as comfortable as possible. The site of the thoracentesis is determined by careful examination of chest films. The goal is dependent aspiration of the fluid with due care taken not to insert the needle too low and risk penetration of the diaphragm and the underlying liver or spleen. Aseptic technique is required. One per cent lidocaine is injected into the skin with a 22-gauge needle, after which an 18-gauge needle is used to infiltrate the tissues of the chest wall, passing over the superior aspect of the rib into the pleural space. A 50-ml syringe with stopcock and drainage tube attached to the sidearm is used for penetration of the chest wall and the pleural space with care being taken to avoid laceration of the underlying lung. The fluid is aspirated and a sample discharged into specimen tubes; the rest of the fluid is discharged into a container for later disposal. Cautious withdrawal of the fluid is necessary when large effusions are present to avoid syncope or the infrequent phenomenon of re-expansion pulmonary edema.

Specimens of pleural fluid are submitted for assays of specific gravity, pH, protein content, and lactate dehydrogenase. Cytologic determination is performed if there is a suspicion of malignancy on the basis of the patient's history. Material is sent for standard cultures if there is a suggestion of infection. Cultures for tuberculo-

sis and fungal organisms are performed only if clinically indicated.

If a diagnosis has not been established, the fluid recurs, and repeat thoracentesis is necessary, a concomitant pleural biopsy with either Cope's or Abrams's needle is done.

Several manufacturers provide kits that contain all of the items necessary for a successful thoracentesis. These items include a sheathed needle, which is withdrawn leaving a small-bore catheter in the pleural space while the aspiration is done, which diminishes the risk of lung laceration.

Persistent effusions may require the placement of a thoracostomy tube. The technique is similar to thoracentesis except that the area of local anesthesia is enlarged and an incision paralleling the intercostal space is made to accept a No. 28 French thoracostomy tube. Scissors are used to dissect through the muscle of the chest wall into the pleural space, with entry through the intercostal space over the top of the rib above the incision to minimize the possibility of an air leak. The thoracostomy tube is sutured in place with 0 silk and is connected to an underwater drainage system for collection of fluid and re-expansion of the lung.

In a few circumstances when a diagnosis is still not established by these measures, thoracoscopy is performed through an indwelling intercostal tube. By using a standard right-angled bronchoscopy connector attached to the end of the tube, the sterilized flexible bronchoscope is passed through the intercostal tube into the pleural space where visceral or parietal pleural lesions can be seen and biopsied under direct vision.

Sclerosis of the pleural space to achieve symphysis between the visceral and parietal pleura in cases of persistent effusion has been accomplished with various agents. I prefer to use tetracycline,* 500 mg to 1 gram in 100 ml of saline instilled through the thoracostomy tube into the pleural space, after which the patient is rotated in both lateral decubitus positions as well as with the head elevated and depressed for 5 minutes each to distribute the sclerosing agent evenly. The tube is then unclamped and reconnected to the underwater drainage system. The volume of fluid generally diminishes rapidly and the tube can be withdrawn the following day. If tetracycline fails to produce sclerosis, we use bleomycin (Blenoxane), 60 units in 100 ml of saline.

It is rarely necessary to do an open thoracotomy with abrasion of the visceral and parietal spaces to provide symphysis.

---

*Although considered to be the treatment of choice by some clinicians, this use of tetracycline is not approved by the U.S. Food and Drug Administration.

I have had no experience with pleural peritoneal shunts for the management of pleural effusion, but they are reported to be successful.

EMPYEMA THORACIS

Pathophysiology

A pleural effusion that becomes infected is an empyema. The diagnosis is established with the findings of bacteria and white blood cells in the pleural fluid and a low pH. As the effusion increases, there will be gradual collapse of the underlying lung and restriction of the thoracic cage. Sepsis may occur.

Etiology

The most common causes of empyema are pneumonia, trauma, or postoperative conditions. Other causes are a secondary infection from intra-abdominal sepsis, atelectasis, and primary mediastinal diseases such as a ruptured esophagus.

Diagnosis

The diagnosis of empyema is based on the clinical assessment of the patient who presents with symptoms similar to those of a pleural effusion but with the addition of fever and chills and a preceding history of pulmonary or abdominal infection. Radiographs of the chest show the presence of a pleural effusion. Lateral decubitus films and echopleurography are of no value. A computed tomographic scan of the thorax occasionally helps to determine the presence of multiple loculated areas of pus, which may require separate drainage.

Treatment

The initial treatment of empyema thoracis is by thoracentesis with the goal of removing the pus, expanding the lung, and obtaining fluid for culture. Antibiotics, such as cefazolin (Ancef), 1 gram every 6 hours, are initiated and altered depending on the culture results. If the patient has persistence or recurrence of the effusion and continues to have signs of infection as evidenced by tachycardia, tachypnea, and hyperpyrexia, a thoracostomy tube should be inserted. If several loculated areas are present, it may be necessary to insert more than one tube.

In cases of chronic empyema in debilitated patients in whom thoracostomy tube drainage is anticipated for a prolonged period, a short portion of rib at the most dependent site of empyema is resected to establish a fistula between the pleural space and the exterior.

If the patient fails to respond to thoracentesis or intercostal tube drainage coupled with antibiotics, thoracotomy is mandatory. This procedure is performed under general anesthesia through a lateral thoracotomy incision with entry into the pleural space through the bed of a resected rib. The liquid and semifluid debris is removed, after which the coagulum on the surface of the lung is meticulously removed. This treatment results in expansion of the lung to fill the thoracic cavity. The debris on the parietal pleura is also removed to allow better respiratory excursion of the ribs. The diaphragm is freed in a similar fashion.

PRIMARY LUNG ABSCESS

method of
SOL KATZ, M.D.
Georgetown University
Washington, D.C.

Because aspiration of bacteria is the common factor in the development of primary lung abscess, the term "aspiration lung abscess" would seem to be more appropriate than "primary lung abscess."

When the aspirate is laden with large numbers of anaerobic organisms and reaches the peripheral portion of the lung, a localized area of pulmonary inflammation ensues that progresses to necrosis and liquefaction. The source of this anaerobic bacterial inoculum is most commonly the oropharynx, especially the gingival crevices in the presence of gingivodental infection, and the gastrointestinal tract. Lung abscess is less commonly encountered in edentulous individuals because there is no gingival crevice.

Dysphagia and conditions that interfere with the cleansing mechanisms of the tracheobronchial tree predispose to the inhalation of infected secretions. Thus, suppressed levels of consciousness may subject an individual to a lung abscess, as in head injury, cerebrovascular accident, alcoholism, general anesthesia, seizure disorders, and drug overdose. Compromise of immunologic defenses, such as in neutropenia, use of corticosteroids, cancer chemotherapy, and acquired immunodeficiency syndrome (AIDS), may lead to lung abscess. Anaerobic organisms may also reach the lung by direct spread from a subphrenic abscess or by hematogenous spread. Prolonged uncoordinated vomiting and disruption of defense barriers such as that caused by use of a nasogastric tube, endotracheal tube, or tracheostomy may encourage aspiration.

In any case of bronchial obstruction such as bronchogenic carcinoma or foreign body, the resulting atelectasis establishes an ideal environment for the growth of anaerobic bacteria. Therefore, the presence of poor oral hygiene and gingivitis in a patient with bronchial occlusion provides the perfect arrangement for the development of a putrid (primary) lung abscess.

Because the infected aspirate composed of saliva, oropharyngeal contents, or gastric juice gravitates to the most dependent part of the bronchial tree, the term bronchial "embolism" readily explains the localization of primary lung abscess. With the patient in the supine position, the superior segment of the lower lobes and the posterior segments of the upper lobes are first met by the aspirate as it descends along the posterior wall of the tracheobronchial tree. The basal segments are encountered next. The more direct course of the right main bronchus explains the more frequent involvement on the right side.

The bacteriology of primary lung abscess has been carefully studied in the past 10 to 15 years as techniques for anaerobic culture became available in most clinical laboratories. At the same time, the taxonomy of anaerobic bacteria was evolving and transtracheal aspiration developed as a method for bacteriologic study. The main anaerobic bacteria normally present in the gingival crevices and oropharynx are also found in aspiration lung abscess and include *Fusobacterium nucleatum, Peptostreptococcus* species, and *Bacteroides melaninogenicus*. Other *Bacteroides* species are less commonly cultured. *Bacteroides fragilis,* which is not usually considered to be an oropharyngeal inhabitant, has been isolated in 5 to 20 per cent of patients with primary lung abscess. Hospital-acquired aspiration lung abscesses are more likely to harbor aerobes such as gram-negative bacilli and *Staphylococcus aureus* as well as the usual anaerobes. Lung abscesses may also be caused by other organisms such as *Mycobacterium tuberculosis, Actinomyces, Nocardia, Klebsiella, Streptococcus pneumoniae* (especially Type III and Type VIII), and *Haemophilus influenzae*. It is common for primary lung abscesses to be polymicrobial.

Because the usual pathogens in lung abscesses are normally found in the mouth or oropharynx, cultures of expectorated sputum are contaminated by these organisms and therefore do not necessarily reflect the contents of the abscess. However, expectorated sputum can be used to detect *M. tuberculosis,* fungi, *Nocardia,* and aerobic pathogens such as staphylococci and gram-negative bacilli. Appropriate specimens for anaerobic cultures are blood, pleural fluid, transtracheal aspirates, transthoracic lung aspirates, and bronchoscopic specimens that are collected with a shielded catheter or a brush for quantitative cultures. Positive blood cultures are obtained in less than 3 per cent of proven anaerobic lung infections. It is thought by most authorities that invasive techniques to obtain material for identification of anaerobes are not indicated when the manifestations of aspiration lung abscess are classic (including putrid sputum).

The early stage of a putrid lung abscess is a localized area of consolidation having an x-ray film appearance similar to that of pneumonia. Pathologically, this inflammation represents gangrenous bronchopneumonia. At times, the area of consolidation is round and sharply defined, which offers a clue to the early detection of lung abscess before liquefaction is established. The consolidation may appear to be quite dense and may continue unchanged for a number of days, thereby differing from ordinary pneumonia. A few small highlights in the dense consolidation suggests the beginning of the phase of liquefaction, which occurs within 1 or 2 weeks after the onset of the illness. Liquefaction then progresses rapidly, and some of the purulent material is discharged through the communicating bronchus, air enters, and the specific sign of abscess—a fluid-containing cavity—appears.

There are several courses after this stage. The necrosis and liquefaction may continue until cavitation replaces the entire area of consolidation. Rapid enlargement of the cavity beyond the original zone of consolidation indicates a ball-valve obstruction for the draining bronchus with the formation of a balloon cavity, which is often associated with perforation into the pleural cavity. When the communicating bronchus is blocked by inflammation, edema, and exudate, the secretions accumulate, the air is absorbed, and the cavity becomes completely filled (blocked cavity). With good drainage the secretions are evacuated, the fluid level is reduced, and pericavity pneumonitis decreases. A diminution in cavity size and complete resolution of the surrounding infection follow. The draining ceases, and the lung may return to normal except for minor distortion of the vascular markings and linear fibrosis.

If the abscess does not disappear in 6 to 10 weeks, irreversible pulmonary changes have usually occurred, which makes cure by medical means unlikely. In some chronic cases, there may not be a fluid level because the cavity is filled with inspissated necrotic debris. This shadow may remain unchanged for many weeks. The chronic abscess is characterized by a rigid fibrous wall, pericavity fibrosis, bronchiectasis, and even epithelization.

THERAPY

Many antibiotics used alone or in combination have been reportedly successful in the treatment of lung abscess. However, for community-acquired aspiration lung abscess, the most successful agents are penicillin G, clindamycin (Cleocin), or metronidazole (Flagyl) plus penicillin. Although penicillin by mouth may give a satisfactory result, the oral route is not preferred and gives a higher failure rate and slower response than aqueous penicillin G given intravenously (8 to 10 million units daily until there is clinical improvement). Foul sputum, when present, usually disappears in a few days, although cough and nonfoul sputum production may continue for longer periods. Fever and subjective improvement occur during the first week, but it takes 1 to 2 weeks for the temperature to become normal. The improvement in the chest film lags behind clinical improvement and may worsen during the first few weeks without being indicative of a therapeutic failure. After the acute phase of intravenous treatment, penicillin may be given orally as penicillin G, penicillin V, ampicillin, or amoxicillin, 500 to 750 mg four times a day. Oral therapy should be continued until there is complete clinical response and the chest film demonstrates a complete resolution or a stable fibrotic lesion, whether it is a scar or a small uninfected cavity. This therapeutic process may last 4 to 8 weeks or, at times, longer.

Although penicillin is preferred by many physicians because it is safe, is inexpensive, and has a long favorable record, it must be appreciated that treatment may fail because of the presence of penicillin-resistant strains of *Bacteroides* and other organisms. For this reason some physicians favor the use of clindamycin initially at an intravenous dose of 600 mg every 8 hours until a clinical response occurs, when oral clindamycin is given, 300 mg four times a day, until the criteria of stability have been achieved.

When metronidazole is selected for therapy, it should be used with penicillin to avoid failures encountered when metronidazole is used alone. Metronidazole, 500 mg orally every 6 hours, combined with high-dose penicillin intravenously as described or, in clinically less severely ill patients, metronidazole plus oral penicillin may be used throughout therapy. Metronidazole plus penicillin is less expensive than clindamycin, and metronidazole broadens the activity against the anaerobes that are penicillin resistant.

Hospital-acquired aspiration lung abscesses are often due to aerobic mixed gram-negative bacilli and *S. aureus* in addition to the usual anaerobes. In this circumstance the choice of antibiotics is best guided by identification of the causative organism and bacterial sensitivity data. For empiric treatment, the physician may select intravenous gentamicin or tobramycin, 1 mg per kg every 8 hours, to cover the aerobic gram-negative bacilli, in addition to penicillin G or clindamycin as described. For *S. aureus,* nafcillin, 2 grams intravenously every 4 hours, should be added to penicillin G or clindamycin. For methicillin-resistant *S. aureus,* neither nafcillin nor clindaymcin is useful and intravenous vancomycin, 1 gram every 12 hours or 500 mg every 6 hours, is used.

When there is a bacteriologically complex infection with multiple organisms, both aerobic and anaerobic, it is not necessary to identify each organism and establish antibiotic sensitivity to outline logical therapy. These organisms often live symbiotically so that the elimination of the major culprits usually destroys the others, even those that are insensitive to the antibiotics being used.

As with an abscess anywhere in the body, appropriate treatment of lung abscess entails adequate drainage coupled with appropriate antibiotic treatment. Chest physiotherapy and postural drainage may improve drainage, as may bronchoscopy. However, the major role of bronchoscopy is to determine the presence of an obstructing lesion such as a foreign body, bronchial stenosis, or bronchogenic carcinoma. Bronchogenic carcinoma with abscess should be suspected in the absence of fever, systemic symptoms, poor oral hygiene, or features that predispose to aspiration. Also suggestive of a malignant lung abscess are an irregular cavity wall with mural nodules and the lack of an infiltrate surrounding the abscess.

Surgery is required in fewer than 10 per cent of patients with lung abscess. The indications for surgery are clinical or roentgenographic deterioration despite good medical management, uncontrollable hemoptysis, benign or malignant bronchial obstruction, suspicion of a necrotizing carcinoma, and peristence of a cavity after 3 months of therapy in the presence of recurrent infection in that segment or lobe. The usual procedure is thoracotomy with lobectomy or occasionally segmentectomy. Critically ill patients or those with poor pulmonary reserve who are considered to have a prohibitively unacceptable surgical risk should undergo pneumonotomy with percutaneous incision and catheter drainage performed thorough an area of pleural symphysis under local anesthesia.

OTITIS MEDIA

method of
COLIN D. MARCHANT, M.D.
Floating Hospital for Infants and Children
Tufts University School of Medicine
Boston, Massachusetts

Acute otitis media is the most common bacterial infection of infancy and childhood. Seventy-five per cent of children will have one or more episodes by age 3 years. In the antibiotic era, complications such as acute mastoiditis and intracranial infections (other than meningitis) are rare. Today, recurrent otitis media and otitis media with effusion (OME) (or serous otitis media) are common management problems.

ACUTE OTITIS MEDIA

Patients typically present with fever and earache after or during an upper respiratory tract infection. Many patients, however, are afebrile, and in young infants slight irritability may be the only evidence of ear pain. In the first few months of life, specific symptoms may not be present or may go unrecognized. Pneumatic otoscopy is the preferred method of diagnosis. Reduced tympanic membrane mobility and opacification and bulging of the eardrum are the most reliable signs. Redness alone is a poor predictor of acute otitis media. Acoustic reflectometry may be a helpful adjunct to confirm the presence of fluid behind the tympanic membrane, but otoscopy is necessary to discern the signs of infection.

Although viral upper respiratory tract infection usually precedes acute otitis media, bacterial pathogens can be isolated in most cases. In infants and children, 70 per cent of middle-ear exudates yield bacterial pathogens (Table 1). *Streptococcus pneumoniae* and *Haemophilus influenzae* are the most common pathogens in adults. In infants, gram-negative enteric bacteria may cause otitis media during the first month of life although very rarely outside the hospital setting.

Approximately 15 years ago, these species were sensitive to amoxicillin and other aminopenicillins. Since then there has been a slow but steady increase in the incidence of beta-lactamase–producing pathogens. Beta-lactamases hydrolyze amoxicillin and other penicillins and render these drugs ineffective. Beta-lactamase–producing strains have been responsible for an increasing rate of bacteriologic failure during therapy with amoxicillin.

Antimicrobial therapy is the mainstay of treatment for acute otitis media. Antihistamines and decongestants do not modify the course of otitis media and are not indicated. An analgesic-antipyretic agent such as acetaminophen (Tylenol, Tempra), 5 to 10 mg per kg per dose, may be given every 4 hours as an adjunct to antimicrobial therapy.

The choice of antimicrobial drug must be made by weighing the relative merits of each drug, including efficacy, patterns of bacterial resistance, nature and incidence of adverse effects, patient history of drug allergy, palatability, and cost. Appropriate drugs and dosages are outlined in Table 2. For many years amoxicillin has been

the drug of choice for initial therapy of otitis media because it has been efficacious and inexpensive and serious side effects have been rare. The slow but steady increase in the incidence of amoxicillin-resistant organisms mandates that we continually re-evaluate this position. It seems prudent to use an alternative drug in situations in which the rate of occurrence of amoxicillin-resistant bacteria is higher than that usually encountered, when symptoms are severe, or when the host may be at increased risk (Table 3).

Within 48 hours of initiating antibacterial therapy, most patients experience reduced fever, irritability, and earache. Patients who have no improvement by this time should be re-evaluated, and diagnostic tympanocentesis and culture should be performed. If amoxicillin was prescribed for initial therapy, an alternative drug should be considered. Otoscopic evaluation at the end of therapy will reveal persistent middle-ear effusion in approximately 70 per cent of cases. If symptomatic response was satisfactory, it is not necessary to treat asymptomatic otitis media with effusion at this time. A second course of antimicrobial therapy is indicated in asymptomatic patients only if the eardrum is opaque, bulging, and immobile.

Complications of acute otitis media, such as mastoiditis, are fortunately rare. Infection of the mastoid air cells accompanies acute otitis media because these spaces communicate with the middle-ear cavity. Thus, opacification of the mastoid air cells can be seen on mastoid plain x-ray films in uncomplicated acute otitis media. However, pain, tenderness and redness of the mastoid area, and high temperature should raise the possibility of acute mastoiditis. Plain x-ray films may reveal loss of trabeculations or subperiosteal abscess formation. *S. pneumoniae, Staphylococcus aureus,* and *Streptococcus pyogenes* are common pathogens; *H. influenzae* is a rare cause of mastoiditis. Acute mastoiditis should be treated with parenteral antimicrobial therapy such as nafcillin (Nafcil, Nallpen, Unipen), 150 mg per kg per day given intravenously in divided doses every 6 hours, or cefuroxime (Kefurox, Zinacef), 75 to 100 mg per kg per day given in divided doses every 8 hours. Myringotomy should be considered and mastoidectomy may be required in complicated cases. Patients who develop facial nerve palsy during acute otitis media should also have a myringotomy performed.

RECURRENT OTITIS MEDIA

Despite adequate therapy of an initial episode of acute otitis media, recurrences often occur days to months afterward. If amoxicillin was pre-

TABLE 1. **Bacteriology of Acute Otitis Media in Infants and Children**

	% of Acute Otitis Media	
Bacterial Species	All Isolates	Beta-Lactamase–Producing Isolates
Streptococcus pneumoniae	30	0
Haemophilus influenzae	22	5
Branhamella catarrhalis	14	9
Streptococcus pyogenes (Group A)	3	0
Staphylococcus aureus	1	1
Sterile/nonpathogens	30	—
Total	100	15

TABLE 2. **Antimicrobial Agents Suitable for Treatment of Acute Otitis Media**

Drug	Dosage	Comments	
		Efficacy	*Safety*
Amoxicillin	40 mg/kg/day divided in 3 doses for 10 days	Increasing bacteriologic failures because of beta-lactamase–producing organisms	Diarrhea, diaper rashes, and maculopapular rashes common to uncommon
Amoxicillin plus clavulanic acid (Augmentin)	40 mg/kg amoxicillin plus 10 mg/kg clavulanic acid/day in 3 divided doses for 10 days	Clavulanic acid inhibits bacterial beta-lactamases and renders amoxicillin effective	Higher incidence of diarrhea than with most other drugs; diarrhea usually tolerable
Trimethoprim-sulfamethoxazole (Bactrim, Septra)	40 mg trimethoprim, 8 mg/sulfamethoxazole/kg/day in 2 divided doses for 10 days	May not eliminate Group A *Streptococcus pyogenes;* nonpenicillin, and therefore resistant to beta-lactamases	Rash, Stevens-Johnson syndrome rare but has been fatal, rare blood dyscrasias
Erythromycin plus sulfisoxazole (Pediazole)	50 mg erythromycin plus 150 mg sulfisoxazole/kg/day in 3 divided doses for 10 days	Nonpenicillin, and therefore resistant to beta-lactamases	Stevens-Johnson syndrome rare but has been fatal
Cefaclor (Ceclor)	40 mg/kg/day divided in 3 doses for 10 days	Less efficacious in vivo than other drugs; resistant to beta-lactamases	Erythema multiforme and serum sickness reactions in 1% (more than amoxicillin); urticaria in 1% (more than amoxicillin)
Cefixime (Suprax)	8 mg/kg/day, either once daily or divided in 2 doses for 10 days	Resistant to beta-lactamases	Limited experience (recently approved)

scribed for the initial therapy and a recurrence occurs 1 to 2 weeks after therapy, an alternative therapy should be considered (Table 2) because there is a moderately increased risk of infection with beta-lactamase–producing organisms. However, the practice of changing drugs with each episode may lead parents to believe that "nothing works" for their child. Parents should be counseled that otitis media is a recurrent disease and that if episodes become too frequent there are other therapeutic options.

Antimicrobial chemoprophylaxis has been shown to decrease the frequency of recurrent otitis media, although precise indications for this therapy are open to debate. Children who have experienced three episodes or more in 18 months benefit from chemoprophylaxis. A more conservative approach would be to require three episodes or more in a 6-month period before starting chemoprophylaxis. Amoxicillin, 20 mg per kg per day given in two divided doses, and sulfisoxazole (Gantrisin), 75 mg per kg per day given in two divided doses, are suitable drugs. Chemoprophylaxis is continued through fall, winter, and spring and then discontinued at the start of the summer season, when the risk of otitis media is lower. If otitis media occurs during the next season, che-

moprophylaxis is restarted. If there is a recurrence during chemoprophylaxis, a course of antimicrobial therapy as outlined in Table 2 is indicated. If amoxicillin is used for chemoprophylaxis, an alternative drug should be used.

If a child continues to have recurrent otitis media despite chemoprophylaxis, insertion of tympanostomy tubes may be of benefit. Tympanostomy tubes have been shown to reduce the frequency of acute otitis media in patients with recurrent episodes. However, few patients require surgery if chemoprophylaxis is faithfully administered.

OTITIS MEDIA WITH EFFUSION (SEROUS OTITIS MEDIA)

Asymptomatic middle-ear effusion, called "otitis media with effusion," is usually diagnosed by the finding of decreased mobility of the tympanic membrane on otoscopic examination. Tympanometry and acoustic reflectometry may be used as alternative diagnostic methods. OME has a marked tendency to resolve spontaneously. All patients with acute otitis media have some fluid in their middle-ear cleft, but 3 months later only 10 per cent of patients still have OME. In asymp-

TABLE 3. **Reasonable Indications for Use of Drugs Resistant to Beta-Lactamases**

1. Probability of amoxicillin-resistant organisms is increased.
   a. Persistent symptoms after 48 hr or more of amoxicillin therapy. *Comment:* most cases will not be caused by beta-lactamase–producing bacteria, but the incidence of infection by these bacteria will be higher than that in untreated acute otitis media.
   b. Patient develops otitis media during amoxicillin therapy or amoxicillin chemoprophylaxis.
   c. Recurrence of acute otitis media within 1 or 2 wk of a previous course of amoxicillin. *Comment:* most cases will not be caused by beta-lactamase–producing bacteria, but the incidence of infection by these bacteria will be higher than in patients not recently exposed to amoxicillin.
   d. Otitis media with purulent conjunctivitis. *Comment:* 80% of cases caused by *H. influenzae;* therefore, the probability of beta-lactamase–positive cases is higher than in acute otitis media alone.
   e. Incidence of beta-lactamase–producing organisms is known to be higher than that in other geographic regions. *Comment:* this is rarely known because very few centers collect systematic data on the microbiology of acute otitis media.
2. Expected benefits of therapy or cost of therapeutic failure is increased.
   a. In immunocompromised hosts.
   b. In infants in the first year of life with high fever.
   c. In patients with severe symptoms, e.g., earache.

tomatic OME in which the onset is unknown, approximately 50 per cent of infections resolve after 2 months of observation.

A mild to moderate degree of hearing impairment accompanies OME, and some children with prolonged OME have measurable deficits in language ability. Moreover, some physicians believe that prolonged inflammation leads to structural changes in the middle ear. For these reasons, intervention should be considered if OME does not resolve spontaneously.

If after 2 to 3 months there has been no resolution, a course of amoxicillin, 40 mg per kg per day given in three divided doses for 14 days, should be tried. This treatment may result in resolution of OME in an additional 15 to 20 per cent of patients. Antihistamines and decongestants have no effect on OME; similarly, use of corticosteroids is not indicated.

If bilateral OME persists despite observation for 4 to 6 months and a trial of amoxicillin, use of tympanostomy tubes should be considered. Hearing acuity usually improves after insertion of tympanostomy tubes, but the tubes are extruded spontaneously in most cases within a year. If OME then recurs, tympanostomy tubes may be reinserted. Adenoidectomy benefits many children and should be performed in the most difficult cases.

CHRONIC OTITIS MEDIA

Perforations of the tympanic membrane and otorrhea frequently accompany acute otitis media. Otorrhea often resolves with the usual oral antimicrobial therapy. Persistent ear drainage may be treated with otic drops such as 2 per cent acetic acid solution, 3 to 4 drops in each ear administered three to four times per day, or Cortisporin Otic Suspension, 3 to 4 drops in each ear administered three to four times per day. Most cases of otorrhea resolve in a matter of weeks; most perforations, especially central perforations, heal spontaneously.

Chronic otitis media is chronic inflammation of the middle ear and mastoid with otorrhea through a perforated eardrum for at least 3 months. *Pseudomonas aeruginosa* and *S. aureus* are the most common pathogens. The site of perforation, not the ear canal, should be cultured after suctioning the external canal. Careful examination after suctioning should be performed to detect cholesteatoma that may be associated with chronic otitis media. A course of oral antimicrobial therapy should be prescribed based on culture and sensitivity results. Daily ear aspiration is often helpful.

The most resistant cases caused by *P. aeruginosa* may require parenteral antimicrobial agents in addition to daily aspiration. Antimicrobial therapy should be guided by the results of sensitivity tests; ticarcillin (Ticar), 100 to 150 mg per kg per day given intravenously in two divided doses, and ceftazidime (Fortaz, Tazicef, Tazidime), 30 to 50 mg per kg per day intravenously in two divided doses, are reasonable choices. Two weeks of therapy is usually sufficient. Ciprofloxacin (Cipro), 500 mg orally twice daily, may be used in adults but it should not be used in children because it has been associated with permanent cartilage lesions in immature dogs.

BACTERIAL PNEUMONIA

method of
GEORGE A. SAROSI, M.D.
The University of Texas Health Science Center at Houston
Houston, Texas

Pneumonia is an inflammatory process involving the lung substance. This inflammation is usually produced by bacteria, but fungi, viruses, and parasites may also be involved. Although it is no longer the feared killer of the elderly, pneumonia remains a serious problem, especially among adults.

For convenience, pneumonias are divided into community-acquired and nosocomial pneumonias. Nosocomial pneumonias are acquired in the hospital, after the patient has been hospitalized for at least 72 hours. All other pneumonias are presumably community acquired.

Pulmonary infections are acquired either by inhalation of the microorganism or by aspiration of the infectious agent from the oropharynx. Because aspiration of pharyngeal content is common and aspiration pneumonias are rare, the amount of material must be large to overwhelm the normal defense mechanisms and precipitate illness. Generally, any maneuver that alters or depresses the normal host defenses increases susceptibility to the development of pneumonia (Table 1).

Understanding of the normal host defense mechanisms and recognition of the events that alter these mechanisms result in clearly defined associations. Pneumonia occurring during an epidemic of influenza A is normally caused by either *Staphylococcus* or pneumococcus. Lower respiratory tract illness that follows contact with sick birds should lead the physician to consider psittacosis, whereas exposure to parturient cats should bring Q fever to mind. Similarly, the patient's age and the season are important clues: an infection occurring in the fall in young people is likely to be caused either by mycoplasma or by the newly recognized chlamydia species, *Chlamydia pneumoniae* (TWAR). Eliciting the history of recent travel or unusual occupation or leisure time activity is essential. Recent travel to the southwestern United States should bring to mind coccidioidomycosis, whereas recent spelunking in Puerto Rico or in the southeastern United States should lead to the consideration of histoplasmosis. Knowledge of the bacteriology of previous cases in one's environment is helpful. In certain locations in the United States, *Legionella pneumophila* is common, whereas in other regions this species is seldom seen.

TABLE 1. **Maneuvers That Alter Normal Pulmonary Defenses**

Site and Abnormality	Maneuver
Upper Airway	
↓ Humidification	Tracheostomy
Alteration of normal bacterial flora	Antibiotics, periodontal disease
Interference with closure of glottis	Seizures, hypoglycemia, inebriation, sedatives
Lower Airway	
↓ Mucociliary transport	Smoking, viral infections, chronic bronchitis, immotile cilia
↓ Cough	Obtundation, decreased respiratory muscle strength
Lung Tissue	
↓ Macrophage function	Smoking, acidosis, cytotoxic drugs
↓ Immunologloblulin	Clonal B cell disease
↓ Cell-mediated immunity	Glucocorticoid therapy, Hodgkin's disease, acquired immunodeficiency syndrome

Individuals whose immune system is altered either by illness or by the administration of glucocorticoids or cytotoxic agents represent an important subgroup. It is necessary to recognize that these patients can develop pneumonia like anyone else in a community, but they tend to have more severe illness or may have atypical presentations. Organ transplant recipients are more susceptible to legionellosis, and tuberculosis is still common in this group. Patients with human immunodeficiency virus infection frequently have *Pneumocystis carinii* pneumonia, but it is extremely important to recall that early during the course of this infection, lobar pneumonias caused by the encapsulated microorganisms *Streptococcus pneumoniae* and *Haemophilus influenzae* are common. Among drug abusers with human immunodeficiency virus infection, tuberculosis should be considered.

Altered mental status, such as that seen in chronic alcoholics, insulin-treated diabetics prone to hypoglycemic attacks, or patients with poorly controlled seizure disorders, predisposes the patients to aspiration pneumonia caused by normally occurring oropharyngeal flora. Pneumonia in hospitalized patients, especially patients in intensive care units, that results from aspiration of gastric contents can be caused by aerobic gram-negative enteric organisms that have colonized the oropharynx, in addition to the usual anaerobes.

Pneumonias occurring in nursing home residents may be identical to those seen in the community at large. However, the less able the patients are to care for themselves, the more likely is the oropharynx colonized by gram-negative enteric organisms. In these patients the frequency of pneumonias caused by these enteric organisms is high, with the pneumonia occurring presumably secondary to aspiration of contaminated oropharyngeal contents.

GENERAL APPROACH TO THE PATIENT

It is important to remember that the definite diagnosis of pneumonia is seldom possible when the illness is first recognized. Every attempt should be made to obtain a good sputum sample. An acceptable sputum sample, when examined by Gram's stain, should show more than 25 neutrophils and fewer than 10 epithelial cells per low-power field (except in neutropenic patients). Examination of such a specimen frequently points to the proper direction, but it is important to realize that even the best sputum specimen can give only a presumptive diagnosis. Sputum should be taken to the laboratory immediately, and cultures should be set up to avoid overgrowth by oropharyngeal organisms, which may obscure the real pathogen. The definite diagnosis of pneumonia can be accomplished only when a pathogen is recovered from either blood cultures or other biologic material from a normally sterile site, such as a pleural effusion. Detection of pneumococcal antigen from serum or urine can also establish the etiology of the infection.

The chest roentgenogram is usually helpful in suggesting the etiologic agent. Lobar or segmental consolidation is usually caused by the pneumococcus, with similar abnormalities seen in pneumonias caused by

H. influenzae, Klebsiella pneumoniae, and *L. pneumophila.* Unfortunately, most roentgenograms show only nonspecific infiltrates. Multiple nodules may be caused by fungi or by *Staphylococcus aureus.* In the final analysis, the chest roentgenogram can only suggest, but seldom establish, the definite etiology.

TREATMENT

Because an initial specific diagnosis is seldom possible, empiric treatment should consist of adequate antimicrobial coverage for the most likely pathogens. There is no single antibiotic that covers *all* possible etiologic agents, so a combination of at least two agents is needed. My empiric treatment for community-acquired pneumonia consists of 500 mg of erythromycin every 6 hours and 2.0 grams of cefonicid (Monicid) once daily, administered intravenously. This combination deals with practically every likely etiologic agent, except for chlamydiae and rickettsia that causes Q fever. If there is a strong epidemiologic reason to suspect either of these two organisms, I add tetracycline, 500 mg every 6 hours. If I strongly suspect that *Legionella* is the likely cause, I increase the dose of erythromycin to 1 gram every 6 hours; the addition of rifampin,* 600 mg every 12 hours,† is recommended by some experts. Because life-threatening legionellosis occurs primarily in recipients of organ transplants, in our hands administration of rifampin has been difficult because of its interaction with cyclosporin A.

When the history is clearly that of an aspiration pneumonia occurring outside of the hospital, my choice is penicillin G, 2 million units every 4 hours for 2 weeks, followed by penicillin V by mouth for another 4 weeks. An acceptable alternative regimen would be clindamycin (Cleocin), 600 mg every 8 hours.

When the pneumonia develops in the hospital, especially if it develops after a prolonged stay in the intensive care unit or after intubation, the offending agent is most likely an enteric organism or a methicillin-resistant staphylococcus. Empiric treatment should include a third-generation cephalosporine, such as cefotaxime (Claforan), ceftizoxime (Cefizox), ceftazidime (Fortaz, Tazicef), for the enteric organisms and vancomycin (Vancocin), 1 gram every 12 hours, for the staphylococcus.‡ If *Pseudomonas aeruginosa* has been plaguing the hospital, it is wise to add an antipseudomonal penicillin such as azlocillin (Azlin), or piperacillin (Pipracil).

Once the etiologic agent has been identified,

---

*This use is not listed by the manufacturer.
†May exceed manufacturer's recommended dose.
‡This is a common "average" dose but it should be based on renal function.

usually because of a positive blood culture, treatment should be changed to the simplest schedule possible that is consistent with adequate coverage. When possible, a single agent should be used.

SPECIAL CONSIDERATIONS

A few words are necessary to reduce confusion and keep hospital costs down. In community-acquired pneumonia, once the initial cultures fail to help and the patient is being given broad-spectrum empiric treatment, no further sputum cultures are needed. All such cultures would show resistant gram-negative rods, which usually have very little to do with the underlying pneumonia.

It is also important to remember that chest roentgenograms take a long time to clear and that the infiltrate may lag behind clinical improvement. If the patient is improving, there is no need to repeat the chest roentgenogram. On the other hand, a single repeat chest film is in order around 6 weeks after start of therapy (when most previously normal chest roentgenograms have returned to normal) to make sure that the pneumonia was not the result of an obstructing endobronchial lesion.

VIRAL RESPIRATORY INFECTIONS

method of
FREDERICK W. HENDERSON, M.D.
*University of North Carolina School of Medicine
Chapel Hill, North Carolina*

Viral respiratory infections are the most common cause of acute illness in persons of all ages. Clinically, symptoms and signs are frequently limited to the upper respiratory tract; in a subset of patients, findings indicative of more generalized involvement of both the upper and lower respiratory tracts are present. When disease of the lower respiratory tract is present, signs and symptoms predominantly reflect involvement of airways (as in croup, bronchitis, bronchiolitis, bronchopneumonia); evidence of diffuse alveolar disease is usually seen only in patients with influenza A virus infections.

In the normal host, viral respiratory infections are self-limited and usually benign. Otitis media and sinusitis are reasonably common bacterial complications of these infections; bacterial pneumonia is an infrequent complication of viral respiratory disease. Children younger than 1 year of age, the elderly, and patients with underlying chronic pulmonary disease, anatomic abnormalities of the respiratory system, cardiac malformations, or chronic heart disease are at increased risk of critical impairment of functional status by viral respiratory infections. Patients with disorders associated with compromised immune function may be at risk for severe or progressive viral infections.

Respiratory syncytial virus (RSV), types A and B influenza viruses, parainfluenza viruses, adenoviruses, rhinoviruses, herpes simplex virus, coxsackieviruses, echoviruses, and coronaviruses are all important causes of acute upper respiratory disease. Most viral lower respiratory tract infections are caused by RSV, the influenza and parainfluenza viruses, and, less frequently, specific serotypes of adenovirus. In hosts with compromised immune function, RSV, parainfluenza virus type 3, and type A influenza virus can cause progressive pulmonary infections. In addition, cytomegalovirus, varicella-zoster virus (VZV), and herpes simplex virus, agents that are infrequently associated with disease of the lower respiratory tract in the competent host, can cause life-threatening disease of the lower respiratory tract in the immunocompromised individual.

Techniques for rapid diagnosis of viral respiratory infections have been developed for several of these agents. The most widely available tests are those for diagnosis of RSV infection.

SPECIFIC TREATMENTS

Three antiviral compounds are available that are active against respiratory disease agents: amantadine (Symmetrel) for type A influenza virus infections, ribavirin (Virazole) for RSV infections, and acyclovir (Zovirax) for herpes simplex and VSV infections. Of these, amantadine and acyclovir can be used prophylactically or therapeutically. A specific human immune globulin preparation (varicella-zoster immune globulin) is available for prophylaxis of VSV infections in immunocompromised hosts.

Influenza Immunization

Patients at risk for severe illness in association with influenza virus infection should be immunized each fall with inactivated influenza vaccine. Groups at risk include the following adults: those with chronic pulmonary or cardiac conditions; residents of nursing homes and other chronic care facilities; those with chronic renal disease, diabetes, or anemia; immunosuppressed patients; and healthy persons older than 65 years of age. Children at risk are those with underlying chronic heart, lung, or kidney disease; diabetes and metabolic diseases; hematologic diseases and malignancies; and disorders associated with immunodeficiency; as well as children receiving long-term salicylate treatment. Household contacts of patients at risk for severe influenza virus disease should be immunized annually because they may transmit influenza to the susceptible person. Influenza immunization is also recommended for health care personnel who have contact with patients in high-risk groups to reduce the likelihood of their transmitting infection to these susceptible persons.

Amantadine

Prophylactic administration of amantadine should be considered for any person for whom influenza immunization is recommended who has not received the required annual dose of influenza vaccine. Amantadine prophylaxis may be initiated when there is clinical or epidemiologic evidence of influenza virus activity within the community, school, work place, or nursing home, and particularly when acute respiratory disease occurs in members of the family of the high-risk patient. Prophylactic use of the drug is recommended for 5 to 7 weeks during periods of high risk of exposure to influenza A infection. Amantadine can also be administered therapeutically to patients with acute type A influenza respiratory disease. The duration of fever and malaise is shortened in persons who begin amantadine treatment early in the course of illness. Amantadine is not effective in persons with acute respiratory disease caused by agents other than influenza A viruses, including influenza B virus.

The dose of amantadine is 100 mg by mouth twice a day in persons older than 9 years of age and younger than 65 years of age. Persons 65 years old and older should receive 100 mg per day. In children younger than 9 years old the dose is 4.0 to 8.0 mg per kg per day (not to exceed 150 mg per day) in two divided doses. The drug is administered for 2 to 5 days, depending on clinical improvement. Amantadine is excreted by the kidney; the interval between doses should be modified in persons with reduced creatinine clearance. Persons with seizure disorders may have an increased risk of seizures when given amantadine; side effects reported most frequently during amantadine treatment are nausea, dizziness, and insomnia.

Ribavirin

Ribavirin (Virazole) is approved for administration to infants with severe disease of the lower respiratory tract caused by RSV. Optimally, rapid diagnostic techniques for RSV should be available in hospitals where use of ribavirin is anticipated. In placebo-controlled clinical trials, ribavirin treatment has been associated with more rapid improvement in clinical status in normal infants and in infants with underlying cardiopulmonary disease who have RSV infections of the lower respiratory tract. However, the magnitude of the differences in rates of clinical resolution of signs and symptoms has been small. The American Academy of Pediatrics now recommends considering ribavirin treatment in hospitalized infants "at high risk for severe or complicated RSV infection," including those with congenital heart disease, bronchopulmonary dysplasia, and other chronic lung diseases; certain premature infants; those with significant immunodeficiency; and hospitalized infants who are severely ill who have lower respiratory tract infections with RSV. Infants with Pa_{O_2} less than 65 mmHg or rising Pa_{CO_2} should be considered candidates for therapy. Treatment might be considered for infants with RSV infection but without severe lower respiratory tract infection who might be at increased risk of progressing to a complicated or severe course because of underlying cardiopulmonary or neurologic disease or very young age (<6 weeks). Ribavirin is administered as an aerosol (20 mg per ml in a nebulizer) via an oxygen hood or tent for 12 to 18 hours a day for 3 to 7 days. A specific small particle aerosol generator is provided by the manufacturer for administration of the drug. The drug is not approved for patients who are using mechanical ventilators because precipitation of the drug in ventilator circuits may cause malfunction. High levels of drug are achieved in respiratory secretions, but ribavirin is not detectable in serum or urine of treated patients; no systemic side effects of aerosol treatment have been identified. Because ribavirin is present in the air in rooms where the drug is being aerosolized, pregnant women should not be involved in the care of children receiving ribavirin because the drug is teratogenic.

Acyclovir

Acyclovir (Zovirax) is active against herpes simplex virus types 1 and 2 and VZV. The drug should be considered in immunosuppressed patients who are infected with HSV or VZV, including those with immunodeficiency diseases, hematologic malignancies, and organ or bone marrow transplants because of the risk of progressive infection, including development of pneumonia. The dose of acyclovir administered intravenously is 15 mg per kg per day* divided in three equally spaced doses. Acyclovir is available for oral administration, but this preparation is not recommended for treatment of uncomplicated upper respiratory tract infections caused by herpes simplex virus in the normal host. Because the drug is eliminated by the kidney, the interval between doses should be increased in persons

---

*Dose must be reduced with renal impairment.

with renal impairment. Output of reasonable volumes of dilute urine should be maintained in all patients receiving acyclovir.

Varicella-Zoster Immune Globulin

This product is effective in preventing or ameliorating varicella infections in immunocompromised patients who lack antibody to VZV and who have been exposed to persons with varicella or zoster infections. High-risk patients should have varicella antibody titers assayed shortly after they are identified as having illnesses that increase their risk of severe varicella infection. Varicella-zoster immune globulin should be administered to seronegative high-risk patients as soon as possible after exposure to VZV.

TREATMENT OF SYMPTOMS ASSOCIATED WITH VIRAL RESPIRATORY INFECTIONS

Fever, malaise, and sore throat associated with viral respiratory infections can usually be controlled satisfactorily with acetaminophen (325 to 650 mg per dose given orally every 4 to 6 hours in adults or 6 to 10 mg per kg per dose in infants and children). Aspirin should not be given to children with febrile respiratory disease during the late fall, winter, or early spring. These patients may have influenza virus infections and may therefore be at increased risk for the development of Reye's syndrome if aspirin is given. For the same reason, aspirin should not be given to children with chickenpox. I rarely recommend topical or systemic antihistamines, decongestants, or cough suppressants for patients with acute respiratory illnesses. Risks associated with their use—drowsiness, jitteriness, rebound nasal congestion, and reduced clearance of lower respiratory tract secretions—probably outweigh any perceived benefit with respect to symptom abatement in most patients. Antihistamines and decongestants do not decrease the risk of developing otitis media, nor do they increase the rate of resolution of middle-ear effusion in patients who develop otitis during acute respiratory illnesses.

VIRAL AND MYCOPLASMAL PNEUMONIAS

method of
W. PAUL GLEZEN, M.D.
Baylor College of Medicine
Houston, Texas

VIRAL PNEUMONIA

Respiratory virus infection can be implicated in the etiology of a large proportion of pneumonia episodes in adults as well as children. Although the death rate attributed to pneumonia has been declining in recent years, the frequency of occurrence has remained high and essentially unchanged. The overall rate has ranged from 1.0 to 1.6 per 100 persons per year, with the higher rates occurring during years when influenza virus epidemics were more intense. These rates can be translated to totals of 2.5 to 3.3 million episodes per year in the United States. The seasonal occurrence of these pneumonia episodes implicates etiologic roles for certain respiratory viruses; 85 per cent of pediatric pneumonia cases have occurred during the relatively discrete outbreaks caused by influenza, parainfluenza, and respiratory syncytial (RS) viruses, whereas 40 per cent of adult pneumonia cases occurred during annual influenza virus epidemics. Knowledge of the seasonal pattern of occurrence of these viruses, their major clinical manifestations, and the usual age distribution for these manifestations aids etiologic assessment of patients with pneumonia. Outbreaks of parainfluenza virus Types 1 and 2 have occurred in the autumn (usually odd-numbered years only) and were accompanied by epidemics of croup in children between 6 and 24 months of age. RS virus epidemics have occurred in winter and were most evident by the common manifestation of bronchiolitis in infants. Influenza epidemics can be charted by frequent bulletins published by public health officials. Influenza epidemics are usually heralded by the increased frequency of febrile respiratory illnesses in school-age children and young adults and come in midwinter after the peak of RS virus activity. Parainfluenza virus Type 3 activity has been greatest in the spring, after activity of the other major viruses has declined.

RS virus is the most common cause of pneumonia in infancy. The illness usually commences with rhinorrhea, low-grade fever, and cough for 2 or 3 days followed by a progressive increase in respiratory rate and development of subcostal and intercostal retractions. The chest roentgenogram reveals scattered peribronchial and perihilar infiltrates, involving multiple lobes. Air trapping may be present. Diffuse interstitial infiltrates may be present, but scattered linear shadows resulting from subsegmental areas of atelectasis are probably more common. Atelectasis of the right upper lobe or middle lobe is not uncommon. Influenza and parainfluenza viruses may give a similar picture but are less likely to produce air trapping than RS virus. Most of these illnesses are self-limited and resolve within 3 weeks. Some adenoviruses (Types 1, 2, 5, and 6) may give a similar clinical picture, but Types 3,

7, and 21 may produce a destructive process that results in obliterative bronchiolitis with permanent damage to the lungs. Measles virus pneumonia in infancy may produce a similar process. Pneumonitis caused by *Chlamydia trachomatis* should be differentiated from viral pneumonias in infants. *C. trachomatis* pneumonitis has an afebrile and indolent course with progressive cough and respiratory distress during 2 to 3 weeks. Infants with this infection usually present between 6 to 12 weeks of age and often have a history of conjunctivitis during the first 2 weeks of life. Influenza viruses are the most common cause of viral pneumonia in adults in civilian populations, but adenovirus Types 4 and 7 have been predominant types in military recruits. Onset usually occurs with fever (temperature up to 39° C) with chills and muscle aches, dry hacking cough, pharyngitis, and conjunctival irritation. Influenza commonly involves the trachea and major bronchi and is accompanied by pneumonitis in about 5 per cent of persons. Influenza pneumonitis may progress rapidly with paroxysmal cough, breathlessness, and thin, bloody sputum. Secondary bacterial invasion is common. The major bacterial pathogens involved are pneumococci, staphylococci, and *Haemophilus influenzae*. Pneumonitis may also be present in approximately 15 per cent of adults with varicella.

Treatment

Ribavirin (Virazole) is a broad-spectrum antiviral drug that is licensed for treatment of RS virus pneumonia and bronchiolitis. The drug is administered by small particle aerosol, which limits its use to hospitalized patients. Use is further limited by cost, so that treatment is recommended particularly for persons who are likely to develop life-threatening infections. Because ribavirin is teratogenic and dispersed throughout the room, health care workers who are pregnant should not prepare or administer it and should avoid rooms where it is being given. Antigen detection by enzyme-linked immunosorbent assay allows rapid identification of infected patients. The patients who are recommended for treatment include infants with congenital heart disease, bronchopulmonary dysplasia, or other chronic lung conditions; infants less than 6 weeks of age; and immunocompromised patients of any age, particularly patients undergoing bone marrow transplantation or patients with acquired immunodeficiency syndrome. Any child presenting with Pa_{O_2} levels less than 65 mmHg or with increasing Pa_{CO_2} levels should be considered for therapy. The drug can be administered successfully through a ventilator, but its use must be monitored closely by trained respiratory therapists. Ribavirin also has been demonstrated to be effective against influenza viruses A and B and parainfluenza viruses. Ribavirin aerosol should be considered for treatment of hospitalized patients with life-threatening infections with these viruses.

Amantadine (Symmetrel), another licensed antiviral drug, is effective against influenza A viruses. The drug is administered orally and can be prescribed for hospitalized patients or ambulatory patients. To have a therapeutic effect, the drug should be started as early as possible in the course of the illness. The dose for children is 5 mg per kg body weight per day administered in two divided doses for 5 days. The total dose should not exceed 150 mg per day for children younger than 10 years of age. For persons aged 10 years or older, the daily dose is 100 mg twice daily. Adults may be given 200 mg as a loading dose to initiate therapy, followed by 100 mg twice daily for 5 days. The dose in elderly patients (older than 65 years) should be 100 mg once daily. Amantadine is not effective for influenza B virus or other respiratory viruses. Amantadine is well tolerated when administered in these dosages, but an occasional patient (about 1 in 20) may complain of nervousness, insomnia, anorexia, or nausea. These symptoms disappear when the drug is stopped. Rimantadine, an analogue of amantadine, should be licensed soon; because of its slower absorption, rimantadine therapy is generally free of the side effects attributed to amantadine. Rimantadine is equally effective for treatment of influenza A virus infections.

Hospitalization is recommended for all infants younger than 4 months of age with lower respiratory tract disease. Only about 10 per cent of patients above that age with viral pneumonia require hospitalization, but bed rest and careful follow-up are recommended until improvement is clinically obvious. Telephone contact, at least, is important during the first few days to watch for signs of bacterial superinfection, which would be indicated by persistence or exacerbation of fever, increased respiratory rate, decreasing appetite, and general deterioration. If any suspicious signs or symptoms occur, the patient should be seen and re-evaluated.

For children we have found certain clinical features to help in differentiating viral infection from bacterial infection. A scoring system has been developed that can assist the physician to decide about initiating antibiotic therapy. The chest x-ray film is scored for features that are characteristic of bacterial or viral pneumonia. Positive scores are applied for features of bacterial infections and negative scores for features of viral infections. The outline for the scoring system is shown in Table 1.

The scores for the chest film are summed and additional positive scores of +1 are added for total white blood cell count of 20,000 per mm^3 or more, absolute polymorphonuclear neutrophil (PMN) count of 10,000 per mm^3 or more, immature PMN count of 500 per mm^3 or more, temperature of 103° F or higher. For hospitalized children 6 months of age or older, another +1 is added. A score of 0 or less usually indicates a viral infection, whereas a score of 1 or more usually indicates a bacterial infection. Viral pneumonias for the common etiologies have yielded average scores ranging from −1.5 to −3.0. In contrast, pneumococcal pneumonias averaged +4.4 and staphylococcal pneumonias averaged +6.3. Pneumonia caused by *H. influenzae* Type b had scores that averaged only +1.5 and may be the most difficult to distinguish from viral infections. Low total white blood cell counts (<5000) were encountered with both influenza virus infections and staphylococcal pneumonias in infants. Because bacterial superinfection may occur during the course of a viral infection, reassessment may be necessary at intervals if the patient's condition is not improving.

When clinical assessment can be combined with methods for rapid detection of viral and bacterial polysaccharide antigens in respiratory secretions, the diagnosis may be clear-cut and treatment can be rationally applied. The presence of a predominant bacterial pathogen in the upper respiratory tree (nasopharynx or trachea) does not establish the diagnosis of bacterial pneumo-

TABLE 1. **Scoring System for Pediatric Chest X-ray Films***

Characteristic	Score
1. Infiltrate	
a. Well-defined lobar, lobular, segmented (rounded)	+2
b. Poorly defined, patchy, lobular, alveolar	+1
c. Interstitial, peribronchial	−1
2. Location	
a. Single lobe	+1
b. Multiple lobes in one or both lungs but as in 1a	+1
c. Multiple sites, perihilar as in 1c	−1
3. Fluid in pleural space	
a. Minimal blunting of costophrenic angle	+1
b. Obvious fluid	+2
4. Abscess, pneumatocele, or bullae	
a. Equivocal	+1
b. Definite	+2
5. Atelectasis	
a. Subsegmental (usually multiple sites)	−1
b. Lobar involving right, middle, or upper lobe	−1
c. Lobar involving other lobes	0

*Developed with Dr. Tuenchit Khamapirad.

nia; however, if clinical features of bacterial infection are present, specific therapy can be directed to the predominant bacteria.

Fluid intake should be encouraged to maintain adequate hydration. Cough depressants are not recommended for children younger than 2 years of age, but an antitussive such as dextromethorphan may be used in older children and adults who are afebrile and have a persistent, nonproductive cough. Aspirin is not recommended for children, but an antipyretic such as acetaminophen may be used for temperatures of 102° F or higher. Antipyretics should not be used routinely at any age because regular use may mask the early signs of bacterial superinfection.

For patients who require hospitalization because of respiratory distress or systemic toxicity, baseline arterial blood gas values should be obtained to assess the need for oxygen therapy. Supplemental humidified oxygen should be administered to maintain the arterial P_{O_2} value between 80 and 100 mmHg. If the P_{CO_2} value climbs to 40 or 45 mmHg, tracheal intubation and ventilatory assistance may be necessary. Bronchodilators should be administered to infants with caution; these medications should be stopped if clear evidence of benefit is lacking. Chest physical therapy is recommended only for patients with lobar atelectasis.

MYCOPLASMAL PNEUMONIA

Mycoplasma pneumoniae is probably the most common cause of pneumonia in school-age children and young adults who are free of chronic underlying conditions. It is rarely seen in infants but is occasionally present in preschool children and older adults. The agent has been responsible for indolent, smoldering epidemics that often begin in summer and peak in autumn. Cases may occur at any time of the year but are unusual from midwinter through spring.

The average incubation period, which usually includes prodromal symptoms, is 18 days. Onset of symptoms is gradual and starts with a scratchy sore throat and intermittent low-grade fever for a few days before a dry cough begins. Cough, malaise, and low-grade fever gradually become more persistent and severe during several more days. On examination of the chest, rales are usually present in both lower lobes, and the chest roentgenogram often shows bilateral patchy infiltrates, usually involving the lower lobes. Cold agglutinin titers of 1:32 or higher support the diagnosis of *M. pneumoniae* infection.

Treatment

Most patients do not require hospitalization for treatment of mycoplasmal pneumonia. Both erythromycin and tetracycline are effective antibiotics. Erythromycin is preferred for children under 10 years of age because of the problem of tetracycline-caused staining of teeth in younger children. Either antibiotic can be used for older children and adults. Usually 7 days of therapy is adequate. Rest at home with plenty of fluids is usually adequate supportive care. Antitussives may be required in some cases, with attention to cautions mentioned earlier. Children with sickle cell disease when they are infected with *M. pneumoniae* may present with a clinical picture similar to that of an acute bacterial pneumonia, and this possibility should be kept in mind when patients with hemoglobinopathies develop pneumonia.

M. pneumoniae infection may be accompanied by nonpneumonic complications such as erythema multiforme, Stevens-Johnson syndrome, central nervous system disorders, and hematologic problems such as hemolysis and thrombocytopenia.

LEGIONELLOSIS
(Pontiac Fever and Legionnaires' Disease)

method of
JOYCE A. KORVICK, M.D.
University of Kentucky School of Medicine and
VA Medical Center
Lexington, Kentucky

Legionellosis refers to disease caused by bacteria belonging to the family Legionellaceae. *Legionella pneumophila* causes two well-defined clinical syndromes: legionnaires' disease and Pontiac fever.

Since the discovery of *L. pneumophila* in 1977, thirteen additional species have been isolated in culture from patients with pneumonia: *L. micdadei, L. bozemanii, L. dumoffii, L. longbeachae, L. jordanis, L. gormanii, L. feeleii, L. hackeliae, L. maceachernii, L. wadsworthii, L. birminghamensis, L. cincinnatiensis,* and *L. oakridgensis*.

CLINICAL SYNDROME

Pneumonia is the most common clinical manifestation of legionnaires' disease. Extrapulmonary manifestations have also been described, including myocarditis, pericarditis, liver abscess, peritonitis, perirectal abscess, cerebral microabscess, hemodialysis fistula infection, pyelonephritis, and prosthetic valvular endocarditis. Symptoms typically include malaise, weakness, chills, dry cough, and fever. Neurologic symptoms range from headache and lethargy to encephalopathy. Watery diarrhea occurs as a prodromal symptom in up to one-half of cases. The degree of illness and severity of pulmonic disease at presentation varies widely. At one extreme, the patient may present with mild cough and slight fever, at the other extreme, with confusion, multisystem failure, and overwhelming pneumonia. The clinical presentation is nonspecific, and specialized laboratory tests are needed for definitive diagnosis. However, the following clues should raise the possibility of legionnaires' disease in the differential diagnosis: (1) Gram's stain of respiratory secretions containing large numbers of neutrophils but few, if any, visible organisms; (2) hyponatremia (serum sodium level less than 130 mEq per liter; (3) failure to respond to beta-lactam or aminoglycoside antibiotics; (4) occurrence in an institution where the potable water is known to be contaminated by *Legionella*. Risk factors include immunosuppression (especially corticosteroids) and cigarette smoking.

Pontiac fever is a nonpneumonic illness. The attack rate is high, and the incubation period is 2 to 4 days. Myalgia, headache, malaise, and fever are presenting symptoms. It is not fatal; recovery usually occurs within 2 days without specific antibiotic therapy. Diagnosis is based on seroconversion to *Legionella* in the context of the clinical syndrome.

DIAGNOSIS

Legionella organisms are faintly staining, gram-negative rods. Direct microscopic evaluation of respiratory secretions is accomplished by a fluorescent antibody stain specific for *Legionella*.

These bacteria are fastidious; they require specialized media for growth (buffered charcoal yeast extract agar). Selective agars have been developed that contain antibiotics and suppress the growth of competing bacteria and dyes that color the *Legionella* colonies. Serologic testing can be a useful adjunct to direct isolation of the organism. However, in most cases this is a retrospective tool requiring serum from both acute and convalescent stages. A DNA probe that identifies *Legionella* in respiratory secretions is now available commercially, but sensitivity and specificity have not been adequately evaluated. A radioimmunoassay for detection of *Legionella* antigen in the urine is also commercially available. Preliminary studies suggest that sensitivity and specificity are comparable to those of the direct fluorescent antibody stain. Urine can be obtained with minimal risk to even the most uncooperative or disoriented patient. At present the test identifies only *L. pneumophila* serogroup 1.

THERAPY

Erythromycin is the drug of choice for legionnaires' disease (Table 1). Controlled trails have never been performed, and this recommendation is based on the lower case/fatality ratio among patients receiving erythromycin during the 1976 outbreak. The duration of therapy is 14 to 21 days. Twenty-one-day therapy is recommended for immunocompromised patients and recipients of transplants. Relapses in this population have occurred with shorter courses of erythromycin.

Combination therapy (erythromycin and rifampin) is recommended in patients with severe disease. Rifampin is very active against *Legionella* but should not be administered alone because of the potential for the development of resistance.

Alternative drugs include doxycycline, trimethoprim-sulfamethoxazole, quinolones, and imipenem. Although no clinical trials have been performed, these antibiotics have been reported to be successful in isolated cases. All have been reported to achieve therapeutic levels in the alveolar macrophage. *Legionella* is an intracellular pathogen, and thus effective anti-*Legionella* agents must penetrate the macrophage to reach their targets.

The majority of patients with *Legionella* prosthetic valvular endocarditis require valve replacement in addition to therapy with erythromycin and rifampin. Two months of intravenous therapy with an additional 6 months of oral therapy is recommended.

TABLE 1. **Antibiotic Therapy for *Legionella* Pneumonia**

Antibiotic	Dose	Route
First Choice		
Erythromycin*	1 gram q 6 hr	Intravenous
(Erythrocin)	500 mg q 6 hr	Oral
Second Choice†		
Ciprofloxacin	750 mg q 12 hr	Oral‡
(Cipro)		
Doxycycline	100 mg q 12 hr	Oral
(Vibramycin, Vivox)		
Imipenem-cilastatin	500 mg q 6 hr	Intravenous
(Primaxin)		
Tetracycline	0.5–1 gram q 6 hr	Oral
(Achromycin, Sumycin)		
Trimethoprim-sulfamethoxazole	160/800 mg q 8 hr	Intravenous
(Septra, Bactrim)	160/800 mg q 12 hr	Oral

*For severe illness combine with rifampin (Rifadin) 600 mg every 12 hr orally.
†Clinical experience is limited with these agents.
‡For severe illness, use intravenous form when available.

SIDE EFFECTS

Side effects of erythromycin include nausea, diarrhea, phlebitis, and ototoxicity, which is reversible on cessation of the antibiotic. Intravenous administration requires large fluid volumes, which may complicate the fluid management of severely ill patients.

Rifampin is available only in the oral form, and thus bioavailability may be decreased in patients with gastrointestinal dysfunction. Rifampin causes nausea, diarrhea, and elevated liver functions, and it interferes with the metabolism of many drugs. Rash, fever, leukopenia, hemolysis, and anemia are rare but have been reported.

Cyclosporine levels must be monitored closely during treatment of legionnaires' disease in recipients of transplants. Erythromycin raises the cyclosporine serum concentration and may lead to nephrotoxicity, whereas rifampin decreases the serum concentration of cyclosporine, which may contribute to rejection of the transplanted organ.

THERAPEUTIC OUTCOME

The patient should respond with a feeling of well-being and decreasing temperature within 5 days of initiation of therapy. The mortality is 5 per cent in patients receiving appropriate therapy and from 24 to 43 per cent in immunocompromised patients.

PULMONARY EMBOLISM

method of
PETER F. FEDULLO, M.D.
VA Medical Center, University of California Medical Center
San Diego, California

Retrospective analysis suggests that pulmonary thromboembolism is responsible for approximately 200,000 deaths in the United States annually. The incidence of fatal plus nonfatal emboli probably exceeds 600,000. The majority of deaths related to pulmonary embolic disease occur either within 1 hour of the acute event or in those in whom the diagnosis is not considered until autopsy.

DIAGNOSIS

It is important to recognize that the clinical presentation of pulmonary embolism, with the exception of massive pulmonary embolic events, is often nonspecific. This is especially true in the elderly and in those with underlying cardiopulmonary disease, in which the manifestations of pulmonary embolism are often obscured. This lack of specificity of clinical symptoms and signs is a major contributing factor in the unnecessary mortality related to the disease. Pulmonary ventilation/perfusion scanning, often interpreted in terms of "probabilities," can provide only two meaningful pieces of information: (1) a normal perfusion scan excludes the diagnosis of pulmonary embolism; (2) a scan characterized by multiple, mismatched, or segmental or larger defects suggests that diagnosis with a high degree (90 per cent) of certainty. Other ventilation/perfusion scan patterns (single defects, matched defects, subsegmental defects, defects associated with corresponding radiographic abnormalities) can neither suggest nor exclude the diagnosis with reasonable certainty. Recent evidence suggests that scan patterns that were once considered to be of "low or intermediate probability" are associated with a clinically unacceptable incidence of angiographically documented pulmonary embolism.

Additional diagnostic procedures, when clinically indicated, must be pursued. Pulmonary angiography remains the "gold standard" for the diagnosis of pulmonary embolism. The diagnosis of acute venous thrombosis, although not confirming that a pulmonary embolic event has occurred, has the same therapeutic implications as a positive pulmonary angiogram. Negative lower extremity studies, however, cannot exclude the diagnosis of pulmonary embolism. Approximately 30 per cent of patients with angiographically documented pulmonary emboli have negative venographic results.

TREATMENT

Prophylaxis

During the past decade, a number of prophylactic methods have been introduced into clinical practice. To apply these methods optimally, the relative risk of thromboembolism must be determined for the individual patient and appropriate prophylaxis applied based on the degree of risk. Factors that increase risk include (1) general surgical procedures lasting longer than 30 minutes, (2) general surgical procedures in patients older than age 40 years, (3) orthopedic procedures of a lower extremity, (4) transabdominal prostatectomy, (5) a prior history of venous thromboembolism, (6) malignancy, (7) obesity, (8) prolonged immobilization, and (9) chronic congestive heart failure.

Low-dose heparin, 5000 units subcutaneously every 12 hours, has proved to be effective in reducing the incidence of venous thrombosis, pulmonary embolism, and fatal pulmonary embolism in patients undergoing abdominal and thoracic surgical procedures. Low-dose heparin should be started 2 hours before surgery and continued until the patient is fully ambulatory. Low-dose heparin prophylaxis is also effective in reducing the incidence of venous thrombosis in the following nonsurgical patients: (1) patients admitted to the hospital with myocardial infarction, respiratory failure, or a prior history of venous thromboembolism; (2) those with obesity, congestive heart failure, or malignancy; and (3) patients who are immobilized for extended periods of time. Low-dose heparin, by accelerating the inhibitory activity of antithrombin III on Factor X, can inhibit thrombus formation without inducing a systemic anticoagulant effect. Although bleeding complications with low-dose heparin are unusual, populations exist in which even this low risk is unacceptable. These include patients undergoing ophthalmic, spinal, or neurosurgical procedures; trauma victims; patients with an underlying bleeding diathesis; and patients with a hemorrhagic stroke. In these patients, the use of intermittent pneumatic compression (IPC) stockings serves as an essentially risk-free and effective alternative. IPC devices also appear to be the prophylactic method of choice in patients undergoing elective knee surgery and in those undergoing urologic procedures. Before placement of IPC devices, noninvasive evaluation of the lower extremities should be performed to exclude the possibility of asymptomatic venous thrombi, which could be dislodged and embolized by the squeezing action of the stockings. The use of IPC is also contraindicated in advanced peripheral arterial disease.

Patients undergoing neurosurgical or genitourinary procedures are considered to be at moderate risk for the development of venous thromboembolism. Patients with multiple medical risk factors are also considered to be at moderate risk. Available studies indicate that the risk of venous thrombosis and its sequelae escalates as risk factors accumulate. Unfortunately, quantitative data about the additive effect of risk factors in specific populations are not available. In these patients, the frequency of subcutaneous heparin can be increased to an every-8-hour schedule or IPC stockings can be added to subcutaneous heparin administered every 12 hours. The combination of heparin-dihydroxyergotamine appears to have an increased prophylactic effect when compared with heparin alone in patients with multiple risk factors. Vasospastic reactions to dihydroxyergotamine can occur but are rare.

High-risk patients include (1) those with a recent history of venous thromboembolic disease who require surgery, (2) those undergoing orthopedic surgery of a lower extremity, and (3) those undergoing extensive abdominal or pelvic surgery for malignant disease. In these patients, low-dose heparin administered every 8 to 12 hours in addition to IPC should be used. In the high-risk orthopedic population, subcutaneous heparin, administered every 8 hours and adjusted to maintain the activated partial thromboplastin time (aPTT), 6 hours after the subcutaneous dose, between 32 and 36 seconds, has also proved to be effective. A strategy of two-step warfarin therapy has proved to be effective in patients undergoing elective hip or knee surgery. Warfarin is administered for 2 weeks before surgery in a dose sufficient to prolong the prothrombin time 1.5 to 3 seconds longer than control and then to 1.5 times control value immediately after surgery. Aspirin has not proved to be effective as a prophylactic agent. Other prophylactic options include low-molecular-weight dextran, alone or in combination with IPC stockings, and oral anticoagulation.

The "intensity" of any prophylactic regimen must be based on the degree of risk in the individual patient. The higher the thromboembolic risk, the more urgent the need for prophylaxis and the higher the acceptable risk of the prophylactic choice. Selection of any regimen depends on the physician's view of safety and efficacy data.

General Measures

Heparin remains the mainstay of therapy for pulmonary embolism not associated with hemodynamic compromise. With a strong suspicion of embolism based on clinical findings and routine laboratory tests, therapy should be instituted immediately, without awaiting diagnostic confirmation, unless anticoagulation places the patient at clear risk.

Three methods of heparin administration have been advocated: continuous intravenous, intermittent intravenous, and subcutaneous. Continuous intravenous administration has become the method of choice despite lack of definitive evidence that it is safer or more effective than the alternative methods. This method maintains more consistent blood levels, allows for simpler monitoring, and makes dosage adjustments easier. In the adult patient, a 10,000-unit bolus should be administered, followed by a continuous infusion of 1000 units per hour; dose adjustments are determined by subsequent aPTT results. It is currently uncertain whether the risk of hemorrhage (the principal complication of heparin therapy) is related to the degree of anticoagulation as reflected by the results of any monitoring assay. Rather, bleeding appears to be principally related to factors such as the coexistence of a focal (duodenal ulcer disease) or systemic (uremia) bleeding predisposition. Current recommendations, although based on incomplete and potentially misleading data, suggest that the aPTT be prolonged to 1.5 to 2.5 times the control value. Because maintenance of the aPTT within a rigidly defined range does not appear to improve either the efficacy or the safety of the drug, frequent dosage adjustments are not necessary once the dose has been reasonably stabilized with aPTTs within this range. The need for daily aPTTs beyond the first 3 or 4 days of therapy remains unclear. Heparin requirements tend to decrease during the course of therapy with a resultant increase in aPTT levels. Heparin "failure" and embolic recurrence are often related to physician practices that lead to suboptimal anticoagulation. These include (1) failure to begin heparin therapy at the time of initial clinical suspicion; (2) low initial bolus and infusion dosing; (3) delay in measuring the initial aPTT; (4) an inadequate bolus and infusion dosing response to a subtherapeutic aPTT; and (5) excessive heparin dose reductions in response to a high aPTT. Platelet counts should be monitored during heparin prophylaxis and full-dose heparin therapy. Therapy is maintained for 7 to 10 days to allow dissolution and/or organization of the embolus to occur. Bed rest is recommended for at least 3 to 5 days to avoid dislodging and embolizing residual lower extremity thrombi.

The decision to use thrombolytic agents must be weighed against the potential complications associated with their use. Despite extensive study and a clear demonstration that these agents can enhance the rate but not the total extent of thrombolysis, it has not been clearly established that their use alters short- or long-term morbidity and mortality associated with pulmonary embolism.

It is in patients with pulmonary embolism associated with hemodynamic compromise that thrombolytic agents may offer a therapeutic advantage. It is essential that the diagnosis of pulmonary embolism be angiographically confirmed. It is also essential that any contraindications to the use of thrombolytic agents be excluded. These agents increase bleeding risk through the induction of a systemic thrombolytic state. Recent surgery or organ biopsy, trauma (including cardiopulmonary resuscitation), recent stroke, severe hypertension, advanced renal or hepatic disease, and diabetic retinopathy are contraindications to their use.

Two agents are currently available: streptokinase and urokinase. The potential role of newer thrombolytic agents, such as tissue plasminogen activator, which may pose less hemorrhagic risk, remains to be established. If the decision to use thrombolytic agents is made, it is essential that there be a clear understanding of the details of therapy. Ideally, the patient should be monitored in an intensive care setting during the period of infusion. Care should be taken to minimize arterial and venous punctures; pressure should be applied to recent puncture sites. A carefully dressed indwelling arterial catheter can be used for pressure measurements and to obtain blood samples. Central venous catheters, if necessary, should be inserted via a brachial approach. Support with other therapeutic modalities, including supplemental oxygen, intravenous fluids, pressor agents, and antiarrhythmics, should not be neglected.

Heparin is discontinued before initiating thrombolytic therapy. Streptokinase, 250,000 units, is infused over 30 minutes. This is followed by 100,000 units per hour for 24 hours by using a constant infusion pump. Before delivery of the loading dose, 100 mg of hydrocortisone and 50 mg of diphenhydramine (Benadryl) can be administered intravenously to reduce the febrile and allergic responses to the streptococcal antigens. Urokinase, 4400 units per kg of body weight, is infused during 10 minutes. This is followed by a maintenance dose of 4400 units per kg per hour for 12 hours. Unlike monitoring during heparin therapy, there is no discrete therapeutic "range" to attain. It is only necessary to determine that a systemic thrombolytic state has been reached. This can be determined by measurement of the thrombin time, euglobulin lysis time, or aPTT. After the infusion, heparin should be restarted when the aPTT falls to 1.5 times the control value. Thrombolytic therapy does not replace heparin therapy; it is used as an adjunct. When used, thrombolytic agents must be followed by a standard course of intravenous heparin therapy.

Emergency pulmonary embolectomy should be considered only if evidence of severe hemodynamic compromise related to embolism is present that does not respond to supportive measures and thrombolytic agents. The mortality with the procedure is high; it should be attempted only if the equipment and expert personnel required for cardiopulmonary bypass and emergency embolectomy are available.

Postembolic Prophylaxis

The rationale for providing long-term protection is clear: to prevent recurrence of venous thrombosis and, therefore, potential recurrence of embolism. Early recurrence rates are sufficiently high to justify a 6-week course of outpatient anticoagulation in all patients who have experienced an embolic episode. The only possible exception includes a situation in which the predisposition to venous thrombosis has been identified and eliminated, lower extremity venous studies and perfusion scan are normal, and the risk with outpatient anticoagulation is high.

Outpatient anticoagulation should be continued for a minimum of 6 weeks. Because persistence of venous outflow obstruction and pulmonary vascular obstruction represent new risk factors, the patient is re-evaluated at 6 weeks with a perfusion scan and impedance plethysmography (IPG). In patients with negative IPG and normal or near-normal perfusion scan, anticoagulation is discontinued. If venous outflow obstruction persists or if the perfusion scan remains abnormal, anticoagulation is continued for an additional 6 to 12 weeks, at which time the patient is re-evaluated. Although persistently abnormal results suggest some risk of recurrence, small but unknown, a patient-interactive decision is made, usually resulting in discontinuation of anticoagulation. There are no firm data to suggest that the benefits of prolonging anticoagulation beyond this time justify the potential risks.

In patients with an irreversible predisposition to venous thrombosis and in those who have had documented recurrent episodes, anticoagulation for an indefinite period is recommended.

Once the decision to provide postembolic prophylaxis is made, two options are available: oral anticoagulation with warfarin sodium or "adjusted" subcutaneous heparin. On the basis of currently available information, the two options appear equally effective and safe if administered and monitored properly. To be effective, the dose of subcutaneous heparin must be adjusted to maintain the middle interval (6 hours after injection) aPTT at 1.5 times control value. In most patients, the dose of heparin approximates 10,000 units every 12 hours. Standard doses of heparin (5000 units every 12 hours) have not proved to be effective as a means of postembolic prophylaxis. The use of subcutaneous heparin provides a simpler in-hospital transition and does not require frequent outpatient monitoring. Available studies do not indicate that osteoporosis is a significant risk. The heparin effect can be interrupted more promptly than the warfarin effect. This method, however, does require the inconvenience of twice daily injections. The individual patient and practical considerations will determine whether this option is a realistic one.

Oral anticoagulation with warfarin sodium should be started at least 5 days before discontinuing intravenous heparin therapy. The decision to use warfarin should be made early, so that the prothrombin time (PT) is in a therapeutic range for several days before heparin is discontinued. An early decision avoids unnecessary prolongation of the hospital stay as well as the need for large loading doses of warfarin. Therapy is usually started with 10 mg of warfarin per day for several days and is then adjusted based on PT results. Recent evidence suggests that maintaining the PT at 1.3 to 1.5 times control value is as effective in reducing recurrence rates as maintaining the PT at 2 times control value as previously recommended. This lower therapeutic target is also associated with a substantially reduced rate of bleeding complications, approaching that attained with the adjusted subcutaneous heparin option.

Interruption of the Inferior Vena Cava

Inferior vena cava interruption is considered for patients with proven embolism if clinical and perfusion scan assessments suggest that an immediate recurrence may be fatal. It is also indicated when significant bleeding or the risk of bleeding contraindicates anticoagulant use. Embolic recurrence is not an absolute indication for interruption as long as a substantial unobstructed pulmonary vascular bed is present and there is no evidence of cardiopulmonary compromise. Heparin, although capable of preventing thrombus propagation, cannot guarantee against early embolic recurrence from residual lower extremity thrombotic material. Recurrent symptoms during the course of therapy may represent fragmentation and distal migration of the original embolic material as organization and lysis occur. Failure with heparin therapy should not occur if adequate anticoagulation has been maintained.

Ligation and plication procedures should be avoided. Anesthesia and surgery pose a significant risk. Recurrence rates through collateral channels are high, and substantial morbidity ensues from subsequent venous stasis. Ligation procedures can result in acute, life-threatening hypotension from the sudden decrease in circulating blood volume. Transvenous intracaval devices (Mobin-Uddin umbrella and Greenfield's filter) can be placed with the use of local anesthesia and guided into position under fluoroscopic monitoring. Greenfield's filter appears to have a higher patency rate than the Mobin-Uddin umbrella and seems to be technically easier to insert. The procedure used, however, should be that with which the vascular surgeon is most familiar. Greenfield's filter can be placed via a percutaneous femoral approach. Before placement, venography must be performed to exclude the presence of asymptomatic femoral or inferior vena cava thrombosis.

Chronic Thromboembolic Pulmonary Hypertension

The prognosis of the patient with pulmonary embolism in whom therapy is properly instituted is excellent. Morbidity after embolism is uncommon because embolic resolution is the rule. On rare occasions, however, resolution of emboli does not occur. If residual pulmonary vascular obstruction is substantial, the patient may present, months or years later, with evidence of pulmonary hypertension or right ventricular failure.

Many of these patients are unable to provide a history of a discrete thromboembolic event. Many are misdiagnosed as having primary pulmonary hypertension or interstitial lung disease. Chest x-ray and electrocardiographic findings are consistent with right ventricular hypertrophy. Pulmonary function tests may be normal, or they may reveal a restricted pattern. Ventilation/perfusion scanning appears to offer a means of differentiating primary pulmonary hypertension (PPH) from large-vessel, thromboembolic pulmonary hypertension (TEPH). In PPH, perfusion scans are normal or demonstrate a mottled pattern; in TEPH, multiple, mismatched, or segmental or larger defects are invariably present. Pulmonary angiography is indicated in those patients with perfusion scans consistent with TEPH because perfusion scanning cannot provide information concerning anatomic extent of disease and often substantially underestimates the true angiographic extent of pulmonary vascular obstruction.

Although these patients should receive chronic anticoagulation therapy and an inferior vena cava filter should be placed to prevent repeat embolization, thrombolytic therapy is not indicated because of the chronic, fibrotic nature of the thrombi. Patients with main or lobar pulmonary artery involvement, documented by angiography or angioscopy, may be candidates for pulmonary thromboendarterectomy. Patients with suspected TEPH should be evaluated at an institution where the staff is familiar with this form of pulmonary hypertension. Unique difficulties complicate the preoperative evaluation and postoperative care of these patients. Surgical intervention involves a true thromboendarterectomy of chronic, endothelialized thrombus rather than an embolectomy. Results in patients with surgically accessible disease (main or lobar pulmonary arteries) have been excellent and have allowed cure of this otherwise fatal form of pulmonary hypertension.

SARCOIDOSIS

method of
ROBERT P. BAUGHMAN, M.D.
University of Cincinnati
Cincinnati, Ohio

Sarcoidosis is a multisystem disease that can present to the physician in several different ways. The most common manifestations are pulmonary, but other organs can be involved. Treatment for sarcoidosis is determined by the level of involvement of the various organs after complete evaluation. There are some absolute indications for therapy, but in most manifestations of the disease, treatment depends on the level of disease activity (Table 1). In addition, therapy if instituted is for acute disease, although some manifestations of the disease need chronic suppressive therapy after acute treatment.

TREATMENT

Acute Disease

For acute disease that is to be treated with systemic steroids, I start with prednisone, 40 mg daily for 2 months followed by 20 mg of prednisone for an additional 4 months. After that point, I try to taper the patient off the steroids. Most patients are treated for a total of 18 to 24 months with some dose of prednisone. After tapering of steroids, the patient is closely watched for signs of recurrence of disease. Relapse, if it occurs, is usually seen between 3 and 6 months of stopping steroids. However, patients may have a delayed relapse, and I follow patients with inactive sarcoidosis every 6 months for the next few years.

Other dose regimens of prednisone have been used, especially the use of alternate-day steroids. This regimen is most successful for the more sensitive manifestations of sarcoidosis, especially hypercalcemia.

Chloroquine has been successfully used in some forms of sarcoid (not listed in manufacturers' directives). It is often used in patients with only skin sarcoid because the drug has fewer side effects than prednisone. The dose ranges from 250 mg twice a day to 200 mg on alternate days. If a patient is taking chloroquine, eye examinations should be performed on a regular basis to watch for the irreversible retinopathy and blindness that are occasionally seen with chloroquine use.

Chronic Disease

For chronic sarcoidosis, once the disease is under control with a higher dosage of prednisone,

TABLE 1. **Manifestations of Sarcoidosis and Requirement for Treatment**

Manifestation	Treatment
Asymptomatic	None
Pulmonary system	None to chronic
Skin	None to chronic
Hypercalcemia	Acute
Eye	Acute
Heart	Chronic
Central nervous system	Chronic

patients are treated with some dose of corticosteroids, usually 5 to 10 mg every other day for years.

Immunosuppressive drugs have been used in some patients with sarcoidosis in an attempt to avoid steroids, although the use of these agents is not listed in the manufacturers' directives. Several drugs have been used, with most experience reported to date being for chlorambucil (Leukeran). Methotrexate (Folex, Mexate), in dosages similar to those used for rheumatoid arthritis, has also been used with success. The drug can be given orally at a dose of 5 to 10 mg weekly to every 2 weeks. It does not appear necessary to achieve neutropenia. Its major drawback seems to be its slow onset of action; it appears to take more than 1 month of therapy before the symptoms of sarcoidosis are significantly relieved.

In patients who are diagnosed incidentally on biopsy, there is no indication for treatment. These patients should be followed for possible disease activity, usually pulmonary symptoms. Patients should be followed by serial examinations and chest roentgenograms for 2 years after initial diagnosis.

Pulmonary Involvement

The lungs are involved in about 90 per cent of patients with sarcoidosis. The extent of disease can vary, ranging from an asymptomatic state to irreversible pulmonary fibrosis and cor pulmonale. In assessing patients with pulmonary sarcoidosis, the use of gallium scan and bronchoalveolar lavage (BAL) fluid obtained during flexible fiberoptic bronchoscopy has recently been studied as a means of assessing patients' need for therapy. Table 2 summarizes a few possible presentations of pulmonary sarcoidosis and how gallium scan and BAL can be useful in deciding about therapy. Gallium uptake in the lung or an increased percentage of T helper lymphocytes in the BAL fluid appears to indicate the same thing, that the patient has active inflammation in the lung. However, the patient's symptoms and pulmonary function tests (especially the lung volume) are a major factor in deciding whether to treat.

Acute pulmonary disease is usually treated with systemic steroids. The use of aerosolized steroids has been suggested, but more information is necessary. If patients show evidence of deterioration of pulmonary function more than 2 years after their initial presentation, or evidence of cor pulmonale, I assume that they have chronic sarcoidosis. I therefore would treat them for chronic disease as first outlined.

Skin Involvement

Erythema nodosum is not disfiguring, but the associated arthralgias can be bothersome. The arthralgias often respond to nonsteroidal agents such as ibuprofen or aspirin. Skin lesions of the face, especially lupus pernio, require specific therapy. If areas of disease are small, creams or intradermal injections may control disease. Chloroquine is useful for skin sarcoidosis, mainly because it is easy to evaluate this drug's efficacy. Some aggressive forms of skin sarcoid, especially lupus pernio, require systemic steroids. Lupus pernio has a high frequency of relapse and can be a troublesome, lifetime manifestation of disease. Methotrexate appears to be a useful drug for this problem.

Hypercalcemia

This unusual but specific problem of sarcoidosis is due to alteration in vitamin D metabolism by the granulomas themselves. In patients with hypercalcemia, increased calcium or vitamin D in the diet or increased sunshine may make the hypercalcemia worse and should be avoided. Steroids are quite effective in treating the hypercalcemia. A recent report suggests that chloroquine can also be useful.

Ocular Involvement

Patients with eye symptoms are best treated in consultation with an ophthalmologist. Slit lamp examination is crucial in determining whether a posterior uveitis is present. If not, and if the patient has only conjunctivitis or anterior uveitis, optic drops of steroids may lead to a good

TABLE 2. **Proposed Treatment Decisions for Patients with Pulmonary Sarcoidosis**

Pulmonary Function Tests	Symptoms	BAL or Gallium Scan	Treatment
Normal	Absent	Positive	Watch
Mildly reduced	Absent	Negative	Watch
Mildly reduced	Present	Positive	Treat
Moderately reduced	Present	Positive	Treat
Moderately reduced	Present	Negative	Treat

response. However, if posterior uveitis or retinitis is present, the patient probably requires systemic steroids.

Cardiac Involvement

Documentation of cardiac disease is often difficult. Patients may present with cardiac arrhythmias or heart failure. In patients with known sarcoidosis, clinical symptoms including palpitations and congestive heart failure may require further work-up. In patients with documented or strongly suspected cardiac sarcoid, the treatment of choice is long-term steroids.

Central Nervous System Involvement

Involvement of the central nervous system usually manifests itself as a cranial nerve palsy; however, diabetes insipidus and seizures are also manifestations. Treatment is usually steroid therapy. It may take several months before any response is noted. In cases in which disease is entirely limited to the brain, radiation therapy has been tried with limited success.

SILICOSIS

method of
DOUGLAS SEATON, M.D.
The Ipswich Hospital
Suffolk, England

Silica, or silicon dioxide, is the most abundant mineral constituent of the earth's crust. As such, it exists in different physical forms, the most common being quartz. Silicosis is a mineral dust disease, or pneumoconiosis, that is caused by inhalation of particles of silica of respirable size. Casual contact with silica dust is insufficient to cause the disease, which requires continued exposure that may arise in the occupations indicated in Table 1. Miners, tunnelers, and quarry workers whose excavations involve the removal of quartz-bearing rock such as sandstone, granite, and slate are at risk, as are workers who cut, crush, finish, or clean such stone. The mouldings used for castings in foundries are made from bonded sand, and the heat of the molten metal that is poured into them produces

TABLE 1. **Some Occupations and Industries Associated with a Risk of Silicosis**

Mining	Manufacture of
Tunneling	Silica flour
Quarrying	Pottery and ceramics
Stone masonry	Glass and enamel
Foundry working	Silica-based abrasives
Sandblasting	Refractory bricks

a fused silica compound that is polished off the casting, a task known as fettling. Fettlers and other foundry workers may also be exposed to silica dust when replacing the silica brick linings of furnaces and kilns. These so-called refractory bricks are produced from sandstone, and persons involved in their manufacture may also develop silicosis. The ceramic industry has traditionally used quantities of silica-containing substances such as crushed flint for the manufacture of china and earthenware pottery, although modern substitutes are now being found. Sandblasting involves the production of a high-speed jet of finally ground sand used for cleaning stone and polishing metal. Safe substitutes such as carborundum are available, and the practice of sandblasting has long been illegal in the European Community but may still be practiced in parts of the United States. Finely ground silica, known as silica flour, may be encountered in the manufacture and use of a wide range of substances including polishes, scouring powders, and toothpaste; it is also used as a filler in rubber and plastics. The glass and enamel industries make use of sand and quartz in polishing or as a component.

CATEGORIZATION AND CLINICAL COURSE

The usual form of silicosis occurs after years of exposure to siliceous dust in an occupational setting and is termed "chronic." The condition is frequently unaccompanied by symptoms or signs and may declare itself only as a chance finding on a routine chest radiograph. At an early stage, various numbers of small nodular opacities are seen in the upper and middle zones of the lungs. This radiographic appearance is similar to that found in simple coal workers' pneumoconiosis (CWP), although the opacities in silicosis tend to get larger as time passes even though exposure may have ceased. The opacities, as well as tending to be larger (3 to 10 mm in diameter), are more dense than those in CWP, and calcification of small nodules may be seen. "Simple" chronic silicosis may progress so that numbers of small opacities aggregate to form larger, more conglomerate shadows. When such opacities exceed a diameter of 1 cm on the radiograph, the condition is referred to as "complicated" chronic silicosis, and progressive massive fibrosis (PMF) is said to be occurring. Such larger opacities, which sometimes cavitate, are associated with fibrosis and distortion of surrounding lung with compensatory emphysema and bullae formation. Pleural thickening is sometimes found, as is so-called eggshell calcification of the hilar lymph nodes, a radiographic sign that is almost pathognomonic of silicosis, although it also rarely occurs in sarcoidosis.

Although there is little functional abnormality in simple chronic silicosis, except perhaps when the small opacities are profuse, silicotic PMF is associated with a mixed restrictive and obstructive impairment of ventilatory capacity and a reduction of diffusing capacity (DL_{CO}). These measurable impairments of lung function are matched by exertional dyspnea, which is often accompanied by cough and production of sputum. Further disease progression may result in respiratory failure with pulmonary hypertension and right-sided heart failure, although such advanced disease is now rare except in settings where dust control legislation does not exist or has been blatantly ignored. Chronic silicosis has a protracted time course lasting many years, but a heavier occupational exposure over a few years may produce a similar but more rapid clinical and radiographic progression that is termed "accelerated silicosis." Heavy occupational exposure to silica dust for a few weeks or months may produce an even more aggressive form of disease called "acute silicosis." In acute silicosis the history is one of accelerating breathlessness and cough, usually culminating in respiratory failure within months. Rather than showing the nodular pattern of chronic silicosis, the chest radiograph shows more diffuse shadowing, often in the middle or lower zones, that may be confused with pulmonary edema or bronchopneumonia if the patient's occupation is overlooked.

The course of silicosis may be complicated by tuberculosis, several epidemiologic surveys having established that this infection is more common in patients with silicosis than in matched control populations. This situation probably exists because the main defense against *Mycobacterium tuberculosis* in the lungs is provided by macrophages, for which silica particles are highly toxic. It follows that this complication is likely to be particularly evident in populations in which tuberculosis is endemic, probably as a result of reactivation of old primary infection. A high index of suspicion is advised in advanced silicosis, in which the cavitation of PMF may be tuberculous rather than ischemic and in which soft-looking infiltrates may be part of a tuberculous process, which requires repeated and regular examination and culture of sputum for diagnosis. Opportunistic mycobacterial infections may also occur in endemic areas, *Mycobacterium avium-intracellulare* and *Mycobacterium kansasii* being important pathogens for patients with silicosis in the southeastern United States. Other complications include pneumothorax, which may occur in any disease associated with fibrosis and bullae formation, and scleroderma, which has been reported to occur with increased frequency in silicosis.

PATHOLOGY

The physicochemical processes by which silica exerts its toxic effects in lung tissue are poorly understood. Crystals of quartz are known to be cytotoxic for lung macrophages that ingest them and cause cellular disruption with release of proteases and other inflammatory and fibrogenic factors. The resultant inflammation causes a characteristic histopathologic response, the hallmark of which is the silicotic nodule, an "onion skin" arrangement of hyalinized collagen, reticulin, and fibroblasts that arises close to respiratory bronchioles and pulmonary arterioles. Both the bronchioles and arterioles may be involved and destroyed as the fibrosis progresses. Particles of silica may be demonstrated in the periphery of these nodules by using polarized light and x-ray defraction techniques, but, in an apparent paradox, the amount of silica demonstrated bears no clear relationship to the extent of the fibrotic reaction found. PMF results in large areas of diffuse and coalescent fibrosis surrounded by silicotic nodules. These lesions may cavitate as a result of avascular necrosis. Although the pathology of accelerated silicosis is primarily similar to that of chronic silicosis, the pathology of acute silicosis is quite different, silicotic nodules being either absent or few in number, the alveolar walls containing a mixed inflammatory cell infiltrate, and the alveolar spaces being filled with thick eosinophilic material that gives a positive periodic acid–Schiff stain reaction. A positive reaction is also found in pulmonary alveolar proteinosis, from which acute silicosis may be histologically distinguished by the presence of interstitial pneumonitis. Macroscopically, the lungs in chronic silicosis are pigmented, with areas of pleural fibrosis and adhesions. The hilar nodes are often enlarged and the cut surface of the lung contains hard, fibrotic nodules. PMF is characterized by coalescence of these lesions, and cavitation may be present.

PREVENTION

Avoidance of exposure to respirable silica dust prevents silicosis, and national and international health agencies are concerned first with making employers and workers aware of the hazards and, when a suitable alternative substance cannot be found, with promoting acceptance of an acceptable and enforceable dust standard. The standard of 100 micrograms per m^3 of respirable quartz, although not ideal, is likely to prevent most severe disease. Dust is removed from the environment by enclosure of processes, by good ventilation, and by use of water suppression where appropriate. When this standard cannot be achieved despite these measures, appropriate breathing equipment (including a suit, headgear, and an isolated supply of clean respirable air) should be provided for the worker. In addition to dust control measures, workers in at risk occupations should be protected by evaluation of chest radiographs, taken at not more than intervals of 4 years, so that early radiographic change can be detected and appropriate measures taken to prevent further exposure. Early radiographic changes that have taken many years of exposure to become manifest are not likely to result in much further deterioration, whereas similar changes that have arisen as a result of relatively short but heavier exposure are likely to continue apace with serious consequences for the patient. Acute silicosis is usually fatal within a matter of a few months.

MANAGEMENT

No treatment influences the progress of silicosis once it has developed, and the usual symptomatic measures include antibiotics for the control of acute respiratory infection, bronchodilators if airflow is limited, oxygen when hypoxemia supervenes, and diuretics in right-sided heart failure. Various other, more specific attempts at treatment have been tried with negative or inconclusive results. These include the inhalation of aluminum powder and the use of D-penicillamine or corticosteroids. A negatively charged polymer, polyvinyl pyridine-N-oxide, when inhaled or injected, may prevent silicic acid from bonding with surface components of lung macrophages and has been shown to protect experimental animals from the effects of silica. It has, however, also been found to be carcinogenic in animals. Whole-lung bronchial lavage has been attempted in acute silicosis but is not known to alter the dismal prognosis of this disease, in which the only present hope of prolonging life may be lung transplantation.

Pulmonary tuberculosis complicating silicosis should be treated according to standard therapeutic guidelines. The earliest effective drug regimens appeared to control tuberculosis about as well in patients with silicosis as in those without the disease. Although controlled trials of modern short-course antituberculous drugs are not available for silicosis, these drugs have nevertheless been shown to be effective in tuberculous patients with CWP and are probably also effective in silicosis. Careful follow-up is mandatory in these patients, as in all patients with tuberculosis. After a 2-month induction course with three or four drugs (rifampicin, isoniazid, ethambutol, pyrazinamide), the physician should be prepared to continue the maintenance drugs (usually rifampicin and isoniazid) for longer than the usual 6- or 9-month course, according to the extent of the disease, its apparent response to treatment, and the compliance of the patient.

HYPERSENSITIVITY PNEUMONITIS

method of
HERBERT Y. REYNOLDS, M.D.
Penn State College of Medicine
Hershey, Pennsylvania

Repeated inhalation of various organic dusts or simple chemicals can cause hypersensitivity pneumonitis, also known as extrinsic allergic alveolitis (Table 1). Colorful, descriptive names for the diseases underscore the frequent occupational nature of exposure. This diagnosis implies that the affected subject has acquired a heightened reactivity to the inciting agent and the inflammatory response is located in the alveolar and interstitial portions of the lung and not in the larger conducting airways, which are usually involved in asthmatic diseases. The distinction is important, for extrinsic, IgE antibody-mediated allergic asthma is also a form of hypersensitivity lung disease and can be caused by airborne organic antigens. Exposure to chemicals such as trimellitic anhydride may also cause asthma.

Although many people can be exposed to these common antigens and many will develop specific serum antibodies to them (precipitins are present in 5 per cent of exposed office workers and 30 to >50 per cent of grain handlers, dairy workers, and pigeon or bird handlers), relatively few manifest symptoms of respiratory disease. Sensitization to an organic dust is often insidious, but repeated exposure can produce lung changes of a lymphocytic alveolitis, yet the subject remains asymptomatic. An alveolitis that persists for several years may not cause detrimental lung function, so physicians must weigh this fact before recommending that a change in job or relocation is necessary. Obviously, unique host susceptibility or resistance influences the individual response; this is especially true for younger subjects. Chronic exposure, however, can result in an interstitial, granulomatous, and fibrotic lung disease that is debilitating.

Clinically, two distinct syndromes can occur:

1. An acute reaction, occurring 2 to 6 hours after heavy exposure, consisting of dyspnea, cough, chills, fever (up to 40° C), transient restrictive impairment of pulmonary function, and leukocytosis. In the absence of a repeat exposure, spontaneous recovery occurs in 12 to 24 hours.

2. With chronic exposure, persistent dyspnea, cough, anorexia, weight loss, and progressive pneumonitis can lead to hypoxemia and restrictive lung function. With time the chest radiograph reveals diffuse reticular shadows in the lung fields, but there is no evidence of adenopathy. In the latter chronic form, the diagnosis can be very difficult and considerable detective work may be necessary. Often a visit to the patient's workplace or home is needed. Positive serum precipitins give a clue to the cause but in themselves do not constitute a diagnosis. Airway challenge with the putative antigen may be required for a cause and effect relationship, especially if occupational exposure and possible compensation or litigation are issues.

THERAPEUTIC APPROACH

In the isolated or sporadic case, establishing a firm diagnosis and a putative cause is difficult. Therapy can be simple by comparison. Avoidance is the best treatment if precipitating circumstances are identified. A perceptive subject may do this instinctively and the disease process ends. Problems develop if exposure persists either by the patient's choice or by necessity. For example, pigeon breeders are often so dedicated to their avocation that they accept the respiratory symptoms rather than forgo the hobby of racing birds. This problem is not unlike the asthmatic who is allergic to animal dander but refuses to give up

TABLE 1. **Some Etiologic Agents in Hypersensitivity Pneumonitis**

Major Antigens	Exposure or Source	Disease
Thermophilic bacteria		
Micropolyspora faeni	Moldy hay	Farmer's lung
Thermoactinomyces vulgaris	Moldy grain	Grain handler's lung
M. faeni, T. vulgaris	Mushroom compost	Mushroom worker's lung
Thermoactinomyces sacchari	Moldy sugar cane (bagasse)	Bagassosis
T. vulgaris, M. faeni	Heated water reservoirs	Humidifier or air conditioner lung
Aureobasidium pullulans		
Other bacteria		
Bacillus subtilis	Water	Detergent worker's lung
Bacillus cereus	Water reservoir	Humidifier lung
True fungi		
Cryptostroma corticale	Moldy bark	Maple bark stripper's lung
Aspergillus clavatus	Moldy malt, barley	Malt worker's lung
A. pullulans and *Graphium* sp.	Moldy redwood dust	Sequoiosis
Mucor stolonifer	Moldy paprika pods	Paprika splitter's lung
Penicillium caseii	Cheese mold	Cheese worker's lung
Penicillium frequentans	Moldy cork dust	Suberosis
Aspergillus spores	Water reservoir	Aspergillosis
Animal proteins		
Avian proteins (serum and excreta)	Pigeons, parakeets	Bird breeder's lung
Chicken feathers, serum	Chickens	Chicken plucker's lung
Turkey feathers, serum	Turkeys	Turkey handler's lung
Duck feathers	Ducks	Duck fever
Rat urine, serum	Rats	Rodent handler's disease
Porcine and bovine pituitary protein	Pituitary snuff	Pituitary snuff-taker's lung
Amebae		
Acanthamoeba castellani	Water	Humidifier lung
Naegleria gruberi	Water	Humidifier lung
Bacterial products		
Lipopolysaccharide	Cotton brac	Byssinosis
Streptomyces verticillus glycopeptides	Bleomycin	Bleomycin hypersensitivity lung (in contrast to fibrosis)
Insect products		
Sitophilus granarius	Contaminated grain	Miller's lung (wheat weevil disease)
Chemicals		
Trimellitic anhydride	Plastics	
Toluene diisocyanate	Polyurethane foam or rubber manufacture	Chemical worker's lung
Methylene diisocyanate		

the household dog or cat. People in agricultural jobs, such as dairy farming and grain handling, may not have a ready option of changing employment. Wearing protective face masks has limited usefulness, so environmental reduction of dust in the work place is a better solution for workers. Prophylactic use of inhaled bronchodilator drugs or corticosteroids is not efficacious. As respiratory symptoms after acute exposure are self-limited and subside in 1 or 2 days, no special treatment, including corticosteroids, is necessary.

With repeated exposures, the acute symptoms gradually diminish with succeeding episodes but are then replaced by chronic and persistent ones that may be more subtle to recognize, such as fatigue, poor appetite, dyspnea, and nonproductive cough. Because this subacute, progressive phase of illness can be associated with restrictive lung function, decreased diffusion capacity, radiologic shadowing, and interstitial fibrosis, patient management is similar to that for other forms of diffuse, interstitial lung disease. After establish-

ment of good baseline pulmonary function parameters, and perhaps an analysis of cells in bronchoalveolar lavage fluid (characteristically, a lymphocytic alveolitis is present, featuring an increased percentage of T suppressor cells over T helper cells, alveolar macrophages with foamy-appearing cytoplasm, and slight elevation of the number of mast cells), a trial of corticosteroid therapy is indicated. Prednisone, 60 mg daily (or 1 mg per kg) given as a single oral dose, is begun and continued for 2 to 3 weeks, then tapered during a 2-week interval to a daily dose of 15 to 20 mg. After an interval of 6 to 8 weeks of therapy, pulmonary function should be reassessed along with patient symptoms, and a judgment should be made about continuing therapy for several more months or reducing it unless a relapse occurs. With avoidance of the antigen and corticosteroid therapy, most patients with chronic disease are improved in 6 to 12 months. Other medications, including bronchodilators, are not indicated.

SINUSITIS

method of
DAVID W. KENNEDY, M.D., and
ALAIN H. SHIKHANI, M.D.
The Johns Hopkins Medical Institutions
Baltimore, Maryland

The nose and paranasal sinuses play a major function in the humidification, filtration, and temperature regulation of inspired air. The sinuses are lined with ciliated stratified columnar epithelium and are continuous with the upper respiratory tract through the sinus ostia. Inflammation causes mucosal edema and increased sinonasal secretion. The inflammatory insult may be an upper respiratory tract infection, an acute exacerbation of allergic rhinitis, dental infection or manipulation, or trauma to the sinuses. If sinus obstruction occurs, the retained secretion results in a milieu that is well suited for bacterial growth. Underlying host factors are also significant in the genesis of sinusitis. General predisposing causes include immunodeficiency, acetylsalicylic acid–asthma–polyposis triad, abnormal mucociliary clearance secondary to ciliary structural abnormalities, as in Kartagener's syndrome, or secretory disturbances such as those in cystic fibrosis. Local anatomic factors are also significant. The importance of severe septal deviation has been generally recognized for some time, but localized abnormalities in the area of the anterior ethmoid–middle meatal area appear to be even more important.

The anterior ethmoid–middle meatal complex (ostiomeatal complex) is a key area in the pathogenesis of sinusitis. The ostiomeatal complex contains the narrow channels that provide for mucociliary clearance and ventilation of the anterior ethmoid, maxillary, and frontal sinuses. Relatively minor swelling of the mucosa in this area may lead to frontal or maxillary sinus obstruction and secondary disease within these sinuses. Indeed, in recurrent frontal or maxillary sinusitis, low-grade lingering infection or an area of anatomic narrowing may often be found in the ostiomeatal complex. This area then leads to recurrent acute episodes of sinusitis. It is therefore imperative that this area be carefully evaluated by diagnostic endoscopy and computed tomography (CT) before surgical intervention is contemplated on one of the major (dependent) sinuses. If such an evaluation reveals an underlying ostiomeatal cause for chronic or recurrent disease, intranasal removal of the cause typically allows the secondary mucosal disease to resolve.

Sinusitis can be classified as acute or chronic on the basis of the duration of the infection. The organisms that have been implicated as primary pathogens in acute sinusitis are *Streptococcus pneumoniae, Haemophilus influenzae,* and *Branhamella catarrhalis.* In contrast, chronic sinusitis is usually associated with anaerobes, most commonly *Streptococcus, Veillonella,* and *Corynebacterium* species. It is important to realize that the bacterial growth on cultures obtained from the nose or nasopharynx and growth on those obtained with sinus aspiration or open antrostomy frequently do not correlate, unless gross purulent discharge is visible through the sinus ostium and is available for culture. Hence the decision about initial management is often a clinical one, based on the history and physical examination. There should be a high index of suspicion for fungal sinusitis (e.g., sinusitis caused by *Aspergillus,* bipolaris, mucormycosis) for nonresponders to antibiotic therapy and for immunocompromised patients.

DIAGNOSIS

The symptoms of acute sinusitis are usually localized to the region of the sinus involved and may include discomfort, pain, headache, and tenderness. In infection of deeper structures such as the posterior ethmoids and sphenoid, symptoms are deep in the head or referred to the occiput. Acute sinusitis is also typically accompanied by systemic signs such as fever, leukocytosis, and lassitude. The symptoms of chronic sinusitis, on the other hand, tend to be more vague and poorly localized. In both types of sinusitis, one may have suppurative rhinorrhea, nasal obstruction, postnasal drainage, and pharyngitis. When a sinus is acutely infected, physical examination may reveal sinus tenderness, erythema and swelling of overlying skin, and a purulent nasal exudate. Transillumination sometimes provides information about the condition of the maxillary and frontal sinuses. Endoscopic examination of the nose and the sinuses with the telescope is the most reliable method to differentiate purulence, mucus, serous fluid, and thickened mucosa. Nasal endoscopy is also critical in the evaluation of the key ostiomeatal area and in identification and biopsy of suspicious lesions.

Complementary to the physical examination are radiologic studies including conventional sinus radiographs and CT scans. The conventional (or plain film) examination usually consists of Water's, Caldwell's, lateral, and basal views of the sinuses. These views give excellent visualization of the frontal and maxillary sinuses and moderately good visualization of the sphenoid. However, plain film radiographs provide poor visualization of the ethmoid sinus as a result of density averaging. Plain films are therefore useful for diagnosing frontal and maxillary sinus disease but are of very limited use in the diagnosis of disease in the important area of the ostiomeatal complex.

The most appropriate method for the diagnosis of ostiomeatal complex pathology is CT, and this radiologic study is necessary to diagnose local underlying causes of recurrent or chronic sinusitis. CT is usually best performed after acute changes have been treated. The scan is performed in the coronal plane without intravenous contrast and is viewed with magnification of the sinus area; window settings are similar to those used to visualize the lung. These parameters optimize demonstration of the fine anatomy of the area and allow not only visualization of gross disease but, more important, identification of minor disease and anatomic obstruction in key areas.

Magnetic resonance imaging is not currently the study of choice for the evaluation of sinus disease. Although magnetic resonance imaging is useful in the differentiation of soft tissue disease, it does not demonstrate the bone, whereas CT allows excellent visualization of the fine bony anatomy and its important anatomic variants. Bony changes may also occur as a result of disease. Inflammatory disease typically expands bone and causes a reactive osteitis, whereas bone destruction is more suggestive of a malignant lesion, although such a lesion may also occur with severe infections and with mucoceles. The use of intravenous contrast during sinus CT is indicated if there may be an intracranial complication.

TREATMENT

Nonsurgical Treatment

Early treatment is medical and consists of the use of antibiotics and decongestants and the avoidance of any exacerbating environmental factors. Oral decongestants such as pseudoephedrine are helpful but should be used with care in hypertensive patients. In older male patients, these drugs may cause urinary retention. A nasal spray (e.g., oxymetazoline) may be added but should be used for no more than 3 to 5 days. A broad-spectrum antibiotic is typically chosen to cover the usual sinus pathogens (*H. influenzae,* *S. pneumoniae,* and *B. catarrhalis*). We favor amoxicillin, 500 mg orally three times daily, or erythromycin, 250 mg four times daily plus a sulfonamide, such as gantrisin, 1 gram orally four times daily, for patients who are allergic to penicillins. Cephalosporins such as cephalexin, 500 mg orally four times daily, or cefaclor, 500 mg three times daily, provide an alternative. Like cefaclor, amoxicillin/clavulanate potassium (500 mg three times daily), covers the beta-lactamase–producing organisms. Time-honored remedies such as inhalation of steam or mist are often not prescribed but may aid both comfort and drainage. Patients with signs and symptoms suggestive of allergic sinusitis and patients with persistent chronic sinusitis are also treated with a nasal beclomethasone (Beconase) inhaler.

If medical treatment fails to relieve the symptoms of maxillary sinusitis or pansinusitis, irrigation may be performed. This method washes out the inspissated material and allows for accurate culture. Irrigation is also performed to allow accurate culture in acute sinusitis when a patient is immunosuppressed or has an underlying immunodeficiency.

Acute ethmoid sinusitis, particularly in children, may lead to periorbital or infraorbital abscess, but such a complication is rare outside the pediatric age group. However, acute frontal and sphenoid sinusitis should be considered to be a medical emergency at any age because of the potential for disease in these sinuses to spread intracranially. Patients with acute symptomatic frontal and sphenoid sinusitis are usually hospitalized and given intravenous rather than oral antibiotic therapy. Failure to improve with medical therapy requires surgical drainage. In the case of acute, poorly responding frontal sinusitis, frontal sinus trephine and irrigation are performed. The irrigation catheter may be left in place for several days. In persistent sphenoid sinusitis, sphenoidotomy is performed.

Whereas acute sinusitis frequently demonstrates a heavy bacterial growth of a predominant pathogen, chronic sinusitis is typically a polymicrobial infection in which anaerobes are often present. Antibiotic therapy is therefore adjusted accordingly, and prolonged therapy (2 to 6 weeks or more) may be required. The prolonged use of topical steroids and short bursts of oral steroid therapy may also help to reduce swelling and relieve ostiomeatal obstruction. Allergic patients also benefit from use of antihistamines and desensitization. Smoke and other environmental pollutants that may be exacerbating factors are to be avoided. Because the most frequent local cause of chronic sinusitis is ostiomeatal disease and the extent of the underlying ostiomeatal pathology may be limited, nasal endoscopy and CT are of particular value in these patients. Endoscopy provides the ability to visualize the middle meatus and adjacent ethmoid structures and to identify areas of persistent infection and edema. It allows the response to medical therapy to be accurately monitored and permits cultures to be performed with precision. This anatomic area also varies widely, and anatomic abnormalities that narrow the ostiomeatal channels and predispose to infection can be identified. CT provides complementary information about the deeper sinuses and ostiomeatal structures. However, when interpreting CT findings it must be remembered that a significant incidence of asymptomatic mucosal thickening is evident on a CT scan.

Endoscopy also provides the ability to accurately visualize disease within the maxillary or sphenoid sinus for an accurate diagnosis of unusual radiographic findings. Maxillary sinuscopy is performed via a cannula inserted sublabially under local anesthesia. Biopsies can be performed and cysts removed. Sphenoid sinuscopy is performed via trocar introduced intranasally or after intranasal sphenoidotomy. The central location of the sinus and the vital structures surrounding it, however, make this a technically demanding procedure that is not without risk.

Surgical Treatment

The importance of managing the underlying problems, whether these are irritation, allergic factors, or structural nasal deformities, cannot be overemphasized. The goal of treatment is restoration of normal ventilation and mucociliary clearance and ultimately reversal of mucosal disease. Although the predominant symptoms and disease are often in the maxillary or frontal sinus, careful endoscopic evaluation and a CT scan frequently reveal underlying disease in the ostiomeatal area. This improved diagnostic accuracy has reduced the need for surgical procedures aimed at the major sinuses. Even when the disease within these sinuses appears to be extensive, the initial approach is often intranasal removal of the underlying ostiomeatal problem. This approach has been termed "functional endonasal surgery" or, when performed under endoscopic visualization, "functional endoscopic surgery."

The channels for sinus ventilation and mucociliary clearance within the ostiomeatal complex are narrow and tortuous. Minor underlying disease in this area may therefore cause extensive secondary changes. Thus localized obstruction in the narrow opening to the frontal recess may give rise to an extensive frontal sinus mucocele. In identifying the relative importance of ostiomeatal disease in chronic or recurrent acute sinusitis, the site of disease is thus more relevant than the extent.

Indications for functional surgery include sinusitis that persists despite adequate medical therapy, and documented recurrent acute sinusitis with related structural or inflammatory abnormalities in the ostiomeatal unit. The functional approach can usually be performed under local anesthesia without external incision and dramatically reduces morbidity compared with standard open surgical techniques. Damage to normal anatomy is minimized, and packing is usually not required. This type of surgery, however, is complicated and requires special skills if the risks to adjacent critical structures are to be minimized. After surgery, the secondarily involved mucosa usually recovers slowly. The extent of surgery performed with this approach varies from a very limited procedure to complete sphenoethmoidectomy with opening of both maxillary and frontal sinuses.

Indications for external sinus surgery include osteomyelitis, orbital complications, intracranial complications, and failure of the functional approach. Numerous techniques for cleaning the different sinuses have been described. The frontal sinus may be approached by an external fronto-ethmoidectomy by using a curvilinear incision in the area of the medial canthus. It can also be approached more completely by an incision across the eyebrows or behind the hairline. In the latter case, the anterior bony wall of the sinus is incised and reflected anteriorly to provide access. The maxillary sinus is typically approached by a sublabial incision (Caldwell-Luc), and the ethmoid by an incision on the side of the nose (external ethmoidectomy). Unfortunately, these procedures, particularly the frontal sinus osteoplasty, may create permanent changes in the sinuses that can be difficult to differentiate radiologically from disease recurrence.

COMPLICATIONS OF SINUSITIS

One of the more common complications of sinusitis, primarily in children, is the spread of ethmoid infection into the orbit. The first indication of orbital involvement is inflammatory edema of the eyelids. Progression of the infection may be rapid with chemosis, ophthalmoplegia, and even visual loss. In the early cellulitic stage of the disease, intravenous antibiotic therapy is appropriate. However, careful evaluation and an orbital CT scan are required to rule out a subperiosteal abscess or intraorbital abscess, both of which require prompt surgical drainage.

Purulent frontal sinusitis may result in extension of the infection through the anterior wall and presentation as a Pott's puffy tumor. Inflammatory sinus disease may also spread intracranially and result in meningitis or epidural, subdural, or brain abscess. The precise incidence of intracranial complications is not known. However, sinusitis is reported to be the source of 35 to 65 per cent of subdural abscesses. It is important to be aware that such complications, although uncommon, are not rare. Intracranial complications are most likely to occur from acute frontal sinus disease but also occur from the sphenoid or, less frequently, the ethmoid sinus. These complications are most common in adolescent patients, and there is male predominance. If there is a clinical suggestion of intracranial spread, lumbar puncture and intravenous contrast CT or magnetic resonance imaging should be performed. Magnetic resonance imaging is more sensitive for identifying early intracranial disease and epidural abscess. If intracranial infection occurs, early surgical drainage of the sinuses is usually performed and, when indicated, can be combined with surgical drainage of the intracranial collection.

STREPTOCOCCAL PHARYNGITIS

method of
NELSON M. GANTZ, M.D.
University of Massachusetts Medical School
Worcester, Massachusetts

Sore throat is the third most common complaint for which people visit a health care provider in the United

States. Despite the frequency of pharyngitis and the numerous articles on the subject, the approach to diagnosis and management remains highly controversial. Some of the controversial issues include the following: When is a throat culture indicated? How best can one differentiate a patient with a sore throat and a positive culture for group A beta-hemolytic *Streptococcus* from a patient who is a streptococcal carrier with symptoms caused by some other organism such as adenovirus? What is the role of rapid antigen detection tests in the diagnosis of group A beta-hemolytic streptococcal pharyngitis? How sensitive is a single throat culture in detecting group A *Streptococcus?* What is the effect of early therapy on the natural course of the disease? Should patients be treated without use of a rapid antigen detection test or a throat culture? What are the best treatment regimens? Should patients have repeat cultures at the end of a course of therapy? How should streptococcal contacts be managed?

A number of organisms have been implicated in pharyngitis, including viruses (adenovirus, coxsackievirus, herpes simplex, influenza, parainfluenza, rhinovirus, cytomegalovirus, and Epstein-Barr), bacteria (group A beta-hemolytic *Streptococcus;* non–group A *Streptococcus,* such as groups B, C, G, and F; *Neisseria gonorrhoeae; Corynebacterium diphtheriae; Corynebacterium haemolyticum;* and *Francisella tularensis*), and *Mycoplasma.* Pharyngitis can be an important feature of secondary syphilis, toxic shock syndrome, Vincent's angina (mixed infection with *Fusobacterium* and *Bacteroides* species), epiglottitis, chronic fatigue syndrome, and infections of the retropharyngeal space. *Haemophilus influenzae,* although frequently (60 per cent) found on a pharyngeal culture, is an unusual cause of pharyngitis. Although *Staphylococcus aureus* and *Streptococcus pneumoniae* are frequently isolated from a patient with a sore throat, these organisms do not cause pharyngitis and should not be treated. *Chlamydia trachomatis* does not appear to cause pharyngitis. However, a new species, *Chlamydia pneumoniae* (TWAR), may be responsible for some cases of pharyngitis. For the clinician, however, the main problem is to determine whether the pharyngitis is caused by group A beta-hemolytic *Streptococcus* or whether the pharyngitis has a nonstreptococcal origin.

EPIDEMIOLOGY

Streptococcal pharyngitis has a peak incidence in the temperate zones during late winter and early spring, with the lowest level in the summer (during August). The organism is transmitted from person to person by large respiratory droplets, and crowding increases the attack rate. Streptococcal disease is most common in school-age children, who are the main source of organisms introduced into a family. The incubation period is 3 to 5 days but can be as long as 3 months. Acquisition of the organisms is often associated with an asymptomatic infection. Food-borne outbreaks caused by group A *Streptococcus* and the other nonstreptococcal organisms result from contamination of the food with the organism by a food handler. Milk and egg products are usually implicated. Strep-

tococcal infection is unusual in children younger than 1 year of age. Specific antibiotic therapy after 24 to 48 hours reduces communicability, and the individual, if symptoms are improved, can return to school or work.

CLINICAL MANIFESTATIONS

Clinical findings are unreliable in predicting the organism that will be identified by antigen detection or throat culture. The classic description of streptococcal pharyngitis in a school-age child consists of an illness with an acute onset, fever, headache, sore throat, pain with swallowing, and painful or enlarged cervical lymph nodes. On examination, the throat is red, tonsils may have exudates (20 per cent), and the cervical lymph nodes are tender and enlarged. Although the presence of pharyngeal exudates, enlarged cervical nodes, temperature higher than 101° F (38.4° C), and a peripheral leukocytosis favors a streptococcal etiology, considerable overlap occurs among all causes of pharyngitis. Moderate throat exudates favor a *Streptococcus* but can occur with adenovirus or *Mycoplasma* infections. The rash of scarlet fever suggests a streptococcal etiology, but a rash can also occur with *C. haemolyticum* infections or with infectious mononucleosis. The presence of cough, hoarseness, diarrhea, conjunctivitis, and a runny nose suggests a nonstreptococcal etiology. Detection of pharyngeal vesicles or ulcers favors a diagnosis of herpes simplex virus or coxsackievirus infection.

DIAGNOSIS

The "gold standard" for diagnosis of group A beta-hemolytic *Streptococcus* is the throat culture, which has a 10 per cent false-negative rate. The isolation of *Streptococcus* on a throat culture does not distinguish an acutely infected patient with streptococcal pharyngitis from a person with another cause for the pharyngitis who is a chronic streptococcal carrier. About one-half of patients with cultures that are positive for group A *Streptococcus* will show a rise in antistreptococcal antibodies, and such patients are at risk for the development of nonsuppurative complications. The other one-half of these patients have elevated streptococcal antibody titers when first seen that do not subsequently increase, and they are streptococcal carriers. Because serologic studies are usually not done when patients present with a sore throat and because other simple tests to detect carriers are not available, all patients with a positive culture are treated as a group. Except for some nasal carriers, chronic carriers are not a major source of spreading the streptococcal organism.

A number of tests to detect streptococcal antigens in the throat have become available and provide an alternative to a throat culture. The tests require 5 to 75 minutes to perform, cost approximately $2 to $3 per test, have a sensitivity of 60 to 90 per cent, and show high specificity. The test is positive only with group A *Streptococcus* and does not detect other streptococcal groups. If the rapid antigen test is positive, the organism is likely to be group A *Streptococcus* and a culture can be omitted. If the rapid antigen test is negative and a streptococcal infection is suspected, a throat culture should be done and treatment should be based on the results. The rapid immunologic tests often fail to identify small numbers of streptococci, which may be associated with a rise in antistreptolysin O titer.

TREATMENT

There are four reasons to treat group A streptococcal pharyngitis. First, therapy begun within 48 hours of the onset of illness can result in a more rapid resolution of fever and symptoms. Second, antibiotic therapy can prevent the development of local suppurative complications such as cervical adenitis, peritonsillar abscess, or retropharyngeal abscess. Third, therapy, even if delayed for 9 days, can prevent acute rheumatic fever but probably not acute glomerulonephritis. Fourth, therapy can decrease the infectivity of the index case. One disadvantage of immediate penicillin therapy is that if therapy is delayed for 48 hours or more, there tend to be fewer late reinfections. Although non–group A beta-hemolytic *Streptococcus* organisms likely cause pharyngitis, the effect of treatment on the clinical course and incidence of sequelae awaits further study.

Because the clinical findings, even when several criteria are met, fail to distinguish a viral from a streptococcal sore throat, the question of whether to take a culture or treat without a culture is controversial. In the setting of a streptococcal epidemic, treatment without a culture is appropriate and is not controversial. In the usual nonepidemic setting, arguments can be made for (1) treating only patients with positive direct antigen tests or cultures (the currently recommended approach), (2) using antibiotic treatment for all patients who have sore throats but no culture, or (3) neither culturing nor treating any patient with a sore throat. The approach adopted depends on the clinician's weighing the rationale for treatment, the various costs to the patient (such as those for cultures and drugs), and the consequences of widespread antibiotic therapy (e.g., drug reactions, bacterial resistance). I suggest that the clinician swab the patient's throat with two swabs for a rapid streptococcal test. If the test is positive, the second swab is discarded and therapy is begun. If the rapid test is negative, the second swab is cultured. Therapy may be instituted pending culture results or may be withheld until the diagnosis is confirmed.

TREATMENT REGIMENS

Penicillin is the drug of choice for streptococcal pharyngitis; most patients may be treated with oral penicillin V. The duration of therapy must be 10 days; 7 days is inadequate. Benzathine penicillin G is an alternative therapy that ensures compliance but is associated with considerable pain at the injection site for both children and adults. Penicillin V is given is a dose of 250 mg orally three or four times a day. In children, a dose of penicillin V of 250 mg orally twice a day is also effective. Benzathine penicillin G is given intramuscularly in a dose of 1.2 million units (900,000 units of benzathine penicillin G and 300,000 units of procaine penicillin G) in a 2-ml injection into the buttocks. Erythromycin is the alternative drug in the United States for penicillin-allergic patients. Children may be given erythromycin estolate, 20 to 50 mg per kg per day orally in two to four divided doses. Adults can be given other erythromycin preparations such as the ethylsuccinate, 250 mg orally four times daily. Erythromycin preparations are better tolerated when they are taken with food. In Japan, more than one-half of group A *Streptococcus* strains are resistant to erythromycin. Other alternative drugs include cephalexin, 250 mg orally four times a day for 10 days, or, rarely, clindamycin. Cephalosporins are contraindicated in patients with an immediate hypersensitivity reaction to penicillin. Drugs such as sulfamethoxazole-trimethoprim, tetracycline, or the new quinolones (e.g., ciprofloxacin or norfloxacin) have no role in treating streptococcal pharyngitis. Adjunctive therapy consists of rest, saline gargles, warm liquids, aspirin or acetaminophen, and lozenges.

The failure rate associated with penicillin is 15 to 20 per cent. The role of pharyngeal penicillinase-producing organisms in contributing to this failure rate is controversial. Clindamycin may be effective for selected patients who fail conventional therapy. In one report, the addition of rifampin, 20 mg per kg per day (600 mg maximum) orally, to the last 4 days of a 10-day course of penicillin was associated with improved bacteriologic cure rates.

There is no indication to treat or culture asymptomatic family contacts unless that member has a history of rheumatic fever. Symptomatic contacts should be cultured and treated.

FOLLOW-UP EVALUATION

Test of cure cultures are not indicated unless a patient is still symptomatic. Only symptomatic patients should be re-treated.

TUBERCULOSIS AND OTHER MYCOBACTERIAL DISEASES

method of
GEORGE M. LORDI, M.D., and
LEE B. REICHMAN, M.D., M.P.H.
University of Medicine and Dentistry
of New Jersey
Newark, New Jersey

Tuberculosis remains an important cause of mortality and morbidity in the United States. In 1986 there was an increase in the number of reported new cases, which reversed the former pattern of annual decreases. Individuals with acquired immunodeficiency syndrome (AIDS) may be partly responsible for recent increases. High rates of new cases are reported from large cities, particularly in younger age groups (middle twenties to middle forties) although the elderly are still the most afflicted. Classification of tuberculosis is based on the concept of tuberculous infection and tuberculous disease stages. Class 1 is characterized by tuberculous exposure with no evidence of infection and the tuberculin skin test not significant. Class 2, tuberculous infection, is defined as exposure with a significant skin test but negative bacteriologic and roentgenographic studies. Positive studies (cultures, smears, x-ray films) constitute tuberculous disease (Class 3). The organism *(Mycobacterium tuberculosis)* is transmitted only by droplet nuclei from an untreated individual with tuberculous disease.

Preventive therapy with isoniazid (INH) is given for tuberculous infection to prevent progression to active disease.

Treatment for tuberculous disease requires the use of a combination of two or more drugs, which is essential to reduce the survival of any drug-resistant strains. Patient compliance is essential. The drugs must be given for an adequate time. Drug susceptibility studies are helpful as a guide to therapy in previously treated patients, those who have failed treatment, and individuals from areas where drug resistance is high.

PREVENTIVE THERAPY: TUBERCULOUS INFECTION

The basis of control of tuberculosis in the United States is preventive therapy with INH. INH is given for 6 months in a single daily dose of 300 mg for adults, and 10 to 14 mg per kg of body weight per day, but no more than 300 mg per day for children. In certain situations, 1 year of treatment is preferred. Preventive therapy is assumed to be successful if tuberculous organisms in foci or scars too small to be seen on chest x-ray films are reduced or eliminated, thereby preventing endogenous reactivation in the future. Protection probably lasts for life.

Because of its hepatotoxicity, particularly after the age of 35 years, INH is not used in everyone who has a significant tuberculin reaction. It is given to patients in whom the risk of tuberculosis is greater than the risk of hepatitis. This group would include all significant reactors under the age of 35 years and all household members and close contacts of persons with active tuberculous disease and significant reactions regardless of age. Children in this contact group are at high risk and are given INH even if tuberculin skin testing is not significant. The test is repeated in 3 months, and INH use is discontinued if the skin test remains nonsignificant. INH is also indicated regardless of age in

1. All newly infected persons (defined as a tuberculin skin test conversion within the past 3 years)

2. Persons with a past history of tuberculosis who have not received adequate chemotherapy

3. Persons with abnormal chest x-ray film (stable but consistent with past tuberculosis; 1 year of therapy required)

4. Persons at increased risk because of special clinical situations such as diabetes mellitus, silicosis, adrenocorticosteroid therapy, immunosuppressive therapy, end-stage renal disease, hematologic malignancy such as Hodgkin's disease, after gastrectomy, and antibodies to human immunodeficiency virus (HIV) (1 year of therapy required for positive test for virus)

Contraindications to the use of INH prophylaxis include age more than 35 years without associated risk factors (just listed), previous adverse reaction to INH, and active or acute liver disease. With regard to pregnancy, preventive therapy is postponed until after delivery.

Monthly monitoring and follow-up are necessary once INH treatment is started. Questionnaire screening for symptoms of adverse effects is useful, with laboratory tests being done only to evaluate signs or symptoms of liver injury. Mild liver function test abnormalities including the elevation of serum transaminase levels occur in 10 to 20 per cent of patients taking INH. Levels more than five times normal are an indication for stopping INH therapy. Persons older than 35 years should have liver function tests before the start of therapy and then periodically during preventive therapy.

TREATMENT OF PULMONARY TUBERCULOSIS: TUBERCULOUS DISEASE

Rifampin, INH, pyrazinamide (PZA), streptomycin, and ethambutol are first line drugs used in the initial therapy of pulmonary tuberculosis. Kanamycin, capreomycin, ethionamide, cycloserine, and para-aminosalicylic acid are considered to be second line drugs and are used in cases of treatment failure, drug resistance, and adverse reactions to first line drugs.

Most patients can be treated on an outpatient basis, with hospitalization reserved for those unable to provide self-care or with severe symptoms.

Our basic regimen for the treatment of pulmonary tuberculosis in adults is a combination of INH, 300 mg per day, rifampin, 600 mg per day for a total of 6 months, with PZA (15 to 30 mg per kg per day, up to 3 grams maximum) given during the first 2 months of the regimen. All drugs can be given in a single daily dose. An alternative acceptable regimen would be to give INH and rifampin alone for 9 months. INH and rifampin should be given as a fixed-dose combination when possible. When available, the fixed-dose combination of INH, rifampin, and PZA should be used.

Ethambutol (15 mg per kg per day) is added to the regimen of INH and rifampin when treating immigrants from areas with a high incidence of primary INH resistance such as Korea, Southeast Asia, and Mexico. If resistance is proved by drug sensitivity studies, therapy is given for a minimum of 12 months. If resistance is not found, ethambutol therapy is discontinued. PZA can still be used during the initial 2 months.

Streptomycin has been used as a third drug in a daily intramuscular dose of 20 to 40 mg per kg per day, to a maximum of 1 gram per day. The total dose should not be more than 120 grams, and continuation of streptomycin beyond 2 months does not seem to change outcome. Injectable treatment may be helpful for the noncompliant patient in that frequent patient visits are required. For the compliant patient, the effectiveness of the regimen is decreased by substituting streptomycin for PZA.

INH is bactericidal and has an important adverse effect—hepatitis. Peripheral neuropathy caused by interference with pyridoxine metabolism is uncommon at the dosage used. However, pyridoxine supplementation is given to patients with seizure disorders and those who are pregnant. Monitoring phenytoin levels may be necessary in epileptics who receive INH because its use results in an increase in the serum phenytoin concentration.

Rifampin is bactericidal and effective against the tuberculous bacillus at all pH levels. Its adverse reactions include rash, hepatitis, and gastrointestinal distress. Thrombocytopenia can occur but is rare. The clearance of many drugs that are metabolized in the liver, such as warfarin, oral hypoglycemics, oral contraceptives, digitalis, and anticonvulsants, is accelerated by rifampin, and diminished serum levels of these can result.

PZA's primary adverse reactions are hyperuricemia and hepatic injury. Gastrointestinal distress is also common, and rash can occur. PZA is bactericidal for intracellular organisms.

Ethambutol is bacteriostatic. Optic neuritis is the most serious side effect, which is uncommon at a daily dose of 15 mg per kg. Manifestations of the optic neuritis include decreased visual acuity and impaired red-green color discrimination.

Ototoxicity with vertigo and hearing loss can occur with streptomycin therapy. Nephrotoxicity may also be a problem. The drug is bactericidal at alkaline pH.

Characteristics of first line antituberculous drugs are summarized in Table 1.

Monitoring of Therapy

Sputum (smear and culture) and symptoms should be evaluated at monthly intervals. Sputum smears should show a reduction in the number of organisms shortly after the start of therapy. Within 2 weeks, the patient can be considered to be noninfectious to others. Sputum conversion to negative occurs in more than 90 per cent of patients within 3 months. If this conversion does not occur, the possibility of drug resistance should be considered and drug susceptibility studies obtained. Monthly smears and cultures are obtained until conversion occurs. In the patient who converts to negative, one additional sputum sample for smear and culture for *M. tuberculosis* is recommended at the end of therapy.

Symptom improvement with weight gain, diminished cough, and lack of fever should be seen in responding patients.

Chest x-ray films are not as valuable as examination of sputum. Serial chest films are not needed. Clearing of x-ray films would confirm sputum conversion. A chest film in the middle and at the end of therapy is sufficient and is helpful in demonstrating progress to the patient.

No routine follow-up is necessary once the usual course of therapy has been completed. The patient can be told to return for follow-up care only if symptoms recur.

Intermittent Drug Therapy

The intermittent administration of antituberculous drugs is as effective as daily administration if doses are adjusted and if an initial daily period of continuous therapy has been given. This type of regimen is indicated mainly for patients who are not compliant. Intermittent therapy should always be part of a directly administered

TABLE 1. **First Line Drugs for *M. tuberculosis* Infections**

Drug	Dosage		Selected Adverse Effects	Comments
	Daily	*Twice Weekly*		
Isoniazid	Adult: 300 mg Children: 10–20 mg/kg (300 mg*)	Adult: 15 mg/kg Children: 20–40 mg/kg (900 mg*)	Hepatitis, hypersensitivity, peripheral neuropathy	Bactericidal; monitor SGOT and SGPT as indicated Fixed-dose combination with rifampin preferred
Rifampin (Rifadin, Rimactane)	Adult: 600 mg Children: 10–20 mg/kg (600 mg*)	Adult: 600 mg Children: 10–20 mg/kg (600 mg*)	Hepatitis, febrile reaction, thrombocytopenia (rare), nausea, vomiting	Bactericidal; monitor SGOT and SGPT as indicated Drug interactions: orange color to secretions (urine) Fixed-dose combination with INH preferred
Pyrazinamide	Adult: 15–30 mg/kg (1–3 grams*) Children: 20–30 mg/kg (2 grams*)		Hyperuricemia, hepatotoxicity, rash, arthralgias, GI distress	Bactericidal and sterilizing; monitor uric acid, SGOT and SGPT Fixed-dose combination with INH and rifampin preferred when available
Streptomycin	Adult: 15 mg/kg (1 gram*) Children: 20–40 mg/kg (1 gram*)	Adult: 25–30 mg/kg Children: 25–30 mg/kg	Nephrotoxicity, eighth cranial nerve damage	Bactericidal in alkaline pH; monitor vestibular function; audiograms; BUN; creatinine 10 mg/kg dose for age >60 yr Adjust dose in renal failure Useful in directly administered therapy
Ethambutol (Myambutol)	Adult: 15 mg/kg (2.5 grams*) Children: 15 mg/kg (2.5 grams*)	Adult: 50 mg/kg Children: 50 mg/kg	Optic neuritis, rash	Bacteriostatic in usual dosage Monitor visual acuity, red-green color discrimination Adjust dose in renal failure

*Maximal dosage.

Abbreviations: SGOT = serum glutamic-oxaloacetic transaminase; SGPT = serum glutamic-pyruvic transaminase; BUN = blood urea nitrogen; GI = gastrointestinal.

treatment program to further ensure compliance. A typical regimen would be to give INH and rifampin with PZA in standard doses for 2 months and then continue rifampin at a higher dosage (15 mg per kg per day with maximum of 900 mg) and INH, 600 mg per day twice weekly for an additional 4 months. Streptomycin can be used as the third drug in this type of program. One gram is given twice a week, and the oral medications are given when the injectable dose is administered.

SPECIAL SITUATIONS

Acquired Immunodeficiency Syndrome

Persons with both HIV and *M. tuberculosis* infection are at increased risk for tuberculous disease. In many patients, the diagnosis of tuberculosis precedes the diagnosis of AIDS. Extrapulmonary involvement, particularly pleural effusion and tuberculous lymphadenopathy, is more common than pulmonary disease.

Tuberculosis in AIDS patients may respond well to standard chemotherapy. The basic regimen of INH, rifampin, and PZA (for the first 2 months) is started whenever acid-fast bacilli are detected. Ethambutol may be added if central nervous system or disseminated disease is suspected.

The optimal duration of therapy is unknown, but a minimum of 9 months of treatment with at least 6 months of therapy after culture conversion is acceptable. Because HIV infection is the most important risk factor for progression of tuberculous infection to disease, a significant tuberculin test in an HIV-infected person is an indication for INH preventive therapy.

Pregnancy

With proper therapy, there is no difference in prognosis between pregnant and nonpregnant patients with tuberculosis. There is also no increased risk of acquiring tuberculosis in pregnancy. Active disease should be treated when diagnosed. No harmful effects on the fetus have been caused by INH, rifampin, or ethambutol. The safety of PZA has not been established in pregnancy. Aminoglycosides such as streptomycin should not be used because of fetal ototoxicity.

Our preferred regimen in the pregnant woman with tuberculosis is the combination of INH and rifampin for 9 months. Pyridoxine is also given.

Breast-feeding is not contraindicated for mothers who are taking antituberculous medication.

Drug Resistance and Treatment Failure

Treatment failure usually occurs in the non-compliant patient and is defined as a failure of sputum conversion to negative after 4 to 5 months of therapy. Cessation of medication or medication's being taken intermittently is usually responsible. Failure also occurs when a patient takes one drug without companion drugs that are required for treatment. Acquired drug-resistant organisms are frequently present and complicate future therapy. Drug susceptibility tests can be used as a guide to a re-treatment program. Re-treatment can be initiated while drug sensitivities are pending, or the patient's initial regimen can be continued until results of susceptibility studies are known. For the patient with resistant organisms, at least two or preferably three drugs to which there is demonstrated or presumed susceptibility are given. When three drugs are given, one should be in injectable form. Twelve to 18 months of therapy is usually necessary. The use of fixed-dose combinations where available ensures that monotherapy cannot be prescribed.

The addition of a single new drug to a failed or failing regimen should never be done.

The use of second line antituberculous drugs is frequently necessary during re-treatment despite their toxicity. The characteristics of second line drugs are summarized in Table 2.

In patients who relapse after completing a course of therapy that included rifampin and INH, the organisms are usually still sensitive and the INH and rifampin regimen can be re-started.

TREATMENT OF EXTRAPULMONARY TUBERCULOSIS

Tuberculous meningitis, tuberculous lymphadenitis, renal tuberculosis, skeletal tuberculosis, tuberculous pericarditis, tuberculous pleural effusion, and tuberculous peritonitis are examples of nonpulmonary sites of tuberculous disease. In miliary tuberculosis, many organs are involved, including the lungs, as a result of a massive hematogenous spread of tubercle bacillus. The typical miliary chest film appearance results.

Diagnosis can be complicated. Microscopic examination of biopsy material and culture of biopsy material for *M. tuberculosis* are usually necessary. The characteristics of pleural, peritoneal, or pericardial fluid obtained by needle aspiration may suggest tuberculosis, but confirmation by biopsy is essential. Renal tuberculosis can be diagnosed by culture of three consecutive morning urine specimens. Lung biopsy may be needed to diagnose miliary tuberculosis. Cerebrospinal fluid culture is valuable in tuberculous meningitis, but treatment must be started before culture results have been received.

The treatment of these types of tuberculosis is not different from the treatment of pulmonary tuberculosis. The 6-month regimen of INH, rifampin, and PZA is considered to be effective as is a 9-month regimen of INH and rifampin. Because many extrapulmonary cases represent AIDS or HIV infection, treatment should last for at least 9 months, or for 6 months beyond culture conversion in the HIV-infected person.

Corticosteroids have been used in tuberculous meningitis in the hope of preventing neurologic sequelae, and steroids have been used in tuberculous pericarditis in the hope of preventing constrictive pericarditis. Doses of 60 to 80 mg of prednisone per day, with tapering during a period of weeks, have been advocated. Efficacy has not been proved in either case.

NONTUBERCULOUS MYCOBACTERIAL DISEASES

The nontuberculous, or atypical, mycobacteria are a diverse group of acid-fast organisms. Many are saprophytes, whereas others can cause disease. *Mycobacterim kansasii* and *Mycobacterium avium-intracellulare* complex can cause chronic pulmonary disease that resembles tuberculosis. These cases usually occur in persons with some type of coexisting lung disease such as chronic obstructive pulmonary disease, pneumoconiosis, or previous tuberclosis. Diagnosis can be difficult; colonization and contamination of specimens must be ruled out.

Disseminated disease caused by *M. avium-intracellulare* complex with involvement of bone marrow, lung, liver, gastrointestinal tract, lymph nodes, and renal tract is seen in patients with AIDS.

Mycobacterium scrofulaceum is a cause of cervical lymphadenopathy in children usually between the ages of 1 and 5 years. Occasional cases of adenopathy have been caused by *M. kansasii* or *M. avium-intracellulare*.

Various organisms are associated with soft tissue, bone, and joint infection. Infection usually occurs when bacteria are introduced after trauma, surgery, or a joint injection.

Nodular, ulcerating skin lesions are caused by *Mycobacterium marinum* after abrasion, trauma

TABLE 2. **Second Line Drugs for *M. tuberculosis* Infections**

Drug	Daily Dosage for Adults and Children	Selected Adverse Effects	Comments
Capreomycin (Capastat sulfate)*	15–30 mg/kg (1 gram†)	Renal toxicity, eighth cranial nerve damage	Monitor vestibular function, audiograms, BUN, creatinine level Use caution in older patients Adjust dose in renal failure
Kanamycin (Kantrex)*	15–30 mg/kg (1 gram†)	Renal toxicity, eighth cranial nerve damage	Monitor vesitbular function, audiograms, BUN, creatinine level Use caution in older patients Adjust dose in renal failure
Ethionamide (Trecator S.C.)	15–20 mg/kg (1 gram†)	Hepatotoxicity, GI distress, hypersensitivity	Monitor SGOT and SGPT Divided doses may help GI distress
Cycloserine (Seromycin)	15–20 mg/kg (1 gram†) 5–15 mg/kg for children	Psychosis, personality changes, convulsions, rash	Monitor via psychologic testing
Para-aminosalicylic acid	150 mg/kg (12 grams†) 200–420 mg/kg for children	GI distress, hypersensitivity, sodium load, hepatotoxicity	Monitor SGOT and SGPT Rarely used

*Safety has not been established in children.
†Maximal dosage.

from handling fish or fish tanks, or swimming pool injury (swimming pool granuloma).

Mycobacterium fortuitum complex includes *M. fortuitum* and *M. chelonei*. These rapidly growing mycobacteria can cause pulmonary disease, soft tissue infections, and postsurgical sternal osteomyelitis.

Treatment

Treatment varies, depending on the organisms involved and the disease caused. Treatment can be difficult.

Surgical excision is the treatment of choice for cervical lymphadenitis. Excisional biopsy is recommended for diagnosis and may be sufficient therapy. If *M. kansasii* is involved, a course of chemotherapy can also be given. A surgical approach is also usually successful for soft tissue and bone infections.

Antituberculous drugs are effective in treating *M. kansasii* infection. Pulmonary disease is treated with a three-drug regimen of INH, rifampin, and ethambutol for 12 to 18 months. However, 9-month short course of therapy has also been successful in some cases.

Pulmonary disease caused by *M. fortuitum* complex is difficult to treat. Resistance is usually present to both first and second line antituberculosis drugs. Antimicrobial agents, not usually effective for mycobacterial infection, may be useful. The resistance patterns of *M. chelonei* and

M. fortuitum vary. Our recommendation for *M. fortuitum* infection is an initial combination of amikacin plus doxycycline or sulfamethoxazole. Our initial recommendation for *M. chelonei* infection is amikacin plus cefoxitin or erythromycin. Changes in regimen depend on susceptibility studies and therapeutic response.

The treatment of pulmonary disease caused by *M. avium-intracellulare* is complicated. The organisms are resistant to commonly used drugs. For disease localized to one lung, resectional surgery (lobectomy or pneumonectomy) can be considered, with chemotherapy given 2 to 3 weeks before surgery and postoperatively for a period of months. Inadequate pulmonary function in many patients prevents use of this approach.

A conservative approach to chemotherapy would be to start a three-drug regimen of INH, rifampin, and ethambutol and to add streptomycin, ethionamide, and/or cycloserine in the patients who does not respond. An alternative would be to start with a five-drug regimen of INH, rifampin, ethambutol, streptomycin, and PZA. In either case, drugs are stopped and added as toxicity or disease progression dictates. Drug susceptibility studies do not seem to be helpful. The aim of therapy is negative cultures for 18 to 24 months. In many patients, therapy will be stopped after 24 months despite positive cultures.

No effective therapy is currently available for disseminated disease caused by *M. avium-intracellulare* in the patient with AIDS.

The Cardiovascular System

ACQUIRED DISEASES OF THE AORTA

method of
JOHN A. MANNICK, M.D., and
LAWRENCE H. COHN, M.D.
*Brigham and Women's Hospital and
Harvard Medical School
Boston, Massachusetts*

Acquired diseases of the aorta are of two types: occlusive disease and aneurysms. Atherosclerosis is the most common cause of both types of disease. An exception is the dissecting aneurysm of the aorta, which is caused by degeneration of the aortic media, a process that also appears to be associated with aneurysms of the ascending aorta. Other less common causes of aortic disease include arteritis, usually giant cell arteritis, which may cause either occlusive disease or aneurysm formation; infection of the aortic wall, which may result in mycotic aneurysms; and trauma, which can cause false aneurysms. Syphilitic aortitis, once a common cause of aortic aneurysm, is now rare in the United States and Europe.

AORTIC OCCLUSIVE DISEASE

Occlusive disease of the aorta is ordinarily most pronounced near the aortic bifurcation and, in most individuals, involves the iliac arteries as well. The earliest manifestation of this form of occlusive disease is intermittent claudication with symptoms involving the muscles of the hip, thigh, and buttock, as well as the calf. However, a sizable minority of patients with aortoiliac disease complain only of calf claudication. In addition to claudication, male patients with aortoiliac occlusive disease may have difficulty in achieving and maintaining an erection because of inadequate perfusion of the internal iliac arteries. Extensive aortoiliac occlusive disease may also cause ischemia at rest or ischemic tissue loss; however, such symptoms are more common when aortoiliac disease is combined with femoral popliteal occlusive disease. The risk factors for aortoiliac occlusive disease are those for atherosclerosis in general and include cigarette smoking, hypertension, elevated serum cholesterol level, and diabetes.

The diagnosis of aortoiliac occlusive disease may be facilitated by segmental lower limb pressure measurements performed with the Doppler flow detector and/or segmental pulse volume recordings or Doppler waveform analysis. The disease is even more likely to be revealed by comparing measurements made at rest with those made after a period of graded exercise, which produces a profound fall in the distal limb pressures in these patients.

Surgical Treatment

The indications for surgery for aortoiliac occlusive disease are disabling claudication and/or resting ischemia manifested by pain at rest, ischemic ulceration, or incipient gangrene. Before surgery, the diagnosis of aortoiliac occlusive disease must be confirmed by angiography, which is usually performed by the transfemoral or transaxillary route.

Preoperative evaluation of the patient who requires surgery for aortoiliac occlusive disease focuses on an assessment of the associated cardiopulmonary disease. Particular attention is paid to evaluation of coronary artery disease, which is clinically evident in approximately one-half of the patients. Symptomatic, unstable coronary artery disease in such individuals may demand extensive preoperative investigation, including cardiac catheterization and coronary angiography. If urgent coronary artery reconstruction is indicated, this should be performed before correction of the aortoiliac occlusive disease. However, patients with milder, stable coronary artery disease can undergo aortoiliac reconstruction without great risk.

The standard operation for correction of aortoiliac occlusive disease is the aortobifemoral bypass graft using vascular bifurcation protheses of Dacron. The operative mortality rate for such procedures is now 2 per cent or less. The long-term results are quite good, with 5-year graft patency of more than 80 per cent in the hands of experienced surgeons. Aortic endarterectomy is ordinarily reserved for those instances in which the lesion is confined to the abdominal aorta, usually the midaortic segment or the upper abdominal aorta. The latter lesions may be of special clinical significance in that they usually involve the orifices of the renal and visceral arteries and therefore may produce symptoms of bowel ischemia, hypertension, or renal insufficiency.

Aortobifemoral grafting is usually performed under general anesthesia with a transabdominal approach through a midline abdominal incision. Incisions in both groins are made as well for exposure of the common femoral artery bifurcations. The graft is anastomosed to the aorta above the occlusive lesions, and graft limbs are brought retroperitoneally down into the groins to reestablish circulation to the lower extremities.

Some elderly and high-risk individuals with ischemia at rest caused by severe aortoiliac occlusive disease may be considered for an alternative procedure such as an axillary bilateral femoral graft rather than a transabdominal aortofemoral bypass. Axillofemoral grafts are probably less stressful than aortofemoral grafts but have a poorer long-term patency and are not commonly indicated in this age of modern anesthetic management.

Balloon Angioplasty

Lesions of aortoiliac occlusive disease that are confined mainly to short segments of the iliac arteries themselves are now managed successfully by balloon angioplasty without surgery. Long-term good results with such angioplasty procedures in the iliac arterial system now approach 70 per cent.

AORTIC ANEURYSMS

Atherosclerotic Aneurysms

Aortic aneurysms occur most often in the infrarenal abdominal aorta. Other common sites of aortic aneurysms, in decreasing order of frequency, include the descending thoracic aorta, the ascending aorta, the thoracoabdominal aorta, and the aortic arch. The usual clinical manifestation of an aortic aneurysm is pain from expansion of the aneurysm. Embolization of clot from the aneurysm contents is a less common clinical presentation.

Infrarenal Abdominal Aortic Aneurysms

The symptoms produced by these common aortic aneurysms are lumbar back pain, occasionally accompanied by sciatic radiation and/or abdominal pain in the epigastrium or midabdomen. Many aneurysms are asymptomatic when detected at physical examination or at the time of x-ray or ultrasound studies of the abdomen. The danger of an aortic aneurysm is principally that of rupture. The size of the aneurysm is directly related to its propensity to rupture, and there is evidence that aortic aneurysms 5 to 6 cm in diameter or larger carry a significant risk of rupture. Rupture can clearly occur in aneurysms less than 5 cm in diameter, but this risk is probably low. Our current policy, therefore, is to operate electively on all abdominal aortic aneurysms measuring 5 cm or more in diameter. We also operate on any symptomatic aneurysms in the 4- to 5-cm range, particularly if the aneurysm is tender to palpation. We also offer surgery to young, low-risk patients with asymptomatic 4-cm aneurysms. The simplest, most accurate method for determining the diameter of an aortic aneurysm is probably ultrasound. Computed tomography (CT) scanning and magnetic resonance imaging (MRI) also give accurate information.

Patients with symptomatic aneurysms should be operated on urgently because of the high risk of imminent rupture. It is our practice to admit these patients to the hospital as soon as the diagnosis is made and to proceed with surgery within 24 hours.

Preoperative evaluation of patients undergoing repair of abdominal aneurysms is similar to that of patients requiring surgery for aortoiliac disease. Again, approximately 50 per cent of patients with aneurysm have clear-cut clinical evidence of coronary artery disease that requires careful preoperative assessment. In certain unusual instances, patients with combined, unstable coronary artery disease and symptomatic abdominal aortic aneurysms may require surgical correction of both problems at the same operation.

We prefer preoperative angiography for all patients undergoing repair of nonruptured aortic aneurysms because angiography gives the best definition of the relationship between the aneurysm and the renal arteries; reveals the status of the celiac, superior, and inferior mesenteric arteries; and gives useful information about the presence of iliac aneurysms and iliac occlusive disease.

Surgical Treatment

Surgery for repair of infrarenal abdominal aortic aneurysms is performed under general anesthesia. The midline transabdominal approach is used most often. The graft inclusion technique is preferred and requires minimal dissection of the aneurysm and the surrounding structures. Common iliac aneurysms, which are present in approximately 25 per cent of patients with infrarenal abdominal aortic aneurysms, should be repaired at the same time. The presence of iliac aneurysms or severe iliac occlusive disease requires the use of an aortic bifurcation prosthesis; otherwise a tube graft is preferred. Woven Dacron is the graft material ordinarily used for aneurysm repair.

In some patients, a retroperitoneal approach to the aneurysm, as popularized by Dr. G. M. Williams of Johns Hopkins School of Medicine, may be appropriate. We have found this approach to be useful for aneurysm repair in patients who have had prior intra-abdominal surgery, particularly on the gastrointestinal tract, where multiple adhesions may make a transabdominal approach to the aorta difficult. We have also found the retroperitoneal approach to be useful in patients whose infrarenal aneurysms extend up to the level of the renal arteries and thus require aortic cross-clamping at the level of the diaphragm. The retroperitoneal approach is not suited for patients with right common iliac aneurysms or for those with a high, narrow costal arch.

The operative mortality rate for infrarenal abdominal aortic aneurysm repair is now approximately 2 per cent in experienced hands. The chief cause of postoperative death is myocardial infarction. Serious postoperative complications include embolization of aneurysm contents into the lower extremities, left colon ischemia from embolization or inappropriate ligation of the inferior mesenteric artery, and renal failure. Modern preoperative and intraoperative monitoring has contributed significantly to reducing the operative mortality for abdominal aortic aneurysm repair during the past decade. We prefer that patients undergoing repair of an aortic aneurysm have peripheral arterial lines and Swan-Ganz catheters inserted preoperatively and that intraoperative fluid management be based on pulmonary capillary wedge pressure measurements. Optimal wedge pressures for each patient can be selected by preoperatively determined left ventricular performance curves. Cardiac stress imposed by cross-clamping of the aorta can be mitigated with appropriate use of vasodilators such as nitroprusside and nitroglycerin.

The good results achieved with elective or urgent repair of intact abdominal aortic aneurysms argue strongly for surgical repair of all abdominal aneurysms more than 5 cm in diameter because survival in patients who reach the hospital with ruptured abdominal aortic aneurysms is still only about 50 per cent in most reported series.

Thoracoabdominal Aneurysms

These aneurysms involve various lengths of the descending thoracic aorta and the upper abdominal aorta and are commonly associated with infrarenal aortic aneurysms as well. Symptoms produced by these aneurysms are those of aneurysm expansion and include epigastric and back pain in the lumbar or lower thoracic regions. CT or MRI scans are useful aids in determining the size and extent of thoracoabdominal aneurysms. Preoperative angiography is also helpful in demonstrating the extent of the aneurysm and the location of the visceral and renal branches in the aneurysm wall. Needless to say, as in patients undergoing abdominal aortic surgery, careful preoperative evaluation of cardiac and pulmonary function is required.

The approach to surgical repair of thoracoabdominal aneurysms is through a thoracoabdominal retroperitoneal exposure, as popularized by Dr. E. S. Crawford of Baylor University. The graft inclusion technique is used, as in the case of abdominal aortic aneurysms; however, openings must be cut in the side wall of the graft and sutured around the orifices of major visceral, intercostal, and renal arteries to re-establish perfusion of these vessels. Precise pharmacologic control of blood pressure is also necessary for repair of these aneurysms because the aorta must be cross-clamped in the supraceliac position. Because the procedure is much more extensive than abdominal aortic aneurysm repair, the mortality rate is proportionately higher, but it is now less than 10 per cent in experienced hands. Complications of thoracoabdominal aneurysm repair, in addition to more customary cardiac and pulmonary problems, include visceral ischemia or necrosis secondary to embolization or inadequate restoration of perfusion to the celiac axis and superior mesenteric arteries; renal failure; and paraplegia or paraparesis from interruption, either permanent or temporary, of the segmental blood supply to the anterior spinal artery from lower intercostal or upper lumbar arterial branches. The risk of the last complication appears to be directly proportional to the length of the thoracic aorta involved with the aneurysm.

Descending Thoracic Aortic Aneurysm

Descending thoracic aneurysms usually arise distal to the left subclavian artery and are the most commonly encountered thoracic aortic aneurysms. Traumatic aortic aneurysms also occur most frequently at this location because the ligamentum arteriosum is an anchoring point of the thoracic aorta and the sheer force of a deceleration injury creates an intimal tear, producing a traumatic aneurysm that is sometimes evident many years after its initiation. Patients with arteriosclerotic aneurysms of the descending thoracic aorta are usually older and have more manifestations of systemic atherosclerosis, including hypertension, and peripheral vascular disease than do patients with other thoracic aneurysms.

The most common clinical presentation is an asymptomatic mass on an x-ray film, although a large aneurysm may produce hoarseness and tracheal tug and may even erode into the pulmonary parenchyma and cause hemoptysis. Rarely, a patient may have an aneurysm large enough to displace or obstruct the esophagus, and dysphagia may be a presenting complaint. Plain chest x-ray films, CT scans, and MRI are valuable in delineating these aneurysms, but aortography is still required to demonstrate the origin and termination of the aneurysm before surgical treatment.

Surgical Treatment

Therapy consists of resection and prosthetic grafting. The aneurysm is visualized through a left thoracotomy performed under general anesthesia, with only the right lung ventilated. As with other aortic aneurysms, the graft inclusion technique is preferred. In very-high-risk patients, an intraluminal, sutureless graft may be used. In this procedure, a simple Dacron tie outside the aneurysm wall around a stented graft is all the fixation that is required. This tie results in shorter aortic clamp time and reduced operating time.

A major risk factor in these operations is inadequate preservation of the arterial supply to the spinal cord and resultant postoperative paraplegia. There is considerable debate about the various available methods of spinal cord protection, but it is now apparent that a bypass technique for perfusion of the lower part of the body during aortic clamping is preferable to simple clamping, excision, and grafting of the aneurysm. Monitoring of spinal cord ischemia is now possible with somatosensory evoked potential measurements, and many surgeons are now using this procedure as an index of spinal cord ischemia during surgery. Despite the use of a bypass for protection of the spinal cord, paraplegia occurs in approximately 5 per cent of all cases.

Ascending Aortic Aneurysms

Aneurysms of the ascending aorta are frequently seen in conjunction with abnormalities of the aortic valve; arteriosclerotic aneurysms are relatively uncommon in this area, although they do occur. Annuloaortic ectasia with dilatation of the aortic valve caused by weakening of the collagen in the aortic wall is one of the most common causes of ascending aneurysms, along with Marfan's syndrome with cystic medial necrosis, particularly in the sinuses of Valsalva. Chronic aortic dissection is also seen in this area much more frequently than in the descending aorta.

The patient with an ascending aortic aneurysm may have an asymptomatic aortic enlargement on an x-ray film or may present with aortic valvular regurgitation or stigmata of Marfan's syndrome. The diagnosis can be confirmed by the echocardiogram, which is an important tool for following patients with small, asymptomatic ascending aortic aneurysms, particularly those associated with Marfan's syndrome. Aneurysms larger than 5 cm in diameter require operation even when asymptomatic. Aortic angiography is again important before surgery to delineate the takeoff of coronary arteries, concomitant aortic valve regurgitation, and proximity of the innominate artery to the aneurysm.

Surgical Treatment

Treatment consists of resection of the aneurysm and replacement with a woven graft while the patient undergoes cardiopulmonary bypass. The type of operation is determined by the pathology in the ascending aorta, specifically, whether the sinuses of Valsalva are involved. If the patient has Marfan's syndrome, it is mandatory to use a one-piece valve-graft conduit that totally excludes the sinuses of Valsalva from the circulation. If, however, the sinuses of Valsalva are not involved and the aneurysm begins above the coronary ostia, a simple supracoronary tube graft is satisfactory. If a valve-graft conduit is used, the right and left coronary arteries must be reimplanted by using a button of aorta around the coronary orifices. Operative mortality in elective cases is about 5 per cent.

Transverse Arch Aneurysms

These aneurysms involve the midtransverse arch and the takeoff of the vessels supporting the cerebral circulation, including the innominate, left carotid, and left subclavian arteries. They are generally fusiform but may occasionally be saccular, thus requiring only a simple excision of the aneurysm without complicated cardiopulmonary bypass techniques. Arch aneurysms may present as an asymptomatic mass on a chest x-ray film, but as they enlarge, they may cause dysfunction of the esophagus, trachea, or recurrent laryngeal nerve. Occasionally, they cause central nervous system symptoms from interference with the cerebral circulation.

Surgical Treatment

Treatment consists of resection of the aneurysm and replacement with a woven prosthetic graft extending from the descending thoracic aorta across the transverse arch to the ascending aorta, with reimplantation of the origins of the cerebral vessels as an island of aorta sutured into the superior aspect of the graft. These techniques are complex and require cardiopulmonary bypass with a period of circulatory arrest or at least low-flow perfusion with profound systemic hypothermia. Hemostasis is often a problem because of the multiple suture lines, difficult exposure, and prolonged cardiopulmonary bypass. The risk of death from these operations varies from 15 to 50 per cent, depending on experience of the operators and the nature of the aneurysm.

Aortic Dissection and Dissecting Aortic Aneurysm

Acute aortic dissection is a sudden, catastrophic event in which the blood leaves the normal true lumen of the aorta through a tear in the intima to dissect the inner from the outer layer of the media. This column of blood is driven by the force of the arterial pressure and strips the inner media from the adventitia for a variable distance along the aorta.

Clinical pathologic manifestations of an aortic dissection are determined by the origin, the path taken by the dissecting hematoma as it progresses between the layers of the aorta, and the obstruction of the orifices of major arteries that arise from the dissected aorta. Dissection may, therefore, cause renal failure, stroke, visceral artery insufficiency, or peripheral ischemia. The most common etiology is probably systemic hypertension in an individual with cystic medial necrosis. It is the mode of death for most patients with Marfan's syndrome. In about 95 per cent of patients, dissections of the aorta arise in one or two locations: (1) in the ascending aorta within several centimeters of the aortic valve in 66 per cent of cases and (2) in the descending thoracic aorta just beyond the left subclavian at the site of the ligamentum arteriosum in about 33 per cent of cases. A small percentage of dissections arise in either the transverse arch or the most distal descending thoracic aorta. Clinical classification of aortic dissection is based on the origin of the dissection because this directs medial and surgical therapy. Thus, the DeBakey classification shows Type I and II dissections originating in the ascending aorta and Type III aortic dissection originating in the descending thoracic aorta.

In the Stanford classification, Type A dissection begins in the ascending aorta and Type B dissection in the descending aorta.

Patients who present with ascending aortic dissection are usually younger than those with descending aortic dissection. The most common presenting symptoms are severe chest pain, which signals the onset of the dissection, and formation of the false channel. The patient often has an expanding mediastinal shadow on a chest x-ray film; a CT scan reliably determines the presence or absence of dissection. Aortography is still required to determine the exact site of origin of the dissection.

Therapy

The natural history of patients with acute aortic dissection in the ascending aorta is extremely poor, with a 95 per cent mortality rate within a relatively short time after the onset of symptoms. Therefore, urgent surgical therapy is indicated for ascending aortic dissection in virtually every case unless the condition of the patient or other systemic disease militates against operation. However, adjunctive medical therapy is important. This includes beta blockade and intravenous antihypertensive medication to control blood pressure before surgery. Surgical therapy consists of placing the patient on cardiopulmonary bypass using femoral artery cannulation, opening the aorta, resecting the dissected aorta to obliterate the origin of the dissection, and inserting a graft to prevent tension of the suture lines of the reconstructed aorta. If the aortic value has been involved, it may be resuspended, and if a coronary artery has been sheared off, it may be anastomosed to the graft by suturing the orifice of the coronary artery into the graft. The distal anastomosis of the graft should be placed into the aorta beyond the dissection whenever possible. Failure to do so leads to a high degree of recurrences of the dissection.

Surgical treatment for descending thoracic aortic dissection is somewhat more controversial. Medical treatment is the cornerstone of therapy for these patients initially and, again, includes antihypertensive drugs and beta blockade to decrease the contractile force of the myocardium. Temporizing may be reasonable with this group of patients as long as no vital structures are compromised or no other complications have occurred. This allows the firming up and scarring of the aortic wall, so that when the patient is operated on in a semielective fashion, the aortic wall can better hold sutures. The sutureless intraluminal graft may be used here as well. Regardless of the timing, most large centers report that surgery for dissection of the descending aorta is usually indicated within the first year after the onset of symptoms because of complications of the dissection and aneurysmal expansion of the dissected aorta. In performing surgery for desending thoracic dissection, attention must be paid to protecting the spinal cord. In most instances, shunting or cardiac bypass through the femoral route is used.

Patients with dissections who have undergone surgical repair should be treated with antihypertensive therapy and beta blockade for the rest of their lives. Mortality rates vary from 5 to 15 per cent after surgery for both ascending and descending thoracic aorta dissection, depending on the extent of the dissection and the local structures or arterial beds that are compromised.

ANGINA PECTORIS

method of
CLARENCE SHUB, M.D.
Mayo Clinic
Rochester, Minnesota

Proper medical management of the patient with angina pectoris should take into account the effects of the disease on the whole person (including physical, psychosocial, and economic aspects). Contributory conditions, for example, anemia, should be treated if possible. An adjustment in lifestyle, including altering risk factors, is often warranted and, depending on individual circumstances, may include cessation of cigarette smoking, weight reduction, dietary and/or drug treatment of hyperlipidemia, and an exercise training program.

DRUG THERAPY

The goal of drug therapy is to minimize the frequency and severity of angina and to improve the patient's functional capacity with as few side effects as possible. A variety of effective drugs are now available. In addition to efficacy and safety, patient compliance and cost must be considered in designing an appropriate medical regimen.

The rationale of antianginal drug therapy is to increase myocardial blood flow or decrease myocardial oxygen demand or both. Factors that increase myocardial blood flow include (1) coronary artery dilatation, (2) enhancement of coronary collateral blood flow, (3) reduction of left ventricular (LV) end-diastolic pressure, and (4) prolongation of diastole by decreasing heart rate, thus increasing coronary perfusion time. Factors that decrease the myocardial oxygen demand include (1) slowing heart rate, (2) decreasing

blood pressure, (3) lessening cardiac contractility, and (4) reducing LV cavity dimension, thereby decreasing LV systolic wall stress.

Currently, three major classes of drugs are available that can be used alone or in combination for the treatment of angina: nitrates, beta blockers, and calcium entry blockers. Multiple drugs are not necessarily better than properly selected monotherapy, increase side effects and cost, and, in some circumstances, may even cause worsening of ischemia.

Nitrates

Nitrates are direct-acting dilators of vascular smooth muscle. By causing venodilatation, nitrates decrease venous return and, thus, LV volume (preload) and LV diastolic pressure.

Nitrates cause coronary vasodilatation, redistribute blood flow to ischemic myocardium, and alleviate coronary artery spasm. Nitrates induce vasodilatation of stenotic coronary segments as long as there is sufficient smooth muscle remaining within the vessel wall. Exertion-related coronary constriction can be reversed or even prevented by nitroglycerin. Whether the predominant effect of nitrates in patients with coronary artery disease is an increase in coronary blood flow or a decrease in oxygen demand, or a varying combination of both, is an academic question that continues to be debated.

Sublingual nitroglycerin (Nitrostat) is an effective, short-acting antianginal agent that works promptly. If symptoms persist despite rest and a second or third dose of nitroglycerin, patients should be advised to contact their physician or a nearby emergency medical facility as soon as possible. Nitroglycerin may be taken prophylactically before an activity that is known to provoke angina. Elderly patients should be warned that at times unpredictable, transient hypotension may occur, especially during hot weather or a hot bath.

Long-acting nitrates may be given sublingually as isosorbide dinitrate (Isordil), orally as isosorbide dinitrate (Sorbitrate or Isordil) or pentaerythritol tetranitrate (Peritrate), via the buccal route (Nitrogard), or transcutaneously. Sublingual nitrates are effective antianginal agents, but their average duration of action (1½ hours) is so short that long-term maintenance dosage is usually impractical. To achieve a significant sustained systemic effect, oral doses of isosorbide dinitrate must be large enough to overcome metabolic degradation by the liver. The effects of single oral doses generally persist for 3 to 6 hours but can last for up to 8 hours. To avoid headaches, nitrate therapy should be started at low doses, for example, 10 mg of isosorbide dinitrate three times a day, and then should be gradually increased, depending on the clinical response, to 20 to 40 mg three times a day. In patients without a history of migraine or other vascular headaches, nitrate headaches are often transient, are relatively mild, and frequently subside during 1 to 2 weeks. Antianginal potency does not seem to diminish despite the disappearance of headaches. A mild analgesic, such as acetaminophen (Tylenol), may be useful during the early phases of therapy. Significant hypotension that occurs during treatment, unless caused by hypovolemia, generally necessitates lowering the nitrate dosage or stopping therapy.

Because of slower, continuous uptake through the skin, the duration of action of cutaneous nitrates (Nitrostat, Nitrol, Nitro-Bid ointment) is considerably extended (6 to 8 hours or more). Certain transdermal preparations (nitropatches, e.g., Transderm-Nitro, Nitrodisc, Nitro-Dur, Deponit) contain special cutaneous delivery systems that permit predictable, nonfluctuating plasma levels of nitrates and can be used once daily. Plasma nitroglycerin concentrations achieved with commonly used nitropatch doses, for example, 2.5 to 10 mg per 24 hours, are relatively low. For approximately 50 per cent of patients, a statistically significant increase in exercise capacity is observed during a 24-hour period after application of 5 to 10 mg of nitropatch. Larger doses, for example, 15 to 30 mg per 24 hours, allow higher plasma concentrations and increased efficacy, but tolerance becomes a potential problem. Development of vascular tolerance to nitrates is variable and unpredictable and can occur even at low doses. Continuous exposure to high levels of plasma nitrates leads to nitrate tolerance, and therapeutic efficacy may be lost very early in treatment at doses of oral isosorbide ranging from 5 to 45 mg. Tolerance to the clinical effects of oral isosorbide dinitrate develops from a sustained dosage of 30 mg four times a day but is not observed when the drug is administered two or three times daily. A daily "nitrate-free interval" of 10 to 12 hours (e.g., overnight) has therefore been advocated to restore nitrate responsiveness. Another drug, such as a calcium entry blocker, can be used during the nitrate-free interval if necessary.

Buccal nitroglycerin (Nitrogard) seems to cause less nitrate tolerance and has a rapid onset of action (within 5 minutes), as well as a sustained action. Most patients benefit from a 1- to 2-mg dose. The initial response parallels that of sublingual nitroglycerin in its timing, hemodynamic changes, and rapid relief of angina. The buccal tablet delivery system allows nitroglycerin to be released steadily across the buccal mucosa. A gel forms around the tablet that keeps it from dissolving. The patient has to learn to eat, drink, and talk without dislodging the tablet. The duration of effect varies but can last for up to 5 hours as long as the tablet remains intact. It can be used on a regular three times daily basis or as needed for angina.

The major advantage of oral nitroglycerin spray (Nitrolingual Spray) (0.4 mg per metered dose) is its ease of administration; for this reason, some patients prefer it to sublingual tablets. The hemodynamic effects of the spray occur within 2 minutes. Unlike nitroglycerin tablets, which tend to undergo chemical degradation over time and require periodic replacement, nitroglycerin spray seems to be protected in its container.

Beta Blockers

In cardiac muscle, beta blockers bind to the myocardial beta-adrenergic receptor (predominantly beta$_1$) and competitively inhibit the binding of catecholamines. Agonist stimulation of adenylate cyclase and the resultant enhancement of calcium influx are thus prevented. Beta blockers may increase LV volume (preload) and end-diastolic pressure, primarily because of their negative inotropic effects. The increased LV volume and end-diastolic pressure caused by beta blockers may be counteracted by the preload-reducing effect of concomitant nitrate and/or diuretic therapy. Patients with severe LV dysfunction may have frank cardiac failure provoked by these agents, and low doses should be used, if used at all. Beta blockers are better tolerated in patients with only mild to moderate LV dysfunction, for example, in patients with an ejection fraction of more than 35 to 40 per cent.

Beta blockers blunt the normal increase in exercise heart rate and systolic blood pressure. The increase in exercise capacity observed with beta blockers is variable and may be offset by changes in peripheral blood flow and an increase in LV diastolic pressure. In general, young to middle-aged adults respond best, especially if there is concomitant hypertension or an excessive heart rate or blood pressure response to exercise.

Beta$_1$-adrenergic blockers are only relatively "cardioselective." As the dose is increased, interaction with beta$_2$-adrenergic receptors also increases so that relatively nonselective effects, such as bronchoconstriction, may also occur. Although a pure beta-adrenergic antagonist produces no receptor stimulation, some agents can occupy beta-adrenergic receptor sites and prevent access by endogenous catecholamines but, at the same time, can cause some degree of receptor stimulation. This latter effect is referred to as partial agonist activity or intrinsic sympathomimetic activity. When basal sympathetic tone is low, the agonist effect predominates and the heart rate may even increase slightly. When sympathetic tone is high, the beta-blocking effect predominates and the adrenergic response is blunted. In some patients with nocturnal or rest angina, sympathetic tone may be low, and angina may actually worsen if a beta blocker with partial agonist activity is given. The reduction by pindolol (Visken) of the exercise heart rate is comparable to that of propranolol. Because pindolol does not appreciably lower cardiac output, it may be preferable in patients with reduced LV systolic function. However, other drugs without negative inotropic effects should be considered first in patients with markedly impaired LV performance.

It can be anticipated that approximately three-fourths of patients who are treated with beta blockers will experience a clinical benefit. Because all beta blockers are about equally effective in the treatment of angina, the choice of a specific drug depends on factors such as side effect profile, coexisting diseases, and duration of action. The negative chronotropic and inotropic actions of beta blockers may also limit the usefulness of these agents, especially in patients with pre-existing bradycardia or reduced LV systolic function.

When treatment is initiated with a beta blocker, a low dose should be used (e.g., 10 to 20 mg three times daily for propranolol [Inderal]) and should be gradually titrated upward, depending on the clinical response. Adverse effects, if any, are often seen within the first several days of treatment. Once a maintenance dosage regimen has been established, a graded exercise test can be considered to document the heart rate and blood pressure response and to ascertain the adequacy of beta blockade. Even relatively short-acting agents, such as propranolol, can be used on a twice daily basis and still retain antianginal effectiveness. Long-acting beta blockers are as effective as propranolol for the treatment of angina. Beta blockers that are currently available, as well as guidelines for administration and dosage, are shown in Table 1. Water-soluble beta blockers reportedly have fewer central nervous system side effects because they do not penetrate the blood-brain barrier as readily as do lipid-soluble agents. However, even water-soluble agents may ultimately be found in cerebrospinal fluid, and all beta-blocking agents have the potential to cause troublesome lethargy and fatigue.

Severe withdrawal symptoms, for example, aggravation of angina, ventricular tachycardia, precipitation of myocardial infarction, and even sudden death (although rare), may occur unpredictably when beta blockers are abruptly terminated in patients with ischemic heart disease. Patients who were taking beta blockers and who undergo general anesthesia may experience involuntary "drug withdrawal" if their medication is not resumed in the early postoperative period. A short-acting intravenous beta blocker, such as esmolol (Breviblock), can be used temporarily until the patient can resume taking oral medications, especially if there is postoperative tachycardia or elevated systemic blood pressure.

For patients with coexistent hypertension, beta blockers lower blood pressure, which may add to their antianginal efficacy. Nonselective beta-blocker drugs may cause an increase in peripheral resistance and may also provoke coronary spasm, especially in patients with variant angina. However, this does not seem to be a common clinical problem.

Calcium Entry Blockers

Calcium entry blockers, which are also referred to as calcium antagonists or calcium channel blockers, are a heterogeneous group of compounds with various dose-dependent effects that have certain common actions on the cardiovascular system. The net effect of these agents on cardiac electrical and mechanical function depends on the complex interaction between the drug's direct effects and the indirect effects of afterload reduction and baroreceptor-mediated reflex sympathetic stimulation. In addition, the hemodynamic effects of a given drug differ depending on LV function, dosage, and method of administration. In addition to lowering myocardial oxygen demand, these agents increase myocardial oxygen supply by lessening coronary spasm, by improving collateral blood flow, and/or by redistributing blood flow to ischemic myocardium. During exercise, mean arterial blood pressure and peripheral vascular resistance are reduced; some agents reduce exercise heart rate as well. The three currently available calcium entry blockers—nifedipine (Procardia, Adalat), verapamil (Calan, Isoptin), and diltiazem (Cardizem)—each have different molecular structures and produce different actions (Table 2). For example, nifedipine produces greater peripheral vasodilation than verapamil or diltiazem, whereas verapamil has a greater tendency to cause decreased myocardial contractility. In vivo, verapamil and diltiazem decrease AV conduction, whereas nifedipine does not. In conscious animals, equipotent doses of diltiazem, verapamil, and nifedipine result in increased LV contractility by nifedipine, a de-

TABLE 1. **Dosages and Selected Pharmacologic Properties of Currently Available Beta-Blocking Agents***

Drug: Generic Name (Trade Name)	Usual Daily Oral Dose (mg)		Cardioselective	ISA‡	Lipid Solubility	Plasma Half-life (hr)	Primary Route of Elimination
	Range	*No. of Daily Doses†*					
Propranolol (Inderal)	160–480	2–4	No	No	High	3.2–6	Hepatic
Nadolol (Corgard)	40–320	1	No	No	Low	12–24	Renal and biliary (90% unchanged)
Timolol (Blocadren)	20–40	2	No	Minimal	Low to intermediate	3–5	Hepatic and renal (20% unchanged)
Metoprolol (Lopressor)	100–450	2–3	Yes	No	Intermediate	3–4	Hepatic
Atenolol (Tenormin)	50–200	1	Yes	No	Low	6–9	Renal (<40% unchanged) and hepatic
Pindolol (Visken)	10–60	3	No	Yes	Intermediate	3–4	Renal (≈40% unchanged) and hepatic
Acebutolol (Sectral)	400–1200	2–4	Yes	Yes	Low	4–6	Hepatic and renal
Labetalol§ (Normodyne or Trandate)	300–1200	3	No	(Yes)‖	Low to intermediate	3–4	Hepatic

*From Shub C, Vlietstra RE, and McGoon MD: Selection of optimal drug therapy for the patient with angina pectoris. Mayo Clin Proc *60*:539–548, 1985. Used by permission.

†Some preparations are now available in long-acting or sustained-release forms or may be administered less frequently for certain indications.

‡ISA = intrinsic sympathomimetic activity.

§Labetalol possesses combined beta-blocking and relatively mild alpha-blocking activity (beta-blocking potency is at least four times the alpha-blocking potency).

‖Partial agonism of beta receptors.

crease by verapamil, and minimal change by diltiazem. Heart rate increases to a variable but mild degree with nifedipine secondary to reflex sympathetic stimulation. In some patients, this effect may be temporary. Heart rate may decrease slightly after administration of verapamil or diltiazem, but the effect is often over-ridden by reflex increases in sympathetic tone. The combination, however, of a beta blocker and diltiazem or verapamil may produce significant bradycardia. All three calcium entry blockers are effective

TABLE 2. **Physiologic Effects of Calcium Entry Blockers (In Vivo)*†**

Effect	Verapamil	Nifedipine	Diltiazem
Vasodilation	Moderate	Marked	Moderate
Decreased contractility‡	None or mild	None	None or mild
Decreased atrioventricular conduction	Mild	None	Mild

*From Shub C, Vlietstra RE, and McGoon MD: Selection of optimal drug therapy for the patient with angina pectoris. Mayo Clin Proc *60*:539–548, 1985. Used by permission.

†In vitro effects may vary depending on complex interaction of direct and indirect reflex-mediated cardiovascular responses.

‡These drugs are best avoided in cases of severe LV failure (see text).

antianginal agents. As assessed by radionuclide techniques, certain calcium entry blockers, especially verapamil, improve ventricular diastolic function in patients with coronary artery disease. Calcium entry blockers are preferable to beta blockers if the patient has known coronary vasospasm or bronchospastic pulmonary diseases, such as asthma or chronic obstructive pulmonary disease.

Nifedipine

The efficacy of nifedipine (Procardia, Adalat) is variable (20 to 100 per cent improvement). The usual oral starting dose of nifedipine is 10 mg three times daily, with gradual upward dose titration based on symptom control and lack of adverse effects. The usual daily maintenance dose of nifedipine ranges from 30 to 120 mg. More side effects are seen at higher doses. The rate, but not the extent, of nifedipine absorption is decreased by concurrent food ingestion. Giving food with nifedipine may blunt the side effects associated with peak vasodilatation. Conversely, very rapid onset of nifedipine action can be obtained by swallowing the liquid contents of a nifedipine capsule. A slow-release preparation of nifedipine appears to cause fewer side effects than the conventional drug. Leg edema may be a troublesome side effect. Another dihydropyridine derivative, nicardipine, has recently become available. Thus far, experience with this agent has been limited.

Verapamil

Verapamil (Calan, Isoptin), taken three or four times a day in total daily doses of 240 to 480 mg, is effective in the treatment of angina, but individual responses also vary. Studies have demonstrated that the half-life of verapamil is prolonged with chronic dosing and that even regular-release preparations can be given twice daily. As an antianginal agent, verapamil (360 mg daily) is comparable to propranolol (240 mg daily). The sustained-release verapamil preparation is as effective as the regular preparation at equivalent total daily doses.* Exercise tolerance may be greater with verapamil than with propranolol. The plasma half-life of verapamil increases with long-term oral therapy, and the frequency of administration can often be decreased from four times daily to three times daily after approximately 1 week of treatment. Constipation occurs in approximately 10 per cent of patients. Leg edema occurs in some patients as well. Patients with mild LV dysfunction appear to tolerate verapamil better than those with severe LV dysfunction. Verapamil should be avoided in patients with overt clinical heart failure unless LV diastolic dysfunction is the predominant abnormality and systolic function is preserved. It should also be avoided in patients with conduction disturbance.

Diltiazem

Diltiazem (Cardizem) at total daily doses of 120 to 360 mg has proved to be effective in the treatment of angina and, in general, is very well tolerated because of the low incidence of side effects. At equal doses, diltiazem is as effective as verapamil in the treatment of angina. A sustained-release diltiazem preparation that can be used twice daily is both effective and well tolerated at daily doses ranging from 240 to 360 mg.

Side Effects

Adverse reactions common to all calcium entry blockers are predictable from their pharmacologic actions and include flushing, hypotension, and headaches (related to vasodilatation). Although these side effects are more frequent with nifedipine, the negative inotropic and dromotropic effects predominate with verapamil and diltiazem, especially with the former.

---

*The sustained-release preparation has been approved only for use in hypertension by the U.S. Food and Drug Administration.

Combination Therapy

Nitrates can be effectively combined with beta blockers. The preload-lowering effect of nitrates offsets the potential deleterious tendency of beta blockers to increase LV volume. Beta blockers may also blunt nitrate headaches. Nitrates can be combined with calcium entry blockers, especially verapamil and diltiazem. The combination of verapamil or diltiazem plus a beta blocker has significant antianginal efficacy but also has a higher frequency of side effects. Nifedipine in combination with a beta blocker provides an additive therapeutic effect with few serious side effects. The beta blocker blunts the reflex tachycardia that may occur with nifedipine. Although the combination of verapamil and beta blockers has been considered to be potentially hazardous (severe bradycardia, atrioventricular (AV) block, hypotension, and/or frank LV failure may occur), verapamil and propranolol have been safely used in combination for carefully selected patients with angina (those who do not have heart failure, severe LV dysfunction, or AV nodal disease). Although the combination of beta blockers and diltiazem is usually well tolerated, marked sinus bradycardia or AV block, or both, may occur. For antianginal effect, the combination of beta blockers with nifedipine, verapamil, or diltiazem is approximately equally effective, although the propranolol-diltiazem combination probably causes the fewest side effects. The use of more than one calcium entry blocker has primarily been reported in patients with variant angina, but the combinations of diltiazem-nifedipine and verapamil-nifedipine (in addition to nitrates) have also been reported in small numbers of patients with refractory angina who were otherwise not candidates for coronary revascularization. An increased incidence of side effects should be anticipated. Lowering the usual dose of each of the calcium entry blockers may be helpful.

The treatment of angina should be individualized according to the patient's specific needs. Angina may occur in patients who have various concomitant disorders, such as hypertension, diabetes, peripheral vascular disease, chronic obstructive pulmonary disease, or arrhythmias, so that no one drug regimen is ideal for all patients in all circumstances (Table 3). Nitrates are both effective and safe to use in patients with angina who have significant LV systolic dysfunction. Because the negative inotropic effects of nifedipine are counteracted by decreased afterload and reflex increases in cardiac sympathetic tone, nifedipine is the calcium entry blocker of choice in patients with severe LV systolic failure. Diltiazem can be used as a second choice.

TABLE 3. **Recommended Drug Therapy (Calcium Entry Blocker versus Beta Blocker) in Patients Who Have Angina in Conjunction with Other Medical Conditions**[*][†]

Clinical Condition	Recommended Drug (Alternative Drug)
Cardiac arrhythmias and conduction abnormalities	
Sinus bradycardia	Nifedipine
Sinus tachycardia (not related to cardiac failure)	Beta blocker
Supraventricular tachycardia	Verapamil or beta blocker
Atrioventricular block	Nifedipine
Rapid atrial fibrillation (with digitalis)	Verapamil or beta blocker
Ventricular arrhythmias	Beta blocker (± group 1 antiarrhythmic agent)
Left ventricular dysfunction	
Congestive heart failure	
Mild (LVEF ≥ 40%)	Nifedipine (verapamil, diltiazem, or beta blockers cautiously)
Moderate to severe (LVEF < 40%)	Nifedipine (cautiously, in combination with other therapy)
Left-sided valvular heart disease[‡]	
Aortic stenosis (mild)[§]	Beta blocker
Aortic insufficiency	Nifedipine
Mitral regurgitation	Nifedipine
Mitral stenosis[‖]	Beta blocker
Miscellaneous medical conditions	
Systemic hypertension	Beta blocker or calcium entry blockers
Severe pre-existing headaches	Beta blocker (verapamil or diltiazem)
COPD with bronchospasm or asthma	Nifedipine, verapamil, or diltiazem (low-dose beta$_1$-selective blocker or beta-ISA)
Hyperthyroidism	Beta blocker
Raynaud's syndrome	Nifedipine
Claudication	Nifedipine, verapamil, or diltiazem (low-dose beta$_1$ blocker or beta-ISA)
Depression	Nifedipine, verapamil, or diltiazem
Neurasthenia or fatigue states	Nifedipine, verapamil, or diltiazem
Insulin-dependent diabetes mellitus	Nifedipine, verapamil, or diltiazem (low-dose beta$_1$ blocker or beta-ISA)

*From Shub C, Vlietstra RE, and McGoon MD: Selection of optimal drug therapy for the patient with angina pectoris. Mayo Clin Proc 60:539–548, 1985. Used by permission.

†Beta-ISA = Beta blocker with intrinsic sympathomimetic activity such as pindolol or acebutolol; COPD = chronic obstructive pulmonary disease; LVEF = LV ejection fraction.

‡Surgical therapy should be considered for patients with severe valvular heart disease; beta blockers are not routinely used in patients with valvular heart disease and LV failure.

§Vasodilators may increase aortic valve gradient, and beta blockers can cause LV failure. Any of these drugs should be used with extreme caution in patients with severe aortic stenosis.

‖If congestive heart failure (associated with normal LV function) occurs in a patient with angina, severe mitral stenosis, and rapid atrial fibrillation, a beta blocker (in combination with digitalis) may be used to reduce the heart rate.

Drug Interactions and Miscellaneous Considerations

In patients taking cimetidine, the dosage of calcium entry blockers or lipophilic beta blockers should be reduced because both drugs are metabolized in the liver. Ranitidine may not decrease hepatic metabolism of these agents as much as cimetidine. Some beta blockers, such as propranolol but not labetalol, have been reported to lower high-density-lipoprotein cholesterol levels and to increase serum triglyceride levels. The long-term effects of these changes on atherosclerotic disease progression are unknown. Metoprolol appears to decrease low-density-lipoprotein cholesterol binding to arterial wall proteoglycans, which in turn may prevent cellular fat deposition. The clinical significance of these observations is still unclear. Gynecomastia has been reported as a rare side effect of calcium entry blocker therapy. Numerous reports have documented a gradual increase (during 7 to 14 days) of serum digoxin levels (by 40 to 77 per cent) in patients using digoxin and verapamil concurrently. The risk of developing digitalis toxicity in these circumstances has been estimated to be approximately 10 per cent. The dosage of digoxin should be decreased by approximately 50 per cent when verapamil therapy is initiated. Measurement of the serum digoxin level after approximately 2 weeks of combined therapy is warranted. Although diltiazem and nifedipine have also been reported to increase serum digoxin levels, the observations have not been as consistent, and the magnitude of the effect is variable.

Other Drugs

Aspirin and other antiplatelet agents such as sulfinpyrazone have shown no consistent antianginal effect. Although aspirin is commonly used in patients with unstable angina or acute myocardial infarction, a reduction in cardiovascular mortality in patients with *stable* angina pectoris remains to be proved. However, even in the absence of supporting data, many physicians still recommend low-dose aspirin, for example, 325 mg daily, because such therapy is usually safe, inexpensive, and well tolerated. For an antiplatelet effect, one children's aspirin tablet (81 mg) daily appears to be as effective as the larger dose. Vasodilator agents such as dipyridamole (Persantine) have shown no consistent beneficial effect in the treatment of angina, and high doses of dipyridamole, in some cases, may even aggravate angina.

CORONARY REVASCULARIZATION

When medical therapy fails to control the symptoms of angina pectoris, coronary angiography should be considered because many patients may benefit from either percutaneous transluminal coronary angioplasty or coronary artery bypass surgery.

SUDDEN CARDIAC ARREST

method of
RICHARD O. CUMMINS, M.D.,
M.Sc., M.P.H.
University of Washington School of Medicine
Seattle, Washington

and

JUDITH REID GRAVES, R.N., E.M.T.-P.
Center for Evaluation of Emergency Medical
Services, Division of Emergency Medical
Services, King County Department
of Public Health
Seattle, Washington

Most readers of *Conn's Current Therapy* are busy office practitioners. For them, the drama and challenge of a cardiac arrest exist as a daily possibility. Cardiac arrest, however, cannot be scheduled like an office visit. Fate may force clinicians to deal with the sudden, unexpected collapse of a patient at any time. A poorly handled resuscitation attempt can make physicians feel as if they have failed as professionals. Public expectations and professional responsibility dictate that physicians know what to do when confronted with this emergency.

To best prepare for managing a cardiac arrest, a physician should participate in a basic life support (BLS) course and in an advanced cardiac life support (ACLS) course, each of which is sponsored by the American Heart Association (AHA). AHA standards require recertification every 2 years; however, after obtaining certification, many physicians fail to recertify. This chapter can serve as a review for physicians who have taken an ACLS course but have not recertified and for physicians who do not practice their resuscitation skills frequently. We strongly recommend that all practicing physicians take at least one formal BLS course and one formal ACLS course, even if circumstances prevent them from maintaining current certification.

The value of an ACLS course comes from its emphasis on psychomotor skills and on the protocol approach to cardiac arrest. The AHA presents the intervention sequences in the form of flow diagrams, or protocol sequences. These AHA protocols have emerged as almost an industry standard. The "recipes" recommended by the AHA are presented for quick review, with mnemonics, in Figures 1 to 6.

The AHA protocols for cardiac arrest may not be the best physiologic approach to cardiac arrest, nor are they the only acceptable approach from a medical or legal perspective. They do, however, provide the consensus recommendations of the multidisciplinary AHA

Standards Conference, last held in 1985 and published 1 year later in the well-known "JAMA Standards" edition of the Journal of the American Medical Association (JAMA *255:*2905, 1986). These same standards are recapitulated in a different format in the *ACLS Textbook*, which is given to all students in an ACLS course. The goal of the 1985 AHA Standards Conference was to recommend approaches that are generally regarded as having the best probability of success, in view of existing scientific data.

Rather than recapitulate the AHA recommendations in this chapter, we comment on aspects of sudden cardiac death of which practicing physicians should be aware, but which are not specifically covered in the AHA training. We make these comments for clinicians who may have to deal with a cardiac arrest in the office and for whom a cardiac arrest "code team" is not immediately available.

DEVELOPMENTS IN EMERGENCY MEDICAL SERVICES: THE CHAIN OF SURVIVAL CONCEPT

The core of the AHA approach to the immediate resuscitation of a person in cardiac arrest is *recognition* that an arrest has occurred, followed by *immediate activation of the emergency medical services (EMS) system.* Once the EMS system has been activated, the rescuer returns to initiate basic cardiopulmonary resuscitation (CPR). This procedure underscores the idea that advanced care, in the form of electrical defibrillation, definitive airway management, and intravenous pharmacology, must be brought to the patient as soon as possible. A physician-rescuer should never forget that the prime chance for a successful resuscitation comes from decreasing the time from the onset of the arrest to the restoration of an effective spontaneous circulation. When additional people in the medical office arrive to help, they can be directed to assist with CPR, to get available ACLS equipment (specific recommendations are made later in this chapter), to activate the resuscitation team (if in a hospital setting), or to activate the EMS system.

A practicing physician can therefore institute in his or her office a "chain of survival," a concept that is being broadly applied on a national and an international basis. The chain of survival has four links: *early access,* to get help; *early CPR,* to buy time; *early defibrillation,* to restart the heart; and *early advanced care,* to stabilize the patient.

Early Access

Early access requires that every community have an efficient emergency medical dispatch system. In many locations this number is *911;* other locations have multiple listings of seven-digit numbers. If a community lacks a 911 system, the family members of high-risk patients

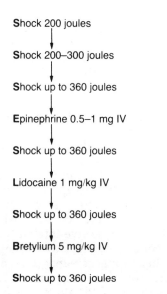

Mnemonic:
Shock, Shock, Shock, Everybody Shock. Little Shock, Big Shock

Figure 1. Ventricular fibrillation. Modified from Eisenberg MS, Cummins RO, and Ho M: Code Blue: Cardiac Arrest and Resuscitation. Philadelphia, W. B. Saunders Co. Blue Book Series, 1987.

should have immediate access, usually through stickers posted on the telephone, of the particular local EMS number. Physicians in their offices can recognize a cardiac arrest easily; however, lay people occasionally become confused by the gasps of a collapsed patient. A community-wide "phone first" program would teach citizens to call 911 immediately and activate the EMS system whenever there is a suspicion of an emergency. From the perspective of emergency personnel, it is certainly better to be told that a suspected cardiac arrest was actually a syncopal episode than to be told that a suspected faint, which had gone unattended for several minutes, was a full cardiac arrest.

Early CPR

Clinicians should be aware that several debates exist about basic CPR. One dispute concerns the mechanism of blood flow that occurs during the

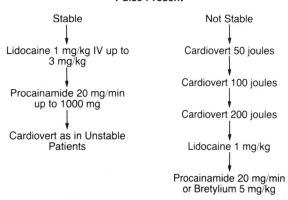

Mnemonic: Pulse and Awake (stable)
              Drug first they take

              Pulse and a Nap (unstable, unconscious)
              First you must Zap

              When shocks cannot win
              Let pharmacy begin

Figure 2. Ventricular tachycardia (VT). Modified from Eisenberg MS, Cummins RO, and Ho M: Code Blue: Cardiac Arrest and Resuscitation. Philadelphia, W. B. Saunders Co. Blue Book Series, 1987.

chest compressions of CPR. Some physicians contend that the chest compressions squeeze the heart between the sternum and the vertebral bodies of the spine; others argue that the blood flow is produced by increased intrathoracic pressure. In this mechanism the chest and all its contents, including the lungs, heart, and great vessels, are like a large sponge, squeezed out with each chest compression. To increase the effectiveness of this squeezing mechanism, several alternative approaches to CPR, including interposed abdominal compressions, high-impulse CPR, and various types of abdominal and chest binders, have been developed. None of these approaches, collectively referred to as "new CPR," have been shown to be significantly better than conventional CPR.

Another issue about conventional CPR has to

Pacer (as soon as possible)
↓
Epinephrine (0.5–1 mg IV)
↓
Atropine 1 mg IV

Mnemonic: Popeye Eats Asparagus

Figure 3. Asystole. Modified from Eisenberg MS, Cummins RO, and Ho M: Code Blue: Cardiac Arrest and Resuscitation. Philadelphia, W. B. Saunders Co. Blue Book Series, 1987.

Epinephrine 0.5–1 mg IV
↓
Memorize the Differential

(includes hypovolemia, cardiac tamponade, tension pneumothorax, pulmonary embolism, acidosis, hypoxia)

Mnemonic: E M D (Epinephrine, Memorize the Differential)

Figure 4. Electromechanical Dissociation (EMD). Modified from Eisenberg MS, Cummins RO, and Ho M: Code Blue: Cardiac Arrest and Resuscitation. Philadelphia, W. B. Saunders Co. Blue Book Series, 1987.

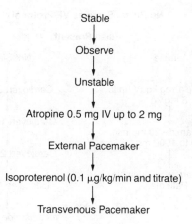

Mnemonic: First Atropine
Then a Pacer Machine

Figure 5. Bradycardia. Modified from Eisenberg MS, Cummins RO, and Ho M: Code Blue: Cardiac Arrest and Resuscitation. Philadelphia, W. B. Saunders Co. Blue Book Series, 1987.

do with the low blood flow that occurs during chest compressions. Laboratory investigators, taking advantage of sophisticated flow meters and improved physiologic instruments, have observed disappointingly low flow through the carotid arteries and the coronary arteries during standard CPR. These flow rates have been observed to be a small fraction (10 to 20 per cent) of normal values. These low flow states may have a negative effect on neurologic recovery from a cardiac arrest. The flows are not high enough to maintain full tissue viability, but they are high enough to support ongoing metabolic processes, and toxic by-products may accumulate. If spon-

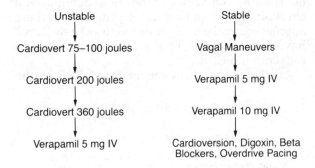

Mnemonic: If there's time, verapamil
If no time, an electric pill

Figure 6. Paroxysmal supraventricular tachycardia (PSVT). Modified from Eisenberg MS, Cummins RO, and Ho M: Code Blue: Cardiac Arrest and Resuscitation. Philadelphia, W. B. Saunders Co. Blue Book Series, 1987.

taneous blood flow returns, these toxic substances induce cascades of severe injury in the brain (socalled reperfusion injury or postresuscitation syndrome). In theory, the low flow, or trickle flow, state of conventional CPR should lead to more negative outcomes.

Observational clinical studies, however, have not reported harmful consequences from conventional CPR, even when the technique is performed by presumably less skilled citizen bystanders. Studies of out-of-hospital cardiac arrest, with a few notable exceptions, have observed a superior survival for arrest victims who receive early, bystander-initiated CPR when compared with victims who receive late CPR performed by the emergency personnel when they arrive.

Even the strongest supporters of widespread citizen training in conventional CPR, however, acknowledge that CPR alone does not defibrillate or resuscitate cardiac arrest victims. It merely buys time until the arrival of the defibrillator and of full ACLS. Conventional CPR may buy time through the mechanism of prolonging ventricular tachyarrhythmias. If arrest victims receive early CPR from bystanders, they are more likely to be in ventricular tachyarrhythmia when the defibrillator-carrying personnel arrive. In addition, some evidence suggests that persons in ventricular fibrillation who receive early CPR are more likely to convert to a spontaneously perfusing rhythm on countershock than persons in ventricular fibrillation who do not receive early CPR.

What is the lesson for practicing office-based clinicians? Certainly they should know CPR themselves, and they should encourage family members and friends of high-risk patients to receive CPR training. (Table 1 presents a review of the basic ABC's for one-person CPR.) In the United States, the term "high risk" may include virtually all men over the age of 50 years and all women over the age of 60 years. Several studies have reported strong reluctance on the part of physicians to discuss the need for CPR training with the relatives of high-risk cardiac patients. Part of this reluctance may be due to the same hesitancy that physicians have to discuss "do not resuscitate" status with the family and friends of people for whom such an approach may be appropriate (discussed in a later section of this chapter). All practicing clinicians should support efforts to increase the percentage of the citizenry trained in BLS. Debate about the mechanism of blood flow during CPR or other subissues should not obscure the fact that receiving CPR training and attempting it on arrest victims improves the chances of survival. It is critical to have early CPR as a strong link in the chain of survival.

TABLE 1. **ABC's: Basic CPR Sequence for One Person*†**

A—Airway

Assess (determine unresponsiveness)
Ask for help
Appropriate positioning for victim and rescuer
Airway open (head tilt/chin lift)

B—Breathing

Breathing normally?
Blow in 2 breaths‡

C—Circulation

Check for a pulse
Call the EMS system
Compress the chest§

Reassess after four cycles of 15 compressions and 2 ventilations

*Modified from Eisenberg MS, Cummins RO, and Ho M: Code Blue: Cardiac Arrest and Resuscitation. Philadelphia, W. B. Saunders Co. Blue Book Series, 1987.

†Note: the adaptations for two-person CPR are (1) two-person compression/ventilation ratio is 5:1; (2) after every fifth compression, stop for 1–1.5 sec to allow ventilation and then immediately resume.

‡Take 1–1.5 sec per ventilation.

§Compression/ventilation ratio is 15:2; compression rate = 80–100/min.

Early Defibrillation

The emphasis on early activation of the EMS system underscores the principle that advanced care, in the form of electrical defibrillation and cardiac pacing, definitive airway management, and intravenous pharmacology, must be brought to the patient as soon as possible. A rescuer should never forget that the prime chance for a successful resuscitation comes from decreasing the time from onset of arrest to restoration of effective spontaneous circulation.

Research has established that early defibrillation is the most important element of advanced cardiac care. Almost 85 per cent of the people who have collapsed in cardiac arrest while wearing a continuously recording monitoring device are in ventricular tachyarrhythmia (either ventricular fibrillation or ventricular tachycardia). No pharmacologic agent has been identified that works acutely as an antifibrillatory agent. Electrical countershock is required to restore coordinated cardiac contractions. Awareness of the importance of early defibrillation has given rise to the principle of early defibrillation, which states that whoever arrives first, in a professional capacity, at the scene of a cardiac arrest should be equipped with a defibrillator. This principle, although supported by a strong clinical rationale, has been difficult to implement with conventional defibrillators. Standard monitor/defibrillators require skill in recognition of rhythm and operation

of the device. The advent of automated external defibrillators has changed the picture immensely. This exciting new technology has considerable implications for the practicing clinician.

Automated external defibrillators are attached to a patient through two adhesive electrode pads. These electrodes serve a dual function to both record the surface electrocardiogram (ECG) and deliver the defibrillatory shock. Microprocessors in the automated defibrillators analyze the ECG signal, and if ventricular fibrillation or rapid ventricular tachycardia is present the devices will either "advise" the operator that a shock is indicated (semiautomatic or shock advisory defibrillators) or will begin to charge and will deliver a shock after appropriate warning sounds and displays.

Unlike many other devices in emergency medicine, automated external defibrillators have been tested extensively, both in vitro (against libraries of cardiac rhythms) and clinically (in numerous field trials). The accuracy of the devices at rhythm analysis has been extremely high. The major errors noted with automated defibrillators in field trials have been omission errors, when the device failed to recognize certain varieties of ventricular fibrillation or ventricular tachycardia. The devices occasionally have trouble discriminating between fine, low-amplitude ventricular fibrillation and asystole. However, no errors of commission (inappropriately delivering a shock to a patient with a viable, nonlethal dysrhythmia) have yet been reported.

Emergency medical technicians (EMTs) have used these devices extensively and have supplied the bulk of the data related to their effectiveness. Training as an EMT requires 110 hours of basic training, plus 4 to 6 hours of training in the use of an automated external defibrillator. Most EMS ambulances in the United States are staffed by personnel trained to the basic EMT level. An EMT is the most likely emergency responder to arrive in a practitioner's office. In addition to EMTs, automated defibrillators have been given to fire fighters and first responders in many states and several large cities, including Seattle, San Francisco, Salt Lake City, New York City, and Miami.

To extend the principle of early defibrillation, recent research has focused on the feasibility of home- and community-based use of automated defibrillators. Individuals who do not normally function as emergency personnel have been trained to operate automated defibrillators in various settings. These settings include the homes of high-risk cardiac patients, large corporate buildings, high-rise office buildings and restaurants, senior care and exercise centers, and wide-body aircraft that fly long international routes. Security personnel at large gatherings also receive such training. These feasibility studies have confirmed that lay people and the family members of high-risk cardiac patients can learn to operate these devices with a minimum of training, that they can remember how to use these devices, with some retraining, for more than 1 year, and that they can successfully use the device in the dramatic moment of the collapse of a family member or office coworker. The long-term contribution of these devices to improving survival from cardiac arrest has not yet been established.

The AHA has recognized the importance of early defibrillation, and in particular, the role of automated external defibrillators in making defibrillation a household word. The AHA has developed a specific training module for automated defibrillation to be added to the ACLS course. It is also offered as a free-standing course. This initiative by the AHA was partly in response to the growing realization that automated external defibrillation has passed the stage in technology development of conceptualization and experimentation and has entered the stage of technology dissemination. Provision of early access to early defibrillation, primarily via automated external defibrillators, will soon become the standard of care.

We strongly recommend that practicing clinicians seriously consider whether automated external defibrillators may solve the dilemma of how to provide early defibrillation for the rare cardiac arrest in the office. Conventional defibrillators are large and expensive and require regular training in recognition of rhythm and operation of the device. Automated external defibrillators are small, relatively inexpensive, and simple to operate. In general, learning to use and operate an automated external defibrillator is easier than learning to perform basic CPR. The devices have a long battery shelf-life and are convenient to store. In several locations, automated external defibrillators have been placed in the hospital on the general medical floors, in evacuation aircraft, and in the offices of dentists, oral surgeons, and other such specialists. The nurses and office staff of a physician's office could be easily trained to operate such devices while awaiting the arrival of emergency personnel. Consequently, we have included an automated external defibrillator in our list of recommended items in an office medical emergency kit (Table 2). There is an increasing likelihood that the emergency personnel who initially arrive will be equipped with an automated defibrillator, which is another reason for physicians to become more

TABLE 2. Recommended Contents of an Office Medical Emergency Kit

General Equipment
Stethoscope
Blood pressure cuff
Three pairs of disposable gloves
Defibrillator/Monitor
Portable, battery-powered, automated (shock-advisory) defibrillator that can display ECG rhythm
Disposable adhesive defibrillator/monitoring electrodes
Airway Adjuncts
Protective face shields (disposable, for mouth-to-mouth ventilations)
Pocket face mask
Bag-valve mask
Oropharyngeal airways (three sizes)
Intravenous Fluid Equipment
One-liter bag of D5W
One-liter of normal saline
Two sets of IV tubing
Needles suitable for initiating IV fluids (16, 18, 20 gauge)
Two IV preparation kits (tourniquets, preparatory solutions, and tape)
Intravenous Medications in Prefilled Syringes
Naloxone, 5 ampules (1-ml ampules, 0.4 mg/ml)
50% dextrose solution, 2 ampules (50-ml ampules, 25 grams, 500 mg/ml)
Atropine, 2 ampules (10-ml ampules, 1 mg, 0.1 mg/ml)
Epinephrine, 4 ampules (10-ml ampules, 1 mg, 0.1 mg/ml)
Sodium bicarbonate, 2 ampules (50-ml ampules, 50 mEq, 8.4% solution, 1 mEq/ml)
Lidocaine, 2 ampules (5-ml ampules, 100 mg, 20 mg/ml, 2% solution)

familiar with these devices. Use of the automated defibrillator by office nurses or clinical assistants will free the physicians to perform other interventions such as endotracheal intubation and intravenous infusions. In many cases, early defibrillation alone may restore a spontaneous rhythm.

Early Advanced Cardiac Life Support

By convention, ACLS care has included three elements: defibrillation, endotracheal intubation, and intravenous medications. Defibrillation, however, should now be considered separate from the usual ingredients of ACLS because with the emergence of automated external defibrillation, even minimally trained rescuers can provide early defibrillation. Whereas formerly BLS and ACLS were separate, the chain of survival concept adds two additional elements: early access, performed by citizens; and early defibrillation, performed by early-responding, first-tier personnel.

Practicing physicians must know what kind of EMS response will take place in their community if a cardiac arrest occurs. In the United States, ACLS for cardiac arrest that occurs outside the hospital is generally provided by paramedics (EMT-Ps). These individuals receive 1000 to 2000 hours of classroom training and field instruction and can provide all elements of ACLS. Studies of prehospital cardiac arrest confirm that ACLS is required to achieve the highest possible survival. Although early CPR and early defibrillation alone may produce many resuscitations, much evidence confirms an incremental value to the rhythm stabilization and definitive airway management performed by ACLS personnel. Unfortunately, paramedic services are expensive and must cover large geographic areas. They are most successful in urban areas where response times are short and the number of calls justifies the expense.

The office practitioner who prepares to handle a cardiac arrest in his or her office must therefore deal with the possibility that ACLS, at least intubation and intravenous medications, may not be available in the community. At the minimum, the responding personnel should be trained in defibrillation, and we encourage all clinicians to inquire about the certification level of the local EMS system. The organization of this system may become even more important from a medicolegal perspective as early defibrillation becomes the standard of care in virtually all communities that meet the minimum requirements for an early defibrillation program.

Must all practitioners be competent in the skills of intubation and starting an intravenous infusion? Legally the answer is clear: practicing physicians are required to maintain competency in only those activities that they perform regularly and that are within their range of training and expertise. A physician who never intubates patients or performs cricothyrotomies is under no legal obligation to attempt such an intervention in an emergency, although the physician's constant imperative to help may impel him or her to try. The practicing clinician should know basic airway management techniques and should be able to inject medications intravenously. Therefore, we recommend competency with the manual techniques of positioning and ventilation (flat on back, chin lift/head tilt, jaw thrust/head tilt, mouth-to-mouth expired air ventilations), and competency with BLS airway management devices. These devices include the oropharyngeal airway, CPR shields (plastic hygienic covers for mouth-to-mouth contact), pocket face masks for mouth-to-mask ventilations, and the bag-valve mask. Supplemental oxygen should be readily available.

By the end of the 1980s, many experts have adopted a largely reductionist viewpoint, which maintained that few medical interventions had an effect on survival after cardiac arrest. Although defibrillation has emerged as the most effective intervention for improving survival, many pharmacologic interventions have fallen into disfavor. Calcium chloride, sodium bicarbonate, and isoproterenol have been of limited effectiveness or even detrimental in most resuscitation attempts. They are no longer mainstays of immediate treatment.

Medications that are still recommended for use in cardiac resuscitation are given, with their doses and indications, in Table 3. The major medications with which an office clinician needs to be immediately familiar are epinephrine, lidocaine, and atropine. More than 90 per cent of the people resuscitated from out-of-hospital cardiac arrest require only CPR, defibrillation, and one or more of these three drugs.

Epinephrine. Epinephrine remains the single most important pharmacologic agent for treatment of cardiac arrest. The vasoconstrictive actions of epinephrine increase diastolic blood pressure and lead to better coronary and carotid artery flow during CPR. If intravenous access cannot be obtained, epinephrine can be injected sublingually or endotracheally. Because of numerous complications and a high failure rate, intracardiac injections of epinephrine are not recommended.

Lidocaine. Lidocaine is the drug of choice in the acute treatment of ventricular premature beats, ventricular tachycardia, and ventricular fibrillation. After successful electrical countershock, lidocaine suppresses ventricular irritability and thus stabilizes the rhythm. Lidocaine works best when injected intravenously in a bolus; however, it can also be administered endotracheally and intramuscularly.

Atropine. As a parasympatholytic agent, atropine accelerates the sinus rate and facilitates conduction at the atrioventricular node. Atropine is useful for the treatment of unstable bradycardias and ventricular asystole. An unstable bradycardia is one with hypotension, chest pain, confusion, decreased mentation, or premature ventricular contractions. Bradycardia that is hemodynamically stable or asymptomatic should not be treated with atropine, especially in the setting of an acute myocardial infarction. If the heart rate accelerates in this setting, myocardial ischemia may be worsened and the area of infarction enlarged.

The Arrival of Emergency Personnel at the Office

Many physicians think that they must continue to be "in charge" of resuscitation efforts after emergency personnel arrive. Legally, as a licensed physician, they remain the senior medical person at the scene. In reality, however, unless

TABLE 3. **Advanced Cardiac Life Suport Drugs: Indications and Dosages***

Drug	Indications	Dosage (Adults)
Isoproterenol (Isuprel)	Symptomatic bradycardia or heart block not responsive to atropine Not indicated in cardiac arrest	2–20 µg/min (1 mg in 250 ml D5W = 4 µg/ml) titrated to heart rate
Lidocaine	VF, VT, PVCs	1.0 mg/kg IV push; may repeat every 10 min with 0.5 mg/kg up to 3 mg/kg; follow with 2–4 mg/min IV drip (1 gram in 250 ml D5W = 4 mg/ml)
Nitroglycerin	Unstable angina, CHF	0.4 mg SL every 5 min up to 3 tablets; 5 µg/min IV, increasing by 5 µg/min every 3–5 min up to 500 µg/min (8 mg in 250 ml D5W = approx 30 µg/ml; use glass container and special administration sets provided)
Nitroprusside (Nipride)	Hypertensive crisis, dissecting aortic aneurysm	0.5–15 µg/kg/min (50 mg in 250 ml D5W = 200 µg/ml)
Norepinephrine, levarterenol (Levophed)	Cardiogenic shock	8–32 µg/min, start at low dose (4 mg in 250 ml D5W = 16 µg/ml)
Procainamide (Pronestyl)	VF or VT not responsive to lidocaine or bretylium	100 mg over 5 min IV up to loading dose of 1 gram followed by 1–4 mg/min IV drip (500 mg in 250 ml D5W = 2 mg/ml)
Propranolol (Inderal)	VF or VT not responsive to lidocaine, bretylium, or procainamide	1 mg/min diluted in 10 ml D5W IV up to 5 mg
Verapamil	PSVT, temporary control of fast atrial flutter or atrial fibrillation	5–10 mg IV over 1 min; may repeat dose in 15–30 min
Atropine	Symptomatic bradyarrhythmia or heart block, asystole (1.0 mg IV)	0.5 mg IV every 5 min up to 2 mg
Bicarbonate	Consider for persistent cardiac arrest and/or return of perfusing rhythm	1 mEq/kg IV, then 0.5 mEq/kg every 10 min
Bretylium (Bretylol)	VF or VT not responsive to lidocaine	5 mg/kg IV push; may repeat in 15-min intervals with 10 mg/kg IV (max of 30 mg/kg)
Calcium chloride	Not indicated in cardiac arrest	
Digoxin (Lanoxin)	Rapid atrial fibrillation	0.5–1.0 mg IV; may repeat 0.25 mg every 2 hr until effect
Dobutamine (Dobutrex)	Short-term inotropic support	2.5–10 µg/kg/min (250 mg in 500 ml D5W = 500 µg/ml)
Dopamine (Intropin)	Cardiogenic shock	2–50 µg/kg/min; start at low dose, 2–5 µg/kg/min (200 mg in 250 ml D5W = 800 µg/ml)
Epinephrine	Asystole, EM dissociation, VF not responding to shocks	0.5–1 mg (10 ml, 1:10,000) IV (or endotracheally or IC); may repeat every 5 min

*Modified from Eisenberg MS, Cummins RO, and Ho M: Code Blue: Cardiac Arrest and Resuscitation. Philadelphia, W. B. Saunders Co. Blue Book Series, 1987.

Abbreviations: VF = ventricular fibrillation; VT = ventricular tachycardia; PVC = premature ventricular contraction; CHF = congestive heart failure; SL = sublingual; PSVT = paroxysmal supraventricular tachycardia; EM = electromechanical.

they are trained specifically in emergency resuscitation techniques, on-scene physicians are generally less skilled in prehospital interventions than the emergency personnel who respond. The emergency personnel are rigidly trained to follow specific protocols and to obtain medical consultations from their base station medical control officer. For cardiac arrest, almost all EMS systems use the "standing orders" approach: personnel are authorized to proceed with their treatment cascades until a predetermined point is reached. They are then required to contact their base station via radio or telephone. EMTs in a defibrillation program are trained to rapidly assume responsibility for airway and continued CPR and to initiate the attachment of the automated defibrillator as fast as possible. In general, field protocols for an EMT-defibrillation program direct three consecutive shocks to patients in ventricular fibrillation, followed by a brief period of CPR and hyperventilation with supplemental oxygen. If ventricular fibrillation persists, emergency personnel deliver additional shocks, usually in stacked sets of three shocks. Rarely does ventricular fibrillation persist after six countershocks. In some systems the field protocols may direct continued shocks as long as ventricular fibrillation persists.

The role of the physician initially on the scene should be one of support as needed rather than leadership. If the responding personnel function at the level of paramedics, they know their equipment and tasks better than office physicians, and they are better at the required psychomotor skills. Most field emergency personnel are skilled professionals who take great pride in their work. Physicians who observe such personnel in action, with their coordinated teamwork, anticipatory actions, and rapid decision-making in critical situations, are invariably impressed.

The physician on the scene should provide the emergency personnel with the patient's chief complaint, age, mechanism of injury, vital signs, pertinent physical findings, and any other information necessary for the resuscitation transfer. This may include intravenous needle size, volume of fluid administered, shocks that have been delivered in the office, medications given, and the patient's response to the medications and shocks. Known allergies, medications, and relevant past medical history should be mentioned. Office-based physicians should not indulge the tasteless compulsion to "act like a doctor" at the scene of a public emergency.

Patients who are successfully resuscitated are transferred to the care of the emergency personnel who, in turn, are under the responsibility of their base station physician. The office physician may want to accompany the ambulance personnel to the hospital. Although this may be appropriate in some circumstances, in general the physician may serve his or her professional role best by attending to the family, friends, and other bystander witnesses to the event. When transfer of care has occurred, the physician should assume immediate responsibility for notification of the family. It is critical to (1) confirm that the patient is indeed who he or she is thought to be, (2) establish the relationship of those present, (3) accurately restate the events leading to the resuscitation, (4) emphasize that a thorough team effort was undertaken, and (5) briefly outline the patient's present condition as best as is known. After allowing for appropriate emotional expression, the physician should inform the family of the immediate disposition of the patient and the identity of the providers who will continue care. A telephone call to the receiving hospital provides a brief report to the emergency physician who assumes responsibility for the patient.

Transcutaneous (External) Cardiac Pacing

In some locations, office practitioners may be surprised to observe the prehospital emergency team arrive not only with automated external defibrillators but also with transcutaneous (or external) pacemakers. These devices have become readily available in emergency departments and hospital critical care units after their initial development and successful use in the 1950s. Poor outcomes have been reported with external pacing for patients with asystole, electromechanical dissociation, and pulseless idioventricular rhythms, primarily because the pacing has been initiated extremely late in the resuscitation attempt. These delays may not occur in an office or in the hospital. The results of external pacing for patients with bradyarrhythmias, however, have been more encouraging. After success with pacing for bradycardia, particularly bradycardias that have been induced by reversible events such as ingestion of drug or cardiotoxic plants and permanent pacemaker failures, several manufacturers have produced and actively marketed transcutaneous external pacemakers for the emergency treatment of bradycardia. In 1990, these devices have become standard equipment in emergency departments, coronary and intensive care units, and some prehospital settings.

"DO NOT RESUSCITATE" AND "DEATH WITH DIGNITY" ISSUES IN OUT-OF-HOSPITAL CARDIAC ARREST

Numerous medical publications have discussed the complex issues of the do not resuscitate (DNR) and terminally ill patient. These issues revolve around questions such as when should CPR be initiated, withheld, or stopped; when are DNR orders appropriate; how valid are living wills; what are acceptable definitions of medical competency and incompetency and legal surrogates and guardianship; what is a "terminally ill" patient; what situations are truly irreversible (no known cure) or irreparable (beyond the reparative state); what are the proper criteria for brain death and for withdrawal of life-sustaining systems? Virtually all of these publications, however, have addressed these issues from the perspective of in-hospital care and have neglected the problem of DNR for out-of-hospital cardiac arrests. The American College of Emergency Physicians, among other groups, has begun to develop guidelines for out-of-hospital DNR patients. The problem is complex and yet must be mentioned, even if superficially, in this chapter.

Consider the situation of a terminally ill patient who has executed a living will in a mentally competent state, with full family agreement. The clinician discharges the patient, to spend the last few weeks of life in the familiar surroundings of home, with the loving support of relatives and friends. What instructions are given to that family regarding the inevitable events? Has a funeral home been selected and notified? Are the physician's DNR orders written, signed, and in the hands of a responsible family member? Physicians seldom provide the family with an exact list of actions to take when they perceive that death is imminent or has occurred. Most specifically, what IS the family to do when death occurs?

Few physicians are aware of the legal obligations and constraints on prehospital care personnel. In many situations, a family member may call 911, not to request emergency care but to report a death. Funeral homes and police cannot pronounce a person dead, so unless the physician has notified the funeral home in advance that he or she is prepared to complete the death certificate, the family members cannot call the funeral home directly. Unfortunately, 911 calls are routed, by protocol, to the emergency dispatcher, who in turn is legally obligated to dispatch emergency personnel. Here the problem becomes even more complex because in most states and locations, with a few notable exceptions, prehospital care personnel are required by state codes to initiate resuscitation efforts. Despite the presentation of a signed living will and despite the protestations of family members, resuscitation efforts must be started once the emergency personnel arrive. The concept of death with dignity is often grossly violated, albeit reluctantly, by all concerned.

Resuscitation efforts can cease when personnel at the level of paramedics arrive because they can make direct verbal contact with the medical control physician, who then takes legal responsibility for death certification (although he or she bases that decision on the information supplied by the paramedics). The most common pattern, however, is arrival of prehospital care personnel who are not at the level of paramedics, and so the resuscitation proceeds.

The American College of Emergency Physicians recommends that all local, regional, and state EMS systems and medical societies establish a comprehensive DNR policy. This policy should be incorporated as part of more comprehensive DNR legislation and should include a valid, legal, and widely recognized form that can be presented to prehospital personnel when they are called to the scene of such a patient. Perhaps even more important, there should be an educational program for patients, their families, and the medical community about appropriate use of EMS in the treatment of the terminally ill. Such efforts will spare the emotions and sensibilities of patients, families members, and emergency personnel, all of whom share the goal of death with dignity.

ATRIAL FIBRILLATION

method of
JAMES D. YATES, M.D.
University of Tennessee Medical Center
Knoxville, Tennessee

DIAGNOSIS

Atrial fibrillation is the most commonly encountered sustained arrhythmia. The diagnostic findings on the electrocardiogram are (1) absence of P waves; (2) disorganized baseline deflections of variable duration, contour, and amplitude; (3) variable atrioventricular (AV) conduction resulting in an irregular ventricular response. If the fibrillation is untreated, the ventricular rate is usually between 120 and 170 beats per minute. The changing stroke volume results in a pulse deficit and variation in systolic pressure on physical examination. The arrhythmia may be chronic and associated with organic heart disease or paroxysmal, sometimes secondary to metabolic or toxic effects (Table 1).

TREATMENT

Rapid Atrial Fibrillation

The decision regarding initial treatment depends on the hemodynamic status of the patient

TABLE 1. **Causes of Atrial Fibrillation**

Rheumatic heart disease
Hypertension
Arteriosclerosis
Hyperthyroidism
Cor pulmonale
Pericardial disease
Lone (idiopathic) atrial fibrillation
Atrial septal defect
Postcardiac surgery
Pre-excitation syndromes
Alcohol (holiday heart)
Pulmonary embolism
Cardiomyopathy

and the clinical setting. If the patient is unstable or angina pectoris is present, immediate electrical cardioversion is indicated. In most situations, the first goal is rate control, which is most reliably achieved with digitalis given intravenously initially and then orally. Increased AV conduction may not be controlled with digitalis alone when sympathomimetic activity is increased, as with exercise, fever, or hyperthyroidism. The addition of a beta blocker or calcium channel blocker may resolve this problem. Propranolol (Inderal) and metoprolol (Lopressor) have the advantage of being available in both oral and intravenous forms. If beta blockade is contraindicated, verapamil (Calan, Isoptin) and diltiazem (Cardizem) have proven efficacy.

Cardioversion

Reversion to sinus rhythm has the potential advantage of increasing cardiac reserve, reducing the risk of pulmonary and systemic emboli, and relieving palpitations. Appropriate patients for cardioversion have atrial fibrillation of short duration (less than 1 year) and left atrial size of less than 4.5 mm. Cardioversion should be considered when predisposing conditions are corrected, as in mitral valve surgery or treated hyperthyroidism. Relative contraindications to cardioversion include age more than 65 years, a ventricular rate less than 70 beats per minute without digitalis, atrial fibrillation of long duration (more than 2 years), early recurrence after previous cardioversion, and marked cardiomegaly. Chemical cardioversion may be attempted with quinidine sulfate, procainamide, or disopyramide phosphate. This treatment is effective in approximately 30 per cent of patients. After 48 hours, if atrial fibrillation persists, digitalis is withheld and electrical cardioversion is performed with 150 to 400 joules of synchronized direct current delivered through anterior-posterior paddles. In elective situations the patient receives anticoagulation therapy for 3 weeks before and for 4 weeks after cardioversion to reduce the risk of thrombolic episodes. The prothrombin time should be maintained at 1.2 to 1.5 times the control value unless a prosthetic valve is present, which dictates higher levels of anticoagulation therapy. Quinidine sulfate or other suppressive therapy is continued on a long-term basis in most situations. Several important new agents are available but are not yet approved for use in atrial fibrillation. These include flecainide (Tambocor), encainide (Enkaid), propafenone (Rhythmol), and amiodarone (Cordarone). Further research and experience are required to determine the place of these agents in treatment (Table 2).

Special Considerations and Precautions

1. Levels of digitalis in blood are not particularly helpful in deciding about dosage and may be misleading. The ventricular response should govern dosage.

2. The development of a regular ventricular response with atrial fibrillation implies that an AV junctional rhythm is present and may indicate digitalis intoxication.

3. Use of digitalis may shorten the recovery period in accessory tracts and dangerously accelerate the ventricular response in Wolff-Parkinson-White syndrome and is therefore contraindicated.

4. Digitalis dosage may require reduction when the drug is given with quinidine, verapamil, flecainide, or amiodarone.

5. Before a Group I antiarrhythmic such as quinidine is given for cardioversion, the AV node must be sufficiently blocked with digitalis to prevent rapid AV conduction as the atrial rate decreases.

6. Patients with atrial fibrillation and a ventricular response less than 70 beats per minute

---

TABLE 2. **Elective Treatment of Atrial Fibrillation***

Reduce Ventricular Response
1. Use digoxin (Lanoxin), 0.5–0.75 mg IV, then 0.25 mg every 2–4 hr until the ventricular rate is controlled, then 0.125–0.25 mg daily orally (usual total digitalizing dose is 0.75–1.25 mg)
2. Add propranolol hydrochloride (Inderal), 1–3 mg IV every 6 hr, or 10–40 mg orally 4 times daily if the ventricular rate cannot be controlled
   or
3. Use metoprolol, 5 mg IV every 12 hr, or 50–100 mg orally every 12 hr
4. If beta blockers are contraindicated, use verapamil (Calan, Isoptin), 3–10 mg IV every 4 hr or 40–120 mg every 6 hr orally
   or
5. Use diltiazem (Cardizem), 30–90 mg every 6 hr orally

Chemical Cardioversion
1. Use anticoagulation (see text)
2. Use quinidine sulfate, 200–400 mg every 6 hr orally
   or
3. Use procainamide, 250–750 mg every 4 hr orally
   or
4. Use disopyramide phosphate, 100–300 mg every 6 hr orally

Electrical Cardioversion
1. Use anterior-posterior paddle placement
2. Use general anesthesia
3. Treat with 150 joules of synchronized direct currect with progressive increase to 400 joules as needed
4. Use maintenance antiarrhythmic therapy

*See special considerations and precautions in text.

without treatment may develop slow sinus rates after cardioversion.

7. When the ventricular rate fails to respond to conventional blocking drugs, particularly in the setting of pulmonary disease, the electrocardiogram should be inspected carefully for evidence of multifocal atrial tachycardia, which may be misdiagnosed as atrial fibrillation.

PREMATURE BEATS

method of
JOHN A. YEUNG-LAI-WAH, M.B., Ch.B.
University of British Columbia
Vancouver, British Columbia, Canada

Premature beats are complexes of ectopic origin that occur relatively early during a baseline rhythm. They can be supraventricular or ventricular. The supraventricular beats may originate from the atrium (premature atrial complexes, PACs) or the junction of the atrioventricular (AV) node and the His bundle (premature junctional complexes, PJCs). The premature ventricular complexes (PVCs), also termed ventricular premature beats or ventricular extrasystoles, arise from a site below the bundle of His.

PREMATURE SUPRAVENTRICULAR COMPLEXES (ATRIAL AND JUNCTIONAL)

Diagnosis

PACs are usually recognized on the electrocardiogram by the presence of a P wave different from that in sinus rhythm, followed by a normal QRS complex. In the presence of PJCs, the ventricle is also activated normally via the His-Purkinje system. The QRS complex is normal, and the P wave may be superimposed on or shortly follow the QRS complex.

Occasionally, early PACs are blocked in the AV node or the His-Purkinje system. There is then an abnormal P wave, usually superimposed on the preceding T wave, with no subsequent QRS complex, mimicking a pause. PACs may be conducted to the ventricles while one of the bundle branches is still refractory. In this case, the QRS complex is wide (PAC with aberrant conduction).

Clinical Features

Premature supraventricular beats occur commonly in individuals who have an otherwise normal heart. They can also be associated with structural heart disease, for example, myocarditis, pericarditis, myocardial ischemia and infarction, and cardiomyopathy. They may be caused by atrial distention secondary to increases in left ventricular end-diastolic pressure. Thus, in unstable cardiac conditions such as myocardial infarction (MI), they may herald heart failure. They sometimes become more frequent during emotional upset or in the presence of medications, in particular, sympathomimetic drugs, alcohol, tobacco, or caffeine.

The most common symptoms associated with PACs and PJCs are palpitations, which become more noticeable when the patient is in a quiet environment. Dizziness is unusual and sometimes results from anxiety and hyperventilation. On occasion, PACs or PJCs may initiate supraventricular tachycardia, atrial flutter, or fibrillation.

Treatment

In general, supraventricular premature beats do not require drug therapy; reassurance is all that is needed. Precipitating factors should be removed if the patient has clearly noticed a cause-and-effect relationship.

When the patient remains symptomatic despite reassurance, an anxiolytic agent or a beta blocker may be tried. When the PACs or PJCs initiate tachycardias, an antiarrhythmic drug such as quinidine or procainamide may be used to prevent the tachycardia. Addition of digoxin or a beta blocker may be required to slow the ventricular response rate.

It is important that blocked PACs (described earlier) not be mistaken for sinus pauses that might erroneously be diagnosed as sinus node dysfunction.

The usual dosage and the adverse effects of antiarrhythmic agents commonly used for premature beats are given in Tables 1 and 2.

PREMATURE VENTRICULAR COMPLEXES

Diagnosis

PVCs are recognized by the presence of an abnormally wide QRS complex different from that in sinus rhythm. It is not preceded by a premature P wave, although it may be preceded by a sinus P wave that occurs at its expected time. The timing of a sinus P wave may or may not be disturbed after the occurrence of a PVC, depending on the retrograde conduction of the impulse to the sinus node.

The term "bigeminy" is used when the PVC alternates with a sinus complex. "Trigeminy" and "quadrigeminy" refer to PVCs after every two and three normal complexes, respectively. PVCs with different morphologies are often described as "multifocal," "multiform," or "polymorphic."

TABLE 1. **Oral Antiarrhythmic Agents**

Vaughan-Williams Class	Generic Name (Trade Name)	Usual Starting Dose (mg)	Usual Maximum Dose (mg)
Ia	Quinidine sulfate (Quinora)	200 q 6 hr	400 q 6 hr
	Quinidine gluconate (Quinaglute)	324 q 8 hr	648 q 8 hr
	Quinidine sulfate, long-acting (Quinidex)	300 q 8 hr	1200 q 12 hr
	Procainamide (Pronestyl)	250 q 4–6 hr	750 q 4–6 hr
	Procainamide, sustained-release (Procan SR, Pronestyl-SR)	500 q 8 hr	1000 q 6 hr
	Disopyramide (Norpace)*	100 q 6 hr	200 q 6 hr
Ib	Mexiletine (Mexitil)	100 q 6 hr	200 q 6 hr
	Tocainide (Tonocard)	400 q 8 hr	600 q 8 hr
Ic	Flecainide (Tambocor)†	100 q 12 hr	200 q 12 hr
	Encainide (Enkaid)†	25 q 8 hr	50 q 6 hr
	Propafenone (Rhythmol)	150 tid	300 tid
II	Propranolol (Inderal)	40 bid	120 bid
	Atenolol (Tenormin)*	25 qd	100 qd

*Dosage reductions are necessary with renal impairment.
†Currently indicated only for severe, life-threatening arrhythmias that cannot be controlled with alternative drugs.

The morphology of impulses from the same site in the ventricle may change, depending on the conduction of the myocardium.

Clinical Features

Frequently, PVCs are asymptomatic and are found when patients are examined for other purposes. Patients who have PVCs may complain of palpitations described as "feeling my heart stop," followed by postextrasystolic "strong beats." They may also complain of pulsations in the neck ("cannon" waves). Frequent PVCs may produce dizziness or difficulty in breathing. In patients who have coronary artery disease, they may precipitate or worsen angina.

PVCs may become worse in the presence of certain medications such as aminophylline or sympathomimetic drugs, electrolyte disturbances, emotional upset, or excessive use of caffeine, alcohol, or tobacco. Exercise may induce an increase in sinus rate and hence may reduce the number of PVCs. In some patients, the number of PVCs may increase. PVCs may increase or decrease in frequency during sleep.

The main concern with PVCs is their potential for initiating life-threatening ventricular tachycardias. Therefore, it is useful to determine whether they are likely to be benign or potentially lethal. This decision is usually influenced by the absence or presence of structural heart disease.

PREMATURE VENTRICULAR COMPLEXES WITHOUT HEART DISEASE

PVCs have been shown to occur in up to 60 per cent of individuals with no structural heart disease, and their prevalence increases with age. Approximately one-third of healthy individuals develop PVCs on exercise. These may occur in pairs or even as brief episodes of nonsustained

TABLE 2. **Common Adverse Effects of Antiarrhythmic Agents**

	Adverse Effects	Effect on Electrocardiogram
Quinidine	Diarrhea, nausea, headache, visual and auditory symptoms, fever, rash, thrombocytopenia, torsades de pointes	Prolongs QRS complex, QT interval
Procainamide	Gastrointestinal symptoms, fever, hypotension, arthralgia, rash, lupus-like syndrome, abdominal cramps, torsades de pointes, agranulocytosis	Prolongs QRS complex, QT interval
Disopyramide	Anticholinergic symptoms, torsades de pointes, heart failure	Prolongs QRS complex, QT interval
Class Ib agents (mexiletine, tocainide)	Gastrointestinal upset, nervousness, tremor, dizziness, loss of balance, sleep disturbance, hepatotoxicity, fever, blood dyscrasias	No change in QRS complex May shorten QT interval
Class Ic agents (propafenone, flecainide, encainide)	Heart failure, aggravation of arrhythmia, sustained ventricular tachycardia, dizziness, blurred vision	Prolong PR interval, QRS complex at low plasma levels
Beta blockers	Bradycardia, AV block, bronchospasm, heart failure, fatigue, worsening of intermittent claudication, impotence, vivid dreams	Prolong PR interval, AV block

ventricular tachycardia (three to six beats). These arrhythmias are often not reproducible on repeat exercise testing and are not predictive of increased cardiac mortality.

Treatment

It is important to reassure patients without heart disease that the presence of PVCs is associated with little or no increase in the risk of cardiac sudden death. Before therapy is initiated, it is useful to explain to the patient that antiarrhythmic drugs have potentially adverse effects, including worsening of arrhythmia, and that it is preferable to avoid medication. If medication is required, we usually start with a beta blocker such as atenolol (Tenormin), 25 to 50 mg once daily. The next drug of choice is a Class Ib or Class Ia antiarrhythmic agent. Class Ib drugs are often preferred because they are unlikely to cause a form of rapid ventricular tachycardia (torsades de pointes) that can occur with Class Ia drugs. Class Ic antiarrhythmic agents such as propafenone, flecainide, or encainide have been found to suppress PVCs in more than 90 per cent of cases. We usually start these drugs in the hospital because they can produce incessant ventricular tachycardia, but this is more likely to occur in patients with decreased ventricular function.

Some patients with normal hearts reproducibly develop sustained ventricular tachycardia during exercise testing. Morphologically the tachycardia is similar to that of isolated PVCs. In general, hemodynamic collapse does not occur during the tachycardia, and the tachycardia sometimes resolves spontaneously with rest. In our experience, these patients have a good prognosis. Tachycardia can usually be prevented with a beta blocker, either alone or in combination with a Class Ia antiarrhythmic agent such as quinidine. Repeat exercise testing is used to evaluate the efficacy of these drugs.

PREMATURE VENTRICULAR COMPLEXES WITH HEART DISEASE

During exercise testing, approximately 50 per cent of patients who have coronary artery disease develop PVCs. These usually occur with a heart rate of less than 130 beats per minute. Complex ventricular arrhythmias have been described in apparently healthy middle-aged men and are associated with the presence of coronary artery disease and subsequent premature death. However, a direct relationship between these PVCs and the episodes of sudden death has not been demonstrated. These arrhythmias may therefore be merely a marker of heart disease. Antiar-

rhythmic therapy has not been shown to reduce fatal events in this group. Therapeutic efforts should therefore be directed to reducing other risk factors such as coronary artery disease, tobacco smoking, hypertension, and hyperlipidemia.

Treatment

During acute MIs, the term "warning arrhythmias" has been used to describe PVCs that are multiform, that occur on the preceding T wave, at a rate of more than five to six per minute, or in salvos of two or more beats. It is noted that they do not occur in about one-half of the patients who develop ventricular fibrillation. Conversely, about one-half of the patients who have warning arrhythmias do not develop ventricular fibrillation. Thus prophylactic intravenous antiarrhythmic therapy is used only in high-risk patients, in most coronary care units that are staffed by well-trained nurses who can deliver prompt emergency treatment. For example, in patients who present within 6 hours of onset of an acute MI, if an antiarrhythmic agent is used, initial treatment consists of an intravenous bolus of lidocaine at a dose of 1 to 2 mg per kg at a rate of 25 to 50 mg per minute, followed by a maintenance infusion dose of 2 to 4 mg per minute. If the initial bolus of lidocaine is ineffective, up to two more boluses of 25 mg may be given at 5- to 10-minute intervals. Maintenance doses should be reduced by one-half in patients with low cardiac output or hepatic disease. Metabolism of the drug is also reduced in older patients and in those who are taking cimetidine or propranolol.

If lidocaine fails to suppress the arrhythmia, procainamide may be used. A loading dose of up to 10 mg per kg may be given at a rate of 30 to 50 mg per minute, up to a maximum loading dose of 1000 mg. The maintenance infusion rate is usually 2 to 4 mg per minute. Constant blood pressure monitoring is required. Sometimes a fall in blood pressure may be caused by peripheral vasodilation rather than myocardial depression.

There is a strong association among the frequency of PVCs, the size of MI and left ventricular function. Patients with complex ventricular arrhythmias are at higher risk of cardiac sudden death. Unfortunately, empiric long-term use of antiarrhythmic agents has failed to achieve a significant decrease in cardiac mortality in these patients. Cardiac electrophysiologic testing is being investigated as a means of identifying patients who are at higher risk of developing ventricular tachycardia and ventricular fibrillation. Beta blockers reduce PVCs during the first year after an acute MI. They are the only class of antiarrhythmic agents that have clearly demonstrated a significant reduction in cardiac mortality in these situations. Type Ic antiarrhythmic agents have been used to suppress PVCs. A recent preliminary report of the use of flecainide and encainide after acute MI suggested that they may increase mortality in patients with PVCs and they should not be used in this setting.

PVCs can occur after surgery, infection, anesthesia, or trauma. They are usually of no prognostic significance.

It is still unclear whether suppression of PVCs associated with chronic cardiac conditions such as chronic valvular disease or cardiomyopathy affects the mortality. Where possible, we perform an exercise stress test. Antiarrhythmic therapy is instituted when arrhythmias are aggravated by exercise or if they produce symptoms such as dizziness, syncope, or shortness of breath. When the arrhythmias are complex, invasive electrophysiologic testing is done.

Amiodarone should not be used for suppression of PVCs unless the patient has had a ventricular arrhythmia. It has many adverse effects, such as pulmonary toxicity, respiratory failure, skin photosensitivity, blue discoloration of skin, and thyroid dysfunction, as well as numerous drug interactions.

GENERAL APPROACH TO MANAGEMENT OF PVCs

Antiarrhythmic drugs can aggravate current arrhythmias or produce new ones. Also, they can cause serious adverse effects such as myocardial depression. These considerations should be carefully weighed against the potential benefits of drug therapy in patients who have PVCs.

Our initial approach is to document the presence of the arrhythmia and to try to correlate it with the patient's symptoms with 24-hour ambulatory recordings. Precipitating or aggravating factors are corrected where appropriate. If the patient has only mild symptoms and no underlying heart disease, and if the PVCs do not occur in long runs, the physician can simply reassure the patient. Drug therapy is not usually indicated except for symptomatic purposes. If antiarrhythmic therapy is required, repeated 24-hour ambulatory monitoring is needed before and after initiation of drug therapy to determine the efficacy of treatment. It is important to realize that there can be considerable day-to-day variation in the number of PVCs in an individual patient. Recent studies have demonstrated that the variation becomes greater if the interval separating two 24-hour recordings is increased. It is suggested that an 85 per cent reduction in the number of PVCs is required to establish drug efficacy (with 95 per cent confidence limits) when the 24-hour recordings are made about 2 weeks apart.

In patients in whom the arrhythmias are aggravated by exercise, serial exercise testing may be used to guide drug therapy.

When new drugs are started or when the doses are changed, 12-lead electrocardiograms are required to monitor the electrophysiologic effects of the drugs. For example, beta blockers may increase the PR interval and induce AV block in susceptible patients; Class Ic antiarrhythmic agents have a marked effect of myocardial conduction and increase the QRS width; and Class Ia antiarrhythmic agents increase the QT interval and produce prominent postpause U waves.

HEART BLOCK

method of
LAWRENCE D. GERMAN, M.D.
Nashville, Tennessee

Heart block denotes failure of conduction in some part of the specialized cardiac conduction system, including the sinoatrial node, the atrioventricular node, the bundle of His, the right and left bundle branches, and the Purkinje fiber system. Conduction block of clinical significance may occur at any one of these anatomic sites.

SINOATRIAL EXIT BLOCK

The diagnosis of sinoatrial exit block is considered when a P wave fails to appear when expected. Because sinoatrial node depolarization cannot be recorded on the standard electrocardiogram (ECG), the differentiation of sinoatrial exit block from complete failure of sinus node depolarization is inferential. In sinoatrial exit block, the sinus node itself depolarizes on time, and the next sinus P wave therefore follows a pause that is an approximate multiple of the sinus cycle length. Complete sinoatrial exit block may be impossible to differentiate from sinus node asystole.

Sinoatrial exit block is part of the sick sinus syndrome and may cause symptomatic bradycardia. Sinoatrial exit block may occur in a variety of clinical settings, especially coronary artery disease, and, when asymptomatic, is of little significance. Sinoatrial exit block may also be the result of heightened vagal tone in some patients. When sinus pauses cause symptoms referable to bradycardia, potentially offending drugs such as beta blockers, calcium channel blockers, and digoxin should be withdrawn if possible. The persistence of symptomatic pauses may require permanent pacing. Treatment strategies in heart block are summarized in Table 1.

TABLE 1. **Treatment Strategies in Heart Block**

Disorder	Treatment
Sinoatrial exit block	
Asymptomatic	None
Symptomatic	Withdraw offending drugs
	Acute: Atropine, 0.6–1 mg
	Temporary pacing
	Chronic: Permanent pacing
First-degree AV block	None
Second-degree AV block	
Mobitz I	
Asymptomatic	None
Symptomatic	Withdraw offending drugs
	Acute: Atropine, 0.6–1 mg
	Chronic: Permanent pacing
Mobitz II	
Asymptomatic	Acute MI: Temprorary pacing
	Chronic: Electrophysiology
	study to localize
Symptomatic	Acute: Temporary pacing
	Isoproterenol, 2–20
	µg/min
	Chronic: Permanent pacing
Complete AV block	
Asymptomatic	Narrow QRS escape: None
Symptomatic	Acute: Temporary pacing
	Isoproterenol, 2–20
	µg/min
	Chronic: Permanent pacing
Bundle branch block	
Asymptomatic	New with acute MI: Temporary pacing
	Chronic: None
Symptomatic	Document correlation between symptoms and AV block

Abbreviations: AV = atrioventricular; MI = myocardial infarction.

BUNDLE BRANCH BLOCK

Abnormalities of atrioventricular conduction may take the form of atrioventricular block, bundle branch block, or both. The significance of bundle branch block depends on factors such as the clinical setting in which it develops and the presence of symptoms suggesting intermittent complete atrioventricular block.

Chronic Bundle Branch Block

Chronic bundle branch block is commonly seen in patients with hypertension or coronary artery disease and may be seen in apparently healthy individuals with no identifiable underlying heart disease. In these settings, chronic bundle branch block has a low probability of progressing to atrioventricular block and does not require treatment. The presence of bundle branch block is more significant in certain conditions, such as myotonic dystrophy and the Kearns-Sayre syndrome, which are associated with a high incidence of syncope and sudden death caused by progressive atrioventricular conduction abnormalities. Invasive studies of atrioventricular conduction may be indicated to demonstrate infranodal conduction abnormalities, and permanent pacing should be considered.

When symptoms suggestive of bradycardia (syncope or presyncope) develop in patients with chronic bundle branch block, an attempt should be made to document an association between the symptoms and transient higher-grade atrioventricular block before assuming a cause-and-effect relationship and recommending permanent pacing. Ambulatory monitoring, transient event monitors, and invasive electrophysiologic studies may be useful.

Acute Bundle Branch Block

When acute myocardial infarction is complicated by the development of left bundle branch block or bifascicular block (right bundle branch block and left anterior or posterior hemiblock), involvement of the conduction system by the ischemic process can be inferred, and temporary pacing should be considered because complete atrioventricular block may occur unpredictably. This is typically seen in acute anterior myocardial infarction.

ATRIOVENTRICULAR BLOCK

Atrioventricular block is traditionally classified into three categories. First-degree atrioventricular block is manifested as a prolongation of conduction between the atria and ventricles (long PR interval) without actual failure of conduction. Second-degree atrioventricular block consists of intermittent failure of atrioventricular conduction together with conducted beats that may display a normal or prolonged PR interval (first-degree block). Third-degree (complete) atrioventricular block is the complete failure of supraventricular impulses to conduct to the ventricles. It may occur intermittently, interspersed with periods of lower-degree atrioventricular block or even normal conduction.

First-Degree Atrioventricular Block

Prolongation of the PR interval may be caused by conduction delays in the atrioventricular node or in the infranodal conduction system (bundle of His and bundle branches). Conduction delay in the atrioventricular node is often the result of drugs (e.g., digoxin, calcium channel blockers) or heightened autonomic (parasympathetic) tone, whereas conduction delay in the infranodal structures is usually the result of pathologic lesions involving the conduction system (fibrosis, infarction, or ischemia). The site of conduction delay in first-degree atrioventricular block cannot be ascertained with certainty from the ECG. Intracardiac recordings are required to measure conduction intervals through the atrioventricular node and the infranodal structures. The site of conduction delay can be inferred, however, from surface ECG recordings based on the morphology of the conducted QRS complex. Abnormalities in atrioventricular nodal conduction alone are usually associated with a normal QRS complex, whereas pathologic processes that involve the infranodal conduction system frequently result in either bundle branch block or intraventricular conduction delay. A normal QRS complex makes a significant pathologic conduction delay in the bundle of His or bundle branches unlikely.

First-degree atrioventricular block itself is not associated with symptoms (unless extreme PR interval prolongation results in atrioventricular asynchrony and reduced cardiac stroke volume) and therefore rarely requires treatment.

Second-Degree Atrioventricular Block

Second-degree atrioventricular block has been classified into two types, designated Mobitz Type I (Wenckebach) block and Mobitz Type II block. In Mobitz Type I second-degree block, the PR interval is prolonged over one or more cycles before failure of conduction. Usually only one P wave fails to conduct, and the succeeding (postpause) P wave conducts with a shorter PR interval than that preceding the dropped beat. This prolongation of the PR interval generally indicates that the atrioventricular node is the site of the block and signifies little likelihood of progression to higher-degree atrioventricular block.

Mobitz II block occurs without prolongation of the preceding PR intervals. This abrupt failure of conduction is generally interpreted as indicating an infranodal site of conduction block, a pathologic process as the cause of conduction failure, and a greater likelihood of progression to higher-degree atrioventricular block.

Two-to-One Atrioventricular Block. A particular variety of second-degree atrioventricular block is 2:1 block. Because there is only one conducted PR interval for every nonconducted beat, it is impossible to classify 2:1 block as either Mobitz I or II. Close observation over time may reveal occasional episodes of 3:2 conduction or similar periods in which several conducted P waves occur successively. The presence of typical Mobitz I or II block during these sequences may allow the 2:1 sequence to be classified by inference. In the absence of such observations, 2:1 block is best classified as such rather than as Mobitz I or II.

The subclassifications of second-degree atrioventricular block is an attempt to localize the pathologic process. An important observation in this regard is the morphology of the conducted QRS complex. Type I conduction with a normal (narrow) QRS complex is almost always associated with intranodal block. Likewise, Type II block with an abnormal (wide) QRS complex is often associated with block below the atrioventricular node. A Wenckebach sequence in the presence of a wide QRS complex does not confirm the atrioventricular node as the site of the block, because Mobitz I conduction has been demonstrated to occur in the infranodal conduction structures. Thus, second-degree atrioventricular block (Mobitz I or II or 2:1 block) with a narrow QRS complex should be differentiated from similar blocks with a wide QRS complex.

In symptomatic patients with second-degree block, correlation between symptoms and episodes of bradycardia must be documented. Patients who are asymptomatic at rest may become symptomatic during exercise if higher-degree atrioventricular block prevents an increase in heart rate. Exercise testing is, therefore, often an important part of the evaluation of patients with second-degree atrioventricular block.

Symptomatic second-degree block caused by increased vagal tone can usually be improved by administration of intravenous atropine in doses of 0.6 to 1 mg. The total dose of atropine can be 2 mg. Second-degree block resulting from infranodal pathology may actually be worsened by administration of atropine, however, if the increase in atrial rate results in higher-degree block. In this situation, intravenous isoproterenol in continuous infusions at a rate of 1 to 4 micrograms per minute may result in improved conduction and acceleration of escape rhythms.

Third-Degree (Complete) Atrioventricular Block

Third-degree atrioventricular block may occur in the atrioventricular node, in which case a narrow QRS escape rhythm is often present at a rate sufficient to prevent the development of major symptoms of bradycardia. Block developing at lower levels is associated with a slower, wide QRS escape rhythm or, occasionally, with no spontaneous escape rhythm. In young people with congenital atrioventricular block who are asymptomatic and have a narrow QRS escape rhythm whose rate increases with exercise, no therapeutic intervention is necessary. Symptoms of syncope or presyncope in a person with third-degree atrioventricular block should prompt serious consideration of permanent pacing. Patients with third-degree atrioventricular block and a wide QRS escape rhythm are rarely asymptomatic and should almost always be considered for permanent pacing.

When new second- or third-degree atrioventricular block complicates the course of acute inferior myocardial infarction, temporary pacing is required, but return of normal conduction without the need for permanent pacing is anticipated. In acute anterior myocardial infarction, transient atrioventricular block may be followed by return of conduction with bundle branch block. When left bundle branch block or bifascicular block remains after transient second- or third-degree block, significant damage to the conduction system has probably occurred and permanent pacing should be considered.

The abrupt development of high-degree atrioventricular block may be treated by intravenous isoproterenol until temporary pacing can be instituted. The potential risks of using isoproterenol in patients with acute ischemic heart disease, in increasing myocardial oxygen consumption and provoking ventricular arrhythmias in patients with ischemic heart disease, must be kept in mind. Transcutaneous external pacing has proved to be a rapid and reliable method in this situation until a transvenous temporary pacing catheter can be placed.

TACHYCARDIA

method of
DOUGLAS L. WOOD, M.D., and
STEPHEN C. HAMMILL, M.D.
Mayo Clinic
Rochester, Minnesota

DIAGNOSIS

Tachycardia is diagnosed electrocardiographically by analysis of single-lead rhythm strips or 12-lead electrocardiograms that are recorded during episodes of rapid beating of the heart. Such recordings may be made in the office, emergency room, or specialized monitoring areas of hospitals. Advanced technology has improved our ability to make electrocardiographic recordings of infrequently occurring and short-lived episodes of tachycardia. Standard Holter monitoring may be used, but telephone transmitters and loop recording devices now make it possible to provide prolonged intermittent electrocardiographic recording for improved diagnostic accuracy. There are circumstances, however, when arrhythmias are sufficiently infrequent or short-lived that electrocardiographic recordings that are made by using these techniques fail to provide the information necessary for accurate diagnosis. In these situations, invasive electrophysiologic studies (EPS) are essential for diagnosis and treatment. EPS is increasingly important in the evaluation

and treatment of arrhythmias, especially when nonpharmacologic treatment is used.

Understanding the mechanism of tachycardia is important for choosing therapy. Narrow complex supraventricular tachycardia may be either atrial fibrillation or flutter or supraventricular tachycardia on the basis of one of several mechanisms. Absence of P waves suggests re-entry within the atrioventricular (AV) node, whereas retrograde P waves with an RP interval longer than the PR interval suggests AV tachycardia that uses an accessory pathway. Wide complex tachycardias are most often ventricular in origin, but it may be difficult to prove the diagnosis on the basis of electrocardiographic recordings alone. The best criteria available are the finding of AV dissociation and a history of cardiac disease. Clearly, diagnosis of the mechanism of tachycardia requires the ability to record the atrial activation sequence accurately. When P waves are not discernible on a rhythm strip or a 12-lead electrocardiogram during tachycardia, the use of esophageal electrodes or the transvenous placement of an intracardiac electrode is helpful in diagnosis and may also provide the potential for immediate control of the arrhythmia by temporary overdrive pacing.

EPS is indicated for the diagnosis and treatment of symptomatic supraventricular tachycardia (especially when initial drug therapy is ineffective), wide complex tachycardias, and sustained ventricular tachycardia, as well as for patients who survive a cardiac arrest. EPS is not clearly helpful in patients with nonsustained ventricular tachycardia.

EMERGENCY TREATMENT

The safest, most effective, and most expedient method for termination of a hemodynamically significant tachycardia is electrical cardioversion. Although administration of intravenous drugs may be helpful, the onset of action of these drugs is sufficiently slow to make them unreliable for emergency treatment of most arrhythmias. Unstable ventricular tachycardia and ventricular fibrillation are best treated with immediate unsynchronized defibrillation. Acute termination of supraventricular tachycardia is also possible with electrical cardioversion when hemodynamics are seriously impaired. In less urgent circumstances, the use of vagal maneuvers may be tried initially while preparations are made to administer an intravenous drug. Patients with narrow complex tachycardias may be treated with intravenous verapamil (Calan, Isoptin), intravenous beta blockers, or intravenous digoxin (Lanoxin). Patients with hemodynamically stable wide complex tachycardias should be treated with lidocaine if it is certain that the tachycardias are ventricular in origin or with procainamide (Pronestyl) if there is doubt about the origin of tachycardia (i.e., possibly aberrantly conducted supraventricular tachycardia or antegrade conduction over an accessory pathway). Verapamil (Calan,

Isoptin) should be avoided especially in patients with wide complex tachycardia. Because most wide complex tachycardias are ventricular in origin, the administration of verapamil is not likely to be helpful, and it often provokes peripheral vasodilation, which causes a reflex increase in the rate of tachycardia. In the circumstance of Wolff-Parkinson-White syndrome with antegrade conduction over an accessory pathway, verapamil may result in acceleration of tachycardia and the development of an unstable arrhythmia or ventricular fibrillation (digoxin and possibly beta blockers have the same effects). Procainamide, however, blocks conduction over an accessory pathway in the antegrade direction, and so it is preferred as the initial therapy in patients with wide complex tachycardia that uses an accessory pathway.

CHRONIC TREATMENT

Several factors influence the therapeutic choice for patients with tachycardia. The frequency and severity of symptoms, the risk of serious hemodynamic consequences (including sudden death), and the safety and efficacy of therapy are important considerations in the selection of an antiarrhythmic drug or other form of therapy. Although antiarrhythmic drugs are still commonly used, improvements in electrical therapy and surgical treatment have made it possible to cure patients with tachycardia surgically or to eliminate the need for drug therapy by implantation of automatic defibrillators, antitachycardia pacemakers, or combinations of devices.

Antiarrhythmic Drug Therapy

Initiation of antiarrhythmic drug therapy (Table 1) may be undertaken as an outpatient regimen in patients with benign arrhythmias and no evidence of heart block or heart disease. However, in patients with potentially lethal or lethal ventricular arrhythmias, especially in the presence of impaired ventricular function, such treatment should be started in the hospital with continuous electrocardiographic monitoring because of the risk of proarrhythmia. Patients with supraventricular tachycardia and underlying heart disease are also better served when they start therapy as an inpatient and are monitored carefully. Assessment of the effectiveness of treatment may be noninvasive, with repeated periods of Holter monitoring with or without exercise testing, but when arrhythmias are associated with serious hemodynamic consequences, invasive EPS is superior to noninvasive monitoring for assessing the potential benefit of any therapy chosen, be it

drug therapy, an antitachycardia pacemaker, an implantable defibrillator, or surgical therapy.

Treatment of Specific Tachycardias

Supraventricular Tachycardia: AV Node Re-entry Tachycardia

Supraventricular tachycardia encompasses a number of different tachycardias that are characterized by a regular tachycardia of 140 to 240 beats per minute, usually associated with a normal QRS complex. The most common mechanism of supraventricular tachycardia is re-entry within the AV node. This tachycardia may be treated initially with vagal maneuvers; if these are unsuccessful, intravenous verapamil is often effective (Table 2). If intravenous verapamil fails to control the arrhythmia, elective cardioversion is safe, quick, and effective. Care should be taken to avoid the combined use of intravenous beta blockers and intravenous verapamil because of increased risk of heart block or heart failure. Patients with frequent episodes of AV node re-entry tachycardia are potentially curable by cryosurgical modification of AV conduction, which eliminates the need for lifelong antiarrhythmic therapy. We prefer surgical therapy to antitachycardia pacing, which has limited ability to prevent recurrences of arrhythmias. In addition, surgical therapy is preferable to catheter ablation because it avoids the need for pacemaker implantation.

When chronic drug therapy is considered for patients with AV node re-entry tachycardia, several drugs may be effective. Digoxin, verapamil, and beta blockers have been used frequently in the past. However, the Class IC antiarrhythmic drugs flecainide (Tambocor) and encainide (Enkaid) (and soon propafenone [Rythmol]) are quite effective in preventing recurrences of AV node re-entry tachycardia by virtue of their ability to prolong refractoriness and slow conduction within the AV node and to reduce the number of atrial and ventricular premature beats that may serve as triggers for the initiation of tachycardia. These drugs appear to be quite well tolerated in chronic therapy in comparison to procainamide, quinidine (Quinidex Extentabs, Quinaglute Dura-Tabs), and disopyramide (Norpace), all of which have a fairly significant potential for the development of noncardiac side effects. However, recent results from the Cardiac Arrhythmia Suppression Trial (CAST) suggest caution in the use of Class IC drugs.

Supraventricular Tachycardia Using an Accessory AV Connection

The next most common form of supraventricular tachycardia is AV tachycardia, which involves

TABLE 1. **Antiarrhythmic Drugs**

Class	Generic Name (Trade Name)	Administration	Dose	Therapeutic Levels (µg/ml)	Use
IA	Procainamide (Pronestyl, Procan SR, Pronestyl SR)	IV, PO	Load; 10 mg/kg; infusion: 1–4 mg/ml; 250–750 mg q 3 hr (procainamide); 500–1500 mg q 6 hr (Procan SR, Pronestyl SR)	4–10	SVT, VPCs, NSVT, VT/VF
	Quinidine (Quinidex Extentabs, Quinaglute Dura-Tabs)	IV, PO	Load: 10mg/kg; quinidine sulfate 200–400 mg q 6 hr; Quinidex Extentabs 300–600 mg q 8–12 hr; Quinaglute Dura-Tabs 324–648 mg q 8 hr	2–4	SVT, VPCs, NSVT, VT/VF
	Disopyramide (Norpace)	PO	100–150 mg q 6 hr	3–6	SVT, VPCs, NSVT, VT/VF
IB	Lidocaine (Xylocaine)	IV	Load: 1 mg/kg; infusion: 1–4 mg/min	2–5	VPCs, NSVT, VT/VF
	Mexiletine (Mexitil)	PO	150–300 mg q 6–12 hr	0.5–2	VPCs, NSVT, VT/VF
	Tocainide (Tonocard)	PO	400–600 mg q 8–12 hr	4–10	VPCs, NSVT, VT/VF
IC	Flecainide (Tambocor)*	PO	50–200 mg q 12 hr	0.2–1	SVT, VPCs, NSVT, VT/VF
	Encainide (Enkaid)*	PO	25–50 mg q 8 hr	NA	SVT, VPCs, NSVT, VT/VF
II	Propranolol (Inderal)	IV, PO	3–5 mg in 1-mg increments; 10–40 mg q 6–12 hr	NA	SVT, VPCs, NSVT, VT/VF
	Esmolol (Brevibloc)	IV	Load: 0.5 mg/kg; maintenance: 0.05–0.2 mg/kg/min	NA	SVT
III	Amiodarone (Cordarone)	PO	Load: 800–1600 mg/day × 10 days; maintenance: 200–400 mg/day	1–2.5	SVT, NSVT, VT/VF
	Bretylium (Bretylol)	IV	Load: 5 mg/kg; maintenance: 1–2 mg/min	NA	VT/VF
IV	Verapamil (Calan, Isoptin, Calan SR, Isoptin SR)	IV, PO	5–20 mg IV; 80–120 mg q 6–8 hr; 240–480 mg/day	NA	SVT, VT
	Digoxin (Lanoxin)	IV, PO	Load: 0.75–1.25 mg; maintenance: 0.125–0.375 mg/day	0.8–2	SVT

*The CAST study found a higher mortality with encainide and flecainide when compared with placebo in patients with VPCs. Because of these findings, these two drugs are now indicated only for severe, life-threatening arrhythmias.

Abbreviations: NA = not available; SVT = supraventricular tachycardia; VPCs = ventricular premature contractions; NSVT = nonsustained ventricular tachycardia; VT/VF = ventricular tachycardia/ventricular fibrillation.

an accessory AV connection (Kent's bundle, Wolff-Parkinson-White syndrome). In most of these tachycardias, the QRS complex is normal because antegrade conduction occurs through the AV node and His-Purkinje system, and retrograde conduction is over the accessory pathway. This condition is often referred to as orthodromic reciprocating tachycardia. Rarely, antegrade con-

TABLE 2. **Antiarrhythmic Drugs for Supraventricular Tachycardia: Comparative Efficacy for Supraventricular Arrhythmias**

Drug	APCs	AF	AVNRT	AVRT(WPW)
Procainamide	+ +	+ +	+	+ +
Quinidine	+ +	+ +	+	+ +
Disopyramide	+ +	+ +	+	+ +
Flecainide	+ + +	+ + +	+ +	+ +
Encainide	+ + +	+ + +	+ +	+ + +
Propafenone	+ + +	+ + +	+ +	+ +
Beta blockers	+	+	+	+
Amiodarone	+ + +	+ + +	+ +	+ + +
Verapamil	0	+	+	+
Digoxin	+	+	+ +	+

Abbreviations: APCs = atrial premature contractions; AF = atrial fibrillation/flutter; AVNRT = AV node re-entry tachycardia; AVRT(WPW) = AV tachycardia (Wolff-Parkinson-White syndrome); 0 = no effect.

duction may occur over the accessory pathway and cause a wide QRS tachycardia (antidromic reciprocating tachycardia) that may be misdiagnosed as ventricular tachycardia.

The acute treatment of narrow complex reciprocating tachycardia is similar to that for AV node re-entry tachycardia. However, care must be taken to avoid drugs that selectively block the AV node and leave the accessory connection unprotected. If digoxin, verapamil, or beta blockers are used in these circumstances, a defibrillator should be nearby in the event that atrial fibrillation occurs and preferential conduction over the accessory pathway follows. If atrial fibrillation is conducted over the accessory pathway, the ventricular response may be extremely rapid, and these patients are at risk of developing ventricular fibrillation. If an intravenous drug is chosen for immediate control of an arrhythmia that uses an accessory pathway in the antegrade direction, intravenous procainamide is preferred because it provides antegrade block in the accessory pathway.

Long-term oral therapy with antiarrhythmic drugs is possible for patients with accessory connections and tachycardia. However, surgical therapy is extremely effective in managing these patients and eliminates the need for lifelong antiarrhythmic therapy. Many patients will consider surgical therapy as first line treatment.

When drug therapy is considered for patients with Wolff-Parkinson-White syndrome, encainide and flecainide are effective because they block conduction in both the accessory pathway and the AV node. In addition, they are well tolerated during long-term use, and because of their long half-lives, dosing is often simpler than it is for patients who are treated with procainamide, quinidine, or disopyramide. Digoxin, verapamil, and beta blockers may be effective in blocking conduction in the AV node, but because they have little effect on the accessory pathway, they should not be used unless EPS or noninvasive testing has indicated that they are extremely likely to be effective without aggravating conduction over the accessory pathway during atrial fibrillation or supraventricular tachycardia. Amiodarone, a Class III antiarrhythmic drug, is effective in patients with Wolff-Parkinson-White syndrome and supraventricular tachycardia that uses an accessory pathway. However, because other drugs are reasonably effective and have a more desirable side effect profile for chronic use, amiodarone is reserved for patients who prove to be refractory to other drugs and who are not candidates for surgical division of their accessory pathway.

Catheter ablation has been used for patients with accessory pathways, but initial experience with this technique indicates that morbidity and mortality are substantial in patients with free-wall accessory pathways, and the likelihood of success is low. The only circumstance in which catheter ablation may help is in a patient with a posterior septal accessory pathway, and its use should be considered to be investigational.

Ectopic Atrial Tachycardias

Ectopic atrial tachycardias may be re-entrant or automatic in origin. Typically, heart rates range from 120 to 220 beats per minute, and vagal maneuvers or drugs like digoxin, verapamil, and beta blockers can be used to increase the level of AV block during tachycardia. Encainide and flecainide appear to be effective in suppressing both atrial re-entry and automatic atrial tachycardias. Quinidine, procainamide, and disopyramide may also be effective in preventing or terminating episodes of ectopic atrial tachycardia. Amiodarone may also be effective in managing these arrhythmias but should be reserved for patients in whom other drugs have either been ineffective or poorly tolerated.

Ectopic atrial tachycardia is also potentially curable surgically. When antiarrhythmic drugs are ineffective and surgery is not an option, catheter ablation of AV conduction and placement of a permanent pacemaker may be extremely helpful, especially when atrial tachycardia has been associated with a severe impairment of ventricular function.

Sinus tachycardia may occur in two circumstances. One form of sinus tachycardia is that related to enhanced autonomic tone in the setting of stress, underlying disease, or the use of sympathomimetic drugs. In these circumstances, patients are bothered by palpitations but have few other associated symptoms, and the tachycardia is often best managed by controlling predisposing factors. Re-entry within the sinoatrial node can cause a paroxysmal sinus tachycardia that can be quite troublesome. This tachycardia may be a form of sick sinus syndrome, and it can be treated with one of a number of drugs, including verapamil, digoxin, beta blockers, or the Class IC drugs encainide and flecainide.

Multifocal Atrial Tachycardia

Multifocal atrial tachycardia is an irregular atrial arrhythmia with several morphologies of P waves at rates of 100 to 240 beats per minute. Most patients have underlying chronic lung disease and in many circumstances, concomitant infection or exacerbation of underlying pulmonary insufficiency requiring increased doses of bronchodilators and sympathomimetic drugs is at the heart of the development of this arrhythmia. In general, treatment includes correction of underlying provocative factors and, where possible, reduction of the dose of bronchodilating drugs. Control of ventricular rate in an acute situation may be accomplished with verapamil; if chronic therapy is required, either verapamil or possibly a Class IC drug may be effective.

Treatment of Ventricular Arrhythmias

Ventricular arrhythmias range from benign to lethal (Table 3). The decision to treat a ventricular arrhythmia depends on the potential risk for sudden cardiac death, the presence of serious hemodynamic consequences associated with the arrhythmias, and the likelihood that a chosen therapy will help in abolishing symptoms or reducing the risk of sudden death with acceptable side effects (Table 4).

Benign ventricular arrhythmias are those that occur in patients without structural heart disease or with only minimal impairment of ventricular function. Such arrhythmias include single premature ventricular contractions in most patients but may occasionally include patients with non-

TABLE 3. **Classification, Characteristics, and Treatment of Ventricular Arrhythmias**

Parameter	Benign	Potential Lethal	Lethal
Risk for death	Low	Intermediate	High
Heart disease	Absent	Present	Present
LV function	Normal	Impaired	Severely impaired
Arrhythmias	VPCs, NSVT	VPCs, NSVT	VF, VT (sustained)
Treatment	Symptoms only	Symptoms; possibly patients with asymptomatic NSVT and heart failure	Treatment mandatory: amiodarone, AICD, endocardial resection, transplantation

Abbreviations: NSVT = nonsustained ventricular tachycardia; VT = ventricular tachycardia; VF = ventricular fibrillation; AICD = automatic implantable cardioverter defibrillator.

sustained ventricular tachycardia. Patients with benign ventricular arrhythmias will not have experienced presyncope or syncope with their arrhythmias.

Patients with potentially lethal arrhythmias almost always have some degree of structural heart disease, and often ventricular function is abnormal. Such patients may have ejection fractions of less than 40 per cent or may have hypertrophic cardiomyopathy. The most common arrhythmia of concern in these patients is nonsustained ventricular tachycardia. Patients with potentially lethal ventricular arrhythmias will not have had symptoms of presyncope or syncope but may be at an increased risk of developing sudden cardiac death.

Patients with lethal ventricular arrhythmias have survived an out-of-hospital cardiac arrest or have experienced sustained ventricular tachycardia, often causing near syncope or syncope. These patients have a high risk of recurrence of the arrhythmias, and their risk for sudden death is high unless an effective antiarrhythmic regimen or some other therapeutic modality can be identified.

Lethal Ventricular Arrhythmias

Patients with lethal ventricular arrhythmias should be aggressively evaluated with electrophysiologic investigations to identify more precisely the mechanism of their arrhythmia and to direct therapy. When an effective antiarrhythmic drug can be identified that prevents the induction of ventricular tachycardia in the electrophysiologic laboratory, the prognosis is excellent. However, when such a drug cannot be identified, patients should be treated with an automatic implantable cardioverter/defibrillator or endocardial resection. In patients with impaired ventricular function (ejection fraction < 40 per cent), response to intravenous procainamide in the laboratory often predicts the response to antiarrhythmic drugs. Failure to respond to procainamide in patients with reduced ventricular function suggests that there is a low likelihood of identifying an antiarrhythmic drug that will successfully prevent induction of tachycardia. In these circumstances, amiodarone prevents induction of ventricular tachycardia in 20 per cent of patients and slows the tachycardia rate in an additional 40 per cent of patients and makes the tachycardia hemodynamically tolerable. However, it is important to identify which patients are at greatest risk of having a fatal recurrence of their ventricular tachycardia. In patients who continue to exhibit nonsustained ventricular tachycardia after a 10-day loading dose of amiodarone, or in patients with inducible ventricular tachycardia that is not slowed by amiodarone, the risk of recurrent arrhythmia is high, and these patients have the greatest likelihood of a fatal recurrence. In these circumstances, endocardial resection or use of an automatic implantable defibrillator is preferred.

Patients who survive ventricular fibrillation that is not associated with an acute myocardial

TABLE 4. **Antiarrhythmic Drugs for Ventricular Tachycardia: Clinical Utility for Ventricular Arrhythmias**

Drug	Efficacy		Negative Inotropy	Proarrhythmic Potential		Adverse Effects Requiring Discontinuation (%)
	NSVT	VT/VF		NSVT	VT/VF	
Procainamide	+ + +	+ +	0	+	+ +	25
Quinidine	+ + +	+ +	0	+	+ +	35
Disopyramide	+ +	+ +	+ + +	+	+ +	35
Mexiletine	+ +	+ +	0	+	+	35
Tocainide	+ +	+	0	+	+	35
Flecainide	+ + + +	+ +	+ +	+	+ + +	15
Encainide	+ + + +	+ +	0	+	+ + +	15
Propafenone	+ + +	+ +	+ +	+	+ +	15
Beta blockers	+ +	+	+ +	+	+	15
Amiodarone	+ + + +	+ + +	0	+	+	35

Abbreviations: NSVT = nonsustained ventricular tachycardia; VT/VF = ventricular tachycardia/ventricular fibrillation; 0 = no effect.

infarction or patients who develop ventricular fibrillation more than 48 hours after a myocardial infarction have an extremely poor prognosis. Such patients should be evaluated with invasive EPS, but they often fail to respond to antiarrhythmic drugs. The automatic implantable defibrillator has proved to be extremely helpful in treating these patients. Improvements in design of the implantable defibrillator and in battery life will lead to an increase in the number of patients treated with the device in the near future. The increasing complexity of these devices will also require that their implantation be performed only in centers with electrophysiologic expertise.

Potentially Lethal Ventricular Arrhythmias

Patients with impaired ventricular function with or without symptoms of heart failure often have nonsustained ventricular tachycardia. When such arrhythmias are associated with symptoms, the decision to treat the arrhythmia is easy, and it is often possible to improve the quality of life of these patients by reducing the frequency of symptomatic nonsustained ventricular tachycardia with antiarrhythmic drugs. In patients with asymptomatic nonsustained ventricular tachycardia, antiarrhythmic drug therapy will not result in symptomatic improvement, obviously, but such therapy is often considered in an attempt to lessen the likelihood of sudden cardiac death. Despite all of the improvements in the management of patients with heart failure, sudden cardiac death continues to account for approximately one-half of the mortality in patients with heart failure, and the presence of nonsustained ventricular tachycardia is often considered to be an independent risk factor for sudden death.

The decision to use antiarrhythmic drugs in patients with asymptomatic nonsustained ventricular tachycardia and heart failure is controversial. Preliminary evidence from retrospective studies suggests that amiodarone used in a low dose is associated with an increase in survival for patients with heart failure and nonsustained ventricular tachycardia. However, large-scale double-blind placebo-controlled trials are necessary before it can be proved that antiarrhythmic therapy with amiodarone specifically reduces the likelihood of sudden cardiac death in patients with heart failure. Although multicenter trials have been designed and are ready for implementation, physicians must make individual decisions regarding treatment of such patients in the absence of available information. Every patient should be carefully evaluated, and if a decision is made to use an antiarrhythmic drug, a drug should be chosen that is likely to suppress non-sustained ventricular tachycardia while avoiding the potential for proarrhythmic effects and aggravation of underlying ventricular dysfunction. Previous empiric use of procainamide, quinidine, and disopyramide has not been associated with a reduction in mortality in patients with heart failure when arrhythmias are asymptomatic. In fact, indiscriminate use of these drugs may increase the risk of sudden cardiac death by proarrhythmic events. Patients with heart failure are more likely to develop proarrhythmic effects with all available antiarrhythmic drugs except amiodarone. In addition, care must be taken when using antiarrhythmic drugs to avoid exacerbation of ventricular dysfunction. Although it is well recognized that flecainide has a negative inotropic effect, recent evidence indicates that encainide may aggravate ventricular function in approximately 10 per cent of patients, and so it should be used carefully. Amiodarone is well tolerated in patients with impaired ventricular function, but its use must be carefully monitored to minimize toxicity for other organs.

Benign Ventricular Arrhythmias

Patients with benign ventricular arrhythmias often require no specific antiarrhythmic therapy and need reassurance alone. In the absence of symptoms, ventricular arrhythmias, including nonsustained ventricular tachycardia occurring in the absence of obvious heart disease or in the absence of significant impairment of ventricular function, are not associated with an increased risk of sudden cardiac death. Therefore, antiarrhythmic drug therapy is not expected to reduce the likelihood of sudden cardiac death and is unnecessary in the vast majority of patients. Only when these arrhythmias are associated with symptoms that are bothersome to patients is it reasonable to consider antiarrhythmic drug therapy. In these circumstances, a drug that is well tolerated and that has a low likelihood of proarrhythmic effects should be considered. Fortunately, when ventricular function is well preserved, most antiarrhythmic drugs are safe. The risk of a proarrhythmic effect with most available antiarrhythmic drugs is less than 10 per cent, and in most cases less than 5 per cent, as long as ventricular function is well preserved. Some patients with symptomatic ventricular ectopy that is not associated with heart disease may feel better when a beta blocker is prescribed, although the frequency of ventricular arrhythmias may not significantly diminish.

Exercise-induced ventricular tachycardia that occurs in younger patients with structurally normal hearts is an unusual but well-described arrhythmia. These patients tend to respond to verapamil, but it is important to exclude the likelihood of significant coronary disease in these patients by appropriate testing before beginning empiric therapy.

CONGENITAL HEART DISEASE

method of
DAVID J. DRISCOLL, M.D.
Mayo Clinic and Mayo Foundation
Rochester, Minnesota

Common forms of congenital heart disease can be grouped into four categories: (1) those resulting in a left-to-right shunt, (2) those resulting in a right-to-left shunt, (3) those causing obstruction to blood flow, and (4) those resulting from abnormal myocardial function.

DEFECTS ASSOCIATED WITH A LEFT-TO-RIGHT SHUNT

Ventricular septal defect, atrial septal defect, patent ductus arteriosus, and atrioventricular canal defects are the most common cardiac defects associated with a left-to-right shunt. Less common defects in this group include aorticopulmonary window, anomalous pulmonary venous return, and arteriovenous fistula. In a left-to-right shunt, oxygenated blood returns abnormally to the systemic venous system or right ventricle without prior gas transfer in the tissues.

Ventricular Septal Defect

Excluding bicuspid aortic valve and mitral valve prolapse, ventricular septal defect is the most common congenital cardiac malformation. A ventricular septal defect can be described anatomically by its location in the ventricular septum. (1) The most common location is in the area of the membranous septum; the so-called perimembranous defect. (2) The supracristal or subaortic defect is located above the crista supraventricularis. (3) The atrioventricular defect is located in the inlet septum. (4) The muscular defect is located in the muscular portion of the septum. Ventricular septal defects range in size from tiny to hemodynamically unimportant to large and life-threatening.

A ventricular septal defect is usually manifested by a holosystolic murmur in the first several weeks of life. The murmur may be absent in the first day or two of life because the normally raised pulmonary vascular resistance of the newborn prevents high-velocity flow of blood through the defect.

A small ventricular septal defect usually produces no symptoms. A moderate to large defect may produce signs and symptoms of congestive heart failure. This condition develops as pulmonary arteriolar resistance falls. It allows an increased flow of blood through the ventricular septal defect into the right ventricle and pulmonary artery, resulting in excessive pulmonary blood flow, left ventricular volume overload, and pulmonary venous hypertension.

The size and importance of a ventricular septal defect can be assessed by clinical examination. A small defect is associated with normal precordial impulses, a loud holosystolic murmur along the left sternal border (frequently associated with a precordial thrill), a normal pulmonary component of the second heart sound, and absence of a diastolic murmur. A moderate-sized defect (i.e., associated with normal or slightly elevated pulmonary artery pressure) is associated with a holosystolic murmur, increased precordial activity, a normal to slightly accentuated pulmonary component of the second heart sound, and a mid-diastolic murmur (caused by increased flow across the mitral valve). A large ventricular septal defect may be associated with a holosystolic murmur, increased activity of the parasternal (right ventricular) and apical (left ventricular) precordial impulses, increased intensity of the pulmonary component of the second heart sound, a mid-diastolic murmur, and evidence of congestive heart failure.

The electrocardiogram and chest radiogram are normal if the defect is small. A moderate-sized defect may be reflected by left ventricular hypertrophy on the electrocardiogram and mild to moderate cardiomegaly with increased pulmonary vascular markings on the chest radiogram. A large defect is associated with biventricular hypertrophy on the electrocardiogram and cardiomegaly with increased pulmonary vascular markings on the chest radiogram.

The presence and location of a ventricular septal defect can be documented by echocardiography. Using Doppler techniques, right ventricular and pulmonary artery pressure can be estimated.

Patients with a repaired or unrepaired ventricular septal defect need bacterial endocarditis prophylaxis. Small defects do not require surgical closure; indeed, many close spontaneously. All large defects resulting in pulmonary hypertension require closure, and this should be done before 1 year of age to prevent the development of irreversible pulmonary vascular obstructive disease. Large defects that have resulted in pulmonary vascular obstructive disease (Eisenmenger's syndrome) must be left open. Defects that are associated with normal to slight elevation of pulmonary artery pressure and cardiac enlargement should be closed, usually before the age of 4 or 5 years.

Atrial Septal Defect

There are four types of atrial septal defects. (1) The secundum defect is most common and is located in the region of the foramen ovale. (2) The ostium primum defect is a form of endocardial cushion defect, is located in the inferior aspect of the atrial septum, and is associated with a cleft in the anterior leaflet of the mitral valve. (3) The sinus venosus defect is located in the cephalad portion of the septum and is usually associated with partial anomalous pulmonary venous return. (4) The coronary septal defect (or defect of the inferior vena cava) is a relatively rare type of atrial septal defect.

Most infants and children with an atrial septal defect are asymptomatic or exhibit mild intolerance of exercise. The presence of the defect is suspected because of a cardiac murmur. Typically, the murmur is a grade 2/6 systolic ejection murmur heard best at the upper left sternal border. The second heart sound is split widely and remains so throughout the respiratory cycle. A tricuspid flow murmur may be heard at the right lower sternal border if the defect is moderate to large. The cardiac impulses at the lower left sternal border may be prominent as a result of right ventricular volume overload. An ostium primum atrial septal defect may be associated with a murmur of mitral regurgitation.

The electrocardiogram frequently exhibits an interventricular conduction delay manifested by an RSR′ pattern in the right precordial leads. If the defect is an ostium primum defect, there is also left axis deviation on the electrocardiogram. The chest radiogram may reveal mild to moderate cardiomegaly, increased pulmonary vascular markings, and a prominent main pulmonary artery segment. The presence, location, and type of atrial septal defect can be confirmed by echocardiographic and Doppler techniques.

All atrial septal defects that produce typical clinical findings or are associated with cardiomegaly should be closed surgically. Usually this is done on an elective basis at about 3 to 5 years of age. The outcome for patients after closure of an ostium secundum defect in childhood is excellent. Patients with an ostium primum defect may have mitral regurgitation or mitral stenosis even after surgical repair. Repair of sinus venosus defects includes correction of the partial anomalous pulmonary venous return. A patient with an atrial septal defect should have bacterial endocarditis prophylaxis both preoperatively and post-operatively. The exception to this rule is the patient who has suture closure of a secundum atrial septal defect. In this case, endocarditis prophylaxis can be discontinued 6 months post-operatively.

Patent Ductus Arteriosus

Normally, the ductus arteriosus closes between birth and 3 days of age. Persistent patency of the ductus arteriosus is more common in infants born prematurely or at high altitude than in full-term infants or those born at sea level.

For full-term infants or children, the presence of a continuous murmur, heard best in the left infraclavicular area, may indicate the presence of a patent ductus arteriosus. The following can mimic the murmur of a patient ductus arteriosus: innocent venous hum, coronary or pulmonary arteriovenous fistula, intracranial arteriovenous malformation or fistula, the combination of a ventricular septal defect and aortic insufficiency, and an aorticopulmonary window. In addition to a continuous murmur, a patient with a patent ductus arteriosus has an increased pulse pressure and may have overactivity of the apical (left ventricular) impulse.

The electrocardiogram usually is normal but may show evidence of left or biventricular hypertrophy if the patent ductus arteriosus is large. The chest radiogram may be normal or reveal cardiomegaly with increased pulmonary vascular markings, depending on the size of the patent ductus arteriosus and the volume of the left-to-right shunt through the defect. The diagnosis of a patent ductus arteriosus can be demonstrated by two-dimensional echocardiography.

With the exception of the rare patent ductus arteriosus associated with irreversible pulmonary vascular obstructive disease, all patients with a patent ductus arteriosus should have it closed. Even a small, hemodynamically insignificant patent ductus arteriosus should be closed because the risk of bacterial endocarditis is greater than the risk of surgical closure of the defect. Endocarditis prophylaxis is necessary preoperatively and for 6 months postoperatively.

Complete Atrioventricular Canal

Complete atrioventricular canal is an endocardial cushion defect in which the inferior aspect of the atrial septum (atrial septal defect) and the inlet portion of the ventricular septum (ventricular septal defect) are absent. In addition, the tricuspid and mitral valves are fused to form a common atrioventricular valve. In essence, the center of the heart is missing. An infant with a complete atrioventricular canal usually has a cardiac murmur and frequently congestive heart failure. The congestive heart failure associated with a complete atrioventricular canal may be severe, resulting in poor feeding, poor weight gain, tachypnea, nasal flaring, intercostal retraction, diaphoresis, and tachycardia. There is an increased right ventricular impulse at the lower left sternal border; a systolic murmur, usually grade 2/6 or greater; and a prominent diastolic flow murmur at the apex. The pulmonary component of the second heart sound is increased, reflecting pulmonary hypertension.

Characteristically, the electrocardiogram reveals a counterclockwise frontal plane loop, left axis deviation, and right and (sometimes) biventricular enlargement. There may be first-degree atrioventricular block and atrial enlargement. The chest radiogram reveals cardiomegaly with increased pulmonary vascular markings. The diagnosis can be confirmed by using echocardiography, and the degree of atrioventricular valve incompetence can be quantitated by Doppler techniques.

In the absence of pulmonary vascular obstructive disease, surgical correction of this malformation is necessary. The operation involves closure of the atrial and ventricular septal defects and division of the common atrioventricular valve to create a "tricuspid" and a "mitral" valve. The quality of the resultant two valves depends on the quality of the original valve tissue. Complete repair should be done before 1 year of age to prevent the development of pulmonary vascular obstructive disease. The operation may be necessary before 3 months of age if significant growth failure and uncontrollable congestive heart failure persist despite appropriate aggressive medical therapy. Patients with complete atrioventricular canal require bacterial endocarditis prophylaxis preoperatively and postoperatively.

DEFECTS ASSOCIATED WITH A RIGHT-TO-LEFT SHUNT

Cyanosis is the predominant feature of patients with congenital cardiac defects associated with a right-to-left shunt. The degree of cyanosis is determined by the volume of pulmonary blood flow and the relative volumes of the right-to-left and left-to-right shunts. Cyanosis in an infant represents a medical emergency because it is critical to ensure stability of pulmonary blood flow and to be certain that adequate sites for mixing of desaturated and saturated blood exist. Although numerous congenital cardiac defects and combinations of defects can produce cyanosis, only four major lesions are addressed. All patients with cyanotic forms of congenital heart disease require endocarditis prophylaxis throughout their lives.

Transposition of the Great Arteries

In transposition of the great arteries, the pulmonary artery originates from the left ventricle and the aorta from the right ventricle. Thus, systemic venous return is directed back to the body via the right ventricle and aorta, and pulmonary venous return is directed back to the lungs via the left ventricle and pulmonary artery. This situation is incompatible with life unless sites exist for mixing of the desaturated and saturated blood. Usually mixing occurs through the patent ductus arteriosus and the patent foramen ovale. For patients with transposed great arteries and an associated ventricular septal defect, mixing can occur through the defect.

Cyanosis usually is the presenting feature in infants with transposition of the great arteries. In addition, the right ventricular impulse at the lower left sternal border may be prominent, and the second heart sound may be single and intensified. A systolic ejection murmur may or may not be present.

In the newborn period, the electrocardiogram is normal or reveals right ventricular hypertrophy. Later, it shows right ventricular hypertrophy. The chest radiogram characteristically reveals cardiomegaly with increased pulmonary vascular markings, but normal heart size and normal pulmonary vascular markings can occur. The diagnosis of transposition of the great arteries and the presence or absence of additional defects (atrial septal defect, patent ductus arteriosus, ventricular septal defect, or pulmonary stenosis) can be confirmed by echocardiographic and Doppler techniques.

The first step in managing an infant with transposition of the great arteries is to ensure that adequate sites exist for intracardiac mixing of the separated circulations. Prostaglandin E_1 can be infused to maintain patency of the ductus arteriosus, allowing mixing at that site. If the ventricular and atrial septa are intact, an atrial septal defect can be created by the balloon septostomy technique of Rashkind and Miller. Definitive repair of transposition of the great arteries can be accomplished by using either an atrial or an arterial switch procedure. The atrial repair is the older of the two techniques and can be accomplished by either Mustard's or Senning's procedure. Both of these procedures redirect systemic and pulmonary venous returns, such that systemic venous return (deoxygenated blood) is directed through the mitral valve, and pulmonary venous return (oxygenated blood) is directed through the tricuspid valve. These operations usually are performed at about 1 year of age. The arterial switch (Jatene) procedure involved transecting both great arteries and reattaching them, such that the aorta is related to the left ventricle and the pulmonary artery to the right ventricle. The origin of the coronary arteries must be transferred to the "new aorta." This operation is performed in the first few days of life.

Tetralogy of Fallot

Tetralogy of Fallot consists of a ventricular septal defect, pulmonary valve and/or subpulmonary stenosis, an aorta that overrides the ventricular septal defect, and right ventricular hypertrophy. In general, the degree of cyanosis is proportional to the severity of the pulmonary stenosis.

Infants and children with tetralogy of Fallot usually present with cyanosis and a systolic ejection murmur. In infants, a patent ductus arteriosus may contribute to the volume of pulmonary blood flow. In this situation, the degree of cyanosis and hypoxia may increase substantially when the ductus closes. If this occurs and profound hypoxemia ensues, the ductus should be reopened with an infusion of prostaglandin E_1.

The electrocardiogram reflects right ventricular hypertrophy, except in newborn infants, in whom it may appear normal. The chest radiogram reveals a heart of normal size with reduced pulmonary vascular markings and a hypoplastic main pulmonary artery segment. The diagnosis can be confirmed by using two-dimensional echocardiography. Cardiac catheterization is necessary to assess the size and distribution of the pulmonary arteries and the number of ventricular septal defects and to exclude anomalies of the coronary arteries.

Complete surgical repair of tetralogy of Fallot consists of relieving the pulmonary stenosis and closing the ventricular septal defect. The optimum age at which this operation should be performed depends on the size of the pulmonary arteries and the degree of hypoxemia. If the pulmonary arteries are of normal or near-normal size and the patient has adequate oxygenation, it is usually performed between 1 and 2 years of age. If the patient has severe pulmonary stenosis and/or unacceptable hypoxemia as an infant, complete repair or a systemic-to-pulmonary artery anastomosis can be performed. The choice of surgical management depends on the size of the pulmonary arteries. If the arteries are too small for complete repair, a systemic-to-pulmonary artery anastomosis should be done using a tradi-

tional or modified Blalock-Taussig anastomosis (subclavian-to-pulmonary artery anastomosis or interposition of a Gore-Tex graft between the subclavian and pulmonary arteries). Patients who require a systemic-to-pulmonary artery shunt are candidates for complete repair of tetralogy of Fallot at a later age.

Truncus Arteriosus

Truncus arteriosus consists of a ventricular septal defect and origin of only one great artery (the truncus) from the heart. This artery arises from the ventricles above the ventricular septal defect. The pulmonary arteries arise from the truncus distal to the origin of the coronary arteries. Interruption of the aortic arch frequently is an associated defect. Usually the pulmonary arteries are unobstructed; hence, pulmonary blood flow is excessive. This results in pulmonary edema, congestive heart failure, and growth failure. If truncus arteriosus is not repaired, death may occur from profound congestive heart failure. If death does not occur, pulmonary vascular obstructive disease will result.

Infants with truncus arteriosus may present with cyanosis or congestive heart failure and/or a cardiac murmur. The apical and right ventricular impulses usually are increased. The second heart sound is increased in intensity, and there may be a systolic ejection murmur and an apical ejection click. There may be a mitral diastolic flow murmur, and if truncal incompetence exists, an early decrescendo diastolic murmur may be audible.

The electrocardiogram reveals right ventricular hypertrophy, and at times left ventricular hypertrophy as well, but in newborns it may be normal. Cardiomegaly and increased pulmonary vascular markings usually are present on the chest radiogram. The diagnosis can be confirmed by echocardiographic and Doppler techniques.

Infants with truncus arteriosus develop significant congestive heart failure, and treatment with digoxin and diuretics is indicated. Surgical repair is necessary before 6 months of age. It includes patch closure of the ventricular septal defect, removal of the proximal pulmonary arteries from the truncus, and interposition of a graft from the right ventricle to the distal pulmonary arteries. Revision of this operation is necessary when the patient outgrows the right ventricular–to–pulmonary artery graft.

Tricuspid Atresia

Tricuspid atresia consists of absence of the right atrioventricular valve. There is no direct communication between the right atrium and right ventricle. Usually there is associated hypoplasia of the right ventricle. An atrial septal defect must exist to allow systemic venous return to exit the right atrium. The aorta and pulmonary arteries can be normally related or transposed. Usually pulmonary or subpulmonary stenosis exists if the great arteries are normally related, but there may or may not be pulmonary stenosis if the great arteries are transposed. The clinical course of these patients depends, to a large extent, on the presence or absence of pulmonary stenosis.

The patient with tricuspid atresia presents during infancy with cyanosis, a murmur, and/or congestive heart failure. Cyanosis predominates in the patients with pulmonary stenosis, and congestive heart failure predominates in those without pulmonary stenosis. A systolic ejection murmur usually is present, and the apical (left ventricular) impulse may be prominent.

The electrocardiogram reveals left axis deviation, and this finding should suggest the diagnosis of tricuspid atresia in a cyanotic infant. The chest radiogram may reveal a heart of normal size and normal or decreased pulmonary vascular markings in patients with pulmonary stenosis, or cardiomegaly with increased pulmonary vascular markings in patients without pulmonary stenosis. The presence of associated lesions can be documented by using echocardiography and Doppler techniques. Cardiac catheterization may be necessary to demonstrate the sources and reliability of pulmonary blood flow and to enlarge the atrial septal defect if it is restrictive.

Initial treatment of infants with tricuspid atresia is directed at optimizing the volume of pulmonary blood flow. Patients with pulmonary stenosis may have insufficient pulmonary blood flow and need a surgically created systemic-to-pulmonary artery shunt. Patients with unobstructed pulmonary blood flow need a pulmonary banding procedure to control the symptoms of congestive heart failure and to prevent the development of pulmonary vascular obstructive disease. Eventual definitive palliation of patients with tricuspid atresia is accomplished by using the modified Fontan operation. In this operation, the atrial septal defect is closed, the pulmonary artery is transected (the proximal stump is oversewn), and the right atrium is connected to the distal portion of the pulmonary artery. The systemic venous return travels from the right atrium directly to the pulmonary artery. The systemic and pulmonary venous systems are now separate, and the ventricular mass receives only pulmonary venous return and ejects it into the aorta. The principles of management of patients with tricuspid atresia

can be applied to patients with other forms of functional single ventricle.

VENTRICULAR OUTFLOW OBSTRUCTION

Pulmonary Valve Stenosis

Pulmonary valve stenosis usually presents with a cardiac murmur in an otherwise asymptomatic infant or child. Occasionally, severe pulmonary stenosis presents as cyanosis in a newborn because of shunting of desaturated blood from the right atrium to the left atrium through a patent foramen ovale.

The murmur of pulmonary stenosis is systolic and of ejection quality. It is best heard along the upper left sternal border and radiates to the lung fields posteriorly. There may be an audible ejection click at the middle to upper left sternal border. With severe pulmonary stenosis the click is inaudible. The second heart sound is normal with mild pulmonary stenosis, more widely split with moderate stenosis, and single with severe stenosis.

The electrocardiogram reveals right ventricular hypertrophy, the degree of which is proportional to the severity of the pulmonary stenosis and the right ventricular pressure. The chest radiogram may show poststenotic dilation of the pulmonary artery. The diagnosis can be confirmed by echocardiography and the transpulmonary gradient estimated with Doppler techniques.

Pulmonary stenosis associated with a transpulmonary gradient of 30 to 40 mmHg or more should be relieved. This can be done most expeditiously by catheter balloon dilation of the valve. The results of this procedure are good, and surgical valvotomy is rarely necessary. The long-term outlook for patients with pulmonary valve stenosis is excellent. Patients with pulmonary stenosis should be given bacterial endocarditis prophylaxis.

Aortic Valve Stenosis

Aortic valve stenosis usually presents with a cardiac murmur in an otherwise asymptomatic infant, child, or adolescent. The exception is the infant with severe aortic stenosis, who may develop severe congestive heart failure with depression of left ventricular contractility.

In addition to a systolic ejection murmur, heard best along the left sternal border and radiating to the right upper sternal border and carotid arteries, an early systolic apical ejection click is frequently present. A precordial and carotid thrill may also exist. The pulse volume in children with aortic valve stenosis who do not have heart failure is usually normal. The apical (left ventricular) impulse may be prominent. Although the presence of aortic stenosis is usually revealed by the physical examination, the severity of the obstruction is difficult to judge on this basis alone.

The electrocardiogram is normal or shows evidence of left ventricular hypertrophy. The presence, absence, or severity of left ventricular hypertrophy, as determined by electrocardiography, correlates poorly with the severity of aortic stenosis. A prominent ascending aorta caused by poststenotic dilation may be evident by chest radiography. The diagnosis of aortic stenosis can be confirmed by using echocardiographic techniques, and the location of this stenosis (valvar, supervalvar, or subvalvar) can be established. The transaortic gradient can be estimated by using Doppler technology.

The indications for and timing of surgery to reduce the degree of aortic stenosis depends to a great extent on the severity of the transaortic gradient. For valvar aortic stenosis, a transaortic gradient of less than 39 mmHg is considered to be mild; 40 to 79 mmHg, moderately severe; and more than 80 mmHg, severe. Patients with a gradient of more than 80 mmHg should have surgery. Some clinicians recommend an operation for patients with a transaortic gradient of more than 60 mmHg. Patients who have symptoms of cardiac syncope or presyncope or evidence of myocardial ischemia should have surgery to relieve the aortic stenosis even if the resting transaortic gradient is as low as 30 mmHg. Aortic valvotomy is not curative and may result in aortic valve regurgitation. Although open surgical valvotomy is the preferred technique, balloon dilation of the aortic valve, albeit still experimental, may be an alternative. Eventually, aortic valve replacement may be necessary for some patients. Operation is recommended for patients with discrete subvalvar aortic stenosis and a gradient of more than 40 mmHg. All patients with aortic stenosis should receive bacterial endocarditis prophylaxis.

Coarctation of the Aorta

Coarctation of the aorta consists of a shelf-like obstruction in the aorta just distal to the origin of the left subclavian artery and opposite the ligamentum arteriosus. Up to 80 per cent of patients with coarctation of the aorta have an associated bicuspid aortic valve. There is a male predominance of coarctation of the aorta. Patients with this condition usually seek medical attention because of a cardiac murmur or upper extremity hypertension. The characteristic physical findings include reduced pulse volume in the lower extremities, upper extremity hypertension, differential blood pressure between the upper and lower extremities, and an apical systolic ejection click (if there is an associated bicuspid aortic valve). Frequently there is a holosystolic apical murmur. The presence of thoracic collateral vessels may be revealed by palpating suprascapular pulsations and by the existence of continuous murmurs heard over the back.

The electrocardiogram is either normal or reveals right ventricular hypertrophy in infancy and left ventricular hypertrophy later on. Poststenotic dilation of the descending aorta and rib notching resulting from thoracic collateral vessels may be apparent by chest radiography. Although the diagnosis of coarctation of the aorta is made on the basis of physical examination, echocardiography and magnetic resonance imaging may be useful to delineate the exact location of the coarctation and to exclude rare situations in which the coarctation is in an unusual position, such as the midthoracic or abdominal aorta.

Surgical repair of coarctation of the aorta is indicated if there is upper extremity hypertension, a significant difference between upper and lower extremity blood pressures, or the presence of thoracic collateral vessels. Except in unusual circumstances, an operation should be done between 1 and 4 years of age. Persistent hypertension and persistent or recurrent coarctation of the aorta are potential postoperative problems. All patients with coarctation of the aorta should receive bacterial endocarditis prophylaxis.

CARDIOMYOPATHY

Dilated (Congestive) Cardiomyopathy

The term "dilated cardiomyopathy" or "congestive cardiomyopathy" encompasses many abnormalities, some of known cause and others idiopathic, that result in reduced myocardial function. Although the etiology of the majority of cases of dilated cardiomyopathy is unknown, it is important to define the specific etiology, if possible, because some cases are treatable. Defects in carnitine metabolism can produce dilated (as well as hypertrophic) cardiomyopathy; this condition is usually reversible with carnitine supplementation. Selenium deficiency is a rare cause of dilated cardiomyopathy and should be sought especially if the patient resides in a geographic location in which the soil is deficient in selenium. Incessant tachycardia can result in cardiomyopathy, and it is important to determine that the cardiomyopathy results from the tachycardia and not vice versa. Occult atrial tachycardia should be suspected in any patient with myocardial dysfunction who consistently exhibits a heart rate greater than 110 to 120 beats per minute, with little variation throughout a 24-hour period. Appropriate treatment of the underlying tachycardia can result in complete resolution of the myopathy.

Hypertrophic Cardiomyopathy

Hypertrophic cardiomyopathy frequently is familial and is associated with sudden, unexpected death. This diagnosis must be considered in patients with a family history of hypertrophic cardiomyopathy or a family history of sudden and unexpected death, particularly at young ages. The diagnosis can be confirmed by echocardiography. The best treatment for hypertrophic cardiomyopathy is unknown.

MITRAL VALVE PROLAPSE AND THE MITRAL VALVE PROLAPSE SYNDROME

method of
HARISIOS BOUDOULAS, M.D., and
CHARLES F. WOOLEY, M.D.
The Ohio State University
Columbus, Ohio

CLASSIFICATION

Subtle gradations may exist between normal mitral valve function and the alterations in mitral valve morphology that result in mitral valve prolapse (MVP). This gray zone or overlap area between normal mitral valve dynamics and minimal to mild mitral valvular dysfunction has contributed to diagnostic difficulties in an era of evolving technology.

"MVP anatomic" refers to patients with a wide spectrum of mitral valvular abnormalities ranging from mild to severe (Table 1). The term "floppy mitral valve" comes from surgical and pathologic studies and refers to expansion of the mitral valve leaflet area, with elongated chordae, a dilated mitral annulus, and characteristic gross and histologic structural changes in the valve leaflets. Symptoms, physical findings, and laboratory abnormalities in these patients are directly related to mitral valvular dysfunction, progressive mitral regurgitation and its complications, and valve surface phenomena such as embolic phenomena or infectious endocarditis.

"MVP syndrome" refers to the occurrence or coexistence of symptoms that result from various forms of neuroendocrine or autonomic dysfunction in patients with MVP in whom the symptoms cannot be explained on the basis of valvular abnormality alone.

This classification is clinically useful and separates

patients whose symptoms are related to progressive mitral valvular dysfunction from patients with MVP and symptoms related to autonomic dysfunction.

DIAGNOSIS

The diagnosis of MVP should be based on the history, physical examination, echophonocardiogram, and Doppler echocardiogram. A family history provides important information because MVP may be inherited and family members may have similar complications. Nonejection systolic clicks of mitral origin, mid to late mitral systolic murmurs, both with well-defined postural auscultatory changes, constitute the typical auscultatory findings in patients with MVP. Echocardiography (M-mode and two-dimensional) interpreted in light of clinical findings is an extremely valuable diagnostic test. Doppler echocardiography may be used to detect the presence of mitral regurgitation and to document the timing and direction of the regurgitant jet in patients with MVP. Color-flow Doppler echocardiography complements pulse Doppler echocardiography.

In general, we are more comfortable when the diagnosis of MVP is based on the auscultatory postural complex with confirmatory echocardiographic findings. Diagnoses based on a subjective interpretation of auscultatory systolic clicks without echophonocardiographic confirmation, or on nonspecific echocardiographic findings without other clinical correlates, have contributed to diagnostic confusion and exaggerated

TABLE 1. **Classification of MVP**

MVP Anatomic	MVP Syndrome
Common mitral valve abnormality with a spectrum of structural and functional changes ranging from mild to severe	Patients with MVP
The Basis for	*Symptom Complex:* chest pain, palpitations, arrhythmias, fatigue, exercise intolerance, dyspnea, postural phenomena, syncope, neuropsychiatric symptoms
Systolic click; mid-late systolic murmur Mild or progressive mitral valvular dysfunction Progressive mitral regurgitation, atrial fibrillation, congestive heart failure Infectious endocarditis Embolic phenomena	*Neuroendocrine or autonomic dysfunction* (high catecholamine levels, catecholamine regulation abnormality, hyper-response to adrenergic stimulation, parasympathetic abnormality, baroreflex modulation abnormality, renin-aldosterone regulation abnormality, decreased intravascular volume, decresed ventricular diastolic volume in the upright position, atrial natriuretic factor secretion abnormality) possible explanation for symptoms
Characterized by a long natural history	
May be heritable or associated with heritable disorders of connective tissue	
Conduction system involvement, possibly leading to arrhythmias and conduction defects	Mitral valve prolapse—a possible marker for autonomic dysfunction

MVP incidence figures. Conversely, because echocardiographic and cineangiographic studies have shown that MVP may occur without external auscultatory phenomena, there must be room for some diagnostic flexibility.

MVP ANATOMIC

Therapy in this group is related to the severity of mitral valvular dysfunction, the severity of mitral valvular regurgitation, and the prevention or treatment of predictable complications.

Severity of MVP and Mitral Regurgitation

Asymptomatic patients with isolated mitral systolic clicks usually have MVP of limited clinical significance, and in most cases this is not a progressive lesion. The prevention of infective endocarditis is the major consideration in these patients (Figure 1).

Patients with mitral systolic click or clicks, mid to late mitral systolic murmurs, and increased mitral valve thickness and valve surface area with increased mitral annulus size usually have MVP with mild to moderate mitral regurgitation. The potential for progressive mitral valvular dysfunction is the major concern in patients in this group. Therapeutic considerations in these patients include prevention of infective endocarditis and the recognition and prevention of progressive mitral valve regurgitation. At present, very little is known about the effects of usual life activities such as heavy labor, physical exercise, or pharmacologic interventions on the progression of mitral regurgitation.

Progressive mitral regurgitation with the development of significant or refractory congestive heart failure usually occurs in the presence of left atrial enlargement that progresses to left atrial failure, with the ultimate development of chronic atrial fibrillation. More acute or subacute forms of mitral regurgitation may be the result of ruptured chordae tendineae occurring in the presence of pre-existing mild or moderately severe mitral regurgitation. Mitral valve surgery should be considered in most patients with congestive heart failure and mitral regurgitation secondary to MVP.

Prevention and Management of Complications

Infective Endocarditis

Patients with MVP are at higher risk for infective endocarditis. In general, these patients should receive antibiotic prophylaxis for diagnostic and therapeutic procedures where bacteremia is a risk. Patients should be encouraged to main-

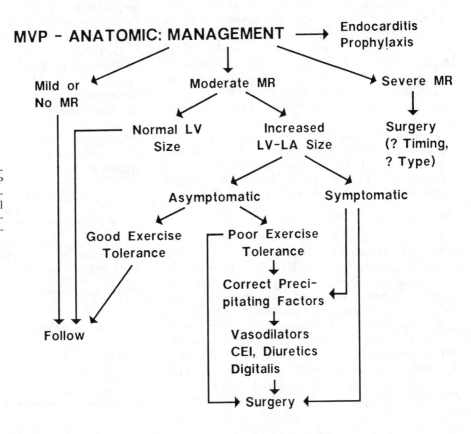

Figure 1. Schematic of management of patients with MVP in relation to the degree of mitral regurgitation. MR = mitral regurgitation, LV = left ventricular, LA = left atrial, CEI = converting enzyme inhibitors.

tain the best possible oral hygiene to reduce potential sources of bacterial seeding because poor dental hygiene, periodontal or periapical infections, or oral mucosal ulcers caused by ill-fitting dentures may induce bacteremia without dental manipulation or procedures. Patients with MVP who develop infective endocarditis should be treated appropriately.

Thromboembolic Complications

Certain patients with anatomic MVP are at risk for embolic events, the embolic source presumably being surface events from the floppy mitral valve involving platelet aggregation or actual thrombi. When atrial fibrillation occurs, thrombi may originate from the left atrium. An increased incidence of MVP in patients with migraine has been suggested for some time. The association of migraine and MVP is especially high in patients with focal cerebral ischemic episodes. It is tempting to speculate that platelets, either by microcirculatory aggregation or by induction of vasospasm in the cerebral circulation, could play an etiologic role in some cases of migraine, especially because migraines may occasionally result in a small infarction. Among the classes of pharmacologic agents that diminish the migraine sequence are antiplatelet drugs such as aspirin and beta-adrenergic blocking drugs. Young women with MVP and a history of thromboembolic complications may be at increased risk for thromboembolic disease, and if it seems otherwise reasonable after a general medical evaluation, we think that it is wise to avoid the use of oral contraceptives. Women who have had clinical manifestations of retinal, cerebral, or peripheral emboli should discontinue oral contraceptive use, abstain from chronic cigarette smoking, and have a careful cardiovascular and hematologic evaluation before long-term anticoagulant or antiplatelet therapy is considered. Chronic anticoagulation should be considered in patients with chronic atrial fibrillation, with or without embolic phenomena.

Congestive Heart Failure

Chronic congestive heart failure in patients with MVP usually results from the progression of mitral regurgitation with left atrial and left ventricular dysfunction. Acute and subacute forms of congestive heart failure may be coincident with, or associated with, the recent onset of atrial fibrillation or ruptured chordae tendineae, or both. Attempts should be made to convert atrial fibrillation to sinus rhythm with antiarrhythmic drugs or cardioversion in patients with a history of recent onset of atrial fibrillation. Therapy with vasodilators, converting enzyme inhibitors, diuretics, and digitalis should be initiated. If atrial fibrillation persists, the ventricular rate should be maintained at 70 to 80 beats per minute at rest and at 90 to 100 beats per minute during routine physical activities. Mitral valve surgery should be considered in patients with mitral regurgitation secondary to MVP complicated by congestive heart failure after their response to intensive medical management has been determined.

MVP SYNDROME

Although individuals with the MVP syndrome may recall chest pain, palpitations, or exercise intolerance dating from childhood or adolescence, most of the symptomatic patients who come to us seeking medical care are young adults in their twenties and thirties, with a peak incidence at approximately 30 years of age. The basic principles of managing patients with the MVP syndrome are listed in Table 2. In our opinion, the single most important noninvasive test and therapeutic step is a carefully taken medical history and a properly performed physical examination. These patients constitute a group at risk for misinterpretation by the physician of the history, physical findings, borderline laboratory test results, nonspecific electrocardiographic changes, or nonspecific echocardiographic changes. Misinterpretation by or bias of the physician may lead to inappropriate, poorly conceived programs of long-term drug therapy, often without clear-cut goals regarding duration of therapy. A careful explanation of the physician's findings, an explanation of what is known about the mechanism of the symptoms, and the best possible answers to the anxious patient's list of questions constitute the cornerstone of long-term management.

Symptoms frequently occur in the presence of acute or gradual increases in the physical or emotional stresses of life. A commonsense ap-

TABLE 2. **MVP Syndrome: General Principles of Management**

Explain and reassure
Avoid volume depletion and the use of diuretics
Avoid catecholamines or other cyclic AMP stimulants
Avoid drugs that may increase adrenergic receptor sensitivity (e.g., thyroxine)
Avoid long-term drug therapy
Use exercise program

Specific Symptoms Requiring Treatment

Chest pain
Fatigue—exercise intolerance
Postural phenomena
Dyspnea
Neuropsychiatric symptoms

proach to stress modification, where possible and feasible, may seem to be too fundamental for the physician to even mention to the patient; however, such an approach may never have occurred to the patient who is attempting to meet demands well beyond his or her capabilities. The re-establishment of order in a patient's chaotic life may be an enormous contribution by the physician and may require assistance from family members, clergy, or a counselor. Undue anxieties, phobias, or panic attacks may form the basis for consultation with an informed psychiatrist.

Patients with MVP syndrome appear to be quite sensitive to volume depletion and manifest postural phenomena such as inappropriate postural-exercise tachycardia, chronic vasoconstriction, and postural hypotension. Women may note an exaggeration of symptoms at the time of menstrual periods. We have found it advisable to avoid or discontinue chronic diuretic therapy in this group of patients; the latter may be particularly important because a diuretic-induced hypokalemia may also contribute to the production or exaggeration of cardiac arrhythmias, which starts a vicious cycle. Prophylactic volume repletion before, during, or immediately after physical exercise may be particularly beneficial to patients with low intravascular blood volume.

The removal of catecholamine and cyclic adenosine monophosphate (AMP) stimulation by abstinence from caffeine, cigarettes, alcohol, and prescribed or over-the-counter drugs containing epinephrine or ephedrine is an important initial step. Agents, such as thyroxine, that may increase sensitivity to catecholamines by modifying the function of beta-adrenergic receptors should be avoided. Small amounts of beta-blocking drugs such as atenolol (Tenormin), 25 to 50 mg, or nadolol (Corgard), 20 to 40 mg, during stressful periods for a short time or as a single dose may be beneficial.

Questions about physical activities, physical fitness, and exercise programs should be addressed. Fatigue and previous exercise intolerance may have resulted in the avoidance of exercise or in very limited attempts to exercise. If there are no serious exercise-induced abnormalities or arrhythmias, enrollment in a cardiac rehabilitation program for aerobic conditioning may be accompanied by gratifying physical, physiologic, and psychologic benefits. Although the precise mechanism of the beneficial effect of exercise is not known, it is suggested that this effect may be mediated by the catecholamine-receptor system because exercise may alter catecholamine levels or adrenergic receptor activity or both.

Treatment of Specific Symptoms

Chest Pain

Management of patients with the MVP syndrome who have severe or incapacitating chest pain may be a source of frustration for patient and physician alike as long as our understanding of its pathogenesis remains limited. Although chest pain in patients with MVP syndrome in many cases may be extracardiac (e.g., chest wall pain), identifying certain patients with MVP who have chest pain associated with coronary artery disease, tachyarrhythmias, or left ventricular diastolic dysfunction may be necessary. Similarly, gastrointestinal causes of chest pain, in particular esophageal causes, should be excluded.

Once this has been accomplished, it is important to educate the patient about the nature of the disorder and chest pain and, especially, to emphasize the positive aspects of the long-term outlook. It is also essential to educate the patient about the factors that may initiate or precipitate chest pain.

In more severe cases, medical management may be indicated. Small doses of a beta blocker may be effective in treating chest pain associated with MVP syndrome. Although the mechanism of action is not clear, beta-blocking agents are known to produce an increase in left ventricular volume, a decrease in left ventricular contractility, and consequently a reduction in papillary muscle tension; the decrease in heart rate after therapy with beta blockers increases the diastolic time, that is, the myocardial perfusion time. It should be emphasized that rigorous controlled studies dealing with the therapy of pain with beta-blocking drugs in MVP syndrome are lacking.

The effect of alpha blockers, calcium channel blockers, and vasodilators on chest pain in patients with MVP syndrome also has not yet been subjected to critical study. Theoretically, these agents should be effective in patients who have chest pain secondary to coronary artery vasoregulatory abnormalities. The effect of other centrally acting sympathetic blocking drugs such as clonidine or antianxiety drugs on chest pain in patients with MVP syndrome has not been subjected to critical evaluation. One unconfirmed study suggested that therapy with digitalis may relieve or abolish chest pain in patients with MVP syndrome.

Fatigue—Exercise Intolerance

If there are no contraindications, enrollment in a cardiac rehabilitation program may be beneficial. Aerobic conditioning may help some patients who present with easy fatigability.

Postural Phenomena

Patients with MVP syndrome appear to be quite sensitive to volume depletion. Postural phenomena may be related to decreased intravascular volume, an abnormal renin and aldosterone response to volume depletion, a hyperadrenergic state, parasympathetic abnormality, or baroreflex receptor abnormality. Diuretic therapy should be avoided in these patients. Liberal sodium and fluid intake in certain patients may be beneficial. Therapy with fludrocortisone acetate (Florinef), 0.1 mg three times daily, may improve symptoms in more severe cases.* Clonidine (Catapres) in low doses (0.3 to 0.4 mg daily) may result in both symptomatic and hemodynamic improvement. The precise mechanisms for the beneficial effect of clonidine remain to be defined. The improvement of sympathetic, parasympathetic, and baroreflex abnormalities may partially account for these beneficial effects.

Dyspnea

There is no specific therapy for patients who present with dyspnea. Again, an exercise program and an explanation about the nature of the symptom and the positive long-term outlook may be beneficial in certain patients.

Neuropsychiatric Symptoms

An explanation to the anxious patient of what is known about the mechanism of symptoms constitutes the best approach. In certain patients with uncontrolled anxiety, panic episodes, or agoraphobia, therapy with psychotropic drugs or psychiatric evaluation may be indicated.

MVP ANATOMIC AND THE MVP SYNDROME

Certain symptoms or phenomena such as arrhythmias-palpitations, syncope-presyncope, or cardiac arrest may be related to autonomic dysfunction and mitral valvular dysfunction and, thus, may occur in both patients with anatomic MVP and those with the MVP syndrome.

Cardiac Arrhythmias-Palpitations

Caffeine or other stimulants such as alcohol, smoking, and sympathomimetic drugs should be avoided in MVP patients with tachyarrhythmias. Supraventricular tachycardia can be suppressed by digitalis, Class IA antiarrhythmic agents, beta-blocking drugs, calcium channel blockers, or combination of these drugs.

Patients with ventricular arrhythmias require

---

*May exceed manufacturer's recommended dose.

individual assessment; those at high risk for severe complications (presyncope, syncope, sudden death) should be identified.

In some cases, when recurrent tachyarrhythmias are refractory to antiarrhythmic drugs or the patient is intolerant of therapy, various pacing devices or automatic defibrillation may be helpful. Catheter ablation and surgical resection play a role in a variety of conditions, including the Wolff-Parkinson-White syndrome with refractory supraventricular tachyarrhythmias, sudden death potential, and recurrent or refractory ventricular tachycardia or fibrillation. Mitral valve surgery in patients with ventricular arrhythmias associated with severe mitral regurgitation and congestive heart failure may result in improvement of the arrhythmias in certain patients.

If palpitations are demonstrated to be related to specific cardiac arrhythmias, the management of cardiac arrhythmias should proceed. If palpitations are related to inappropriate sinus tachycardia during routine daily activities, small amounts of beta-blocking drugs may be beneficial.

Syncope-Presyncope

In view of the wide variety of disorders that can result in syncope, it is clear that effective treatment demands accurate diagnosis. Therapy for the patient with syncope varies from simple maneuvers, such as avoiding precipitating factors, to more direct forms of therapy, including potent antiarrhythmic drugs or cardiac pacemakers. For the patient with vasodepressor or vasovagal syncope, avoiding the precipitating factors (e.g., by lying down when venipuncture is attempted) may be sufficient. For the patient with arrhythmic syncope, control of cardiac arrhythmias with antiarrhythmic drugs, a cardiac pacemaker, or surgery may be necessary. For the patient with syncope related to orthostatic hypotension, increased sodium and fluid intake should be advised; in certain patients, therapy with fludrocortisone acetate may improve symptoms. Therapy with clonidine has been reported to improve some of the orthostatic symptoms. In patients with syncope of unknown origin, attempts to define the underlying causes should be continued. In patients with combined causes of syncope, the underlying pathophysiologic mechanisms should be corrected.

Cardiac Arrest

Patients with MVP and a history of cardiac arrest (survivors following cardiopulmonary resuscitation for ventricular fibrillation or asystole) should undergo a thorough cardiovascular evaluation to define the potential participating mechanisms before selection of the most appropriate therapy for the cardiac arrhythmias.

MVP: SPECIAL CONSIDERATIONS

Childhood

The prognosis in children with MVP appears to be good, although complications related to prolapse may occur. Diagnostic evaluation and therapy are similar to those described for adults. It is emphasized that diagnosis of MVP in children should be based mostly on auscultatory findings and not only on minor echocardiographic findings. We think that it is wise to follow children with MVP every 2 years even when they are asymptomatic.

Pregnancy

Few studies have dealt with pregnancy in patients with MVP. Available data and clinical experience suggest that complications are not anticipated and that the frequency of intrapartum complications is no greater in MVP patients than in patients with no cardiac disorder. Because of the expansion of intravascular volume during pregnancy, symptoms related to a low circulating blood volume or volume depletion responses in symptomatic patients with MVP syndrome are less evident during pregnancy.

Family history is important because patients may have complications similar to those of their mothers. On rare occasions, aortic root dilatation may occur in patients with MVP. Thus, during the echocardiographic evaluation, special attention should be given to the aortic root because patients with aortic root dilatation may be at a higher risk for aortic rupture or dissection during pregnancy.

Although recent information suggests that antibiotic prophylaxis is not needed for routine, uncomplicated vaginal deliveries, data are limited; antibiotic prophylaxis, however, should be given for any complicated delivery.

Sympathomimetic drugs (often used in premature labor), dehydration, volume depletion, and blood loss may precipitate or initiate symptoms in patients with MVP. Thus, sympathomimetic drugs should be used with great caution if they are absolutely necessary for obstetric reasons, and every effort should be made to avoid volume depletion and dehydration.

Athletics

Firm data on which to base a judgment for recommendations for athletes with MVP are not yet available. Despite the high prevalence of MVP in the general population, sudden death in competitive athletes with isolated MVP has not been reported. There are no data to demonstrate that strenuous exercise in patients with MVP predisposes to death that otherwise would not have occurred, or that withdrawal from competitive athletics will prolong life. The best approach at present for recommendations to athletes should be based on common sense, good clinical judgment, and appropriate exercise testing. Recommendations and advice need to be balanced between restricting activity unduly and reducing the chance of injury from participation in athletics.

It is important in each case to define the severity of MVP, mitral regurgitation, the aortic root size, the presence of cardiac arrhythmias, and symptomatology, if present. In general, asymptomatic patients who have MVP without or with mild mitral regurgitation, with normal left ventricular size and function, with normal aortic root size, with normal exercise tolerance, and without cardiac arrhythmias can participate in all competitive athletics. Patients with aortic root dilatation require further evaluation before a decision can be made about low-intensity participation in sports.

The long-term prognosis in patients who have MVP and normal left ventricular size and function, with ventricular or supraventricular arrhythmias detected with exercise testing or ambulatory monitoring, is unknown. Certain arrhythmias, however, may create symptoms and are dangerous. These arrhythmias in general are characterized by a very rapid heart rate, such as atrial flutter, atrial fibrillation, or ventricular tachycardia, or a very slow heart rate, such as atrioventricular block or profound sinus bradycardia. Patients who have suspected cardiac arrhythmias and who are being considered for competitive athletics should have long-term ambulatory monitoring, if possible during the type of exercise performed, and an exercise test.

Patients with a history of palpitations should be carefully evaluated to exclude any significant arrhythmia before permission is given to participate in competitive sports.

Syncope may be related to or result from a life-threatening condition; thus, a complete evaluation is indicated to define the cause of syncope.

CONGESTIVE HEART FAILURE

method of
GARY S. FRANCIS, M.D.
University of Minnesota
Minneapolis, Minnesota

Even the definition of congestive heart failure provokes considerable controversy. It is above all a clinical syndrome that can complicate virtually any form of heart disease, and it has at least two components: cardiac dysfunction and reduced exercise tolerance. The most common causes of congestive heart failure in the United States are as follows:

1. Coronary artery disease with destruction of contractile muscle tissue
2. Systemic hypertension
3. Chronic alcoholism
4. Diabetes mellitus
5. Idiopathic dilated cardiomyopathy
6. Valvular heart disease

Of course, these etiologic factors may coexist with each other, particularly coronary artery disease, hypertension, and diabetes mellitus. In the United States an estimated 400,000 individuals develop heart failure annually; it is thus the most common inpatient diagnosis of patients older than age 65 years. The therapy is closely related to the etiology. For example, patients with acute aortic insufficiency and infective endocarditis are managed by urgent valve replacement, whereas patients with idiopathic cardiomyopathy are treated with diuretics and vasodilators. This discussion will focus on patients with congestive heart failure caused by a large, dilated heart. Treatment of both acute and chronic heart failure will be considered.

ACUTE CONGESTIVE HEART FAILURE (PULMONARY EDEMA)

Patients with acute pulmonary edema are usually unable to give a detailed history because of breathlessness. They commonly come to the emergency room in acute respiratory distress, diaphoretic, somewhat cyanotic, and unable to lie down or give more than two or three words of history at a time. The differential diagnosis includes acute exacerbation of chronic obstructive lung disease and acute asthma. Arterial blood gas analyses, a portable chest x-ray film, and an echocardiogram (when the patient is stable) are extremely useful to confirm the diagnosis of heart failure.

Low-flow oxygen via Venturi's mask (40 to 60 per cent) should be initiated and adequate oxygenation ensured by obtaining arterial blood gas measurements. If adequate oxygenation cannot be accomplished with a mask or if severe carbon dioxide retention occurs, the patient may have to be intubated and mechanically ventilated.

Morphine sulfate should be given in doses of 2 to 5 mg intravenously every 15 minutes to alleviate anxiety and to further reduce venous pressure. Because of possible respiratory depression and hypotension, morphine should be used with great care. The total dose should not exceed 15 mg. If respiratory depression occurs, naloxone, 0.4 mg, should be given intravenously every 2 to 5 minutes as necessary.

Furosemide (Lasix), 40 mg intravenously, should be administered. If the blood urea nitrogen level is raised, large intravenous doses of furosemide (>100 mg) may be necessary. Oral furosemide is poorly absorbed in acute heart failure. Sublingual nitroglycerin (Nitrostat) is also useful in the early stages of pulmonary edema. If the systolic blood pressure is 90 mmHg or higher, nitroprusside (Nipride) should be started at 10 to 15 micrograms per minute. Fifty milligrams of nitroprusside should be mixed in 250 ml of 5 per cent dextrose in water to a concentration of 200 micrograms per ml. The dose should be rapidly increased as needed to control breathlessness, not to allow the systolic blood pressure to go below 90 mmHg. Nitroprusside in excess of 300 micrograms per minute is rarely necessary. The infusion should be maintained for 24 to 48 hours, with close attention paid to blood pressure, arterial blood gas levels, urine output, electrolyte values, and renal function. Nitroprusside has a balanced effect on arterial resistance and venous capacitance. It reduces the systolic wall tension on the heart and lowers pulmonary capillary wedge pressure. Nitroprusside is particularly valuable because of its immediate onset of action and extremely short half-life. Toxicity is rare.

Acute pulmonary edema occasionally occurs in the setting of rapid atrial fibrillation or atrial flutter. Rather than trying to slow the atrial arrhythmia with intravenous digoxin, electrical cardioversion is preferred. Immediate restoration of normal sinus rhythm, rather than gradual slowing of the ventricular response, is desirable in acute pulmonary edema.

Patients who present with hypotension and acute pulmonary edema have a grave prognosis. Restoration of blood pressure becomes an immediate goal. Dopamine (Intropin) (500 mg in 500 ml of 5 per cent dextrose in water [1000 micrograms per ml]) should be administered at 5 to 20 micrograms per kg per minute to restore blood pressure to a systolic level of 90 to 100 mmHg. Dopamine in doses of less than 2 micrograms per kg per minute may cause additional arterial dilation and lowered blood pressure, so large doses are necessary to promote a "pressor" effect. Dopamine enhances myocardial contractility directly and produces peripheral vasoconstriction related to alpha-adrenergic receptor activation in peripheral arteries. When hypotension and acute pulmonary edema coexist, insertion of a Swan-Ganz pulmonary artery catheter and an arterial catheter is strongly encouraged. Cuff blood pressure measurements are notoriously inaccurate in patients with severe hypotension. Once blood pressure is restored (systolic blood pressure > 100 mmHg), nitroprusside can be added to dopamine, 15 to 300 micrograms per minute, to augment cardiac output and further reduce pulmonary capillary wedge pressure. The combination of dopamine and nitroprusside can usually maintain circulatory homeostasis once blood pressure is stable. Dopamine use is limited by tachycardia and arrhythmias.

Dobutamine (Dobutrex) (500 mg in 500 ml of 5 per cent dextrose in water [1000 micrograms per ml]) markedly improves cardiac output but has little or no peripheral vasoconstrictor activity. It usually does not restore blood pressure in patients with severe hypotension. However, dobutamine is appropriate therapy for severe heart failure if blood pressure is adequate (systolic blood pressure > 90 mmHg). The usual dose of dobutamine is 3 to 20 micrograms per kg per minute; as with dopamine, its use is limited by tachycardia and arrhythmias. Dobutamine is sometimes added to nitroprusside to augment cardiac output.

The therapy for acute pulmonary edema, perhaps more than any condition, must be tailored to the individual patient's needs. Table 1 offers useful therapies, but success is predicated on a firm understanding of the pathophysiology of acute heart failure and of the pharmacology of the various agents.

CHRONIC HEART FAILURE

As in acute heart failure, a thorough search for etiologic factors should be performed. Almost always, an electrocardiogram, chest x-ray film, and echocardiogram are required, in addition to a careful history and physical examination. Cardiac catheterization is frequently necessary. I generally also perform an exercise test to assess the degree of disability.

Nearly all patients should follow a regimen that includes a low-sodium diet (2 grams), a diuretic (furosemide, 20 to 40 mg per day), and a vasodilator (Table 2). There is now firm evidence that vasodilator therapy improves survival, even in patients with Class II and III heart failure. The role of digitalis is less clear, and I reserve it for patients with an obviously dilated heart, an S_3 gallop, and resting tachycardia. I prefer to begin therapy with furosemide and a vasodilator regimen, and I add digitalis later if the patient does not improve. Because furosemide tends to promote hypokalemia, supplemental potassium (20 to 40 mEq per day) is usually necessary.

One vasodilator regimen that has been shown to improve survival is hydralazine (Apresoline), 300 mg per day in divided doses, with isosorbide dinitrate (Sorbitrate or Isordil), 40 to 60 mg three times per day. Experience indicates that patients with large, dilated hearts respond best to vasodilator therapy. If peripheral edema or pulmonary congestion recurs, metolazone (Zaroxolyn), 2.5 to 10 mg, should be added to furosemide on a temporary basis, usually for 1 or 2 days. Patients should be instructed to weigh themselves daily and to use metolazone or an extra dose of furosemide on those days that they note a gain in weight (2 to 3 pounds) or feel edematous or congested.

Converting enzyme inhibitors may also be used as first line vasodilator therapy, and they have been shown to prolong survival. Captopril (Capoten) should be started at 6.25 mg every 8 hours and should be titrated to 25 to 50 mg three times per day. The blood urea nitrogen level may rise,

TABLE 1. **Treatment of Acute Pulmonary Edema**

Generic Name	Trade Name	Route of Administration	Average Dose	Limiting Factors	Comments
Furosemide	Lasix	IV	40–100 mg		Correct hypokalemia
Oxygen		Venturi's mask	50–60%	CO_2 narcosis	Monitor blood gas levels
Morphine sulfate		IV	2–5 mg q 10–15 min	Respiratory depression	May reverse respiratory depression with naloxone, 0.4 mg q 2–5 min
Nitroprusside	Nipride	IV	15–300 µg/min	Hypotension	May be combined with dopamine if BP is stable
Dopamine	Intropin	IV	3–20 µg/kg/min	Tachycardia, arrhythmias	Use only for hypotension or combine with nitroprusside if BP is stable
Dobutamine	Dobutrex	IV	3–20 µg/kg/min	Tachycardia, arrhythmias	Not useful for hypotension
Nitroglycerin	Nitrostat	SL	1/150 grain	Hypotension	May repeat q 5–10 min if BP is stable
Heparin		SC	5000 q 8 hr	Bleeding, thrombocytopenia	

Abbreviations: SL = sublingual; BP = blood pressure.

TABLE 2. **Treatment of Chronic Congestive Heart Failure**

Generic Name	Trade Name	Starting Dose	Maintenance Dose	Limiting Factors	Comments
Furosemide	Lasix	40 mg/day	40–100 mg/day	Hypokalemia	
Metolazone	Zaroxolyn	2.5 mg		Dehydration, hypokalemia	Should be used as intermittent supplement
Captopril	Capoten	6.25 mg tid	6.25–50 mg tid	Hypotension, cough, rash, hyperkalemia	Renal function and K$^+$ level should be monitored
Enalapril	Vasotec	2.5 mg bid	2.5–10 mg bid	Hypotension, cough, rash, hyperkalemia	Renal function and K$^+$ level should be monitored
Hydralazine	Apresoline	25–75 mg qid	300 mg/day	Lupus, hypotension, nausea, vomiting, edema	Dose is highly variable
Isosorbide dinitrate	Isordil, Sorbitrate	10–20 mg tid	10–60 mg tid	Headache, hypotension	Headaches usually respond to acetaminophen (Tylenol)
Digoxin	Lanoxin		0.125–0.375 mg/day	Toxicity	

which usually responds to a reduction in diuretic dose. Captopril should be avoided in patients who have recently undergone vigorous diuresis or who are severely hyponatremic (serum sodium level < 130 mEq per liter) because precipitous hypotension may ensue. Asymptomatic hypotension that is induced by converting enzyme inhibitors need not be treated, but symptomatic hypotension usually responds to leg raising or careful rehydration. Converting enzyme inhibitors should probably not be used in patients with systolic blood pressures less than 80 mmHg, although this decision must be individualized. Enalapril (Vasotec) can be used instead of captopril if desired; captopril and enalapril appear to be equally effective. The usual starting dose of enalapril is 2.5 or 5 mg twice daily, and the dose should be increased to 10 mg twice daily over several weeks as maintenance therapy. Potassium and diuretic therapy can frequently be reduced when using converting enzyme inhibitor therapy. Potassium-sparing agents should be avoided in patients taking angiotensin-converting enzyme inhibitors because of potentially dangerous hyperkalemia, except under unusual circumstances. The most frequent complications of the use of converting enzyme inhibitors are hypotension, nonproductive cough, rash, and renal insufficiency. Renal function and serum electrolyte levels should be monitored 1 week and sometimes sooner after initiating converting enzyme inhibitor therapy for heart failure. If the blood urea nitrogen or serum creatinine levels rise after starting this therapy, a reduced diuretic dose frequently improves these abnormalities without the need for reducing the dose of converting enzyme inhibitor. Clinical improvement sometimes requires 3 to 4 weeks of therapy. These agents have had a positive influence on the treatment of congestive heart failure, are generally well tolerated, and

are effective in all degrees of severity of heart failure.

Digitalis (digoxin) is still widely used to treat heart failure. The usual dose is 0.25 mg daily but will vary according to renal function. Loading doses are rarely necessary for chronic heart failure. Unlike the situation with vasodilator therapy, it is not known if digoxin improves survival in patients with heart failure. Except for patients with rapid atrial fibrillation, long-term clinical benefit from digoxin therapy has remained controversial. Monitoring serum digoxin levels is not routinely necessary unless toxicity or a subtherapeutic response is suspected. I use digoxin in patients with large, dilated hearts and an S$_3$ gallop.

Ventricular arrhythmias are common in patients with heart failure. To date there are no controlled data to indicate that treatment of these arrhythmias prolongs survival. Symptomatic ventricular arrhythmias should be treated, but this has proved to be a difficult task, may require the use of multiple antiarrhythmic drugs, and should be based on electrophysiologic studies. This problem is an important one that will require a large, randomized controlled trial to solve.

INFECTIVE ENDOCARDITIS

method of
CLAUDIA R. LIBERTIN, M.D.
Loyola University Medical Center
Maywood, Illinois

Infective endocarditis is a microbial infection of the cardiac valves and endocardium. In the preantibiotic era, infective endocarditis was considered a uniformly fatal disease. Surgical advances and aggressive antibiotic therapy have reduced its mortality, although the mortality rate is still 14 to 21 per cent.

Infective endocarditis has been classified in two ways. One method of classification is based on the divisions of acute, subacute, and chronic time relationships determined by the onset of symptoms. The acute form of endocarditis traditionally progressed in days or weeks, the subacute form evolved in weeks to months, and the chronic form existed for greater than 6 months. However, since the use of antibiotic therapy the chronic form is extremely rare. The other classification arranges divisions by the infecting microorganism. Each organism has specific implications for the rapidity of the infectious process and for the presence or absence of underlying heart disease. Infections caused by *Staphylococcus aureus, Streptococcus pneumoniae, Neisseria gonorrhoeae,* and group A streptococci most frequently have a fulminant course. Often there is severe destruction of the cardiac valves, which were normal prior to the infection. Infections caused by the viridans group of streptococci or *Staphylococcus epidermidis* run a more indolent course and occur on deformed heart valves or prostheses, and valvular damage evolves more slowly. Since classification by the infecting organism can be useful in therapy for suggesting the antibiotic regimen to be used, it is the scheme most commonly adopted.

Infective endocarditis tends to originate at areas of turbulence, such as on deformed valves or at sites of damaged endocardium. Endocarditis tends to occur in areas of high pressure. For example, endocarditis is more frequent on the left side of the heart. Approximately 70 per cent of patients with endocarditis have evidence of pre-existing structural cardiac abnormalities. High-risk patients are those with prosthetic cardiac valves, aortic stenosis or insufficiency, patent ductus arteriosus, mitral insufficiency, or ventricular septal defect. Patients undergoing hyperalimentation with a right-sided heart indwelling catheter are similarly at risk. Those at intermediate risk for infection are patients with mitral stenosis and prolapse, tricuspid valve disease, hypertrophic obstructive cardiomyopathy, tetralogy of Fallot, and calcific aortic sclerosis. In the remaining 30 per cent of patients, no underlying heart disease may be found or known.

The spectrum of infective endocarditis has changed significantly within the past 30 years. This is explained by the increasing number of patients with prosthetic heart valves, the problem of intravenous drug abuse, the occurrence of antibiotic-resistant, nosocomial infections, and the widespread use of antibiotics that replace normal host flora with unusual organisms. Prosthetic valve endocarditis occurs in approximately 1 to 5 per cent of patients who receive such prostheses. With the advent of this procedure, early-onset prosthetic valve endocarditis (occurring within 2 months of surgery) was frequent and often fatal. Mortality associated with it was reported to be as high as 50 per cent and often resulted from intraoperative contamination with nosocomial bacteria, especially *S. epidermidis.* Now, with the use of prophylactic antibiotic therapy and improvement in surgical techniques, early-onset prosthetic valve endocarditis has become less common. The incidence of late-onset prosthetic valve endocarditis (occurring at least 2 months after surgery) has remained constant. Late-onset prosthetic valve endocarditis is caused by the same microorganisms that cause native valve endocarditis.

DIAGNOSIS

The presence of endocarditis is often difficult to identify and should be based on careful physical examination and the general clinical presentation of the patient rather than on individual symptoms and signs. Any organ system can first manifest symptoms or signs of endocarditis. A nonspecific history such as a fever, anorexia, and weight loss may suggest endocarditis. Therefore, careful serial physical examinations are necessary to detect the development of a new organic murmur, embolization, or cardiac compromise. Rarely are peripheral cutaneous manifestations such as petechiae and splinter hemorrhages seen. Osler's nodes and Janeway's lesions are seen in only 20 to 40 per cent of cases. Splenomegaly is found in as few as 5 to 15 per cent of all endocarditis patients. Consequently, suspicion of the disease process must be high to make the diagnosis. The most helpful laboratory tests include those revealing anemia, increased erythrocyte sedimentation rate, and red blood cells on urinalysis.

The definitive diagnosis of infective endocarditis is made by isolating the infecting microorganism. Three separate blood cultures should be collected within a 24-hour interval from patients who have not received antimicrobial therapy within the prior 2 weeks. This number of blood cultures is adequate for isolation of the etiologic agent in at least 96 per cent of previously untreated patients with infective endocarditis. Collection of an additional two or three separate blood cultures may be necessary in previously treated patients or in those with endocarditis due to fastidious microorganisms. Blood cultures need to be repeated during therapy to document clearance of the microorganism as well as 1 and 2 months after the cessation of therapy because of the possibility of relapse.

Determinations of minimum inhibitory concentrations as well as minimum bactericidal concentrations need to be done on the infecting microorganism. The role of the serum bactericidal titer (SBT) to guide the choice and dosage of antibiotics for patients with infective endocarditis is uncertain. The principal problem has been the lack of a standard method for determining the SBT. It is suggested that a peak SBT equal to or greater than 1:64 correlates with cure. However, lower titers do not correlate with treatment failures. Consequently, concerns remain about the reliability of SBT monitoring in infective endocarditis patients, and this technique is seldom used.

Although echocardiography is a relatively nonspecific and insensitive method of diagnosing infective endocarditis, it is an important part of the patient assessment, particularly in surgical candidates. A combined M-mode and two-dimensional echocardiogram (with Doppler evaluation) is useful for detecting valvular incompetence, fistulas, annular ring abscesses, ruptured chordae tendinae, and prosthetic valve dehiscence. However, the absence of a vegetation does not exclude the diagnosis of infective endocarditis.

TREATMENT

General Principles

No single regimen exists for the management and treatment of all patients with infective endocarditis. However, the following general principles will be helpful.

Establish the Microbiologic Diagnosis. Before starting antimicrobial therapy, the microbiologic diagnosis should be established by obtaining three separate blood cultures drawn approximately 10 to 15 minutes apart. Since the majority of patients with infective endocarditis have a subacute course, antimicrobial therapy does not need to be expeditious. Once the microorganism has been cultured in the laboratory, antimicrobial therapy can be started before the in vitro susceptibility data are available. Failure to secure the diagnosis may prolong hospitalization, increase cost, result in iatrogenic complications related to inappropriate therapy, and lead to possible recurrence of the infection. On the other hand, if the patient presents acutely or if the microbiologic diagnosis has been established, therapy should be initiated promptly.

Empiric Antimicrobial Regimens Should Be Used in Acute Cases. This therapy should be initiated only after three separate sets of blood cultures have been obtained. The antimicrobial regimen should definitely include a combination of antibiotics effective against streptococci, staphylococci, and enterococci in native valve endocarditis. Penicillin, a semisynthetic penicillin (such as nafcillin), and gentamicin or vancomycin and gentamicin (in penicillin-allergic patients) are reasonable choices. In individuals with acute prosthetic valve endocarditis, the regimen should include antibiotics effective against coagulase-negative staphylococci, *S. aureus,* streptococci, and gram-negative nosocomial pathogens. A combination of vancomycin and gentamicin is adequate empiric therapy in early-onset prosthetic valve endocarditis. These regimens should be adjusted when the microorganism is identified and when in vitro susceptibilities are known.

Obtain Early Consultation from Cardiovascular Surgery. Patients with infective endocarditis may require emergency cardiac valve replacement. In particular, patients with aortic valve infective endocarditis or prosthetic valve endocarditis may have acute insufficiency or valve dehiscence in association with cardiac decompensation. Immediate surgical intervention may be necessary.

Daily Physical Examination Should Be Performed. Subtle changes in findings, such as blood pressure and cardiac auscultation, may precede cardiac decompensation. The hemodynamic status is important in determining the need for and the timing of cardiac valve replacement.

Portal of Entry Should Be Identified. The microorganism causing endocarditis may suggest the portal of entry. For example, viridans streptococci commonly arise from the oral cavity; dental roentgenograms are appropriate for identification of an abscess. *Streptococcus bovis* is associated with colonic lesions; consequently, proctoscopy and a colon roentgenogram are warranted. These procedures should be conducted while the patient is receiving antibiotics for endocarditis.

Repeat Blood Cultures During and After Therapy. Blood cultures should be repeated 48 to 72 hours after the initiation of therapy to establish clearance of the microorganism. Persistent bacteremia is suggestive of a myocardial or peripheral abscess, inappropriate antimicrobial therapy, or an error in the choice of the parenteral antibiotic. Since most relapses occur within the first 2 months after the completion of therapy, repeat blood cultures at that time are also warranted.

Instruct Patient in Prophylaxis for Infective Endocarditis Prior to Dismissal. Transient bacteremia occurs after a variety of different invasive procedures. Even though the effectiveness of antibiotic prophylaxis has not been fully documented, proposed recommendations by the American Heart Association have been made.

Therapy of Specific Types of Endocarditis

Approximately 75 per cent of cases of native valve infective endocarditis are caused by gram-positive microorganisms. Recently, relatively uncommon causes of endocarditis have been identified because of improved microbiologic techniques. The incidence of culture-negative endocarditis is generally less than 1 to 4 per cent. Common causes of culture negativity are the previous use of antibiotics, fastidious organisms, right-sided endocarditis, and noninfective endocarditis. In general, parenteral administration of antibiotics by either intravenous or intramuscular routes will give good bactericidal drug levels in the blood. Drug doses may need to be adjusted for renal function; the following recommendations assume normal renal function.

Streptococcal Endocarditis. Penicillin G or ampicillin, often combined with an aminoglycoside, such as streptomycin or gentamicin, remains the cornerstone of therapy for endocarditis caused by streptococci (Table 1). *Streptococcus viridans* and *S. bovis* are very sensitive to penicillin with minimum inhibitory concentrations of less than 0.1 microgram per ml. Most viridans streptococci are susceptible at this level. Dosage recommendations vary, but penicillin G, 12 million units per day intravenously as a continuous drip or given in divided doses every 4 hours, is adequate.

TABLE 1. **Treatment Regimens for Native Valve Infective Endocarditis Caused by Gram-Positive Cocci**

Organism	Regimen
Viridans streptococci, *Streptococcus bovis* (MIC < 0.1 µg/ml)	1. Penicillin G, 10–20 million U total/day, given as continuous drip or divided into 4-hr doses IV for 4 wk 2. Penicillin G, as above; plus streptomycin, 15 mg/kg/day IM, divided into 2 equal doses, every 12 hr for 2 wk 3. For penicillin-allergic patients: cefazolin (Ancef, Kefzol), 1–2 grams every 8 hr for 4 wk; or vancomycin (Vancocin), 30 mg/kg/day IV, divided into 2–4 equal doses for 4 wk
Enterococcus faecalis and other penicillin-resistant streptococci (MIC > 0.5 µg/ml)	1. Ampicillin, 1–2 grams IV every 4 hr for 4–6 wk; plus gentamicin (Garamycin), 3 mg/kg/day, divided into 3 equal doses every 8 hr for 4–6 wk; or streptomycin, 15 mg/kg/day divided into 2 equal doses every 12 hr for 4–6 wk 2. For penicillin-allergic patients: vancomycin, 30 mg/kg/day total IV, divided into 2 equal doses, every 12 hr for 4–6 wk; plus gentamicin or streptomycin, as above
Staphylococcus aureus	1. Nafcillin (Nafcil) or oxacillin (Prostaphlin), 2 grams IV, every 4 hr for 4–6 wk after defervescence; plus gentamicin, 3–5 mg/kg/day IV, in 3 equal doses, every 8 hr for first 3 days 2. Cefazolin, 2 grams IV, every 8 hr for 4–6 wk after defervescence; plus gentamicin, as above 3. Vancomyin, 30 mg/kg/day IV in 2–4 equal doses, every 8 hr for 4 wk after defervescence; plus gentamicin, as above

Abbreviation: MIC = minimum inhibitory concentration.

Four weeks of therapy with appropriate doses of penicillin should be effective. Because the combination of an aminoglycoside with penicillin results in synergistic killing of streptococci, streptomycin (7.5 mg per kg every 12 hours) or low-dose gentamicin (1 mg per kg every 8 hours) for 2 weeks with intravenous penicillin has been successful in the treatment of streptococcal endocarditis. This regimen is as curative as penicillin alone, with relapse rates of approximately 1 per cent. Contraindications for aminoglycoside use include renal insufficiency and auditory or vestibular disorders. Patients not able to be identified or evaluated for eighth nerve toxicity also should be excluded from the short-course regimen. Some viridans streptococci have minimum inhibitory concentrations to penicillin between 0.1 and 0.5 microgram per ml. For these organisms no definitive guidelines exist. However, higher levels of penicillin G (20 million units per 24 hours) or vancomycin are advisable, combined with an aminoglycoside for the first 2 weeks of a 4-week antibiotic regimen. For patients with prosthetic valve endocarditis due to these same organisms, 6-week therapy with penicillin or vancomycin is recommended, combined with an aminoglycoside for the first 2 weeks if feasible. Penicillin-allergic patients may be treated with vancomycin or a cephalosporin, provided a history of allergy does not include anaphylaxis.

Enterococcal Endocarditis. Enterococci are relatively resistant to penicillin G in minimum inhibitory concentrations of 1 to 4 micrograms per ml. The source of infection is often the genito-urinary tract. Because of the relative resistance, penicillin G or ampicillin must be combined with an aminoglycoside for the duration of therapy. Until recently, low-dose gentamicin (1 mg per kg every 8 hours) would have been synergistic in all cases of endocarditis. During this decade, however, high-level gentamicin- and streptomycin-resistant strains have been found with minimum inhibitory concentrations of 500 micrograms per ml and 2000 micrograms per ml or greater, respectively. The presence of this high-level aminoglycoside resistance implies the absence of synergy when combined with penicillin. Resistance to streptomycin does not confer resistance to gentamicin, and vice versa. However, high-level resistance to gentamicin does negate the synergistic benefits of tobramycin, netilmicin, amikacin, kanamycin, and sisomicin. Therefore, high-level susceptibility testing of gentamicin and streptomycin is warranted to select the aminoglycoside for therapy. A 4- to 6-week course of combination therapy is ideal. Patients allergic to penicillin should be treated with the combination of vancomycin and gentamicin for the same amount of time.

Staphylococcal Endocarditis. Because patients infected with *S. aureus* are often acutely ill, urgent initiation of antibiotics is appropriate. The antibiotics of choice are the semisynthetic penicillins, nafcillin and oxacillin, in a dose of 2 grams every 4 hours. If the minimum inhibitory concentration of penicillin G is less than 0.1 microgram per ml, then penicillin G will be equally effective. On the other hand, if the bacterial strain is found to be

TABLE 2. **Treatment Regimens for Prosthetic Valve Endocarditis Caused by Staphylococci**

Organism	Regimen
Methicillin-resistant staphylococci	Vancomycin,* 30 mg/kg/day IV, in 2 equal doses for a minimum of 6 wk; plus rifampin,† 300 mg PO every 8 hr for a minimum of 6 wk; plus gentamicin,* 1 mg/kg IM or IV every 8 hr for the initial 2 wk
Methicillin-sensitive staphylococci	Nafcillin or oxacillin, 2 grams IV every 4 hr for a minimum of 6 wk; plus rifampin,† 300 mg PO every 8 hr for a minimum of 6 wk; plus gentamicin,* 1 mg/kg IM or IV every 8 hr for the initial 2 wk

*Vancomycin and gentamicin doses must be modified appropriately in patients with renal failure. Serum concentrations of vancomycin and gentamicin should be monitored and doses adjusted.

†Rifampin is recommended for therapy of infections with coagulase-negative staphylococci. Its use in coagulase-positive staphylococcal infections is controversial. Rifampin may increase the amount of warfarin sodium required for antithrombotic therapy.

resistant to methicillin (and consequently to all other semisynthetic penicillins and cephalosporins), vancomycin therapy is indicated. A 4- to 6-week course of antibiotics is recommended and may have to be longer if an initial delay in clinical response occurs or complications arise. Because low-dose gentamicin (1 mg per kg per dose every 8 hours) in combination with a semisynthetic penicillin may lead to more rapid killing of staphylococci, gentamicin for the first 3 days may be beneficial; evidence of increased efficacy beyond this time is lacking. The benefits of such use of aminoglycosides must be weighed against their potential toxicities. Cases of native valve, prosthetic valve, and addict-associated endocarditis should be considered individually because of differences in their prognosis and approach.

Gram-Negative Endocarditis. Endocarditis caused by gram-negative bacteria is relatively rare. Appropriate therapy depends on the in vitro susceptibility of each organism. *Pseudomonas aeruginosa,* most commonly seen in intravenous drug addicts, requires combination therapy with an antipseudomonal penicillin or cephalosporin combined with tobramycin for a duration of 6 weeks.

Fastidious Organisms. The HACEK group of organisms, which includes *Haemophilus* species, *Actinobacillus actinomycetemcomitans, Cardiobacterium hominis, Eikenella corrodens,* and *Kingella kingae,* rarely cause endocarditis. In general, these organisms are sensitive to ampicillin, which may be combined with an aminoglycoside for 4 to 6 weeks of therapy. Nutritionally deficient streptococci are fastidious organisms that require pyridoxal supplementation for growth. Blood culture Gram's stains show gram-positive cocci, but the organisms fail to grow on agar plates without addition of a staphylococcal streak or pyridoxal supplementation. Penicillin or vancomycin combined with an aminoglycoside is recommended for 4 to 6 weeks of therapy. If the strain is penicillin resistant, vancomycin should be used.

Prosthetic Valve Endocarditis. Coagulase-negative staphylococci and *S. aureus* together account for approximately half of the total cases of prosthetic valve endocarditis. The microbiology of early-onset prosthetic valve endocarditis (less than 2 months postoperatively) differs from that of late-onset prosthetic valve endocarditis. In the former type, resistant organisms such as gram-negative rods, fungi, and staphylococci are more common. As in any case of endocarditis, antibiotic therapy is guided by the susceptibility of the infecting organism. For the treatment of methicillin-resistant staphylococci in the presence of a prosthetic valve (Table 2), vancomycin and rifampin (300 mg orally every 8 hours) are given for a minimum of 6 weeks, with gentamicin use

TABLE 3. **Prophylactic Therapy for Infective Endocarditis**

Indication	Low-Risk Patients	High-Risk Patients	Low-Risk Penicillin-Allergic Patients
Procedures involving the oral cavity, respiratory tract, and endoscopies	2 grams oral penicillin V 60 min before procedure followed by 1 gram penicillin V 6 hr later	1–2 grams ampicillin plus 1.5 mg/kg gentamicin IV or IM 30 min before procedure, followed by 1 gram oral penicillin V 6 hr later	1 gram oral erythromycin 60 min before procedure, followed by 500-mg dose 6 hr later
Procedures involving genitourinary or gastrointestinal tract	3 grams oral amoxicillin 60 min before procedure followed by 1.5-gram dose 6 hr later	1–2 grams ampicillin plus 1.5 mg/kg gentamicin IV or IM 30 min before procedure; repeat regimen 8 hr later	Substitute 1 gram vancomycin IV for ampicillin; no following dose needed

limited to the initial 2 weeks of therapy. Prosthetic valve endocarditis caused by methicillin-susceptible, coagulase-negative staphylococci should be treated with a semisynthetic penicillinase-resistant penicillin (nafcillin) in combination with rifampin (300 mg orally every 8 hours) and gentamicin.

Management of Complications

Congestive heart failure is the most common serious complication of infective endocarditis and is a leading cause of death. In patients with hemodynamic compromise, prompt valve replacement should be considered, regardless of the duration of preoperative antibiotic therapy. Similarly, most patients with multiple major emboli should undergo valve replacement or débridement. However, in the absence of severe congestive heart failure or major embolic events, a complete course of antibiotics should be attempted before cardiac valve replacement is considered.

Other complications of infective endocarditis include arrhythmias, renal failure, mycotic aneurysms, neurologic complications, and splenic abscesses. Medical management for each of these situations should be tailored to the individual situation. For example, a patient with atrioventricular block may require transvenous pacemaker insertion for the extravalvular extension of the infection. The development of S. aureus pericarditis may need prompt surgical drainage or pericardiectomy. A patient with a splenic abscess will need splenectomy. The recurrence or persistence of fever, which may complicate management, may be related to intravenous administration-related phlebitis, metastatic abscess formation, drug fever, uncontrolled valvular infection, or nosocomial infections at other sites.

Prophylactic Therapy

Conclusive proof of the efficacy of chemoprophylaxis for endocarditis is lacking and the choice of an optimal prophylactic regimen is controversial. Nevertheless, the recently revised recommendations by the *Medical Letter,* British Society, and American Heart Association are basically similar. Standard prophylaxis is 2 grams of oral penicillin V 60 minutes before the procedure, with 1 gram 6 hours later (Table 3). Patients with prosthetic valves are given a combination of ampicillin and gentamicin parenterally 30 minutes before the procedure. A second dose of 1 gram of penicillin V should be given orally 6 hours after the procedure. Penicillin-allergic patients are given 1 gram of oral erythromycin 1 hour before the procedure followed by 500 mg 6 hours later. For gastrointestinal or genitourinary procedures, parenteral ampicillin and gentamicin are given 30 minutes before the procedure and a repeat dose is given 8 hours later in high-risk patients. Vancomycin and gentamicin are used in penicillin-allergic patients. In low-risk patients, an oral regimen of amoxicillin (3 grams) is given orally 60 minutes before the procedure, followed by 1.5 grams 6 hours later. Continued antibiotic therapy beyond the second dose is unnecessary because the bacteremia is transient.

HYPERTENSION

method of
CHARLES P. TIFFT, M.D.
Boston University School of Medicine
Boston, Massachusetts

Hypertension is one of the most common reasons that individuals seek outpatient care. Hypertension management requires follow-up at regular intervals and thus may be considered a facilitator of routine health care by encouraging regular interaction with a health care provider. Hypertension may be defined as a sitting systolic blood pressure higher than 139 mmHg, a diastolic blood pressure higher than 89 mmHg, or both. This classification system is based on the average of two or more readings on two or more occasions.

At present, there are approximately 65 million individuals with abnormally elevated blood pressure in the United States. Of these, a little over two-thirds have diastolic blood pressure between 90 and 104 mmHg and may be considered to have mild hypertension. This mildly elevated blood pressure is not a minor problem because 60 per cent of the morbid complications in hospital patients attributable to hypertension occur in patients with mild hypertension. Unfortunately, treatment of these hypertensives does not eliminate the risk of cardiovascular complications. On the other hand, treatment may reduce the rate of some of them. One of the major problems facing physicians today is whether or not to treat mild hypertension with pharmacotherapy.

EVALUATION OF THE HYPERTENSIVE

A medical history should be taken, comprising a family history of cardiovascular disease, including hypertension; a personal history of cardiovascular or renal disease, as well as known cardiovascular risk factors; a history of alcohol, sodium, and fat intake; and any significant weight gain. A history of antihypertensive therapies may be extremely helpful in planning a program based on success or failure and side effects in the past. A common error is not to ask for this information vigorously enough.

The physical examination should include measurement of the blood pressure in both arms while the patient is sitting, and preferably in the standing position in addition. Repeated measurements to estimate the blood pressure are suggested. The use of proper technique cannot be overemphasized. Height and weight can be used to determine whether obesity may be a contributing factor. An examination for carotid, abdominal, and flank bruits should be performed, as well as a general vascular examination, including pulses and aortic enlargement. A check for dependent edema should be made. Funduscopic examination should search for arteriolar narrowing, arteriovenous compression, and hemorrhages and exudates, as well as disk edema. A careful cardiac examination is always indicated. The abdomen should also be checked for renal enlargement. A simple baseline neurologic examination should be performed.

The evaluation appropriate for each individual depends on factors such as age, severity of the hypertension, and cost of the evaluation. A simple battery of tests such as a complete blood count; urinalysis; serum creatinine, calcium, and potassium levels; and plasma glucose, uric acid, and total cholesterol levels, as well as the high-density-lipoprotein cholesterol level, should be performed. If the individual is male, recent recommendations include testing the fasting total triglyceride level to estimate the low-density-lipoprotein cholesterol level. Females require the presence of an additional cardiovascular risk factor before estimation of the low-density-lipoprotein cholesterol level is suggested on the initial evaluation. A baseline electrocardiogram should be done, but a cardiac echocardiogram demonstrating diastolic function and wall thickness should be individualized because of its additional cost. A chest x-ray film is not generally suggested but may be required for reasons other than the hypertension.

Screening for secondary hypertensions (Table 1) is usually not appropriate during the initial evaluation, with the exception of the tests previously mentioned. The following is a brief introduction to the evaluation for secondary hypertension. A history of sweating, palpitations, and headache suggests the need for pheochromocytoma testing, and 24-hour urinary creatinine and metanephrine excretion tests or a clonidine suppression test may be considered before adrenal computed tomography scanning or magnetic resonance imaging. Abrupt onset of hypertension with an abdominal or flank bruit that extends into diastole suggests renovascular hypertension. In this case, waiting for the results of the initial laboratory evaluation makes sense. Invasive evaluation with arteriography is best performed with the blood pressure controlled and should be reserved for those hypertensives who would have either surgery or transluminal angiodilatation if a suitable lesion were found. Renal ^{99m}Tc diethylenetetraminepentaacetic acid scanning before and after administration of captopril may be useful in those in whom proceeding to arteriography seems risky. Striae, truncal obesity, and glucose intolerance may indicate glucocorticoid excess, in which case a dexamethasone suppression test may be appropriate.

Unprovoked or easily provoked hypokalemia may be caused by primary or secondary aldosteronism, vom-

TABLE 1. Causes of Hypertension

Idiopathic or essential hypertension

Renal hypertension
  Parenchymal
    Pyelonephritis
    Glomerulonephritis
    Interstitial nephritis
    Diabetic nephropathy
    Connective tissue disease
    Renal tumors (juxtaglomerular cell tumor, hypernephroma, Wilms's tumor)
    Renal cysts and polycystic kidneys
    Developmental abnormalities (Ask-Upmark kidney)
    Other (amyloidosis, gouty nephritis, hematomas)
  Obstructive—hydronephrosis
  Renovascular
    Renal artery atherosclerosis
    Fibrous stenosis of renal arteries
    Thrombotic or embolic occlusion
    Other diseases (tumors, inflammation, pseudoxanthoma elasticum)
  Renoprival
    Renal failure
    Anephric state

Adrenal hypertension
  Mineralocorticoid
    Primary aldosteronism
    Idiopathic aldosteronism
    DOC hypertension
    18-Hydroxy-DOC hypertension
    Hydroxylation deficiency syndromes
  Pheochromocytoma
  Cushing's disease
  Adrenogenital syndrome

Other endocrinopathies
  Myxedema
  Hyperparathyroidism
  Acromegaly

Coarctation of the aorta

Toxemia of pregnancy

Neurogenic hypertension
  Increased intracranial pressure (brain tumors, hematomas)
  Neuroblastomas
  Neuropathies (polyneuritis, porphyria, lead poisoning, tabes)
  Spinal cord transection
  Encephalitis
  Bulbar poliomyelitis
  Diencephalic syndrome
  Acute porphyria
  Lead poisoning

Drug-induced hypertension
  Oral contraceptives, estrogens
  Monoamine oxidase inhibitors with tyramine
  Sympathomimetics (e.g., amphetamines, cold remedies)

Other hypertension
  Hypercalcemia
  Carcinoid syndrome
  Licorice excess

Abbreviation: DOC = deoxycorticosterone.

iting, or diarrhea. After a careful history is taken, the physician may determine the upright or stimulated plasma renin activity, which is low in most cases of primary aldosteronism. On the basis of results, further testing may be warranted. Hypothyroidism may be associated with diastolic hypertension. Hyperthyroidism may cause systolic hypertension as may severe anemia, complete atrioventricular block, large arteriovenous fistula, and aortic valvular insufficiency.

Many drugs may be associated with or may worsen hypertension. Examples include oral contraceptives used therapeutically and occasionally estrogen used for replacement therapy; sympathomimetics found in weight loss preparations and in oral and nasal spray cold remedies; alcohol; nonsteroidal anti-inflammatory agents and steroids; and the immunosuppressive cyclosporin A. Reducing the dosage or stopping the use of the offending drug usually reverses the hypertension in this form of secondary hypertension.

REVIEW OF THE INTERVENTION TRIALS

To convince a patient that he or she requires drug therapy, the practitioner needs to understand the salient findings of the major intervention trials that are performed in hypertensives. The following paragraphs review these briefly.

The Hypertension Detection and Follow-Up Program enrolled 10,940 hypertensives in a trial in which the usual community care was compared with specialized care at centers that included free medication, home visits when necessary because of missed clinic appointments, and enhanced triage for other health-related problems. Thus, immersion in health care was tested, rather than the effect of antihypertensive therapy alone. This trial involved 7825 mild hypertensives (diastolic pressure 90 to 104 mmHg) aged 30 to 69 years, including a significant number of black hypertensives; participants included males and females. Blood pressures were determined as recommended in clinical practice, which helped to make this trial's participants similar to those who are seen throughout the United States today.

The results of this trial show that persons of both sexes, both races, and all ages and levels of hypertension studied benefited from therapy. This information should not be interpreted on the basis of the statistical results alone because these results reflect only some of the effects of drug therapy, as well as immersion in the health care system that this study provided.

A reduction of 32 per cent in fatal and nonfatal strokes was observed in mild hypertensives who were treated with special care (1.5 versus 2.2 strokes per 100 individuals treated per 5 years). Overall, there was a 26 per cent reduction in all cardiovascular causes of death with the special treatment and a 20 per cent reduction in deaths related to coronary heart disease. Thus, this trial is the first one to suggest that treatment of hypertension may reduce coronary deaths.

This trial included enough hypertensives to allow estimation of the relative benefits of this form of therapy in the various subsets of mild hypertensives. For black women, black men, and white men, 5-year death rates were lower with special treatment. This

means a reduction in 5-year death rates per 100 individuals treated of 2.0, 2.4, and 1.0 deaths, respectively. The white women showed results that may be predicted based on the known epidemiologic risk. Approximately 1000 white women aged 30 to 49 years would need to be treated for 5 years to prevent two deaths. Even more problematic is that these data are based on the results of treatment of all types of hypertensives, not just mild hypertensives.

One important point that should be made is that this study shows convincingly that a marked reduction in risk may be obtained by treating the black hypertensive in this fashion. In addition, this result was found to be independent of socioeconomic status, which is a significant new finding in this population of high-risk hypertensives.

The Australian National Blood Pressure Study included approximately 3427 hypertensives with a diastolic blood pressure of 95 mmHg or more and no higher than 109 mmHg after a series of screening visits. Placebo therapy was given and allowed easier interpretation of the data than in the Hypertension Detection and Follow-Up Program. This trial showed no convincing benefit of treating blood pressure between 95 and 100 mmHg. In fact, when the blood pressure was reduced with medication to the same level achieved with placebo therapy (48 per cent of the placebo group had blood pressure of 95 mmHg or less after 3 years of follow-up), the trial's end-point rate was higher than with placebo therapy. On the other hand, this trial does support the use of therapy for diastolic blood pressure between 100 and 104 mmHg. After 3 years of follow-up, a significant reduction in total trial end points was demonstrated in the total group: death, stroke, angina, congestive heart failure, and so on. In addition, smokers benefited particularly from therapy. This trial provided no information about the treatment of diastolic blood pressure between 90 and 95 mmHg.

The Medical Research Council Trial was a clinical trial of mostly mild hypertensives who had a baseline systolic blood pressure of less than 200 mmHg and a diastolic blood pressure of 90 to 109 mmHg. The trial included more than 17,000 subjects aged 35 to 64 years from general practices, who were treated with placebo or active therapy for an average of 5.5 years. This trial was the first to compare thiazide diuretic–based therapy and beta-blocker–based therapy in a controlled fashion.

Strokes were reduced with active treatment (1.4 versus 2.6 per 1000 patient-years). Treatment did not reduce coronary events (5.2 versus 5.5 per 1000 patient-years). All-cause mortality was reduced in men (7.1 versus 8.2 per 1000 patient-years) but was actually higher in women who received active treatment (4.4 with treatment versus 3.5 per 1000 patient-years with placebo). The thiazide diuretic appeared to reduce the stroke rate more effectively than the beta blocker, whereas myocardial infarctions tended to be reduced more with beta-blocker treatment. Smoking appeared to interfere with the protective effect of propranolol in reducing strokes. One stroke was prevented for every 850 treated hypertensives.

The Metoprolol Atherosclerosis Prevention in Hypertension Study was not a placebo-controlled trial but was a carefully performed study that compared thiazide- to metoprolol-based therapy in middle-aged men who had a mean serum cholesterol level of 244 mg per dl and of whom one-third were smokers. The results showed an impressive difference in overall mortality (−22 per cent) and cardiovascular mortality (−27 per cent) in favor of metoprolol. Smokers also received benefit from the beta blocker, which has not been found in studies with other beta blockers. This study, along with others, suggests that thiazides may not be the best initial therapy for certain hypertensives.

Reduction of the risk of stroke appears to be continuous as the blood pressure is lowerered. By contrast, a few studies suggest that coronary mortality may be reduced only with a reduction in diastolic blood pressure to 85 mmHg, and further reduction may be associated with a higher mortality. I am generally happy to achieve a blood pressure reduction to below 90 mmHg except when there is a strong history of stroke. Clearly, more information on the optimal blood pressure level is needed.

Because of the results just outlined, many physicians prefer to individualize their approach based on the family history of cardiovascular disease, the lipid profile, and the smoking status and likelihood of smoking cessation, as well as the patient's age, sex, and race. For example, in a mildly hypertensive white woman who is 35 years old, smoking cessation is preferable to antihypertensive therapy. One concern is that an individual who is not given pharmacologic therapy may feel that the medical problem is not significant. Thus patient education is extremely important, especially in our mobile society, where the patient may see a number of health care providers in a short time.

INITIAL THERAPY WITH NONDRUG MEASURES

I believe that all hypertensive individuals initially require nondrug therapy. From the outset, the hypertensive should be told that these approaches may be helpful, but not necessarily in everyone.

Sodium restriction may be successful when the intake is already high. Approximately one in three hypertensives may respond to a 2-gram (88 mEq) sodium restriction, which means that two in three do not respond. Many individuals curtail their sodium intake before they appear for care, but it still may be helpful for them to see a dietitian because much of the sodium in foods today is hidden. The consultation could also include advice regarding a heart-healthy diet. If after a few weeks to a month there is no appreciable effect on the blood pressure, the physician could consider liberalizing the sodium restriction. If diuretic therapy is used later on, a high-sodium intake could exacerbate and a low-sodium intake could lessen the tendency toward hypokalemia. In addition, sodium restriction may potentiate the effect of almost all of the antihypertensive

agents in use today and allow the total dosage of antihypertensive medication to be reduced.

Weight loss in patients who are overweight may also reduce blood pressure. Patients expect the practitioner to suggest weight loss, but unfortunately, the success of this modality is limited by the inability to maintain a reduced body weight. Significant weight loss may also improve an adverse lipid profile and impaired glucose tolerance and thus can be recommended for reasons other than blood pressure control. The weight gain that may occur after smoking cessation tends to be moderate and should not be used as an excuse for the hypertensive to continue smoking because the interaction of hypertension and cigarette smoking leads to at least a doubling of the cardiovascular risk.

Excessive alcohol intake may interfere with compliance with therapy and may elevate the blood pressure in some hypertensives. As in detecting sodium-sensitive hypertensives, there is no way to identify alcohol-sensitive individuals other than by evaluating the cessation or reduction in intake. Screening tests for alcohol excess, such as those for gamma-glutamyl transpeptidase level or red blood cell mean corpuscular volume, may be useful. One risk of challenging the patient is that the hypertensive will drop out of care. Thus the practitioner needs to individualize the approach used and to consider the simultaneous use of other supportive measures available in the community. Hypertensives who enjoy alcohol should be asked to limit their intake to two regular beers, 8 ounces of wine, or 2 ounces of distilled spirits daily.

Behavioral approaches have been shown to have moderate short-term success in controlling mild hypertension. These approaches include biofeedback, various forms of meditation and yoga, and relaxation. The combination of various approaches may have an additive effect but requires an additional time commitment. I have not found that these approaches are useful in the long term and thus recommend that individuals using them agree to more frequent follow-up. Acupuncture has been inadequately studied to date and cannot be recommended.

Dynamic exercise training may reduce blood pressure in a number of ways, one of which is a reduction in weight. The lowering of blood pressure does not necessarily depend on weight loss, but because many hypertensives are overweight, this form of nondrug therapy may be especially useful. In addition, regular exercise may improve the lipid profile and help reduce smoking. Vigorous walking or mild aerobics performed for 20 to 40 minutes three to four times weekly may be adequate for most patients. Based on preliminary reports, it is possible that less exercise may be adequate and that more exercise may not be as effective. Compliance remains a major problem, and again, long-term follow-up has not been reported. On the other hand, properly advised and graduated, regular exercise fits the heart-healthy lifestyle generally recommended for the hypertensive.

Mineral supplementation has been a popular subject in the recent lay press and has resulted in many questions from patients with hypertension. Epidemiologic evidence suggests that higher potassium intake may be associated with reduced hypertension, as well as with fewer strokes in the general population. Potassium chloride supplementation in hypokalemic, thiazide-treated hypertensives has reduced blood pressure slightly. At present, however, there is not sufficient evidence to warrant potassium supplementation as a nondrug therapy for the hypertensive individual. The practitioner should remember that hyperkalemia may be dangerous, silent, and more common in those with renal insufficiency or those taking concomitant converting enzyme inhibitors.

Low-calcium intake has been linked to hypertension, but the data indicating a beneficial effect of calcium on blood pressure do not support the use of supplements for the average hypertensive. Even less information is available to support the use of magnesium supplementation in the otherwise healthy hypertensive.

Reducing the total fat content in the diet and the total cholesterol intake to less than 250 to 300 mg daily may be appropriate for the majority of hypertensives who have a total serum cholesterol level higher than 200 mg per dl, but a reduced fat intake and an increased intake of polyunsaturated fat have not been definitively shown to reduce blood pressure. The role of omega-3 fatty acid supplementation in the treatment of hypertension is currently under investigation. At present, there is no evidence to support its use other than in the form of whole fish as part of a prudent diet.

Garlic and onion extracts probably cause no significant harm but have not been shown to have an appreciable effect on blood pressure.

INITIAL DRUG THERAPY OF HYPERTENSION

Initial therapy of hypertension has evolved over the past 30 years from a limited number of options to at least six classes of drugs from which to choose. The available antihypertensive agents and their major side effects are outlined in Tables 2 and 3, respectively.

Originally, thiazides were the best choice for therapy; later, beta blockers were added to the initial step. More recently, converting enzyme inhibitors and calcium channel entry blockers have been added. Although they are not listed in the 1988 report of the Joint National Committee on Detection, Evaluation, and Treatment of Hypertension, I also consider the centrally acting agents and the selective alpha blockers as initial therapy in mild hypertension. I believe that tailoring the antihypertensive plan to the patient's lifestyle and other medical conditions requires that all of these classes of drugs be considered as options. This is discussed in more detail later.

Thiazide diuretics have the advantages of widespread, long-term experience in the intervention trials and relatively low to moderate cost even with potassium supplementation. Their side effects are well known and include the metabolic changes of increased uric acid, glucose, calcium, cholesterol, and triglyceride levels, as well as decreased potassium and magnesium levels. Weakness, muscle cramps, and palpitations may occur, and sexual dysfunction is apparently much more common than was previously thought. Thiazide diuretics potentiate the effects of other antihypertensive agents and are available in rational combination formulations to enhance compliance. They are probably the most effective antihypertensive agents studied so far for reducing the risk of stroke. For this reason, I use thiazide diuretics in hypertensives with a previous stroke or a strong family history of stroke. Lower doses, such as 12.5 to 25 mg hydrochlorothiazide daily, are probably as effective as the previously used higher doses and have fewer metabolic side effects.

The treatment of asymptomatic hypokalemia in the thiazide-treated hypertensive remains a hotly debated issue. I tend to treat mild hypokalemia even in the asymptomatic patient when the plasma potassium level remains below 3.5 mEq per liter and aim for levels of serum potassium closer to 4 mEq per liter when the individual has known or suspected coronary disease, has had premature ventricular contractions on a previous electrocardiogram, or is an exerciser. I have not found that recommending a higher-potassium diet is effective in many cases. If potassium supplementation is used in a diuretic-treated hypertensive, the replacement salt should be in the form of potassium chloride, not potassium citrate or bicarbonate.

Loop diuretics may be required when the hypertensive is allergic to thiazide diuretics or when the serum creatinine level is above 2.5 mg per dl. The loop diuretics may elevate the blood sugar level less than the thiazide diuretics and thus may be preferable when trying to avoid oral

TABLE 2. **Antihypertensive Drugs***

Type of Drug	Usual Minimum Dose† (mg)	Usual Maximum Dose† (mg)
Diuretics		
Thiazide and related sulfonamide diuretics		
Bendroflumethiazide	2.5	5
Benzthiazide	12.5–25	50
Chlorothiazide	125–250	500
Chlorthalidone	12.5–25	50
Cyclothiazide	1	2
Hydrochlorothiazide	12.5–25	50
Hydroflumethiazide	12.5–25	50
Indapamide	2.5	5
Methyclothiazide	2.5	5
Metolazone	1.25	10
Polythiazide	2	4
Quinethazone	25	100
Trichlormethiazide	1–2	4
Loop diuretics		
Bumetanide‡	0.5	4
Ethacrynic acid‡	25	100
Furosemide‡	20–40	320
Potassium-sparing agents		
Amiloride	5	10
Spironolactone	25	100
Triamterene	50	150
Adrenergic Inhibitors		
Beta-adrenergic blockers§		
Acebutolol	200	1200
Atenolol	25	150
Metoprolol	50	200
Nadolol	40	320
Penbutolol sulfate	20	80
Pindolol‡	10	60
Propranolol hydrochloride‡	40	320
Propranolol, long-acting	60	320
Timolol‡	20	80
Centrally acting alpha agonists		
Clonidine‡	0.1	1.2
Clonidine TTS (patch)‖	0.1	0.3
Guanabenz‡	4	64
Guanfacine hydrochloride	1	3
Methyldopa‡	250	2000

hypoglycemic or insulin therapy. These agents usually require twice daily dosing, may cause disturbing polyuria, and are no more effective than thiazides when used in the usual dosages that do not cause volume contraction. I reserve their use for hypertensives who require diuretic therapy and are not candidates for thiazide diuretics.

Potassium-sparing diuretics generally add little to blood pressure control, but they may help in maintaining potassium levels in those who become hypokalemic, and they do not exacerbate glucose intolerance or precipitate gout. Higher doses of amiloride or spironolactone may have significant antihypertensive effects in certain low-renin hypertensives or those who may have primary aldosteronism. Older age, renal insuffi-

ciency, diabetes, and concomitant converting enzyme inhibitor or potassium supplementation may lead to hyperkalemia. These patients require careful monitoring early after initiation of therapy and periodically thereafter. Spironolactone may cause nausea, sexual dysfunction, gynecomastia, and menorrhagia; amiloride may cause nausea.

Methyldopa may be given twice daily and has been widely used in the intervention trials. Sedation, orthostatic intolerance, and sexual dysfunction are frequent; hepatotoxicity, acute febrile reactions, and hemolytic anemia are much less common. This agent may be given intravenously and remains useful for inpatient use. Because of extensive clinical experience with it, methyldopa remains the drug of choice in women

TABLE 2. **Antihypertensive Drugs*** *Continued*

Type of Drug	Usual Minimum Dose† (mg)	Usual Maximum Dose† (mg)
Peripheral-acting adrenergic antagonists		
Guanadrel sulfate‡	10	100
Guanethidine monosulfate	10	100
Rauwolfia alkaloids		
Rauwolfia (whole root)	50	100
Reserpine	0.1	0.25
Alpha₁-adrenergic blockers		
Prazosin hydrochloride‡	1–2	20
Terazosin hydrochloride	1–2	20
Combined alpha- and beta-adrenergic blockers		
Labetalol‡	200	1800
Vasodilators		
Hydralazine‡	50	300
Minoxidil‡	2.5	80
Angiotensin-Converting Enzyme Inhibitors		
Captopril‡	25–50	300
Enalapril maleate	2.5–5	40
Lisinopril	5	40
Calcium Antagonists		
Diltiazem hydrochloride¶	60	360
Nifedipine¶	30	180
Nitrendipine	5	40
Verapamil‡	120	480
Verapamil SR (long-lasting)	120	480
Nicardipine¶	60	120

*Adapted from The 1988 Report of the Joint National Committee on Detection, Evaluation, and Treatment of High Blood Pressure. Arch Intern Med *148*:1023–1038, 1988. U.S. National Institutes of Health Publication No. 88–1088, May 1988.

†The dosage range may differ slightly from the recommended dosage in the *Physicians' Desk Reference* or the package insert.

‡This drug is usually given in divided doses twice daily.

§Atenolol, metoprolol, and acebutolol are cardioselective; pindolol and acebutolol have partial agonist activity.

‖This drug is administered as a skin patch once weekly. Larger doses of loop diuretics may be required in patients with renal failure.

¶This drug is usually given in divided doses 3 or 4 times daily.

who require antihypertensive therapy while planning to become pregnant.

Clonidine, guanabenz, and guanfacine are centrally acting agents that decrease central sympathetic outflow by stimulating central alpha receptors. These agents may cause sedation, dry mouth, and increased sexual dysfunction when their dosages are increased, but I find that they are well tolerated at lower doses. Clonidine is available in a once weekly transdermal patch formulation, which avoids or reduces the need for oral medication and may be useful for those who easily forget to take medication but can be visited weekly, for example. This formulation may be helpful for the patient who is unable to take oral medication in the immediate postoperative period but requires a few days for therapeutic blood levels to develop. Clonidine may help to reduce the craving for nicotine and thus seems a reasonable choice for smokers who attempt to stop smoking.

The selective alpha blockers prazosin and terazosin cause few central nervous system side effects and little sexual dysfunction and may be the most beneficial drugs for lipid profiles. Although these agents may cause some sodium retention, tachyphylaxis has not been reported in the control of blood pressure. Side effects such as headache, palpitations, and malaise may occur, but these drugs are generally well tolerated. Orthostatic intolerance may occur occasionally. The rare first-dose syncope may best be avoided by not giving concomitant diuretics at the initiation of therapy and by giving the first dose at bedtime in the lowest available dose. One of the most common errors in the use of selective alpha blockers is the failure to titrate the drug to an adequate dose.

Beta blockers are available with properties such as relative cardioselectivity, water and fat solubility, intrinsic sympathomimetic activity (ISA), and membrane stabilization. Knowledge of

TABLE 3. **Adverse Drug Effects***†

Drugs	Selected Side Effects‡	Precautions and Special Considerations
Diuretics§		
Thiazide and related sulfonamide diuretics	Hypokalemia, hyperuricemia, glucose intolerance, hypercholesterolemia, hypertriglyceridemia, sexual dysfunction, weakness	May be ineffective in renal failure; hypokalemia increases digitalis toxicity; may precipitate acute gout; may cause an increase in blood levels of lithium
Loop diuretics	Hypokalemia and hyperuricemia	Effective in chronic renal failure
Potassium-sparing agents	Hyperkalemia	Danger of hyperkalemia or renal failure in patients treated with an ACE inhibitor or a nonsteroidal anti-inflammatory drug; may increase blood levels of lithium
Spironolactone	Gynecomastia, mastodynia	Interferes with digoxin immunoassay
Triamterene	—	—
Amiloride	—	—
Adrenergic Inhibitors		

Beta-adrenergic blockers‖
  Acebutolol
  Atenolol
  Metoprolol
  Nadolol
  Penbutolol sulfate
  Pindolol
  Propranolol hydrochloride
  Timolol
	Bronchospasm, peripheral arterial insufficiency, fatigue, insomnia, sexual dysfunction, exacerbation of congestive heart failure, masking of symptoms of hypoglycemia, hypertriglyceridemia, decreased HDL cholesterol (except for pindolol and acebutolol)	Should not be used in patients with asthma, COPD, congestive heart failure, heart block (greater than first degree), and sick sinus syndrome; use with caution in insulin-treated diabetics and patients with peripheral vascular disease; should not be discontinued abruptly in patients with ischemic heart disease

Centrally acting adrenergic inhibitors Clonidine	Drowsiness, sedation, dry mouth, fatigue, sexual dysfunction	Rebound hypertension may occur with abrupt discontinuance, particularly with prior administration of high doses or with continuation of concomitant beta-blocker therapy
Clonidine TTS (patch)	Same as for clonidine; localized skin reaction to the patch	—
Guanabenz	Same as for clonidine	Same as for clonidine
Guanfacine hydrochloride	Same as for clonidine	Same as for clonidine
Methyldopa	Same as for clonidine	May cause liver damage and Coombs's-positive hemolytic anemia; use cautiously in elderly patients because of orthostatic hypotension; interferes with measurements of urinary catecholamine levels
Peripheral-acting adrenergic inhibitors		
Guanadrel sulfate	Diarrhea, sexual dysfunction, orthostatic hypotension	Use cautiously because of orthostatic hypotension
Guanethidine monosulfate	Same as for guanadrel	Same as for guanadrel
Rauwolfia alkaloids	Lethargy, nasal congestion, depression	Contraindicated in patients with history of mental depression; use with caution in patients with history of peptic ulcer
Reserpine	Same as for rauwolfia alkaloids	Same as for rauwolfia alkaloids
Alpha$_1$-adrenergic blockers Prazosin hydrochloride	First-dose syncope, orthostatic hypotension, weakness, palpitations	Use cautiously in elderly patients because of orthostatic hypotension
Terazosin hydrochloride	Same as for prazosin hydrochloride	Same as for prazosin hydrochloride

TABLE 3. **Adverse Drug Effects***† *Continued*

Drugs	Selected Side Effects‡	Precautions and Special Considerations
Combined alpha- and beta-adrenergic blockers		
Labetalol‖	Bronchospasm, peripheral vascular insufficiency, orthostatic hypotension	Should not be used in patients with asthma, COPD, congestive heart failure, heart block (greater than first degree), and sick sinus syndrome; use with caution in insulin-treated diabetics and patients with peripheral vascular disease
Vasolidators	Headache, tachycardia, fluid retention	May precipitate angina pectoris in patients with coronary artery disease
Hydralazine	Positive antinuclear antibody test	Lupus syndrome may occur (rare at recommended doses)
Minoxidil	Hypertrichosis	May cause or aggravate pleural and pericardial effusions; may precipitate angina pectoris in patients with coronary artery disease
ACE Inhibitors	Rash, cough, angioneurotic edema, hyperkalemia, dysgeusia	Can cause reversible, acute renal failure in patients with bilateral renal arterial stenosis in a solitary kidney; proteinuria may occur (rare at recommended doses); hyperkalemia can develop, particularly in patients with renal insufficiency; rarely can induce neutropenia; hypotension has been observed with initiation of ACE inhibitors, especially in patients with high plasma renin activity or in those receiving diuretic therapy
Calcium Antagonists	Edema, headache	Use with caution in patients with congestive heart failure; contraindicated in patients with second- or third-degree heart block
Verapamil	Constipation	May cause liver dysfunction
Diltiazem hydrochloride	Constipation	May cause liver dysfunction
Nifedipine	Tachycardia	—
Nitrendipine	Tachycardia	—

*Adapted from The 1988 Report of the Joint National Committee on Detection, Evaluation, and Treatment of High Blood Pressure. Arch Intern Med *148*:1023–1038, 1988. U.S. National Institutes of Health Publication No. 88–1088, May 1988.

†Sexual dysfunction, particularly impotence in men, has been reported with the use of all antihypertensive agents.

‡The listing of side effects is not all-inclusive, and health practitioners are urged to refer to the package insert for a more detailed listing.

§See Table 2 for a list of these drugs.

‖Sudden withdrawal of these drugs may be hazardous in patients with heart disease.

Abbreviations: ACE = angiotensin-converting enzyme; HDL = high-density lipoprotein; COPD = chronic obstructive pulmonary disease.

the first three of these properties may help in tailoring beta-blocker therapy. Cardioselective beta blockade causes less protracted insulin-induced hypoglycemia and hypertension and less reflex bradycardia compared with blockade with a nonselective beta blocker. If bronchospasm occurs with a beta blocker, patients receiving selective agents are easier to treat, but I tend to avoid beta blockade in those who are prone to broncho-spasm. Beta blockers with ISA may be more neutral in their effect on the lipid profile and cause less bradycardia than non-ISA beta blockers. Water-soluble beta blockers such as atenolol and nadolol accumulate in the presence of renal insufficiency.

Beta blockers have been shown to be cardioprotective during and after certain acute myocardial infarctions. Their effectiveness in preventing the first myocardial infarction remains controversial and has been demonstrated only with the use of metoprolol in high-risk men at this time. Smoking may interfere with the antihypertensive efficacy of beta blockers. In different studies, smoking has also been demonstrated to reduce the benefits of propranolol and possibly atenolol, but not of metoprolol. This emphasizes how important smoking cessation is for the hypertensive patient.

The side effects of the beta blockers are well known and include bronchospasm, fatigue, exacerbation of congestive heart failure, exacerbation of peripheral vascular insufficiency or coolness of extremities, and central nervous system side effects. It is of interest that hypotension and orthostatic intolerance are uncommon with beta-blocker treatment. On the other hand, the calming effect of beta blockade may be helpful to some hypertensives, and coronary symptoms and migraine may be reduced with this therapy.

Angiotensin-converting enzyme inhibitors have no central nervous system side effects and appear not to worsen sexual performance, pulmonary function, or metabolic parameters. Nausea, headache, and rash are the most common side effects. A cough can be quite bothersome to a small percentage of individuals. These drugs may be useful in treating congestive heart failure but require caution and a reduced dosage when used in renal insufficiency because they are excreted by the kidney. Hyperkalemia may occur in this setting, and the chance of developing rash and agranulocytosis increases when captopril is used in the presence of renal insufficiency, other immunologic diseases, or both. The use of these drugs in the presence of bilateral tight renal artery stenoses or in a functionally single kidney with renal artery stenosis may result in reversible renal failure. Other antihypertensive agents may also worsen renal insufficiency with blood pressure reduction, but this effect appears to be more dramatic with the angiotensin-converting enzyme inhibitors. Although proteinuria may be reduced with their use, it is still not known whether angiotensin-converting enzyme inhibitors are better than standard therapy to halt the progression of renal failure in diabetes and other proteinuric states.

Hypotension may occur when angiotensin-converting enzyme inhibitors are added to a diuretic. If the diuretic is not withheld in the usual manner for a day or so before initiating therapy, the patient should probably be warned of the possibility of hypotension and the drug should be started at bedtime. I generally try to start all nondiuretic antihypertensive therapies at bedtime to avoid side effects and initial or first-dose orthostatic intolerance.

The calcium channel blockers are the most recent addition to the list of agents that are appropriate for initial therapy of mild hypertension. These agents have the advantages of also treating coronary disease and preventing migraine. They do not cause metabolic abnormalities or central nervous system side effects, nor do they worsen peripheral vascular insufficiency, pulmonary function, or sexual performance. They are available in longer-acting formulations by slow-release or osmotic pump technology, which will make therapy easier for the hypertensive. Headache, flushing, localized edema, and constipation are their major side effects. Any pedal edema that may occur is extravascular; plasma volume has actually been found to be decreased in this setting. Verapamil and diltiazem may occasionally worsen cardiac conduction, but this is uncommon in otherwise healthy hypertensives.

One common error in treating hypertension is to use an inadequate dose of an antihypertensive agent before concluding that the agent is not effective for a given patient. I try not to increase the dosage of a given nondiuretic to the point where bothersome side effects occur, accepting the fact that in some individuals a higher dosage could have achieved control. The medication can always be tried again at a higher dosage if required, and the greater the push to higher doses, the greater the incidence of side effects that upset the patient and make it more difficult to introduce additional agents. Obviously, the more a hypertensive patient can participate in deciding when to discontinue titration, the easier this becomes. I usually titrate the drug dosage to a little more than one-half of the accepted maximum before considering an additional drug if there has been a moderate response or an alternative drug if there has been no appreciable response. In mild hypertensives I often try an alternative medication before resorting to combinations of drugs.

ADDITIONAL DRUG THERAPY OF HYPERTENSION

Diuretics may always be added to the agent selected as the first drug. Combinations of nondiuretic agents may also be effective. It does not make sense to combine two agents from the same class, such as centrally acting agents and a beta blocker or, in certain hypertensives, high doses of a centrally acting agent and a selective alpha blocker. Patients with coronary heart disease may experience worsening of cardiac conduction when a beta blocker and diltiazem or verapamil are combined, but this risk is reduced in an otherwise healthy hypertensive.

Reserpine remains a useful agent to be added

to a diuretic in a low dose. This drug may cause sedation and nasal stuffiness, depression, and sexual dysfunction, and may aggravate peptic disease, yet it is tolerated by many patients. It is available in combination preparations and tends to be inexpensive, which may be necessary in certain circumstances. Periodic removal of the reserpine and observation of the hypertensive patient while alternative therapy is given can unmask any depressive action that the agent may have slowly caused. This problem appears to be less common with the lower dosages used presently.

Hydralazine is a useful vasodilator to be added as a third agent when a centrally acting agent, reserpine, or a beta blocker is used to prevent reflex tachycardia. I tend not to use hydralazine as a second agent even though other physicians have found it to be useful in the elderly. Hydralazine may cause tachycardia; aggravate angina pectoris, headache, and malaise; and cause a lupus syndrome. The last is more common when higher doses are given, especially in black persons, who have a higher probability of metabolizing hydralazine at a slower rate. The hydralazine-related lupus syndrome is uncommon at the currently recommended doses.

Minoxidil may be a useful vasodilator to be added as a third or fourth agent in treating patients with refractory hypertension. It may also be useful in low doses as a third agent in treating men with moderate hypertension. Minoxidil may cause reflex tachycardia and thus may aggravate coronary disease if the reflex heart rate response is not blocked by beta blockade or a centrally acting agent. The use of minoxidil may transiently alter the T waves on the electrocardiogram, making interpretation of coronary symptoms difficult. Fluid retention and hirsutism may limit the acceptance of the drug, and pericardial effusions, pleural effusions, or both may occasionally become serious problems, necessitating cessation of the drug.

OVERVIEW OF TREATMENT OF HYPERTENSION WITH OTHER MEDICAL PROBLEMS

The large number of antihypertensive agents that are presently available allows the practitioner to tailor therapy based on patient preference and other medical problems or needs. The following is an incomplete overview of approaches to these different clinical situations.

Noncompliance

Noncompliance with the prescribed regimen is a major obstacle in obtaining adequate control of blood pressure. Once or twice daily medication appears to have the most success in achieving this goal. Fortunately, antihypertensive agents from each drug class are now available for once or twice daily administration. The addition of slow-dissolution and osmotic pump formulations of shorter-acting antihypertensives increases the number of options available while simultaneously decreasing the side effects when more constant drug blood levels are obtained. The hypertensive should be asked about problems in taking the medication as prescribed, as well as whether any significant side effects occur. If cost is a major problem, sensitivity to this issue is important, but it may limit the options in choosing medications free of side effects. I find it helpful to compare the cost of a loaf of bread or even of the pack of cigarretes that the patient may still be consuming to the cost of daily medication. The least expensive medications include thiazide diuretics without potassium-sparing agents or supplements, reserpine, hydralazine, and some generic drugs. One problem is the confusion created by the different sizes, shapes, and colors of the generic drugs that some patients obtain from different pharmacies and from different suppliers to the same pharmacy, depending on the price quoted that month or quarter.

Sexual Dysfunction

Sexual dysfunction is a major reason for noncompliance as well as for discontinuing antihypertensive care. Because almost 10 per cent of hypertensive men receiving placebo therapy may have sexual dysfunction, it is helpful to remove the antihypertensive drug, if possible, for a trial period. Thiazide diuretics have been associated with at least a 20 per cent rate of sexual dysfunction. For this reason, it makes sense to discontinue the use of these agents if possible. I have found that return of sexual function may take some time. The centrally acting agents may need to be discontinued, being tapered as one would a beta blocker. The converting enzyme inhibitors, selective alpha blockers, and calcium channel blockers, followed by the beta blockers, have the lowest possibility of causing or worsening sexual dysfunction. Finally, one must remember that there are causes of sexual dysfunction other than antihypertensive therapy, and referral for intensive urologic evaluation may be appropriate both diagnostically and therapeutically.

Dyslipidemia

One recent concern about the selection of antihypertensive therapy has been the choice of drug for the patient who has a higher risk of cardio-vascular disease because of elevated plasma lipid levels. The selective alpha blockers and the centrally acting agents are most promising, whereas the converting enzyme inhibitors, calcium channel blockers, and directly acting vasodilators may be neutral. Although the non-ISA beta blockers may reduce high-density-lipoprotein cholesterol levels, beta blockers are effective in certain acute and post–myocardial infarction patients, and metoprolol has been found to be more effective than thiazide-based therapy in reducing myocardial infarction death rates in high-risk Scandinavian men.

Coronary Heart Disease

Blood pressure should be controlled in hypertensives with coronary heart disease. Some would argue for control between 85 and 89 mmHg diastolic blood pressure because patients with lower treated diastolic blood pressures may have a higher mortality. I generally reduce the blood pressure with beta-blocker– or calcium channel blocker–based therapy to below 150 mmHg systolic and to 80 to 88 mmHg diastolic. If low-dose thiazides are required, I prefer to maintain the serum potassium level above 3.8 mEq per liter if possible.

Congestive Cardiac Failure

Blood pressure should be vigorously controlled in patients with congestive cardiac failure. A diuretic followed by the cautious addition of a converting enzyme inhibitor is the most promising treatment. A selective alpha blocker or vasodilator with nitrates may also be useful but could be associated with tachyphylaxis. Selective alpha blockers do not cause tachyphylaxis when used in the hypertensive patient who does not have congestive heart failure. The centrally acting drugs and dihydropyridine calcium channel blockers that do not have the potential to reduce cardiac output are also appropriate choices. The hypertensive should be questioned regarding compliance with drug therapy and sodium intake, and for the possibility of using competing agents such as nonsteroidal anti-inflammatory drugs.

Left Ventricular Hypertrophy

The presence of left ventricular hypertrophy heralds a poor prognosis for the hypertensive. Methyldopa and the other centrally acting agents, reserpine with a thiazide diuretic, beta blockers, converting enzyme inhibitors, calcium channel blockers, and, more recently, prazosin have been shown to reduce the hypertrophied left ventricular mass.

Diabetes Mellitus

Thiazide diuretics may aggravate glucose intolerance, as previously noted; the other classes of antihypertensive agents tend not to cause this problem. Diabetic hypertensives may also have lipid abnormalities and sexual dysfunction, which would require modification of their treatment regimen, as previously outlined. If a beta blocker is required, a selective one may be preferable, as noted earlier. Orthostatic intolerance may develop in long-standing diabetics with neuropathy and may be exacerbated by the centrally acting agents and the selective alpha blockers. The role of the converting enzyme inhibitors in retarding renal failure still requires clarification.

Isolated Diastolic or Combined Hypertension in the Elderly

The older patient with diastolic hypertension has been shown to benefit from blood pressure reduction. Between 15 and 35 per cent of older hypertensives may have overestimation of their blood pressure by indirect cuff sphygmomanometer compared with direct arterial measurement. This problem may be more frequent in those with severely elevated blood pressures, those with other atherosclerotic vascular diseases, and those who have a palpable but pulseless radial artery when the blood pressure cuff is insufflated to a pressure above the auscultated systolic blood pressure (a positive Osler's maneuver).

The older hypertensive with isolated diastolic or combined systolic and diastolic hypertension is responsive to diuretic therapy but may be at higher risk than younger patients for volume contraction, azotemia, glucose intolerance, and complications related to hypokalemia. This hypertensive responds well to the centrally acting agents but may also be susceptible to possible central nervous system side effects. Calcium channel blockers appear to be effective and are tolerated when the side effect of constipation is acceptable or manageable. The selective alpha blockers reduce blood pressure while maintaining cerebral blood flow. Treatment with both beta blockers and converting enzyme inhibitors is effective and tolerated by the older hypertensive. Thus, the therapeutic options available for this patient are less limited than was previously thought.

The elderly hypertensive should be treated with reduced initial doses of an antihypertensive drug and should probably be monitored more frequently during the early stages of therapy. Postural measurement of blood pressure should be part of the routine, as well as careful questioning about expected and unexpected side effects that could impair the patient's lifestyle. It may also be useful to question the spouse, a relative, or another interested third party about how the patient seems to be doing with the current treatment program. In addition, certain elderly hypertensives may benefit from enhanced social support.

Isolated Systolic Hypertension in the Elderly

Systolic hypertension is a major contributor to cardiovascular complications in the elderly, but intervention data on the risks and benefits of treatment are lacking. For this reason, I cautiously initiate a trial of therapy in all elderly hypertensives with isolated systolic hypertension who do not have concomitant cardiovascular disease or target organ damage. This conservative approach is especially indicated for those with systolic blood pressure between 160 and 178 mmHg. When the systolic blood pressure is equal to or higher than 180 mmHg, I attempt to reduce it toward or below 160 mmHg with one or more therapies. The results of therapy should include a global evaluation of the patient until the benefits of therapy have been clearly shown. A more aggressive approach is indicated in elderly hypertensives with complications of hypertension or other cardiovascular disease that would benefit from blood pressure reduction.

Black Race

Black hypertensives have a much higher risk of cardiorenal failure than white hypertensives and have clearly been shown to benefit from standard thiazide-based therapy. Thiazide diuretics are effective in all dose ranges. Beta blockers may be less effective as monotherapy in blacks, but more than half of those treated may have a reasonable response. To achieve a response in a black individual, higher doses of a beta blocker are not required if the individual is a responder. Black persons who respond to a beta blocker do so at the same dosage as white persons. The converting enzyme inhibitors are moderately useful, but their effectiveness is enhanced with the addition of a thiazide diuretic. Other agents, such as selective alpha blockers, centrally acting agents, and especially calcium channel blockers, are effective.

Exercise

Regular exercise may have a salutary effect on hypertension but may not be adequate to reduce

TABLE 4. **Causes of Refractory Hypertension***

1. Nonadherence to therapy

2. Drug-related causes
   a. Doses too low
   b. Inappropriate combinations (e.g., two centrally acting adrenergic inhibitors)
   c. Rapid inactivation (e.g., hydralazine)
   d. Effects of other drugs
      i. Sympathomimetics
      ii. Antidepressants
      iii. Adrenal steroids
      iv. Nonsteroidal anti-inflammatory drugs
      v. Nasal decongestants
      vi. Oral contraceptives

3. Associated conditions
   a. Increasing obesity
   b. Alcohol intake of more than 1 oz of ethanol a day
   c. Renal insufficiency
   d. Renovascular hypertension
   e. Malignant or accelerated hypertension
   f. Other causes of hypertension

4. Volume overload
   a. Inadequate diuretic therapy
   b. Excess sodium intake
   c. Fluid retention from reduction of blood pressure
   d. Progressive renal damage

*Adapted from The 1988 Report of the Joint National Committee on Detection, Evaluation, and Treatment of High Blood Pressure. Arch Intern Med 148:1023–1038, 1988. U.S. National Institutes of Health Publication No. 88–1088, May 1988.

the blood pressure to a desired level. It is important not to decrease exercise tolerance in patients who exercise to help control their hypertension, as well as in those whose work requires them to do physical labor. Diuretics do not impair exercise tolerance, but they may cause problems related to possible volume contraction and electrolyte imbalance, including hypokalemia. Beta blockers improve exercise tolerance in those with coronary heart disease but may decrease it in those without such disease. Some hypertensives who exercise only moderately do not find that beta blockers impair their exercise tolerance. Antihypertensive agents that generally do not impair exercise tolerance include the selective alpha blockers, calcium channel blockers, converting enzyme inhibitors, centrally acting agents, combined alpha-beta blockers, and possibly long-term pindolol. Either a reduction or an increase in antihypertensive medication may become necessary if a patient begins or discontinues an exercise program, respectively.

Asthma

In the hypertensive with asthma, control of the bronchospastic condition with medications that include the sympathomimetic agents achieves better control of the hypertension. Combined di-

TABLE 5. **Intravenous Antihypertensives Used for Hypertensive Emergencies**

Drug	Dose (IV)	Onset	Side Effects
Hydralazine	10–20 mg	10 min	Tachycardia, angina, headache, GI upset
Sodium nitroprusside	0.5–10 µg/kg/min infusion	Seconds	Nasal stuffiness, GI upset, confusion, muscle twitching, thiocyanate excess, methemoglobinemia
Nitroglycerin	5–100 µg/min infusion	2–3 min	Headache, tachycardia, GI upset, methemoglobinemia
Diazoxide	50- to 150-mg bolus 15- to 30-mg mini-boluses	1–2 min	Hypotension, tachycardia, angina, hyperglycemia
Trimethaphan	1–4 mg/min	1–5 min	Delayed reversal, ileus, Foley's catheterization required
Phentolamine	5- to 10-mg bolus	1–2 min	Hypotension, tachycardia, nasal stuffiness
Labetalol	2 mg/min infusion 20–80 mg/10 min bolus	5–10 min	Heart block, asthma, orthostatic hypotension
Enalaprilat	1.25-mg bolus	15 min	Hypotension, rash, angioedema, hyperkalemia
Verapamil	10-mg slow bolus	2–10 min	Heart block
Methyldopa	250- to 500-mg short infusion	0.5–1 hr	Sedation, fever, hemolysis, hepatitis

Abbreviation: GI = gastrointestinal.

uretic and steroid use may provoke profound hypokalemia. Calcium channel blockers have replaced beta blockers in most asthmatic hypertensives with coronary heart disease. Beta blockers are to be avoided. In the rare cases in which they are necessary, the lowest possible dose of a selective beta blocker should be used. In patients without coronary heart disease, the centrally acting agents, selective alpha blockers, converting enzyme inhibitors, and diuretics are appropriate, in addition to the calcium channel blockers. The occasional cough that may result from treatment with the converting enzyme inhibitors appears not to be caused by bronchospasm and is reversible on discontinuation of the agent.

Migraine

In the patient with migraine and hypertension, other causes of the headache should be ruled out when appropriate. Drug dependence may be a complicating factor in some hypertensive patients with migraine. Ergot derivatives may elevate blood pressure. For this reason, the patient's

blood pressure response should be monitored when initiating therapy. Beta blockers and calcium channel blockers are both effective in reducing the frequency of migraine attacks while simultaneously lowering elevated blood pressure and thus should be considered first when selecting therapy.

REFRACTORY HYPERTENSION

Various combinations of drugs should be effective in controlling hypertension in most patients. Those whose hypertension cannot be controlled with therapy require a systematic evaluation for noncompliance, volume overload, other complicating medical disorders including alcoholism, possible drug interactions, and secondary hypertension (Table 4). Evaluation for secondary hypertension should be the last step in this process. Home blood pressure monitoring may be helpful in discovering office hypertension and is less costly than ambulatory monitoring. I tend to treat office hypertension especially if there is any suggestion of target organ damage or if the in-

TABLE 6. **Oral Antihypertensives Used for Hypertensive "Urgencies"**

Agent	Usual Oral Dose	Onset	Side Effects
Nifedipine	10-mg oral or "bite and swallow"; repeat as needed	10–20 min	Tachycardia, flushing, hypotension
Captopril	12.5–25 mg	20–30 min	Hypotension
Clonidine	0.1–0.2/hr up to three doses	30 min	Sedation, dry mouth

dividual has other cardiovascular risk factors. Therapy is individualized based on the patient's tolerance of antihypertensive therapy.

HYPERTENSIVE URGENCIES AND EMERGENCIES

It is relatively uncommon today to see malignant phase hypertension with diastolic blood pressure of 130 mmHg or more and hemorrhages, exudates, and/or disk edema unless one practices in a clinical setting that is underserved or where many patients do not comply with therapy. A more common presentation is markedly elevated blood pressure with chest pain, congestive heart failure, headache, or no symptoms at all. Because many therapeutic options are available, it is most important to treat the whole person and not the blood pressure alone. Before treatment is initiated, the practitioner should have a preconceived plan to achieve the immediate goal of blood pressure reduction and should know what blood pressure will be appropriate in 12 to 24 hours. Oral therapy should not be delayed and should be initiated as soon as possible unless minute-to-minute control seems necessary.

Severe hypertension with mental status or neurologic changes with or without disk edema, aortic dissection, subarachnoid hemorrhage, recent vascular surgery, anticoagulation, or a thrombolytic state should prompt a reduction in blood pressure by parenteral means. The intravenous agents that are useful to reduce blood pressure are outlined in Table 5. The goal in the initial phase of treatment should be a reduction of approximately 10 per cent in mean blood pressure in the individual with malignant or accelerated hypertension. Zealous blood pressure reduction should be avoided. In situations where bleeding is a concern, blood pressure should be reduced to normal, if possible, while the patient is observed for signs of poor perfusion or worsening neurologic status. In patients with aortic dissection, the blood pressure should be lowered to below normal if the patient can tolerate it. Intravenous nitroprusside, with or without beta blockade when needed to control the heart rate, is often easiest to use because of the smooth blood pressure control achieved with dose titration, the short duration of action, and nurses' familiarity with the drug. Other agents may be satisfactory substitutes, depending on the clinical situation.

Even mild hypertension associated with preeclampsia or eclampsia should be promptly treated with parenteral or intramuscular hydralazine while stabilizing the pregnant patient for delivery. Cerebral hemorrhage is a major concern in this hypertensive condition of pregnancy.

I am not certain how far to lower the blood pressure in acute myocardial infarction, thrombotic stroke, or intracerebral hemorrhage. In acute myocardial infarction, I generally treat the pain first, and then use intravenous nitroglycerin or nitroprusside with an acute intravenous beta blocker if possible. In the hypertensive states associated with thrombotic stroke or intracerebral hemorrhage, I attempt to reduce the blood pressure moderately while observing the patient for any deterioration associated with blood pressure reduction.

Severely elevated blood pressure without associated symptoms should not generally necessitate parenteral therapy. In this situation, oral captopril, oral or "bite and swallow" nifedipine, or oral clonidine "loading" with observation of the patient for a few hours may be adequate to initiate blood pressure reduction safely. Some information about these approaches is outlined in Table 6. All patients who are discharged for outpatient follow-up should have their postural blood pressure determined before discharge. In my experience, follow-up blood pressure monitoring usually is necessary within 1 or 2 days to allow for drug adjustment. Although acute administration of oral or paste formations of nitroglycerin may lower blood pressure, I have not found this form of therapy helpful in planning longer-term management.

The most common error in the management of these urgent situations is to overtreat the hypertension when standard one- or two-drug oral dosing would have reduced it in a more evenly controlled fashion without the risks associated with more rapid blood pressure reduction.

ACUTE MYOCARDIAL INFARCTION
method of
G. WILLIAM DEC, M.D.,
PATRICK T. O'GARA, M.D.
Massachusetts General Hospital

and

GREGORY D. CURFMAN, M.D.
New England Journal of Medicine
Boston, Massachusetts

Acute myocardial infarction continues to be one of the most common and vexing clinical problems that general internists and primary care physicians must confront. This year, nearly 1.5 million Americans will have a myocardial infarction, and 540,000 (36 per cent) of them will die. More than 300,000 of these deaths will occur before the patients are able to reach a hospital. By comparison, the next two most common causes of death in the United States are cancer (460,000 deaths) and accidents (92,000 deaths).

Despite the magnitude of the problem, a steady downward trend in the age-adjusted death rate from coronary artery disease has been observed during the past 25 years. The mortality from this disease reached a peak of 240 deaths per 100,000 population in 1962. Since that time, it declined to 150 per 100,000 population in 1984, a decrease of nearly 38 per cent in 22 years. Current figures suggest that this downward trend is continuing. Although part of this decline can be attributed to advances in medical care, changes in lifestyle resulting in modification of coronary risk factors also appear to have made an important contribution. Most physicians would agree that prevention of myocardial infarction is a more reasonable goal than attempts to intervene at a time of crisis. Nevertheless, until our society becomes much more serious about preventing coronary disease, physicians must be prepared to deal with acute coronary events as they arise.

Our understanding of the pathogenesis of acute myocardial infarction has been increased considerably by the recognition that nearly all infarctions are precipitated by the formation of a thrombus in an epicardial coronary artery. This concept is not new, Herrick having elaborated on it as early as 1912, but serial visualization of the coronary arteries by arteriography has now firmly documented the presence of a thrombus in a large majority of infarct-related coronary arteries. In many instances, the thrombus may arise from hemorrhage into or rupture of an unstable atherosclerotic plaque. The activation of platelets at the site of the unstable plaque undoubtedly plays an important part in the formation of a thrombus. Although focal spasm in a coronary vessel may also contribute to the obstruction of blood flow, spasm as the sole mechanism of obstruction is unusual. The ability to modify the process of coronary thrombosis with fibrinolytic and antiplatelet agents has markedly changed our therapeutic approach to acute myocardial infarction. Recent studies have also helped to clarify the role of coronary angioplasty in the management of patients with acute infarction.

In this article, we focus principally on the treatment of acute myocardial infarction, and we emphasize developments that have occurred during the last 5 years. Little is said about diagnosis. Because the treatment of myocardial infarction is evolving rapidly, some of the information presented here may be outdated by the time of publication. Such is the price of progress.

PREHOSPITAL MANAGEMENT

In part because of denial or misinterpretation of symptoms, delays of several hours or more are common before patients with acute myocardial infarction arrive at a hospital. Because more than 50 per cent of patients who die of acute myocardial infarction succumb before they reach a hospital, the potential benefit of emergency transport systems could be substantial. Stimulated in part by studies performed in Seattle, Washington, a growing number of U.S. cities have developed medical transportation systems for the rapid management of out-of-hospital cardiac emergencies, including myocardial infarction and its complications. Mobile coronary care units (CCUs) are now usually equipped for the intravenous administration of lidocaine and other cardiovascular drugs, continuous cardiac monitoring, and electrical cardioversion. Radio communication with the nearest hospital can alert the staff to the patient's arrival.

One of the most important recent additions to the mobile CCU is the automatic external defibrillator. By means of adhesive electrodes attached to the patient's chest, this device analyzes the cardiac rhythm and detects the presence of ventricular fibrillation. When this arrhythmia is identified, the defibrillator automatically delivers up to three 200-joule shocks. The survival rate, as measured by the percentage of patients with out-of-hospital ventricular fibrillation who are eventually discharged from the hospital, is approximately 30 per cent with this device. This figure contrasts with a 19 per cent survival rate when standard defibrillators are used. In the light of these encouraging results, the automatic external defibrillator is being used more widely in ambulances and other emergency transport vehicles.

GENERAL TREATMENT MEASURES

The Coronary Care Unit

All patients in whom the diagnosis of acute infarction is suspected with reasonable certainty should be admitted to a CCU. Studies performed in the late 1960s that raised questions about the efficacy of the CCU in improving the survival of patients with acute infarction are not applicable to the CCU of today. The state-of-the-art CCU should be equipped for continuous monitoring of the electrocardiogram and for invasive hemodynamic evaluation. Equipment should be available for the delivery of supplemental oxygen, for transvenous and external emergency cardiac pacing, and for electrical cardioversion. The staff should be experienced in the intravenous administration of thrombolytic agents. Facilities should also be available for echocardiographic and radionuclide imaging studies for patients in whom these procedures are indicated.

For uncomplicated patients, the stay in the CCU need be no longer than 48 to 72 hours in most instances. Patients can then be transferred to an intermediate care area. Patients in whom the diagnosis of acute infarction is being entertained, but is of low probability, can be admitted directly to an intermediate care area for evaluation and monitoring.

Relief of Pain, Fever, and Anxiety

Analgesia and sedation are important early goals of treatment because they can diminish tachycardia and thereby reduce myocardial oxygen demand. The mainstay of pain relief is morphine sulfate in a dose of 2 to 8 mg intravenously, which may be repeated at 10- to 15-minute intervals as required. Occasional patients may need even larger doses for complete relief. The side effects of morphine include hypotension, respiratory depression, nausea, and vomiting. Respiratory depression can be attenuated with naloxone in a dose of 0.1 to 0.2 mg intravenously.* Patients who cannot tolerate morphine can be treated with meperidine, 25 to 50 mg intravenously, which can be repeated at intervals of 10 to 15 minutes.

A low-grade fever may occur as a consequence of necrosis of myocardial tissue or associated pericarditis. Tylenol or aspirin, 650 mg orally every 4 to 6 hours, is the agent of choice. In some patients, pericarditis, which is most likely to occur on days 2 to 5 after a transmural infarction, may respond better to indomethacin, 25 to 50 mg every 8 hours. It is important to distinguish the pain of pericarditis, which may be exacerbated by respiration or changes in body position, from that of recurrent myocardial ischemia. Both problems can be associated with re-elevation of the ST segments on the electrocardiogram.

Relief of anxiety is best accomplished by the administration of diazepam, 2 to 10 mg orally every 6 to 8 hours. The importance of this comfort measure, which can help to reduce sympathetic stimulation of the heart and peripheral vessels, should not be underestimated.

Diet and Activity

During the first 24 hours, the diet should consist of caffeine-free liquids and bland, soft solids. Thereafter a 4-gram-sodium, cholesterol-lowering diet (less than 30 per cent of total calories from fat and less than 10 per cent from saturated fat) is recommended. Total calories should range from 1200 to 1800, depending on body weight and individual energy needs. A stool softener, such as docusate sodium, 100 mg orally, should be administered daily to prevent constipation. Before discharge from the hospital, the patient should receive dietary counseling from a regis-

tered dietitian. The principal dietary goals are to reduce the blood cholesterol level to less than 200 mg per dl and to achieve ideal body weight. Sodium restriction to 4 grams daily may be necessary if hypertension or heart failure is present.

During the first 48 hours, rigid enforcement of bed rest is neither necessary nor desirable in patients with no complications. Stable patients should be permitted to use a bedside commode within the first 24 hours, and they should be allowed to dangle their legs and sit in a chair after 24 hours. If the patient is free from complications after 48 to 72 hours, supervised walking may begin. The heart rate should be monitored by telemetry, and it should not be permitted to exceed the heart rate at rest by more than 20 per cent. The occurrence of ventricular arrhythmias or ST segment deviations during ambulation can also be detected with the use of telemetry.

Oxygenation and Electrolytes

In patients who are suspected clinically of being hypoxemic because of pulmonary congestion or coexisting pulmonary disease, arterial blood gas levels should be measured while the patient is breathing room air. Although administration of oxygen has become standard practice in many CCUs, patients who are not hypoxemic do not require supplemental oxygen. Mild hypoxemia usually responds to oxygen delivered at a rate of 2 to 4 liters per minute by nasal prongs or mask. More severe hypoxemia may require more intensive evaluation and higher concentrations of inspired oxygen. In no case should hypoxemia in a patient with acute infarction be left untreated. Patients with anemia (hematocrit of 25 ml per dl or less) may be candidates for transfusion to improve the oxygen-carrying capacity.

Serum electrolyte levels should also be measured on admission to the CCU, and hypokalemia should be corrected to a level above 4.0 mEq per liter. Patients who have been taking diuretics may be deficient in magnesium, and the serum concentration of this cation should be measured if ventricular arrhythmias are present.

Anticoagulation

The purpose of systemic anticoagulation in patients with acute infarction is to prevent the formation of thrombi in the ventricular chambers and in the veins of the lower extremities. Standard anticoagulants, such as heparin, do not appear to be effective for the dissolution of coronary artery thrombi. Two-dimensional echocardiography has disclosed left ventricular mural

---

*It may be necessary to use larger doses.

thrombi in approximately 30 per cent of patients with anteroapical myocardial infarction, but patients with inferior infarction appear to have a much lower incidence. Recent studies have shown that both deep venous and intraventricular thrombi can be prevented by the administration of heparin, 12,500 units subcutaneously every 12 hours. Although lower doses of heparin may prevent deep venous thrombosis, they may not be effective in preventing intraventricular thrombi. Early ambulation of the patient is also helpful in preventing deep venous thrombosis. In patients who are treated with a thrombolytic agent, the combination of aspirin and intravenous heparin should be used routinely (see later), and therefore subcutaneous heparin should be omitted.

The efficacy of long-term oral anticoagulation in preventing systemic embolization after myocardial infarction is an unsettled question. On the basis of current information, the following approaches seem reasonable. If two-dimensional echocardiography performed before hospital discharge reveals the presence of a mural thrombus in a patient with an anterior infarction, the patient should be treated with warfarin to maintain the prothrombin at one and one-half to two times the control value for 6 months. Some physicians prefer to treat all patients with anterior infarction with warfarin for 6 months, as long as there are no contraindications to systemic anticoagulation. Warfarin is not recommended routinely in patients with inferoposterior infarcts because they appear to be at much lower risk of mural thrombosis. Whether antiplatelet agents are effective in preventing late systemic embolization is unknown.

Length of Hospital Stay

The recommended length of hospitalization for patients with uncomplicated myocardial infarction has been shortened progressively during the past three decades. Patients with no complications are now frequently discharged after 7 to 10 days. A recent study has suggested that patients treated effectively with thrombolytic therapy may be safely discharged on the third hospital day. This recommendation is unrealistic for most patients, however, and our view is that most patients without complications should remain in the hospital for 1 week. Occasional patients who are clinically stable and have successfully completed an exercise test with no evidence of ischemia or arrhythmias may be discharged on day 5, as long as careful outpatient follow-up is planned. Patients with important clinical complications, such as heart failure, persistent arrhythmias, or recurrent ischemia, must remain in the hospital

until these problems have been successfully managed.

EARLY TREATMENT OF ACUTE MYOCARDIAL INFARCTION

The urgent management of acute myocardial infarction has changed rapidly over the past decade. Several approaches to coronary artery reperfusion have been proposed and evaluated in a vast array of studies involving thousands of patients. Although certain treatment issues have been resolved, many problems remain that require further study through properly designed prospective trials. The currently available reperfusion therapies include thrombolysis, direct coronary artery angioplasty, and coronary artery bypass surgery. The ultimate goals of reperfusion therapy are limitation of infarct size, preservation of left ventricular function, and reduction of short- and long-term mortality.

Thrombolytic Therapy

Administration of a thrombolytic agent should now be routinely considered for properly selected patients with acute myocardial infarction. In particular, patients who present to the hospital within 3 to 4 hours of the onset of pain compatible with myocardial ischemia and who display ST segment elevation of greater than 0.1 mV in at least two contiguous leads on the electrocardiogram should be considered for pharmacologic thrombolysis. As of this writing, patients with ST segment depression (or those with unstable angina pectoris) are not routinely considered candidates for such therapy. Although some debate remains, thrombolytic treatment should be offered to patients with either anterior or inferior infarction. For anterior infarction, there is no doubt that successful thrombolysis can be beneficial. Most investigators and clinicians also now agree that a patient with an inferior infarction, particularly one associated with precordial ST segment depression or with inferior ST segment elevations of more than 0.3 mV, should be given thrombolytic therapy. For selected patients who present as late as 6 hours after the onset of pain, lytic therapy can still be considered, especially if pain, ST segment elevation, or both have persisted and there is no evidence of extensive Q wave development.

Thrombolytic therapy should not be administered before a physician evaluates the patient in the hospital. Absolute contraindications to its use include recent major surgery, a history of gastrointestinal or genitourinary bleeding, a previous cerebrovascular accident (intracerebral hemorrhage, thrombotic stroke, or transient ischemic attack), prolonged cardiopulmonary resuscitation with external cardiac massage, uncontrolled hypertension (systolic pressure higher than 180 mmHg, diastolic pressure higher than 110 mmHg), and a hemorrhagic diathesis. The stool must be examined for occult blood immediately on presentation. Relative contraindications are age more than 75 years, diabetic retinopathy with neovascularization, and altered mental status.

Several thrombolytic agents have been studied intensively in numerous multicenter trials. They include streptokinase, recombinant tissue plasminogen activator (rt-PA), anisoylated plasminogen–streptokinase activator complex (APSAC), single-chain urokinase plasminogen activator (scu-PA, prourokinase), and urokinase (Table 1). Investigations are currently proceeding with mutant forms of rt-PA and with complexes of plasminogen activators coupled with monoclonal antifibrin antibodies. Potent antiplatelet agents, such as monoclonal antibodies directed against specific membrane receptors, are also under study. In the United States, however, the present therapeutic choice lies between streptokinase and rt-PA.

Streptokinase is a nonenzymatic protein derived from beta-hemolytic streptococci that complexes with plasminogen to form an active conjugate that, in turn, liberates plasmin from plasminogen. A loading dose is required because of the presence of circulating antibodies produced as a consequence of previous streptococcal infections. Streptokinase is not fibrin specific and therefore causes a decrease in the concentration of systemic fibrin and fibrinogen, with corresponding increases in fibrin(ogen) breakdown products.

Streptokinase can be delivered subselectively to the site of the thrombus in the coronary artery. The recommended dose for intracoronary use is 2000 to 4000 units per minute over 1 hour, up to a maximum of 250,000 units. Its efficacy can be assessed by coronary arteriography during or after the infusion. Patency of the infarct-related artery can be expected in approximately 60 to 80 per cent of cases. Such therapy, however, is not widely applicable because it demands the immediate availability of a catheterization facility,

TABLE 1. **Thrombolytic Agents***

Agent	Fibrin Selectivity	Systemic Lytic Effect	Dose	Half-Life (min)	Adverse Effects/Comments
Streptokinase	0	+ + + +	IC: 2000–4000 U/min for 60 min up to 250,000 U (a bolus of 20,000 U may be given)		Bleeding, allergic reactions, hypotension Inexpensive
			IV: 1.5 million U over 1 hr	23	
Recombinant tissue plasminogen activator (rt-PA), single chain	+ + + +	+	IV: 6-mg bolus, 54 mg over first hr, 20 mg over second hr, 20 mg over third hr	5	Bleeding Expensive
Anisoylated plasminogen–streptokinase activator complex (APSAC)	+	+ + + +	IV: 30 U over 2–5 min	90	Side effect profile similar to that of streptokinase No maintenance infusion necessary ? lower incidence of reocclusion
Single-chain urokinase plasminogen activator (scu-PA, prourokinase)	+ + + +	+	Optimal dose, either alone or in combination with rt-PA, not known	7	May be best used in synergistic combination with rt-PA Expensive
Urokinase	0	+ + +	IC: 4000–6000 U/min for 2 hr; average total dose, 500,000 U		
			IV: ? 1.5 million U bolus, then 1.5 million U over 90 min; ? 2.0 million U over 5–15 min	16	Optimal IV dose has not been established Not antigenic

*Adapted with permission from Marder VJ and Sherry S: The New England Journal of Medicine, *318*, 1512, 1988. *Symbols*: 0 = none; + + + + = highest.

highly trained operators, and skilled support staff.

Although it has not enjoyed great popularity in the United States, intravenously administered streptokinase has been shown in several European and South Pacific clinical trials to improve left ventricular function and to decrease mortality after acute myocardial infarction. Reported rates of patency restoration in the infarct-related artery have ranged from 31 to 76 per cent. The drug is administered as a continuous intravenous infusion of 1.5 million units over 1 hour. The resulting systemic lytic effect persists for as long as 24 hours after the infusion, and great care must be taken to minimize the risk of hemorrhage during this period.

Tissue plasminogen activator, in contrast to streptokinase, is a fibrin-specific substance that activates plasminogen bound to a fibrin thrombus, theoretically resulting in the release of plasmin at the level of the clot. Indeed, tissue plasminogen activator causes far less derangement of the hemostatic system than streptokinase, as manifested by significantly less reduction in the concentration of fibrin and fibrinogen. Because of its short half-life (5.7 minutes), whatever systemic effects tissue plasminogen activator may have should resolve within 30 minutes of its discontinuation. The widespread clinical application of tissue plasminogen activator has followed the introduction of recombinant DNA technology for its production (rt-PA).

The approved intravenous dose of rt-PA is 100 mg given over 3 hours. Usually 60 mg is delivered over the first hour (6-mg bolus, 54-mg infusion), 20 mg over the second hour, and 20 mg over the third hour. Patency of the occluded vessel is restored in 60 to 75 per cent of cases. Several studies have indicated that treatment with rt-PA can limit the size of the infarct, preserve left ventricular function, and reduce mortality. When compared directly with streptokinase, rt-PA previously proved to be more efficacious in restoring vessel patency, whether given early (within 3 hours) or late (3 to 6 hours) after the onset of ischemic pain. However, more recent studies suggest that patency rates with rt-PA and streptokinase may be more nearly equal.

Despite its relative specificity for fibrin, it should be noted that the risk of significant bleeding with rt-PA remains substantial. This risk is compounded by the routine use of adjunctive anticoagulant or antiplatelet therapy (see later) and by the frequent placement of intra-arterial and intravenous sheaths. Bleeding is most common at the site of vascular access, although intracranial and visceral hemorrhages occur rarely. As with all other thrombolytic agents, the treating physicians must remain vigilant for any hemorrhagic complications that may occur in association with rt-PA.

APSAC is chemically synthesized from a complex of streptokinase and plasminogen by placing an anisoyl group at the active site of the plasminogen molecule. This anisoyl group temporarily blocks plasminogen's fibrinolytic activity. The complex, when given in small doses, displays modest specificity for fibrin. Activation occurs by a process of gradual deacylation (over 90 to 105 minutes), and the longer half-life of the complex allows the administration of a single intravenous bolus. This agent may be associated with a lower rate of acute reocclusion of the vessel. Clinical trials, conducted largely in Europe, have reported reperfusion rates in the 50 to 80 per cent range, with corresponding improvements in ventricular function and mortality. APSAC is given as a 30-mg bolus over 4 to 5 minutes, a dose at which systemic fibrinolysis occurs with production of a lytic state for a minimum of 12 hours. It has not yet been approved for clinical use in the United States.

scu-PA is a direct plasminogen activator and is itself converted to urokinase by plasmin. Urokinase is a serine protease that also activates plasminogen directly. scu-PA displays high specificity for fibrin and may eventually find its greatest use in the synergistic enhancement of the thrombolytic potency of rt-PA. Urokinase, when given intravenously as a bolus of 1.5 million units followed by a continuous infusion of 1.5 million units over 90 minutes, may produce effects similar to those of 70 mg rt-PA in regard to vessel patency, left ventricular function, and early mortality. However, it produces a systemic lytic state like that observed with streptokinase. Urokinase has also been given by the intracoronary route in doses ranging from 4000 to 6000 units per minute for up to 2 hours, with an average dose of 500,000 units. scu-PA has not yet been approved for clinical use; urokinase has not been widely used in the treatment of acute myocardial infarction.

Having decided to administer thrombolytic therapy, the physician must determine which agent, intravenous streptokinase or rt-PA, is preferable. There is no absolutely right answer. rt-PA gained initial favor in the United States primarily because of early reports of its relatively greater efficacy in restoring the patency of the infarct-related artery. More recent studies suggest that reperfusion rates with intravenous streptokinase and rt-PA, given in conjunction with aspirin and heparin, are more nearly equal. Both agents, especially when administered within 3 hours of symptom onset, definitely improve short- and long-term survival rates.

Secondary concerns about the choice of a thrombolytic agent include the desirability of avoiding a systemic lytic state, nonfibrinolytic side effects, and cost. Clearly, rt-PA causes less derangement of the coagulation system; yet, clinical bleeding complications remain problematic. The fibrinolytic effects of rt-PA should theoretically dissipate within 30 minutes of its discontinuation, whereas a systemic lytic state persists for as long as 24 hours after streptokinase administration. In contrast to rt-PA, streptokinase is associated with a variety of side effects, such as allergic reactions (cross-reactivity caused by previous streptococcal infections), fever, nausea, vomiting, and hypotension. These problems occur, in the aggregate, with a frequency of 10 to 20 per cent. The routine prophylactic use of antihistamines or corticosteroids is not recommended. Streptokinase is also not likely to be effective if given a second time between 10 days and 6 months of its initial administration because of the production of antistreptokinase antibodies. Finally, rt-PA is nearly 20 times more expensive than streptokinase, a difference in cost that continues to spark great controversy.

We cannot categorically recommend one agent over the other for all patients with acute myocardial infarction. Rather, we advise the physician to exercise judgment based on the exigencies of the particular case.

Adjunctive Measures

Patients receiving rt-PA should be given simultaneously a 5000-unit bolus of heparin, followed by a continuous intravenous infusion of heparin at a rate sufficient to keep the activated partial thromboplastin time at one and one-half to two times control values. The use of heparin in a patient being treated with streptokinase is more problematic; a conservative approach would dictate that the activated partial thromboplastin time fall to less than twice the control value before heparin is added. In practice, however, its simultaneous delivery has been accepted, usually without an initial bolus. Aspirin (160 to 325 mg per day) should be administered to all patients receiving thrombolytic therapy and continued indefinitely unless contraindicated by bleeding.

Other measures to alter the balance of myocardial oxygen supply and demand are always essential. Sublingual nitroglycerin (0.4 mg) should be given immediately, as dictated by the systemic blood pressure, to ascertain whether the myocardial injury might respond to the nitrate-induced changes in coronary tone, collateral flow, and ventricular preload. Nitroglycerin can also be administered safely as a continuous intravenous infusion (25 to 500 micrograms per minute) with careful monitoring of the blood pressure. Intravenous administration of beta-blocking agents is also beneficial because they may improve survival and decrease the incidence of recurrent infarction and ischemia. In the United States, only the cardioselective agent metoprolol has been approved for such use. Metoprolol is given in three equal intravenous doses of 5 mg, separated by 2 to 5 minutes, with close observation of the patient. Contraindications to its use include second- or third-degree atrioventricular block, first-degree atrioventricular block (PR interval longer than 0.24 second), bradycardia of less than 50 beats per minute, congestive heart failure, hypotension (systolic blood pressure less than 95 mmHg), and asthma. If the patient tolerates the full 15-mg loading dose, metoprolol should be continued orally beginning 6 to 8 hours later, first as 50 mg twice daily and advancing to 100 mg twice daily as tolerated. Other oral beta-blocking agents can be substituted if necessary. The goals of such therapy are a resting heart rate near 60 beats per minute and a systolic blood pressure in the range of 110 to 120 mmHg. Although the calcium channel antagonists have not been demonstrated to limit infarct size, they can be extremely helpful measures in controlling blood pressure or alleviating coronary vasospasm. Patients who demonstrate persistent injury, hemodynamic instability, or both may benefit from intra-aortic balloon counterpulsation.

Post-Thrombolytic Care

Under even the best circumstances, only 75 per cent of patients achieve reperfusion with thrombolytic therapy. Clinical markers of reperfusion are somewhat imprecise. These indicators include resolution of chest pain, return of ST segment elevation to baseline, and the appearance of particular ventricular arrhythmias (frequent, late-cycle premature ventricular beats or accelerated idioventricular rhythms). Such ventricular arrhythmias do not presage ventricular fibrillation. None of these criteria alone can predict successful reperfusion; the occurrence of all three is usually required. Reperfusion is typically accompanied by a higher and earlier rise (8 to 12 hours) of the myocardial-specific creatine kinase level than is observed in patients who do not receive thrombolytic therapy. Unfortunately, 10 to 20 per cent of patients who achieve successful reperfusion experience early reocclusion.

Given the fact that a high-grade coronary artery stenosis remains at the site of a previous thrombotic occlusion in the vast majority of patients, and the fact that reocclusion may be most closely related to the severity of the stenosis, it seems logical to perform selective percutaneous transluminal coronary artery angioplasty (PTCA) immediately or soon (within 48 hours) after reperfusion. However, on the basis of several recently completed clinical trials, the routine, empiric use of PTCA, either early (18 to 48 hours) or late (7 to 10 days) after infarction, is no longer recommended. PTCA, or revascularization surgery where appropriate, should be undertaken when recurrent ischemia, whether spontaneous or exercise induced, intervenes during the hospital course. "Rescue" PTCA, which is performed immediately after a failed course of thrombolytic therapy, can be undertaken by highly skilled operators when signs of continuing myocardial injury and hemodynamic instability persist. The associated risks of bleeding and other complications (e.g., ventricular arrhythmias, repeated reocclusion, vessel dissection) are higher under such circumstances.

Direct or Primary Percutaneous Transluminal Coronary Artery Angioplasty

This term refers specifically to the use of PTCA, without thrombolytic therapy, as a direct, first line intervention in the management of patients with acute myocardial infarction. PTCA under these circumstances can be performed in patients for whom thrombolysis is contraindicated and in those who display ST segment depression (as well as elevation) on the electrocardiogram. The results of the procedure compare favorably with those of thrombolytic therapy when performed by highly skilled operators. Obviously, the risk of bleeding is lower than with thrombolysis. Patency of the vessel may be restored with a higher frequency (85 per cent), and the size of the residual coronary artery lumen, coronary blood flow, and ventricular function may be better than can be achieved with the use of thrombolytic agents. New mechanical devices under investigation, such as endovascular stents, atherectomy catheters, and laser probes, will continue to expand the role of PTCA. Nevertheless, only a few centers can accomplish direct PTCA within the time frame (2 to 3 hours from symptom onset) necessary for optimal results. The requirements of a dedicated, continuously available catheterization laboratory, highly skilled operators, and on-call technical personnel make such an approach inappropriate for widespread application.

Coronary Artery Bypass Surgery

Coronary artery bypass graft (CABG) surgery in the treatment of acute myocardial infarction suffers from the same constraints as PTCA. The necessary resources for CABG surgery for pa-

tients who develop acute myocardial infarction outside the hospital must be mobilized quickly. Nevertheless, because of improvements in surgical and anesthetic techniques, and in the techniques of myocardial preservation at the time of surgery, the operative mortality for properly selected patients (less than 6 hours from onset of pain) may be as low as 2 per cent at selected centers. CABG surgery can be undertaken urgently for patients who develop acute coronary occlusion during the course of coronary angiography or PTCA; its safety and efficacy can be enhanced by placement of a "bail-out" perfusion catheter across the obstruction (when feasible) and by placement of an intra-aortic balloon for temporary hemodynamic support. Some centers are now using percutaneous cardiopulmonary bypass in the catheterization laboratory to maximize hemodynamic support. The risk of perioperative myocardial infarction is higher when CABG surgery is undertaken for failed or complicated PTCA, but it is still acceptable. CABG surgery can also be performed after successful thrombolysis for patients who have recurrent ischemia but whose coronary anatomy is not suitable for PTCA.

POSTINFARCTION ISCHEMIC SYNDROMES

The development of signs and symptoms of recurrent ischemia after acute myocardial infarction is an ominous event. Given the associated increase in both morbidity (heart failure and arrhythmias) and mortality, an aggressive treatment approach is warranted. Ischemia can occur in many different forms; it may be accompanied by angina, or it may be silent. It may arise from the zone of the infarct or from noncontiguous myocardial segments. Reinfarction or infarct extension can ensue, with the attendant risk of progressive ventricular dysfunction, heart failure, and death.

The pathogenesis of postinfarction ischemia is similar to that of the original infarct. Acute coronary artery reocclusion, usually by a platelet-fibrin thrombus or, less frequently, by an intimal flap created at the time of the initial manipulation of the vessel, complicates the course of 10 to 20 per cent of patients who achieved initial reperfusion with thrombolysis, PTCA, or both. Further instability of the underlying atherosclerotic plaque with rupture, or propagation of a subtotally occlusive thrombus, can also precipitate recurrent ischemia. Coronary vasospasm may also complicate matters, leading to a further increase in coronary vascular resistance and a decrement in coronary artery blood flow. Precipitants of ischemia not related to the plaque must always be sought and corrected. These include inappropriate tachycardia or hypertension, anemia, fever, thyrotoxicosis, hypoxemia, and the use of medications that may have deleterious consequences, such as sympathomimetics for bronchospasm.

Detection of postinfarction ischemia must always rely on a high index of suspicion. Chest pain must be carefully evaluated and, when possible, distinguished from other common causes of chest pain in the postinfarction patient, especially pericarditis. New ischemic electrocardiographic changes, most frequently involving the ST segment and the T wave, can aid in the diagnosis. These changes may be observed in the zone of the infarct or at a remote site. The latter phenomenon has been referred to as "ischemia at a distance," an event that presages an even worse prognosis. Even in the absence of new electrocardiographic changes, pain of a nature and quality similar to that associated with the original infarction should be interpreted as having an ischemic origin until proved otherwise.

The absence of chest pain does not exclude the presence of recurrent ischemia. Actually, postinfarction patients may more often have asymptomatic than symptomatic ST segment and T wave changes on continuous electrocardiographic recordings. For this reason, the telemetry monitor tracings that are now a routine feature of both coronary care and intermediate care surveillance should be carefully screened for the presence of both arrhythmias and electrocardiographic repolarization abnormalities. Finally, in the absence of documented ischemia in the convalescent period, the potential for recurrent ischemia or reinfarction can be assessed by predischarge, submaximal exercise testing, preferably in conjunction with radionuclide imaging.

It has also been shown that patients with a non–Q wave infarct are at high risk for recurrent ischemia. Although the hospital mortality is lower for these patients than for those with a Q wave infarct, patients with a non–Q wave infarct are more likely to have recurrent ischemia and reinfarction. Therefore, the non–Q wave infarct should be considered to be an incomplete event that leaves behind susceptible myocardium. The search for ischemia, be it spontaneous or provoked with exercise testing, should be an aggressive enterprise in patients with non–Q wave infarctions.

Infarct extension complicates the course of as many as 10 per cent of patients with acute myocardial infarction. It may be distinguished from postinfarction angina by the presence of prolonged pain or persistent electrocardiographic changes. Infarct extension occurs in the zone of

the original infarct and depends for its diagnosis on a re-elevation of the myocardial-specific fraction of creatine kinase (CK-MB). Extension may occur more frequently in patients who display an early CK-MB rise (less than 15 hours), during the first infarction in overweight women, in diabetics, or in patients with non–Q wave infarcts. Infarct extension may explain the progressively downhill course of many patients who develop cardiogenic shock.

Management of Postinfarction Myocardial Ischemia

In the absence of any obvious contraindication (advanced age, underlying medical illness), the management of a patient with a postinfarction ischemic syndrome should be aggressive, with a view toward prompt coronary angiography and revascularization. Concomitant medical therapy is also essential.

The general measures of oxygen administration, analgesia, relief of anxiety, antipyresis, correction of anemia (hematocrit greater than 30 per cent), and withdrawal of offending medications are as vital here as they are for the initial event. Nitroglycerin should be given sublingually (0.4 mg) and the dose repeated as many as two more times over 15 minutes, as tolerated by the blood pressure, should pain or electrocardiographic changes persist. Although nitrates are not recommended for the patient with a completed infarct, they play an important role in the treatment of postinfarction ischemia. They are available in sublingual, oral, transmucosal, and transcutaneous preparations, but they must be administered in such a way as to avoid nitrate tolerance (Table 2). In general, nitrates remain most effective when the patient is exposed to them for the shortest time possible over the course of 24 hours. Delivery of isosorbide dinitrate orally or 2 per cent nitroglycerin ointment transcutaneously every 4 to 6 hours, for example, is no longer recommended. A nitrate "holiday" is preferable. Alternative approaches include the use of sublingual isosorbide dinitrate (half-life, 1 to 2 hours) at 4- to 6-hour intervals, oral isosorbide dinitrate on a three-times-daily basis, or 2 per cent nitroglycerin ointment applied every 6 to 8 hours, but withdrawn for at least 6 hours during every 24-hour period.

Despite the well-documented tolerance that develops with the nonparenteral forms of nitrates, enthusiasm surrounds the intravenous use of nitroglycerin for angina or ischemic electrocardiographic changes that are refractory to more conventional medical measures. Nitroglycerin administered intravenously can promptly relieve ischemia, both when first instituted and when its

TABLE 2. **Commonly Used Nitrate Preparations***

Agent	Dosage	Onset of Effect (min)	Duration of Effect
Sublingual NTG	0.3–0.6 mg	2–5	10–30 min
Sublingual ISDN	2.5–10 mg	3–15	1–2 hr
Oral ISDN	5–40 mg	15–30	3–6 hr
2% NTG ointment	½–2 in	20–60	3–8 hr

*Adapted from Frishman WH: Pharmacology of the nitrates in angina pectoris. Am J Cardiol 56:81, 1985. Used by permission.
Abbreviations: NTG = nitroglycerin; ISDN = isosorbide dinitrate.

dose is increased, even after several hours of a constant infusion. It is generally well tolerated, although it should be avoided in hypotensive patients (systolic blood pressure less than 95 mmHg), particularly those with right ventricular infarction. Intravenous nitroglycerin is usually begun at a dose of 25 micrograms per minute and increased thereafter in 25-microgram increments. Doses of several hundred micrograms per minute are not uncommon. Continuous monitoring of the systemic blood pressure with an indwelling radial artery catheter is recommended when the dose of intravenous nitroglycerin exceeds 150 micrograms per minute. Problems with its prolonged use in large doses include methemoglobinemia and ethanol intoxication. The latter reaction occurs because most commercially available forms of nitroglycerin for intravenous use are prepared with ethanol as a diluent.

Beta blockade occupies a prominent place in the management of patients with myocardial infarction (Table 3). The use of metoprolol intravenously in the acute phase, either alone or as an adjunct to reperfusion therapy, has been dis-cussed. Such therapy may limit the size of the infarct, reduce the frequency of reinfarction, and improve survival. For those patients not receiving a beta blocker who develop a postinfarction ischemic syndrome, the addition of such an agent to the medical regimen can be beneficial. Beta-adrenoreceptor blockade can improve the ratio of oxygen supply to demand by counteracting those perturbations that lead to an increase in myocardial oxygen demand, such as tachycardia and hypertension. In general, a shorter-acting agent (propranolol or metoprolol), especially one that can be given intravenously, is preferred in the acute setting. Pindolol, because of its intrinsic sympathomimetic activity, should be avoided. In patients with important bronchospastic lung disease, selection of a cardioselective agent (beta$_1$ blocker) may be advisable. Infusions of the ultra-short-acting cardioselective agent esmolol may prove helpful in those situations where beta blockade might be beneficial but also potentially dangerous, such as in patients with depressed ventricular function or bronchospasm.

The calcium channel antagonists have made a

TABLE 3. **Commonly Used Beta-Adrenoreceptor Antagonists***

Agent	Relative Beta$_1$ Selectivity	Lipophilicity	ISA	Elimination Half-Life (hr)	Potency Ratio (Propranolol = 1)	Dose
Propranolol	0	+++	0	3.5–6.0	1	IV: 0.25-mg test dose, then increments of 1.0 mg up to 0.15 mg/kg total PO: 40–80 mg qid
Metoprolol	+	++	0	3–7	1	IV: 5-mg bolus q 5 min up to 15 mg total PO: 50–100 mg bid
Atenolol	+	+	0	6–9	1	PO: 50–100 mg qd
Nadolol	0	+	0	14–25	1	PO: 40–80 mg qd
Pindolol	0	++	+	3–4	6	PO: 15–20 mg tid
Timolol	0	+	0	3–4	6	PO: 10–20 mg bid
Esmolol	+	+	0	9 min	1	IV: 500 µg/kg bolus over 1 min; then infusion of 50 µg/kg/min; repeat bolus of 500 µg/kg can be given 5 min later and the infusion increased to 100 µg/kg/min; maximum dose, 200 µg/kg/min

*Adapted from Frishman WH, Kaftka KR, and Meltzer AH: Anti-anginal agents. Part 1. β-Blockers. Hosp Formul 21:62, 1986. Used by permission.
Abbreviation and symbols: ISA = intrinsic sympathomimetic activity; 0 = none; + = low; ++ = moderate; +++ = high.

substantial contribution to the treatment of patients with ischemic heart disease (Table 4). For patients with postinfarction ischemic syndromes, the addition of a calcium channel antagonist to the medical regimen can often provide salutary effects. Diltiazem, for example, in a dose of 90 mg four times daily, has proved to be effective in reducing the incidence of reinfarction in patients with non–Q wave infarctions. It is not yet known whether nifedipine and verapamil may have the same effect. Of the three agents, nifedipine is the most potent coronary and peripheral arterial vasodilator. It can be given orally or the contents of a capsule (10 mg) can be aspirated into a sterile syringe and administered sublingually. Nifedipine is particularly useful when systemic hypertension coexists with postinfarction ischemia. Verapamil is used most frequently when supraventricular tachycardia (paroxysmal supraventricular tachycardia, atrial flutter, atrial fibrillation) precipitates or complicates myocardial ischemia. It is also a potent antihypertensive agent. Verapamil is given intravenously in 5- to 10-mg boluses (0.075 to 0.15 mg per kg) to treat supraventricular tachycardia. The dose can be repeated in 15 to 30 minutes if necessary.

All of the previously mentioned agents can lower the blood pressure, the nitrates least effectively. However, the nitrates can lower ventricular preload (venodilatation), and the possible subsequent fall in cardiac output can be deleterious. The beta blockers, given in combination with diltiazem or verapamil, can produce conduction system disturbances ranging from profound sinus bradycardia to high-grade atrioventricular block. The beta blockers and the calcium channel antagonists, especially verapamil and nifedipine, can impair ventricular contractile performance when used in combination, and caution must be exercised lest heart failure ensue.

Heparin and aspirin are standard adjunctive therapies to thrombolysis, with or without PTCA.

Aspirin is continued indefinitely (160 to 325 mg per day). Most experts now recommend that heparin be continued for at least 5 days after successful reperfusion. If postinfarction ischemia occurs thereafter, heparin should be reinstituted as a bolus of 5000 units followed by a continuous infusion to keep the activated partial thromboplastin time at one and one-half to two times the control value unless contraindications to its use exist. Such contraindications include bleeding and a previously documented heparin-induced thrombocytopenia.

For patients with postinfarction ischemia who fail to respond to these aggressive medical measures, intra-aortic balloon pumping (IABP) should be instituted as quickly as possible. IABP frequently results in resolution of ischemia (pain, ST segment deviations) within minutes and allows subsequent coronary angiography and PTCA or CABG surgery to be performed under more stable conditions. Vascular access is the chief problem associated with institution of IABP. Anticoagulation with heparin and prophylactic cephalosporin (or vancomycin in the allergic patient) antibiotic coverage should be provided as long as the balloon is in place.

Coronary angiography and revascularization therapy are the next steps in the management of patients with postinfarction ischemia. The decision to proceed with these interventions must always be tempered by the expected outcome, the age of the patient, and the presence of other severe medical problems. Definition of the coronary anatomy with angiography should guide the appropriate choice for revascularization. In certain patients—for example, those with acute thrombotic reocclusion after initially successful reperfusion therapy—re-treatment with a thrombolytic agent via the intracoronary or intravenous route would be reasonable.

When appropriate, PTCA should be directed at the culprit lesion; stenoses in other coronary

TABLE 4. **Calcium Channel Antagonists***

Agent	Dosage	Onset of Action	Peak Effect	Half-Life	Negative Inotropy	Bradycardia, AV Block
Nifedipine	PO: 10–40 mg tid or qid	20 min	1–2 hr	4 hr	0†	0
	SL: 10–20 mg q 4 hr	3 min				
Diltiazem	PO: 30–120 mg tid or qid	15 min	30 min	4 hr	+	+
Verapamil	IV: 5–10 mg (0.075–0.15 mg/kg)	2 min	3–5 min	Less than 30 min	+	+ +
	PO: 80–120 mg tid or qid	2 hr	3–4 hr	8–12 hr‡	+	+ +

*Adapted from Singh BN: Clinical pharmacology of calcium antagonist drugs. Cornell Postgraduate Course on Calcium Antagonists. New York, Medcom, 1982, p. 5.

†Nifedipine can cause left ventricular dysfunction when used in combination with beta-blockers. It also exerts negative inotropic effects in patients with pre-existent heart failure.

‡Half-life of verapamil increases with consecutive doses.

Abbreviations and symbols: AV = atrioventricular; SL = sublingual; 0 = none; + = mild; + + = moderate.

arteries should not be approached at this time. The patient can return for elective PTCA of the other lesions, as dictated by their severity or functional importance, in several weeks. Alternatively, angiography may reveal coronary lesions that would best be treated with CABG surgery, such as left main coronary artery disease, three-vessel disease, or coronary lesions that would not be amenable to PTCA because of their morphologic characteristics (their length or the presence of residual thrombus) or location (lesions at bifurcations, angulated or tortuous position). Finally, it should be recognized that CABG surgery performed urgently for postinfarction ischemia is associated with a higher rate of perioperative infarction and death than elective operation.

CARDIAC ARRHYTHMIAS

Ventricular Arrhythmias

If searched for carefully, ventricular arrhythmias are ubiquitous early after acute myocardial infarction. Virtually all patients experience *ventricular premature beats* (VPBs). In the past, VPBs were treated with an antiarrhythmic agent only if they were considered to be harbingers of malignant ventricular arrhythmias. These so-called warning VPBs included those that were frequent, multifocal, repetitive, or early ("R-on-T phenomenon"). We now realize that VPBs can trigger ventricular tachyarrhythmias even if they lack these features. This fact has led to the widespread prophylactic use of antiarrhythmic agents, especially lidocaine, in patients with acute infarction. Prophylactic therapy has been shown to reduce the incidence of ventricular fibrillation, although the effect on mortality is uncertain. It is our practice to treat with lidocaine all patients under age 75 years in whom infarction is strongly suspected, beginning with a loading intravenous bolus of 1.5 mg per kg, followed 10 minutes later by a second bolus of 0.5 mg per kg. A continuous intravenous infusion is then started at a dose of 2 to 4 mg per minute (approximately 50 micrograms per kg per minute). These dosages should be reduced by approximately 50 per cent in patients with advanced congestive heart failure or liver disease. Because the half-life of lidocaine increases during continuous intravenous infusion, it may be necessary to reduce the rate of the infusion after several hours to avoid late toxicity. In view of the high incidence of toxicity in patients over age 75 years, we do not usually treat these patients prophylactically with lidocaine. Toxic manifestations include paresthesia, lassitude, somnolence, confu-

sion, slurred speech, diplopia, and seizures. We usually continue prophylactic treatment for 48 hours and then taper the drug in the absence of breakthrough arrhythmias.

In patients who continue to have frequent or complex VPBs despite treatment with lidocaine, or in those who are intolerant of lidocaine, procainamide is a useful alternative. The average loading dose is 1000 mg intravenously, which should be given over 30 to 45 minutes. The blood pressure must be monitored carefully during the administration of the loading dose to avoid hypotension. A maintenance intravenous infusion should then be started at a rate of 2 to 4 mg per minute (approximately 50 micrograms per kg per minute).

The occurrence of *ventricular tachycardia* during the early hours after acute infarction has been reduced, but not eliminated, by the prophylactic use of antiarrhythmic agents. The treatment of this arrhythmia depends on its hemodynamic consequences. Patients who are unconscious should be electrically cardioverted immediately. Because this arrhythmia is often quite sensitive to electrical energy, the magnitude of the initial direct current shock should be 10 to 50 joules. Anteroposterior placement of the electrodes may reduce the energy level required for cardioversion. If the initial shock is unsuccessful, the energy level should be increased by 25 to 50 joules for each subsequent shock. "Thumpversion," striking the patient on the sternum with the fist, sometimes terminates ventricular tachycardia, but this maneuver is not a reliable form of treatment and should never be performed in a patient who is awake.

If the patient is conscious, time is usually available for a trial of pharmacologic cardioversion. The drugs of choice are lidocaine or procainamide, administered intravenously in the doses indicated previously. An alternative is bretylium tosylate, 5 to 10 mg per kg, given by intravenous infusion over 3 to 5 minutes. If the arrhythmia is converted, a maintenance infusion of 1 to 2 mg per minute should be started. The principal side effect of bretylium is orthostatic hypotension, which limits its usefulness. If drug therapy fails and electrical cardioversion is to be performed on a conscious patient, methohexital sodium, 50 to 100 mg, or diazepam, 5 to 10 mg intravenously, should be administered first. Hypokalemia, hypomagnesemia, and hypoxemia should be searched for and corrected in all patients who have had ventricular tachycardia.

When ventricular tachycardia occurs (or recurs) 2 or more weeks after infarction, it is often an indication either that myocardial ischemia is present or that the infarct is large and that considerable hemodynamic compromise is present. In such patients, the arrhythmia may recur and may be difficult to suppress with drugs. The first step in management is to treat congestive heart failure, ischemia, hypoxemia, fever, or electrolyte imbalance if any of these problems are present. Even when these complications have been alleviated, specific antiarrhythmic therapy is often required. The selection of an effective antiarrhythmic agent or a combination of agents is often a painstaking empiric process, which can be guided in part by the use of ambulatory electrocardiographic (Holter) monitoring, invasive electrophysiologic testing, or both. Recent data suggest that effective suppression of arrhythmia documented by these techniques does not necessarily predict a better long-term prognosis after acute infarction. Cardiologic consultation is recommended to assist in management. Because a separate chapter in this volume is devoted to the treatment of tachyarrhythmias, only the high points of antiarrhythmic therapy are mentioned here.

Antiarrhythmic agents have been classified into four groups on the basis of their physiologic properties. Class I antiarrhythmic agents, which block the fast sodium channel in the myocardial cell membrane, are the mainstay of treatment of recurrent ventricular tachycardia. These agents are subdivided into Classes A, B, and C. Class IA drugs (quinidine, procainamide, disopyramide), which prolong the duration of the action potential, are the agents used most commonly, although disopyramide has fallen into disfavor because of its troublesome side effects of urinary retention and congestive heart failure. Drugs in this class can worsen ventricular arrhythmias (proarrhythmia) in approximately 10 per cent of patients. Class IB drugs (phenytoin, tocainide, mexiletine), which shorten the duration of the action potential, are considered to be second line drugs because, as a general rule, they tend to be less effective than Class IA agents. The powerful new Class IC agents (flecainide, encainide, lorcainide, propafenone), which slow electrical conduction, show great promise, but their use may be restricted because of their prominent proarrhythmic effects. Among the Class IC agents, only flecainide and encainide have been approved for general use at the time of this writing. Recent data suggest that they should be used with caution after acute infarction because of their proarrhythmic effects.

Class II agents, the beta-adrenergic receptor antagonists, are almost never used alone in the treatment of recurrent ventricular tachycardia but are sometimes used in combination with Class I agents.

Class III agents, such as amiodarone, block potassium channels. Amiodarone is effective in preventing recurrent ventricular tachycardia, but it is used only when all other drugs have failed because of its many serious side effects, including pneumonitis, hepatitis, corneal deposits, and thyroid disturbances. Oral dosing is complicated because of its long onset of action, variable pharmacokinetics, and long half-life. Amiodarone is seldom useful for the urgent management of ventricular arrhythmias because of its prolonged loading period.

Class IV agents (verapamil, nifedipine, diltiazem), the slow calcium channel antagonists, have little use in the treatment of ventricular arrhythmias.

An important question, as yet unanswered, is whether patients with acute infarction should routinely undergo ambulatory electrocardiographic monitoring or invasive electrophysiologic testing in an attempt to disclose or induce ventricular arrhythmias. A large clinical trial is currently in progress to answer this important question. Until the data are available, it is our practice to perform ambulatory monitoring only on those patients who have displayed frequent or complex VPBs during hospitalization. Antiarrhythmic therapy is instituted if nonsustained or sustained ventricular tachycardia is detected. We reserve invasive electrophysiologic testing for those patients who have had recurrent, sustained ventricular tachycardia. Invasive testing in these patients is used to aid in the selection of an antiarrhythmic agent. New information may soon lead to modification of these approaches.

Accelerated idioventricular rhythm is a slow form of ventricular tachycardia, with rates that vary between 60 and 110 beats per minute. This arrhythmia, which is more common in patients with inferior infarction, usually develops when the underlying sinus rate decelerates and the rate of depolarization of an ectopic ventricular focus increases. Because the arrhythmia is usually transient and intermittent, it often does not cause hemodynamic instability. If it is sustained, however, the loss of a synchronized atrial contraction may reduce the cardiac output. The arrhythmia should then be treated by suppressing the ventricular focus with standard doses of lidocaine or by increasing the sinus rate with atropine (0.5 mg intravenously). Because accelerated idioventricular rhythm is sometimes associated with more malignant forms of ventricular tachycardia, some physicians choose to treat it whenever it is detected. Whichever approach is followed, patients with this arrhythmia require careful monitoring of the cardiac rhythm.

Ventricular fibrillation, the most common cause

of death in patients with acute infarction before hospitalization, is still a threat after admission to the CCU. As with ventricular tachycardia, the incidence of ventricular fibrillation has been sharply reduced, but not eliminated, by the prophylactic use of lidocaine. When it does occur, the treatment is immediate electrical defibrillation with 200 to 360 joules of direct current energy. The success of defibrillation depends critically on the time interval between the onset of fibrillation and delivery of the first shock. Therefore, speed is essential. "Quick-look" electrodes, which can both detect the cardiac rhythm and deliver the shock, are useful to confirm rapidly the presence of the arrhythmia in unmonitored patients. In contrast to ventricular fibrillation, asystole does not respond to electrical defibrillation. This problem should instead be treated with epinephrine, 0.5 to 1 mg, administered either intravenously or via the endotracheal tube in the absence of an intravenous line. This agent occasionally causes fine ventricular fibrillation to appear, and an attempt to defibrillate is then appropriate. External or transvenous pacing can also be attempted, but asystole is notoriously difficult to treat successfully, and the mortality rate is high.

In patients with small infarcts and good left ventricular function, the occurrence of ventricular fibrillation during the early hours after infarction does not usually portend a poor prognosis. Electrical defibrillation, if performed promptly, is usually successful, and the arrhythmia does not tend to recur as long as defibrillation is followed by treatment with standard doses of lidocaine or procainamide. By contrast, ventricular fibrillation in patients with large infarcts and pump failure is often difficult to treat and does tend to recur. Electrolyte imbalance, myocardial ischemia, and hypoxemia should be corrected, and every effort should be made to improve cardiac pump function. Bretylium tosylate, 5 to 10 mg per kg intravenously over 3 to 5 minutes, is sometimes helpful in suppressing the arrhythmia. Despite these interventions, the prognosis of these patients is often poor because of the extensive damage to the myocardium that is usually present.

Supraventricular Arrhythmias

Sinus bradycardia occurs more commonly in patients with inferoposterior rather than anterior infarction because of the enhancement of vagal tone that may accompany infarction of the inferoposterior wall. Marked sinus bradycardia in this setting usually responds well to treatment with atropine, 0.5 mg intravenously. Paradoxical bradycardia and hypotension, mediated by vagal stimulation, are rare complications that have been reported in patients with acute infarction who have received nitroglycerin. Here, too, atropine is the drug of choice. Marked sinus bradycardia in a patient with an anterior infarction may be caused by ischemia or infarction of the sinus node (sick sinus syndrome). Atrial pacing may be required if severe bradycardia persists after a trial of atropine.

Sinus tachycardia is common in patients with acute infarction as a consequence of fever, pain, or anxiety, all of which may be associated with enhanced sympathetic tone. Sinus tachycardia that persists after these three problems have been treated should encourage the physician to look carefully for evidence of congestive heart failure, another common and worrisome cause of sinus tachycardia. A patient with sinus tachycardia should not be treated with a beta-adrenergic receptor blocking agent until it is certain that heart failure is not present. In patients with persistent sinus tachycardia and no evidence of heart failure, treatment with propranolol or metoprolol, 1 to 10 mg intravenously, is indicated to slow the heart rate to less than 90 beats per minute and thereby reduce myocardial oxygen demand.

The new onset of *atrial fibrillation* in acute myocardial infarction may be caused by congestive heart failure, pericarditis, atrial infarction, pulmonary emboli, or coexisting severe chronic obstructive pulmonary disease. The treatment of choice is digoxin, 0.5 to 1 mg intravenously, to slow the ventricular response rate to less than 90 beats per minute. Additional doses of digoxin (0.25 mg) may be given hourly until the target heart rate has been achieved or a total dose of 1.5 mg has been administered over 18 to 24 hours. Patients may occasionally, but not consistently, revert to sinus rhythm after treatment with digoxin. Verapamil, 5 to 10 mg intravenously, is an effective alternative to digoxin for rate control, but it should not be used if congestive heart failure is present. If the ventricular response rate is rapid and the patient is hemodynamically unstable, electrical cardioversion may be required to restore sinus rhythm. The patient should be premedicated with methohexital sodium, 50 to 100 mg, or diazepam, 5 to 10 mg intravenously, and supplemental oxygen should be given by face mask. The electrodes should be positioned anteriorly and posteriorly, and the countershock should be synchronized with the R wave of the electrocardiogram. The initial energy level should be 150 joules. If the first shock is not successful in restoring sinus rhythm, the energy level of each subsequent shock should be increased by 25 joules.

Atrial flutter and *supraventricular tachycardia* are uncommon in patients with acute infarction, and their treatment is discussed elsewhere in this volume.

Conduction Disturbances

Complete (third-degree) atrioventricular (AV) block can occur in patients with anterior or inferoposterior infarction, but the mechanisms and prognosis of heart block are different, depending on the anatomic location of the infarct. In patients with inferoposterior infarction, heart block is usually caused by the simultaneous occurrence of ischemia of the AV node and enhancement of vagal tone. Third-degree block may alternate with periods of Mobitz Type I (Wenckebach) second-degree block and periods of first-degree block. A stable junctional or ventricular escape mechanism may be present, and the need for temporary pacing depends on the rate and stability of the escape mechanism and the hemodynamic condition of the patient. Many physicians choose to place a temporary pacemaker in all patients with inferoposterior infarction complicated by complete heart block. Heart block is usually reversible in inferoposterior infarction, and AV nodal conduction often reappears spontaneously within 5 to 10 days. A permanent cardiac pacer is usually not required, although patients with inferoposterior infarction complicated by complete heart block usually have larger infarcts and reduced long-term survival compared with patients who do not have this complication.

When complete AV block complicates acute anterior infarction, the conduction disturbance is usually caused by an extensive infarct that has damaged both the right and left bundle branches. The prognosis is poor, even if temporary ventricular or AV sequential pacing is instituted immediately, because of the presence of severe pump dysfunction. The occurrence of complete AV block may be foreshadowed by periods of Mobitz Type II second-degree block, and therefore the latter conduction disturbance is considered to be an indication for the institution of temporary pacing.

The appearance of new *bifascicular block* also carries a substantial risk of progression to complete heart block. Bifascicular block can be manifested as right bundle branch block and left anterior fascicular block, right bundle branch block and left posterior fascicular block, or alternating right and left bundle branch block. Because complete AV block may appear suddenly in patients with bifascicular block, a temporary pacemaker should be inserted prophylactically. Alternatively, an external temporary pacing device can be kept on standby for immediate use if complete heart block appears. With recent modifications in its design, the external temporary pacer has proved effective in maintaining the cardiac rhythm until a temporary transvenous pacer can be placed. Because complete heart block occurs in no more than 30 per cent of patients with bifascicular block, the availability of an external temporary pacer obviates the need for a prophylactic transvenous pacer in approximately two-thirds of patients with bifascicular block. Placement of a permanent ventricular pacer is indicated in patients with bifascicular block only if transient or sustained complete heart block occurs. Patients with new unifascicular block (such as right bundle branch block or left anterior fascicular block) have little risk of developing complete heart block, and temporary pacing is not indicated.

HEMODYNAMIC ABNORMALITIES ASSOCIATED WITH ACUTE MYOCARDIAL INFARCTION

Hemodynamic abnormalities are the rule, not the exception, during the early phases of acute myocardial infarction. The principal determinants of cardiac performance, namely, preload, afterload, and contractility, are all affected to varying degrees. Left ventricular preload, as measured by pulmonary capillary wedge pressure, may be inappropriately low because of hypovolemia, the administration of morphine sulfate, or excess vasomotor tone. Alternatively, preload may be abnormally elevated in patients with pulmonary congestion, as the failing left ventricle relies on Starling's mechanism to maintain cardiac output. Afterload may be inappropriately elevated in the setting of depressed cardiac output and high sympathetic tone. Contractility is always impaired in the zone of the infarction and may be further compromised by associated myocardial ischemia in border zones between normal and infarcted tissue. The severity of the hemodynamic abnormality depends on the extent and location (anterior usually greater than inferior) of the infarction, as well as the presence or absence of mechanical complications such as acute mitral regurgitation, rupture of the interventricular septum or free wall, and the extent of pre-existing left ventricular dysfunction.

It is useful for the clinician to categorize patients during the early phases of acute infarction into subgroups on the basis of the degree of hemodynamic impairment. We have generally found the classification system of Forrester and associates (Table 5), which is based on invasive measurement of cardiac index (normally >2.2 liters per minute per M^2) and pulmonary capil-

TABLE 5. **Hemodynamic Classification of Forrester and Associates***

Subset	Clinical Findings	Hemodynamic Definition	Mortality (%)	Suggested Intervention
I	No pulmonary congestion or peripheral hypoperfusion	PCW < 18 CI > 2.2	2.2	Beta-adrenergic blockade if no contraindications exist
II	Isolated pulmonary congestion	PCW > 18 CI > 2.2	10.1	Diuretics, correction of hypoxemia
III	Isolated peripheral hypoperfusion	PCW < 18 CI < 2.2	22.4	Repletion of vascular volume
IV	Pulmonary congestion and peripheral hypoperfusion	PCW > 18 CI < 2.2	55.5	Diuretics, vasodilators, sympathomimetic agent with positive inotropic effects, circulatory assistance

*Modified, by permission from Forrester JS, Diamond G, Chatterjee K, et al: The New England Journal of Medicine, *295;* 1404, 1976.

Abbreviations: PCW = pulmonary capillary wedge pressure (mmHg); CI = cardiac index (liters/min/M²).

lary wedge pressure (normally <18 mmHg), to be the most useful for patient management and prognostication. Quantification of these two variables defines four hemodynamic subgroups: those with normal perfusion and no pulmonary congestion (normal cardiac index and pulmonary capillary wedge pressure), those with normal perfusion but pulmonary congestion (normal cardiac index and elevated pulmonary capillary wedge pressure), those with diminished systemic perfusion but no pulmonary congestion (reduced cardiac index and normal pulmonary capillary wedge pressure), and those with diminished perfusion and pulmonary congestion (reduced cardiac index and elevated pulmonary capillary wedge pressure). Although this classification scheme is useful, it must be recognized that patients often change from one category to another with therapy and sometimes even spontaneously. These four hemodynamic subsets generally reflect the clinical status and prognosis, and the aim of hemodynamic therapy is to achieve normal values for the cardiac index and pulmonary wedge pressure.

Invasive Hemodynamic Monitoring. Patients with clinically uncomplicated acute myocardial infarction do not need or benefit from routine invasive monitoring. These patients can be managed by careful clinical evaluation, which should consist of continuous electrocardiographic monitoring of heart rate and rhythm; frequent measurement of systemic arterial blood pressure by cuff; careful and repeated auscultation of the lung fields for evidence of pulmonary congestion; cardiac examination to detect ventricular or atrial gallops, murmurs, or pericardial rubs; assessment of the pulmonary vasculature by chest x-ray film; assessment of systemic perfusion (urinary output,

mental status, perfusion of extremities); and arterial blood sampling for Po_2, Pco_2, and pH when metabolic acidosis or hypoxemia is suspected.

We undertake invasive hemodynamic monitoring in the following settings: (1) persistent low-output state, unexplained hypotension, or shock; (2) recurrent or refractory pulmonary congestion or edema; (3) appearance of a new systolic heart murmur associated with hemodynamic instability; (4) persistent or recurrent ischemic chest pain refractory to conventional analgesics and requiring intravenous nitroglycerin; (5) extensive right ventricular infarction with hypotension; (6) evaluation of the response to intravenous vasoactive drugs or IABP; and (7) unexplained persistent sinus tachycardia. The goal of hemodynamic monitoring should always be to achieve a cardiac index and a pulmonary capillary wedge pressure as close to normal as possible. Whenever invasive monitoring is undertaken, it should be discontinued as soon as it is feasible to reduce the risk of infection.

Hypotension

During the early prehospitalization phase of acute myocardial infarction, hypotension is common and usually associated with hypovolemia (Forrester Class III). Hypotension associated with bradycardia most commonly accompanies infarction of the inferior or inferoposterior wall and usually responds to the intravenous administration of atropine (0.6 to 1 mg) and elevation of the legs. Hypotension associated with tachycardia is particularly common in patients who have received diuretics before the infarction. Marked diaphoresis, reduction of fluid intake, or vomiting may all contribute to the development of hypovolemia.

Even if the effective vascular volume is normal, relative hypovolemia may be present because ventricular compliance is reduced during the early stages of acute infarction. A pulmonary wedge pressure as high as 18 to 20 mmHg may be needed to provide sufficient preload for optimal ventricular performance. In the absence of pulmonary rales, the patient should be placed in the reverse Trendelenburg position. Atropine (a total dose not to exceed 2 mg) should be administered if sinus bradycardia is present. If hypotension persists, crystalloid solution should be administered intravenously, beginning with a bolus of 100 ml of 5 per cent dextrose in normal saline and followed by a maintenance infusion of 100 to 200 ml per hour. The patient should be carefully observed and the infusion discontinued when systolic blood pressure rises above 90 to 100 mmHg, if the patient develops dyspnea, or if pulmonary congestion develops or increases.

Recognition of hypovolemia is of particular importance in hypotensive patients because improvement in circulatory function can be readily achieved by augmentation of vascular volume. Because of the poor correlation between pulmonary capillary wedge pressure and jugular venous pulse or central venous pressure, hypovolemia may be frequently overlooked without invasive hemodynamic monitoring. Exclusion of hypovolemia as the cause of hypotension requires documentation of a depressed cardiac index despite a pulmonary wedge pressure of more than 18 mmHg.

Administration of vasoactive agents such as dopamine is indicated in the management of hypotension that persists after correction of hypovolemia and excessive vagal tone. We generally administer dopamine at doses of 2.5 to 10 micrograms per kg per minute by constant intravenous infusion and adjust the dosage, depending on the blood pressure response. When there is clinical evidence of excessive vasodilatation, an uncommon occurrence in the absence of fever or sepsis, phenylephrine (Neo-Synephrine) is the agent of choice.

The Hyperdynamic State

Patients with uncomplicated myocardial infarction often have excessive activation of the sympathetic nervous system because of pain and anxiety. The hemodynamic profile of a patient with a hyperdynamic state includes an increased heart rate, arterial hypertension, and elevation of the cardiac index in the presence of a normal or low pulmonary capillary wedge pressure.

Other causes of sinus tachycardia, such as fever, infection, persistent pain, pericarditis, or congestive heart failure, should be excluded before treatment with a beta-adrenergic blocking agent is undertaken. Propranolol is usually the drug of choice in this setting, beginning with 0.25 to 0.5 mg intravenously and increasing the dose to 1 mg if necessary. Additional doses can be administered every 5 to 10 minutes until the heart rate is less than 80 beats per minute or a total of 0.2 mg per kg has been given. When the heart rate and blood pressure have reached optimal levels, oral propranolol can be given at a dose ranging from 40 to 160 mg per day. We have recently begun using esmolol, an ultra-short-acting beta blocker, in patients in whom the use of beta-adrenergic blockage may be accompanied by adverse effects. Such patients include those with a history of congestive heart failure, a large, evolving anterior myocardial infarction, or pre-existing first-degree AV block. Esmolol should be administered intravenously in a 500 microgram per kg loading dose over 1 minute, followed by an infusion at 50 micrograms per kg per minute. The dosage can be increased by repeating the loading dose and increasing the infusion rate in 50 micrograms per kg per minute increments every 5 to 10 minutes. Most patients do not require doses in excess of 100 micrograms per kg per minute.

Pulmonary Congestion and Acute Pulmonary Edema

A mild to moderate degree of pulmonary congestion is common in patients with acute myocardial infarction. The patient complains of dyspnea and orthopnea; objective findings often include tachypnea, bibasilar pulmonary rales, an audible or palpable third heart sound, mild to moderate hypoxemia on arterial blood gas examination, and radiologic evidence of mild to moderate pulmonary venous hypertension. Therapy should be aimed at ensuring adequate arterial oxygenation and relieving pulmonary venous congestion. Reduction in the pulmonary capillary wedge pressure not only relieves pulmonary congestion but also reduces left ventricular volume, wall tension, and myocardial oxygen consumption, and it may improve subendocardial myocardial perfusion. A diuresis can often be initiated by the intravenous administration of furosemide, 20 to 40 mg. Higher doses may be necessary in patients who previously required diuretic therapy. Excessive diuresis must be avoided because it can cause a low-output state as a result of underfilling of the left ventricle, as well as electrolyte abnormalities, particularly hypokalemia. Vasodilator therapy with organic nitrates or sodium nitroprusside may also be used as an adjunct to diuretics, particularly when mitral regurgitation or systemic hypertension accompanies pulmonary venous congestion. Long-acting nitrates, particularly oral isosorbide dinitrate (10 to 40 mg orally every 3 to 4 hours), or 2 per cent nitroglycerin ointment (a patch of 0.5 to 2 inches applied cutaneously every 4 to 6 hours during the day) are useful agents.

Acute pulmonary edema is characterized by severe respiratory distress, expectoration of frothy pink sputum, tachycardia, hypertension, and cool, clammy, diaphoretic skin because of excessive activation of the sympathetic nervous system. Acute pulmonary edema is most commonly caused by extensive damage to the left ventricle, which may occur after a first myocardial infarction or as the result of multiple infarctions. Other causes of acute pulmonary edema include diminished compliance of the left ventricle with relatively normal systolic contraction (diastolic heart failure); persistent or intermittent acute mitral regurgitation caused by papillary muscle dysfunction or rupture; or profound left ventricular ischemia associated with a small or modest degree of myocardial necrosis. Regardless of the cause, rapid and marked elevation of the pulmonary capillary wedge pressure (exceeding 25 mmHg) characterizes the hemodynamic picture in acute pulmonary edema after myocardial infarction. Assessment of the left ventricular ejection fraction by radionuclide techniques is often critical in determining the etiology of the acute pulmonary edema.

The principles of management of acute cardiogenic pulmonary edema include maintenance of adequate gas exchange and a stable cardiac rhythm; correction of hypotension, if present; and rapid lowering of the pulmonary capillary wedge pressure. Frequent measurement of arterial blood gases is essential to ensure adequate gas exchange. High concentrations of oxygen (60 to 100 per cent by Ventimask or rebreathing mask) should be tried initially, and endotracheal intubation should be considered for patients who are unable to maintain an arterial Po_2 greater than 60 mmHg, who develop progressive elevation of Pco_2, or who exhibit significant respiratory or metabolic acidosis. Mechanical ventilation should be supplemented with positive end-expiratory pressure to maintain adequate oxygenation with the lowest possible oxygen concentration in the inspired air. Hemodynamic monitoring may be required to determine the optimal amount of positive end-expiratory pressure.

After adequate oxygenation has been restored, the next goal of therapy should be the rapid reduction of pulmonary capillary wedge pressure.

Initial treatment generally consists of nitrates, given intravenously, transdermally, or sublingually. Nitrates produce pharmacologic phlebotomy through their peripheral venodilator effects, shift blood volume to the extrathoracic space, and rapidly decrease pulmonary venous return and thus pulmonary capillary wedge pressure. Improvement in left ventricular function may also result from a decrease in afterload and improved oxygenation of ischemic zones of myocardium. Morphine sulfate should also be administered in small doses (1 to 5 mg intravenously) to calm the agitated patient and produce moderate venodilation. Potent loop diuretics, such as intravenous furosemide (20 to 40 mg) or ethacrynic acid (50 mg), should be given early in the treatment of pulmonary edema, but they may take 20 to 60 minutes to produce a diuresis. The dose of intravenous diuretics should be doubled if the initial response has been suboptimal after 45 to 60 minutes. Sodium nitroprusside may be of use in severely hypertensive patients or in those with significant mitral regurgitation or ventricular septal rupture. We do not use digitalis glycosides or aminophylline as a general routine. Rotating tourniquets and phlebotomy are reserved for patients with severe renal insufficiency and those whose response to high doses of intravenous diuretics remains inadequate. Inotropic and vasodilator therapy in the management of acute pulmonary edema is discussed in the section on cardiogenic shock.

Cardiogenic Shock (Low-Output, Hypotensive Syndrome)

Cardiogenic shock is a syndrome characterized by severe, prolonged tissue hypoperfusion associated with hypotension (systolic blood pressure usually $\leq$ 90 mmHg) and marked reduction in cardiac output. Cardiogenic shock results from severe impairment of left ventricular systolic function caused by a loss of muscle mass or after the development of mechanical complications, such as acute mitral regurgitation, rupture of the interventricular septum or free wall of the left ventricle, ventricular aneurysm, or right ventricular infarction. Cardiogenic shock is usually associated with damage to 40 per cent or more of the left ventricle. This syndrome may be precipitated by a small infarction in a patient with previous myocardial damage or by a single massive infarction. At autopsy, approximately 70 per cent of patients with cardiogenic shock demonstrate three-vessel coronary artery disease, usually including the left anterior descending artery. Almost all such patients are found to have thrombosis of the artery that supplies the region of recent infarction. Profound impairment of ventricular performance results in ongoing myocardial ischemia and necrosis as a consequence of systemic hypoperfusion and inadequate coronary artery blood flow. A vicious cycle is thereby created, and mortality often exceeds 80 per cent.

Severe underperfusion of various end organs caused by depressed cardiac output (cardiac index < 2.2 liters per minute per M^2) often results in progressive dysfunction. Renal failure, hepatic dysfunction, gastrointestinal bleeding secondary to ischemia, and lactic acidosis are common during the terminal stages of cardiogenic shock. Cardiac arrhythmias are also frequent accompaniments. Cardiogenic shock is more common in elderly patients, in those with diabetes, in patients with previous myocardial infarction, and in those with infarction of the anterior wall. Early thinning and stretching of necrotic myocardium (infarct expansion) may contribute to acute ventricular dilatation and precipitation of the shock syndrome. It does not appear that the location of the infarction is an independent contributor to the development of shock beyond the extent of the myocardial damage itself.

The clinical features of cardiogenic shock include moderate to profound vasoconstriction with cool, clammy skin and peripheral cyanosis; oliguria with urine output of less than 30 ml per hour; mental obtundation; a systolic blood pressure of 90 mmHg or less; and a narrow pulse pressure. Blood pressure should be determined directly from an intra-arterial catheter because cuff pressures may underestimate the true pressure by 10 to 25 mmHg as a result of intense vasoconstriction. Cheyne-Stokes respirations are particularly common in elderly patients or after the use of narcotic analgesics.

Hemodynamic findings include a low mean arterial pressure, depressed cardiac index, elevated pulmonary capillary wedge pressure, elevated systemic vascular resistance, and a widened AV oxygen difference. The cardiac index is below 2.2 liters per minute per M^2, and the pulmonary capillary wedge pressure exceeds 18 mmHg and often averages 25 mmHg (Forrester Class IV). Systemic vascular resistance is usually elevated and generally exceeds 2000 dyne-seconds per cm^5. Left ventricular function, as assessed by radionuclide ventriculography, shows severe contractile dysfunction with a global ejection fraction almost always less than 30 to 35 per cent.

The prognosis is extremely poor, with an 80 to 90 per cent hospital mortality. Survivors often have evidence of continued heart failure and cardiac arrhythmias, and the probability of long-term survival is low. The prognosis appears to be more favorable in patients under the age of 50, in those with single-vessel coronary artery disease, and in those in whom subsequent coronary artery revascularization is able to salvage a substantial amount of viable myocardium. The latter group of patients often has large areas of reversible [201]Th perfusion defects, confirming the presence of nonfunctional, but viable, ischemic myocardium.

Management of cardiogenic shock has the following objectives: (1) improve ventricular systolic contractile performance; (2) maintain adequate systemic blood pressure and sustain perfusion to vital organs; (3) reduce pulmonary congestion; (4) preserve viable but ischemic areas of myocardium; and (5) limit the size of the myocardial infarct. At times, however, these goals are at odds with each other. Frequently, it is necessary to use vasopressor agents to support blood pressure, which may lead to further ischemia in a zone of jeopardized myocardium and may, in fact, extend the size of the infarct. Likewise, alpha-adrenergic agonists, although useful in supporting blood pressure, may further decrease left ventricular systolic performance because of further elevation in afterload. Optimal management requires a constant balancing of the risks and benefits of therapy and continuous reassessment of hemodynamic changes after institution of new therapies.

The management of patients with cardiogenic shock should begin with general supportive measures. Relief of ongoing ischemic pain, as well as anxiety, should be accomplished with the use of small doses of analgesics such as morphine, 2 to 4 mg intravenously every 5 to 10 minutes. Electrolyte disturbances, fever, nausea and vomiting, and acid-base abnormalities (particularly acidosis) should be treated. The optimal left ventricular filling pressure should be established for each patient. The pulmonary capillary wedge pressure should usually average 18 to 20 mmHg; relative hypovolemia may exist when lower values are present. A small increase in the filling pressure may help improve cardiac output by means of Starling's mechanism.

Adequate ventilation and oxygenation should be maintained and frequently re-evaluated by measurement of arterial blood gases. Oxygen should be administered by nasal cannula or face mask to maintain an arterial Po_2 higher than 70 mmHg. Endotracheal intubation and mechanical ventilation may be necessary temporarily to achieve adequate oxygenation and reduce the work of breathing.

Continuous electrocardiographic monitoring is essential because arrhythmias may contribute to the low-output state. Because the ischemic ventricle is more susceptible to the myocardial depressant effects of antiarrhythmic agents, the need for administration of these drugs and their dosages must be carefully reviewed and monitored to avoid adverse effects. Transvenous ventricular pacing or, preferably, AV sequential pacing may be necessary in patients with persistent bradycardia or AV block. Whenever pacing is undertaken, every attempt should be made to preserve AV synchrony.

Invasive hemodynamic monitoring using a pulmonary artery thermodilution catheter, as well as an indwelling intra-arterial catheter, is essential as an adjunct to careful clinical assessment. Accurate, up-to-date hemodynamic data permit the selection of specific pharmacologic agents and other therapeutic interventions. They also facilitate the diagnosis of other causes of cardiogenic shock, such as mitral regurgitation, acute ventricular septal rupture, hypovolemia, or right ventricular infarction (Table 6).

Specific therapeutic interventions may include pharmacologic agents (loop diuretics, intravenous vasodilators, vasopressor drugs, and positive inotropic agents); mechanical circulatory assistance (IABP or, rarely, left or right ventricular assist devices); coronary artery reperfusion by thrombolysis, PTCA, or CABG; and cardiac surgery for the correction of mechanical complications of the acute infarction. Vasopressors, vasodilators, and positive inotropic agents all have a role in the management of patients in shock. Frequently, drugs that raise systemic vascular resistance and augment left ventricular contractility are required to maintain adequate mean arterial pressure and coronary perfusion. Agents that have mixed alpha- and beta-adrenergic agonist properties, such as norepinephrine (Levophed) and moderate to high doses of dopamine, are particularly useful in this setting. In high doses, both agents can produce severe peripheral vasoconstriction and further impair cardiac output because of excessive afterload. Agents that have both inotropic and vasodilatory properties, such as dobutamine and amrinone, may also be useful in the management of cardiogenic shock that has failed to respond to either dopamine or norepinephrine.

Vasodilators are assuming an increasingly important role in the acute management of cardiogenic shock. Many studies have reported hemodynamic improvement in patients who have marked elevation of systemic vascular resistance and pulmonary capillary wedge pressure. Afterload reduction may also benefit patients with shock caused by severe mitral regurgitation or ventricular septal defect. An intravenous vasodilator such as sodium nitroprusside is usually chosen and the dose titrated so that the systemic blood pressure does not fall below 90 mmHg. Vasodilators are not useful when severe hypotension is present, but they may be used in combination with vasopressor agents to balance the positive inotropic effect with an appropriate degree of peripheral vasodilatation. Systemic vascular resistance should be calculated frequently during administration of these agents to maximize their effectiveness.

Progress has been made over the past decade in reducing the exceedingly high mortality associated with cardiogenic shock. Most approaches aim to decrease the size of the infarct and to prevent the development of cardiogenic shock. Myocardial reperfusion is most rapidly accomplished through the use of an intravenous thrombolytic agent. Even when cardiogenic shock has developed, thrombolytic therapy or primary coronary angioplasty may result in improved left ventricular function and survival. Although the impact of prompt reperfusion (<4 hours) on the incidence of cardiogenic shock has not been adequately studied, growing numbers of reports have documented the reversal of shock in patients treated with thrombolytic agents. Recent data suggest that mortality may be decreased in patients treated with successful coronary angioplasty for cardiogenic shock. Short periods of circulatory support, both pharmacologic and mechanical using the IABP, may be required despite successful reperfusion until areas of myocardial "stunning" recover sufficiently to support adequate contractile function. Stunned myocardium is potentially viable but temporarily nonfunctional because of acute ischemia. Although the management of cardiogenic shock has improved and mortality has decreased, it is clear that prevention through early reperfusion and limitation of infarct size is far preferable to medical or surgical management once shock has occurred.

Treatment

Inotropic Agents

DIGITALIS GLYCOSIDES. Although digitalis is known to increase myocardial contractility and oxygen consumption in hearts of normal size, it may result in a decrease in heart size, wall tension, and myocardial oxygen consumption in patients with heart failure and a dilated heart. Digitalization is relatively ineffective in severe acute heart failure after myocardial infarction. Although the issue remains controversial, ventricular arrhythmias may be worsened by digitalis, particularly when given during the first 6 to 8 hours after acute infarction, and especially in the setting of hypokalemia, hypothyroidism, advanced age, or hypoxemia. Mortality has been

TABLE 6. **Principal Causes of Shock After Acute Myocardial Infarction***

| Pathophysiologic Abnormality | Diagnostic Evaluation | | | Guides of Management | Prognosis |
	Clinical	Hemodynamic	Noninvasive		
Hypovolemia	Clear lungs on chest film	BP < 100 PCW < 15 CI < 2.2	Vigorous LV function	Rapid but cautious volume expansion until PCW 15–18 mmHg	Very good
Right ventricular infarction	Inferior myocardial infarction on electrocardiogram	BP < 100 RA pressure ≥ PCW Reduced PA and RV pulse pressure CI < 2.2	Dilated RV with RVEF ≤ 0.30, LVEF generally > 45, inferior and/or posterior LV dysfunction	Volume expansion if PCW < 15 mmHg, inotropic support, maintain atrial transport	Good unless severe LV dysfunction coexists
Cardiogenic shock	Pulmonary rales, S₃ gallop, pulmonary congestion on chest x-ray film	BP < 90 PCW > 18 CI < 2.2 Elevated SVR	LVEF ≤ 0.40 Marked regional LV wall motion abnormalities	Inotropes and/or vasopressors to maintain BP > 90 and CI approx. 2 liters/min/M² Vasodilators and diuretics to keep PCW < 18 IABP support	Poor, mortality 80%; early reperfusion (PTCA, TPA) may improve outlook
Acute mitral regurgitation	Holosystolic murmur at apex, pulmonary rales, S₃ gallop, pulmonary congestion on chest x-ray film	PCW > 18 with large V waves CI < 2.2 SVR elevated BP < 90	LVEF may be high, normal, or depressed, depending on extent of infarction	Vasodilators and inotropes, IABP, prompt MVR	Surgical mortality 30–40%; medical mortality 80%
Acute ventricular septal rupture	Shock syndrome, rales, S₃ gallop, holosystolic murmur at LLSB, thrill in 50%	BP < 90 O₂ "step-up" from RA to RV or PA	Left-to-right shunt by first-pass RVG, LVEF, and RVEF are variable; two-dimensional echocardiography should visualize defect; Doppler confirms shunt	Vasodilators and inotropes, IABP Early VSD closure	Surgical mortality 40–50%; medical morality 80–85%; outlook better with anterior myocardial infarction

*Adapted from Shah PK and Swan HJC: Complications of acute myocardial infarction. *In* Parmley WW, Chatterjee K (eds): Cardiology: Philadelphia, J. B. Lippincott, 1988. Used by permission.

Abbreviations: PCW = pulmonary capillary wedge pressure; CI = cardiac index (liters/min/M²); SVR = systemic vascular resistance; BP = blood pressure; LVEF = left ventricular ejection fraction; RVEF = right ventricular ejection fraction; LV = left ventricle; RV = right ventricle; RA = right atrium; IABP = intra-aortic balloon pump; PA = pulmonary artery; JVP = jugular venous pressure; PTCA = percutaneous transluminal coronary angioplasty; TPA = tissue plasminogen activator; VSD = ventricular septal defect; MVR = mitral valve replacement; LLSB = lower left sternal border; RVG = radionuclide ventriculogram.

shown to be greater in patients treated with digoxin after infarction, but this finding may be entirely explained by the confounding variables associated with its use (i.e., refractory supraventricular arrhythmias or progressive heart failure). When it is used, it should be administered intravenously at an initial dose of 0.5 mg. Additional doses of 0.25 mg should be given as needed until a total dose of 1 to 1.5 mg has been administered over 18 to 24 hours. The serum digoxin level should be measured and kept between 1 and 2 ng per ml. Levels higher than 2 ng per ml are frequently associated with digoxin toxicity, although lower levels do not exclude the presence of toxicity when digoxin sensitivity exists, particularly in the elderly or in patients with advanced heart failure. Digoxin-toxic rhythms are myriad and may include ventricular bigeminy, trigeminy, multifocal premature ventricular beats, paroxysmal junctional rhythms, heart block, and ventricular tachycardia or fibrillation. Treatment of toxicity should include discontinuation of the drug, correction of hypokalemia if present, and antiarrhythmic therapy when indicated.

DOPAMINE. Dopamine represents one of a variety of short-acting, intravenous, inotropic agents that have proved useful in the management of persistent heart failure and cardiogenic shock (Table 7). Dopamine has a variety of hemodynamic effects mediated through direct stimulation of cardiac beta$_1$-adrenergic receptors, peripheral alpha-adrenergic receptors, and dopaminergic receptors, as well as through the release of endogenous norepinephrine from sympathetic nerve endings. The type of receptor that is stimulated depends on the dose. At relatively low

TABLE 7. **Comparative Effects of Vasodilators and Positive Inotropic Agents in the Treatment of Heart Failure**

Agent	Drug Class	Dosage	Hemodynamic Effects				Indications	Adverse Effects
			HR	BP	PCW	SVR		
Dopamine	Beta-adrenergic agonist	2.5–5 µg/kg/min (low dose)	↑	↑	—	↓	Oliguria, borderline hypotension	Cardiac arrhythmias, tachycardia
		5–20 µg/kg/min (high dose)	↑↑	↑↑	↑	↑	Hypotension	Limb ischemia in patients with peripheral vascular disease, myocardial ischemia
Dobutamine	Beta-adrenergic agonist	5–15 µg/kg/min	—↑	—↓	↓↓	↓↓	Refractory heart failure, low cardiac output	Cardiac arrhythmias, myocardial ischemia
Amrinone	Phosphodiesterase inhibitor	0.75 mg/kg bolus 5–10 µg/kg/min maintenance infusion	—↑	—↓	↓↓	↓↓	Low cardiac output, refractory heart failure	Nausea, vomiting, diarrhea, thrombocytopenia (2%), increased ventricular ectopy, liver function abnormalities
Nitroglycerin (IV)	Smooth muscle relaxant	25–1000 µg/min	—↑	—↓	↓↓	↓↓	Preload reduction in heart failure, ongoing myocardial ischemia	Headache, nausea, hypotension, particularly with right ventricular infarction or hypovolemia, methemoglobinemia
Nitroprusside	Smooth muscle relaxant	10–500 µg/min	—↑	↓	↓↓	↓↓↓	Pulmonary edema with normal or hypertensive blood pressure, refractory heart failure, low output in conjunction with dobutamine	Thiosulfate toxicity, intrapulmonary shunting, excessive hypotension
Captopril (PO)	Converting enzyme inhibitor	6.75–50 mg tid	—	↓—	↓↓	↓↓	Chronic low-output failure	Hypotension, proteinuria, rash, cough, dysgusia, deterioration in renal function
Enalapril (PO)	Converting enzyme inhibitor	2.5–20 mg qd	—	↓—	↓↓	↓↓	low-output failure	Hypotension, angioedema, hyperkalemia, deterioration of renal function

Abbreviations and symbols: HR = heart rate; BP = blood pressure; PCW = pulmonary capillary wedge pressure; SVR = systemic vascular resistance; —, no change; ↑, small increase; ↑↑, moderate increase; ↓, small decrease; ↓↓, moderate decrease; ↓↓↓, marked decrease.

doses (0.5 to 2 micrograms per kg per minute), dopaminergic stimulation causes vasodilation of renal, mesenteric, coronary, and cerebral arterioles and increases in blood flow. With doses between 2 and 5 micrograms per kg per minute, an increase in stroke volume and cardiac output mediated by stimulation of beta$_1$ receptors as well as peripheral vasodilation may be observed. At higher doses (5 to 20 micrograms per kg per minute), alpha-adrenergic vasoconstriction is observed. Although helpful in supporting systemic blood pressure, vasoconstriction may cause tissue hypoxemia, as well as elevation of the left ventricular filling pressure, as a result of excessive afterload. Ventricular and supraventricular arrhythmias may occur when doses exceed 10 micrograms per kg per minute. It should be recognized that there is marked individual variation in the dose response to this agent, and it is essential that the lowest dose that produces an optimal hemodynamic and clinical response be chosen.

DOBUTAMINE. Dobutamine is a synthetic catecholamine that is principally a beta-adrenergic agonist, produces minimal alpha-adrenergic stimulation, and does not cause release of endogenous norepinephrine. It has potent positive inotropic and chronotropic effects, but it does not produce significant vasoconstriction even at very high doses. It does not alter renal blood flow, but it does cause redistribution of mesenteric and renal blood flow in favor of coronary and skeletal vascular beds. Dose-related increases in stroke volume and cardiac output, and decreases in left ventricular filling pressure, may be seen in patients with acute and chronic heart failure. Several studies have demonstrated that dobutamine is preferable to dopamine in the treatment of patients with severe refractory heart failure because of its favorable effects on pulmonary capillary wedge pressure and its use as a vasodilator. Although equivalent doses of dobutamine produce fewer arrhythmias and less tachycardia than dopamine, the lack of alpha-adrenergic stimulation makes this agent ineffective as a vasopressor and inappropriate as the sole treatment for systemic hypotension. Like dopamine, dobutamine should be administered beginning at a low dose (2 to 5 micrograms per kg per minute), and the dose should be increased rapidly under close hemodynamic monitoring. The dose should be increased up to 15 micrograms per kg per minute or until improvement in cardiac output, pulmonary capillary wedge pressure, and clinical status has been achieved. The dose should be reduced if systolic blood pressure exceeds 110 to 120 mmHg, the heart rate exceeds 110 beats per minute, arrhythmias develop, or ST segment monitoring documents further ischemia. The combination of dobutamine and dopamine has been useful in the management of patients with cardiogenic shock. Moderate doses of both agents have been shown to maintain arterial blood pressure better, with fewer deleterious effects on pulmonary capillary wedge pressure, than higher doses of either agent alone.

NOREPINEPHRINE (LEVOPHED). Norepinephrine is a potent alpha-adrenergic agonist that produces arteriolar and venous constriction. It has relatively modest beta-adrenergic agonist properties. It may be useful in transiently maintaining adequate arterial pressure in severely hypotensive patients, but it often results in a decrease in cardiac output and a decline in blood flow to peripheral tissues, especially during long-term use. It is particularly useful in the treatment of conditions associated with excessive vasodilatation, particularly anaphylaxis and sepsis with high cardiac output. In patients with cardiogenic shock, it is useful when systemic arterial blood pressure is below 80 mmHg and the systemic vascular resistance is normal (1200 dyne-seconds per cm^5) or reduced. Dopamine is usually a better first choice, but its use may be limited by excessive tachycardia. Norepinephrine is particularly useful when combined with direct-acting vasodilators such as low intravenous doses of nitroglycerin or sodium nitroprusside. We prefer this approach because combination therapy tends to avoid excessive peripheral vasoconstriction and may lead to a decrease in left ventricular filling pressure. Norepinephrine is usually begun at a low infusion rate (1 to 4 micrograms per minute) and increased to achieve optimal hemodynamic effects. Excessive peripheral vasoconstriction or arrhythmias often limit its use.

AMRINONE. Amrinone, like aminophylline, is a phosphodiesterase inhibitor. Amrinone is relatively specific for Type III phosphodiesterase, which is found in cardiac and vascular smooth muscle. It has powerful positive inotropic properties but is also a potent vasodilator with balanced effects on preload and afterload. It increases cardiac output, reduces left ventricular filling pressure, and decreases systemic vascular resistance, and is particularly useful in patients with refractory heart failure. Amrinone is not a vasopressor; blood pressure is usually unaffected but may fall. In patients in whom preload falls dramatically, frank hypotension may occur; it may be treated by decreasing the dose or replacing volume. Heart rate typically increases by 5 to 10 per cent. Amrinone is more effective than either dopamine or dobutamine in lowering pulmonary capillary wedge pressure and is intermediate between nitroprusside and dobutamine in its effects as a vasodilator and an inotropic agent. Therapy should be initiated with a bolus of 0.75 mg per kg followed by an infusion of 5 to 10 micrograms per kg per minute. An additional bolus of 0.75 mg per kg may be given 15 to 30 minutes after the first to achieve maximum hemodynamic effects. A maximal dose of 18 mg per kg per 24 hours is recommended. Adverse effects include nausea, vomiting, hypotension, fever, and occasional thrombocytopenia. Ventricular arrhythmias are also frequently exacerbated.

Vasodilators

Vasodilator therapy plays an important role in the management of patients whose infarction has been complicated by persistent heart failure, hypertension, or mechanical complications. Agents vary in their ability to reduce preload through venodilation and afterload through arteriolar dilation. Reduction of afterload results in improvement in forward stroke volume and cardiac output, and reduction of preload leads to decreases in pulmonary capillary wedge and right atrial pressures. By improving cardiac performance, vasodilators decrease myocardial oxygen demand, decrease heart size, and improve subendocardial blood flow. Careful hemodynamic monitoring is essential when vasodilator therapy is instituted early after myocardial infarction to prevent hypotension. Vasodilators alone or in combination with IABP may help to provide the hemodynamic stability necessary to undertake cardiac catheterization in patients with mechanical complications and to prepare the patient for surgery. The rapidly changing hemodynamics during acute infarction require that therapy be initiated with agents that can be administered intravenously, have a rapid onset of action (1 to 2 minutes), and have a short half-life (2 to 4 minutes). Nitroglycerin and sodium nitroprusside are the drugs of choice for initial stabilization.

NITROGLYCERIN. Nitroglycerin is a rapidly acting vasodilator whose principal hemodynamic benefit is preload reduction through venodilation. At high intravenous doses, it also decreases afterload. Arteriolar dilation with nitroglycerin is critically dependent on preload because the observed decrease in afterload diminishes as pulmonary capillary wedge pressure falls. Nitroglycerin administered by the intravenous route is preferred by many clinicians in the setting of acute infarction and heart failure because of its potent anti-ischemic effects and its ability to reduce the size of the infarct. The drug has also been shown in experimental studies to limit coronary steal (the diversion of blood flow from ischemic to nonischemic myocardium), which occurs to a greater degree with nitroprusside. Intravenous infusion of nitroglycerin should begin

at 20 micrograms per minute, and the dose should be increased by increments of 10 to 20 micrograms per minute every 5 minutes until the desired effect (either improvement in hemodynamics or relief of ischemic chest pain) has occurred or arterial blood pressure has declined to unacceptable limits.* Adverse effects of nitroglycerin include hypotension, reflex tachycardia, severe headaches caused by cerebral vasodilation, increased intraocular pressure in patients with glaucoma, methemoglobinemia, and ethanol intoxication (ethanol is the vehicle for most intravenous nitroglycerin preparations). Paradoxical bradycardia has also been reported but is usually responsive to atropine. Tachyphylaxis may develop during prolonged infusion.

SODIUM NITROPRUSSIDE. Sodium nitroprusside produces rapid, balanced vasodilation of both arterioles and venules. This drug has been studied more than any other vasodilator during acute myocardial infarction and has proven benefits in the management of severe heart failure with or without cardiogenic shock. Its beneficial effects are most pronounced in patients with marked elevation of filling pressures and in those with either mitral regurgitation or ventricular septal defect. Hemodynamic benefits include a decrease in systemic vascular resistance, pulmonary capillary wedge pressure, and myocardial oxygen consumption, as well as an improvement in left ventricular ejection fraction. Nitroprusside may improve cardiac output in patients with cardiogenic shock, provided that the diastolic blood pressure and coronary perfusion pressure are maintained—either through the concomitant use of inotropic agents, particularly dobutamine, or by mechanical circulatory support with IABP. Therapy should begin with a low dose (10 to 20 micrograms per minute), and the dose should be rapidly increased every 5 to 10 minutes up to a total dose of 15 micrograms per kg per minute. The dose should be titrated either to achieve a fall in pulmonary capillary wedge pressure to 15 to 18 mmHg or until an unacceptable drop in systemic blood pressure has occurred, generally below 90 mmHg. Adverse effects of nitroprusside therapy include excessive hypotension, reflex tachycardia, the potential for worsening myocardial ischemia, thiocyanate toxicity (particularly in the presence of renal insufficiency), worsening hypoxemia caused by intrapulmonary shunting, and methemoglobinemia.

ORAL VASODILATORS. A variety of oral vasodilators are available for the treatment of patients with persistent heart failure after myocardial

---

*This dose exceeds the dosage recommended by the manufacturer.

infarction. Oral and transdermal nitrates are useful in producing venodilation and are effective in patients with high filling pressures and low cardiac output. They reduce pulmonary capillary wedge pressure without reducing cardiac output. Nitrate tolerance has become increasingly recognized in patients with angina pectoris and probably also occurs in those with congestive heart failure. A drug-free period of at least 6 to 8 hours daily should be used when nitrate preparations are given on a long-term basis.

Although short-term therapy with hydralazine or prazosin may be useful, tolerance continues to be a major problem with these two agents, and sustained improvement in functional capacity is uncommon. It is our current recommendation to use converting enzyme inhibitors for the treatment of chronic heart failure. Captopril, enalapril, and lisinopril have been extensively studied and proved effective in long-term management. Because converting enzyme inhibitors have been shown to decrease or prevent myocardial infarct expansion, it is hoped that the later development of dilated cardiomyopathy and heart failure may be significantly reduced by early treatment. All converting enzyme inhibitors decrease both preload and afterload. We initiate therapy with captopril using a small dose (6.25 mg twice daily) and titrate the dose upward on the basis of the patient's blood pressure. Orthostatic hypotension is particularly common in patients with impaired ventricular function and must be sought through frequent monitoring of orthostatic vital signs. A dose-response curve for these agents has not been established, and the optimum dose has never been quantified.

Intra-Aortic Balloon Counterpulsation. This method has proved to be an effective temporizing measure in the management of cardiogenic shock. The intra-aortic balloon can be inserted percutaneously and advanced into the aorta through the femoral artery. Phased balloon pulsation is synchronized with the electrocardiogram. The balloon is inflated at the time of aortic valve closure to produce augmentation of the diastolic pressure, and deflation occurs just before the onset of systole to produce systolic unloading. A 10 to 20 per cent increase in cardiac output is generally achieved, and the augmentation in diastolic coronary blood flow often results in improvement in myocardial ischemia.

The principal uses for IABP are (1) temporary support for patients with cardiogenic shock that is unresponsive to medical management; (2) short-term stabilization of patients in preparation for diagnostic studies such as cardiac catheterization or correction of mechanical lesions, including mitral regurgitation or ventricular sep-

tal rupture; (3) stabilization of patients who have extensive areas of jeopardized myocardium that are nonfunctional but still viable before coronary revascularization; (4) treatment of persistent myocardial ischemia that has failed to respond to medical therapy; and (5) treatment of refractory recurrent ventricular tachycardia. Counterpulsation unfortunately does not reduce overall mortality in patients with cardiogenic shock unless surgical correction of a mechanical lesion or revascularization can be performed. Patients least likely to benefit from intra-aortic balloon support during acute myocardial infarction are those with depressed left ventricular function caused by previous myocardial infarctions; those with extensive areas of infarction but little reversible ischemia; those in advanced stages of shock with evidence of end-organ hypoperfusion, such as oliguria or acidosis; and patients with significant peripheral vascular disease. We recommend this procedure for relatively young patients in cardiogenic shock who have no significant peripheral vascular disease or aortic regurgitation and who fail to show hemodynamic improvement after a short-term (30 to 120 minutes) trial of vasodilator and inotropic pharmacologic support. Early cardiac catheterization and surgical intervention are advised whenever possible. Patients who are unsuitable candidates for surgery should be weaned from balloon support after a stabilization period of 2 to 5 days. During this period, any areas of stunned myocardium will have had time to recover systolic function, and cardiac performance may improve sufficiently to support the circulation.

Complications of IABP may occur in up to 20 to 25 per cent of patients when either the percutaneous or the surgical insertion technique is used. These complications are principally vascular and include limb or abdominal ischemia, damage to the femoral or iliac arteries, and aortic dissection. Infection is a risk when the device remains in place for a prolonged period, as are hemolysis, thrombocytopenia, and embolization. We treat all patients with heparin intravenously. Antibiotic treatment with a cephalosporin is given while the balloon is in place.

Right Ventricular Infarction

Infarction of the free wall of the right ventricle may occur in as many as 30 to 40 per cent of patients with acute inferior or posterior myocardial infarction but produces important hemodynamic abnormalities in only about 5 per cent. The four clinical findings that suggest right ventricular infarction are acute inferior infarction, elevation of the jugular venous pressure (>7 cmH$_2$O), clear lung fields, and hypotension. A Kussmaul's sign (an inspiratory fall of more than 10 mm in systemic blood pressure) with little evidence of pulmonary congestion is present in approximately 70 per cent of cases. The electrocardiogram, in addition to revealing acute inferior wall injury, often shows ST segment elevation in the right precordial leads (V$_{3R}$ or V$_{4R}$).

Whenever right ventricular infarction is suspected, the diagnosis should be confirmed by bedside catheterization of the right side of the heart, which typically shows elevation of right atrial and right ventricular end-diastolic pressures but little elevation in right ventricular systolic pressure. The pulmonary capillary wedge pressure is usually normal or only slightly elevated because left ventricular damage is usually not severe enough to produce profound left ventricular dysfunction. Other hemodynamic findings may include a steep right atrial Y descent, Kussmaul's sign, a dip-and-plateau pattern during diastolic filling in the right ventricular pressure tracing, and a diminished pulse pressure in the pulmonary artery. Many of these hemodynamic abnormalities may suggest the presence of pericardial tamponade, constrictive pericarditis, or acute massive pulmonary thromboembolism. Noninvasive assessment of right ventricular function (with the use of gated blood pool imaging or bedside echocardiography) may be helpful in differentiating these entities. In approximately 25 per cent of patients, right atrial pressures may be nearly normal initially and may become elevated later in the course of the infarction or after volume infusion.

The hypotension observed with right ventricular infarction is usually caused by inadequate left ventricular filling resulting from right ventricular dysfunction. Volume expansion with crystalloid or colloid, often requiring 2 to 5 liters within 24 hours, is the initial treatment and increases right ventricular preload and cardiac output. Frequently, volume expansion alone does not correct the hypotension adequately, and inotropic support using dopamine or dobutamine may be required. Bradyarrhythmias and AV block are commonly observed and may further worsen the cardiac output through the loss of atrial contraction. With appropriate and aggressive therapy, survival rates in excess of 80 per cent can be expected.

MECHANICAL COMPLICATIONS AFTER ACUTE MYOCARDIAL INFARCTION

Acute Mitral Regurgitation

Acute mitral regurgitation may occur because of transient papillary muscle dysfunction secondary to myocardial ischemia or from rupture of the papillary muscle itself. Less commonly, rupture of one or more of the 120 chordae tendineae may occur. Although the anterolateral papillary muscle receives a dual blood supply from the left anterior descending and circumflex arteries, the posteromedial papillary muscle has less reliable perfusion from the posterior descending branch of the dominant coronary artery. Consequently, dysfunction of the posteromedial papillary muscle is approximately five times more common than dysfunction of the anterolateral papillary muscle.

The diagnosis of papillary muscle dysfunction may be made by physical examination or hemodynamic findings. Typically, a new systolic apical murmur that varies in intensity from Grade I to Grade III over VI is present and may be intermittent or persistent. Large V waves are seen on the pulmonary capillary wedge pressure tracing. Intermittent pulmonary edema, hypotension, or frank shock may occur rapidly and resolve quickly during periods of papillary muscle ischemia. Therapy of papillary muscle dysfunction includes anti-ischemic medications such as intravenous nitroglycerin, beta blockers, or calcium channel blockers. In addition, the coronary anatomy should be defined through early catheterization when hemodynamically significant mitral regurgitation is present. Intravenous vasodilators or circulatory support using IABP may also be of use.

Partial or complete rupture of a papillary muscle is a rare complication occurring in approximately 1 per cent of patients, but it accounts for 5 per cent of the deaths from myocardial infarction. Rupture typically occurs between 3 and 7 days after transmural infarction but has been reported in up to 20 per cent of cases within 24 hours of onset of the infarction. The posteromedial papillary muscle is most frequently involved, and the location of the infarct is usually inferior. Unlike ventricular septal rupture, which is seen with extensive transmural infarctions, papillary muscle rupture may occur with a relatively small or subendocardial infarction, and the extent of coronary artery disease may be modest. Single-vessel disease is present in approximately 50 per cent of patients. The sudden onset of severe pulmonary congestion and a loud (Grade III to VI) holosystolic apical murmur characterize the initial presentation. Pulmonary edema, hypotension, and frank cardiogenic shock often ensue, and 70 per cent of patients succumb within 24 hours of presentation if appropriate stabilization cannot be achieved. Occasionally, a systolic murmur may be brief, or even completely absent, when cardiac output is markedly depressed and little turbulent blood flow is occurring.

It is often difficult to differentiate acute mitral regurgitation from acute ventricular septal rupture because both conditions are characterized by the development of acute pulmonary edema, hypotension, and a new, loud holosystolic murmur. Catheterization of the right side of the heart at the bedside helps to differentiate these conditions and permits appropriate hemodynamic monitoring during pharmacologic therapy. Two-dimensional echocardiography should be promptly undertaken because it frequently visualizes a flail mitral leaflet. The presence of severe mitral regurgitation can be confirmed by a Doppler study. Papillary muscle rupture can be differentiated from ventricular septal rupture by several features given in Table 6. Medical therapy has little role in the management of papillary muscle rupture other than temporary support until surgery can be undertaken. IABP should be promptly initiated and diuretic, vasodilator, and inotropic drugs administered. Sodium nitroprusside in combination with dobutamine or moderate doses of dopamine has proved to be particularly effective in the short-term management of these patients. Early surgical correction of acute mitral regurgitation by mitral valve replacement can alter the natural history of this catastrophic complication, and a success rate of 60 to 70 per cent may be achieved.

Rupture of the Interventricular Septum

Rupture of the interventricular septum is reported to occur in approximately 1 per cent of patients with acute infarction and is responsible for 3 to 5 per cent of all infarct-related deaths. The size of the perforation may range from 1 to several centimeters; the magnitude of the left-to-right shunt and the extent of hemodynamic deterioration determine the likelihood of survival. Septal rupture appears to be slightly more common in anterior and anterolateral than inferior and posterior infarctions. Rupture of the septum occurs most frequently near the apex after anterior infarction, and perforation occurs in the basal portion of the septum in inferior infarctions. Multivessel coronary artery disease is present in almost all patients. Septal rupture has a peak incidence on days 3 to 5 after infarction, but it may occur as early as 24 hours or as late as 2 weeks afterward. Left-to-right shunting through the perforation produces volume overload of the right ventricle, increased pulmonary blood flow, and a marked fall in systemic venous blood flow and cardiac output.

The most prominent physical finding of acute septal rupture is a new, harsh, loud (Grade III to VI) holosystolic murmur, which is heard best at the lower left sternal border but may radiate throughout the precordium. A palpable thrill is present in approximately 50 per cent of cases. Findings of right ventricular volume overload, including tricuspid regurgitation, moderate to marked elevation of the jugular venous pressure, and a right ventricular heave, help to differentiate this condition from acute mitral regurgitation. Catheterization of the right side of the heart should be performed as quickly as possible to confirm the diagnosis and define the magnitude of the left-to-right shunt. An oxygen "step-up" of more than 10 per cent from the right atrium to the right ventricle or the proximal pulmonary artery confirms the diagnosis. Echocardiography using microbubble contrast, Doppler echocardiography, or first-pass radioventriculography all may be used to confirm the presence of a ruptured septum.

Medical management of acute septal rupture should be instituted before definitive surgical repair. The mortality of patients not undergoing repair approaches 50 per cent at 1 week and 80 per cent by 8 weeks. IABP should be undertaken immediately after confirmation of the diagnosis to stabilize the patient. Vasodilator therapy using nitroprusside is often effective but generally cannot be used before balloon pump insertion because of the presence of systemic hypotension. Whenever possible, cardiac catheterization should be performed to define the coronary anatomy, identify coexisting mitral valve disease, and assess ventricular function. Aggressive surgical treatment may result in a 50 to 75 per cent short-term survival rate as long as cardiogenic shock and pulmonary or renal dysfunction are absent.

Rupture of the Free Wall of the Left Ventricle

Rupture of the free wall of the infarcted left ventricle results in approximately 10 per cent of hospital deaths after acute myocardial infarction. This catastrophic complication is more frequent in women and in patients of both sexes in their seventh or eighth decade of life. Transmural infarction is almost always present, and the infarct-related artery is totally occluded, with little collateral circulation. Rupture of the free wall is most frequently seen in patients with hypertension. It is uncommon after right ventricular infarction and occurs with equal frequency after inferior and anterior infarctions. The peak incidence is between days 3 and 8, but rupture may occur within 24 hours or as late as 3 weeks afterward. Rupture is usually preceded by thinning and dilation of the necrotic zone of myocardium (i.e., infarct expansion) and usually occurs at the junction between infarcted and normal myocardium. Early ambulation, anti-inflammatory drugs such as corticosteroids or indomethacin, and anticoagulant therapy are suspected, but unproven, contributors to cardiac rupture. A variety of studies have failed to show any relation between thrombolytic therapy during acute myocardial infarction and an increased risk of cardiac rupture.

Cardiac rupture usually presents with the development of sudden, profound right heart failure and shock and rapidly proceeds to electromechanical dissociation. Most patients experience tearing chest pain. Survival, which is unusual, depends on prompt recognition of this complication, urgent hemodynamic stabilization, and, most important, immediate surgical repair. Pericardiocentesis may provide temporary relief of cardiac tamponade.

Occasionally, rupture of the left ventricular free wall may be accompanied by the development of a pseudoaneurysm caused by containment of the hemopericardium by adhesions between the pericardium and the epicardium. Pseudoaneurysms are composed of organized hematoma and pericardium, lack any original myocardial fibers, communicate with the true left ventricular cavity through a narrow neck, and may become quite large over time, often equaling the size of the left ventricular cavity itself. They frequently contain mural thrombi and are prone to embolization. Clinical manifestations are similar to those seen with a true aneurysm. Pseudoaneurysms are prone to rupture, with catastrophic consequences. The diagnosis is easily made by echocardiography or left ventriculography using a contrast medium. Surgical repair is recommended even in asymptomatic patients, regardless of the size of the pseudoaneurysm, to prevent subsequent rupture and death.

Left Ventricular Aneurysm

A true ventricular aneurysm is a circumscribed, noncontractile outpouching of the left ventricle composed of fibrous tissue and necrotic myocytes. Aneurysms of various size develop in 10 to 38 per cent of patients with transmural myocardial infarctions and are most frequently observed after anterior infarction when there is total occlusion of the infarct-related artery and few collateral blood vessels. Aneurysms may vary widely in size, usually have a wide base that helps to distinguish them from pseudoaneurysms, and are frequently lined by mural thrombi. The systolic dyskinesia seen with aneurysms results in ineffective forward stroke volume because of wasted contractile energy during systolic bulging. Mortality is up to six times higher than that

in patients without aneurysms. Although rupture almost never occurs during the first few weeks, progressive congestive heart failure or life-threatening ventricular tachyarrhythmias are frequently seen with aneurysms. The incidence of systemic emboli is low (<5 per cent) despite a high frequency of mural thrombi. The diagnosis should be suspected in patients with severe refractory heart failure, recurrent ventricular tachyarrhythmias, a dyskinetic, displaced left ventricular impulse on physical examination, persistent ST segment elevation in an area of old infarction, or an abnormal bulge of the cardiac silhouette on the chest film. Two-dimensional echocardiography or radionuclide ventriculography serves to confirm the diagnosis.

Surgical aneurysmectomy is the treatment of choice but should be reserved for those patients whose symptoms are not controlled by medical management. A successful outcome depends on the preservation of contractile function in the nonaneurysmal portion of the ventricle. Surgical aneurysmectomy, usually combined with coronary revascularization, may result in considerable functional improvement in carefully selected patients. Electrophysiologic mapping should be undertaken before resection of the aneurysm in patients with recurrent ventricular tachyarrhythmias. Anticoagulation therapy should be considered in all patients in whom a mural thrombus has been documented.

RISK STRATIFICATION AFTER ACUTE MYOCARDIAL INFARCTION

The principal goal of risk stratification after acute infarction is the development of a management strategy for the individual patient. A low-risk status implies a risk of cardiac death of 2 per cent or less during the first year after discharge from the hospital, with a small probability of recurrent infarction or new-onset angina. Patients who are placed in the lowest-risk category require few medications other than aspirin (300 mg orally daily) and prophylactic nitroglycerin, and they should be candidates for early return to work and resumption of normal physical activities. In contrast, patients in the intermediate- or high-risk categories (to be defined) require more aggressive medical management and frequently need invasive evaluation to determine the coronary anatomy and ventricular function.

The initial assessment of risk begins with the determination of whether the patient's clinical course is complicated or uncomplicated. Approximately 15 to 30 per cent of patients experience congestive heart failure, ventricular arrhythmias, or postinfarction angina while they are in the hospital. These patients should be considered high risk on the basis of these clinical predictors. However, 70 to 85 per cent of patients have an uncomplicated hospital stay and should undergo further diagnostic studies before discharge to determine their risk for subsequent cardiac events.

Three characteristics have been clearly identified as predictive of increased risk during the first year infarction: myocardial ischemia, which may be either symptomatic or silent and may occur at rest or during exercise; depression of the left ventricular ejection fraction; and ventricular arrhythmias that persist beyond the initial 12 to 24 hours. Each has been identified as an independent risk factor for morbidity and mortality. Myocardial ischemia and impaired ventricular function are stronger predictors of subsequent mortality than ventricular arrhythmias.

Survival after hospital discharge is related to the presence or absence of myocardial ischemia, the frequency and magnitude of the ischemia, and the extent of underlying coronary artery disease. Inducible ischemia in the presence of multivessel disease has been shown to have a poorer prognosis than ischemia associated with single-vessel disease. This is not surprising because patients with multivessel disease have a higher rate of cardiac events in the first year than patients with single-vessel disease, regardless of the left ventricular ejection fraction or other variables.

The value of a submaximal (low-level) exercise test before discharge in patients with uncomplicated myocardial infarction has been studied extensively over the past 15 years. Both the safety and the predictive value of this test have been conclusively demonstrated. Most clinical studies indicate that patients who demonstrate ST segment depression (either silent or with angina pectoris) during low-level exercise testing have a higher incidence of reinfarction, unstable angina, and cardiac death than patients who have been able to perform at least 4 METS of exercise without ST segment depression. Although there is general agreement that ST segment depression during testing predicts a poorer prognosis, the importance of the degree of this depression remains uncertain. Myocardial imaging with [201]Th is frequently performed in conjunction with low-level exercise testing to enhance the sensitivity and specificity of the test. Nuclear imaging techniques are particularly useful in patients with pre-existing electrocardiographic abnormalities such as left bundle branch block or left ventricular hypertrophy, in those receiving antiarrhythmic agents or digitalis, and in patients with repolarization abnormalities in areas beyond the area of acute infarction. Patients whose thallium scan identifies perfusion defects in more than one region of the heart, delayed redistribution within or remote from the infarct itself, or abnormal uptake of radioisotope by the lungs on predischarge testing should be considered at risk for sudden death, recurrent infarction, and unstable angina during the next year. Patients who demonstrate myocardial ischemia beyond the original infarcted area or evidence of reversible ischemia in addition to fixed scarring in an infarcted area, particularly a subendocardial infarct, should undergo coronary arteriography. Those patients in whom no myocardial ischemia is detected on low-level exercise testing should undergo maximal exercise testing in 6 to 8 weeks to determine their need for anti-ischemic medications.

In addition to determining whether myocardial ischemia is present, a predischarge exercise test is helpful in documenting the ischemic threshold, that is, the product of heart rate and blood pressure, or workload, at which ischemia is seen. Those patients with evidence of ischemia at a low workload or heart rate, or who demonstrate hemodynamic instability, such as a fall in blood pressure during exercise testing, should also undergo coronary arteriography to determine the extent of coronary artery disease.

Ambulatory (Holter) monitoring has been used increasingly for the detection of silent myocardial ischemia after infarction. Ischemia detected by such monitoring is usually also detected during exercise testing, particularly if thallium scintigraphy is used. Only those patients in whom ischemia is observed at a low workload during exercise testing have evidence of frequent, prolonged episodes of ischemia during Holter monitoring. Furthermore, silent ischemia detected by Holter monitoring is rarely observed when none can be produced during exercise testing. Therefore, low-level exercise testing appears superior to Holter monitoring for predischarge evaluation and management of both painful and silent myocardial ischemia.

The left ventricular ejection fraction, measured with the patient at rest, is the single best predictor of the outcome after acute myocardial infarction. The ejection fraction can be measured noninvasively by radionuclide ventriculography or two-dimensional echocardiography. Not all patients, however, need necessarily undergo such studies. Assessment of ventricular function is indicated in patients with persistent signs of heart failure on physical examination or chest x-ray films; those in whom frequent premature ventricular beats are seen; patients with marked limitation of exercise capacity, a fall in blood pressure, or an ischemic response during low-level exercise testing; or those with a large infarct in whom beta-blocker therapy is being considered. In patients whose ejection fraction is between 25 and 45 per cent, coronary arteriography should be performed if myocardial ischemia has been demonstrated because these patients can ill afford to lose any remaining functional myocardium. Therapy with a converting enzyme inhibitor should also be considered, regardless of the presence or absence of symptoms, in light of the growing body of knowledge suggesting that these agents may decrease the likelihood of subsequent cardiac dilation.

Studies have indicated that frequent or complex VPBs, occurring either at rest or during exercise, are independent risk factors for sudden death. Precisely what constitutes complex rhythm disturbances remains uncertain. Ventricular arrhythmias remain a particularly ominous finding when left ventricular dysfunction or provokable myocardial ischemia is also present after infarction. Given the random variability of ventricular ectopy, the unproven benefits of successful suppression of ventricular arrhythmias in the postinfarction setting, and the known proarrhythmic effects of all currently available antiarrhythmic agents, routine Holter monitoring is not indicated in all postinfarction patients. It should be undertaken in patients with a left ventricular ejection fraction below 40 per cent, those with evidence of myocardial ischemia during low-level exercise testing, and those with complex ventricular ectopy during the late phase of hospitalization.

The treatment of complex ventricular ectopy remains controversial. Patients who demonstrate sustained or recurrent, nonsustained ventricular tachycardia should usually receive antiarrhythmic therapy. Invasive electrophysiologic testing is usually not warranted when adequate suppression of nonsustained ventricular tachycardia can be documented by ambulatory electrocardiographic monitoring. However, those patients with symptomatic ectopy or ventricular arrhythmias that persist despite antiarrhythmic therapy may benefit from electrophysiologic testing. This issue remains undecided, and management must be individualized for each patient. In patients with persistent, complex ventricular arrhythmias and adequate left ventricular function, exercise testing should be undertaken to determine the presence and extent of reversible myocardial ischemia. When myocardial ischemia can be documented, coronary arteriography should be performed because coronary revascularization may result in improved survival and aid in the suppression of the arrhythmia.

SECONDARY PREVENTION AFTER ACUTE INFARCTION

Prevention of a second infarction and other cardiovascular events in patients who have had a first infarction has been the subject of considerable research. Both changes in lifestyle and treatment with a variety of drugs have been investigated as possible preventive measures.

The evidence is compelling that cessation of cigarette smoking promptly reduces the risk of a second myocardial infarction. Above all else, the physician should strongly encourage current smokers who have had a first infarction to quit. Patients whose blood cholesterol level is above 220 mg per dl, especially when the high-density-lipoprotein level is below 40 mg per dl, should be instructed to follow a cholesterol-lowering diet. The blood cholesterol level should not be measured until 4 to 6 weeks after infarction because the measurement may be inaccurate in the setting of the acute illness. If a 3- to 6-month trial of dietary therapy is not effective in reducing the blood cholesterol level below 200 mg per dl, drug therapy should be considered. Because of its efficacy and relative lack of side effects, lovastatin is currently emerging as the drug of choice. The daily dose is 20 to 80 mg orally, depending on the degree of hypercholesterolemia and the specific response to therapy.

Many physicians recommend that their patients engage in a structured program of physical activity after myocardial infarction, and the evidence suggests that regular exercise of a low to moderate level may prevent recurrent infarction and improve survival. Such programs should be undertaken only after the patient has completed a graded exercise test and a safe level of exercise has been defined. Walking, easy jogging, and bicycling, alone or in combination, are convenient forms of aerobic exercise for postinfarction patients.

Among the many drugs that have been studied for efficacy in secondary prevention, beta-adrenergic receptor blockers and antiplatelet agents have received the most attention. On the basis of a large body of evidence, many physicians choose to treat all patients after infarction with a beta-receptor blocker, usually propranolol, 20 to 80 mg orally two or three times daily, or metoprolol, 50 to 100 mg orally twice daily. Other physicians prefer to reserve beta-blocker therapy for patients at high risk, such as those who have multivessel coronary disease and angina pectoris. Our practice is to treat all postinfarction patients who do not have contraindications to the use of beta-adrenergic blockers. We favor this approach in part because of recent studies showing that beta-blocker therapy is cost effective for patients at all levels of risk.

Individual studies of antiplatelet therapy after myocardial infarction have produced mixed results. Nevertheless, a recent meta-analysis of 25 studies involving 29,000 patients suggests that antiplatelet therapy may reduce the incidence of subsequent vascular events after infarction. Aspirin is the agent of choice, but the most effective dose remains in doubt. In the absence of definitive information, we use 325 mg daily or every other day, depending on the patient's ability to tolerate the drug. We do not routinely administer dipyridamole with aspirin because of lack of evidence of an additive effect.

REHABILITATION AFTER MYOCARDIAL INFARCTION

method of
W. DOUGLAS WEAVER, M.D.
University of Washington
Seattle, Washington

The goal of cardiac rehabilitation is to characterize the sequelae associated with acute myocardial infarction and then apply interventions that will return the patient to full physical capabilities and to work, if appropriate.

THE PERIOD OF EARLY RECOVERY

It is now helpful to classify patients with acute infarction into those with Q wave infarcts and those with non–Q wave infarcts on the basis of the electrocardiogram (ECG). Only patients with ST segment elevation and chest pain have been shown consistently to benefit from thrombolytic therapy. The benefit is greatest in those with ST segment elevation in multiple locations (e.g., inferior and anterior), is somewhat less when changes are present only in the anterior location, and is less still with inferior ST segment changes—an inaccurate finding but one that is statistically correlated with the area of myocardium at risk. Patients with ST segment elevation usually develop Q waves on the ECG. Patients with non–Q wave infarction have similar morbidity and mortality after hospital discharge and should, therefore, be assessed for catheterization, angioplasty, and coronary surgery in the same way as patients with Q wave infarction.

FOLLOW-UP OF PATIENTS RECEIVING THROMBOLYTIC THERAPY

With the use of thrombolytic therapy, recovery of the patient has changed dramatically. There is a small subset of individuals in whom chest pain rapidly resolves and who are, therefore, left with minimal evidence of acute infarction. The patient with symptoms of fatigue and lethargy that last for 3 to 5 days after the event—who was typical of the era before thrombolytic therapy—is now far less common. Some patients appear to be totally recovered, even by the second day after the event.

The greatest difficulty in rehabilitation and recovery is a change of focus from determining residual myocardial function to understanding which, if any, intervention should be made subsequent to thrombolytic therapy. Of the patients who have coronary arteries recanalized with thrombolytic therapy, 60 to 70 per cent have high-grade coronary narrowing in the affected vessel caused by a residual thrombus and an atherosclerotic plaque. In addition, symptoms of recurrent ischemia are relatively common after thrombolytic therapy. Before hospital discharge, 5 to 25 per cent of patients show evidence of either recurrent infarction or ischemia. Chest pain and other evidence of ischemia in the early recovery phase are now relatively common compared with the prethrombolytic era. In addition, continuous monitoring of the ECG has shown that many episodes of ischemia do not include symptoms of chest pain (silent ischemia). This ECG finding is indicative of residual ischemia and prognostic of future coronary events.

One of the first questions that should be addressed is how to identify patients with significant residual coronary stenosis who are at risk for recurrent infarction. Should all patients undergo coronary angiography, and if so, when?

Three large trials have shown no benefit of emergent catheterization and percutaneous transluminal coronary angioplasty performed immediately after thrombolytic therapy. These well-controlled studies failed to demonstrate improved residual left ventricular function in patients who underwent emergent coronary angioplasty compared with patients who were evaluated and who underwent angioplasty, if indicated, 2 to 3 days later. In fact, there was higher morbidity, a greater requirement for emergent coronary surgery, and a trend toward even higher mortality in patients undergoing these emergent procedures.

An even more important question, just recently answered, is whether asymptomatic patients after thrombolytic treatment should undergo catheterization and angioplasty electively before hospital discharge. The recently completed thrombolysis in myocardial infarction (TIMI II) study failed to show any benefit in the routine angiographic assessment of asymptomatic patients after thrombolytic therapy. There was no reduction in mortality or in the incidence of recurrent infarction in patients undergoing routine catheterization and angioplasty compared with the results in patients treated conservatively, that is, with diagnostic angiography and angioplasty performed only in patients who have recurrent episodes of chest pain or evidence of ischemia on exercise testing before hospital discharge. Instead, the findings from this large, well-conducted trial suggest that clinical decisions should be dictated by continued evidence of ischemia rather than simply treating anatomic changes.

One recent study has suggested that patients without angina, heart failure, or arrhythmia after thrombolytic therapy can be evaluated in as few as 3 days after the acute myocardial infarction, using submaximal exercise testing (target heart rate of 140 beats per minute or symptoms). Patients who fail to show evidence of ischemia (normal ECG and no redistribution on thallium myocardial perfusion scans) can be discharged at that time, with little risk of subsequent ischemic events. By contrast, patients with recurrent chest pain or those who fail to augment blood pressure or who develop ST segment abnormalities with exercise should be considered for further diagnostic studies and coronary angioplasty or surgery if significant underlying coronary disease persists.

Clearly, in this new era of treatment for acute myocardial infarction, many questions are still to be answered. However, all approaches are aimed at earlier hospital discharge. To effect this, patient education and enhancement of activity must occur, even on the first day. Coronary care unit patient activity protocols are often helpful. Patients cannot be treated in a systematic fashion, but those who tolerate higher levels of activity in the first 3 days must be permitted to do so. Hypertension should be treated, and activities that cause increases in arterial diastolic blood pressure should be avoided because they may increase the likelihood of infarct expansion.

Cholesterol

Disorders in lipid metabolism need to be characterized during acute hospitalization, and a plan for appropriate treatment should be initiated at that time. Cholesterol screening should occur for all patients on the day after admission for acute myocardial infarction. A simple total cholesterol determination is adequate as a preliminary screen. A patient whose cholesterol level is higher than 200 mg per dl should have a determination of fasting low-density-lipoprotein (LDL) cholesterol, high-density-lipoprotein (HDL) cholesterol, and triglyceride levels. In those with no abnormality, determination of apoprotein B is indi-

cated. Most studies have shown that up to 85 per cent of patients with acute myocardial infarction have some underlying abnormality in lipid metabolism. Interventions aimed at lowering LDL cholesterol and raising HDL cholesterol have caused marked reductions in cardiac events after acute myocardial infarction. Treatment may even reverse the atherosclerotic process.

Beta Blockers

Several studies have shown that the use of beta blockers after acute myocardial infarction results in a reduction in the incidence of sudden cardiac death and recurrent myocardial infarction in the 1 to 2 years after the initial event. Unfortunately, accurate ways to identify the 3 to 4 per cent of patients who benefit most from this treatment are yet to be demonstrated.

Prognostic studies have shown that advanced age and severe left ventricular dysfunction, as reflected by the presence of heart failure, a remote history of myocardial infarction, and a reduced left ventricular ejection fraction, are indicators of mortality after acute myocardial infarction. In addition, the presence of frequent (more than 10 premature ventricular contractions per hour) ventricular ectopy or ventricular tachycardia recorded during Holter monitoring 1 to 2 weeks after the acute event or evidence of recurrent chest pain or electrocardiographic evidence of myocardial ischemia during treadmill testing and ambulatory monitoring is also an indication of subsequent cardiac events. Unfortunately, neither test is highly sensitive or specific in identifying individuals at risk who should be considered for pharmacologic or surgical treatment.

Calcium Channel Blockers

These agents should not be given routinely to all patients recovering from acute myocardial infarction. Several large studies with each of the currently available drugs failed to show any reduction in the incidence of recurrent infarction or sudden death after recovery from acute myocardial infarction. One study even suggested that the use of these drugs in patients with reduced left ventricular function (ejection fraction < 0.40 or heart failure) may actually be associated with increased mortality. These drugs should be reserved for patients with angina or hypertension. One beneficial characteristic of calcium channel blockers is that they do not elevate LDL cholesterol, unlike most beta blockers.

Unless contraindications exist, the wealth of evidence suggests that one tablet of aspirin daily or every other day is useful to prevent myocardial infarction and should be utilized. Although fish oils are undergoing extensive evaluation, their routine use after coronary thrombosis cannot now be recommended.

Exercise Testing

The exercise test, using both low and standard work-level protocols, can be extremely helpful not only in identifying ischemia but also in measuring levels of exercise performance after acute infarction. With the trend toward earlier hospital discharge, the exercise test can indicate which activities can be safely undertaken when the patient returns home. A standard exercise test should also be done before resumption of full activities and again at 6 and 12 months after the index event. Up to 25 per cent of patients who have had coronary angioplasty have recurrent stenosis in the first year. The exercise test can be used to help re-evaluate these patients.

Low-level exercise testing can also be helpful in evaluating patients after myocardial infarction. Those who develop signs of ischemia or symptoms of angina are at far higher risk for recurrent cardiovascular events, including death, within the following year.

Standard exercise testing done 3 weeks after acute infarction can also be helpful in assessing performance, as well as in enhancing patients' perceptions of their physical disabilities. Those who exhibit near-normal tolerance become far more physically active after testing. However, the resumption of other activities, such as sexual intercourse and lifting, is more favorably influenced by counseling by the physician or nurse.

Supervised Exercise Programs

One of the major benefits of supervised exercise programs is their educational component, which allows modification of risk factors. The group setting also provides reassurance to the patient. Perhaps the most important attribute of supervised programs is their ability to deliver emergency care if an untoward event occurs during exercise. In supervised exercise programs, an ECG rhythm strip can be recorded, either continuously or intermittently, by using a monitor-defibrillator. Exercise test data provide the ability to prescribe specific levels of activity before enrollment in such programs. During supervised exercise, it is recommended that patients reach 70 to 85 per cent of their maximal heart rate to stimulate aerobic metabolism. Maximal exercise activity levels are to be discouraged because they may place the patient at risk for severe ischemia

or cardiac arrest. The consensus is that patients who exercise regularly are at less risk for sudden cardiac death and recurrent ischemic events. By contrast, the risk of sudden cardiac death is 6 to 160 times higher during exercise than during sedentary activities. These results indicate that the safest setting in which to perform exercise after acute myocardial infarction is a supervised exercise program. Patients who want to exercise routinely and achieve high target rates should be strongly encouraged to use these programs. There is some evidence that these programs should not be initiated until 3 to 4 weeks after acute infarction.

The exercise program usually consists of a 5- to 10-minute warm-up period followed by 15 to 30 minutes of aerobic or endurance exercise. This may consist of walk and run sequences, as well as bicycle exercise or swimming. Leg exercise (brisk walking) is recommended over arm exercise because there is less of a decrease in blood pressure with isotonic compared with isometric exercise.

Unsupervised Exercise

Despite the proliferation of supervised programs, the majority of patients exercise without supervision after discharge from the hospital. With this in mind, it is important to prescribe specific levels of exercise and to monitor patient performance during several office visits in the first 6 months after infarction. The exercise test can help to determine the patient's maximal heart rate. Patients can be taught to monitor their heart rate and should be advised not to exceed levels higher than 70 per cent of maximum. Walking should be advised as an initial exercise with a goal of 2 miles a day within 8 weeks after hospital discharge.

There is now greater emphasis on allowing patients to return to work earlier. The fast pace and economic environment of the business world do not permit many patients to maintain their position at work if they are disabled for 2 to 3 months after hospital discharge. The exercise test can be used to determine when the patient can return to normal activity. In many patients, thrombolytic therapy results in a small infarction. Clearly, many of these patients, who have no evidence of ischemia, may return to work, at least part-time, as early as 1 to 2 weeks after hospital discharge.

All these findings point to the fact that each patient must be assessed individually and recommendations must be made on the basis of the resultant left ventricular function, infarct size, persistent ischemia, and the level of exercise performance as measured by treadmill testing.

Patient Education

With the decline in number of days of hospitalization, physicians must place more emphasis on both screening and modifying risk factors. A discussion with the spouse should take place regarding dietary recommendations, sexual counseling, and the need for the family to prepare a plan should another emergency occur. This discussion, with both the patient and the spouse, should include recognition of symptoms and knowledge of when and whom to call if cardiac symptoms occur. The spouse should be advised to learn the techniques of cardiopulmonary resuscitation. Although the prevalence of cardiac arrest should not be exaggerated to avoid alarm, the ability of the spouse to treat this disorder, if it does occur, should be emphasized. Most cardiac arrests (more than 70 per cent) occur at home, and it is likely that family members will witness the event. They must know whom to call and the importance of using the basic techniques of chest compression and ventilation before arrival of the emergency medical system providers. It is evident, after training hundreds of spouses, that families are far more comfortable after being trained in such a course of action than when they do not know what to do should an emergency occur.

PERICARDITIS

method of
E. WILLIAM HANCOCK, M.D.
Stanford University
Stanford, California

ACUTE PERICARDITIS

Nonspecific Etiologies

The initial management of nonspecific or viral acute pericarditis is partly based on the presenting differential diagnosis because acute pericarditis usually presents with chest pain as the predominant symptom. Hospitalization is usually indicated, unless idiopathic or viral pericarditis is clearly the most likely diagnosis, and the patient is not in severe discomfort. Initial symptomatic therapy is best carried out with a nonsteroidal anti-inflammatory drug (NSAID) such as aspirin, 650 mg orally every 4 hours, or indomethacin (Indocin), 25 to 50 mg orally three times daily. Analgesics such as codeine, 30 to 60 mg

orally every 4 to 6 hours, or propoxyphene hydrochloride (Darvon), 32 to 65 mg orally every 4 to 6 hours, may be used in addition when the pain is unusually severe and persistent.

Administration of adrenal corticosteroids should be avoided, if possible, in the treatment of acute pericarditis because of a tendency to relapse when their use is discontinued, sometimes followed by a chronic relapsing course and a risk of corticosteroid dependency. In unusually severe cases in which a combination of NSAIDs and analgesics has been ineffective, a 7- to 14-day course of prednisone may be indicated. Prednisone should be given initially in a dose of 60 mg daily, reduced to 40 mg daily after 2 days, to 20 mg daily after 2 more days, and tapered more slowly thereafter. In patients with chronic relapsing pericarditis who experience recurrent symptoms when prednisone is reduced or discontinued, the tapering process should be extended for a period of 4 to 6 months.

Specific Etiologies

If the etiology of acute pericarditis is known, the treatment of the underlying disease assumes primary importance. Bacterial infective pericarditis should be treated with antibiotics in the same manner as systemic infections because antibiotics pass readily from the circulating blood into the pericardial space. Pericarditis related to rheumatic diseases such as rheumatoid arthritis or systemic lupus erythematosus requires administration of corticosteroids more frequently than do idiopathic cases. Pericarditis in patients who are undergoing chronic dialysis may call for more frequent dialysis, a shift from peritoneal dialysis to hemodialysis, or a shift from systemic to regional heparinization.

Pericardiectomy is rarely indicated for relief of the symptoms of acute pericarditis but may be resorted to occasionally in the chronic relapsing syndrome or in dialysis patients. An exception is purulent pericarditis, where an anterolateral parietal pericardiectomy is often indicated to provide adequate drainage and to prevent constriction, even though cardiac tamponade may be adequately relieved by pericardiocentesis initially.

PERICARDIAL EFFUSION

Echocardiography is normally indicated in patients with pericarditis because pericardial effusion occurs frequently in virtually all of the etiologies. Diagnostic studies of the pericardial fluid provide useful information, particularly in neoplastic and specific infectious cases. However, the greatest importance of pericardial effusion is its capacity to cause cardiac tamponade. Cardiac tamponade results from an abnormally positive pressure within the pericardial fluid that therefore compresses the heart. The increase in intrapericardial fluid pressure is accompanied by a similar elevation of central venous pressure (CVP), which is therefore distinctly elevated in cardiac tamponade, with only rare exceptions. Although cardiac tamponade is sometimes defined in terms of a reduction in systemic arterial pressure or cardiac output, it is actually a hemodynamic continuum in which the earliest clinically detectable abnormality is a rise in CVP. When the CVP has risen to approximately 10 mmHg because of pericardial fluid under increased pressure, a relatively small additional increase in the volume of fluid can raise the intrapericardial pressure inordinately and cause a critical reduction in cardiac output and systemic arterial pressure. Removal of pericardial fluid is therefore indicated when the CVP becomes distinctly elevated to prevent the emergence of cardiac tamponade. However, removal of pericardial fluid for purely diagnostic purposes when the CVP is normal is not indicated in most circumstances because of the low yield of specific diagnoses.

Pericardial fluid may be removed by a needle tap (pericardiocentesis) or by a surgical procedure (pericardiostomy). The choice depends on the circumstances and the experience of the physicians involved. In surgical conditions, such as traumatic or postoperative hemopericardium, a pericardiostomy is preferable, whereas in medical conditions, such as idiopathic, viral, neoplastic, or dialysis-related pericardial effusion, a pericardiocentesis is usually preferable.

Pericardiocentesis should be done, if possible, in facilities that permit simultaneous measurements of intracardiac, intrapericardial, and systemic arterial pressures. Echocardiography should also be used to assess the size and predominant location of the fluid. A catheter should be left in the pericardial space for continuous percutaneous drainage for at least 24 hours. Recurrent pericardial effusion, particularly in neoplastic cases, may be treated with instillation of tetracycline,* 500 mg in 30 ml of normal saline, into the pericardial space to promote inflammatory obliteration of the pericardial space.

CONSTRICTIVE PERICARDITIS

Constrictive pericarditis presents its greatest challenge in the area of diagnosis. Chronic cases

---

*The use of tetracycline as a sclerosing agent is not listed as an approved indication by the manufacturer.

develop insidiously and may simulate noncardiac conditions because of the prominence of pleural effusion or ascites as the presenting clinical feature. Recognition of elevated jugular venous pressure is the key to early diagnosis. Subacute cases, by contrast, often present with active pericarditis and pericardial effusion. Here the key is to demonstrate that a peel of constricting tissue is present on the surface of the heart (visceral pericardium); this often requires a hemodynamic study during pericardiocentesis, in which it is shown that the CVP remains elevated even after reduction of the intrapericardial pressure to normal by removal of the pericardial fluid. Constrictive pericarditis normally requires the surgical procedure of pericardiectomy for its effective treatment. Surgery is indicated if the CVP is approximately 10 mmHg or more and if diuretics are required to control fluid retention.

PERIPHERAL ARTERIAL DISEASE
method of
JAMES S. T. YAO, M.D., PH.D.
Northwestern University Medical School
Chicago, Illinois

OCCLUSIVE ARTERIAL DISEASE

Acute Ischemia

Sudden onset of pain, paresthesia, and coldness in a pulseless leg constitute the diagnosis of acute arterial occlusion. Common causes of sudden arterial occlusion are embolization, thrombosis of an atherosclerotic artery, or popliteal aneurysm. Acute thrombus of an atherosclerotic artery or an aneurysm must be differentiated from embolic occlusion. A history of claudication favors the diagnosis of arterial thrombosis, whereas sudden onset of pain in an otherwise normal extremity is characteristic of acute embolic occlusion. Table 1 shows the common causes of acute arterial ischemia. Most embolic occlusions caused by a cardiac source occur in major arterial bifurcations; thus, severe acute ischemia involving the entire leg is common. In contrast, atheromatous emboli, such as from atherosclerotic plaques or proximal aneurysms, are microemboli in origin. These emboli are too small to cause major artery occlusion and are commonly manifested by the so-called purple toe syndrome. Occasionally, a petechia-like lesion is seen in the skin of the leg.

Treatment

Once the diagnosis is established, heparin sodium should be administered intravenously to

TABLE 1. **Etiology of Acute Arterial Ischemia**

1. Embolic occlusion
   A. Cardiac source
      i. Acute myocardial infarction
      ii. Atrial fibrillation
      iii. Sinoatrial disease
      iv. Left ventricular aneurysm
      v. Atrial myxoma
      vi. Paradoxical emboli
   B. Noncardiac source
      i. Atheromatous emboli
      ii. Emboli from a proximal aneurysm
      iii. Mycotic aneurysm
         a. Drug addiction
         b. Endocarditis
      iv. Diagnostic and therapeutic procedures
         a. Percutaneous transluminal balloon angioplasty
         b. Intra-aortic balloon
2. Thrombotic occlusion
   A. Arteriosclerosis obliterans
   B. Thromboangiitis obliterans
   C. Aneurysm
   D. Drug-induced disease
      i. Ergotism
      ii. Dopamine
3. Aortic dissection
4. Hematologic disorders

prevent propagation of the thrombotic process. Pain relief and protection of the limb by avoiding local heat are helpful. In a typical case of acute embolic occlusion from the heart, arteriography is rarely needed. If there is doubt, especially in patients with evidence of atherosclerotic disease in the contralateral limb, arteriography is helpful to differentiate thrombosis from embolization. A Doppler examination helps to confirm the diagnosis and to determine the viability of the limb. For acute embolization, the treatment of choice is embolectomy using Fogarty's balloon catheter. This relatively simple procedure can be done under local anesthesia with minimal morbidity. The onset of ischemia from acute thrombosis usually is insidious. Therefore, treatment can be instituted in a less urgent manner, using intravenous heparin followed by an elective femoral bypass procedure to relieve ischemia. Arteriography is needed in acute thrombosis to define the distal anatomy for distal anastomosis. Recently, thrombolytic therapy, especially urokinase, has received much attention. This mode of therapy is costly and is not without complications. Thrombolytic therapy, however, can be used as an alternative procedure if there are contraindications to surgery.

Chronic Ischemia

Depending on the extent of occlusion, patients with chronic occlusive arterial disease may present with mild ischemia, such as intermittent claudication to severe ischemia manifested by pain at rest or tissue loss (e.g., ulcer or gangrene). Diagnosis is easily made by pulse examination. A noninvasive test such as Doppler flow examination or systolic pressure measurement helps to (1) confirm the diagnosis, (2) locate the site of occlusion, and (3) classify the degree of ischemia objectively.

In adults over the age of 40 years, the most common etiology of chronic occlusive arterial disease is arteriosclerosis obliterations. Table 2 lists the etiologies of chronic occlusive arterial disease. In young adults with intermittent claudication, popliteal cystic degeneration or popliteal artery entrapment must be suspected.

Treatment

The plan of treatment depends on the site of occlusion and the presenting symptoms. Arteriography is needed if patients are to be considered for interventional therapy or surgical treatment. In patients who have superficial femoral artery occlusion with mild claudication, conservative management is the treatment of choice. In these patients, arteriography is seldom necessary. Doppler examination is all that is needed to determine the degree of ischemia and to monitor the progress of the disease by repeat measurement of ankle systolic pressure. By contrast, patients with limb-threatening ischemia such as pain at rest or tissue loss require arteriography and definitive treatment.

Exercise, abstinence from tobacco, weight loss, and better control of diet, hypertension, and diabetes mellitus constitute conservative treatment in patients with mild ischemia. It is universally agreed that oral vasodilating agents are ineffective. Recently, the use of pentoxifylline (Trental), a drug to increase erythrocyte flexibility and improve the microcirculation, was claimed to be effective in controlled trials in a dose of 400 mg three times orally. However, our experience, as well as that of others in treating intermittent claudication with this drug, has been disappointing.

Therapeutic intervention depends on the degree of ischemia. Disabling claudication is defined as the inability to work; in these patients, intervention may become necessary. Whether the

TABLE 2. **Etiology of Chronic Arterial Ischemia**

1. Arteriosclerosis obliterans
2. Fibromuscular dysplasia
3. Thromboangiitis obliterans (Buerger's disease)
4. Takayasu's arteritis
5. Abdominal aortic coarctation
6. Radiation injury
7. Popliteal artery entrapment syndrome
8. Popliteal cystic degeneration
9. Arteritis (systemic and infectious)

patient is a candidate for percutaneous transluminal balloon angioplasty (PTLA) or surgery depends on the arteriographic findings. The PTLA technique, pioneered by Grüntzig, is now a standard procedure for short segmental stenosis of either the iliac artery or the superficial femoral artery. Long-term patency of an iliac stenosis is much greater than that of the superficial femoral artery. In the presence of total occlusion of the unilateral iliac artery, a femorofemoral crossover graft is an effective surgical procedure with minimal morbidity and a short hospital stay. For an extensive aortic lesion or bilateral iliac artery occlusion, aortofemoral bypass grafting using a Dacron bifurcation graft provides satisfactory long-term patency.

Severe ischemia such as pain at rest or tissue loss requires arteriography and immediate intervention. In combined lesions (aortoiliac and femoropopliteal), correction of the proximal lesion must be done before femoropopliteal or femorotibial bypass surgery. In many instances, correction of proximal lesions alone is often sufficient to alleviate the ischemic symptoms. In severe ischemia as a result of femoropopliteal or infrapopliteal occlusive disease, either the reversed saphenous vein or the in situ saphenous vein graft is the procedure of choice. With better angiographic and surgical techniques, it is now possible to place distal anastomoses of these grafts into either the posterior tibial or dorsalis pedis arteries at the ankle level. In patients with previous vein surgery or coronary bypass graft surgery in whom an autogenous vein is not available, the use of prosthetic grafts such as the polytetrafluoroethylene graft may be necessary. When these prosthetic grafts are placed below the infrageniculate arteries, heparinization during the immediate postoperative period followed by long-term warfarin (Coumadin) is often needed to maintain graft patency in these patients.

As a result of the in situ vein graft technique, treatment of ischemia by lumbar sympathectomy is now virtually nonexistent. Many patients who were thought to be nonreconstructable can now be revascularized by this technique. Recently, laser and atherectomy devices have emerged as percutaneous techniques adjunctive to PTLA in the treatment of arterial occlusive disease. The role of these devices, however, remains unclear, and further trials are needed to establish their effectiveness.

Other than atherosclerotic occlusion, unusual ischemia from Buerger's disease or a variety of collagen arteritis may also cause ischemia. Most of these patients are not candidates for surgical intervention. Treatment is often directed to correction of the underlying medical conditions and abstinence from tobacco use.

In young adults, diagnosis of popliteal artery entrapment or cystic adventitial degeneration is often facilitated by arteriography and infusion computed tomography (CT) scanning. Once the diagnosis is confirmed, a posterior surgical approach to the popliteal fossa either to divide the anomalous tendon or to decompress the cyst results in dramatic relief of symptoms.

VASOSPASTIC DISEASE

Acrocyanosis, livedo reticularis, and Raynaud's phenomenon are commonly seen in young women. A typical attack of Raynaud's phenomenon consists of cyclic discoloration of the finger, proceeding from white to blue to red. The attack is often precipitated by exposure to cold or emotional stress. The episodic spasm is often accompanied by numbness or paresthesia. In contrast, acrocyanosis or livedo reticularis is often painless and persistent. This vasospastic disease is a result of spasm of small arteries or arterioles without actual occlusion. Raynaud's phenomenon can be primary (Raynaud's disease) or secondary to a wide variety of diseases. Table 3 shows the multiple causes of hand ischemia. Distinction between Raynaud's phenomenon and disease depends on the extent of the work-up. In patients with hand ischemia, a careful history including occupational, pharmacologic, and medical inquir-

TABLE 3. **Etiology of Upper Extremity and Hand Ischemia**

1. Occupational causes
   A. Vibratory tools
   B. Hypothenar hammer syndrome (carpenters, electricians)
2. Pharmacologic causes
   A. Ergot poisoning
   B. Dopamine-induced ischemia
   C. Beta blockers
   D. Chemotherapeutic agents
3. Atherosclerosis
4. Arteritis
   A. Collagen disease
   B. Takayasu's arteritis
   C. Giant cell arteritis
   D. Buerger's disease
5. Blood dyscrasia
   A. Cold agglutinins
   B. Cryoglobulins
   C. Polycythemia
6. Thoracic outlet syndrome
7. Congenital arterial wall defect
8. Trauma
   A. Iatrogenic catheter injury
   B. Frostbite
9. Radiation injury
10. Renal transplantation and related problems
    A. Azotemic arteriopathy
    B. Hemodialysis shunts
11. Aneursym of the upper extremity

ies will help guide the work-up. The use of non-invasive tests, especially finger systolic pressure measurement, also helps to uncover organic lesions accounting for Raynaud's phenomenon. In selected cases, especially when proximal arterial lesions are suspected, arteriography including that of the innominate artery to the fingers is needed to establish the definitive diagnosis. For patients suspected of having thoracic outlet compression, positional exposure with the arm in abduction–external rotation or hyperabduction is needed to demonstrate the compression.

Treatment

Treatment is directed to the underlying cause of the ischemic symptoms. If no proximal lesion or systemic disease is found, symptomatic control can be achieved by not smoking, and wearing warm or heated gloves. In addition, if symptoms are severe or troublesome, using a calcium blocker such as nifedipine (Procardia), 10 to 20 mg three times a day, may be helpful. Sympathectomy is often not indicated or needed. In proximal lesions such as an atherosclerotic plaque, thoracic outlet compression, with or without aneurysm of the axillary-subclavian artery, requires appropriate surgical procedures to eliminate the source of embolization. In occupational disease, a change of job or a decrease in working intensity is required to relieve ischemic symptoms. Unlike lower extremity ischemia, amputation is often not needed in these patients.

ARTERIAL ANEURYSMS

The most common location of arterial aneurysms is the abdominal aorta. At present, aortic aneurysm ranks as the fifteenth cause of death in the United States. If untreated, the aneurysm expands in size and ruptures, or compresses the surrounding structure and, not infrequently, causes severe ischemia by thrombosis or distal embolization. Most aneurysms are atherosclerotic in origin; therefore, they often occur in men older

TABLE 4. **Etiology of Nonatherosclerotic Aneurysm**

---

1. Chronic trauma
   A. Thoracic outlet compression (cervical rib)
   B. Hypothenar hammer syndrome
2. Behçet's disease
3. Congenital arterial wall defect
   A. Pseudoxanthoma elasticum
   B. Ehlers-Danlos syndrome
4. Fibromuscular dysplasia (media degeneration)
5. Electrical burn
6. Mycotic etiologies
7. Infectious etiologies
8. Congenital arteriovenous malformation

---

than age 50. In young adults, aneurysm may be infectious, mycotic, or caused by unusual arterial lesions (Table 4).

A family history of aneurysm is not uncommon, and evidence of aneurysm should be sought in family members. Also, aneurysms are frequently multiple, so the discovery of one aneurysm should call for a search of other locations. The combination of aortic and popliteal aneurysms is common, and the popliteal pulse should be carefully examined in all patients with aortic aneurysm. Diagnosis of aortic aneurysm is often aided by an ultrasound or infusion CT scan. Of these two tests, the ultrasound scan is the better screening procedure. Once aortic aneurysm is suspected, an infusion CT scan is often definitive to confirm the diagnosis and determine the extent and dimension of the aneurysm. Arteriography is seldom needed and is often nondiagnostic. However, it should be done in patients with suspected extension to the suprarenal aorta or in those who have renovascular hypertension, visceral ischemia, or evidence of peripheral arterial occlusive disease.

Treatment

All aneurysms regardless of size, once confirmed by radiologic techniques, should be considered for surgery. The use of size (5 cm) for decision-making is appropriate only in those who are poor surgical risks. In patients who are not candidates for surgery, the size of the aneurysm can be followed by interval examination using infusion CT scan. Before surgery, careful evaluation of the extracranial carotid artery and the coronary artery reserve is mandatory. Patients with a history of myocardial infarction or angina must be evaluated by thallium scan and, if positive, by coronary arteriography. In patients with significant coronary artery disease, coronary revascularization is needed before aortic surgery.

Surgical treatment for infrarenal aortic aneurysm is straightforward. Either Dacron tube graft replacement or an aorto-bi-iliac or bifemoral Dacron graft is used, depending on the extent of involvement of the iliac artery. For peripheral aneurysms affecting the femoral or popliteal artery, similar surgical principles are also applicable. Short prosthetic graft replacement is often performed for common femoral aneurysm. For popliteal aneurysm, the aneurysm is often excluded from the circulation by proximal and distal ligation followed by a bypass graft using either autogenous vein or a prosthetic graft. Removal of the aneurysm is often hazardous because of involvement of the surrounding structures.

Visceral arterial aneurysm, especially splenic aneurysm in young women, requires surgical treatment. Splenic aneurysms are most likely to rupture during the third trimester of pregnancy; therefore, routine resection is recommended in women of childbearing age. Aneurysms of the renal, superior mesenteric, or celiac arteries require surgical treatment only if the aneurysm exceeds 2 cm in size. Most of these aneurysms are discovered during radiologic examination for other causes, and many of these are asymptomatic.

DEEP VEIN THROMBOSIS AND THROMBOPHLEBITIS

method of
DENNIS F. BANDYK, M.D.
The Medical College of Wisconsin
Milwaukee, Wisconsin

The pathophysiology of venous thrombosis is based on *Virchow's triad* of hypercoagulability, venous stasis, and endothelial injury. Risk factors that promote components of the triad have been recognized to predispose to the development of acute deep venous thrombosis (Table 1). The population most at risk includes the elderly (older than 60 years), postoperative patients (particularly after hip and knee surgery), spinal cord injury and stroke patients, patients with disseminated malignancy, and those with a prior episode of venous thromboembolism.

As many as one-half of the patients with thrombotic occlusion of one or more veins of the lower limb venous system may be asymptomatic. Clinical signs are common when thrombus formation is extensive. The classic signs and symptoms are edema, pain, tenderness, cyanosis, warmth, and prominence of superficial veins. Tenderness on posterior calf compression (Pratt's sign) and on passive dorsiflexion of the foot (Homan's sign)

TABLE 1. **Risk Factors for the Development of Acute Deep Venous Thrombosis**

Hypercoagulability
  Malignancy
  Oral contraceptives
  Polycythemia
  Thrombocytosis
  Antithrombin III deficiency
  Protein-C and protein-S deficiency

Venous stasis
  Immobility
  Varicose veins
  Advanced age
  Congestive heart failure
  Obesity

Endothelial injury
  Trauma
  Recent surgery
  Systemic infections

TABLE 2. **Clinical Conditions That Mimic Symptoms and Signs of Deep Venous Thrombosis**

Pain
  Ruptured Baker's cyst
  Subfascial hematoma
  Ruptured plantaris muscle
  Nerve entrapment
  Myalgia or myositis

Edema
  Congestive heart failure
  Lymphedema
  Extrinsic compression caused by
    Trauma
    Hematoma
    Malignancy
  Prolonged dependency

Inflammation
  Cellulitis
  Lymphangitis
  Subcutaneous fat necrosis

may be seen. Even if symptoms are present, they are not reliable indicators of the presence or location of thrombus in the deep veins of the lower limb. A number of clinical conditions can mimic the pain, edema, and inflammation of acute deep venous thrombosis (Table 2). The fallibility of clinical diagnosis requires the use of objective testing methods to confirm or exclude the diagnosis in patients with suspected venous disease. A noninvasive diagnostic technique should be used initially because these methods are accurate (sensitivity and specificity more than 90 per cent) in detecting occlusive thrombi in the iliac, femoral, and popliteal veins. Acceptable modalities include venous duplex scanning, impedance plethysmography, phleborheography, and continuous-wave Doppler examination. Nonocclusive thrombi or thrombosis involving calf, profunda femoris, and internal iliac veins may not be detected by these methods. Contrast venography, the current standard for the documentation of acute deep venous thrombosis, should be used when noninvasive testing is not available or its interpretation is equivocal. Adequate visualization of the femoral and iliac veins may require femoral injection of contrast material, and up to 4 per cent of patients with normal studies can develop deep venous thrombosis after venography.

Venous thrombosis most frequently occurs in the soleal venous sinuses of the calf and at the valves of tibial veins. Thromboembolism from these sites rarely produces significant pulmonary embolism because of the small size of the thrombi and the high (80 per cent) spontaneous lysis rate of thrombus isolated to the calf veins. Ambulation appears to facilitate lysis, and immobility promotes propagation of thrombus into the proximal popliteal and femoral veins. Thrombus formation in these larger veins, especially with involvement of the iliac veins, predisposes to life-threatening pulmonary embolism (incidence of 30 to 40 per cent). Other sequelae of deep venous thrombosis include the destruction of venous valves with the development of the post-thrombotic syndrome and an increased risk of recurrent thrombosis. Four clinical syndromes of venous thrombosis must be accurately diagnosed and treated by the clinician: (1) acute deep venous thrombosis, (2) recurrent deep venous thrombosis, (3) calf vein thrombosis, and (4) superficial thrombophlebitis. Rational management of venous thromboembolic disease requires an awareness of the patients at risk, the use of objective diagnostic criteria to confirm the location and extent of thrombosis, and implementation of therapy to minimize acute and long-term morbidity.

ACUTE DEEP VENOUS THROMBOSIS

The extent and location of lower limb venous thrombosis may vary. Thrombosis commonly involves both the muscular veins of the calf and more proximal veins, including the popliteal, superficial femoral, and iliofemoral venous segments. Extensive thrombus formation and propagation can occur and produce complete venous outflow obstruction, marked fluid sequestration in the limb, and the development of gangrene (phlegmasia cerulea dolens). This condition is rare (1 per cent of acute deep venous thrombosis) and is more prevalent in patients with disseminated malignancies. An accurate clinical diagnosis of iliofemoral venous thrombosis can be made in massively swollen, cyanotic lower limbs, a condition that occurs more commonly on the left side. Deep venous thrombosis may also involve the major veins of the upper extremity and superior vena cava. Acceptable therapy for acute deep venous thrombosis, confirmed by noninvasive diagnostic modalities or venography, includes use of standard anticoagulants, thrombolytic therapy, prevention of pulmonary embolism by vena cava interruption (transvenous filter placement, plication, ligation), and rarely, thrombectomy.

Anticoagulant Therapy

Anticoagulation to prevent extension of thrombosis and pulmonary embolism is the treatment of choice for established deep venous thrombosis. Therapy is initiated with heparin as an intravenous bolus followed by a continuous infusion because bleeding complications are less than with intermittent bolus therapy (Table 3). The partial thromboplastin time is checked after 4 hours of heparin administration, and the dosage is adjusted to prolong the level to one and one-half to two times control values. Subtherapeutic levels are managed by infusion of an additional intravenous bolus (5000 units). The majority of patients require 1000 to 1500 units per hour of heparin, although larger doses may be required

TABLE 3. **Dosage Schedules for Anticoagulants and Thrombolytic Agents for Venous Thromboembolism**

Agent	Amount	Monitoring Tests
Heparin		
Loading dose	100 U/kg as an IV bolus	
Maintenance dose	1000–1500 U/hr by continuous infusion	PTT, platelet count
Prophylaxis	5000 U/SC 2 hr before surgery and every 12 hr until ambulatory	
Warfarin sodium		
Loading dose	10 mg PO	
Maintenance dose	2.5–10 mg PO each day	Prothrombin time
Streptokinase		
Loading dose	250,000 IU over 30 min	
Maintenance dose	100,000 IU for 72 hr	Thrombin time (two to three times control values), PTT, fibrinogen
Urokinase		
Loading dose	4400 IU/kg over 10 min	
Maintenance dose	4400 IU/kg/hr × 12 hr	Thrombin time, PTT, fibrinogen

Abbreviation: PTT = partial thromboplastin time.

initially in patients with extensive iliofemoral venous thrombosis. Failure to prolong the partial thromboplastin time despite the use of increasingly large doses of heparin can occur in patients with congenital hypercoagulable states such as antithrombin III or protein-C deficiency. If these conditions are suspected, warfarin sodium (Coumadin Sodium) therapy should be instituted immediately. While the patient is receiving heparin, the partial thromboplastin time should be checked twice daily until the level has stabilized in the therapeutic range, and daily thereafter. Routine testing of urine and stool for blood is performed daily, as is determination of the hematocrit. Platelet counts should be measured on alternate days to detect heparin-induced thrombocytopenia, an acquired immune complex disease that can result in further thrombosis involving both the venous and arterial circulations.

For the first few days, the patient should be confined to bed, with the legs elevated above the level of the right atrium to facilitate the reduction of limb edema. The knees should be flexed 20 to 30 degrees to avoid the popliteal vein obstruction that occurs with full extension. As swelling abates, the patient may ambulate in moderate-compression elastic stockings fitted to the below-knee level. Intramuscular injections and analgesics that affect platelet function must be avoided during anticoagulant therapy.

Prophylaxis for rethrombosis is begun on the sixth day of heparin therapy with the oral administration of warfarin sodium. Warfarin is prescribed daily thereafter at an adjusted dosage to prolong the prothrombin time to 18 to 20 seconds (one and one-half times the control value). Heparin and warfarin therapy should be overlapped for at least 4 days because the therapeutic value of the prothrombin time may be prolonged as a result of the heparin effect. With the prothrombin time in the therapeutic range for 3 days after oral warfarin therapy, the heparin infusion can be discontinued. Of note, *deep venous thrombosis during pregnancy* is managed with intravenous heparin followed by long-term subcutaneous heparin therapy (10,000 to 20,000 units every 12 hours).

With the commencement of oral anticoagulation, the patient's medications should be reviewed to avoid the possibility of synergistic or antagonistic actions. Patients must be specifically instructed to avoid platelet-active analgesics (aspirin, ibuprofen) and to use acetaminophen (Tylenol) for relief of pain. Before discharge from the hospital, patients should be encouraged to walk and be fitted with below-knee elastic stockings with a 20 mmHg gradient. Therapy with warfarin sodium should be continued for a minimum of 4 months, and longer if associated pulmonary embolism (for 6 months) or a hypercoagulable state has been detected (for life). Oral anticoagulation is monitored with weekly determinations of the prothrombin time for the first month and every second week to monthly thereafter.

Thrombolytic Therapy

The administration of fibrinolytic agents that actively dissolve clot is an accepted alternative to the use of heparin. The goal of thrombolytic therapy is to clear all thrombus, with the hope that venous valve function will be preserved and late circulatory and skin changes of the postthrombotic syndrome will not develop. There is no evidence that thrombolytic therapy is superior to anticoagulant therapy for the prevention of pulmonary embolism in patients with acute deep venous thrombosis of the lower limb. Careful patient selection is paramount for rational use of thrombolytic therapy. Patients with unexplained deep venous thrombosis of the lower limb or "effort thrombosis" of the subclavian vein and no serious concomitant disease are ideal candidates. Venous duplex scanning or contrast venography must be performed to confirm the diagnosis before institution of therapy. The major complication of thrombolytic therapy is hemorrhage from arterial and venous puncture sites; therefore, all arterial lines should be removed and patients should not be given intramuscular injections.

Streptokinase and urokinase are approved exogenous plasminogen activators that initiate measurable activity of the body's natural fibrinolytic system. Therapy should be implemented with a loading dose followed by a maintenance dose administered through a peripheral venous line by a constant infusion pump. The recommended dosage schedule is sufficient to produce a systemic fibrinolytic state (thrombin time greater than twice normal) in the majority (90 per cent) of patients (see Table 3). Before and during therapy (3 to 4 hours after initiation and twice daily thereafter), the following tests should be performed: hematocrit, thrombin time, partial thromboplastin time, prothrombin time, and fibrinogen. The thrombin time is a sensitive and reproducible test that measures the effect of fibrinolysis and of the products of fibrinolysis on coagulation time. A level higher than twice the control value during drug infusion is recommended to ensure that fibrinolysis is continuing. If the thrombin time after 4 hours of streptokinase administration is not significantly prolonged compared with the control level, the infusion should be discontinued because excessive resistance caused by antibodies is present.

The duration of therapy is individualized to the patient. Most patients require 3 days of therapy. Venous imaging should be used to monitor the effect of therapy. If no thrombolysis is observed after 24 hours, streptokinase or urokinase administration should be stopped and heparin therapy initiated in the dose and manner previously outlined. If partial thrombolysis is detected and no major bleeding complication has occurred, thrombolytic therapy should be continued for another 1 to 3 days or until complete dissolution of the thrombus is observed (by venous imaging or contrast venography). Anticoagulants and antiplatelet agents must be avoided during thrombolytic therapy because of their associated risk of hemorrhage. Physical handling of the patient should also be minimized, with needle punctures for laboratory monitoring confined to compressible vessels. At the conclusion of thrombolytic therapy, contrast venography should be performed. To prevent rethrombosis, heparin and warfarin should be administered in the dosage schedule previously outlined. The thrombin time should be less than twice the control value before anticoagulant therapy is initiated.

Therapy When Anticoagulants and Thrombolytic Therapy Are Contraindicated

Absolute contraindications to the use of heparin or fibrinolytic agents in patients with objectively confirmed deep venous thrombosis include recent injury involving the central nervous system, the presence of an active bleeding source such as duodenal ulcer or colon carcinoma, or the presence of a bleeding diathesis. In these circumstances, therapy is directed to the prevention of pulmonary embolism by vena cava interruption or, in patients with phlegmasia cerulea dolens, improvement of lower limb venous hemodynamics with thrombectomy.

Transcutaneous placement of a filter (Kimray-Greenfield) in the inferior vena cava below the level of the renal veins is the most appropriate method for preventing massive pulmonary embolism. This procedure is performed with fluoroscopic control under local anesthesia, commonly using a percutaneous technique via the right common femoral vein or right internal jugular vein. The availability of this technique and technical improvements in catheter delivery hardware have virtually abolished the necessity for vena cava interruption by direct surgical access. Circumstances in which vena cava interruption should be considered include pulmonary embolism in spite of adequate heparin therapy (1 to 2 per cent incidence), patients with severe pulmonary hypertension and iliofemoral venous thrombosis, and hemorrhage during heparin therapy that requires blood transfusion. The last complication is most likely to occur in female patients, the elderly (>60 years), patients who have recently undergone surgery, those with thrombocytopenia, and those in whom large doses of heparin have been administered.

Venous thrombectomy is not superior to anticoagulant or thrombolytic therapy for the treatment of deep venous thrombosis. Thrombectomy and fasciotomy may be indicated in cases of phlegmasia cerulea dolens that are not responsive to heparin anticoagulation and when contraindications to thrombolytic therapy are present. The need for thrombectomy is rare, but improvement in venous outflow from the lower limb can be accomplished by exposing the femoral vein in the groin, clearing the proximal iliac venous segment with Fogarty's balloon catheter, and extracting thrombus from the distal venous system by sequential wrapping from the toes to the thigh with an elastic bandage. Construction of a temporary arteriovenous fistula and concomitant heparin administration are essential components of the procedure designed to maintain iliac vein patency.

RECURRENT DEEP VENOUS THROMBOSIS

Symptoms of recurrent deep venous thrombosis may mimic those of post-thrombotic syndrome.

Diagnosis requires objective testing by either venous duplex scanning or contrast venography. Patients with confirmed recurrent, active venous thrombosis should receive anticoagulant therapy (heparin followed by oral warfarin sodium), as outlined previously, and oral anticoagulants are prescribed for 1 year. If a patient develops recurrent venous thrombosis despite anticoagulant therapy, testing for a hematologic abnormality (antithrombin III or protein-C deficiency, platelet function abnormality, abnormal plasminogen) should be performed. If a hypercoagulable state is identified, oral anticoagulation should be prescribed for life.

CALF VEIN THROMBOSIS

The diagnosis of calf vein thrombosis can be made accurately only with contrast venography, or with venous duplex scanning if performed by an experienced vascular technologist. Patients who are confined to bed should be treated with continuous intravenous heparin, as described for acute deep venous thrombosis. After the initial 10 days of heparin therapy, warfarin sodium is administered orally for 6 weeks. The development of calf vein thrombosis can be decreased in patients undergoing surgery by perioperative administration of low-dose heparin (see Table 3) or the application of external pneumatic compression garments on the lower limbs.

In patients who are ambulating normally, venography does not need to be performed, but serial noninvasive testing (every 2 days until symptoms abate) should be performed to determine whether propagation into the proximal femoropopliteal venous segment has occurred. This diagnostic approach has been shown to be effective in the ambulatory outpatient.

SUPERFICIAL THROMBOPHLEBITIS

This condition is usually a nonbacterial inflammation of the superficial veins precipitated by the presence of thrombus in the lumen. The most common cause in the upper extremities is the intravenous infusion of fluid with an acidic pH; in the lower extremities, it is typically associated with primary or secondary varicose veins. The symptoms and signs of superficial thrombophlebitis include tenderness, erythema, and induration in the subcutaneous tissues overlying a vein that frequently can be palpated as a firm chord. The thrombus can extend into the deep system, particularly if the saphenous vein is involved at the saphenofemoral junction, the lessor saphenopopliteal junction, or the perforator vein. Up to 30 per cent of patients develop concomitant deep venous thrombosis, and pulmonary embolism occurs in 2 to 4 per cent. Noninvasive diagnostic testing (duplex scanning or Doppler flow detection) should be used to confirm the presence of superficial vein thrombosis and to identify extension into the deep system.

In the lower limb, the optimal treatment for superficial thrombophlebitis uncomplicated by deep venous thrombosis is excision of the thrombosed varicose veins. This procedure, which can usually be performed under local anesthesia, significantly shortens the period of disability and reduces the likelihood of recurrence. In the upper extremity or when surgical therapy cannot be considered, anti-inflammatory agents such as phenylbutazone (Butazolidin),* 200 to 400 mg daily in divided doses, or indomethacin (Indocin), 50 to 150 mg daily in divided doses, should be instituted. Bed rest is to be avoided, as it contributes to stasis and may promote further thrombosis. Resolution may take 7 to 14 days. When symptoms persist or the process extends toward the saphenofemoral junction, surgery or anticoagulation is recommended. External elastic support stockings or bandages should be provided for comfort as the process subsides.

---

*Manufacturer states that this drug should be used only when other nonsteroidal agents have been ineffective.

The Blood and Spleen

APLASTIC ANEMIA

method of
KRISTINE C. DONEY, M.D.
Fred Hutchinson Cancer Research Center
Seattle, Washington

Aplastic anemia is a disease characterized by bone marrow failure that results in peripheral blood pancytopenia. If neutropenia and thrombocytopenia are severe, patients with aplastic anemia can be at acute risk of death from infection or bleeding. Initial care, therefore, consists of expeditiously (1) establishing the diagnosis, (2) assessing the need for transfusion support, (3) treating infection, and (4) determining the therapeutic options available to reverse the marrow failure.

DIAGNOSTIC CRITERIA

To confirm the diagnosis, a complete blood count, including a white blood cell differential and a reticulocyte count, should be done, as well as a bone marrow aspirate and biopsy. Both routine morphologic studies and cytogenetic analysis should be performed on the bone marrow sample. Established criteria for severe aplasia include any two of the following three peripheral blood findings: (1) a granulocyte count of less than 500 per mm³, (2) a corrected reticulocyte count of less than 1 per cent, and (3) a platelet count of less than 20,000 per mm³. In addition, the marrow must be hypocellular, with lymphoid cells usually being predominant. If cytogenetic analysis reveals a clonal abnormality, the patient is considered to have a myelodysplastic syndrome and not aplastic anemia.

ETIOLOGY

A careful history should be obtained to determine a potential etiology of the patient's aplasia. In the majority of cases no specific association is found, and the patient is considered to have "idiopathic" disease. However, aplastic anemia has been associated with (1) other hematologic disorders, (2) drugs, (3) infections, especially viral illnesses, (4) irradiation, (5) exposure to certain organic chemicals, and (6) rarely, pregnancy. Drug-induced marrow aplasia can occur either as an idiosyncratic reaction or in a dose-related manner. All prescription and over-the-counter medications taken by a patient should be reviewed for any possible association with aplasia. All nonessential medications should be discontinued immediately.

HUMAN LEUKOCYTE ANTIGEN TYPING

Histocompatibility (human leukocyte antigen, HLA) typing should be done as rapidly as possible on all patients and their immediate family members (siblings and parents). Patients who have a genotypically or phenotypically HLA-identical family member are candidates for bone marrow transplantation as primary therapy. Transfusion support of these patients is different from support of patients who are candidates for immunosuppressive therapy, as will be discussed.

TRANSFUSION SUPPORT

Platelet Transfusions

Because patients with aplastic anemia usually require long-term transfusion therapy, every effort should be made to limit transfusions to delay platelet alloimmunization. Platelet transfusions are provided based on (1) the platelet count and associated platelet function and (2) the presence and severity of bleeding. We routinely transfuse any patient with a platelet count of less than 5000 per mm³. Patients with higher platelet counts are transfused if they have evidence of significant bleeding (e.g., gastrointestinal, genitourinary, or intracerebral hemorrhage). Patients whose only evidence of bleeding is petechiae or ecchymoses are not routinely transfused. Drugs known to interfere with platelet function are also avoided if possible.

Several strategies to prevent platelet alloimmunization have been evaluated in limited transfusion trials in leukemic patients, with conflicting results. The applicability of these results to patients with aplastic anemia who are being transfused in the absence of potentially immunosuppressive chemotherapeutic agents is unknown. Single-donor apheresis platelets, from either random or HLA-matched donors, have been used to limit antigen exposure. Leukocyte-poor blood products can also be obtained. By using special filters, 99 per cent of contaminating leukocytes that express both Class I and Class II HLA antigens that stimulate the immune response can be removed. At present, these approaches should be considered to be experimental.

Platelet transfusions are provided as pooled random donor platelets or as single-donor apheresis products, depending on the resources of the local blood bank. We routinely use platelets from pooled random donors until there is evidence of refractoriness to these products. Single-donor platelets from community donors who are matched for all or most of the patient's major HLA antigens are then used. If a patient is not being considered for a transplant, platelet transfusions from a family member may also be considered. If the patient is a candidate for bone marrow transplantation, platelet transfusions from family members should be avoided to prevent sensitization to minor histocompatibility antigens that may prevent engraftment.

Red Blood Cell Transfusions

The hematocrit at which patients with aplasia become symptomatic from anemia depends on the rapidity of onset of the anemia, the age of the patient, and intercurrent medical problems. Packed red blood cell transfusion requirements must therefore be determined on an individual basis. The risk of alloimmunization and the probability of a long-term red blood cell transfusion requirement, with its attendant risk of iron overload, must be weighed against the need to provide the patient with a "buffer" if bleeding occurs because of thrombocytopenia. In general, we maintain an otherwise asymptomatic patient at a hematocrit of 25 to 30 ml per dl.

Granulocyte Transfusions

Prophylactic granulocyte transfusions are of no proven benefit. For persistently neutropenic patients who have a documented infection unresponsive to appropriate antibiotics, therapeutic granulocyte transfusions can be considered. Uniform criteria for selecting the best granulocyte donors have not been established. In general, for patients who are eligible for marrow grafting, community granulocyte donors are used. For patients who are not eligible for marrow grafting or who have received a marrow transplant, family members may also be suitable donors. The duration of therapy is usually determined by the clinical response of the patient, the duration of neutropenia, and the availability of donors. Daily granulocyte transfusions are administered for a minimum of 10 to 14 days. Further granulocyte infusions are not recommended in the absence of clinical improvement.

ANTIBIOTIC THERAPY

Afebrile, neutropenic patients are not treated with prophylactic antibiotics. Neutropenic patients who develop temperatures above 38.5° C are cultured and immediately given empiric broad-spectrum antibiotics. We use a combination of a semisynthetic penicillin with activity against pseudomonas and a third-generation cephalosporin. Our current regimen includes mezlocillin (Mezlin), 3 grams every 4 hours intravenously,* and ceftizoxime (Cefizox), 2 grams every 8 hours intravenously (adult doses). We avoid intramuscular injections to prevent infection or bleeding at the injection site. Specific antibiotic coverage, based on culture sensitivities, can be instituted if a pathogen is identified. For febrile, neutropenic patients with no identifiable pathogen, broad-spectrum therapy is continued for 10 to 14 days.

If patients remain persistently febrile despite an adequate course of broad-spectrum antibiotics and no

*This dose may exceed the manufacturer's recommended dose.

pathogen has been identified, an empiric trial of amphotericin B (Fungizone) is given. The duration of this therapy is determined by the response of the patient. If the patient does not defervesce and shows no other evidence of improvement clinically, amphotericin is discontinued after a several-day course. If, however, the patient does improve, a full course of amphotericin is administered. For patients who do have positive fungal cultures, amphotericin is also given. First, a test dose of 1 mg of amphotericin B is given intravenously. If it is tolerated, therapeutic doses of 0.5 to 1 mg per kg per day intravenously are administered. A total dose of 1 to 2 grams of amphotericin is administered, depending on the organism being treated.

TREATMENT

Bone Marrow Transplantation

If HLA typing of the patient and the family is done while the diagnosis of aplastic anemia is being confirmed, treatment options can be determined quickly. If the patient does have a genotypically or phenotypically HLA-identical family member and meets the age requirement for transplantation, he or she should be immediately referred for marrow grafting. Most transplant units accept patients less than 40 years of age. We currently accept patients up to 55 years of age if an HLA-matched donor is available. Age restrictions for marrow donors also vary among institutions. All marrow donors must be in good general health.

Bone marrow transplantation offers the best chance of cure for patients who have a suitable syngeneic or allogeneic, HLA-matched, related donor. We treat our transplant patients in laminar airflow rooms and prophylactically administer both oral nonabsorbable antibiotics and intravenous broad-spectrum antibiotics. These measures are aimed at decreasing both the risk of infection and the incidence of severe acute graft-versus-host disease (GVHD). The major risks of transplantation include graft rejection, acute and chronic GVHD, infection, and interstitial pneumonia.

In Seattle, conditioning for transplantation consists of a 7-day regimen of alternate-day doses of cyclophosphamide (Cytoxan) and antihuman thymocyte globulin (ATG). Four doses of cyclophosphamide are administered intravenously on days 7, 5, 3, and 1 before transplantation. Each dose is 50 mg per kg (total dose is 200 mg per kg). Three doses of ATG are given intravenously on days 6, 4, and 2 before transplantation, each dose being 30 mg per kg (total dose is 90 mg per kg). Twenty-four hours after completion of the conditioning regimen, the marrow is infused (day 0). An attempt is made to infuse a minimum marrow cell dose of 2×10^8 cells per kg of recipient body weight. Post-transplant immunosuppression used as prophylaxis for acute GVHD consists of a combination of methotrexate and cyclosporine (Sandimmune). Methotrexate is given on day 1 after marrow infusion at a dose of 15 mg per M² intravenously followed by doses of 10 mg per M² intravenously on days 3, 6, and 11. Cyclosporine is initiated on the day before marrow infusion and is administered at an initial dose of 1.5 mg per kg intravenously twice daily. Each cyclosporine dose is infused over 1 to 4 hours. Cyclosporine therapy is continued intravenously until the patient can tolerate oral medications, at which time it is administered at a dose of 6.25 mg per kg orally twice daily until day 50. After day 50, it is tapered by 5 per cent per week. Cyclosporine doses are frequently altered based on patients' renal function and cyclosporine levels. After a patient has been conditioned for the transplant, family members can be used as platelet or granulocyte donors. After transplantation, the marrow donor (if HLA matched with the patient) is often the best source of platelet support.

Immunosuppressive Therapy

If no suitable marrow donor is identified, immunosuppressive therapy should be considered as de novo therapy. Immunosuppressive therapy for aplastic anemia has included ATG or antihuman lymphoblast globulin as a single agent or in combination with corticosteroids or androgenic steroids. Two prospectively randomized, controlled studies have shown immunosuppressive therapy to prolong survival significantly compared with traditional supportive care with transfusions and androgenic steroids. Although the precise mechanism of action of ATG in aplastic anemia is unknown, it is hypothesized that ATG may act on suppressor T lymphocytes that are inhibiting normal stem cell growth and differentiation.

Although ATG is commercially available, immunosuppressive therapy should not be administered by individuals unfamiliar with its potential side effects. Excellent blood bank support is also needed because different ATG batches have varying titers of antiplatelet antibodies and patients may require intensive platelet transfusion support.

In Seattle, our current immunosuppressive regimen consists of the following three drugs: ATG (Atgam), 15 mg per kg intravenously daily for 10 days; methylprednisolone sodium succinate (Solu-Medrol), 0.5 mg per kg intravenously daily for 10 days concurrently with the ATG; and oxymetholone (Anadrol), 3 mg per kg orally daily

for 3 months, beginning 48 hours after completion of ATG therapy. Each dose of ATG is infused over 4 to 10 hours, depending on patient tolerance. No patient should receive ATG therapy before being skin tested to determine possible hypersensitivity to this horse serum preparation. Methylprednisolone is given with the ATG to ameliorate the acute side effects of ATG, which include fever, rash, and arthralgias. Antihistamines are also often necessary in addition to the corticosteroid therapy. Additional short courses of methylprednisolone may be necessary for patients who develop symptomatic serum sickness. Oxymetholone is administered to only those patients with normal hepatic function.

Data in the literature suggest that concurrent use of very-high-dose corticosteroids with ATG can result in an increased frequency of response, which also occurs earlier than if ATG is administered alone. Our experience with this high-dose corticosteroid regimen has failed to confirm these observations. We have therefore discontinued using the high-dose corticosteroid regimen.

The time to response after immunosuppressive therapy is variable. We evaluate patients for evidence of marrow recovery 3 months after initiation of ATG therapy. Patients with improved peripheral counts are followed without further therapy. Long-term follow-up is necessary because a minority of these responding patients have recurrence of their aplasia and require retreatment with a second or even a third course of ATG. Some patients also have evidence of evolution to another hematologic disease (e.g., paroxysmal nocturnal hemoglobinuria or acute leukemia). For patients who have no evidence of hematologic improvement at 3 months, secondary therapy is considered.

Secondary Therapy

Unrelated Donor Transplants

We do not routinely offer a second course of ATG to patients who fail their first course. We prefer to try to identify an unrelated, HLA-matched marrow donor for the patient using the National Marrow Donor Program. This computerized search for an unrelated donor begins when the immunosuppressive therapy is initiated. If a donor is identified, a patient can be offered an unrelated-donor transplant once immunosuppressive therapy fails. Because of the increased risk of marrow graft rejection, the conditioning regimen for patients receiving marrow from unrelated donors includes total body irradiation. Currently, we condition these unrelated-marrow transplant recipients with cyclophosphamide, 50 mg per kg intravenously daily for 2 days followed by total body irradiation, 200 cGy fractions daily for 6 days. Prophylaxis against acute GVHD consists of the same regimen of cyclosporine and methotrexate described earlier for the related-donor transplants.

Androgenic Steroids

If patients have no other therapeutic options, androgens can be administered. Oxymetholone, 3 mg per kg orally, is given daily. Side effects include fluid retention, virilization, acne, hypertension, and sexual and hepatic dysfunction. These patients should be monitored regularly with liver function studies. A 2- to 3-month trial is usually necessary to assess the response adequately.

Investigational Agents

Growth Factors

The factor of current interest is recombinant granulocyte-macrophage colony-stimulating factor. We are using it in patients with aplasia who are to receive immunosuppressive therapy or who have had graft failure after marrow transplantation. Our current dose schedule is 240 micrograms per M^2 intravenously daily for 14 days. Preliminary data suggest that this factor has little or no effect on increasing the level of circulating red blood cells or platelets, and the degree of granulocyte proliferation is proportional to the marrow myeloid reserves.

PROGNOSIS

Historically, 60 per cent of patients with aplastic anemia who were treated with supportive care alone died within 4 months of diagnosis. In contrast, for patients who are transplanted shortly after diagnosis (when they are untransfused) from related, HLA-matched donors, actuarial survival rates are 90 per cent at 10 years. For transfused patients with HLA-matched marrow donors, long-term survival ranges from 50 to 80 per cent. Long-term survival of 50 to 75 per cent can be achieved with ATG therapy. Too few unrelated-donor transplants have been performed to assess long-term survival, but early results are encouraging.

IRON DEFICIENCY ANEMIA

method of
BERNARD J. DREILING, M.D., and
MARTIN H. STEINBERG, M.D.
*University of Mississippi School of Medicine
and VA Medical Center*
Jackson, Mississippi

INCIDENCE AND CAUSE

Iron deficiency is the most common cause of anemia. Although the etiology may differ, this is true not only of people in underdeveloped countries but of those in affluent societies as well. The incidence in the United States and Canada is similar: 3 to 5 per cent in males and 20 to 25 per cent in females. In early childhood, iron deficiency usually results from dietary lack. In adolescent girls, in addition to menstrual loss, accelerated growth contributes to the high incidence of iron deficiency. In premenopausal women, iron deficiency is most often secondary to menorrhagia and the increased iron cost of pregnancy and childbirth. In men and postmenopausal women, iron lack implies blood loss and usually results from gastrointestinal tract bleeding. Although extensive evaluation may not be warranted in children, adolescents, and premenopausal women, iron deficiency in adult men and postmenopausal women demands a search for a lesion responsible for blood loss. Finally, a rare cause or contributing factor to anemia is malabsorption of iron in patients with celiac disease or after gastric surgery with Billroth's type II intestinal bypass.

PRESENTATION AND DIAGNOSIS

Iron deficiency evolves slowly and progresses through several stages before overt anemia ensues. Whether symptoms occur in the preanemic stage is controversial. Body iron is ubiquitously distributed but is most concentrated in red blood cells, muscle, and the reticuloendothelial storage pool. The sensitivity of the laboratory parameters of iron status varies with the degree of iron lack. In the early stage of storage iron depletion, the serum ferritin level falls and the transferrin level rises. The second stage of iron deficient erythropoiesis is characterized by a fall in serum iron and transferrin saturations, accumulation of red blood cell protoporphyrin, hypochromia, and microcytosis. It is only in the final stage of iron deficiency, when storage iron is absent, that the hemoglobin level and hematocrit fall. With the almost universal use of automated blood counts, it has become apparent that an elevated red blood cell distribution width (RDW) precedes microcytosis and anemia in evolving iron deficiency. In fact, it has been suggested that an isolated high RDW indicates iron deficiency perhaps two-thirds of the time.

Although it is widely believed that serum iron, transferrin, and ferritin determinations are highly reliable in diagnosing iron deficiency, a diagnostic problem all too frequently arises when iron deficiency and the anemia of chronic disease (infection, inflammation, or malignancy) coexist. Clues to the presence of such a combined anemia are an elevated RDW, anemia more severe than that generally seen with chronic disease alone, and a serum ferritin level in the low normal range (30 to 100 micrograms per liter). The only reliable guide to the presence or absence of iron deficiency in such patients may be the final arbiter: bone marrow stained for iron.

THERAPY

Oral Iron Therapy

Once the cause of iron deficiency has been determined, and eliminated where feasible, the physician is obliged to correct the anemia and restore body storage iron. Unfortunately, the choice of therapy has been made needlessly difficult. The forty-third edition of the *Physician's Desk Reference* lists 79 oral iron preparations. Although almost all of them work, there is little evidence that preparations containing multiple hematinics offer any advantage over simple ferrous salts. Although the addition of high doses of ascorbic acid facilitates iron absorption, it does so at the expense of additional gastrointestinal side effects. Although sustained-release forms of iron reduce the side effects of iron therapy, there is a parallel reduction in the amount of iron absorbed. With the use of enteric-coated tablets, the reduction of iron absorption may be profound. All too often, generic prescriptions for iron tablets result in patients receiving enteric-coated rather than simple iron salts. To be certain that prescriptions are not filled with a pill that has a slow dissolution time, the phrase "not enteric coated" should be added to the prescription.

Simple ferrous salts are by far the least costly, safest, and most effective form of therapy, and in most instances are well tolerated. The most widely prescribed ferrous sulfate tablet contains 60 mg of elemental iron. In the usual dosage of a 300-mg tablet thrice daily, 180 mg of elemental iron is presented to the intestinal tract and approximately 40 to 50 mg is absorbed. This should result in an increased marrow production rate of two to three times normal and a daily hemoglobin response of 0.2 to 0.3 gram per dl or 1.5 to 2.0 grams per dl per week, depending on the magnitude of the original anemia.

Maximal iron absorption occurs when iron tablets are taken 1 to 2 hours before meals and again at bedtime. Bioavailable iron is reduced by approximately 50 per cent when taken with meals and by as much as 90 per cent when taken with cow milk and tea. Although controversy exists about the frequency of gastrointestinal side effects, the major problems with oral iron therapy are nausea, epigastric distress, and heartburn. These symptoms typically occur within 1 hour after ingestion, are more prevalent in adults than in children, seem to be dose related, and can be ameliorated by giving iron with meals, by reducing the dosage to one or two tablets daily for a time, by prescribing a liquid preparation of ferrous sulfate, or by using a sustained-release form of iron. Because there is seldom urgency in correcting iron deficiency, there is no harm and some merit in the preceding alternative approaches. It matters little if it takes a bit longer to restore a state of iron balance. When smaller doses are given, fewer patients are made ill by the therapy. The treatment of iron deficiency anemia in adults

is a simple matter. The more important issue is to uncover the source of blood loss and to manage it appropriately.

In children, the recommended dose is 2 mg of elemental iron per kg given thrice daily. Because liquid preparations are more often used in the young, to avoid temporary staining of the teeth children are encouraged to drink liberal amounts of liquid or to brush the teeth after administration. Finally, acute iron intoxication is the second most common cause of death from poisoning (after aspirin) in children less than 5 years of age. The minimum lethal dose of ferrous sulfate for a child is approximately 3 grams or the amount in 10 iron sulfate tablets. Needless to say, all iron preparations must be kept out of reach of young children.

Response

The nonhematologic consequences of iron deficiency (e.g., pica, fatigue, irritability, and anorexia) respond promptly to iron therapy, often within 24 to 48 hours. Reticulocytosis is evident by day 4, peaks in 7 to 10 days, and increases two to three times over the basal level. After 1 week of treatment, the hemoglobin level should increase by 0.1 to 0.3 gram per dl daily, the risk being directly proportional to the severity of the anemia. The response is considered to be suboptimal if there is less than a 0.1 gram per dl daily increment in the hemoglobin level or if the hemoglobin level is not fully restored after 6 to 8 weeks of iron therapy. Once the anemia is corrected, it is generally recommended that iron supplements be continued for 3 to 6 months until stores are replenished. The adequacy of storage iron can then be determined by monitoring the serum ferritin level, which approximates the amount of storage iron. One microgram per liter of serum ferritin corresponds to 10 mg of storage iron. Consequently, iron should be continued until the serum ferritin level exceeds 50 micrograms per liter.

Failure to Respond

The majority of patients with iron deficiency respond to iron therapy when it is given properly. However, occasional patients do not respond as expected. By far the most common cause of failure is poor patient compliance, suspected by the failure of stools to change color during the course of iron therapy. Taking time to explain to the patient the importance of iron therapy significantly reduces many of these treatment failures. Other causes of so-called refractory iron deficiency anemia are relatively infrequent.

Incorrect diagnosis is most often caused by the anemia of chronic disease or thalassemia minor;

serum ferritin measurement, hemoglobin electrophoresis, and marrow iron staining may be necessary to identify these causes of microcytosis. An unsuspected combined deficiency or a dual cause of anemia may limit the response to iron alone. Occasional patients bleed in excess of the amount of iron given. Because a patient receiving an optimal iron dosage can absorb 40 to 50 mg of iron daily, a whole-blood loss in excess of 80 to 100 ml per day would be required, an amount that should be detected easily.

Intestinal malabsorption of iron, although exceedingly uncommon, may occur in patients who have undergone partial gastrectomy with duodenal bypass (gastrojejunostomy) and in patients with diseases of the upper small intestine such as celiac disease. Malabsorption may be confirmed by performing an oral iron absorption test. The serum iron level is measured before and again 60 and 120 minutes after administering 100 mg of elemental liquid ferrous sulfate. A rise of less than 100 micrograms per dl above the basal serum iron level suggests malabsorption, warrants further investigation, and usually necessitates parenteral iron therapy.

Parenteral Iron Therapy

Although there are circumstances in which parenteral iron therapy is justified, it must be emphasized that repair of the iron deficiency is no more rapid than with an optimal oral regimen. In addition, it is more costly and potentially hazardous. Four indications for parenteral therapy are an absolutely unreliable patient, intractable side effects of iron pills, documented intestinal malabsorption, and uncontrollable blood loss, as seen in some patients with hereditary hemorrhagic telangiectasia or inflammatory bowel disease.

The only parenteral iron preparation available in the United States is Imferon, an iron-dextran complex that contains 50 mg of iron per ml and can be administered intramuscularly or intravenously. When the intramuscular route is used, the iron is given in the upper outer buttock by a deep zigzag injection in 2-ml daily or twice weekly doses until the full course of therapy has been given.

It is now apparent that a more convenient way to administer Imferon is by giving the total calculated dose in a single intravenous infusion by diluting the total quantity of iron-dextran in 500 ml of normal saline. To minimize the risk of anaphylaxis, the infusion is started at a rate of 10 drops per minute for the initial 10 minutes, with Solu-Cortef, epinephrine, and diphenhydramine (Benadryl) available should anaphylaxis

occur. If no untoward reactions occur, the remainder can be infused during a 6-hour period. A simple formula for calculating the total dose (mg Fe) required follows:

$$\text{mg Fe} = \text{Hb deficit (grams/dl)} \times \text{body weight (lb)} + 1000 \text{ (replenishment of stores)}$$

The most common adverse effects of parenteral iron are pain at the injection site, arthralgias, and fever, sometimes accompanied by leukocytosis, adenopathy, and splenomegaly hours to days after Imferon administration. Anecdotal cases of aseptic meningitis, reactivation of quiescent rheumatoid arthritis, and stillbirth have also been reported.

Transfusion

Although the main objective of iron therapy is to avoid transfusion of blood, and although the rationale for transfusion based on predetermined hemoglobin concentrations and hematocrits (e.g., 10 grams per dl and 30 per cent, respectively, for surgical patients) is fading, there are situations where anemia threatens to compromise the function of vital organs. No single laboratory measure replaces good clinical judgment as a basis for decisions regarding transfusion. If there is evidence of impaired pulmonary function, inadequate cardiac output, myocardial ischemia, or cerebrovascular or peripheral circulatory disease, transfusion of packed red blood cells may be cautiously undertaken. Iron deficiency anemia typically develops slowly, and its treatment need not be aggressive.

AUTOIMMUNE HEMOLYTIC ANEMIA

method of
RICHARD J. DAVEY, M.D.
National Institutes of Health
Bethesda, Maryland

Autoimmune hemolytic anemia (AIHA) is the accelerated destruction of red cells caused by pathologic autoantibody. This accelerated destruction may be rapid and profound, with severe and life-threatening symptoms, or it may be more modest, with only a nominal decrease in the normal red cell life span of 110 to 120 days.

Modest reductions in red cell life span may not be noticed by the patient or clinician. The normal bone marrow is capable of a tenfold increase in the production of red cells in response to anemic stress. Therefore, low-grade immune hemolysis may be fully compensated by an increased production of red cells, with an elevated reticulocyte count being the primary indicator that increased red cell turnover is occurring.

Symptomatic anemia develops when the rate of hemolysis exceeds the ability of the marrow to respond, or when the marrow becomes depleted of the necessary substrates to sustain the accelerated rate of red cell production. If immune hemolysis is suspected, the most helpful confirmatory test is the direct antiglobulin test (DAT), also known as the direct Coombs's test. The presence of immunoglobulin or complement components on the red cell membrane in combination with anemia and an elevated reticulocyte count is strong evidence of an immune hemolytic process. The major varieties of immune hemolysis are primary and secondary AIHA, immune hemolytic anemia secondary to drugs, cold agglutinin disease (CAD), and paroxysmal cold hemoglobinuria (PCH). A more detailed classification of these disorders is shown in Table 1.

PRIMARY AND SECONDARY AUTOIMMUNE HEMOLYTIC ANEMIA

AIHA mediated by warm-reacting autoantibodies can be either primary (idiopathic) or secondary to diseases such as chronic lymphocytic leukemia, lymphocytic and histiocytic lymphomas, systemic lupus erythematosus, and acquired immunodeficiency syndrome. AIHA is an uncommon disorder, with an incidence of about 1 in 80,000. Idiopathic AIHA is seen in all age groups, with women being affected more than men (about 60 to 40). Secondary AIHA parallels the age and sex distribution of the underlying disorder.

The etiology of AIHA is unclear. The observation that the disease is often seen in association

TABLE 1. **Classification of Autoimmune Hemolytic Anemias**

Autoimmune Hemolytic Anemia—Warm-Reactive Antibody
  Primary (idiopathic)
  Secondary
    Lymphoproliferative disorders (chronic lymphocytic leukemia, lymphomas)
    Connective tissue disorders (systemic lupus erythematosus)

Drug-Induced Immune Hemolytic Anemia
  Red cell autoantibody type (methyldopa)
  Immune complex type (quinidine)
  Drug absorption (hapten) type (penicillin)
  Membrane modification type (cephalosporin)

Cold Agglutinin Disease
  Primary (idiopathic)
  Secondary
    Lymphoproliferative disorders
    Infections (infectious mononucleosis, *Mycoplasma pneumoniae*, postviral syndrome)

Paroxysmal Cold Hemoglobinuria
  Primary (idiopathic)
  Secondary
    Syphilis
    Postviral syndrome

with disorders of the immune system suggests a defect in normal immune function—a loss of the ability to differentiate "self" from "nonself." There is evidence that AIHA may be related to an impairment in normal T suppressor lymphocyte function, thus allowing unrestrained B cell activity and the production of abnormal antibodies.

A small number of IgG molecules (<50) are found on the red cells of normal individuals. This number increases as the cell ages, leading to speculation that membrane-bound IgG plays a role in the removal of senescent red cells from the circulation. As the number of cell-bound IgG molecules increases (>200), the likelihood of immune hemolysis correspondingly increases. In the typical case of AIHA, large numbers of IgG molecules are found on the red cell surface, usually of the IgG subclasses IgG1 and IgG3. There are well-documented cases, however, when no hemolysis is seen, although many thousands of molecules are on the red cell and the DAT is strongly positive. There is evidence that anti-idiotype antibodies against the red cell autoantibody may block or otherwise modify the events that would otherwise lead to immune hemolysis of the cell. This phenomenon may also be related to the subclass of the IgG autoantibody that is being produced. Subclasses IgG2 and IgG4 are not associated with severe hemolysis. Conversely, hemolysis is almost always found when IgG3 is present. Immune hemolysis cannot be predicted with as much certainty when the most common subclass, IgG1, is present.

Although the immunoglobulin class of autoantibody in warm AIHA is almost always IgG, examples of warm-reactive IgM and IgA autoantibodies have been reported and should be considered when "DAT-negative" immune hemolytic anemia is encountered.

Diagnosis

Patients with AIHA present with weakness, dizziness, pallor, jaundice, and moderate splenomegaly. If the anemia is severe, hemoglobinuria, fever, palpitations, chest pain, and syncope may be prominent. If AIHA is suspected, it is imperative that a thorough search be made for an implicated drug or for a potentially treatable underlying disorder.

Laboratory findings that support the diagnosis are spherocytes on the peripheral blood smear, reticulocytosis, hyperbilirubinemia (indirect), low or absent serum haptoglobin, and elevated serum lactate dehydrogenase. Thrombocytopenia may indicate that immune destruction of platelets is also occurring, an association known as

Evans's syndrome. The direct antiglobulin test detects IgG and complement components on the red cell and is positive in the vast majority of patients with AIHA; however, this test is not diagnostic. The DAT can be positive in other disorders and in normal individuals. Conversely, AIHA can be DAT negative under unusual circumstances (e.g., IgA autoantibodies). The indirect antiglobulin test, if positive, indicates the presence of red cell auto- or alloantibodies in the serum of the patient. This usually indicates that sufficient red cell autoantibody is being produced to maximally coat the red cells, with additional autoantibody being present in the serum.

Treatment

Treatment of AIHA is effective in the majority of patients; however, various published series have reported a mortality rate between 14 and 38 per cent. The initial steps in the treatment of AIHA are well established. If the disease is not controlled after these efforts, then one or more of several secondary treatments may be considered.

Initial treatment of the disease is with a corticosteroid, usually prednisone. The starting dose of prednisone should be in the range of 1 to 1.5 mg per kg per day. Larger doses are not more effective. About 80 per cent of patients will respond to this regimen with a decrease in hemolysis, a rise in hemoglobin, and an improvement in symptoms. If no response is seen after 3 weeks of high-dose prednisone, the treatment should be considered a failure. The mechanism of action of prednisone is not known. Steroids may interfere with the binding of antibody to the red cell surface, may delay the clearance of antibody-coated red cells, or may reduce the rate of synthesis of the abnormal autoantibody.

In patients who have responded to prednisone with a stabilization of hematocrit, a schedule of tapering the drug should be initiated. The dose should be reduced over 4 to 6 weeks to 30 mg per day, then reduced by 5 mg every 4 weeks until a level of 10 to 15 mg per day is reached. At that point either a very slow tapering of the dose or alternate-day therapy should be considered. If a relapse occurs, the dose should be increased to the previous dose and tapering should be reinstituted after the hemolysis stabilizes. If the prednisone dose cannot be lowered to below 15 mg per day without relapse, splenectomy should be considered. Although some patients can be maintained on low-dose, alternate-day prednisone for several years, most will eventually require splenectomy.

Splenectomy will result in improvement in symptoms in a majority of patients (about 60 per cent) who have failed with prednisone. Splenectomy not only eliminates the primary site of red cell destruction but also removes a major organ where antibodies are produced. It may permit the lowering of an unacceptably high maintenance dose of prednisone to one that is within tolerable limits. Relapses after splenectomy are common, however, and may occur months to years after the procedure.

As initial treatment of AIHA, all patients should be given a trial of steroids, followed by splenectomy if necessary. Failure of this initial regimen leads to a consideration of secondary treatments. Intravenous gamma globulin* (IVIgG) is effective in some patients if it is given in a sufficient dose. Initial studies with this therapy were disappointing, but more recent work has shown that large doses (0.5 to 1.0 gram per kg per day for 5 days)† often result in a sustained response. It is thought that IVIgG blocks the Fc gamma receptor on reticuloendothelial system (RES) macrophages, thus blocking RES removal of sensitized red cells.

Immunosuppressive drugs such as azathioprine* (Imuran) (125 mg per day) and cyclophosphamide (Cytoxan) (100 mg per day) given for up to 6 months will result in improvement in 40 to 50 per cent of patients, but side effects (e.g., marrow suppression) must be carefully monitored. Splenic irradiation has been advocated for those in whom splenectomy is contraindicated. Platelets coated with vinca alkaloids have been used as an experimental treatment in patients with AIHA. These platelets are ingested by RES macrophages, thus reducing the number and activity of these phagocytic cells. Plasma exchange is generally not useful, although it may temporarily lower plasma antibody levels. A summary of treatment modalities of AIHA is found in Table 2.

Transfusion

Transfusing patients with AIHA poses difficult challenges for both the clinician and the blood bank. The autoantibodies formed by these patients are directed against red cell membrane structures that are common to almost all human red cells, often being serologically identified as reacting with basic components of the Rh red cell antigen system. All donor red cells are usually incompatible with the patient's serum in the cross-match. Minor variations in the serologic strength of the incompatibility among units are usually of no consequence and should not be used

---

*This use is not listed in the manufacturer's directive.

†This dose exceeds that recommended by the manufacturer for approved uses.

TABLE 2. Treatment of Autoimmune Hemolytic Anemia—Warm Antibody Type

Primary Treatments
1. Prednisone: Starting dose of 1–1.5 mg/kg/day (60–100 mg) with slow taper to 10–15 mg/day depending on response*
2. Splenectomy: For relapses or failures on prednisone
3. Transfusion: Do not withhold incompatible transfusions if necessary for life-threatening anemia*

Secondary Treatments
1. Immunosuppressive drugs†: Azathioprine, cyclophosphamide
2. Intravenous gamma globulin† (IVIgG): 0.5–1 gram/kg/day for 5 days
3. Plasma exchange: Temporary benefit only
4. Vinca-loaded platelets: Experimental

*See text.
†This use is not listed in the manufacturer's directive.

as a primary guide in selecting units for transfusion. Red cells transfused to these patients can be expected to survive no better but also *no worse* than the patient's own red cells. The transfusion of red cells incompatible with the patient's autoantibody should not be withheld in the case of severe symptomatic anemia, especially if there has been insufficient time for the effect of other therapies to be fully evaluated.

The major risk of transfusion in these patients is that one or more red cell alloantibodies may be masked by the stronger autoantibody. Blood bank reference laboratories are usually able to identify these alloantibodies through the use of sophisticated serologic techniques, but the clinician should be especially cautious in transfusing patients with AIHA who have been exposed to red cell products in the past. Some transfusion medicine specialists recommend transfusing patients with red cells that are phenotypically matched with those of the patient for antigens in the Rh, Kell, and Kidd systems to prevent the development of dangerous alloantibodies in these systems.

Drug-Related Immune Hemolytic Anemia

Many drugs have been etiologically associated with warm-antibody AIHA. The patient with the onset of AIHA should be questioned closely for a history of prescription or over-the-counter drug ingestion. The mechanisms of drug-induced immune hemolysis fall into the following categories:

1. *Drug-induced red cell autoantibody (e.g., alpha-methyldopa [Aldomet]).* The antibody that is produced in response to the drug is not directed against the drug but against red cell membrane components. The antibody is identical in its characteristics to the autoantibodies seen in idiopathic warm AIHA. About 15 per cent of patients receiving alpha-methyldopa will develop a posi-

tive DAT, whereas about 1 per cent will have hemolytic anemia. It has been suggested that alpha-methyldopa may alter the function of T suppressor lymphocytes, thus allowing B lymphocytes to elaborate pathologic antibody.

2. *Immune-complex mechanism (e.g., quinidine).* An immune complex of drug and antidrug antibody is formed in the plasma. This immune complex activates complement on the surface of the otherwise uninvolved red cells, leading to accelerated destruction of the sensitized cells.

3. *Drug absorption (hapten) mechanism (e.g., penicillin).* The drug or drug components bind directly to the red cell surface. Therefore, antidrug IgG antibody that binds to the drug is also bound to the red cell, leading to the cell's immune destruction.

4. *Membrane modification mechanism (e.g., cephalosporins).* The drug alters the red cell membrane so that other proteins are nonspecifically absorbed. Although the DAT is positive, immune hemolysis is rarely seen with this mechanism.

A given drug can cause a positive DAT and red cell hemolysis by more than one of these mechanisms. If a patient is taking a drug that has been implicated in causing AIHA, the drug should, of course, be stopped. This will usually result in prompt improvement in the hemolysis and stabilization of the hematocrit. In some cases, such as the immune hemolysis associated with alpha-methyldopa, reversion of the DAT to normal may take several months.

COLD AGGLUTININ DISEASE

Hemolytic anemia that results on exposure to cold and symptoms related to intermittent occlusion of the microvasculature compose the syndrome of CAD. The primary (idiopathic) form of CAD is a disease found primarily in the elderly. CAD can also be secondary to several infectious diseases (e.g., infectious mononucleosis) and to lymphoproliferative disorders.

Cold-reactive red cell autoantibodies can be detected in the plasma of most individuals if serologic reactions are conducted at 4° C. These IgM antibodies usually have anti-H, anti-I, or anti-i specificity and are of no clinical importance. On occasion, however, these autoantibodies can be active over a wide thermal range, with agglutination of red cells occurring at temperatures approaching 37° C.

The pathologic IgM cold agglutinins of CAD usually have anti-I specificity. The antibodies activate complement, resulting in the deposition of C3b molecules on the red cell surface. These red cells adhere to the C3b receptors on RES macrophages and are removed from the circulation. The chronic hemolytic anemia of CAD is usually not as severe as that seen in warm AIHA, but acute exacerbations with hemoglobinuria can occur, usually associated with exposure to cold temperatures.

Patients with CAD also have symptoms (aside from those of anemia) related to ischemia of areas of the body exposed to cold. Pallor and acrocyanosis of the fingers, toes, nose, and ears are common and are thought to be secondary to red cell agglutination in the microvasculature of these areas. Raynaud's phenomenon is often seen. The spleen is only slightly enlarged in most cases.

Laboratory findings include autoagglutination of blood samples that are allowed to cool after being drawn, a cold agglutinin of high titer reacting at a temperature of at least 30° C or higher in serologic tests, and red cells that are coated with C3 but not IgG. Compatible cross-matches can usually be obtained if all serologic tests are conducted at 37° C or if a cold autoabsorption procedure is carried out prior to cross-matching.

Treatment of cold agglutinin disease consists primarily of avoidance of the cold. Patients should be advised to protect exposed areas and, in more severe cases, to consider changing their residence to a warmer climate. Other treatments are generally unsatisfactory. Steroids, immunosuppressive drugs, and splenectomy are less effective than in warm-antibody AIHA and should be used only with considerable caution. Plasma exchange has been used with some success as a temporary measure to lower plasma IgM levels during an acute hemolytic episode.

PAROXYSMAL COLD HEMOGLOBINURIA

This unusual disorder is caused by a biphasic hemolytic antibody that reacts with the patient's red cells at low temperatures, with subsequent complement fixation and cell lysis when the cells are returned to physiologic temperatures. PCH was originally thought to be related to syphilis, but it is now recognized that it also follows many types of viral infections. Often PCH cannot be related to any distinct antecedent event. Patients experience acute paroxysms characterized by fever, chills, abdominal and back pain, and hemoglobinuria. Exposure to cold often precipitates an acute attack, but symptoms can develop in the absence of such an exposure.

The bithermic hemolysis test (Donath-Landsteiner test) is essential for the diagnosis of PCH. The patient's serum is incubated with test red cells in ice for 30 minutes, incubated at 37° C for 30 minutes, and then observed for the presence of hemolysis. The pathologic red cell antibody that is responsible for this bithermic hemolysis is anti-P.

Treatment of PCH is generally supportive. The patient should be instructed to avoid the cold and should be screened for syphilis and treated if necessary. Acute postinfectious PCH often resolves spontaneously. Short courses of steroids may be beneficial during acute attacks of the illness but are not recommended for long-term therapy. Transfusion of either the P or P^k blood types avoids the offending antibody, but these blood types are very rare. In the absence of these types, transfusions of cross-match–compatible, P-positive units can be given through a blood warmer.

NONIMMUNE HEMOLYTIC ANEMIA
method of
WILLIAM N. VALENTINE, M.D.
Center for Health Sciences
University of California, Los Angeles
Los Angeles, California

Although moderate shortening of the normal life span of red blood cells occurs in many patients, the term "hemolytic anemia" is usually reserved for syndromes in which hemolysis is substantial and plays a meaningful role in the pathogenesis of clinical and hematologic manifestations. In actuality, anemia is not always present because normal bone marrow can compensate for premature destruction of erythrocytes by increasing the production of red cells about six to eight times. If hemolysis exceeds the capacity for compensation, anemia is inevitable.

The nonspecific hallmarks of hemolysis are persistent reticulocytosis, polychromasia of red blood cells on stained blood films, erythroid hyperplasia of marrow, and sometimes an increase in plasma lactate dehydrogenase level and jaundice. The latter, when present, is caused by increased catabolism of hemoglobin and the resultant increase in indirectly reacting bilirubinemia. Purely hemolytic jaundice is never associated with bilirubinuria or with elevation of the directly reacting fraction of serum bilirubin. The latter may occur, of course, as a concomitant of hemolytic syndromes from causes other than hemolysis per se (e.g., biliary obstruction with pigment stones, transfusion-induced hepatitis, microinfarcts of liver in sickle cell anemia). Splenomegaly is a common, but not universal, accompaniment of chronic hemolysis. One notable exception occurs in the adult with sickle cell anemia. Although infants and young children present with splenomegaly, repeated splenic infarction commonly results in what may be termed an "autosplenectomy" by the time of adulthood. In a subset of hemolytic syndromes, hemolysis may be largely intravascular. If it is sufficiently marked, hemoglobinemia and overt hemoglobinuria may be present. The latter must be clearly differentiated from hematuria. The nonspecific hallmarks of hemolysis may be mimicked during a regenerative response to anemia of other etiology (e.g., hemorrhage, hematinic therapy). If the hemorrhage is internal, overt bleeding may be absent and resorption of hematomas may be accompanied by hyperbilirubinemia and jaundice. Ineffective erythropoiesis, such as that accompanying a variety of refractory anemias with cellular bone marrow, including pernicious anemia, folate deficiency, and the thalassemia syndromes, may also, when marked, be associated with jaundice, anemia, and elevation of the plasma lactate dehydrogenase level. These manifestations are secondary to intramarrow death of partially hemoglobinated, nucleated erythroid precursors never destined to reach the circulation, a form of intramarrow red blood cell precursor hemolysis. Other clinical and laboratory features point to the correct diagnosis.

CLINICAL EVALUATION

Hemolytic anemia whose pathogenesis lies in immunologic mechanisms is described elsewhere and will not be discussed further here. Management of the nonimmune hemolytic anemias rests squarely on their expeditious and correct diagnosis, and the latter is directed by answers to several pertinent questions.

Is the hemolysis of infectious or toxic origin? Life-threatening sepsis with hemolytic organisms such as *Clostridium perfringens* obviously requires prompt diagnosis and heroic measures. Hemolysis accompanies red blood cell parasitism with plasmodia in malaria. Severe lead poisoning is associated with marked hemolytic anemia, as is the much rarer exposure to arsine gas. Hemolysis also may result from spider and snake bites and, more rarely, from bee stings. However, in all of these situations, the clinical picture is dominated by systemic and local manifestations, and in most instances the history, physical examination, and pertinent laboratory findings point early to the correct diagnosis. The diagnosis of red blood cell parasitism may, however, be obscure, particularly in areas where its incidence and the index of suspicion are low.

Is the hemolysis predominantly intravascular, or is it mediated by the reticuloendothelial system? If the hemolysis is ongoing, the serum haptoglobin, a protein-binding free hemoglobin, is essentially undetectable. If the hemolysis is sufficiently marked, frank hemoglobinuria is noted; if it is milder, hemoglobin passing the renal filter is taken up by tubular epithelium, whose shed cells in centrifuged urinary sediment stain positively for iron. Hemosiderinuria and hemoglobinuria both reflect intravascular hemolysis. Intravascular hemolysis occurs in microangiopathic syndromes with diffuse lesions in the microvasculature, with defective cardiac prostheses, in patients with glucose-6-phosphate dehydrogenase (G6PD) deficiency during hemolytic episodes, in the comparatively rare syndrome of paroxysmal nocturnal hemoglobinuria, and in certain rare, unstable hemoglobinopathies.

In reticuloendothelial-mediated hemolysis, red blood cells are prematurely destroyed by phagocytic macrophages. The serum haptoglobin level may be moderately low, but the haptoglobin does not disappear.

Hemoglobinuria, hemosiderinuria, and iron deficiency are not part of the picture. This is the case in sickle cell disease and other major hemoglobinopathies; in hereditary spherocytosis, elliptocytosis, and other syndromes caused by defective erythrocyte membranes; in hemolysis associated with most red blood cell enzymopathies other than G6PD deficiency; and in the rare abnormality of hereditary acanthocytosis.

Is the syndrome hereditary or acquired? A family history of anemia, jaundice, early cholelithiasis, painful crises, red urine, splenomegaly, or splenectomy may direct the diagnostic regimen toward the hereditary syndromes. Ethnic derivation and a history of lifelong symptoms have obvious implications.

Is the pathogenic abnormality intracorpuscular or extracorpuscular? In all hereditary syndromes with the exception of the abetalipoproteinemia of hereditary acanthocytosis, the pathogenic defect is intracorpuscular; in all acquired hemolytic anemias with the exception of paroxysmal nocturnal hemoglobinuria, it is extracorpuscular.

Is the hemolysis episodic or chronic? In many of the manifold variants of G6PD deficiency, hemolytic episodes occur only with oxidant stresses such as ingestion of certain antimalarial drugs, nitrofurantoin, sulfanilamide, or, with some variants, fava beans. Infections and surgical stress may also produce episodic hemoglobinuria in deficient persons. In other syndromes, such as hereditary spherocytosis, jaundice may wax and wane, and anemia occasionally worsens rapidly as a result of transient marrow failure during certain myelosuppressive viral infections (the so-called self-limited aregenerative or aplastic crises).

Are there telltale morphologic abnormalities on the stained blood film? Although sophisticated evaluation of red blood cell morphology may require consultative assistance, its importance in directing diagnosis and management renders it mandatory that the necessary evaluation be obtained from the laboratory or a specialist. The stained blood film, properly evaluated, yields more valuable clues than any other single laboratory procedure. The small, round, densely staining "spherocyte," lacking the normal zone of central pallor, when present in substantial numbers and in the absence of a positive Coombs's test strongly suggests hereditary spherocytosis. The spherocyte, a cell whose surface area is relatively small for its volume, lyses at concentrations of hypotonic saline, leaving normal erythrocytes intact. The osmotic fragility test therefore provides laboratory confirmation of spherocytosis. The test is rendered more sensitive in doubtful cases if whole blood is sterilely incubated at 37° C for 24 hours before testing. Small numbers of spherocytes may be present in clostridial sepsis, in hemolytic episodes occurring in G6PD-deficient persons, and together with elliptocytes in certain hemolytic forms of hereditary elliptocytosis.

Cells appearing as targets on stained blood films are present in all the major hemoglobinopathies. Hemoglobins S, C, D, and E are mutants found in large numbers of persons. Hemoglobins S and C are encoded by genes arising in Africa, the latter having a much more circumscribed distribution in West Africa. Hemoglobin D[Punjab] is found in large numbers in persons from Pakistan and northwest India. Hemoglobin E has a wide distribution in Burma and parts of Southeast Asia. "Target cells" are also common in thalassemia; in certain forms of liver and biliary disease; and, to a lesser extent, after splenectomy and in marked iron deficiency.

Irreversibly "sickled cells" on the stained blood film indicate sickle cell anemia or syndromes involving the simultaneous inheritance of hemoglobins S and C (SC disease), S and D^{Punjab} (SD disease), or S and beta-thalassemia. They are not seen in persons heterozygous for hemoglobin S.

"Schistocytes" are fragmented, traumatized red cells. When present, they suggest microangiopathic anemia or the "Waring Blender" syndrome occurring with defective cardiac prostheses.

"Heinz bodies" are inclusions of denatured hemoglobin. They occur particularly in hemolysis accompanying G6PD deficiency and in certain rare, unstable hemoglobinopathies. Because of the efficiency of the pitting function of the normal spleen, they are often inconspicuous except in splenectomized subjects.

"Acanthocytes" are irregularly shaped cells with pseudopod-like or finger-like projections. They are seen most prominently in hereditary acanthocytosis, a rare syndrome caused by genetically determined abetalipoproteinemia.

"Stomatocytes" appear on stained blood films to have a slit, or mouth-like, zone of central pallor. They can be artifacts of preparation, but they occur in a subset of hemolytic syndromes caused by defective cell membranes and grossly abnormal fluxes of the cations Na$^+$ and K$^+$.

"Elliptocytes" are oval or sausage-shaped red blood cells. They are associated with both a benign abnormality lacking hemolysis and an overtly hemolytic disorder.

Is the hemolysis caused by direct red blood cell trauma? Red blood cells may be severely damaged and fragmented when passing through a damaged microvasculature. In the latter case, the erythrocyte may be forced through partially occluded areas where endothelium is disrupted and fibrin networks abound. Diffusely damaged microvasculature is associated with the syndrome of thrombotic thrombocytopenic purpura and, at times, with malignant hypertension, acute glomerulonephritis, and widespread metastatic, neoplastic emboli. Trauma may likewise accompany defective valvular prostheses in the heart and other surgical complications such as incomplete epithelialization of repaired septal defects. The intracardiac battering of red blood cells that can be associated with these abnormalities may cause hemolysis in the "Waring Blender" syndrome.

MANAGEMENT

Syndromes Secondary to Infections and Toxins. Treatment is focused on the underlying disease: administration of appropriate antibiotics and/or antimalarials, support of blood pressure, maintenance of fluid balance, and prompt therapy of special complications. Transfusions may or may not be necessary in individual cases. The diagnosis of lead poisoning mandates removal of the patient from the toxic environment and may require treatment with lead-chelating agents.

Prevention of Hemolytic Episodes. When clinically significant G6PD deficiency is present, the patient should be advised to avoid medications and agents known to produce oxidant stress and to precipitate hemolysis. Although many medications have been doubtfully or even erroneously incriminated in the production of hemolytic episodes, a number of them are firmly established. These include sulfonilamide (but not all sulfa-containing medications), furadandin, acetanilid, the antimalarials primaquine and pamaquine, and trimethoprim-sulfamethoxazole (Bactrim). Ingestion of fava beans provokes hemolysis in some G6PD deficiency syndromes but not in others. There are more than 300 reportedly different G6PD variants (some may prove to be identical), and their phenotypic clinical manifestations differ widely in different genotypes. Hemolytic episodes may be precipitated by oxidant stress in patients with certain rare, unstable hemoglobinopathies and rare erythroenzymopathies other than G6PD deficiency. When drug-induced hemolysis is suspected, prompt withdrawal of all potentially involved medications is indicated.

Transfusions. Transfusions are overused and should be avoided except for specific indications. The latter include rapidly worsening anemia, clinical or electrocardiographic evidence of myocardial ischemia, obtundation believed to be related to anemia, infectious complications, the possibility of surgery, and, at times, pregnancy. The well-known potential complications of transfusion—hepatitis and other viral infections, transfusion reactions, development of alloantibodies after repeated transfusions, and ultimately iron overload—constitute contraindications if the patient is stable and if a reasonable quality of life is being maintained. In short, the patient, and not an arbitrary hemoglobin level, is the object of treatment. Exchange transfusion may prove necessary in newborns with kernicterus-threatening hyperbilirubinemia secondary to hemolysis. The use of exchange or other transfusions in the management of painful crises or the acute chest syndrome in patients with sickle cell syndromes also requires sophisticated evaluation and is frequently controversial. Transfusion in the splenic sequestration syndrome sometimes encountered in young children with sickle cell anemia is an emergent and potentially life-saving measure. In general, when transfusion is indicated, packed red blood cells are the modality of choice. Transfusions in patients with paroxysmal nocturnal hemoglobinuria may present a special problem. Reactions caused by transfused plasma that contains components of the complement system may occur in some patients with this disorder. In this case, recipient (not donor) cells undergo lysis. When it occurs, all subsequent transfusions should be with saline-washed red blood cells. (Recipient cell lysis is one of the few indications for this procedure.) Such cells must be administered shortly after washing to ensure viability.

Splenectomy. Splenectomy as an emergency procedure may be lifesaving in splenic sequestration crises occurring in young children with sickle cell anemia. Although the morphologic abnormalities persist, splenectomy is clinically curative in the great majority of patients with hereditary spherocytosis. Jaundice abates, reticulocyte counts markedly decrease, and the erythrocyte life span measured with ^{51}Cr labeling of red blood cells is nearly normal. In a subset of these patients, some evidence of hemolysis persists. Although this has often been ascribed to residual accessory spleens, only rarely does it appear to be the case. Whether or not splenectomy is recommended in the mildest compensated cases is controversial. It is the author's belief that in the absence of contraindications, the procedure has genuine benefit chiefly in ameliorating the likelihood of later cholecystitis and cholelithiasis. The patient must share in the decision. If it is not contraindicated, when cholecystectomy is necessary in patients with this disorder, splenectomy may simultaneously be performed. Results of splenectomy are gratifying in most cases of hemolytic elliptocytosis and in certain cases of hemolytic syndromes characterized by stomatocytosis. The procedure is usually ineffective in the G6PD deficiency syndromes and in microangiopathic hemolytic anemias. In patients with pyruvate kinase deficiency, and probably in other hemolytic erythroenzymopathies involving anaerobic glycolysis, splenectomy is indicated only when comfortable existence requires frequent transfusions. After the procedure, hemolysis remains severe and reticulocytosis may often be increased, but a partial benefit in the form of diminished or eliminated transfusion requirements and an increase of 1 to 3 grams per dl in hemoglobin may be distinctly worthwhile. In the most severe syndromes, splenectomy may be lifesaving.

Cholelithiasis and Cholecystectomy. In all chronic hemolytic anemias, the increased amount of bilirubin continuously presented to the liver and excreted in bile sharply increases the incidence of pigment stone formation, cholecystitis, and biliary obstruction, all of which may appear at an early age. Surgical management is frequently indicated. Simultaneous splenectomy should be considered only in those syndromes where its value is substantiated. In patients with sickle cell syndromes, avoidance of hypoxia during and after surgery is of great importance.

Iron, Folate, and Corticosteroids. Iron administration is contraindicated except where iron deficiency is documented. Normally there is no deficiency, and especially when transfusions have been necessary, iron stores are replete and perhaps excessive. Exceptions are the hemolytic syndromes characterized by intravascular hemolysis, hemoglobinemia, hemoglobinuria, and/or hemosiderinuria. Renal loss of hemoglobin in these circumstances is often a cause of associated iron deficiency that requires appropriate treatment (300 to 900 mg of ferrous sulfate per day). Corticosteroids have no place in the management of the syndromes discussed here, with the possible exception of the rare syndrome of thrombotic thrombocytopenic purpura.

Chronic hemolysis increases folate requirements, and folate in doses of 1 mg per day is a rational supplement. This may modestly increase the hemoglobin level and may provide some protection against the aregenerative crises discussed in the next section. We favor the routine administration of such supplements in patients with ongoing hemolysis of any etiology.

The "Aplastic" or "Aregenerative" Crisis. In any chronic hemolytic syndrome, transient acute marrow suppression may occur in the course of an illness that is usually attributed to a parvovirus. Marrow temporarily becomes hypoplastic, reticulocytopenia intervenes, the serum bilirubin level falls, and cytopenia becomes evident. Neutropenia and thrombocytopenia rarely become sufficiently severe to cause clinical manifestations, but in the presence of substantial hemolysis, anemia rapidly worsens and often becomes symptomatic. The crisis is self-limited, ordinarily lasting for 7 to 12 days. Afterward, marrow activity surges back, heralded by returning reticulocytosis and correction of cytopenia. During the period of marrow suppression, transfusion may or may not be required.

Special Considerations. Certain hemolytic syndromes have prominent accompaniments of clinical significance. Paroxysmal nocturnal hemoglobinuria may be associated in some patients with marrow hypoplasia, with a hypercoagulable state and widespread thrombotic phenomena, and sometimes with a variety of underlying myeloproliferative syndromes. Hemolysis in thrombotic thrombocytopenic purpura accompanies a greatly diminished platelet count, bleeding, and fluctuating, often severe, neurologic manifestations. The sickle cell syndromes are not only hemolytic but manifest a large array of vaso-occlusive problems discussed elsewhere. The patient with microangiopathic anemia has underlying diffuse disease of the microvasculature and sometimes metastatic neoplasia. The presence of marked intracardiac red blood cell trauma with defective prostheses may require replacement of the latter by the cardiac surgeon.

PERNICIOUS ANEMIA AND OTHER MEGALOBLASTIC ANEMIAS

method of
RALPH CARMEL, M.D.
*University of Southern California School of Medicine
Los Angeles, California*

The optimal management of megaloblastic anemia requires one to be certain of the specific vitamin deficiency involved (folate versus cobalamin) and to establish as precisely as possible the specific disorder responsible for that deficiency. This ensures that the right vitamin is given, that the route and duration of therapy are appropriate, that the underlying process is managed properly and, if possible, reversed, that appropriate information is given to the patient, and that pertinent common complications are anticipated. Megaloblastic anemia can occur in disorders unrelated to cobalamin or folate deficiency, but those are rare and will not be considered here.

Serum levels of cobalamin (vitamin B_{12}) and folate usually identify the specific vitamin deficiency, although exceptions may occasionally occur. Several general diagnostic principles may be applied. First, atypical or subtle expressions of deficiency, especially of cobalamin, may be more common than we think. The most important atypical presentation to consider may be minimal or even absent megaloblastic anemia. For example, "pernicious anemia," although a hematologic term, actually refers to a gastroenterologic entity: the malabsorption of cobalamin caused by absence of gastric intrinsic factor secretion. There may be no anemia, or the anemia may be normocytic rather than macrocytic. Thus, a patient may have "pernicious anemia" and yet may not be anemic. Furthermore, cobalamin deficiency may produce serious neurologic symptoms with few or no hematologic abnormalities.

Second, cobalamin deficiency virtually always arises because of gastric or intestinal disease. It is almost never caused by poor diet and certainly never by malnutrition of only a few weeks' or even a few months' duration. Thus it should not be attributed to a dietary cause until malabsorption has been excluded. Therefore, tests of cobalamin absorption, like the Schilling test, are central to the evaluation of all cases of cobalamin deficiency.

On the other hand, folate deficiency frequently has a dietary basis. Alcohol contributes to many, if not most, cases of dietary folate deficiency. Therefore, alcoholism, often otherwise unsuspected, should be considered whenever dietary folate deficiency is diagnosed. Malabsorptive diseases and drug-induced disorders should also be considered.

TREATMENT OF VITAMIN DEFICIENCY

General Principles

The initial goal is to determine whether the deficiency is of cobalamin or folate (or both) in order to avoid using the wrong vitamin in therapy. The chief danger arises from the fact that the hematologic abnormalities of cobalamin deficiency can respond transiently to doses of folic acid as small as 0.1 mg. Neurologic abnormalities of cobalamin deficiency, however, do not respond to folate. As a result, neurologic dysfunction can progress, or may appear for the first time, while the hematologic changes improve with folate therapy and become masked. This danger underscores the twin necessities of making certain that the diagnosis is correct and of monitoring the patient's response after treatment.

Fortunately, emergency treatment is rarely required. Therefore, there is ample time to obtain the necessary tests first, especially the vitamin levels. It is usually advisable (and quite safe) to defer therapy for a few days until the vitamin deficiency has been satisfactorily identified. Many of the diagnostic abnormalities are blurred once the patient is treated, and it may sometimes be difficult to retrace one's diagnostic steps if treatment is given prematurely.

Urgent therapy is generally needed in only two situations. One is severe or deteriorating neurologic disease, where cobalamin therapy should be started as soon as the appropriate tests have been obtained. The longer the neurologic abnormalities go untreated, the greater the risk of irreversibility or incomplete reversibility.

The second situation in which urgent therapy may be needed is when severe anemia exists. The urgency of this situation must be tempered by two considerations. Because reticulocytosis takes several days to develop, vitamin therapy does not affect the blood count for some time. Immediate "shotgun" therapy is therefore useless in extreme situations. If the clinical situation is so severe that the anemia truly requires immediate reversal, blood transfusion is needed. However, the more important consideration is that the clinical picture rather than the blood count must determine the urgency of the situation and the need for transfusion. Megaloblastic anemia is a chronic process that develops slowly, which allows compensatory adjustments to the low blood count. As a result, hemoglobin levels as low as 4 or 5 grams per dl are usually well tolerated. Symptoms are often limited to fatigue and inability to tolerate exertion. Simple bed rest may be all that is needed while waiting for vitamin replacement to produce the desired effect.

Blood transfusion, with all its risks, should be avoided whenever possible. Only serious cardiopulmonary or cerebral symptoms or the risk of decompensation because of coexisting serious disease compromising those systems warrants transfusion. Because plasma volume is often increased, volume overload must be avoided and any transfusion should be given slowly, with re-evaluation after each unit of blood is administered.

Cobalamin Deficiency

There are three goals in treating cobalamin deficiency. The first is to reverse the sequelae of the deficiency. The megaloblastic anemia can be reversed with as little as 1 to 10 micrograms of cobalamin, but larger doses are usually used. Injections are usually given intramuscularly, although subcutaneous injection is preferable if the patient is thrombocytopenic. A single 100- or 1000-microgram injection produces full hematologic remission, as long as there are no coexisting complicating disorders that might blunt the hematologic response. Whether larger amounts are necessary to reverse neurologic deficits is unknown. Nevertheless, it is common practice to treat neurologic symptoms of cobalamin deficiency with more frequent injections, at least in the beginning, than are used to treat hematologic abnormality.

With such therapy, the patient quickly feels better even before the blood count rises. Other manifestations of deficiency, like glossitis, also respond quickly.

The second goal of treating cobalamin deficiency is to prevent relapse. If the disorder that produced the deficiency can be reversed, its reversal accomplishes that goal. However, most underlying causes of cobalamin deficiency are not reversible and therefore require regular, permanent vitamin supplementation. The daily requirement seems to vary among individuals but usually approximates 1 to 2 micrograms per day. Adequate maintenance is best achieved with monthly intramuscular injections of 100 or 1000 micrograms. Variable fractions of these relatively large injected doses are retained. I prefer to use the 1000-microgram dose; even though much more of it is immediately excreted than with the 100-microgram injection, a larger absolute amount of cobalamin is retained. The larger dose thus provides a better margin, and it is not much more expensive than the 100-microgram dose.

In unusual circumstances where injections are refused or for some reason impossible to administer, oral maintenance therapy can be used. Even if the specific intrinsic factor–mediated absorptive process for cobalamin is impaired, diffusion allows a tiny fraction of the oral dose (less than 1 per cent) to be absorbed. Thus, daily oral ingestion of at least 100 micrograms may be adequate maintenance even in malabsorption, although the patient's status obviously requires careful, regular monitoring. As a rule, however, oral therapy is advisable only in those rare patients whose deficiency is dietary in origin. Once adequate repletion has occurred, such patients can take oral supplements of 10 micrograms daily if they choose not to discontinue their limited diet. A gel preparation of cyanocobalamin for nasal instillation has recently become available, but it provides no known advantage over the oral form and is expensive.

The third goal of treating cobalamin deficiency is to replenish the depleted body stores. Although unreplenished patients do not seem to do worse than replenished ones (as long as daily requirements are regularly met), it seems prudent to provide a "safety net" both for those unsuspected patients who have higher daily requirements and for those patients who fail to continue regular supplementation.

Although many regimens can achieve all three goals satisfactorily, and although little evidence exists for recommending one over another, my approach is to begin with a series of about 15 intramuscular injections of 1000 micrograms of cobalamin spread over a 2-month period.* Thereafter, adequate maintenance can be achieved by monthly injections of 1000 micrograms* of cobalamin. Infrequently, patients may complain of symptoms like fatigue before the end of the monthly interval. Although the explanation for this complaint is unclear, it may represent a faster cobalamin turnover rate and warrants the attempted use of more frequent maintenance injections. Finally, many patients can be taught self-injection, thus saving the time and expense of office visits. However, this self-injection should not prevent periodic follow-up by the physician.

It bears re-emphasis that the proper long-term management of cobalamin deficiency has less to do with doses, routes, and schedules than with patient education and compliance.

Several forms of cobalamin are available for replacement therapy. The most widely used form is cyanocobalamin. This stable but nonphysiologic cobalamin is converted to metabolically active cobalamins in the body. A more physiologic

---

*These dosages exceed the manufacturer's recommended dosage.

form, and one that is also better retained in the body after injection, is hydroxocobalamin. This form is preferred by many European physicians because fewer injections are required, but it is not widely used in the United States and is somewhat more expensive than cyanocobalamin.

Cobalamin has no known toxicity even in very large doses. The excess is rapidly excreted in the urine, and stores cannot become overloaded. Allergic reactions are infrequent and seem to be caused by the preservative in the parenteral solution. If recurrences occur, they usually can be prevented by changing to a different preparation (e.g., from another manufacturer). Autoantibody to cobalamin-binding proteins may occasionally appear in patients who take depot preparations of cobalamin or hydroxocobalamin. Unusually high serum cobalamin levels may result, but there seem to be no adverse clinical effects. Finally, frequent sudden death after therapy of severe megaloblastic anemia was reported long ago, but this finding has not been substantiated. As long as one avoids fluid overload, such as with excessive blood transfusion, and manages complicating problems like congestive heart failure appropriately, the prognosis is excellent. As mentioned earlier, most patients tolerate even severe anemia surprisingly well; my approach has been to do as little as possible beyond providing standard, prudent medical care while waiting for cobalamin replacement to take effect.

Folate Deficiency

The goals of therapy of folate deficiency and the responses obtained are very similar to those described for cobalamin deficiency.

As little as 0.1 mg folic acid can ultimately reverse the megaloblastic anemia caused by folate deficiency. The widely available formulations usually contain 1 mg of folic acid, and such doses are optimal. Unless there is a drug-induced or hereditary metabolic block, folic acid is the preferred form, and the more expensive formyl-tetrahydrofolic acid (folinic acid) should not be used.

Replacement therapy can be and usually is achieved orally. Unlike cobalamin deficiency, which is almost always malabsorptive in origin, folate deficiency is usually produced by dietary insufficiency (with or without coexisting alcohol abuse). Parenteral therapy is needed only if oral doses cannot be absorbed. However, even folate deficiency due to malabsorption can often be treated with oral folic acid. In such cases, higher doses (e.g., 2 to 5 mg twice daily) are advisable, and serum levels and the patient's response should be monitored.

Unlike cobalamin deficiency, whose underlying cause is usually irreversible, folate deficiency often need not be treated indefinitely. A 3- or 4-week course of 1 mg of folic acid daily generally suffices to reverse the megaloblastic anemia and replete tissue stores. If the underlying cause (e.g., inadequate diet or a malabsorptive disorder) has been corrected, it is sufficient simply to recheck the patient's folate status with a serum folate level determination and a blood count several months after folate replacement has been completed. If the underlying disorder is not reversible, therapy with 1 mg of folic acid daily or every other day can be maintained indefinitely.

Folic acid is nontoxic even in large doses. Rarely, children with seizure disorders, who may become folate deficient with hydantoin therapy, have been reported to suffer increased seizures if the folate is given parenterally. The only truly serious toxicity of therapy, however, occurs when folic acid is given in error to a patient with cobalamin deficiency.

TREATMENT OF THE UNDERLYING DISORDER

Identifying the underlying disorder that produced the vitamin deficiency is almost as important as treating the deficiency itself. Such identification allows treatment of the underlying disorder if it is reversible (e.g., antibiotics for the bacterial overgrowth in the small bowel that produced the cobalamin malabsorption or counseling for the alcoholism that contributed to the dietary folate insufficiency). If the underlying disorder is reversed, periodic monitoring is advisable because the disorder may recur.

Even if the underlying disorder is not treatable, its correct identification has important clinical benefits. Informed decisions can be made about the route of vitamin replacement and its duration. Identification of the underlying disorder allows reliable prognostic information to be given to the patient. Careful attention to early recognition of known complications also becomes possible. For example, hypothyroidism, iron deficiency, and gastric cancer all occur with increased frequency in patients with pernicious anemia and may develop at any time. Because of the increased risk of gastric cancer in patients who have pernicious anemia, the issue of preventive screening has arisen. The consensus at this time is that annual endoscopy or barium studies are not worthwhile. Nevertheless, part of the regular follow-up of patients with pernicious anemia must include testing stool for occult blood and questioning the patient about dyspeptic symptoms.

FOLLOW-UP AND PATIENT EDUCATION

Many important benefits accrue from careful follow-up. Assessing whether a full clinical re-

TABLE 1. Suggestions for Avoiding Common Errors in the Management of Megaloblastic Anemia

Diagnosis

Remember that vitamin deficiency can be present without megaloblastic anemia.

Pay attention to even mildly subnormal serum vitamin levels.

Obtain both serum folic acid and cobalamin levels before treatment.

Always establish why the patient became cobalamin deficient or folate deficient.

Do not automatically equate cobalamin deficiency with pernicious anemia.

Cobalamin deficiency is malabsorptive in origin until proved otherwise; it is very rarely dietary in origin.

Therapy

Avoid shotgun therapy or preparations of multiple hematinics unless the patient is known to need all of them (a rare event).

Avoid at all costs treating with the wrong vitamin; if in doubt, restudy the patient completely.

Transfusion should be guided solely by symptoms and the clinical setting, not by laboratory results such as the blood count.

A single injection without follow-up is never appropriate for treating cobalamin deficiency.

Avoid oral cobalamin therapy unless there are specific reasons for using it rather than parenteral therapy.

Discuss the nature of the disorder fully with the patient to make sure that it and the duration of therapy are well understood.

Monitor the patient's response to therapy.

---

sponse occurred is the most obvious benefit and provides the ultimate proof of the correctness of the diagnosis of deficiency. It also permits the uncovering of coexisting disturbances that are often not diagnosable until the megaloblastic anemia has been reversed. The major example of the latter case is iron deficiency, which can occur in nearly one-half of the patients with pernicious anemia but may be unrecognizable until the vitamin deficiency has been treated.

The patient often feels better within 24 hours of beginning therapy, even before the blood count has risen (reticulocytosis does not begin until the second or third day). However, the best objective hallmarks of an adequate response to cobalamin or folate replacement are a peak reticulocytosis after 7 days and the full normalization of the blood count no later than 6 to 8 weeks after beginning therapy, no matter how severe the initial anemia was. The failure of these events to occur indicates a suboptimal response, either because the diagnosis and therapy were incorrect or because coexisting disorders prevented a full response.

Neurologic symptoms of cobalamin deficiency may not always be fully reversible. However, it takes several months and sometimes as long as a year to obtain maximal recovery. Even when neurologic dysfunction cannot be reversed by cobalamin therapy, it should cease to progress. Any evidence of progression despite therapy calls for evaluation for coexisting neurologic disease.

During follow-up, appropriate testing to establish the underlying disorder can be completed (e.g., the various Schilling tests in cobalamin-deficient patients). Follow-up also permits a fuller explanation of the diagnosis and prognosis to the patient. For example, patients with pernicious anemia and other irreversible disorders often fail at first to appreciate the permanent nature of their cobalamin malabsorption. All too often, as a result, they may discontinue the injections of cobalamin once they feel better. Follow-up provides the opportunity to explore more fully the patient's and family's understanding of the disease and to address any questions that they may have. It is particularly helpful to re-emphasize to the patient the gastrointestinal origin of many of the disorders, in contrast to the cured hematologic or neurologic expressions of the deficiency.

Follow-up should include education of the folate-deficient patient about diet. Emphasis must be given not only to the appropriate foods but also to their methods of preparation. Folate is a labile vitamin. Storage, cooking, or canning often destroys much of its activity. Increased intake of fresh vegetables may be helpful. Finally, follow-up also permits exploration of delicate issues like alcoholism that may be denied or deferred at the time of acute illness.

THALASSEMIA

method of
JACQUES A. BOLLEKENS, M.D., and
EDWARD J. BENZ, JR., M.D.
Yale University School of Medicine
New Haven, Connecticut

PATHOPHYSIOLOGY: BASIC MECHANISMS OF HEMOGLOBIN SYNTHESIS

The sequential expression of the different globin genes is responsible for the production of specific types of hemoglobins at different stages of development. At about 12 weeks of gestation there is a transition from embryonic to fetal hemoglobin, followed at 38 weeks by the switch to adult hemoglobin. Hemoglobin production occurs in bone marrow erythroblasts. The stable accumulation exclusively of fully formed hemoglobin tetramers in normal development can be achieved only when the production of alpha-like and beta-like globins by the globin gene clusters (alpha genes on chromosome 16; beta-like genes on chromosome 11) is balanced at all times.

Thalassemia syndromes result from deficiencies in the production of either alpha (alpha-thalassemia) or beta (beta-thalassemia) globin chains. The disease becomes manifest when production of the affected globin is required during development. For alpha globin, symptoms thus occur during gestation. Because beta globin is not required before birth, beta-thalassemia is asymptomatic for 6 to 12 months after birth.

An obvious consequence of the biosynthetic defect in thalassemia is the microcytosis and hypochromia caused by the decrease in the amount of normal hemoglobin tetramer in each red blood cell. However, the major pathology in the thalassemias is caused by the imbalance of alpha and non–alpha chain accumulation. Aggregation of the unaffected chains produced in normal amount occurs because the surplus chains are unable to find a heterologous counterpart. The aggregates precipitate in cells because the individual chains and aggregates are far less soluble than the normal heteromeric tetramers. In beta-thalassemia the precipitated alpha globin forms inclusion bodies that damage the red blood cell membrane and cause cell death (ineffective intramedullary erythropoiesis) and decreased red blood cell survival because of uptake in the splenic reticuloendothelial system (splenomegaly). A dramatic expansion of the bone marrow compartment also results from erythropoietin stimulation of further ineffective erythropoiesis. The marrow overgrowth leads to cortical thinning, pathologic fractures, and deformities of bones. Hypersplenism worsens the anemia by causing increased trapping of the formed elements of the blood. An increase in plasma volume, a consequence of the marrow and splenic expansion, also lowers the effective level of hemoglobin.

In alpha-thalassemic fetuses, excessive gamma globin forms tetramers ($gamma_4$ = hemoglobin Bart's) in the fetal and neonatal period; excess beta globin ($beta_4$ = hemoglobin H) accumulate after birth. Hemoglobin Bart's and hemoglobin H are somewhat more soluble and (for the same degree of imbalance) result in a milder ineffective erythropoiesis than is seen in beta-thalassemia. These tetramers, however, behave like variant hemoglobins in that they exhibit abnormal O_2 binding and sensitivity to oxidant stress (see later).

The alpha globin gene is duplicated. The most common genetic lesions causing alpha-thalassemia are deletions. There is a good correlation between the number of abnormal alpha globin loci and the clinical presentation. Loss of all four globin genes results in a lethal intrauterine condition, hydrops fetalis. In these fetuses, only hemoglobin Bart's can form; this hemoglobin has a massively left-shifted O_2 dissociation curve that effectively ablates O_2 delivery to tissues. Deletion of three alpha loci produces a chronic hemolytic anemia of moderate severity called hemoglobin H disease. Hemoglobin A production is sufficient for survival, but hemoglobin H behaves like a mildly unstable, oxidant-sensitive hemoglobin variant, causing hemolysis. There are no symptoms when only one (alpha-thalassemia-2) or two loci (alpha-thalassemia-1) are deleted. The latter condition is detected by hypochromia and microcytosis. Identical syndromes can arise from point mutations that inactivate the alpha loci.

Severe forms of alpha-thalassemia are common in Asians and in Mediterranean populations. In black (African) populations, severe disease is almost never seen, even though the alpha-thalassemia-2 deletion is extremely common (5 to 15 per cent gene frequency). In black persons, the virtual absence of chromosomes on which both alpha globin loci are inactivated explains this discrepancy in the incidence of mild and severe alpha-thalassemia.

In beta-thalassemia, clinically significant disease is seen only when both beta globin alleles are affected by the same mutation (homozygosity) or by two distinct forms of mutation (double heterozygosity). Analysis of globin chain production or direct globin gene analysis in an affected patient and in his or her kindred indicates whether the expression of each of the two affected genes is completely absent ($beta^0$-thalassemia) or partially reduced ($beta^+$-thalassemia). A large number of different molecular lesions of the gene, mostly point mutations, can be responsible for these two alternatives.

Thalassemia syndromes are commonly graded according to the severity of the anemia. Severe anemia presenting in the first 6 to 9 months after birth (thalassemia major) is usually caused by inheritance of two seriously impaired beta globin alleles. No symptomatic disease is usually seen in the heterozygous state; inheritance of a single defective allele gives rise to a mild hypochromic and microcytic anemia (thalassemia minor). Under certain circumstances, the "homozygous" state has a milder than usual presentation, for example, when there is a relatively mild reduction in globin synthesis attributable to one or both thalassemic alleles, when there is a higher than usual compensatory increase in gamma chain production, or when the co-inheritance of alpha-thalassemia decreases the net imbalance and alpha and beta globin synthesis. This condition is termed "thalassemia intermedia." These patients exhibit stigmata of anemia, hemolysis, and marrow expansion but do not require chronic transfusions for survival.

DIAGNOSIS

The diagnosis of severe thalassemia usually presents few difficulties. The family history in a compatible ethnic background (Italian, Greek, black, Asian, North American) frequently offers a solid lead. Strongly suggestive of thalassemia major or thalassemia intermedia are physical findings of microcytic anemia associated with jaundice, bony deformities, and splenomegaly with onset during the first 2 years of life. Hydrops fetalis often presents as polyhydramnios and fetal distress during the second trimester.

The blood morphology often shows a number of characteristic features that distinguish thalassemia from iron deficiency. For the same level of anemia, thalassemic peripheral blood shows a more pronounced microcytosis with significant anisocytosis and *relative* hypochromia, punctate basophilic stippling, and a high percentage of target cells (up to 30 per cent). The latter two phenomena are less dramatically expressed in iron deficiency. The reticulocyte count is not always a distinctive element; because of the intramedullary destruction, it is often lower than expected for the degree of hemolysis: 2 to 8 per cent. In hemoglobin disease the diagnosis can be made by in vitro precipitation of hemoglobin H with brilliant cresyl blue.

Analysis of red blood cell indices and iron parameters is usually sufficient for the diagnosis. Beta-thalassemia trait (beta-thalassemia minor) is recognized by mild anemia (hematocrit > 30) with dramatically low mean corpuscular volume (<75 fl) values and near-normal mean corpuscular hemoglobin concentration values, accompanied by erythrocytosis (red blood cells > 5 × 10^6 per mm^3), a normal serum iron level, normal total iron-binding capacity, and normal ferritin level. A microcytic blood picture is also seen in cases of congenital sideroblastic anemia, but the usual dimorphic picture and the higher degree of transferrin saturation in this disorder suggest a search in the marrow for ringed sideroblasts. If the evidence is not conclusive, hemoglobin electrophoresis, including a quantitative search for the elevation of hemoglobin A_2 and F levels characteristic of beta-thalassemia, clarifies the diagnosis.

In most heterozygotes, an increased percentage of hemoglobin A_2, often accompanied by an increase in hemoglobin F, constitutes an unequivocal confirmation of the diagnosis of beta-thalassemia. Rare forms of beta-thalassemia (e.g., delta-beta-thalassemia) do not cause elevated hemoglobin A_2 levels. Alpha-thalassemia trait can be completely silent or similar to beta-thalassemia trait, except for an absence of changes in hemoglobin A_2 or F levels.

Iron deficiency can mask thalassemia by decreasing the hemoglobin A_2 level. Coexisting thalassemia trait may thus be overlooked in an iron-deficient individual. If microcytic anemia does not respond completely to iron therapy, hemoglobin electrophoresis should be (re)considered.

The prenatal diagnosis of beta-thalassemia can now be accomplished with a high degree of safety and reliability. Fetal blood sampling is no longer necessary. Direct study of beta globin genes is now performed on fetal cell DNA obtained by amniocentesis after 14 weeks of gestation or by chorionic villus biopsy anytime in the first trimester, using gene mapping, oligonucleotide hybridization, or linkage of parental DNA markers.

The large variety of DNA sequence defects that can cause thalassemia render these analyses laborious and time-consuming. Many mutations must be screened to achieve useful predictability. One solid improvement in recent years has been the tailoring of the searches within each ethnic group; surveys have shown that in a given group three or four mutations account for the great majority of serious cases. A recent advance has been the introduction of the polymerase chain reaction, a technique that amplifies specific DNA sequences effortlessly and rapidly, obviating the need for cell culture and markedly increasing the sensitivity, precision, and rapidity of DNA diagnosis. Direct sequence determination of the mutant gene can now be offered as a clinical laboratory test in centers possessing this technology.

THERAPY

Beta-Thalassemia

In heterozygous alpha- or beta-thalassemias, close monitoring of the hematocrit is necessary during pregnancy to avoid a harmful drop, but patients are otherwise asymptomatic. Genetic counseling is mandatory.

Transfusion Therapy

In beta-thalassemia, major red blood cell transfusion is the mainstay of supportive therapy. Transfusions should be administered in sufficient quantity and frequency to achieve a hemoglobin level of *at least* 9.3 grams per dl; this level partly suppresses the erythropoietic drive. A regimen that maintains the mean hemoglobin above 10.5 to 11 grams per dl reduces marrow expansion, leading to a reduction in plasma volume and thus in the amount of blood required to achieve the same level of hemoglobin, especially in splenectomized patients. Bony changes are arrested or even regress, splenomegaly is retarded or recedes, growth improves, and improved physical activity can be expected. The increased transfusional iron load is partially compensated for by decreased gastrointestinal iron absorption. A nearly complete suppression of erythropoiesis is obtained with the "supertransfusion" regimen (hemoglobin level above 12 grams per dl). Major treatment centers currently differ with regard to the optimal level to be sought. *Most* experts maintain patients in the 9.5 to 11 grams per dl range.

With regard to initiation of chronic transfusions, one can safely follow the recommendations of the guide of Cooley's Anemia Foundation: Transfusion should be started for a persistent and otherwise unexplained fall in hemoglobin below 7 grams per dl. Patients with higher hemoglobin levels may also require chronic transfusions if there is significant growth impairment, serious bone changes, or progressive splenomegaly. A maintenance hemoglobin level above 10.5 to 11 grams per dl in nonhypersplenic patients is recommended. Frequent (one or two weekly) transfusions of small quantities of red blood cells provide the most "physiologic" support, but the psychologic burden is usually too high for children. In general, transfusions of about 15 ml per kg at 3- to 5-week intervals prove more manageable for patients and families. Transfusion records should be kept to measure the annual mean hemoglobin level and the annual blood consumption.

A complete genotype of the patient's red blood cells should be established before any transfusion treatment occurs; this information simplifies later identification of the involved antigens should isoimmunization occur. Only fresh ABO- and Rh(D)-compatible, cross-matched blood should be given. We advocate continuous monitoring for isoantibodies to critical red blood cell antigens, using indirect antiglobulin testing. When patients develop febrile reactions during transfusions, filters retaining the leukocytes should be installed or red blood cells frozen in glycerol used instead. If this is unsuccessful, washing the red blood cells is the next option. Aspirin taken before the transfusion often reduces the reaction. Increased transfusion requirements should alert the physician to possible hypersplenism, or (especially after splenectomy) alloimmunization, or the presence of an accessory spleen. In addition to the careful screening of donor blood for hepatitis B surface antigen, patients should be immunized early for hepatitis B. When titers drop to low levels, booster immunizations are suggested.

The danger of human immunodeficiency virus infection acquired from blood transfusion depends on the incidence of the disease in the donor pool but is favorably influenced by the intensity of the donor blood screening program; the latter has considerably diminished the risk of human immunodeficiency virus in the United States. Newer screening methods using the polymerase chain reaction will lower this risk even further.

Splenectomy

Massive splenomegaly is usually avoided or delayed by a proper hypertransfusion regimen. However, splenic sequestration of donor cells can eventually cause an excessive transfusion requirement, prompting splenectomy. A 50 per cent or greater increase in the transfusion requirement over a 1-year period is the major indication for surgical removal of the spleen. A transfusion requirement of more than 200 ml per kg per year of packed red blood cells is also an indication for splenectomy if there is no serologic evidence of isoimmunization. Significant leukopenia and thrombocytopenia by splenic trapping are other indications, but these rarely occur without the aforementioned increase in the red blood cell requirement.

Splenectomy significantly increases the risk of overwhelming sepsis, especially in young children. The encapsulated pneumococcus is the responsible organism in two-thirds of the cases. The other two most frequent pathogens are *Haemophilus influenzae* and *Neisseria meningitidis (meningococcus)*. *Yersinia enterocolitica* or *Yersinia pseudotuberculosis* is also found, especially in patients undergoing deferoxamine mesylate treatment. (The latter organisms use the iron bound to the chelator.) Because the risk of infection is greatest if patients are splenectomized during infancy, one should attempt to defer the operation until the age of 6 years.

Polyvalent pneumococcal vaccine should be administered 1 month before splenectomy. Many experts advocate the administration of oral penicillin V (250 mg per day) as prophylaxis after the procedure for at least 2 years in children less than 10 years old. Trimethoprim-sulfamethoxazole is an alternative in case of allergy. Parents should be instructed to seek immediate medical attention when significant fever develops ($>102°$ F°). Such patients are at risk for a fulminant course leading to death within 6 hours. Broadspectrum antibiotics should be given immediately, even before the results of any laboratory investigations are obtained. Splenectomized patients undergoing invasive procedures (e.g., dental work, endoscopy) should be given prophylactic penicillin (or alternative drugs in allergic patients, as stated earlier) for 24 hours before and after the procedure.

Treatment of Iron Overload

Each unit of blood contains approximately 250 mg of iron. A typical hypertransfusion regimen encumbers each patient *each year* with an average of four times the normal total body iron burden. There is no compensatory mechanism of sufficient magnitude to eliminate this burden; even a decrease in intestinal absorption, as seen in other cases of iron overload, does not suffice in this setting. Indeed, many transfused thalassemic patients continue to absorb dietary iron because the negative feedback regulation is suppressed, probably by signals from the expanded erythropoietic drive. By the time these patients reach adolescence, their iron stores have risen to toxic levels (transfusional hemosiderosis).

Before effective iron chelation therapy was developed, the dramatic multiorgan toxicity of iron was the major determinant in the fatal progression of the disease. The complications have a more subtle presentation in patients maintained on chelation therapy. Hemosiderosis causes the most striking clinical dysfunction in the endocrine organs, liver, and heart.

One common endocrinologic complication is glucose intolerance. Insulin-dependent diabetes mellitus occurs in a smaller group. Laboratory evidence of primary hypothyroidism, hypoparathyroidism, and other endocrinopathies can often be detected in the absence of symptoms; digoxin refractoriness in such patients should lead one to suspect hypocalcemia on this basis. One should be alert to diminished adrenal reserves during periods of metabolic stress in these patients. Delayed puberty is quite common and is probably the result of iron deposition in the hypothalamus. Retarded growth in hypertransfused patients is less striking in the early years but becomes pronounced at puberty. The exact mechanism is unclear.

Hepatic toxicity can lead to cirrhosis, but progression to symptomatic liver disease before the era of sustained chelation therapy was unusual because of the superseding onset of lethal cardiac complications. Subclinical cardiac dysfunction usually begins in the early teens; it is detectable by the reduced ejection fractions in exercising patients or by wall motion anomalies. Onset of clinical symptoms usually begins with arrhythmias or pericarditis, followed by congestive failure in the late teens and death at around the age of 20 years.

The iron chelator deferoxamine mesylate (Desferal) became a potentially effective therapy when it was shown that a continuous subcutaneous or intravenous infusion markedly improved urinary iron excretion in comparison to previous intramuscular injection regimens. When given as a continuous infusion in high enough doses in *most* patients, the drug maintains a negative iron balance despite continuing blood transfusions. When started (before 5 to 8 years of age) these regimens are *probably* effective in delaying cardiac disease, potentially prolonging survival.

In the presence of a significant iron burden before the onset of therapy, complete reversibility of the lesions by deferoxamine cannot be expected. If therapy is started after 10 years of age, progressive cardiac dysfunction continues in many patients. Cardiac disease may not be completely prevented unless deferoxamine is started before 5 years of age. Early initiation of therapy is thus advocated.

Iron overload should be documented first in candidates for iron chelation by a deferoxamine test. The 24-hour urinary iron excretion after injection of 500 mg deferoxamine should exceed 1 mg to consider chelation therapy (or the serum ferritin level should be above 1000 ng per ml). Another option is to start the deferoxamine therapy at the same time as the transfusions.

A small infusion pump is used to administer a dose of about 40 mg per kg per day over a period of 10 hours into the abdominal subcutaneous fat, with rotation of the infusion sites. Local swelling caused by the hypertonicity of the solution can be prevented by increasing the volume of water for the delivery of a given dose. Local allergic reactions (pruritus, hyperemia) can be suppressed by adding hydrocortisone (up to 2 mg per ml) to the solution or by using topical diphenhydramine. A number of cases of severe arrhythmias and severe congestive heart failure have been temporarily reversed with high-dose (15 mg per kg per hour for 10 hours) deferoxamine through a central venous catheter.

The drug is generally well tolerated. Anaphylactic reactions are rare and can be treated with desensitization. A number of patients treated with high-dose intravenous deferoxamine developed optic and acoustic neuritis, with only partial reversibility. Although these complications were reported by only one group, periodic vision and hearing tests are advocated. If the abnormalities disappear after discontinuation of the drug, the treatment can be cautiously reinitiated.

Iron overload causes depletion of vitamin C. This deficiency inhibits iron release from the reticuloendothelial cells. Sudden availability of vitamin C can lead to a massive, abrupt release of iron, a situation that can cause serious cardiotoxicity. It is therefore advisable to start exogenous vitamin C administration only *after* the first cycle of treatment with deferoxamine. The dose should be about 5 mg per kg, should not exceed 100 mg per day when deferoxamine is given, and should be given only while the deferoxamine infusion is actually in progress. Ascorbate can be replaced by oranges (75 mg per orange) or orange juice (50 mg per 100 ml).

The major problem with deferoxamine therapy is noncompliance because of the inconvenience of using the pump. Regular monitoring and psychologic support are important for the success of the treatment. In addition to specialized assistance from social workers and child psychologists, patient advocacy associations can help the patient cope with the emotional burden of the disease. There is reason to hope that the inconvenience of the present chelation therapy will disappear in the near future. Phase II clinical trials with a promising oral chelator (1,2-dimethyl-3-hydroxy-pyrid-4-one) are under way in the United Kingdom.

An innocuous practice that, according to some reports, reduces oral iron absorption is regular tea drinking.

Thalassemia Intermedia

A number of patients with homozygous beta-thalassemia do not develop a debilitating anemia. These patients should not be started on a lifelong transfusion regimen. Generally, when the hemoglobin level rises above 8 grams per dl, patients lead a normal life; under 7 grams per dl, complications inevitably arise. Regardless of the steady-state hemoglobin level, the patient should be watched closely for signs of bone marrow expansion, increasing spleen size, or growth retardation. These are all indications to initiate the same hypertransfusion regimen used to treat thalassemia major. If the fall of the mean hemoglobin to uncomfortably low levels parallels an increase in spleen size, splenectomy should be considered. Hypertransfusion can be delayed or avoided by splenectomy in some cases. This intervention can be combined with a cholecystectomy if gallstones are present, as it is frequently the case in patients with chronic hemolysis.

The hyperplastic marrow in thalassemia intermedia stimulates intestinal iron absorption, resulting in iron overload. Deferoxamine therapy should probably be started when the ferritin level rises above normal; one or two subcutaneous infusions a week generally suffice. Deferoxamine therapy is stopped during pregnancy, and a regular transfusion regimen during this period should be considered. The avoidance of iron-rich meats (liver and spleen) and cereals and regular drinking of a cup of tea are advocated as dietary measures.

Other complications of chronic hemolysis are (relative) folate deficiency, gallstones, leg ulcers, and, rarely, compression syndromes. Vitamin deficiency can be avoided by a daily supplement of 1 mg of folic acid. Patients should be evaluated promptly for symptoms suggestive of cholecystitis. In addition to local treatment of leg ulcers, leg elevation and peroral zinc sulfate are useful. Resistant cases benefit from a high transfusion regimen. Radiotherapy may be needed to treat spinal cord compression from marrow expansion in vertebrae.

Alpha-Thalassemia

Often no treatment is necessary with this disorder. The homozygous form is usually lethal in utero. Cases have been described of neonates who were kept alive with exchange transfusions. Patients with hemoglobin H disease usually present with moderate anemia. They should be monitored for worsening of the anemia during infections. If it is persistent and is associated with increasing splenomegaly, splenectomy should be considered; as in other forms of unstable hemoglobin level, a substantial increase in red blood cell survival and in hemoglobin level often follows removal of the spleen. Another characteristic in common with unstable hemoglobin variants is the sensitivity of hemoglobin H to oxidant stress; drugs such as sulfonamides exacerbate the effect of the infection in worsening the anemia. Oxidant drugs should thus be avoided in this disease. Folic acid supplements are indicated, as in other cases of chronic hemolysis. Iron overload is a considera-

tion in these patients, by analogy to patients with beta-thalassemia intermedia.

EXPERIMENTAL THERAPY

Bone Marrow Transplantation

Stem cells with an extensive self-renewal capacity can replenish erythroid and other hematopoietic progenitor compartments in the bone marrow. Bone marrow transplantation in a patient with thalassemia cures the disease by replacing stem cells harboring defective globin genes with normal cells. This curative therapy is associated with significant mortality and morbidity resulting from the toxicity of the conditioning regimen and from the pancytopenia and acute and chronic graft-versus-host disease after the procedure. Because of the immediate risks, only a few centers have systematically used this therapeutic option in the last decade. The largest experience has been accrued by Lucarelli et al. (In Bone Marrow Transplantation: Current Controversies. New York, Alan Liss, 1989, pp. 359–366): In 191 patients who underwent allogeneic bone marrow transplantation, a mortality of 10 per cent was found in those less than 7 years of age and a mortality of 20 per cent in those from 8 to 15 years. Organ hemosiderosis is considered the age-related risk factor. Relapse occurred in 13 per cent of the younger patients and 5 per cent of the older ones. Moderate to severe graft-versus-host disease was present in 5 per cent of patients less than 7 years of age and in 13 per cent of the older group. In coming years, improvement could occur from tailoring marrow-conditioning and immunosuppressive prophylactic regimens.

It is believed that if a patient has a human leukocyte antigen–matched sibling, marrow transplantation could be considered in the earlier years. The risks of this curative therapeutic modality must be weighed against the lifelong burden of hypertransfusion regimens and iron-chelating therapy. This balance may be shifted in the near future by the introduction of oral chelating agents and by improvement in the transplantation regimens.

Activation of Fetal Globin Synthesis

In a limited number of patients, gamma globin chain expression was stimulated by the use of the chemotherapeutic agent 5-azacytidine. The increased gamma chain synthesis resulted in a significant decrease in the transfusion requirement that lasted for several days after discontinuation of the drug. Initially, the effect of the drug was thought to be mediated by the DNA-hypo-methylating activity of this agent, as gamma globin gene expression was inversely correlated with the methylation status of gamma globin gene DNA. Kinetic studies and analogous effects with cell-cycle–specific agents (hydroxyurea and cytosine arabinoside) with no direct demethylating activity suggested that cell selection and reprogramming of globin gene regulation occurred independently of direct demethylating activity. The uncertainty about the (carcinogenic) side effects resulting from long-term use of these drugs has limited this therapy to adult patients with advanced disease in the controlled setting of experimental trials in few centers. Until more information about long-term toxicity and optimized regimens is available from these studies, this therapy should be still be considered experimental.

Gene Transfer

Several centers are investigating the biologic mechanisms necessary to achieve the long-term goal of correcting the defective genes in the stem cells of a thalassemic patient. At present, the most efficient system for transferring globin genes in hematopoietic stem cells is the retroviral vector.

Recent research has defined the DNA control elements that must be introduced with the structural globin sequences in retroviral vectors for controlled, abundant expression.

Several important problems must be solved before gene transfer systems can be applied in a curative mode to human thalassemic, hematopoietic stem cells. No definite time frame for the introduction of gene therapy in thalassemia can be anticipated at this moment.

SICKLE CELL DISEASE

method of
HAROLD ZARKOWSKY, M.D.
Washington University School of Medicine and
St. Louis Children's Hospital
St. Louis, Missouri

Sickle cell disease includes homozygous sickle cell anemia and those doubly heterozygous sickle hemoglobinopathies in which the gene for sickle hemoglobin production is paired with another abnormal gene for beta-globin chain production. Most common among the latter are sickle cell–hemoglobin C and sickle cell–beta-thalassemia (S-thal). Although the gene for sickle hemoglobin is present in many ethnic and racial groups worldwide, in the United States sickle cell disease primarily affects black persons, among whom the frequency of the sickle gene is 8 per cent, that of the hemoglobin C gene is 4 per cent, and that of the beta-thalassemia gene is 0.8 per cent. Hence, about 1 in 600 black infants has sickle cell anemia. There are two forms of S-thal: S-beta^0-thal, in which no hemoglobin A is produced, and S-beta$^+$-thal, in which up to 20 per cent of the hemoglobin is A. Sickle cell anemia and S-beta^0-thal are the most clinically severe, followed by sickle cell–hemoglobin C and S-beta$^+$-thal. Within each of the conditions comprising sickle cell disease, there is a great range in the incidence of recurrent acute events and in the development of major organ failure. A number of factors have been associated with modification of the clinical severity of sickle cell anemia. These include percentage of fetal hemoglobin, alpha-thalassemia genotype, beta-globin haplotype, and in vitro adhesiveness of sickle cells to endothelial cells, and the state of sickle cell hydration and deformability. The clinical expression of sickle cell disease is likely the result of a complex interplay of molecular and physical factors.

COMPREHENSIVE CARE

Because there is no cure or specific therapy for sickle cell disease, continuity of patient care, emphasis on health maintenance and preventive measures, and social support are the key elements in reducing mortality and improving the health status of patients with sickle cell disease. The goal is an ongoing educational and preventive health program that helps to reduce the complications of sickle cell disease and helps the patient to cope with the chronic illness.

Comprehensive care requires the early diagnosis of sickle cell disease because penicillin prophylaxis is the most effective therapy in reducing mortality and morbidity in young children with sickle cell anemia. Although autoinfarction of the spleen is a delayed sequela of impaired blood flow through the spleen, functional asplenia can occur as early as 4 to 6 months of age in infants with sickle cell anemia and S-beta^0-thal. Splenic incompetence in handling pneumococcal bacteremia puts the infant with sickle cell anemia at a 25 per cent risk of succumbing to pneumococcal sepsis or meningitis. Pneumococcal bacteremia has been reported in nearly 10 per cent of children with sickle cell anemia less than 3 years of age. Penicillin prophylaxis, 125 mg twice daily (at ages 4 months to 3 years) and 250 mg twice daily after age 3 years, markedly reduces the incidence of serious pneumococcal infection. Although pneumococcus-related deaths are far less likely in infants with sickle cell–hemoglobin C and S-beta$^+$-thal, it is recommended that all children with sickle cell disease receive penicillin prophylaxis. The duration of this prophylaxis is under study. Discontinuing penicillin prophylaxis at age 5 years has been recommended because the incidence of serious pneumococcal infection in older children who have not received this prophylaxis is extremely low. However, it is not known whether the prophylaxis increases the age range of susceptibility.

The impact of penicillin prophylaxis is felt only if the diagnosis of sickle cell disease is made within the first 6 months of life. Many states have adopted cord blood screening programs as the most effective method for early diagnosis. If newborn screening has not been performed, all infants at risk for sickle cell disease should be tested by age 4 to 6 months.

Immunization with multivalent pneumococcal vaccine should be given at age 2 years and repeated at 5 years. Children with sickle cell anemia are also at increased risk for *Haemophilus influenzae* infection, so that conjugated vaccine should be given at age 18 months. Immunization before these ages is not recommended because the vaccines do not produce consistent and effective antibody titers. However, if vaccines are developed with proven effectiveness at earlier ages, they should be used.

Hematologic abnormalities develop as the percentage of fetal hemoglobin declines after birth. Patients with sickle cell anemia usually maintain a hemoglobin concentration between 6 and 8.5 grams per dl, whereas in sickle cell–hemoglobin C the average hemoglobin concentration is 10.5 grams per dl. Iron therapy should be instituted only when there is laboratory evidence of iron deficiency (low iron saturation or low ferritin level). The need for folic acid supplements is controversial. The leukocyte count is usually elevated (12,000 to 15,000 leukocytes per mm^3), and this must be considered when evaluating patients for bacterial infection.

Both the chronic anemia and the fear of precipitating vaso-occlusive events often restrict the activity of patients with sickle cell disease. Although strenuous exercise must be avoided, children should be encouraged to participate in physical education activities at school. Both children and adults can establish their own tolerance levels.

Delayed growth of children with sickle cell disease is observed in early childhood. Although they eventually achieve height within a normal range and full sexual maturation, about 25 per cent of children with sickle cell anemia and S-beta^0-thal suffer markedly delayed growth and delayed puberty. There is no good explanation for this delay, and no therapeutic intervention has proved to be effective. Extra support by health care providers is necessary to help the teenager cope with this additional insult to the self-image.

The potential for chronic lung damage from recurrent infarction makes it particularly important to advise patients against cigarette smoking. Patients should also be educated to seek prompt care for high fever and symptoms of acute anemia.

CARE IN ACUTE EVENTS

The predominant pathophysiologic process in sickle cell disease is vaso-occlusion. It is not understood what initiates or propagates vaso-occlusion to a degree that results in a clinically evident episode.

Painful Episodes

The most common vaso-occlusive event is the painful episode (or crisis), presenting as bone or abdominal pain. In infancy the painful episode often involves the hands, feet, or both and is associated with swelling. After infancy the back, long bones, and sternum are the most frequent painful sites, and usually there are no clinical signs. When swelling, tenderness, and warmth are present, it may be difficult to distinguish bone infarction from infection. Infarction is a far more common occurrence, and usually the tenderness and swelling are diffuse rather than localized. There is no single test to differentiate infection from infarction. Radionuclide scans of bone are expensive and difficult to interpret, and plain radiographs are of no value. The combination of skeletal findings, temperature, and degree of leukocytosis should be included in the evaluation. If osteomyelitis or septic arthritis is suspected, every effort should be made to obtain the bacteriologic etiology by blood culture or aspiration.

The management of painful episodes is symptomatic, with the use of analgesics and comfort measures. Hydration is an important consideration, but fluid administration must be placed in proper perspective. Some patients may become dehydrated as a painful episode evolves because of reduced fluid intake and the hyposthenuria of sickle cell disease. However, the dehydration is not associated with plasma hypertonicity leading to red blood cell dehydration and increased sickling. Fluid therapy should correct any dehydration that is present. Otherwise, the objective is to maintain adequate hydration, which should be accomplished with oral fluids when possible. Intravenous fluid intake should be monitored carefully. Excessive fluid administration has resulted in pulmonary edema and hyponatremia.

Analgesics are given to provide optimal pain relief. "Optimal" means that the therapy does not lead to oversedation, depression of respirations, vomiting, or severe nausea. A combination of sedation and decreased respiratory effort can lead to atelectasis, pulmonary infarction, or pneumonia. Most painful events can be managed at home. Patients prefer this method to emergency room visits, and it gives them a sense of control that is often lost in the hospital setting. Treatment of mild pain begins with acetaminophen or aspirin. If the pain is not controlled, oral codeine is the preferred narcotic. Patients and parents of children should be given clear guidelines in the use of analgesia at home and instructed to seek hospital management when the pain is not sufficiently alleviated by codeine.

The narcotic of choice for severe pain requiring parenteral administration is morphine, 0.1 to 0.15 mg per kg per dose. It can be administered subcutaneously, intramuscularly, or intravenously. Occasionally, patients obtain relief from one injection of morphine and in 3 to 4 hours feel that the pain can be controlled with oral codeine at home. If a second injection of morphine is required, it is best to admit the patient to a hospital or to a comfortable short-stay area. An extended stay in a busy emergency room is not appropriate. Morphine is usually given every 3 to 4 hours. All parenteral narcotics must be given on a fixed schedule rather than as needed. If the patient is asleep or heavily sedated, the regularly scheduled dose should not be given. It is best to re-evaluate the pain medication every 24 hours. When the pain has diminished, the physician should gradually decrease the dose of parenteral narcotics but maintain the same interval. When the patient has gradually been weaned to about 50 per cent of the initial total daily parenteral dose, a change to codeine should be attempted. The duration of severe painful episodes can be 7 to 10 days.

Demerol should never be used in patients with a seizure disorder. Drugs reputed to potentiate the analgesic effect of narcotics are of limited value, and phenothiazines are potentially harmful because they may provoke seizures during parenteral narcotic therapy. Oxygen therapy is of no benefit unless hypoxemia is present.

Pain perception, for which we use analgesic therapy, is only one aspect of the pain pathology. The patient suffers and may demonstrate "pain behavior." Suffering and pain behavior are managed with sympathetic care and meticulous attention to analgesic therapy. Most patients prefer to be in a quiet, darkened room with little intrusion by nursing or medical personnel. For about 20 per cent of the patients with sickle cell anemia and S-beta^0-thal, painful episodes are recurrent and severe. These patients account for most of the hospital admissions and emergency room visits. The full resources of the psychosocial support system are necessary to help the patients. Their families must also be included in any counseling effort.

Splenic Sequestration Crisis

Sudden, massive pooling of blood in the spleen can occur in infants with sickle cell anemia, which results in a profound decrease in the hemoglobin concentration to 1 to 2 grams per dl and massive splenomegaly. Hypovolemic shock and death occur unless the condition is recognized and plasma expanders and red blood cells are promptly administered. There is no need to achieve the patient's baseline hemoglobin concentration because within 24 to 48 hours most of the sequestered red blood cells return to the circulation. Less severe splenic sequestration crises occur and can be seen in older patients with sickle cell–hemoglobin C or sickle cell anemia whose spleens have not become fibrotic from repeated infarcts. There is moderate splenic enlargement and a decrease in hemoglobin concentration of 2 to 3 grams per dl.

The fear of repeated and potentially fatal sequestration crises has led to the recommendation that splenectomy be peformed after the first or second sequestration crisis. Alternatively, a 1- or 2-year schedule of chronic red blood cell transfusions can be instituted. This treatment eliminates the risk of sequestration crisis, but once the transfusions are discontinued, the infant may be at risk again.

Aplastic and Hemolytic Crises

Aplastic crises are the result of a transient depression in red blood cell production. The red blood cell aplasia is associated with infections, most notably with parvovirus, and may last for up to 2 weeks. The onset of the anemia is more gradual than in a sequestration crisis, and the reticulocyte count is reduced. The degree of anemia depends on the duration of the depressed erythropoiesis and the patient's red blood cell survival. Patients with sickle cell anemia and S-beta^0-thal are most likely to sustain a severe decrease in hemoglobin concentration because the hemolytic rate is greater than that in other sickle cell disease conditions.

The decision to transfuse with packed red blood cells is based on the patient's symptoms, extent of anemia, and evidence of erythropoietic recovery. Serial observations are often necessary to determine whether transfusion or close observation is necessary. The severely anemic patient with an aplastic crisis has an expanded blood volume. Therefore, small transfusions of packed cells must be given slowly (5 ml per kg during 4 hours) to prevent circulatory overload. In some patients, a partial exchange transfusion may be necessary to restore an adequate red blood cell mass.

Hemolytic crises are more difficult to define. Typically, the patient has a decreased hemoglobin concentration, but the reticulocyte count is not depressed. It is difficult to determine whether these hematologic values represent a recovery from an aplastic crisis or evidence of an accelerated hemolytic state. Most often, a falling hemoglobin concentration without a change in reticulocyte count is seen in patients with bacterial infections.

Hepatic Events

A mildly elevated serum bilirubin concentration is commonly seen in sickle cell disease. Episodes of severe hyperbilirubinemia exceeding 40 mg per dl may be caused by viral hepatitis, common bile duct obstruction, or acute hepatic crisis. Gallstones are found in more than 50 per cent of adults with sickle cell anemia. It is controversial whether gallstones, detected by an incidental examination, should be removed. Most hematologists prefer to recommend cholecystectomy only in patients experiencing symptoms associated with gallbladder disease. However, it is sometimes difficult to attribute recurrent right upper quadrant pain to gallbladder disease or to the sickling process. Acute hepatic crises rarely lead to severe hepatic necrosis. Management is supportive, and red blood cell transfusions should be considered.

Priapism

Prepubertal boys and adult men may experience repetitive, painful erections lasting for less than a few hours or prolonged, painful erections lasting for periods ranging from days to weeks. Acute, prolonged priapism can lead to impotence, and several surgical approaches have been developed to treat priapism and prevent impotence. However, all surgical techniques have complications and sometimes fail to prevent impotence, so most hematologists prefer conservative management. Treatment begins with intravenous hydration and administration of parenteral narcotics. Because prompt improvement rarely occurs with these measures, transfusions are routinely given. The goal is to reduce the percentage of sickle cells below 50 per cent. This can be accomplished by partial exchange transfusion or repeated transfusions over several days. Even when detumescence begins within a few days, complete resolution may take weeks.

Stroke

Cerebral infarction secondary to occlusion of large and medium-sized cerebral arteries occurs in about 10 per cent of children with sickle cell anemia. Although complete neurologic recovery may occur in some patients, the risk of a subsequent stroke is 60 to 70 per cent. Repeated strokes can have devastating effects on neurologic and intellectual function. A chronic transfusion program that maintains the percentage of sickle cells below 30 per cent is effective in preventing the recurrence of strokes and is the recommended practice. How long the transfusion program must be maintained is not known, except that 1 to 2 years is not sufficient. Some hematologists stop the transfusions at 4 years, but other feel that a longer period is necessary and add chelation therapy with deferoxamine to prevent iron overload. There are no data that can be used to compare the recurrence rate and neurologic sequelae of these two approaches.

Acute Chest Syndrome

The acute chest syndrome is characterized by fever, cough, pulmonary infiltrates, and chest pain. The term acknowledges the difficulty in distinguishing between pneumonia and pulmonary infarction in patients with sickle cell disease. The acute chest syndrome can appear several days after the onset of a painful episode. Antibiotics are recommended for all patients and are continued until clinical findings are convincing for the diagnosis of pulmonary infarction. The choice of empiric antibiotic therapy depends on the age of the patient. When *H. influenzae* infection is a concern in young children, ceftriaxone is the antibiotic of choice. For older patients, ampicillin should be adequate. Consideration should be given to adding erythromycin because of the frequency with which mycoplasma pneumonia is associated with the acute chest syndrome. It is not uncommon for fever to persist for several days after appropriate antibiotic coverage has been administered.

When there is concurrent severe anemia, red blood cell transfusions should be given. Partial exchange transfusion is necessary when there is rapid progression of the disease and respiratory insufficiency.

Acute Febrile Episodes

The use of penicillin prophylaxis or pneumococcal vaccination does not mitigate the seriousness of unexplained febrile (>38.8° C) illnesses in children with sickle cell anemia less than 4 years of age. Blood cultures should be obtained and intravenous antibiotics promptly administered. Antibiotic coverage for pneumococcus is most important, but *H. influenzae* must also be considered, for which the use of ceftriaxone is recommended.

The evaluation of older children with fever or younger children with low-grade fever (temperature <38.5° C) must be individualized. A patient who appears to be toxic must receive aggressive treatment with intravenous antibiotics regardless of age.

SPECIAL PROBLEMS

Pregnancy

In adolescence, girls should be counseled regarding the increased morbidity of pregnancy combined with sickle cell disease, including the high rates of spontaneous abortion, premature delivery, and intrauterine growth retardation. It is appropriate to offer these adolescents genetic counseling and to stress the value of sickle cell testing of the partner and the newborn infant. Medically, barrier methods are the safest form of contraception, but compliance is often inadequate. There is no evidence that low-dose estrogen oral contraceptives pose a greater thrombotic risk to girls or women with sickle cell disease than to their normal counterparts.

The improved medical care of pregnant women with sickle cell disease has eliminated the excessive mortality that was previously reported. This experience suggests that all pregnant women with sickle cell disease should receive obstetric care at a high-risk obstetric center.

A recent study randomized pregnant women with sickle cell anemia into two groups: one received prophylactic red blood cell transfusions, and the other received such transfusions only for medical or obstetric emergencies. The only benefit to the patients receiving prophylactic transfusions was a reduction in painful episodes. Medical and obstetric complications were no different between the two groups, nor was there any statistical difference in perinatal outcome between them. This study shows that routine prophylactic red blood cell transfusion is not indicated in pregnant women who receive obstetric care at specialized clinics.

Surgery

Patients with sickle cell disease undergoing surgery have benefited from improved perioper-ative management, with careful attention to the state of hydration and administration of oxygen during surgery and in the immediate postoperative period. The role of preoperative red blood cell transfusions is debatable. Previously, a minimum hemoglobin concentration of 10 grams per dl was considered necessary in healthy individuals. In stable, chronically anemic individuals, surgery can be safely performed with a hemoglobin concentration of 8 grams per dl. The same is true for patients with sickle cell disease, and we have had excellent outcomes without preoperative transfusion. Many physicians advocate an entirely different approach, namely, reducing the percentage of sickle cells to less than 30 to 40 per cent before surgery. For elective procedures, this requires several transfusions during the 3 to 4 weeks before surgery. Partial exchange transfusion is the only way to reduce the percentage of sickle hemoglobins before emergency surgery.

NEUTROPENIA

method of
DAVID C. DALE, M.D., and
WILLIAM P. HAMMOND, M.D.
University of Washington
Seattle, Washington

An adequate supply of neutrophils is a critical component of the host defense system. The absolute blood neutrophil count (the total white blood cell count × the percentage of neutrophils) is a measure of the number of neutrophils freely flowing in the circulation. The total supply consists of the circulating and marginal neutrophil pools in the blood, the marrow neutrophil reserves, and the capacity of the marrow to produce new white blood cells. Normally, the absolute count remains relatively constant; the normal range is 2000 to 7500 cells per mm³ (95 per cent confidence limits).

The term "neutropenia" is used to describe a reduction in the number of blood neutrophils. For practical purposes, neutropenia may be described as "mild" if the neutrophil count is 1000 to 2000 cells per mm³, as "moderate" if the count is 500 to 1000 cells per mm³, and as "severe" if the count is below 500 cells per mm³. These subdivisions are important because the consequences of neutropenia vary dramatically, depending on the degree to which the count is reduced.

Neutropenia can occur as an isolated abnormality or as part of a broader defect in the host defense system. When neutropenia is the sole abnormality and is mild or moderate, there is little increase in susceptibility to infections. When neutropenia is severe or occurs with other abnormalities (e.g., lymphocytopenia, monocytopenia, hypogammaglobulinemia, or damaged mucous membranes or skin), susceptibility to infections is severe. Transient severe neutropenia, lasting for 1 to 2 days, may be well tolerated. If it is more protracted, fever and bacterial infections from surface microorganisms are likely. When antibiotics are given to such patients, colonization of the skin and intestinal tract by antibiotic-resistant bacteria, yeast, or fungi often follows.

CLINICAL PRESENTATION

When patients become severely neutropenic, they usually develop evidence of inflammation and infection within a few days. They usually present with fever, oral ulcers, upper respiratory tract symptoms, or skin infections. Less often, they have symptoms of sinusitis, otitis, pneumonia, peritonitis, or bacteremia. Patients with severe, chronic neutropenia often have dental complaints because of gingivitis or periodontitis.

DIFFERENTIAL DIAGNOSIS

Neutropenia may be acute or chronic, congenital or acquired. Drugs (i.e., cytotoxic agents or drugs causing neutropenia or agranulocytosis by an idiosyncratic reaction) are the most frequent cause of acute neutropenia. Acute viral infections (e.g., the viral exanthems, infectious mononucleosis, infectious hepatitis, or cytomegalovirus infection) are other common causes. Neutropenia also occurs with overwhelming bacterial infections, particularly in patients with pre-existing hematologic disorders (e.g., folate deficiency with alcoholism, marrow damage from radiation or tumors, or pernicious anemia). Acute neutropenia may be the presenting feature of acute leukemia, aplastic anemia, or other marrow failure states.

Chronic neutropenia occurs as a congenital disorder, but these cases are rare. More commonly, chronic neutropenia is caused by an immunologic disorder (e.g., isoimmune neonatal neutropenia, autoimmune neutropenia, systemic lupus erythematosus, or other collagen vascular diseases), splenic sequestration (e.g., rheumatoid arthritis or Felty's syndrome, sarcoidosis, cirrhosis), or a hematopoietic stem cell disease (e.g., the myelodysplastic-preleukemic syndrome). Human immunodeficiency virus infection is another important cause of chronic neutropenia.

MANAGEMENT

Focus

Concern should be directed principally to patients with moderate or severe neutropenia. Mild neutropenia generally has few clinical consequences and should be simply observed.

Patients presenting with fever and neutropenia, with or without a localized area of inflammation, deserve urgent attention. Ordinarily, they should be hospitalized for diagnosis and treatment. After a thorough physical examination, with particular attention to the oropharynx, lungs, abdomen, and perianal areas, blood cul-

tures should be done. Microbiologic cultures from other areas of suspected infection should be obtained. A chest x-ray film and x-ray films of other areas of suspected inflammation are usually indicated.

Patient Isolation and Hygiene

It is a common practice in many hospitals to isolate patients with severe neutropenia in private rooms and to require visitors and staff to wear mask and gowns. Isolation with ultraviolet lamps and laminar airflow rooms is used in some facilities. Although these procedures can be shown to delay the occurrence of infections in some settings, their value is limited because most infections come from the patient's own surface organisms. To avoid colonization by new, potentially antibiotic-resistant microorganisms, the most important factors are thorough handwashing by staff before and after examining patients, use of gloves for handling patients' blood or secretions, judicious use of antibiotics, and avoidance of exposure to others with obvious infections. Attention to good nutrition and personal hygiene (i.e., regular bathing and good mouth, dental, and skin care) is important in maintaining the barrier functions of the skin and mucous membranes.

Antibiotics*

Antibiotic therapy for the febrile neutropenic patient is continually evolving with the development of better drugs and the changing antibiotic sensitivities of the infecting organisms. The search continues for ideal broad-spectrum antibiotics that can be used as single agents and are nontoxic and nonallergenic. Three single agents have been evaluated recently. They are ceftazidime (Fortaz, Tazicef, Tazidime), 2 grams intravenously every 8 hours, cefoperazone (Cefobid), 2 to 4 grams intravenously every 12 hours, and imipenem-cilastatin (Primaxin), 0.5 to 1 gram intravenously every 6 hours. Response rates are usually very good; about 80 per cent of severely neutropenic cancer patients receiving chemotherapy either become afebrile or improve significantly when given these agents. In some centers, a combination of drugs, such as cefoperazone or imipenem-cilastatin (same dosages) plus mezlocillin (Mezlin), 4 grams intravenously every 8 hours, or piperacillin (Pipracil), 3 grams intravenously every 4 hours, is preferred. The combination of cefoperazone, imipenem-cilastatin, mez-

---

*Doses given for all antibiotics are for adults with normal renal function.

locillin (same dosages), or ticarcillin (Ticar), 3 grams intravenously every 4 hours, with an aminoglycoside such as tobramycin (Nebcin), 3 to 5 mg per kg per day intravenously divided every 8 hours, or amikacin (Amikin), 15 mg per kg per day intravenously every 8 hours, is used in other centers. The aminoglycosides have the disadvantage of causing nephrotoxicity, which is often greater if the patient is concomitantly receiving other nephrotoxic drugs. It is important to be prepared to change antibiotics for the febrile neutropenic patient as soon as the results of microbial cultures, particularly the blood cultures, are available. In many centers, infections caused by gram-positive organisms, usually staphylococci, have recently been increasing. For these infections, a semisynthetic penicillin such as nafcillin (Nafcil, Unipen), 2 grams intravenously every 4 hours, or vancomycin (Vancocin), 1 gram intravenously every 12 hours, may be indicated.

Most severely neutropenic patients who do not have fever or a recent infection should be managed without antibiotics. For some patients with chronic neutropenia and recurrent infections, chronic oral antibiotic therapy may be helpful. Trimethoprim-sulfamethoxazole or a beta-lactamase–resistant penicillin such as cloxacillin (Tegopen) is often used. Chlorhexidine (Peridex) mouth rinse (0.12 per cent solution) may be used for short-term treatment of gingivitis.

Antifungal Therapy

Most patients with severe neutropenia and fever become afebrile within 72 hours of beginning broad-spectrum antibiotic therapy as just outlined. Those who do not should be re-examined thoroughly, repeat cultures should be obtained, and antifungal therapy should be considered. It is common practice in many centers to treat severely neutropenic patients who remain febrile when taking broad-spectrum antibiotics for more than 3 to 5 days with amphotericin (Fungizone),* 0.25 to 1 mg per kg per day intravenously. Nystatin throat lozenges and vaginal suppositories are useful adjunctive measures for patients with oral or vaginal candidiasis.

Antiviral Therapy

Some viral infections, particularly with herpes simplex virus and cytomegalovirus, may become activated in patients with severe neutropenia, particularly when neutropenia occurs in patients

---

*The manufacturer recommends a 1-mg test dose infused slowly.

with defects in cellular immunity. Therapy with acyclovir (Zovirax), 5 mg per kg intravenously every 8 hours, or ganciclovir, 5 mg per kg intravenously every 8 hours (investigational), is useful for these patients.

Neutrophil Transfusions

Supportive therapy with neutrophils collected from normal persons can temporarily improve host defenses for severely neutropenic patients. The utility of neutrophil transfusions is limited by the number of cells that can be collected and the short life span of the transfused cells. Neutrophil transfusions are of proven benefit in patients with documented infections who have not responded to antibiotics and who can be predicted to have their neutrophil counts recover within 2 or 3 weeks. For most patients, this form of supportive therapy is not necessary.

SPECIFIC TREATMENT FOR NEUTROPENIA

Observation and Withdrawal of Toxic Drugs

If neutropenia is caused by recent therapy with a cytotoxic drug, marrow recovery in a few days to a few weeks is expected. If an idiosyncratic reaction to a drug is suspected, all drugs should be stopped except those that are essential. Marrow recovery usually occurs within 7 to 10 days. If neutropenia is caused by a viral or bacterial infection, it should resolve as the patient recovers from the infection.

Chemotherapy

The diagnosis of acute leukemia or other primary bone marrow disorders is usually made from examinations of the blood and bone marrow. With chemotherapy to induce a remission, improved neutrophil production usually occurs. The use of cytotoxic drugs for immune neutropenia generally is not indicated.

Bone Marrow Transplantation and Immunotherapy with Antithymocyte Globulin

These therapies are useful for patients with aplastic anemia. The diagnosis is usually based on the finding of pancytopenia and hypocellular bone marrow. Bone marrow transplantation may also be of benefit to patients with immunodeficiency syndromes and congenital neutropenia and may be helpful in sustaining remissions in some forms of leukemia.

Corticosteroids and Other Steroidal Hormones

Because corticosteroids may increase the risk and mask the signs of infections, and because they are of no benefit in the vast majority of neutropenic patients, they should not be given without specific indications. Occasional patients with chronic idiopathic neutropenia or immune-mediated neutropenia (e.g., lupus erythematosus or proven immune neutropenia) may benefit. This can usually be determined only with a short trial in the individual patient. In these instances, the use of alternate-day or intermittent therapy is recommended to lower the risk of infectious complications. Androgen therapy alone is infrequently beneficial for patients with aplastic anemia but is of no value for most patients with neutropenia. These drugs cause masculinization, increased libido, and toxic hepatitis.

Lithium Carbonate Therapy

Lithium carbonate (usually 600 mg three times daily) causes an increase in blood neutrophil numbers in normal individuals and has been tried in a variety of neutropenic disorders. Although lithium accelerates marrow recovery slightly after chemotherapy, its therapeutic value is limited. Only rarely have patients with chronic neutropenia been reported to benefit from this therapy. Lithium causes nephrogenic diabetes insipidus, thyroid disorders, dermatitis, tremors, and other neurologic sequelae.

Gamma Globulin Therapy

Intravenous gamma globulin has been shown to elevate neutrophil counts in children with autoimmune neutropenia, but most of these children recover without this or other specific therapies. Its use in adults with idiopathic neutropenia has been limited. This therapy is expensive and should still be regarded as experimental.

Splenectomy

The spleen serves to trap effete red blood cells and may sequester neutrophils under some clinical circumstances. In some diseases (e.g., myelofibrosis and chronic granulocytic leukemia) splenic production of neutrophils contributes substantially to the blood neutrophil count. At present, there is no accurate method to determine if the spleen causes neutropenia. The decision to remove the spleen should never be based solely on the number of the blood neutrophils. Splenectomy to treat neutropenia should be limited to patients with both splenomegaly and frequent infections (e.g., some patients with Felty's syndrome or hairy cell leukemia). Splenectomy generally is not indicated for neutropenia in sarcoidosis, infectious mononucleosis, or hepatitis.

Nutritional Therapies

Patients with folic acid or vitamin B_{12} deficiency may have neutropenia, and their neutrophil counts increase dramatically with the appropriate therapy. Occasional patients receiving chronic intravenous therapy develop copper deficiency, and the associated neutropenia responds to copper therapy.

Experimental Therapies

Recently, specific hormones have been identified that stimulate neutrophil production in humans. These hormones are called colony-stimulating factors and interleukins. Granulocyte colony-stimulating factor increases the number of blood neutrophils; granulocyte-macrophage colony-stimulating factor increases the number of neutrophils, monocytes, and eosinophils. The interleukins appear to stimulate cell production at an early stage and to have lesser effects on the blood counts. These factors may soon be available to accelerate marrow recovery in patients with drug-induced neutropenia and bone marrow transplantation, and as primary therapies for severe congenital or acquired neutropenia.

HEMOLYTIC DISEASE OF THE NEWBORN

method of
GARY R. GUTCHER, M.D.
Medical College of Virginia
Richmond, Virginia

The term *"hemolytic disease of the newborn"* (HDN) is generally used as if it were synonymous with only isoimmune hemolytic diseases. Although isoimmune hemolytic diseases do account for the majority of cases of HDN, the relative decrease in the severe manifestations of problems related to the Rh blood group requires a heightened awareness on the part of physicians of the other causes outlined in Table 1. All of these conditions are characterized by the production of bilirubin from red blood cell destruction to a degree that overwhelms the excretory system. This is in contrast to those causes of neonatal hyperbilirubinemia that result from delayed or blunted excretion.

As the classic example of HDN, the Rh antibody

TABLE 1. **Causes of HDN and Overproduction of Bilirubin**

1. **Isoimmunization**
   Rh, ABO, anti-c, anti-E, anti-Kell, anti-Duffy, anti-M

2. **Spherocytic Diseases (Membrane Defects)**
   Spherocytosis, elliptocytosis, stomatocytosis, pyknocytosis

3. **Nonspherocytic Diseases (Enzyme Defects and Hemoglobinopathy)**
   Glucose-6-phosphate dehydrogenase deficiency, pyruvate kinase deficiency, alpha-thalassemia trait

4. **Drug-Induced**
   High-dose water-soluble vitamin K

5. **Infection**
   Bacterial sepsis
   Viral (especially intrauterine): cytomegalovirus, rubella, coxsackievirus B, and herpesvirus
   Syphilis
   Protozoan (toxoplasmosis, malaria)

6. **Inborn Errors of Metabolism**
   Galactosemia

7. **Microangiopathic**
   Disseminated intravascular hemolysis, hemangioma (Kasabach-Merritt syndrome), severe arterial stenosis (renal, aortic)

system provides the model for other forms of isoimmune disease. The Rh blood group has three antigenic groupings (Cc, Dd, Ee) on the surface of the erythrocyte. Rh "positivity" is conferred by the presence of D, and Rh "negativity" by its absence. Although modified by the closely aligned Cc-Ee antigens, an individual's Rh status is predominantly determined by the presence or absence of a "big" D from at least one parent. Approximately 15 per cent of the caucasian population but only 5 per cent of American black persons are Rh negative.

Throughout the pregnancy of an Rh-negative mother who is carrying an Rh-positive fetus, fetomaternal transplacental transfusions will initiate a response of both an anti-D IgM (saline, or complete) antibody and an anti-D IgG (incomplete) antibody. IgG is capable of crossing the placenta, sensitizing the fetal Rh-positive cells, and initiating destruction and clearance of erythrocytes by the fetal reticuloendothelial system (RES). The severity of the ensuing disease is in large part, then, determined by the degree of sensitization (leak) and the ability of the fetal RES to process the erythrocytes. To the extent that subsequent sensitizations are "primed," each succeeding Rh-positive fetus in an Rh-negative woman will be more severely affected. Table 2 delineates the manifestations and mechanisms involved in this process.

Unlike the Rh system, which is limited to primate erythrocytes, the ABO blood group antigens are also present in foods and bacteria. Thus, previous exposure to blood products is not the prerequisite that it is in Rh disease. A maternal blood group O sets the stage for an isoimmune response to fetal A or B antigen. Fetal antigen A is more sparsely distributed on erythrocytes than is fetal B. This may account for the relatively less severe manifestations of O-A incompat-

ibility when compared with O-B. Though generally not associated with erythroblastosis fetalis, ABO isoimmune hemolytic disease can produce unpredictable and severe degrees of hyperbilirubinemia.

As indicated earlier, the decline in Rh disease as a result of prophylactic immune therapy (see later) has resulted in the relative increase in isoimmune diseases secondary to other blood group antigen incompatibilities: anti-c, anti-E, anti-Kell, anti-M, and anti-Duffy. The diagnosis and nonimmune therapy of these diseases are identical to those of the Rh model.

ANTENATAL MANAGEMENT

All pregnant women should be screened early (first visit) with blood group typing and antibody screening (indirect Coombs's test). The diagnosis should be suspected in a setup (maternal Rh-negative or O type) and confirmed when specific antibody titers exceed 1:8. When the titers are 1:8 or lower, monthly retesting is indicated. When they are higher than 1:8, closer evaluation by amniocentesis is required.

Amniocentesis is performed with ultrasonographic guidance. The fluid (free of meconium or blood) may be scanned in a recording spectrophotometer and the peak optimal density (above baseline) at 450 nm, called the delta OD_{450}, is plotted against gestational age on semilogarithmic paper. The normative reference zones of Liley classify patients into Zone I (normal, no action); Zone II, declining (abnormal, no action without other compromising data); and Zone II, rising/Zone III (abnormal, intervene). The general scheme is depicted in Table 3. Once the need for amniocentesis is determined, referral to fetomaternal specialists is indicated, as the management becomes quite complex, involving intra-

TABLE 2. **Clinical Features of HDN**

Manifestation	Mechanism
1. Hemolysis	Erythrophagocytosis in RES Induction of enzymes degrading heme and globin Hyperbilirubinemia (in infant)
2. Erythropoiesis—peripheral blood reticulocytosis and normoblastemia	Enhanced in response to ongoing hemolysis Extramedullary hematopoiesis in liver, spleen, and skin ("blueberry muffin")
3. Anemia	Exhausted erythropoiesis
4. Hydrops fetalis—edema, anasarca	Anemia Decreased oncotic pressure Increased portal venous pressure Heart failure
5. Other (e.g., hypoglycemia)	Pancreatic cell hyperplasia secondary to in utero amino acid (alanine) stimulation

TABLE 3. **Utilization of Liley Graph Plot**
of Delta OD$_{450}$

Delta OD$_{450}$	Action
Zone I	Repeat every 2 to 3 wk
Zone II, falling	Repeat every week
Zone II, rising/ Zone III	Intervene ≤33 wk: intrauterine transfusion >33 wk: assess pulmonary maturity and consider delivery

uterine transfusion and/or early, premature induction of delivery.

For those infants requiring intrauterine transfusion, ultrasonographic guidance of a radiopaque catheter permits the intraperitoneal infusion of cytomegalovirus-negative, O-negative, washed, packed erythrocytes. The volume of blood infused is empirically calculated as

$$[\text{Gestational age (in weeks)} - 20] \times 10 \text{ ml}$$

Close fetal monitoring is used in decisions to slow or terminate the infusion as indicated. Peritoneal lymphatics will assimilate more than 90 per cent of the cells. The procedure will need to be repeated every 2 to 3 weeks. Failure to assimilate is an ominous sign. Because of the development of high-resolution sonography and enhanced operative skills, the intraperitoneal technique is being replaced by the direct intravascular infusion technique.

Other forms of therapy purported to alter the maternal immune response have been proposed, using a variety of agents. None have worked consistently. On the other hand, anti-D globulin (RhoGAM), which was introduced nearly 20 years ago, has proved to be an effective prophylactic immunotherapy. In documented maternal Rh-negative/neonatal Rh-positive situations, 300 micrograms is given intramuscularly within 72 hours of delivery. If there is some question or delay in defining the neonatal blood type, the Rh-negative mother should receive RhoGAM anyway, since nearly two-thirds of the infants will be Rh positive. Furthermore, although less effective, administration of RhoGAM up to 4 weeks later may be helpful and should *not* be withheld. These generous recommendations are made despite a reported persistent, disappointing so-called failure rate of RhoGAM. These failures are typically the result of errors in the accurate diagnosis of blood type (maternal or infant) or errors of omission (failure to administer at all times when sensitization may occur, such as amniocentesis, placenta previa or abruptio placentae, ectopic pregnancy, or spontaneous abortion). Furthermore, sensitization may occur early in

pregnancy, so that current recommendations are for a prophylactic dose at 28 weeks' gestation in all unsensitized women. The recommendations for RhoGAM administration are outlined in Table 4.

NEONATAL MANAGEMENT

The mainstay of neonatal management remains the exchange transfusion. Exchange transfusions are advocated for three general reasons:

Anemia. When present at birth, there should be a partial exchange with packed erythrocytes for hematocrits less than 30 ml/dl.

Rapidly Rising Serum Bilirubin. When this occurs at any time, whole blood should be utilized to remove sensitized cells from the circulation in an effort to blunt the peak bilirubin attained.

Elevated Bilirubin. An exchange transfusion using whole blood should be given at any time when the bilirubin exceeds some threshold level above which the risk of bilirubin encephalopathy is unacceptable.

A body of evidence suggests that the first and third types of exchange transfusions described are beneficial; no such supportive data exist for the second indication. In any event, as the accurate measurement of bilirubin is fraught with problems, any assessment of the rate of rise should be based on several bilirubin determinations, not just two.

The exchange transfusion is conducted under the same clean/sterile conditions as for the insertion of umbilical catheters. For all infants, approximately twice the calculated blood volume (80 to 100 ml per kg) is projected to exchange about 85 per cent of circulating blood. When the removal of bilirubin (especially at high levels) is the object, then "priming" the patient with 1 gram per kg of 25 per cent salt-poor albumin will help scavenge tissue-bound bilirubin into the

TABLE 4. **Recommendations for Rh Immune**
Globulin (RhoGAM)

Status	Action
Every Rh-negative unimmunized woman with:	
Rh-positive baby delivered	240–300 μg
Abortion*	50 μg
Amniocentesis*	240–300 μg
28 wk completed gestation*	240–300 μg
Massive transplacental hemorrhage (known Rh-positive fetus)	240–300 μg/25 ml estimated bleed
Every Rh-negative, weakly immunized† pregnant woman with Rh-positive baby delivered (Rh antibody by Autoanalyzer only)	240–300 μg

*Unless father is known to be Rh negative.
†May not be effective.

circulation if given 30 minutes to 1 hour prior to the exchange. When a longer time elapses, the effect may not be as good, as the albumin will rapidly re-equilibrate to the extravascular space. When cardiorespiratory status is precarious, the potential for decompensation with a rapid volume expansion may argue against this practice. For infants with HDN weighing 2500 grams or more at birth, any with a bilirubin level of 20 mg/dl or more (or $\geq$ 15 mg/dl if over 72 hours) should be undergo exchange transfusion. For those under 2500 grams, the birth weight in 100-gram increments may serve as a guide (e.g., 15 mg/dl at 1500 grams). Sepsis, hypoxia, and acidemia require exchange at lower levels, but good guidelines are lacking. In infants weighing more than 1500 grams, exchange transfusion utilizing specially designed kits, catheters, and stopcocks can be accomplished via a single umbilical vein catheter, alternatively removing and infusing blood. Because this causes rapid fluctuations in blood volume and pressure, for infants weighing less than 1500 grams simultaneous infusion and withdrawal from two sites (so-called isovolemic transfusion) may be less traumatic when the risk of pressure-dependent hemorrhage (intracranial) is of real concern. The current relatively infrequent need for exchange transfusions suggests referral of the patient to units and/or physicians familiar with the technique.

Phototherapy with blue or white lamps producing 6 to 13 microwatts per cm^2 from irradiance at 420 to 480 nm bandpass is effective in producing photoproducts more rapidly excreted than native bilirubin. However, in the face of severe hemolysis, the impact on serum bilirubin may not be easily discernible. Here, phototherapy is an *adjunctive* therapy only.

Not only the irradiance per area just noted is important but also the total area of bilirubin-rich skin exposed. Thus the infant should have a *minimally* sized diaper to shield gonads and collect excreta. Periodically "rolling" the infant to expose new skin to the lamps is helpful.

In mild cases, phototherapy alone may be sufficient. Complications of the treatment include increased insensible water loss and dehydration, loose stools, photosensitized rash, and tanning. In order to prevent retinal damage, some type of eye patch is used. These are occasionally dislodged, with the potentially severe complications of airway occlusion (nares) or corneal abrasion. When used in severe cases, phototherapy may produce the bronzed baby syndrome, resulting from the complex photodegradation of bilirubin in the presence of the cholestasis caused by hepatic extramedullary hematopoiesis and hepatocellular damage.

Even if the disease is mild with respect to hyperbilirubinemia, hemolysis may be brisk. Moreover, in severe cases, exchange transfusions may mask the underlying destruction of erythrocytes and erythrocyte precursors outside the circulation. Consequently, late anemia may result at 4 to 6 weeks of age. Sequential assessment is necessary to decide on the need for simple transfusion. Hematocrits may fall below 20 ml/dl, and treatment should largely be based on symptoms. The earliest is generally poor feeding, followed by resting tachypnea and tachycardia and diaphoresis.

HEMOPHILIA AND VON WILLEBRAND'S DISEASE

method of
CRAIG S. KITCHENS, M.D.
VA Medical Center
Gainesville, Florida

Patients with heritable disorders of coagulation may present as "free bleeders," a term sensitive enough to include most persons with von Willebrand's disease or a deficiency of one of the plasma coagulation proteins but not specific enough for modern medicine. Current therapy of these disorders is based on the establishment of a precise diagnosis that dictates the specific therapy in specific clinical conditions for a specific patient. In addition, as these disorders are heritable, the correct diagnosis assists the care of the patient throughout life and confirms or denies that diagnosis in his or her kindred.

Precise diagnosis depends in part on evidence garnered by the history and physical examination but is confirmed by specific laboratory tests. The history and physical examination justify the practitioner's decision as to which patients should be subjected to further laboratory testing. This chapter is limited to a discussion of von Willebrand's disease and a congenital deficiency of Factor VIII (hemophilia A), Factor IX (hemophilia B), or Factor XI (hemophilia C) (Table 1). Congenital deficiencies of Factor I (fibrinogen), Factor II (prothrombin), Factors V, VII, X, XII, and XIII, and acquired deficiency of any factor, although each just as precise a diagnosis with its specific therapy, are beyond the scope of this review.

Clinical suspicion is key in leading the primary care physician to the correct diagnosis. Table 2 gives clues as to which patients and their clinical manifestations should cause suspicion. Hemorrhagic events are clearly linked to the degree of deficiency in persons lacking Factors VIII or IX. Ironically, the *lack* of hemorrhagic manifestations, absence of joint destruction, and a seemingly negative family history in the milder forms of hemophilia may prove to be dangerous because of the occult nature of this disorder. Lack of clinical

TABLE 1. **Characteristics of Hemophilia and von Willebrand's Disease**

Disorder	Degree	Activity of Factor* (%)	Prolonged PTT	Prolonged BT	Genetics	Comments
Factor VIII deficiency	Severe	<1	Always	No	Sex-linked	Lifelong, obvious disease
	Moderate	1–5	Usually	No	Sex-linked	Bleeding and hemarthrosis with trauma
	Mild	5–25	Usually	No	Sex-linked	Bleeding usually only with trauma or surgery; disease process often occult
Factor IX deficiency	Severe	<1	Always	No	Sex-linked	Lifelong, obvious disease
	Moderate	1–5	Usually	No	Sex-linked	Bleeding and hemarthrosis with trauma
	Mild	5–25	Usually	No	Sex-linked	Bleeding usually only with trauma or surgery; disease process often occult
Factor XI deficiency		1–50	Usually	No	Autosomal	Highly variable; often precipitated by surgery or aspirin administration
von Willebrand's disease, common variety (Type I)		30–70	Occasionally	Usually	Autosomal	Mucocutaneous bleeding; hemarthrosis rare

*Activity of the patient's factor compared with normal pooled plasma, which is defined as 100% activity.
Abbreviations: PTT = partial thromboplastin time; BT = bleeding time.

suspicion of an underlying heritable coagulation disorder can lead to either an operation, with resultant massive postoperative hemorrhage, or, in an actively hemorrhaging patient, the failure to consider such a diagnosis. Indeed, in my professional experience, fatal or serious hemorrhage is more common in mild forms than in severe forms. The patient, family, and practitioner are aware of the hemorrhagic potential of the severe types; that of the milder types is rarely suspected. In addition, it appears that the combined frequency of all the milder forms is about the same as that of the severe types, namely, approximately 1:10,000. Factor levels in Factor VIII deficiency and Factor IX deficiency are constant (within the degree of

TABLE 2. **Clinical Manifestations Helpful for Diagnosis of Hemophilia and von Willebrand's Disease**

Manifestations of Severe Deficiency of Either Factor VIII or Factor IX

Positive family history 75% of the time; spontaneous mutation in 25%
Diagnosis established by age 2 years
Spontaneous hemarthroses: knee, elbow, ankle, wrist, shoulder, hip
Destruction of these joints, resulting in limp or other dysfunction
Family history of bleeding in a sex-linked pattern (e.g., maternal uncles, maternal grandfathers, and male siblings)
Extensive medical history and frequent emergency room visits
Frequent soft tissue hemorrhage; bleeding after circumcision
Extensive bleeding after trauma or surgery

Manifestations of Moderate Deficiency of Either Factor VIII or Factor IX

Family history typically negative, except under close scrutiny
Diagnosis may be delayed until second or third decade
Hemarthrosis rare and usually occurs only with trauma; joint deformity rare
Soft tissue hemorrhage frequent
Postoperative bleeding severe; frequently delayed 24–72 hr
Bleeding after dental extractions

Manifestations of Mild Deficiency of Either Factor VIII or Factor IX

Family history typically appears negative; disease occult
Diagnosis may be made at any age
Joint disease and joint deformity rare
Hemorrhage after trauma or surgery, usually delayed 24–72 hr
Bleeding after dental extractions, particularly if aspirin prescribed

Manifestations of Factor XI Deficiency

50% of patients are of European Jewish extraction
Family history may be positive in an autosomal dominant fashion
Diagnosis may be made at any age
Hemorrhage often follows surgery, dental extractions, or trauma; often precipitated by aspirin administration

Manifestations of von Willebrand's Disease (Type I)

Family history usually positive in autosomal dominant fashion (e.g., equal number of males and females and no skipped generations)
Diagnosis may be made at any age
Frequent childhood epistaxis
Bleeding after dental extractions, particularly if aspirin is prescribed
Bleeding after shaving and with minor cuts and abrasions
Serious or fatal bleeding unusual

laboratory variability), both in an individual patient over time and in his or her kindred. Accurate diagnosis and all the events that hinge on it depend on the primary care physician's suspicion and confirmation of the diagnosis.

Although the severity of symptoms and the degree of deficiency of either Factor VIII or Factor IX correlate well, such is not the case in Factor XI deficiency. A patient experiencing a slight hemorrhage may have 1 per cent of normal Factor XI levels, whereas another patient having a major postoperative hemorrhage may have 20 per cent of normal activity.

Attempts to correlate clinical manifestations with laboratory parameters in von Willebrand's disease are even more surely doomed to failure. I expect and prepare for the worst in an attempt to deal with this fact. With the exception of those rare patients with homozygous von Willebrand's disease (Type III, Factor VIII levels, and von Willebrand's factor levels 0 to 3 per cent of normal and having very long bleeding times; see Table 3), there is no correlation between hemorrhagic manifestations and laboratory findings. In fact, the consistency of these test results over time in an individual with von Willebrand's disease is poor. Any of these test results may change, even though the hemorrhagic potential may not. The consistency among family members is even poorer. Accordingly, there is no laboratory test or tests that are pathognomonic for either the presence or absence of von Willebrand's disease.

Factor VIII serves as a cofactor and Factor IX serves as an enzyme in the coagulation cascade. Deficiency of either results in slow and defective generation of thrombin and, hence, impaired hemostasis. The greater the deficiency, the more severely impaired is coagulation, which can be manifested clinically by hemorrhage and, in the laboratory, by a prolonged partial thromboplastin time (PTT). However, because the PTT is not extremely sensitive to levels of either Factor VIII or Factor IX, and because reagents used in the PTT vary in their ability to detect a partial deficiency of either of these factors, the PTT should *not* be depended on to exclude hemophilia as a diagnostic possibility: A nor-

mal PTT does not exclude mild hemophilia A or B. In addition, the PTT cannot be relied on to follow therapeutic replacement levels of these factors. Rather, specific measurement of plasma levels of these factors is in order for both diagnostic and therapeutic purposes.

TREATMENT

Treatment principles are based on the fact that if bleeding is caused by the deficiency of a given coagulation factor, replacement of that factor leads to improved or even normal hemostasis. Factor replacement is typically achieved by infusion of plasma products, either cryoprecipitate or Factor VIII concentrate in Factor VIII deficiency; Factor IX concentrate in Factor IX deficiency; fresh-frozen plasma (FFP) in Factor XI deficiency; and cryoprecipitate in von Willebrand's disease. A new product not derived from blood or blood products, 1-deamino-8-D-arginine vasopressin (DDAVP) (Stimate), a vasopressin analogue, is probably the agent of choice in the common type (Type I) of von Willebrand's disease and mild Factor VIII deficiency; it is not efficacious in Type II or Type III von Willebrand's disease, in severe deficiency of Factor VIII, or in deficiency of either Factor IX or Factor XI.

The *degree of factor replacement* is dictated by the seriousness of the clinical situation. One may not wish to replace totally (i.e., to 100 per cent level of activity) the deficient factor because (1) excessive factor is no more hemostatic than sufficient factor, (2) the cost is excessive, and (3) these products are limited worldwide so their use must be distributed among all patients.

A unit of Factor VIII, IX, or XI is defined as the amount of that factor in 1 ml of normal human plasma. In clinical medicine, I assume

TABLE 3. **Types of von Willebrand's Disease**

Type	Abnormality	Occurrence	Factor VIIIc*	Factor VIII$_{RAg}$†	Bleeding Time	Multimeric Analysis of Factor VIII
I	Heterozygous deficiency of Factor VIII molecule	Common	30–70%	30–70%	6–20 min	Normal distribution
II	Heterozygous abnormality of Factor VIII molecule	Rare	70–150%	70–150%	>20 min	Absence of high-molecular-weight forms
III	Homozygous deficiency of Factor VIII molecule	Rare	<3%	<3%	>20 min	Absence of all forms

*Factor VIIIc refers to that part of the Factor VIII molecule involved in blood coagulation.

†Factor VIII$_{RAg}$ (also known as von Willebrand's factor) refers to the part of the Factor VIII molecule measured by immunologic methods.

that an adult patient has a plasma volume of 3000 ml. If the baseline level of Factor VIII is 0 per cent, infusion of 1500 units of Factor VIII should result in an initial therapeutic level of 50 per cent, whereas infusion of 3000 units would increase the Factor VIII level from 0 per cent to 100 per cent. Because the volume of distribution of Factor VIII appears to be the plasma volume, calculation (which is actually an estimate) of the amount of Factor VIII to be infused is simple. The volume of distribution for Factor IX behaves more like twice the plasma volume, so roughly twice as much Factor IX is needed to achieve a desired level. For instance, 3000 units of Factor IX infused into a patient with 0 per cent Factor IX results in a therapeutic plasma level closer to 50 per cent than to 100 per cent. The volume of distribution of Factor XI is roughly the plasma volume.

The *frequency of infusion* is determined by the half-life of the factor. For Factor VIII, this is approximately 8 to 12 hours, and for Factor IX it is 12 to 24 hours. For Factor XI, the half-life is 60 to 80 hours, long enough that it allows Factor XI levels to accumulate from therapeutically infused FFP. This is fortunate because FFP is the only therapeutic source of Factor XI. Aggressive treatment with FFP is more cumbersome than the infusion of concentrates that are available for replacement of either Factor VIII or Factor IX.

The *duration of infusion* is difficult to determine with certainty. For some events, such as early treatment of a simple hemarthrosis, a single infusion suffices. In contrast, infusion may be needed for 10 to 14 days after a complicated surgical procedure.

Infusion of DDAVP typically doubles or triples the native Factor VIII level in patients with moderate hemophilia; for instance, the Factor VIII level can be raised from 8 per cent to approximately 20 per cent after such infusion. If such levels are thought to be sufficient for the clinical situation, the use of DDAVP is strongly encouraged. DDAVP is administered intravenously, at a dose of 0.3 microgram per kg in 50 ml of saline over 30 minutes every 12 to 24 hours.

These therapeutic guidelines are just that; factor levels, both peak and trough, must be determined by precise factor assay. Based on the results, the dosage, frequency, and duration of therapy can be monitored and modified accordingly.

Therapeutic decisions are less clearly made in von Willebrand's disease, as there is no good correlation between clinical bleeding and either Factor VIII levels or bleeding times, although both usually improve after successful therapy.

Most authorities agree that Factor VIII concentrate, although highly effective in hemophilia A, is not effective in von Willebrand's disease. Cryoprecipitate is thought to be the superior source of von Willebrand's factor, the absence of which is probably more important than the modest degree of Factor VIII clotting activity seen in the common type (I) of von Willebrand's disease. Usually 5 to 10 bags (1 bag being defined as the cryoprecipitate prepared from 1 unit [300 ml] of FFP) of cryoprecipitate are administered every 8 to 12 hours. DDAVP is efficacious and safe to use in Type I von Willebrand's disease. It is administered as previously described.

Although patients with heritable disorders of coagulation are at risk for bleeding in almost any conceivable fashion, place, or time, certain hemorrhagic events are characteristic of these disorders. These will be addressed separately.

Hemarthrosis

Bleeding into joint spaces is characteristic of severe classic deficiency of either Factor VIII or Factor IX. It is the most common hemorrhagic event in hemophiliacs. When it occurs spontaneously (or with trauma so minimal that it is not recalled by the patient), deficiency of the factor is usually total. Hemarthrosis is extremely rare in von Willebrand's disease and Factor XI deficiency. The joints most commonly involved include (in descending order) the knee, elbow, ankle, wrist, shoulder, and hip. Other joints bleed far less often. In my experience, ankle bleeds can be almost totally eliminated by the use of boots. Repeated bouts of either untreated or undertreated hemarthroses lead to the joint destruction (hemarthropathy) characteristic of severe hemophilia. Individuals with moderate and mild hemophilia bleed in the joints only after trauma or overusage, such as with jumping or falls.

Because joint bleeds are common, patients become knowledgeable about their nature. They initially perceive bleeding in the joint by a peculiar warm, tingling sensation rather than pain. It is axiomatic that early bleeds can be treated more easily than established bleeds. Accordingly, patients who direct their own care often promptly infuse themselves with factor at home, at the job site, or even in school to stop the joint bleed and to alleviate the progression of pain. This can be done so rapidly and easily that little productive time is lost. Patients have taught me how little factor may be required for hemostasis. If their bleeds are treated promptly, some patients can control a hemarthrosis with as little as 300 to 400 units of factor, which raises their plasma factor level to only 10 per cent. Such infusion obviously is not only less expensive for the patient, society, or both but also makes good medical sense. Factor replacement is the mainstay of therapy for joint bleeds. Splints, joint aspiration, and casts have no place in the modern treatment of acute hemarthrosis. With proper training, the patient can treat the vast majority of hemarthroses without consultation with the physician. The frequency of hemarthrosis varies enormously even within a given patient. Some patients experience spontaneous hemarthrosis twice a week for months for some time and then experience it once every month or so. The reason for this disparity in frequency is unknown.

Most joint bleeds respond to a single infusion of factor sufficient to raise the level to 10 to 20 per cent. The notable exception is hemarthrosis of the hip joint, which is rather rare but does require several days of aggressive replacement therapy.

Chronic joint bleeds lead to joint destruction. Definitive surgical management of chronic hemarthropathy is outside the scope of this review. Occasionally, rather than having a random distribution of joint bleeds, a patient may experience repeated bleeds in a single joint. Synovium in the affected joint may become extremely hypertrophic, inflamed, and boggy. In addition, because of the hypervascularity of the synovium, the bleed may become more frequent, perpetuating a vicious cycle. These joints often respond favorably to surgical synovectomy.

Soft Tissue Bleeds

These bleeds are the second most common bleeding manifestation and, again, are limited generally to hemophiliacs rather than affecting patients with von Willebrand's disease. Key to the management of soft tissue bleeds is recognition of potential damage from the bleed. For instance, an abdominal or chest wall bleed may be spectacular but is not dangerous to the patient. By contrast, a much smaller bleed in the neck could compromise the airway. Soft tissue bleeds are often initiated by trauma but can be spontaneous. Bleeding often occurs between fascial planes. Three types of soft tissue bleeds require special discussion. The first of these is the *retropharyngeal hematoma,* which can dissect between fascial planes in the retropharyngeal area, with resultant obstruction of the airway. This hemorrhage is rather rare but is important because of its danger. A sore throat or difficulty in breathing in a hemophiliac should raise this possibility. Replacement therapy should be aggressive, with peak levels of 100 per cent and trough levels of 50 per cent maintained for a minimum for 5 to 7

days. Prompt therapy obviates the need for surgical manipulation. The second soft tissue hemorrhage of importance is *other hemorrhages in the mouth and throat area.* These can occur in the tongue, floor of the mouth, or anterior neck. They should be treated as aggressively as retropharyngeal bleeds. The third important soft tissue bleed is the *gastrocnemius bleed,* which is extremely painful, as it dissects between the two heads of the gastrocnemius muscle into the leg as a result of the forces of gravity and pressure. Because of the pain, the patient hyperextends the ankle to shorten the length of the gastrocnemius. If this bleed is not aggressively treated, the muscle deformity becomes chronic and the patient walks on the toes of the affected leg, the classic equine gait. In my experience, the development of equine gait is often the first major orthopedic event in a downhill, domino-type progression of joint disease. Accordingly, gastrocnemius bleeds should be aggressively identified by the painful swelling of the leg and the characteristic posture that the patient assumes. I treat this bleed with peak and trough levels of 80 per cent and 40 per cent, respectively, for at least a week, during which time aggressive physical therapy is provided to allow the patient to walk with the heel flat, bearing the body's full weight.

Genitourinary Bleeding

Menometrorrhagia, and especially menorrhagia, may occur in patients with bleeding disorders. Because most hemophiliacs are males, excessive menstrual bleeding is unusual in hemophilia except in patients with severe deficiency of Factor XI. Such symptoms may be bothersome in females with von Willebrand's disease and may, in fact, be a presenting feature leading to a hemostatic diagnosis. Excessive menstrual bleeding often responds to hormonal treatment, such as with birth control pills. Pregnancy ameliorates bleeding in von Willebrand's disease, so routine delivery is rarely a hemostatic problem even without specific therapy.

Spontaneous, nontraumatic urinary bleeding of renal origin is frequently encountered in hemophiliacs and occasionally in patients with von Willebrand's disease. It is almost never associated with structural lesions such as those seen in nonhemophiliacs. Accordingly, exhaustive examinations for neoplastic growths, stones, or abscesses are rarely productive. This is one hemorrhagic episode for which epsilon-aminocaproic acid is contraindicated for fear of causing obstructive uropathy from clotted blood. If hematuria is spontaneous, it may be treated with aggressive factor replacement, although in my experience this rarely shortens the natural history of the event. Often no therapy is as effective; the bleeding stops in about 1 week.

Retroperitoneal Hemorrhage

This is a rare but classic hemorrhagic event in hemophiliacs, representing the second leading cause of hemorrhagic death. It is unusual in von Willebrand's disease. This hemorrhage should always be considered in the hemophiliac who is hypotensive and tachycardic and has mild abdominal pain. Because of the almost limitless size of the retroperitoneal area, patients can bleed to death internally before any physical findings direct the unsuspecting clinician to retroperitoneal bleeding. If the diagnosis is entertained, prompt, aggressive replacement therapy should be given, aiming for peak levels of 100 per cent. After full replacement, radiographic examination with either computed tomography or ultrasound establishes the diagnosis. Full replacement therapy for approximately 1 week is in order. Surgical exploration is not indicated.

Gastrointestinal Bleeding

In contrast to genitourinary bleeding, gastrointestinal bleeding is usually associated with a structural lesion. This bleeding is common in both hemophiliacs and patients with von Willebrand's disease. More often than not, peptic ulcer disease, neoplastic growths, or the like underlie this hemorrhagic manifestation. Replacement therapy should be given, aiming for peak levels of 50 per cent. During replacement therapy, diagnostic radiography or endoscopic procedures should be performed, as in other patients.

Epistaxis

Epistaxis is rare in hemophiliacs without trauma but is characteristic of von Willebrand's disease, particularly in the first two decades of life. Epistaxis in patients with von Willebrand's disease can be easily corrected with administration of either cryoprecipitate or DDAVP. Surgical treatment is rarely, if ever, of benefit.

Central Nervous System Bleeding

This is the rarest of the classic bleeds of hemophilia or von Willebrand's disease but is the leading cause of hemorrhagic death. It may be spontaneous but more often is associated with trauma, including that which appears trivial. At the first suspicion of an ongoing central nervous system hemorrhage, full replacement to 100 per cent factor levels is mandatory before further investigation. After full replacement, radiographic or other investigations to establish the presence or absence of central nervous system bleeding should take place. At no time should these investigations take place before the prompt replacement of 100 per cent factor levels in these patients. The clinician and patient must have a high suspicion of, appreciation of, and respect for central nervous system bleeding.

Other Special Considerations

Trauma. The hemophiliac who has sustained significant trauma should immediately receive total factor replacement. No lesion, whether a fracture or a gunshot wound, or one from an automobile accident, can improve until factor replacement has been done. After factor replacement and other acute resuscitative measures, the patient should be treated like any other trauma patient. The patient is at such high risk for bleeds from multiple sites that replacement should be done based on suspicion alone. The physician must *not* insist on waiting for hemorrhage to become so established that the physical or radiographic examination detects an advanced hemorrhage, which is then far more dangerous and resistant to therapy.

Surgery. Modern aggressive replacement therapy for hemophiliacs has enabled these patients to enjoy the full benefits of modern surgery. Far too often in the past, surgical procedures were performed on hemophiliacs too late and too emergently to achieve acceptable results. It is our belief that hemophiliacs or patients with von Willebrand's disease without an inhibitor can undergo any surgical procedure, and the decision to perform these procedures should be based on the same indications or contraindications used in other patients. Patients prepared appropriately before surgery experience no more morbidity and mortality than otherwise normal patients undergoing a similar operation. Surgical hemostasis is perfectly normal with appropriate aggressive control of the underlying disease. Recent consecutive clinical series have demonstrated no excessive morbidity and mortality in hemophiliacs undergoing the full gamut of modern surgical procedures.

Dental Procedures. These procedures can be performed in patients with hemophilia or von Willebrand's disease as simply as in other patients. Preventive dentistry and restorative work should be aggressively maintained. Usually, only minimal amounts of factor replacement are necessary, aiming for peak and trough levels of approximately 20 per cent and 10 per cent, respectively.

Some authorities have combined this low-level replacement with administration of epsilon-aminocaproic acid; I have found that this adds little more than the variability of another drug. Partial replacement therapy should be continued for 4 or 5 days after the procedure.

General Medical Care. As in any chronic condition, the maintenance of optimal health is beneficial. Accordingly, patients should receive good dental care, be kept up-to-date on immunizations, and keep themselves in trim physical condition.

Safety of Replacement Therapy. Before the availability of modern replacement therapy, the length and quality of life of the hemophiliac or patient with von Willebrand's disease were severely compromised. Some studies indicated that the average age at death in severe hemophilia was 8 years. Because surgical therapy was impossible, patients were also at risk of dying of processes that usually do not lead to death in this century, such as appendicitis or mild trauma. In the second half of this century, with the advent of better diagnostic and therapeutic resources, patients who have a heritable bleeding disorder expect a nearly normal life span. However, confounding factors have recently appeared. The first of these is the unacceptably high incidence of transfusion-associated hepatitis, mostly caused by hepatitis B and non-A, non-B hepatitis. Nearly all multiply transfused patients have a mild, persistent form of liver disease characterized by chronic, stable, but mild elevations of serum transaminase levels. The vast majority do not progress to chronic active hepatitis. About 10 per cent of these patients develop cirrhosis and hepatic failure. More recently, of course, has been the specter of acquired immunodeficiency syndrome (AIDS) associated with administration of contaminated blood product concentrates prepared approximately between 1979 and 1983. The vast majority of patients transfused with these products during that time now test positive for human immunodeficiency virus, and many will develop AIDS, with its attendant prognosis. Safer blood products are now either commercially available or being prepared. Such progress will no doubt brighten the future of hemophiliacs, as will further therapeutic developments for AIDS.

Comprehensive Care. The concept of comprehensive care for the patient with a heritable bleeding disorder has had a great positive impact on these patients and their families (Table 4). Health care providers attuned to the hemophiliac's needs are quick to offer prophylactic care and psychosocial support and have become accustomed to easing the socioeconomic burden of the disorder. For instance, health insurance or employment may pose difficulties for a hemophiliac. However, support groups, including lay organizations such as the National Hemophilia Foundation, have proved effective in combating not only the medical aspects of the disease but also its socioeconomic and psychologic impacts on the patient and the family. Health care providers should help patients with heritable bleeding disorders to make contact with such support organizations.

Inhibitors. Inhibitors directed against a factor develop in approximately 7 to 10 per cent of patients with hemophilia A and in a smaller number of those with hemophilia B. This dreaded situation makes replacement therapy with factor concentrate either impossible or extremely difficult. Appropriate therapy for this unfortunate situation is beyond the scope of this review. Most such patients should receive expert consultation for further assistance.

TABLE 4. **Impact of Comprehensive Health Care on Hemophiliacs***

Outcome Data	Before	After	% Change
Patients performing self-infusion (home care)	514	2517	+ 390
Average days/yr lost from work or school	14.5	3.9	− 73
Average hospital admission/yr	1.9	0.22	− 88
Average days/yr spent as inpatient	9.4	1.6	− 83
Percentage of unemployed adults	36	9.4	− 74

*Modified from data from the National Hemophilia Foundation.

PLATELET-MEDIATED BLEEDING DISORDERS

method of
CAROL COLA, M.D., and
JACK ANSELL, M.D.
University of Massachusetts Medical School
Worcester, Massachusetts

Bleeding secondary to platelet disorders is typically mucosal. Epistaxis, gingival bleeding, hematuria, menorrhagia, and gastrointestinal bleeding are common manifestations. Petechiae and occasionally ecchymoses comprise the usual cutaneous findings. Platelet-related bleeding may result from thrombocytopenia or from qualitative platelet defects.

THROMBOCYTOPENIA

When evaluating a patient with a reduced platelet count, it is essential to categorize the mechanism of the thrombocytopenia as decreased production, increased destruction, sequestration, or dilution. Bone marrow aspiration remains the most clinically useful means of discriminating between decreased production and peripheral destruction or sequestration.

Decreased Platelet Production

Decreased platelet production may result from primary bone marrow failure such as in aplastic anemia, or thrombopoiesis may be exogenously suppressed by toxins, drugs, radiation, or sepsis. Myelophthisic processes are those characterized by replacement of normal marrow such as by metastatic tumor, fibrosis, or granulomatous disease. Acute leukemias cause thrombocytopenia as the malignant clone usurps the marrow space and abnormal stem cells lead to defective thrombopoiesis. Finally, ineffective thrombopoiesis may result from various deficiency states, such as vitamin B_{12} or folate deficiency, or from the disordered growth that is characteristic of myelodysplastic syndromes.

The management of patients with thrombocytopenia secondary to decreased platelet production should include treatment of the underlying cause and withdrawal of any possible offending agents. As in any patient with significant thrombocytopenia, antiplatelet agents and anticoagulants should be avoided. In the setting of active bleeding, platelets should be transfused to attain a level of 60,000 to 70,000 per microliter. This level is usually adequate to achieve hemostasis. If bleeding persists or if the hemorrhage is life-threatening, additional platelets can be given, but efforts should be made to identify other causes of bleeding.

The risk of spontaneous bleeding, including central nervous system bleeding, increases significantly when the platelet count falls below 50,000 and especially below 20,000 per microliter. Prophylactic platelet transfusions are generally indicated when the platelet count falls below 20,000 per microliter, provided that the thrombocytopenia is caused by decreased production.

Random donor platelets should be transfused in a dose of 1 unit per 10 kg of body weight. The platelet count should be repeated 24 hours after transfusion to assess the response and to determine whether further transfusions are necessary. If an adequate response is not achieved, the platelet count should be checked 1 hour after the next transfusion. Failure to demonstrate an increase in the platelet count 1 hour after transfusion suggests destruction of transfused platelets secondary to alloimmunization. This occurs in approximately 30 to 50 per cent of patients re-

quiring long-term platelet support. The use of single-donor platelets decreases exposure to alloantigens. Once alloimmunization has occurred, the use of human leukocyte antigen–compatible platelets may provide a response to the transfusion. If this fails, however, patients are considered platelet refractory, and further platelet transfusions are reserved for the setting of active bleeding.

The parameters cited here are intended to serve as general guidelines. Because of the problem of alloimmunization, prophylactic platelet transfusions are not performed in certain situations. For example, persistently thrombocytopenic patients with terminal illnesses managed only with supportive care may have platelet transfusions reserved for the treatment of bleeding.

Increased Platelet Destruction

Immune Thrombocytopenic Purpura

In contrast to the disorders cited earlier, a number of conditions exist in which thrombocytopenia is caused by increased platelet destruction. Such destruction may result from either an immunologic or a nonimmunologic cause. Immune thrombocytopenia is often idiopathic or may be associated with a variety of other disorders. Idiopathic or immune thrombocytopenic purpura (ITP) can be acute or chronic. The former occurs typically in childhood, and the latter occurs in adulthood (Table 1). Chronic ITP is characterized by the insidious onset of mucocutaneous hemorrhage. It is most commonly seen in young women. The platelet count typically falls between 20,000 to 100,000 per microliter, although lower counts may be seen. Splenomegaly is unusual in ITP. Its presence should heighten the suspicion that another disorder exists. ITP may be associated with several other maladies, including systemic lupus erythematosus, lymphoproliferative disorders, sarcoidosis, and thyroid disease.

The majority of patients with ITP have IgG antiplatelet antibodies. Antibody-coated platelets fall victim to the macrophages of the reticuloendothelial system. The spleen is the major source of antibody production and the primary site of platelet destruction.

Only 10 to 20 per cent of patients with chronic ITP recover spontaneously. Corticosteroid administration generally constitutes initial therapy. Prednisone is given at a dose of 1 to 1.5 mg per kg of body weight; sometimes 2 mg per kg is necessary before an adequate response is achieved. The platelet count usually begins to rise within 7 days of the beginning of treatment and peaks in 2 to 4 weeks. A corticosteroid trial should usually be given for a minimum of 3 to 4

TABLE 1. Clinical Features of the Acute and Chronic Forms of ITP

Feature	Acute (Predominating in Children)	Chronic (Predominating in Adults)
Age of onset	2–6 yr	20–40 yr
Sex predilection	None	3 females to 1 male
Presentation	Sudden	Insidious
Preceding illness	Common	Unusual
Onset of bleeding	Abrupt	Insidious
Serious bleeding	Uncommon	Uncommon
Palpable spleen	Rare	Rare
Platelet count	$<20,000/\mu l$	$20,000–80,000/\mu l$
Clinical course	2–6 wk	Months to years (fluctuating)

weeks; it should be given for 6 weeks if an inadequate but partial response is achieved in 4 weeks. When a favorable plateau has been attained, a gradual reduction of the steroid should begin. Patients who cannot maintain an adequate platelet count without continued high-dose prednisone therapy should be considered for splenectomy. After splenectomy, the platelet count quickly increases in about 80 per cent of patients. Of these, two-thirds maintain a normal count. About one-third of patients suffer a relapse within 16 months and require reinstitution of corticosteroids. In some patients who fail to achieve a sustained response to corticosteroids or who depend on high doses, observation rather than splenectomy may be considered if a reasonably safe platelet count is maintained (e.g., greater than 50,000 per microliter).

From 15 to 30 per cent of patients fail with both corticosteroid therapy and splenectomy. In these patients, a variety of other modalities may be tried. Intravenous administration of gamma globulin at a dose of 400 mg per kg of body weight produces a rise in platelet count at least in part by competitively blocking the Fc receptors of splenic macrophages. Daily infusions over 3 to 5 days may be necessary to achieve a response. The duration of the response is variable, sometimes lasting for 2 to 3 weeks. This treatment may be used to raise the platelet count acutely in preparation for surgery or similar invasive procedures. Danazol, a synthetic androgen, also has demonstrated efficacy in the management of refractory ITP.* The initial dose is 400 to 800 mg per day in two divided doses. About 50 per cent of patients respond, with an improvement in platelet count occurring in 1 to 3 weeks. Within 1 to 3 months, most patients exhibit a decrease in antiplatelet antibody level, reflecting the androgen's ability to suppress antibody formation. Danazol acts synergistically with steroids. Responses can usually be maintained as long as an

adequate dosage is continued. Danazol may not be as well tolerated by women as by men because of its mild androgenic effects.

Plasmapheresis may be used to lower antibody levels, but very few patients with chronic ITP respond to this maneuver; in addition, the response is limited to 1 to 3 weeks. Antineoplastic drugs have also been used in the treatment of ITP. Vincristine and vinblastine can both increase the platelet count within 1 to 2 weeks. However, responses are usually transient, and maintenance therapy is limited by cumulative neurotoxicity.

ITP patients with active bleeding present a special challenge. Platelets should be transfused without delay, but autoantibodies limit the usefulness of transfusional support. Concurrent gamma globulin infusion or vigorous plasmapheresis may be efficacious in slowing the consumption of transfused platelets. If hemostasis is not readily achieved, emergency splenectomy should be considered.

The acute form of ITP, primarily a disease of children, can also be seen in adults. It is characterized by the abrupt development of thrombocytopenia, often preceded by a viral illness 1 to 3 weeks earlier. Unlike chronic ITP, acute ITP typically resolves spontaneously within the first 6 months and often within the first 2 months. As in chronic ITP, corticosteroids constitute the initial therapy, although many children are simply observed. Prednisone is begun at a dose of 2 mg per kg of body weight. It is quickly tapered once the platelet count exceeds 20,000 per microliter. Patients with serious bleeding are again managed with platelet transfusions administered concurrently with gamma globulin. Occasionally, life-threatening hemorrhage develops, necessitating emergency splenectomy. However, in acute ITP, dangerously low platelet counts seldom persist longer than 1 to 2 weeks, regardless of therapy.

Acquired Immune Deficiency Syndrome and ITP

There is a syndrome of ITP associated with human immunodeficiency virus (HIV). Clinically,

---

*Danazol is an approved drug but this use is not listed by the manufacturer.

this syndrome is indistinguishable from classic chronic ITP. It is characterized by increased megakaryocytes in the bone marrow, peripheral destruction of antibody-coated platelets, negative antinuclear antibodies, and a positive response to corticosteroids, splenectomy, or both. The syndrome can be seen in HIV-positive individuals with or without clinical acquired immune deficiency syndrome (AIDS). Furthermore, the development of ITP in an asymptomatic, HIV-positive individual does not portend more rapid progression to AIDS. The etiology of HIV-associated ITP is not yet clearly established, but evidence suggests that immune complexes are responsible for the platelet destruction.

The treatment of HIV-associated ITP is similar to the standard treatment for classic ITP. At present, there is insufficient evidence to determine whether immunosuppressive measures such as the administration of corticosteroids or the performance of splenectomy accelerates the progression of HIV infection to AIDS. Prednisone therapy has been complicated by the development of oral candidiasis and the activation of latent herpes simplex virus infection. Given these results, some physicians administer corticosteroids at considerably lower doses than those used in classic ITP, starting with 30 to 40 mg of prednisone per day and quickly tapering to 10 to 15 mg per day. Others avoid corticosteroids entirely and advocate the use of alternative therapeutic modalities such as danazol or high-dose gamma globulin. The most appropriate initial form of management remains to be determined.

Drug-Induced Thrombocytopenia

Drug-induced thrombocytopenia may be the result of myelosuppression or increased platelet destruction. The latter mechanism is immune mediated. In the prototypic situation, the drug interacts with a plasma protein, forming a hapten-antigen complex that elicits an antibody response; the resulting immune complex innocently binds to the platelet membrane, resulting in its selective destruction. Alternatively, the antibody may interact with the drug bound to a platelet-associated antigen. The antibody-coated platelets then fall victim to complement-mediated lysis or may be ingested by splenic macrophages.

Numerous agents have been implicated in drug-induced immune thrombocytopenia. The most common culprits are quinidine, quinine (including tonic water), gold salts, sulfonamides and their derivatives, and heparin. Although exposure to a new medication may elicit this response within several days, one cannot exonerate a medication that has been taken for years. A careful history should, however, reveal ingestion of the causative agent within 24 hours of the onset of symptoms.

Although ecchymoses and petechiae are the initial manifestations, the clinical course may quickly progress to generalized purpura and fulminant hemorrhage. Any patient presenting with unexplained, significant thrombocytopenia should have all medications withdrawn, if possible. Once the offending drug is cleared from the system, bleeding abates as the thrombocytopenia gradually resolves. Recovery of a normal platelet count may take 10 to 14 days.

Drug-induced thrombocytopenia is typically associated with increased platelet-associated IgG. Although the diagnosis is usually made clinically by excluding other causes of thrombocytopenia, and by removing the offending drug and observing the platelet count rise, confirmatory in vitro tests may be performed. These tests entail incubating normal platelets with patient serum in the presence and in the absence of the implicated drug, and then assessing the antibody binding.

Heparin-Induced Thrombocytopenia

Heparin-induced thrombocytopenia causes special problems and merits additional mention. Not uncommonly, a mild decrease in the platelet count may be seen 2 to 5 days after heparin therapy begins. This is a nonimmunologic and transient effect. However, a far more severe reaction may be caused by heparin-induced antibodies that appear 6 to 14 days after heparin therapy begins. The antibodies appear to be directed against heparin-platelet complexes. In this situation, however, the interaction between antibodies and drug-platelet complexes may lead to in vivo platelet aggregation and may result in major arterial thromboses in addition to thrombocytopenia. Therefore, when immune-mediated, heparin-induced thrombocytopenia is suspected, all heparin administration, including low-dose subcutaneous heparin and intravenous line flushes, must immediately be stopped. Platelet transfusions are relatively contraindicated because they may precipitate thrombosis. The diagnosis can sometimes be confirmed by performing platelet aggregation studies on normal platelets incubated with patient serum in the presence or absence of heparin. Once heparin has been withdrawn, the thrombocytopenia gradually resolves over the course of several days. If an alternative form of anticoagulation is required, various options may be considered. Warfarin can be started, but it does not provide effective anticoagulation for the first few days. When an immediate effect is desired, the antiplatelet agent dextran may be administered intravenously. Finally, low-molecular-weight heparin, the subject of ongoing clinical trials, may be considered. Standard heparin is composed of a heterogeneous mixture of polysaccharide molecules of varying molecular weights. The low-molecular-weight forms have been shown to interact less with platelets while retaining their anticoagulant activity. Low-molecular-weight heparin has been used successfully in some patients but not in others with heparin-induced thrombocytopenia. Once a diagnosis of heparin-induced thrombocytopenia has been established, the patient must not be rechallenged with standard heparin in the future because even trace amounts of the drug may lead to thrombocytopenia and recurrence of arterial thrombosis.

Post-Transfusion Purpura

Post-transfusion purpura is another form of immune-mediated thrombocytopenia. This syndrome is characterized by fulminant thrombocytopenic purpura with an onset 5 to 12 days after transfusion of blood to a patient with a history of transfusions or prior pregnancies. The platelet count abruptly falls to less than 10,000 per microliter; the risk of life-threatening hemorrhage is high. In most cases, the patient's own platelets lack the Pl^{A1} antigen, a component of platelet membrane glycoprotein IIIa, which is present in 97 per cent of the general population. The pathophysiology of this syndrome is poorly understood, but evidence suggests that transfusion exposure of a Pl^{A1}-negative recipient to a Pl^{A1}-positive donor leads to massive destruction of the patient's own Pl^{A1}-negative platelets. The presumption is that, at an earlier time, these patients had produced complement-activating antibody directed against this antigen as a result of either paternal Pl^{A1} antigens, fetal Pl^{A1}-positive platelets that entered the maternal circulation, or Pl^{A1} alloantigens from a prior transfusion. Then, during storage of donor blood to be transfused, some of the Pl^{A1} antigens are eluted from the platelets to the plasma. During the subsequent transfusion, these free antigens may bind to the patient's Pl^{A1}-negative platelets and lead to platelet destruction by the preformed Pl^{A1} antibody.

Anti-Pl^{A1} antibodies are readily detectable in patient serum. The treatment of choice for this catastrophic syndrome is plasma exchange. One to four exchanges, with removal of 5 to 10 units of plasma each, are usually required. If apheresis is not immediately available, intravenous gamma globulin may be used as a temporizing measure. Corticosteroids have not been shown to be effective.

When a recently transfused patient presents with unexplained thrombocytopenia and active bleeding, emergency transfusion with fresh Pl^{A1}-positive blood should be done to stabilize the patient while the diagnosis is established. Transfusion reactions are frequent, and the first unit should be given slowly under observation for signs of anaphylaxis. Transfusion of platelets from Pl^{A1}-negative donors is ineffective.

The possibility of recurrence with a vigorous anamnestic response years later exists. For this reason, future transfusions should be restricted to blood from Pl^{A1}-negative donors, preferably from siblings or other human leukocyte antigen–compatible individuals, or, if possible, autologous donation.

Thrombotic Thrombocytopenic Purpura

Thrombotic thrombocytopenic purpura (TTP) is a nonimmune disorder that results in thrombocytopenia. The syndrome is composed of microangiopathic hemolytic anemia, consumptive thrombocytopenia, fluctuating neurologic manifestations, fever, and renal insufficiency. The pathologic findings are widespread hyaline thrombi in the microvasculature. TTP may be triggered by an infectious process, pregnancy, a connective tissue disorder, a malignancy, or certain drugs, including mitomycin, oral contraceptives, and cyclosporine. However, 90 per cent of these cases are idiopathic. The clinical course may be acute, chronic, or relapsing. Rarely, TTP may occur as a familial disorder.

The hemolytic anemia and thrombocytopenia are severe. Median platelet counts range from 8000 to 40,000 per microliter. Examination of the peripheral blood smear reveals schistocytes, reticulocytes, and occasional nucleated red blood cells.

The preferred treatment is plasma exchange, using fresh frozen plasma as the replacement solution. Response rates are between 70 and 90 per cent. The response to therapy is best monitored by following the patient's clinical condition, platelet count, and serum lactate dehydrogenase level, values of which indicate the adequacy of plasmapheresis. If the major manifestations are thrombotic rather than hemorrhagic, antiplatelet agents are given adjunctively. In refractory cases, other modalities that have yielded some success include splenectomy combined with antiplatelet agents and high-dose corticosteroids, azathioprine combined with prednisone, and weekly intravenous vincristine.

Disseminated Intravascular Coagulation

Disseminated intravascular coagulation (DIC) is another example of a nonimmune process that leads to consumptive thrombocytopenia. This topic is addressed in a separate chapter. Management entails treatment of the underlying cause, as well as supportive measures that may include transfusion of fresh-frozen plasma, cryoprecipitate, and platelets.

Thrombocytopenia Associated with Infection

Thrombocytopenia associated with infection may be multifactorial. As noted earlier, an element of myelosuppression may be present. Additionally, sepsis may trigger DIC, leading to consumptive thrombocytopenia. Sepsis without DIC may also lead to platelet destruction. Circulating immune complexes may bind to platelets and promote their destruction. Alternatively, platelets may be cleared from the circulation by interacting with endothelial surfaces damaged by the infectious process. Septicemic patients are particularly prone to develop thrombocytopenia. More than two-thirds have platelet counts of less than 150,000 per microliter; one-third have counts of less than 50,000, regardless of whether or not DIC coexists. Therapy primarily entails treatment of the underlying infection. Platelet transfusions may be necessary if bleeding ensues or if the thrombocytopenia is sufficiently profound to put the patient at risk for life-threatening hemorrhage. It is prudent to assume that the survival of the transfused platelets is also curtailed by the septic process.

Hypersplenism

Another cause of thrombocytopenia is splenic sequestration, or hypersplenism. In a normal individual, approximately 30 per cent of the total platelet population traverses the spleen at a given instant. This platelet pool serves as a reservoir. Under adrenergic stress, these platelets are expelled into the circulation and produce a transient thrombocytosis. In a patient with splenomegaly, platelet sequestration is increased. Typically, the platelet count falls to 50,000 to 100,000 per microliter. However, virtually the entire pool of sequestered platelets can be mobilized by adrenergic stimuli. Hemorrhage is unusual. If the platelet count is less than 50,000 per microliter and an invasive procedure is planned, platelets should be transfused. The usual dose is increased 1.5- to 2-fold to compensate for the portion that is sequestered.

Dilutional Thrombocytopenia

Thrombocytopenia secondary to platelet loss occurs in situations involving massive hemorrhage and blood replacement, or during extracorporeal perfusion. When brisk bleeding occurs, the replacement of lost blood with packed red blood cells devoid of viable platelets leads to thrombo-cytopenia that is proportional to the number of units transfused. Severe thrombocytopenia may be avoided by transfusing an appropriate quantity of platelets after every 10 to 12 units of packed red blood cells.

When patients undergo surgery assisted by extracorporeal perfusion, a 30 to 50 per cent reduction in the platelet count typically occurs and may persist for a few days. The etiology is presumed to be physical damage to platelets by the perfusion apparatus, leading to the formation of microaggregates that are cleared by the perfusion filters or the lungs. Platelet transfusions may be used to rapidly correct the thrombocytopenia in those patients who experience bleeding after cardiopulmonary bypass.

QUALITATIVE PLATELET DISORDERS

The disorders cited earlier are all characterized by thrombocytopenia. Alternatively, platelet-associated bleeding may ensue when platelets are adequate in number but are abnormal in quality. The qualitative defects may be congenital or acquired. They may be categorized according to the facet of platelet function that is impaired: adhesion, secretion, aggregation, or procoagulant activity.

Congenital Disorders of Platelet Function

When a breach in the normal vascular endothelium occurs, platelets stick to the subendothelium in a process called adhesion. Plasma von Willebrand's factor (VWF), a component of the Factor VIII complex, forms bridges between the platelet and subendothelial collagen. The platelet surface receptor for VWF resides in a specific membrane protein called glycoprotein Ib. Defective platelet adhesion results from a deficiency or abnormality of VWF or from a deficiency of glycoprotein Ib. The former, known as von Willebrand's disease, is discussed in detail elsewhere. The latter, known as Bernard-Soulier syndrome, is an autosomal recessive disorder characterized by unusually large platelets on smear, a normal or slightly decreased platelet count, a prolonged bleeding time, and bleeding manifestations that are variable and often severe. Platelet transfusions are indicated in the presence of bleeding or for prophylaxis before invasive procedures.

Once adhesion has occurred, the stimulated platelets begin the complex process of secretion and aggregation. It is via this process that additional platelets are recruited by products of secretion to interact with each other and form aggregates. The complexity of the platelet aggregatory process makes it susceptible to a multitude of possible derangements. Disorders of platelet secretion are referred to as thrombocytopathies. They are characterized by moderate mucosal bleeding and excessive bleeding with surgery. The bleeding time is usually prolonged, although occasionally normal, and may be strikingly prolonged after aspirin ingestion. Secretion defects may result either from a faulty secretory mechanism, as seen with disorders of prostaglandin metabolism, or from a deficiency of storage granule contents (e.g., storage pool disease). On a hereditary basis, both of these disorders are unusual, but acquired secretory defects account for the majority of drug-induced platelet defects. Platelet transfusion, again, is reserved for bleeding or for prophylaxis before an invasive procedure. Recently, desmopressin acetate has been shown to be somewhat effective in correcting the bleeding time, although its mechanism of action in this case is unclear (see the next section).

Defects in aggregation mark the next category of congenital qualitative platelet disorders. Fibrinogen molecules constitute the major interplatelet bridges in the process of aggregation. Glanzmann's thrombasthenia is a disorder marked by defective aggregation. This autosomal recessive disorder is one of the rarest congenital bleeding disorders. The thrombasthenic platelets fail to bind fibrinogen because of a deficiency of the glycoprotein IIb-IIIa complex. Thus, they fail to aggregate. A similar defect may be seen with another rare congenital disorder called afibrinogenemia because of the lack of fibrinogen for the interplatelet bridges.

Finally, platelet function is intimately associated with the coagulation cascade. Platelet granules contain several coagulation factors, and the platelet membrane provides the phospholipid surface on which a number of key coagulation enzymatic reactions proceed. Rare congenital bleeding disorders have been described in which the primary abnormality is limited to the loss of platelet procoagulant activity.

Patients with congenital qualitative platelet disorders may be managed with platelet transfusions. One should reserve this therapeutic intervention for situations involving significant hemorrhage or for prophylaxis against bleeding when an invasive procedure is planned. Platelet transfusions are not given during asymptomatic periods because of the risk of alloimmunization with repeated transfusion.

Acquired Disorders of Platelet Function

Platelet function defects may also be acquired and these probably account for the majority of qualitative defects. Categorization according to functional derangement is not as helpful in understanding the pathophysiology of acquired defects as it is in congenital disorders because several facets of platelet function are often affected at once.

Abnormal platelet function is a common complication of uremia, with the degree of dysfunction tending to parallel the progressive accumulation of metabolic products in the blood. The defect is primarily in adhesion, although decreased platelet thromboxane A_2 production and enhanced inhibitory prostaglandin production by the vascular endothelial cells may also contribute. The mainstay of therapy is dialysis to remove toxic metabolites that poison platelet function. In the presence of bleeding or in preparation for an invasive procedure, the synthetic vasopressin analogue 1-deamino-8-D-arginine vasopressin (desmopressin acetate) should be administered intravenously (0.3 microgram per kg of body weight over 30 minutes). Desmopressin acetate effects the release of high-molecular-weight forms of VWF from endothelial cells to support platelet adhesion. Its effects may be seen within 1 hour and persist for several hours. The dose may be repeated in 8 to 12 hours, but the response is less with repeated infusions, presumably because of the exhaustion of endothelial stores of VWF. Nonetheless, desmopressin acetate can be most helpful in providing transient improvement in platelet function and thereby allowing invasive procedures to be performed. The administration of cryoprecipitate is another means of improving platelet function. Its effects on the bleeding time are seen within 4 hours and may last for up to 24 hours. Again, the beneficial response may be mediated by VWF, which is a component of cryoprecipitate.

Acquired disorders of platelet secretion, such as storage pool deficiency, may develop as a complication of various autoimmune diseases including systemic lupus erythematosus, autoimmune hemolytic anemia, and chronic ITP. They may also develop transiently during cardiopulmonary bypass because of the activation of platelets and the consequent granule release that may occur in the perfusion apparatus. Patients with myelodysplastic syndromes or myeloproliferative disorders may have acquired storage pool deficiency on the basis of platelet dyspoiesis. By far the most common cause of a secretory defect is the use of drugs. Aspirin irreversibly acetylates cyclo-oxygenase, the enzyme necessary for production of prostaglandin endoperoxides and thromboxanes. Nonsteroidal anti-inflammatory agents other than aspirin may also inhibit thromboxane synthesis, but their effects are usually reversible, leading to more transient and less

TABLE 2. **Drugs That Interfere with Platelet Function**

Classification	Examples
Antibiotics	Penicillin and derivatives, nitrofurantoin, hydroxychloroquine
Antihistamines and antitussives	Diphenhydramine and others, glyceryl guaiacolate
Anti-inflammatory agents	Aspirin and other nonsteroidal anti-inflammatory agents, corticosteroids
Antithrombotic agents	Heparin, dextran
Calcium channel blocking agents	Verapamil and others
Diuretics	Furosemide
Serotonin antagonists	Reserpine, cyproheptadine
Sympathetic blocking agents	Alpha blockers (e.g., phentolamine), beta blockers (e.g., propranolol)
Tranquilizers and antipsychotic agents	Phenothiazines and derivatives, tricyclic antidepressants
Vasodilators	Sodium nitroprusside, nitroglycerin
Xanthine derivatives	Theophylline, caffeine, dipyridamole
Miscellaneous	Clofibrate, ethanol

severe functional impairment. Other drugs, including corticosteroids, dextrans, and ethanol, have also been shown to interfere with the secretory mechanism.

Drugs may also impair platelet function primarily by interfering with aggregation (Table 2). When given in high doses, the penicillins and the cephalosporins can impair aggregation, presumably by coating the platelet membranes. Blockade of platelet receptors for adenosine diphosphate and VWF has been demonstrated. The functional deficit may occur within 24 hours of the start of the therapy and generally peaks in 3 to 5 days. The effect may persist for 1 to 2 weeks after the antibiotic is discontinued.

Acquired defects in platelet aggregation may also be seen in patients with dysproteinemias. Although the mechanism is poorly characterized, the presumption is that the paraprotein interferes with reactions occurring on the platelet membrane surface. Platelet procoagulant activity is also impaired in these disorders.

Finally, platelet aggregation may be inhibited by the proteolytic products of fibrin and fibrinogen degradation. These degradation products may be increased in the setting of DIC, liver disease, or fibrinolytic therapy.

DISSEMINATED INTRAVASCULAR COAGULATION

method of
JOHN J. BYRNES, M.D.
University of Miami School of Medicine
Miami, Florida

Disseminated intravascular coagulation (DIC) is a clinicopathologic syndrome that may occur secondary to a variety of disorders. The primary disorder causes either endothelial cell injury or the release of coagulant material into the circulation. Thrombin is formed through either the intrinsic or extrinsic coagulation pathway in excess of the capacity of normal counter-regulatory activities such as antithrombin III. Excessive intravascular activation of thrombin leads to formation of fibrin, which deposits as microthrombi in the smaller vessels of the circulation. In the process, fibrinogen and Factors II, V, VIII, and XIII are consumed. Platelets are trapped in the fibrin meshwork. In addition, exposure of platelets to thrombin causes their aggregation, which contributes to thrombocytopenia. Thrombin in lesser concentrations causes secretion of platelet granules, which leads to a functional defect of platelets remaining in the circulation. Fibrinolysis occurs as plasminogen is activated to plasmin in response to intravascular fibrin deposition. Plasmin also degrades fibrinogen and Factors V, VIII, and XIII, which causes even more severe depletion of coagulation factors. Degradation products of fibrinogen and fibrin inhibit fibrin polymerization and platelet-platelet interaction, further interfering with hemostasis. Consequently, a hypocoagulable state may result from the depletion of hemostatic elements, whereas inhibitors of hemostatic mechanisms, such as fibrin degradation products, exacerbate the hemorrhagic diathesis. Conversely, a hypercoagulable state may ensue because of activated procoagulant factors in the circulation and the depletion of counter-regulatory factors such as antithrombin III and protein-C and protein-S.

The clinical presentation of DIC may be either acute and fulminant or low grade and chronic depending in large part on the initiating process. Thrombotic or hemorrhagic clinical manifestations may predominate in a given patient or both manifestations may occur simultaneously. In general, hemorrhagic problems more often complicate acute DIC, whereas chronic DIC is more frequently associated with thrombotic disorders. In acute DIC the precipitating disorder generally is flagrant and often catastrophic; common etiologies of intravascular coagulation are given in Table 1. Dysfunction of multiple organs or generalized bleeding complicates an already difficult situation. On the other hand, chronic DIC is more subtle and may be manifest long before or after the underlying disorder. Recurrent thromboses may be the clue that prompts the search for the occult cancer.

Hemorrhagic manifestations seen with DIC reflect associated trauma or breaches in skin or mucosal integrity that may be relatively minor. Organ systems

TABLE 1. **Etiologies of Intravascular Coagulation**

Disseminated

Infections
  Gram-negative sepsis
  Meningococcemia
  Rocky Mountain spotted fever
  Postsplenectomy sepsis
Hypotension-shock
  Of any etiology
Obstetric complications
  Abruptio placentae
  Amniotic fluid embolism
  Retained dead fetus
  Saline-induced abortions
Malignant disorders
  Mucin-producing adenocarcinomas, especially
    prostatic and gastric adenocarcinomas
  Promyelocytic leukemia
Injuries
  Extensive tissue damage
  Brain trauma
  Burns
  Snake bite
Metabolic disorders
  Hyperthermia
  Acidosis
Immunologic disorders
  Hemolytic transfusion reaction
  Anaphylaxis

Localized

Vascular malformations
  Giant hemangioma
  Aortic aneurysm

that are often involved are the skin, gastrointestinal tract, lungs, and brain. Continued bleeding from sites of minor trauma such as venipunctures is typically seen. As previously mentioned, hemostatic failure is due to the depletion of coagulation factors and platelets accompanied by the accumulation of inhibitors of hemostatic mechanisms.

Thrombotic manifestations of DIC can result from widespread microthrombus formation leading to impaired perfusion of multiple organs. Fulminant DIC can lead to occlusion of the terminal arterioles in the skin and thus to necrosis of digits, nose, and ears, and occasionally diffuse skin infarction (purpura fulminans). Renal dysfunction may be extreme and may result in complete renal failure. Involvement of cerebral microvessels often produces nonfocal dysfunction or seizures. Occlusions in the pulmonary microcirculation may be manifest as the respiratory distress syndrome. The clinical syndrome in cancer patients of recurrent or migratory venous thromboses, Trousseau's syndrome, is due to the hypercoagulable state resulting from chronic low-grade DIC. Frequently, nonbacterial thrombotic endocarditis is associated, which leads to systemic emboli as well.

The laboratory picture of DIC may be unmistakable or subtle. In acute DIC, the platelet count is low, 50 per cent of the time less than 50,000 per microliter; the prothrombin time (PT) and partial thromboplastin time (PTT) are prolonged; and the fibrinogen level is below normal. Fibrinogen levels may be normal if the patient initially had elevated levels because of preg-

nancy or because of a response to infection. Fibrin (and fibrinogen) degradation products are a hallmark of the disorder and can be measured by rapid and simple latex particle agglutination assays or the staphylococcal clumping test. A simple latex particle agglutination technique may also be used to detect specific cross-linked fibrin degradation products, D-dimer, which indicate fibrin clot lysis. Impaired microvascular blood flow by fibrin strands leads to fragmentation of red blood cells, and microangiopathic hemolytic anemia may ensue, especially in severe acute DIC. Characteristic schistocytes and helmet cells appear in the blood smear. Laboratory parameters such as reticulocytosis, elevated levels of bilirubin and serum lactate dehydrogenase, and depletion of haptoglobin indicate intravascular hemolysis. In chronic DIC, fibrin degradation products are present but the PT and PTT may or may not be prolonged; the PTT may actually be shorter than normal because of activated factors and depletion of antithrombin III.

TREATMENT

In all instances successful resolution of DIC depends ultimately on successful management of the initiating process. Thus, the first priority is dealing with the initiating process. It is also important that supportive measures to maintain adequate blood pressure, hemoglobin concentration, oxygenation, and acid-base and electrolyte balances are pursued to minimize organ damage consequent to the impaired microvascular perfusion. Therapeutic intervention aimed at the coagulation disorder must be considered in the full clinical context, and the risks of therapy must, as usual, be weighed against the potential benefit. If there is only laboratory evidence of DIC but no significant hemorrhage or thrombosis, specific measures other than addressing the underlying process are not required. If bleeding is the predominant clinical problem, factor replacement with fresh-frozen plasma (FFP), cryoprecipitate, and platelet transfusion should be used to replenish diminished levels. Two to four units of FFP daily is generally adequate. A platelet count of at least 50,000 per microliter should be maintained if there is significant bleeding. Cryoprecipitate may be required in severe DIC to obtain a fibrinogen level higher than 100 mg per dl. If despite these measures the bleeding continues and the initiating process persists, disrupting the actions of thrombin with heparin should be considered. A continuous infusion of 600 to 1000 units per hour is generally recommended, with subsequent empiric adjustment. If this treatment is successful, the bleeding should diminish and the platelet count and fibrinogen level should increase.

When thrombotic complications resulting in

severe organ hypoperfusion occur, anticoagulation with heparin should also be considered if the activating process cannot be terminated. In adults, a loading dose of heparin 5000 units followed by the continuous intravenous infusion of 1000 units per hour is usually given to start. Adjustment of the dose of heparin is determined by the clinical and laboratory response. Improvement in organ perfusion and a rising fibrinogen level and platelet count with diminished signs of intravascular hemolysis point to a satisfactory response. If both thrombotic and bleeding manifestations occur simultaneously, FFP and platelets should be given concomitantly with heparin treatment. FFP also serves to replenish antithrombin III and proteins-C and -S. Often, less oozing from venipunctures is also seen as platelets regain hemostatic effectiveness. It must be realized that there are no properly controlled studies demonstrating the effectiveness of heparin in DIC or studies demonstrating the optimal dosing and modification. The evidence for effectiveness is limited to case reports. Specific contraindications to the use of heparin are DIC associated with head trauma or intracerebral hemorrhage.

Several circumstances require particular mention. Acute promyelocytic leukemia is associated with the release of lysosomal granule contents from the promyelocytes into the circulation, thus activating the coagulation cascade. Cytolysis caused by treatment of the leukemia releases even more granule contents into the circulation, which causes acceleration of the DIC. It has been common practice to treat the DIC prophylactically with heparin before embarking on chemotherapy. The thrombocytopenia is due partly to the leukemia, and platelet transfusions are usually required despite control of the DIC.

Acute DIC in pregnancy is caused most often by abruptio placentae. Mild DIC is common in patients in whom abortion is induced by intra-amniotic injection of hypertonic saline; severe DIC is relatively uncommon. In most obstetric patients, management of acute DIC consists of removing the products of conception and supportive care. Transfusions are used to replace clotting factor in patients with significant bleeding. The role of heparin remains controversial, and there are no control studies. However, several reports demonstrated the effectiveness of heparin in controlling bleeding manifestations when there was an unavoidable delay in the resolution of the underlying cause.

Certain disease states are associated with the consumption of platelet and clotting factors at localized anatomic sites. These states include aortic aneurysm, large hemangiomas (Kasabach-Merritt syndrome), and certain renal disorders including hyperacute allograft rejection. The laboratory values are often compatible with disseminated consumption (DIC). The risk of not recognizing the limited nature of the disorder is that inappropriate therapy may be given for a presumed "disseminated" state. If surgery for an aortic aneurysm is to be done, stabilization of hemostasis is best obtained initially. Most patients with chronic DIC of this nature respond to treatment with heparin and factor replacement. A new approach to the treatment of surgically unresectable hemangiomas is to purposefully thrombose the vascular channels by using a fibrinolytic inhibitor.

Chronic low-grade DIC associated with venous thromboses such as in Trousseau's syndrome requires treatment with full-dose heparin, a loading dose of 5000 to 10,000 units followed by continuous intravenous infusion of 1000 to 2000 units per hour. After resolution of the venous thrombosis, 5000 units of heparin should be given subcutaneously every 8 or 12 hours to prevent recurrence; warfarin sodium (Coumadin) is not as effective in this setting.

THROMBOTIC THROMBOCYTOPENIC PURPURA AND THE HEMOLYTIC UREMIC SYNDROME

method of
JOHN J. BYRNES, M.D.
University of Miami School of Medicine
Miami, Florida

Thrombotic thrombocytopenic purpura (TTP) most often afflicts relatively young adults who are otherwise healthy. Platelets agglutinate and form microthrombi in arterioles and capillaries throughout the body. The cause of this agglutination is poorly understood; it appears that von Willebrand's factor participates in the process. Several other abnormalities of plasma factors have been described, but the pathogenetic significance of each is not clear. Endothelial injury, recanalization of the thrombi, endothelial cell proliferation, and microaneurysm formation ensue. The consumption of platelets results in thrombocytopenia, and the thrombi disrupting the microcirculation cause fragmentation of red blood cells, which gives the characteristics of microangiopathic hemolytic anemia (MAHA). Disturbance in the microcirculation of the brain is readily manifest as symptoms and clinical findings. The unpredictable distribution of lesions leads to a diversity of neurologic manifestations. Impaired perfusion of the kidneys generally results in renal dysfunction, although it is often not severe. Other organs variably manifest clinical or laboratory abnormalities early in the disease. The triad of thrombocytopenia, fragmentation hemolysis, and waxing and waning, bizarre neurologic abnormalities is highly indicative of TTP. In addition, the high incidence of renal impairment and fever at presentation has been noted. This pentad of findings has been popularized as constituting the syndrome. However, the patient with TTP may be virtually asymptomatic or may suffer from failure of virtually every organ system. Without effective treatment, the disorder is fatal because of progressive multiple organ failure or bleeding into the brain.

The outlook for patients with TTP was extremely poor until the beneficial effect of infusion of whole blood or plasma was recognized. A plasma factor, which is still poorly characterized, can neutralize abnormal platelet agglutination. A satisfactory clinical response to plasma therapy occurs in more than 70 per cent of patients. Eventually, the syndrome passes, and the plasma requirement abates. However, relapses or recurrent episodes can occur.

EVALUATION BEFORE INSTITUTING THERAPY

Alternative disorders with consumptive thrombocytopenia and MAHA may resemble TTP and should be excluded. Disseminated intravascular coagulation often has to be considered. However, the clinical setting is generally not appropriate for disseminated intravascular coagulation, and the fibrinogen level is typically normal in TTP. Furthermore, there is usually little or no evidence of coagulation factor consumption, fibrin deposition, or fibrinolysis. The prothrombin time and partial thromboplastin time are usually normal; the thrombin time, however, may be slightly prolonged. The hemolytic uremic syndrome (HUS) resembles TTP in many features but should be considered separately (see later section). The HELLP syndrome of pregnancy—*h*emolysis with schistocytes, *e*levated *l*iver enzymes, and *l*ow *p*latelets—is probably a variant of eclampsia. During the peripartum period, either HUS or the HELLP syndrome may be confused with TTP. Furthermore, there is an association of TTP with pregnancy. Severe vasculitis can resemble TTP; systemic lupus erythematosus, especially with cerebritis, can mimic TTP in many clinical features. Malignant hypertension can cause platelet consumption and fragmentation hemolysis, often with associated neurologic disturbance. Occasionally, these disorders and TTP cannot be distinguished and empiric treatment for both must be considered.

The question of a tissue biopsy often arises to establish the diagnosis more firmly. TTP must be treated promptly. Biopsies in TTP, even in fulminant disease, have a substantial percentage of false negatives. Thus, the biopsy result does not change the management; therapy should be instituted without delay.

It is important to assess the patient clinically and with laboratory measurements so that the response to therapy can be evaluated and adjustments can be made accordingly. The rapid reversibility of neurologic manifestations is often remarkable. Laboratory parameters that are especially important to follow are the platelet count, hematocrit, and the serum lactate dehydrogenase (LDH) level. The serum LDH level reflects the combined hemolysis and other tissue injury, and as such, it is an excellent guide to the patency of the microcirculation and a good indicator of disease activity. These studies should be obtained daily during the acute phase of management. Cardiovascular and renal status must be evaluated for the ability to handle the plasma volume challenge that ensues with therapy.

TREATMENT

I generally recommend an initial infusion of the equivalent of one plasma volume during 24 hours. Most patients with TTP can tolerate plasma infusion of this magnitude with an occasional pharmacologic stimulation of diuresis if a positive fluid balance develops. If the cardiac or renal function does not permit vigorous plasma infusion, arrangements for plasmapheresis must be made promptly. Treatment is preferably carried out in an intensive care setting because the central nervous, cardiac, pulmonary, and renal systems may malfunction. Strict attention to fluid balance is necessary, including daily weighing of patients; central hemodynamic pressure measurements are often required for optimal management.

Some patients have a reversal of the syndrome with the infusion of only a few units of plasma; most patients require much more. The daily dose of plasma and the duration of the requirement are separately variable. The amount of plasma necessary to control the disorder and the duration must be empirically determined for each patient. Plasma should be infused during 24 hours at a rate of 40 ml per kg daily until the patient's clinical status has stabilized, that is, that the central nervous system and other organ dysfunction has reversed, the platelet count is rising, the LDH level is approaching normal, and hemolysis is minimal. As the patient improves, the rate of plasma infusion should be gradually tapered. When the platelet count returns to normal, the plasma infusion is discontinued. Thereafter, if the platelet count falls substantially, plasma therapy must be resumed.

If the cardiac or renal status does not permit vigorous plasma infusion or if the patient does not respond to the infusion of one plasma volume daily, plasmapheresis is recommended. The effectiveness of plasma infusion often is evident within 48 hours. Plasmapheresis should be calculated to provide at least a 75 per cent plasma volume exchange. The replacement fluid is always plasma. Plasmapheresis is continued daily until the patient's clinical status has stabilized.

Occasionally, larger volume exchanges are necessary.

Some physicians advocate using plasmapheresis immediately if the patient presents with severe neurologic impairment. Partial removal of the platelet-agglutinating factor, in addition to its neutralization by plasma infusion, may be useful. A comparative trial of plasma infusion versus plasmapheresis is under way in Canada. Because plasma infusion is more available and less costly, this is an important issue to settle. If plasmapheresis is planned, plasma infusions should be instituted while arrangements for plasmapheresis are being made. Plasma infusions can be given between episodes of plasmapheresis. After a satisfactory clinical response is obtained and plasmapheresis is discontinued, plasma infusions are resumed at a rate that is tolerated by the patient and then are slowly tapered. If the patient starts to relapse, the frequency of plasma infusions should be increased. If this does not control the relapse, then plasmapheresis should be resumed.

Antiplatelet agents have been used in the treatment of TTP. In general, I do not recommend their use, especially if the patient is severely thrombocytopenic. Their effectiveness in TTP is marginal and they handicap the platelets' ability to prevent hemorrhage. Clinical experience suggests that patients with TTP are more likely to suffer bleeding complications if antiplatelet agents are used.

Corticosteroids are often used. They have an apparently beneficial effect, although this is not proved, especially when used in conjunction with other effective modalities. Because of this potentially ancillary benefit I generally give prednisone, 1 to 2 mg per kg daily or equivalent. This agent is gradually stopped when the patient is in remission.

The requirement for plasma therapy generally lasts 1 week or more but may be extended for many months in some patients. Various therapeutic modalities have been used in attempts to end the requirement. There are a number of reports of the disorder's abating after the administration of agents such as vincristine, cyclophosphamide, or azathioprine.* There are also reports of TTP's resolution after splenectomy. If the course is becoming protracted, I recommend the administration of vincristine (Oncovin) in standard dosage, 1.4 mg per M², not to exceed 2 mg final dose, be given intravenously. This treatment can be repeated weekly, with the usual precautions. I consider splenectomy in a patient who

---

*This use is not approved for vincristine, cyclophosphamide, or azathioprine by their respective manufacturers.

responds poorly to continued plasma therapy and in whom several attempts to terminate the process with vincristine administration have failed.

Some physicians may be tempted to give platelet transfusions to a severely thrombocytopenic patient, especially if surgery is being contemplated. Several instances of severe neurologic deterioration and death immediately after platelet transfusion have been recorded. I believe that platelet transfusions in TTP are extremely hazardous and of unlikely benefit.

In all patients with TTP, a search for an exacerbating inflammatory process or associated illness should be undertaken because addressing such problems may help to alleviate the disorder. Some patients have a recurrence of TTP precipitated at the time of a subsequent illness. Therefore, any patient who recovers from TTP should be closely monitored, especially during illness.

There are reports of the occurrence of TTP secondary to chemotherapy. Several patients have apparently benefited from plasma therapy, and the same therapeutic recommendations hold. However, because several reports were associated with chemotherapy regimens containing vinca alkaloid, use of these agents in TTP in this setting would not seem to be advisable.

THE HEMOLYTIC UREMIC SYNDROME

HUS is characterized by microangiopathic hemolytic anemia, thrombocytopenia, and acute renal failure. As in TTP, microvascular thrombi are responsible and von Willebrand's factor appears to participate in the platelet agglutination. In contrast with TTP, the kidneys are virtually the only organ involved, but severely so. In children the syndrome often is preceded by an episode of pneumonia or gastroenteritis. There is seasonal prevalence as well as small clusters of cases. Verotoxin produced by a strain of Escherichia coli has been implicated in HUS. In adults, HUS occurs even more sporadically. Associations with pregnancy and chemotherapy (especially that containing mitomycin) have been reported.

Treatment

Because of the resemblance of HUS to TTP, similar plasma therapy is often applied. Plasmapheresis rather than plasma infusions is generally the necessary mode of therapy because of oliguria or anuria. However, in childhood HUS plasmapheresis has been shown *not* to be better than good supportive care. A number of adults with HUS have been reported to have responded to plasmapheresis. Because HUS is a more self-limited and less life-threatening disorder than

TTP, it is difficult to draw firm conclusions about the effectiveness of therapy; most patients survive and improve as long as the complications of acute renal failure are adequately managed. I consequently recommend supportive care in childhood HUS and plasmapheresis in adult HUS if the disorder cannot be clearly differentiated from TTP or if the thrombocytopenia, which is an indicator of active thrombi formation, persists for more than 3 days. The same guidelines for plasmapheresis are used as those described for TTP; plasma infusions generally cannot be given. Regeneration of renal function, which is usually the critical issue, is more likely to be complete in children than in older adults.

HEMOCHROMATOSIS AND HEMOSIDEROSIS

method of
CORWIN Q. EDWARDS, M.D., and
JAMES P. KUSHNER, M.D.
University of Utah College of Medicine
Salt Lake City, Utah

HEMOCHROMATOSIS

Hemochromatosis is one of the most common heritable disorders in humans. It is transmitted as an autosomal recessive trait, and homozygosity for hemochromatosis occurs with a frequency of about 5 per 1000 in the caucasian population. About 10 to 13 per cent of the population are heterozygotes. The abnormal gene and its product have not been identified, but the gene is linked to the HLA-A locus on the short arm of chromosome 6. Not all homozygotes develop clinical manifestations of hemochromatosis, but usually those who do are men in the fifth decade of life or older.

Hemochromatosis results in accumulation of excessive iron in most organs. The most common symptoms are weakness, weight loss, arthralgias, right upper quadrant abdominal pain, palpitations, loss of libido or impotence, and polyuria/polydipsia. Homozygotes can be detected by routine screening blood tests of iron stores before iron-induced organ damage occurs. The most effective screening test is the transferrin saturation test (serum iron concentration divided by total iron-binding capacity). A value greater than 62 per cent, measured after an overnight fast, strongly suggests the homozygous condition.

Prolonged body iron overload causes gray or bronze hyperpigmentation of skin, liver disease, hepatomegaly, splenomegaly, arthropathy of metacarpophalangeal joints or knees, supraventricular or ventricular cardiac arrhythmias, congestive heart failure, testicular atrophy, loss of midline body hair, or loss of menses at a young age. Rarely, young hemochromatosis homozygotes develop severe endocrinopathy and life-threatening cardiac arrhythmias between ages 20 and 40, but most affected individuals are diagnosed between ages 40 and 60 years.

The diagnosis of iron overload can be made by measuring the serum iron concentration, percentage of saturation of transferrin, and serum ferritin concentration. It is advisable to perform a liver biopsy in affected individuals to document hepatic iron loading and to search for histologic evidence of fibrosis or cirrhosis. This information is important in determining the desirable rate of treatment (see the later discussion) and the prognosis. The presence of fibrosis or cirrhosis creates a lifelong risk of developing a hepatoma even if hepatic iron stores are depleted by therapy.

Treatment

The treatment of choice is rapid-sequence phlebotomy therapy. Individuals with heavy liver iron overload, signs of liver failure, life-threatening cardiac arrhythmias, or congestive heart failure should be treated by removal of 500 ml of whole blood every 3 or 4 days. This is continued until the hematocrit drops to and remains at about 32 ml per dl for 2 weeks in a row. Iron deficiency can be documented by finding very low values for the transferrin saturation and the serum ferritin concentration. Patients detected by screening tests may serve as blood donors if the liver biopsy specimen shows no evidence of hepatitis or other transmissible diseases and if they are otherwise acceptable as donors.

As a group, men with hemochromatosis have 2.5 times as much iron as affected women. Men require removal of 26 to 125 units (mean, 68 units) to induce iron-limited erythropoiesis, whereas women require removal of 8 to 42 units (mean, 25 units). After rapid-sequence phlebotomy therapy is completed, the individual enters the maintenance phase of therapy. This involves lifelong removal of 1 unit of whole blood every 2 to 6 months. If this is not performed, excess iron may reaccumulate.

The prognosis and survival of each individual correlate directly with the adequacy of phlebotomy therapy and with the presence or absence of hepatic cirrhosis and diabetes mellitus. Survival of iron-depleted individuals is five times greater than survival of those who do not undergo iron depletion therapy. Individuals who adhere to a lifelong schedule of phlebotomy therapy and who do not have cirrhosis or diabetes at the time of diagnosis have a normal life expectancy. Heart failure, liver failure, hepatomegaly, and skin pigmentation may be reversible by rapid iron depletion, but hepatic cirrhosis, arthropathy, diabetes, hypogonadism, and hypothyroidism usually do not resolve. Sometimes it is not possible to be certain if an individual is a homozygote with modest iron overload or a heterozygote with larger than usual iron stores. In such cases, it is advisable to deplete iron stores with weekly phlebotomies.

It seems reasonable to measure the serum ferritin concentration at yearly intervals during maintenance phlebotomy therapy. A rising serum ferritin concentration suggests that hepatic iron stores are increasing. In this event, phlebotomy therapy should be more frequent to maintain the ferritin concentration in the low-normal range (less than 100 ng per ml). Treatment should be given as needed for failure of other organs: liver failure, ascites, heart failure, cardiac arrhythmias, diabetes, arthritis, and hypogonadism. Some physicians prescribe folic acid, 1 mg by mouth daily, during rapid-sequence phlebotomy. Usually, however, no supplements are required.

Brothers and sisters of affected individuals are the relatives who are most likely to have hemochromatosis. They should be screened by measuring the percentage of saturation of transferrin and the serum ferritin concentration. If the results suggest the presence of hemochromatosis, liver biopsy is indicated and phlebotomy therapy should proceed as discussed earlier. Siblings with complete human leukocyte antigen identity to a proband can be assigned the homozygous genotype—even if not iron loaded at that time—but such typing is expensive. The most practical screening tests are the percentage of saturation of transferrin and the serum ferritin concentration.

HEMOSIDEROSIS

Organ iron overload (hemosiderosis) can be caused by processes other than hemochromatosis. Chronic transfusion therapy that is used to correct anemias not resulting from blood loss is the most common cause of hemosiderosis. Each unit of transfused packed red blood cells contains about 200 mg of iron, and a massive iron load can occur after 1 or 2 years of chronic transfusion therapy. The clinical and laboratory findings in patients with transfusion-induced iron overload closely resemble those in patients with hereditary hemochromatosis. Death may occur as a result of iron-related heart disease or liver failure.

It is advisable to deplete the excessive iron stores of these individuals, but phlebotomy therapy obviously is not practical. The only available effective therapy is iron chelation with deferoxamine, which is a product of *Streptomyces pilosus*. Deferoxamine is not absorbed adequately from the gastrointestinal tract and must be administered parenterally. Deferoxamine has an ex-

tremely high avidity for iron and enters cells, where it binds iron in the cellular chelatable iron pool. The deferoxamine-iron complex is then excreted in the urine and in bile.

Deferoxamine produces the greatest iron excretion when administered as a continuous intravenous infusion, but this approach is rarely practical. Continuous subcutaneous infusion of deferoxamine is nearly as effective as continuous intravenous infusion and does not require intravenous access. Intramuscular injections of deferoxamine are far less effective and are painful because of the large volume necessary. The most practical method of administering deferoxamine is a nightly 12-hour subcutaneous infusion. This method can produce 65 to 70 per cent as much iron excretion as continuous intravenous administration. The deferoxamine is administered by using an infusion pump and a pediatric scalp vein needle placed subcutaneously on the abdomen or thigh.

The amount of iron excreted varies with the dosage of deferoxamine used. A dose of 2 grams nightly is effective for most adults. Two grams of deferoxamine costs $22 to $24. Many types of infusion pumps can be purchased from medical supply outlets at costs ranging from $300 to $1,500.

An inexpensive infusion pump capable of holding a 10-ml syringe serves well because about 8 ml of sterile, injectable, nonbacteriostatic water is required to dissolve 2 grams of the lyophilized powder. Home nursing services, available in many large cities, can help patients and relatives with preparation of the deferoxamine for injection, programming of the infusion pump, and insertion of the subcutaneous infusion needle into the anterior abdominal wall for the first few days.

Serial measurements of the serum ferritin concentration are a simple way to monitor the efficacy of chelation therapy. If deferoxamine-induced iron excretion is not greater than or equal to the rate of transfusional iron loading, higher doses of deferoxamine (3 or 4 grams nightly*) can be tried. It is also advisable to infuse 1 gram of deferoxamine intravenously with each unit of packed red blood cells administered.

Long-term subcutaneous deferoxamine therapy may cause rash, pruritus, mild discomfort at the infusion site, or cataract formation. Slit lamp examination may be performed at 1- to 2-year intervals. The potential risk of cataract formation seems to be preferable to the option of not treating transfusional iron overload, which may cause life-threatening heart or liver injury.

---

*May exceed manufacturer's recommended dose.

HODGKIN'S DISEASE: CHEMOTHERAPY

method of
JAY MARION, M.D.
Washington University
St. Louis, Missouri

Hodgkin's disease is a lymphoreticular malignancy that usually presents with painless lymphadenopathy. Preceding the diagnosis, the patient may also be aware of systemic symptoms such as generalized malaise, fatigue, and anorexia. Three such constitutional symptoms have been associated with a reduction in survival and thus have special significance. These have been titled "B symptoms" and include

1. Unexplained weight loss of more than 10 per cent of the body weight in 6 months
2. Night sweats
3. Unexplained increases in temperature above 38° C

It is essential to document the presence or absence of B symptoms and to include the appropriate suffix to the numerical stage when discussing a patient with Hodgkin's disease. This anatomic staging system, which was developed at the Ann Arbor Conference in 1971, is widely accepted by clinicians who treat Hodgkin's disease (Table 1). It is a functional staging system because the usual pattern of spread in Hodgkin's disease is predictable and nonrandom. There is usually orderly spread via lymphatic channels to contiguous lymph node chains. Hematogenous spread does not usually occur until the disease has involved the spleen.

Approximately 70 per cent of all patients with Hodg-

TABLE 1. **Hodgkin's Disease: Ann Arbor Staging System**

Stage	Characteristics
I	Involvement of a single lymph node region (I) or of a single extralymphatic organ or site (I_E).
II	Involvement of two or more lymph node regions on the same side of the diaphragm (II) or localized involvement of an extralymphatic organ or site and of one or more lymph node regions on the same side of the diaphragm (II_E).
III	Involvement of lymph node regions on both sides of the diaphragm (III), which may be accompanied by localized involvement of an extralymphatic organ or site (III_E), or by involvement of the spleen (III_S), or both (III_{SE}).
IV	Diffuse or disseminated involvement of one or more extralymphatic organs or tissues, with or without associated lymph node enlargement. Involvement of the liver or bone marrow is always considered Stage IV.
Note:	Unexplained increase in temperature > 38° C (>100.5° F), night sweats, and/or weight loss > 10% of body weight in 6 mo preceding diagnosis are defined as systemic symptoms and denoted by the suffix letter B. Asymptomatic patients are denoted by the suffix letter A.

kin's disease can be cured. Radiation therapy has curative potential in early-stage disease, and combination chemotherapy is similarly effective in advanced-stage disease. Because the initial therapy chosen depends on the stage of the disease, the outcome is affected by the accuracy of the staging process. Thus, after a diagnosis of Hodgkin's disease is made, further studies are usually indicated to allow for the appropriate staging of the patient. Exhaustive staging studies, however, should not be undertaken in all patients as a matter of routine. Invasive staging studies, such as laparotomy, should be performed only in patients in whom a change in stage would result in a change in initial therapy. There remains much controversy regarding the role of aggressive staging procedures in various subsets of patients.

TREATMENT

Patients with early-stage Hodgkin's disease (Stages I and II) are usually managed with radiotherapy alone. Stage IIIA patients who have only minimal disease in the upper abdomen at laparotomy may also be managed primarily with radiotherapy. Some Stage I and II patients who have bulky adenopathy or multiple sites of disease are best managed with a combination of radiotherapy and chemotherapy. Patients with more advanced disease (Stages IIIB and IV) are usually offered chemotherapy for primary management. Such treatment is almost always given with curative intent.

Chemotherapy

Effective chemotherapeutic regimens in Hodgkin's disease include combinations of drugs that have different mechanisms of action, nonoverlapping toxicity, and proven efficacy in that disease. The landmark studies at the National Cancer Institute (NCI) in the late 1970s demonstrated that more than 50 per cent of patients with advanced Hodgkin's disease could be cured with a combination of four chemotherapeutic agents: nitrogen mustard, vincristine, procarbazine, and prednisone (MOPP) (Table 2). It remains the standard with which all other regimens are compared. A recently published 20-year update of the NCI data demonstrated an 84 per cent complete response rate with MOPP. Sixty-six per cent of the complete responders have remained free of disease for more than 10 years after treatment. However, although MOPP has revolutionized the management of advanced Hodgkin's disease, it has not turned out to be a panacea. At least 15 per cent of patients do not achieve a complete remission, and approximately 30 per cent of complete responders ultimately relapse. MOPP is also associated with significant and sometimes lasting

TABLE 2. **Chemotherapy Regimens for Hodgkin's Disease**

Agent	Dose (mg/M^2)	Days and Route
MOPP		
Nitrogen mustard	6	1 and 8 IV
Vincristine (Oncovin)	1.4	1 and 8 IV
Procarbazine	100	1–14 PO
Prednisone	40	1–14 PO
Repeat every 28 days		
BVCPP		
Carmustine (BCNU)	100	1 IV
Vinblastine	5	1 IV
Cyclophosphamide	600	1 IV
Procarbazine	100	1–10 PO
Prednisone	60	1–10 PO
Repeat every 28 days		
ABVD		
Doxorubicin (Adriamycin)	25	1 and 15 IV
Bleomycin	10*	1 and 15 IV
Vinblastine	6	1 and 15 IV
Dacarbazine (DTIC)	375	1 and 15 IV
Repeat every 28 days		
MOPP-ABV Hybrid		
Nitrogen mustard	6	1 IV
Vincristine (Oncovin)	1.4	1 IV (maximal dose 2.0 mg)
Procarbazine	100	1–7 PO
Prednisone	40	1–14 PO
Doxorubicin (Adriamycin)	35	8 IV
Bleomycin	10*	8 IV
Vinblastine	6	8 IV
Repeat every 28 days		

*Dose in U/M^2.

toxicity. This acute toxicity almost always includes nausea and vomiting, which can be variably controlled with antiemetic regimens. Myelosuppression is also common; a sliding scale of dose reduction for cytopenias that is built into the regimen must be strictly followed. Potential delayed toxic complications of MOPP include infertility and secondary malignancy.

Infertility. Infertility is a well-defined, long-term complication of MOPP chemotherapy. Because many patients with Hodgkin's disease are of reproductive age, this is not a minor toxicity. MOPP has been shown to produce profound, lasting impairment of fertility in the majority of men. This regimen also induces ovarian failure in the majority of premenopausal women. The closer a woman is to natural menopause, the more likely it is that she will develop premature ovarian failure. Women who retain fertility after MOPP chemotherapy appear to have normal pregnancies and children.

Secondary Malignancy. Patients with cured Hodgkin's disease have a small but increased risk of developing acute leukemia. This is usually a myeloid leukemia and is often preceded by a refractory anemia or another myelodysplasia. Chromosomal abnormalities are commonly found in the leukemic cell lines. The interval between completion of treatment and the appearance of leukemia is approximately 5 to 8 years. The overall incidence of acute leukemia in patients with cured Hodgkin's disease is approximately 3 to 4 per cent. The subgroup of patients who are treated with both radiotherapy and MOPP chemotherapy are at higher risk than those who are treated with either modality alone. The incidence of solid tumors in cured Hodgkin's disease patients does not appear to be increased.

Alternative Chemotherapeutic Regimens. Because MOPP alone is unable to cure approximately 40 per cent of patients with Hodgkin's disease and is associated with significant toxicity, there has been an impetus to develop alternative chemotherapeutic regimens. Several other drugs with proven efficacy in Hodgkin's disease are theoretically non–cross-resistant with the agents i MOPP. Such drugs (doxorubicin, bleomycin, carmustine, dacarbazine, lomustine, and vinblastine) have been used in various combinations as initial and salvage therapies in Hodgkin's disease (Table 2). The combination of doxorubicin (Adriamycin), bleomycin, vinblastine, and dacarbazine (ABVD) has been shown to produce complete remissions in approximately 30 to 60 per cent of patients who fail to respond to MOPP. Acute toxicity with ABVD is similar to that experienced with MOPP (nausea, vomiting, alopecia, and cytopenias). ABVD, however, is less often associated with infertility and the induction of secondary malignancies, and thus has been used as an alternative to MOPP for initial therapy. Comparative trials suggest that it is therapeutically equivalent to MOPP. ABVD may thus be the therapy of choice in patients with advanced Hodgkin's disease who desire to maintain fertility. However, this regimen must also be given with caution because it is associated with long-term cardiac toxicity (doxorubicin) and pulmonary toxicity (bleomycin).

Guidelines for Administration. The optimal number of chemotherapy cycles required to attain a durable, complete remission varies from patient to patient. The usual practice is to offer a minimum of six cycles of MOPP, or its equivalent, to patients with advanced Hodgkin's disease. The response to therapy should be monitored during treatment, and patients should receive two cycles after the documentation of a clinical complete remission. Maintenance therapy after these additional two cycles has not been shown to improve survival. The importance of administering full doses of chemotherapy in a timely fashion cannot be overemphasized. Dose reductions, if necessary, should follow the established protocol guidelines.

New Directions. Attempts are underway to improve both the initial and salvage therapies available to patients with advanced Hodgkin's diseases. The goal is to provide more effective and less toxic chemotherapeutic regimens. Alternating the use of MOPP and ABVD as initial therapy in selected patients with advanced disease is common but has not been clearly demonstrated to be superior to using MOPP alone. Other "hybrids" of MOPP and ABVD regimens are also being investigated as primary therapy. Autologous and allogeneic bone marrow transplantation has been demonstrated to be an effective salvage therapy for a small percentage of patients with refractory disease. The role of bone marrow transplantation in these patients is presently being defined through cooperative trials.

HODGKIN'S DISEASE: RADIATION THERAPY

method of
NANCY PRICE MENDENHALL, M.D., and
RODNEY R. MILLION, M.D.
University of Florida College of Medicine
Gainesville, Florida

Radiation is the single most effective agent available in the treatment of Hodgkin's disease. The success of radiation treatment depends on three factors: the relative radiosensitivity of Hodgkin's disease in comparison with the radiation tolerance of associated normal tissues, a predictable pattern of tumor spread, and technical advances in the field of radiation therapy that allow comprehensive treatment of all areas involved or at risk for tumor involvement. Cure is achieved in at least two-thirds of patients treated for Hodgkin's disease, and attention must be paid to sequelae of successful treatment. Treatment goals are not only relapse-free survival and survival but also survival without complications of treatment. Treatment alternatives include radiation therapy alone, chemotherapy alone, and a combination of the two modalities. Because of the effectiveness of combination chemotherapy in the salvage setting, a treatment plan resulting in lower relapse-free survival rates may be selected in order to avoid adverse complications of chemotherapy or combined-modality therapy without compromising a patient's overall chance of survival. In addition to Ann Arbor staging, other factors including bulk of disease (more or less than one-third of the maximum intrathoracic diameter for mediastinal lesions) number of sites of involvement (more or fewer than four), and degree of splenic involvement (more or fewer than five nodules) may be used to define three general risk groups. The low-risk group includes Ann Arbor Stages IA, IB, and IIA without other risk factors and is treated with radiation therapy alone with a high degree of success (Table 1). The intermediate group includes Ann Arbor Stages IA, IB, and IIA with bulky mediastinal disease, IIA with more than four sites of involvement, IIB, and IIIA$_1$ with minimal (fewer than five nodules) or no spleen involvement. The intermediate group may be treated with combined modality therapy or with radiation therapy alone with chemotherapy reserved for salvage with equal changes of overall survival. The high-risk group includes Stages IIIA$_1$ with extensive spleen involvement, IIIA$_2$, IIIB, IVA, and IVB and should be treated with combined-modality therapy or occasionally with chemotherapy alone, when the bone marrow is extensively involved.

TREATMENT RECOMMENDATIONS AND RESULTS

Treatment for all patients is individualized, but basic guidelines are shown in Table 1 along with expected 10-year relapse-free, absolute, and cause-specific disease-free survival rates.

Special Considerations

Older patients tolerate laparotomy and combination chemotherapy less well than younger patients. Consequently, there is a tendency to rely on clinical rather than pathologic staging in patients 60 years of age or older and to rely on radiation therapy except in advanced disease, when chemotherapy is mandated. Musculoskeletal defects from the use of radiation therapy in children have led to increased reliance on combination chemotherapy in children and the use of lower doses and more limited radiation treatment volumes.

Technical Aspects of Radiation Therapy for Hodgkin's Disease

Successful radiation therapy requires treatment of all clinically involved lymph nodes and all nodal and extranodal regions at risk for subclinical involvement. The anatomic position and extent of the lymphatic regions at risk in most patients necessitate treatment of very large fields and large volumes of normal tissues. Potential acute complications in normal tissues incidentally treated necessitate sequential irradiation of segments of the entire treatment volume; fractionation, protraction, and limitation of the radiation dose; careful tailoring of the radiation portals with individualized blocks made of Lipowitz's metal; and careful matching of the treatment portals to avoid overdosage through overlapping fields or underdosage in areas between fields.

TABLE 1. **Hodgkin's Disease: Treatment Recommendations and Results Achieved at the University of Florida**

Stage	Treatment	10-Year Survival Rate* (%)		
		Relapse-Free	Absolute	Cause-Specific
Low-risk				
IA, IB, IIA, IIB—no poor prognostic factors	MTNI or TNI	90	82	93
Intermediate-risk				
IA, IB, IIA, IIB–large mediastinal mass or	MTNI or TNI	60	86	83
>4 sites involved	CB	80	78	78
IIIA$_1$	TNI	80	80	80
IIIA$_{1S}$—minimal	TNI	50	90	80
	CB	100	75	75
High-risk				
IIIA$_{1S}$—extensive	CB	67	63	60
IIIB	CB	40	40	40
IV	CH	20	29	32
III, IV†	alt. CB or alt. CH	67–85	77–100	nd

*In relapse-free survival, only disease relapse was counted as an event. For absolute survival, death from any cause counted as an event. For cause-specific survival, deaths due to Hodgkin's disease or treatment-related causes (i.e., complications of treatment or secondary leukemia) were counted as events.

†Three-year results from Stanford University trials (Rosenberg SA and Kaplan HS, Int J Radiat Oncol Biol Phys 11:5–22, 1985).

Abbreviations: MTNI = modified total nodal irradiation; TNI = total nodal irradiation; CB = combined modality with radiation therapy and chemotherapy; CH = chemotherapy alone; alt. CB = chemotherapy alternating with segments of irradiation; alt. CH = alternating chemotherapy regimens; nd = no data.

Treatment Volumes

Involved-field irradiation refers to the treatment of only the site of clinical involvement. *Extended-field irradiation* refers to treatment of the site of clinical involvement plus elective treatment of contiguous, clinically uninvolved lymph node areas. *Total nodal irradiation* refers to treatment of all nodal and extranodal areas commonly involved in Hodgkin's disease, including the mantle, para-aortic, spleen, and pelvic fields; in some clinical settings, the liver is also treated. *Modified* or *subtotal nodal irradiation* differs from total nodal irradiation only in that the pelvic volume is not treated. *Comprehensive lymphatic irradiation* refers to treatment of Waldeyer's ring, mantle, and whole abdomen and is used more often in the treatment of non–Hodgkin's lymphoma, in which mesenteric node involvement is common.

The *Waldeyer's ring* treatment volume includes not only the lymphoid tissue in the tonsil, base of tongue, and nasopharynx, which is rarely involved in Hodgkin's disease but also, more important, the preauricular, postauricular, occipital, submaxillary, submental, upper jugular, and spinal accessory lymph nodes, which are not optimally treated in the mantle field. Waldeyer's ring fields are treated through opposed lateral portals when clinically involved or when subclinical involvement is suspected because of upper cervical lymphadenopathy or bulky involvement of midneck nodes.

The *mantle* is an irregularly shaped volume that includes the cervical, supraclavicular, infraclavicular, axillary, mediastinal, and hilar lymph nodes. When indicated, treatment of the whole lung, hemilung, or whole heart is incorporated into the mantle. Opposed anterior and posterior fields are used. The lower border of the mantle is approximately at the bottom of T10 when there is either minimal or no mediastinal disease. Custom blocks made of Lipowitz's metal shield the lung parenchyma, larynx, humeral heads, and portions of the mandible and parotid glands. When there is extensive mediastinal involvement with masses greater than one-third of the maximum intrathoracic diameter, subcarinal or hilar node involvement, or pleural effusion, consideration must be given to an *extended mantle field* including the hemilung or whole lung; if there is gross pericardial involvement or pericardial effusion, consideration must be given to treatment of the whole heart.

The *para-aortic volume* includes all para-aortic and paracaval lymph nodes between the aortic bifurcation and the bottom of the mantle field. The celiac axis nodes are incidentally covered. The para-aortic volume is treated through opposed anterior and posterior fields, matched (with an appropriate gap) to the mantle fields superiorly, the pelvic fields at the bottom of L$_4$ inferiorly, and the spleen field(s) laterally.

The *spleen treatment volume* includes the spleen and the splenic hilar nodes. When the spleen has been removed, a small field may be treated for coverage of the splenic hilum, which can be identified by clips placed at laparotomy. When the spleen is extensively involved or there is known liver involvement, the liver may be treated in a separate field.

The *pelvic volume* includes the femoral nodes and the common, external, and internal iliac nodes. The pelvic volume is treated through opposed anterior and posterior fields. The superior border is at the bottom of L4, matched, with an appropriate gap, to the bottom of the para-aortic fields. A customized block made of Lipowitz's metal shields the midline structures not at risk, including the ovaries after oophoropexy and the iliac wings. In males, special anterior and posterior testicular shields are used to decrease the dose of internally scattered radiation to the testicles from the pelvic fields. An *inverted Y treatment volume* combines the para-aortic and pelvic volumes. A *spade volume* is an abbreviated inverted Y that does not treat the femoral or pelvic lymphatics below the common iliac nodes.

Special Technical Features

The mantle is technically one of the most difficult treatment volumes used in radiation therapy and should be undertaken only by an experienced radiotherapist. Because doses are modest and the setup for the large, irregularly shaped mantle fields is quite difficult, a physician checks the setup each day in the treatment room, and daily port films are taken to verify adequate coverage of all target areas. If an area is missed, the dose is made up with a boost. Because of the potential for overdosage from overlapping of the sequential matched segmental fields, visually verifiable gaps on the skin between the adjacent fields are maintained.

Attention must be given to the position of the left kidney when treating the spleen and to para-aortic treatment volumes. If more than two-thirds of the left kidney must be included in these fields, consideration should be given to laparotomy with splenectomy. When the liver or whole abdomen must be treated, special kidney blocks are placed at 1500 cGy.

Time-Dose Factors

When radiation therapy alone is used, the dose delivered at the University of Florida is 3500 cGy to clinically involved areas and 3000 cGy to clinically uninvolved areas. Many institutions use doses 15 to 25 per cent higher. The overall time required for total nodal irradiation, including a planned break prior to pelvic irradiation, is 4 months; for modified total nodal irradiation the time is approximately 2 months. For particularly bulky disease treated with radiation therapy alone, an additional 250 cGy may be delivered. Doses in patients receiving six courses of chemotherapy are usually reduced to 3000 cGy for clinically involved sites and 2500 cGy for uninvolved sites. No dose reduction is made in adults receiving only three courses of chemotherapy. In children receiving four to six courses of chemotherapy, doses may be limited to 2500 cGy for clinically involved sites and 1500 to 2000 cGy for uninvolved sites.

Patients are treated 5 days a week and all fields are treated each day. The daily dose depends on the site and treatment volume. The standard mantle receives 160 to 170 cGy per day; the daily dose is reduced to 150 cGy when the whole heart is incorporated into the mantle volume and to 100 cGy when a hemilung or whole lung is included. The Waldeyer's ring, spleen, para-aortic, and pelvic fields receive 160 to 170 cGy per day. When the liver is treated, the daily dose is 150 cGy per day. When the whole abdomen is treated, the daily dose is 100 cGy per day.

To decrease acute normal-tissue toxicity and to allow for field reduction after tumor shrinkage, particularly in patients with large mediastinal masses, a split-course technique is used, in which the mantle and upper abdominal segments are each divided into two parts and treated in alternating, ping-pong fashion. As opposed to split-course techniques in carcinomas, this approach has not been associated with decreased control rates.

Sequencing and Modifications of Radiation Therapy in Combined-Modality Therapy

Three courses of chemotherapy may be used prior to definitive radiation therapy to shrink bulky mediastinal disease or reduce failure rates in Stage II patients with more than four sites of involvement. In this setting, radiation doses are not decreased, but the mantle treatment volume is usually significantly reduced so that more lung parenchyma may be shielded. In Stage III patients (excluding A_1 with minimal or no spleen disease) there is a high risk of failure in an extranodal site with total nodal irradiation, so six courses of chemotherapy are given. The radiation therapy may be sandwiched between the third and fourth courses of chemotherapy, delivered after completion of chemotherapy, or delivered in an alternating fashion with two courses of chemotherapy followed by mantle irradiation, two more courses of chemotherapy followed by upper abdominal irradiation, and a final two courses of chemotherapy followed by pelvic irradiation. The disadvantage of sandwich therapy is the relatively long period of time during completion of modified or total nodal irradiation after three courses of chemotherapy when some clinically involved areas receive neither chemotherapy nor radiation therapy. When total nodal irradiation is attempted after delivery of six courses of chemotherapy, it is often not possible to complete the sequential segments of irradiation because of marrow compromise, and there are often long treatment delays during the irradiation. The alternating approach has the advantages of induction chemotherapy prior to consolidative irradiation of all commonly involved areas. During the planned 2-month splits between the segments of irradiation, the patient is continuously treated with chemotherapy.

POTENTIAL SIDE EFFECTS AND COMPLICATIONS

Acute Side Effects

Expected side effects of treatment include transient hair loss, xerostomia, and skin reaction associated with the mantle and Waldeyer's ring fields, and nausea associated with the upper abdominal fields. Hair loss is particularly noticeable in the occipital region and preauricular regions in all patients and in the beard and anterior chest of men. Partial regrowth is usually observed within 2 to 4 months of treatment. Transient xerostomia occurs in all patients because of incidental parotid irradiation. The degree of recovery of normal salivary function is related to the patient's pretherapy salivary output, with complete resolution of symptoms of xerostomia usually observed in young patients and partial resolution in older patients. The skin reaction observed in the supradiaphragmatic fields is usually limited to mild erythema and occasional patchy, dry desquamation along tangentially irradiated surfaces; after completion of radiation therapy, a lanolin-, vitamin E-, or aloe-based lotion will provide symptomatic relief. The nausea and vomiting associated with para-aortic and splenic irradiation can be controlled with standard antiemetics such as prochlorperazine maleate (Compazine), promethazine HCl (Phenergan), metoclopramide HCl (Reglan), or chlorpromazine HCl (Thorazine) capsules or suppositories. Nausea and vomiting occasionally are observed with mantle irradiation, when the inferior mantle border is lowered to accommodate whole lung or heart irradiation. Because of the extensive bone marrow treated with total nodal irradiation, hemograms and platelet counts should be monitored weekly throughout the course of treatment, and more often when counts

begin to fall. When radiation therapy alone is given, the sequential treatment of segments of the irradiation volume allows for sufficient recovery so that few patients require treatment interruptions for bone marrow recovery. When combined-modality therapy is used, treatment interruptions are frequently required. Generally, radiation therapy is withheld until the white blood cell count is higher than 2000 per mm^3 and the platelet count is higher than 50,000 per mm^3.

Subacute Side Effects

Fatigue and loss of energy are common complaints during and after irradiation. Although most patients are able to continue their routine activities during treatment, it is often 4 to 6 months after completion of treatment before the patient is back to his or her normal baseline energy level. Except for prolonged lymphocytopenia, which may last up to a year after treatment, blood cell counts usually return to baseline values within several months following treatment.

Within 1 to 4 months after completion of mantle irradiation, some patients experience Lhermitte's syndrome, usually characterized by an electric shock sensation associated with neck flexion; this is transient and is not associated with late or permanent neurologic sequelae of treatment.

Patients with Hodgkin's disease have a propensity to develop herpes zoster. Although some patients have a preceding history of herpes zoster, the outbreak usually occurs within 2 years of successful treatment of Hodgkin's disease; when the outbreak occurs more than 2 years following therapy, it may be associated with recurrence of Hodgkin's disease. Usually the herpes zoster infection is confined to a single dermatomal distribution and is self-limited. The pain associated with the herpetic outbreak is often excruciating, is unresponsive to anti-inflammatory or narcotic medications, and may precede the appearance of the typical vesicular lesions by a week. Acyclovir may ameliorate the course of the viral outbreak and should certainly be used if the outbreak is in a critical area or if there is any sign of dissemination.

Radiation pneumonitis occurs in less than 5 per cent of patients, usually in those who had extensive mediastinal disease, and most often within 2 to 4 months after mantle irradiation. It is characterized by a dry, hacking cough with an infiltrate confined to the radiation portals on chest roentgenogram. Symptoms may precede radiographic signs and may also include fever and shortness of breath. Although radiographic changes are usually confined to previous radiation portals, the process can extend outside the previous field and diffusely involve the lung. In patients who received combined-modality therapy, pneumocystic pneumonia must be ruled out. Rapid improvement is usually seen with the initiation of steroids (60 to 100 mg of prednisone daily), but some cases are not responsive. Early diagnosis and treatment are essential, as most fatalities have been associated with delay in therapy, often for histologic confirmation of the diagnosis. Prednisone may mask radiation pneumonitis, as some cases in patients receiving combined-modality therapy have been associated with steroid withdrawal. It is important to withdraw steroids slowly after treatment for radiation pneumonitis (over a period of several months), as rapid withdrawal has been associated with reactivation of the pneumonitis which may not be responsive to reinitiation of steroids.

Acute pericarditis occurs in 2 to 5 per cent of patients (usually those who had extensive mediastinal and pericardial disease) 4 to 6 months after mantle irradiation. Most patients are asymptomatic, and the diagnosis is based on plain chest roentgenograms; the condition usually resolves over a period of months without therapy. Occasionally, the patient may develop typical signs and symptoms of pericarditis including pleuritic or ischemic chest pain, shortness of breath, pericardial friction rub, paradoxic pulse, and electrocardiographic changes. Nonsteroidal anti-inflammatory medications and steroids may be effective. The patient must be observed for increasing pericardial effusion and possible tamponade, in which case emergent pericardiocentesis can be lifesaving.

Late Complications

Potential late complications include hypothyroidism, sterility, pulmonary fibrosis, cardiac damage, transverse myelitis, nephritis, growth abnormalities, and second malignancies.

Approximately 25 per cent of patients who receive mantle irradiation will develop hypothyroidism; periodically, thyroid functions are measured, and replacement thyroid hormone is prescribed even for asymptomatic patients who show only elevated levels of thyroid-stimulating hormone. With ovarian transposition to midline position at laparotomy and special testicular shields to decrease the dose of indirect radiation to the testicles from internal scatter during pelvic irradiation, sterility due to irradiation is unusual. It is important, prior to beginning pelvic irradiation in a patient who has undergone oophoropexy, to verify midline ovarian position, however, as

the ovaries may detach and return to the normal anatomic position. Symptomatic pulmonary fibrosis may occur in patients in whom large mediastinal masses preclude shielding of adequate lung parenchyma; with current dose recommendations and either shrinking-field technique with radiation therapy alone or the use of chemotherapy for shrinkage of the tumor prior to definitive radiation therapy, the risk of clinically significant pulmonary damage is less than 5 per cent. Rarely, fibrotic lung that results in infectious or hemodynamic problems may be resected. The risk of radiation fibrosis is increased with the use of bleomycin. Constrictive pericarditis is an uncommon complication of mantle irradiation, usually occurring only in patients with extensive mediastinal disease with pericardial involvement in whom high doses of radiation were delivered to the whole heart. Pericardiectomy may be necessary in severe cases. Whether the risk of coronary artery disease is increased by mantle irradiation is unknown. Transverse myelitis is a rare but catastrophic complication of irradiation, usually related to poor technique in matching opposing and abutting fields; there is no known effective treatment for myelitis. Radiation nephritis occurs rarely and may be avoided with proper technique or splenectomy. If radiation nephritis results in hypertension and the contralateral kidney is functional, consideration may be given to nephrectomy.

The use of radiation therapy in children often results in hypoplastic development of the irradiated tissues and significant subsequent musculoskeletal defects, which may also contribute to psychosocial problems. The younger the child, the more significant the subsequent growth abnormalities will be. Common sequelae include a "skinny neck" and shortened interclavicular distance secondary to mantle irradiation, posterior left abdominal wall deficit from treatment of the spleen field(s), and shortened sitting height secondary to irradiation of the mantle and para-aortic fields.

Patients treated with radiation therapy alone for Hodgkin's disease do not appear to be at an increased risk over the general population for developing leukemia. There is approximately a 7 per cent risk of leukemia in patients treated with MOPP (Mustargen, Oncovin, procarbazine, and prednisone) chemotherapy; patients receiving combined-modality therapy do not appear to be at a significantly increased risk over those receiving chemotherapy alone. Although there appears to be an increased risk of second solid malignancies in patients receiving radiation therapy for Hodgkin's disease compared with the general population, many of the reported malignancies are not in the previous radiation fields and are clearly related to other risk factors, such as cigarette smoking. Large numbers of patients have not been observed beyond the expected latency period for radiation-induced malignancies (5 to 30 years), and the risks due to inherent genetic deficiencies are not defined, so the relationship between second solid malignancies and the use of radiation in the treatment for Hodgkin's disease is not clear.

NEW DIRECTIONS

As survival is in excess of 80 per cent, the emphasis in low- to intermediate-risk patients is on reduction of the late sequelae of treatment by reduction of the radiation dose and volume through shrinking-field techniques and the use of preirradiation chemotherapy and by the search for effective drug combinations that will be less leukemogenic and have less cardiopulmonary toxicity in combination with radiation. The emphasis in high-risk patients is improvement in survival rates through more effective combinations and sequencing of drugs and radiation. The role of ablative therapy followed by autologous bone marrow transplantation in patients with an extremely poor prognosis is also being investigated.

ACUTE LEUKEMIA IN ADULTS

method of
KENNETH B. MILLER, M.D.
Tufts University School of Medicine
Boston, Massachusetts

The acute leukemias are a group of neoplastic disorders characterized by the proliferation and accumulation in the bone marrow and peripheral blood of immature hematopoietic cells. These malignant cells gradually replace and inhibit the growth and maturation of normal erythroid, myeloid, and megakaryocytic precursors. If untreated, the acute leukemias are usually fatal within weeks to months. The leukemias are broadly divided into two groups on the basis of cell type. The myeloid leukemias (acute myelogenous leukemia [AML]) are more common in adults and the lymphoid leukemias (acute lymphoblastic [ALL]) are more common in children.

ACUTE MYELOGENOUS LEUKEMIA

The introduction of effective antileukemic chemotherapy and advances in supportive care have dramatically changed the management and prognosis of AML. The possibility of a long-term disease-free response, or even cure, for patients with AML is now a realistic goal.

Initial Evaluation and Diagnosis

The diagnosis of acute leukemia is usually readily apparent on reviewing the peripheral blood smear and examining the patient. Patients typically present with a brief history of progressive fatigue, pallor, and easy bruisability. Lymphadenopathy and splenomegaly, when present, are more suggestive of ALL than AML. The peripheral blood smear reveals a decreased platelet count and circulating blast count. As part of the initial evaluation and before beginning therapy, a bone marrow aspirate and biopsy should be performed to confirm the diagnosis and for cytogenetic studies, immunologic and biochemical markers, and histochemical stains. These studies are important to differentiate the subtypes of leukemia and provide important prognostic and clinical information. The immunologic and biochemical markers are necessary to characterize biphenotypic leukemias, to differentiate subsets of the lymphoid and myeloid leukemias, and to plan therapy. Cytogenetic studies, by use of high-resolution banding techniques, have identified specific chromosome abnormalities that are associated with distinctive morphologic and clinical features. For instance, the presence of the Philadelphia chromosome in ALL is associated with a poor prognosis, whereas an inversion of chromosome 16 in the acute myelomonocytic M-4 variant is a favorable prognostic variable. Alterations of chromosomes 7, 8, and 11 are associated with a prior myelodysplastic syndrome or preleukemic condition and a probable poor response to chemotherapy.

Before starting chemotherapy, special attention should be paid to renal, liver, and cardiac function. The anthracycline antibiotics, daunorubicin and doxorubicin, that are included in the standard induction regimens must be used cautiously in patients with underlying heart disease. Patients with impaired liver function require a reduction in the dose of cytosine arabinoside (ara-C). The serum electrolyte levels should be monitored closely, especially the serum potassium level. A partial thromboplastin time, prothrombin time, and screen for disseminated intravascular coagulation (DIC) should be evaluated before starting induction chemotherapy, and any abnormalities should be addressed and corrected. Before beginning standard intensive induction therapy, efforts should be made to correct any underlying medical problems. Despite the sense of urgency felt by many patients and physicians with regard to the diagnosis and treatment of the acute leukemias, it is the rare patient who requires emergent therapy. Patients can usually be supported with blood products, hydroxyurea, and antibiotics while preparations are being made to provide adequate emotional and medical support.

The use of surgically placed implantable venous access devices has greatly facilitated the care of patients with acute leukemia. Indwelling catheters (e.g., Hickmans, Cooks, or Infusaports) should be placed before beginning therapy. At our institution we restrict the access and care of these implantable catheters to a limited number of specially trained personnel. These catheters can be left in place for months for the infusion of chemotherapy, blood products, and antibiotics. Patients and their families should be instructed in the care and maintenance of these devices.

Allopurinol, 300 mg per day, should be administered to all patients before starting induction chemotherapy and discontinued when there is documented bone marrow aplasia. The rapid lysis of cells also requires that the patient be adequately hydrated to prevent the development of a tumor lysis syndrome.

Induction Therapy

Induction chemotherapy is administered as the initial therapy to eradicate all detectable leukemia and to induce a complete remission, which is defined the absence of leukemic cells in the peripheral blood and bone marrow and the return of normal bone marrow function. A complete remission is required for a long-term or durable response.

The complete remission rate in AML is between 50 and 70 per cent. The factors that determine the outcome of the remission induction include the histologic subtype (French-American-British [FAB] type), age of the patient, performance status, organ involvement, and white blood count at presentation. Age more than any other factor correlates with the outcome of remission induction therapy. The complete remission rate for patients younger than the age of 40 years is 60 to 75 per cent; in individuals older than 60 years it is 30 to 40 per cent. Older patients do not have more resistant leukemia but tolerate the side effects associated with intensive induction chemotherapy poorly. The lower remission rate reflects the increased number of deaths related to infections, bleeding, or toxicity of the chemotherapy.

Patients are usually maintained in a private room and are given a low-bacteria, cooked food only, diet. Medical personnel are instructed to wash their hands carefully before examining the patient. Laminar airflow rooms or strict reverse isolation precautions are not required. Live plants or flowers are discouraged in patients' rooms to prevent exposure to fungal or unusual pathogens. Patients are instructed in the importance of oral and perianal hygiene. To prevent the development of oral candidiasis, nystatin oral suspension, 5 ml swish and then swallow, or clotrimazole troches are routinely started on the first day of induction therapy and are continued until a patient leaves the hospital. The use of prophylactic absorbable and nonabsorbable antibiotics remains controversial. However, we routinely use trimethoprim-sulfamethoxazole or norfloxacin prophylactically to decrease the incidence of common bacterial infections.

A number of induction regimens are presently available that give similar results. Virtually all remission induction regimens use ara-C, by a continuous 24-hour infusion for 7 to 10 days, together with an anthracycline antibiotic, daunorubicin (Cerubidine), intravenously for 3 days. The addition of oral 6-thioguanine does not appear to increase the remission induction rate meaningfully. Patients older than 60 years generally receive a 25 per cent reduction in the daunorubicin dose. The aim of induction therapy is to induce bone marrow aplasia. At our institution, patients younger than 50 years receive 7 days of ara-C at 100 mg per M^2 and 3 days of daunorubicin at 45 mg per M^2, followed by 3 days of high-dose ara-C, 2 grams* per M^2 every 12 hours for six doses. High-dose ara-C is an active compound with a number of unique and disturbing side effects. All patients given high-dose ara-C receive steroid eye drops to prevent a chemical conjunctivitis. A neurologic examination is performed before each dose, and the high-dose ara-C is withheld if there is any evidence of neurologic toxicity. Patients between the ages of 50 and 60 years receive the same dose of daunorubicin and 10 days of standard-dose ara-C without the 3 days of high-dose ara-C. Patients older than the age of 60 years receive 30 mg per M^2 of daunorubicin and 7 days of standard-dose ara-C. A bone marrow aspirate and biopsy are performed 7 to 10 days after completing induction chemotherapy. If there is residual leukemia, a second, attenuated course of induction chemotherapy is administered, 2 days of daunorubicin and 5 days of continuous-infusion ara-C at the standard 100 mg per M^2 dose.

The induction chemotherapeutic agents uniformly produce profound and prolonged neutropenia. The nadir granulocyte count occurs 7 to 10 days after completing therapy. Almost all patients develop a fever during their induction.

---

*Dosage may exceed manufacturer's recommended dose.

A source for the fever should be sought in every patient. However, despite repeated cultures and investigations a documented infection is found in fewer than one-third of the patients. Frequently overlooked sources for infection include periodontal and perirectal abscesses.

The infectious complications in the neutropenic patient with acute leukemia can usually be managed with one of the new semisynthetic penicillins (ticarcillin, piperacillin) or a third-generation cephalosporin (ceftazidime) in combination with an aminoglycoside. The sensitivities and prevalence of bacterial infections at each individual hospital are important in guiding the clinician in the choice of antibiotics. The most common infecting organisms include *Escherichia coli*, *Staphylococcus aureus*, *Klebsiella*, and *Pseudomonas*. *Staphylococcus epidermidis* infections are also frequent because of the expanded use of implantable venous access devices. Vancomycin should be started if a line infection is suspected. A disturbing trend has been the development of fungal infections in patients who are given multiple broad-spectrum antibiotics. Fungi, including *Candida* and *Aspergillus*, are rarely cultured by the usual techniques. The use of empiric antifungal therapy remains controversial; however, if no infectious site is found and fevers persist for 3 to 5 days after the initiation of broad-spectrum antibiotics, amphotericin B,* 0.5 mg per kg daily, should be started. It must be emphasized that the choice of antibiotics should be guided by the sensitivities and prevalence of bacterial infections at the local institution rather than the results of large international studies. The duration of antibiotic therapy is also controversial. At our institution, antibiotics are continued until the patient is no longer febrile and has more than 500 neutrophils per mm³.

Nausea and vomiting during induction therapy should be treated with antiemetics. Persistent diarrhea in these patients is worrisome. A cause of the diarrhea should be investigated, including stool cultures for enteric pathogens and *Clostridium difficile*, even if the patient has not been taking broad-spectrum antibiotics. However, opiates should be used cautiously to treat the diarrhea. The nutritional needs of the patient should be closely monitored, and total parenteral nutrition or other nutritional support should be started early if the oral intake falls. Mucositis can be a severe problem. Patients frequently require narcotics to control the discomfort associated with the mucositis. Acylovir is added if herpetic mucositis is suspected and is continued until the mucositis resolves.

---

*The manufacturer recommends a 1-mg test dose infused slowly.

Transfusion Support

The importance of the blood bank in the care of patients with acute leukemia cannot be overstated. The availability of platelets and red blood cells during induction therapy has decreased many fatal bleeding complications. Platelet and red blood cell transfusions are administered prophylactically in an attempt to keep the platelet count above 15,000 per mm³ and the hematocrit above 30 ml per dl. Approximately 50 per cent of patients become refractory to random donor platelets. These patients may then respond to HLA-matched single-donor platelets. Prophylactic granulocyte transfusions are not routinely administered to the neutropenic adult patient. Moreover, studies suggest that granulocyte transfusions may be dangerous for both the recipient and the donor. Adverse effects include pulmonary reactions, fever, and the transmission of viral infections. Some studies have suggested a role for granulocyte transfusions in the neutropenic patient with documented bacterial sepsis that is unresponsive to appropriate antibiotics. However, this event is rare because of presently available antibiotics. A granulocyte transfusion has not been recommended to any adult neutropenic patient in our institution in the last 10 years.

A course of induction therapy usually lasts about 30 days. If 7 to 10 days after completing therapy the bone marrow has no residual leukemic cells, no further chemotherapy is administered, and bone marrow aspirates are repeated every 7 to 10 days to monitor recovery. Remission induction failures are usually due to death from bleeding or infections. Documented chemotherapy-resistant disease occurs in fewer than 15 per cent of all patients. Despite the advances in supportive care and chemotherapy, most adults with acute leukemia still ultimately relapse and die of their disease. In an effort to prevent leukemia relapse, intensive postremission induction regimens are administered.

Consolidation and Maintenance Therapy

Consolidation therapy is a form of intensive therapy given to patients who are in a complete remission. The drugs and doses used are similar to those for induction therapy. Most centers use some form of intensive postremission consolidation therapy to prevent relapse. We start consolidation therapy for all patients under the age of 65 years within 1 month of attaining a complete remission. Three cycles of consolidation are administered. The first cycle is 3 days of daunorubicin (45 mg per M²) and 7 days of ara-C (100 mg per M² by continuous intravenous infusion); the second cycle is high-dose ara-C (2 grams per M^{2*}) every 12 hours for eight doses plus 2 days of VP-16 (100 mg per M^2 intravenously); the third cycle is a repeat of the first cycle. This intensive consolidation regimen is associated with prolonged periods of neutropenia and thrombocytopenia. The drug doses are not adjusted for nadir leukocyte or platelet counts. Patients require platelet support and are frequently hospitalized with fevers and neutropenia. Consolidation therapy is administered either in the hospital or on an outpatient basis. Consolidation therapy is completed within 4 months.

Maintenance therapy is low-dose chemotherapy that is usually given on an outpatient basis for many months to years. Maintenance therapies range from single agents to complicated multidrug regimens. The importance of a prolonged maintenance therapy phase is unclear. At our institution, maintenance therapy has been abandoned in favor of the three cycles of intensive consolidation. The use of intensive consolidation therapy has translated to an increase in the number of long-term disease-free survivors. Thirty to 40 per cent of patients treated with intensive consolidation are alive, not receiving therapy, and disease free at 3 to 5 years. Most of these patients may be "cured" of their AML.

Special Therapeutic Conditions and Problems

Elderly patients with AML tolerate intensive chemotherapy poorly. Despite a dose reduction for all patients older than 60 years of age, 25 to 35 per cent of elderly patients still die from complications of therapy and not because of chemotherapy-resistant disease. Therefore, at our institution we critically evaluate all patients older than 65 years with regard to their ability to tolerate an intensive chemotherapy regimen. Moreover, patients with intercurrent medical problems such as diabetes, chronic obstructive lung disease, and congestive heart failure have a higher mortality and morbidity during induction therapy. An alternative approach for these patients is a prolonged, 14- to 21-day infusion of low-dose ara-C. One effective regimen uses 21 days of ara-C, 20 mg per M^2, by continuous intravenous or subcutaneous infusion. The complete remission rate with this regimen is between 30 and 60 per cent. Similar results have been reported with attenuated courses of the standard induction regimen. The value of postremission therapy in elderly patients remains unclear.

Prior Myelodysplastic Syndrome

Leukemia that is associated with a prior myelodysplastic syndrome or that is secondary to prior chemotherapy or radiation therapy remains a difficult problem. These patients tolerate induction and consolidation therapy poorly. High-dose ara-C (2 to 3 grams per M^2 for 10 to 12 doses*) has been reported to produce complete remissions in selected patients; however, most of these remissions were short-lived. The options for effectively treating these patients with chemotherapy are limited. If they are eligible, these individuals should be referred for an allogeneic bone marrow transplant early in the course of the disease.

Central Nervous System Leukemia

Central nervous system (CNS) leukemia occurs in fewer than 5 per cent of patients with AML. There has been no detectable benefit of CNS prophylaxis on survival. Patients presenting with a white blood cell count higher than 75,000 per mm^3 or the monocytic variant of acute leukemia have a higher risk of CNS disease. These patients should have lumbar puncture performed at the time of attaining a complete remission. Patients with meningeal signs or cranial nerve abnormalities should be evaluated for overt CNS leukemia earlier in the course of the disease. With overt CNS leukemia, an Ommaya reservoir should be placed to facilitate the administration of intrathecal methotrexate or ara-C. The need for additional cranial irradiation is unclear. Patients who present with CNS leukemia have an overall poorer prognosis.

Hyperleukocytosis Syndromes

Patients with AML who present with more than 70,000 per mm^3 circulating myeloblasts require emergency therapy. Sludging by the leukemic blasts results in an increased blood viscosity and the formation of blast cell microthrombi. The hyperleukocytosis syndrome rarely occurs in patients with ALL and chronic lymphocytic leukemia, possibly because of the normal distensibility of the leukemic cell in these disorders. The lung and brain are most severely involved in the hyperleukocytosis syndrome. Patients develop hypoxia and respiratory distress associated with diffuse infiltrates seen on chest x-ray film. Care should be taken to rule out a pseudohypoxia and hypoglycemia resulting from the consumption of oxygen and sugar by the blasts while the blood is being transported to the laboratory. The CNS

---

*This dose may exceed the manufacturer's recommended dose.

*This dose may exceed the manufacturer's recommended dose.

involvement results from thrombosis, hypoxia, and hemorrhage. The symptoms of CNS leukostasis can progress within hours from headache to coma. Treatment must be prompt and directed to reducing the number of circulating leukemic blasts rapidly. Leukapheresis and hydroxyurea (2 grams per M orally every 12 hours*) should be started as soon as possible. To treat the increased blood viscosity, the hematocrit should be maintained in the 25 to 30 ml per dl range until induction chemotherapy starts.

Disseminated Intravascular Coagulation

Patients with acute myeloblastic leukemia may develop DIC during therapy. DIC is particularly common in the acute promyelocytic variant (FAB classification M-3). These patients frequently present with a prolonged prothrombin time and partial thromboplastin time and low serum fibrinogen level. During induction therapy with the rapid lysis of the leukemic cells, the DIC worsens. Heparin has been recommended to treat the DIC. However, the decision to use heparin should be made on an individual basis. In general, we administer heparin to patients with acute promyelocytic leukemia who do not have major organ involvement related to bleeding. Heparin is given as a continuous infusion, without an initial bolus, at 10 units per kg per hour. In addition, we replace the clotting factors with fresh frozen plasma and fibrinogen. Platelets are administered to maintain the platelet count between 20,000 and 50,000 per mm³. Heparin is stopped when there are no circulating leukemic cells. Although the prophylactic use of heparin in these patients may be a benefit, there are no prospective controlled studies evaluating its use, and many centers therefore prefer to support these patients with blood products alone.

Treatment of Relapsed Disease

The treatment of relapsed acute leukemia is difficult. Patients who relapse while being treated have a poor prognosis. Some of these patients may respond to chemotherapeutic regimens using amsacrine or other anthracyclines in combination with high-dose ara-C or VP-16. Although a second remission is possible, these remissions are usually of short duration. At this point an allogeneic bone marrow transplant offers the only hope, albeit small, of a lasting remission. However, patients who relapse while not receiving chemotherapy usually respond to their primary induction regimen. Patients who relapse within 18 months of attaining a complete remission

---

*This dose may exceed the manufacturer's recommended dose.

should be considered to be not curable with standard chemotherapy. These patients should then be considered for alternative forms of therapy. These patients have disease that is not responsive to chemotherapy and, if eligible, should be considered for a bone marrow transplant at this point.

Bone Marrow Transplantation

A promising new approach for patients in first remission in AML is the use of autologous bone marrow transplantation. Patients in complete remission have their bone marrow harvested and frozen. High-dose chemotherapy with or without radiation therapy is administered, followed by the infusion of the autologous bone marrow. Some centers purge the marrow with chemotherapy or antibodies to eliminate any residual leukemic cells. The importance, or even need, of purging is unclear. Preliminary studies from a number of centers suggest that patients who undergo autologous transplantation in first remission or early second remission may have a prolonged remission. The timing of the transplant, patient selection, and long-term survival of these patients remain to be determined. This approach, however, may provide an alternative for allogeneic bone marrow transplantation for older individuals and patients without an HLA-matched donor.

The use of allogeneic bone marrow transplantation in adults with AML is rapidly changing. Allogeneic bone marrow transplantation is available for more adult patients because of advances in the prevention and management of acute and chronic graft-versus-host disease, viral and opportunistic infections, and the development of a national HLA bone marrow transplant registry for nonrelated donors. The timing of an allogeneic transplant remains controversial. A number of studies have compared HLA-matched allogeneic bone marrow transplantation and chemotherapy for adults with acute leukemia in first remission. After bone marrow transplantation, there was a significant decrease in the incidence of leukemic relapse. The decreased leukemic relapse rate, however, did not translate into a statistically significant survival advantage. More patients were cured of their leukemia but died as a consequence of the transplant. The toxicity of bone marrow transplantation is age related. Patients older than the age of 35 years develop more fatal complications. At our institution, we recommend an allogeneic transplant for all patients in second remission under the age of 50 years with an HLA-compatible donor. An allogeneic bone marrow transplant is recommended in first-remission patients with a prior myelodysplastic syndrome, preleukemic condition, or secondary leukemia.

Summary

The use of intensive induction and consolidation therapy has resulted in a median remission duration of 16 to 24 months. Approximately 20 to 40 per cent of patients remain in remission while having no therapy at 3 to 5 years. Most of these patients are probably cured of acute leukemia. Allogeneic or autologous transplantation should be considered for all high-risk patients.

ALL IN ADULTS

ALL in adults is an uncommon disease and accounts for approximately 10 to 25 per cent of all adult acute leukemias. Adult patients with ALL have a poor prognosis, in contrast to the 65 to 75 per cent cure rate in children. The adult patients tend to present with poor prognostic variables including a greater proportion of the T cell subtype, a 20 to 30 per cent incidence of the Philadelphia chromosome, and a higher proportion of morphologically undifferentiated and biphenotypic leukemias.

The induction therapy for ALL consists of vincristine, 2 mg per week for 3 weeks, prednisone, 60 mg per M^2 orally for 21 days, and daunorubicin, 45 mg per M^2 intravenously on days 1, 2, and 3. The complete remission rate with this regimen is between 60 and 80 per cent. Patients then receive 9 to 12 months of alternating chemotherapy using cytoxan, vincristine, methotrexate, prednisone, L-asparaginase, and adriamycin. All patients receive intrathecal prophylaxis with methotrexate once a month. The use of postremission consolidation and intensification has not shown to be of clear benefit in adult ALL patients. Poor prognostic features include advanced age, elevated presenting white blood cell count, abnormal cytogenetics, and a prolonged time to attain a complete remission. ALL in the adult is a more heterogeneous disease than that in children. The 5-year disease-free survival in adults is 25 to 35 per cent.

Relapsed Acute Lymphocytic Leukemia

Patients with ALL who relapse are reinduced with the same drugs used to achieve the initial remission. Approximately 50 per cent of patients achieve a second remission. Patients who relapse while being given maintenance therapy have a poor prognosis. Although a second remission is possible, it is usually short. These patients should be considered for bone marrow transplantation. However, even with transplantation their prognosis is poor. In contrast, patients who relapse while receiving no therapy usually attain a durable second remission. Autologous or allogeneic transplantation has produced long-term disease-free survival in these patients and is a controversial alternative to standard chemotherapy. At our institution, we consider all patients with relapsed ALL as high risk and recommend bone marrow transplantation. Patients who fail to respond to the induction regimen receive moderate- or high-dose methotrexate (200 mg per M^2 escalating to 2 grams per M^2) followed by L-asparaginase (10,000 units) 24 hours later. Subsequent therapy includes alternating cycles of ara-C and VP-16 and methotrexate, L-asparaginase, and prednisone.

Adult patients with ALL have a median remission duration of 16 to 24 months with chemotherapy alone. The timing of autologous and allogeneic transplantation remains to be determined but should be considered early for high-risk patients.

ACUTE LEUKEMIA IN CHILDHOOD

method of
ARNOLD I. FREEMAN, M.D., and
GERALD M. WOODS, M.D.
The Children's Mercy Hospital
Kansas City, Missouri

There are two major families of acute leukemia, acute lymphocytic leukemia (ALL) and acute nonlymphocytic leukemia (ANLL), which is also known as acute myelocytic leukemia. Recently, acute leukemia with evidence of both myeloid and lymphocytic differentiation in the same patient has been identified and termed "mixed lineage leukemia."

DIAGNOSIS

The diagnosis of acute leukemia is established primarily by bone marrow examination. In the French-American-British (FAB) classification, there are three subtypes of ALL, whereas there are seven subtypes of ANLL (Tables 1 and 2). Cell surface markers establish the diagnosis and distinguish ALL from ANLL. Special stains often help to identify lineage: the peroxidase stain is generally positive in myeloid series and the nonspecific esterase stain is positive in cells of the monocytic series. Cytogenetics also often helps to separate ALL from ANLL and may delineate the subtype.

Diagnostic techniques, support systems, and treatment regimens are changing so rapidly that all children with acute leukemia should be referred to a pediatric oncology center. In some situations co-management with a pediatric oncology center is feasible, but at least the initial evaluation and the plan of therapy should be instituted at such a center.

ACUTE LYMPHOCYTIC LEUKEMIA

This type of leukemia accounts for approximately 80 per cent of childhood leukemia. Its peak incidence occurs at age 3 to 4 years.

TABLE 1. **FAB Classification of Acute Lymphocytic Leukemia**

Cytologic Features	L1 (80%)	L2 (15–20%)	L3 (1–2%)
Size (cell size)	Small cells predominate	Large and heterogeneous	Large and homogeneous
Nucleus			
Nuclear chromatin	Homogeneous	Variable and heterogeneous	Finely stippled and homogeneous
Nuclear shape	Regular, some clefting	Irregular; clefting and indentation common	Regular: oval to round
Nucleoli	Small and inconspicuous	One or more present, often large	Prominent; one or more vesicular
Cytoplasm			
Amount	Scanty	Variable; often abundant	Moderately abundant
Basophilia	Slight	Variable; occasionally prominent	Deep
Vacuolation	Variable	Variable	Generally prominent

Approximately 80 per cent of ALL falls within the B cell lineage and the remaining 20 per cent in the T cell lineage. Immune markers, cytogenetics, and molecular probes have helped to classify B cell lineage ALL:

1. B cell lineage leukemias
   a. "Early B cell" ("null cell," generally positive for common ALL antigens (CALLA): 60 per cent of ALL
   b. Pre–B cell (cytoplastic immunoglobulin): 15 to 20 per cent of ALL
   c. B cell (surface immunoglobulin): 1 to 2 per cent of ALL
2. T cell lineage leukemias: 15 to 20 per cent of ALL

Prognosis

1. High leukemic white blood cell count (blast count at diagnosis) remains the single most important and widely accepted prognostic feature. The higher the blast burden, the worse the prognosis.

2. Age is also important. Infants less than 1 year of age have a substantially worse prognosis. They are 90 per cent CALLA negative and have a variant of ALL. Children and teenagers older than age 10 years also have a somewhat worse prognosis.

3. Patients presenting with lymphoma and leukemia (i.e., those presenting with large, bulky tumors in nodes or in liver and spleen) have a worse prognosis.

4. Children with translocations in the leukemic cells also have a worse prognosis. Examples are: t(9:22), t(8:14), and t(4:11).

5. Children who do not achieve complete remission quickly with induction chemotherapy also have a poorer prognosis.

Treatment

It should be kept in mind that successful therapy over-rides prognostic features and that with continued advances in treatment, these prognostic features may become historical curiosities.

Conceptual Basis

The outlook for a child presenting with ALL has improved enormously within the last generation. Now the overall cure rate is approximately 70 per cent. Therefore the goal is *cure*.

Successful therapy involves the use of effective, multiple drugs and the recognition that leukemic sanctuaries exist, particularly in the central nervous system (CNS) and to a lesser extent in the testes, which require specific therapeutic maneuvers.

TABLE 2. **FAB Classification of Acute Nonlymphocytic Leukemia**

	FAB Category	Predominant Cell
M-1	Acute undifferentiated myelogenous leukemia*	Predominantly myeloblasts; may have minimal evidence of myeloid differentiation
M-2	Acute differentiated myelogenous leukemia*	Myeloblasts with azurophilic granules and promyelocytes (total > 50%) and myelocytes
M-3	Acute promyelocytic* leukemia	Predominantly promyelocytes
M-4†	Acute myelomonocytic leukemia	Promyelocytes, myelocytes, promonocytes, and monocytes
M-5a	Acute monoblastic‡ leukemia	Monoblasts (undifferentiated)
M-5b	Acute differentiated‡ monocytic leukemia	Monoblasts, promonocytes, and monocytes (differentiated)
M-6	Acute erythroleukemia	50% are erythroblasts, 30% of nonerythroid cells are blasts
M-7	Acute megakaryoblastic leukemia	Predominantly megakaryoblasts, undifferentiated and often difficult to diagnose

*Myeloperoxidase positive.
†M-4 is often positive for both myeloperoxidase and esterase stains.
‡Nonspecific esterase positive.

Also, there is now an effort to tailor treatment by using more aggressive therapy for the higher-risk patients with ALL. With such therapy, these children have a 60 to 70 per cent chance for cure. This therapy necessitates use of cell surface markers and cytogenetics to classify the disease according to risk factors. It also necessitates having qualified support systems, such as infectious disease services, nutritional support, transfusion support, and intensive care units, because of the severe complications resulting from these aggressive regimens.

In standard or lower-risk leukemia, the treatment is less aggressive and there are fewer complications.

Treatment phases for ALL include:

1. In the *induction phase,* in approximately 4 weeks there is complete remission of the disease so that there is *no* evidence of leukemia.

2. *Intensification* generally follows induction. In this phase, there is more intensive therapy than that during induction, with the objective of eradicating the small numbers of leukemic cells remaining in the body.

3. The *maintenance phase,* which is a poor term, follows intensification. Here, attempts are made to eradicate small numbers of leukemic cells over a longer time. It is rationalized that this continuation therapy given over protracted periods may be more effective in destroying leukemic cells that are dividing slowly.

4. The *CNS phase* generally extends from induction through intensification and at least part of maintenance. In standard and intermediate-risk ALL, this phase is composed of intrathecal chemotherapy.

Treatment of standard ALL and intermediate-risk ALL used by the authors outside of a national protocol setting is as follows.

Induction. Vincristine, dexamethasone, and L-asparaginase are used and achieve a complete remission in approximately 95 per cent of patients. Vincristine is given once weekly for 4 weeks at 1.5 mg per M^2 (maximum of 2 mg). L-Asparaginase is given twice weekly for 3 weeks at 10,000 units per M^2. Intramuscular L-asparaginase is used because of the lower incidence of severe allergic reactions, including anaphylaxis, when it is given by this route compared with the intravenous route. Dexamethasone, at a dose of 6 mg per M^2 by mouth in three divided doses for 4 weeks, is used in place of prednisone because it penetrates better into the CNS. The dose is then tapered over 1 week.

Intensification. Methotrexate is infused at 1 gram per M^2 during 24 hours with hydration (3000 ml per M^2 during 24 hours). Hydration is continued for 72 hours. Methotrexate is followed by L-asparaginase, 10,000 units per M^2 intramuscularly, given once at 48 hours (24 hours after completion of methotrexate treatment). Also, leucovorin neutralization is used at 15 mg per M^2 intravenously, starting at 48 hours and given every 6 hours three times. Methotrexate is used to penetrate into sanctuaries such as the CNS, testes, liver, spleen, and bone marrow. L-Asparaginase is used because it has been shown to improve the prognosis when administered as intensification early in therapy. Also, these two agents are combined because of synergism. This regimen is given at week 6 after diagnosis provided that blood cell counts are adequate and the patient is in complete remission. It is then repeated every 2 weeks for a total of six occasions.

If there is mucositis, methotrexate levels in the serum are measured and additional leucovorin is administered. Complete blood cell counts and chemistries are monitored.

Maintenance. A standard maintenance therapy includes daily oral 6-mercaptopurine, 50 mg per M^2 by mouth daily, and weekly oral methotrexate, 20 mg per M^2. Pulses of a single dose of vincristine given intravenously with dexamethasone for 7 days at a dose of 6 mg per M^2 per day each month are also used. During this week, 6-mercaptopurine and methotrexate are discontinued. Maintenance therapy is given to complete 2 full years (i.e., approximately 20 months of maintenance). Complete blood cell counts and chemistries are monitored.

Central Nervous System Prophylaxis. Triple intrathecal therapy (methotrexate, cytosine arabinoside, and hydrocortisone) is used from induction through intensification and through approximately 8 months of maintenance; that is, triple intrathecal therapy is given for 1 year. The dose is calculated and based on age rather than body surface area because this more accurately reflects the size of the CNS compartment (Table 3). A total of 15 doses of intrathecal chemotherapy is administered.

Because of substantial toxicity to the CNS, including a reduction in IQ (which is worse in patients younger than 5 years of age), radiation as CNS prophylaxis is *not* used in this group of patients with a relatively favorable prognosis.

TABLE 3. **Dosage in Triple Intrathecal Chemotherapy**

Drug	Dose (mg)				
	<1 yr	1–2 yr	2–3 yr	3–10 yr	>10 yr
Methotrexate*,†	6	8	10	12	15
Hydrocortisone*	6	8	10	12	15
Cytosine arabinoside*	12	16	20	24	30

*Dissolve in Elliot's B solution or preservative-free saline.
†Preservative-free formulation.

Relapse

Bone Marrow Relapse (During Chemotherapy).

These children can readily achieve remission. Eighty-five per cent will achieve a second complete remission with oral prednisone, 40 mg per M^2 daily, vincristine, 1.5 mg per M^2 weekly (maximum 2 mg per M^2), L-asparaginase, 10,000 units per M^2 intramuscularly twice weekly, and daunorubicin (Cerubidine), 45 mg per M^2 intravenously once weekly. After a second remission, when feasible, these children should receive a bone marrow transplant. In this situation approximately one-third of patients are "salvaged." HLA-matched sibling bone marrow donors are used most often. However, recently computer-matched HLA donors have also been used or less than complete HLA-matched sibling donors, termed "mismatched bone marrow transplant donors."

An alternative approach has been the use of aggressive chemotherapy retreatment. Here, long-term cure rates appear to be improving and now may reach 10 or 15 per cent.

Bone Marrow Relapse After Cessation of Chemotherapy.

In children who have successfully completed chemotherapy and have received no treatment for more than 1 year, when they experience a bone marrow relapse there is a salvage rate of approximately 25 to 30 per cent. Intensive chemotherapy programs are generally used for these patients.

Extramedullary Relapse

CENTRAL NERVOUS SYSTEM. For isolated CNS relapse, it has been our practice to re-treat these patients intensively with triple intrathecal chemotherapy given weekly until the cerebrospinal fluid contains no cells. This treatment is followed by triple intrathecal chemotherapy on a monthly schedule.

At the same time, systemic reinduction with vincristine (Oncovin), steroids, and high-dose intravenous therapy such as methotrexate and cytosine arabinoside (Cytosar-U) is administered. Note that high-dose cytosine arabinoside, 3 grams per M^2, is not administered simultaneously with intrathecal chemotherapy because of CNS toxicity. After approximately 3 months of such a program, cranial or craniospinal radiation therapy is administered.

An alternative approach is the use of an intraventricular reservoir such as the Ommaya reservoir to administer chemotherapy into the ventricular spinal fluid. Again, craniospinal radiation is also used after intensive intravenous and intraventricular chemotherapy.

Salvage rates of approximately 25 to 30 per cent may be expected.

TESTICULAR RELAPSE. Methotrexate at a dose of 1 gram per M^2 has been shown to substantially decrease the chances for testicular relapse. Routine testicular biopsies during therapy or at the end of therapy to detect residual leukemia in the testes are of little or no benefit and do not appear to be indicated.

After the development of isolated testicular relapse, reinduction therapy, re-treatment of the CNS, and intensive intravenous therapy should be used, as should testicular radiation therapy.

Long-Term Complications

Unfortunately, cranial radiation has been associated with a reduction in IQ of approximately 10 to 12 points. Losses are greater in the younger child. Second primary cancers also have been seen in the irradiated sites. For these reasons, radiation should be avoided when feasible; however, in some high-risk ALL patients, it may still be needed.

ACUTE NONLYMPHOCYTIC LEUKEMIA

These leukemias account for 15 to 20 per cent of childhood leukemia. The FAB classification is used.

In general, treatment for ANLL in childhood parallels that in adults and should be intensive. We have treated M-5 pure (monocytic) leukemia separately because of its different biologic behavior.

The two principal agents on which therapy of ANLL has been based are daunomycin and cytosine arabinoside. There is little evidence that treatment, if intensive, needs to be continued beyond 6 months.

Standard induction therapy generally consists of cytosine arabinoside, 100 mg per M^2 daily as a continuous intravenous infusion for 7 days, and daunomycin, 45 mg per M^2 as an intravenous push daily on the first 3 days. Approximately 80 per cent of children achieve a complete remission.

After complete remission, four or five intensification courses are given. At present, high-dose cytosine arabinoside, 3 grams per M^2 every 12 hours, is generally used for at least one of these intensification courses. This course is often given as Capizzi-type regimen with 2 days (four doses) of high-dose cytosine arabinoside followed by L-asparaginase and then repeated 1 week later. Consolidation therapy (repeating the same drug program as during induction) is also often used. Other agents frequently employed include mitoxantrone (DHAD), amsacrine (m-AMSA*), and etoposide (VP-16).

Except for M-5, two or three doses of intrathe-

---

*Investigational drug.

cal chemotherapy are generally sufficient for CNS prophylaxis, and cranial radiation therapy is not needed. This may be because continuous intravenous cytosine arabinoside achieves 35 per cent of plasma levels in the cerebrospinal fluid and high-dose cytosine arabinoside (3 grams per M^2) achieves significant levels in the cerebrospinal fluid. Thus intravenous therapy is effective for CNS prophylaxis.

The use of bone marrow transplants in first line therapy remains controversial. Cure rates of 50 to 60 per cent are seen with transplants, but some select chemotherapy regimens are approaching a 50 per cent cure rate. With the considerable long-term toxicity after bone marrow transplant, these differences do not appear to be sufficient to justify bone marrow transplant in all patients with ANLL. Certain high-risk subgroups are an exception and at present merit immediate transplantation.

After bone marrow relapse, approximately 40 to 50 per cent of patients are successfully reinduced into complete remission. In this situation, bone marrow transplant offers the only viable avenue for cure.

The bone marrow aplasia, with resultant infections, gut toxicities, and other toxicities, is so profound after chemotherapy of ANLL that highly sophisticated support systems must be in place.

CHRONIC MYELOCYTIC LEUKEMIA

Philadelphia chromosome–positive chronic myelocytic leukemia (CML) is occasionally seen in childhood, mostly in the teenage years. It accounts for 1 to 3 per cent of childhood leukemias. It is managed like adult CML (more fully described in another chapter of this book). At present, bone marrow transplantation offers the only chance for cure. Recently, interferon therapy has shown some impressive early results.

Juvenile CML

Juvenile CML is a rare type of leukemia that accounts for less than 1 per cent of childhood leukemia. The term CML is a misnomer. This leukemia is most likely a variant of a myelodysplastic syndrome or ANLL. Cytogenetically, monosomy 7 may be seen.

The characteristic presentation includes high white blood cell count, large spleen, low platelet counts, high fetal hemoglobin level, altered immunoglobulin, and increased level of muramidase.

Treatment of juvenile CML has been uniformly disappointing, with survival of less than 1 year.

The recommended therapy now is bone marrow transplantation.

SUPPORT SYSTEMS

Treatment of Infections

Infectious complications account for approximately 90 per cent of deaths from leukemia, primarily because of the lack of functioning neutrophils and likely monocytes, which results from marrow replacement by leukemic cells or from marrow ablation by chemotherapy.

Antibiotics with broad-spectrum coverage are needed to treat the neutropenic febrile patient. With the widespread use of central lines such as the Hickman catheter, staphylococcal epidermitis has become the most common infection. We therefore use vancomycin, which is highly effective against this organism, and ceftazidine as our initial antibiotic regimen. Identification of the infecting organism may necessitate a different antibiotic. Alpha-hemolytic streptococcal sepsis appears to be increasing in prevalence. Again, vancomycin is the antibiotic of choice.

If a fever is unresponsive for 5 to 7 days, we add amphotericin B. With documented deep-seated fungal infections, protracted therapy with this antimicrobial agent is required.

Pneumocystis carinii pneumonia may complicate the course of therapy whether or not there are adequate numbers of neutrophils. Trimethoprim-sulfamethoxazole (Septra, Bactrim) given prophylactically (5 mg per kg per day of trimethoprim) in two divided doses three times weekly helps to prevent this type of pneumonia. Recently, pentamidine as an aerosol has been shown to prevent *Pneumocystis* pneumonia and may even be more effective than trimethoprim-sulfamethoxazole.

For overt *Pneumocystis* pneumonia, trimethoprim-sulfamethoxazole is administered in therapeutic doses. Trimetrexate has also been shown to be effective.

Fluids

When there is rapid destruction of a large leukemic burden, for example, during induction therapy, particularly in children with a high white blood cell count or a lymphoma-leukemia syndrome, an enormous release of purines occurs, leading to the formation of uric acid. Uric acid is not soluble in acid urine, and uric acid nephropathy may result. To prevent this nephropathy, the following measures are important: hydration with twice maintenance (3000 ml per M^2 per 24 hours); the use of allopurinol, 300 mg per M^2 per day by mouth; and the use of sodium bicarbonate intravenously or by mouth to keep the urine pH *above* 7.0.

Nutrition

Maintenance of adequate nutrition is important, particularly for the ability of these children to fight infections. If oral caloric intake is insufficient, we have utilized nasogastric tube feedings. If this approach is not feasible, we have used central hyperalimentation.

Lines

Indwelling right atrium catheters are commonly used for administration of antibiotics, chemotherapy, and nutritional support and for blood sampling. They have proved to be a mixed blessing to these patients in that their use has reduced the number of injections but has also led to a substantial incidence of line infections and even sepsis. The incidence of infections appears to be higher with more aggressive treatment regimens and resultant profound neutropenia. Fastidious care of these catheters is indicated and appears to decrease the chances for infection.

Blood Products

Anemia is common in these patients either because of disease or because of chemotherapy. Radiated packed red blood cells may be given at 10 ml per kg if the patient's hemoglobin concentration is higher than 5 grams per dl. If the patient's hemoglobin concentration is less than 5 grams per dl, smaller volumes of red blood cells are given so as not to overload the cardiovascular system. We attempt to keep the hemoglobin concentration above 9 grams per dl.

Radiated platelets may also be used (approximately 6 units per M^2). In view of infection and platelet consumption, we attempt to keep platelet count above 30,000 per microliter. Attempts to maintain platelets depend to some extent on the stage of disease. Soon after diagnosis, platelet transfusions are used more aggressively, whereas this may not be true later in the disease.

Psychosocial Support

These children and their families are subjected to enormous stress. Out-of-pocket financial losses are substantial. Marital stress and divorce are common. Even in children who are cured, these families worry greatly. The children, when possible, should be managed as outpatients and kept at home. A team approach is critical. Oncologic nurse-practitioners, psychologists, social workers, and parent advocates, as well as the pediatric oncologist, are all important parts of this support system.

THE CHRONIC LEUKEMIAS

method of
ROBERT PETER GALE, M.D., Ph.D.
UCLA School of Medicine
Los Angeles, California

and

KENNETH A. FOON, M.D.
Roswell Park Memorial Institute
Buffalo, New York

CHRONIC MYELOGENOUS LEUKEMIA

Chronic myelogenous leukemia (CML) is a hematologic neoplasm characterized by the proliferation and accumulation of myeloid cells and their progenitors. Malignant transformation in CML typically occurs in a pluripotent stem cell capable of giving rise to granulocytes, monocytes and macrophages, red blood cell (RBC), megakaryocytes and platelets, and B lymphocytes. Less often, T lymphocytes are involved. Although the transformed cell in CML is pluripotent, the major manifestation of the disease is increased granulopoiesis. About one-half of affected persons also have increased platelet levels; RBC elevation is rare.

More than 90 per cent of persons with CML have the Ph^1 chromosome. This usually results from a translocation between chromosomes 9 and 22 designated t(9;22). Occasionally, a third or even a fourth chromosome may be involved; these situations are referred to as complex translocations. Recent molecular studies indicate that these translocations result in the activation of the *abl* proto-oncogene by recombination with a gene on chromosome 22 designated *bcr* for "breakpoint cluster region." The precise mechanism whereby the activation of *abl* leads to CML is unknown.

CML is a biphasic disease characterized by chronic and acute phases. About 50 to 75 per cent of cases have an intermediate accelerated phase. The chronic phase of CML can be envisioned as a preleukemia in that cell differentiation is normal or nearly normal. Consequently, the major objective of therapy for this phase of CML is to control granulocyte (and occasionally thrombocyte) production. This can be achieved by drugs or with interferon (see later). The acute phase, in contrast, is characterized by a block of differentiation resembling acute leukemia. Several forms of the acute phase have been identified, including myeloid and B lymphoid. Less often, the acute phase can be dominated by erythroblast or megakaryoblast proliferation. An acute phase involving T lymphocytes is rare. About 90 per cent of cases of acute phase CML are myeloid or lymphoid; the usual ratio is 2:1. Recent detailed studies suggest that many cases of acute phase CML are of mixed phenotype. Transition to the acute phase is often accompanied by further cytogenetic changes in the leukemia clone, including a second Ph[1] chromosome, isochromosome 17, trisomy 8, or trisomy 19. Therapy for acute-phase CML resembles that for acute leukemia but is usually unsuccessful; death occurs within about 3 months to 1 year.

Survival of persons with CML is determined predominantly by the duration of the chronic phase. Median survival is 3 to 4 years in most studies. The likelihood of transformation to the acute phase is about 10 per cent in the first year after diagnosis, increasing to 20 to 25 per cent per year thereafter. It is important to realize that this risk is constant after the first year. Consequently, in persons with CML for 4 or 5 years, the risk of transformation to the acute phase in the succeeding year is no greater than it was 3 or 4 years earlier. This consideration mandates a relatively conservative therapeutic strategy in most instances, even with an increasing duration of disease. Several factors at diagnosis are correlated with the duration of the chronic phase, including sex (female > male), white blood cell (WBC) count (low > high), percentage of blood or bone marrow blasts (low > high), and spleen size (small > large). Although prognostic factor analyses distinguish subpopulations of persons with different prognoses, they are not sufficiently precise to predict the course of individual patients.

The accelerated phase represents a transition between the chronic and acute phases. In some instances, there is no accelerated phase; the transition to the acute phase is abrupt. However, most persons have a 3-month to 1-year period in which their disease is increasingly difficult to control. Although there is no uniform definition of the accelerated phase, common factors include fever, weight loss, a requirement for increasing doses of cytotoxic drugs, anemia, basophilia, and thrombocytopenia or thrombocytosis. Cytogenetic analyses may indicate new abnormalities in the accelerated phase, such as a second Ph[1] chromosome, isochromosome 17, trisomy 8, trisomy 19, or other structural or numerical abnormalities.

Therapy

Chronic Phase

The therapeutic strategy in the chronic phase is to control the extent of proliferation of the malignant clone, as measured by the WBC level. This is typically achieved with cytotoxic drugs, most often with busulfan (Myleran) or hydroxyurea (Hydrea).

Busulfan is an alkylating drug that is cell cycle nonspecific. Therapy is usually initiated with doses of 4 to 6 mg per day for about 2 to 4 weeks or until the WBC count is about 15×10^9 per liter. Treatment is then discontinued and the WBC count monitored (because it may continue to decrease after discontinuation of treatment). There is also usually regression (or resolution) of splenomegaly and other clinical features associated with CML. Some persons achieve a stable WBC count after this regimen and require no additional therapy for several months. Others require reinstitution of busulfan immediately to maintain the WBC count at less than 15×10^9 per liter. The usual maintenance dose of busulfan is 2 mg per day. Persons with busulfan-induced control of the WBC count do not achieve true remission (as in acute myelogenous leukemia, AML) because most, if not all, myeloid cells are produced by the neoplastic clone and retain the Ph[1] chromosome.

Busulfan therapy is associated with few adverse effects. Gastrointestinal toxicity is rare. Amenorrhea and sterility can occur, so busulfan is best avoided in treating prepubertal patients. Increased skin pigmentation is a rare complication of busulfan therapy, as is pulmonary fibrosis. Severe bone marrow suppression is the most serious adverse consequence of busulfan therapy. The blood count should be carefully monitored and therapy promptly interrupted when there is a suggestion of bone marrow failure. Because busulfan is associated with pulmonary fibrosis, it is best avoided in persons who are potential bone marrow transplant candidates.

Hydroxyurea is also commonly used to treat chronic phase CML. Hydroxyurea is a cell-cycle–active alkylating drug. The usual initial dose is 1 to 2 grams (20 mg per kg) twice daily.* This results in a prompt decrease in the WBC count. The dose is usually reduced to 1 to 2 grams once daily when the WBC count is 25 to 50×10^9 per liter and then adjusted to maintain the WBC count at about 10 to 15×10^9 per liter. In contrast to busulfan, hydroxyurea must be given continuously to control the WBC level; unmaintained remissions are not achieved. Also, as with busulfan, myeloid cells in persons who respond remain Ph[1] chromosome–positive, indicating their origin from the leukemia clone.

Adverse side effects of hydroxyurea are rare. Mild nausea can be decreased by postprandial administration. Skin or nail changes and fever are less common. As indicated, hydroxyurea is preferred in potential transplant recipients be-

---

*This dose may exceed the dose recommended by the manufacturer.

cause, unlike busulfan, it is not associated with pulmonary fibrosis. Hydroxyurea is particularly useful when it is necessary to decrease the WBC count rapidly from levels more than 100×10^9 per liter. In this instance, it is important to prevent uric acid nephropathy by administering hydration, allopurinol, and possibly corticosteroids.

Other drugs are rarely used to treat chronic phase CML. There are relatively few data regarding cytarabine, anthracyclines, mercaptopurine, or 6-thioguanine. Nor are there sufficient data to evaluate drug combinations such as cytarabine and 6-thioguanine or busulfan and mercaptopurine.

Persons with CML unresponsive to busulfan or hydroxyurea may respond to other alkylating drugs, such as melphalan or cyclophosphamide, or to drug combinations. Sometimes it is necessary to switch to these drugs when platelet levels are low because they are less suppressive of thrombopoiesis than busulfan. There are limited trials of intensive chemotherapy in chronic phase CML. The object of this approach is to achieve hematologic remission without the Ph^1 chromosome. In most instances this approach is unsuccessful, and it is not widely used.

Interferon. There are also recent reports of therapy of chronic phase CML with interferon—usually interferon-alpha.* Interferon treatment can result in control of the WBC count and platelet level over several weeks. The usual initial dose is 2 to 5 million units per M^2 per day, either daily or every other day, until the WBC count is about 10 to 15×10^9 per liter; a maintenance dose is then selected. Interferon therapy, in contrast to busulfan and hydroxyurea, decreases the proportion of myeloid cells with the Ph^1 chromosome. Decreases exceeding 50 per cent occur in about 30 per cent of cases; some persons (<10 per cent) may become Ph^1 chromosome negative. Usually these changes are transient, lasting for several weeks to a few months. However, some cases (<5 per cent) remain Ph^1 chromosome negative for 1 year or more. It is not known whether these cytogenetic changes result in improved survival; randomized trials are in progress.

Transplantation. Recently, bone marrow transplants were performed in chronic phase CML. The usual donor is an HLA-identical sibling. This results in about 50 per cent 3-year leukemia-free survival. The results are best in persons less than 25 to 35 years of age. There are also controversial data indicating that results are superior when the duration of the chronic phase is less than 1

year. Because CML cannot be cured with chemotherapy and probably not with interferon, it seems reasonable to recommend transplantation in persons less than 50 years of age. The optimal timing is not known, but a delay of about 1 year is not unreasonable. Transplants from donors other than HLA-identical siblings, such as unrelated, HLA-matched persons, result in about 25 per cent 3-year leukemia-free survival. Although imperfect, the long-term results are superior to those of chemotherapy. Consequently, this approach should be considered in young persons with CML. The results of autotransplants in CML are poor and are presently considered investigational.

Splenectomy. Splenectomy is of no value in the routine management of chronic phase CML, and controlled trials indicate no impact on survival. However, splenectomy may be useful in certain patients, such as those with progressive splenomegaly unresponsive to drugs and radiation and those in whom severe thrombocytopenia (from hypersplenism) prevents appropriate chemotherapy. Severe anemia (from hypersplenism) may also respond to splenectomy.

Radiation. There is little role for radiation therapy in chronic phase CML. Radiation is sometimes used to reduce chemotherapy-unresponsive splenomegaly, other tumor masses, or splenic infarction. It may also be useful in persons with splenomegaly in whom the risk of surgery is high.

It should be noted that although most therapies of chronic phase CML attempt to control the WBC level, to reduce the proportion of Ph^1 chromosome–positive cells, or both, no data convincingly show an impact on the duration of the chronic phase or on survival.

Acute Phase

Chemotherapy. Therapy of acute phase CML is difficult and is not curative. As indicated, several forms of the acute phase have been distinguished, including myeloid, lymphoid, megakaryocyte, and erythroid. Cases of acute phase CML in which the cells contain the enzyme terminal deoxynucleotidyl transferase (TdT) may respond to therapy with vincristine and prednisone. These are usually, but not always, lymphoid acute phase. When this therapy is successful (about 50 per cent of TdT-positive cases), a second chronic phase is achieved. Some persons receive 24 Gy of central nervous system radiation at this point because the disease resembles acute lymphocytic leukemia, but there are no convincing data showing that this is useful. The second chronic phase lasts for a median of 3 to 6 months and is terminated by a second acute phase, which is usually resistant to further therapy.

Treatment of TdT-negative (usually myeloid)

---

*This is an approved drug but this use is not listed by the manufacturer.

acute phase CML is even less successful. Regimens used to treat AML are often given, but the remission rate is less than 25 per cent and the median survival is less than 3 months. Another approach is to attempt to control the WBC count with hydroxyurea or cytarabine, either alone or combined with mercaptopurine or thioguanine. This can prolong survival by a few months but is not curative.

Interferon is ineffective in acute phase CML.

Transplantation from an HLA-identical sibling results in 10 to 15 per cent 3-year leukemia-free survival; this is the only curative approach to acute phase CML.

Persons with megakaryoblastic acute phase CML are difficult to treat and may develop severe hemorrhagic complications. Platelets sometimes respond to short courses of high-dose busulfan (10 mg twice daily for 5 days*) or to uracil mustard. It is also possible to reduce platelet levels rapidly but temporarily by plateletpheresis.

The prognosis of persons with acute phase CML is poor, with median survival of less than 1 year. There are no long-term survivors, except for transplant recipients. Consequently, the therapeutic approach should be palliative, predominantly to control levels of WBC and platelets, to prevent complications of leukostasis and thrombocytosis.

CHRONIC LYMPHATIC LEUKEMIAS
Chronic Lymphocytic Leukemia

Chronic lymphocytic leukemia (CLL) is a hematologic neoplasm characterized by proliferation and accumulation of mature-*appearing* but *biologically immature* lymphocytes. CLL is the most common leukemia in the United States and Europe, accounting for approximately 30 per cent of all cases; it is extremely rare in the Orient. CLL typically occurs in persons over 50 years (median age, 60 years); occasionally, it develops in young adults or even children. CLL affects males twice as often as females.

In most instances, CLL results from malignant transformation of a B lymphocyte; a small proportion of cases (<5 per cent) involve T lymphocytes. CLL is a clonal disease; the cells express a single immunoglobulin light chain, either kappa or lambda, on the cell surface membrane. More sophisticated techniques confirm clonality by showing unique immunoglobulin-idiotype specificities, a single pattern of glucose-6-phosphate dehydrogenase activity, clonal chromosomal abnormalities, and immunoglobulin gene re-

arrangements. Persons with T cell CLL may also have clonal chromosomal abnormalities and clonal rearrangements of T cell antigen receptor genes.

Most cytogenetic abnormalities in CLL involve chromosome 12 or 14. Trisomy 12 is usually the only abnormality in early disease; in advanced disease, it occurs in combination with other chromosome changes. According to one study, survival of persons with trisomy 12 as the sole abnormality is no different from survival of those with normal karyotypes; persons with additional cytogenetic abnormalities have poorer survival.

Clinical Features

Hypogammaglobulinemia occurs in approximately 50 per cent of patients with CLL. Infections, particularly with encapsulated microorganisms, are a frequent cause of morbidity and mortality. Their incidence is related to the degree of hypogammaglobulinemia. Persons with CLL may develop features of autoimmunity. For example, autoimmune hemolytic anemia occurs in 10 to 25 per cent of patients some time during the course of the disease. Some persons develop either idiopathic thrombocytopenic purpura or neutropenia related to autoantibodies to platelets or neutrophils, respectively. Rarely, patients develop a syndrome resembling pure red blood cell aplasia; this is most commonly associated with T rather than B CLL. It is important to distinguish these autoimmune causes of anemia from those related to bone marrow infiltration for accurate disease staging (see later).

The clinical course of CLL is variable; many patients are older (median age, 60 years) and have only elevated lymphocyte levels or asymptomatic lymphadenopathy or splenomegaly; others have complicating medical disorders. These patients may require no specific treatment and are unlikely to die of leukemia. In contrast, occasional persons with CLL may present with lymphoma-like symptoms or features of bone marrow failure, including severe anemia and thrombocytopenia. These persons have a rapid, progressive course, with a median survival of less than 2 years. Most patients with CLL fall into an intermediate group that does reasonably well for several years without therapy, eventually requiring specific treatment. Ideally, one should use prognostic factors to determine the patient's prognosis so as to design optimal therapeutic strategies. In 1975, Rai and coworkers proposed a five-stage staging system for CLL, shown in Table 1 (Rai KR, Sawitsky A, Cronkite EP, et al: Clinical staging of chronic lymphocytic leukemia. Blood 46:219–234, 1975). Recently, the Rai classification was modified into three groups: Stage 0, Stages I and II, and Stages III and IV. Another

---

*This dose may exceed the manufacturer's recommended dose.

TABLE 1. **Staging Systems for Chronic Lymphocytic Leukemia**

Rai Staging System

Stage	Criteria	Median Survival (mo)
0	Lymphocytes > 15 × 10⁹/liter Bone marrow > 40% lymphocytes	>150
I	As above, with lymphadenopathy	100
II	Blood and bone marrow lymphocytes plus liver and/or spleen enlarged, with or without lymphocytes	70
III	Blood and bone marrow lymphocytes plus anemia (Hb < 11 grams/dl)	20
IV	Blood and bone marrow lymphocytes plus thrombocytopenia (platelet level < 100 × 10⁹/liter)	20

Binet Staging System

Group	Criteria	Median Survival (mo)
A	No anemia or thrombocytopenia; fewer than three of the following five areas involved: axillary, inguinal cervical (unilateral or bilateral) lymph nodes, liver, spleen	>100
B	No anemia or thrombocytopenia; three or more involved areas	80
C	Anemia (Hb < 10 grams/dl) and/or thrombocytopenia (platelet level < 100 × 10⁹/liter)	20

Abbreviation: Hb = hemoglobin.

staging system is that of Binet (Table 1), in which patients are divided into Stages A, B, and C based on criteria that are similar (but not identical) to those of the Rai system (Binet JL, Auguier A, Dighiero G, et al: A new prognostic classification of chronic lymphocytic leukemia derived from a multivariate survival analysis. Cancer 48:198–216, 1981). This system is also useful and closely resembles the modified Rai staging system. The Rai system is more commonly used in the United States; the Binet system is used in other countries.

Therapy

Persons with CLL commonly develop hypogammaglobulinemia, which may be severe. Prophylaxis with intravenous immunoglobulin can prevent or modify bacterial infections; it is being investigated for the treatment of immune thrombocytopenia and anemia that develop in CLL.

Immune-mediated hemolytic anemia, thrombocytopenia, and neutropenia are generally treated with prednisone. Persons who fail to respond may require splenectomy. Chemotherapy may be required to control the underlying disease. Rare persons with CLL develop a hyperviscosity syndrome and require plasmapheresis, corticosteroids, or chemotherapy. Persons with CLL may develop a hypermetabolic state and hyperuricemia, particularly after therapy; these are usually treated with hydration and allopurinol.

One unresolved question in the treatment of CLL is when to initiate therapy. There are no data indicating that therapy of persons with only an elevated leukocyte count and lymphadenopathy prolongs survival. When limited lymph node enlargement causes symptoms, local or systemic therapy may be initiated. Most physicians initiate systemic therapy when patients develop anemia, thrombocytopenia, or massive hepatosplenomegaly. Three classes of therapeutic agents are commonly used: alkylating agents, corticosteroids, and radiation.

Chlorambucil (Leukeran) is the drug most commonly used to treat CLL. It is an aromatic derivative of nitrogen mustard that is absorbed orally. The standard dose of chlorambucil is 0.08 to 0.12 mg per kg of body weight per day; it may also be given at a dose of 0.4 to 1 mg per kg once every 2 to 4 weeks. Response rates to chlorambucil are about 60 per cent, with 10 to 20 per cent complete remissions. Responses may take several months to achieve. Cyclophosphamide (Cytoxan), 50 to 100 mg per M² orally daily or 300 mg per M² orally for 5 days every month, is probably as effective as chlorambucil and can be given intravenously or orally. Corticosteroids are used to control leukocytosis and to treat immune-mediated hemolytic anemia and thrombocytopenia. The usual dose is 30 to 60 mg per M² of body surface area per day. Corticosteroids should not be used alone to treat CLL except for autoimmune hemolytic anemia and thrombocytopenia, or in advanced disease unresponsive to other therapies. Prednisone is often given with chlorambucil. Often prednisone is started 1 to 2 weeks before chlorambucil is begun. Fludarabine monophosphate is also effective in CLL. In recent studies, partial and complete responses were reported in almost 50 per cent of patients resistant to standard therapies. 2-Deoxycoformycin (pentostatin), an adenosine deaminase inhibitor, also has activity in CLL. Both fludarabine and pentostatin are investigational.

The role of multidrug chemotherapy in CLL is controversial. As indicated, corticosteroids are often included in combination with chlorambucil, but convincing data that this increases the response or improves survival are not available.

Combination therapy with cyclophosphamide (300 mg per M² orally days 1 to 5 every month or 800 mg per M² on day 1 every month intravenously), vincristine (1 mg per M² intravenously on day 1 every month), and prednisone (40 mg per M² orally days 1 to 5 every month) (CVP) is used in advanced disease. Response rates are comparable to those of chlorambucil or chlorambucil with or without prednisone; there may be a role for this combination in persons resistant to chlorambucil. Recent reports suggest that adding doxorubicin on day 1, 25 mg per M² to CVP improves survival. Other chemotherapy combinations are being investigated but cannot be recommended at present.

Whole-body irradiation is proposed as a therapy for advanced CLL. This approach has severe hematologic toxicity, and responses are no better than those achieved with chemotherapy. Despite these limitations, whole-body irradiation may be useful in persons resistant to chemotherapy. Local irradiation is used to treat lymphadenopathy compromising vital organs and painful bone lesions. Splenic irradiation is also used to treat painful splenomegaly, progressive lymphocytosis, anemia, and thrombocytopenia.

There is no role for splenectomy in the routine therapy of CLL. However, it may be useful for hemolytic anemia, thrombocytopenia, pancytopenia, and painful splenomegaly. Splenectomy may lead to a sustained improvement in previously depressed hematologic parameters in persons with hypersplenism.

In summary, persons with low-stage disease (Stage 0, I, or A) have not been convincingly shown to benefit from treatment. Initial therapy for persons requiring treatment is usually chlorambucil or cyclophosphamide, with or without prednisone, given as pulse therapy every 2 to 4 weeks. Combinations of other chemotherapeutic agents should be reserved for more advanced disease. Persons with intermediate-stage disease (Stage I, II, or B) have comparable response rates to chlorambucil and CVP. Persons with advanced disease (Stage III, IV, or C) respond favorably to CVP with low-dose doxorubicin, but this combination cannot be recommended until these data are confirmed.

MAINTENANCE THERAPY. Another unanswered question in the therapy of CLL is whether maintenance chemotherapy is useful. Currently, there is little evidence that maintenance chemotherapy in CLL improves survival, although one large study suggested that 18 months of treatment prolonged survival in persons with Stage III and IV CLL.

Prolymphocytic Leukemia

Prolymphocytic leukemia (PL) is characterized by a leukocyte count of more than 100×10^9 per liter in which prolymphocytes predominate. Extensive spleen involvement is common, as are hepatomegaly and bone marrow infiltration; lymphadenopathy is usually absent or minimal. The disease is typically aggressive and responds poorly to therapy. The median age of persons with PL is approximately 60 years, and there is a strong male predominance. The etiology is unknown.

Clinical Features

Typically, the presenting features are fatigue, weakness, and weight loss. Fever unassociated with infection is also common. Some persons experience abdominal pain and early satiety from massive splenomegaly. The outstanding physical sign is spleen enlargement; hepatomegaly may also be prominent. Lymphadenopathy is absent or modest. Rare persons have petechiae and purpura from thrombocytopenia.

The leukocyte count exceeds 100×10^9 per liter and is composed predominantly of prolymphocytes. There is often anemia, with hemoglobin level less than 12 grams per dl, and thrombocytopenia with a platelet level less than 150×10^9 per liter. Some persons have granulocytopenia.

Therapy

PL is typically aggressive, with a rapid downhill course. Combination chemotherapy including cyclophosphamide, doxorubicin, vincristine, and prednisone is often used (doses described above); complete remissions are reported. Splenic irradiation is also used to treat PL. The role of splenectomy has not been clearly defined, but it is reported to be successful in rare patients.

Hairy Cell Leukemia

Hairy cell leukemia accounts for 1 to 2 per cent of the leukemias diagnosed annually. It affects males five times more often than females. The median age is approximately 50 years. In the United States, most patients are caucasian; a minority are black, Oriental, or Hispanic. Hairy cell leukemia is typically a clonal proliferation of B lymphocytes.

Clinical Features

The onset of symptoms is usually insidious; the most common presenting complaints are weakness and fatigue. One-third of patients tend to bleed with easy bruising; one-third have recent recurrent infections. Abdominal discomfort from an enlarged spleen is common. Some persons have weight loss, fever, and night sweats. Splenomegaly is the most common physical finding at diagnosis; 10 to 90 per cent of persons have massive spleen enlargement. Approximately 10 per cent of patients have lymphadenopathy, and 20 per cent have hepatomegaly with abnormal liver function tests. Most persons present with mild to moderate normochromic, normocytic anemia secondary to replacement of the bone marrow by leukemia cells and to hypersplenism. Approximately 20 per cent of patients have a leukemia phase. Eighty per cent of affected persons have neutropenia, and 50 per cent have fewer than 100×10^9 platelets per liter. Qualitative platelet abnormalities are common.

Therapy

Approximately 10 per cent of persons with hairy cell leukemia never require treatment. They are usually older and have only modest splenomegaly and granulocytes levels of 1×10^9 per liter or more. The remainder ultimately require therapy. First line therapy for hairy cell leukemia is splenectomy. It is reported that spleen size does not predict the response to splenectomy. In approximately two-thirds of patients, platelets return to normal levels; this response also does not correlate with spleen size but rather with the degree of bone marrow replacement by hairy cells. It is suggested that those with extensive replacement of bone marrow by hairy cells might benefit from alternative therapies. The response to splenectomy is complete in approximately 40 per cent of persons, with normalization of blood counts. Usually a small percentage of hairy cells persist in the blood. After splenectomy, approximately one-half of patients show disease progression several months to more than 10 years later. Until recently, persons with progressive disease received chlorambucil. This improves erythrocyte and platelet levels but not granulocyte levels. Other therapies include fluoxymesterone (Halotestin), oxymetholone, and intensive combination chemotherapy; these are not currently recommended.

Newer therapies are active in hairy cell leukemia. Low doses (2 million units per M^2 three times weekly with interferon-alfa-2b or 3 million units daily with interferon-alfa-2a) induce partial or complete remissions in 90 per cent of cases. Because less than 5 per cent of persons become resistant to interferon, and because 90 per cent have normalization or near normalization of blood counts, most live normal lives without blood transfusions, bleeding, or infections. Toxicity at these low doses is usually restricted to mild

fatigue and malaise. Many persons with good partial remissions or complete remissions can discontinue interferon for periods of 1 to 3 years; they respond again when the disease progresses.

2-Deoxycoformycin is also effective in hairy cell leukemia. Treatment with 4 mg per M^2 intravenously every 2 weeks produces complete and partial remissions in over 90 per cent of cases. 2-Deoxycoformycin leads to a more rapid and more complete response than interferon-alpha. Toxicities include rash, diarrhea, nausea, and vomiting; these reactions are generally mild at these doses. Recent data suggest that 2-deoxycoformycin causes profound immunosuppression. A randomized trial of 2-deoxycoformycin versus interferon-alpha is under way.

In summary, splenectomy is recommended in persons who are good surgical candidates and whose bone marrow is not diffusely replaced by hairy cells. Interferon-alpha is recommended if splenectomy is not chosen or if it fails. 2-Deoxycoformycin is available only for experimental studies.

Adult T Cell Leukemia and Lymphoma

Adult T cell leukemia and lymphoma (ATL) is a T cell lymphoproliferative syndrome first described in Japan and later identified in the United States, the Caribbean, and other countries. ATL is characterized by pleomorphic, neoplastic cells with membrane features of mature T helper lymphocytes and is often rapidly fatal.

Clinical Features

Presenting features include lymphadenopathy, hepatomegaly, splenomegaly, cutaneous infiltration with neoplastic T cells, hypercalcemia (with or without lytic bone lesions), and interstitial pulmonary infiltrates. Development of ATL is associated with infection by human T cell lymphotrophic virus-1 (HTLV-1). The median age of persons with ATL is approximately 40 years. They typically present with an elevated leukocyte count ranging from 5 to 100 $\times 10^9$ per liter. There are circulating malignant lymphocytes in most cases; anemia and thrombocytopenia are uncommon. The onset of symptoms is typically acute, with rapidly rising cutaneous lesions, as well as lymphadenopathy, hypercalcemia, or both.

Therapy

Treatment with combination chemotherapy including doxorubicin results in complete clinical remission in many persons. However, the duration of response is typically only 12 months. Relapses often occur at the sites of initial disease;

new sites include the skin, liver, and central nervous system.

Cutaneous T Cell Lymphoma

Cutaneous T cell lymphoma (CTCL) consists of mycosis fungoides and Sézary's syndrome. These disorders are malignant proliferations of T lymphocytes of the helper phenotype in which the initial clinical presentation is in the epidermis.

CTCL is an uncommon malignancy in the United States, with approximately 1500 new cases per year. It occurs twice as often in males as in females; it is less frequent in black than in caucasian persons. The median age at diagnosis is 55 years. Initial skin lesions are clinically and histologically nonspecific, and it may take up to 10 years before the diagnosis is confirmed. Median survival after histologic diagnosis is approximately 10 years.

Clinical Features

Most persons with CTCL progress through distinct cutaneous stages, beginning with a premycotic," erythematous, or eczematoid stage, followed by an infiltrative "plaque" stage and finally the "tumor" stage. The course of this progression is variable but commonly lasts for many years.

Sézary's syndrome is characterized by pruritus, generalized exfoliative erythroderma, and abnormal hyperconvoluted mononuclear cells in the peripheral blood. Its biologic features are similar to those of the other forms of mycosis fungoides; currently, these entities are considered CTCL. Most patients with generalized erythroderma have circulating "Sézary's" cells in varying numbers; 25 per cent of those in the plaque or tumor stage also have circulating Sézary's cells.

Therapy

Four therapeutic modalities can produce remissions in most persons with CTCL: topical nitrogen mustard; photochemotherapy with psoralen and ultraviolet A light; radiotherapy, particularly whole-body electron beam therapy; and systemic chemotherapy. However, cure is uncommon and is achieved only in early disease.

Topical nitrogen mustard is useful in persons in the early cutaneous stages. In more advanced stages, this approach is used to supplement other therapies directed against lymph node or visceral disease. The approach to whole-body therapy is to apply 10 mg of nitrogen mustard diluted in 60 ml of tap water daily. This is continued for up to 12 months in persons who respond. The frequency of application is reduced to every other day for an additional 1 to 2 years; therapy is discontinued

after 3 years in persons whose cutaneous lesions completely disappear.

Psoralen is a phototoxic furocoumarin activated by ultraviolet A light and binds covalently and reversibly to DNA. Ultraviolet A light penetrates only the upper part of the dermis. A 60 per cent complete remission rate is reported with psoralen; persons with generalized erythroderma and tumors have lower response rates than those with plaque disease. Psoralen is usually given at a dose of 0.6 mg per kg orally 2 hours before ultraviolet A light therapy. Treatments are initially given three times per week. After resolution of cutaneous lesions, maintenance therapy may be given every 2 to 4 weeks indefinitely.

Electron beam therapy produces complete remissions in 80 per cent of cases, with a median duration of 1.5 years. Twenty per cent of responders remain relapse free at 3 years, and few relapse. Typical treatment is with 4 Gy per week up to a total dose of 30 to 36 Gy (rad) in 8 to 9 weeks.

The most extensive experience with single-agent chemotherapy is with alkylating agents, including nitrogen mustard, cyclophosphamide, and chlorambucil. Response rates of 60 per cent with 15 per cent complete remissions are reported. Similar results are reported with methotrexate, bleomycin, and doxorubicin. Single-agent therapy does not cure CTCL. Combination drug therapy produces objective responses in more than 80 per cent of persons and complete responses in approximately 25 per cent. The duration of remission varies, with a median of about 1 year. Although the objective response rate is slightly higher than that with single agents, the superiority of combination therapy is not convincing. There are no reports of long-term disease-free survival after combination chemotherapy. Some data suggest that combinations of chemotherapy with whole-body electron beam therapy may be superior to standard approaches.

Experimental therapy includes interferon-alpha; a 50 per cent response rate is reported. Preliminary data suggest that 2-deoxycoformycin and 13-cis-retinoic acid may be active. Leukapheresis, alone or combined with oral psoralen, followed by leukapheresis and exposure ex vivo to ultraviolet A light, is also promising.

T Gamma Lymphoproliferative Disease (Large Granular Lymphocytic Leukemia)

Recently, a new T cell lymphoproliferative disorder termed "chronic T gamma lymphoproliferative disease" or "large granular lymphocytic leukemia" was recognized. This disease typically follows a chronic course characterized by lymphocytosis with bone marrow infiltration, neutropenia, and recurrent infections. The median age of affected persons is 60 years; virtually all are caucasian.

Clinical Features

The typical clinical presentation is that of recurrent pyogenic bacterial infections secondary to granulocytopenia. Also common is fatigue from anemia; the platelet level is normal. One-half of patients have minimal to moderate splenomegaly, approximately 20 per cent have hepatomegaly, and fewer than 10 per cent have lymphadenopathy. A small percentage have hypogammaglobulinemia, and approximately one-third have hypergammaglobulinemia. Skin infiltration is rare.

In this disease, T gamma lymphocytes infiltrate the bone marrow, spleen, and liver. Lymphocytosis of T gamma lymphocytes is common; in one-half of cases, lymphocyte levels are more than 10×10^9 per liter. Bone marrow lymphocytosis ranges from 30 to 75 per cent; some persons have reduced myelopoiesis. Approximately one-half of patients have severe granulocytopenia, with fewer than 5×10^9 granulocytes per liter.

Therapy

Most persons do not require specific therapy, although they may need supportive therapy for anemia and antibiotics for bacterial infections. Chemotherapy with single alkylating agents such as chlorambucil or cyclophosphamide, or combination chemotherapy with alkylating agents, vincristine, and prednisone, is used to treat progressive disease. Although chemotherapy is usually not effective, some patients benefit. Interferon-alpha is not effective. Some persons are treated by splenectomy or splenic irradiation without benefit. Because this disease appears to represent a spectrum from almost benign to aggressive malignancy, it is impossible to recommend a specific therapeutic approach. Clearly, many persons do not require chemotherapy and can be followed for many years with support only.

MALIGNANT LYMPHOMA
(Non-Hodgkin's Lymphomas)
method of
STEPHEN J. FORMAN, M.D., and
AUAYPORN P. NADEMANEE, M.D.
City of Hope National Medical Center
Duarte, California

The non-Hodgkin's lymphomas (NHL) are a heterogeneous group of lymphoid malignancies characterized by a natural history ranging from indolent to aggressive. The treatment approach to the NHL patient depends on the histology and stage of the lymphoma. The etiology of NHL is unknown. Individuals with congenital or acquired immunodeficiency syndrome and those who are immunosuppressed are at increased risk of developing NHL, including those who have received cyclosporine A after organ transplantation (kidney, heart). Similarly, patients with autoimmune diseases (Sjögren's syndrome, celiac sprue, inflammatory bowel disease) are predisposed to the development of NHL even in the absence of immunosuppressive therapy. In addition, specific clonal cytogenetic translocations have been noted in certain lymphomas, suggesting genetic alterations as a possible etiology.

Most patients with NHL present with either localized or generalized lymphadenopathy. The involved lymph nodes are usually rubbery and painless and may fluctuate in size, especially in low-grade lymphomas. About 20 per cent of the patients may have "B" symptoms of fever, night sweats, and weight loss. However, the presence of B symptoms does not have the same prognostic significance as in Hodgkin's disease.

The diagnosis and classification of NHL can be made only by biopsy. Although needle aspiration of lymph nodes may suggest a diagnosis, this technique does not yield sufficient tissue to classify lymphomas accurately. In addition, the histologic slides should be reviewed by an expert hematopathologist to confirm the diagnosis and to subclassify the lymphomas because the treatment depends on the specific cell type. Additional studies including cell surface marker studies, immunoglobulin gene rearrangements, and cytogenetics can further refine the diagnosis.

There are at least five different pathologic classifications of NHL. Rappaport's classification, which emphasizes an important relationship between the histologic patterns of the involved node and the prognosis, has been used most commonly. Recently, a new classification system, the Working Formulation (Table 1), which defines subtypes of NHL according to morphology, clinical features, and prognosis, has been widely accepted. It divides NHL into low-, intermediate-, and high-grade categories, which have clinical relevance in designing therapeutic plans and predicting the prognosis.

Once the diagnosis of NHL is established, patients require clinical staging evaluation, including a complete blood count; chemistry profiles; chest x-ray film; computed tomography scan of the chest, abdomen, and pelvis; and bone marrow aspiration and biopsy. Lymphangiography and staging laparotomy are reserved for selected patients with clinical Stage I disease when local irradiation with curative intent is being considered and the discovery of intra-abdominal disease would alter the treatment.

GENERAL PRINCIPLES OF TREATMENT

As in other tumors, the staging and histologic classification of the disease determine the appropriate therapy. The ultimate goal in the manage-

TABLE 1. **Classification of NHL**

Rappaport Classification	Working Formulation
	Low Grade
Diffuse lymphocytic, well differentiated	ML, small lymphocytic
Nodular, poorly differentiated lymphocytic	ML, follicular, predominantly small cleaved cell
Nodular, mixed lymphocytic-histiocytic	ML, follicular, mixed small cleaved and large cell
	Intermediate Grade
Nodular histiocytic	ML, follicular, predominantly large cell
Diffuse lymphocytic, poorly differentiated	ML, diffuse small cleaved cell
Diffuse mixed lymphocytic-histiocytic	ML, diffuse, mixed small and large cell
Diffuse histiocytic	ML, diffuse large cell
	High Grade
Diffuse histiocytic	ML, large cell immunoblastic
Lymphoblastic convoluted/nonconvoluted	ML, lymphoblastic
Undifferentiated, Burkitt's and non-Burkitt's	ML, small noncleaved cell

Abbreviation: ML = malignant lymphoma.

ment of many lymphomas is the achievement of complete remission, as it is only these patients who can be cured. In general, patients who are treated for malignant lymphoma respond rapidly; the signs and symptoms of the disease regress usually within the first weeks of treatment with either radiation therapy, or chemotherapy. Patients with indolent lymphoma respond to therapy when it is clinically indicated but are often not cured. Nevertheless, they have a prolonged natural history and may require repeated treatment over the course of many years. By contrast, patients with intermediate- and high-grade lymphomas require aggressive therapy early in the course of their disease. Patients who either relapse or fail to respond adequately to therapy usually succumb to lymphoma within the first year after diagnosis.

In general, patients with malignant lymphoma are treated with multiagent chemotherapy of varying intensity, depending on the age and condition of the patient, the histology, and the clinical characteristics. Several clinical presentations even warrant emergent management. Patients who present with large mediastinal masses may have signs and symptoms related to the superior vena cava syndrome or airway obstruction. Sometimes it is difficult to obtain adequate tissue, as the emergent symptoms require the initiation of either chemotherapy or radiation therapy to shrink the tumor, allowing for a safer biopsy at a later time. In addition, some patients may present with neurologic symptoms secondary to spinal cord compression that also require urgent intervention with either surgery, chemotherapy, or radiation therapy to prevent serious neurologic sequelae.

The chemotherapeutic regimens are designed to treat these tumors with agents that have different mechanisms of action to eliminate all malignant cells and prevent the emergence of

resistance. For most patients, treatment is given for 6 to 10 months, with reassessment of the disease at 3 months after initiation of therapy. This allows the physician to determine the adequacy of the response, particularly in the intermediate- and high-grade lymphomas. Patients who have not achieved a complete remission after three or four cycles of therapy have a poor prognosis and may be considered for early autologous marrow transplantation.

Some patients, after extensive staging, are found to have only limited disease and sometimes can be cured with radiotherapy to the involved or extended field area. Some studies have noted that the results of chemotherapy in such patients are just as effective as those of radiotherapy, and with less chance of systemic relapse.

Although the lymphomas generally present as nodal disease, some patients, particularly those with small noncleaved cell lymphoma (SNCL) or lymphoblastic lymphoma are at high risk for the development of central nervous system (CNS) relapse and should receive prophylaxis (intrathecal methotrexate, cranial irradiation) to prevent this complication. Treatment programs designed to treat both the systemic disease and the CNS have resulted in cures in many patients. The most effective therapy consists of systemic treatment with drugs such as high-dose methotrexate and high-dose cytosine arabinoside, which can penetrate the blood-brain barrier. An additional approach is to use concomitant intrathecal methotrexate for at least five doses.

Because these tumors are often sensitive to chemotherapy, rapid lysis of tumor cells may follow the initiation of treatment. This rapid response can lead to serious complications such as uric acid nephropathy, hyperkalemia, hyperphosphatemia, and hypocalcemia with resulting fever, hypotension, and possibly oliguric renal failure. Therefore, all patients receiving chemotherapy for these histologies should be treated with allopurinol and hydration, particularly during the first course of therapy while the tumor burden is high. Once the tumor has been controlled, subsequent courses of therapy are usually not associated with these complications.

The major side effect of chemotherapy, in addition to nausea and vomiting, is myelosuppression. Patients whose granulocyte count falls to less than 1000 per mm^3 as a consequence of chemotherapy are at risk for infection. Therefore, the blood count should be monitored on a weekly basis during chemotherapy. Fever should be treated urgently with systemic antibiotics, usually in the hospital, and the patient should receive blood transfusions and platelet transfusions to treat anemia and prevent bleeding. As expected, older patients with high-grade histologies do not tolerate therapy as well as do younger ones. Usually the chemotherapy-induced pancytopenia is self-limited and the blood count returns to normal within 10 to 14 days, so that cycles of chemotherapy can be given regularly every 4 to 5 weeks. It is best to allow the blood counts to return to normal before initiating the next course so that full doses of chemotherapy can be administered. An exception to this rule is the patient who presents with extensive bone marrow involvement and pancytopenia as a consequence of this lymphoma. This patient should receive full-dose therapy at the beginning of treatment, with aggressive management of the resulting infectious and bleeding complications until the marrow has been cleared of tumor cells and the blood counts return to normal.

In addition to the pancytopenia, there are other side effects of chemotherapy that must be monitored, most of which are usually self-limited. Two medications, however, can have irreversible side effects and must be monitored more closely during the course of therapy. Doxorubicin (Adriamycin) in doses of more than a total of 550 mg per M^2 is associated with a high incidence of cardiomyopathy, and the ejection fraction should be assessed during therapy to determine that it is not being altered by this drug. Patients with previous radiation therapy to the heart area or with coronary artery disease are probably at greater risk for this complication. Bleomycin (Blenoxane) in total doses greater than 300 mg per M^2 can lead to pulmonary infiltrates, as well as possible fibrosis and respiratory failure. Pulmonary dysfunction can be assessed by measuring the diffusion capacity as part of formal pulmonary function studies. The drug should be omitted in patients who show decreases in the diffusion capacity during therapy. An acute clinical picture with pulmonary infiltrates, cough,

and fever can be managed successfully with prednisone in most patients. The drugs used in the treatment of malignant lymphoma and their major side effects are noted in Table 2.

TREATMENT

Low-Grade Lymphoma

Low-grade lymphoma accounts for approximately 50 per cent of all NHL. The median age at diagnosis is 50 to 60 years, and it is uncommon for the diagnosis to be made during the first two decades of life. Most patients present with disseminated disease with a high incidence of bone marrow involvement. Nevertheless, the median survival is more than 8 years. Spontaneous regression occurs during the first year after the diagnosis in 5 to 23 per cent of the patients and may persist for variable periods. Histologic transformation into aggressive large cell lymphoma occurs during the course of disease and is associated with an accelerated clinical course and a poor prognosis. If a change in histology is suspected on clinical grounds, biopsy confirmation is mandatory and treatment should be altered accordingly.

After complete staging, less than 10 per cent of all patients will remain in Stage I or II. In these cases, involved-field irradiation is the treatment of choice. Relapse-free survival in 50 per cent or more of these patients at 5 to 10 years has been reported from several centers. Relapses can occur either locally in unirradiated lymph nodes or in extranodal sites. There is no clear benefit of adjuvant chemotherapy after radiotherapy in patients with Stage I and II low-grade lymphoma.

Management of advanced Stage III and IV low-grade lymphoma is controversial and can be individualized based on the bulk, symptoms, and biologic behavior of the disease. Initial treatment may vary from aggressive combined modality therapy to no initial treatment (Table 3). In general, these diseases are highly treatable, but they are probably not curable with current approaches. Moreover, in spite of advanced disease at presentation and the inability to induce long-term remission, patients may survive for many years with active disease. Although deferring initial therapy under the close supervision of an experienced hematologist may be appropriate for selected asymptomatic patients, systemic therapy is indicated in symptomatic patients. Prospective trials comparing single-agent chemotherapy, combination chemotherapy, whole-body irradiation, and combined modality therapy have shown similar rates of complete remissions, disease-free

TABLE 2. **Major Side Effects of Chemotherapeutic Agents Used in Treatment of Lymphoma**

Drug	Administration	Side Effects
Cyclophosphamide	Intravenous	Nausea, vomiting, alopecia, cystitis, cytopenia
Doxorubicin	Intravenous	Nausea, vomiting, alopecia, cytopenia, extravasation reaction, cardiomyopathy (>550 mg/M^2)
Vincristine	Intravenous	Peripheral neuropathy, ileus
Prednisone	Intravenous or oral	Diabetes, increased gastric acid, pneumocystis infections, psychosis, osteoporosis, hypertension, cushingoid appearance
Bleomycin	Intravenous	Pulmonary fibrosis (>300 mg/M^2)
Methotrexate	Intravenous	Mucositis, nephrotoxicity
VP-16 (etoposide)	Intravenous	Pancytopenia
Cisplatin	Intravenous	Nausea, vomiting, renal insufficiency, hearing loss, fluid and electrolyte disturbances
Cytosine arabinoside	Intravenous	Nausea, vomiting, alopecia, pancytopenia
Procarbazine	Oral	Nausea, pancytopenia, CNS effects

survival, and median survival. A randomized trial comparing no initial therapy with aggressive combined modality treatment with Pro-MACE-MOPP (see Table 3) followed by total nodal irradiation for patients with Stage III and IV disease is being conducted at the National Cancer Institute. Preliminary results indicate that a longer duration of remission and increased disease-free survival can be achieved with ProMACE-MOPP plus total nodal irradiation. However, longer follow-up is required for definitive conclusion.

TABLE 3. **Chemotherapy Regimens for Treatment of NHL**

Low Grade	Intermediate Grade	High Grade
Single-Agent Chemotherapy Cyclophosphamide Chlorambucil	*First Generation* C-MOPP CHOP COMLA BACOP	*L17M Protocol* Induction, consolidation, maintenance therapy for 2 yr and intrathecal methotrexate
Combination Chemotherapy CVP C-MOPP CHOP ProMACE-MOPP	*Second Generation* m-BACOD ProMACE-MOPP COP-BLAM I	*Stanford Protocol* Cyclophosphamide, doxorubicin, vincristine, prednisone, L-asparaginase, 6-methylprednisolone, methotrexate for 52 wk
	Third Generation MACOP-B COP-BLAM III ProMACE-cytaBOM	*NCI Regimen* Cytoxan, Adriamycin, vincristine, prednisone alternating with methotrexate infusion and intrathecal methotrexate for 6–15 cycles
	High-dose therapy and ABMT	High-dose therapy and ABMT

Abbreviations:
CVP = cyclophosphamide, vincristine, and prednisone
C-MOPP = cyclophosphamide, vincristine, procarbazine, and prednisone
CHOP = cyclophosphamide, doxorubicin, vincristine, and prednisone
COMLA = cyclophosphamide, vincristine, methotrexate, leucovorin, and cytosine arabinoside
BACOP = bleomycin, doxorubicin, cyclophosphamide, and vincristine
m-BACOD = methotrexate, bleomycin, Adriamycin, cyclophosphamide, vincristine, and dexamethasone
ProMACE-MOPP = prednisone, methotrexate, Adriamycin, cyclophosphamide, VP-16, nitrogen mustard, vincristine, procarbazine, and prednisone
MACOP-B = methotrexate, Adriamycin (doxorubicin), cyclophosphamide, vincristine, prednisone, and bleomycin
COP-BLAM = cyclophosphamide, vincristine, prednisone, bleomycin, Adriamycin (doxorubicin), Matulane (procarbazine)
CytaBOM = cytarabine, bleomycin, vincristine, and methotrexate

Intermediate-Grade Lymphoma

The terms "diffuse large cell lymphoma" and "aggressive lymphoma" are commonly used for these types of NHL. Over the past decade, the prognosis of patients with large cell lymphoma has improved significantly as a result of advances in the design of combination chemotherapy regimens. Now up to 60 per cent of patients with advanced stage of large cell lymphoma can be cured with multiagent chemotherapy. Three generations of chemotherapy regimens for treatment of aggressive large cell lymphoma have evolved in the past decade. The first-generation combination regimens (see Table 3), CHOP, MOPP, C-MOPP, BACOP, and COMLA, produced a complete remission rate of about 50 to 60 per cent, and a survival plateau was achieved in approximately 30 per cent of patients. The second-generation regimens, COP-BLAM, ProMACE-MOPP, M-BACOD, and m-BACOD, which are characterized by an increased number of drugs and increasing treatment intensity, resulted in a complete remission rate of over 70 per cent and a 2-year disease-free survival in excess of 50 per cent. In addition, the majority of the patients who attained a complete remission remained alive and free of disease.

The third-generation regimens introduced the concept of alternating non–cross-resistant drug combinations that used alternative modes of drug administration, greater incorporation of agents with different mechanisms of action, and frequent, intense administration. These regimens, COP-BLAM III, MACOP-B, and ProMACE-CytaBOM, have produced at least 80 per cent complete remission, with survival plateaus occurring in about 65 per cent of patients. However, the treatments are extremely intense and toxic, with significant treatment-related morbidity and mortality. Consequently, special consideration should be given when treating older patients with these regimens.

For patients with Stage I and II diffuse large cell lymphoma, combination chemotherapy, with or without radiation therapy, is recommended. Complete remission rates of 98 per cent are reported, with a 5-year disease-free survival rate exceeding 80 per cent. Radiation therapy alone also produces excellent results in Stage I disease when the pathologic stage is confirmed by staging laparotomy. However, the use of chemotherapy can eliminate the need for staging laparotomy because the procedure causes significant morbidity in elderly patients.

Despite the improvement in chemotherapy, patients with aggressive large cell lymphoma relapse and die with progressive disease. Several prognostic factors, including poor performance status, large, bulky masses (10 cm or larger), multiple extranodal sites, and elevated lactate dehydrogenase values, have been shown to influence the response rate and duration and are associated with poor survival. Only 20 per cent of the patients with these poor prognostic factors are alive at 5 years despite aggressive therapy. Our current approach to these patients is to administer high-dose chemotherapy and total body irradiation followed by autologous bone marrow transplantation (BMT) after initial chemotherapy-induced remission in an attempt to prevent relapse and thereby improve the disease-free survival.

High-Grade Lymphoma

Lymphoblastic Lymphoma

Lymphoblastic lymphoma (LBL) is a clinical entity characterized by an increased incidence in young men, a predilection for mediastinal involvement, and a high incidence of bone marrow and CNS involvement during the course of the disease. Morphologically, the disease is indistinguishable from acute lymphoblastic leukemia (ALL), and its natural history is similar to that of ALL. The treatment approach should be identical to that of ALL and should include intensive induction, consolidation, and maintenance therapy, as well as CNS prophylaxis. Excellent results have been reported from the investigators at Stanford University and at Memorial Sloan-Kettering Hospital (see Table 3). By using this treatment approach, about 50 per cent of the patients with LBL can be expected to be cured. However, the prognosis of those who present with bone marrow or CNS involvement is poor. In these cases, allogeneic BMT from a human leukocyte antigen–identical sibling is recommended.

Small Noncleaved Cell Lymphoma

SNCL is characterized by an aggressive clinical course; a high incidence of bone marrow, CNS, and extranodal involvement; brief median survival; and low rates of long-term survival. A rapid tumor response with tumor lysis syndrome occurs frequently after initiation of therapy. Therefore vigorous hydration, alkalinization, and allopurinol should be given before treatment. Debulking surgery has a therapeutic role in the treatment of SNCL because the tumor burden has been recognized as an adverse prognostic factor. The treatment strategy for SNCL is similar to that for LBL and should include an intensive multiagent chemotherapeutic regimen consisting of high-dose cyclophosphamide, doxorubicin, vincristine, prednisone, midcycle high-dose methotrexate, and intrathecal methotrexate. Three-year survival of 60 per cent has been reported with this approach. Patients with bulky disease, elevated serum lactate dehydrogenase levels, and bone marrow and CNS involvement are at high risk of treatment failure, and an alternative innovative approach should be considered.

Human Immunodeficiency Virus–Related Lymphoma

An increase in the incidence of NHL has been noted as a major clinical manifestation of the acquired immunodeficiency syndrome (AIDS). According to the Centers for Disease Control, the occurrence of diffuse, aggressive, intermediate- or high-grade NHL in an individual who is seropositive for the human immunodeficiency virus (HIV) is considered to be a criterion that would be diagnostic of AIDS.

Several studies at many institutions have shown that approximately 70 per cent of the lymphomas develop in individuals with a high-grade histology (small noncleaved cell or large cell immunoblastic), with the remaining 30 per cent being of intermediate grade (diffuse large cell lymphoma). In addition, it has been noted that unlike most lymphomas, which present as nodal disease, HIV-related lymphoma presents at unusual extranodal sites, including the skin, lungs, anus, and rectum. CNS involvement, even as a primary manifestation, has been described in these patients. An analysis of the surface immunoglobulin of these lymphomas indicates that almost all of them are B cell restricted, suggesting a B cell derivation.

The prognosis for these patients with high-grade lymphoma is quite poor, with relapses either during or shortly after completion of therapy. It has also been noted that patients with HIV-related lymphoma do not tolerate the toxicity of aggressive chemotherapeutic regimens. Lymphoma in these patients can be the primary manifestation of disease or can arise after other diseases (i.e., opportunistic infections or AIDS-related complex) have been noted. It has been suggested that all patients presenting with lymphoma of high-grade histology who have associated risk factors be tested for the presence of HIV antibody.

Recurrent Lymphoma

The prognosis of patients with refractory or relapsing lymphoma is extremely poor. Patients with large cell or high-grade lymphoma who fail to achieve a complete remission with first line therapy usually die within 12 months. Salvage chemotherapy with single-agent or combination regimens has produced a poor response ranging between 10 and 30 per cent with a brief median

TABLE 4. **Indications for High-Dose Therapy and Autologous Bone Marrow Transplantation (ABMT) for Lymphoma**

1. Drug-sensitive relapse in high- or intermediate-grade lymphoma
2. Patients with high- or intermediate-grade lymphoma who achieve only partial remission with standard-dose chemotherapy
3. Consolidation therapy of intermediate- or high-grade lymphoma with poor prognostic features after standard chemotherapy-induced remission

duration of response. Thus, long-term survival is unlikely with salvage therapy, regardless of the histologic grade.

Recently, two effective salvage regimens, DHAP (dexamethasone, high-dose cytarabine, cisplatin) and MIME (methyl-GAG, ifosfamide, methotrexate, etoposide) have been reported to produce higher response rates—31 and 24 per cent complete response and 60 and 63 per cent overall response rates. Responses were seen in both aggressive and low-grade lymphoma. The median duration of the complete response was 15 months for aggressive and 16.5 months for low-grade lymphoma. However, long-term follow-up will be necessary to determine the curative potential of these regimens.

Autologous Bone Marrow Transplantation

The rationale for high-dose chemotherapy or chemoradiotherapy with autologous bone marrow transplantation (ABMT) for the treatment of NHL is based on the importance of dose intensity and the steep dose-response curve characteristic of NHL (Table 4). The early published experience demonstrated a low cure rate when ABMT was performed in advanced, bulky, and refractory disease. Patients with gross, bulky tumors resistant to second line chemotherapy are unlikely to benefit from ABMT. In contrast, patients who have a drug-sensitive relapse with minimal disease at the time of ABMT or who have had their second or subsequent remission may have a 50 to 60 per cent chance of achieving a long-term, disease-free survival. Patients who achieve only a partial response to first line therapy are rarely cured with further conventional therapy; high-dose therapy and ABMT have been reported to induce long-term remission in this group. Overall survival of 75 per cent at 24 months has been reported. Because bone marrow involvement complicates the use of ABMT, bone marrow purging of residual tumor cells with monoclonal antibodies or chemotherapy, or substituting peripheral stem cells for bone marrow, has been used successfully for these patients.

MYCOSIS FUNGOIDES

method of
RICHARD T. HOPPE, M.D.
Stanford University Medical Center
Stanford, California

Mycosis fungoides (MF) is a cutaneous lymphoma of T lymphocyte origin that has a variable clinical course. Despite its generally long natural history, MF eventually becomes symptomatic in most patients, therapy is required, and death may ensue. MF is an uncommon malignancy; approximately 400 new cases and 100 to 200 deaths are reported each year in the United States. This lymphoma is most common in older males. The median age of onset is about 60 and the male/female ratio is 2:1. The etiology of MF is unclear. Chemical exposure, chronic antigen stimulation, and viral causes have been proposed. A few cases of MF in association with human T cell lymphotrophic virus I infections have been reported.

DIAGNOSIS

The diagnosis of MF is often difficult and may be established only after the disease has been present and symptomatic for many years. The typical light microscopic features of MF include a polymorphous upper dermal infiltrate that is intimate with the epidermis and has atypical mononuclear cells. These atypical mononuclear cells have hyperconvoluted ("cerebriform") nuclei, and monoclonal antibody staining reveals that they have the cell surface characteristics of helper T cells. Some of these cells must be present in the epidermis as either scattered individual cells or small clusters (Pautrier's microabscesses) in order to establish a definitive diagnosis. Biopsy studies on multiple occasions are indicated when the diagnosis of MF is suspected clinically but previous biopsy results were only suggestive of that diagnosis. Since the cellular infiltrate of this disease is located in the upper dermis and epidermis, shave biopsies are generally preferable to punch biopsies in order to provide a large surface of epidermis for examination.

CLINICAL APPEARANCE

The cutaneous lesions of MF are variable in appearance. Some patients present with poikilodermatous patches characterized by variable atrophy and telangiectasia. Other patients present with well-demarcated erythematous scaling patches or infiltrated plaques. It is common for disease to arise initially in the bathing trunk distribution that includes the lower abdomen, upper thighs, and buttocks. The lesions of MF are generally intensely pruritic, and pruritus is often the main presenting complaint. Some patients may present with or develop frank cutaneous tumors, which may become secondarily ulcerated and infected.

Occasional patients will present with generalized erythroderma, often accompanied by marked skin atrophy. Some patients with erythroderma have abnormal cells circulating in the peripheral blood that are identical to those found in the dermal and epidermal infiltrates of the disease. These patients often have palpable lymphadenopathy and splenomegaly as well, and this constellation of findings is referred to as Sézary's syndrome. These patients usually experience severe generalized pruritus.

STAGING

In staging MF, the most important considerations are the extent of skin involvement, the presence of lymph node involvement, and the presence of visceral disease. Table 1 summarizes the TNM (tumor, node, metastases) system for staging MF. Skin involvement characterized as limited plaque implies patches or plaques involving less than 10 per cent of the total skin surface. Generalized plaque disease indicates that patches or plaques involve more than 10 per cent of the skin surface. Tumorous involvement implies frank cutaneous tumors, and erythroderma indicates total skin erythema.

Staging studies completed in these patients should include a thorough history and physical examination with careful mapping of cutaneous lesions. Examination of the skin should also include careful evaluation of the scalp, palms, soles, fingernails, and toenails. Lateral and posteroanterior chest radiographs, a complete blood cell count, and serum chemistry studies are indicated both to rule out extracutaneous involvement by MF and also to evaluate for the presence of other pathology. Patients with palpable lymphadenopathy should undergo lymph node biopsy. If lymph node biopsy shows involvement by MF, other staging studies should be utilized to determine the extent of extracutaneous disease. Most commonly, lymphangiography and computed tomographic scanning of the abdomen and pelvis are helpful in this setting. If any of these

TABLE 1. **TNM Staging System for Mycosis Fungoides**

T1 — Limited plaque. Patches or plaques covering less than 10% of the total skin surface
T2 — Generalized plaque. Patches or plaques covering 10% or more of the total skin surface
T3 — Tumorous. One or more cutaneous tumors
T4 — Erythroderma. Total skin erythema, with or without cutaneous tumors
N0 — No palpable lymph nodes
N1 — Palpable lymph nodes. If a biopsy is done, light microscopic appearance of specimen may be consistent with reactive changes or dermatopathic lymphadenitis, but not with actual involvement by MF
N2 — Palpable lymph nodes that have been biopsied, specimen reveals MF microscopically
M0 — No evidence of visceral involvement
M1 — Visceral involvement present. Should be documented by biopsy

	Stage of MF*			
N Stage	*T1*	*T2*	*T3*	*T4*
N0	IA	IB	IIB	IIIA
N1	IIA	IIA	IIB	IIIB
N2	IVA	IVA	IVA	IVA

*Any T, N with M = 1 is Stage IVB.

studies suggest visceral involvement, biopsy documentation is warranted. Other cancers are common in patients of this age group and may account for abnormal findings of these examinations. The most common site of identifiable extracutaneous MF is in lymph nodes, and the most common visceral sites are the lungs and liver.

TREATMENT

Cutaneous Therapy

The potential for curative treatment of MF is controversial. However, most patients are symptomatic because of pruritus or are unhappy with the cosmetic deformities associated with the disease, and treatment is usually indicated. At the time of initial diagnosis, it is reasonable to use aggressive cutaneous treatment in order to clear the skin. With this approach, some patients will in fact achieve complete skin clearance, some of these will maintain clearance for variable periods of time, and occasional patients will have no evidence of return of disease activity. Furthermore, it appears that when disease on the skin can be kept at a minimal level, the likelihood that the patient will develop extracutaneous disease is exceedingly small. The topical treatment modalities utilized in this situation include topical chemotherapy with nitrogen mustard, photochemotherapy with psoralens and ultraviolet (PUVA) radiation, and total skin electron beam therapy.

Topical nitrogen mustard may be utilized either in an aqueous solution or in an ointment base in a concentration of 10 to 20 mg per dl. Patients generally apply the topical nitrogen mustard to the entire cutaneous surface, sparing only the eyelids. Intertriginous areas are treated more sparingly. Cutaneous lesions are slow to respond with this therapy, and complete response, if it occurs, may require more than a year of daily treatment. It is recommended that therapy be continued during a maintenance period of 1 to 2 years following complete skin clearance.

Therapy with PUVA consists of oral 8-methoxypsoralen followed by exposure to long-wavelength ultraviolet (UVA) light. The psoralens intercalate with DNA, which, on exposure to UVA, forms cross-links that inhibit DNA replication. Generally three treatments per week are given until moderate clearing has been achieved. Maintenance programs are then introduced with two treatments per week, and, subsequently, gradually tapering schedules are initiated, with treatments ultimately given as infrequently as once every 4 to 6 weeks. Generally, if treatment is discontinued completely, the disease recurs.

Total skin electron beam therapy provides the greatest likelihood of skin clearance. Electrons are a form of ionizing irradiation that penetrate to a specific depth, depending upon their energy. Electrons of appropriate energy can be used; these penetrate the skin for only several millimeters, and special techniques of treatment permit entire cutaneous therapy. Treatments are administered 4 days a week for about 9 weeks (total dose 30.00 to 36.00 Gy). About 80 per cent of patients will achieve complete skin clearance with this treatment. However, 50 to 75 per cent of patients who complete this therapy will have a later recurrence. Often, however, only minimal disease is present at this point, and it can be treated effectively with either topical nitrogen mustard or PUVA. The side effects of total skin electron beam therapy are more marked than those that occur with the other two topical modalities. Temporary hair loss, temporary loss of sweat gland function, and long-term skin dryness are common.

Recommendations for Cutaneous Treatment. In patients who present with the limited plaque phase of skin involvement, treatment with topical nitrogen mustard is a reasonable first line therapy. Although the time to skin clearance is quite prolonged, as many as 50 per cent of patients will achieve a complete response. Even in those who do not achieve a complete response, there is usually a significant improvement in disease with resolution of most symptoms. If the disease fails to respond to topical nitrogen mustard or progresses during therapy, institution of total skin electron beam therapy is appropriate. Patients who present with generalized plaque disease in which there is only a minimally infiltrative component and who have a long history of disease without recent progression may be treated in a similar fashion. However, in the presence of very infiltrated plaques or if there is a history of recent progression, total skin electron beam therapy is a preferable first choice of treatment. The majority of patients treated in this fashion will achieve a complete response. However, since subsequent relapse is common, it may be beneficial to institute a program of maintenance treatment with topical nitrogen mustard immediately following the completion of electron beam therapy.

Patients who present with tumorous involvement are treated initially with total skin electron beam therapy. In addition, supplemental small-field irradiation with low energy x-rays to individual tumor lesions is indicated. After completion of irradiation, topical nitrogen mustard is used as a maintenance therapy.

Patients who present with erythroderma are difficult to manage inasmuch as their skin is often atrophic and very sensitive to any type of

TABLE 2. **Five-Year Results of Treatment for Patients with Cutaneous Disease**

	Nitrogen Mustard (101 Patients)		Electron Beam Therapy (170 Patients)	
Extent of Disease	Survival (%)	Freedom from Relapse (%)	Survival (%)	Freedom from Relapse (%)
Limited plaque	92	32	92	55
Generalized plaque	66	10	73	25
Tumorous	—	—	39	5

therapy. Low-exposure PUVA therapy can be successful in achieving gradual skin clearance. If either topical nitrogen mustard or electron beam therapy is utilized, the concentration or daily dose of these agents must be reduced.

Palliative Management of Skin Lesions. Frequently, despite the use of total cutaneous therapies, individual lesions develop that may be refractory and symptomatic. Local topical measures that may be helpful in this setting include topical corticosteroids, small-field irradiation with either low-energy x-rays or electrons, or more intensive localized treatment with higher concentrations of nitrogen mustard (i.e., 50 mg per dl).

Management of Extracutaneous Disease

The median survival of patients who develop extracutaneous disease is only 1 year. Systemic therapies, while occasionally achieving responses, seldom achieve complete responses, and remissions are generally brief. When extracutaneous sites are clinically localized (i.e., localized adenopathy), local field megavoltage irradiation can achieve a very good palliative and symptomatic response. Generalized systemic disease is usually treated with combination chemotherapy using agents such as cyclophosphamide, doxorubicin (Adriamycin), vincristine, and prednisone (CHOP).

An uncommon form of systemic disease is Sézary's syndrome, which is incurable but usually requires treatment for relief of symptoms (i.e., pruritis). Daily treatment with chlorambucil and prednisone in addition to monitoring white blood cell counts is often successful in achieving palliative responses. When the disease becomes resistant to this approach, more intensive chemotherapy programs may be initiated, but response is unpredictable.

PROGNOSIS

Prognosis is related to the extent of skin involvement, presence of extracutaneous disease, the type of therapy administered, and other factors such as age and intercurrent disease. The median survival of large groups of patients may be greater than 10 years, but is very dependent upon the initial extent of disease and the treatment programs utilized. Table 2 summarizes our results of treatment at Stanford, using topical nitrogen mustard or electron beam therapy in patients with disease limited to the skin.

MULTIPLE MYELOMA
method of
DANIEL E. BERGSAGEL, M.D.
Ontario Cancer Institute
Toronto, Ontario, Canada

The question of whether a patient has myeloma often starts with the discovery of an M protein (M for monoclonal) in the serum or urine. In a screening study of 10,000 Swedish subjects over the age of 25, about 1 per cent were found to have a serum M protein. The majority were asymptomatic and were classified as having monoclonal gammopathy of unknown significance (MGUS). These patients are well and require no therapy. Patients with symptomatic myeloma have a median survival of about 30 months and thus do not accumulate in the population. The prevalence of the two disorders in a population of 100,000 is about 582 for MGUS and 30 for symptomatic myeloma. Patients with symptomatic myeloma should be treated immediately; those with MGUS should be re-evaluated every 6 months because about 2 per cent per year progress to develop plasma cell myeloma.

PATIENT EVALUATION

The evaluation of a patient with an M protein is outlined in Table 1. For IgG M proteins and IgA peaks greater than 20 grams per liter, the serum electrophoresis strip is an accurate method of measuring the M protein, whereas radial immunodiffusion is less reliable. With IgA M proteins less than 20 grams per liter, the peak may be poorly defined, and the immunoglobulin is measured more accurately by nephelometry. About 60 per cent of myeloma patients excrete a light chain in the urine. The urine dipstick test for protein is designed to detect albumin and often fails to detect light chains. The electrophoresis pattern of concentrated urine should be determined. The usual lesion caused by light chain deposits in the renal tubules

TABLE 1. **Evaluation of Patients with M Protein**

1. Measure the M protein by the following methods:
   Serum electrophoresis—measure M protein and albumin in grams per liter
   Urine protein—measure grams of protein excreted per 24 hours
2. Establish monoclonality of the M protein by immuno-electrophoresis
3. Hematology: hemoglobin, leukocyte and platelet counts, differential counts
4. Marrow: per cent plasma cells in marrow differential; may need to sample more than one site, since marrow plasmacytosis may be spotty
5. Biopsy of solitary lytic lesion; extramedullary plasmacytoma; skin nodules; enlarged lymph nodes
6. Evaluate renal function: serum creatinine; creatinine clearance; electrophoresis of concentrated urine to distinguish between tubular and glomerular proteinurea patterns
7. Complete skeletal survey, including skull, ribs, vertebrae, and long bones; identify lytic lesions and osteoporosis
8. Serum calcium
9. Serum beta₂-microglobulin
10. Labeling index of marrow plasma cells (if available) for distinguishing progressive from indolent myeloma
11. Myelogram if there is paraspinal mass or signs and symptoms of spinal cord or nerve root compression; send cerebrospinal fluid to laboratory for cytospin, cell count, and protein assays
12. Special tests: serum viscosity; check for cryoglobulins; plasma volume; rectal biopsy (search for amyloid); check joint effusions for amyloid

results in the excretion of large amounts of light chains, which migrate in the globulin region, plus some albumin. Damage to the glomerulus by deposits of amyloid or light chains results in the nonspecific leakage of all serum proteins into the urine. The glomerular urine electrophoresis pattern resembles that of serum. The bone lesions demonstrated in the skeletal survey are important in directing radiation therapy. Large lytic lesions should be irradiated before a pathologic fracture occurs. Back pain, associated with diffuse osteoporosis and vertebral collapse, usually responds better to chemotherapy than to radiation, unless a distinct lytic lesion can be identified.

Myelomatous lesions in ribs or vertebrae may extend beyond the bone and form paraspinal masses, which can be visualized on vertebral radiographs. These plasma cell tumors may invade the spinal canal through an intervertebral foramen and cause spinal cord compression; paraspinal masses should be irradiated as soon as they are discovered, before neurologic complications develop. The increased bone resorption associated with plasma cell myeloma often exceeds the capacity of the kidney to excrete calcium. As a result, about one-third of patients present with symptoms of hypercalcemia (nausea, vomiting, constipation, polyuria, thirst, and mental confusion), and another one-third develop hypercalcemia during the course of the disease. Patients immobilized by bone pain are especially vulnerable to this complication. Beta₂-microglobulin (B_2m) is the light chain of the major histocompatibility complex of the cell membrane. The release of this protein into the blood is increased in active tumors with increased cell turnover. B_2m is normally excreted in the urine; renal failure leads to rising serum levels. Serum B_2m has proved to be a useful measurement for gauging the activity of plasma cell neoplasms; levels in the normal range (less than 3.0 mg per liter) are associated with indolent tumors (MGUS and asymptomatic, stable myeloma), whereas elevated levels indicate a more active tumor, with increased cell turnover, and possibly renal failure. The determination of the proportion of plasma cells in the DNA synthesis phase of the cell cycle (labeling index) with tritiated thymidine or bromodeoxycytidine is another useful means of distinguishing indolent from aggressive myeloma. Patients with symptomatic myeloma requiring treatment usually have plasma cell labeling indices of greater than 0.4 per cent.

STAGING

Patients with symptomatic myeloma can be staged on the basis of the important prognostic factors. Those with a hemoglobin of less than 85 grams per liter, hypercalcemia, more than three lytic bone lesions, or a greatly increased M protein (more than 70 grams per liter of IgG, more than 50 grams per liter for IgA, or more than 12 grams per 24 hours of light chain proteinuria) have a high myeloma cell mass and a poor prognosis. A simpler and more useful staging system is based on serum B_2m and albumin levels. Stage 1 patients with serum B_2m levels of 6.0 mg per liter or less, and serum albumin (by electrophoresis) of 30 grams per liter or more, have the best prognosis. Stage 2 patients have a serum B_2m of more than 6.0 mg per liter, and a serum albumin of 30 grams per liter or more. Stage 3 patients, with the worst prognosis, have both an elevated serum B_2m of more than 6.0 mg per liter and albumin reduced to less than 30 grams per liter.

TREATMENT OF SYMPTOMATIC MYELOMA

General Measures

First, pain should be relieved and the patient ambulated. This requires the effective use of analgesics, and irradiation of painful lytic lesions identified by the patient and the skeletal survey. For painful rib lesions we often use a single dose of 800 cGy; for larger lytic lesions in vital areas, such as vertebrae or long bones, doses of 2000 to 3500 cGy are administered. The patient should be encouraged to get out of bed, if only to walk to the bathroom, as soon as the pain has been adequately controlled. It is important to preserve muscle strength and reduce bone resorption by putting some stress on the skeleton. All patients should make special efforts to drink at least 3 liters of fluid a day so that the increased amount of calcium and light chains can be excreted by the kidneys. Dehydration favors the development of renal failure and hypercalcemia and the formation of tubular casts that further compromise renal function.

Initial Chemotherapy

Melphalan and prednisone are the drugs of choice as the initial form of chemotherapy. I start with a melphalan (Alkeran) dose of 9 mg per M^2 (0.25 mg per kg) before breakfast daily for 4 days every 4 to 6 weeks, along with 100 mg of prednisone in one dose with breakfast for 4 days. The melphalan should be administered in one dose at least 30 minutes before breakfast (giving melphalan with food significantly reduces the absorption of this drug). Blood counts should be repeated weekly. When an effective dose has been administered, the leukocyte and platelet counts will fall to a nadir at about 3 weeks, with recovery by the fourth to sixth week.

If a significant fall in the leukocyte and/or platelet count is not observed, the next course of melphalan should be increased by 2 mg per day and, if necessary, increased by an additional 2 mg per day in subsequent courses, until a definite, transient fall in leukocyte and/or platelet count occurs, to indicate that adequate amounts of melphalan have been absorbed. Most patients can tolerate repeat courses of melphalan and prednisone every 4 weeks, but some will have delayed marrow recovery. If the leukocyte or platelet count has not begun to rise by the fourth week, the next course should be delayed by 1 or 2 weeks to prevent the development of cumulative hematologic toxicity. Some patients are distressed by the acute stimulatory effects of prednisone (hyperactivity, insomnia, dyspepsia); in these patients the prednisone can be discontinued; although prednisone does increase the response rate in myeloma, it has not been shown to improve survival.

With this therapy, 46 per cent of patients will respond with a fall in the serum and/or urine M protein to reach a stable plateau (at less than 50 per cent of the initial serum M protein concentration or at less than 10 per cent of the initial urinary M protein excreted per 24 hours), with relief of bone pain, weight gain, and improved performance status. An additional 10 per cent will become asymptomatic but will not achieve a sufficient fall in the M protein to qualify as responders, and 44 per cent will progress and require alternate forms of therapy.

Attempts to improve therapy by adding vincristine and other alkylating agents to melphalan and prednisone have failed to improve survival. There is some evidence that combining doxorubicin (Adriamycin) with alkylating agents may lead to a marginal improvement in survival.

There is no benefit in continuing therapy after a stable response has been achieved. My practice is to continue treatment with melphalan and prednisone as long as the M protein level continues to decline. After the M protein level reaches a stable plateau that persists for 4 months, I discontinue therapy but continue to see the patient at 2-month intervals to follow the course of the disease. It is impossible to monitor the management of a myeloma patient without a chronologic record (flow sheet) of changes in weight, serum M protein and albumin measured by serum electrophoresis, 24-hour urine protein, serum calcium, serum creatinine, blood counts, serum B_2m, and repeated skeletal surveys, along with a record of the treatment administered to the patient. Patients who achieve a stable response will remain in remission for a median of 10 to 12 months after treatment is stopped, but some will not show signs of progression for 3 years or more. Patients must be monitored carefully so that treatment can be restarted at the first sign of relapse (i.e., a progressive increase in serum and/or urinary M protein), preferably before bone pain signals progressive bone disease.

Patients treated in this way with melphalan and prednisone will survive for a median of 30 months. Those whose disease progresses despite melphalan/prednisone induction therapy have the poorest prognosis, with a median survival of 15 months; responders have a median survival of 48 months; and those who do not achieve a response but remain stable without progression also survive well, with a median of 49 months.

Second Line Therapy

The prognosis for patients whose disease is primarily resistant to melphalan and prednisone is poor, and only about 10 per cent will respond to alternate therapy. Patients whose disease responds initially to melphalan/prednisone therapy but then progresses despite reinstituted therapy have a better prognosis; about 25 to 30 per cent will respond to second line therapy.

If the disease progresses when the patient is receiving melphalan/prednisone therapy, I change to cyclophosphamide (Cytoxan), 500 mg (intravenously or orally) once a week, combined with prednisone, 100 mg with breakfast, on alternate days. This treatment gives the patient the advantage of high-dose prednisone, which is well tolerated without signs of hypercorticism when administered on alternate days, and also a change in the alkylating agent to cyclophosphamide in a schedule that is well tolerated, even by patients with pancytopenia.

Patients whose disease progresses during

weekly cyclophosphamide and prednisone therapy, with clear progression of bony disease, are difficult management problems. Bone pain is best treated with irradiation, and when there are widespread lesions this may require half-body irradiation. Some patients may also respond to 4-day infusions (using venous catheter access to a large vein) of vincristine (Oncovin) and doxorubicin (Adriamycin) and 4-day courses of dexamethasone (Decadron). The treatments used at this stage of the illness require considerable clinical experience and are best administered at centers where physicians have experience in the use of wide-field irradiation and intensive chemotherapy and have access to the required supportive care.

MANAGEMENT OF SPECIAL PROBLEMS

Solitary Osseous Plasmacytomas

About 3 per cent of patients present with apparently solitary osteolytic lesions. These patients require a needle aspirate or biopsy from the lytic lesion to establish the diagnosis, since marrow aspirations from other sites will not show a plasmacytosis. Solitary lesions should be treated with irradiation, using a dose of about 3500 cGy. About one-third of these patients will have an M protein, and this should disappear completely following irradiation. Persistence of the M protein means that myeloma cells persist, probably outside of the irradiated area. These patients must be followed carefully because in the majority the disease will eventually progress to multiple myeloma.

Extramedullary Plasmacytomas

About 3 per cent of patients present with extramedullary plasmacytomas, usually in the nasopharynx or paranasal sinuses. Since the usual spread of these tumors is to the regional lymph nodes, the radiation field should include the regional nodes whenever possible. We use a radiation dose of 3500 cGy. One-third of these patients will have an M protein, which should disappear following irradiation. If the M protein persists along with residual tumor, the residual tumor should be resected; the M protein will often disappear if the tumor can be resected. Extramedullary plasmacytomas can usually be controlled by local irradiation and surgical resection. Melphalan and prednisone therapy can be used for those cases that are not controlled by local measures.

Hypercalcemia

Because hypercalcemia develops frequently in myeloma patients, the serum calcium should be measured once a week in hospitalized patients and on every follow-up visit. This complication can usually be controlled in myeloma patients with a combination of hydration (using normal saline to promote the excretion of calcium, whenever possible), corticosteroids, and chemotherapy for the myeloma.

Anemia

A low hemoglobin concentration in a myeloma patient may be partially dilutional, as the plasma volume expands to accommodate the serum M protein. Red cell transfusions are not indicated and may be harmful for patients with an expanded plasma volume, especially if this is associated with hyperviscosity. The common causes of anemia, such as bleeding, should be ruled out. The usual cause is marrow failure associated with the myeloma. If anemia persists and requires transfusions in a myeloma patient whose disease is otherwise controlled by chemotherapy, I try fluoxymesterone (Halotestin), 5 mg three times a day with meals.* This treatment is often effective in raising the hemoglobin concentration slowly, but it must be continued for 3 to 6 months before the full effect is achieved.

Renal Failure

Constant encouragement of the patient to drink 3 liters of fluid a day will do much to retard the development of renal failure. The occasional patient who presents with acute renal shutdown requires emergency treatment to clear light chains from the plasma and renal tubules. Plasmapheresis is 10 times more effective than dialysis in accomplishing this. During this emergency treatment one should also attempt to reduce the production of light chains by the myeloma cells. Melphalan should be administered with great caution, because toxicity is greatly increased when the drug cannot be excreted into the urine. In this situation I use intravenous cyclophosphamide (Cytoxan), 500 mg per week, and prednisone, 100 mg per day or every other day.

Infections

Infections occur frequently in myeloma patients and are the most common cause of death. All fevers must be monitored carefully and antibiotics administered immediately for suspected infections. Neutropenic patients who develop a fever should be hospitalized for intravenous an-

---

*This use is not listed in the manufacturer's directive.

tibiotic therapy. Myeloma patients do not mount an adequate antibody response to organisms such as the pneumococcus; thus repeat infections with the same strain of pneumococcus are common. Consideration should be given to administering prophylactic penicillin to myeloma patients who have been treated for a pneumococcal infection.

EXPERIMENTAL THERAPY

Attempts to eliminate all myeloma cells with intensive chemotherapy, such as high-dose melphalan, and allogeneic or twin marrow transplantation have failed to cure patients but have succeeded in inducing prolonged remissions. Interferon has been found to reduce the self-renewal capacity of myeloma colony-forming cells and is being tested for its capacity to prolong remissions induced by other agents.

POLYCYTHEMIA VERA AND OTHER POLYCYTHEMIC CONDITIONS

method of
HARRIET S. GILBERT, M.D.
Albert Einstein College of Medicine
Bronx, New York

Polycythemia vera (PV) is one of a group of chronic myeloproliferative disorders (MPD) involving the pluripotential hematic precursor cell. The syndromes composing MPD are low-grade hematologic malignancies characterized by monoclonal proliferation of a precursor cell that maintains its pluripotentiality and its capacity for commitment, differentiation, and maturation into the hematic populations normally derived from this cell. The result of this intrinsic growth disturbance is an expansion of the bone marrow organ throughout the medullary cavity and a reactivation of hematopoiesis in extramedullary sites that are usually active only during fetal development. The resulting panmyelosis produces increased levels of some or all circulating hematic cell progeny, as well as myeloid metaplasia of the spleen and liver. The phenotypic expression of MPD is highly variable, and nomenclature of the syndromes is based on the predominant manifestation of the proliferative process. Although they result from the same intrinsic lesion of the hematic precursor cell and share many features, the phenotypic expressions of MPD pose sufficiently different problems in diagnosis and management to justify subclassification into three variants known as PV, essential thrombocythemia (ET), and myeloid metaplasia (MyM). Erythrocythemia is the predominant manifestation of PV at the inception of the disease. With time, PV may change its phenotype, and the proliferative, erythrocythemic phase may be followed by a spent phase in which erythroid activity wanes in the absence of therapy and manifestations of MyM predominate. This phase is known as postpolycythemia MyM. Some patients develop progressive compromise of bone marrow function with myelofibrosis or myelodysplasia, or both. At this stage hematopoiesis becomes ineffective and bone marrow failure supervenes.

Notwithstanding the malignant nature of PV, the last four decades have seen a remarkable increase in survival from 2 years in untreated patients to a life expectancy that does not differ from that of an age-matched population without PV. This has been achieved by two strategies: reduction of the increased red cell mass by phlebotomy to reduce blood viscosity and inhibition of hematopoiesis by myelosuppressive agents. Several important observations have emerged from randomized clinical trials to evaluate these therapeutic approaches. It was found that the choice of therapy has less effect on survival than on the type of complication. Patients treated with phlebotomy show an increase in thrombotic events during the first 4 years of their course, and those managed with myelosuppression have an increased incidence of malignancy after the fourth year. Malignant transformation is related to both dose and agent, and administration of alkylating agents is associated with an earlier leukemic transformation than that seen with radioactive phosphorus. Extensive statistical analysis has failed to associate an elevated platelet count with a high risk of thrombotic complications. The incidence of late thrombotic events in patients treated with myelosuppression is increased so that the overall thrombosis-free cumulative survival is comparable in the phlebotomized and myelosuppressed groups.

These findings have prompted modifications in the therapy of PV in which there is a greater reliance on phlebotomy, avoidance of alkylating agents, more sparing use of radioactive phosphorus, the introduction of antiaggregating platelet therapy to prevent thrombosis, and the use of less mutagenic myelosuppressive agents, such as hydroxyurea, when myelosuppression is indicated. As survival has improved, the late complications of PV have become more of a problem. The demonstration that myelofibrosis is a reactive phenomenon rather than an intrinsic manifestation of MPD has stimulated investigations into its pathophysiology, but approaches to prevention of fibrosis and myelodysplasia have not been found, and these late, life-threatening complications of MPD still pose a difficult problem in management.

DIAGNOSIS

A diagnosis of PV requires demonstration of an absolute increase in circulating red cells in the presence of other stigmata of panmyelosis. Adherence to rigorous diagnostic criteria serves to distinguish PV from the myriad of disorders that can produce an elevated hematocrit. Most hematocrit elevations result from a reduction in circulating plasma volume rather than an absolute increase in erythrocytes. Acute dehydration is readily appreciated clinically, but a chronic, low-grade state of dehydration may be overlooked. This state may result from smoking or ingestion of caffeine or diuretics. These cause a diminution in plasma volume that is easily reversed and can be detected by hematocrit determinations before and after 72 hours of abstention. The presence of a persistently elevated hematocrit without obvious explanation necessitates direct measurement of red cell mass and plasma volume by isotope dilution to distinguish between relative and absolute polycythemia. Erythrocyte indices should be assessed prior to this determination, and if microcytosis is present, iron deficiency should be sought and corrected to elicit masked erythrocytosis. Blood volume determinations should be performed prior to phlebotomy, since the reactive changes in bone marrow proliferation induced by phlebotomy can be confused with stigmata of MPD.

Relative Polycythemia. Patients with a normal red cell mass and reduced intravascular plasma volume outnumber those with absolute erythrocytosis by a ratio of more than 5:1. The prototype is a young or middle-aged male smoker who presents with a hematocrit below 60 per cent and multiple nonspecific complaints, including headache, fatigue, dizziness, paresthesias, dyspnea, and epigastric distress. He is of stocky habitus, plethoric, and hypertensive and often has hypercholesterolemia, hypertriglyceridemia, and hyperuricemia. Patients with relative polycythemia are prone to cardiovascular disease, and their management should be directed at correction and prevention of coronary risk factors and elimination of any agents that further reduce the plasma volume, including phlebotomy.

Isolated Erythrocytosis. Documentation of an absolute increase in red cell mass to levels 25 per cent in excess of the predicted value requires further diagnostic evaluation to distinguish between isolated erythrocytosis arising from an abnormality affecting only the erythroid precursors and erythrocythemia as part of the panmyelosis of PV. One of the most significant stigmata of MPD is splenomegaly. If this organ is not readily palpable, a spleen scan is recommended to detect subclinical enlargement. An enlarged spleen combined with absolute erythrocytosis fulfills the criteria for a diagnosis of PV. Other criteria of diagnostic value are leukocytosis greater than 12,000 per mm³, neutrophilia above 7000 per mm³, a direct basophil count above 65 per mm³, a platelet count above 400,000 per mm³, increased leukocyte alkaline phosphatase activity, and an unsaturated serum vitamin B_{12}–binding capacity over 2200 pg per ml. In the absence of splenomegaly, at least two of these abnormalities should be present to fulfill the diagnostic criteria. All patients with absolute erythrocytosis should have an assessment of the adequacy of tissue oxygenation by measurement of arterial oxygen saturation and content, as well as oxygen affinity of hemoglobin. Tissue hypoxemia may be responsible for isolated erythrocytosis or may coexist with PV. Recognition of compensatory erythrocytosis is essential for proper management, since patients who have compensatory erythrocytosis require extra oxygen-carrying capacity and have different criteria for hematocrit reduction.

Causes of inappropriate erythrocytosis due to increased erythropoietin elaboration from hypoxic renal tissue or from tumors or hyperplasias of extrarenal tissues that elaborate erythropoietin inappropriately should be sought by appropriate testing, since many of these conditions are remediable. Patients with idiopathic or unclassified erythrocytosis should be observed carefully and restudied periodically for further clues to the nature of the erythrocytosis. Management should be restricted to manipulation of the circulating red cell mass with phlebotomy.

TREATMENT

The mainstay of therapy for PV is phlebotomy. The objective of this therapy is to maintain the hematocrit at levels of 45 per cent or less with the rationale that uncontrolled erythrocythemia with its attendant hypervolemia and hyperviscosity is the main contributory factor in the thrombotic and hemorrhagic complications of PV. These risks may be compounded further by qualitative platelet abnormalities. The presence of circulating platelet aggregates and degranulated platelets attests to in vivo hyperfunction of the platelet population. The normal stimulatory effect of phlebotomy on hematopoiesis is preserved and even exaggerated in PV. This response includes an increase in platelet count and the appearance of circulating platelets with increased hemostatic activity. The increased incidence of thrombosis during the first 4 years of a phlebotomy regimen may be attributable to this effect and suggests a role for platelet-deaggregating therapy. However, this approach was rejected when a randomized study comparing high-dose aspirin, 300 mg three times daily, combined with dipyridamole (Persantine), 75 mg three times daily, with radioactive phosphorus supplemented with phlebotomy not only failed to show a reduction in thrombotic complications but produced an increased incidence of gastrointestinal hemorrhage. However, in contrast to the results with high doses of deaggregating agents, patients treated with low-dose aspirin (325 mg or less per day) showed a complete absence both of thrombotic events and of significant hemorrhagic complications in two studies.

Phlebotomy and Platelet-Antiaggregating Therapy

The combination of phlebotomy and low-dose aspirin is an efficacious regimen for most patients in the erythrocythemic phase of PV and is the treatment of choice at the time of diagnosis. Every patient with proven PV should have an initial series of phlebotomies to restore the hematocrit to between 40 and 45 per cent, a level that provides maximal cerebral blood flow. A phlebotomy of 500 ml should be performed every second or third day until this result is achieved. The number of phlebotomies required depends upon the degree of elevation of the red cell mass.

Replacement of plasma or fluids is unnecessary, as the patient quickly reconstitutes his or her blood volume if oral hydration is maintained. Several phlebotomies may be required before a decrease in hematocrit occurs. In elderly patients or in those with cardiovascular disease, smaller phlebotomies of 350 ml are preferable to avoid abrupt changes in blood volume. Prior to or at the time of the first phlebotomy the patient should be placed on a regimen of acetylsalicylic acid at a dose of 325 mg a day. A buffered form of acetylsalicylic acid or concomitant administration of antacids is recommended. In addition to its prophylactic function, this dose of aspirin produces prompt relief of symptoms attributable to small vessel stasis, such as erythromelalgia and transient ischemic attacks. Allopurinol (Zyloprim), 300 mg once a day, should be prescribed, regardless of the serum uric acid level, to reduce the excessive load of uric acid that results from increased nucleoprotein turnover. Blocking the conversion of hypoxanthine to uric acid reduces the risk of secondary gout and urate stones or nephropathy. Pruritus, related to release of histamine from basophils, may be relieved by the antihistaminic cyproheptadine (Periactin) in doses of 4 to 16 mg, as needed. The severe itching that is induced by bathing, showering, or undressing can be attenuated by administration of 4 to 8 mg of cyproheptadine 30 minutes before exposure to the precipitating event.

After restoration of a normal hematocrit, the patient should be seen at 6-week intervals to assess the rate at which the hematocrit increases. Some patients display relatively indolent erythropoiesis, and the hematocrit may be kept at normal levels with four to six phlebotomies a year. Management with phlebotomy and aspirin should be employed in such patients, as well as in those with isolated erythrocytosis and in patients with polycythemia vera who are of childbearing age. Hypoferremia is an unavoidable consequence of the phlebotomy regimen but is rarely symptomatic except for producing pica manifested by a craving for crisp green vegetables (lettuce and celery) and ice. Erythrocyte indices are invariably hypochromic and microcytic. Iron replacement should not be given, since it will produce an increase in hematocrit and increase the phlebotomy requirement. A normal diet is appropriate, and no attempt to limit iron-containing foods should be made. Reactive thrombocytosis may occur following the initial series of phlebotomies. This increase in platelet count will be superimposed upon any elevation present prior to phlebotomy but is transient, and the platelet count usually returns to the prephlebotomy level within several weeks. Once the degree of ery-

throid and other proliferative activity and the need for phlebotomy have been assessed, visits may be reduced to every 8 to 10 weeks and phlebotomies of 500 ml performed as needed to maintain the hematocrit between 40 and 45 per cent. Aspirin should be continued at a dose of 325 mg each day unless the platelet count falls below normal or the patient has significant hemorrhagic complications. Concomitant administration of other drugs with platelet/antiaggregating effects, such as nonsteroidal anti-inflammatory agents or antihistaminics, should be avoided to lessen the risk of hemorrhage. If these are indicated, aspirin should be discontinued during their administration.

Myelosuppressive Therapy

Myelosuppressive therapy should be reserved for treatment of proliferative manifestations other than erythrocythemia and used only when these become symptomatic. The most common indication is splenomegaly of sufficient degree to cause early satiety, abdominal discomfort on a mechanical basis, splenic infarction, and a hypermetabolic state manifested by weight loss, diaphoresis, and fever. These symptoms usually occur when the patient enters the phase of postpolycythemic MyM. Indications for myelosuppression during the polycythemic phase include a history of thrombotic events in a patient of advanced age (over 70 years) with risk factors for thrombosis; patients with extreme thrombocythemia (over 2 million per microliter) and symptoms of small vessel stasis; or inability to implement a phlebotomy regimen due to inadequate veins or adverse reactions to blood volume reduction. Myelosuppression can be achieved readily in MPD with a variety of agents, and the selection of an agent rests more on the nature of its potential toxicity than on its ability to produce the desired therapeutic effect.

Hydroxyurea (Hydrea). This agent is a nonalkylating myelosuppressive that inhibits DNA synthesis by inhibition of ribonucleoside diphosphate reductase. Prior experience with hydroxyurea has been confined to treatment of malignancies in patients with short life expectancies relative to that of PV, and in this setting mutagenesis has not been observed. The chronic nature of PV and the short-lived effect of hydroxyurea usually require continuous administration over many years. In a cohort of patients treated with hydroxyurea for a median of 5 years, there has been no increased incidence of leukemia or other malignancies, but the incidence of late-onset leukemia and cancer that is characteristic of other myelosuppressive agents remains to be determined. Until this information is available, hydroxyurea is the myelosuppressive agent of choice because of the theoretical absence of mutagenesis confirmed by short-term experience and the well-established increased incidence of leukemia and cancer produced by radioactive phosphorus and alkylating agents.

An initial dose of 1 gram per day produces a response in 80 per cent of patients without untoward myelosuppression. As the spleen shrinks and the platelet count is reduced, the dose may be adjusted downward to 500 mg per day. If no effect is observed in 3 weeks, the dose may be increased to 1.5 grams per day. The blood count should be monitored frequently until an efficacious regimen is found. Since hydroxyurea induces a megaloblastic blood picture and has less effect on hematocrit levels than on platelet and leukocyte counts, supplementary phlebotomy is usually required. Toxicity is minimal at the doses employed for PV and is limited to rash, gastrointestinal intolerance, and fever.

Once the objective of myelosuppressive therapy has been achieved and the patient's disease activity is stabilized, it is useful to discontinue hydroxyurea administration to determine the rate at which the spleen enlarges or thrombocythemia recurs. In those patients with more indolent disease, it may be possible to interrupt chemotherapy for many months. In view of the dose-related mutagenicity of other agents, this would be preferable to continuous therapy. Unfortunately, maintenance treatment is usually required, since blood counts return to pretreatment levels within 2 weeks after therapy is discontinued.

Radioactive Phosphorus. Radioactive phosphorus (^{32}P) is a strong beta-ray emitter that irradiates the bone marrow both directly by isotope uptake and indirectly through uptake of the phosphate by surrounding bone. It is an excellent myelosuppressive agent, and it was particularly effective in controlling erythropoiesis and megakaryopoiesis in the large doses employed before its mutagenicity was appreciated. However, with the dose limitations imposed to deal with this toxicity, supplementary phlebotomies are frequently required, and splenomegaly may not respond. It has been recommended for the treatment of patients over the age of 70 because of their relatively short life expectancy, but in a physiologically young patient of 70 years with an expected survival of 13 years, disease duration will extend well beyond the 4-year period after which malignant transformation begins to occur. There may be an indication for the use of ^{32}P in elderly patients with thrombocythemia and a history of thrombosis and in patients who cannot tolerate hydroxyurea. The agent should be given intravenously in an initial dose of 2.7 mCi per M^2 (up to a total dose of 5 mCi). If after 12 weeks suppression is inadequate, a second treatment at a 25 per cent dose escalation and a limit of 7 mCi may be given. A third dose may be administered at 24 weeks, if necessary, but if this is ineffective another agent should be employed. The action of ^{32}P is slow, and its full effect is seen after 3 months. Responsive patients may have remissions of 6 months to a year. Patients in whom thrombocythemia shows only a partial response can be managed with phlebotomy and platelet-antiaggregating agents to minimize the amount of radiation administered.

Interferon.[*] The antiproliferative properties of recombinant human interferon-alpha may have an application in the treatment of PV, since early experience has shown that control of thrombocythemia, leukocytosis, and the splenomegaly of myeloid metaplasia can be achieved and maintained with doses that produce minimal side effects. An induction dose of 3.5 million units per M^2 of body surface area of interferon-alpha-2b given daily by subcutaneous injection for 20 weeks produced control of proliferative activity and significant reduction in spleen size, which persisted as dosage was reduced and finally discontinued. The ability to obtain cytoreduction with this biologic response modifier may avoid the problem of leukemogenicity posed by other myelosuppressive agents. Until further investigation establishes the efficacy of interferon as a first line agent, its use in polycythemia vera is reserved for patients whose proliferative disease activity is life-threatening and cannot be controlled by conventional cytoreductive therapy.

Anagrelide. This compound is a quinazolin originally developed to inhibit platelet aggregation. In humans anagrelide causes a dose-dependent decrease in platelet numbers at doses below those required for sustained inhibition of aggregation. At these doses, even prolonged administration of anagrelide for more than 3 years has had no effect on the numbers of other cell types in the circulation and no other evidence of chronic toxicity. Clinical trials have demonstrated a reduction in platelet count to below 600,000 per microliter and maintenance of platelets within the physiologic range in 80 per cent of patients with MPD and thrombocythemia. Side effects have been mild and transient. The platelet-lowering effect of anagrelide is transient and completely reversible, requiring chronic administration for control of thrombocythemia. This agent is undergoing extensive premarketing clinical trials. Because anagrelide is not myelosuppres-

---

*This use is not listed by the manufacturer.

sive and has no known mutagenic or leukemogenic effects, if these studies confirm effectiveness without significant toxicity, this drug may offer a valuable alternative to myelosuppressive therapy in the management of high-risk patients with PV and thrombocythemia.

Management of Complications

Thrombotic and hemorrhagic complications are managed in the same way as in the nonpolycythemic population. If medically indicated, anticoagulants may be employed. Platelet/antiaggregating agents should be withheld in patients with hemorrhagic manifestations. Surgical morbidity and mortality are increased in PV, and elective surgery should be avoided. When surgery is indicated, the blood volume should be restored to normal with phlebotomy. Platelet/deaggregating therapy should be introduced on the fourth or fifth postoperative day if there is no postoperative bleeding to prevent thrombotic complications secondary to the reactive thrombocytosis that may follow surgery.

Postpolycythemia MyM is often complicated by anemia. At this stage iron or folate deficiency should be sought and corrected. Splenomegaly is accompanied by an expansion of the plasma volume, and in some patients the anemia is primarily dilutional. Measurement of the red cell mass is useful, as it may reveal normal or even increased levels of circulating red cells combined with marked hydremia. The use of diuretics may partially correct this state and relieve any symptoms of circulatory overload that are present. An absolute reduction in red cell mass may result from decreased erythropoiesis or shortened red cell survival. In the latter case, the patient may benefit from shrinkage of the spleen with hydroxyurea as described earlier.

Patients who have hypersplenism with shortened red cell survival sufficient to require transfusion therapy may benefit from corticosteroid therapy. Androgens may stimulate erythropoiesis and are worthy of a trial. Response is slow to occur, and therapy should be continued for 6 months. Splenectomy may benefit selected patients with postpolycythemic MyM in whom there is evidence of hypersplenism. Thrombocythemia is an absolute contraindication to splenectomy and must be corrected with myelosuppressive therapy before surgery in order to avoid a life-threatening postoperative thrombocythemia. Evidence of low-grade disseminated intravascular coagulation is also a contraindication to splenectomy.

Acute leukemia develops in 1 to 2 per cent of PV patients treated with phlebotomy alone and in 10 to 20 per cent of patients treated with myelosuppressive agents. Acute nonlymphocytic leukemia is the most common type, but acute lymphoblastic or biphenotypic leukemias occur in one-third of cases. Acute leukemia complicating MPD shows a poor response to conventional therapy. Thus, younger patients should be offered the opportunity to harvest and cryopreserve bone marrow during the polycythemic phase of their disease to permit aggressive chemotherapy and autologous bone marrow transplant if acute leukemia develops.

Choice of Therapy

The patient with PV presents a challenge in management, for the benefits conferred by proper treatment are dramatic in terms of improved survival and well-being. Customizing management to accommodate the factors of age, disease duration, previous and present complications, disease phenotype, and disease activity can afford the patient a long and uncomplicated course. The dilemma of myelosuppression versus phlebotomy and platelet-antiaggregating therapy remains. However, equipped with the knowledge that the use of myelosuppression can be avoided or minimized in many patients and that a potentially nonmutagenic chemotherapeutic agent is now available, the physician can meet the challenge of treatment with greater optimism and expectation of even longer survival and fewer complications for the patient.

PORPHYRIA

method of
CLAUS A. PIERACH, M.D.
University of Minnesota, Abbott-Northwestern Hospital
Minneapolis, Minnesota

The porphyrias are a group of diseases that have in common disturbances of the heme biosynthetic pathway. Their clinical presentation varies widely, as does their therapy. Thus, a good knowledge of their biochemical background is required not only to arrive at the specific diagnosis but also to select effective therapy. There is no single screening test to exclude or include all porphyrias. Testing for porphyrias with neurologic involvement requires measurement of delta-aminolevulinic acid and porphobilinogen, whereas the diagnosis of porphyric skin disease rests on increased levels of porphyrins, whether in the serum, urine, or feces. Figure 1 shows the distribution of heme precursors in the clinically most important porphyrias. Slight elevations of levels of porphyrins

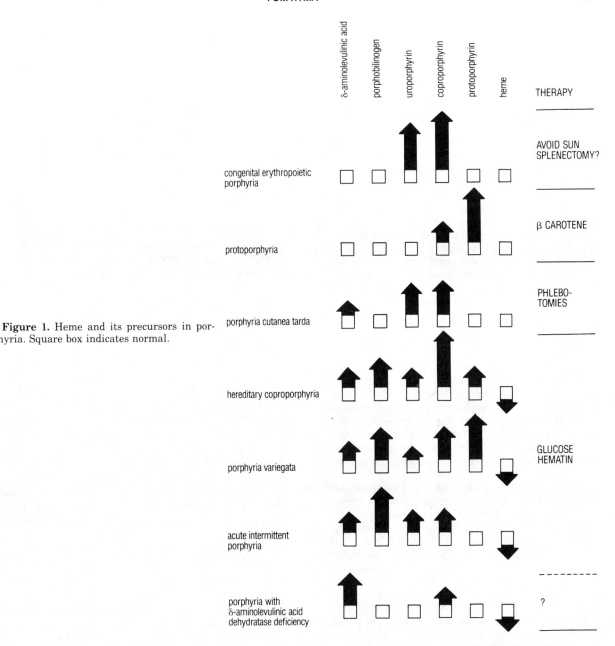

Figure 1. Heme and its precursors in porphyria. Square box indicates normal.

alone do not permit the firm diagnosis of a porphyria because they are often found in patients with liver disease. It is a fairly frequent mistake to call an undiagnosed disease porphyria on the basis of a small elevation in the level of a single porphyrin. The misdiagnosis of coproporphyria is not uncommon because coproporphyrin is often excreted in amounts slightly above normal. Similarly, porphyrias with neurologic involvement are occasionally assumed to exist if screening tests such as the Watson-Schwartz test or Hoesch's test are considered to be positive when a reddish color develops during the test, a not infrequent occurrence in patients with liver disease (caused by excessive amounts of urobilinogen). Strict adherence

to the test procedure and experience in test interpretation are absolutely necessary. It is most difficult to rediagnose a patient who has been erroneously labeled as having porphyria.

All porphyrias are characterized by specific enzyme deficiencies and therefore are best diagnosed by measurement of these enzyme levels. Although these deficiencies have been proved to exist, their routine clinical use is presently limited to measurement of porphobilinogen deaminase, the critical enzyme in acute intermittent porphyria. The enzymatic deficiencies generate characteristic patterns for heme precursors, which permit classification of patients (Figure 1).

It is of great importance to differentiate between

porphyrias with skin involvement and those with neurologic manifestations. Acute intermittent porphyria is the only porphyria with no skin involvement (except for the rare porphyria with delta-aminolevulinate dehydratase deficiency). Variegate porphyria and hereditary coproporphyria involve both the skin and the nervous system, although not necessarily at the same time. The porphyrias with neurologic involvement (acute intermittent porphyria, variegate porphyria, and hereditary coproporphyria) are inducible because they are sensitive to certain drugs, infections, and starvation. The list of inducing drugs is long and will never be complete because new drugs are continuously introduced. Patients are at risk in taking any drug whose induction potential is unknown. The most dangerous drugs in this context are barbiturates, sulfonamides, and anticonvulsants (except bromides). Seizures and epilepsy present a difficult problem in patients with an inducible porphyria. Status epilepticus can be interrupted with intravenous diazepam. A detailed list of safe and unsafe drugs may be found in the chapter on porphyria by Kappas A, Sassa S, Galbraith RA, et al. The Porphyrins. *In* Scriver CR, Beaudet AL, Sly WS, et al (eds): *The Metabolic Basis of Inherited Disease.* New York, McGraw-Hill, 1989, pp. 1305–1365.

Porphyria cutanea tarda seems to occur in two different forms (clinically identical): familial and sporadic. All other porphyrias have a well-recognized genetic background, which is important in counseling and family screening. The rare porphyria with delta-aminolevulinate dehydratase deficiency and the equally rare congenital erythropoietic porphyria are autosomal recessive; the other porphyrias are autosomal dominant.

The dermatologic symptoms are directly related to the presence of porphyrins in the skin and present as light sensitivity, ulcerations, hyper- and hypopigmentation, and skin fragility. The porphyrias with neurologic involvement sometimes occur in life-threatening attacks, often provoked by the use of unsafe drugs, infection, negative caloric balance (intentional weight loss), or premenstrually, but often without an identifiable inducer. Hepatic involvement in protoporphyria can lead to liver failure and may necessitate liver transplantation. Dermatologic symptoms in porphyria cutanea tarda develop only if some liver damage is present, most commonly caused by alcohol abuse (although liver disease alone does not lead to porphyria).

ACUTE INTERMITTENT PORPHYRIA, HEREDITARY COPROPORPHYRIA, AND VARIEGATE PORPHYRIA

Prophylaxis, clinical presentation in an attack, and treatment are alike in these inducible porphyrias, and probably also in porphyria with delta-aminolevulinate dehydratase deficiency (with which too little experience exists). To prevent attacks, patients and their physicians must respect the drug list and avoid using unsafe compounds. This guideline, however, can and must be modified when a patient's life is endan-

gered. Thus it would not be wise to withhold potentially lifesaving drugs just because they are not on the list of safe drugs. This can be very important when considering chemotherapy or other interventions where no options may exist. Under these circumstances, it is advisable to measure porphyrin precursor levels periodically. If these levels remain close to baseline, the danger of a porphyric attack is probably not imminent, and the drug in question may be continued.

The most frequent symptom of a patient with a porphyric attack is abdominal pain. In addition, weakness, restlessness, constipation (at times with an ileus), and urinary retention can develop quickly. Seizures, ascending paralysis, and coma are most ominous signs, often heralding death. Mortality was previously around 80 per cent at this stage, but with newer treatment, it is now far lower. Recovery, although often rather prolonged, is mostly complete. Signs during an attack most often include tachycardia, hyporeflexia, and, in advanced cases, the syndrome of inappropriate antidiuretic hormone secretion. There is always excessive excretion of porphobilinogen (except in porphyria with delta-aminolevulinate dehydratase deficiency), and the Watson-Schwartz test or Hoesch's test is positive during an attack. These test results are useful for clinical diagnosis but not necessarily for genetic studies.

The first step in managing a patient with a porphyric attack is to eliminate the inducing drugs and circumstances. A high-carbohydrate diet has proved to be of help, probably by producing a heme-sparing effect; 400 grams per day of glucose or other carbohydrates should be given, intravenously, if necessary. Other nutrients may be considered in the long run (total parenteral nutrition, if necessary) but are no substitute for carbohydrates. A prophylactic effect of a carbohydrate-rich diet is unproved, and patients should be advised to eat regular, well-balanced meals and to stay as close as possible to their ideal weight. Exercise is a good method of weight control, should that become necessary.

If a patient does not improve or at least stabilize clinically within a day, hematin therapy should be started. A dose of 2 to 4 mg per kg twice daily for 3 days has been found to be helpful and should be instituted early because the attack may otherwise progress to the point of no return. Because the course of an attack is unpredictable, corrective measures must be taken early. The mode of action of hematin is unclear, but two possible explanations can be discussed. The first is that hematin inhibits the induction of delta-aminolevulinate synthase, the rate-limiting enzyme, thus stopping porphyrogenesis and preventing the formation of potentially toxic intermediaries in the heme pathway. The second explanation is that a deficient heme pool is replenished. The current commercially available hematin preparation (Panhematin) is a lyophilized product that must be reconstituted immediately before strictly intravenous injection. The solution is not stable, and there is evidence that decay products act as pro- and anticoagulants. Thus clotting factors (platelet count, prothrombin time, partial thromboplastin time) should be checked periodically, and concomitant administration of anticoagulants should be avoided. A newer preparation as heme-arginate (Normosang) is not yet available in the United States, but it seems to be stable and virtually free from side effects. The clinical course of an attack can be assessed at the bedside by considering tachycardia, hyporeflexia, and simple spirometry (peak flow, forced vital capacity in 1 second). Worsening of these observations indicates progression of the attack.

Pregnancy creates a slightly higher risk of a porphyric attack, but this reason should not be sufficient for an abortion. Genetic counseling is advisable for all women with porphyria, but because most porphyric problems are currently treated with great success, family planning should rarely hinge on this disease. Oral contraception in patients with an inducible porphyria may precipitate an attack and should generally be avoided; however, there is a small group of patients with fairly regular premenstrual exacerbation of their porphyria who do better with oral contraceptives. Thus, the decision on whether to use or avoid them is difficult. A newer approach to this problem is the administration of a luteinizing hormone-releasing hormone analogue.

Acute Intermittent Porphyria

This is the most common and probably the most serious of the inducible porphyrias. It is rarely (if ever) symptomatic before puberty. The critical enzyme is porphobilinogen deaminase, which is readily measured in red blood cells and is well suited for family studies. Precautions must be taken to avoid inducing drugs and circumstances. The skin is not affected. Existence of a more subacute, chronically symptomatic form is unproved. Treatment should start immediately with carbohydrates—for example, glucose. If the patient does not improve or stabilize within a day, hematin should be given (see earlier). The newer preparation of heme-arginate may make the decision to treat an attack with hematin even easier because it is virtually free from side effects.

Hereditary Coproporphyria

Skin and neurologic symptoms may occur, either together or separately. The drug list must be respected. Skin manifestations are often minor and may require only avoidance of sunlight. During a porphyric attack, the Watson-Schwartz test is positive. For family screening, measurement of fecal coproporphyrin levels is suitable. The critical enzyme, coproporphyrinogen oxidase, is not yet measured routinely. Treatment of an attack is as outlined earlier. Because small elevations of coproporphyrin levels are fairly common, the diagnosis of coproporphyria is difficult at times and occasionally must be questioned.

Variegate Porphyria

Again, skin and neurologic symptoms may occur, either together or separately. Treatment and prophylaxis are the same as those for hereditary coproporphyria. As mentioned previously, the critical enzyme, protoporphyrinogen oxidase, is not yet assayed routinely. For family screening, measurements of fecal copro- and protoporphyrin are suitable (protoporphyrin is not water soluble and thus is not found in urine).

PORPHYRIA CUTANEA TARDA

This is the most common porphyria. There are no neurologic symptoms or attacks, and although the drug list for the inducible porphyrias is not applicable, this porphyria is sensitive to certain drugs, such as alcohol, estrogens, and hepatotoxins. Liver disease, often caused by alcohol abuse, is common, and hepatocellular carcinoma is occasionally found. Sclerodermoid changes are fairly common, as are milia and a violaceous hue. Elevated uroporphyrin levels are found in serum, urine, and stool. The critical enzyme, uroporphyrinogen decarboxylase, is not yet measured routinely. If the level of this enzyme is unknown, urinary uroporphyrin measurements must be used for family screening (there is also a common sporadic form). Treatment consists of elimination of the causative substances, most often alcohol. In addition, remission can be induced by phlebotomy, in which 6 to 10 units of blood is removed over 3 to 5 months to avoid anemia. If this cannot be done, low-dose chloroquine may be tried (125 mg twice weekly).

PROTOPORPHYRIA

This porphyria is characterized at times by marked sensitivity to sunlight, with edema formation and intense itching. In addition, liver disease related to hepatic protoporphyrin deposits may be present and must be looked for because the disease can be life-threatening and may require liver transplantation. Beta-carotene (30 to 300 mg per day) often gives excellent protection from the sun (but does not ameliorate protoporphyric liver disease, for which cholestyramine may be tried). High fecal protoporphyrin levels, together with normal urinary porphyrin and precursor excretion, are virtually diagnostic and are suitable for family screening because the incriminated enzyme, ferrochelatase, is not yet assayed routinely.

CONGENITAL PORPHYRIA (GÜNTHER'S DISEASE)

This autosomal recessive porphyria is rare and can be diagnosed in infancy because the large amounts of uroporphyrin stain the diapers red. The children are sensitive to the sun, and deformations are common (short fingers, acral scars, alopecia, erythrodontia), as is anemia. Milder forms are seen occasionally. Sunlight must be avoided. The frequently present anemia occasionally responds well to splenectomy.

THERAPEUTIC USE OF BLOOD COMPONENTS

method of
ROBERT M. KENNEY, M.D., and
JAMES P. CROWLEY, M.D.
Brown University School of Medicine
Providence, Rhode Island

The recognition that acquired immunodeficiency syndrome (AIDS) could be transmitted by blood transfusion has led to increased concern about the safety of blood transfusion. Moreover, there is a growing national consensus that blood transfusions are often given without firm indications and that a substantial amount of blood use in the United States is unnecessary. Nevertheless, blood transfusion remains a cornerstone of modern medicine, and approximately 20 million transfusions of blood components are administered to patients annually in the United States.

The indications for blood transfusion presented in this chapter and in Table 1 are situations in which transfusion is reasonable. By no means are these situations meant to be the only ones in which a transfusion is justifiable. For each patient, the balance between risk, benefit, and alternatives has to be assessed individually.

ALTERNATIVES TO HOMOLOGOUS BLOOD

For elective procedures that are likely to require blood, blood conservation begins with the evaluation of the patient for surgery. The possibility of transfusion should be discussed with the patient and the alternatives to homologous blood transfusion presented. Most patients preparing for elective surgery can donate autologous blood if surgery is scheduled sufficiently far in advance.

Additional blood conservation techniques have been applied to the surgical patient. Preoperative hemodilution is frequently used in patients undergoing cardiopulmonary bypass operations. This "fresh whole blood" provides the patient with a readily available blood source containing red blood cells (RBC), platelets, and plasma proteins without the risk of a homologous transfusion. Moreover, intraoperative administration of 1-deamino-8-D-arginine vasopressin (DDAVP) at the time of heparin reversal in patients undergoing cardiopulmonary bypass surgery has been shown to reduce blood loss during the first 24 hours after surgery in patients undergoing valve replacement with or without coronary artery bypass. Blood conservation during and after surgery may also include intraoperative salvage of shed blood. The salvaged blood may be washed and concentrated or occasionally reinfused without additional processing.

BLOOD COLLECTION, STORAGE, AND PROCESSING

Whole blood (WB) (450 ml) is collected from donors and stored in an anticoagulant-preservative solution. Most of these solutions contain sodium citrate as the anticoagulant and dextrose and phosphate as the preservative. A unit of blood may be stored as WB or fractionated into components such as RBC, plasma, cryoprecipitate, and platelets. A single unit of blood can therefore benefit several patients. WB is separated into RBC and platelet-rich plasma by "soft centrifugation." The platelet-rich plasma is separated into plasma and platelets by a second "hard centrifugation." The platelet concentrate is suspended in 50 to 60 ml of plasma and allowed to "rest" for 1 or 2 hours. A platelet concentrate contains approximately 6×10^{10} platelets. Plasma removed from the platelet concentrate may be frozen and stored at or below $-18°$ C for up to 1 year as fresh-frozen plasma (FFP). Cryoprecipitate may be stored at or below $-18°$ C for up to 1 year.

BLOOD COMPONENT THERAPY

Whole Blood

WB provides an oxygen (O_2)-carrying capacity equivalent to that of RBC, volume expansion, and stable plasma coagulation factors. Processing

TABLE 1. Components and Derivatives Commonly Available for Transfusion Therapy and Indications for Their Use

Available Components	Indications	Approximate Volume	Average Adult Dose	Infusion Rate/Filter
Whole blood	Massive acute blood loss exceeding 25% of BV	500 ml	Varies	Up to 100 ml/min
Whole blood, modified	Exchange transfusion			
Red blood cells	Hgb < 8.0 with symptomatic chronic anemia	250 ml	Varies	1–2 hr
Leukocyte-poor red cells	Hgb < 9.0 in patient with heart or lung disease			
Centrifuged	Massive acute blood loss exceeding 25% of BV	200 ml		140-μm or less filter for all red cell components
Saline washed	O₂ extraction > 50% or mixed venous O₂ saturation < 50%	200 ml		
Frozen-deglycerolized		180 ml		
Filtered		220 ml		
Platelets: random donor	Platelets < 20,000/μl except in patient with idiopathic thrombocytopenic purpura	60 ml/U	6–8 U	Transfused over approximately 1 hr
Platelets: single donor	Platelets < 50,000/μl in actively bleeding patient	300 ml		
Platelets: HLA matched	Intraoperative platelets < 100,000/μl for operation in critical area (brain, spinal cord)	300 ml		
Platelets: washed				140-μm filter
Platelets: leukocyte poor	Bleeding time > 15 min in bleeding patient			
	Platelet dysfunction syndrome (congenital or acquired in bleeding patient)			
Fresh-frozen plasma	PT > 16 sec or PTA < 45% in bleeding patient	220 ml	4 U	Approximately 5 ml/min
Single-donor plasma	APTT > 55 sec in bleeding patient	220 ml		140-μm filter
	Emergency reversal of coumarins and indandiones			
	Selective deficiency states			
Cryoprecipitate	Hemophilia A (Factor VIII deficiency)	15 ml/bag	10 bags	170-μm filter; approximately 5 ml/min
	Von Willebrand's disease			
	Uremic bleeding			
	Hypofibrinogenemia, disseminated intravascular coagulation			
	Factor XIII deficiency			
	Localized surgical hemostasis ("fibrin glue")			
Granulocytes	PMNs < 500/μl, serious infection unresponsive to antibiotics			
	Neonatal neutropenia			

Available Derivatives	Indications	Approximate Volume	Average Adult Dose	Infusion Rate/Filter
Intravenous immune globulin	Immune globulin deficiency	50 ml	400 mg/kg	See package insert
	Idiopathic thrombocytopenic purpura			Drip chamber
	Kawasaki's disease (not approved by FDA)			
Albumin	Hypovolemic shock	250 ml	Varies	Drip chamber
5%	Severe hypoalbuminemia	50 ml		
25%	Acute liver failure			
	Severe burns (after first 24 hr)			
	Therapeutic plasma exchange			
Clotting factor concentrates	See section of book on hemophilia	Varies	Varies	See package insert

Abbreviations: BV = blood volume; Hgb = hemoglobin; PT = prothrombin time; PTA = plasma thromboplastin antecedent (Factor XI); APTT = activated partial thromboplastin time; PMN = polymorphonuclear neutrophil; FDA = U.S. Food and Drug Administration.

and testing of blood generally delay its availability for transfusion for 24 hours. Therefore, even the "freshest" WB is unlikely to provide appreciable platelet function. The plasma associated with WB is depleted in labile (V, VIII) clotting factors.

Red Blood Cells

In most circumstances, packed RBC is the appropriate component for patients who require blood. One unit of RBC increases an adult's blood hemoglobin concentration by approximately 1 gram per dl. This relationship is generally satisfactory in determining the quantity of blood to transfuse. However, if a more precise estimate is required, a detailed calculation may be made based on the blood volume (for adults, approximately 70 ml per kg), the desired increase in hemoglobin, and the quantity of hemoglobin in a unit of RBC.

The amount of O_2 delivered to the tissue per unit time is the amount of blood delivered to the tissues per unit time (cardiac output) times the amount of O_2 dissolved in arterial blood (arterial O_2 content). The cardiac output is the amount of blood delivered per ventricular contraction (stroke volume) times the number of contractions per unit time (heart rate). The O_2 content of arterial blood is the product of the hemoglobin concentration, the amount of O_2 hemoglobin can carry (O_2-binding capacity), and the degree to which the hemoglobin is saturated with O_2 (O_2 saturation). The degree of hemoglobin saturation is determined by the Po_2 and the hemoglobin dissociation curve. The hemoglobin dissociation curve is influenced by pH, CO_2, temperature, and the level of intracellular 2,3-diphosphoglycerate (DPG). The intracellular DPG level, in turn, is influenced by the enzymes of the glycolytic pathway.

The amount of O_2 extracted from the blood per unit time is the difference between the arterial and mixed venous (pulmonary artery) O_2 concentrations times the cardiac output. The amount of O_2 required to maintain aerobic metabolism varies with the metabolic activity of the patient. The arteriovenous O_2 difference is a measurement of the extent to which cardiac output keeps pace with the metabolic needs of the patient. The body has a tremendous reserve of O_2-carrying capacity. If patients are using this reserve to meet their O_2 needs without compromising vital organs, they do not need to be transfused. Making a decision about when to transfuse requires an appreciation for the compensatory mechanisms available, as well as an understanding of the signs and symptoms suggesting that these mechanisms are being taxed.

With most patients, a deficit in the usual work capacity is not appreciable until the hemoglobin concentration falls to 7 grams per dl or less. An increased intracellular level of DPG is an important compensation for chronic anemia. When the hemoglobin level is decreased by half (from 14 to 7 grams per dl), the reduction of O_2 delivery is only 30 per cent instead of the 50 per cent predicted based on the decreased hemoglobin level. Cardiovascular compensation generally does not occur in the resting patient until the hemoglobin level falls to 7 grams per dl or less. Signs of cardiovascular compensation include tachycardia and "flow murmurs." Angina pectoris and high output failure may appear if coronary oxygen flow is unable to keep pace with the myocardial demand. If this occurs at a hemoglobin level of more than 7 grams per dl in the resting patient, it is usually a sign of intrinsic cardiovascular disease. In severe anemia (hemoglobin level less than 5 grams per dl), coronary O_2 delivery may be so impaired as to lead to reduced ventricular function and congestive heart failure. In some patients, cardiac failure may not occur until the hemoglobin level drops to as low as 2 grams per dl. Many factors, including fever, inflammation, nutrition, and thyroid status, influence the O_2 requirements of the patient. Therapeutic modalities that should be considered before transfusing include reducing activity to decrease the O_2 needs of the patient; increasing the inhaled O_2 concentration, which can marginally increase the arterial O_2 saturation; fluid replacement, which can markedly improve the cardiac output and O_2 delivery if the patient is hypovolemic; and treating the underlying cause of anemia.

Acute blood losses of 20 to 30 per cent of a patient's blood volume can generally be tolerated without RBC transfusions provided that the patient receives prompt fluid replacement with crystalloid with or without colloid solutions. In many patients with an acute blood loss, exact quantitation of the amount of blood lost is impossible. In this situation, a drop in blood pressure or an increase in heart rate may be the measurable indicator of blood loss. A therapeutic trial of crystalloid is appropriate to assess the need for a transfusion. If crystalloid is insufficient to maintain the blood pressure, transfusion may be indicated. Patients with chronic anemia and normal cardiovascular function generally do not require transfusion until their hemoglobin level falls below 8 grams per dl and approaches 7 grams per dl. For many patients, it is more appropriate to teach them to adjust to the limitations associated with the anemia than to institute a program of chronic transfusion. In the patient with known heart or respiratory disease, it is more difficult to determine the appropriate time to transfuse. In many of these patients, it is reasonable to transfuse when the hemoglobin level drops below 9 grams per dl. Erythropoietin may further enhance the ability of patients with chronic anemia to make blood, particularly that associated with renal failure.

In selected clinical situations, it is appropriate to administer RBC in a form other than packed RBC. For patients with repeated or severe febrile reactions, leukocyte-poor RBC are appropriate. These may be prepared by centrifugation, washing, or filtration. The last method is associated with leukocyte removal approaching 99.5 per cent and minimal loss of RBC. For these reasons it is preferred. Washed red cells are indicated for patients with IgA deficiency or severe allergic reactions.

All RBC components transfused should be compatible with the patient's plasma. In emergency transfusions, type O RBC are used. If the patient is a child or a premenopausal woman, Rh-negative RBC should be used. In nonemergency situations, the patient's serum is tested for antibodies (antibody screen) and blood is selected that lacks any clinically significant antibodies present in the patient's serum. A patient with a negative antibody screen has an extremely high (99.9 per cent) probability of being compatible with ABO-compatible RBC, which is the basis for the "type and screen" protocol used in many transfusion services. All RBC components should be transfused through either a standard 140-micrometer or a microaggregate (20- to 40-micrometer) blood filter. Isotonic sodium chloride (0.9 per cent USP) may be mixed with the blood to reduce its viscosity and improve the flow rate. A unit of blood should generally be administered to an adult within 1 to 2 hours. Patients with cardiac disease or fluid overload should be transfused more slowly and may require premedication with a diuretic. If blood has to be infused rapidly, adults may tolerate flow rates of up to 1.5 ml per kg per minute, although at these extreme rates a drop in the ionized calcium level may be expected. An 18-gauge needle or catheter is a reasonable size for routine transfusions.

Platelets

For patients with thrombocytopenia diagnosed on the basis of bone marrow hypoplasia, an inverse relationship exists between platelet count and bleeding time. When the platelet count falls below 100,000 per microliter, the bleeding time increases, approximately doubling at a level of 50,000 per microliter. This relationship does not hold for thrombocytopenia associated with accelerated platelet destruction accompanied by active production in conditions such as idiopathic thrombocytopenic purpura (ITP). In these patients the bleeding time is shorter than would be predicted by the platelet count, and platelet transfusions can generally be avoided. The platelets in these patients are larger, younger, and apparently more functional. In patients with platelet dysfunction, bleeding times are prolonged beyond what would be predicted on the basis of the platelet count.

The most influential study associating bleeding with platelet counts in leukemic patients was conducted by the National Cancer Institute in the early 1960s. Increased hemorrhage was observed with counts below 20,000 per microliter, which led to the recommendation that patients with counts below this value be prophylactically transfused. However, the risk of serious bleeding did not accelerate significantly until the count fell below 5000 per microliter. In thrombocytopenia associated with bone marrow hypoplasia, the risk of bleeding is greatly influenced by other factors, such as medications, fever, infection, liver disease, or disseminated intravascular coagulation (DIC). These factors should be taken into consideration when prophylactic transfusions are considered for thrombocytopenia. In the absence of risk factors, prophylactic transfusions may be appropriate with platelet counts below 5000 to 10,000 per microliter. In the presence of risk factors, it is reasonable to raise this threshold to 20,000 per microliter. It is generally recognized that a patient with a platelet count of more than 50,000 per microliter without any associated platelet dysfunction does not benefit from prophylactic platelet transfusion. It is usually safe to perform invasive procedures under these circumstances. An exception might be surgery in a critical area such as the brain or spinal cord, in which the potential consequences of even a minor hemorrhage might be severe.

Platelet dysfunction may be congenital or acquired. Both DDAVP and cryoprecipitate have corrected the bleeding time and improved hemostasis for some patients with platelet dysfunction and von Willebrand's disease. For these patients, a therapeutic trial of DDAVP is justified. If the bleeding time is corrected, the preoperative use of DDAVP is warranted. DDAVP should be avoided in patients with Type IIb von Willebrand's disease because of its propensity to cause thrombocytopenia and thrombosis.

Based on availability, most patients transfused with platelets receive pooled, random donor platelets. The usual adult dose is 6 to 8 units, or approximately 1 unit per 10 kg of body weight. Alternatively, platelets collected by automated pheresis may be used. One platelet pheresis component may supply an equivalent number of platelets to 6 to 8 units of random donor platelets. Pheresis platelets have the advantage of minimizing donor exposure. When inventories permit, platelets are chosen to be ABO identical to the patient. Often sufficient quantities of ABO-identical platelets are unavailable, and platelets are chosen so that the associated plasma is compatible with the patient's RBC. When feasible, Rh-negative patients are transfused with Rh-negative platelets. Rh sensitization is rare but should be avoided in Rh-negative, premenopausal women. Rh-immune globulin may be used prophylactically to reduce the possibility of sensitization when premenopausal, Rh-negative women must be transfused with Rh-positive platelets. Refractoriness to platelet transfusions is generally due to human leukocyte antigen (HLA) antibodies. For approximately two-thirds of these patients, HLA-matched platelets provide an adequate therapeutic response. For the patient who does not respond to HLA-matched platelets, platelet cross-matching can increase the response rate to approximately 80 to 90 per cent.

For neonates with isoimmune thrombocytopenia or older patients with severe allergic reactions or IgA deficiency, washed platelets are indicated. For patients in whom volume is an important consideration, platelet concentrates may be made low in volume by centrifugation and plasma removal. Patients with repeated or severe febrile reactions to platelets may benefit from leukocyte-poor platelets prepared by either filtration or centrifugation. Platelets must be given through a blood filter with a standard 170- to 220-micrometer pore size. Platelets must not be transfused through a microaggregate filter. Generally, platelets are transfused into adults over approximately 1 hour, although they may be transfused more rapidly if this is tolerated. Flushing the infusion line with 20 to 50 ml of saline is usually permissible unless the patient is saline or volume restricted. Transfusion through needles as small as 25 gauge does not appear to be harmful to platelets.

In addition to observing whether bleeding decreases after the transfusion, it is important to determine whether the transfusion resulted in the expected rise in platelet count. Each platelet concentrate is expected to increase the platelet count by 5000 to 10,000 per microliter in an adult or, expressed per M^2 of body surface area (BSA), approximately 15,000 per M^2. The most widely accepted index of platelet response is the 1-hour "corrected count increment" (CCI). A 15-minute count may be substituted for the 1-hour count if it is more convenient.

$$CCI = \frac{\text{post-transfusion count} - \text{pretransfusion count} \times BSA\ (M^2)}{\text{count of platelets given}\ (\times\ 10^{11})}$$

If the patient is not in septic shock and the CCI is below 7000 to 10,000 per microliter, the patient is likely to have antibody-mediated destruction, involving either platelet autoantibodies or alloantibodies. Most alloantibodies are HLA antibodies. If the 1-hour CCI is greater than 10,000 per microliter but less than that at 18 to 24 hours, platelet consumption is likely and may be caused by fever, splenomegaly, sepsis, DIC, or active bleeding. If both the 1-hour and 18- to 24-hour CCI values are higher than 10,000 per microliter, the response is categorized as adequate in terms of the platelet increment. If the patient has a low 1-hour CCI on two or more occasions, the patient can be considered to be refractory to random donor platelets.

Plasma

FFP contains normal quantities of plasma proteins. It is separated from the RBC within 6 hours of collection and frozen at $-18°$ C or less. Single-donor plasma (SDP) is a comparable product that differs primarily in its content of labile clotting factors. SDP may be prepared from WB any time up to 5 days after expiration of the unit. Plasma contains numerous proteins with myriad functions, including oncotic pressure, transport, coagulation, fibrinolysis, complement, and humoral immunity. In many cases, specific derivatives of plasma are available that provide the specific proteins in a more concentrated, less infectious form. When appropriate, these derivatives should be used instead of plasma. Transfusion of plasma is indicated only to replace multiple clinically significant clotting factors that cannot be replaced by safer alternatives. Despite its widespread use, few specific indications justify FFP administration.

Coumarin drugs, including warfarin (Coumadin), function as anticoagulants by blocking the oxidation of vitamin K. Oxidized vitamin K acts as a cofactor in the carboxylation of glutamic acid residues on Factors II, VII, IX, and X, as well as protein-C and protein-S. Reversal of the effects of these drugs by the administration of vitamin K_1 may be achieved within approximately 6 to 12 hours. If patients are bleeding briskly or require immediate surgical intervention, FFP or SDP can be transfused. Plasma (FFP or SDP) may also be useful for hypercoagulable patients with antithrombin III deficiency, either congenital or acquired (severe hepatic dysfunction, contraceptive use, nephrotic syndrome, DIC). These patients may require replacement if they are undergoing surgery or treatment with heparin for thrombosis.

The pathophysiology of thrombotic thrombocytopenic purpura is not known. In its acute form it consists of the triad of microangiopathic hemolytic anemia, renal dysfunction, and fluctuating neurologic dysfunction. Untreated, it has an extremely high mortality. Therapeutic plasma exchange using FFP as replacement fluid has achieved remission rates of about 80 per cent.

Plasma selected for transfusion should be compatible with the RBC of the patient. It does not have to be cross-matched. Rh-negative plasma is generally given to Rh-negative patients. Plasma should be administered through a standard 170-micrometer blood filter. A transfusion rate of 5 ml per minute is reasonable in an adult, although faster rates are possible if they are tolerated. Most transfusions should be completed within 1 to 2 hours.

Cryoprecipitate

Cryoprecipitate was developed as a source of concentrated Factor VIII and revolutionized the care of patients with hemophilia A. Cryoprecipitate contains appreciable quantities of fibrinogen and fibronectin in addition to Factor VIII. Each bag of cryoprecipitate prepared from a single donation of WB contains approximately 100 units of Factor VIII activity. With the development of commercial Factor VIII concentrates, the use of cryoprecipitate decreased dramatically up to recent years, when concern over the safety and supply of Factor VIII concentrates prompted a resurgence of its use. Usage of cryoprecipitate may decrease again as monoclonally purified and eventually recombinant Factor VIII concentrate becomes more readily available.

Cryoprecipitate is an excellent source of von Willebrand's factor. In patients with von Willebrand's disease who are unresponsive to DDAVP or in patients with Type IIb von Willebrand's disease, cryoprecipitate is the therapy of choice for patients who require intervention. It is also useful in managing bleeding in uremic patients unresponsive to DDAVP. Cryoprecipitate is the best source of fibrinogen and is the product of choice when fibrinogen is depleted or nonfunctional, as in selected patients with DIC, obstetric complications, or congenital fibrinogen deficiency. A bag of cryoprecipitate contains approximately 250 mg of fibrinogen. Cryoprecipitate

may be used as a source of Factor XIII in deficient patients when volume is a consideration. If cryoprecipitate is used as "fibrin glue," it should be prepared from autologous plasma when collection of autologous blood is possible.

Cryoprecipitate is stored frozen. It is thawed at 37° C and pooled immediately before use. In general, any ABO type cryoprecipitate can be given to any patient. Only when massive quantities of cryoprecipitate are used does the ABO type become important. Cryoprecipitate should be administered through a standard 170-micrometer blood filter. It may be administered to adults at a rate of 5 ml per minute, or faster if tolerated. After transfusion, the infusion set may be rinsed with 20 to 30 ml of sterile normal saline.

Granulocytes

Extreme granulocytopenia (absolute granulocyte count < 500 per microliter) is associated with severe bacterial infection. Although granulocyte transfusions have gone out of vogue, they may be valuable for neutropenic patients who do not respond to antibiotics. In the infected neutropenic patient, the decision to administer a granulocyte transfusion should depend in part on the institution's experience with severely neutropenic patients, as well as on the ability of the blood center to provide daily granulocyte concentrates that are highly concentrated and leukocyte compatible. Septic neonates with an absolute neutrophil count of less than 3000 per microliter during the first week of life or subsequently of less than 1000 per microliter, and with decreased marrow reserves of neutrophils, may benefit from granulocyte transfusions. In the noninfected neutropenic patient, prophylactic granulocyte transfusions are generally considered to be of marginal value.

Granulocyte donors should be selected to be ABO compatible with the patient. If the patient has been sensitized to white blood cells, the granulocytes should be from a compatible donor optimally selected by leukocyte cross-matching and HLA matching. Granulocytes should be collected daily in large numbers (preferably 2 to 3 × 10^{10} for an adult and 0.5 to 1 × 10^9 per kg for a neonate) by a method shown to produce functional cells. They should be transfused as soon as possible after collection. Granulocytes are administered with a 170-micrometer filter. They must not be transfused through a microaggregate filter. They should generally be transfused slowly over 2 to 4 hours while the patient is closely monitored. Reactions are common and include severe pulmonary reactions. Premedication (with diphenhydramine, meperidine, or both) may lessen the side effects, and premedication with steroids and nonaspirin antipyretics may be indicated to reduce or prevent a febrile reaction. Amphotericin B may exacerbate pulmonary reactions, and it is prudent to administer it at a different time of day than the granulocyte transfusion.

DERIVATIVE TRANSFUSION THERAPY (SELECTED TOPICS)

Plasma derivatives are derived from plasma pooled from many donors. The plasma undergoes various fractionation and purification procedures, resulting in derivatives such as coagulation concentrates, albumin, and gamma globulin preparations. This section discusses albumin and intravenous immune globulin. Other chapters of this book cover the use of and indications for coagulation concentrates.

Albumin

Albumin constitutes 60 per cent of the plasma protein and provides approximately 80 per cent of the oncotic pressure of plasma. Albumin is also a major transport protein and complexes with unconjugated bilirubin, drugs, and metabolites. It is prepared by fractionation of pooled plasma and is available as 5 and 25 per cent solutions, of which approximately 96 per cent of the protein content is albumin. Albumin is pasteurized and is not known to transmit hepatitis or AIDS.

Albumin may be indicated as part of the fluid replacement in therapeutic plasma exchange or added to packed cells as part of an exchange transfusion protocol for neonates. In each of these situations, albumin is used to replace an acute, massive loss of plasma. In therapeutic plasma exchange, albumin may be supplemented by normal saline, which may substantially reduce the cost of the procedure. Patients with shock and low (<2.5 grams per dl) albumin levels may respond better to albumin replacement than to crystalloid therapy alone. For patients with severe edema and fluid overload, albumin may have a role in conjunction with diuretics to mobilize the fluid.

Albumin is infused with a standard infusion set with a drip chamber. Use of a filter is not required. In general, albumin may be infused as rapidly as tolerated by the patient. When the blood volume is not reduced, rates of 2 to 4 ml per minute for 5 per cent albumin and of 1 ml per minute for 25 per cent albumin may be used. The patient should be closely monitored for signs of fluid overload. Adverse reactions to albumin are rare but have been reported.

Intravenous Immune Globulin

Intravenous immune globulin (intravenous IgG) preparations are prepared by cold alcohol fractionation of pooled plasma. The main clinical indication for intravenous IgG is replacement therapy in patients deficient in IgG. Although some differences exist between intravenous IgG preparations from different manufacturers (Sandoglobulin, Gammagard, Gamimune-N), they generally contain at least 98 per cent IgG, mostly in the monomeric form, with subclass distributions present in proportions approximating those of normal plasma. The preparations have slightly different functional specifications when evaluated by in vitro assays. Intravenous IgG is not known to transmit hepatitis or AIDS. All of the preparations are expensive. Whether they are cost effective remains to be determined.

Although intravenous IgG has been used in several autoimmune conditions, the only disease for which it is specifically approved by the U.S. Food and Drug Administration is ITP. In most patients with ITP, high-dose intravenous IgG can cause a prompt increase in the platelet count. In acute ITP of childhood, intravenous IgG increases the platelet count sooner than prednisone, and remissions at 60 and 120 days are more frequent than those in patients treated with prednisone alone. Adults with acute ITP often undergo splenectomy soon after their diagnosis. Intravenous IgG may be able to eliminate the need for splenectomy in some patients. In patients with diseases such as diabetes mellitus, peptic ulcer disease, or osteoporosis, intravenous IgG may avoid the exacerbation of disease by steroids. Intravenous IgG may also help to reduce steroid use during pregnancy and to increase the platelet count before delivery. Adults with chronic ITP who fail to respond to splenectomy may benefit from intravenous IgG. Although intravenous IgG is not approved for Kawasaki's disease, pediatric patients treated with intravenous IgG and aspirin have a decreased incidence of aneurysms. Patients with autoimmune neutropenia and infections may also benefit from intravenous IgG.

The preparations of intravenous IgG vary in their packaging, concentration, and recommended dosages. Package inserts should always be consulted before infusion. Infusion should begin at a slow rate (often 0.01 to 0.02 ml per kg) according to the manufacturer's instruction. The patient should be closely monitored for signs of anaphylactic reaction.

ADVERSE REACTIONS TO BLOOD TRANSFUSION

method of
CAROL A. BELL, M.D.
Brotman Medical Center
Culver City, California

Transfusion of blood or blood components is intended to correct deficits in red blood cells, white blood cells, platelets, or coagulation factors. These therapies are effective but temporary, and although they are generally safe, there is always an unavoidable risk of either immune- or non–immune-mediated adverse consequences (Table 1). These consequences vary from mild to fatal or may involve long-term morbidity. The risk of infection increasingly outweighs the danger of immune reactions. Because there is no zero-risk transfusion, the risk/benefit ratio must strongly favor the benefit. The risks of transfusion and alternatives to transfusion should be discussed with the patient, and these discussions should be documented.

Transfusion of red blood cells is used to increase the oxygen-carrying capacity of the blood. However, the red blood cell normally functions far below its potential. There is increasing scientific evidence that tissue oxygen perfusion is adequate at hemoglobin levels of 7 grams per dl in many patients. Hypovolemia may be treated with other volume expanders such as crystalloids, synthetic colloids, albumin, or plasma protein fraction which do not have the same risk of infection and can reduce the number of red blood cells needed.

TABLE 1. **Classification of Transfusion Reactions**

Immune Mechanisms
1. Acute catastrophic intravascular hemolysis
2. Delayed hemolysis
3. Nonhemolytic febrile
   a. Leukoagglutinins
4. Allergic
   a. Urticaria
   b. Asthma
   c. Noncardiogenic pulmonary edema (leukoagglutinins)
5. Graft-versus-host disease

Nonimmune Mechanisms
1. Vascular overload
2. Embolism
   a. Air
   b. Tissue particles and fat
3. Infections
   a. Bacterial sepsis
   b. Syphilis
   c. Parasitic infections
      i. Malaria
      ii. Chagas's disease
      iii. Babesiosis
   d. Viral infection
      i. Hepatitis B
      ii. Non-A, non-B hepatitis
      iii. Cytomegalovirus or Epstein-Barr virus
      iv. Human immunodeficiency virus 1
      v. Human T cell lymphotrophic virus I

Before elective surgery, consideration should be given to autologous blood transfusion. With current anticoagulants, blood may be stored in a refrigerator for 42 days, which may allow the patient to donate as many as 3 or 4 units for his or her own surgery. In addition, using preoperative hemodilution or intraoperative salvage of shed blood further reduces dependence on red blood cells. Conservative use of blood products reduces the potential for transfusion reactions.

Acute transfusion reactions can be defined as any untoward reactions occurring while blood or its components are infusing or in the 2 to 3 hours after transfusion. Delayed reactions occur days to weeks or months later and, in the case of human T cell lymphotrophic virus I (HTLV I) infection, years later.

ACUTE REACTIONS TO BLOOD TRANSFUSION

The symptoms of acute transfusion reaction can be quite variable and may not correlate with the actual clinical severity of the reaction. Therefore, it is prudent to assume that every immediate reaction may be caused by acute intravascular hemolysis and to stop the infusion immediately and keep the intravenous line open with normal saline so that further therapy may be given if necessary.

Acute Catastrophic Intravascular Hemolysis

Acute catastrophic transfusion reactions are almost always caused by ABO incompatibility resulting from human error in identifying the blood specimen drawn for cross-match or in identifying the patient at the time of infusion. These reactions account for the majority of the transfusion fatalities, approximately 15 to 20 per year. The ABO blood group is unique because of the obligatory antibodies—anti-A, anti-B, or both—present in the recipient's plasma. These antibodies are hemolytic because they activate the classic complement pathway. Red blood cell lysis is massive, producing hemoglobinemia and hemoglobinuria. The antigen-containing stroma from the lysed, incompatible red blood cells produces renal cortical necrosis with oliguria or anuria. Less commonly, other red blood cell antibodies, such as anti-C, anti-S, anti-Kell, or anti-Duffy[a], may cause intravascular hemolysis. These antibodies, unlike anti-A or anti-B, are present in patients who have been previously transfused and immunized only after many transfusions; for that reason, acute hemolytic reactions to these antibodies are less common.

Acute intravascular hemolysis is usually heralded by fever and chills, followed by hypotension, disseminated intravascular coagulation (DIC), renal failure, shock, and death. DIC produces generalized oozing from mucous mem-

411

branes, venipunctures, and operative wounds. Other symptoms of acute hemolysis include pain at the site of the infusion, chest or flank pain, nausea, vomiting, and dyspnea.

Not all patients exhibit all the signs or symptoms given in Table 2, but fever occurs in 80 per cent of cases. Unfortunately, the patient who is under anesthesia does not show the early symptoms of fever or chills, or feel pain, so that the first signs of a major transfusion reaction are hypotension, generalized oozing from the surgical field, and hemoglobinuria. For this reason, transfusion during general anesthesia should be kept to a minimum. Because shock is a frequent symptom of serious reactions, the unwary physician may compound the disaster by administering more incompatible blood in the mistaken belief that the shock is hypovolemic shock.

Acute hemolytic reactions are dose related and are more likely to be fatal if not recognized promptly and the administration stopped. The blood filter and intravenous tubing should be changed because they contain a further 50 ml of incompatible blood. The volume of incompatible blood that may be fatal can be as little as 200 ml. Children can be seriously affected by even smaller volumes.

When a transfusion reaction is suspected, the blood must be stopped but the intravenous line kept open with normal saline (0.9 per cent NaCl). The paperwork identifying the blood and the patient should be immediately checked because clerical error is the most common cause of an ABO-incompatible transfusion. A blood specimen is taken to check for hemoglobinemia, and a urine specimen is obtained to document urinary output and to check for hemoglobinuria. A direct Coombs's test is performed to detect sensitized donor cells. However, after massive hemolysis this test may be negative because all the incompatible cells have been destroyed. The therapy is summarized in Table 3. The most important goal is to keep the patient well hydrated, while avoiding congestive heart failure, to preserve renal function. Hypotension should be treated with 5 per cent albumin and intravenous crystalloids to maintain renal perfusion.

Increased hydration and diuresis should be

TABLE 2. Signs and Symptoms of Acute Hemolytic Transfusion Reaction

Mild, Early	Major, Late
Fever	Chest pain
Chills	Dyspnea
Flank pain	Hemoglobinuria
Hypotension	Oliguria, anuria
Impending sense of doom	Generalized oozing
	Shock

TABLE 3. Treatment of Intravascular Hemolytic Transfusion Reaction

Symptoms	Treatment

Hemoglobinuria, oliguria	1. Prevention of renal failure
	  a. 1000 ml 0.9% NaCl/hr for 2–3 hr
	  b. Diuretic: furosemide, 40 mg IV, or ethacrynic acid, 50 mg IV
	  c. Maintain urine flow at 100 ml/hr for 6–8 hr or until hemoglobinuria clears

Generalized diffuse bleeding	2. Treatment of DIC a. Cryoprecipitate—6 units with six platelet concentrates as needed for prolonged partial thromboplastin time and thrombocytopenia; repeat in 30 min if clotting is not achieved
Hypotension, shock	3. 5% albumin with adequate saline infusion to maintain systolic pressure above 100 mmHg

maintained until hemoglobinuria is cleared, which may require as long as 24 hours, depending on the volume of incompatible blood. Diuretics that promote renal blood flow, such as furosemide or ethacrynic acid, are preferred to older osmotic diuretics such as mannitol. The volume of saline administered must be adequate to support the diuretic agent and the amount of concurrent albumin infused, so that urine flow is 100 ml per hour and congestive heart failure is avoided. Vasopressors such as dopamine are to be avoided because they cause vasoconstriction and may diminish renal blood flow. If DIC is present, treatment requires cryoprecipitate, which replaces Factor VIII and fibrinogen, fresh-frozen plasma (FFP) to replace other coagulation factors, and platelets. Treatment of DIC with heparin is fraught with hazard in the already bleeding patient. When DIC appears, the consumption of coagulation factors is beyond the point of heparin therapy, and replacement therapy is necessary to replace the factors already consumed. For the adult, 6 units of cryoprecipitate, administered in conjunction with six platelet concentrates, is often effective. The dose of each can be repeated in 30 minutes if bleeding persists, and this therapy is usually satisfactory. Although the platelet count and partial thromboplastin time can be monitored, the cessation of clinical bleeding is the important indicator of the adequacy of therapy.

Delayed Hemolytic Reactions

Red blood cell antibodies may fade with time, so that pretransfusion screening or the crossmatch will not show incompatibility. For that reason, it is advisable to provide patients with a card listing the identified antibody. Red blood cell antibodies that are weak may increase in titer after transfusion of antigen-positive red blood cells. The secondary immune response occurs in 24 hours to 10 days, and with the increase in titer, the incompatible cells are coated with antibody and sequestered in the reticuloendothelial system, usually in the spleen. This extravascular red blood cell destruction is slow and may be asymptomatic, except for failure to achieve and maintain expected elevations in hemoglobin level (1 gram per unit of packed red blood cells) in the absence of bleeding. Antibodies in the Rh system, anti-E and anti-C, are commonly involved. If destruction is more rapid, there may be mild, transient elevations in the bilirubin level (1.5 to 3 mg per dl) in the first 6 to 8 hours posttransfusion, with an increase in the indirect fraction. In some cases, as with anti-Kidd, there may be abrupt intravascular hemolysis at 7 to 10 days post-transfusion of all the Kidd-positive units given. The hemoglobinuria is alarming but often asymptomatic, although oliguria can occur. Increased hydration should be maintained to clear the urine hemoglobin rapidly.

Hemolysis Caused by Transfused Antibody

The previous discussion has described hemolysis of donor red blood cells by patient antibodies. Of less importance is the hemolysis of *patient* red blood cells by anti-A or anti-B found in ABO group–incompatible frozen plasma or cryoprecipitate. (Donors of these products are screened for other immune antibodies, so they are usually not a consideration.) The relative volume of frozen plasma or cryoprecipitate to the patient's blood volume makes these reactions of somewhat less clinical significance. However, in infants or children under 5 years of age, these reactions can produce mild to moderate intravascular hemolysis and fever or chills. The reactions are usually recognized immediately and should be treated by adequate hydration.

Nonhemolytic Febrile Reactions Caused by Leukocyte Antibodies

The most common transfusion reaction symptom is fever, with or without chills. Because it is a symptom of intravascular hemolysis, it cannot be ignored, but in many cases no direct cause is identified. Fever that begins 45 minutes after the transfusion has started or in the first hour post-transfusion is characteristic of a leukoagglutinin reaction caused by antibodies to granulocytes. This type of reaction is often preceded by severe

chilling before the abrupt rise in temperature to 104° or 105° F. Leukoagglutinins are seen in multiply transfused patients or after pregnancy. They may be present without prior transfusion or pregnancy in patients with acute myelogenous leukemia. Treatment consists of acetaminophen (Tylenol), 650 mg orally, repeated in 3 to 4 hours. Future blood components may need to be saline washed to decrease leukocyte exposure. If the antibody titer is high, frozen, deglycerolized red blood cells should be given to minimize the granulocyte exposure. Both products increase the cost of transfusion three to five times. In 50 per cent of cases, a single febrile reaction is not repeated, so that it is not necessary to provide the more expensive component. For patients with strong leukoagglutinins, transfusion of platelet concentrates with the included buffy coat is a serious problem. Filters that remove granulocytes are now available for both red blood cell products and platelets. The negatively charged fibers in these filters attract granulocytes (but not lymphocytes) to them. The decrease in granulocytes is frequently efficient enough to prevent further febrile reactions. For patients who continue to have leukoagglutinin reactions, premedication with acetaminophen may be necessary. In general, premedication is avoided because it may obscure the very symptoms used to recognize a transfusion reaction (Table 4).

In rare cases, multiply transfused patients (e.g., thalassemics) develop severe leukoagglutinates that aggregate in the pulmonary circulation, causing noncardiac pulmonary edema and acute respiratory distress. These reactions may respond to high doses of steroids (e.g., prednisolone, 80 to 160 mg intravenously) in addition to acetaminophen, 650 mg orally. Symptoms usually clear in 12 to 24 hours, and the chest x-ray is clear in a few days. Further transfusion should be given slowly and the patient premedicated with steroids. Fevers that persist for many hours to days post-transfusion are not likely to be caused by transfusion, and some other source should be identified.

Reactions Caused by Platelet Antibodies

Antibodies to platelets occur in patients immunized to platelet antigens by previous trans-

TABLE 4. **Treatment of Nonhemolytic Febrile Reactions**

Symptom	Therapy
Leukoagglutinins	Acetaminophen, 650 mg PO every 3–4 hr; repeat once
Noncardiac pulmonary edema	Prednisone, 80–200 mg IV Acetaminophen, 500-mg suppository
Bacteremia	Cefoxitin, 1–2 grams IV every 6 hr

fusion or pregnancy. Allo-anti-Pl[A1] in a patient negative for this antigen destroys infused platelets approximately 1 week post-transfusion, resulting in thrombocytopenic purpura. In infants, reactions are severe, and death from intracranial hemorrhage is common. Plasma exchange, which reduces the amount of platelet alloantibody, is occasionally successful. The plasma exchanged is 1 to 1.5 plasma volumes, and the exchange is repeated two or three times over several days. Because anti-Pl[A1] is usually IgG antibody, which easily re-enters the vascular space from the extravascular compartment, plasma exchange is often of limited benefit. The half-life of IgG antibody is 45 days, so that the antibody usually fades if not restimulated. Donors with high-titer anti-Pl[A1] in their plasma can provoke an immediate response of fever, rash, or purpura in the transfusion recipient who is Pl[A2] positive.

Complications of Massive Transfusion

In addition to the expected risks of post-transfusion infection and hemolysis, massive transfusion has additional risks related to volume. Large volumes of refrigerated blood with a core temperature of 10° C infused rapidly may provoke arrhythmias, particularly if administered through a central line. In-line blood warmers reduce this risk. Massive amounts of citrate anticoagulant have a theoretical potential for causing citrate toxicity and metabolic acidosis. However, if the patient can be kept warm, citrate has a minimal risk. The patient in hypovolemic shock is initially in metabolic acidosis; as the patient is resuscitated with fluids and transfusion, he or she usually develops compensatory respiratory alkalosis. Citrate-induced hypocalcemia is uncommon, although the risk is greater in exchange transfusion of infants because of their small blood volume. Treatment with calcium gluconate often creates more problems than it solves. For infants it is wise to remove some of the anticoagulant from the blood bag before the exchange or to use saline-washed red blood cells.

When more than 1 volume of blood and components is infused, there is potential dilution of labile coagulation factors and platelets by the stored blood. Based on prolongation of the prothrombin and partial thromboplastin times, a platelet count of less than 50,000 per mm³, and clinical bleeding or generalized oozing, therapy with FFP, cryoprecipitate, and platelets should be instituted. Stored bank blood has decreased amounts of labile Factors VIII and V and no functional platelets. Stable Factors VII, IX, X, XI, XII, and fibrinogen remain in adequate amounts even with storage. Thus massive trans-

fusion with stored blood reduces the levels of the labile factors. The differential diagnosis of dilution coagulopathy and DIC in the massively transfused patient is frequently a problem and may be resolved by measuring the patient's plasma fibrinogen level. Transfused components contain and therefore provide fibrogen, whereas DIC consumes it. In addition, when platelet counts are below 30,000 per mm³, DIC is more likely to be present. In the patient with prolonged hypovolemic shock, both dilution coagulopathy and DIC may be present, one superseding the other. Coagulation factors may be replaced with FFP, but the 250-ml volume for each unit limits the amount that can be given without inducing congestive heart failure and pulmonary edema. Cryoprecipitate contains Factor VIII and fibrinogen and is 50 ml per unit. Four cryoprecipitate units provides 1 gram of fibrinogen. Initial therapy for either dilution coagulopathy or DIC is eight cryoprecipitates with six to eight platelet concentrates, repeated in 30 to 60 minutes until bleeding is controlled. The partial thromboplastin time and the platelet count can be monitored to assess therapy.

Allergic Reactions

Urticaria is the mildest reaction. Hives, skin blotches, or generalized itching appears after the patient is exposed to the donor plasma containing specific IgE antibody to a substance to which the recipient is allergic. These reactions are much less likely to occur when packed red blood cells with diminished plasma volume are transfused.

The unit should be discontinued because of the potential for producing an asthma attack in the atopic patient. Antihistamines are given, such as diphenhydramine (Benadryl), 50 mg intravenously or orally, or tripelennamine, 50 mg orally. An urticarial response is seldom repeated with subsequent transfusions. However, urticaria associated with fever often heralds a leukoagglutinin reaction, which requires treatment as previously described.

Anaphylactic reactions may occur in patients who are IgA deficient (1 in 800 of the population) and who have developed anti-IgA antibodies. These patients may have anaphylactic reactions not only to red blood cells but also to platelets, FFP, cryoprecipitate, and albumin. Symptoms include flushing, dyspnea, hypotension, or retrosternal pain 10 to 15 minutes after the transfusion has begun. In the mildest form, only hives appear. Reactions become progressively worse with further transfusions. Treatment includes prednisolone, 80 mg intravenously; epinephrine, 1:1000, 0.4 ml given subcutaneously or intravenously; and antihistamines (Table 5). Future transfusions require saline-washed or frozen, deglycerolized red blood cells, which have no remaining plasma. If plasma products are required, specific donors who are themselves IgA deficient are available in many large blood centers, through the American Association of Blood Banks, or through American Red Cross rare donor files.

NONIMMUNE TRANSFUSION REACTIONS

Vascular Overload

Vascular overload is the most common nonimmune reaction, occurring in 10 to 15 per cent of transfused patients. The margin for venous vascular expansion is only 10 per cent, which is critical in the chronically anemic patient or the patient with a small blood volume. Even packed red blood cells can produce congestive heart failure. Patients with compensated anemia transfused immediately before surgery may develop congestive heart failure with positioning (e.g., elevation of the legs, as in pelvic surgery). Symptoms of vascular overload in the monitored patient consist of premature ventricular contractions or frank arrhythmias, which can progress to ventricular tachycardia and death. There may be abrupt rises in systolic blood pressure of 50 to 100 mmHg, dyspnea, and overt congestive heart failure. Treatment is diuresis using furosemide, 40 mg intravenously, repeated in 2 hours if necessary. If pulmonary edema is not controlled, phlebotomy and rotating tourniquets may be necessary. Symptoms may be relieved within 3 to 4 hours by aggressive treatment but tend to recur within hours. Therefore the patient should be monitored for 6 to 8 hours after the transfusion and further furosemide given if necessary.

Embolism

Embolic phenomena are uncommon complications with transfusion because all blood products, including platelets, plasma, and cryoprecipitate, must be administered through a 170-micrometer blood filter. Leukoagglutinates that form with the storage of red blood cell products have not been proved to cause pulmonary perfusion problems, and 40-micrometer filters are not necessary for routine transfusion. Microfilters are necessary in surgical procedures that bypass the lungs because these microemboli may produce small strokes.

There is increasing emphasis on intraoperative salvage of blood. With some equipment there is the potential for air embolus because the suction device is in direct communication with the circulation. Such salvage pumps are no longer manufactured, but this older equipment may still be in use. In most cases, a collecting canister is between the environment and the circulation, and therefore traps potential air emboli. Air embolism under anesthesia may produce hypotension and cardiac arrest. In the conscious patient, air embolism produces chest pain and ill-defined anxiety. It is treated by placing the patient in Trendelenberg's position on the left side so that the air bubble remains in the right ventricle until the heartbeat reduces the bubble to microscopic particles.

Nonimmune Hemolysis

Nonimmune causes of hemolysis are caused by mechanical injury to red blood cells such as by addition of medications to blood bags, fragmentation of cells by extracorporeal pump oxygenators, injury of red blood cells by microwave blood warmers, or warming with water temperatures above 40° C. The symptoms are hemoglobinemia and hemoglobinuria. Mechanical destruction of red blood cells, as with pump oxygenators, may produce marked hemoglobinemia and hemoglobinuria, but rarely with renal shutdown, DIC, and shock, as seen in immune hemolysis. These reactions are easily avoided by not adding medications to blood and by using blood warmers that are in line with sensor alarm systems. If mechanical hemoglobinuria occurs, the patient should be hydrated to maintain a urine flow rate of 100 ml per hour until hemoglobinuria clears. Hemoglobin alone does not cause cortical necrosis, whereas the stroma with foreign antigen, as seen in immune hemolysis, does.

Infection

The blood donor's skin is prepared with Betadine, and although the procedure is aseptic, it is not sterile, and bacteria may grow in the collected blood. Blood and its components are natural media for bacterial growth. This unhappy event is prevented by storing these components in properly monitored refrigerators that keep the temperature at 1° to 6° C. Contamination of the blood

TABLE 5. **Treatment of Allergic Reactions**

Symptom	Therapy
Urticaria	Diphenhydramine, 50 mg IV or PO, or tripelennamine, 50 mg PO
Asthmatic attack	Diphenhydramine, 50 mg IV
Anaphylaxis	Epinephrine, 1:1000 0.4 ml SC; prednisone, 80 mg IV; in IgA anaphylaxis use negative donors

product can also occur when the blood bag is hooked to the intravenous tubing. FFP or cryoprecipitate can be contaminated during thawing by the water in the warming bath, a natural source for *Pseudomonas*. Platelets stored at room temperature must be transfused within 5 days; longer storage periods have produced several incidents of transfusion sepsis with death.

To prevent significant bacterial growth, blood products should be infused within 4 hours, limiting the time the bag is at room temperature and reducing the opportunity for significant bacterial growth. If vascular overload is a clinical problem, so that blood must be infused over a longer time, the unit should be aliquoted, so that only a small volume of blood is allowed to be at room temperature and the remainder is kept properly refrigerated.

Postoperative drainage devices are available with suction tubing that drains surgical areas into collection bags, which are then inverted and the blood reinfused into the patient. These collection containers should not be allowed to remain at room temperature for more than 2 to 3 hours, and the blood should be reinfused rapidly to prevent potential transfusion sepsis. It is desirable to wash red blood cells collected in this manner to remove fat and other cellular or surgical debris.

Transfusion sepsis produces a fulminant reaction that is usually rapidly fatal. Severe hypotension, chills, and dyspnea often precede the development of fever, nausea, and vomiting. Bacterial reactions must be prevented because treatment is seldom successful. Blood should never be stored in medicine refrigerators on the ward because the interior temperature is often warmer than the 1° to 6° C required, and bacterial growth can occur. If a bacterial reaction is suspected, the transfusion should be stopped immediately. The blood bank should immediately prepare and read a Gram's stain, culture the blood or platelet bag, and take blood cultures from the patient. Therapy consists of an intravenous antibiotic such as cefoxitin, if the organism is unidentifiable, and high-dose steroids. Blood pressure should be maintained with dopamine.

TRANSFUSION-TRANSMITTED DISEASE

Infection after transfusion can never be totally prevented, despite detailed interviewing of donors and an increasing array of tests performed on the donated blood.

Hepatitis

Before 1972, the major post-transfusion infection was hepatitis B, but with uniform testing of blood for hepatitis B surface antigen, hepatitis B has been reduced to 10 per cent of cases. Ninety per cent of cases are due to non-A, non-B (NANB) hepatitis, for which there is no specific serologic test. Approximately one-half of the patients with NANB hepatitis develop chronic active hepatitis, which ends in cirrhosis in 10 per cent. In an effort to exclude potential carriers of this unidentified virus, so-called surrogate tests were instituted in 1987.

These tests are anti–hepatitis B core and alanine aminotransferase. Although 5 to 8 per cent of donated blood is therefore discarded, these two tests are expected to decrease NANB hepatitis by only 30 per cent. The incidence of NANB hepatitis, which was 8 per cent, is expected to decrease to 2 per cent, or 1 in 50 tranfusions. NANB hepatitis may produce only mild malaise, and the patient is not jaundiced in 90 per cent of cases, so that the diagnosis may be difficult to make. Treatment of the acute illness, if recognized, is supportive. The patient should be followed with periodic alanine aminotransferase determinations for 1 or 2 years. If liver enzyme levels remain intermittently elevated, the patient should be referred for long-term follow-up.

Cytomegalovirus

The herpetic viruses, cytomegalovirus (CMV) and Epstein-Barr virus, are widespread in the population with over 50 per cent having antibodies by their twentieth year. These viruses are so common that they are almost normal components. The viruses are carried in the monocytes and lymphocytes of whole blood. Rarely, they produce postpump perfusion syndrome, a serum sickness type of illness originally noted after open heart surgery.

Immunosuppressed patients or premature infants weighing less than 1200 grams may develop clinically significant CMV illness post-transfusion. In adults, this may be a reactivation of a latent virus infection. CMV infection in neonates may be received from seropositive mothers rather than from blood transfusion. Although seroconversion may occur, it does not always indicate disease. Symptoms in these premature infants may include respiratory distress, pallor, and, rarely, death. In the immunosuppressed adult, CMV pneumonia or hepatitis may prove to be fatal. For these patients, blood products from previously screened CMV-negative donors are available. Because of the many sources for infection, seronegative blood products may not prevent the infection.

Post-Transfusion Syphilis

Syphilis is almost never transmitted by transfusion because the current complex testing of donated blood for disease results in refrigeration of blood products for 36 to 48 hours before release, and the treponeme does not survive. Although donor blood is tested for reaginic antibodies to syphilis, 80 to 90 per cent of positive results are biologic false reactions.

Malaria

Malaria is occasionally transmitted in whole blood or red blood cells because the parasite is intracellular. Donors who are at high risk because of their place of origin, or who are receiving suppressive therapy, are excluded from donating. In areas of the world where malaria is endemic, a chemoprophylactic agent is often added to the blood bag to kill the parasite. The incubation period depends on the type of malaria but is usually 2 to 3 weeks, followed by paroxysmal fevers. Treatment for most types of malaria is chloroquine for 3 days. Falciparum malaria is frequently resistant to chloroquine and should be treated with sulfadoxine-pyrimethamine (Fansidar), 500 mg by mouth daily for 3 days.

Other Uncommon Post-Transfusion Infections

Chagas's disease is rarely transmitted in the United States; however, many donors from South and Central America and Mexico have antibodies to the causative organism, suggesting that they have been infected. The risk to recipients is considered to be limited at the present time. Babesiosis has been transmitted from donors of Cape Cod, where the disease is transmitted by mosquitoes.

Human Immunodeficiency Virus

Human immunodeficiency virus (HIV) can be transmitted via blood transfusions from high-risk individuals or their sexual partners. Serologic testing for anti-HIV, which began in the spring of 1985, is 99 per cent effective in excluding infectious donors. This test, combined with intensive interviews of potential donors, further diminishes the risk by excluding donors with high-risk behavior who have not yet developed the antibody—the so-called window period of 6 to 12 weeks. Although 82,604 cases of acquired immunodeficiency syndrome had been reported by the beginning of 1989, only 1.8 per cent of these cases have been associated with transfusion. Almost all exposures are caused by transfusions given before 1985. Published estimates of disease transmission by transfusion vary from 1:40,000 to 1:250,000. Eighty per cent of hemophiliacs are HIV positive as a result of exposure by coagulation factors. Use of heat-treated Factor VIII has begun to reduce this percentage. Clinical trials of recombinant Factor VIII, which does not have the infectious potential, are now in progress.

Anti–Human T Cell Lymphotrophic Virus I

The major blood banking organizations—the American Association of Blood Banks, American Red Cross, and Council of Community Blood Centers—have instituted testing of blood components for the retrovirus HTLV I. In southern Japan, where the virus is endemic, there has been a high incidence of adult T cell leukemia in people with antibodies to HTLV I. In the Caribbean, there has been an association of anti–HTLV I with tropical spastic paraparesis. No direct transmission by transfusion has been demonstrated, although in Japan when blood donations were screened to exclude HTLV I positives, the incidence of post-transfusion seroconversion also declined. However, seroconversion has not been associated with either T cell lymphoma or spastic paresis. Initial studies in the U.S. donor population indicate that 6 in 10,000 donors have confirmed antibody. Anti–HTLV I is usually associated with intravenous drug abuse. It is expected that only red blood cell products and platelets carry the virus, and that FFP and cryoprecipitate do not, because the U.S. population of hemophiliacs has not been shown to have the antibody. Because the incubation period for T cell leukemia or lymphoma is as long as 30 years, it may be difficult to prove that the disease has been prevented by anti–HTLV I screening.

Creutzfeldt-Jakob Disease

This slow virus disease has been transmitted with corneal transplants from patients who had received human growth hormone. No cases of post-*transfusion* Creutzfeldt-Jakob disease have been reported, but persons who have received human growth hormone are permanently prevented from donating blood.

Graft-Versus-Host Disease

Cellular blood products, red blood cells, platelets, and granulocytes contain immunocompetent lymphocytes that have the potential to produce graft-versus-host disease in the immunosuppressed adult or premature infant. This disease is usually fatal, either acutely or in the long term. It can be prevented by irradiating blood products with a dose of 1500 to 3000 rad before transfusion.

Adverse immune consequences of transfusion can often be treated successfully. Infectious consequences can be treated in some cases, but in the case of acquired immunodeficiency syndrome and HTLV I infection, prevention is the only course: prevention by serologic screening of the donated blood and by reducing the use of blood products.

Section 6

The Digestive System

BLEEDING ESOPHAGEAL VARICES

method of
DUANE G. HUTSON, M.D.
Miami, Florida

The problem of bleeding from gastroesophageal varices can be categorized as one requiring immediate or long-term control. Achieving immediate control represents the more formidable problem, since the first episode is associated with a mortality of 30 to 80 per cent. Some plan for long-term control is mandatory, since bleeding recurs in 70 per cent of cases and is associated with a 50 per cent mortality for each recurrence. The debate regarding immediate control centers around immediate operative intervention versus nonoperative control. For long-term management, the major issue is the use of sclerotherapy versus various shunting procedures. Both of these areas remain controversial.

MANAGEMENT OF ACUTE EPISODES

Diagnosis

A careful history and physical examination will most often identify the presence of cirrhosis and the suspicion of portal hypertension, but the fact that 50 per cent of patients with gastroesophageal varices and hemorrhage bleed from a nonvariceal source complicates the problem. The key to the diagnosis is endoscopy of the upper gastrointestinal tract, which identifies the source of bleeding in 67 per cent of cases. Endoscopy should be done as early as possible, but if it is delayed, it should be performed during the quiescent period rather than waiting for recurrent hemorrhage, at which time the procedure may be technically impossible. If the bleeding is massive enough to preclude the use of endoscopy, treatment with lavage or vasopressin (Pitressin) should be instituted in the hope that sufficient control can be obtained to allow definitive endoscopic evaluation. If this is unsuccessful, however, visceral angiography should be considered. Angiography is not particularly effective in identifying bleeding from varices but may identify nonvariceal sources such as duodenal ulcers. If these maneuvers fail to identify the source of bleeding, operative intervention is indicated in most cases. Prolonged delays in attempting to make a diagnosis should be avoided because survival following massive transfusions with repeated episodes of hypotension is unlikely.

Resuscitation and Monitoring

Since blood loss in these patients is often massive, a large-bore catheter should be placed even though there is no evidence of bleeding at the time of examination. A setting that permits careful monitoring of vital signs is mandatory. Unstable patients with massive bleeding are best managed in an intensive care unit.

Frequent hemodynamic assessments are essential in all patients, since hematocrit changes may lag behind such parameters as pulse rate and blood pressure. Careful hemodynamic monitoring requires the placement of a Swan-Ganz catheter, which is mandatory in patients with signs of hemodynamic instability. Fluid administration is continuously adjusted as indicated by the measurements of cardiac output and wedge pressures.

The key to fluid replacement in these patients is the use of whole blood. The use of salt and fluid should be limited because of the tendency to the development of ascites. The goal should be minimal fluid and minimal salt. The use of diuretics for maintaining urinary output in most patients is condemned; however, this condition is an exception to this concept. If the patient is hemodynamically stable and the urinary output marginal, the use of small doses of diuretics is appropriate, since increasing the fluid load often leads to ascites rather than urinary output.

Hematologic Monitoring

A battery of coagulation tests, including a prothrombin time, should be ordered on admission. If the prothrombin time is low, vitamin K (phytonadione), 10 to 25 mg intramuscularly, should be given. If severe, hypoprothrombinemia may be treated with 2 to 3 units of fresh-frozen plasma (FFP) given over 3 hours. Massive transfusions may lead to a deficiency in platelets and the labile Factors V and VIII, which are deficient in bank blood. Thus, 1 unit of FFP and 1 to 2 units

419

of platelet concentrate should be given for every 5 units of bank blood.

General Supportive Measures

Aspiration pneumonia is a frequent complication and can be minimized by the liberal use of an endotracheal tube. Its use is required in all patients who are massively bleeding or comatose and in those patients requiring endoscopy or balloon tamponade. Nutritional support should begin early and is best provided by a glucose solution at a concentration that allows for adequate calories (25 calories per kg) without excessive fluid volume. If a protracted course is expected, a solution with high concentration of branched chain amino acids and low concentrations of aromatic amino acids (HepatAmine) should be added. There is some evidence to suggest that prolonged coma in these patients is detrimental; therefore, the gastrointestinal tract should be cleared of blood by the use of saline enemas. Lactulose, 60 to 120 ml daily in divided doses, can be added if needed.

CONTROL OF BLEEDING

Gastric Lavage

Lavage with iced saline or tap water should be the first approach, since it is simple and relatively free of complications and effectively controls bleeding in 30 per cent of cases. A standard nasogastric (NG) tube should be left in place for monitoring of further bleeding episodes and repeated irrigation. Its presence does not promote bleeding.

Vasopressin

Vasopressin produces a decrease in splanchnic blood flow and portal vascular resistance resulting in a decrease in portal pressure of 25 to 30 per cent. This reduction in portal pressure results in control of hemorrhage in 50 per cent of patients. The continuous peripheral intravenous infusion is as effective as the selective intra-arterial infusion and more effective than intermittent infusions. The side effects are rather profound and relate to generalized vasoconstriction. Vasopressin produces severe coronary artery constriction and hypertension. Extravasation into the subcutaneous tissue may produce gangrene, and the antidiuretic effect may produce hyponatremia. Unusual complications such as necrosis of the tongue have been seen. Because of its cardiac effects, continuous electrocardiographic monitoring is mandatory and the presence of coronary artery disease is a contraindication to its use. The usual dose is 0.2 to 0.4 unit per minute as a continuous intravenous infusion.*

High doses (0.8 unit per minute) have been used with careful monitoring. Profound bradycardia and severe peripheral vasoconstriction may be seen with these doses. Despite these problems, the drug is quite safe in low doses and with adequate monitoring.

Balloon Tamponade

Balloon tamponade is the modality suggested following failure of irrigation and vasopressin. The conservative use of the device relates to a 39 per cent complication rate associated with its use. These include severe problems such as aspiration, esophageal rupture, and stenosis. The Sengstaken-Blakemore triple-lumen tube is most commonly used but requires placement of an NG tube above the inflated esophageal balloon to aspirate secretions. The Minnesota tube provides a fourth lumen for aspiration of secretions, thus eliminating the need for a second tube. We believe that all patients should be intubated prior to use of these devices.

Placement can be either oral or nasal; however, the nasal route is better tolerated. Its position in the stomach is verified by the injection of air and auscultation over the gastric area. The gastric balloon is inflated with 50 ml of air, and a chest film is taken. If in proper position, the gastric balloon is fully inflated and placed on traction. Adequate traction can be obtained by the use of a football helmet with an attached face mask. If the bleeding is not controlled by the gastric balloon, the esophageal balloon should be inflated to a pressure of 25 to 40 mmHg. Occasionally, respiratory distress will develop with the use of this tube; should this occur, the tube should be immediately transected so as to deflate the balloons. For this purpose a pair of heavy scissors should be attached to the bed.

If bleeding is controlled over a period of 24 hours, the esophageal balloon may be deflated. The gastric balloon may be deflated if continued control is noted over the next 6 hours. Continuous tamponade should not be continued for more than 36 hours. This technique controls bleeding in 70 per cent of patients; however, bleeding recurs in approximately one-half of these cases.

Emergency Endoscopic Sclerotherapy

It is difficult to get a clear idea as to the usefulness of this procedure in the patient with

---

*This use of vasopressin is not listed by the manufacturer.

active bleeding. There is little question that in experienced hands the procedure can be performed in the presence of active bleeding and that immediate control can be gained. This probably represents an exceptional circumstance and requires the skills of an experienced endoscopist.

Percutaneous Transhepatic Obliteration of Varices

The coronary vein represents a major direct conduit between the portal vein and the gastroesophageal area. This arrangement permits catheterization by the percutaneous transhepatic route and successful obliteration of this vessel as well as associated collaterals in 80 per cent of cases. The materials used to produce thrombosis are gelatin foam, sodium tetradecyl sulfate, and wire coils. Despite this technical feat, the procedure is rarely used because of a 65 per cent rebleeding rate noted on long-term follow-up. In addition, portal vein thrombosis occurs in 36 per cent of patients, often producing acute hepatic failure. The procedure may be tried in a high-risk patient in whom other conservative measures have failed.

Emergency Nonshunting Procedure

The use of a direct operative approach to the bleeding varix is advocated in those cases in which conservative measures fail. Most are disappointing. Transesophageal ligation of varices through the left side of the chest is associated with a rebleeding rate of 33 per cent and an operative mortality of 30 per cent. The 5-year survival is a discouraging 5 per cent. If the approach is transabdominal and a devascularization is added to transection of the esophagus, the figures improve somewhat. The use of various stapling devices such as the EEA or the Russian SPTV has been advocated for esophageal transection. If the transections are combined with ligation of the coronary vein and a limited devascularization of the lower esophagus, the rebleeding rate can be reduced to 20 per cent; however, the operative mortality is 30 per cent. The Japanese have had considerable success with Sugiura's procedure (esophageal transection and gastric devascularization) for control of acute variceal hemorrhage, but this has not been duplicated in the United States. The choice of patients for these various procedures is not clear but probably depends on the interest and expertise of the surgeon involved.

Emergency Shunts

All shunting procedures effectively control variceal hemorrhage but are associated with an operative mortality of 20 per cent in Child's Class A patients and of 80 to 90 per cent in Child's Class C patients. The use of emergency shunts as the initial mode of therapy in the low-risk group is suggested by some investigators, but this approach is not widely accepted. The procedure chosen most often depends upon the interest and expertise of the surgeon involved, since there are no definitive studies identifying the most appropriate procedure in an individual patient. The end-to-end portacaval shunt is the procedure most commonly used, since it effectively controls bleeding and can be constructed with considerable facility. A side-to-side portacaval shunt is more appropriate, if the anatomy permits, since it tends to control ascites—which is common during this period of resuscitation—and can be reversed if the patient becomes chronically encephalopathic. The interposition mesocaval shunt is also commonly used. It is relatively easy to construct, controls bleeding, and can be easily reversed if chronic encephalopathy develops. Long-term patency of this shunt, however, is questioned by some investigators. The distal splenorenal shunt is not generally recommended in acute emergencies because of the time required for its construction and the problem of postoperative ascites. It is, however, the procedure of choice in a relatively stable patient who has maintained portal perfusion of the liver. If this procedure is considered, preoperative panhepatic angiography is essential to identify the anatomy and the status of perfusion of the liver. If perfusion through the portal vein is minimal or reversed, the procedure is not indicated. Preoperative panhepatic angiography is recommended in all cases, if readily available, since it will identify those conditions such as splenic or portal vein thrombosis that alter the surgical approach.

LONG-TERM CONTROL OF BLEEDING

Prevention of recurrent variceal hemorrhage is dependent upon either an endoscopic or an operative procedure. Although medical control of recurrent hemorrhage is desirable, the use of propranolol (Inderal) has been ineffective and is of historic interest only. Presently, sclerotherapy is the procedure most often employed, and there is considerable evidence to support its use.

Portacaval Shunt

This time-honored procedure effectively controls recurrent hemorrhage in 90 per cent of patients and is still extensively used. Dissatisfaction with the procedure developed because of the high incidence of encephalopathy reported by most investigators and the fact that survival following the operation is no different from that reported with medical management. This was thought to be related, at least in part, to the fact that the procedure produces sudden and total diversion of portal flow. This fact prompted the development of the distal splenorenal shunt (DSRS). It remains the procedure of choice, however, if portal perfusion is either reversed or minimal or if the patient has intractable ascites.

Distal Splenorenal Shunt

The DSRS procedure avoids sudden diversion of portal blood flow and is the procedure of choice when portal perfusion of the liver has been maintained. It controls recurrent hemorrhage in 90 per cent of patients and is associated with a 5 per cent incidence of chronic clinical encephalopathy. The development of collaterals over time will convert many of those selective shunts into a central shunt; however, the incidence of encephalopathy remains low at the 10-year level. This most probably relates to the slow development of this conversion. Preoperative panhepatic angiography is essential in order to demonstrate the direction of portal flow as well as patency and position of the splenic and renal veins.

Sclerotherapy

There is little question that sclerotherapy has become the procedure of choice for long-term control of hemorrhage from esophageal varices. The technique varies but consists of the injection of a sclerosing agent directly into a varix or into the adjacent tissues. The initial injection is followed by a series of injections that are continued until all varices have been obliterated. This is followed by annual endoscopic evaluation and by sclerosis of recurrent varices. This technique obliterates varices in 90 per cent of patients. Recurrent hemorrhage occurs in 20 to 30 per cent of patients, a figure that is significantly less than the 60 to 70 per cent recurrence reported in untreated patients. A randomized series comparing sclerotherapy with the DSRS suggests that survival is improved with the use of sclerotherapy as the initial form of treatment followed by a DSRS in those who rebleed. The complication rate is an acceptable 10 to 20 per cent per patient and consists of fever, ulceration, strictures, and aspiration. Despite the present enthusiasm for this procedure, adequately controlled long-term studies are presently unavailable; therefore, whether this procedure will stand the test of time is not known.

CHOLECYSTITIS AND CHOLELITHIASIS

method of
EDWARD C. SALTZSTEIN, M.D., and
LEO C. MERCER, M.D.
Texas Tech University School of Medicine
El Paso, Texas

Gallstones and diseases resulting from them are among the most common clinical entities encountered by physicians in the United States. An estimated 10 per cent of the population, or more than 20 million Americans, have gallstones, with 800,000 new cases reported annually. The majority of patients with stones have supersaturated bile, and the precipitation of cholesterol from solution forms the nidus for stones in the gallbladder. Other factors that may cause precipitation of cholesterol are bacteria, fungi, intestinal reflux, and stasis of bile.

Anomalous anatomy is more frequent in the extrahepatic biliary ductal system than anywhere else in the body, and a thorough knowledge of the anatomy is essential to avoid operative injury, especially to the common bile duct. From a surgical standpoint, the origin of the cystic duct and cystic artery is not important in cholecystectomy; if one ligates and/or divides only those structures identified as going to the gallbladder, the incidence of injury (particularly to the common bile duct) is minimized.

DIAGNOSIS

In many patients, gallstones are not symptomatic and are diagnosed during a general evaluation or in the course of an evaluation for other problems. When biliary tract stone disease is suspected, a history to elicit symptoms supporting the diagnosis is taken. Classically, patients present with colicky or constant right upper quadrant pain that radiates to the back. A temporal relationship between food and pain exists in which eating aggravates pain, and an intolerance of fatty foods may be particularly evident. Up to 80 per cent of gallbladder patients are female, and a history of multiple pregnancies is frequent. A history of dark urine, light stools, or both suggests common duct obstruction. Pertinent physical findings include varying degrees of right upper quadrant and epigastric tenderness and rebound tenderness. Bowel sounds may be depressed, and jaundice may be present.

The differential diagnosis includes other right upper quadrant inflammatory processes, particularly hepatitis, pancreatitis, and peptic ulcer disease. These possibilities should be evaluated when history and physical examination are performed.

Important x-ray and laboratory studies to establish the diagnosis are ultrasonography, radionuclide imaging, and liver function studies. When the diagnosis is not readily apparent, helpful studies are oral cholecystography, duodenal drainage analysis, and endoscopic retrograde cholangiopancreatography.

Abdominal Roentgenography

Abdominal films are of benefit if radiopaque stones are visualized (15 per cent of biliary calculi) or if an "air cholangiogram" is seen (pathognomonic of a biliary-enteric fistula).

Ultrasonography

Ultrasonography is accurate in defining biliary calculi in 95 per cent of cases, and false-positive results are rare. It is usually the only diagnostic tool required, and with ultrasonographic evidence of stones, one can proceed with cholecystectomy. Ultrasonography may also demonstrate stones in the common bile duct and can demonstrate the size of the duct as well as pancreatic abnormalities.

Radionuclide Imaging

^{99m}Tc-labeled iminodiacetic acid (IDA) scanning "lights up" the liver, gallbladder, extrahepatic ducts, and duodenum in the normal person. Nonvisualization of the gallbladder strongly supports a diagnosis of acute cholecystitis, whereas visualization rules it out. Visualization of the radionuclide in the intestine rules out complete ductal obstruction (and therefore cholangitis). In general, the diagnosis of acute cholecystitis can be made by the history and physical findings, plus the demonstration of stones by ultrasonography. In this situation, radionuclide imaging may be useful to rule out other conditions, such as amebic liver abscess.

Liver Function Studies

Because of the increased morbidity and mortality associated with delayed or untreated cholangitis, the presence of jaundice must be ascertained in patients with symptomatic biliary calculi. The combination of right upper quadrant pain, fever, and jaundice (Charcot's triad) represents cholangitis until proved otherwise. Liver function studies are indicated to assist in distinguishing between hepatitis and obstructive jaundice. Further diagnostic studies (radionuclide imaging, percutaneous transhepatic cholangiography) and subsequent prompt surgical decompression of the common duct may be required.

Serum Amylase Level Determination

Because hyperamylasemia, pancreatitis, or both complicate biliary calculi in up to 25 per cent of cases, serum amylase level determinations should be done routinely.

TREATMENT

Asymptomatic Gallstones

Conflicting evidence exists regarding the likelihood that patients with asymptomatic stones will develop symptoms (10 to 50 per cent). However, there appears to be no significant increase in mortality when treatment (cholecystectomy) is delayed until the onset of symptoms. The deaths that do occur usually involve elderly patients with known stones who develop acute cholecystitis requiring emergent surgery. Recent successful experience in managing patients with diabetes indicates that diabetes per se does not increase the complication rate of acute cholecystitis and therefore is not an absolute indication for cholecystectomy in the asymptomatic patient.

Symptomatic Stones—Biliary Colic and Acute Cholecystitis

Biliary colic results from contraction of the smooth muscle of the gallbladder, extrahepatic ducts, or both, that is believed to be related to intermittent obstruction by stones. Anticholinergic drugs such as dicyclomine hydrochloride (Bentyl) or Donnatal may be tried to relieve smooth muscle spasms, and a low-fat diet may be instituted.

It is generally agreed that cholecystectomy is indicated for symptomatic biliary calculi. The risk of elective surgery is extremely low and eliminates the risk of urgent surgery for subsequent acute cholecystitis, particularly in the elderly patient. After a general evaluation to determine the operative and anesthetic risks, patients can be brought to the hospital the day of surgery. Prophylactic antibiotics are indicated in patients over age 60 years, those with choledocholithiasis, and those with diabetes. However, we routinely give perioperative antibiotics to all patients, using cefazolin (Ancef), 1 gram intravenously every 8 hours for a total of three doses. Operative cholangiography of the transcystic duct should accompany cholecystectomy to identify common duct stones (both their number and location), to prevent unnecessary duct explorations, and to identify anatomic variations and possibly avoid operative ductal injury. When common duct stones are identified by intraoperative cholangiography, common duct exploration with stone removal and large T tube drainage is indicated. A No. 14 French or larger T tube to facilitate fluoroscopically controlled basket retrieval of possibly retained stones should be used. Almost all patients have their drains removed, are afebrile, and are able to eat the day after cholecystectomy, and more than one-half of our patients are discharged home 24 hours postoperatively.

Acute calculous cholecystitis results from obstruction of the cystic duct, with subsequent edema of the gallbladder, relative vascular insufficiency, and secondary infection. Infection occurs via overgrowth of organisms in the gallbladder bile, via lymphatics, and possibly by translocation of colon organisms. Patients present with constant pain and an elevated temperature. The white blood cell count is not necessarily elevated. We start to administer antibiotics empirically (without culture) on the basis of the organisms likely to be found (enteric organisms, most commonly *Escherichia coli*), using piperacillin (Pipracil), 2 grams intravenously every 6 hours. Narcotics, such as morphine and meperidine, are contraindicated because they cause contraction of the sphincter of Oddi and mask symptoms that are important to follow in evaluating the success of therapy.

Although clinical resolution of acute cholecystitis can be obtained in more than 85 per cent of patients with antibiotics, nasogastric suction, and possibly anticholinergic drugs, prompt cholecystectomy is generally the preferred treatment. Surgery as soon as the diagnosis is made (by ultrasonography with or without radionuclide imaging) and the patient is appropriately resuscitated is safe, greatly reduces the hospital stay, avoids observation for possible failure to respond to nonsurgical therapy, and is not associated with increased technical difficulty. Forty per cent of our patients are discharged within 24 hours and 60 per cent within 48 hours of surgery for acute cholecystitis.

Although this practice is controversial, we also operate on patients with biliary hyperamylasemia, pancreatitis, or both as soon as the diagnosis is made. Cholecystectomy, intraoperative cholangiography, and common duct exploration as necessary are performed.

ALTERNATIVE AND NEW THERAPIES

The role of medical dissolution of gallstones, if any, has not been defined. Chenodeoxycholic acid increases the bile acid pool and slowly dissolves cholesterol gallstones. However, the treatment is prolonged (1 to 2 years) and expensive. Further, on cessation of therapy, the bile returns to its previous lithogenic state, and more than 30 per cent of patients re-form stones in 5 years. Because cholecystectomy is such a safe and effective procedure, treatment with agents that increase the bile acid pool should probably be reserved for patients who have small stones (less than 2 cm) in functioning gallbladders and who are prohibitive risks for surgery.

The efficacy of extracorporeal shock wave lithotripsy (ESWL) in selected patients is becoming apparent. Early studies on patients with one to three radiolucent gallstones with a total stone mass of 30 mm or less and with functioning gallbladders showed complete disappearance of

stone fragments in up to 90 per cent at 12 months. ESWL is noninvasive and therefore of interest as an alternative to cholecystectomy. There is concern over the consequences of stone fragments passing into the extrahepatic ductal system, but there are now reports of successful treatment by ESWL of small numbers of patients with retained stones and other complex biliary tract stone disease. The data from several centers in the United States are accumulating to confirm and expand the initial reports from Germany.

Another experimental technique is the instillation, via a percutaneous catheter into the gallbladder, of a potent lipid solvent, methyl tertbutyl ether, that solubilizes the cholesterol in cholesterol stones, causing dissolution within hours. The safety of this technique has not been established. It is of interest as an alternative to cholecystectomy because it can be done on an outpatient basis under local anesthesia.

Each of these three therapies preserves the gallbladder. Of concern is the likelihood of gallstone recurrence after therapy and the unknown effects of preservation of a chronically diseased organ. In addition, none of these therapeutic options are now applicable to the nonfunctioning gallbladder (the more seriously ill patient). Cholecystectomy remains the procedure of choice for the vast majority of patients with biliary calculi. It is safe, definitive, and well tolerated, with minimal morbidity and brief hospitalization (and therefore reduced cost).

ACALCULOUS CHOLECYSTITIS

Acute and chronic inflammatory disease of the gallbladder occurs without stones. Acalculous cholecystitis occurs in less than 5 per cent of adult patients in the United States and in a somewhat larger percentage in children. It is frequently seen as a complication of burns, sepsis, cardiovascular disease, major surgery, prolonged illness, or conditions that may result in significant inactivity of the gut with biliary stasis, and especially in patients receiving total parenteral nutrition. Antomic variations causing kinking of the cystic duct may be involved.

Acalculous cholecystitis should be considered in patients who develop signs and symptoms of cholecystitis and in whom ultrasonography does not reveal stones. Ultrasonography may reveal a thickened gallbladder wall. The accuracy of radionuclide imaging is questionable in these cases, but nonvisualization of the gallbladder supports the diagnosis.

Although a small percentage of patients may respond to nasogastric suction, anticholinergic drugs, and antibiotics, prompt cholecystectomy to prevent progression to gangrene and rupture and to prevent further compromise of the underlying medical condition is indicated.

CIRRHOSIS

method of
FRANK L. IBER, M.D.
Loyola University and Edward Hines, Jr. VA Hospital
Chicago, Illinois

Cirrhosis is a chronic usually progressive liver disease characterized clinically by failure of liver cell function and portal hypertension. Histological examination is valuable in establishing the etiology but is infrequently essential to diagnose cirrhosis. Portal hypertension usually can be identified by endoscopy or barium swallow (for esophageal varices), sonography or other imaging (to establish enlarged portal veins or collaterals).

ETIOLOGY OF CIRRHOSIS

Common etiologies
  Alcohol
  Chemical exposure
  Medicinal agents
  Hepatitis B
  Non-A, non-B hepatitis
  Schistosomiasis
  Primary biliary cirrhosis
  Chronic active hepatitis
Uncommon etiologies
  Delta hepatitis
  Iron storage disease
  Copper storage disease
  Alpha$_1$-antitrypsin deficiency

Although the diagnosis of cirrhosis is relatively easy, establishing the etiology is more difficult. Removing the causes of injury (e.g., toxin or alcohol) or controlling a harmful effect (e.g., of steroid treatment of autoimmune cirrhosis) improves survival of patients.

TREATMENT

Permanent removal of the cause of cirrhosis is the mainstay of treatment; if this is not possible, many specific therapies exist that intermittently or partially control new hepatic damage. A large number of nonspecific measures that reduce disability are useful. Many complications of cirrhosis, including ascites, malnutrition, infection, and variceal hemorrhage, can be effectively treated to avoid incapacitation and death.

Nonspecific Treatment

The goals of this approach are to delay and reduce disability caused by cirrhosis and its complications. Diet, appropriate activity, and avoidance of new liver damage are all effective. The ultimate nonspecific therapy for the final stage of cirrhosis is *transplantation.*

Diet. The diet should be nutritious and contain about 20 per cent excess of calories, protein, and most trace nutrients. Hence the inactive 70-kg person should eat at least 2500 kcal daily with at least 1 gram per kg protein. If the patient is unable to eat this amount, feeding at least one-third of the daily food as breakfast and adding evening snacks is effective. There should be no restriction of fat. All cirrhotics metabolize sodium poorly, so salty foods, condiments, and added salt should be avoided. Dietary supplements are appropriate when there is specific malnutrition, in alcoholics for 1 month after drinking stops or longer if drinking continues, and in jaundiced subjects. Alcoholics need a multivitamin with minerals and often require extra magnesium and zinc; these requirements may be identified by serum measurements. Patients with jaundice need parenteral vitamin K (5 mg menadione intramuscularly monthly) and oral supplements of 10,000 units of vitamin A, 50,000 units of vitamin D, and 400 units of vitamin E as long as the jaundice continues. Almost all patients who are taking diuretics or those with diarrhea caused by lactulose need oral potassium supplements as determined by serum potassium levels. A common dose is 40 mEq per day.

Activity. Activity should be undertaken daily with a goal of preserving muscle mass and exercise tolerance short of producing extreme fatigue. Regular and increasing walking or noncompetitive exercises (aerobics) often increase work tolerance even in the face of progressive liver disease. Additional rest to avoid extreme fatigue should be encouraged, with 10 hours in bed and a rest period in the middle of the day often required.

Potential Injurious Agents. Agents such as alcohol, new medications, health store macrosupplements of nutrients, and extensive solvents that are used in certain hobbies should be avoided. The patient should ask the physician about the possible hepatic effects of treatments, query physicians at work about agents at the work place, and avoid new chemical exposures. In alcoholic patients, blood or urine tests for alcohol at the time of routine visits to the physician have been found to be valuable in detecting and confronting the problem of surreptitious alcohol use. All patients should be tested for hepatitis B; the patients who have not acquired this infection should be immunized with recombinant vaccine. Patients who are exposed to crowds should also receive influenza and pneumococcal immunization.

Useful Office Information. Information should be acquired on all patients, particularly those doing well. Patients should keep a diary of weight with weekly recordings. Sudden weight gains may indicate new ascites or raised plasma volume, which increases the risk of hemorrhage. Suitable patients can be given furosemide (Lasix), 40 mg in a single dose, if weight increases by 3 pounds. At a minimum, patients should visit the physician yearly. On each visit, the patient's weight and a sample of handwriting (or the trail-making test, which is provided by the manufacturers of lactulose), as well as liver chemistries, electrolytes, and creatinine, should be obtained. The blood alcohol level is also measured in alcoholic patients. A test for occult blood should be done. A barium esophagogram or endoscopy should be obtained each year; after varices appear, endoscopy is required yearly to determine the likelihood of bleeding. If these tests have been performed regularly, early complications are often identified and effectively treated without the need for hospitalization. When clinical deterioration is encountered, a prompt search for occult infection, gastrointestinal bleeding, and hepatocellular carcinoma (by alpha-fetoprotein) should be undertaken.

Therapies for Specific Diseases

Alcoholic Liver Disease. This liver disease improves with total abstinence from alcohol and adequate oral nutrition; in most patients this therapy is all that is required. In severe cases of acute injury with both malnutrition and jaundice, intravenous alimentation with 1000 ml of 3 to 5 per cent amino acids seems to be beneficial, usually continued until eating is possible or for a maximum of 1 month. In these same cases, treatment with oral oxandrolone (Anavar), 20 mg per day for 1 month, has improved survival and is used in malnourished patients. I do not currently use either propylthiouracil, 300 mg daily for 3 or 4 months, or colchicine, 1 mg daily, to treat these patients. To facilitate alcohol withdrawal, I use diazepam (Valium) as needed for a maximum of 1 week. Disulfiram (Antabuse), 250 mg per day, is occasionally used in conjunction with other therapy for alcoholism with no detrimental effects on the liver. Some form of therapy for alcoholism is essential, the most effective treatment for alcohol abstinence being the program of Alcoholics Anonymous.

Hepatitis B. Hepatitis B in its viral replicative stage (identified by HBs, HBe antigens and DNA in the serum) has been arrested by treatment with alpha-interferon. A dose of 10,000 units three times weekly for 16 weeks has been used.

Idiopathic Chronic Active Hepatitis. This hepatitis, which occurs often with cirrhosis, may be discerned by immunologic markers such as antinuclear antibody and anti–smooth muscle antibody and has a typical biopsy pattern. The illness is highly responsive to prednisone, 20 mg per day, with biochemical and clinical improvement apparent in 1 or 2 months. For chronic management, azathioprine (Imuran) is added in a dose of 50 mg per day and the dose of prednisone is reduced to 10 mg per day. Treatment should be continued for 1 year after biochemical stability is achieved and then should be slowly discontinued.

Biliary Cirrhosis. Treatment with colchicine, 1 mg per day, and, more recently, methotrexate, 25 mg intravenously weekly, has been found to be effective. Pruritus is best treated with cholestyramine (Questran), by taking a 9-gram dose both before and after breakfast and additional doses with each subsequent meal. Bone loss is a major incapacitating problem and should be treated prophylactically with extra calcium equivalents (to 1 pint of milk daily) and sufficient oral or intramuscular vitamin D to maintain normal serum 25-hydroxyvitamin D_2 levels. Typically, 100,000 IU of oral vitamin D is required daily, or this dose of intramuscular vitamin D_2 monthly. This cirrhosis in its late stages is one of the most frequent reasons for liver transplantation.

Hemochromatosis. Recognized by an increased serum ferritin level and an elevated iron content of the liver, hemochromatosis is treated by repeated phlebotomies of 500 ml each. The frequency of phlebotomy is weekly or twice weekly if the hemoglobin can regenerate this quickly. After a few weeks, weekly or twice monthly phlebotomy is used.

Wilson's Disease. Recognized by a low serum ceruloplasmin level, raised liver copper concentration, and a Kayser-Fleischer corneal ring, Wilson's disease is treated with oral penicillamine, 2 to 3 grams per day.

Hepatic Schistosomiasis. Biopsy and large egg loads in the stool in patients from endemic areas indicate hepatic schistosomiasis. Praziquantel is used for treatment. The Parasitic Disease Drug Service (Atlanta, Ga., 404–329–3654) can provide up-to-date information on useful drugs and their availability and on newer diagnostic tests.

TREATMENT OF COMPLICATIONS OF CIRRHOSIS

Ascites

Ascites, or edema, in liver disease rarely requires urgent intensive treatment. Severe restriction of respiration, nonreducible umbilical hernias, and variceal bleeding are the only clear indications for urgent treatment. In such circumstances, a large (3 to 6 liters) paracentesis is the most reliable treatment, but about two-thirds of the removed volume will recur in 48 hours and require removal again. All other cases are managed with dietary sodium restriction and diuretics. Treatment of ascites is required for many months, so the diet selected should be one that can be followed at home and should include 4 grams of sodium chloride (70 mEq) per day or less. The diuretic of choice is spironolactone (Aldactone), starting at 150 mg per day in three divided doses and increasing if needed to 600 mg per day. The progress of diuresis should be followed by measuring body weight at least three times weekly; weights should be recorded in a diary. The goal of safe diuresis is a weight loss of 0.5 to 2 pounds per day and can most rapidly be predicted by obtaining urine sodium values on a single sample in the middle of the day. A negative sodium balance must be attained; if the diet includes 4 grams of sodium chloride (70 mEq), the urine loss must be at least 100 mEq per liter (about the same as per 24 hours) to attain weight loss. Values less than this require more spironolactone or addition of furosemide, 40 mg in the morning, with doubling each 2 days until the desired effect is obtained. A 2- to 4-hour period of supine rest assists diuresis. Potassium supplements are almost always required (40 mEq per day is a typical dose), and assays of serum electrolytes and creatinine levels are needed weekly during the first month and monthly thereafter. Water restriction is required if the serum sodium level is less than 125 mEq per liter and should be kept to a maximum of 1000 ml of fluid per day. Nonsteroidal anti-inflammatory drugs are to be avoided because they precipitate hepatorenal syndrome. Patients who develop elevation of the creatinine level before diuresis occurs or who are refractory may be candidates for the surgical placement of a LeVeen-type peritoneovenous shunt. A consultation with a physician who is experienced in treating chronic ascites with such devices, at least by phone, usually predicts accurately whether the treatment will be effective.

A frequent complication of ascites is spontaneous bacterial peritonitis, which should be suspected if fever, clinical deterioration, failure of diuresis, or onset of hepatic encephalopathy occurs and which is verified by diagnostic paracentesis. The characteristic finding is more than 250 polymorphonuclear cells per mm³ in the fluid. Many fluids have small numbers of bacteria, pH less than 7.25, or an elevated lactate dehydrogen-

ase level. Treatment is undertaken on the basis of the elevated ascites white blood cell count and consists of intravenous cefoxitin (Mefozin) or cefamandole (Mandol). Combinations with aminoglycosides are more toxic in the cirrhotic patient and are to be avoided.

Hepatorenal syndrome frequently occurs in patients with ascites who are undergoing diuresis or who hemorrhage. Diminishing renal output, rising creatinine levels, and no urine sediment are the prominent features. Treating infections, restoring blood volume, and removing diuretic and nonsteroidal anti-inflammatory drugs from treatment may lead to reversal of the syndrome. A fluid challenge of 500 ml of saline with 25 grams of albumin, while urine output is monitored, is used to identify plasma volume depletion.

Hepatic Encephalopathy

Hepatic encephalopathy is disordered central nervous system function produced by materials from the intestine reaching the brain through portal systemic shunts. In cirrhosis, these shunts are mostly through collateral portal venous channels. Toxins that have some role include ammonia, mercaptans, eight-carbon fatty acids, and a gamma-aminobutyric acid–like material. All seem to be produced by bacteria acting on dietary protein in the small and large intestines.

Treatment is highly effective when the hepatic encephalopathy is mild, but when the patient cannot be aroused it is disappointing. In about one-half of the cases, a precipitating cause is found that on removal leads to prompt improvement. Gastrointestinal bleeding, occult infection, unrecognized potassium depletions, and central nervous system depressant drugs are common precipitants; fluid and electrolyte imbalance, anoxia, and additional liver disease are precipitants less frequently associated with a dramatic response.

All patients are provided nonspecific treatment, with the intensity of each measure proportional to the severity of the encephalopathy. Some dietary protein restriction is usually used: a diet free of meat, eggs, and dairy products (i.e., a diet of approximately 20 grams of protein; fruit; and vegetables) is readily obtained and used in most patients able to eat. Lactulose, 30 ml of a 50 per cent solution by mouth (or gastric tube if the patient cannot cooperate) three to five times on the first day and three times daily thereafter, is useful. A diarrhea will result, and the electrolyte losses, often high in potassium, need to be replaced. If these measures do not lead to improvement in 48 hours, antibiotics are added. Oral neomycin, 1 gram every 24 hours, is sufficient, but almost any antibiotic alone or in combination capable of suppressing gut flora is effective. Nutrition should be adequate, and intravenous alimentation (including protein) is given if needed, with no danger of worsening the coma. Special amino acid preparations, such as combinations with high concentrations of branched chain amino acids, are of no special benefit. Unresponsive patients should have a careful review of the diagnosis, including computed tomography. If the patient is unconscious for 4 days because of liver encephalopathy, cerebral edema ensues and produces death by medullary herniation. In patients who are awaiting transplantation or who are expected to recover liver function, intravenous mannitol to lessen swelling, hyperventilation, and even a cranial decompression based on monitoring intraventricular pressures have been lifesaving. Recurrent liver encephalopathy produces a permanent basal ganglion disease called non-Wilsonian hepatolenticular degeneration.

Bleeding Esophageal Varices

Bleeding esophageal varices are best treated by planning that the event may occur. Endoscopy can now predict which varices are likely to bleed (extent, size, presence of vessels on varices), and these patients are subjected to closer follow-up to avoid increased plasma volume. The weight should be monitored three times weekly and each 2 to 3 pounds of weight gain should be reversed with diuretics. Prophylactic propranolol (Inderal) therapy is recommended for patients who have extensive varices with endoscopic markers of probable bleeding.

Gastrointestinal bleeding may be with hematemesis, melena, or occult from varices, but the source must be identified, usually by endoscopy. Resuscitative measures must be promptly undertaken, and sclerotherapy to eradicate the bleeding vessel must be considered. Sclerotherapy destroys three to five varix columns with each treatment, and four to seven treatments at weekly intervals are required to eradicate the varices and the possibility of bleeding. Once eradicated, varices seldom recur for 1 year. For patients who have not bled or patients who are unwilling to undergo sclerotherapy, treatment with propranolol seems to be effective. The dose of 80 mg twice daily is used for the indefinite future. Portacaval shunts are used for patients with low operative risk (Child's A classification: no major jaundice, malnutrition, ascites, encephalopathy, or coagulopathy) and recurrent variceal hemorrhage.

DYSPHAGIA AND ESOPHAGEAL OBSTRUCTION

method of
THOMAS J. PULLIAM, M.D., and
JOEL E. RICHTER, M.D.
Bowman Gray School of Medicine
Winston-Salem, North Carolina

Dysphagia is derived from the Greek roots *dys* (with difficulty) and *phagia* (to eat). Dysphagia encompasses the symptoms that include either difficulty in initiating a swallow or the sensation that food, liquids, or both are hindered in their passage from mouth to stomach. It is important to differentiate dysphagia from odynophagia (pain with swallowing), although it is often difficult to separate the two clearly.

It is useful to consider dysphagia in two separate categories: oropharyngeal (entry or transfer) dysphagia and esophageal (transport) dysphagia. In addition, the entirely different symptom complex of globus hystericus must be considered and initially excluded. Globus is a functional complaint that is not associated with a true swallowing disorder. These patients can swallow normally but complain of having a "lump" in the throat that is usually constant and not related to the act of swallowing. True dysphagia almost always indicates the presence of organic disease and merits investigation to define the underlying pathologic process.

Oropharyngeal (transfer) dysphagia implies difficulty in propelling the food bolus from the mouth into the upper esophagus. Normal initiation of swallowing is accomplished automatically by a series of finely tuned neural and muscular events modulated by the swallowing center in the brain stem. Oropharyngeal dysphagia occurs when there is a weakness of the pharyngeal musculature or failure of successful coordination between the tongue, pharynx, and upper esophageal sphincter (UES). Anything that affects the brain stem's swallowing center or the afferent or efferent nerves that modulate the process (cranial nerves V, VII, IX, X, and XII) can cause oropharyngeal dysphagia. Neuromuscular diseases are responsible for approximately 80 per cent of these cases (Table 1). For a few of these diseases, specific therapy is available: corticosteroids for dermatomyositis, neostigmine for myasthenia gravis, and levodopa for Parkinson's disease. Unfortunately, specific therapy is not available for most of the diseases responsible for oropharyngeal dysphagia. Modification of the nature and consistence of the diet may be helpful in some patients. In the most severe cases, nasogastric feeding tubes or gastrostomy tubes (surgical or endoscopic) may be required to manage these patients.

Esophageal (transport) dysphagia is produced by diseases that interfere with the transport of solids and liquids through the esophagus. The peristaltic wave takes approximately 8 seconds to pass from the UES to the esophagogastric junction. Transport is quite efficient, and the primary peristaltic wave is followed by waves of secondary peristalsis that sweep the esoph-

TABLE 1. Abnormalities Causing Oropharyngeal Dysphagia

Neuromuscular Diseases
Central nervous system (CNS)
  Cerebrovascular accident (brain stem or pseudobulbar palsy)
  Parkinson's disease
  Wilson's disease
  Multiple sclerosis
  Amyotrophic lateral sclerosis
  Brain stem tumors
  Tabes dorsalis
  Miscellaneous congenital and degenerative disorders of the CNS
Peripheral nervous system (PNS)
  Bulbar poliomyelitis
  Peripheral neuropathies (diphtheria, botulism, rabies, diabetes mellitus)
Motor end plate
  Myasthenia gravis
Muscle
  Muscular dystrophies
  Primary myositis
  Metabolic myopathy (thyrotoxicosis, myxedema, steroid myopathy)
  Amyloidosis
  Systemic lupus erythematosus

Local Structural Lesions
Inflammatory (pharyngitis, abscess, tuberculosis, syphilis)
Neoplastic
Congenital webs
Plummer-Vinson syndrome
Extrinsic compression (thyromegaly, cervical spinal hyperostosis, lymphadenopathy)
Surgical resection of the oropharynx

Motility Disorders of the UES
Hypertensive UES (globus, spasm)
Hypotensive UES (esophagopharyngeal regurgitation)
Abnormal UES relaxation
  Incomplete relaxation (cricopharyngeal achalasia, CNS lymphoma, cricopharyngeal bar)
  Premature closure (Zenker's diverticulum?)
  Delayed relaxation (familial dysautonomia)

agus clean of any retained food or liquid. The three major mechanisms causing this form of dysphagia are esophageal motility disorders, mechanical obstruction of the esophageal lumen (extrinsic or intrinsic), and inflammation of the esophageal mucosa (Table 2).

DIAGNOSTIC EVALUATION

History

When Schatzki first described the lower esophageal ring that now bears his name in 1959, he stated that a strong suspicion of the correct diagnosis could be obtained from a careful and extensive history in 80 to 85 per cent of patients with dysphagia. Figure 1 is a suggested algorithm for the evaluation of patients with dysphagia. After obtaining a general medical history, including medications used, a detailed history of swallowing should emphasize the duration of the symptoms and the types of foods and liquids that cause them. It

is important to ascertain whether the problem is constant or intermittent and if the dysphagia has been progressive. The presence of other esophageal symptoms should be addressed: heartburn, a sour taste in the mouth, sore throat, odynophagia, and a sensation of food sticking, with an attempt to localize the perceived level of obstruction. In addition, changes in voice, sleep habits, and eating habits should all be thoroughly evaluated. The presence of chest pain or new respiratory symptoms may also be helpful in tracing dysphagia to an esophageal etiology.

Physical Examination

A thorough physical examination, with emphasis on the head, cranial nerves, oropharynx, neck, and thorax, is necessary in the complete evaluation of the patient with dysphagia. Positive physical findings may include cervical and supraclavicular lymphadenopathy caused by metastases or swellings in the neck resulting from a dilated esophagus or esophageal diverticulum. Watching the patient swallow may also be useful. Those with oropharyngeal dysphagia may demonstrate aspiration or nasal regurgitation. However, the yield of positive findings from the physical examination is quite low. The diagnostician must therefore rely primarily on coupling the complete history with judicious use of the multiple available diagnostic tests.

TABLE 2. Causes of Esophageal Dysphagia

Neuromuscular (Motility) Disorders
Most common
  Achalasia
  Scleroderma
  Nutcracker esophagus
Other
  Other collagen vascular diseases
  Chagas's disease
  Chronic idiopathic intestinal pseudo-obstruction
  Diffuse esophageal spasm

Intrinsic Mechanical Lesions
Most common
  Peptic stricture
  Lower esophageal rings
  Carcinoma
Other
  Esophageal webs
  Esophageal diverticula
  Benign tumors
  Foreign bodies

Extrinsic Mechanical Lesions
Vascular compression (dysphagia lusoria)
Mediastinal abnormalities (e.g., aneurysms, goiter, tumor)
Cervical osteoarthritis

Mucosal Inflammation
Most common
  Reflux esophagitis
  Infectious esophagitis (candida, herpes)
Other
  Pill-induced ulcers
  Caustic burns (lye ingestion)

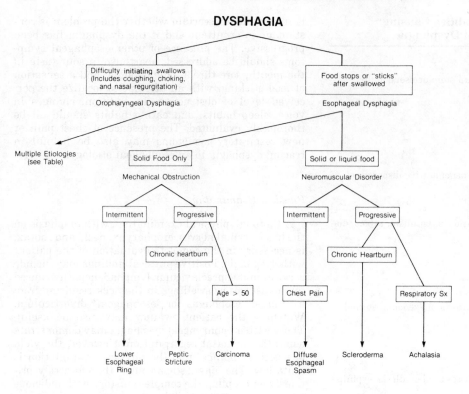

Figure 1. Algorithm for evaluation of patients with dysphagia.

Diagnostic Studies

The four major studies used in diagnosing dysphagia are the contrast esophagram, esophagogastroscopy, esophageal manometry, and continuous pH monitoring.

Contrast Esophagram. Barium swallow should be *the initial test* performed in most patients who complain of dysphagia. Barium outlines irregularities in the esophageal lumen, defines sites of anatomic obstruction, and assesses liquid transit. In cases where esophageal perforation is suspected, the water-soluble contrast material meglumine diatrizoate (Gastrografin) is usually substituted. When oropharyngeal dysphagia is suspected, a barium cine-esophagram shows how the barium bolus is organized by the oropharyngeal musculature before the swallow. Pharyngeal motility is so swift that rapid-sequence cinefilming is' necessary to study this area adequately. Instead of barium in a liquid slurry, barium-impregnated marshmallows or tablets can be given to define problems with swallowing solids more effectively.

Esophagogastroscopy. Upper gastrointestinal endoscopy is probably used most often to explain unclear radiologic findings in the esophagus. Endoscopy can also be used to evaluate radiologically inapparent lesions that are causing persistent swallowing difficulties. Lesions that are identified can be further defined by brushing for cytology, biopsy techniques for histology, and still or video photography. Fiberoptic endoscopes also have a variety of therapeutic applications, including dilation of esophageal strictures or removal of foreign objects from the proximal gastrointestinal tract.

Esophageal Manometry. With the development of small intraluminal transducers and low-compliance infusion systems, it is now possible to measure both normal and abnormal pressures and disturbances precisely in peristalsis. Currently, the major role of esophageal manometry in patients with dysphagia is to diagnose esophageal motility disorders, particularly achalasia. In our laboratory, more than 50 per cent of patients presenting with dysphagia have an abnormal esophageal motility study. If the contrast esophagram fails to reveal a definite abnormality or mechanical obstruction, manometry should be the next diagnostic procedure. Provocative testing is an optional portion of the manometric study. These tests bring out or reproduce subjective symptoms that may be esophageal in origin. The two most commonly used provocative tests are the acid infusion (Bernstein's) and edrophonium (Tensilon) tests.

Continuous pH Monitoring. Esophageal pH monitoring for 24 hours is a helpful tool in the diagnosis of gastroesophageal reflux disease (GERD). Today many commercial systems featuring microcomputer data collection and analysis devices are in widespread use. This technology allows the patient freedom of movement while the study is conducted under conditions that are as nearly physiologic as possible. By convention, the pH probe is placed 5 cm above the manometrically defined lower esophageal sphincter (LES). Reflux is defined by a drop in the intraesophageal pH to less than 4. This study may be helpful in the evaluation of dysphagia if the contrast esophagram and endoscopy indicate that GERD is at the root of the symptoms.

SPECIFIC COMMON ETIOLOGIES: DIAGNOSIS AND TREATMENT

Esophageal Diverticula

General. The three major types are Zenker's diverticula, midesophageal diverticula, and epiphrenic diverticula. Zenker's diverticula arise posterolaterally between the cricopharyngeus and inferior pharyngeal constrictor muscles. These lesions invariably present with high dysphagia even when the diverticulum is quite small. Although the pathogenesis of Zenker's diverticulum is not clear, it is most likely a pulsion diverticulum resulting from the intermittent incoordination of pharyngeal contraction and cricopharyngeal relaxation. The midesophageal diverticulum is typically an acquired diverticulum arising from traction forces caused by an intrathoracic inflammatory process (tuberculosis, fungal infection, or prior surgery). Most midesophageal diverticula are asymptomatic. The epiphrenic esophageal diverticulum is typically a pulsion diverticulum. These diverticula are found in the lower third of the esophagus, most frequently 5 to 10 cm proximal to the gastric cardia, and usually arise from the right posterolateral wall. They are often associated with other esophageal disorders (hiatal hernia, diffuse esophageal spasm, achalasia, esophagitis, or eventration of the diaphragm).

Symptoms. The symptoms produced by esophageal diverticula have two components: (1) those caused by the underlying diverticula (dysphagia, regurgitation, vomiting, and aspiration) and (2) those caused by accumulation and putrefaction of food within the diverticulum (halitosis, bad taste, regurgitation, and local pain). If the diverticulum is small, the symptoms are vague and usually consist of mild dysphagia alone. With time, the pulsion diverticulum grows and the symptoms just noted may develop to varying degrees.

Diagnosis. Barium esophagram is the best study for diagnosing an esophageal diverticulum. If aspiration is suspected, barium remains the contrast material of choice because it is fairly inert and does not cause a pneumonitis if aspirated. Esophagoscopy is not necessary and may be contraindicated, as the risk of perforation increases with instrumentation. Before any surgery, all patients should have manometry because esophageal diverticula (particularly epiphrenic) may recur after simple resection if the associated motility disorder is not treated.

Treatment. Surgical intervention is the only effective treatment. Surgery is indicated for troubling symptoms and for diverticula complicated by perforation, bleeding, aspiration, foreign body impaction, abscess formation, or esophagopulmonary or vascular fistulas. For small Zenker's diverticula, cricopharyngeal myotomy may suffice. For larger diverticula, myotomy is usually combined with diverticulopexy or diverticulectomy.

Peptic Strictures, Barrett's Esophagus, and Gastroesophageal Reflux Disease

General. A benign stricture is a narrowing of the esophagus caused by either edema and inflammation (reversible stricture) or fibrous scar tissue (true stricture). Most commonly, these strictures are secondary to reflux esophagitis (peptic stricture) and are located in the distal esophagus near the LES. Barrett's columnarlined epithelium (or Barrett's esophagus) is associated with ulcerations and stricturing in the esophagus. These strictures may be found in the distal or midesophagus near the *new* squamocolumnar junction. This condition represents the most severe consequences of chronic GERD.

Symptoms. Strictures cause obstructive symptoms of variable severity, depending on the degree of luminal narrowing and the length of the stricture. With time, the frequency of dysphagia usually increases, and the size of the offending food bolus decreases. As a result, patients frequently indicate that they have gradually changed their diet in accordance with their symptoms. A history of long-standing heartburn and/or use of antacids or H_2 blockers is a good clue to the possibility of peptic stricture.

Diagnosis. The barium esophagram is the first test used in diagnosing esophageal strictures. The use of a barium marshmallow or tablet helps to identify relatively mild strictures that are usually *missed* at endoscopy. Endoscopy with brushings and biopsy must be done to exclude the possibility of carcinoma and to evaluate the mucosa for Barrett's esophagus or esophagitis. Continuous pH monitoring can help to assess the severity of GERD and the efficacy of therapy.

Treatment. Therapy is directed at dilation of the stricture and treatment of the underlying reflux disease.

Esophageal dilation becomes necessary once the patient is symptomatic or when the luminal diameter is less than 1 cm. Initial management involves the use of mercury-filled, flexible rubber dilators. Generally, tapered Maloney's dilators are used, although some clinicians prefer the blunt, rounded Hurst's dilators. The technique involves placing the patient in the upright sitting position with adequate pharyngeal anesthesia. Dilation may be done in the lateral decubitus position as well, especially if the patient requires intravenous sedation. After adequate cleansing, the dilators are lubricated and passed orally with the patient swallowing to allow passage through the UES. The weight of the dilator coupled with gentle pressure from the operator usually carries the dilator through the narrowed esophageal segment. Three or four dilators progressing in No. 2 French diameter increments are passed in each session. We usually begin with a No. 30 French diameter dilator (1.0 cm) and progress to as large as No. 50 (1.7 cm) to No. 60 (2.0 cm) French dilator over several sessions. If the rubber dilators cannot be passed easily because of tortuous esophageal anatomy or a tight stricture, the thermoplastic (Savary's) dilators can be used. These tapered-tip dilators are passed over a guidewire in a progressive fashion, as described previously. This procedure usually requires the use of fluoroscopy to reduce the risk of esophageal perforation. Serial dilation may be required in some patients. Some practitioners prefer a regular schedule of dilation, but we prefer to dilate only when symptoms recur.

After adequate dilation, the GERD needs to be vigorously treated. The severity and the response of symptoms direct the type of therapy used. Phase I antireflux measures include elevation of the head of the bed on 6- to 8-inch blocks; use of antacids with alginic acid (Gaviscon); avoidance of foods (chocolate, ethanol, peppermint, fatty foods, and citrus fruits) and medications (calcium channel blockers, anticholinergics, and nitrates) that may aggravate reflux disease; timing the evening meal to occur at least 3 hours before retiring; and avoidance of tight-fitting garments, bending, stooping, or lifting. Phase II measures center on the addition of round-the-clock H_2 blockers. Promotility agents such as metoclopramide (Reglan), 10 mg orally 30 minutes before meals and at bedtime, or bethanechol (Urecholine), 25 mg orally four times a day, may be added if symptoms persist. Phase III antireflux measures (surgery) are reserved for the 5 to 10 per cent of patients with intractable GERD and its complications (ulceration, bleeding, or aspiration). The most satisfactory antireflux procedures are Hill's or Nissen's transabdominal fundoplication or Belsey's transthoracic repair.

A final word about Barrett's esophagus. The potential for malignant changes in the columnar epithelium is real but controversial. Presentation because of cancer-induced symptoms likely overestimates the risk. The true prevalence of carcinoma in a Barrett's esophagus is 4 to 47 per cent (average, 10 per cent). However, recent studies suggest incidence rates of 1 in 81 to 1 in 441 cases per person-year of follow-up. Most authorities suggest annual or biannual endoscopic examinations with multiple biopsies to ensure appropriate cancer surveillance.

Tumors: Benign and Malignant

General. Esophageal tumors giving rise to dysphagia are most commonly malignant. Other lesions of the esophageal wall that may cause dysphagia or obstruction include congenital cysts, reduplications, and benign tumors. The most common benign tumor is the leiomyoma, with lipomas, squamous papillomas, epithelial cysts, and inflammatory pseudotumors being much less common. Many of these tumors (especially leiomyomas) may be multiple. Carcinomas of the proximal esophagus are generally of squamous histology and consist of either squamous carcinomas or adenocarcinomas in the distal esophagus. Adenocarcinomas of the gastric fundus may present with dysphagia caused by submucosal upward extension. These tumors may also present with a picture resembling achalasia.

Symptoms. Benign tumors and cysts are usually asymptomatic and are discovered incidentally during routine barium upper gastrointestinal tract studies performed for unrelated symptoms. Progressive dysphagia of relatively short duration, typically beginning with solid foods but rapidly progressing to include liquids and even swallowed secretions, should make the clinician think of carcinoma. Other clues pointing to a malignant lesion include an age over 40 years, a history of excessive ethanol and tobacco use, and weight loss. Constant pain localized to the substernal region is an unfavorable sign indicating local tumor invasion into adjacent structures. Late in the disease, severe cough, dyspnea, and aspiration with secondary pneumonia may result from severe esophageal obstruction or an acquired tracheoesophageal fistula.

Diagnosis. The barium esophagram shows irregularities of the esophageal wall and luminal narrowing. The tumor may appear as a stricture, mass, or plaque. Esophageal dilation is not common proximal to a stenosing malignant lesion. It is important that the gastric cardia and fundus be evaluated well. Endoscopy with brushings and multiple biopsies is necessary when an esophageal tumor is suspected. Brush cytology is positive in 95 per cent of cases, and biopsy is positive in approximately 70 per cent of cases when cancer is present.

Treatment. An attempt should be made to resect distal localized lesions. Computed tomography scanning is useful in defining those patients who may have operable disease. For most other patients, radiation therapy is the treatment of choice. Squamous malignancies are more radiosensitive than adenocarcinomas. Controlled trials of combined radiation therapy and chemotherapy are under way, but the results are not yet available. Malignant strictures may be dilated with the same technique used for benign strictures, and with equal safety. Patients whose esophageal lumens cannot be kept open by dilation or who have tracheoesophageal fistulas may be helped by endoscopic placement of a wire-reinforced polyvinyl prosthesis that keeps the lumen patent and seals off the fistula. Five-year survival for patients with esophageal carcinoma is still less than 5 per cent. Therefore, palliative therapy is the goal in most patients.

Webs and Rings

General. Schatzki's B rings occur just above a hiatal hernia at the junction between the squamous esophageal and columnar gastric epithelia. Their etiology is unknown but may be chronic reflux changes. The proximal side of the ring is lined with squamous epithelium, and the underside is lined with columnar epithelium. The A rings are muscular rings that arise in the distal esophagus and are lined completely with squamous epithelium. These rings are caused by contractions of hypertrophic, circular muscle tissue in the distal esophageal body. They occur most commonly in children and are changeable in location. Esophageal webs are thin mucosal membranes that grow across the lumen of the esophagus. Webs may be found at any level in the esophagus but are most common in the cervical area or midesophagus. Cervical webs are frequently associated with iron deficiency anemia (Patterson-Kelly syndrome or Plummer-Vinson syndrome) and pernicious anemia.

Symptoms. Most patients with webs and rings are asymptomatic. However, symptomatic patients have the classic complaint of intermittent dysphagia for solid foods, particularly bread and steak. This pattern may persist for years and may occur most often when the patient is experiencing unusual psychologic stress. Occasionally, patients present with sudden esophageal obstruction caused by impaction of meat on an esophageal ring. Dysphagia is the rule if the luminal diameter is less than 13 mm but is unlikely if the diameter is larger than 20 mm.

Diagnosis. Barium studies are the best method for identifying webs and rings. Cine-esophagrams with lateral and oblique views most often detect the presence of webs. In defining the anatomy of more subtle esophageal rings, it may be necessary to give a solid barium bolus (pill or marshmallow). Lower esophageal rings usually appear as thin, symmetric narrowings at the esophagogastric junction and are nearly always associated with hiatal hernias. Endoscopy with possible biopsy may be performed to rule out carcinoma or short peptic strictures. An association between hypopharyngeal cancers and webs has been reported.

Treatment. Webs are usually quite friable and may break apart during endoscopy. If needed, mercury-weighted rubber dilators can also be used. Rings require dilation with blunt rubber dilators. If symptoms persist after repeated peroral dilations, pneumatic dilation (as applied for achalasia) can be used.

Food Impaction and Foreign Bodies

General. Most ingested foreign bodies that become impacted consist of poorly chewed food masses, animal bones, or inorganic objects. Most swallowed foreign objects do not linger in the esophagus but proceed into the stomach and usually are excreted with the feces. Coins are the major exception; they tend to lodge high in the esophagus around the level of T1. Food impaction occurs with poor mastication, alcohol or drug intoxication, strictures (benign or malignant), esophageal motility disorders, or a combination of these factors. Foreign body impaction occurs most frequently in children and in the mentally ill.

Symptoms. The symptoms of foreign body or food impaction include dysphagia, severe and acute odynophagia, coughing, gagging, and choking caused by aspiration. The victim or observers may report attempts to clear the obstruction by vomiting or ingesting water. Once the impaction has cleared, a foreign body sensation may persist for a long period if mucosal or submucosal damage has occurred. When esophageal perforation occurs, the patient usually becomes dyspneic, diaphoretic, shocky, and febrile while experiencing severe substernal and epigastric pain radiating to the back. However, asymptomatic esophageal perforations can occur. Subcutaneous crepitance may indicate trapping of air in the mediastinum or soft tissues of the thorax.

Diagnosis. Plain films of the neck and chest, including lateral views, should be done to look for evidence of perforation and bony or metallic objects. A limited amount of contrast medium (preferably water soluble) can be introduced to define the extent and nature of the obstruction. Endoscopy can then be performed if needed to visualize and relieve the obstruction.

Treatment. If esophageal perforation, hemorrhage, or sepsis is not present, nonsurgical means of relieving the obstruction may be attempted. It is essential to intubate the patient if there is any potential for airway compromise or aspiration during the impaction-clearing procedures. Initially, glucagon (1 to 2 mg intravenously over 1 to 2 minutes), nitrates, or anxiolytics may relax the LES or smooth muscles of the esophageal body enough to allow passage of the impaction. Once in the stomach, most boluses pass freely through the remainder of the gastrointestinal tract. The exceptions are sharp or jagged objects that may perforate the gastrointestinal tract as they pass along. Meat tenderizers should be avoided, as they have been reported to cause esophageal perforation. If the impaction does not clear easily, fiberoptic or rigid endoscopy may be required. The bolus can be broken up and removed piecemeal, by using the grasping forceps, an endoscopic snare, or a polyp-retrieving device. The bolus should never be pushed ahead blindly toward the stomach. Once the impaction has cleared, it is essential to survey the esophagus with contrast radiography to exclude perforation and with endoscopy to define the nature of the underlying obstruction.

Achalasia

General. Achalasia was the first clinically recognized esophageal motility disorder. Although obstruction was initially believed to result from spasm of the gastric cardia (hence the name "cardiospasm"), manometric techniques have shown the true nature of the disease. The lower esophageal sphincter has abnormally high pressures associated with absent or incomplete relaxation with swallowing. In fact, "achalasia" means failure of relaxation. Aperistalsis of the esophagus is typical, along with striking esophageal dilation. Chronic *Trypanosoma cruzi* infection (Chagas's disease) and adenocarcinoma of the stomach also may present with the clinical, radiologic, and manometric findings of achalasia.

Symptoms. The symptoms of achalasia can be subtle. The onset is insidious, with patients complaining of progressive, painless dysphagia for both liquids and solids. Frequently, the dysphagia is worse when the patient is under stress or is forced to eat more rapidly than usual. A recent study reported that the average interval from onset of symptoms to initial appropriate treatment was more than 8 years. These patients may display ingenious or bizarre techniques to compensate for their disease. Rapid postural movements combined with Valsalva's maneuver force the contents in the esophageal lumen down into the stomach, using the transmission of hy-

draulic forces. Regurgitation of undigested food lacking an acid taste is common. Regurgitation may be complicated by aspiration and chronic pulmonary symptoms including wheezing, coughing, and choking. Some persons may induce regurgitation before bedtime to minimize their tendency to aspirate. Weight loss is gradual, although often quite dramatic.

Diagnosis. Achalasia can be diagnosed by examining a plain chest film. Radiographic findings suggesting achalasia include an air-fluid level within the esophagus, absence of gastric air bubbles, a widened mediastinum, and the thin, curving line of the dilated esophageal wall in the right upper mediastinum. The barium esophagram shows the characteristic features of achalasia: a smoothly tapered narrowing of the distal esophagus ("bird beaking"), a fluid level in the proximal esophagus, and, in advanced cases, a "sigmoid" esophagus. Manometry must be performed to confirm the diagnosis of achalasia. The characteristic manometric findings are absence of peristalsis in the esophageal body, incomplete LES relaxation with swallowing, hypertensive LES (usually >30 mmHg), and elevated intraesophageal pressure greater than gastric pressure. Endoscopy must be performed to rule out malignancy. The closed LES should open easily with gentle pressure applied by the endoscope. If firm resistance is encountered, an organic stricture or malignancy should be suspected. It is essential to get a good retroflexed view of the gastric cardia to exclude intragastric malignancy.

Treatment. Patients with early achalasia and no weight loss may receive symptomatic relief with medical therapy: nifedipine, 10 to 20 mg orally before meals, or isosorbide dinitrate, 20 to 30 mg orally before meals. More severe cases are treated by disruption of the LES, either by pneumatic dilation or by surgical intervention (Heller's myotomy). Pneumatic dilation is done after adequate intravenous sedation has been given and a nasoesophageal tube has been used to decompress the esophagus. The balloon dilator is passed into the esophagus so that it straddles the LES. The balloon is inflated to a pressure of 15 pounds per in^2 for 1 minute. The balloon is deflated and removed. An esophagram with Gastrografin is performed to rule out perforation. If no perforation is present, the patient is observed for 6 to 24 hours and released. If the dysphagia recurs, repeated dilation may be performed up to two or three times. If the achalasia remains refractory to this therapy, Heller's myotomy should be considered. Young children with achalasia or adults with associated epiphrenic diverticula or large hiatal hernia may best be treated initially with surgery.

Scleroderma

General. Involvement of the esophagus occurs in 75 to 85 per cent of patients with scleroderma. Fibrous connective tissue replaces the smooth muscle in the wall of the lower two-thirds of the esophagus. There is loss of peristalsis and tone in the lower esophageal sphincter, with resultant severe GERD.

Symptoms. Patients presenting with progressive dysphagia for solids and liquids with an associated history of severe heartburn should have scleroderma excluded. Symptoms and signs of skin changes, Raynaud's phenomenon, arthralgias, and myalgias coupled with dysphagia suggest underlying scleroderma.

Diagnosis. The barium esophagram shows a distended distal esophagus with free flow through the LES. Manometry demonstrates weak to absent distal esophageal peristalsis, low to absent LES pressures, and normal UES pressure and peristalsis. Manometry is more sensitive than contrast radiography in detecting early esophageal scleroderma.

Treatment. Management of esophageal scleroderma is directed at the GERD. Dilation may be necessary if severe acid reflux results in an esophageal stricture.

Motility Disorders: Diffuse Esophageal Spasm, "Nutcracker" Esophagus, and Nonspecific Esophageal Motility Disorder

General. Diffuse esophageal spasm is a clinical syndrome characterized by symptoms of substernal chest pain, dysphagia, or both caused by a generalized disorder of esophageal motility in which normal peristalsis is interrupted by simultaneous, nonpropulsive contractions. Repetitive, prolonged, high-pressure and spontaneous contractions and LES abnormalities are associated features. Nutcracker esophagus is characterized by high-pressure (>180 mmHg) esophageal contractions with normal peristaltic progression. Nonspecific esophageal motility disorders encompass a broad spectrum of manometric abnormalities whose true clinical significance remains to be discovered. These disorders are defined by any combination of the following: increased nontransmitted contractions, triple-peaked contractions, retrograde contractions, low-amplitude (<30 mmHg) contractions, isolated incomplete LES relaxation, and peristaltic waves of prolonged duration (>6 seconds).

Symptoms. Intermittent dysphagia for both solids and liquids is the classic symptom of an esophageal motility disorder. Angina-like chest pain can also be seen with these motility disorders, causing great concern for both the patient and the physician. Cardiac catheterization may be required to distinguish esophageal motility disorders from coronary artery disease.

Diagnosis. Although barium cine-esophagrams may reveal abnormalities in peristalsis and tertiary contractions, the best test for diagnosing these motility disorders is esophageal manometry. Patients are usually asymptomatic when their motility disorders are defined. Provocative testing with edrophonium may reproduce the patient's symptoms of chest pain, dysphagia, or both.

Therapy. Nitrates and calcium channel blockers have been used to treat motility disorders, but their effectiveness in long-term trials is disappointing. Anticholinergic compounds such as dicyclomine hydrochloride (Bentyl), 10 to 20 milligrams orally 1 hour before meals and at bedtime, may be efficacious in some individuals. Others may improve with antidepressant medications such as trazodone (Desyrel), 150 mg orally once a day. For significant debility caused by dysphagia, chest pain, or odynophagia, pneumatic dilation or "long" esophagomyotomy extending from the LES to the level of the aortic arch may be necessary in rare cases.

Infectious Esophagitis

General. Esophageal infections are rarely seen in healthy persons. However, the esophagus is the most common site of gastrointestinal infection in the immunocompromised patient. In view of the multitude of immunocompromised patients with acquired immunodeficiency syndrome, neoplasms and leukemias, allograft transplants, and those receiving either chemotherapy or immunosuppressive drugs, it is important for the clinician to have a basic understanding of the major pathogens infecting the esophagus. Bacterial infections do occur, although the most common organisms are opportunistic fungi (candida) and viruses (herpes simplex virus and cytomegalovirus).

Symptoms. The major symptoms of infectious esophagitis are dysphagia, odynophagia, and noncardiac chest pain. Often the patient is unable to tolerate swallowing because of the significant pain that arises, which results in marked weight loss. Bleeding from infectious esophageal ulcers can also occur.

Diagnosis. Barium swallow may suggest the presence of mucosal disease. However, the procedure of choice is endoscopy with brushings and biopsy. Endoscopic findings may be characteristic (i.e., whitish plaques with candida and punctate "volcano ulcers" with herpes), although when the infection is advanced, the picture becomes less clear. Specimens should be obtained for potassium hydroxide smear and for fungal and viral culture. Cytology using silver and immunofluorescent stains or Papanicolaou's technique should be obtained.

Treatment. Oral doses of nystatin (Mycostatin), 100,000 to 500,000 units every 2 to 4 hours ("swish and swallow"), or clotrimazole (Mycelex) troches, 10 mg dissolved slowly every 4 to 5 hours, may be effective with mild candidal esophagitis. In more advanced cases, systemic therapy with ketoconazole (Nizoral), 200 mg per day orally for 1 to 2 weeks, is effective. Systemic parenteral therapy with amphotericin B (Fungizone) in a low dose for a short course (0.15 to 0.5 mg per kg total dose) is reserved for advanced cases that are refractory to oral therapy. Herpes simplex virus type 1 infections should be treated with intravenous acyclovir (Zovirax) at a dose of 6.5 mg per kg administered every 8 hours for 1 week.* Cytomegalovirus infections have been reported to have a 75 per cent response rate to the use of ganciclovir intravenously at a dose of 5 mg per kg every 12 hours for 2 weeks.

Pill-Induced Ulcers

General. Some medications are caustic to the esophageal mucosa and may actually produce esophageal ulcerations. Examples include tetracycline, potassium chloride tablets, iron preparations, steroids, nonsteroidal anti-inflammatory agents, and quinidine. Older patients are at particular risk, as well as those with esophageal motility disorders, impaired consciousness, and intrinsic or extrinsic esophageal luminal narrowing.

Symptoms. Dysphagia and odynophagia are prominent symptoms. The medications ingested seem to "hang up" as they are swallowed. A burning sensation may also be noted.

Diagnosis. Barium swallow may demonstrate an esophageal ulcer or a luminal narrowing that may predispose to the formation of a pill-induced ulcer. Endoscopy is performed to confirm the findings of contrast radiography. Pill-induced ulcers are usually seen at the level of the aortic arch or the most distal esophagus.

Treatment. Patients taking potentially caustic medications should ingest them in the sitting position with large amounts of water. Once injury has occurred, the offending medication should be discontinued. Antacids, H_2 blockers, or sucralfate (Carafate), given in a slurry at a dose of 1 to 2 grams orally twice a day, help the ulcer to heal.

---

*The usual dose is 5 mg per kg infused over 1 hour every 8 hours.

DIVERTICULA OF THE ALIMENTARY TRACT

method of
HARRIS R. CLEARFIELD, M.D.
Hahnemann University
Philadelphia, Pennsylvania

Diverticula are often asymptomatic but may produce symptoms if they distend with food or liquid and compress the lumen (Zenker's and epiphrenic diverticula), harbor sufficient organisms to produce a bacterial overgrowth syndrome (jejunal diverticula), become inflamed, or bleed (Meckel's and colonic diverticula).

ESOPHAGEAL DIVERTICULA

Hypopharyngeal Diverticula

The hypopharyngeal diverticulum (Zenker's diverticulum) is found in approximately 2 per cent of patients presenting with dysphagia, and the majority of cases occur in patients beyond the seventh decade of life. The diverticulum generally protrudes between the cricopharyngeus muscle (superior esophageal sphincter) and the inferior constrictor muscle. Small diverticula are asymptomatic, but progressive enlargement can occur as a result of food-induced stretching. The opening to the diverticulum may become larger than the lumen of the esophagus, so that food and liquid preferentially enter the diverticulum and subsequently spill over into the lumen, and the progressively enlarging diverticulum may exert sufficient pressure on the esophagus to produce dysphagia. Inadequate or uncoordinated relaxation of the superior sphincter has been postulated to result in sufficient pharyngeal pressure to force mucosa through the muscle bundles to form the diverticula, but more recent manometric studies have cast doubt on this hypothesis. Symptoms include cervical dysphagia, coughing while eating, bad breath from the fermenting food, a lump in the neck caused by the enlarging diverticulum, and nocturnal wheezing resulting from aspiration. Medications may also accumulate in the diverticulum, causing erratic absorption. These symptoms may be suggestive, but barium upper gastrointestinal tract x-ray films usually establish the diagnosis. Flexible endoscopy should be avoided if this diverticulum is suspected because perforation may occur.

Treatment

No treatment is needed for asymptomatic diverticula, but those producing symptoms often require surgery. A myotomy of the superior esophageal sphincter is advocated for small diverticula; larger lesions are generally resected.

Midesophageal Diverticula

Midesophageal diverticula were once thought to represent a fibrotic "pull" or "traction" from an adjacent mediastinal inflammatory reaction, but this theory has been largely replaced by the observation that many diverticula are associated with motility abnormalities, such as achalasia or esophageal spasm. The diverticula are usually small and wide-mouthed, so that food trapping rarely occurs and symptoms are unusual. If chest pain is associated with these diverticula, esophageal motility studies should be performed. No treatment is usually required for the diverticula.

Epiphrenic Diverticula

Epiphrenic diverticula occur in the distal esophagus and are thought to result from high pressure generated by a motility disorder of the lower esophageal sphincter or distal esophagus, such as achalasia or esophageal spasm. Most diverticula are asymptomatic, but an occasional diverticulum may progressively distend and begin to trap food and secretions, leading to dysphagia, substernal discomfort, or vomiting (often nocturnal). The diagnosis is usually established by barium upper gastrointestinal tract x-ray films. The outpouching may be mistaken for an esophageal ulcer.

Treatment

No treatment is required for small, asymptomatic outpouchings, but detailed motility studies should be performed for larger diverticula. Symptomatic diverticula associated with esophageal spasm or achalasia may respond to pharmacologic therapy, such as nitrites or calcium channel blockers. If surgery is required, diverticulectomy should be combined with a procedure directed to the underlying motility disorder, such as a lower esophageal myotomy.

SMALL INTESTINAL DIVERTICULA

Duodenal Diverticula

Duodenal diverticula are quite common, exceeded in frequency only by colonic diverticula. They usually occur within the "C loop," often adjacent to the ampulla of Vater, and are rarely found on the lateral wall of the duodenum. The diverticula increase in frequency with advancing age and are usually composed of mucosa without muscle fibers, which suggests that they are the result of duodenal pressure, but congenital diverticula may also occur. They are described more frequently by barium upper gastrointestinal tract x-ray films than by endoscopy because the narrow or slit-like ostia are easily missed during the endoscopic examination. Because the x-ray films are usually obtained as a result of upper abdominal symptoms, it is tempting to ascribe such symptoms to the presence of the diverticula. However, it is difficult to establish a correlation between these frequently encountered diverticula and a variety of dyspeptic or aerophagic complaints. Preliminary reports suggest that dysfunction of the sphincter of Oddi may result from the presence of periampullary diverticula. There appears to be an increased incidence of common duct stones in these patients, with a higher percentage of pigment stones than would be expected. This observation has been attributed to low sphincter pressure, which permits access of bacteria to the common duct. Additional information regarding the relationship of duodenal diverticula to common duct stones is required.

Treatment

Duodenal diverticula rarely produce symptoms and therefore usually require no therapy. Upper gastrointestinal tract bleeding, brisk rather than occult, may occur in patients with these diverticula, but efforts should be made to define some other more likely cause. A causal relationship between diverticula and bleeding should be established only with convincing endoscopic or angiographic findings. The management of the bleeding is similar to that of other causes of upper gastrointestinal tract hemorrhage, with emphasis on monitoring hemodynamic status, blood replacement, and exploration when supportive measures fail. The diverticula located adjacent to the ampulla pose special difficulties. Diverticular perforation and abscess are even more uncommon and probably require computed tomography scan, ultrasonography, or surgical exploration to establish the diagnosis.

Small Intestinal Diverticula

Jejunal and ileal diverticula are uncommon and are thought to be primarily of the acquired type. They tend to occur on the mesenteric border of the small bowel, where blood vessels penetrate from the serosal surface, thus creating a potential weak area in the musculature. Multiple large diverticula, usually jejunal, may permit sufficient bacterial overgrowth to result in a malabsorption syndrome. This complication may be associated with a more generalized bowel motility disorder, such as scleroderma. The symptoms are those of other malabsorption syndromes and include megaloblastic anemia secondary to vitamin B_{12} or folate deficiency, steatorrhea, diarrhea, weight loss, and fat-soluble vitamin deficiency. Jejunal diverticula have also been associated with intestinal pseudo-obstruction, although the retrospective nature of the published reports does not permit an estimate of the frequency of this relationship. The diverticula appear to be a manifestation of the pseudo-obstruction rather than the cause. The generalized nature of the small bowel motility disorder in these patients is illustrated by such associated findings as esophageal dysmotility, the CREST syndrome (calcinosis cutis, Raynaud's phenomenon, esophageal dysfunction, sclerodactyly, and telangiectasia), and degenerated smooth muscle cells consistent with a visceral myopathy. True mechanical obstruction has also been reported as a result of diverticulitis (sometimes with perforation), volvulus, or adhesions.

Treatment

The bacterial overgrowth of small bowel diverticulosis often responds to antibiotic therapy. Tetracycline, 250 mg four times daily, or metronidazole (Flagyl), 250 mg three or four times daily for 7 to 10 days, may be effective. Unfortunately, relapse is common, and some patients benefit from 1 week of antibiotic therapy each month. Pharmacologic agents to increase small bowel motility, such as bethanechol (Urecholine), may be helpful. Vitamin B_{12}, folic acid, and fat-soluble vitamins should be provided, and dietary fat and milk products should be reduced. Resection of the small bowel containing the diverticula has been suggested for patients with chronic symptoms, but this may prove to be ineffective if the diverticula are the result of a generalized neuropathic or myopathic process. Surgery should be reserved for acute complications, such as bleeding, diverticulitis, or volvulus. It is therefore important to consider an associated motility disturbance in patients with symptomatic small bowel diverticula.

Meckel's Diverticula

Meckel's diverticulum represents the failure of the intestinal end of the primitive yolk duct (vitelline duct) to close completely. The diverticulum usually occurs on the antimesenteric surface of the ileum, approximately 60 to 80 cm from the ileocecal valve, but it may occur as far as 200 cm proximal to the valve. It is usually several centimeters in size; diverticula measuring up to 10 cm have been described. The majority of the diverticula are asymptomatic. The major complications of bleeding, inflammation, and obstruc-

tion are seen most commonly in infants and young children, with a male predominance. *Bleeding* generally results from the presence of ectopic gastric mucosa within the sac, a finding in approximately 60 to 70 per cent of symptomatic patients. The acid production leads to ulceration and bleeding from within or adjacent to the diverticulum. The bleeding is more frequently maroon or red than tarry and is more likely to be brisk than occult. *Obstruction* can result from volvulus or intussusception and may be of the closed-loop type. *Inflammation* of the diverticulum (diverticulitis) is less common than appendicitis because of the diverticular wide neck, which permits the fecal stream to exit easily. The mobility of the ileum decreases the likelihood that the inflammation will be sealed off, increasing the likelihood of perforation should diverticulitis occur. The presence of painless, massive lower gastrointestinal tract bleeding in an infant or child should suggest the possibility of Meckel's diverticulum. Bowel obstruction or peritonitis in this age group should also raise this suspicion. Although less common, the preceding complications can also occur in adults. The *diagnosis* of Meckel's diverticulum is rarely made by barium small bowel examination, although this study may be useful in selected patients to exclude other disorders. The ^{99m}Tc pertechnetate isotope is taken up by Meckel's diverticula containing gastric mucosa and may be helpful for establishing the diagnosis, but a negative examination does not exclude the possibility. Mesenteric angiography may be useful during active bleeding; intestinal obstruction is diagnosed on the basis of clinical and radiographic criteria; and peritonitis in an infant or child should suggest appendicitis or diverticulitis.

Treatment

The treatment of bleeding from Meckel's diverticula requires blood replacement, localization of the bleeding point if possible by isotope scan or angiography, and diverticulectomy if the lesion can be identified. Occasional patients, both young and old, may bleed intermittently, posing diagnostic problems if the preceding localizing efforts prove to be fruitless. Bowel obstruction requires immediate surgery, and inflammation of a diverticulum usually requires exploration. An incidental Meckel's diverticulum discovered during abdominal surgery for some other disorder should be removed if there is no contraindication.

DIVERTICULAR DISEASE OF THE COLON

Diverticula occur in two rows on either side of the colon, with a distinct clustering in the sigmoid colon. Although diverticula may also be observed in the proximal colon, it is most unusual for patients to have right-sided or transverse colon diverticula in the absence of sigmoid involvement. The frequency of diverticula formation is almost directly related to age, so that the condition is found in approximately 50 per cent of individuals in their ninth decade of life.

The diminished frequency of diverticula among individuals from Africa, Asia, and certain areas of South America has been attributed to a high-fiber diet, which tends to decrease transit time in the gut, to increase stool frequency, and to result in softer, larger stools. This is an attractive hypothesis, but recent studies indicate difficulty in distinguishing normal persons from those with diverticulosis on the basis of stool weight and frequency. Another theory regarding the causes of diverticula relates to the high sigmoid pressure observed in patients with the irritable bowel syndrome. This is the basis of the supposition that increased intraluminal pressure forces the mucosa to protrude through the relatively weak areas of the colonic musculature adjacent to the blood vessels that penetrate from the serosal surface. This explanation seems reasonable, but diverticula have been found in patients with no history of irritable bowel symptoms. A convincing explanation for the development of colonic diverticula is not yet available.

Diverticulosis

Uncomplicated diverticula do not produce symptoms, but in patients with the irritable bowel syndrome, colonic diverticula may be revealed by barium enema examination or colonoscopy. Treatment, therefore, is not directed to the diverticula but focuses on the predominant symptoms, such as pain, diarrhea, or constipation. Consider therapy with a high-fiber diet or psyllium preparations (Metamucil, Konsyl) for constipation, antispasmodic medications such as tincture of belladonna or dicyclomine (Bentyl) for crampy pain, or antidiarrheal agents such as loperamide (Imodium) or diphenoxylate (Lomotil). Patients with diverticula and the irritable bowel syndrome should not be informed that they have diverticular disease or diverticulitis because these labels may induce added anxiety and create confusion for physicians who may subsequently evaluate the patients.

Diverticular Bleeding

Diverticula are one of the major causes of massive colonic hemorrhage. The bleeding is usually painless and rarely accompanies clinical di-

verticulitis. It is thought to result from the presence of an inspissated diverticular fecalith that erodes or ulcerates into an adjacent penetrating artery. The close relationship of the diverticula to these arteries explains why bleeding may be more severe than that encountered from an arteriovenous malformation (AVM). Although it has been stated that right-sided diverticula are more prone to bleed than sigmoid diverticula, colonoscopic examinations suggest that AVM is a more common cause of bleeding from the right colon. The bleeding site (but not the cause) may be established by a technetium isotope bleeding study or by angiography, but these studies must obviously be performed during the bleeding episode. Cleansing of the colon with a lavage solution (GoLYTELY, Colyte) can be safely accomplished during the bleeding episode if hemodynamic stability can be achieved, permitting a colonoscopic examination that can often determine the site of bleeding and the cause (diverticula, AVM, or neoplasm).

Treatment

It is more important to determine which segment of the colon is the site of bleeding (sigmoid, left, transverse, or right colon) than to identify the specific diverticulum at fault. Isotope studies, angiography, and urgent colonoscopy are time-consuming, and the bleeding may be brisk. Thus it is necessary to monitor hemodynamic stability (pulse rate, blood pressure, urine output) closely while the patient is in various imaging laboratories. The most common cause of death during gastrointestinal hemorrhage is inadequate blood replacement. If the bleeding segment is identified and hemodynamic stability cannot be maintained with 3 or 4 units of blood, surgical intervention and segmental colonic resection are required. If major hemorrhage continues and the bleeding site cannot be established, a subtotal colectomy with ileorectal anastomosis should be considered. A "blind" left-sided colectomy in such patients may be disastrous if the bleeding originates from the right colon. If diverticular bleeding stops with conservative measures, elective surgery need not be considered because there is a reasonable possibility that bleeding will not recur.

Diverticulitis

Diverticulitis results from a microperforation of a single diverticulum, usually into pericolic tissues. The inflammatory reaction is generally walled off by surrounding omentum or adjacent bowel loops but may progress to an abscess or phlegmon (marked cellulitis without pus). If the inflammatory process is not sealed, a free perforation may rarely occur. Diverticulitis usually involves the sigmoid colon, but instances of right-sided diverticulitis have been encountered.

The patient usually complains of left lower quadrant or suprapubic pain, which may be accompanied by back pain, nausea, vomiting, dysuria, or fever. Gross rectal bleeding is unusual. Physical examination generally reveals tenderness over the left lower area, suprapubic area, or both. Muscle guarding or rebound tenderness may be elicited.

An obstruction series may provide little information, but a sigmoid obstruction secondary to edema and inflammation may occur, or a partial small bowel obstruction may result from a segment of distal jejunum or proximal ileum that becomes surrounded by the pericolonic inflammatory reaction. An ultrasound study of the left lower quadrant may demonstrate an abscess, although overlying bowel gas may pose interpretation problems. A computed tomography scan of the abdomen may also prove useful in determining the presence of an abscess, but it may be unremarkable if performed early in the course of the disease. An elevated white blood cell count has little localizing value but can be useful in distinguishing between the irritable colon (normal count) and diverticulitis (usually elevated count). A urinalysis may reflect the presence of a colovesical fistula (ask the patient about the passage of gas during urination) or cystitis secondary to an adjacent inflammatory reaction. Blood cultures should be obtained.

Sigmoidoscopy and colonoscopy should be avoided during the acute process so that free perforation secondary to air insufflation can be avoided. Contrast x-ray films of the colon should be deferred for the same reason. Imaging studies can often be performed after 7 to 10 days of therapy. The barium enema may show a fistula, partial obstruction, or evidence of an extrinsic mass effect. Colonoscopy is less useful for the diagnosis of recent diverticulitis but can be helpful in the differential diagnosis. There are, however, occasions when imaging studies are required during the acute process if other diseases, such as ischemic colitis, cannot be excluded with reasonable confidence.

The differential diagnosis may include the irritable bowel syndrome, but the presence of fever, leukocytosis, and/or peritoneal signs should suggest an inflammatory reaction. Ovarian pathology, appendicitis (the appendix may extend down into the pelvis), inflammatory bowel disease, and ischemic colitis should be considered. A confined perforation of a colonic carcinoma is more difficult to exclude during the acute process. Even the surgeon may have problems making the diagnosis during emergency exploration because the surrounding inflammatory reaction may be intense. A colon neoplasm can usually be diagnosed by colonoscopy or barium enema when the inflammation has subsided.

Complications include fistulas to the bladder, small bowel, or vagina. Free perforation, abdominal abscess, partial or complete obstruction of the small or large bowel, and septicemia may occur. Another serious complication of diverticulitis is spread of the bacteria through the portal vein to the liver, leading to pylephlebitis (pus in the portal vein) and suppurative liver abscesses.

Treatment

Immediate treatment for most cases requires hospitalization. The bowel should be kept at rest and intravenous fluids given. Nasogastric suction should be used if peritonitis or obstruction is present. Because the inflammatory reaction is largely extraluminal, nonabsorbable antibiotics, such as neomycin, are no longer used. Parenteral broad-spectrum antibiotic coverage against aerobic and anaerobic bacteria should be provided. An aminoglycoside, such as gentamycin (Garamycin), 1.5 mg per kg every 8 hours if renal function is normal, is often combined with clindamycin (Cleocin), 600 mg every 6 hours or 900 mg every 8 hours, or ampicillin, 2 grams every 6 hours, but single-drug therapy with cefoxitin (Mefoxin), 2 grams every 8 hours, may also be used. Other antibiotic combinations have also been effective. Aminoglycoside blood levels should be closely monitored to prevent nephrogenic and ototoxic complications.

If the patient fails to improve, as judged by the white blood cell count, fever status, and abdominal findings, surgical intervention may be required. A one-stage procedure with resection of the inflamed bowel and reanastomosis is more often performed now, but a staged procedure with a diverting colostomy is preferable if significant peritonitis or infection is present in the area of the anastomosis or if the anastomosis cannot be accomplished without tension.

If the patient responds to medical therapy, the diet is gradually advanced, but the patient should be instructed to avoid small, hard particles, such as seeds, nuts, corn, and fish bones, to prevent their entrapment in diverticula. It is also prudent to avoid constipation by increasing the fiber content of the diet, using either bran cereals or psyllium products such as Konsyl or Metamucil. Elective resection of the sigmoid colon after the diverticulitis has resolved was once advocated, but current experience indicates that approximately 50 per cent of patients have no further symptoms. A recurrence of diverticulitis, however, should suggest consideration of surgery in view of the potential complications.

ULCERATIVE COLITIS

method of
KIRON M. DAS, M.D., Ph.D.
University of Medicine and Dentistry
of New Jersey
Robert Wood Johnson Medical School
New Brunswick, New Jersey

Ulcerative colitis is a chronic inflammatory disease of unknown etiology, affecting the mucosa of the rectum and a variable length of colon. It is characterized by rectal bleeding and diarrhea during exacerbation, which usually undergoes remission with treatment. The pathogenesis of the disease is considered to be an autoimmune process where specific autoantibodies develop to colonic epithelial cell components. The common age of onset is during the second and third decades of life, although it can become manifest as early as the neonatal period or after 60 years of age. There is no difference in sex distribution. There is a significantly higher incidence among the family members, particularly first degree blood relatives. The diagnosis is usually made on the basis of clinical symptoms and the demonstration of a uniformly involved mucosal inflammation by sigmoidoscopy. The diagnosis is supported by chronicity; negative stool examinations for bacteria, viruses, and parasites capable of causing colitis; and the characteristic findings on proctoscopy, colonoscopy, mucosal biopsy, and barium enema.

There is no medical cure for ulcerative colitis. Medical therapy, however, does offer comfort to at least 80 per cent of these patients and improves their lives. Surgery can provide a cure but requires the very high price of total colectomy and ileostomy. Newer surgical procedures creating either a continent ileostomy or one of several types of ileoanal anastomoses may be more appealing cosmetically. These techniques, however, are still evolving, and their results are not always completely satisfactory. The aims of medical therapy are to maintain nutritional status, to provide symptomatic relief, and, it is hoped, to reverse the bowel inflammation itself.

SUPPORTIVE TREATMENT

There is no specific diet for ulcerative colitis. Patients should be encouraged to eat well and maintain an adequate caloric intake with whatever food they prefer and can tolerate. They need to avoid only those foods that clearly provoke symptoms. Some patients may be consistently lactose intolerant; others may find that alcohol provokes diarrhea or that spices aggravate their symptoms. During an acute exacerbation, excess dietary roughage, although not contraindicated, may precipitate bleeding from a friable colonic mucosa or may increase the number of bowel movements. Roughage, however, is helpful in patients with constipated colitis usually due to left-sided or distal colon involvement.

Patients with ulcerative colitis often find that their overall food intake is limited because of diarrhea, anorexia, or abdominal pain, and thus they may suffer a variety of nutritional deficiencies, compounded by gastrointestinal protein, fluid, and blood loss. Anemia, electrolyte and fluid deficiencies, and evidence of malnutrition must be corrected during the initial phases of the medical treatment, particularly in patients with moderately severe disease who have hypoalbuminemia and anemia. The most aggressive efforts to reverse nutritional disturbances have focused on various regimens of parenteral hyperalimentation. While this approach may certainly reverse specific deficiencies and maintain body protein, it has no role as primary therapy for acute exacerbations of disease. Oral preparations, if tolerated, may have a similar supportive role. Parenteral nutrition or oral supplements are useful in acute episodes of illness by maintaining hydration and potassium supplement and nutritional intake until the disease undergoes remission.

Psychotherapy

General emotional and psychologic support is very helpful. No specific emotional disorder is prominent in the ulcerative colitis group; however, individual psychotherapy and group and family therapy can be beneficial, particularly in children and adolescents.

SULFASALAZINE THERAPY

The most commonly prescribed medication for ulcerative colitis is sulfasalazine (Azulfidine; S.A.S.-500), a drug that was developed by linking a sulfonamide and a salicylate by an azo (N=N) bond. This drug has been used for over 40 years, and its effectiveness in treating mild ulcerative colitis and in preventing relapse has been amply confirmed in randomized controlled trials. Unfortunately it is of little or no benefit in 20 to 30 per cent of patients with ulcerative colitis.

Pharmacokinetics

Studies have shown the patterns of absorption, metabolism, and excretion of sulfasalazine in patients with ulcerative colitis and Crohn's disease are the same as those in healthy subjects.

Absorption and Metabolism. The metabolic pathway of sulfasalazine is depicted in Figure 1. Only

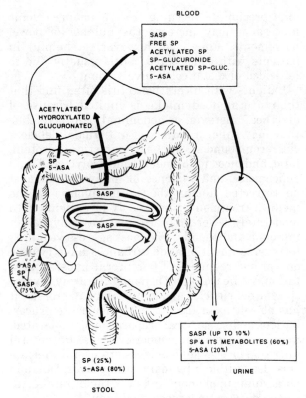

Figure 1. Metabolic pathway of sulfasalazine. Numbers in parentheses indicate percentage of administered dose normally absorbed, metabolized, or excreted. SASP, sulfasalazine; SP, sulfapyridine; 5-ASA, 5-aminosalicylic acid. (From Das KM and Sternlieb I: Salicylazosulfapyridine in inflammatory bowel disease. Am J Dig Dis *20:*971–976, 1975. Used by permission of Plenum Publishing Corporation.)

20 to 30 per cent of an oral dose of sulfasalazine is absorbed from the upper gastrointestinal tract. When the bulk of an orally administered dose of sulfasalazine arrives in the colon, bacterial action causes cleavage to its active metabolites sulfapyridine (SP) and 5-aminosalicylic acid (5-ASA). Azo reduction by intestinal flora has been shown to be the major metabolic route for a number of other azo compounds and can be accomplished by most strains of bacteria. Therefore, concomitant administration of antibiotics may influence the metabolism of sulfasalazine. In addition, sulfasalazine breakdown may be reduced if transit time of the drug is shortened, a condition that can occur in diarrheal states caused by large-bowel disease such as ulcerative colitis or colonic Crohn's disease or following ileal resection.

The foregoing observations on the role of bacteria in sulfasalazine metabolism, combined with clinical evidence, led to the prediction that sulfasalazine would be a useful agent in ulcerative colitis or colonic Crohn's disease, but not in disease limited to the ileum. The clinical relevance of this point is discussed later.

Excretion. Most of the sulfasalazine absorbed from the small intestine is excreted into the bile without being metabolized in the liver. About 1 to 10 per cent of the ingested sulfasalazine is excreted unchanged in the urine. Most of SP and only a negligible amount of the 5-ASA that is liberated by bacterial action are absorbed from the colon. Absorbed SP is metabolized in the liver and excreted by the kidney as SP and its metabolites. Individuals vary genetically in their rate of SP metabolism in the liver, which may affect steady-state serum concentrations. The capacity to acetylate SP is dependent on individuals' being slow or fast acetylators. The latter group acetylates the drug fast and excretes quickly. The combination of slow acetylation and slow hydroxylation causes the serum SP to rise to twice the normal level and these patients are prone to side effects as discussed later.

Drug Interactions. Sulfasalazine, but not SP or 5-ASA, inhibits absorption of folic acid by competitive inhibition of the jejunal brush border enzyme folate conjugase, which hydrolyzes folate polyglutamate to the monoglutamate form essential for intestinal absorption. Administration of folic acid is therefore helpful, especially when a large dose (more than 3 grams per day) of sulfasalazine is given. Cholestyramine and ferrous sulfate combine with sulfasalazine and prevent its absorption from the small intestine. Concurrent administration of sulfasalazine and digoxin may reduce the bioavailability of digoxin by about 25 per cent.

Clinical Use and Dosage

Several randomized controlled trials have established the effectiveness of sulfasalazine therapy in mild to moderate cases of symptomatic ulcerative colitis at a dosage of 3 to 4 grams per day. Although about one-third of placebo-treated patients show improvement, about three-fourths of patients with ulcerative colitis are expected to improve with sulfasalazine. Although studies have shown sulfasalazine to be effective in mild to moderate cases of ulcerative colitis, it appears that concomitant steroid therapy is superior for rapid improvement of an acute attack. However, the effectiveness of sulfasalazine (not of steroids) for maintenance of remission in ulcerative colitis has been shown in several studies. One showed that 86 per cent of patients with quiescent ulcerative colitis who were given 2 grams per day of sulfasalazine remained symptom-free compared with less than 20 per cent of patients on placebo. The usual initial dose is 3 to 4 grams per day. A few patients will respond better to doses up to 6 grams per day but at the cost of possible side effects, unless they are fast acetylators. The drug can be continued indefinitely at a dose of 1.5 to 2 grams per day as prophylaxis in patients with ulcerative colitis who have gone into remission.

Side Effects

The incidence of the side effects related to sulfasalazine in different series ranges from a low of 5 per cent to as high as 55 per cent. Side effects are frequent during the initial 6 to 8 weeks of treatment, but in patients on long-term therapy, the incidence is 12 per cent. Some side effects such as rash, fever, and hepatitis are due to a hypersensitivity reaction. Most of the others seem to be dose related and reflect total serum SP concentration and slow acetylator phenotype. Side effects are more frequent with a daily dose of 4 grams or more. Total SP concentrations usually in excess of 50 micrograms per ml serum may be manifested through one or another adverse reaction. Commonly observed toxic reactions include nausea, vomiting, anorexia, headache, fever, rash, arthralgia, anemia with reticulocytosis due to increased red blood cell fragility or folic acid deficiency, leukopenia, thrombocytopenia, asthmatic bronchitis, and decreased sperm motility with infertility in young men. Recently, sulfasalazine was found to induce exacerbation of ulcerative colitis after oral or rectal administration probably related to 5-ASA moiety.

Desensitization

Although numerous reports have documented the side effects of sulfasalazine, few have considered desensitization to the medication, which can be accomplished easily and effectively. This is clinically important because of the established value of sulfasalazine in preventing relapses. In one study, 26 of 28 patients with inflammatory bowel disease who suffered toxic effects from sulfasalazine were successfully desensitized. After temporarily stopping the drug for 1 to 2 weeks, side effects usually subside, allowing its readministration in gradually increasing doses, starting with 0.25 or 0.5 gram daily and then gradually increasing the dose by one-half a tablet (250 mg) every week until the final dose of 2 to 3 grams is achieved. A history of agranulocytosis or frank hemolysis and hepatitis during sulfasalazine treatment contraindicate desensitization. Other reports confirm successful desensitization of patients to sulfasalazine starting with an even smaller dose.

Mode of Action

The mechanism of beneficial effects of sulfasalazine in ulcerative colitis is still not clear. For a long time it was unknown whether the clinical efficacy of sulfasalazine resided in the unsplit sulfasalazine or in its metabolites. Recent studies in patients with distal colitis using sulfasalazine, SP, and 5-ASA demonstrate that both sulfasalazine and 5-ASA are clinically effective, but SP is not. It is thought that sulfasalazine serves as a vehicle for the delivery of active metabolites, especially 5-ASA, to the colon in higher concentrations than can be achieved by oral administration of 5-ASA alone.

5-ASA may be topically active through an antiinflammatory effect or by inhibiting prostaglandin production. The improved transportation of sodium and water in the colon by sulfasalazine is independent of mucosal prostaglandin production. Improvement may be related to an antidiarrheal effect observed in patients treated with sulfasalazine. Abnormal immunologic functions observed in patients with inflammatory bowel disease revert to normal following treatment with sulfasalazine alone. During treatment with sulfasalazine, 5-ASA, or steroids, there is decreased release of prostaglandins E_2 and F_2, thromboxane A_2, and prostacyclin metabolites from the rectal mucosa. Sulfasalazine and 5-ASA block the synthesis of several products of the lipoxygenase pathway related to inflammatory cellular response. The beneficial action of sulfasalazine and its metabolites may be related to one or more of these effects.

Pregnancy and Nursing

Sulfasalazine crosses the placenta. Mean concentrations in cord serum are approximately one-half those in maternal serum. Despite the exposure of the fetus to sulfasalazine and its metabolites there is no evidence of fetal harm. The concentration of sulfasalazine in milk may be as high as 30 per cent of that found in the maternal serum. The concentration of free SP is as much as 50 per cent of that in maternal serum, whereas 5-ASA concentration is negligible. There appears to be no harm to the fetus or evidence of kernicterus related to this exposure. The evidence suggests that sulfasalazine can be used to treat ulcerative colitis during pregnancy. There is no evidence suggesting that therapy must be stopped near the time of delivery or that use by a nursing mother will harm the infant. However, reduction of dose to 1.5 grams per day seems appropriate.

5-AMINOSALICYLIC ACID (MESALAMINE) THERAPY

Pharmacokinetic studies suggest that 5-ASA is probably the important therapeutic moiety of sulfasalazine and that SP is related to most of the side effects. 5-ASA, like aspirin, when given orally, is exclusively absorbed from the upper small intestine, and only a small amount reaches the site of inflammation in the colon. This shortcoming has been corrected by the development of a timed-release capsule containing 5-ASA, which avoids small bowel absorption and is capable of reaching the terminal ileum/colon, thus avoiding side effects related to the sulfonamide component. 5-ASA enema preparations (2 to 4 grams per enema) have been developed for patients with distal colitis and proctitis. Suppositories containing 5-ASA will also soon be available.

Enema Treatment

A study of 5-ASA enemas confirmed that 5-ASA is poorly absorbed from the colon. The retrograde spread of an enema is volume dependent. A comparison of 4-ASA (4-aminosalicylic acid [para-aminosalicylate; PAS]) (2 grams) and 5-ASA (2 grams) enemas in mild to moderately severe distal colitis showed that about 80 per cent of the patients in both groups improved clinically and sigmoidoscopically after 2 weeks. Another controlled study showed that 4-ASA enemas (1 to 2 grams) were superior to placebo. However, early reports suggest that more than one-half of the patients experience flare-up following stoppage of treatment with these salicylate enemas, and therefore the treatment may need to be continued for an indefinite period.

Rowasa (Reid-Rowell) is the first 5-ASA enema preparation approved by the U.S. Food and Drug Administration. Each enema contains 4 grams of mesalamine in 60 ml of suspension. The enema can be given as a retention enema once or twice a day for patients with proctitis and proctosigmoiditis.

Oral Treatment

To overcome the rapid absorption of 5-ASA, several slow- or delayed-release preparations have been manufactured. Other azo compounds have also been synthesized using a carrier other than SP. At present several mesalamine preparations are close to being approved. They all have different formulations.

Asacol (Tillot) is a tablet of mesalamine covered with an acrylic polymer that is soluble at pH 7 and above. 5-ASA is released in the lower ileum and in the colon. Pentasa (Marion) is a preparation of mesalamine in 1-mm granules individually coated with an ethylcellulose membrane with amphionic properties. The microgranules are available in the small intestine, and up

to 53 per cent of the dose is excreted in the urine. Thus this preparation appears well suited for treatment of small bowel disease and possibly colonic disease.

The most extensively studied new azo compound is azodisal sodium (olsalazine or Dipentum) in which two 5-ASA molecules are linked together by an azo bond. Like sulfasalazine, only a small amount of intact olsalazine is absorbed from the small intestine, and of this a considerable amount enters the enterohepatic circulation without being split. The half-life is considerably longer than that for sulfasalazine. Sulfasalazine and olsalazine are distributed somewhat differently in the body. The concentrations of 5-ASA in the feces are doubled when sulfasalazine is replaced by the equivalent dosage of olsalazine.

Clinical Use, Tolerance, and Toxicity

Mesalazine (Asacol) and olsalazine have been given to large numbers of patients; Pentasa is being clinically evaluated in the United States. About 75 per cent of patients with mild to moderately severe ulcerative colitis improved, with partial to complete remission, when treated over a 6-week period with either Asacol (4.8 grams per day) or olsalazine (up to 4 grams per day). However, when Asacol and olsalazine were given to sulfasalazine-intolerant patients, it was necessary to stop treatment because of side effects in 24 and 14 per cent of patients, respectively.

The most common side effect of olsalazine is watery diarrhea, which appears to be dose dependent and occurs in one-third of patients taking a 4-gram dose. Common side effects of asacol are muscle aches, headache, and dizziness in about one-third of the patients. Bloody diarrhea with fever, nausea, and abdominal cramps has been described with both 5-ASA preparations.

CORTICOSTEROID THERAPY

Clinical Use

Corticosteroids given orally, parenterally, or by enema are beneficial in the treatment of either limited or extensive ulcerative colitis that is unresponsive to sulfasalazine alone or of disease that initially is more severe. Local rectal instillations are useful for distal ulcerative colitis. When there is more extensive involvement, systemic administration is necessary.

For distal ulcerative colitis, hydrocortisone enemas (Cortenema) may be given once or twice daily until significant clinical improvement is achieved, which may require 3 to 6 weeks or longer. Treatment is then tapered to one enema at bedtime, then to one every other night, and then discontinued. The foam (Cortifoam) is easier to tolerate but is effective only for localized proctitis. The enemas contain 100 mg of hydrocortisone; the foam, 90 mg. Advances are being made in the development of topical corticosteroid therapy, which results in minimal systemic corticoid side effects. Tixocortol pivalate and beclomethasone dipropionate enemas have been extensively studied but are not yet approved for distal ulcerative colitis therapy.

Oral therapy is usually initiated with 30 to 60 mg of prednisone daily. This dose is continued for approximately 10 to 14 days and then decreased by 5 mg every 7 to 10 days. The dose can be given as a single morning dose or in two divided doses; reducing the evening dose helps minimize side effects. If there is a relapse, the prednisone dose will need to be increased again. Once disease control is achieved, the tapering process is resumed. Corticosteroids do not have a prophylactic role in ulcerative colitis and should be discontinued in patients with quiescent disease.

In patients with severe symptoms, parenteral hydrocortisone therapy can be beneficial. Hydrocortisone (300 mg daily) is preferred for patients who have received corticosteroids prior to hospitalization. It can be given as a continuous intravenous infusion or every 6 to 8 hours for 5 to 7 days. Once maximal benefit is achieved, oral prednisone is substituted.

Pharmacology and Adverse Effects

Oral corticosteroid absorption in severe colitis may be delayed, but total absorption is normal. Intravenous therapy results in higher and more prolonged plasma levels than the oral route. The mechanism by which corticosteroids exert their clinical usefulness is also unknown. The toxicity of corticosteroid therapy at the doses used to suppress active ulcerative colitis is appreciable. Adverse effects include facial mooning, acne, ecchymoses, petechial bleeding, striae, hirsutism, infection, hypertension, peptic ulcer, bone abnormalities, emotional disturbances, and many others. These complications generally resolve with the withdrawal or reduction of the dose and with specific therapy for the complications.

Pregnancy. Corticosteroids are well known to cause fetal abnormalities in animals. Studies in humans, however, have failed to demonstrate significant harmful effects. Fetal complications are more common when the mother's disease is active and untreated than when she is treated with corticosteroids during pregnancy.

ANTIBIOTIC THERAPY

Antibiotics do not have a role as primary therapy for ulcerative colitis. On the contrary, they may affect intestinal bacteria, disturbing the metabolism of sulfasalazine, and may cause *Clostridium difficile*–associated colitis. The toxin of this organism may induce or aggravate the underlying ulcerative colitis.

IMMUNOSUPPRESSIVE THERAPY

Azathioprine (Imuran)* or 6-mercaptopurine (Purinethol)* may be helpful in a rare case, but they have little role in the usual patients with ulcerative colitis. Their toxic side effects, which include infection, pancreatitis, and the potential development of malignancy, generally outweigh their benefits. Cyclosporin A has not been especially successful in the few patients in whom it has been used.

APPROACH TO THE PATIENT

The first step in choosing therapy is to make a global assessment of the disease activity and to exclude any specific pathogen(s) by appropriate stool cultures. There is no uniform measurement of disease activity available. A simple activity index one can follow is to ascertain the disease to be *in remission* when the patient has 2 or 3 bowel movements per day without any mucus and blood; *mild* when there are 4 to 6 stools daily, including minimal rectal bleeding and mucus; *moderate* when there are 7 to 9 stools daily with rectal bleeding, mucus, anorexia, or nausea and some weakness; *severe* when there are 10 or more stools daily with mucus and blood and one or more of the following signs of colitis are present: abdominal tenderness, pulse rate greater than 100 beats per minute, and a body temperature above 37.5° C. The disease is *fulminant* when the patient has 10 or more bowel movements daily with significant bleeding plus a body temperature higher than 38° C, anemia, hypoalbuminemia, or colonic dilatation on plain abdominal x-ray films (greater than 6 cm in diameter).

The appearance of the rectal mucosa at proctoscopy adds important objective information for the assessment of disease activity. Mild to moderate colitis activity is indicated by a red mucosa that is finely granular and easily friable and has a vascular pattern obliterated by edema. Spontaneous bleeding, prominent ulcerations, or mucosal sloughing indicates more severe activity. The proctoscopic appearance may be more severe

---

*This use is not listed in the manufacturer's directives.

than the clinical colitis activity and may help predict a flare-up of disease in the near future indicating the need for prompt therapy. In addition, improvement of the rectal mucosa may lag behind clinical recovery during therapy. This should mandate slower reduction of drug doses to prevent disease recurrence. Occasionally, in a patient with chronic ulcerative colitis, especially after receiving topical steroids, the rectal mucosa may appear relatively spared and may not accurately reflect the total colitis activity.

Mild to Moderate Disease Activity

Ambulatory patients with mild to moderate ulcerative colitis activity should be given sulfasalazine initially at a dose of 1.5 grams per day, slowly increasing to 3 to 4 grams per day, if tolerated. Since most patients will achieve a good response within 2 to 3 weeks, this time period seems reasonable before drawing conclusions regarding effectiveness. Patients who cannot tolerate sulfasalazine may benefit from one of the newer preparations without SP such as Asacol,* olsalazine, or Pentasa.*

Those who fail therapy with sulfasalazine or who are very uncomfortable will generally require the addition of steroids. Topical therapy may be used for distal colitis; hydrocortisone enemas for disease distal to the splenic flexure; or foam when disease is confined to the rectum (proctitis). Topical therapy is given once or twice daily for 2 to 4 weeks, at which time a clinical response should be observed. Therapy is then continued once before bedtime until remission is achieved, usually over the subsequent 3 to 6 weeks, and then may be reduced to alternate nights for several weeks. Assuming the patient remains well, topical agents can then be discontinued, with sulfasalazine continued as a maintenance dose of 1 to 2 grams per day. Patients with proctosigmoiditis refractory to topical steroid therapy may benefit from topical salicylate enemas as described previously. If the response to topical therapy is inadequate or there is more extensive colonic disease, prednisone, 30 to 60 mg per day orally, will be required. This dose is continued for 7 to 14 days and then tapered over approximately 2 months as the symptoms improve. The continuation of high doses of prednisone for prolonged periods is not recommended. Intramuscular adrenocorticotropic hormone (ACTH) gel occasionally can be used (40 to 80 units daily) to supplement sulfasalazine in patients with milder disease activity when a long course of oral prednisone is unnecessary.

---

*Investigational drugs, not yet approved.

A variety of preparations, including antidiarrheals, anticholinergics, tranquilizers, and analgesics, may be of symptomatic benefit. However, these agents should be avoided as much as possible because of side effects and possible toxic dilatation of the colon with high doses.

A trial of avoidance of lactose and raw vegetables may also be worthwhile during a flare-up. Proper nutritional balance, supplemental vitamins and iron, and adequate rest are important, but strict bed rest is not necessary.

Severe to Fulminant Disease Activity

The patient with severe activity will generally require corticosteroids and often hospitalization. Oral feedings should be encouraged if they are tolerated, but very ill patients will require bowel rest or even nasogastric suction. Intravenous fluids and electrolytes will be required to ensure adequate hydration. If a full diet will not be reinstituted within 10 to 14 days, total parenteral nutrition should be considered. If there is any suspicion of a suppurative complication, antibiotics are given after all appropriate cultures are collected. Sulfasalazine alone is generally not helpful. Its onset of action is slow, and it may be poorly tolerated owing to the side effects of gastric intolerance. If tolerated, I prefer oral suspension (rather than tablets) of sulfasalazine (about 3 grams per day). Oral prednisone can be used as previously described. If this has failed to induce improvement by 10 to 14 days or if oral intake is not tolerated, parenteral therapy will be necessary. ACTH (120 units daily) or hydrocortisone (300 mg daily) is given as a continuous intravenous infusion or 100 mg three times daily. Intravenous ACTH is preferred for the patient not already on steroid therapy. After 7 to 10 days of intravenous infusions, therapy is continued with 30 to 60 mg of oral prednisone. Once prednisone is tapered, sulfasalazine is added to the medical regimen if it has not already been started. Hydrocortisone enemas may also be useful, especially when the patient is on a lower prednisone dose (10 to 20 mg daily). This may allow continued reduction of the prednisone and reduced overall corticosteroid side effects. Patients who do not improve with vigorous medical therapy should be considered for surgery. This is especially true for patients with complications such as profuse bleeding or toxic megacolon and is mandatory when there is a free colonic perforation.

In the ill hospitalized patient, twice daily physical examinations and frequent abdominal radiographic observations are necessary. Toxic megacolon or perforation may develop quickly and without obvious clinical signs in these very ill patients on high doses of steroids. Toxic megacolon may be induced by diagnostic procedures such as a barium enema or colonoscopy or by hypokalemia, hypomagnesemia, or anticholinergic, antidiarrheal, or analgesic therapy. Avoiding these procedures, correcting the deficiencies, and eliminating the offending drugs are essential. Failure to improve after 48 to 72 hours of intensive therapy or deterioration is an indication for early surgery; prolonging the medical therapy significantly increases the overall mortality and morbidity.

Remission

Once disease activity has subsided, withdrawal of steroids must be attempted; sulfasalazine is continued indefinitely. Unfortunately, some patients are not able to be withdrawn from steroids without a flare-up of their disease. A continued requirement of more than 15 mg daily of prednisone for more than 1 year is a relative indication for surgery.

CANCER SURVEILLANCE

The risk of colon cancer in ulcerative colitis begins to increase after 8 years among those with extensive disease. The cumulative risk of cancer by 20 years is about 12 per cent or 32 times the risk of cancer in a normal population. The risk is also higher among those with disease confined to the left colon, but its onset appears delayed about 10 years.

Patients with continuous symptoms are at risk for cancer and have a poor quality of life, and their general health is at risk. They should be encouraged to undergo total colectomy. The cancer issue is but one more indication for surgery.

Patients who are relatively well but at risk for cancer should be in a continued surveillance program. These patients require annual colonoscopy, including multiple colonic biopsies. Surgery may be indicated if definite high-grade dysplasia is noted, especially if associated with a mass lesion. These patients are at very high risk or may already have cancer. Lower grades of dysplasia require close observation, with repeat colonoscopy and biopsy at 6-month intervals.

CROHN'S DISEASE

method of
WILLIAM J. TREMAINE, M.D.
Mayo Clinic
Rochester, Minnesota

Crohn's disease is a chronic inflammatory disorder of unknown cause that can involve any portion of the digestive tract from the mouth to the anus. Most commonly, the disease affects the colon, the terminal ileum, or both areas. Histologically, lesions develop as areas of focal inflammation adjacent to epithelial crypts that progress to transmural inflammation, fissures, and ulcers. In addition to the direct involvement of the digestive tract, there may be coexistent inflammation in the joints, skin, eyes, and liver. The clinical course of the disease is unpredictable, with exacerbations and remissions of varying duration. This unpredictability makes it difficult to determine the efficacy of different therapies.

MANAGEMENT

Nutrition

Diet. Food intolerances occur four times as often in patients with Crohn's disease as in healthy individuals, particularly for vegetables, cereals, and dairy products. Patients should be encouraged to eat a balanced diet and to avoid only those foods that clearly cause symptoms. Careful attention should be paid to maintaining nutrition, particularly in children, as growth failure in Crohn's disease is caused mainly by malnutrition. Lactose intolerance is particularly common and should be looked for, either by a trial of a lactose-free diet and assessment for improvement in symptoms or by a lactose breath hydrogen test. There is no need to avoid milk products unless there is evidence of intolerance. For patients who have steatorrhea, caused either by previous resections of portions of the terminal ileum or by extensive disease, dietary fat should be restricted to 40 to 60 grams per day. In the presence of steatorrhea, hyperoxaluria may occur because of decreased intraluminal binding of oxalate to calcium and increased absorption. Patients who have hyperoxaluria should avoid foods that are high in oxalate such as rhubarb, grapefruit, tea, and cola beverages. High-fiber foods should be avoided if there are strictures of the bowel with partial obstruction.

Vitamin and Mineral Supplements. A water-soluble multiple vitamin should be taken daily by patients with restricted diets. Vitamin B_{12}, 100 micrograms intramuscularly, should be given monthly to patients who have had 60 cm or more of the terminal ileum resected or who have active disease involving this amount or more of the ileum; the patient can be instructed in self-administration. Calcium carbonate or calcium gluconate, in a dose of 1.5 grams per day or more, and vitamin D, in a dose of 50,000 units per week or more, should be given to prevent osteoporosis and osteomalacia in patients with steatorrhea who have laboratory evidence of calcium or vitamin D malabsorption. After treatment for 1 month, the doses of calcium and vitamin D should be adjusted, as determined by urinary calcium and serum vitamin D levels. Serum magnesium levels should be monitored in patients with short bowels and replaced with oral magnesium sulfate, if tolerated, or given by intramuscular injection. Folic acid should be given orally as a tablet, 1 mg per day, to patients who have low serum folate levels. Patients who have extensive small intestinal disease or who have undergone major small intestinal resections are at risk for vitamin E deficiency, which can cause progressive neuromuscular disease; serum vitamin E levels should be monitored in these patients, and low levels should be treated with oral supplements of 200 mg two times a day or more. Deficiencies of vitamins A and K are rare except in patients with short-bowel syndrome. The serum level of vitamin A and the prothrombin time should be monitored or prophylactic treatment should be given in these patients.

Supportive Therapy

Education and Emotional Support. Patients and their families may not have heard of Crohn's disease until the diagnosis has been made. A knowledgeable physician can explain the disease to them, and excellent literature for the patient can be obtained from the National Foundation for Ileitis and Colitis (NFIC), 444 Park Ave. South, New York, N.Y. 10016–7374. Patients benefit from the ongoing care of a physician during times of active disease and during remission. There are also local chapters of the NFIC where patients can share experiences with other patients and gain support. Psychiatric illness is a result, not a cause, of Crohn's disease, and these patients more commonly have psychiatric problems, particularly depression, than other medically ill patients. Antianxiety and antidepressant medications may be indicated in some patients, but in most the best solution is to bring the underlying disease under control.

Diarrhea. The most common symptom of Crohn's disease, diarrhea, usually improves with treatment of the inflammatory disease (see later). Mild symptoms may be controlled with a bulk agent such as psyllium (Metamucil, Hydrocil, Perdiem Fiber), one or two teaspoons one to two times a day, or methylcellulose (Citrucel), one tablespoon one to three times a day. Diphenoxylate with atropine sulfate (Lomotil), 2.5 to 5 mg one to four times daily, or loperamide (Imodium), one to eight tablets per day, can be used for the temporary relief of mild symptoms. For more troublesome diarrhea, deodorized tincture of opium, 6 to 10 drops two to six times a day, can be used. These antidiarrheal agents should not be used in patients who have severe diarrhea caused by

colonic disease because of the risk of precipitating toxic megacolon.

Patients who have undergone one or more resections of the terminal ileum (usually less than 100 cm total) can have bile acid (cholerrheic) diarrhea caused by the inadequate resorption of bile from the terminal ileum with direct stimulation of fluid secretion from the colonic mucosa by the bile acids. These patients usually have postprandial watery diarrhea, which can be controlled with cholestyramine (Questran), 2 to 4 grams two to four times a day, or colestipol (Colestid), 5 grams one to four times a day. These anion exchange resins also bind fat-soluble vitamins and a number of other medications, so that the lowest effective dose should be used. Cholestyramine and colestipol should not be used in patients who have steatorrhea; instead, a low-fat diet is the treatment.

Treatment of Active Disease

Anti-Inflammatory Therapy. A number of different medications are used, alone or in combination, for the treatment of inflammation.

SULFASALAZINE. Sulfasalazine (Azulfidine) is the first line treatment for mild or moderately active Crohn's disease when there is involvement of the colon, with or without ileal involvement. Sulfasalazine requires bacterial action for breakdown to its components, sulfapyridine and 5-aminosalicylic acid. It is not effective for the treatment of small bowel disease alone, probably because of the lack of breakdown of the drug there. Sulfasalazine should be started in a dose of 1 gram per day (500 mg two times a day) and gradually increased over 1 week to a final dose of 3 to 4 grams per day in divided doses, although some patients may be able to tolerate 5 or 6 grams per day. The complete blood count should be checked after 1 week to look for drug-induced hematologic problems (hemolysis, leukopenia, thrombocytopenia, or pancytopenia). Folic acid can be given prophylactically in a dose of 1 mg per day as a tablet, or the serum folate level can be monitored periodically to look for drug-induced folate deficiency. Up to 45 per cent of patients develop dose-related adverse reactions such as nausea, vomiting, or headaches with high-dose therapy; these reactions usually resolve with a reduction of the dose. After 6 weeks of treatment, about 45 per cent of patients show improvement.

5-AMINOSALICYLIC ACID. Mesalamine (5-aminosalicylic acid) accounts for the majority of the anti-inflammatory action of sulfasalazine, and it has few side effects when administered as an enema or orally. Mesalamine enemas (Rowasa) are available in a 4-gram dose for the treatment of distal ulcerative colitis. They may also be useful for the treatment of distal Crohn's colitis, although they have not been approved for this indication. Several forms of oral mesalamine are used in Europe and in Canada for the treatment of inflammatory bowel disease, but so far, none of these oral preparations have been approved for use in the United States.

CORTICOSTEROIDS. Corticosteroids are the first line treatment for Crohn's disease in patients with severe symptoms or with only ileal involvement, and they are adjunctive treatment for patients with mild or moderate symptoms. Adrenocorticotropic hormone is probably no more effective than oral or intravenous steroids. Alternate-day therapy with steroids does not usually give satisfactory results when the disease is symptomatic, but it is sometimes effective when the symptoms subside and the dose is being tapered. Patients who have severe symptoms with abdominal pain, diarrhea, and fever should be given no medication orally and should be treated with prednisolone, 30 to 60 mg intravenously, or with hydrocortisone (Solu-Cortef), 200 to 400 mg per day in divided doses, until symptoms improve. Prednisone, 30 to 60 mg per day in divided doses, can be used when the patient with severe symptoms has improved and is no longer barred from taking oral medication, and doses of 20 to 40 mg per day can be started in patients with less severe symptoms. The response to prednisone should be seen in 3 to 7 weeks. With improvement, the dose should be tapered gradually over the subsequent 2 to 3 months to the lowest dose that controls the symptoms, and the prednisone should be discontinued, if possible. Prednisone usually can be given as a single morning dose in patients who are taking 30 mg or less to minimize insomnia. Hydrocortisone enemas as a solution (Cortenema) or as a foam (Cortifoam) can be used in patients with distal colonic disease, with one enema taken at bedtime if the patient has good anal continence.

METRONIDAZOLE. For patients with mild to moderately active colitis or ileocolitis who are intolerant of sulfasalazine or in whom sulfasalazine has not been effective, metronidazole (Flagyl), 20 mg per kg (250 to 500 mg three or four times a day) as an initial dose, may be helpful. As symptoms improve, the dose can be tapered gradually, often to 10 mg per kg per day. This drug has been particularly useful when perianal involvement is present. Metronidazole may be used in combination with prednisone to achieve a steroid-sparing effect, although there are no studies to support this strategy. The most worrisome side effect of metronidazole is peripheral neuropathy, manifested by burning paresthesias in the toes and feet and sometimes in the hands. These paresthesias usually resolve with discontinuation of treatment, although full resolution may take months.

OTHER ANTIBIOTICS. A number of other antibiotics have been used in Crohn's disease, such as tetracycline, 250 to 500 mg orally every 6 hours, amoxicillin, 250 to 500 mg every 6 hours, trimethoprim-sulfamethoxazole (Bactrim, Septra), double strength 160 mg/800 mg twice a day, or ciprofloxacin (Cipro), 750 mg every 12 hours for 10 to 14 days. These are likely to be effective in relieving symptoms caused by microabscess formation as a complication of Crohn's disease, rather than in treating the actual disease process. However, controlled studies to confirm the efficacy of these treatments have not been done.

6-MERCAPTOPURINE AND AZATHIOPRINE. These drugs are usually reserved for patients with chronic severe disease that cannot be controlled with other forms of treatment, or for patients whose high doses of steroids cannot be tapered because of a resulting flare in symptoms. 6-Mercaptopurine (Purinethol) and its derivative, azathioprine (Imuran), have similar biologic effects, and either one may be used in a dose of 50 to 100 mg per day in adults or 25 mg per day in children. Neither should be used as a single initial agent in Crohn's disease, as they may take up to 4 months to produce a response. The major drawbacks of these drugs are the serious side effects (bone marrow suppression, fever, and pancreatitis) that occur in 10 per cent of patients and the small risk of inducing malignancy, either carcinoma or lymphoma. The hemoglobin, white blood cell count, and platelet count should be monitored weekly during the first month and then monthly or bimonthly while the patient is taking one of these drugs.

Nutritional Therapy

ENTERAL NUTRITION. Two randomized studies have shown elemental feedings (Vivonex) to be as effective as prednisone in inducing a remission in Crohn's disease, although the remissions may not last as long. A trial of elemental feeding for 3 to 4 weeks as the sole source of calories, along with prednisone, can be considered in patients who have not responded to sulfasalazine, prednisone, or metronidazole. The volume should be calculated for the patient's ideal body weight and with 1 kcal per ml (e.g., Vivonex HN), usually 1500 to 2500 ml per day of the preparations is needed. The expense (from $700 to $950 for 3 weeks) and taste fatigue are major drawbacks.

CENTRAL PARENTERAL NUTRITION. Two randomized studies showed no added benefit of bowel rest in the induction of remission in Crohn's disease. Central hyperalimentation is particularly helpful in the stabilization of the malnourished patient with obstructive symptoms before surgical resection; 3 weeks of therapy is usually needed to achieve improvement in protein stores.

Medical Treatment During Remission

No medication has been shown to be effective in maintaining a remission in patients with Crohn's disease. Likewise, no medication has been shown to reduce the rate of recurrence in patients who have undergone surgical resection of all evidence of disease.

Surgery

More than 60 per cent of patients with Crohn's disease require one resection, and more than one-half need a second operation. The physician must be careful not to err either in sending the patient for surgery before a reasonable trial of the medical options or in delaying surgery when the disease is refractory to treatment. The indications for surgery are (1) chronic obstruction caused by stricture, (2) uncontrollable diarrhea caused by enteroenteric fistulas, (3) free perforation and intra-abdominal abscess, (4) massive bleeding, (5) toxic megacolon, and (6) intractable symptoms caused by a limited area of involvement. Stricturoplasty, in which a stricture is opened horizontally and closed vertically, without resecting bowel, has recently been shown to be effective in patients with obstructive symptoms caused by multiple skip areas.

Treatment During Pregnancy

There are theoretical concerns about the use of corticosteroids or sulfasalazine during pregnancy. Fortunately, neither drug has caused significant problems when used in pregnant women with Crohn's disease. Either drug may be used to control active disease. As neither drug prevents relapses of inactive disease, prednisone and sulfasalazine should be discontinued in the asymptomatic patient. Both may be used in the nursing mother, if indicated. Sulfasalazine temporarily lowers the sperm count in men and may cause infertility. Azathioprine, 6-mercaptopurine, and metronidazole should be avoided during pregnancy. Nutritional treatment in pregnant patients with Crohn's disease should be prompt and aggressive and may be administered as enteral or parenteral hyperalimentation.

Extraintestinal Manifestations

Joint, skin, mouth, and eye symptoms are much more common with colonic involvement than when the disease is confined to the small intestine.

Arthritis. Peripheral arthritis is the most common extraintestinal problem and occurs in about one-fourth of patients. The joint symptoms usually parallel the activity of the bowel disease, and the most effective therapy is to control the bowel inflammation. In addition to reducing intestinal inflammation, sulfasalazine probably acts directly to reduce joint inflammation. A nonsteroidal anti-inflammatory drug such as naproxen (Naprosyn), 250 mg three or four times a day, is also helpful.

Spondylitis. Ankylosing spondylitis and sacroileitis occur in human leukocyte antigen (HLA)-B27–positive patients and do not follow the course of the bowel disease. Therapy is directed at the joint disease and includes the use of sulfasalazine, nonsteroidal anti-inflammatory drugs, and physical therapy.

Skin and Oral Manifestations. Erythema nodosum occurs in about 10 per cent of patients who have colonic involvement and in 4 per cent of patients with only small bowel disease. It occurs synchronously with the activity of the bowel disease and resolves with treatment of the bowel inflammation. Pyoderma gangrenosum occurs in less than 2 per cent of patients. It is treated with high-dose systemic steroids and usually improves as the bowel symptoms resolve, although in some cases it persists despite remission or resection of the involved bowel. Apthous stomatitis occurs in about 10 per cent of patients, usually along with other extraintestinal symptoms, and resolves with control of the bowel disease.

Eye Manifestations. Eye symptoms caused by conjunctivitis, recurrent episcleritis, or uveitis occur in more than 10 per cent of patients with colonic disease and are rare with ileal involvement alone. Topical steroid drops can be used under the direction of an ophthalmologist. The symptoms are usually synchronous with the bowel disease activity.

Hepatobiliary Abnormalities. Cholesterol gallstones are common in patients who have extensive terminal ileal disease or who have undergone terminal ileal resections because of the diminished bile acid pool. Cholecystectomy is the treatment of choice for symptomatic gallstones. Primary sclerosing cholangitis occurs rarely in association with Crohn's disease, and treatment of Crohn's disease has no effect on the liver disease. So far, no medical therapy has proved to be effective.

Urinary Tract Abnormalities. Nephrolithiasis occurs in 5 to 10 per cent of patients because of dehydration caused by chronic diarrhea, as well as increased colonic oxalate absorption. Prophylactic therapy for the calcium oxalate stones was discussed earlier. Right ureteral obstruction with hydronephrosis occurs because of contiguous inflammation in the overlying terminal ileum and colon and may require temporary stenting of the ureter.

IRRITABLE BOWEL SYNDROME

method of
SIMON K. LO, M.D., and
WILLIAM J. SNAPE, JR., M.D.
*Harbor-UCLA Medical Center, Torrance,
    California*
*UCLA School of Medicine, Los Angeles,
    California*

The irritable bowel syndrome (IBS) is a gastrointestinal tract motility disorder that is usually, but not always, accompanied by abdominal pain. Although its pseudonyms are spastic colon or mucous colitis, IBS involves not only the colon but also the small intestine. In addition, patients frequently experience symptoms suggestive of biliary, gastric, esophageal, and even urinary bladder origin. Mucosal inflammation is not present in IBS.

The classic clinical features of IBS are chronic abdominal pain associated with diarrhea, constipation, or alternating bowel habits. Other associated symptoms may include dyspepsia, abdominal bloating, early satiety, nausea, vomiting, fatigue, and headache. Emotional stress may exaggerate the symptoms, although its causal role in IBS is uncertain. This common problem is responsible for 40 to 70 per cent of referrals to gastrointestinal specialists. Approximately 20 per cent of seemingly healthy individuals experience typical IBS symptoms.

DIFFERENTIAL DIAGNOSIS

The differential diagnosis for conditions simulating IBS with diarrhea include parasitic disorders (giardiasis), infection (bacterial, tuberculous), diet-related disorders (celiac sprue, lactose or sorbitol intolerance), idiopathic inflammatory diseases (ulcerative colitis, Crohn's disease, collagenous colitis), and chronic laxative abuse. Problems that simulate IBS with constipation include idiopathic (intestinal pseudo-obstruction), neurologic (adult Hirschsprung's, diabetes mellitus), hormonal (hypothyroid), muscular (scleroderma), and anatomic (rectal outlet obstruction) abnormalities of the gastrointestinal tract.

ETIOLOGY

IBS is a heterogenous group of motility and afferent sensory disorders of the gastrointestinal tract whose pathogenesis is still undefined. Conceptually, the etiology for the motility disturbance may be independent of the cause of the abdominal pain.

Underlying factors that are believed to cause this motility disturbance include alterations that are humoral (increased response to stimulation by cholecystokinin or decreased response to inhibition by vasoactive intestinal peptide), myogenic (increased slow-wave pattern of three cycles per min), and neural (decreased afferent neural input, altered cerebral response to stress). Mucosal irritation from an increased intraluminal concentration of bile acid may also alter motility. Any of these factors may lead to focal or generalized hypermotility, increased segmenting nonpropulsive contraction, or enhanced propulsion. Factors contributing to increased pain include altered afferent input from the gut, altered cerebral interpretation of normal stimuli, and exaggerated spasm or distention of a segment of the gut. Despite a lower threshold for abdominal pain, patients with IBS have an increased somatic pain threshold. Although patients frequently feel bloated, increased intestinal gas content is unusual.

DIAGNOSIS

The diagnosis of IBS is made principally by exclusion. Every effort should be made to balance between under- and over-testing for more serious diseases. The most important clues to the diagnosis of IBS are chronicity and the lack of systemic problems such as weight loss and gastrointestinal bleeding. Initial laboratory tests should include complete blood cell count, stool guaiac test, electrolyte assays, glucose levels, and liver and thyroid profiles. Stool examination for ova, parasites, bacteria, and *Clostridium difficile* toxin, and mucosal biopsy may be required in cases with diarrhea. Abdominal radiograph or computed tomography scan, barium enema, colonoscopy, upper gastrointestinal tract and small bowel x-ray films, anorectal manometry, or radiopaque markers transit study may be done depending on the clinical presentation.

TREATMENT

Therapeutic outcome is influenced greatly by the rapport between physician and patient. It is crucial that the physician is understanding and provides support. Education of the patient should emphasize the benign, non–life-threatening, but chronic, nature of the IBS. Dietary manipulation is an integral aspect of therapy. A trial of a lactose-free diet, avoidance of gas-producing foods like onions and wheat, and reduction of intake of fatty foods, sorbitol, and coffee should be attempted. Any food that clearly aggravates the patient's symptoms should be eliminated. A high-fiber diet may alleviate constipation, but the patient should be warned of possible increased flatulence during the first 6 to 8 weeks of therapy. Moderate exercise, use of a heating pad applied to the abdomen, and wearing comfortable, nonrestraining clothing may also be tried.

TABLE 1. **Drug Therapy for Motility Disturbance of the Gastrointestinal Tract**

Motility Problem	Drug Group	Example of Agent	Dose (PO)
Constipation with increased contractility	Bulk fiber	Psyllium	1 Tbsp tid
	Antispasmodic	Dicyclomine	20–40 mg tid
	Calcium channel blocker*	Nifedipine	20 mg tid
	Nitrate*	Isosorbide	20 mg tid
Diarrhea	Bulk fiber	Psyllium	1 Tbsp tid
	Opioids	Loperamide	2 mg tid
	Bile acid binder	Cholestyramine	1 pack qid
	Calcium channel blocker*	Nifedipine	20 mg tid
	Alpha$_2$ agonist*	Clonidine	0.1 mg bid
	Gut hormone*	Somatostatin	†
Constipation with decreased contractility	Bulk fiber	Psyllium	1 Tbsp tid
	Cholinergic	Bethanechol	25 mg tid
	Stimulant	Bisacodyl	5–15 mg/day
	Dopamine antagonist*	Metoclopramide	10–20 mg tid
	Acetylcholine releaser*	Cisapride	10–20 mg tid

*Agents that have been used infrequently or inadequately examined but that have theoretical benefits. Some are not available in the United States or are not approved by the U.S. Food and Drug Administration for their use in IBS.

†Subcutaneous doses of 50 µg bid to 150 µg tid have been used for other diarrheal disorders.

Psychotherapy results in mixed, but mostly positive, results. A good doctor-patient relationship is probably the key ingredient to its success.

Pharmacologic therapy is directed at three aspects of the disease: motility disturbance, anxiety, and pain. There have been a dearth of controlled trials that show convincing evidence of effective therapy of the IBS symptom complex, which probably reflects the heterogeneity of the disease.

Drugs that alter motility of the gastrointestinal tract should be categorized according to the three major patterns of motility disturbance: (1) increased contractility but poor propagation, that is, constipation; (2) increased contractility with increased propagation, that is, diarrhea; and (3) decreased motility, that is, constipation (Table 1). Drugs used for diarrhea may decrease symptoms through an effect on mucosal absorption or motility. Although single-agent therapy should be tried initially, the lack of a dramatic response frequently leads to multiple-drug regimens. Once a therapeutic regimen leads to suppression of symptoms, long-term use of the regimen is expected. Recurrence of symptoms is common after withdrawal of an effective drug therapy.

Sedatives and tranquilizers have been studied alone or in combination with antispasmodics for treatment of abdominal pain and constipation with some positive effects. Addition of fiber may have further increased benefit. Occasional and short-term symptomatic use of tranquilizers may be reasonable, but long-term use for IBS treatment should be discouraged. If the patient demonstrates depression or another neuropsychiatric disorder, appropriate antidepressants or other anxiolytic drugs may be tried.

Pain control in severe IBS cases is difficult.

Pain may not be relieved even if the associated motility problem is corrected. Although narcotics frequently suppress painful symptoms, they may affect overall management negatively because of their constipating, emetic, and habit-forming effects. Nonsteroidal analgesics may cause gastritis or ulcer and further complicate management. Therefore, except for the most unusual cases, even occasional use of analgesics other than acetaminophen should be discouraged.

HEMORRHOIDS, ANAL FISSURE, AND ANAL FISTULA AND ABSCESS

method of
SAMUEL B. LABOW, M.D.
North Shore University Hospital
Cornell University Medical College
Great Neck, New York

HEMORRHOIDS

Hemorrhoids are vascular cushions composed of a complex of veins and arterioles supported by smooth muscle and elastic tissue. These vascular cushions are present in all persons and are normally situated in three distinct locations in the anal canal: the right anterior quadrant, the right posterior quadrant, and the left lateral quadrant. There are two types of hemorrhoids: those above the dentate line covered by mucosa (internal hemorrhoids) and those at the outer edge of the anal canal covered with modified squamous epithelium (external hemorrhoids). These two types of hemorrhoids are separated by the dentate line in the middle of the anal canal. The different location and covering of internal and external hemorrhoids (mucosa versus squamous epithelium) account for their different potential symptoms. Internal hemorrhoids frequently present with bright red rectal bleeding during bowel movements, with blood on the tissue and possibly in the bowel. Internal hemorrhoids may also prolapse with bowel movements, sometimes reducing spontaneously and in other cases requiring manual reduction. In some patients the internal hemorrhoids may be chronically prolapsed. In this situation, patients frequently have bleeding and a discharge of mucus between bowel movements. External hemorrhoids are often a source of pain because of edema or thrombosis of the external hemorrhoidal vessels. Thrombosed external hemorrhoids may erode through the anoderm and cause bleeding.

Treatment

Asymptomatic hemorrhoids, regardless of their size, do not require therapy. Symptomatic internal hemorrhoids may be treated by medical management, injection therapy, local destruction or hemorrhoidectomy. Symptomatic external hemorrhoids may be managed by medical therapy, minor office surgery for thrombosed external hemorrhoids, or hemorrhoidectomy.

Medical Management

Medical management requires the use of a high-fiber diet with supplemental bran or psyllium seed preparations to avoid constipation. The use of warm sitz baths and nonsteroidal antiinflammatory drugs may help alleviate the acute symptoms of edematous external hemorrhoids. Suppositories and steroid ointments have no proven effect in the management of these symptoms.

Injections of Sclerosing Solutions

The use of a sclerosing solution such as 5 per cent phenol in cottonseed oil or quinine urea hydrochloride can provide symptomatic relief for bleeding and minimally prolapsing internal hemorrhoids. From 0.5 to 2 ml of the sclerosing solution is injected into the submucosal plane above the dentate line. The advantages of this procedure are its ability to treat all symptomatic internal hemorrhoids at one time, the relative lack of discomfort, the almost immediate cessation of bleeding, and the ability to be used in patients with hemorrhagic diatheses. Its major disadvantage is its temporary nature, with results usually lasting for periods ranging from 6 months to 3 or 4 years. Repeat injections can be given as needed within 2 to 3 weeks if symptoms persist or recur.

Local Destruction

Because of the absence of pain receptors in the overlying mucosa, internal hemorrhoids can be destroyed as an office procedure without the use of anesthesia. The advantage of these procedures over injection therapy is the possibly permanent elimination of internal hemorrhoids. These procedures include rubber band ligation therapy, cryotherapy, infrared photocoagulation, and laser therapy. Of these procedures, rubber band ligation therapy is the oldest and still the most widely used. Although each of the other therapies has its proponents, to date there is no documented evidence of increased efficiency with any of them.

Rubber Band Ligation. This can be performed rapidly and easily as an office procedure, with no preparation and minimal discomfort to the patient. Hirschman's or other type of anoscope is inserted into the anal canal, and a single internal hemorrhoid is identified. A grasping forceps is passed through the barrel of the ligator, the internal hemorrhoid is grasped approximately 1 cm above the dentate line and drawn into the barrel of the ligator, and the rubber band is released. The tourniquet effect of the rubber band is usually complete within 3 to 5 days, at which time the internal hemorrhoid and rubber band are passed with a bowel movement, leaving a clean ulceration of the rectal mucosa at the hemorrhoid site. This area normally heals completely within 2 to 3 weeks, at which time another treatment can be performed. Normally, four to six treatments are required for the most effective results. Severe pain after the procedure is rare. Severe bleeding occurs on rare occasions and can be controlled by electrocoagulation or suture ligature in the office or hospital. Complications of the procedure can be minimized by ligating only one hemorrhoid at a time.

Subcutaneous Injection

Thrombosed external hemorrhoids frequently occur without any precipitating factors. The patient has a sudden onset of severe pain and swelling at the anal verge. Examination reveals a large, edematous, tender external hemorrhoid with a hard lump in its center. Although this is a self-limiting problem that usually resolves within 1 to 2 weeks, more rapid resolution can be achieved with minor office therapy. The involved external hemorrhoid is injected subcutaneously with 1 per cent lidocaine with 1:100,000 epinephrine. An ellipse of skin is excised and the clot removed. A pressure dressing can be applied for a short time. To prevent rapid recurrence of the problem, an ellipse of skin must be excised rather than a simple skin incision made. Postoperative care usually requires several sitz baths a day and a small piece of cotton dressing for several days. Local care is discontinued as soon as healing has occurred.

Hemorrhoidectomy

In patients who cannot be rendered asymptomatic by office therapy or who have persistent symptoms from painful, edematous external hemorrhoids, hemorrhoidectomy is the procedure of choice. It can be performed under general, spinal, or caudal anesthesia or by combined intravenous sedation and local anesthesia. The use of intravenous sedation combined with local anesthesia allows optimum relaxation of the anal sphincter, with the added benefit of improved hemostasis resulting from the use of low-dose epinephrine in the local anesthetic. The internal and external hemorrhoids are excised in each quadrant. An elliptic incision of the skin over the external hemorrhoid, and of the mucosa over the internal hemorrhoid, is followed by dissection of the hemorrhoidal vessels from the underlying internal and external sphincters. The apex of the hemorrhoidal complex is then suture ligated for hemostasis. The external wound can then be either left open or closed with a running fine suture. The benefit of closing the external wound appears to be more rapid healing, probably at the cost of increased postoperative discomfort. The most common postoperative problems associated with hemorrhoidectomy are pain and urinary retention. Severe restriction of the patient's fluid intake during and after surgery can usually reduce the incidence of urinary retention. Severe postoperative hemorrhage is usually rare and can occur up to 2 weeks after surgery. Control requires resuture ligation of the bleeding site.

ANAL FISSURE

A fissure is a tear of the anoderm of the anal canal distal to the dentate line, usually over the distal portion of the internal sphincter. Fissures are usually considered to be traumatic, resulting possibly from constipation, diarrhea, or any other form of anal trauma. Fissures usually occur in the midline posteriorly and, less frequently, in the midline anteriorly. A fissure that is not in the midline should raise concerns about other pathologies such as Crohn's disease, leukemia, or venereal disease, including syphilis. An acute fissure is usually superficial, whereas a more chronic fissure is frequently deeper, with possible exposure of the underlying internal sphincter and the presence of a skin tag (sentinel tag) at the outer edge of the fissure. Pain is the most common symptom associated with a fissure, starting either immediately or up to several hours after a bowel movement and lasting for periods ranging from minutes to hours. A fissure is frequently associated with bright red rectal bleeding at the time of the bowel movement. A fissure can usually be identified by gentle separation of the buttocks, with exposure of the fissure at the anal verge. If it is not visualized in this fashion, 5 per cent lidocaine (Xylocaine) ointment can be applied to the anal canal with a cotton-tipped applicator, after which a gentle digital and anoscopic examination can be performed to confirm its presence. A fissure usually has a clean, well-delineated margin. In the absence of this appearance, further evaluation for possible Crohn's disease, syphilis, tuberculosis, or leukemia should be considered.

Treatment

Conservative therapy usually allows healing of most anal fissures. The patient is advised to use a psyllium preparation (e.g., Metamucil, Hydrocil, Konsyl) twice daily and a lubricating suppository at bedtime and after bowel movements. Sitz baths are recommended twice a day. Fissures that respond to conservative therapy usually heal within 2 to 4 weeks. Those that fail to respond require surgery. Symptomatic relief and healing may be obtained by a lateral sphincterotomy of the internal sphincter. This procedure can be performed under local anesthesia in the office or under combined intravenous sedation and local anesthesia in an ambulatory surgical unit. When performed in an ambulatory surgical unit, lateral sphincterotomy may be combined with excision of the fissure. The patient is maintained on therapy with a psyllium preparation and sitz baths postoperatively until healing occurs. The early postoperative complications relate primarily to pain, urinary retention, and occasional bleeding. Late postoperative complications, although rare, include difficulty in controlling flatus and occasional mucus discharge.

ANAL FISTULA AND ABSCESS

Most perianal abscesses and fistulas originate as an infection of the crypts and glands at the dentate line. On occasion, they may be related to other etiologies, such as inflammatory bowel disease. The infection originates in the glands at the base of the crypts and extends into the intersphincteric space. Most often, the infection extends from this point down to the perianal skin and presents as a perianal abscess. On rare occasions, the abscess is confined to the intersphincteric space and presents as an intramuscular abscess of the anal canal. Alternatively, it extends cephalad as a superlevator abscess or through the external sphincter as an ischiorectal abscess. The patient usually presents with a history of increasing rectal and anal pain, frequently unrelated to bowel movements and sometimes associated with chills and fever. On examination, there are perianal edema, erythema, and tenderness. In the less common intramuscular abscesses, there may be minimal findings in the perianal area but exquisite tenderness is present on digital examination, usually with an area of induration and fluctuance.

Treatment

Regardless of the initial presenting findings, the abscess should be drained immediately; drainage should not be delayed until the abscess "points." This can be performed under local anesthesia, with a cruciate incision into the abscess cavity followed by excision of each of the corners of the cruciate incision, leaving a wide-open drainage tract. Abscesses that are not amenable to simple drainage under local anesthesia should be drained immediately in the operating room under anesthesia, as previously described for hemorrhoidectomy. In an otherwise healthy patient, antibiotic therapy has little or no place in the management of perianal abscesses. After drainage, the patient should use sitz baths two or three times a day and should be re-evaluated in 3 or 4 weeks. At this time, approximately one-third of the patients have had spontaneous healing of their abscess and fistula, and two-thirds have formed a chronic fistula in ano. The latter group of patients present with an opening at the drainage site on the perianal skin and possibly with continuing purulent drainage. A tract is frequently palpable on digital examination to the dentate line, where a prominent crypt is noted. Anoscopic examination may also reveal a prominent crypt at the dentate line, possibly with a small amount of purulent drainage. Some patients who had spontaneous drainage of their perianal abscess will have a mature fistula in ano at the time of their initial examination.

With rare exceptions, such as patients with Crohn's disease, surgery is the only form of therapy available to eradicate a fistula in ano. Surgery requires a fistulotomy—the opening of the fistula tract from the internal opening at the dentate line to the external opening on the perianal skin. Depending on the direction of the fistula tract through the sphincter muscles, this procedure requires division of a variable portion of the internal and external sphincters. This can have a potentially significant impact on the patient's continence after surgery, particularly with fistulas that extend deeply through the sphincter muscles. Continence after surgery may also be a problem in women with fistulas anteriorly, where the sphincter mechanism is often thinned. In either of these cases, a staged procedure, with the use of a seton, can minimize the potential for extensive sphincter damage or incontinence. The use of a seton requires a partial fistulotomy, with a portion of the sphincter mechanism being left intact and encircled by a nonabsorbable suture. This suture slowly migrates distally through the remaining sphincter muscle while allowing minimal retraction of the divided muscle. The seton can be removed in 6 to 9 weeks as an office or day operative procedure. Postoperative complications associated with surgery usually include difficulty in controlling gas or possibly liquid stool, depending on the extent of sphincter injury caused by the initial abscess and by surgery. Perianal fistulas secondary to Crohn's disease are best managed by treatment of Crohn's disease rather than of the fistula. Surgical therapy for these fistulas is frequently associated with delayed or nonhealing wounds and with possible continence problems.

GASTRITIS

method of
WILLIAM S. HAUBRICH, M.D.
*University of California, San Diego,
School of Medicine*
La Jolla, California

Gastritis can be broadly defined as inflammation of the stomach, but the term, used in a casual way, surely would be near the top of any list of overused diagnostic terms. For most patients who are merely dyspeptic, "upset stomach" would be more apt. A bona fide diagnosis of gastritis requires endoscopy and, in some cases, biopsy; inflammation in the gastric mucosa is not reliably evident in radiographic contrast films. Unfortunately, it is often difficult to satisfactorily reconcile even endoscopic and biopsy findings with a given patient's symptoms. Nonetheless, gastric mucosa is liable to inflammatory reaction and, bearing in mind these disclaimers, there are several forms of gastritis for which therapy can be considered.

PATCHY ERYTHEMA OF THE GASTRIC MUCOSA

This probably is the single most frequently reported finding at gastroscopy. But often gastroscopic observation is liable to exaggerated interpretation. A few patches of redder than usual mucosa, especially in the prepyloric antrum, are seldom significant. No therapy is required. The prudent clinician looks elsewhere for a cause of the patient's dyspepsia.

EROSIVE GASTRITIS

This is the most commonly encountered form of gastric mucosal injury, and the usual cause is exposure to a noxious chemical agent, either a drug or alcohol. Notoriously injurious to the gastric mucosa in susceptible persons are aspirin and other nonsteroidal anti-inflammatory drugs (NSAIDs). The reaction can be as mild as mere erythema or as severe as extensive ulceration. Fortunately, gastric mucosa is capable of healing rapidly, once the noxious agent is removed. Treatment, first and foremost, is withdrawal of the imputed offender.

However, often the patient cannot manage well without aspirin or NSAIDs. In most cases, if a satisfactory substitute cannot be found, palliative therapy, using one or another of the measures described below, will suffice to allay the patient's dyspepsia, even when the NSAID therapy is cautiously continued.

True *corrosive* gastritis is seldom encountered. Concentrated acids or alkalis, when deliberately or inadvertently swallowed, wreak havoc mainly in the esophagus.

REFLUX GASTRITIS

Bile and pancreatic juice, normally abundant in the duodenum, are potentially injurious to gastric mucosa when it is exposed by reflux. Reflux of duodenal content occurs normally but is abated by the barrier of the intact pylorus and by prompt clearing from the stomach. Endoscopic evidence of bile-stained fluid entering the stomach from the duodenum is *not* to be construed as evidence of reflux gastritis. Of more concern is the circumstance wherein the pylorus has become distorted (as after pyloroplasty) or ablated (as after antrectomy) or when gastric emptying is impaired. Even in these instances, a degree of mucosal reaction is to be expected and should not precipitate a hasty decision for further surgical intervention. Palliative treatment, with watchful waiting, should be the rule. Cholestyramine (Questran), once suggested as a remedy for bile-reflux gastritis, has been found ineffective and is no longer recommended.

HEMORRHAGIC GASTRITIS (STRESS ULCERATION)

The pathogenesis here, insofar as it is understood, is principally hemodynamic. Any inflam-matory component is probably secondary to the vascular lesion. The condition is observed usually in patients subject to the stress of hypovolemia. The typical locale is the intensive care unit. Bleeding is common and covers a broad spectrum of severity, from little more than a few flecks of blood issuing from an indwelling nasogastric tube to exsanguinating hemorrhage.

The risk of hemodynamic injury to gastric mucosa in any stressed patient is sufficient to warrant consideration of preventive measures. Needless to say, the most effective preventive or therapeutic measures are those undertaken to relieve the injurious stress. These include correction of hypovolemia, restoration of circulatory perfusion, and control of sepsis.

The injured mucosa suffers from back-diffusion of hydrogen ions, so it makes sense to inhibit or counteract gastric acid secretion. Thus, the use of H_2 receptor antagonists or antacids, as described later, is well advised. Another approach is to bolster mucosal resistance. Sucralfate (Carafate) seems to be helpful in this way. Experimental evidence suggests that prostaglandins, especially those of the E type, recently made available for clinical use, are even more specifically beneficial in allaying mucosal injury. Therapy, when the lesion becomes evident, is a stepped-up version of these preventive measures.

Hemorrhage consequent to stress ulceration can be life-threatening. Such circumstance calls for more vigorous measures. Endoscopically guided cautery by heater probe, electrocoagulation, or laser therapy can be tried, but often the lesions are so numerous and widespread that cautery is futile. In extreme instances, emergency total gastrectomy may be necessary.

INFECTIOUS GASTRITIS

The stomach is notably resistant to bacterial infection, and this is rarely a problem, with one important exception. Recent investigation has shown that gastric mucosa, particularly in older patients, can harbor the organism *Campylobacter pylori* (a species distinct from *C. jejuni* that is well known to cause enteritis). The relation between *C. pylori* infection and gastritis or mucosal ulceration is not yet clear, but if mucosal inflammation is associated with infection by curved bacilli, as evident in silver-stained biopsy sections, then more specific therapy can be considered. Interestingly, *C. pylori* is eradicated more efficiently by bismuth (readily available as the subsalicylate in the form of Pepto-Bismol, 30 ml or two tablets—about 500 mg three times daily for 5 to 7 days), than by more conventional antibiotic agents. When prescribing bismuth, remember to tell the patient to expect to see black stools. Evidence is yet insufficient to promote bismuth as rational therapy in all cases of gastritis, but its easy availability, apparent safety, and low cost are commendable features.

An exceedingly rare form of infection in the stomach is phlegmonous gastritis, a suppuration involving the entire stomach wall. This occurs in a setting of sepsis, typically streptococcal, and requires intensive, parenteral penicillin therapy.

GASTRIC MUCOSAL ATROPHY

This is mentioned here because often it is referred to as "atrophic gastritis." The lesion, however, is primarily a disintegration of gastric epithelium, caused by a yet incompletely understood immune reaction. Any inflammatory component is secondary. Gastric mucosal atrophy is significant when it is attended by deficiency of intrinsic factor and impaired absorption of vitamin B_{12}. The treatment is that for vitamin B_{12} deficiency (see p. 321).

GENERAL METHODS OF TREATMENT

With the possible exception of *C. pylori* infection, as just noted, there is no specific therapy for the various types of gastritis. Hence, the following are offered as generally applicable measures. Just as reaction in gastric mucosa ranges widely from mild to severe, so the intensity of treatment should be modulated accordingly.

Diet

Most patients with symptomatic gastritis will have blunted appetite and some nausea; therefore, they are amenable to prescription of a light, soft diet. When nausea is severe and attended by vomiting, food should be withheld, and parenteral fluid and electrolyte supplements will be required.

Antacids

These agents constitute first line therapy and often are the only medication required. Antacids combine with H^+ in the lumen of the stomach, thus preventing the potentially injurious back-diffusion of acid. Antacids should be given in liquid form (diluted if necessary to facilitate delivery through a nasogastric tube) and in ample volume (one can hardly give too much or too frequently). An average antacid dose (e.g., Mylanta-II) would be 15 ml every 1 or 2 hours. The only drawbacks to the use of antacids are the necessity for frequent dosage and lack of compli-

ance by the patient. A minor side effect of magnesium-containing antacids is diarrhea. This is easily corrected by substituting aluminum hydroxide (e.g., Alternagel).

H_2 Receptor Antagonists

Gastric acid secretion can be effectively inhibited by cimetidine (Tagamet), ranitidine (Zantac), and famotidine (Pepcid), and by this means back-diffusion of H^+ is reduced. Moreover, for severely ill patients these agents can be given intravenously. Continuous intravenous infusion, rather than repeated boluses, is recommended for both efficacy and reduced cost.

If cimetidine is chosen, the usual schedule calls for an initial intravenous "priming" dose of 300 mg and then a steady infusion of 37.5 to 75 mg per hour, dissolved in the running fluid. If the patient has an indwelling nasogastric tube, the stomach contents can be aspirated from time to time and checked for pH. The aim is to keep the pH above 4; the running dose of cimetidine can be regulated accordingly.

Patients less acutely ill can be given medication orally: cimetidine, 300 mg every 6 hours; ranitidine, 150 mg every 12 hours; or famotidine, 20 mg every 12 hours. If medication is being used prophylactically, the frequency of doses can be halved.

Antacids and H_2 receptor antagonists are compatible, although—as in the case of the person who wears both belt and suspenders—the combination may amount to more caution than is necessary.

If antacids or H_2 receptor antagonists are administered in such a way as to totally eliminate gastric acid secretion in the stomach of an acutely ill patient, there is a risk of complication by nosocomial infection, that is, pneumonitis resulting from aspiration of bacterially contaminated gastric juice. This does not happen often, but because of the possibility, care should be taken to avoid unduly vigorous therapy.

Other Measures

Another approach is to use measures for bolstering mucosal defense. This involves agents that are said to confer "cytoprotection."

Sucralfate can be given orally, 1 gram (one tablet) every 4 to 6 hours on an empty stomach, for both prevention of mucosal injury and therapy. While efficacy is not always certain, safety is assured. Following is a simple and useful technique for administering sucralfate to a patient with an indwelling nasogastric tube. Place a tablet of sucralfate (1 gram) in the empty barrel of a 60-ml syringe. Replace the plunger and draw up 20 ml of water. Let the syringe stand with its tip up for about 5 minutes, gently shaking the syringe occasionally. The tablet will disintegrate, forming a sucralfate suspension that can be injected through the nasogastric tube. This can be repeated every 3 or 4 hours.

Prostaglandins of the E type can be administered orally. Recent trials suggest a dose of 100 to 200 micrograms four times daily. This class of agents is now available as misoprostol (Cytotec). Prostaglandins are welcomed as a useful addition to the armamentarium of agents available for the prevention and treatment of gastritis.

ACUTE AND CHRONIC VIRAL HEPATITIS

method of
RICHARD B. SEWELL, M.D.
Austin Hospital, University of Melbourne
Melbourne, Australia

ACUTE VIRAL HEPATITIS

Acute viral hepatitis refers by convention to cases of acute hepatic cell necrosis caused by the hepatitis A, hepatitis B, delta hepatitis, and non-A, non-B hepatitis agents. Other viral infections, including infectious mononucleosis and cytomegalovirus, may produce hepatitis and should be considered in the appropriate clinical setting. If serologic evidence of viral infection is absent, consideration should be given to causes such as alcohol, drug-induced hepatitis, and extrahepatic cholestasis. The majority of cases of acute viral hepatitis are subclinical, especially in children, and are only recognized by coincidentally measured elevations of serum transaminases. Hepatitis A virus (HAV) causes type A hepatitis, is usually acquired by the fecal-oral route, and has an incubation period of 20 to 50 days. Hepatitis B virus (HBV) causes type B hepatitis and is acquired by percutaneous introduction or by close personal contact; it has an incubation period of 28 to 150 days. Delta hepatitis virus (HDV) causes type D hepatitis and is a small, defective RNA virus dependent on HBV for its replication. Non-A, non-B (NANB) hepatitis is caused by three or more viruses that have not been unequivocally identified, although serologic tests for identification of two NANB hepatitis agents are likely to become available in the near future. It can be spread by percutaneous introduction, with either a short or a long incubation period, or by personal contact in the "sporadic" form. Hepatitis A is usually uncomplicated and never runs a chronic course. Hepatitis B is self-limited and uncomplicated in 90 per cent of cases. Delta hepatitis is more often associated with a severe and sometimes fulminant outcome. Hepatitis NANB tends to produce a mild disease; when acquired following blood transfusion, there is a significant (10 to 40 per cent) incidence of indolent chronic liver disease or cirrhosis. Clinical severity tends to increase with age.

Treatment

Standard treatment is conservative and has little effect on the course of acute viral hepatitis. The patient should be observed and monitored for potential acute complications and to ensure that chronic disease does not develop. Initial blood should be taken for biochemistry, including standard liver function tests, and serology, including tests for hepatitis B surface antigen (HBsAg) and IgM anti-HAV. The main purposes are confirming the diagnosis, planning protection of contacts, and predicting fulminant hepatitis.

Hospitalization. The patient can usually be managed at home. Hospitalization is reserved for patients at risk of developing complications, particularly fulminant hepatic failure, those requiring special diagnostic procedures, and those who cannot be adequately isolated and cared for at home. Dehydration, altered consciousness, prolonged prothrombin time, and bruising or development of ascites warrant hospitalization.

Bed Rest. Although bed rest has not been proved to alter the course of the illness, it is usually advised while the patient is symptomatic. Patients should not work while jaundiced and during the postictal malaise (usually 1 to 4 weeks). Activity should be increased in parallel with clinical improvement.

Diet. The choice of diet is at the discretion of the patient. Fluid input should be maintained. A low-fat, high-carbohydrate diet is usually acceptable. Abstinence from alcohol is advisable for 3 to 4 months. If parenteral nutrition or fluids are necessary, the patient should be hospitalized.

Drugs. There is generally no place for drugs in most cases of hepatitis. If medication is given, allowance should be made for altered, and usually impaired, drug metabolism. Special care is required for drugs that may precipitate encephalopathy, including sedatives and analgesics. Corticosteroids are not indicated and in hepatitis B may predispose to chronicity.

Isolation. Patients with hepatitis A are most infective prior to the development of jaundice but can shed the virus for up to 2 weeks from its onset; they should be isolated while potentially infectious and special care should be taken to prevent fecal-oral contamination. Patients with hepatitis B or NANB do not require isolation. These patients should be advised about routes of hepatitis spread; those with hepatitis are potentially infectious until serum antibodies appear. Blood and body fluids are potentially infectious. Toothbrushes, razors, and so forth should not be shared. Sexual intercourse need not be disallowed, but a condom is advised, and the partner should be vaccinated. For the patient hospitalized with hepatitis B, NANB, or D, the institutional guidelines for handling the patient's blood and secretions should be carefully followed.

Patient Contacts. Those in close contact with a patient who develops acute hepatitis A should generally receive normal immunoglobulin; if the contact already has anti-HAV antibodies, immunoglobulin is not indicated. Immunoglobulin is not officially recommended for contacts of patients with NANB hepatitis. Close contacts of a patient with hepatitis B (e.g., spouse, sexual partner, children under 5 years) should be vaccinated if they are HBsAg negative and antibody negative.

Convalescence and Recovery. In the typical patient, improvement is evident by the end of the second or third week of illness. The period of convalescence should be approximately twice the symptomatic period. Follow-up biochemical studies (bilirubin and transaminase) should be performed initially at weekly and then at monthly intervals until recovery is complete. Prior to return to work and usual routines, the patient should be free of symptoms, with normal serum bilirubin and transaminase.

A gradual return to full activity should be planned. If HBsAg remains positive for 3 months or if transaminase abnormalities persist, follow-up studies must be continued to check for possible progression to chronic hepatitis.

Relapses. Relapses occur in 5 to 10 per cent of patients. They may be mildly symptomatic or there may be only an increase in serum transaminases or bilirubin. Treatment is as for the initial episode. Subsequent recovery is usually complete.

Complications

Prolonged Cholestasis. Occasionally prolonged cholestasis may complicate the convalescent phase despite symptomatic improvement. Jaundice may persist for up to 6 months. Treatment is usually unnecessary, although cholestyramine may be used. If the diagnosis is in doubt, cholangiography or needle biopsy of the liver should be performed. Laparotomy is to be avoided.

Fulminant Hepatitis. Fulminant hepatic failure is a rare complication of acute viral hepatitis, more common with hepatitis B and NANB hepatitis than with hepatitis A. There is a high mortality rate (70 to 90 per cent); however, if recovery occurs, liver function and architecture return to normal. Management is best undertaken in a specialized intensive care unit, with careful observation and monitoring of vital functions. The major causes of death are related to the development of hepatic encephalopathy, gastrointestinal bleeding, and renal failure.

The goal of therapy is to provide support while hepatic regeneration occurs. Careful monitoring of cardiovascular, renal, respiratory, hematologic, hepatic, and neurologic function is mandatory. Impending hepatic encephalopathy is treated with neomycin and lactulose. Hypoglycemia may impair consciousness and is treated with 10 per cent dextrose infusion. Mannitol may be required if signs of cerebral edema develop. Protein intake should be stopped and nutrition maintained enterally or parenterally. Coagulation studies determine the need for replacement therapy with fresh frozen plasma, clotting factor concentrates, or platelets. Heparin is ineffective. Prophylactic histamine$_2$ (H$_2$) antagonists decrease the incidence of complicating gastrointestinal bleeding. Corticosteroid therapy is not recommended.

A number of temporary hepatic support systems have been tried. These include exchange blood transfusions, plasmapheresis, cross-circulation, extracorporeal pig liver perfusion, hemodialysis, and charcoal column hemoperfusion. There is no clear-cut evidence that any of these measures are of value in improving survival.

When there is access to a center performing liver transplantation, early consultation during Stage I or II of hepatic precoma is recommended, particularly in NANB hepatitis, which has a poor prognosis.

Hepatitis During Pregnancy. In women of lower socioeconomic backgrounds, the clinical course may be more severe. Therapeutic abortion may add risk to the mother and does not alter the course of the illness. There is no evidence that hepatitis produces congenital malformations; however, there is evidence of transmission of HBV and NANB to the infant when infection occurs in the third trimester.

Aplastic Anemia. Bone marrow hypoplasia is a rare complication of acute viral hepatitis.

CHRONIC VIRAL HEPATITIS

Chronic Hepatitis B

Persistent infection with HBV for more than 6 months occurs in up to 10 per cent of patients following hepatitis B, regardless of the initial severity. Liver biopsy shows that approximately one-third of patients have chronic active hepatitis and two-thirds have chronic persistent hepatitis. In other cases, chronic viral hepatitis is not preceded by a clearly recognizable acute attack. Cirrhosis may be present, and hepatocellular carcinoma represents a late event. Patients with chronic hepatitis B often have serum markers of viral replication, such as serum HBV DNA, Dane particles, hepatitis B e antigen (HBeAg), and DNA polymerase. These patients convert from HbeAg positive to anti-HBe at the rate of about 10 per cent per year. In addition to losing markers of viral replication, HBeAg seroconversion is usually accompanied by normalization of transaminases. HBsAg seroconversion, on the other hand, occurs rarely. Care should be taken in giving HBV-positive patients blood or blood products since a minute inoculum of HDV may induce severe disease.

Delta Agent. The delta agent (HDV) is a small, incomplete RNA hepatitis virus that is dependent on coexisting hepatitis B infection for its replication. It is highly virulent, and parenteral transmission may occur simultaneously with exposure to HBV or as a superinfection in a hepatitis B carrier. Both fulminant hepatitis and progressive liver disease occur with HDV infection. No specific therapy is available. Serologic evidence of delta agent should be sought in relapse of chronic hepatitis B.

Clinical Relapse. This can occur during spontaneous conversion from HBeAg positive to negative and is marked by increasing fatigue and raised serum transaminase values. It may occur due to additional HDV infection. Rarely, spontaneous reactivation from HBeAg negative to positive has been described. Clinical deterioration may mark development of hepatocellular carcinoma.

Treatment

The patient must be counseled about personal infectivity, and close family and sexual contacts should be considered for hepatitis B vaccination. Alcohol excess should be avoided since this may potentiate the HBV damage. Antiviral therapy should be considered particularly in a patient likely to transmit the disease.

Corticosteroid Therapy. Although immunosuppressive therapy is of proven benefit in *autoimmune* chronic active hepatitis, corticosteroid therapy may have deleterious effects in chronic hepatitis B. Viral replication is increased by steroid therapy. Prednisolone should be considered only in HBeAg-negative chronic hepatitis B when the patients are symptomatic and the bi-

opsy shows severe chronic active hepatitis. In these cases the drug should be given for 3 to 6 months and withdrawn if there is no improvement. Small trials have shown that immunostimulant substances are not successful in therapy.

Antiviral Therapy. Results have been encouraging in trials using the antiviral agents adenine arabinoside and soluble adenine arabinoside monophosphate, which inhibit viral DNA polymerase. Viral replication ceases while the patients are on therapy; in some, the effect is sustained, and seroconversion from HBeAg to anti-HBe occurs. Similar improvement has been noted in some patients treated with various interferons. Studies with these and other antiviral agents are continuing, but as yet they are not available for routine clinical use.

Chronic Non-A, Non-B Hepatitis

Chronic hepatitis occurs in more than 50 per cent of patients with NANB hepatitis following blood transfusion and less commonly after sporadic infection. Liver biopsy will disclose chronic persistent hepatitis in 30 per cent, chronic active hepatitis in 60 per cent, and cirrhosis in 20 per cent of these cases. The course of NANB is characterized by relapses and remissions, especially in transaminases. Regular supervision is necessary, and in the absence of controlled studies, prednisolone cannot be recommended.

Complications

Hepatic encephalopathy, variceal hemorrhage, ascites, renal failure, and bacterial infections may complicate chronic hepatitis and cirrhosis following both hepatitis B and NANB hepatitis. Hepatocellular carcinoma may develop in both cirrhotic and noncirrhotic carriers of hepatitis B and possibly NANB hepatitis. Resection is possible in less than 1 per cent, and chemotherapy with doxorubicin (Adriamycin) induces remissions in around 20 per cent of cases.

PREVENTION

Hepatitis A. Personal hygiene and proper sanitation are mandatory. Separate toilet facilities are desirable. Bedding and clothing should be autoclaved or separately laundered. General handling of food or water by patient or contacts should be prevented. The use of disposable crockery and cutlery is encouraged. Because virus shedding in stools begins at least 2 weeks before the illness, quarantine is unlikely to influence the spread of disease in the community.

Hepatitis B. High-risk groups include certain hospital and dental staff (e.g., oncology, hemodialysis-transplantation, gastroenterology, intensive care units, diagnostic laboratories, surgical units), staff in institutions for the mentally handicapped, patients receiving blood and blood products, drug addicts, male homosexuals, and the families of chronic carriers (Table 1). For high-risk hospital personnel, a program of continuing education concerning hepatitis transmission, monitoring of clinical practices, and regular serologic surveillance for hepatitis B is recommended.

Disposable material and equipment must be used whenever possible; nondisposable equipment should be sterilized by autoclaving for 15 minutes, boiling for 20 minutes, or exposing to dry heat for 1 hour. Equipment that cannot be heat sterilized should be disinfected with sodium hypochlorite (60 grams per 9 liters of water) or 2 per cent glutaraldehyde. The wearing of gloves and protective clothing by medical and dental staff is advised when they are working in a field contaminated with blood or other body fluids. All blood donors must be screened for HBsAg. Blood products should be used sparingly and only for specific indications.

Transmission of HBV from mother to neonate

TABLE 1. **Prevalence of HBV Exposure and Annual Hepatitis B Attack Rates in Different Groups***

Group	Prevalence of HBV Markers (%)	Annual Attack Rate (%)
Health Care Workers		
Dialysis staff	34–39	3–11
Oral surgeons	30	5
Staff of custodial institutions	22–33	13–20
Surgeons	23–28	5
Nurses in high-risk units	7–47	1–11
Blood bank workers	6–26	1–2
Laboratory technicians	11–26	1–3
Physicians (general)	12–19	2
Dentists (general)	14–15	2
Surgical house officers	10–17	4–10
Nurse (general)	5–21	1
High-Risk Patients		
Dialysis patients	42–59	3–14
Hemophiliacs	76–96	13–20
Institutionalized Persons		
Mentally retarded	50–90	1–10
Prisoners	42	5–10
Other Groups		
Homosexual men	60–68	12–19
Intravenous drug users	50–71	4–33
Household contacts of HBsAg carriers	26–61	2–5
Promiscuous heterosexuals	15–31	2–5
Military	7–20	0.5–12
General U.S. Population	5–10	0.1

*Reprinted from Mulley AG, Silverstein MD, and Dienstag JL, by permission of The New England Journal of Medicine, *307*, 651, 1982.

is the most common route of infection. The risk to the infant of an HBeAg-positive carrier mother of becoming a chronic HBsAg carrier is about 90 per cent. Carrier risk to infants of HBV carriers who have anti-HBe antibodies is low (5 to 10 per cent), but acute hepatitis may occur. HBsAg screening of mothers whose likely prevalence of HBV carriage is relatively high is probably cost effective. Infants of all HBV carriers should receive combined active/passive vaccination as soon as possible after birth.

Non-A, Non-B Hepatitis. Most transfusion-related hepatitis is NANB hepatitis. Exclusion of paid donors and those with a past history of hepatitis will reduce the risk. Exclusion of blood from volunteer donors who have serum glutamic-pyruvic transaminase levels greater than 2.25 times the standard deviation above the mean will reduce the incidence of NANB hepatitis about one-third while excluding less than 2 per cent of blood donors. Prevention of post-transfusion NANB hepatitis awaits identification of the viruses involved and development of reliable screening tests.

Immune Globulin

Hepatitis A. Immune serum globulin (ISG) is effective in preventing or modifying hepatitis A. The dose recommended by the United States Public Health Service Advisory Committee on Immunization Practices is 0.06 ml per kg administered once, as soon as possible after exposure, to people in close contact with patients with acute type A hepatitis, especially in households, institutions for the mentally retarded, and prisons. It is not recommended in the postexposure situation for casual contacts in schools, hospitals, offices, and factories, unless an overt epidemic develops.

ISG may be effective prophylactically in individuals traveling to tropical and developing countries. The recommended dose is 0.06 ml per kg at 4- to 6-month intervals, unless the period of exposure is less than 3 months, in which case it can be given in a dose of 0.02 ml per kg immediately before the visit.

Hepatitis B. Hepatitis B immune globulin (HBIG) is prepared from persons who have high titers of antibody to HBsAg. The United States Public Health Service Advisory Committee recommends that HBIG, 0.06 ml per kg, be administered within 24 hours of parenteral (needle stick) exposure to HBsAg-positive blood and again 1 month later. Active vaccination should be commenced immediately as well.

All infants born to HBsAg-positive mothers (especially those positive for HBeAg) should be given HBIG (total dose 0.5 ml) within 24 hours of birth, followed by vaccination. It is not currently recommended that HBIG be given to sexual contacts of acute type B hepatitis patients.

Although there is a theoretical risk of immune complex disease if HBIG is given to an HBsAg-positive individual, this has not been reported, and it is not necessary to test the recipient prior to treatment.

Non-A, Non-B Hepatitis. Although one study indicated that ISG in standard doses appears to offer significant protection against NANB hepatitis, other studies failed to confirm this, and firm recommendations cannot be given.

Vaccination

Hepatitis A. Vaccines against this virus are under development but are not yet available.

Hepatitis B. A successful immunization trial against acute hepatitis B using inactivated HBsAg prepared from the plasma of asymptomatic carriers (Heptavax B, Merck) led to licensing for its clinical use in the United States in 1982. Most side effects recognized to date have been mild. Although the vaccine is made from human serum, purification includes steps to inactivate all known pathogens, including the slow viruses, and three separate studies have excluded any association between the vaccine and the acquired immunodeficiency syndrome. A similar vaccine has been prepared and used in France (Pasteur, Hevac B).

The high cost and limited availability of these first-generation vaccines require that priorities for immunization be ascertained. Strategies will differ between countries. In countries with a high incidence of HBsAg carriage and vertical transmission, an immunization program should be directed at infants and young children. Hepatitis B vaccine and HBIG can be given simultaneously without diminishing the efficacy of either, and infants born to HBsAg-positive mothers should receive both at birth.

In developed countries, immunization should be offered to high-risk groups. It is believed that protection will last for at least 5 years. Injection should be given into the deltoid. Seroconversion is lower with increasing age and in the immunocompromised; a check for HBs antibody is recommended in these groups, if not in all subjects. The most cost-effective way of immunizing a high-risk, high–previous exposure group is to perform serologic testing for hepatitis B markers and to immunize only those who are not immune. In contrast, a high-risk, low–previous exposure group will be most effectively protected by immunization without prior testing.

Alternative vaccines using recombinant DNA technology are now available, and synthetic vaccines have shown encouraging results with the added benefit of superior safety. The lower cost of these second- and third-generation vaccines should eventually allow an immunization program worldwide.

MALABSORPTION SYNDROMES
method of
CHARLES M. MANSBACH, II, M.D.
The Health Science Center
University of Tennessee, Memphis
Memphis, Tennessee

"Malabsorption" is a generic term that covers both malabsorption and maldigestion. Most commonly this term is used to refer to the impaired assimilation of dietary fat. This is because excessive fat excretion (>5 per cent of the intake of at least an 80-gram fat diet) is the most commonly used indicator of malabsorption. Levels of protein and carbohydrates, which are also malabsorbed concomitantly with fat, are usually not measured in the stool. Protein malabsorption is difficult to assess because of large amounts of protein normally excreted into the bowel each day. Assessment is further complicated by abnormal leakage of protein into the bowel in certain disease states. Carbohydrate malabsorption is also difficult to study because of sources of amylase other than the pancreas, the effective surface digestion of carbohydrates, and the colonic bacterial transformation of malabsorbed carbohydrates to noncarbohydrate products. Specific absorption defects of amino acids and carbohydrates, with the exception of lactase deficiency, are rare. Therefore, excessive fat excretion remains the best indicator of malabsorption and maldigestion.

Malabsorption should be considered in anyone with unexplained weight loss; production of stools suggestive of steatorrhea; the development of osteomalacia and/or a low serum calcium level; the development of a prolonged prothrombin time in the absence of liver disease; iron deficiency anemia not caused by blood loss, especially if it is difficult to control by oral iron replacement; and the development of lactase insufficiency in adulthood. The development of any of these symptoms should suggest, first, the establishment of the malabsorptive state and, second, the definition of the disease causing the malabsorption. Although there are screening tests for malabsorption in common use, such as the D-xylose test or the bentiromide (Chymex) test, the 72-hour fecal excretion of fat coupled with a known fat intake remains the most secure way to establish the problem. A qualitative test of stool fat may also be used in which the stool is examined for fat globules with the aid of Sudan III before and after being heated with acidic acid.

Physical signs to be looked for include evidence of muscle wasting, edema, tetany, bruises and ecchymoses, and glossitis or cheilosis.

The establishment of the etiology leading to malabsorption is crucial because therapy is directed in each instance to a specific diagnosis. If the diagnosis is correct and the treatment is appropriately tailored, reduction in stool output and weight gain are to be expected.

FAT MALDIGESTION CAUSED BY LIPASE DEFICIENCY

The most common cause of malabsorption is lipase deficiency. This occurs when lipase excretion from the pancreas into the duodenum is less than 10 per cent of normal output. The majority of cases are caused by chronic pancreatitis, usually because of excessive ethanol intake. Other causes of chronic pancreatitis include hypertriglyceridemia, the rare familial form, cystic fibrosis, and the idiopathic form. Gallstone-caused acute pancreatitis does not lead to the development of the chronic form. Not all cases of chronic pancreatitis are associated with abdominal pain. Completely painless pancreatitis is well known. There are no tests to reveal subtle abnormalities of the pancreas. The most sensitive test in common use in the United States is the secretin infusion test. Secretin is infused intravenously, which stimulates pancreatic fluid and bicarbonate output into the duodenum. Both of these substances are measured while gastric contents are aspirated. Seventy per cent of the pancreas must be destroyed before the secretin test becomes abnormal. Particularly useful in establishing the diagnosis of chronic pancreatitis is the finding of pancreatic calcification on a flat plate of the abdomen. The use of computed axial tomography can increase the chances of identifying this important phenomenon. The development of diabetes without a family history and/or low serum trypsin-like immunoreactivity is also helpful to establish the diagnosis.

Treatment. The treatment of the malabsorptive symptoms of chronic pancreatitis must often be individualized to optimize the results. First, attention needs to be paid to the lipase content of the preparations used. The formulations with the highest lipase content are Creon, Ilozyme, Ku-Zyme HP, Festal, Cotazym, and Pancrease. Second, the two major obstacles to adequate replacement therapy are destruction of the digestive enzymes by acidic gastric contents and delivery of enzymes to the duodenum either before or after the arrival of food. Some of the preparations used, such as Creon and Pancrease, contain the digestive enzymes in microspherulated form. These microspheres are designed to retain and protect the digestive enzymes from inactivation by acidic gastric contents by releasing them only in a more alkaline environment. This principle, although sound, does not work in all patients.

Pancreatic replacement tablets or capsules should be given with meals. Giving them before meals will likely inactivate the preparation in the stomach and/or deliver the enzymes to the duodenum before the arrival of food. It is a good idea to give additional capsules 0.5 to 1 hour postprandially to help ensure that pancreatic enzymes will continue to be delivered to the duodenum during the later stages of digestion. If the patient's symptoms are not improved with this regimen alone, a different pancreatin preparation can be tried—for example, switching from one with microspheres to one without them. If the patient remains symptomatic, the most common cause of continued problems is gastric acidic inactivation of the pancreatin. Therefore, an H_2 antagonist such as cimetidine (Tagamet), ranitidine (Zantac), famotidine (Pepcid), or nizatidine (Axid) should be given 0.5 to 1 hour before meals. Antacids should not be used in this setting. The still unresponsive patient may be helped by increasing the number of tablets or capsules further. Compliance with the prescribed regimen is crucial to success. The patient's adherence to scheduled therapy should be regularly checked. Even under the best conditions, a disappointingly small amount of active enzyme is delivered to the duodenum.

Fat-soluble vitamins are usually not malabsorbed in chronic pancreatitis. This is because they do not require digestion before absorption. However, one may occasionally see symptoms of vitamin deficiency caused by poor intake, usually in the setting of chronic alcoholism. In these cases, vitamin supplementation can be given. Approximately 50 per cent of patients with chronic pancreatitis have an abnormal Schilling's test for vitamin B_{12} absorption. Rarely, however, do these patients manifest clinical symptoms of vitamin B_{12} deficiency. Adequate pancreatic replacement therapy leads to restoration of vitamin B_{12} absorption.

Some patients demonstrating malabsorption from chronic pancreatitis continue to have the abdominal pain associated with this condition. These patients may also be helped by pancreatic replacement therapy. Pain relief is helpful in maintaining weight because some patients decrease their food intake in an attempt to avoid pain. Pain relief with enzyme supplementation therapy may require more capsules or pills than are given under normal conditions. In these cases, the development of hyperuricemia and hyperuricosuria should be considered, especially in patients with a history of gout. The presence of complicating factors in chronic pancreatitis, such as the development of a pseudocyst or carcinoma of the pancreas, should also be considered in these individuals.

Narcotics should be avoided if possible, in treating the pain of chronic pancreatitis because chemical dependence in this situation is common. If dependence does develop, the narcotic should be withdrawn. In this setting the use of clonidine may be useful to reduce the symptoms of withdrawal.

It is important to note that the abdominal pain associated with chronic pancreatitis tends to wane over the years. In some patients, however, surgery is required for relief. Operations on the pancreas should be done only by a surgeon skilled in these procedures. In no case is pain relief always expected. Glandular destruction continues even after adequate surgical ductular drainage. Surgical therapy may consist of distal pancreatectomy with pancreaticojejunostomy for those patients who have a demonstrated pancreatic ductular stricture with proximal ductular dilatation or in whom pancreatic stones have been identifed. In other patients with multiple strictures of the pancreatic duct, Puestow's procedure (longitudinal pancreaticojejunostomy) may be performed. Other patients may develop a strictured common bile duct, which, if persistent, must be bypassed. Endoscopic retrograde pancreatography is crucial in these settings. Celiac ganglionectomy or celiac block has been performed, but their use for pain control is, at best, uncertain. Some physicians advocate 95 per cent pancreatectomy as a last resort. These individuals are invariably left with diabetes as an outcome and require insulin replacement or the new approach of islet cell transplantation. Supplementation with digestive enzymes is always required.

MALDIGESTION CAUSED BY BILE SALT DEFICIENCY

Bile acids are secreted from the liver conjugated to the amino acids glycine or taurine. They aggregate above a certain concentration to form micelles. These micelles have an exterior that is hydrophilic and an interior that is hydrophobic. The products of fat digestion are presumed to be found in the interior of the bile salt mixed micelle. This property of bile salts optimizes fat absorption and is especially important for the absorption of vitamin D. Without any bile acids, approximately 50 per cent of dietary fat can be absorbed. This percentage can be increased by maximizing the intake of polyunsaturated fatty acids, which, in the absence of bile acids, interact better with water than do saturated fatty acids.

BILIARY DRAINAGE

If bile is drained from the intestinal tract, the bile salt pool is quickly lost and the liver is stimulated maximally to synthesize bile acids. One way in which bile may be drained from the liver is the placement of a T tube in the bile duct, which enables bile to flow out of the long arm of the tube. In certain instances in which palliation for inoperable obstructive jaundice is desired, nasobiliary drainage or transhepatic drainage of the bile ductular system can be performed. When a transhepatic tube is placed internal drainage may be possible, thus restoring bile drainage to the intestinal tract.

If malabsorption becomes a problem, a diet rich in polyunsaturated fats should be eaten or medium-chain triglyceride (MCT) oil should be substituted for normal dietary fat. The fatty acids of MCT are 8 to 10 carbons in length. They are essentially water soluble and thus do not require bile acids for absorption. On absorption they go to the liver, where they are oxidized (which is not the normal fate of newly absorbed long-chain fatty acids). Patients who use MCT oil should be observed for the development of essential fatty acid deficiency.

BACTERIAL OVERGROWTH

In this condition, bacteria, usually in the upper intestine, deconjugate bile acids that have reduced solubility at the slightly acidic pH present in the upper intestine. The precipitated bile acids are passively absorbed and therefore deplete the lumen of the bile acids necessary for optimal fat absorption. In addition, enzymes released by the bacteria hydrolyze portions of the luminal surfaces of absorptive cells, which, in turn, become dysfunctional. The bacteria primarily responsible for these abnormalities are anaerobes. The diagnosis is made by intubating the duodenum and finding more than 10^5 bacteria per ml. Alternatively, an increase in the amount of deconjugated bile acids in duodenal fluid is also diagnostic. These patients may have increased breath hydrogen in the fasting state and increased amounts of hydrogen appearing in the breath shortly after ingesting the poorly absorbed sugar, lactulose. An increase in breath ^{14}C from ingested ^{14}C-labeled xylose may also be found. These breath tests are not specific and also depend on adequate gastric emptying.

Identification of the cause of the increase in intestinal bacteria is important because treatment varies depending on the diagnosis made. An upper gastrointestinal series with small bowel follow-through enables the diagnosis of multiple intestinal diverticuli, Crohn's disease, and potentially impaired gastrointestinal motility to be made. Scleroderma and diabetes, especially in the presence of peripheral neuropathy, are systemic diseases that may be associated with impaired intestinal motility. Achlorhydria may also be associated with this problem. It remains to be determined if the new, powerful gastric proton pump inhibitors such as omeprazole become associated with the development of this syndrome. A cologastric fistula is best diagnosed by barium enema. Surgical correction of the fistula is warranted.

Treatment. Treatment begins with tetracycline, 250 mg four times a day for 10 days. If the patient does not improve, metronidazole (Flagyl) should be given, 250 mg three times a day. If still no improvement is observed, other antibiotics that are effective against anaerobes may be given. Successful treatment should be followed by no antibiotic therapy until symptoms recur. For motility disturbances, a prokinetic drug such as metoclopramide (Reglan) or cisapride should be given. Serum folate levels are usually increased in this condition. If the vitamin B_{12} level is low, this vitamin should be replaced parenterally.

IMPAIRED BILE SALT REABSORPTION

The most common cause of this problem is intestinal resection. As little as 30 cm of the most distal ileum, including the ileocecal valve, can be associated with significant malabsorption of bile salts. Usually the resection is caused by Crohn's disease, which itself usually does not lead to bile acid malabsorption. Either stenotic Crohn's disease or resection of the ileocecal valve may result in bacterial contamination of the distal intestine. Excessive bile acid loss to the colon may result in diarrhea without the presence of steatorrhea. This is usually seen in ileal resections of 30 to 60 cm. Dihydroxylated bile salts cause the colon to secrete salt and water. A diagnosis of impaired bile salt reabsorption can be made by finding an increased proportion of bile salts conjugated with glycine compared to taurine or an increase in the amount of $^{14}CO_2$ excreted into the breath after ^{14}C-labeled bile salts are given by mouth.

Treatment. Oral replacement of bile salts increases the diarrhea. Bile acid binders, such as cholestyramine (Questran) or colestipol (Colestid) should be given as one packet or one scoop (4 grams) before meals and at bedtime. The dose should be reduced if the patient becomes constipated.

For larger resections, especially those greater than 100 cm, vitamin B_{12} malabsorption can be expected, as well as more significant steatorrhea. In this setting, the diarrhea results from excessive fat in the stool rather than from the secretory stimulation of excessive bile acids in the colon. Although bile acid binders usually do not work

in this condition, they should be tried first. If they are not successful, a diet low in fat, but with the proportion of fat eaten being high in polyunsaturates, should next be tried. MCT oil may also be used to provide calories. Four ounces of MCT oil equals 1000 calories.

MALABSORPTION SECONDARY TO PRIMARY INTESTINAL DISORDERS

The reasons for malabsorption are especially well documented in gluten-sensitive enteropathy (GSE). These include (1) a decreased intestinal surface area secondary to villous atrophy; (2) reduced amounts of the hormone cholecystokinin-pancreozymin (CCK-PZ) in the duodenum, resulting in poor CCK-PZ release on stimulation by food, which reduces the quantities of bile salts and lipase in the upper intestine after meals; (3) immature cells at the surface of the intestine that are unable to perform adequately the absorptive and transport functions of mature intestinal cells; and finally (4) the secretory state induced by these immature cells, which normally secrete chloride. This last reason results in an enlarged fluid volume in the upper intestine and reduces the effective concentration of bile acids, which in turn reduces the number of micelles available for lipid solubilization.

A small bowel biopsy is crucial for the specific diagnosis. Villous flattening can be seen in GSE, collagenous sprue, immunoglobulin deficiencies, nodular lymphoid hyperplasia, and tropical sprue. Atrophy may be seen in intestinal irradiation and chronic intestinal ischemia. It may also be seen in Whipple's disease. A small bowel series may be abnormal, demonstrating the disordered motility pattern or small bowel edema secondary to hypoalbuminemia. Nodules may be identified in nodular lymphoid hyperplasia. A specific diagnosis is necessary so that treatment may be appropriately directed.

GLUTEN-SENSITIVE ENTEROPATHY

This disorder, also called celiac sprue, is probably an immunologic disorder caused by exposure of the intestine to gluten, which is found in wheat, rye, barley, and oats. Histologic examination of the intestine demonstrates cryptal hypertrophy and an increase in inflammatory cells including plasma cells. Lymphocytes are seen infiltrating the abnormal-appearing surface cells.

Treatment. Dietary treatment of malabsorption secondary to GSE consists of avoiding all products containing gluten. Careful reading of the contents of all foods bought in cans or boxes is required. Information on gluten exclusion may be obtained from the Celiac Sprue Society and gluten-free recipes from books such as *Luncheon with Laurie* (Rock Hill, SC, Carpenter). Clinical improvement is expected within 1 to 2 weeks, but intestinal histologic improvement lags. If there is no improvement, the patient should be hospitalized to be certain that an adequate gluten exclusion diet is being eaten. If still no improvement is apparent, the patient should be tested for pancreatic insufficiency or intestinal bacterial overgrowth as complicating factors. The establishment of the diagnosis is important because this is a lifelong problem that requires significant dietary changes. The diagnosis is based on the significant clinical improvement on dietary therapy. Usually the patient, once improved, has a dietary indiscretion that leads to recurrence of symptoms.

TROPICAL SPRUE

Patients who spend more than 1 month in a tropical area where the disease is endemic may be suspected of having this disease. Not all tropical areas are involved. The intestinal histology of this condition is similar to that of GSE. Vitamin B_{12} and folate levels are often reduced.

Treatment. Patients should be given oral folate replacement, 5 mg per day, followed in 1 week by tetracycline therapy, 250 mg four times a day. Improvment is quicker if folate is replaced. Folate should be given for 1 month and tetracycline for 6 months. This regimen prevents relapses from occurring.

COLLAGENOUS SPRUE

In this condition, excessive collagen deposition is seen underneath the epithelial cells of the small intestine. There is no good treatment, although corticosteroids may be tried. The diarrhea may be decreased by reducing the amount of fat in the diet and increasing the percentage of polyunsaturated fatty acids in the fat eaten. MCT oil may be used. A low-calcium diet may also be helpful. Total parenteral nutrition (TPN) may be required to maintain the patient's weight.

RADIATION ENTERITIS

After abdominal irradiation, diarrhea is common and may be treated by diphenoxylate hydrochloride with atropine sulfate (Lomotil) or loperamide (Imodium). This acute radiation-induced diarrhea is usually self-limiting. Many months or years later chronic radiation enteritis may ensue. This is secondary to mucosal atrophy caused by the arteritis induced by the radiation.

Treatment. A low-fat diet with a high proportion of polyunsaturated fatty acids may be tried. MCT oil and a low-calcium diet may also be helpful. TPN may be necessary.

CHRONIC ISCHEMIC BOWEL DISEASE

This disease is caused by a decreased blood supply to the intestine. At least two of the arteries supplying the intestine need to be stenosed to ensure the diagnosis. Patients complain of abdominal cramps after eating and learn to decrease food intake to avoid pain causing weight loss. Diarrhea may be present.

Treatment. Treatment of the disease consists of angioplasty or surgical revascularization. Treatment of the diarrhea is similar to that of radiation enteritis.

SHORT-BOWEL SYNDROME

In this condition, usually caused by surgical resection, the surface area of the intestine is greatly reduced, with reduction in the contact time of nutriments with the intestinal mucosa. If the resection is recent, small oral feedings should be started because enteric nutrition helps to induce adaptation (hypertrophy of the remaining intestinal mucosa). Adaptation is not as great in the proximal intestine after distal resection as it is in the distal intestine after proximal resection.

Treatment. Chemically defined diets, especially those containing casein hydrolyzates, should be used. Those containing crystalline amino acids should be avoided because small peptides are absorbed better than amino acids. These formulations may have to be diluted to avoid the effects of their high osmolar content. Multiple small feedings may be needed. Vitamin and mineral supplements are important and should be given by mouth if possible. Magnesium oxide is preferred to magnesium citrate or magnesium hydroxide because the latter may enhance intestinal motility and thus further shorten the contact time. Calcium supplements should not be given with meals because the calcium may bind to fatty acids, reducing the likelihood of absorbing both the calcium and the fatty acids. In distal resections, vitamin B_{12} malabsorption is expected. This vitamin should be given parenterally. Folate and other water-soluble vitamins should be given by mouth. TPN may also be required.

DEFECTS IN DELIVERING ABSORBED LIPIDS TO THE SYSTEMIC CIRCULATION

Absorbed split triglycerides are resynthesized in the intestinal mucosa to triglycerides, which are transported out of the intestine into the lymph in chylomicrons. Lymph collects in the thoracic duct, which joins the general circulation. The chylomicrons have on their surface apolipoproteins that direct their delivery to specific bodily sites. Beta-lipoprotein synthesis is required for triglyceride transport out of the intestinal absorptive cell.

IMPAIRED LIPOPROTEIN SYNTHESIS

Abetalipoproteinemia is a condition in which the intestine cannot synthesize beta-lipoprotein. The diagnosis is suggested by finding excessive fat in intestinal cells after an overnight fast. Serum cholesterol and triglyceride levels are low. The patients are usually young when first seen and may manifest neurologic and red blood cell abnormalities, as well as growth deficiencies and steatorrhea. Reinfusion of beta-lipoproteins is not curative.

Treatment. Treatment consists of instituting a low-fat diet with a high proportion of polyunsaturated fatty acids. MCT oil is usually required for caloric supplementation.

ABNORMAL LYMPHATIC DRAINAGE

Abnormal lymphatic drainage may be seen in a variety of conditions that impede the normal flow of lymph, such as retroperitoneal fibrosis, lymphoma, metastatic carcinoma, idiopathic lymphangiectasia, and severe right-sided heart failure. Intestinal biopsy reveals club-shaped villi caused by the dilated lymphatics.

Treatment. Treatment should be directed to the specific problem. Chemotherapy for lymphomatous involvement is helpful, as is decortication of patients with constrictive pericarditis. Severe congestive heart failure may respond to appropriate therapy. In conditions such as retroperitoneal fibrosis or intestinal lymphangiectasia, where no specific treatment is available, diarrhea may be greatly reduced by a low-fat diet, with MCT oil as caloric supplementation. Fat-soluble vitamins should be given. Over the long term, these patients should be observed for essential fatty acid deficiency.

WHIPPLE'S DISEASE

Whipple's disease is uncommon but is invariably fatal if not treated. It is found most often in middle-aged to older men. In addition to diarrhea and wasting, these patients usually have arthritis or arthralgias. They may also have fever and lymphadenopathy. The diagnosis is established by small intestinal biopsy, which demonstrates many periodic acid–schiff (PAS)-positive macrophages infiltrating the lamina propria. In patients with the acquired immunodeficiency syndrome, infection with *Mycobacterium avium-intracellulare* may produce a similar picture. These organisms may be distinguished from the Whipple bacterium by electron microscopy or by acid-fast stains.

Treatment. It is important to treat patients with antibiotics that cross the blood-brain barrier to prevent central nervous system manifestations of Whipple's disease, which are usually irreversible and occur later in the course of the disease. Trimethoprim-sulfamethoxazole (Bactrim, Septra) may be given, or streptomycin and penicillin for 10 days, followed by tetracycline, 250 mg four times a day. Patients receiving tetracycline alone are at risk for central nervous system disease. Treatment should be continued for 1 year to prevent relapses. Clinical improvement is usually rapid (1 to 2 weeks). The rare patient who does not improve on this regimen may require chloramphenicol. Severely malnourished individuals may require TPN or other caloric supplements. Repeat intestinal biopsies should show a reduction in the number of PAS-positive macrophages. However, a few macrophages may exist for up to 25 years after successful treatment.

POSTGASTRECTOMY SYNDROMES

Weight loss and malnutrition are often seen after gastrectomy, especially if significant amounts of the stomach have been removed. The reduced gastric receptive relaxation leads to early satiety and a decrease in food intake. Reduction in food intake may also be caused by fear of inducing the dumping syndrome. In this condition, hyperosmolar food is "dumped" into the small intestine more quickly than normal, which induces water secretion into the intestinal lumen to lessen the osmotic load. This reaction may be great enough to induce hypotension with a feeling of faintness. Patients usually learn to lie down when these symptoms appear. Symptoms of hypoglycemia may also be found 2 to 4 hours after meals. This condition is caused by excessive insulinemia for the amount of glucose present in the blood. Symptoms of the early dumping syndrome are usually ameliorated by having the patient eat small, dry meals followed later by liquids. Reduction in carbohydrate intake usually reduces the late manifestations of dumping.

Patients with Billroth II resections are likely (50 per cent) to have steatorrhea. Steatorrhea is seen less often in patients with Billroth I resections or with a parietal cell vagotomy. The steatorrhea results from the poor synchronization of food and pancreaticobiliary secretions. This is because food is placed directly into the jejunum. The amount of CCK-PZ in the jejunal mucosa is much lower than in the duodenum, reducing its output, which further impairs digestion and absorption of the meal. Absorption sites for calcium and iron are also bypassed in patients with gastrojejunostomies.

Treatment. If the patient is symptomatic, pancreatin may be given with meals. If a blind loop syndrome develops as a result of obstruction of the afferent loop, surgical reconstruction should be performed. If this is not possible, treatment with tetracycline is usually efficacious. After gastrectomy, previously silent lactase deficiency or GSE may become clinically manifest. It should be treated appropriately. Bacterial overgrowth may also result from low acid output in the stomach. In this condition, tetracycline should be given. In young or middle-aged patients, osteoporosis is expected as the patient ages. Careful attention to vitamin D and calcium supplementation in the intervening years is helpful.

PARASITIC INFECTION

The most common parasite associated with steatorrhea in the United States is *Giardia lamblia*. Contaminated water, even from mountain streams, is the usual cause. The reason for the malabsorption in this condition is not clear. The cysts of *Giardia* can be demonstrated in the stool, but only 50 per cent of the time. Duodenal intubation to demonstrate trophozoites free in the lumen greatly increases the yield. The best way to identify *Giardia* is on the surface of the intestine. After biopsy of the small bowel, the luminal surface of the biopsy is applied to a glass slide and stained. Giardiasis is especially common in patients with acquired immunodeficiency syndrome and may be reacquired after treatment.

Treatment. Metronidazole* (Flagyl), 250 mg three times a day for 7 to 10 days, or quinacrine (Atabrine), 100 mg three times a day for 5 to 7 days, is effective therapy for this condition. Patients with the acquired immunodeficiency syndrome may have *Isospora belli* infection or cryptosporidosis.

EOSINOPHILIC GASTROENTERITIS

In this condition the eosinophils, which are normally present in the lamina propria of the gastrointestinal tract, infiltrate the glands of the stomach or crypts of the small intestine. This may result in nodulation, which may be identified

---

*This use is not listed by the manufacturer.

on gastrointestinal x-ray examination. Biopsy of the small bowel is helpful.

Treatment. Patients respond rapidly to prednisone, which should be begun at a dose of 20 to 30 mg per day for 7 to 10 days, followed by a tapering dose. Patients who relapse may need additional treatment. If a partial response is seen, therapy may be continued at a dose of 10 to 15 mg per day of prednisone.

CARBOHYDRATE AND PROTEIN MALABSORPTION

The complex carbohydrates seen in starch require breakdown by amylase secreted by the salivary glands, followed by breakdown by amylase secreted by the pancreas. This breakdown partially digests these complex sugars, with final digestion being accomplished by specific hydrolases present at the luminal surface of the small intestine. The final result is the production of monosaccharides that are absorbed by specific transport mechanisms present in the intestinal mucosa. In addition to these complex carbohydrates, disaccharides such as lactose and sucrose require hydrolysis before absorption.

LACTASE DEFICIENCY

Lactase deficiency is the most common malabsorptive condition in the United States. This enzyme is localized to the tips of villi and normally disappears after weaning. However, in people of Northern European extraction and in certain tribes in Africa, lactase levels persist at a high level throughout life. Even in these individuals, after gastroenteritis, which reduces the height of villi, transient lactase deficiency may result. The symptoms occur rapidly after the ingestion of lactose-containing foods such as milk. They include abdominal bloating, cramps, and passage of gas. Acidic diarrhea may also occur, resulting from the increased osmolar load that passes into the colon. Usually the diagnosis is made most simply by having the patient avoid dairy products for 2 weeks and observing the effect on the symptoms. If symptoms persist and lactase deficiency is suspected, a lactose tolerance test or a breath hydrogen test after ingestion of lactose may be performed.

Treatment. Patients who continue to drink milk may do so if the lactose in the milk has been reduced either by lactase enzyme (Lactaid) treatment or by buying currently available lactose-reduced milk, which is available at most stores. The amount of milk or other dairy products that can be ingested by these patients must be individualized because tolerance of lactose varies. Yogurt, especially natural vanilla yogurt, may be a good source of calcium for patients who cannot tolerate any milk products. Calcium and vitamin D supplementation may be required for severly affected individuals.

SELECTIVE ABSORPTION DISORDERS

Rarely, patients are congenitally unable to absorb glucose and galactose. Manifestations of diarrhea are first seen in infancy and result from the congenital absence of the specific transporter of these monosaccharides. Fructose should be substituted for glucose and galactose (the mono-saccharides of sugar).

Several congenital defects in amino acid absorption also exist. Hartnup's disease and cystinuria are the ones most commonly seen. Protein deficiencies do not result from these rare entities because di- and tripeptides containing the neutral amino acids not absorbed in Hartnup's disease or basic amino acids, malabsorbed in cystinuria, are adequately absorbed.

ACUTE PANCREATITIS

method of
JOAQUIN S. ALDRETE, M.D.
The University of Alabama
Birmingham, Alabama

"Acute pancreatitis" is a term that includes a wide spectrum of pathologic conditions involving the pancreas and the peripancreatic spaces. In some instances, the devastating effects of severe acute pancreatitis involve other organ systems, as in the respiratory or renal failure often seen in these patients. The morphologic changes observed in the pancreas vary from mild edema to total necrosis. Thus, the clinical course of acute pancreatitis can vary from a mild, self-limiting illness to a relentlessly lethal process. Therefore, the therapeutic approaches to acute pancreatitis are dictated by the variety of functional and morphologic changes.

The exact etiopathogenesis of acute pancreatitis remains elusive. Some etiologic factors, such as the presence of biliary lithiasis, alcohol abuse, and hyperlipoproteinemia, can be established in some patients. However, at the subcellular level, the exact mechanism by which these or any other possible etiologic factors cause the disease remains to be elucidated.

CATEGORIZATION

Because the clinical manifestations, treatment, and outcome of patients with acute pancreatitis vary so much, some form of categorization is essential. The more relevant one, from the clinician's point of view, categorizes the cases into *mild acute pancreatitis*, char-

TABLE 1. **Acute Mild Pancreatitis**

Morphologic changes: Edema of pancreatic cells, mild interstitial inflammation, no necrosis, minimal amount of fluid in the peripancreatic spaces

Symptoms: Mild epigastric pain, nausea, vomiting

Signs: Mild epigastric tenderness, no peritoneal irritation, no jaundice, mild tachycardia, no obvious hemodynamic changes

Diagnostic investigation: Amylase in serum and urine (elevated level); ultrasound scan to assess biliary system

Treatment: Nothing by mouth, IV fluids, cholecystectomy if indicated

Expected evolution and prognosis: Rapid recovery in most cases, >90% survival rate

acterized by interstitial edema and mild inflammation of the pancreas; *moderate acute pancreatitis*, characterized by diffuse inflammation with focal areas of necrosis in the pancreas; and *severe acute pancreatitis*, characterized by extensive necrosis of the pancreatic parenchyma extending into the peripancreatic spaces, often complicated by local or systemic sepsis, renal failure, respiratory failure, hemorrhage of the pancreas, and hemodynamic instability. Whether these categories of acute pancreatitis occur as sequential stages or independently of each other remains a matter of speculation (Tables 1, 2, and 3).

DIAGNOSIS

Symptoms and Signs

All patients with moderate to severe pain in the midabdomen should be suspected of having acute pancreatitis, and their serum amylase level should be measured. When it is elevated (usually more than 150 IU), the diagnosis of acute pancreatitis is highly prob-

TABLE 2. **Acute Moderate Pancreatitis**

Morphologic changes: Severe diffuse edema, focal necrosis of the acinar epithelium with gross focal but minimal necrosis visible in the pancreas, small amount of fluid in the peripancreatic spaces

Symptoms: Moderate to severe epigastric pain, nausea, vomiting

Signs: Tachycardia, mild abdominal distention, mild peritoneal irritation, tachycardia, no other hemodynamic changes

Diagnostic investigation: Amylase in serum and urine (elevated level); ultrasound scan to assess biliary system, CT scan to assess pancreas

Treatment: Nothing by mouth, IV fluids, antibiotics (?), cholecystectomy if indicated

Expected evolution and prognosis: Improvement in 3–5 days in 70% of patients; 30% progress to severe necrotizing pancreatitis

TABLE 3. **Acute Severe Pancreatitis**

Morphologic changes: Severe inflammation of the pancreas with partial or total necrosis of the organ; necrosis usually extends to the peripancreatic spaces; hemorrhage throughout the pancreas (hemorrhagic pancreatitis) can occur in addition in 10–15% of cases

Symptoms and signs: Severe epigastric or diffuse abdominal pain, nausea, and vomiting; signs of peritoneal irritation may or may not be present; nausea and vomiting, mental confusion, abdominal distention; a mass may be palpable, and high fever can be present; tachycardia, hypotension, and shock can occur in some extreme cases associated with systemic sepsis

Diagnostic investigation: Amylase in serum and urine (elevated levels); electrolyte disturbances, reduced Ca, reduced K, and reduced Na, raised BUN and raised creatinine, reduced Hct. CT scan of the abdomen to assess extension of pancreatic necrosis

Treatment
    Nonoperative: Nothing by mouth, IV fluids and antibiotics, respiratory support and hemodialysis as needed, intensive care, parenteral nutrition

    Operation indicated:
      1. Signs of pancreatic abscess (air bubbles on CT scan)
      2. Uncertain diagnosis; extensive necrosis within or surrounding the pancreas
      3. Lack of improvement after 3 days of supportive treatment with signs of pancreatic necrosis on CT scan

Abbreviations: Ca = calcium; K = potassium; Na = sodium; BUN = blood urea nitrogen; Hct = hematocrit.

able. The findings on physical examination can vary from none or mild epigastric tenderness to prostration and shock. Obviously, the patients with severe forms of pancreatitis have the most noticeable physical findings. These patients can appear to be acutely ill and dehydrated; fever is not uncommon. Tachycardia may be present; hemodynamic instability is present in patients who have bleeding or systemic sepsis. The abdomen may be distended, with decreased or absent bowel sounds. Palpation may reveal a tender epigastric mass or just diffuse, generalized tenderness. True abdominal rigidity is uncommon.

Laboratory Tests

The elevation of the serum amylase level is the main diagnostic clue to acute pancreatitis. The magnitude of this elevation is not in direct proportion to the severity of the disease; it simply indicates an increase in the production of the amylase enzyme by the pancreas, which is assumed to be caused by acute pancreatitis. Serum amylase measurements 24 hours after the onset of a mild attack of acute pancreatitis may reveal normal levels.

Amylase is normally cleared by the kidney at a rate of only about 3 ml per minute, and the amylase/creatinine clearance ratio is about 2.5 per cent. In acute pancreatitis, the amylase cannot be totally reabsorbed by the renal tubule. Defective tubular reabsorption may exist, leading to an increase in urinary

amylase excretion, amylase clearance, and the amylase/creatinine clearance ratio. These measurements are also considered useful in diagnosing acute pancreatitis in questionable cases of hyperamylasemia.

Plain Film Radiographs

Plain film radiographs of the chest are often (70 per cent) abnormal in patients with severe pancreatitis. The most common findings are pleural effusions, left lower lobe consolidation, and widened mediastinum. Plain film radiographs of the abdomen are nonspecific for acute pancreatitis; however, fluid levels and dilatation of the duodenum, gastric dilatation, and generalized intestinal ileus are often found in patients with severe pancreatitis.

Ultrasonography

Ultrasonography can detect both focal and generalized pancreatic enlargement, which may be associated with acute pancreatitis. Ultrasonography is also useful to detect pancreatic pseudocysts and the presence of biliary lithiasis.

Computed Tomography

The image of the acutely inflamed pancreas, as assessed by computed tomography (CT), can vary from normal to greatly disrupted. CT also assesses the involvement of or damage to the peripancreatic spaces; however, it has been estimated that one-third of the patients with acute pancreatitis have a normal-appearing pancreas by CT. Pancreatic enlargement can be noted in two-thirds of the cases, diffuse enlargement in 55 per cent, and focal enlargement in 45 per cent. Blurring of the margins of the pancreatic gland, decreased CT density of the gland, and fluid collections in the peripancreatic spaces are almost always found in moderate or severe pancreatitis. More specifically, in severe necrotizing or hemorrhagic pancreatitis, the CT image of the pancreas is almost always abnormal. Because of the lack of uniformity in the terminology used, it has been difficult to establish firmly how the radiologic descriptions correlate with the different stages of the severe forms of acute pancreatitis, as observed at operation. Terms such as "phlegmon," "pancreatic pseudocyst," "pancreatic fluid collection," and "pancreatic abscess" have, unfortunately, been used indiscriminately by clinicians and radiologists alike, and fulfillment of the capabilities of the imaging procedures in acute pancreatitis has been curtailed by this lack of uniformity in terminology and description. As these imaging procedures are used more frequently, the terminology is becoming more uniform and relevant to the operative findings. The information obtained on CT scans is the most important basis for the decision-making process, indicating the appropriate and timely operative therapy of patients with severe acute pancreatitis.

Endoscopic Retrograde Cholangiopancreatography

Endoscopic retrograde cholangiopancreatography (ERCP) can cause acute pancreatitis; therefore, most expert reviews state that ERCP is contraindicated in the acute phase of this disease. In a few cases of recurrent acute pancreatitis, ERCP can guide effective therapy, but it should be done only after the serum amylase level is normal and the patient has been completely free of symptoms for at least 15 days. These restrictions greatly limit its usefulness.

TREATMENT

General Principles

Although the majority of patients with mild to moderate pancreatitis require a short period of hospitalization without intensive care, patients with severe necrotizing pancreatitis cannot always be identified in the early stages of the disease. Therefore, patients with abdominal pain and hyperamylasemia should be admitted to the hospital.

There is no specific treatment for acute pancreatitis; the traditionally recommended therapeutic maneuvers are based on the principle that the requirements for pancreatic function should be kept at an absolute minimum as the first step in arresting whatever processes are producing the disease. Therefore, before taking specific therapeutic measures, it is essential to discuss a therapeutic concept for acute pancreatitis (Figure 1). This therapeutic concept involves two main areas: the general supportive therapy of the patient, and the operative treatment to correct specific complications or eliminate possible etiologic factors. The supportive measures include restoration and maintenance of the intravascular vol-

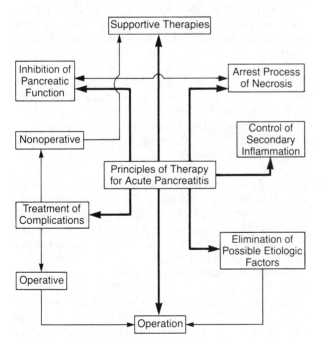

Figure 1. Therapeutic concept of acute pancreatitis.

ume, correction of electrolyte disturbances, and adequate nutritional support, as well as support for failing systems or organs, including mechanical ventilation and hemodialysis when needed.

The general supportive and operative therapies should be complemented by efforts to inhibit pancreatic function, such as nasogastric intubation and administration of anticholinergics, glucagon, or cimetidine. However, none of these agents have proved effective in significantly inhibiting pancreatic secretion in humans. Other experimental approaches designed mainly to arrest the process of necrosis through inactivation of pancreatic enzymes by administering fresh frozen plasma, aprotinin, or soybean trypsin inhibitor; inducing cytoprotection with prostaglandins; and decreasing the inflammatory response with corticosteroids do not affect the course of acute pancreatitis in humans. The recently available synthetic analogue somatostatin (octreotide acetate) appears to be the most promising method of inhibiting pancreatic secretion and function, but its clinical effectiveness has not yet been proved objectively.

Attempts to control secondary inflammation or to interrupt the pathogenesis mechanism, mostly comprising the administration of antibiotics, antacids, heparin, plasmin, low-molecular-weight dextran, and vasopressin, have also been made, but without impressive results.

The treatment of well-identified complications is the only specific therapeutic measure that can be applied to patients with acute pancreatitis; it can vary from correction of electrolyte and fluid imbalances to more invasive measures, such as ventilatory support and hemodialysis. Operative treatment should be reserved for the treatment of etiologic agents, such as biliary lithiasis, and well-identified complications, such as pancreatic pseudocysts, pancreatic abscess, and the removal of necrotic tissue.

Treatment of Mild and Moderate Pancreatitis

Most of these patients show mild dehydration; therefore, intravenous fluids should be given as soon as they are admitted to the hospital. Because most of them receive a nasogastric tube, losses through the tube should be replaced on a volume-for-volume basis, usually with normal saline. Serum electrolyte levels should be checked, and all deficiencies should be corrected. These patients should not be given alimentation directly through the gastrointestinal tract; in fact, removal of gastric juice through nasogastric suction has been advocated as one way to inhibit pancreatic secretion. Sedatives and analgesics should be given as needed. There is no proof that prophylactic antibiotics are useful for these types of pancreatitis; however, wide-spectrum antibiotics, such as cefoxitin, are often used on the empiric premise that they may prevent sepsis in the presence of mild pancreatic necrosis.

As previously noted, a synthetic analogue of somatostatin to inhibit pancreatic function appears promising. It is hoped that the results of trials with this new drug, currently under way, will confirm its effectiveness. As a general rule, the patient should not be given anything by mouth until the amylase level has returned to normal. Most patients with mild to moderate pancreatitis recover from the acute attack within 2 to 5 days; their improvement should be noticeable within 48 hours after admission to the hospital. If it is not, the possibility of a more severe form of the disease should be considered and evaluated with an abdominal CT scan. Once the amylase level returns to normal the nasogastric tube can be removed, and a liquid diet can be given and increased as tolerated to a soft diet. At this point, a decision should be made in regard to cholecystectomy in patients with biliary lithiasis. We recommend elective cholecystectomy during the same hospital admission, or no later than during the next 3 weeks.

Nonoperative Management of Severe Acute Pancreatitis

Because of their more severe and persistent symptoms and signs, most patients with severe acute pancreatitis can be diagnosed at the time of admission or shortly thereafter. Such patients require close observation and intensive nursing care. Their pain is often severe and requires narcotic analgesics. They should be given a nasogastric tube and intravenous fluids to correct fluid and electrolyte imbalances. There is general agreement that prophylactic antibiotics should be given to these patients; cefoxitin and ampicillin are commonly selected. Because gastroduodenal stress ulcerations with bleeding are common complications, they should be prevented by the administration of one of the H_2 receptor antagonists.

Patients with severe pancreatitis may experience severe hemodynamic instability. In many cases, insertion of invasive monitoring devices, such as needles in a radial artery and Swan-Ganz catheters in the pulmonary artery, are justified. When oliguria occurs, a low dose of dopamine, 3 to 5 micrograms per kg per minute, should improve the patient's hemodynamics and, consequently, the renal output. Renal failure occurs frequently in patients with severe pancreatitis, is related to hypovolemia, and is usually prere-

nal. Acute tubular necrosis or cortical necrosis can occur; these conditions can best be prevented by maintaining adequate intravascular volume. When renal failure is established despite the use of diuretics (furosemide), hemodialysis should be promptly instituted. Metabolic complications such as hypoglycemia and hyperglycemia, as well as hypocalcemia, can develop in patients with severe pancreatitis. They should be recognized and treated.

Respiratory failure is common and is indistinguishable from other causes of adult respiratory distress syndrome; therefore, in patients who are seriously ill, serial measurements of arterial blood gases should be done. A falling Po_2 is always a worrisome sign; endotracheal intubation and mechanical ventilation should be promptly established when respiratory failure appears inevitable. Positive end-expiratory pressure is helpful to maintain adequate Po_2 in hypoxemic patients who require high fractional expiratory oxygen concentrations (FI_{O_2} more than 50 per cent). Some of these patients require prolonged respiratory support on a ventilator. When they improve, they should be weaned from the ventilator slowly, with close observation and guidance by improvements in Po_2, compliance, tidal volume, and vital capacity.

Once it is recognized that a patient has severe acute pancreatitis, a central line should be inserted and intravenous hyperalimentation begun. Such patients will probably not be able to eat for at least 3 weeks, and adequate nutritional support is essential.

The use of peritoneal lavage, with catheters such as those used for peritoneal dialysis, has been advocated by many authors as an effective method to treat or ameliorate the effects of severe acute pancreatitis. However, several prospective randomized studies have not documented the efficacy of peritoneal lavage in diminishing the mortality or morbidity of these patients. Furthermore, although the rationale for peritoneal lavage is that "toxins" freely floating in the peritoneal cavity are diluted or removed by this method, it is clear that pancreatic necrosis occurs primarily in the lesser sac and usually extends into the retroperitoneal space, rather than into the free peritoneal cavity. It appears unrealistic to think that lavaging the free peritoneum can reduce or eliminate necrosis located in a separate peritoneal compartment.

Needle aspiration done blindly or under radiologic guidance should be avoided in patients with suspected pancreatic necrosis, even if they have fluid. The problem is the thick necrotic tissue that does not drain even through large catheter tubes. In our experience, this procedure usually offers no diagnostic or therapeutic benefits and, not uncommonly, contaminates an area of pancreatic necrosis that was previously uninfected.

Operative Treatment of Severe Pancreatitis

It is essential to recognize that in patients with acute necrotizing pancreatitis, hemorrhagic pancreatitis, or both, operative treatment can only be directed at the complications of the disease. It does not interrupt the pathogenesis of the necrotic or hemorrhagic process affecting the pancreas.

The decision on when to operate on a patient with severe pancreatitis remains difficult. Once the surgeon is convinced that there is extensive necrosis in the pancreas and peripancreatic tissues, based on the CT scan of the abdomen and the deteriorating clinical condition of the patient, serious consideration should be given to operating promptly to remove the necrotic tissue. Similar indications for surgery are applicable to "enlarging pancreatic pseudocysts" (>10 cm in diameter), which in the acute stage are actually fluid collections frequently associated with extensive necrosis in the pancreas and peripancreatic tissues. Nonspecific indications for operation, or operations to drain the gallbladder or place a tube gastrostomy or tube jejunostomy for feeding purposes, usually do not benefit the patient. Uncertainty about the diagnosis and the possibility or other abdominal catastrophes, such as infarcted bowel or perforated viscus, can also indicate the need for operation. Once the decision to operate has been made, a serious commitment is implied on the part of the surgeon to continue the intensive nonoperative treatment. There is also a strong possibility of repeated operations to remove and drain persistent necrotic tissue. The operation is done through a subcostal, often bilateral, incision. The free ascitic fluid is aspirated, the abdomen is carefully evaluated, and then the lesser sac is entered and the pancreas and its surroundings are examined. Then the necrotic tissue is carefully removed. This is best accomplished by "scooping out" the tissue, rather than by doing a formal pancreatectomy, which, in most cases, is nearly impossible because the anatomic margins have been destroyed by the necrotic process. Several closed system–type drains are left to irrigate and drain the area continuously. The continuous irrigation keeps the catheters open and removes the loose debris, but the thick residual necrotic tissue can be directly removed only at reoperation.

When infection appears in the necrotic tissue, a pancreatic or peripancreatic abscess, or both, develop. This abscess should also be treated by open drainage, packing, and removal of the necrotic tissue, sometimes leaving the lesser sac and pancreatic bed wide open into the open incision.

Extreme care should be taken to drain the complete area of necrosis and to avoid erosion or intrusion into one of the neighboring blood vessels. Often the process of necrosis obliterates most of the minor blood vessels in and around the pancreas; the entire lesser sac is packed with gauze rolls and left completely open. The dressings are changed under sterile conditions, preferably in the operating room, where the necrotic tissue can be débrided manually. The thickness of the necrotic material is the best confirmation that percutaneous drainage or needle aspiration is not totally effective in removing this thickened, often "sticky," necrotic tissue. In fact, two or three more operations are sometimes needed to complete its removal.

When the CT scan shows moderate pancreatic necrosis and fluid collections that measure 5 cm or less in diameter, aspiration or intervention is usually not needed. Follow-up CT scans eventually show spontaneous resolution of most of these "pseudocysts." However, when these fluid collections are more than 6 cm in diameter, they are often associated with extensive pancreatic necrosis that requires operation, as described earlier. Some patients with segmental pancreatic necrosis do not require operation during the acute phase, but their fluid collection becomes a pancreatic pseudocyst that usually measures 6 cm or more and often becomes symptomatic. Such patients should be treated by internal drainage of this well-established, noninfected cyst into a defunctionalized limb of jejunum (Roux-en-Y method).

CHRONIC PANCREATITIS

method of
MICHAEL G. SARR, M.D., and
JON A. VAN HEERDEN, M.D.
Mayo Clinic and Mayo Foundation
Rochester, Minnesota

Chronic pancreatitis is a difficult management problem for physicians and surgeons alike. Not only does chronic progressive pancreatic injury affect both pancreatic endocrine and exocrine functions, but associated inflammatory and fibrotic changes within and around the pancreas may lead to biliary and duodenal obstruction, may cause structural damage in surrounding organs, and may induce a debilitating, chronic pain syndrome. Because no single treatment is appropriate in all patients and because many proposed medical and surgical therapies remain controversial, the spectrum of chronic pancreatitis presents as a diverse and fascinating disease process.

ETIOLOGY

Throughout the world, the most common cause of chronic pancreatitis is chronic, persistent alcohol abuse. This effect of alcohol, although still poorly understood from the standpoint of pathogenesis, is well known to be a dose-related phenomenon. However, the detrimental effect of alcohol on the pancreas appears to vary in different individuals; some individuals may consume equal or greater daily amounts of alcohol and yet exhibit few, if any, pancreatic parenchymal changes. Other causes of chronic pancreatitis are much less common; these include a hereditary pancreatitis, an idiopathic form, and possibly forms of persistent pancreatic injury related to a partial anatomic, structural, or functional obstruction to the egress of pancreatic exocrine secretion into the duodenum. Whether the consequences of gallstone disease can lead to chronic pancreatitis is unclear. Although a direct causal relationship between gallstones and acute (gallstone) pancreatitis is undisputed, it is unclear whether the related, intermittent passage of gallstones through the ampulla into the duodenum, or chronic choledocholithiasis, can injure the ampulla and induce a chronic progressive pancreatic injury.

SYMPTOMS

The clinical spectrum of chronic pancreatitis is quite diverse. In some patients, the disease process remains subclinical and asymptomatic. Progressive pancreatic destruction may eventually lead to pancreatic endocrine insufficiency and diabetes mellitus or to pancreatic exocrine insufficiency and maldigestion (steatorrhea). Pancreatic insufficiency usually occurs when pancreatic enzyme production has fallen to 10 per cent or less of its capacity. Rarely, this exocrine insufficiency may give rise to vitamin B_{12} malabsorption. Pain syndromes may manifest as repeated episodes of acute abdominal pain (chronic relapsing pancreatitis) or as the progressive development of a chronic debilitating pain syndrome with associated narcotic analgesic addiction. The pain usually has a boring epigastric quality that radiates to the back and prevents sleep and productive function in society. The patient with chronic pancreatitis may, at times, present with upper gastrointestinal hemorrhage from esophagogastric varices, which are secondary to splenic vein thrombosis (sinistral or left-sided portal hypertension). The common denominators in most of these varied presentations are the presence of destruction and inflammation within the pancreas superimposed on the setting of chronic alcoholism.

DIAGNOSIS

The diagnosis is usually not difficult and should be highly suspect in most patients with these symptoms. Radiographic imaging techniques aid in confirming the clinical impression. Diffuse pancreatic calcifica-

tions seen on plain radiographs are relatively specific but are present in only approximately one-third of patients. Computed axial tomography or ultrasonography may reveal an enlarged gland with surrounding inflammatory changes, but, in the absence of calcification, this picture does not necessarily signify chronic pancreatitis. Endoscopic retrograde cholangiopancreatography (ERCP) provides one of the best objective means of confirming the diagnosis. Changes of primary and secondary pancreatic ductal irregularity, narrowing or saccular dilatations ("chain-of-lakes" appearance), associated pseudocysts, and pancreatic ductal stones are pathognomonic, and virtually all patients harbor some form of these changes on ERCP. Pancreatic function tests, such as Lund's meal, the secretin stimulation test, or the bentiromide and pancreolauryl tests, can usually document the presence of pancreatic exocrine insufficiency in advanced cases. Demonstration of abnormalities of exocrine secretion in less-advanced cases is less reliable.

TREATMENT

Management of the patient with chronic pancreatitis must assume a supportive role because the pancreatic damage is in large part irreversible. Discontinuation of all alcohol ingestion (in an attempt to prevent further glandular injury) and enrollment of the patient in some form of alcoholic rehabilitation program should be foremost. From a practical standpoint, treatment addresses the symptoms and complications that may arise.

Endocrine and Exocrine Insufficiency

Generally, about 90 per cent of the pancreatic parenchyma must be destroyed before pancreatic insufficiency is evident. Endocrine insufficiency manifests as diabetes mellitus and is treated as such with dietary modifications, oral hypoglycemics when possible, or, in a few selected patients, daily insulin administration. Insulin requirements are less than those in most spontaneous diabetics and in contrast to genetic diabetes, these patients have no tendency toward ketoacidosis, are seldom resistant to insulin, and are often thin and malnourished. Exocrine insufficiency is best managed by oral pancreatic enzyme replacement with sufficient doses of Viokase, Pancrease, or Cotazym with each meal to improve the maldigestion and the associated malabsorption and steatorrhea.

Pain

Pain remains the most difficult complication of chronic pancreatitis to treat effectively. All attempts at nonoperative management should be exhausted before surgical intervention is considered. The acute episodes of chronic relapsing pancreatitis are managed expectantly as for acute pancreatitis. However, when chronic pain becomes established, a multidisciplinary approach is necessary. Pancreatic pain can become debilitating and may be difficult or impossible to manage with non-narcotic analgesics. Nevertheless, every effort should be made to avoid use of narcotic analgesics. The introduction of narcotics sets the stage for a secondary drug dependency and addiction, which compounds the problem and makes it more difficult to differentiate visceral pain from narcotic withdrawal. Some investigators have provided evidence that oral pancreatic enzyme replacement therapy may ameliorate (not relieve) the pain of chronic pancreatitis in some patients by a still controversial feedback regulation of pancreatic exocrine function. Use of percutaneous celiac plexus block in an attempt to block afferent visceral pain fibers from the pancreas may provide transient relief (3 to 6 months) in a small percentage of patients and should be entertained. In some patients, the chronic pain syndrome is refractory to all the treatment modalities mentioned, and surgical therapy should be considered. Most investigators believe that the chronic pain from chronic pancreatitis eventually resolves; however, this resolution may take years and the physician must weigh the risks of operative intervention and its expected benefits and limitations against the quality of life of the patient and whether or not he or she can function satisfactorily.

When surgical therapy is necessary, the surgeon's principal concern should be the status of the pancreatic duct on ERCP (or on a good computed axial tomographic scan). If the pancreatic duct is dilated (>7 mm), a ductal drainage procedure is indicated. This usually entails opening the pancreatic duct for *its entire length* and anastomosing the "filleted" duct to a Roux-en-Y limb of jejunum—the so-called lateral pancreaticojejunostomy (Puestow's procedure). This is a safe procedure with little morbidity or mortality, and good results can be expected in about 80 per cent of patients. This procedure relieves the associated pancreatic ductal hypertension (the possible cause of the pain), preserves pancreatic endocrine function, and allegedly preserves exocrine function by preventing further pancreatic parenchymal destruction. Attempts to promote better pancreatic ductal drainage by operative or endoscopic sphincterotomy or by distal pancreatectomy and distal pancreaticojejunostomy (Duval's procedure) alone are doomed to failure because of associated pancreatic ductal stones or multiple strictures.

When the pancreatic duct is not dilated (small duct or parenchymal disease), a formal pancreatic resection may be undertaken. Such ablative procedures should be avoided when possible because they sacrifice pancreatic endocrine and exocrine functions, are technically demanding, are accompanied by significant morbidity and mortality, and are far from uniformly successful. The preservation of endocrine or exocrine function is not as important in patients with overt pancreatic insufficiency but can be an important consideration in the poorly compliant alcoholic patient who may be rendered diabetic and dependent on parenteral insulin and oral pancreatic enzyme replacement postoperatively. Pancreatic resection should be directed at the major site of glandular involvement. This operation usually entails resection of the head of the gland (pancreaticoduodenectomy or Whipple's procedure), resection of the body and tail of the gland (distal or 80 per cent subtotal pancreatectomy), or, in selected patients, resection of the entire pancreas (total pancreatectomy). These procedures carry a definite morbidity (approximately 20 per cent) and mortality (1 to 4 per cent), which must be acknowledged by both surgeon and patient. Such pancreatic resections give satisfactory long-term pain relief in 60 to 80 per cent of patients. Previous attempts at autotransplanting the islets of Langerhans (islet cell autotransplantation) from the resected pancreas to the spleen or liver have generally proved to be unsuccessful.

Surgical pancreatic denervations, an extension of the percutaneous celiac plexus block, were designed as a more complete denervation of the pancreatic parenchyma by interrupting visceral afferent pain fibers. Many modifications have included transthoracic greater and lesser splanchnic neurotomies and transabdominal celiac and superior mesenteric ganglionectomies, but the long-term results in general have been disappointing. Recently, some interest has been generated by encouraging preliminary results with other forms of complete pancreatic denervation by autotransplanting the body and tail of the gland into the pelvis; however, the long-term success remains unknown.

Inflammatory Complications

The progressive fibrosing reaction of chronic pancreatitis may cause a cicatrixing obstruction of either the proximal duodenum or the intrapancreatic portion of the common bile duct, which requires operative relief in the form of an enteric or biliary bypass. Pancreatic pseudocysts are not uncommon complications of chronic pancreatitis and, if symptomatic, are indications for operative intervention to provide enteric drainage and relief of symptoms. The peripancreatic inflammatory changes have been associated with visceral artery aneurysms (splenic or gastroduodenal arteries) that can rupture and bleed into the stomach or into the pancreatic duct (hemosuccus pancreaticus). Similarly, splenic vein thrombosis may occur and lead to left-sided or sinistral portal hypertension, gastric varices, and intragastric hemorrhage necessitating curative splenectomy.

The best treatment of chronic pancreatitis is prevention. Chronic pancreatitis should be considered to be a medical disease until the patient proves to be a chronic medical failure or develops a serious complication; only then should surgical intervention be entertained.

PEPTIC ULCER

method of
JAMES H. LEWIS, M.D.
Georgetown University Medical Center
Washington, D.C.

The pathogenesis of peptic ulcer disease (PUD) is multifactorial, and it is important that any therapeutic approach to ulcer healing address those factors that may be associated with an increased risk of PUD. These factors include continued smoking, the use of aspirin and other nonsteroidal anti-inflammatory drugs (NSAIDs), and certain underlying diseases (e.g., chronic lung disease, chronic renal failure, hyperparathyroidism). The relationship between PUD and environmental or emotional stress remains largely unproved, although most clinicians continue to recommend stress reduction techniques for selected patients. Similarly, diet therapy has never been shown to significantly alter the course of duodenal ulcer (DU) disease and has been relegated to a position of minor importance. The Ingle-finger diet (three regular meals daily with avoidance of a bedtime snack or any foods or beverages that cause symptoms) seems the most sensible.

The natural history of PUD is one of recurrent exacerbations and remissions. Although the overall incidence of DU appears to be declining, the complication rate from ulcer disease has remained relatively constant, despite the introduction of the H$_2$ blockers and other new ulcer agents. Whether or not PUD ever eventually "burns itself out" after one or more decades (as has been suggested) is not known with any certainty. As a result, ulcer disease should be regarded as a chronic disorder and treated accordingly.

The role played by *Campylobacter pylori* in the pathogenesis of ulcer disease and its inherent tendency to relapse remains controversial. *C. pylori* is currently regarded as an important cause of nonerosive gastritis, which is found in most (but not all) patients with PUD, and which has been associated with many instances of

ulcer relapse. However, since *C. pylori* is also seen in approximately 20 per cent of asymptomatic individuals (nearly all of whom harbor unsuspected nonerosive gastritis), the relationship between the organism and dyspeptic symptoms has not been fully defined. Nor has the issue of whether to look for and/or treat *C. pylori* infection been settled, as will be discussed.

TREATMENT
Duodenal Ulcer
Short-Term Therapy

Several dozen pharmacologic agents have been developed for the treatment of DU. These drugs fall into four general categories: (1) acid-neutralizing agents, (2) antisecretory drugs, (3) mucosal protective compounds, and (4) compounds with both antisecretory and mucosal protective properties (Table 1). No clinically important differences exist in the ability of any of the currently available agents to heal ulcers acutely or to relieve ulcer symptoms. Between 60 and 80 per cent of DUs heal endoscopically at 4 weeks. Continuing therapy for an additional 2 or 4 weeks will increase healing to 90 per cent or more. Even ulcers treated with placebos heal 25 to 60 per cent of the time depending on geographic location.

Since healing and symptom relief are similar regardless of which agent is prescribed, the remaining factors that govern the rational choice of ulcer therapy must center on the issues of drug safety (adverse effects and drug interactions) and patient acceptability (compliance and cost) as discussed later.

TABLE 1. **Ulcer-Healing Drugs**

Class	Examples
Acid neutralizing	Antacids
Antisecretory	
H$_2$ receptor antagonists	Cimetidine, ranitidine, famotidine, nizatidine
Muscarinic receptor antagonists	
Nonselective	Anticholinergics
Selective	Pirenzepine*
Gastrin antagonists	Proglumide*
Tricyclic antidepressants	Trimipramine*
Cell activation inhibitors	
Calcium entry blockers	Verapamil,* nifedipine*
Proton pump inhibitors	Omeprazole*
Mucosal protective	
Sulfated disaccharides	Sucralfate
Bismuth compounds	De-Nol,* Pepto-Bismol*
Licorice derivatives	Carbenoxolone,* Caved-S*
Antisecretory-cytoprotective	
Prostaglandins E$_1$, E$_2$	Misoprostol,* enprostil*

*Not approved by the U.S. Food and Drug Administration for ulcer treatment.

Antacids

Antacids are a time-honored therapy for peptic ulcer disease but are inconvenient because of a dosing schedule that generally calls for 30 to 60 ml of a liquid suspension to be taken 1 and 3 hours after meals and at bedtime. Even the use of lower acid-neutralizing capacity products or tablet antacid regimens requires dosing at least four times daily. Bowel dysfunction is common, with diarrhea resulting from magnesium-containing preparations and constipation from aluminum-containing products. Mineral and electrolyte disturbances, variable sodium content, the ability to interfere with the absorption of numerous drugs (including cimetidine, ranitidine, digoxin, tetracycline, and isoniazid), and the fact that the cost of therapeutic amounts of many antacids can be more expensive than other classes of agents are several additional reasons why antacids are currently unattractive to many patients as well as physicians.

H₂ Blockers

These agents reduce acid secretion through competitive inhibition of the H_2 receptor on the parietal cell. Tens of millions of patients have been treated with cimetidine (Tagamet) and ranitidine (Zantac), and the safety and compliance profiles that have emerged for each drug are excellent. Short-term healing rates and symptom reduction are virtually identical for the two medications. The compounds are, however, structurally dissimilar, cimetidine having an imidazole ring and ranitidine a furan ring. This chemical difference probably accounts for many, if not all, of the important potential clinical differences that have become apparent between the two drugs. Famotidine (Pepcid) and nizatidine (Axid) are the two newest agents in this class. Both possess a thiazole ring structure. However, clinical experience continues to be limited in comparison with cimetidine and ranitidine, and the complete safety profiles of famotidine and nizatidine remain to be defined. Neither agent appears to offer any advantages in terms of clinical efficacy, safety, or compliance as compared with ranitidine.

Perhaps the most important distinction to be made among the H_2 blockers is the potential for cimetidine to inhibit the hepatic cytochrome P-450 mixed-function oxidase (MFO) system. The result of this MFO inhibition is a reduction in hepatic clearance, leading to an increased serum concentration of many drugs, including warfarin, theophylline, phenytoin, benzodiazepines, lidocaine, and propranolol. In some patients these increased blood levels may result in clinically evident toxicity: e.g., bleeding from warfarin; arrhythmias, diarrhea, and convulsions from theophylline; nystagmus, ataxia, and confusion

from phenytoin; and so on. Ranitidine, famotidine, and nizatidine have at most only one-tenth the affinity of cimetidine to inhibit the P-450 MFO system, and suspected instances of drug interactions are very rare.

The antiandrogenic effects seen with cimetidine (impotence, gynecomastia, and breast tenderness) generally do not occur unless the drug is taken in large doses for long periods of time (e.g., in Zollinger-Ellison syndrome). Ranitidine is not antiandrogenic and has been used successfully in patients with these cimetidine-induced antiandrogenic effects. Both famotidine and nizatidine appear to be devoid of antiandrogenic side effects. Headaches are probably the most commonly reported side effect seen with ranitidine and famotidine. Mental confusion has been reported with all four drugs, but it anecdotally appears to be more common in cimetidine recipients, especially those with multiple organ failure in an intensive care unit setting.

None of the currently available H_2 blockers is intrinsically hepatotoxic, although mild hepatic dysfunction and rare instances of overt hepatitis have been reported for all four agents. The incidence and clinical severity of hepatitis appear similar for cimetidine and ranitidine. Instances of hepatitis were identified during clinical trials of both famotidine and nizatidine, and the true incidence of hepatic injury remains to be defined for these two newer H_2 blockers. There are no reports of hepatitis from the intravenous use of these drugs. The potential use of cimetidine in the prevention of hepatic injury from acute acetaminophen overdose remains theoretical and investigational. No instances of acetaminophen-induced liver injury have been reported in volunteers or patients receiving ranitidine or the newer H_2 blockers.

Each H_2 blocker is effective when used twice daily, and all have been approved for use as a single bedtime dose to control nocturnal acid and improve patient compliance. The move to bedtime dosing (800 mg cimetidine; 300 mg ranitidine; 40 mg famotidine; and 300 mg nizatidine) is based in part on the pioneering work on vagotomy conducted more than 40 years ago by the American surgeon Lester Dragstedt. His studies suggested that nocturnal acid secretion is most important in terms of ulcer pathogenesis. Recent studies indicate that taking the H_2 blocker just after the evening meal may be an even more effective means of controlling acid and healing ulcers in smokers and in patients with large ulcers.

Other Antisecretory Drugs

Anticholinergics are not suited for primary therapy of peptic ulcer disease because of inferior healing rates and unwanted side effects. Their role is presently confined to that of adjunctive therapy in certain patients with the Zollinger-Ellison syndrome and other hypersecretory states that are poorly controlled with H_2 blockers. But even here, newer agents (e.g., omeprazole) may soon make this role obsolete.

Tricyclic antidepressants are not officially approved for use in peptic ulcer disease, but they have been successfully employed in ulcer patients requiring psychotropic drug therapy. Whether or not their effects are additive to those of H_2 blockers or other agents remains speculative. *Pirenzepine* is a drug with selective antimuscarinic and tricyclic antidepressant properties that is in use outside of the United States. Clinical experience has not demonstrated any advantages over H_2 blockers.

Omeprazole, a substituted benzimidazole, is a potent inhibitor of the H^+/K^+ ATPase (proton) pump of the parietal cell. It has been recommended for use in Zollinger-Ellison syndrome and for short-term treatment of severe reflux esophagitis that is unresponsive to other therapy. Omeprazole was not recommended by the U.S. Food and Drug Administration (FDA) Gastrointestinal Drugs Advisory Committee for uncomplicated peptic ulcer disease because it was not thought to offer any distinct advantage over the H_2 blockers in terms of healing or pain relief at the 20-mg dose over a 4-week period, and because of potential safety concerns. Gastric carcinoid tumors developed in rats during long-term toxicity trials, presumably the result of achlorhydria-induced hypergastrinemia. The carcinogenic potential of omeprazole and its long-term safety profile in patients with non–Zollinger-Ellison syndrome disorders have not been defined. Its use in refractory PUD is currently under consideration.

Mucosal Protective Drugs

A number of agents that heal ulcers through mechanisms other than inhibition or neutralization of gastric acid have been termed "mucosal protective." *Sucralfate* (Carafate), the aluminum salt of sucrose octasulfate, is a coating agent that is thought to enhance mucosal defenses. It has been in use for more than 17 years in various countries and has proved to be an excellent alternative therapy for short-term treatment of DUs. Although some patients have complained of slower initial pain relief compared with H_2 blockers, overall healing efficacy and symptom reduction at the end of 4- to 8-week trials are not significantly different from those of other agents.

Constipation is the most commonly reported side effect with sucralfate, the result of the high aluminum content of the compound. Since su-cralfate is very poorly absorbed, no systemic side effects are expected. However, it may interfere with the absorption of other agents, such as tetracycline and phenytoin. Accordingly, it should not be given concomitantly with other drugs and should be taken at least 30 minutes prior to meals to avoid being bound to food. Although initially designed to be given as 1 gram four times daily, twice daily regimens may be equally effective but are not currently approved by the FDA.

Synthetic *prostaglandin* analogues of the E_1 and E_2 classes remain investigational for the treatment of DU in the United States. Although healing efficacy is similar to that of the H_2 blockers, no clinical advantages over these or other agents have emerged, and concerns about safety (e.g., diarrhea and abdominal cramps in 15 to 39 per cent of recipients and the potential abortofacient effects of misoprostol [Cytotec]) continue to delay FDA approval for use in PUD. However, misoprostol was recently approved for short-term prevention of NSAID-induced gastric (but not duodenal) ulcers, as will be discussed later.

Combination Ulcer Therapy

Antacids are widely prescribed with H_2 blockers and other agents to help control ulcer symptoms, although they are usually unnecessary for this purpose. Only a few studies have examined the usefulness of two or more therapeutically active agents taken together to promote ulcer healing. In one well-controlled trial, no advantage was found for the combination of cimetidine plus sucralfate (both given four times a day) compared with either agent used alone. It is doubtful that any other combination would be of additional benefit. Combination therapy for bleeding ulcers or refractory ulcers has not been well studied.

Follow-up

In contrast to gastric ulcers, it is generally not necessary to document healing of a DU following short-term therapy. If ulcer symptoms remain well controlled throughout the course of treatment, most physicians do not repeat the endoscopy or upper gastrointestinal tract series, even though it is well known that there is a poor correlation between symptoms and the presence or absence of the ulcer after therapy with H_2 blockers. On the other hand, if the symptomatic response at the end of therapy is not satisfactory, or if an ulcer relapse is suspected, it may be useful to document healing (or nonhealing) to help determine the direction that future therapy or additional diagnostic evaluation should take.

Prevention

Endoscopic studies have consistently revealed that up to 80 per cent of healed ulcers will relapse endoscopically within 1 year after therapy is withdrawn. This relapse rate is virtually the same, regardless of whether healing is accomplished with antacids, H$_2$ blockers, sucralfate, omeprazole, pirenzepine, or other agents and no matter how long the acute therapy is extended prior to being discontinued. The one exception appears to be bismuth compounds, which are associated with significantly lower relapse rates after acute healing than occur after treatment with H$_2$ blockers. This has been attributed to the eradication of *C. pylori* infection and resolution of the accompanying gastric (and possibly duodenal) inflammation.

Since most DUs remain in remission only during the time that active therapy is being administered, a number of long-term treatment approaches have been developed. The most commonly employed method utilizes a low dose of an H$_2$ blocker (usually half of the nocturnal dose used for short-term healing, e.g., cimetidine, 400 mg; ranitidine, 150 mg; famotidine, 20 mg; or nizatidine, 150 mg) given daily at bedtime. One-year DU relapse rates can be reduced from 80 per cent to 20 or 30 per cent using these agents, with the relapse rate for patients on ranitidine thought to be somewhat lower than that for cimetidine. Much less information and clinical experience is available for other agents. Maintenance therapy with sucralfate, 1 gram twice daily, is effective but currently lacks FDA approval for this indication. Antacids given several times throughout the day have been shown to be as effective as other agents. However, they are not effective when given only at bedtime and are not recommended by this author for patients with a severe underlying ulcer diathesis.

Continuous daily maintenance therapy is not necessary or indicated for all patients with PUD. Those with either a first time, uncomplicated DU or no important relapse risk factors (Table 2) can usually be followed expectantly. If a symptomatic ulcer relapse occurs, these individuals are often

TABLE 2. Predictors of Ulcer Relapse

Strongly Associated

Cigarette smoking
Poor compliance with maintenance therapy
Incomplete healing after initial therapy
Acid hypersecretion
Continued use of nonsteroidal anti-inflammatory drugs
Prior ulcer complications (e.g., bleeding)
Presence of *C. pylori* infection

Possibly Associated

Family history of ulcer disease
Psychologic stress
Alcohol ingestion

treated with full-dose therapy for several weeks (intermittent therapy). Patients who develop frequent symptomatic relapses or who have a history of an ulcer-related complication such as hemorrhage or obstruction become candidates for continuous daily maintenance therapy with H$_2$ blockers (Figure 1).

A small number of patients will experience a "breakthrough" relapse while on maintenance therapy. These relapses tend to be clinically mild, relatively easy to reheal, and less likely to be associated with ulcer complications compared with relapses that develop in individuals not receiving preventative therapy.

Just how long maintenance therapy can or should be continued is unclear at this time. To date, the longest controlled maintenance trials conducted with H$_2$ blockers have lasted only 5 to 6 years. However, cumulative relapse rates suggest that an ulcer that remains healed during the first year of maintenance therapy will continue to do so during subsequent years. Few adverse side effects from long-term continuous administration of the H$_2$ blockers in maintenance doses have been observed or are expected. While some individuals have expressed concern that gastric cancer might develop from prolonged exposure to these agents, this complication remains more theoretical than practical, as it has not been borne out in experimental or clinical studies.

For patients in whom chronic (perhaps several years and even possibly lifelong) maintenance therapy is recommended but is not acceptable for reasons such as cost, compliance, or the potential for long-term side effects, consideration should be given to a surgical means of ulcer prevention. Highly selective (proximal) vagotomy has been favored over more conventional operations (vagotomy and pyloroplasty or antrectomy) in some European centers. Although it has a lower perioperative and postoperative morbidity and mortality rate compared with more conventional operations, it also has a higher recurrence rate and has fallen out of favor with many U.S. surgeons. Nevertheless, its recurrence rate of 2 to 3 per cent per year compares quite favorably with an annual relapse rate of 20 to 30 per cent for medical therapy.

Gastric Ulcer

Short-Term Therapy

The same drugs used in DU therapy are used to treat gastric ulcers (GU), but the healing rates are generally 10 to 25 per cent lower than those observed for DU, reflecting, in part, differences in the pathophysiology of the two conditions. In European trials, omeprazole has been shown to

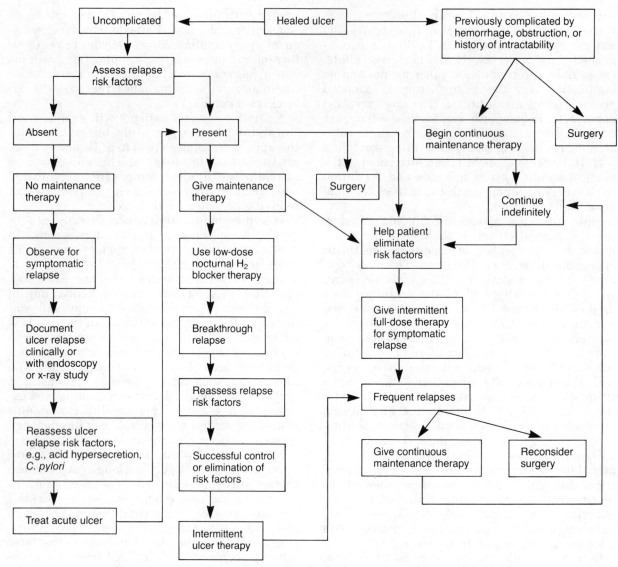

Figure 1. Prevention of peptic ulcer relapse.

have superior GU healing rates compared with H$_2$ blockers, but its use is not indicated for this indication in the United States.

The risk of a non–drug-related GU being malignant (approximately 1 to 3 per cent) mandates that all GUs be followed endoscopically or radiographically until they heal completely. A combination of endoscopically directed biopsies and brushings for cytologic findings can accurately exclude malignancy in over 99 per cent of cases and should be obtained early in all patients in whom the endoscopic or radiographic findings are equivocal or suspicious for gastric cancer.

Most benign GUs can be expected to heal after 6 to 8 weeks of therapy with an H$_2$ blocker. For some others, up to 15 weeks may be required for healing, depending on their size. It should be remembered that even a malignant GU can par-

tially heal on therapy. Therefore, any GU that does not heal completely on an intensive medical regimen after an appropriate length of time (e.g., 8 to 12 weeks for ulcer diameter < 2.5 cm and 12 to 15 weeks for an ulcer > 2.5 cm) should be seriously considered for surgery.

NSAID-Related Gastroduodenal Injury

Approximately 20 per cent of chronic NSAID users develop either a GU or DU, the majority of which are asymptomatic. The analgesic effects of aspirin and other NSAIDs may mask the pain of an ulcer and represent one possible reason for the poor correlation between NSAID injury and symptoms. These patients, however, remain at increased risk for ulcer-related complications such as hemorrhage and perforation with continued NSAID use. Healing of NSAID-related ulcers can be accomplished by using H_2 blockers, sucralfate, or misoprostol in standard doses, despite the continued administration of the NSAID.

The only agent currently approved by the FDA for the prevention of NSAID-induced ulcers is misoprostol. It is indicated, however, for only short-term (e.g., 3-month) protection of GUs at a dose of 100 to 200 micrograms four times daily with meals and at bedtime. Secretory diarrhea and abdominal cramps develop in some patients, and relief of NSAID-related pain was not significantly different from placebo in controlled trials. The drug is contraindicated in pregnancy and in women of childbearing potential unless they are using effective contraception. Postmenopausal bleeding has been reported to some older women.

Many unanswered questions remain about which course of action is best to minimize NSAID injury and about defining which NSAID users might benefit most from preventive therapy.

Refractory Ulcers

Approximately 10 to 25 per cent of DUs remain unhealed after 4 to 8 weeks, regardless of the agent employed. Noncompliance with the prescribed treatment regimen, cigarette smoking, the continued use of NSAIDs, and gastric acid hypersecretion are the most common reasons why ulcers fail to heal. Several early reports of "cimetidine-resistant" DUs that were subsequently responsive to ranitidine have appeared. However, in most instances the initial treatment period was only 4 to 6 weeks. This may have been too short a time to label an ulcer as truly "resistant," and it is equally as likely that continued treatment with cimetidine for an additional 2 to 4 weeks would have resulted in the same rate of healing as was accomplished by switching to ranitidine. Actual "resistance" to an active agent due to genetic or other factors is thought to be exceedingly rare.

If, however, an ulcer is judged to be refractory to a standard course of H_2 blocker therapy, treatment options include (1) continuing the same drug at the same or a higher dose, (2) adding a second agent such as sucralfate or an anticholinergic, or (3) switching to a completely different class of agent, e.g., omeprazole. In our unit many patients with refractory ulcers have been found to have idiopathic hypersecretion of acid. We have had good success treating these patients with increased doses of H_2 blockers to keep the basal acid output below 10 mEq per hour.

Special Circumstances

Ulcer Disease in Pregnancy. Pregnancy is normally associated with a lower incidence of DU relapse and ulcer complications than is the nonpregnant state, although some patients may require treatment during gestation. Although no ulcer-healing drug is approved for use during pregnancy, antacids and sucralfate are probably safe, especially after the first trimester. The H_2 blockers may be used if the expected benefits are thought to outweigh the possible risks. These agents, however, are excreted in breast milk and are not recommended for nursing mothers.

Ulcer Disease in Children. The same drugs used in adults may be used to heal PUD in children, recognizing that there is far less experience with these agents in the younger age groups.

Treatment of *Campylobacter pylori* Infection

C. pylori continues to command increasing attention as an important factor in the pathogenesis and relapse of PUD. However, it remains controversial whether to look for or attempt to eradicate the organism. It is thought that with the future widespread availability of noninvasive diagnostic techniques such as the carbon-labeled urea breath test or newer serologic tests that have recently been developed, the indications for initial detection and the need for post-treatment follow-up will be met with less skepticism.

At present, treatment of *C. pylori* is best accomplished with the combination of a bismuth compound (e.g., Pepto-Bismol, two tablets or 30 ml four times daily on an empty stomach) for a total of 21 days plus one or even two antibiotics administered concomitantly for the final 10 to 14 days (e.g., amoxicillin, 500 mg three or four times daily; tetracycline, 500 mg four times daily; and/or metronidazole, 250 to 500 mg three times daily). Approximately 80 per cent of cases are treated effectively with this regimen, but relapse rates of *C. pylori* infection can be high, the possible result of reinfection from unsuspected family members who transmit the organism by fecaloral or respiratory droplet routes.

Side effects of bismuth generally are only cosmetic (e.g., black stools and darkening of the tongue), but encephalopathy is reported with prolonged use. Antibiotics in this setting have been associated with the usual hypersensitivity reactions and *Clostridium difficile*–related colitis (even among those receiving metronidazole). Thus, the decision to treat *C. pylori* with these agents must take such risks into account. Since ulcers have been shown to heal quite well with H_2 blockers, despite the presence or persistence of *C. pylori* infection, treatment of *C. pylori* is not necessary if the therapeutic response to conventional ulcer therapy is satisfactory. However, if dyspeptic symptoms persist after treatment with

H_2 blockers or if ulcer relapses are frequent when therapy is discontinued, the knowledge that *C. pylori* is present may provide for a reasonable treatment alternative.

TUMORS OF THE STOMACH

method of
ROBERT S. NELSON, M.D.
The University of Texas
M. D. Anderson Cancer Center
Houston, Texas

A wide variety of tumors, both benign and malignant, may be encountered in the stomach. The benign lesions can remain asymptomatic or produce life-threatening complications.

BENIGN TUMORS

Epithelial Tumors

These tumors are represented by gastric adenomas and hyperplastic polyps, which comprise 9.8 and 38.4 per cent, respectively, of all benign gastric tumors. Adenomas are true neoplasms and can undergo malignant degeneration, especially the villous types. Hyperplastic polyps are seldom associated with malignancy. Both types are frequently multiple; in such cases, malignancy of the nonpolypoid mucosa can occur in adenomatous polyposis. In other more specific forms of gastrointestinal polyposis, such as juvenile polyposis or Peutz-Jeghers and Gardner's syndromes, the tumors generally tend to be benign, although six cases of malignancy have been reported in Peutz-Jeghers syndrome. Diagnosis of these patients can be made with considerable accuracy by endoscopic polypectomy and biopsy, and when polyps are small or few in number, all of them can be removed. Follow-up is especially important in adenomatous polyposis, and if there are no medical contraindications, such patients probably should have total gastrectomy because of the malignant potential of these polyps.

Mesenchymal (Nonepithelial) Tumors

Leiomyomas are by far the most common tumor in this group and represent 1 to 3 per cent of all gastric tumors. They project into the lumen submucosally but may occasionally ulcerate and bleed. In the nonulcerated tumors biopsy is difficult, but needle aspiration may be positive. Histologically, the small endoscopic biopsy specimens are sometimes difficult to distinguish from leiomyosarcoma. All leiomyomas should be re-moved surgically when diagnosed. Many undiagnosed leiomyomas remain asymptomatic throughout life.

Pseudolymphomas, or inflammatory lymphoid hyperplasia, may be large or small, ulcerated or nonulcerated. Even after complete surgical removal of pseudolymphomas, patients should be followed at intervals because occasionally they develop true lymphoma. In our experience, one of three patients with pseudolymphoma develops lymphoma over a period of years, and there are similar reports in the literature. Other rare lesions are neurogenic and vascular tumors, as well as lipomas (rare) and fibromas. Depending on their size and growth rate, these mesenchymal tumors may cause bleeding, pain, or even obstruction (if they are large enough). Unlike the epithelial tumors, few of them can be removed at endoscopy, although biopsy is usually possible. Surgical removal is necessary in the majority of cases.

MALIGNANT TUMORS

Malignant Lymphoma

Gastric lymphoma is the most common tumor believed to originate in the gastrointestinal tract, constituting 3 to 8 per cent of all malignant gastric lesions. The vast majority are non-Hodgkin's lymphomas. The symptoms, as well as the gross x-ray and endoscopic findings, may be indistinguishable from those of adenocarcinoma, so histologic identification is essential for diagnosis. This is true especially because primary gastric lymphoma may be treatable without surgery if the diagnosis can be made at endoscopy. This can be done in approximately 92 per cent of patients. If the lesion is extensive (and many are, with submucosal extension) or the patient is a poor surgical risk, medical means are the best approach, with an excellent chance of obtaining a response.

Biopsy specimens should be submitted for immunoperoxidase staining, and at least 10 specimens should be obtained. If gross involvement is minimal, surgery may still be considered the treatment of choice. However, gross observations may be misleading because lymphoma generally involves the stomach submucosally over a large area. If medical treatment is primary, chemotherapy followed by radiation therapy is the proper form of management. Chemotherapy always involves a combination of drugs. It has become quite effective, and long-term follow-up on our service has recorded a number of asymptomatic patients with continuing negative gross and biopsy results.

Other Primary Malignant Tumors

Leiomyosarcoma has already been mentioned in connection with leiomyoma. Surgical resection at the time of diagnosis is the treatment of choice because neither chemotherapy nor radiation therapy has much value. Rarer primary malignant tumors include unusual types of sarcoma, squamous carcinoma, choriocarcinoma, and malignant vascular tumors. In the last category, Kaposi's sarcoma may produce several gross types of gastric tumors, which are often susceptible to chemotherapy. Carcinoid may develop as primary gastric tumors. Metastases are fairly frequent, but carcinoid syndrome is unusual. The latter complication can now be treated with somatostatin with good results.

METASTATIC TUMORS

The most common sources of metastatic disease of the stomach are carcinoma of the breast and bronchus, and melanoma. Other tumors that may rarely produce gastric metastases are those of the testis, thyroid, uterus, ovary, and pancreas. Gross appearances vary from submucosal nodules to projecting, ulcerating tumors. Ulcerating tumors frequently bleed and may be a threat to life. Diagnosis can be made with certainty only by endoscopy and biopsy. In general, treatment focuses on the primary tumor.

Carcinoma of the Stomach

The incidence of adenocarcinoma of the stomach has been slowly declining in the United States, but the most recent projections show a probability of 20,000 gastric cancer deaths for 1989. Factors influencing the incidence of this malignancy include diet and heredity (minor), as well as changes in the mucosa such as atrophy secondary to various causes. Increased survival time is directly related to early diagnosis and adequate resection. In Japan, where the incidence remains high, early cancer is diagnosed with increasing frequency, and survival is improving. The failure to obtain early diagnosis in the United States is related to patient delay (often for more than 7 months) and failure to prove cancer histologically by endoscopy and biopsy during work-up.

Symptoms are not diagnostic, and there appears to be a strong tendency in many areas of the world to regard "dyspepsia" as a group of symptoms that should first be treated by standard antacid therapy and disregarded if symptoms subside. X-ray films, if not of the air-contrast type, can also be deceiving, particularly in the diagnosis of ulcers and "gastritis." It goes without saying that anything that appears to resemble a tumor on radiologic examination requires biopsy, but in ulcers or minor mucosal changes, biopsy is also imperative. On the gastrointestinal service of a cancer hospital, a number of patients are seen every year in whom failure to make a histologic diagnosis at the earliest possible moment may have jeopardized survival. In a few cases, endoscopic biopsy was inadequate and poor or little follow-up was performed. Multiple biopsies with brush cytology, if available, should be the rule. In what appear to be submucosal infiltrations, repeat biopsies in the same area to reach the submucosa are frequently rewarding. In recent years, a number of antigen tests have been studied as possible laboratory indicators of gastric cancer (carcinoembryonic antigen, fetal sulfoglycoprotein antigen [FSA]), but these are nonspecific and have not helped in differential or early diagnosis.

In short, if early diagnosis is desired, we must revise our ideas about long-term treatment of undiagnosed dyspepsia and be more objective. A number of recent studies in the U.S. literature indicate that early gastric cancer can be diagnosed and treated, with improved results in this country. This is truly a necessity because radiation therapy and chemotherapy, although extensively used, have been ineffective. Surgical results have improved, but only in relation to earlier diagnosis and better technique. It is hoped that more basic studies of the cancer cell in relation to response to various agents will be rewarding in the future.

CANCER OF THE LARGE BOWEL

method of
WAYNE H. SCHWESINGER, M.D.
University of Texas Health Science Center
San Antonio, Texas

Colorectal cancer continues to be a major source of morbidity in Western countries, with little change noted in its incidence or in the associated death rate during the past three decades. It is now estimated that 151,000 new cases of colorectal cancer will be diagnosed in the United States in 1989. More than 1 in every 20 Americans will be afflicted with this neoplasm. During the same period, 61,300 patients are expected to die from colorectal cancer, corresponding to an overall mortality of more than 50 per cent. This represents far more cancer deaths than from any other cancer except carcinoma of the lung.

Nonetheless, adenocarcinoma of the large bowel is a relatively slow-growing tumor, with a growth period frequently ranging from 4 to 6 years before symptoms develop. It is therefore realistic to expect that substantial improvements in outcome will eventually be achieved. In particular, improved methods for detection before the onset of symptoms would allow definitive therapy to be instituted before the tumor has progressed to an advanced incurable stage.

EPIDEMIOLOGY AND ETIOLOGY

The incidence of colorectal cancer is highest in North America and Western Europe and lowest in Africa, Asia, and South and Central America. It is a disease of advancing age, with two-thirds of the patients being more than 50 years of age, and with an incidence that peaks in the seventh and eighth decades of life. Both sexes appear to be affected nearly equally, but current ethnic studies suggest that the incidence among Hispanics is substantially lower than among U.S. caucasian or black persons.

Little is definitely known about the specific etiology of colorectal cancer. Both environmental and genetic factors appear to be capable of influencing its development. Of the environmental factors, diet is likely to be most important. There is a growing, although not unequivocal, body of evidence to suggest that high animal fat content in the diet promotes carcinogenesis, perhaps by inducing increases in the intraluminal concentrations of secondary bile acids or peroxidized fatty acids. Both of these substrates are capable of damaging colonocytes and, in the proper circumstances, can induce an abnormal proliferative response. Also, diets low in fiber content appear to enhance the risk of colorectal cancer, presumably by slowing intestinal transit and allowing prolonged exposure of mucosal cells to endogenous fecal carcinogens.

The role of genetics in colorectal cancer is most striking in the gastrointestinal polyposis syndromes. In familial polyposis and Gardner's syndrome, 50 per cent of first-degree relatives inherit the trait and all family members so affected ultimately develop colorectal cancer if the colon is not prophylactically resected. More recently, other dominantly inherited gene defects have been identified that are associated with an increased susceptibility to adenocarcinoma but are not related to the polyposis syndromes. Thus, more of the total cancer burden may be caused by primary genetic factors than had previously been appreciated. This may explain the observation that at least 25 per cent of patients with colorectal cancer have a family history of the disease.

Other important risk factors have also been identified. Patients with chronic ulcerative colitis, especially those with extensive colonic involvement, are estimated to have a cumulative cancer risk ranging from 3 to 12 per cent after 15 years of disease. This range exceeds the expected incidence in the normal population by more than three times and continues to rise in subsequent decades. Crohn's colitis is also associated with an increased risk of both colorectal and small bowel cancers, but the increment is not as high as with ulcerative colitis.

The presence of an index colorectal neoplasm should suggest the possibility that another neoplasm is present. In patients found to have one colorectal cancer, a synchronous or second cancer is present about 5 per cent of the time when the initial diagnosis is made. Metachronous cancers develop during the follow-up period in another 2 to 5 per cent of patients. Adenomas are found in more than one-third of patients with colorectal carcinoma.

Nearly all colorectal cancers appear to originate in neoplastic polyps, except in patients with inflammatory bowel disease. Thus, colonic polyps should be considered to be precursors to malignancy even though most remain benign throughout life. The actual malignant potential of polyps is determined by their histology and their size, factors that are often interrelated. Villous adenomas are much more likely to contain foci of invasive carcinoma (9 to 12 per cent) than tubular adenomas (3 per cent). And regardless of their histology, small polyps with a diameter of less than 1 cm carry only a low cancer risk, probably under 1 per cent. In polyps measuring 2 cm or more, the risk increases markedly to more than 15 per cent for villous adenomas and to more than 7 per cent for tubular adenomas.

In an individual polyp, a proliferative nidus of carcinoma in situ is considered invasive once it penetrates the muscularis mucosae. Malignant growth then proceeds by direct extension through the bowel wall and ultimately by metastasis into regional lymphatics and visceral veins. At the time of initial diagnosis, 40 per cent of patients with colorectal cancer have lymphatic involvement.

LOCATION AND PRESENTATION

The segmental distribution of colorectal cancer generally parallels that of benign adenomas. Both have shifted proximally during the past several decades, with right-sided colon carcinomas gradually becoming more common; they now account for 25 per cent of the total. Still, nearly 55 per cent of new lesions are located in the rectum and sigmoid colon. The anatomic location and the stage of the disease are generally responsible for the specific clinical manifestations of colorectal cancer. Early cancers at any location are asymptomatic and associated only with the presence of occult blood in the stool. More advanced cancers located in the right colon are commonly associated with anemia and abdominal pain. A bulky mass may also be palpable. Lesions of the left colon are more likely to cause alterations in bowel habits ranging from subtle reductions in stool caliber to obstipation and cramping, often together with hematochezia. Bright red rectal bleeding and production of mucus with tenesmus are more typical of rectal tumors.

DIAGNOSTIC EVALUATION

Symptomatic patients suspected of having colorectal tumors should undergo a thorough history, as well as a physical examination that includes a careful digital evaluation of the rectum. In at least 10 per cent of patients with colorectal cancer, the tumor is palpable within the rectal vault. Total colonscopy should be performed after optimal preparation, and primary lesions localized and biopsy performed. This approach also ensures accurate identification of synchronous cancers or polyps, which might necessitate changes in the therapeutic strategy. If colonoscopy is unsuccessful or impractical, air contrast barium enema can be used together with proctoscopy or flexible sigmoidoscopy to localize primary and secondary lesions of the large bowel. Laboratory studies are generally obtained to evaluate the clinical condition of the patient, but they provide little direct information concerning the diagnosis of cancer. An elevated hepatic alkaline phosphatase level is a relatively sensitive but nonspecific marker of liver metastases. An elevated level of carcinoembryonic antigen generally is found when either a large primary tumor or metastatic involvement is present. It should return to normal in the early postoperative period if resectional therapy is successful.

Other tests are available for selected use in special circumstances. Hepatic metastases may be characterized by the radionuclide scan, computed tomography, or preoperative and intraoperative ultrasonography. Computed tomography can also define the extent of adjacent tissue involvement by large rectal tumors. This baseline study is especially helpful in patients being considered for preoperative pelvic irradiation. In patients being considered for hepatic resection or portal infusion of chemotherapeutic agents, preoperative angiography is mandatory. Intravenous pyelography is sometimes used to define the course of the ureters and to identify areas of obstruction.

SCREENING

Asymptomatic individuals known to be at increased risk for colorectal neoplasms should be screened using measures such as fecal occult blood testing, air contrast barium enema, or colonscopy. High-risk patients who are candidates for screening include first-degree relatives of patients with familial polyposis, Gardner's syndrome, or hereditary nonpolyposis colon cancer. In addition, patients with long-standing ulcerative colitis, or with Crohn's disease and involvement of the large bowel, are at risk and should have multiple endoscopic biopsies of random areas within the colon, with careful histologic examination specifically for the presence of moderate to severe dysplasia. Surveillance should continue at regular intervals as determined by the activity of the inflammatory disease. Patients with colorectal polyps should also be followed with colonoscopy because they have a risk of cancer nearly three times that of the normal population. Even when benign polyps are endoscopically removed, the likelihood of recurrence is 30 to 40 per cent, a finding that mandates continued long-term surveillance after polypectomy.

Because the risk of colorectal cancer begins to increase in the general population after age 40, the American Cancer Society has recommended a modified screening program for all asymptomatic individuals: (1) men and women over age 50 years should have a stool blood test every year; (2) men and women over age 50 should have annual sigmoidoscopic examinations until two consecutive examinations are normal and thereafter every 3 to 5 years; and (3) men and women over age 40 should have a digital rectal examination every year.

Fecal occult blood testing uses guaiac-impregnated paper to test for the presence of peroxidase from hemoglobin. As a screening modality, it is an acceptably sensitive but relatively nonspecific test that appears to be most accurate when used by individuals eating a meat free diet who have abstained from aspirin, anti-inflammatory drugs, vitamin C, and iron tablets. It is customary to recommend two samples from each of three consecutive stools and to consider any single positive test to be indicative of the need for further endoscopic or radiologic testing. In several studies in which this approach was used, it appeared that the majority of colorectal cancers could be detected at an early, asymptomatic stage. Whether widespread use of this approach can affect overall mortality or can be justified on the basis of cost-benefit calculations remains to be determined.

TREATMENT

The only effective curative strategy for colorectal cancer is complete operative removal. In general, this means resection of the primary tumor with an adequate margin of normal tissue (at least 5 cm) and wide excision of a segement of the subjacent mesentery, which includes regional lymphatic and vascular structures. Intestinal continuity is then restored whenever possible. The specific therapy for cancer localized to the cecum or right colon is radical right hemicolectomy with a concurrent anastomosis of the terminal ileum to the mid-transverse colon. Tumors of the sigmoid colon can be adequately managed with a radical sigmoid resection and an anastomosis of the descending colon to the rectum. Low rectal lesions, within 8 cm of the anal verge, commonly require abdominoperineal resection, with wide excision of the pelvic soft tissues and anal musculature and a descending colostomy.

When adjacent organs or tissues are involved they may be included in an en bloc resection, if this is anatomically feasible. A solitary metastatic cancer in distant organs, such as the liver or lung, may also be resected if the primary tumor appears to be otherwise controlled. Approximately 20 per cent of the patients with solitary liver or lung metastases that are resected live for 5 years.

Neither the methods nor the results of curative surgery have changed greatly in the past 30 years. In general, 90 per cent of patients are explored, but in only 70 per cent is resection ultimately performed with curative intent. The operative mortality ranges from 5 to 9 per cent, accounted for, in part, by the advanced age of many patients and the presence of serious concomitant medical illnesses.

Long-term survival is proportional to the stage

of tumor progression at the time of diagnosis. Clinical staging using the modified Dukes's classification provides reasonable but imprecise guidelines for the prognosis. For Stage A lesions, confined to the mucosa or submucosa, the cumulative 5-year survival is 95 per cent; for Stage B lesions, involving muscle with or without invasion of adjacent structures, survival is approximately 60 per cent; for Stage C lesions with regional lymph node involvement it is 35 per cent; and for Stage D lesions with distant metastases it is 5 per cent or less.

When definitive surgical treatment is used and fails, the patterns of failure are variable. The distribution of recurrent lesions may be single or multifocal because multiple mechanisms of spread can occur. Liver metastases are a common cause of treatment failure and appear as a component of failure in more than 50 per cent of the failure group. Local recurrence is another common mode of failure, especially in tumors of the rectum. There is a strong correlation between local recurrence and penetration of the tumor through the full thickness of bowel wall. Peritoneal seeding and extra-abdominal metastases to the lung, bone, or brain are less commonly seen. The majority of failures (70 to 75 percent) are noted within 3 years of presumably curative surgery. Once they are detected, mean survival is generally less than 10 months.

Many patients who are deemed incurable can benefit from a more limited palliative procedure to avoid bleeding, pain, perforation, or local extension. Palliative procedures may include internal or external bypass of lesions or wedge resection when possible. Recent results with palliative laser surgery for partial ablation of advanced rectal tumors suggest that this approach offers another reasonable but limited option in patients with nearly obstructing or uncontrollably painful cancers.

Adjuvant therapy with irradiation and chemotherapy has not been demonstrated to have a significant effect on survival in patients with colon cancer. However, both preoperative irradiation and postoperative irradiation appear to have some benefit when used adjunctively for primary cancers in the rectum. Studies of the use of these and other measures in colorectal cancer are ongoing.

INTESTINAL PARASITES

method of
D. W. MacPHERSON, M.D.
McMaster University
Hamilton, Ontario, Canada

Intestinal parasites are common infections. The majority of them can be diagnosed by examination of stool specimens. A number of other parasitic infections that initially infect the gastrointestinal system are not evident by this examination. In these infections, humans are usually a dead-end host for the parasite or eggs are not produced (i.e., *Toxocara canis, Trichinella spiralis, Anisakis* species, *Angiostrongylus* species, *Echinococcus granulosus,* and *Echinococcus multilocularis*). These infections must be diagnosed by means other than stool examination and are not dealt with here. The prevalence of intestinal parasites is usually proportional to the local socioeconomic and sanitary conditions. It is estimated that at least one-quarter of the world's population have one or more intestinal parasites. In developed nations, 5 to 10 per cent of the population may be carrying a parasite in the stool, usually a protozoan. The intestinal protozoa are single-celled organisms that can multiply within the gut. The helminths (worms) are multicellular and, with only a few exceptions, do not multiply within the human host. Eosinophilia is associated with helminth rather than protozoal infections. Worms have a definite life span and therefore, without reinfection or treatment, are eventually cleared by the host. The concept of a parasite burden with worms correlates with the risk of human morbidity. Light infections are usually asymptomatic. It is also recognized that many persons may have intestinal protozoa without symptoms. When standards of personal and community hygiene are high, the public health risk and the risk of person-to-person transmission are low. Asymptomatic individuals with light worm infections may not require specific treatment. Knowledge of the life cycle of the organism, its potential for causing disease, and the public health implications of the infection direct the need for specific medical management.

TREATMENT

The majority of drugs described here are licensed and available in the United States and Canada. Some drugs are approved for certain infections but not for others. Some agents manufactured outside of the United States, but not approved, can be obtained by contacting the Parasitic Disease Drug Service of the Centers for Disease Control (CDC) in Atlanta, Georgia (telephone: 404–639–3670). In Canada, restricted drugs can be obtained by approval of the Bureau of Drugs, Health Protection Branch, Ottawa (telephone: 613–993–3105).

Summaries for drug therapy for protozoa (Table 1) and helminths (Table 2) follow.

Protozoan Infections

Three protozoal organisms account for the majority of symptomatic infections in this group: *Giardia lamblia, Cryptosporidium* species, and *Entamoeba histolytica* (see the separate chapter on amebiasis).

Giardia lamblia

Giardiasis is the most commonly diagnosed protozoal infection. It has a cosmopolitan distri-

TABLE 1. **Drug Therapy for Intestinal Protozoan Parasites***

Parasite	Drug	Adult Dose†	Pediatric Dose†	Availability
Balantidium coli	Tetracycline‡	500 mg qid × 10 days	10 mg/kg qid × 10 days (max 2 grams/day, not for use in patients less than 7 yr old)	
	or iodoquinol‡	650 mg tid × 20 days	40 mg/kg/day in three divided doses × 20 days (max 2 grams/day)	Yodoxin (Glenwood, Inc.), others
	or metronidazole	750 mg tid × 5 days	35–50 mg/kg/day in three divided doses × 5 days	Flagyl (Searle), others
Blastocystis hominis	Not definitely shown to be a pathogen; no therapy proved effective			
	Iodoquinol	As per *B. coli*	As per *B. coli*	
	or metronidazole	750 mg tid × 10 days	As per *B. coli* × 10 days	
Cryptosporidium species	None proved effective Spiramycin§	1 gram tid × 21 days or more		Rovamycin (Rhone-Poulenc, Montreal, Canada)
Dientamoeba fragilis Not definitely shown to be a pathogen	Iodoquinol	As per *B. coli*	As per *B. coli*	
	or tetracycline	As per *B. coli*	As per *B. coli*	
	or difetarsone‖	500 mg tid × 10 days	<1 yr: 50 mg/kg once daily 1–3 yr: 250 mg bid 4–5 yr: 250 mg tid 6–10 yr: 500 mg bid >10 yr: adult dose × 10 days	Bémarsal (Poulenc)
Entamoeba histolytica	See separate chapter on amebiasis			
Giardia lamblia	Quinacrine HCl	100 mg tid × 5 days	2 mg/kg tid × 5 days (max 300 mg/day)	Atabrine (Winthrop-Breon)
	or metronidazole‡	250 mg tid × 7 days or 2 grams qhs × 3 days	5 mg/kg tid × 7 days or <25 kg: 35 mg/kg 25–40 kg: 50 mg per kg >40 kg: adult dose; once daily for 3 days	Flagyl (Searle), others
	or furazolidone	100 mg qid × 10 days (tablets)	2 mg/kg qid × 10 days (suspension)	Furoxone (Norwich Eaton)
Isospora belli	Trimethoprim-sulfamethoxazole‡ (TMP-SMX)	TMP 160 mg + SMX 800 mg qid × 10 days, then bid × 3 weeks; one tablet daily may be needed for chronic suppression		Bactrim (Roche), Septra (Burroughs Wellcome), others
	or pyrimethamine‡	50–75 mg/day × 28 days; then 25 mg/day for chronic suppression		Daraprim (Burroughs Wellcome)

*Adapted from the medical literature, previous editions of this book, and *The Medical Letter*.
†All recommended drugs are given orally.
‡Considered investigational for this indication by the U.S. Food and Drug Administration (FDA).
§Not approved for this indication by the FDA.
‖Not available in the United States; see Bureau of Drugs, Health Protection Branch, Ottawa, Canada.

TABLE 2. **Drug Therapy for Intestinal Helminths***

Parasite	Drug	Adult Dose†	Pediatric Dose†	Availability
Ascaris lumbricoides	Pyrantel pamoate	11 mg/kg in a single dose (max 1 gram)	Same as adult dose	Antiminth (Pfizer)
	or mebendazole	100 mg bid × 3 days	>2 yr: same as adult dose	Vermox (Janssen)
	or piperazine citrate	75 mg/kg/day × 2 days (max 3.5 grams/day)	Same as adult dose	Antepar (Burroughs Wellcome), others
Capillaria philippinensis	Mebendazole‡	100 mg bid × 20 days	Same as adult dose	
	or thiabendazole‡	25 mg/kg/day × 30 days (max 3 grams/day)	Same as adult dose	Mintezol (Merck)
Enterobius vermicularis (pinworm)	Pyrantel pamoate	As per *Ascaris*; repeat in 2 weeks	Same as adult dose	
	or mebendazole	100 mg in a single dose; repeat in 2 weeks	>2 yr: same as adult dose	
Hookworms *Necator americanus* *Ancylostoma duodenale*	Mebendazole	As per *Ascaris*	Same as adult dose	
	or pyrantel pamoate‡	As per *Ascaris* × 3 days	Same as adult dose	
Hermaphroditic intestinal flukes *Fascioplopsis buski*	Praziquantel‡	25 mg/kg tid × 1 day	Same as adult dose	Biltricide (Miles)
	or niclosamide‡	2 grams (4 × 500-mg tablets), well chewed as a single dose	11–34 kg: two tablets 35–40 kg: three tablets >40 kg: adult dose, well chewed, single dose	Yomesan (Miles)
Heterophyes heterophyes	Praziquantel‡	As per *F. buski*	Same as adult dose	
Metagonimus yokogawai	Praziquantel‡	As per *F. buski*	Same as adult dose	
Hermaphroditic liver flukes *Clonorchis sinensis* *Opisthochoris viverrini*	Praziquantel‡	As per *F. buski*	Same as adult dose	
Fasciola hepatica	Praziquantel‡	25 mg/kg tid × 5–8 days	Same as adult dose	Biltricide (Miles)
	or bithionol‡	30–50 mg/kg on alternate days for 10–15 doses	Same as adult dose	Parasitic Disease Service, Centers for Disease Control, Atlanta, Georgia
Paragonimus westermani	Praziquantel‡	25 mg/kg tid × 2 days	Same as adult dose	
	or bithionol‡	As per *F. hepatica*	Same as adult dose	
Schistosomiasis flukes *Schistosoma mansoni*	Praziquantel	20 mg/kg tid × 1 day	Same as adult dose	
	or oxamniquine	American strains: 15 mg/kg × 1 day	10 mg/kg bid × 1 day	Vansil (Pfizer)
		African strains: East: 15 mg/kg bid × 1 day Egypt and South Africa: 15 mg/kg bid × 2 days	Same as adult dose	

TABLE 2. **Drug Therapy for Intestinal Helminths*** *Continued*

Parasite	Drug	Adult Dose†	Pediatric Dose†	Availability
Schistosoma japonicum *Schistosoma haematobium* *Schistosoma mekongi* *Schistosoma intercalatum*	Praziquantel	As per *S. mansoni*	Same as adult dose	
Tapeworms *Taenia saginata* *Taenia solium* *Diphyllobothrium* spp. *Dipylidium caninum* *Hymenolepis diminuta*	Niclosamide	As per *F. buski*	Same as *F. buski*	Yomesan (Miles)
	or Praziquantel‡	10–20 mg/kg once	Same as adult dose	
Hymenolepis nana	Praziquantel‡	25 mg/kg once	Same as adult dose	Biltricide (Miles)
	or niclosamide	Single 2 gram dose (four tablets), followed by 1 gram (two tablets) daily for 6 days (well chewed)	<34 kg: single 1 gram dose (two tablets) followed by 0.5 gram (one tablet) daily × 6 days 35–40 kg: single 1.5 gram dose (three tablets) followed by 1 gram (two tablets) daily × 6 days >40 kg: adult dose (well chewed)	Yomesan (Miles)
Strongyloides stercoralis	Thiabendazole	25 mg/kg bid × 2 days (max 3 grams day)	Same as adult dose	Mintezol (Merck)
	or mebendazole§, ‖	500 mg/day in divided doses × 21 days		Vermox (Janssen)
Trichostrongylus spp.	Thiabendazole‡	As per *S. stercoralis*	Same as adult dose	
	or pyrantel pamoate‡	As per *Ascaris*	Same as adult dose	Antiminth (Pfizer)
Trichuris trichiura	Mebendazole	As per *Ascaris*	Same as adult dose	
	or difetarsone¶	As per *D. fragilis* (Table 1)	As per *D. fragilis* (Table 1)	Bémarsal (Poulenc)

*Adapted from the medical literature, previous editions of this book, and *The Medical Letter*.
†All recommended drugs are given orally.
‡Considered investigational for this indication by the FDA.
§Moderate success with high-dose mebendazole. Albendazole and ivermectin have also been effective.
‖For disseminated strongyloidiasis, continue therapy for at least 5 days. In the immuncompromised patient, it may be necessary to continue therapy or to use other agents (see footnote §).
¶Not available in the United States; see Bureau of Drugs, Health Protection Branch, Ottawa, Canada.

bution. The majority of persons infected are asymptomatic. The usual symptoms include diarrhea with bloating, excessive gas and flatulence, fatigue, and weight loss. Malabsorption occurs rarely.

Studies have not shown any adverse outcome if asymptomatic infections in children are not treated. The concept of not treating asymptomatic individuals (except those who affect public health, such as food handlers) remains controversial.

Cure rates of 53 to 92 per cent have been reported with quinacrine HCl (Atrabrine, mepacrine), the drug of choice approved by the U.S.

Food and Drug Administration (FDA) for the treatment of giardiasis in the United States. The lower cure rate was seen in young children who did not tolerate the medication. Common side effects include cramping, headache, and dizziness. Yellow discoloration of the skin and sclera, vomiting, fever, exfoliative dermatitis, and toxic psychosis may also occur.

Metronidazole (Flagyl) is not an FDA-approved drug for the treatment of giardiasis in the United States. It is as effective as and better tolerated than quinacrine HCl. Short courses (3 days) are as effective as longer ones and are easier in treating children. Adverse effects include cramping, nausea, a metallic taste or dryness in the mouth, dark urine, and a disulfiram-like reaction if taken with alcohol. Metronidazole is mutagenic for bacteria and carcinogenic in rodents. No such problems have been documented in humans. Teratogenicity has not been found in pregnant women treated inadvertently with metronidazole. Tinidazole, a similiar imidazole agent, has an equal cure rate when administered as a single dose giving excellent compliance but is not approved in the United States or Canada.

Both quinacrine HCl and metronidazole taste bitter and are poorly accepted by young children. Hiding the taste in a gelatin capsule, or giving the drug in sweet food like ice cream or jam, may improve acceptance.

Furazolidone (Furoxone), a nitrofurantoin derivative, is available in tablet and suspension forms. It is the only antigiardial drug supplied in liquid form and hence is useful in treating young children and infants. Cure rates of 89 to 92 per cent have been reported. Adverse effects include nausea and vomiting, diarrhea, fever, and rash. A disulfiram-like reaction may occur if furazolidone is taken with alcohol. Furazolidone is a monoamine oxidase inhibitor and may cause hemolysis in patients with glucose-6-phosphate dehydrogenase deficiency.

Cryptosporidium Species

Cryptosporidiosis is caused by a coccidian parasite that was once thought to be a zoonosis limited to animal handlers and veterinary students. It has since been shown to have a worldwide distribution, causing watery, nonbloody diarrhea with severe abdominal cramping and occasional fever. Children are most commonly infected, but household contacts, international travelers, and the immunocompromised are also at increased risk. Immunocompetent patients have a self-limited infection but may be quite ill during its course. In immunocompromised individuals, especially those with the acquired immunodeficiency syndrome (AIDS), cryptosporidiosis is a severe, chronic, and debilitating cause of diarrhea. Daily stool volumes of more than 10 liters may occur. Cryptosporidiosis may be associated with death in this group. Dozens of drugs have been investigated, but none have been shown to result in a parasitologic cure or to influence the outcome. In one open study in a small number of patients, spiramycin was suggested to be useful in immunocompromised patients. This finding has not been confirmed in follow-up studies. Symptomatic and supportive care is indicated for both immunocompetent and immunocompromised patients. Total parenteral nutrition may be required in AIDS patients. Recent reports using somatostatin, and its synthetic analogue octreotide, have shown some promise in the management of AIDS-associated diarrhea.

The following two protozoan infections are documented enteropathogens but are rare even in well-defined risk groups.

Balantidium coli

This is the only ciliated protozoan recognized to cause disease in humans. It is a common organism in pigs, and this contact is usually part of the clinical picture when disease is present. This organism may cause diarrhea and colitis. The recommended drug for treatment is tetracycline, with iodoquinol and metronidazole being alternative choices.

Isospora belli

This coccidian parasite is common in the tropics but is also seen in situations that favor fecal-oral contamination. Hence, international travelers, male homosexuals, and institutionalized individuals are the individuals usually infected. The trimethoprim-sulfamethoxazole combination is the most effective treatment for this infection. Some authors have also recommended pyrimethamine alone in sulfa-allergic patients.

A number of other bowel protozoa are found frequently in stool examinations. At least two of these may be emerging as potential pathogens, but definite evidence is still lacking.

Dientamoeba fragilis

D. fragilis is an intestinal flagellate frequently seen in children and may be associated with Enterobius vermicularis (pinworm) infection. Anecdotal reports of anorexia, recurrent diarrhea, cramping, and even colitis have appeared. Although tetracycline and iodoquinol are the recommended drugs, cure rates are low. These drugs are often contraindicated in the usual age group being treated. Difetarsone (Bémarsal), a pentavalent organic arsenical available as an emergency release drug in Canada, achieves parasitologic cure rates of 95 per cent with minimal side effects.

Blastocystis hominis

B. hominis, recently classified as a protozoan, may cause gastrointestinal disturbances. Several short anecdotal reports have suggested that when present, especially in large numbers, B. hominis may cause abdominal pain, bloating, and diarrhea. No treatment has definitely been shown to influence the clinical outcome. Iodoquinol and metronidazole have been suggested for the treatment of symptomatic patients, with no other identified cause, who have large numbers of this organism in their stools. Recently, travelers with diarrhea who were taking trimethoprim-sulfamethoxazole prophylactically were found to have a lower incidence of *B. hominis* in their stool specimens compared with similar travelers with diarrhea who were not taking this drug.

Nonpathogenic Protozoa

These organisms are found frequently in children in day care centers (20 to 30 per cent), in homosexual males (50 to 70 per cent), and in the institutionalized, mentally disadvantaged patient (25 to 50 per cent). These organisms include *Entamoeba hartmanni, Entamoeba coli, Endolimax nana, Iodamoeba butschlii, Chilomastix mesnili, Trichomonas hominis, Enteromonas hominis,* and *Retortamonas intestinalis.* No evidence of pathogenicity for these organisms has been found. Treatment for these parasites is not recommended even for public health reasons.

Helminthic Infections

Nematodes (Roundworms)

E. vermicularis, Ascaris lumbricoides, hookworms, *Trichuris trichiura,* and *Strongyloides stercoralis* are common geohelminths, indicating that, in general, a period of soil incubation is required before they become infectious for humans. As a result, these nematode infections are usually imported or occur in areas of the country where soil and socioeconomic conditions facilitate transmission of these organisms.

Enterobius vermicularis (Pinworm). Pinworm is a ubiquitous infection that occurs at a higher rate in North American children than in those of developing nations. The eggs require a short period of incubation and are usually infectious when passed with the stool. Hence, children and their adult household contacts are commonly infected. Single-dose treatments, repeated once at 2 weeks, with mebendazole (Vermox) or pyrantel pamoate (Antiminth) are effective and well tolerated.

If reinfection does occur, additional methods may be required to control it: bathing in the morning, with keen attention to nail care; wearing well-fitting undergarments and pajamas for sleeping; changing bed linens; and treating the entire family. A tendency to excessive disinfection of the home should be discouraged, as it is unlikely to prevent additional infections and may lead to unnecessary fear of parasites.

Note that *D. fragilis* may be associated with *E. vermicularis* infection. Up to five pinworm paddles may have to be collected to exclude pinworm infection in a compatible clinical setting. A similar number of tests are required to confirm eradication of infection with *E. vermicularis.*

Ascaris lumbricoides (Roundworm). This adult worm (approximately 15 cm long) is rarely confused with other worms. It is easily treated with a number of agents. Pyrantel pamoate, given in a single dose, is about 100 per cent effective and is relatively free of side effects. Mebendazole is equally effective when given over 3 days. Piperazine citrate, administered over 2 days and on an empty stomach, is also effective but potentially more toxic. When mixed infections are present, ascariasis should be treated first, as some drugs may stimulate worm migration, resulting in an obstructed viscus or other ectopic worm syndromes. Because of the size of these worms and the possibility of luminal obstruction, the aim of treatment is eradication, not reduction of the worm burden.

Hookworm Infections. The human hookworms, *Necator americanus* and *Ancylostoma duodenale,* cannot be distinguished by egg morphology in the stool specimen. Both infections respond well to a 3-day course of mebendazole or pyrantel pamoate. Light infections are usually clinically inapparent and are not associated with anemia, and so may not need to be treated. Heavy infections may be a cause of marked anemia and protein-losing enteropathy. Measures to correct the anemia should be used concurrently with therapy.

Strongyloides stercoralis. This intestinal parasite is so well adapted to the human host that it is able to autoinfect and can persist for the lifetime of the host. Diminished immunity from any cause may be associated with hyperinfection and lethal systemic dissemination. Thiabendazole (Mintezol) given for 2 days in uncomplicated infections or for at least 5 days in disseminated cases is the drug of choice. The drug is 60 to 90 per cent effective. Nausea, vomiting, headache, and dizziness are common side effects. Mebendazole is better tolerated but requires higher than standard doses to be effective. When persistent immunosuppression is present, monthly 2-day treatment with thiabendazole may reduce the worm load and prevent hyperinfection. Thiabendazole is not marketed in Canada but is available through designated tropical medicine and infectious disease centers.

Trichuris trichiura (Whipworm). Whipworm infection has a worldwide distribution but is most common in poor rural communities and areas lacking sanitary facilities. Most infected persons are asymptomatic. Again, light infections in asymptomatic persons do not require therapy. Mebendazole has a cure rate of 70 to 90 per cent and reduces the egg load by 90 to 99 per cent. Difetarsone has also been shown to be effective.

Trichostrongylus Species. This parasite is common in the Middle East and Far East. The infection is usually of low intensity, and the patients are often asymptomatic. Heavy infections may produce gastrointestinal symptoms and should be treated. Thiabendazole is the drug of choice, but because of its toxicity, most physicians prefer to try pyrantel pamoate first. Both drugs are considered investigational treatments for this infection.

Capillaria philippinensis. Capillariasis is endemic in Southeast Asia. It is characterized by a severe gastroenteritis that in untreated cases has been associated with a 10 to 30 per cent mortality. Treatment requires aggressive nutritional support. Thiabendazole and the less toxic drug mebendazole have both been used successfully to treat this infection. Prolonged courses and high doses are required to prevent relapse.

Cestodes (Tapeworms)

The tapeworms for which humans are, or can be, the definitive host are diagnosed by finding eggs in the stool or occasionally by passing an active worm segment. *Taenia saginata* (beef tapeworm) and *T. solium* (pork tapeworm) cannot be distinguished on the basis of egg morphology. A single dose of niclosamide (Yomesan) is the treatment of choice. Because of the risk of regurgitated or ingested *T. solium* eggs causing cysticercosis, some authors suggest a magnesium sulfate purge 2 hours after treatment to ensure passage of the entire worm. This also reduces the risk of environmental contamination with the eggs. The fish tapeworms (*Diphyllobothrium latum, D. pacificum, D. dentriticum*), the dog tapeworm (*Dipylidium caninum*), and the rat tapeworm (*Hymenolepis diminuta*) are also treated with a single dose of niclosamide. Alternative drug therapy with praziquantel (Bitricide) is effective but is not approved for these infections. *Hymenolepis nana* (dwarf tapeworm) is the only cestode in which humans can act as both the intermediate and definitive hosts, maintaining a constant cycle of infection. It is treated with a single dose of praziquantel or with niclosamide for 6 days.

Trematodes (Flukes)

Schistosoma Species. *Schistosoma mansoni* is the most common cause of intestinal schistosomiasis imported into North America. *S. japonicum* from East Asia, *S. mekongi* from Southeast Asia, and *S. intercalatum* from Central Africa are rarely seen. The treatment of choice for these schistosomes and for urinary schistosomiasis (*S. haematobium*) is a 1-day course of praziquantel. This drug is effective and usually well tolerated. Occasional gastrointestinal upset does occur. In the United States praziquantel is approved for treatment of all forms of schistosomiasis, but in Canada, authorization is required. Oxamniquine (Vansil, Mansil) is an alternative drug for the treatment of *S. mansoni*. Electroencephalographic changes and seizures have been described with use of this drug. African strains of *S. mansoni* require higher doses of oxamniquine for effective treatment than do strains from South America or the Caribbean.

Other Intestinal Flukes. *Fasciolopsis buski, Heterophyes heterophyes,* and *Metagonimus yokogawai* are imported infections rarely seen in North America. The majority of patients have no symptoms, and the infections are detected only on routine stool screening. Praziquantel is the current treatment of choice. Niclosamide (in the same dose as that for taeniasis) is an alternative drug for the treatment of *F. buski.*

Liver Flukes. *Clonorchis sinensis* and *Opisthorchis viverrini* (Oriental liver flukes) are common stool findings from immigrants from Southeast Asia. *Fasciola hepatica* is occasionally reported in Canada and the United States. The eggs of the lung fluke (*Paragonimus westermani*), usually found in sputum, may also be found in stools. Praziquantel is the drug of choice for all of these fluke infections but is considered to be investigational. Bithionol (Bitin), alternative therapy for *F. hepatica* and *P. westermani*, is also an investigational drug. It is available through the CDC.

Follow-up Stool Examinations

Sufficient time must be allowed for clearance of intestinal contents and for regeneration of the parasite after treatment before repeat stool examinations are done. For the protozoa, this may be as short as 1 week. The tapeworm and fluke examinations should be repeated after 3 or 4 months. The test for cure of pinworm infections is five pinworm paddles collected on consecutive mornings.

Metabolic Disorders

BERIBERI
(Thiamine Deficiency)

method of
RICHARD W. VILTER, M.D.
University of Cincinnati College of Medicine
Cincinnati, Ohio

Classic beriberi is rare in the United States except in the chronic alcoholic. (Alcoholic beverages not only add thiamine-free calories but also interfere with absorption of thiamine provided by other foods.) Beriberi may occur occasionally, however, in persons with diseases that predispose them to increased nutritional requirements, such as hyperthyroidism, malignant disease, or malabsorption syndromes, as well as in pregnant and lactating women. A recent survey of healthy, free-living, elderly Americans revealed little evidence of thiamine deficiency. In the Orient, beriberi occurs in adults who are dependent for calories on vitamin-poor polished rice. An infantile form presenting as acute cardiac failure, aphonia, pseudomeningitis, convulsions or vomiting, constipation, and failure to thrive (Shoshin beriberi) also occurs in infants with thiamine-deficient mothers. Because thiamine is involved in carbohydrate metabolism, mainly as a codecarboxylase of alpha-keto acids such as pyruvic acid and, to a lesser extent, as a cotransketolase in the pentose phosphate pathway, long-term use of unsupplemented intravenous glucose solutions or mixtures used for intravenous hyperalimentation may precipitate a thiamine deficiency state. Psychoneurotic symptoms, peripheral neuritis, edema, heart failure (usually of the high output type), and Wernicke's encephalopathy (ophthalmoplegia, nystagmus, ataxia, and global confusion) are the classic manifestations of thiamine deficiency. Thiamine-dependent beriberi, a rare hereditary metabolic abnormality requiring much more than the usual thiamine allowance, has been described in association with thiamine-responsive anemia.

PREVENTION

A diet rich in meat, dairy products, cereals, and vegetables, particularly legumes, prevents beriberi even in the chronic alcoholic. Ingestion of bread or rice enriched with the B complex vitamins affords a large measure of protection. In pregnant women and in persons with systemic diseases that limit the appetite or interfere with proper absorption of vitamins from the gastrointestinal tract, 2 to 5 mg of thiamine a day, usually prescribed in capsule form or as an intramuscular injection with other members of the vitamin B complex, prevents the deficiency state. The dietary allowance of thiamine that prevents the manifestations of deficiency is approximately 0.5 mg for each 1000 calories. The Food and Nutrition Board of the National Research Council recommends 1.0 to 1.1 mg of thiamine daily for women, 1.2 to 1.4 mg daily for men, and 0.3 to 1.2 mg daily for infants and children. Pregnant or lactating women should have an additional 0.4 to 0.5 mg per day.

TREATMENT

Patients with peripheral neuritis caused by a lack of thiamine should abstain from alcohol; should follow a diet that is rich in meat, vegetables, cereals, dairy products, and fruit; and should be given thiamine, 5 mg four times daily by mouth or parenterally. In addition, a multiple-vitamin capsule should be taken several times a day, because it is almost certain that a patient deficient in one of the B complex vitamins is deficient in all of them. An anaphylactic reaction occasionally occurs when thiamine is given intravenously.

Analgesics may be necessary to relieve the painful burning of the feet and legs. Acetylsalicylic acid or acetaminophen and codeine are usually sufficient, but occasionally meperidine (Demerol) may be necessary. Hyperesthetic feet and legs, the usual sites of the most severe neuropathy, should be protected from the bedclothes by a cradle; when foot drop develops, the feet should be supported by a footboard at the end of the bed or by light splints to avoid contractures.

As soon as the pain allows, physiotherapy should be started; it should be passive at first and then active as muscles begin to function. Convalescence is prolonged, particularly in the chronic alcoholic, and may take 6 months or longer. Damaged nerves regain function slowly. Dead nerves never recover.

Patients with heart disease resulting from beriberi should be confined to absolute bed rest

493

because even mild activity may bring about sudden death. A diet low in salt and residue and rich in protein and B complex vitamins is important. If patients cannot eat such a diet, tube feedings may be necessary until the most acute stage of the disease has passed. It is customary to give an initial dose of 25 to 50 mg of thiamine intravenously, followed by an oral dose of 5 mg four times daily. Administration should be continued parenterally if the patient cannot take medication orally. Larger doses, especially when administered parenterally, are excreted rapidly in the urine. The other vitamins of the B complex should be administered as described for peripheral neuritis. Congestive heart failure is managed in the usual fashion with diuretics and digitalis, which may be helpful after the thiamine deficiency has been alleviated. Occasionally, thiamine therapy alone may be sufficient to induce massive diuresis. Convalescence may be prolonged, but if the patient recovers and remains on an adequate diet thereafter, there will usually be no noticeable residual effects of cardiac damage. Alcoholic cardiomyopathy (low-output failure) is a frequent complication and interferes with a dramatic response to thiamine and with eventual recovery.

DIABETES MELLITUS IN ADULTS

method of
MARK E. MOLITCH, M.D.
Northwestern University Medical School
Chicago, Illinois

Diabetes mellitus affects approximately 2.5 per cent of the population, although perhaps an equal percentage have diabetes but are undiagnosed. The prevalence is increasing because of an increasing incidence of non–insulin-dependent diabetes mellitus (NIDDM), as well as a declining mortality rate. The prevalence of NIDDM rises with age, the peak level occurring between the ages of 45 and 65 years.

The introduction of insulin in the 1920s resulted in the decline of diabetic ketoacidosis as the major cause of death in people with diabetes. It quickly became apparent that diabetes resulted in long-term complications that produced far greater morbidity and mortality. At present, deaths related to the long-term complications of diabetes make diabetes the seventh leading cause of death. In addition, at all ages of onset, the life expectancy of a diabetic individual is only about two-thirds of that of the general population.

About 5 to 10 per cent of the total population of people with diabetes have insulin-dependent diabetes mellitus (IDDM). IDDM is thought to be an autoimmune disease that destroys the insulin-producing beta cells of the islets of Langerhans, eventually causing virtual cessation of insulin production. Although most persons develop IDDM during childhood, a substantial number develop it during their twenties and thirties. Onset after 40 years of age is uncommon. Therefore, among adults with diabetes, there is a considerable number with IDDM, with onset either in childhood or in adulthood.

Most adults have NIDDM, which usually develops after the age of 40. In this disorder there is both tissue resistance to the action of insulin and defective insulin production, so that insulin cannot be hypersecreted sufficiently to overcome this resistance. Patients with severe hyperglycemia are resistant to insulin, and their islet cells cannot continue to hypersecrete it, so that insulin levels may be quite low. Obesity, present in 80 to 90 per cent of people with NIDDM, contributes additional resistance to the action of insulin, which is reversible with weight loss.

CONTROL OF BLOOD GLUCOSE

Relationship of Control to Complications

The exact relationship between the abnormal metabolic milieu of diabetes and the morphologic changes that result in the long-term complications of the disease remains to be clarified. Hypotheses include (1) alterations in the sugar alcohols sorbitol and myoinositol, which result in impaired intracellular phosphoinositide metabolism; (2) nonenzymatic glycosylation of proteins that alter function, especially in vessel walls; (3) acceleration of atherosclerosis, in part caused by elevation of low-density lipoproteins (LDL) and reduction of high-density lipoproteins (HDL); and (4) increased basement membrane thickness.

Many patients suffer few or even no complications despite more than 25 to 30 years of diabetes that has not been well controlled. Conversely, in other patients, complications abound with diabetes of much shorter duration. Obviously, there is some genetic substrate that influences the rate of progression and the types of complications that develop in any individual. Family longevity, exercise, stress, diet, underlying lipid abnormalities, smoking, hypertension, and possibly other risk factors also are important. Even within the same individual, different types of complications may proceed at vastly different rates.

Studies attempting to determine whether the control of blood glucose levels affects the development or progression of the long-term complications of diabetes have almost all focused on IDDM. At present, the limited data available suggest, but certainly do not prove, that such control may make a difference in IDDM. The Diabetes Control and Complications Trial is an ongoing, 5- to 9-year, multicenter study of 1400 patients with IDDM that will answer this question. It is clear already, however, that intensive insulin therapy, which is necessary for the achievement of near-normoglycemia, carries with it an approximately threefold increased risk of severe hypoglycemia. Although the benefits and risks of trying to achieve near-normoglycemia in patients with IDDM will be clarified by the mid-1990s by the Diabetes Control and Complications Trial, it is not yet clear whether the data will be able to be extrapolated to people with NIDDM. The only study that attempted to show the benefit of treatment on the complications that developed in people with NIDDM was the University Group Diabetes Program study, done in the late 1960s. Although the "headlined" conclusions from that study had more to do with the possible cardiac effects of tolbutamide, it should also be remembered that this study showed no benefit of diabetes control on the development and progression of complications. Much of the possible benefit of tight control that has been reported from the previously mentioned studies has to do with the microvascular complications of diabetes (i.e., retinopathy and nephropathy). Whether any benefit may accrue to the macrovascular complications such as coronary artery, peripheral vascular, or cerebrovascular diseases is still unknown.

The issue of when intervention must be initiated in an attempt to alter the development of long-term complications is a vexing one. We have long known that people with NIDDM may often go for years with undetected hyperglycemia before the clinical diagnosis of diabetes is made. Such patients may present for the first time with an already established complication, such as gangrene of a toe. The metabolic abnormalities that eventually result in long-term complications take years to progress to the point where such complications become clinically recognized. It is not known whether intervention to prevent complications must begin early after the onset of disease, before there is any evidence of complications (primary intervention), or whether intervention can be useful even after complications have developed (secondary intervention). Furthermore, the degree of metabolic control needed to alter the development of complications is not known.

Setting Treatment Goals

The most reasonable course to take with patients is, first, to establish treatment goals. One goal to be achieved in all patients is clinical well-being, that is, the elimination of fatigue, polyuria, nocturia, thirst, blurred vision, or undesired weight loss. A second goal is the avoidance of hypoglycemia. This goal must be considered on an individual basis. A young person may tolerate mild hypoglycemia quite well; therefore, occasional episodes may be acceptable as long as they do not occur while the patient is driving or in other life-threatening situations. Severe episodes that require the assistance of another person or that result in seizures or loss of consciousness are never acceptable. On the other hand, even mild hypoglycemia may be significant for the older patient, who may have underlying cardiac or cerebrovascular disease. In such individuals, hypoglycemia may trigger arrhythmia, stroke, or seizure. Even mild hypoglycemia must be avoided in such patients.

Therefore, blood glucose levels should be maintained that result in minimal symptoms related to hyper- or hypoglycemia. Glucose levels in the postprandial period that are generally less than 200 to 250 mg per dl usually achieve the first purpose. The older the patient, the higher the renal threshold for glucose, so that higher levels may not cause glycosuria with resultant polyuria and polydipsia. To establish a level that avoids fatigue and provides optimal energy is more difficult, and, again, there is considerable interindividual variability. A normal postprandial plasma glucose level is generally less than 140 mg per dl. Using the criteria for diagnosing diabetes of the National Diabetes Data Group, a plasma glucose level of more than 200 mg per dl 2 hours after a glucose load during a glucose tolerance test is considered to be diagnostic of diabetes, levels between 140 and 200 mg per dl being thought to reflect impaired glucose tolerance. Although the criteria for fasting plasma glucose levels suggest that a level of more than 140 mg per dl is considered to be unequivocally abnormal, it is clear from a variety of studies that a level of more than 115 mg per dl is associated with distinct impairment of insulin secretion. Therefore, an ideal goal is normoglycemia, with a fasting plasma glucose level of less than 115 mg per dl and a 2-hour postprandial plasma glucose level of less than 140 mg per dl. Acceptable goals are a fasting glucose level of less than 140 mg per dl and a postprandial glucose level of less than 200 mg per dl. It should be understood that these "acceptable" goals are based on patient well-being rather than documented proof that such levels prevent or alter the development of long- or short-term complications. More stringent goals should be set with the patient only after careful discussion of the uncertain nature of the benefits, the very real risks of hypoglycemia, and the considerable demands that more frequent blood glucose monitoring and more intensive therapy will place on the patient, family, and staff. Whenever hypoglycemia is encountered in such therapy, however, careful consideration should be given to setting less stringent blood glucose treatment goals.

Monitoring

Urine Testing

Glucose. In recent years, it has become apparent that even doubly voided urine specimens are inaccurate reflections of the simultaneous blood glucose level. Furthermore, the renal threshold for glucose gradually increases with age, so that individuals 60 to 70 years of age may well have negative urine tests for glucose when their blood glucose levels are more than 300 mg per dl. For these reasons, urine testing is gradually being replaced by self-monitoring of blood glucose (SMBG), even for people with NIDDM.

Ketones. Urine testing for ketones is still necessary for patients with IDDM when blood glucose levels are more than 250 mg per dl and when these patients become ill.

Self-Monitoring of Blood Glucose

Techniques. SMBG is a technique in which the patient obtains a drop of blood via finger prick with a spring-loaded lancet device and places the drop on a plastic strip that holds a pad impregnated with glucose oxidase and a color reagent. The strip is then blotted to remove the remaining blood cells, and the plasma penetrates the reagent pad. After a certain time period, the patient compares the color with a color chart or inserts the strip in a light reflectance meter to obtain a digital readout of the glucose level. New variations on this theme with new meters are continually being developed.

Accuracy. With SMBG, it is predominantly plasma glucose that is being measured. Capillary and venous plasma glucose levels are very similar in the fasting state, but in the postprandial state, capillary levels may be 10 to 15 per cent higher. Overall, the methods are reasonably accurate, so that readings within 15 per cent of the true plasma glucose level are considered to be excellent, and they certainly suffice for guidance in making therapeutic decisions. However, the accuracy of SMBG is strongly dependent on the technique, patients with poor technique having quite variable results. Teaching of the technique by a skilled diabetes educator is of paramount importance. The patient must also be taught how to calibrate the meter, do routine maintenance, and check the accuracy via control solutions. It should also be remembered that on hospital inpatient services, nurses who do not perform this test all the time may achieve quite inaccurate results.

Use. SMBG allows patients and physicians to obtain a glucose reading at any time of the day, which allows unprecedented control and flexibility of patient management and lifestyle. The need to perform SMBG is strongly dependent on the management modalities used. SMBG can also be performed any time the patient feels ill or is experiencing what may be a hypoglycemic reaction.

Glycosylated Hemoglobin

Via a series of chemical reactions, glucose can attach irreversibly to hemoglobin in direct proportion to the circulating blood glucose level. Because the red blood cells survive in the circulation for about 120 days, the amount of hemoglobin that becomes glycosylated reflects the state of diabetes control for the preceding several weeks. It is important to check with the laboratory being used for glycosylated hemoglobin (also known as "hemoglobin A1c") measurement to be sure that a rapidly changing, intermediate moiety is excluded from the final measurement.

Changes in glucose control result in changes in glycosylated hemoglobin levels within 2 to 3 weeks, but a steady state is not reached until 2 to 3 months later. In patients being seen for diabetes management every 2 to 4 months, glycosylated hemoglobin measurements therefore reflect control of the diabetes for the preceding interval and provide an objective confirmation of SMBG reporting. If there is a great discrepancy between the two, it is likely that the technique used in SMBG is poor or that the patient is falsifying the SMBG data. The latter possibility can be checked by using one of the new reflectance meters containing a memory (some store more than 300 values) or by examining the data for preferences for certain digits.

Therapeutic Approaches

Diet

Diet remains the cornerstone of management of both IDDM and NIDDM. Three main forms of dietary manipulation are used in the management of diabetes: (1) alterations in the total number of calories eaten to achieve normal body weight; (2) alterations in the composition of those calories to effect better glucose control and lower cholesterol levels; and (3) alterations in the timing of consumption of those calories to match the use of other therapeutic modalities, such as exercise, oral hypoglycemic agents, and insulin. The diet needs to be individualized for each patient by a dietitian experienced in diabetes management to achieve compliance. This involves assessing current eating practices and then determining what types of alterations are practical and how they fit into the patient's lifestyle. Continued adjustment and follow-up by the dietitian are critical. Preprinted tear sheets of diet plans are insufficient.

New nutritional guidelines on the composition of the diet and new exchange lists were developed by the American Diabetes Association and the American Dietetic Association in 1986 on the basis of newer information regarding the relationships between the various food groups and blood glucose and cholesterol levels.

Calorie Reduction. Because 80 to 90 per cent of people with NIDDM are overweight, and because this excess weight contributes an additional burden of insulin resistance, weight loss is a major goal for many patients. A balanced reduction in caloric intake combined with increased exercise remains the preferred method of weight reduction for the person with diabetes. This approach can be supplemented by the use of support groups, behavior modification, and other forms of counseling. Very-low-calorie (500 to 800 kcal per day) diets can cause a more rapid weight loss but usually result in a gradual return to the baseline weight once normal eating resumes. However, if a patient does choose to follow such a diet, during the period of very-low-caloric intake dosages of insulin or oral hypoglycemic agents must usually be reduced markedly and the patient followed carefully. Once weight loss is accomplished, continued dietary counseling is important to achieve stabilization and to prevent regaining weight.

One potential area of concern is the weight gain that often accompanies major improvements in diabetes control. When diabetes is poorly controlled, the body is inefficient at handling incoming calories and spills many of them into the urine as glucose. As the body becomes more efficient in handling these calories, during better control of diabetes, if food intake remains the same, these excess calories will be stored as fat. Thus, careful attention to diet with restriction of caloric intake is important when making changes in other aspects of the therapeutic plan.

Carbohydrates. In an effort to reduce fat intake and lower the cholesterol level (see later), the carbohydrate portion of the diet has been increased to 50 to 60 per cent of total calories. Uncommonly, such a high-carbohydrate diet may reduce HDL cholesterol levels and increase triglyceride levels. Therefore, the effects of such diets must be monitored.

The carbohydrates used in the diet should be almost exclusively complex (e.g., starches), rather than simple sugars such as sucrose. This diet results in a more gradual and lower increment in blood glucose levels after meals. Small amounts of sucrose (<5 per cent of carbohydrate calories) may be added to the diet judiciously. Foods high in soluble fiber may help to lower blood glucose and cholesterol levels and their intake should be encouraged, but only to the point where they do not hinder other aspects of dietary compliance. At this point, there does not appear to be substantial benefit to adding purified fiber supplements to aid in diabetes control.

Some foods that appear to have the same complex carbohydrate content result in higher blood glucose levels after being eaten. This has given rise to what has been termed the "glycemic index" of foods. However, this index was based on eating such foods separately from other foods. When carbohydrates with a low, medium, and high glycemic index are added to fats and proteins to make up a normal "mixed" meal, these differences in glycemic index appear to be lost.

Fats. Because of concern about the role of saturated dietary fat in determining serum LDL cholesterol levels and the development of atherosclerosis, it has been recommended that the total proportion of fat in the diet be limited to less than 30 per cent of total calories, with saturated fat being less than 10 per cent of total calories and total cholesterol content limited to less than 300 mg per day. If normal LDL cholesterol levels are not achieved with such a diet and otherwise optimal diabetes treatment, total fat should be limited to less than 25 per cent and 200 to 250 mg of cholesterol or to less than 20 per cent total fat and 100 to 150 mg of cholesterol. Additional hypolipidemic agents may also need to be prescribed.

In some poorly controlled diabetic individuals, triglyceride levels may rise to more than 1000 mg per dl, which raises the danger of acute pancreatitis. In such individuals, aggressive pharmacologic treatment of the diabetes combined with a 10 to 15 per cent fat diet may be necessary to reduce the triglyceride values to less dangerous levels.

Protein. The remainder of the caloric intake, about 12 to 20 per cent, is protein. Generally, non–red-meat sources are recommended to avoid saturated fats.

Alcohol. Alcohol is calculated as a fat in the diet, yielding 7 kcal per gram (kcal = 0.8 × "proof" × number of ounces ingested). The other components of a drink and mixers also add calories. Current recommendations allow for a drink with a meal. However, excessive alcohol intake can (1) inhibit gluconeogenesis by the liver, which aggravates hypoglycemia when insufficient food is eaten; (2) worsen hypertriglyceridemia by augmenting fatty acid and triglyceride synthesis while impairing hepatic fatty acid oxidation; (3) impair compliance with the diabetes management regimen; and (4) impair glucose tolerance. Alcohol in any amount can cause a disulfiram (Antabuse)-like reaction (usually limited to facial flushing) in patients taking first-generation oral hypoglycemic agents, especially chlorpropamide.

Sweeteners. Nutritive and non-nutritive sweeteners are acceptable for use by people with diabetes, although sweeteners with substantial calories (fructose, sorbitol) must have their calories calculated as part of the total caloric allowance. Although aspartame (Nutrasweet) is a nutritive sweetener containing phenylalanine and aspartic acid, it is 180 to 200 times sweeter than sucrose, so the small amounts used for sweetening can usually be ignored. Despite protests to the contrary, aspartame has proved to be safe in general use. Although the use of these artificial sweeteners should not be generally encouraged, if it is thought that they will help dietary compliance, their use is acceptable.

Meal Timing. The timing of meals has particular importance in the patient taking insulin. The peak absorption of nutrients may be timed to coincide with the peak time of action of injected insulin (see later). Between-meal and bedtime snacks may thus be necessary. Because postprandial rises in the blood glucose level may be prolonged in patients with NIDDM, spacing of meals at least 4 to 5 hours apart without snacks may also be beneficial.

Exercise

Regular exercise, when it can be done, has many potential benefits for the person with diabetes. During exercise, the increase in glucose oxidation and in the metabolic rate results in more rapid burning of calories and weight loss. This may, however, precipitate hypoglycemia in someone receiving oral hypoglycemic agents or insulin who cannot decrease endogenous insulin secretion, as the normal person does. This continued presence of insulin impairs the hepatic glycogenolysis and gluconeogenesis needed to restore blood glucose levels. Thus, a lowered insulin dose or increased caloric intake may be necessary.

Hypoglycemia may also develop if the exercise occurs within an hour of insulin injection and the insulin has been injected into the exercising limb. This is because of the more rapid distribution of the injected insulin that results from the increased blood flow. Occasionally, hypoglycemia may arise several hours after exercise in such a person because of the replenishment of muscle glycogen stores.

Exercise increases insulin sensitivity and results in improved glucose tolerance even after the period of exercise. Regular exercise may cause a decrease in LDL cholesterol and an increase in HDL cholesterol levels and may also decrease

elevated blood pressure. Exercise may also have a beneficial effect on the cardiovascular system, perhaps countering some of the adverse effects of diabetes.

In the patient with IDDM whose diabetes is poorly controlled, peripheral use of glucose is decreased, hepatic glucose output is increased, and lipolysis is already enhanced. When such a person exercises, hepatic glucose output increases further and lipolysis rises, which results in increased blood glucose and ketone levels. Thus, exercise should not be done if the individual's pre-exercise blood glucose level is more than 250 mg per dl and if ketonuria exists (Table 1).

Oral Hypoglycemic Agents

Oral hypoglycemic agents are effective only in patients with some endogenous insulin secretion, that is, in most patients with NIDDM and in none with IDDM.

Pharmacology. The mechanisms of action of these drugs are still not completely understood. They facilitate the secretion of insulin from the pancreas by lowering the glucose threshold at which insulin is secreted. In the patient with markedly impaired basal insulin secretion and marked fasting hyperglycemia, insulin levels may actually rise. This facilitation of basal insulin secretion results in lowered hepatic glucose output. In peripheral tissues, these drugs also appear to enhance insulin action at receptor and postreceptor sites.

Currently, six oral hypoglycemic agents are

TABLE 1. **Strategies to Avoid Hypoglycemia or Hyperglycemia with Exercise in Individuals Taking Insulin***

Food
Eat 1–3 hr before exercise.
If exercise is prolonged, take supplemental carbohydrates every 30 min.
Increase food intake after exercise, depending on intensity and duration of exercise.

Insulin
Take insulin > 1 hr before exercise if injecting it into the exercising area.
Decrease insulin dose before exercise if not increasing food.
Adjust subsequent insulin doses if subject to delayed hypoglycemia.

Blood glucose monitoring
Monitor blood glucose before and after exercise, as well as during exercise if > 1 hr duration.
Delay exercise if glucose > 250 mg/dl and/or if ketonuric.
Learn individual glucose responses to different types of exercise.

---

*Modified from Horton ES: Role and management of exercise in diabetes mellitus. Diabetes Care *11*:201, 1988. Reproduced with permission of the American Diabetes Association, Inc.

available in the United States (Table 2). They are usually divided into two categories based on their time of availability in this country, that is, first- and second-generation medications. The medications are different in method of metabolism and excretion, duration of action, and potency. The second-generation medications, glyburide and glipizide, are considerably more potent than those of the first generation, both on a milligram-for-milligram basis and clinically. Many patients who do not respond to the older agents do respond to these newer medications, and many who become secondary failures with the first-generation drugs again respond to the second-generation drugs.

University Group Diabetes Program Study. This multicenter study was designed to determine the effects of treatment with tolbutamide, insulin, and phenformin (a now abandoned oral agent with a different structure and mechanism of action) on the long-term complications of NIDDM. One outcome of this study was the finding that tolbutamide was associated with an increased risk of death from cardiovascular causes. This study has been widely criticized, and its results have been questioned by many. These results have not been duplicated by other evaluations of tolbutamide or other oral agents. At present, most diabetologists feel comfortable using oral agents in appropriately selected patients with NIDDM, although many avoid using tolbutamide because of the results of the University Group Diabetes Program Study.

Clinical Use. The oral agents should be used only in patients with NIDDM who fail to attain satisfactory blood glucose levels despite dietary and exercise interventions. The best candidates for therapy are those with disease of less than 5 years' duration, with fasting plasma glucose levels between 140 and 225 mg per dl, with continued adherence to diet, and, if taking insulin, with a requirement of less than 40 units per day.

Choosing among the different agents is a matter of personal preference, and becoming confident in the use of two or three of them is recom-

mended. I prefer to start giving new patients one of the two second-generation drugs, especially if the fasting blood glucose level is more than 180 mg per dl, because of their potency. During therapy, patients must be monitored for secondary failure, which is generally caused by poor dietary adherence.

Use with Insulin. Because the oral agents can enhance the action of insulin, it seemed natural to try to use these agents and insulin together. Controlled studies suggest, however, that for most patients such combined use has little benefit. In some patients, the addition of an oral agent to insulin therapy may permit reduction of the insulin dose. However, two drugs are now being used instead of one, and both medications have potential side effects. In general, there is little indication for the use of both medications together.

Side Effects. The side effects of these medications are uncommon. Jaundice, rashes, and agranulocytosis are rare. The first-generation agents, especially chlorpropamide, can occasionally cause a mild disulfiram-like reaction (usually limited to facial flushing) with alcohol ingestion. Chlorpropamide also may cause a syndrome of inappropriate antidiuretic hormone secretion, which results in water intoxication.

The first-generation agents are ionically bound to albumin and cause displacement of other drugs from binding sites on protein; the converse is also true. Thus, these medications may potentiate the action of dicumarol and barbiturates. Conversely, the action of the first-generation agents may be potentiated by sulfonamides, salicylates, phenylbutazone, and clofibrate. The two newer drugs are not bound to albumin in this fashion and have few drug-drug interactions.

Transient, mild, between-meal hypoglycemia may occur with the second-generation drugs because of their potent effect in stimulating insulin production. More rare is prolonged, severe hypoglycemia that requires hospitalization and continued glucose supplementation. This severe hypoglycemia occurs most often with chlorpro-

TABLE 2. **Oral Hypoglycemic Agents Used in the Management of Diabetes**

Generic Name	Brand Name	Dose Range (mg)	Doses Per Day	Tablet Sizes (mg)
First generation				
Tolbutamide	Orinase	500–3000	2	250, 500
Chlorpropamide	Diabinese	100–750	1	100, 250
Tolazamide	Tolinase	100–1000	1–2	100, 250, 500
Acetohexamide	Dymelor	250–1500	1–2	250, 500
Second generation				
Glyburide	Micronase, Diabeta	1.25*–20	1–2	1.25, 2.5, 5
Glipizide	Glucotrol	2.5*–40	1–2	5, 10

*Especially geriatric patients.

pamide and glyburide, perhaps because of their particularly long half-lives.

Insulin

All patients with IDDM must receive insulin. Patients with NIDDM are candidates for insulin therapy if they do not respond adequately to dietary therapy alone or to dietary therapy plus oral hypoglycemic agents. In addition, even for patients who normally require oral agents or who can be managed with diet alone, insulin may be necessary for treatment when they develop hyperosmolar, nonketotic coma, ketoacidosis, or acute illness; when they become pregnant; or when they need surgery.

Types of Insulin. Insulin may be of beef, pork, beef-pork mixture, or human origin. Because human insulins have declined in price, cause less fat atrophy, generate fewer antibodies, and cause less insulin allergy, they have now become the usual insulin for initiating chronic therapy and for intermittent use (e.g., with hyperalimentation, during pregnancy, and perioperatively). However, if a patient is doing well with nonhuman insulin, there is no need to switch to human insulin. Human insulins tend to have a slightly shorter duration of action than beef or pork insulin, perhaps caused in part by a lower titer of antibodies with their use.

Insulins can be modified with either zinc or protamine to prolong their biologic half-lives (Table 3). Regular (crystalline), or unmodified, insulin is the shortest-acting form, with an onset of action within 30 to 60 minutes, a peak action at 2 to 5 hours, and a total duration of action 5 to 8 hours after subcutaneous injection. Semilente has a slightly longer action spectrum. Neutral protamine Hagedorn (NPH) insulin usually has an onset of action within 1 to 1½ hours, a peak at about 8 to 12 hours, and a total duration of about 24 hours. Lente insulin generally has a similar action spectrum. However, with both of these intermediate-acting insulins, there is a great deal of individual variability in response.

Thus, in many individuals, the action peaks at 6 to 10 hours after injection and lasts for only 12 to 16 hours. In such individuals, two injections per day are clearly necessary. In other persons, NPH and Lente may have greatly prolonged action, with little activity within the first 6 to 10 hours, a modest peak at 14 to 18 hours, and a total duration of 24 to 30 hours. Ultralente insulin and protamine zinc insulin (PZI) have a total duration of action of about 24 to 36 hours and are almost peakless insulins.

Patients should be instructed to look at their insulin bottles before taking each dose to detect any deterioration in the insulin. Frosting of the bottle or precipitation in clumps may occur, especially with human insulins and with NPH. This deterioration may be lessened by storing the bottles in the refrigerator.

Insulin Regimens. Insulin therapy can usually be initiated on an outpatient basis. Instruction in insulin administration should be coupled with that for SMBG and diet by experienced nurse-educators and dietitians. Some patients respond well to a single injection of an intermediate-acting insulin given before breakfast. This regimen is, perhaps, the simplest when initiating insulin, especially in someone with NIDDM. It is safest to begin with a relatively low dose, such as 10 to 15 units. Often, however, NPH and Lente do not give a full 24-hour duration of action, as determined by SMBG, and a second dose before supper or bedtime may be needed. Even when two doses are used, SMBG done before meals may reveal elevated glucose levels at lunch and/or bedtime, indicating the need to add regular insulin to each dose of NPH/Lente (a "split/mixed" regimen). A rule of thumb in patients using this regimen is to take two-thirds of the insulin in the morning and one-third before supper. At each of these times, two-thirds of the insulin given is intermediate acting (NPH or Lente) and one-third is short acting (regular or Semilente). In fact, 70:30 per cent fixed mixtures of NPH and regular insulin are available commercially for

TABLE 3. **Types of Insulin**

Insulin	Modifier	Onset* (hr)	Peak* (hr)	Duration* (hr)
Short acting				
Regular	None	0.5–1	2–5	5–8
Semilente	Zinc	1.0–1.5	3–8	8–16
Intermediate acting				
NPH	Protamine	1–1.5	6–14	18–28
Lente	Zinc	1–2.5	6–14	18–28
Long acting				
PZI	Protamine, zinc	4–8	None	24–36
Ultralente	Zinc	4–8	None	24–36

*Considerable interindividual variation for these times.

TABLE 4. **Example of Insulin Algorithm in Intensive Insulin Therapy***

Glucose Level (mg/dl)	Breakfast Insulin (U)†	Lunch Insulin (U)	Supper Insulin (U)	Bedtime Insulin (U)
<80	4	3	6	
81–120	5	4	7	
121–160	6	5	9	
161–200	7	6	11	1
201–240	9	7	13	2
241–300	11	8	15	3
301–360	13	10	17	4
>360	15	12	20	5

*This is an example only. Each patient's algorithm must be individually developed and adjusted.

†Regular insulin. NPH/Lente is also given at supper or bedtime. Alternatively, Ultralente could be given instead of NPH/Lente.

patients who have difficulty mixing insulin. The patient's actual insulin needs may be quite different, of course, and are based on SMBG results. Patients mixing regular insulin with NPH, Lente, or Ultralente should be aware that if the insulins are left together in the syringe for more than 5 to 15 minutes, the excess protamine or zinc may bind the regular insulin and convert some of it to the longer-acting form. Thus, patients should inject the mixture immediately after mixing it.

Intensive Insulin Therapy. "Intensive insulin therapy" is the name given to techniques designed to achieve near-normoglycemia. Insulin may be given as a continuous subcutaneous insulin infusion via an insulin pump and a needle left in the subcutaneous tissue for 24 to 48 hours or via multiple (three or more) daily injections. With continuous subcutaneous insulin infusion, a basal rate is chosen that can be varied at different times of the day. Subsequently, boluses of insulin are given via the pump before each meal.

With multiple daily injections, regular insulin is given as separate injections before each meal, and an intermediate-acting insulin is given at supper or bedtime. Alternatively, Ultralente can be given to provide a constant background of insulin, and regular insulin can be given again at each meal.

With all of these methods, the premeal dose of insulin is based on the glucose level obtained at that time via SMBG, the anticipated amount of food to be eaten at that meal, and the anticipated amount of exercise to be done over the next several hours. The insulin dose is adjusted according to an algorithm developed for the individual patient. An example is given in Table 4.

Intensive insulin therapy is generally used in people with IDDM, whose blood glucose levels usually are more labile than those with NIDDM. It takes a great deal of effort on the part of the patient and an experienced staff to develop and

continually modify the algorithm and for the patient to adhere to this regimen. SMBG at least four times a day is mandatory. When the goal of treatment is near-normoglycemia, the risk of hypoglycemic reactions increases almost threefold (see later).

Lipodystrophy. Impurities in older insulin preparations occasionally caused atrophy of the subcutaneous fat at injection sites. This is rarely a problem with the newer insulins, especially the purified pork and human preparations. Hypertrophy of the fat at the injection site is still common because of the lipogenic and antilipolytic effects of the insulin. This may be avoided by rotating insulin injection sites. Because of this effect, however, direct injection of human insulin into previously atrophied sites may cause them to fill in.

Insulin Allergy. Insulin allergy has become even more rare now that most patients are started with human insulin, although it still occurs. It is usually manifested by diffuse urticaria and pruritus. In patients in whom insulin therapy is mandatory, several steps must be taken, usually on an inpatient basis, by an allergist with emergency equipment available. First, if the insulin used is not human, the human form should be substituted. Second, if the insulin used was NPH, regular insulin should be tried to be sure that the allergic reaction was not caused by the protamine in the NPH. Third, the dose of regular insulin initially tried should be 0.001 unit given intradermally. If there is no reaction, desensitization can be done by increasing the dose at tenfold increments at 20- to 30-minute intervals.

Patients may also experience a local hypersensitivity reaction at the injection site. Usually this can be managed with antihistamines and disappears after several weeks. Sometimes a local reaction may occur with cold insulin that has just been taken out of the refrigerator. This may be avoided by warming the insulin to room temperature before injection.

Insulin Resistance. Insulin resistance is rare and is caused by the development of antibodies that bind the insulin sufficiently to impair its action. By definition, a patient is considered to be insulin resistant when he or she needs to use more than 200 units per day in the absence of infection. This type of resistance is different both from the tissue resistance to the action of insulin occurring in NIDDM and obesity and from the rare form of resistance caused by disorders of the insulin receptor associated with the skin condition known as acanthosis nigricans. With insulin resistance mediated by antibodies, insulin should be switched to the human form. Rarely, glucocorticosteroids may need to be given to reduce the antibody titers.

MANAGEMENT OF COMPLICATIONS

Acute Complications

Hypoglycemia

Hypoglycemia results from an imbalance in the amount of food eaten, the amount of insulin or oral hypoglycemic agent used, and the amount of exercise performed. Mild, interprandial hypoglycemia occasionally occurs with oral agents and may be avoided by decreasing the dose. More severe, prolonged hypoglycemia may occur with chlorpropamide and glyburide and usually requires hospitalization.

With insulin treatment, hypoglycemia occurs with increasing frequency the lower the target blood glucose goals. Hypoglycemia is usually seen when a meal is delayed or when exercise is done that has not been planned for by decreasing the prior insulin dose or increasing food intake.

The two regulatory hormones most important in countering hypoglycemia are glucagon and epinephrine. People with IDDM commonly lose their glucagon response to hypoglycemia after about 5 years of diabetes; people with NIDDM do so less commonly. Subsequently, people with IDDM may lose their epinephrine response to hypoglycemia as a result of autonomic neuropathy or the use of beta-adrenergic blocking medications to treat hypertension. Loss of both glucagon and epinephrine responses makes these individuals quite susceptible to hypoglycemic reactions. Furthermore, loss of the epinephrine response results in loss of the early warning signs of hypoglycemia, such as tachycardia, sweating, and anxiety. Because of this unawareness, the first sign of hypoglycemia is confusion. Thus, these persons are at risk for a severe reaction for two reasons: (1) they can become confused quickly, so that they do not eat the food that is necessary to stop the reaction, and (2) they have lost their endogenous counter-regulatory mechanisms to reverse their hypoglycemic state, and they will not recover until their injected insulin dissipates. Beta blockers are, therefore, contraindicated in patients with IDDM who may be prone to hypoglycemia.

Education is the key to prevent hypoglycemia. All patients should wear a Medic-Alert identification bracelet or necklace or similar identification. Patients must avoid delaying meals and should prepare for exercise by decreasing their insulin dose or increasing their food intake. All patients prone to hypoglycemia should carry a readily absorbable simple sugar with them at all times to treat a reaction.

For the unconscious patient, 1 mg of glucagon can be administered subcutaneously or intramuscularly by a family member or friend; glucagon injection kits are available for this purpose. The patient with unawareness of hypoglycemia faces considerable danger from hypoglycemia and should raise target glucose goals. Patients should be instructed to stop driving and eat if they feel hypoglycemic. Because it takes about 30 to 45 minutes for cerebral function to return to normal after eating, they should not resume driving before this time. Patients with unawareness of hypoglycemia should either eat before driving or check their blood glucose levels before driving routinely. There is no excuse for a patient's having an automobile accident while hypoglycemic.

Diabetic Ketoacidosis

Ketoacidosis occurs in patients with IDDM because of an inadequate amount of insulin, usually in the face of increased counter-regulatory hormone levels resulting from stress, commonly an infection. People with NIDDM can also develop ketoacidosis in the face of great stress, such as sepsis or a myocardial infarction, but it is usually not as severe.

Education of patients is important in preventing ketoacidosis. A typical mistake patients make is to omit their insulin when they vomit because of a gastroenteritis. Patients can often abort an episode of ketoacidosis by telephoning their physician promptly, so that by careful testing of urine ketones and SMBG, extra doses of regular insulin can be taken every 4 to 6 hours. However, some patients are too ill to be managed at home, and hospitalization is necessary. In the hospital, intravenous fluids to correct dehydration, bicarbonate for severe acidosis (pH < 7.1), intravenous insulin, and other supportive treatment may be needed. (See Chapter "Diabetes Mellitus in Children and Adolescents.") At the end of an insulin infusion, it is important to give regular insulin subcutaneously and never to omit an insulin dose if blood glucose levels are low. A smaller dose may be needed, but if the dose is omitted altogether, the stress state may push the patient into ketoacidosis.

Nonketotic Hyperglycemic Hyperosmolar Coma

This state occurs in the patient with NIDDM and is also usually precipitated by an underlying illness. High mortality continues to be associated with this condition, usually because of the underlying precipitating illness. Rehydration with intravenous fluids is important, but attention must be paid to the cardiac status to avoid congestive heart failure in older patients. Intravenous insulin can be given as for ketoacidosis, but bicarbonate is not necessary unless there is a supervening lactic acidosis. When acidosis is present in a severely hyperglycemic patient with NIDDM, it is important to quantify serum ketones (serial dilutions of serum can be tested at the bedside with Ketostix or Acetest tablets) to determine whether the patient is suffering from lactic acidosis or ketoacidosis.

Chronic Complications

Retinopathy

Diabetes is the leading cause of new blindness between the ages of 20 and 74 years in adults in the United States. By 25 years after being diagnosed, more than 90 per cent of people with IDDM and 75 per cent of people with NIDDM have some retinopathy. However, in 80 per cent of eyes, the disease is confined to "background" retinopathy. In 5 per cent of people with background retinopathy alone, the edema may involve the macula and result in impaired vision. Laser photocoagulation may delay or prevent reduction in visual acuity when this occurs.

Of the individuals with IDDM for 20 years and retinopathy, 20 to 40 per cent progress to proliferative retinopathy. For individuals with NIDDM, this figure is 4 to 6 per cent. Laser photocoagulation has proved to be remarkably successful in retarding or preventing the progression from preproliferative to proliferative retinopathy. Vitrectomy can also be performed to remove vitreous hemorrhages and scar tissue.

Routine annual visits to an ophthalmologist are necessary to assess the development and progression of retinopathy so that timely intervention can be arranged. Such visits may also be used to detect the presence of glaucoma, for which such patients are at slightly increased risk, and cataracts, for which such patients are at twofold increased risk.

Nephropathy

Diabetic nephropathy develops in over one-third of people with IDDM and in 5 to 10 per cent of those with NIDDM by 20 to 25 years' duration of the disease. The earliest signs of renal impairment are the development of proteinuria (>0.3 gram per 24 hours) and microscopic hematuria, usually beginning about 15 to 20 years after the onset of disease. Hypertension commonly begins at this time as well. The glomerular filtration rate (GFR) begins to decline within a year or two after the onset of proteinuria, with a relatively linear rate of fall. However, the rate of fall for each individual is highly variable. Because interventions may alter this rate of fall in the GFR, yearly determinations of the creatinine clearance and 24-hour protein excretion are indicated after about 10 years of diabetes or in the patient found to be hypertensive.

Aggressive treatment of hypertension, maintaining diastolic pressures less than 90 mmHg, has been shown to be effective in slowing the decline in GFR. Although some preliminary studies suggest that angiotensin-converting enzyme inhibitors may provide additional benefit, there are no controlled studies suggesting that they are better than other antihypertensive agents in controlling blood pressure and affecting glomerular filtration. Because beta blockers block the ability of epinephrine to raise glucose levels in the event of hypoglycemia, they should be avoided in most patients taking insulin and are contraindicated in patients with IDDM undergoing intensive insulin therapy.

Thiazide diuretics often cause hypokalemia, which may impair insulin secretion and thus reduce glucose tolerance in the patient with NIDDM. Potassium supplementation is thus necessary. However, patients with NIDDM and mild renal insufficiency may have hyporeninemic hypoaldosteronism, which results in hyperkalemia. In such patients, potassium supplements may not be necessary and may, indeed, be harmful. Angiotensin-converting enzyme inhibitors may also cause hyperkalemia in the patient with hypoaldosteronism. Careful determination of electrolyte levels and renal function is important when using these medications. Thiazides may also cause an increase in LDL cholesterol levels.

A reduction in dietary protein to 0.6 gram per kg of ideal body weight may also prove to be beneficial in slowing the fall in the GFR in patients with all forms of renal insufficiency. Although this has not been well documented in diabetic nephropathy, there is no reason to suspect that it does not hold true for this entity. The hypothesis that protein restriction may influence the progression of renal disease is currently being

TABLE 5. **Diabetic Neuropathy**

Neuropathy Type	Manifestations	Nerve Structure Involved
Polyneuropathy	Sensory loss and sometimes pain in feet and hands	Nerve terminals
Radiculopathy	Sensory loss and pain in dermatome distribution	Nerve root
Mononeuropathy	Sensory loss, pain, and weakness in mixed nerve distribution	Mixed cranial or spinal nerve
Amyotrophy	Weakness, muscle atrophy, pain	Nerve terminal on muscle
Autonomic	Visceral disease	Autonomic nerves

tested in a large, prospective, controlled multicenter trial.

When renal failure does develop, patients with diabetes tend to do less well than those without diabetes. Patients clearly do best after transplantation, and it appears that they fare better with chronic ambulatory peritoneal dialysis than with hemodialysis.

Neuropathy

By 20 years' known duration of diabetes of either type, almost 50 per cent of patients have neuropathy. There are many different types of neuropathy (Table 5), with peripheral, symmetric polyneuropathy being the most common.

Peripheral Neuropathy. This type of neuropathy causes loss of sensation in the feet and hands and leads to painless injury. Because of the usually concomitant vascular disease, such injuries heal slowly, allowing the development of infection. Poor blood supply hinders healing and the delivery of adequate concentrations of antibiotics, and amputation may be the result. The infected foot ulcer usually contains three to six types of organisms, usually including anaerobes. Aggressive treatment with intravenous, broad-spectrum antibiotics with anaerobic coverage, bed rest to avoid pressure on the ulcer, and debridement of necrotic tissue are all necessary to avoid amputation. Patient education with respect to foot care and avoidance of injury is critical in preventing such amputations.

Occasionally, the most pressing aspect of peripheral neuropathy is pain. This pain sometimes responds to treatment with a tricyclic antidepressant such as amitriptyline, 75 mg at bedtime, and a phenothiazine such as perphenazine,* 4 mg three times daily, or fluphenazine,* 1 mg three times daily. Carbamazepine* may also be helpful. Recently, a topical ointment containing capsaicin, the active ingredient in hot peppers, has been found to ameliorate the pain in some patients, probably by depleting nerve terminals of substance P, a pain neurotransmitter.

Loss of sensation may occasionally lead to the

development of Charcot's arthropathy in the foot. Multiple small fractures occur, leading to joint deformity and further trauma. The foot and ankle may swell, with shortening and widening. Initially, this may present as an acute swelling with erythema and may be confused with osteomyelitis or cellulitis.

Radiculopathy. Radiculopathy occurs when a spinal nerve root is affected, causing loss of sensation and pain along the affected dermatome. Occasionally, it may present as abdominal or chest pain.

Mononeuropathy. A mixed spinal or cranial nerve may also be affected, causing pain, loss of sensation, and weakness in its distribution. Cranial third and sixth nerve palsies fall into this category. Radiculopathy and mononeuropathy are probably caused by occlusion of the vasa nervorum. Return of some or all function over several months is the rule.

Amyotrophy. Amyotrophy is of uncertain etiology and causes weakness and wasting of muscles in the pelvic girdle in association with weight loss. Although there is little sensory involvement, pain may be significant. Partial to complete reversibility over several months is the rule.

Autonomic Neuropathy. Autonomic neuropathy involves nerves to the viscera and may be quite disabling. Patients with evidence of cardiac neuropathy, evidenced by resting tachycardia and failure of the heart rate to change normally with breathing, upright posture, or Valsalva's maneuver, are at increased risk of arrhythmias perioperatively and merit close cardiac monitoring in this setting.

Esophageal motility may be affected. Gastroparesis diabeticorum (delayed gastric emptying) may result in a mismatch between the therapeutic timing of insulin's peak action and the absorption of food. A delay in insulin administration may be helpful. Nausea, early satiety, and vomiting of undigested food may be presenting complaints. Small meals and metoclopramide (Reglan), 10 mg before meals and at bedtime, are helpful. Uncontrolled diarrhea may be another manifestation of gastrointestinal neuropathy. Steatorrhea is present in 30 to 50 per cent of

---

*This use is not listed by the manufacturer.

patients with diarrhea. Bacterial overgrowth is occasionally present, and some improvement may be seen in certain patients receiving rotating antibiotics. Some patients also respond to clonidine. Metoclopramide, given for gastroparesis, may worsen diarrhea.

Bladder neuropathy is common, leading to stasis and repeated urinary tract infections. Indwelling catheters should be used only as a last resort in an effort to avoid infections. Bethanecol, 25 to 100 mg every 6 to 8 hours, may be helpful in some patients.

Impotence is present in about 50 per cent of diabetic men by age 50 and is caused by neuropathy or vascular disease. Psychogenic causes and medications used for hypertension also need to be considered. Recently, direct injections of papaverine and phentolamine into the penis of men with neuropathic impotence have resulted in satisfactory erections lasting for up to 1 hour. When such medications are ineffective, prosthetic implants may be indicated.

Orthostatic hypotension can be a severe problem because of lack of vascular constriction and an increase in heart rate on assuming the upright posture. Treatment consists of expanding the intravascular fluid volume with the mineralocorticoid 9-alpha-fludrocortisone (Florinef), wearing support stockings, and elevating the head of the bed at night to avoid supine hypertension.

Diabetic neuropathic cachexia is a syndrome, usually occurring in older men, consisting of painful polyneuropathy, depression, impotence, and marked weight loss. Spontaneous recovery is the rule after about 1 year, although antidepressant therapy may speed this improvement. It is not clear whether depression is the root cause, brought on by the painful neuropathy and resulting in impotence and weight loss, or whether it is a distinct syndrome.

Macrovascular Disease

Coronary Artery Disease. This disease is the single most common cause of death in adults with diabetes in the United States. Myocardial infarctions are more commonly pain free in people with diabetes, perhaps as a result of coexisting cardiac sensory neuropathy. Patients commonly present with congestive heart failure from their infarction. People with diabetes who have an acute myocardial infarction are three times more likely to have a fatal outcome, and long-term survival is reduced by about 50 per cent compared with those without diabetes. Angina pectoris and congestive heart failure are also increased two- to fourfold in people with diabetes. Angiography generally reveals more extensive disease than exists in the matched nondiabetic patient. Pa-

tients with diabetes do not appear to be at increased risk, however, from coronary artery bypass surgery or angioplasty.

Cerebrovascular Disease. The risk of stroke is increased two- to sixfold in people with diabetes and is generally of the ischemic occlusive type rather than hemorrhagic.

Peripheral Vascular Disease. Intermittent claudication occurs five times more frequently in people with than in people without diabetes. Often there are multiple lesions rather than a single occluding lesion, rendering bypass surgery and angioplasty more difficult. As discussed earlier, when occlusive vascular disease is combined with peripheral neuropathy, foot ulcers may develop that become infected and ultimately amputation is required. At present, diabetes accounts for 40 to 50 per cent of all nontraumatic amputations in the United States. It has been estimated that these figures could be reduced by 75 per cent by proper education of patients.

DIABETES MELLITUS IN CHILDREN AND ADOLESCENTS

method of
RODNEY A. LORENZ, M.D.
Vanderbilt University
Nashville, Tennessee

DIAGNOSIS

The diagnosis of diabetes mellitus in childhood is rarely difficult and can usually be made on the basis of the history and confirmed by simple laboratory procedures. Most patients present with symptoms related to hyperglycemia and glycosuria, that is, polyuria, polydipsia, and weight loss despite normal appetite. This constellation of symptoms occurs with blood glucose levels consistently above the renal threshold for glucose, normally 160 to 180 mg per dl. Therefore a random blood glucose level generally exceeds 200 mg per dl, and further diagnostic studies are not needed.

Although this presentation is most common, the severity of the disease at diagnosis varies from asymptomatic disease to ketoacidosis and coma. It now appears that insulin-dependent diabetes mellitus (IDDM), which accounts for more than 95 per cent of the cases in children, usually results from gradual autoimmune destruction of the pancreatic islets over a period of weeks to years. Symptoms occur only when the insulin-producing capacity falls to about 10 per cent of normal. Thus occasional asymptomatic individuals are identified by urinalysis done as part of a routine health examination, and others are detected when relatively mild symptoms are recognized by parents. Still others present when an intercurrent illness precipitates an insulin-resistant state and rapid development of ketoacidosis.

The child with few or no symptoms and either glycosuria or hyperglycemia is best approached by determining the fasting glucose level. Diagnosis of diabetes in these circumstances requires a fasting glucose level higher than 140 mg per dl on two occasions. However, levels of 100 to 140 mg per dl are probably abnormal in children and should be followed by repeat determinations every few months. Formal glucose tolerance testing in children is rarely indicated.

A prediabetic state may be suggested by sophisticated procedures such as determination of the presence of antibodies to insulin or pancreatic islet cells, or an acute insulin response to intravenous glucose. Because no safe method of preventing progression to full-blown diabetes is known, there is no clear advantage in detecting this early stage of disease, and these methods remain research procedures.

Causes of diabetes in childhood other than autoimmune islet destruction account for less than 5 per cent of cases. These include other pancreatic diseases (e.g., cystic fibrosis) and non–insulin-dependent diabetes mellitus (NIDDM). NIDDM may occur in nonobese children, especially in certain kindreds with clear dominant inheritance. Recent reports have described a group of black children whose presentation resembles that of IDDM but whose subsequent clinical course suggests NIDDM. The true nature of this disorder remains to be clarified.

TREATMENT

Because the vast majority of children and adolescents with diabetes have the insulin-dependent variety, the remainder of this chapter addresses the treatment of IDDM. Acute and chronic phases of treatment can be considered separately. The goals of acute management are (1) restoration of metabolic equilibrium, (2) establishment of insulin requirements for chronic therapy, and (3) education of the patient and family for home management of diabetes. Although a minority of children present to our service in ketoacidosis, this is a life-threatening condition that requires expert management, preferably in an intensive care setting. Therefore, treatment of ketoacidosis is described first.

Management of Diabetic Ketoacidosis

Diabetic ketoacidosis (DKA) may be diagnosed in the presence of hyperglycemia (a glucose level usually higher than 300 mg per dl), elevated ketone levels in urine and serum, and acidosis (arterial pH less than 7.25 or serum bicarbonate level less than 15 mEq per liter). Patients generally describe recent polyuria and polydipsia. Anorexia, abdominal pain, and vomiting are common and, in the context of high urine output,

contribute to the dehydration evident on physical examination. Tachypnea or Kussmaul's respirations are noted. There may be abdominal distention, tenderness, or both. With further progression, there may be orthostasis, hypotension or shock, and coma.

The pathophysiology of DKA suggests the major elements of therapy, that is, fluids to correct dehydration, electrolytes to correct existing deficits and imbalances, and insulin to reverse hyperglycemia and ketogenesis. Careful monitoring of total fluid balance, blood pH and chemistries, vital signs, and the patient's neurologic status is essential. Precipitating causes, such as infection or nonadherence to prescribed insulin therapy, must be sought.

Fluid Therapy

All patients with DKA are dehydrated. The rationale of fluid therapy is (1) to improve blood volume and circulatory stability, (2) to correct total body fluid deficits, and (3) to correct slowly, as in any other form of hyperosmolar dehydration. Total body fluid deficits can be estimated from recorded weights, when available. Alternatively, the physician can assume that severe DKA (pH < 7.1) reflects a fluid loss of at least 10 per cent of body weight, and mild DKA (pH > 7.2) reflects a 5 per cent loss. The total fluid required is calculated by adding to the deficit the amount required for daily maintenance (1500 ml per M^2 of body surface area) plus ongoing urinary losses.

Therapy is initiated with 10 to 20 ml per kg of normal saline (up to 1 liter) over 0.5 to 1 hour for volume expansion. This can be initiated as soon as the clinical diagnosis of DKA is made and is continued while awaiting laboratory data to confirm the diagnosis and help plan subsequent therapy. Subsequent fluid infusion rates can be calculated to correct one-half of the total body fluid deficit in the first 8 to 12 hours and the remainder by 24 to 48 hours. A primary concern is to avoid too rapid correction, which may result in cerebral edema. Once adequate blood pressure and tissue perfusion are established and the pH is higher than 7.1, there is little justification for rapid correction. Total fluid volume of more than 4 liters per M^2 per day should be avoided. We do not allow oral intake until acidosis is corrected because of the high likelihood of vomiting. Once the patient can tolerate oral fluids, intravenous fluid rates can be adjusted downward accordingly. Ketonuria may continue for 1 or 2 days after resolution of the acidosis.

Electrolytes

Because glucosuria is accompanied by excessive excretion of sodium and potassium, patients with DKA usually have total body deficits of both, which may be especially severe in the individual with several weeks or months of polyuria before diagnosis. These deficits can be assumed to exist regardless of serum levels on admission.

Fluid and electrolyte therapy is further complicated by hyponatremia and by shifts of water and electrolytes between body compartments. The serum sodium level is often low at admission because of the osmotic effect of hyperglycemia. As the hyperglycemia is corrected, the sodium level should rise. The presence of an initially normal or elevated sodium level in the face of hyperglycemia indicates a more severe hyperosmolar state and a need for slower correction (i.e., during 48 hours). A serum sodium level that remains low during correction suggests excessive free water administration and the risk of cerebral edema as a result of fluid shifts.

Acidosis promotes movement of potassium from intracellular to extracellular compartments. Correction of acidosis and cellular glucose uptake promote transfer of potassium into the intracellular compartment. The net effect of correction of DKA is to the lower serum potassium level, sometimes dramatically.

Based on the preceding considerations, a simplified protocol for electrolyte therapy is to follow the initial bolus of normal saline with half-normal saline, given at a rate determined by volume requirements. Once the serum potassium level is known to be in the normal range, potassium is added to rehydration fluids at a concentration of 40 mEq per liter and then adjusted according to frequent monitoring. Rarely, as much as 80 mEq per liter of potassium chloride is required to maintain normal serum potassium levels. Many authorities have suggested giving potassium as the phosphate salt to help correct phosphate deficits and to avoid the hyperchloremia that develops if chloride is the only anion given. Giving potassium phosphate does correct hypophosphatemia, but it has not been associated with demonstrable clinical benefits and has occasionally caused hypocalcemia. For these reasons, we continue to use potassium chloride.

The use of bicarbonate in DKA remains controversial. Excessively rapid correction of acidosis can cause potentially fatal central nervous system acidosis and increases the risk of hypokalemia. Therefore we give sodium bicarbonate only if the initial arterial pH is less than 7.1. The amount of bicarbonate given is calculated to correct one-half of the base deficit by the following formula:

$$\frac{\text{Anion gap}}{10} \times \text{kg body wt} = \text{mEq NaHCO}_3$$

The bicarbonate is infused slowly during 4 to 6 hours and can be stopped once the pH exceeds 7.1. An alternative approach we use is to substitute sodium lactate for sodium chloride. Lactate is a weak buffer that is metabolized to bicarbonate and thus helps to correct acidosis gradually while avoiding the administration of excess chloride.

Insulin

Insulin is best given as an intravenous infusion. Beginning with a priming dose of 0.1 unit per kg, the infusion is started at a rate of 0.1 unit per kg per hour and is subsequently adjusted according to the blood glucose level monitored hourly, aiming for a blood glucose decrement of 50 to 100 mg per dl per hour. Correction of hyperglycemia is generally quite predictable and is quickly responsive to changes in the insulin infusion rate. When the blood glucose level approaches 250 mg per dl, intravenous fluids are changed to include 5 per cent glucose, and the insulin infusion rate is adjusted to achieve and maintain a blood glucose level of about 150 mg per dl, thereby minimizing glucosuria and urinary water losses as well as the risk of hypoglycemia.

The insulin infusion can be prepared by adding regular insulin to normal saline (e.g., 1 unit per ml), to be piggybacked onto other intravenous fluids and given by infusion pump. This allows independent adjustment of the insulin infusion rate and the total fluid rate. Some insulin adheres to the plastic tubing, but if 50 to 100 ml of the insulin-containing fluid is allowed to run through the tube, binding is saturated and the amount of insulin delivered to the patient is relatively constant.

Monitoring

Frequent monitoring is a key to successful management of DKA and is individualized according to the severity of the situation. Initially, vital signs are monitored hourly (or more frequently), along with pH and glucose. Serum electrolyte levels are obtained every 1 or 2 hours until the pH reaches about 7.2; at this point, the frequency of monitoring can be gradually decreased. Changes in the rate or composition of fluid therapy may necessitate more frequent monitoring after the change. Repeated assessment of the patient's neurologic status is essential for the first 24 hours because of the uncommon occurrence of cerebral edema, often several hours after correction of acidosis. Subtle changes in the level of consciousness are often the first sign of impending cerebral edema. Total fluid balance must be watched carefully. Surgical consultation is appropriate for severe or persistent abdominal pain.

Complications of DKA

Hypoglycemia and hypokalemia as complications of DKA can be prevented by frequent monitoring and careful adherence to the procedures previously outlined. Mild cerebral edema may occur in many patients. It has not been possible to relate the rare development of clinically significant cerebral edema to specific aspects of therapy, such as fluid composition or rate of administration. Nevertheless, it stands to reason that excessively rapid correction of hyperosmolarity may be a contributing cause. Therefore, special care should be exercised in the management of patients whose initial sodium level is normal or high, indicating more severe hyperosmolarity, and in patients with long periods of dehydration, hyperosmolarity, or both before initiation of therapy. Evidence of cerebral edema is an indication for beginning osmotherapy (e.g., mannitol) and obtaining a diagnostic computed tomography scan. Even more rarely, patients may develop acute arterial or venous thrombosis or embolism during correction of DKA. These events are manifested by acute effects in the distribution of the affected vessels, in contrast to the more gradual development of symptoms seen in cerebral edema.

Initiation of Chronic Insulin Therapy

Subcutaneous insulin administration may be considered when acidosis is corrected, fluid deficits are largely replaced, and the patient is able to tolerate oral intake. It is important to give the first subcutaneous insulin injection 20 to 30 minutes before stopping the insulin infusion to avoid rapid development of hyperglycemia before the subcutaneous insulin takes effect. The change from intravenous to subcutaneous therapy is conveniently done when the usual insulin dose is given (i.e., at breakfast or supper).

The first step in initiating chronic insulin therapy is to estimate the total daily insulin requirement, which in most newly diagnosed patients approximates 0.5 unit per kg per day. Patients who are mildly symptomatic may require less. The insulin can be divided initially into four to six doses per day of regular insulin, while monitoring the blood glucose level before giving each dose so as to adjust the amounts given. A more efficient method is to begin immediately with a mixture of regular and intermediate-acting insulin (i.e., NPH or Lente), given before breakfast and supper. A useful guideline is to begin with two-thirds of the total daily dose at breakfast, with two-thirds of that as NPH and one-third as regular. The remaining one-third of the total daily dose is divided equally between NPH and regular at supper. Blood glucose is monitored before meals, at bedtime, and once during the night to guide adjustments in these doses according to the individual patient's response.

Initial Patient Education

Chronic management of IDDM is shared by the patient, the family, and the health professional team and is most successful when the patient and family are committed to the goals of therapy, exercise initiative in daily management, and possess the necessary skills. Care of the newly diagnosed patient is therefore incomplete without an educational program designed to promote the patient's acquisition of appropriate knowledge, skills, and attitudes. Realistically, however, the educational process cannot be completed during the first few days, both because of the volume of material to be learned and because the patient's and family's emotional state may impede efficient learning. Thus the goal for the first few days is to teach "survival skills," the minimal essentials of daily management required for home care. The basic pathophysiology of diabetes, accurate administration of insulin, blood glucose testing, the basics of dietary therapy, and the recognition and treatment of hypo- and hyperglycemia should be thoroughly taught in the initial program of education.

The educational process may take many forms but usually requires a team of professionals with expertise in diabetes management. Participation by a knowledgeable physician, nurse, and dietitian is essential, and a social worker or psychologist is often a useful addition. Organized programs are available in many communities and may include inpatient or outpatient individual or group instruction. Adequate time must be allowed for instruction, evaluation of the patient's learning, and reinstruction when necessary.

Chronic Management of IDDM

Chronic management of IDDM has multiple goals: (1) maintenance of normal growth and development, (2) integration of effective diabetes care with a lifestyle that is as close as possible to normal, (3) prevention of acute and chronic complications, and (4) gradual transfer of responsibility from parents to child, leading to the development of a productive adult fully prepared to meet the challenge of living with diabetes. These objectives are not likely to be reached consistently by a haphazard, crisis-oriented approach. In most settings, the comprehensive, systematic program of regular education and care required is best delivered by a professional team able to devote considerable time to the effort. The diabetes management system includes insulin, diet, monitoring of metabolic status, exercise, education, and psychologic support. The details of the approach to each of these components are greatly influenced by the specific blood glucose targets agreed on by the patient and the professional team.

Insulin

Conventional insulin therapy for diabetic children consists of two daily injections of mixtures of intermediate and short-acting insulins (e.g., NPH and regular). Injections are given 30 minutes before meals unless the blood glucose level is already low. Starting with the proportions outlined earlier, doses are adjusted for the individual patient. By using the guidelines in Table 1, adjustments to the usual dose are made in response to consistent patterns noted in the patient's daily glucose monitoring. It is generally best to change only one part of the dose at one time and to change by no more than 10 per cent of the total daily dose. After 2 to 3 days, the response to the new dose can be assessed. We avoid insulins premixed in fixed proportions so that doses of short- and intermediate-acting insulin can be adjusted separately. It must be emphasized that the patient's preferred lifestyle and dietary pattern should determine the specifics of the insulin dose, rather than strict guidelines for insulin use dictating when the patient should eat. Many families can be taught to make these adjustments independently.

During the weeks after diagnosis, blood glucose control may be maintained relatively easily with low insulin doses. This so-called honeymoon period may reflect some endogenous insulin production and may last for up to 12 months. Thereafter, most children require doses of 0.6 to 1.2 units per kg per day, increasing to 1.5 units per kg per day or more during adolescence.

The relevance of newer, intensive insulin therapy methods to children remains questionable. These methods use insulin pumps or more frequent injections coupled with blood glucose–based adjustments of each insulin dose to approx-imate "physiologic" insulin delivery in an attempt to achieve blood glucose levels close to normal. Application of intensive insulin therapy to children has at least two problems. First, these methods are not successful when imposed on an unwilling patient; few children or adolescents are adequately motivated independently of their parents. Second, blood glucose levels approaching normal are associated with a higher risk of hypoglycemia. One must consider carefully whether the child is emotionally and intellectually prepared to deal with this risk.

Two modifications of the preceding conventional protocol may be useful for many families, however. The first is to instruct patients to supplement, insulin doses with additional regular insulin, either according to the blood glucose level indicated at that time or in anticipation of deviations from the usual day's activities. An example of such a schedule is given in Table 2. A second modification of conventional therapy is to give the evening NPH insulin at bedtime rather than with the evening meal. This approach is sometimes effective in patients whose fasting glucose level is high despite being near normal during the evening and in the middle of the night. In such patients, increasing the supper dose of NPH may lead to nocturnal hypoglycemia before adequate control of the fasting glucose level is achieved.

Most authorities recommend the use of human insulin as the most pure preparation available, although no clear long-term advantage over animal insulins has been demonstrated. We have not systematically changed insulins in patients who are doing well. Because of potential pharmacokinetic differences, insulin should be changed under medical supervision.

Diet

Few children with diabetes achieve adequate control of blood glucose level without consistent attention to diet, and excellent control is probably impossible without excellent dietary management. The goals of dietary management are to develop with the patient and family a meal plan that ensures (1) a nutritionally balanced intake sufficient for normal growth and maintenance of weight for height within normal limits, (2) con-

TABLE 1. **Guidelines for Routine Insulin Dose Adjustments By Using Two Daily Injections of Mixed Insulin**

Condition	Adjustment		
Fasting glucose level outside target range	Change	p.m.	NPH/Lente
Before-lunch glucose level outside target range	Change	a.m.	Regular
Before-supper glucose level outside target range	Change	a.m.	NPH/Lente
Bedtime glucose level outside target range	Change	p.m.	Regular

TABLE 2. **Adjusting Insulin Doses According to Measured Blood Glucose Level**

Blood Glucose Level (mg/dl)	Change in Dose of Regular Insulin (U)
Below 80	−1
150–200	+1
200–250	+2
250–300	+3

sistent caloric intake from day to day, with adjustments for unusual exercise or other conditions, and (3) consistent distribution of intake throughout the day so as to match the timing of exogenous glucose availability with insulin effects.

Total caloric requirements for diabetic children with modest glucosuria are equivalent to those of normal children. The best guide to caloric needs is a careful history of the previous intake obtained by a dietitian. Formulas used to estimate caloric needs yield an average that may be appropriate for a population but inappropriate for any individual. Caloric needs may change dramatically, such as during and after the adolescent growth spurt. Therefore, the meal plan should be reviewed with the dietitian annually and adjusted to the patient's weight gain and appetite. Dietary excesses are a common cause of hyperglycemia, and reliance on increasing the insulin doses alone to control hyperglycemia may result in iatrogenic obesity.

Current recommendations for nutrient content of the diet are 50 to 60 per cent of calories from carbohydrate, 15 to 20 per cent from protein, and 30 per cent or less from fat. Several acceptable methods are used to teach patients how to select from a variety of foods while achieving their nutritional goals. An experienced dietitian should select the system most suitable for an individual patient. Weighing and measuring food is a useful way of learning to estimate portion sizes accurately, but this need not be maintained indefinitely.

Distribution of feedings throughout the day on a consistent schedule is an important part of the prevention of hypoglycemia. We recommend three main meals with snacks in midmorning and midafternoon, and at bedtime. The bedtime snack is thought to be essential for prevention of nocturnal hypoglycemia. Older children often object to the morning snack because it sets them apart from their peers at school. In these instances, the insulin regimen can sometimes be tailored to minimize the need for a snack, or a snack that can be quickly consumed can be chosen, such as 8 ounces of milk.

Monitoring

Consistent monitoring of the metabolic status is the key to successful diabetes management because it provides feedback that guides decisions about all other components of the regimen. Blood glucose testing with reagent strips made for home use is the preferred method, although useful information can be obtained from urine glucose testing in the occasional patient who refuses to monitor blood glucose levels. Numerous products for blood glucose testing with acceptable accuracy are available. Many patients prefer to use one of the meters that provide a digital interpretation of the blood glucose level, although with practice and effort, some patients can perform visual readings with equal accuracy. It is essential that patients be carefully trained in the use of these products, and the accuracy of their glucose determinations must be assessed at the time of initial training and at regular intervals thereafter (e.g., annually). An experienced nurse educator can be helpful with practical aspects of this technique.

As a general principle, the more frequently testing is done, the more information is available and the more appropriate decisions can be made. On the other hand, there are practical limits to the frequency of testing. We recommend a minimum of two tests daily, usually at the time of insulin injections. Most patients can also test at bedtime without much difficultly. Tests at noon can be done on weekends to obtain information about that time of day without disrupting the school day. Patients who are striving to achieve normal or near-normal glucose levels should test before each meal, at bedtime, and occasionally during the night.

Specific blood glucose targets should be discussed with the patient and family. We recommend that patients aim for a premeal blood glucose level consistently in the range of 80 to 180 mg per dl. These levels can be achieved with moderate effort by most patients and are associated with few symptoms of diabetes. We do not recommend attempting to maintain normal glucose levels in children who are fully dependent on exogenous insulin, pending conclusive evidence regarding the risks and benefits of this approach.

In addition to daily monitoring of blood glucose levels, the overall quality of metabolic control is assessed by following growth and weight gain over the long term and by assessing glycated hemoglobin for the short term (2 to 3 months). Glycated hemoglobin measures provide an index of average blood glucose levels that is objective, not influenced by meals or fasting, and cannot be acutely manipulated by the patient. It provides a reliable check for patients' inaccuracy or fabrication of daily monitoring results. Because of variability in the methods of assaying glycated hemoglobin levels, each patient must be compared with the local laboratory's normal range. Any diabetic child whose glycated hemoglobin is within 1.5 per cent of the upper limit of normal is in good to excellent control, unless symptoms or home blood glucose testing indicate problems not reflected in the measure of average glucose.

Exercise

Exercise has benefits for the diabetic child in addition to those relevant to all children. Exercise acutely increases glucose use and decreases the blood glucose level; especially when performed on a regular basis, exercise increases insulin sensitivity. For both reasons, consistent exercise is most advantageous for diabetic children. Rather than give an exercise "prescription," we encourage patients to practice active lifestyles and engage in organized sports, and encourage parents to limit television time. In many communities, organized athletic programs are available for almost any age and level of athletic prowess.

Exercise that is inconsistent poses a problem, as it increases the risk of hypoglycemia. Families should be taught that the basic meal plan is designed for a typical day's activity level. Extra food should be taken for extra exercise (e.g., an extra snack for each hour of moderate to heavy exercise). Extended episodes of heavy exercise (e.g., a day-long bicycle ride) may be followed by hypoglycemia as late as 12 to 18 hours after the exercise, perhaps because of glycogen depletion, acute increases in insulin sensitivity, or both. Patients beginning a program of serious physical training are well advised to increase the frequency of their blood glucose monitoring, especially just before and after bouts of exercise.

Some patients use exercise in place of insulin for its acute blood glucose–lowering effects. This strategy may be particularly useful for the patient who is trying to lose or avoid gaining weight. In patients who are hyperglycemic and ketotic, however, heavy exercise may actually cause further metabolic deterioration. These patients should not exercise until steps have been taken to improve their metabolic state.

Education and Psychosocial Support

The many psychosocial impacts of diabetes in children present difficult challenges to the health professional team. Different issues assume importance over the duration of the illness and as the child develops. The most immediate impact is the intrusion on daily activities and loss of spontaneity in lifestyle. The requirements of the regimen set the child apart from peers and even family members. Separation from peers and body image concerns become most salient during early adolescence. Later, identity formation and independence from parents are potential sources of conflict. The older adolescent may be concerned about the impact of diabetes on future adult life.

Transient symptoms of mild depression, similar to those of a grief reaction, are common during the first 6 to 12 months. Denial of the disorder, expressed as nonadherence to the regimen and leading to conflict with parents, is frequently seen. Inaccurate reporting or fabrication of glucose test results is so common that it can almost be regarded as a normal developmental phenomenon. Any pre-existing psychologic dysfunction is likely to be aggravated. Each child's response is different and changes over time, along with his or her ability to understand and cope with the illness.

Thus it is essential that the child and family interact regularly with a professional team that is sensitive to these issues and prepared to offer an ongoing program of education and support tailored to individual needs. Assistance from a social worker, psychologist, or counselor is often helpful. It is becoming increasingly apparent that family cohesiveness and adaptability are important influences and that, whenever possible, the entire family should be involved in the care and support of the diabetic child.

Prevention of Acute Complications

Prevention of hypoglycemia and ketoacidosis is an important goal for all patients and is largely an educational task. Patients should be able to recognize the signs and symptoms of both conditions, understand their causes, and know and practice preventive measures. Prevention of hypoglycemia is largely a matter of consistent adhering to the basic regimen, anticipating those circumstances likely to cause hypoglycemia, and making appropriate adjustments, such as extra food for extra exercise. However, when the blood glucose level is maintained close to normal, occasional episodes of mild hypoglycemia are inevitable. The diabetic child should always have access to a source of sugar. Commercial products for treating hypoglycemia, such as glucose tablets, are available in standard 5- to 10-gram doses and are preferable to candy or ordinary food. School authorities must be educated about the potential for hypoglycemia and its management. The occurrence of severe hypoglycemia (e.g., loss of consciousness, seizure) is frightening for families and indicates a need for careful review of the circumstances to identify the causes. The treatment of choice is immediate injection of 0.5

to 1.0 mg glucagon. Family members should be taught the use of glucagon for severe episodes, and a glucagon emergency kit should be kept at home at all times.

For all practical purposes, prevention of DKA depends on adequate treatment of diabetes during intercurrent illness, a common precipitating factor. The primary goal is to prevent dehydration leading to DKA. Patients are taught special sick-day rules. Insulin should always be given on such days, even when oral intake is reduced, because of the insulin resistance that often accompanies significant illness. Blood glucose levels must be tested more frequently than usual, as often as every 3 or 4 hours, and each urine void should be tested for ketones. Results are used to guide the composition of oral intake and the dose of insulin. If the blood glucose level remains below 180 mg per dl, fluids may contain carbohydrates; above 180 mg per dl, sugar-free liquids are used. If the blood glucose level exceeds approximately 250 mg per dl, the insulin dose is supplemented with regular insulin in amounts up to 10 per cent of the total daily dose, given as often as every 3 or 4 hours until the glucose level drops. Patients should be given specific guidelines regarding the amounts of clear liquids to be consumed. The presence of significant ketonuria or vomiting indicates a need for immediate contact with the physician. Antiemetics should be used with caution and for short periods only. Attempts to control vomiting with antiemetics for more than a few hours sometimes delay the recognition and treatment of DKA. Repeated episodes of DKA indicate a failure of the diabetes management system and are usually related to nonadherence, poor technique, or significant psychosocial disturbance. Children who exhibit this problem should have a careful review of their diabetes care practices and should be referred for psychologic evaluation.

Prevention of Chronic Complications

The development of chronic complications is one of the most devastating and frustrating features of IDDM. Affected individuals are at high risk of visual loss, renal failure, painful neuropathy, amputations, and accelerated cardiovascular disease. The average life expectancy is reduced by about one-third. The pre-eminent controversy in clinical diabetes today is whether maintenance of blood glucose levels closer to normal prevents or delays these complications. Although there is evidence suggesting that the degree of metabolic control is associated with the risk of complications, conclusive evidence may be available only at the completion of clinical trials now under way. Therefore the potential benefits of tight control must be balanced humanely against the potential risks (e.g., hypoglycemia) and the rigorous demands of the regimen required to achieve such control. Ideally, a well-educated patient and family are active participants in making these decisions.

Despite the controversy regarding the pathogenesis of chronic complications, their associated morbidity can be reduced by consistent use of currently available methods. Timely detection of advanced retinopathy permits laser photocoagulation and prevents blindness. Careful planning of pregnancy so that excellent metabolic control can be maintained throughout gestation has been shown to reduce morbidity and mortality greatly among infants of diabetic mothers. Aggressive treatment of hypertension appears to retard the progression of nephropathy. Thorough education regarding foot care can prevent lower extremity amputations. Therefore, once the duration of diabetes exceeds 5 years in a postpubertal patient, routine care should include an annual formal ophthalmologic examination and urinalysis for proteinuria. All young women with diabetes should be counseled about family planning and the special care required for a successful diabetic pregnancy. Blood pressure should be assessed on every visit.

HYPERURICEMIA AND GOUT

method of
DAVID F. GIANSIRACUSA, M.D.
University of Massachusetts Medical Center
Worcester, Massachusetts

Gout is a clinical syndrome that occurs only in humans. It is caused by hyperuricemia, excessive accumulation of monosodium urate in joints and soft tissues, excessive urinary excretion of uric acid, or all three. Manifestations include (1) recurrent attacks of acute arthritis, (2) chronic deforming, erosive tophaceous arthritis, (3) deposition of monosodium urate (MSU) crystals in the kidneys (urate nephropathy), (4) uric acid urolithiasis, and (5) acute uric acid crystallization in renal tubules called acute hyperuricemic (or uric acid) nephropathy.

Hyperuricemia is a requisite for the development of gout. Defined in physicochemical terms, hyperuricemia is the level above which urates are no longer soluble. At 37° C, the saturation concentration of urate is 7 mg per dl. In most laboratories, this corresponds to a serum urate level of approximately 7.5 to 8 mg per dl.

Hyperuricemia occurs as a result of diminished urinary excretion of uric acid or excessive biosynthesis. Underexcretion is responsible for approximately 90 per cent of gout. It results from polygenic factors that diminish renal clearance of uric acid, acquired renal diseases, and/or ingestion of drugs including diuretics (particularly thiazides), low-dose salicylates, ethanol (which also increases the biosynthesis of uric acid), and toxins such as lead that impair renal excretion.

Overproduction of uric acid is defined as a urinary uric acid excretion rate in 24 hours of more than 600 mg on a purine-restricted diet or 1000 mg on a regular diet. Overproduction may result from diseases such as psoriasis, sarcoidosis, and myelo- and lymphoproliferative diseases in which increased cell turnover leads to excessive synthesis of uric acid. In a small percentage of gout patients, overproduction results from primary enzymatic abnormalities that increase de novo synthesis of uric acid; these include deficiencies of hypoxanthine-guanine phosphoribosyltransferase and glucose-6-phosphate dehydrogenase and increased activity of phosphoribosylpyrophosphate synthetase. Inherited enzymatic abnormalities should be considered in young men and premenopausal women with marked hyperuricemia, hyperuricosuria, gouty arthritis, and/ or uric acid urolithiasis, as well as in gout patients with a strong family history of the syndrome.

Evaluation of the patient with hyperuricemia includes assessment of diet, body weight, alcohol consumption, salicylate and thiazide use, hypertension, cardiovascular disease and risk factors, volume status, presence of tophi, renal function, 24-hour urinary uric acid excretion, and a family history of gouty arthritis, renal stones, and renal disease.

CLINICAL FEATURES OF GOUTY ARTHRITIS

Acute gouty arthritis is characterized by the abrupt onset of exquisite pain, tenderness, swelling, and erythema most commonly affecting a single joint. The arthritis generally occurs after 10 years or more of asymptomatic hyperuricemia. Men in their fourth through sixth decades of life and postmenopausal women are most commonly affected. Attacks often occur at night and may be associated with inflammation of the surrounding tendons and bursae, often simulating joint sepsis or cellulitis. Approximately 50 per cent of patients experience their first attack in the metatarsal phalangeal joint of the great toe (podagra). Other peripheral joints (midfoot, ankles, knees, fingers, wrists, and elbows) may be involved in a monarticular or migratory fashion. Attacks may be precipitated by minor trauma, physiologic stress, or ingestion of ethanol, salicylates, or uric acid–lowering agents. Approximately 10 to 15 per cent of attacks are polyarticular. Women, more frequently than men, manifest polyarticular gout. Even if untreated, acute attacks are usually self-limited, lasting for 3 to 7 days, after which the patient becomes asymptomatic and the joints return to normal; this is referred to as the intercritical period. With the passage of time, attacks become more frequent and prolonged and may eventually result in chronic, persistent gout with palpable tophi on examination and/or erosions on radiographs. Elderly women treated with thiazide diuretics may develop tophaceous gout in osteoarthritic interphalangeal finger joints with little or no preceding inflammation.

DIAGNOSIS OF GOUTY ARTHRITIS

The diagnosis of gouty arthritis is established unequivocally by demonstration of needle-shaped MSU crystals within polymorphonuclear leukocytes in synovial fluid under the polarizing light microscope. The MSU crystals parallel to the axis of light are yellow when viewed with a first-order red compensator under the polarizing microscope. To maximize the yield of MSU crystals (1) the most recently inflamed joint(s) should be aspirated, (2) examination of multiple synovial fluid samples may be necessary, (3) local anesthetics that dissolve urate crystals should not be mixed with the synovial fluid samples, and (4) a centrifuged pellet should be examined.

In the absence of MSU crystal identification, a presumptive diagnosis of acute gout is based on the clinical findings of a self-limited (3- to 10-day) monarticular arthritis in an appropriate individual and joint; a response to colchicine within 48 hours; at least a 7-day asymptomatic interval between attacks, during which time the joint is normal; and hyperuricemia.

Because acute gouty arthritis is an intensely inflammatory joint disease, and because MSU crystals may be present in septic synovial effusions, it is critical that the synovial fluid be evaluated with Gram's stain and culture to exclude bacterial joint infection.

TREATMENT

Asymptomatic Hyperuricemia

Treatment of patients with asymptomatic hyperuricemia with pharmacologic agents is not justified except in the overexcreter of uric acid (24-hour urinary uric acid excretion more than 1000 mg), in which allopurinol is used to prevent urolithiasis.

Arguments against treating asymptomatic hyperuricemia with uric acid–lowering (hypouricemic) therapy are several: (1) of the 5 per cent of the population with hyperuricemia, less than one-fifth develop gout; (2) effective therapy is available for the treatment of gout; (3) hypouricemic therapy requires lifelong treatment, which incurs an expense and potential risks; (4) asymptomatic hyperuricemia does not appear to affect renal function adversely until possibly the serum urate level exceeds 13 mg per dl in men and 10 mg per dl in women; and (5) although hypertension, obesity, hyperlipidemia, alcohol abuse, and atherosclerosis are prevalent in series of gout patients, hyperuricemia is not an independent risk factor for coronary artery disease.

In the individual with asymptomatic hyperuricemia, as in the patient with gout, coronary artery disease risk factors should be minimized and the ingestion of fat, alcoholic beverages, and foods rich in purines (sardines, anchovies, liver, and sweetbreads) should be moderated.

Gouty Arthritis

Treatment goals for gouty arthritis are to (1) provide analgesia and terminate the acute attack, (2) prevent recurrent attacks, and (3) prevent and/or improve erosive, tophaceous arthritis. Agents used are anti-inflammatory, prophylactic, or hypouricemic drugs. Anti-inflammatory agents do not lower serum urate levels, and uric acid–lowering agents do not have anti-inflammatory activity. Altering the dose of uric acid–lowering drugs may actually precipitate an attack of gouty arthritis or aggravate an ongoing one. Educating the patient about the natural history of the disease and the appropriate use of pharmacologic agents is of critical importance.

The earlier an acute attack of gouty arthritis is treated, the more rapidly the inflamed joints respond. Joint aspiration and immobilization, plus administration of analgesics including nonsteroidal anti-inflammatory drugs (NSAIDs), acetaminophen, and, for severe attacks, narcotic analgesics, generally provide some degree of pain relief. Suppression of inflammation with NSAIDs, colchicine, corticosteroids, and/or corticotropin provides further symptomatic improvement.

To treat acute gouty arthritis, NSAIDs are generally given in high doses for the first 2 or 3 days and then tapered. Indomethacin (Indocin) traditionally has been considered the NSAID of choice, but essentially any of the nonsalicylate NSAIDs may be prescribed (Table 1). Side effects and drug interactions of NSAIDs are given in Table 2. Because of the severe side effects of phenylbutazone (Butazolidin) and the availability of potentially less toxic NSAIDs, phenylbutazone is rarely used at this time. Elderly patients, especially those with cardiac and renal disease, are particularly vulnerable to serious gastrointestinal bleeding, renal function impairment, and central nervous system side effects from NSAIDs.

Oral colchicine may be effective if treatment is begun within several hours of the onset of the acute gouty attack. It is given as 0.5 or 0.6 mg every hour until (1) significant control of inflammation is achieved, (2) gastrointestinal side effects including nausea, vomiting, cramping abdominal pain, and diarrhea develop, and/or (3) a maximum of 6 mg is given. No more than 6 to 8 mg should be given in the first 24 hours, followed by a week without colchicine.

Colchicine may also be given intravenously and is particularly useful in patients who have gastrointestinal bleeding or heart failure or who require oral anticoagulants. From 2 to 3 mg may be infused initially, followed by 0.5 to 1 mg 8 to 12 hours later, not to exceed a total dose of 4 mg in 48 hours, followed by 7 days without colchicine.

TABLE 1. NSAIDs Used to Treat Acute Gouty Arthritis

Class/Generic Name	Brand Name	Daily Dose (mg)
Propionic Acids		
Ibuprofen	Advil, Nuprin, Motrin	400–800 mg tid
Naproxen	Naprosyn	250–500 mg bid–tid
Fenoprofen	Nalfon	300–600 mg qid
Ketoprofen	Orudis	50–75 mg tid
Flurbiprofen	Ansaid	100 mg bid–tid
Indoleacetic Acids		
Indomethacin	Indocin	25–50 mg tid–qid
Sulindac	Clinoril	150–200 mg bid
Tolmetin sodium	Tolectin	400 mg 3 to 5 times daily
Fenamic Acids		
Meclofenamate	Meclomen	50–100 mg qid
Oxicams		
Piroxicam	Feldene	10–20 mg qd
Phenylacetic Acid		
Diclofenac sodium	Voltaren	50–75 mg bid

Intravenous colchicine, which is extremely irritating to soft tissues, may cause a chemical thrombophlebitis associated with the infusion and tissue necrosis if extravasation occurs. Colchicine administered intravenously should be diluted in 20 ml of normal saline and infused over 10 to 20 minutes in a well-running intravenous line. Intravenous administration minimizes gastrointestinal side effects.

TABLE 2. Side Effects and Drug Interactions of NSAIDs Used to Treat Acute Gouty Arthritis

All NSAIDs
  Dyspepsia, nausea, vomiting, diarrhea, constipation, gastric mucosal erosions and ulcerations
  Renal function impairment, nephrotic syndrome, acute renal failure, interstitial nephritis, hypertension, fluid retention
  Platelet dysfunction
  Headache, drowsiness, dizziness, vertigo, tinnitus, depersonalization reaction, depression
  Liver function abnormalities
  Aggravation of bronchial asthma, angioedema, and/or urticaria
  Displacement of warfarin sodium, oral hypoglycemic agents, and anticonvulsants from protein-binding sites

Phenylbutazone
  Fever, rash, hepatitis, gastrointestinal bleeding, perforation, salt and fluid retention, and, rarely, aplastic anemia

Indomethacin
  Hyperkalemia; excretion inhibited by probenecid

Because colchicine is excreted by the liver and kidneys, it should not be used in patients with significant liver disease, renal disease, or both. Doses should be reduced in elderly patients even if no evidence of renal impairment is reflected by the serum creatinine level.

Systemic reactions to colchicine include myelosuppression, disseminated intravascular coagulation, myopathy, neuropathy, and injury to renal, hepatic, and nervous tissue.

Corticosteroids may be required to treat acute gouty arthritis if contraindications exist to the use of other agents. After joint infection has been excluded, corticosteroid therapy may be administered as corticotropin (ACTH), 40 to 80 units intramuscularly or 20 units intravenously every 12 to 24 hours for 1 to 3 days; or as oral, intramuscular, or intravenous systemic corticosteroids (30 mg of prednisone or its equivalent, tapered over 6 days); or as a single intra-articular administration of 10 to 40 mg of a long-acting preparation such as methylprednisolone acetate (Depo-Medrol). Because some patients experience a rebound flare of gout after initially responding to corticosteroids, prophylactic colchicine or low doses of NSAIDs (see the next section) should be given during and for several days after the corticosteroid treatment.

Prophylactic Therapy Against Acute Gouty Arthritis

Prophylactic therapy against recurrent attacks of gouty arthritis is generally recommended for individuals who have experienced a particularly severe attack or two or more attacks per year. For patients with normal renal and hepatic function, oral colchicine, 0.5 or 0.6 mg once or twice a day, is generally effective. As an alternative, low doses of NSAIDs, generally one-half of the usual therapeutic dose, may provide effective prophylaxis.

Uric Acid–Lowering Therapy

The decision to use these medications is controversial; some physicians recommend hypouricemic therapy after the first attack of gouty arthritis. Others contend that because only certain individuals with one attack develop other manifestations of gout, and because hypouricemic therapy involves daily, lifelong use of medication, which incurs expense and creates a potential for side effects and serious toxic reactions, uric acid–lowering therapy should be confined to specific clinical indications, as shown in Table 3.

Two types of uric acid–lowering agents are available: (1) the uricosuric drugs probenecid

TABLE 3. **Specific Indications for Uric Acid–Lowering Therapy**

1. Frequent, disabling attacks of gouty arthritis in spite of prophylactic therapy
2. Tophaceous gout (identified by physical examination or erosions on radiographs)*
3. Uric acid urolithiasis*
4. Recurrent calcium oxalate renal stones in the setting of hyperuricosuria*
5. Marked overproduction of uric acid (24-hour urinary excretion on a normal diet in excess of 1000 mg)*
6. Before cytotoxic therapy for lymphoproliferative and myeloproliferative diseases to prevent acute uric acid nephropathy*

*Allopurinol is the indicated agent.

(Benemid) and sulfinpyrazone (Anturane), which increase urate clearance, and (2) the xanthine oxidase inhibitor allopurinol (Zyloprim), which blocks uric acid production. The goal of hypouricemic therapy is to reduce the serum urate level below 6 mg per dl, and, for overproducers, to reduce 24-hour urinary uric acid excretion rates below 750 mg. Because the institution of uric acid–lowering therapy may precipitate an attack of gout, hypouricemic agents should not be started or the dose changed during and for several weeks after resolution of an attack. Prophylactic therapy should always be administered in conjunction with a uricosuric drug or allopurinol and should be continued for at least 6 months after the serum urate level is controlled below 6 mg per dl or for 6 months after resolution of tophi. Once uric acid–lowering therapy is instituted for appropriate indications, it is maintained for life.

Uricosuric agents may be prescribed for patients who experience recurrent attacks of gouty arthritis in spite of prophylactic therapy. To take a uricosuric agent, a patient must have normal renal function (creatinine clearance more than 50 ml per minute) and must excrete less than 700 mg of uric acid per day. With treatment, adequate fluid intake to ensure more than 1 liter of urine output per day and occasional alkalinization of the urine to achieve a pH of 6.0 to 6.5 are indicated to prevent uric acid renal stone formation.

Probenecid, available in 500-mg tablets, is given initially at a dose of 250 mg twice daily. The dose is increased by 500 mg every 1 to 2 weeks until the serum urate level is controlled below 6 mg per dl; this is generally achieved with a dose of 1.5 to 3 grams per day in three divided doses. Probenecid interferes with the excretion of indomethacin, as well as that of chlorpropamide and other sulfonylureas. Side effects of probenecid are infrequent, the most common being headache, nausea, and anorexia. Rarely, nephrotic syndrome, hepatic necrosis, and aplastic anemia occur.

Sulfinpyrazone, available in 100-mg tablets, is started at a dose of 50 mg twice daily and is then increased by 100 mg each week to achieve a serum urate level below 6 mg per dl, generally 200 to 400 mg daily in three or four divided doses. Sulfinpyrazone is generally well tolerated; the most common adverse reactions are dyspepsia, rash, and aggravation of peptic ulcer disease. Rarely, toxic hematologic reactions such as aplastic anemia occur. Because sulfinpyrazone inhibits platelet function, it may be the preferred uricosuric agent to treat gout patients with coronary risk factors.

Allopurinol, by decreasing both serum urate and urinary uric acid levels, is the hypouricemic drug of choice in patients with uric acid overproduction, urolithiasis, or tophaceous gout; in patients with renal insufficiency who require uric acid–lowering therapy; and in patients with lymphoproliferative or myeloproliferative disease to prevent acute hyperuricemic (uric acid) nephropathy associated with cytotoxic therapy (see Table 3). Allopurinol is started at a dose of 100 mg a day and increased every 2 to 4 weeks by 100 mg to reduce the serum urate level below 6 mg per dl, which generally requires a maximal dose of 300 mg per day. Because allopurinol is rapidly metabolized to oxypurinol, which has a half-life of 18 to 30 hours, allopurinol may be given once a day. In renal insufficiency, the dose must be reduced considerably (100 mg per day or less). Allopurinol reduces the metabolism of warfarin sodium, 6-mercaptopurine, and azathioprine; therefore, the doses of these medications must be appropriately reduced. Potential toxicities of allopurinol include severe allergic reactions, nausea, diarrhea, fever, leukopenia, hepatic injury, interstitial nephritis, hypersensitivity angiitis (vasculitis), and a rash that may evolve into exfoliative dermatitis or toxic epidermal necrolysis. Serious side effects most commonly occur when allopurinol is prescribed in the presence of renal insufficiency, particularly in the setting of thiazide diuretic therapy, which further impairs the excretion of the metabolite oxypurinol.

In the patient with severe tophaceous gout, combined allopurinol and uricosuric therapy may be necessary. In some of these patients, surgical débridement and excision of tophi may be helpful.

HYPERLIPOPROTEINEMIA

method of
ERNST J. SCHAEFER, M.D.
Tufts University School of Medicine
Boston, Massachusetts

Elevated plasma or serum cholesterol and/or triglyceride levels are associated with increased levels of lipoproteins. Increased plasma low-density lipoprotein (LDL) cholesterol levels and decreased high-density lipoprotein (HDL) cholesterol levels are associated with the development of atherosclerosis, and severe hypertriglyceridemia with circulating chylomicrons in the fasting state is associated with recurrent pancreatitis.

LIPOPROTEIN METABOLISM

Cholesterol is a sterol that is an important constituent of membranes and a precursor of various hormones as well as bile acids. The very properties that make this molecule important for membranes (i.e., its insolubility in aqueous media) also cause it to promote atherosclerosis in the artery wall when present in excess. About 70 per cent of the cholesterol in the blood stream has one fatty acid attached to it (known as "cholesteryl ester"). Humans consume about 400 mg of cholesterol per day in the diet, and absorption from the intestine varies between 30 and 70 per cent of the amount ingested. Triglyceride or triacylglycerol is a molecule composed of three fatty acids attached to a glycerol backbone. Humans consume about 20 to 150 grams of fat or triglyceride per day. Triglyceride is broken down into fatty acids in the intestine by lipases in the presence of bile acids. Fatty acid absorption in the intestine is very efficient (more than 90 per cent of the amount ingested). Humans can synthesize both cholesterol and triglyceride.

Lipoproteins are round particles composed of cholesterol, triglyceride, phospholipid, and protein. Chylomicrons are very large, triglyceride-rich (90 per cent by weight) particles made in the intestine in response to a fat-rich meal. On entry into the plasma, the chylomicron triglyceride content is rapidly depleted by lipoprotein lipase, an enzyme that is located on the surface of endothelial cells in the capillary bed. This enzyme, in the presence of a protein activator (apolipoprotein C-II) and albumin, removes fatty acids from the glycerol backbone of triglyceride. Fatty acids are stored as triglyceride in the fat cell. During the lipolytic process, chylomicron remnants are formed, which are taken up by the liver. In normal individuals, chylomicrons are not present in fasting plasma. When chylomicron catabolism is impaired, severe hypertriglyceridemia occurs, and such particles can be deposited in various tissues, including the liver and pancreas. Such deposition causes an enlarged, fatty liver and pancreatitis as a result of intracellular release of pancreatic lipase. Chylomicrons are not thought to be atherogenic particles because they contain very little cholesterol and are too large to be filtered into the arterial wall. However, accumulations of chylomicron remnants are probably atherogenic.

Very-low-density lipoproteins (VLDLs) are triglyceride-rich (60 per cent by weight) lipoproteins that are made by the liver. VLDL is the major carrier of plasma triglyceride in normal individuals in the fasting state. After VLDL enters the plasma, its triglyceride content is rapidly depleted by lipolytic enzymes to form LDL. In certain instances, especially in the setting of hypertriglyceridemia, VLDL is removed from the plasma without being converted to LDL. In other instances, especially in the setting of hypercholesterolemia, LDL may be produced directly by the liver. There is debate as to whether VLDL particles are atherogenic. Patients with elevated triglyceride levels caused by increased VLDL often have decreased HDL levels, and this lipid pattern is often observed in patients with premature coronary heart disease (CHD). Small, cholesterol-rich VLDL particles are probably atherogenic.

LDL particles are cholesterol rich (60 per cent by weight) and are the major carriers of plasma cholesterol in normal individuals. About 70 per cent of LDL is removed from the blood stream by the liver, and about 70 per cent of all LDL catabolism occurs via LDL receptor-mediated uptake. Dietary saturated fat (especially myristic and palmitic acids) and dietary cholesterol both down-regulate LDL receptor activity, which results in increased plasma LDL cholesterol levels. LDL particles are known to be atherogenic and are deposited in the arterial wall.

HDL particles are protein rich (50 per cent by weight). They are synthesized directly in both the liver and the intestine. In addition, HDL constituents are derived from components (proteins and lipids) shed from the surface of chylomicrons and VLDL during lipolysis. HDL has been shown to promote removal of free cholesterol from cholesterol-laden cells. The free cholesterol in HDL is rapidly esterified. It can then remain with the HDL particle or be transferred to other lipoproteins, such as chylomicron or VLDL remnants, by transfer proteins. HDL is catabolized mainly by the liver and appears to play a major role in reverse cholesterol transport. There is currently debate as to whether an HDL receptor exists. Moreover, the precise role of HDL in protecting against atherosclerosis remains to be defined.

DIAGNOSIS OF LIPOPROTEIN DISORDERS

In 1985 a National Institutes of Health Consensus Conference panel concluded that elevated blood cholesterol levels (specifically, increased LDL cholesterol) were associated with premature CHD and that lowering LDL cholesterol levels was associated with a decreased risk of developing CHD. In addition, the panel concluded that the blood cholesterol levels of many Americans were undesirably high because of an excessive intake of dietary saturated fat and cholesterol. The panel recommended identification and treatment of individuals whose cholesterol levels were above the seventy-fifth percentile of normal. In 1987, the adult treatment panel of the National Cholesterol Education Program (NCEP), sponsored by the National Heart, Lung, and Blood Institute, released its guidelines for the diagnosis and treatment of elevated blood cholesterol levels in individuals older than 20 years of age; the guidelines focused on elevated LDL cholesterol.

Total plasma or serum cholesterol levels can be measured in the nonfasting state as well as in the fasting state. For screening programs, finger stick methodology is now available. A total cholesterol level below 200 mg per dl has been classified as desirable and should be rechecked in 5 years. A cholesterol level of 200 to 239 mg per dl is in the borderline category, and a level of 240 mg per dl or more is in the high-risk category. To proceed further with individuals in the borderline category, it is necessary to obtain information about the presence of CHD or CHD risk factors. CHD has been defined as prior myocardial infarction or angina. Other CHD risk factors include male sex, a family history of premature CHD (defined as myocardial infarction or sudden death in a parent or a sibling before age 55 years), cigarette smoking, hypertension, decreased HDL cholesterol level (below 35 mg per dl, confirmed by repeat measurement), diabetes mellitus, a history of cerebrovascular or peripheral vascular disease, and severe obesity (defined as 30 per cent or more above ideal body weight).

If the patient has a cholesterol level in the borderline category in the absence of CHD or two or more CHD risk factors, dietary information (see later) should be given to the patient and the cholesterol level should be rechecked in about 1 year. For the patient in the borderline cholesterol category with CHD or two or more CHD risk factors, or for the patient in the high-risk cholesterol category, a lipoprotein analysis is recommended. An alternative approach is to measure lipoprotein levels in all patients with cholesterol values of 200 mg per dl or greater. I prefer the latter approach because patients in the borderline category may be misclassified if their HDL cholesterol level is not measured. Alternatively, HDL cholesterol can be measured in the nonfasting state, but it may be 2 to 4 mg per dl lower than when measured in the fasting state.

To measure lipoprotein levels, the patient should be instructed to fast for at least 12 hours, except for water. Total cholesterol and triglyceride levels in plasma or serum are measured. Plasma levels are 3 per cent lower than serum levels. HDL cholesterol is also measured in the supernatant fraction after the other lipoproteins have been precipitated. Ideally, laboratories should obtain coefficients of variation for these assays of 3 per cent or less and should participate in a standardization program linked to the Centers for Disease Control Lipid Research Clinics program. To calculate the VLDL cholesterol level, the triglyceride level is divided by 5. The LDL cholesterol level is then calculated by subtracting the VLDL and HDL cholesterol levels from the total cholesterol level. This calculation is not valid if the triglyceride level is higher than 400 mg per dl. For an approximate measure of the LDL cholesterol level in patients with triglyceride levels higher than 400 mg per dl, the triglyceride level should be divided by 6 for levels up to 1000 mg per dl and by 8 for levels higher than 1000 mg per dl. Precise measurement of LDL cholesterol levels in these latter categories requires ultracentrifugation.

An LDL cholesterol level of less than 130 mg per dl has been classified as desirable, a level of 130 to 159 mg per dl as borderline, and a level of 160 mg per dl or more as high risk. An LDL cholesterol level of 160 mg per dl represents approximately the seventy-fifth percentile for middle-aged Americans. An LDL cholesterol level higher than 225 mg per dl is above the ninety-fifth percentile for all age and sex groups, and an HDL cholesterol level less than 27 mg per dl is below the fifth percentile for all age and sex groups. Triglyceride levels higher than 250 mg per dl, with VLDL cholesterol levels higher than 50 mg per dl, have been classified as elevated. A triglyceride level greater than 320 mg per dl is above the ninety-fifth percentile for all age and sex groups. Severe hypertriglyceridemia is characterized by triglyceride levels greater than 1000 mg per dl. In this latter category, chylomicrons are almost invariably present, as assessed by lipoprotein electrophoresis. It is important to confirm the presence of elevated levels by repeat determinations. Acute infections and myocardial infarction are known to affect plasma lipid levels, so patients should have these levels checked more than 6 weeks after such illnesses.

Secondary Causes

Secondary causes of hypercholesterolemia should be ruled out before initiating dietary and drug therapy. Secondary causes of an elevated LDL cholesterol level include hypothyroidism, obstructive liver disease, and nephrotic syndrome. Rarer secondary causes include dysproteinemia and porphyria. Secondary causes of hypertriglyceridemia include excess alcohol intake, diabetes mellitus, renal insufficiency, use of beta-blocker medication, and estrogen therapy. Rarer causes include glycogen storage disease and lipodystrophy. Secondary causes of HDL deficiency include hypertriglyceridemia, diabetes mellitus, renal insufficiency, use of beta-blocker medication, male sex, obesity, and use of progestins and anabolic steroids.

TREATMENT

Hypercholesterolemia (Elevated LDL Level)

Hypercholesterolemia is defined as an elevated plasma cholesterol level (240 mg per dl or higher) in the setting of a normal triglyceride level. Rarely, patients in this category have markedly elevated HDL cholesterol levels but normal LDL cholesterol levels. These patients do not require therapy. Most hypercholesterolemic patients have elevated LDL cholesterol levels (160 mg per dl or higher, Type IIA hyperlipoproteinemia), as previously defined. The most common forms of these disorders have either an autosomal dominant or a polygenic mode of inheritance without xanthomas. Therefore it is worthwhile to screen family members. Some of these patients can be treated with dietary therapy alone, but many require medication in addition to diet. Before using medication, dietary therapy (see later) should be tried for at least 6 months. Drugs should be initiated in all patients who maintain an LDL cholesterol level higher than 190 mg per dl after dietary therapy, with the goal being to lower the LDL cholesterol level to less than 160 mg per dl. In addition, in patients with CHD or two or more CHD risk factors, drugs should be initiated after dietary treatment if the LDL cholesterol level remains higher than 160 mg per dl after dietary therapy, with the goal being to lower the LDL cholesterol level to less than 130 mg per

dl. Patients should be encouraged to continue the dietary treatment even after receiving medication.

Anion exchange resins (see later) are currently the drugs of choice for the treatment of elevated LDL cholesterol levels. Patients who cannot tolerate these agents should be given niacin (see later). Both of these agents have been shown to reduce the incidence of CHD in prospective studies but are difficult for many patients to tolerate. A new medication, lovastatin, which inhibits hydroxymethylglutaryl coenzyme A (HMG CoA) reductase, the rate-limiting enzyme in cholesterol biosynthesis, is now available. This medication (see later) is extremely effective in lowering the LDL cholesterol level and is well tolerated by most patients. However, its long-term safety and efficacy in reducing the incidence of CHD have not yet been demonstrated. Current experience with the agent indicates excellent safety after at least 5 years of use. If its efficacy in reducing the incidence of CHD is established, this agent will become the drug of choice for reducing LDL levels. Lovastatin is currently the drug of choice in patients who are unable to tolerate either resins or niacin or who do not achieve an adequate LDL cholesterol reduction with these other agents. Probucol (see later) is another agent that is available for lowering cholesterol levels. This is a third line agent that is generally well tolerated. Probucol lowers LDL cholesterol levels modestly but also lowers HDL cholesterol levels significantly. Long-term efficacy data on reduction of the risk of CHD are not yet available for this agent. For this reason, I rarely use it. The combination of resins and niacin is extremely effective, as are the combinations of resin and lovastatin and of niacin and lovastatin. However, all these agents have side effects (see later) that require careful follow-up of the patient.

Occasionally, patients present with marked hypercholesterolemia (level often higher than 400 mg per dl, with LDL cholesterol levels well above the ninety-fifth percentile) and tendinous xanthomas. These patients are heterozygotes for classic familial hypercholesterolemia (autosomal dominant mode of inheritance) and often develop CHD before the age of 50 years. Homozygotes with this disorder are very rare, can develop CHD in their teens, and have been shown to have a variety of LDL receptor defects. Heterozygous patients almost invariably require treatment with medication in addition to diet. Moreover they often require two medications used in combination. In children with this disorder (cholesterol levels higher than 300 mg per dl), I use low doses of resin. After puberty these patients are treated in the same manner as adult patients with elevated LDL cholesterol levels. Homozygotes with familial hypercholesterolemia generally require plasma exchange every 2 weeks. Some of these patients respond to medication but do not achieve adequate reductions in LDL cholesterol levels. Those patients who do respond should continue to receive medication in addition to plasma exchange.

Hypercholesterolemia and Hypertriglyceridemia (Elevated VLDL and LDL Levels)

Combined elevations of plasma cholesterol levels (higher than 240 mg per dl) and triglyceride levels (higher than 250 mg per dl) are commonly observed. One form of this disorder, known as "familial combined hyperlipidemia," is an autosomal dominant disorder in which affected family members may have elevations of both plasma cholesterol and triglyceride levels (associated with VLDL cholesterol levels higher than 50 mg per dl and LDL cholesterol levels higher than 160 mg per dl, Type IIB hyperlipoproteinemia) or elevations of either one alone. These patients have overproduction of VLDL and LDL, and those with hypertriglyceridemia have some delayed VLDL clearance as well. Screening of family members is worthwhile. Some patients with this lipid pattern can be treated with dietary therapy alone (alcohol abstention, weight reduction, and an exercise program are also important). For patients who maintain an LDL cholesterol level higher than 190 mg per dl or for those whose LDL cholesterol level is higher than 160 mg per dl in the presence of CHD or two or more CHD risk factors after 6 months of dietary therapy, the drug of choice is niacin. For patients who are not candidates for this agent or who cannot tolerate it, the combination of resin and gemfibrozil can be used. Resins should not be used as the only agents in these patients because they elevate triglyceride levels. For patients who cannot tolerate the combination or obtain an inadequate response, lovastatin should be used. The combination of gemfibrozil and niacin can also be used.

Rarely, patients in this category may have dysbetalipoproteinemia or Type III hyperlipoproteinemia associated with a marked increase in cholesterol-rich VLDL of abnormal beta-migrating electrophoretic mobility. These patients may have palmar xanthomas (yellow creases in the palms) and tuberoeruptive xanthomas, especially on the elbows. This disorder is associated with genetic abnormalities in apolipoprotein E and with delayed clearance of chylomicron remnants and VLDL, as well as excess hepatic VLDL production. Diagnosis is not essential except for research purposes because the treatment is the same as that for other patients with combined elevations of cholesterol and triglyceride levels.

Hypertriglyceridemia (Elevated VLDL Level)

Hypertriglyceridemia is defined as a triglyceride level higher than 250 mg per dl in the setting of a normal LDL cholesterol value (Type IV hyperlipoproteinemia). These patients often have decreased HDL cholesterol levels. Patients with elevated triglyceride levels may have familial hypertriglyceridemia, an autosomal dominant disorder. These patients have overproduction of hepatic triglyceride and may have defective VLDL catabolism as well. All patients with hypertriglyceridemia should be treated with dietary therapy. Emphasis should be placed on caloric restriction in overweight patients and abstinence from alcohol, as well as a regular program of exercise. An attempt should be made to switch patients who are on beta-blocker medication to other agents, such as calcium channel blockers, that do not raise triglyceride levels. The goal of therapy is reduce triglyceride levels to less than 200 mg per dl and to raise the HDL cholesterol level to more than 40 mg per dl. Patients in this category are not covered by the new NCEP guidelines, and yet they are among the ones most commonly observed in any survey of patients with premature CHD. In one large recent primary prevention study (the Helsinki Heart Study), about 8 per cent of the subjects had elevated VLDL cholesterol and normal LDL cholesterol levels. In this study, subjects in this category who received gemfibrozil had a lower incidence of CHD prospectively than subjects in this category who received a placebo. The question is whether such patients should be treated with medication if dietary therapy fails to normalize their triglyceride levels. Our practice is to treat such patients with medication if they have established CHD or a definite family history of CHD. The medication of choice is niacin. For patients who cannot tolerate this agent or who are not candidates for the drug, gemfibrozil should be used.

Severe Hypertriglyceridemia

Severe hypertriglyceridemia is defined as a triglyceride level higher than 1000 mg per dl in plasma obtained from a patient after a 12- to 14-hour overnight fast. Patients can be subclassified further on the basis of lipoprotein electrophoresis into those who have both chylomicrons and excess VLDL present (Type V hyperlipoproteinemia) or those in whom only chylomicrons are present (Type I hyperlipoproteinemia). The former pattern is much more common, and these patients are often middle-aged, overweight individuals who commonly have concomitant adult-onset Type II diabetes mellitus and hyperuricemia. These patients have delayed clearance of triglyceride-rich lipoproteins of either intestinal or hepatic origin and increased hepatic production of VLDL. These patients may have arthritis, paresthesias, or dry eyes and mouth, as well as emotional lability. Family members of these patients often have moderate hypertriglyceridemia. Treatment with diet is very important (dietary fat should be restricted to less than 20 per cent of calories), as is weight reduction via calorie restriction, abstinence from alcohol, and avoidance of estrogens, beta blockers, and thiazide diuretics. An exercise program is also recommended. In the diabetic patient, careful control of glucose levels is important. These patients are at high risk of developing recurrent pancreatitis and may present with eruptive xanthomas and lipemia retinalis. If dietary and other therapies are not effective in lowering the triglyceride levels to less than 500 mg per dl, the drug of choice is gemfibrozil. If additional triglyceride reduction is required or if patients cannot tolerate this agent, fish oil capsules should be used. In patients without diabetes, niacin can be used as well. Gemfibrozil is the single most effective triglyceride-lowering agent in this category of patient.

Occasionally, patients with severe hypertriglyceridemia are children or young adults and are not obese or diabetic. These rare patients often have chylomicrons as their major lipoprotein band on electrophoresis. They may have a deficiency of the enzyme lipoprotein lipase or of its activator protein (apolipoprotein C-II) and have a striking inability to catabolize chylomicrons. Treatment consists of dietary fat restriction to less than 20 grams per day. Niacin and gemfibrozil are generally not effective in these patients, but a trial of therapy is indicated. In my experience, fish oil capsules (see later) are effective in lowering triglyceride levels in some patients in this group.

HDL Deficiency

HDL deficiency is defined as an HDL cholesterol level less than 35 mg per dl in the presence of normal VLDL and LDL cholesterol levels. Dietary therapy is recommended for these patients to optimize their LDL cholesterol levels. For overweight patients, caloric restriction is indicated. An exercise program is also important, as is cessation of smoking. Patients taking beta-blocker medication should be switched to lipid neutral medications if possible. For patients with established CHD with HDL deficiency that is still present despite attempts to use the previously described measures, niacin therapy can be used. In patients who cannot tolerate niacin or who do not obtain an adequate response, gemfibrozil should be used.

Patients with Coronary Heart Disease

In such patients, efforts should be made to optimize levels of plasma lipids and lipoproteins. My goals in these patients, in addition to smoking cessation and control of hypertension, body weight, and glucose level, are to reduce LDL cholesterol levels to less than 130 mg per dl, to raise HDL cholesterol levels to more than 40 mg per dl, and to lower triglyceride levels to less than 200 mg per dl. In a recent 2-year study of hypercholesterolemic post–coronary artery bypass patients, use of the combination of niacin and colestipol was associated with marked reductions in LDL cholesterol levels and with significantly less progression of angiographically documented coronary atherosclerosis compared with the placebo group. However, many CHD patients cannot tolerate these agents. I do not hesitate to use lovastatin in such patients because one can achieve similar LDL cholesterol reductions, along with modest decreases in triglyceride levels and increases in HDL cholesterol levels with this agent.

Pregnant Women

Patients who become pregnant should immediately stop use of all lipid-lowering medications until after pregnancy and nursing are completed. Women who are attempting to conceive should also stop medication. Pregnant women who have severe hypertriglyceridemia and who have had pancreatitis should be treated with marked dietary fat restriction (less than 20 grams per day). If these measures are unsuccessful in reducing triglyceride values to less than 1000 mg per dl, fish oil capsules should be tried.

Children

All children above the age of 2 years should be treated with diet if their LDL cholesterol levels are higher than 130 mg per dl. Children with LDL cholesterol levels higher than 225 mg per dl while eating an LDL-reducing diet are candidates for therapy with low doses of resin (see later). After puberty, adolescents should be treated in the same manner as adults.

Diabetic Patients

Patients with Type I diabetes generally have normal lipid levels if their glucose levels are well controlled. In contrast, patients with Type II diabetes frequently have elevated triglyceride levels and decreased HDL cholesterol levels. Occasionally, these patients may have elevated LDL cholesterol values. Attempts should be made to optimize their lipid levels, as for CHD patients, because these patients are at high risk for developing clinically significant atherosclerosis. In addition to glucose control and modification of diet and lifestyle, gemfibrozil is useful for lowering triglyceride levels and raising HDL levels, and cholestyramine or lovastatin can be used to control LDL cholesterol levels.

Dietary Management

Dietary therapy should be initiated in all patients with an LDL cholesterol level of 160 mg per dl or greater and in patients with levels of 130 mg per dl or greater if CHD or two or more CHD risk factors are present. Target levels for therapy in these two groups are identical to initiation levels. The current recommendation is to provide the patient initially with pamphlet information and counseling, and then to determine if the patient has reached the target levels. Excellent pamphlets can be obtained from the local American Heart Association affiliate or the NCEP Program (telephone 301–951–3260), which provide information about the NCEP Step 1 diet. The goal of this diet is to reduce dietary fat to less than 30 per cent of calories, dietary saturated fat to less than 10 per cent of calories, and dietary cholesterol to less than 300 mg per day. Such a diet has been recommended as prudent for the entire population by both the American Heart Association and the U.S. Surgeon General. Achieving optimal weight and exercising regularly are also recommended. These latter measures are often more effective in lowering triglyceride levels than cholesterol levels.

If the patient has not reached target levels within 3 months, referral to a trained registered dietitian is recommended for implementation of the Step 2 diet. This diet is designed to reduce dietary fat to less than 25 per cent of calories, saturated fat to less than 7 per cent of calories, and dietary cholesterol to less than 200 mg per day. In general, physicians should allow 6 months to determine whether target levels can be achieved with dietary therapy alone. Use of dietitians is encouraged, but the physician should also emphasize the importance of diet as the cornerstone of therapy. In our experience, this stepwise approach may be too cumbersome and lengthy for many patients to adhere to, and direct referral to a dietitian with implementation of the Step 2 diet is preferable. The same diet is used for all forms of hyperlipoproteinemia.

Some guidelines about the NCEP Step 2 diet follow. The use of fresh vegetables (as long as they are not prepared with saturated fat) and fruits is encouraged, as are cereals except for granola or "natural cereals" containing coconut oil. The use of skim milk, egg whites, and nonfat or low-fat yogurt products is encouraged, and the use of eggs, cheeses, and other dairy products such as butter, whole milk, cream, and ice cream is discouraged. Sherbet can be used. The oils that are lowest in saturated fat include rapeseed (canola), safflower, and sunflower oils. Soft margarine made from these oils should be used instead of butter. Foods containing palm or coconut oil should be avoided. Most breads are fine except for croissants and muffins. Fish is fine, as is white meat turkey or chicken meat without the skin. Lobster, crab, clams, and mussels are fine, but shrimp should be eaten only occasionally because of its high cholesterol content. Patients can occasionally eat lean beef (round) or extra lean ham. Spaghetti and macaroni are fine, but pizza, quiche, cookies, cakes, pies, chocolate, and french fries should be avoided unless they have been specially prepared.

Some authorities have recommended the use of a high-monounsaturated-fat diet instead of a high-polyunsaturated-fat diet or a high-carbohydrate, low-fat diet. It has been shown that monounsaturated fats are as effective in lowering LDL cholesterol levels as are polyunsaturated fats, compared with saturated fat, and have the advantage of not lowering HDL cholesterol levels. In addition, some studies suggest that polyunsaturated fats act as cocarcinogens when used in experimental animals in large amounts in the diet. Therefore the current recommendations are that polyunsaturated fat intake not exceed 10 per cent of caloric intake and that no limitation be placed on monounsaturated fats. Studies suggest that a saturated fatty acid (stearic acid) found in beef and chocolate does not raise LDL cholesterol levels. It should be noted, however, that these food products contain more palmitic acid than stearic acid, and palmitic acid definitely raises LDL cholesterol levels. It should also be noted that a major source of monounsaturated fat in the U.S. diet is meat. The emphasis of the NCEP Step 1 and Step 2 diets on lowering dietary saturated fat and cholesterol intake is appropriate because these are the dietary constituents that raise LDL cholesterol levels in the blood stream. The NCEP Step 1 and Step 2 diets are lower in monounsaturated fat content than the current U.S. diet (about 15 per cent of calories as saturated fat and monounsaturated fat and 6 per cent of calories as polyunsaturated fat). In patients with severe hypertriglyceridemia, dietary fat should be restricted to less than 20 per cent of calories.

Drug Therapy

Drug therapy is indicated after at least a 6-month trial of diet in all patients with LDL cholesterol levels higher than 190 mg per dl, with the goal of reducing LDL cholesterol levels to less than 160 mg per dl. Drug therapy is also indicated after dietary therapy in patients with LDL cholesterol levels higher than 160 mg per dl if CHD or two or more CHD risk factors are present, with the goal of reducing the LDL cholesterol level to less than 130 mg per dl. Medications used for lipid reduction include anion exchange resins, niacin, fibric acid derivatives, HMG CoA reductase inhibitors, fish oil capsules, and probucol.

Anion Exchange Resins

The resins bind bile acids in the intestine, which prevents their reabsorption and promotes their fecal excretion. This process causes conversion of more cholesterol to bile acids in the liver, depletion of the cholesterol content in hepatocytes, and up-regulation of liver LDL receptor activity. This process, in turn, leads to enhanced catabolism of plasma LDL resulting in reductions in plasma LDL cholesterol levels. The most common side effects are constipation, abdominal cramps, and distention. Less common effects include flatulence, nausea, vomiting, heartburn, and anorexia. These agents often increase plasma triglyceride levels and interfere with the absorption of digoxin, thyroxine, warfarin sodium (Coumadin), phenobarbital, phenylbutazone, beta blockers, chlorothiazide, tetracycline, and potentially other agents. Therefore such medications must be given either 1 hour before or 4 hours after the use of resins. Decreased levels of folate and of fat-soluble vitamins have been reported with chronic use of fairly high doses of resin. Therefore annual measurements of the prothrombin time, as well as of folate, retinol, and alpha-tocopherol levels, are reasonable. Deficiencies of these nutrients are extremely rare in patients on resins.

Two different resins are available. Cholestyramine (Questran) comes in packets containing 4 grams of active compound, and colestipol (Colestid) comes in similar packets containing 5 grams of a different resin. Both agents have similar efficacy and side effects. Cholestyramine has an orange-like flavor and has extra filler, whereas colestipol is tasteless. Both agents also come in containers from which patients can scoop the powder. One packet is equal to one scoop, and the price of scoops is substantially less than the price of packets. Cholestyramine is also available as a bar (one bar is equal to one packet). The packets or scoops of powder must be mixed with water or juice and thoroughly stirred before use. Patients can try either resin formulation to see which they prefer. Some authorities recommend using resins in a dose of one or two packets orally four times per day. It has been shown that resin is equally effective if given in a comparable dose twice a day. I start by giving the patient one packet or scoop twice a day and increase the dose to two scoops twice a day. Many patients can tolerate this regimen and achieve LDL cholesterol reductions of 15 to 20 per cent. If constipation develops, it can be treated with psyllium (Metamucil), 1 teaspoon orally twice daily, which may lower LDL cholesterol further. In a large prospective study (Lipid Research Clinics Study) in asymptomatic middle-aged men with elevated LDL cholesterol levels, the use of cholestyramine during a 7-year period resulted in a 12 per cent reduction in LDL cholesterol levels in the drug group and a 19 per cent lower rate of development of CHD compared with a placebo group. Subjects receiving the drug were supposed to use six packets per day, but the average subject used three and one-half; four and one-half packets per day were used in the placebo group. Clearly, long-term compliance is a problem with this agent. Those subjects in the study who actually took 24 grams per day of cholestyramine sustained a 35 per cent reduction in LDL cholesterol levels. In my experience, using lower doses (16 grams per day of cholestyramine) markedly increases compliance. In children with marked hypercholesterolemia under the age of 5 years, I use one-half packet or scoop of resin twice daily; in children between the ages of 5 and 10 years, I use one scoop twice daily; and in older children and adults, I use two scoops of resin twice daily. In patients who develop vomiting, the drug should be discontinued immediately.

Niacin

Niacin or nicotinic acid, when used in pharmacologic doses of 2 to 3 grams per day, decreases the production of VLDL and LDL and increases HDL cholesterol levels. Triglyceride levels are decreased by approximately 30 per cent and LDL cholesterol levels by about 20 per cent, and HDL cholesterol levels are increased by about 20 per cent. In a large prospective study (the Coronary

Drug Project), use of niacin in a dose of 3 grams per day in patients with previous myocardial infarction was associated with a 10 per cent reduction in total cholesterol and a 20 per cent reduction in prospective CHD incidence during a 5-year period compared with the placebo group. Fifteen years after initiation of the trial and 9 years after completion of the study and termination of medication, subjects who had been taking niacin had an 11 per cent lower mortality than those who had been taking a placebo. Responses are quite variable. Niacin is available as an over-the-counter medication in 50-, 100-, 250-, 500-, and 1000-mg tablets. The drug is started at a dose of 100 mg orally twice daily with meals and gradually increased during a 2-week period to 1 gram orally twice daily. Three times daily dosing may reduce adverse reactions. Doses of either 1 gram orally three times daily or 1.5 grams orally twice daily with meals can also be used. Some authorities use even higher doses, but the incidence of side effects increases markedly. I recommend using no more than 2 grams per day for most patients. Almost all patients have initial problems with flushing, but this effect decreases with time. Aspirin or nonsteroidal anti-inflammatory compounds decrease the flushing and may have to be used for the first month of therapy, or whenever niacin is stopped for even short periods. Long-acting or delayed-release niacin can also be used. The drug may also cause gastritis and should not be taken on an empty stomach, but after 1 month I switch the patient to regular niacin. There is evidence that long-acting niacin is less effective and is associated with more gastrointestinal side effects than regular niacin. Niacinamide has no lipid-lowering effect and cannot be used in place of niacin.

All patients receiving niacin should have baseline liver enzymes, glucose, and uric acid levels measured. These parameters need to be monitored in all patients initially every 6 weeks for the first 6 months, and then every 3 to 6 months. Contraindications to niacin use include peptic ulcer, liver disease, and hyperuricemia (although the last problem can be treated with allopurinol). Niacin should not be used in diabetic patients unless they are taking insulin and one is prepared to increase the dose of insulin. There is a significant incidence of liver enzyme level elevation in patients taking niacin, and if these levels increase to greater than three times the normal mean, the drug should be discontinued. Other side effects include dry skin, dry eyes, postural hypotension, and, rarely, acanthosis nigricans.

Fibric Acid Derivatives

The fibric acid derivatives gemfibrozil (Lopid) and clofibrate (Atromid-S) are extremely effective triglyceride-lowering agents and are generally well tolerated. These agents decrease VLDL and HDL cholesterol synthesis and enhance VLDL cholesterol degradation. Clofibrate is used less frequently than gemfibrozil because it is less effective in lowering triglyceride levels and because excess mortality was associated with its use compared with placebo in the World Health Organization Study. In this large prospective primary prevention study in middle-aged, hypercholesterolemic men, subjects taking clofibrate had 8 per cent lower cholesterol levels and a 21 per cent lower incidence of CHD during a 5-year period compared with the placebo group but had higher mortality. Clofibrate is known to promote lithogenic bile and to cause gallstones. In another study with clofibrate (the Coronary Drug Project), no increases in mortality were observed (even at the 15-year follow-up), but only a 6 per cent reduction in cholesterol levels and a 10 per cent decrease in prospective CHD incidence were observed during 5 years compared with the results achieved with a placebo. In contrast, in a recent large prospective primary prevention study in middle-aged, hypercholesterolemic men (the Helsinki Heart Study), the use of gemfibrozil at a dose of 600 mg orally twice daily was associated with a mean 9 per cent lower total cholesterol level, a 35 per cent lower triglyceride level, a 9 per cent lower LDL cholesterol level, a 10 per cent lower HDL cholesterol value, and a 34 per cent lower incidence of CHD compared with the results achieved with a placebo. Gemfibrozil appears to be less lithogenic than clofibrate. No major adverse effects were noted with gemfibrozil in the Helsinki study.

Gemfibrozil is generally well tolerated. Occasional gastrointestinal side effects are noted, as are rare liver enzyme level elevations and changes in hematologic test results. Muscle cramps and increased creatine phosphokinase (CPK) levels are observed in about 1 per cent of cases; therefore CPK monitoring is warranted. Allergic skin reactions also occur rarely. The drug is contraindicated in patients with renal insufficiency or liver disease. It is available in 300-mg capsules and 600-mg tablets. The standard dose is 600 mg orally twice daily. The drug potentiates the action of Coumadin, so that patients taking both agents may have to have their Coumadin dose reduced by 50 per cent. A new fibric acid derivative, fenofibrate, may soon be available in the United States. This agent is substantially more effective in lowering LDL cholesterol than either clofibrate or gemfibrozil and has been used in Europe for a long time. In patients with normal LDL cholesterol levels, gemfibrozil is the drug of choice for lowering triglyceride levels.

Lovastatin

Lovastatin (Mevacor) inhibits HMG CoA reductase, the rate-limiting enzyme in cholesterol biosynthesis, which results in reduced intracellular cholesterol levels, up-regulation of LDL receptor activity, enhanced plasma clearance of LDL, and decreased LDL cholesterol levels in plasma. The drug may also decrease VLDL and LDL hepatic production. The drug is available in 20-mg tablets. The starting dose is 20 mg orally per day in the evening, and the maximal dose is 40 mg orally twice daily. Reductions of approximately 20 per cent in LDL cholesterol are observed with 20 mg per day, 30 per cent with 40 mg per day, and about 40 per cent with 80 mg per day. Some patients obtain a maximal effect with a dose of 20 mg orally twice daily. The drug is generally well tolerated. There is about a 1 per cent incidence of significant liver enzyme level elevation and a similar incidence of significant CPK level elevation and muscle cramping. Both of these side effects necessitate discontinuation of the drug. Other reported side effects include headaches, decreased sleep duration, insomnia, nausea, fatigue, and rashes. Other HMG CoA reductase inhibitors will soon be available in the United States. One of these, pravastatin, does not cross the blood-brain barrier, so that the potential central nervous system side effects of lovastatin, such as headaches, decreased sleep, and insomnia, may be reduced.

It is recommended that patients taking lovastatin have their liver enzyme and CPK levels monitored at baseline and every 6 weeks for the first year, and every 3 to 6 months thereafter. Elevations in CPK levels, myalgia, and rhabdomyolysis have usually occurred in patients treated concurrently with niacin, gemfibrozil, or immunosuppressive agents. An annual eye examination is recommended to rule out the development of cataracts, although there is no evidence at present that this agent causes cataract formation in humans at the dose levels used. In contrast to other effective LDL-lowering agents (resins and niacin), lovastatin is generally well tolerated by most patients. If long-term safety is established and efficacy in CHD reduction is demonstrated, HMG CoA reductase inhibitors will become the drugs of choice for LDL reduction.

Fish Oil Capsules

Fish oil capsules are effective triglyceride-lowering agents in patients with severe hypertriglyceridemia in whom sufficient triglyceride reduction has not been achieved with other agents. Fish oil capsules contain 1 gram of fish oil, which is almost entirely fat. These capsules contain as much saturated fat as they do omega-3 fatty acids. The capsules that we use are obtained from Bronson Pharmaceuticals (LaCanada, Calif.; 800–521–3322) and, based on our own analysis, contain the least saturated fat and the most omega-3 fatty acids of all commercially available capsules that we have tested. Moreover these capsules (SuperEPA) are much less expensive than some of the other heavily advertised products. The starting dose is three 1-gram capsules orally twice daily, which may have to be increased to five capsules twice daily. In some studies, 30 to 40 grams per day has been used. Ten capsules per day is a low dose compared with clinical trials. These capsules can be used in combination with any other lipid-lowering drug. They are generally well tolerated. They cause a modest increase in bleeding time and occasional gastrointestinal distress and may cause a fishy odor when the patient belches. Fish oil capsules may increase LDL cholesterol levels and may also increase glucose levels in diabetic subjects.

Probucol

Probucol (Lorelco) is a potent antioxidant compound that is incorporated into both LDL and HDL particles. It enhances LDL clearance by non–receptor-mediated mechanisms and decreases HDL production. The drug is available in 250- and 500-mg tablets, and the dose is 500 mg orally twice daily. The drug lowers LDL cholesterol levels by about 10 to 15 per cent and HDL cholesterol levels by about 20 per cent. Some authorities recommend its use as a second- or third-line drug in the treatment of familial hypercholesterolemia. However, in my view, this drug cannot be recommended until its efficacy in CHD reduction has been documented because of its adverse effects on HDL cholesterol levels. Probucol is generally well tolerated but may cause diarrhea, flatulence, abdominal pain, and nausea and may prolong the QT interval on the electrocardiogram.

Combination Therapy

The combination of resins and niacin is extremely effective in lowering LDL cholesterol and triglyceride levels and in raising HDL cholesterol levels. The combination of lovastatin with either resins or niacin is even more effective in lowering LDL cholesterol levels. However, the incidence of significant liver enzyme level elevation is quite high with the niacin-lovastatin combination. The combination of resins and gemfibrozil is effective in lowering triglyceride and LDL cholesterol levels and in raising HDL cholesterol levels. The combination of lovastatin and gemfibrozil is extremely effective in lowering triglyceride and LDL cholesterol levels and in raising HDL cholesterol levels, but the incidence of myositis and CPK elevation is about 7 per cent. Therefore patients taking this combination of drugs need to be carefully monitored.

OBESITY

method of
ROLAND L. WEINSIER, M.D., Dr.P.H.
*The University of Alabama at Birmingham
Birmingham, Alabama*

In the absence of better standards, 1959 Metropolitan Life Insurance Company weight-height data (Table 1) are frequently used to estimate relative degrees of overweight. Because of controversy about acceptability of the higher reference weights of the 1983 tables, the earlier data are still used. They offer reasonable estimates of desirable weights for adults. A value of 20 per cent or more above the desirable weight is considered to be overweight and constitutes an established health hazard. Body mass index (BMI) = weight (kg)/height (M²). Obesity is generally defined as a BMI greater than 25. A BMI of 26.4 for men and 25.8 for women corresponds to 20 per cent above the desirable weight for height, as shown in Table 1.

TREATMENT

The International Congress on Obesity established therapeutic guidelines for professional weight control programs that call for the combined use of diet, physical activity, and behavior modification with emotional support in an interdisciplinary program.

The diet should be based on a sound scientific rationale, should be safe and nutritionally adequate, and should be practical and effective for long-term weight control. One diet program that meets these guidelines is referred to as "time-calorie displacement" (TCD). The TCD diet emphasizes foods that are low in caloric density, are high in bulk, and require relatively more time to eat. The caloric densities of the food groups are shown in Table 2. As an example of the extremes of caloric density and eating time, 2400 kcal from the fat group (e.g., 9 ounces of butter or oil) requires less than 5 minutes to ingest. By contrast, 2400 kcal as raw vegetables (represented by approximately 30 pounds of salad) requires more than one-third of one's waking hours to consume. The actual diet prescription, in which patients are encouraged to "lean to the left" of the spectrum by relying heavily on vegetables and fruits, is shown in Table 3. Each patient is prescribed a specific number of vegetable, fruit, starch, milk, meat, and fat servings per day. This allows food choices similar to those provided by

TABLE 2. **Spectrum of Caloric Density of Various Food Groups (cal/oz)**

Low-Calorie High-Bulk Slow-Eating	Lean Left			High-Calorie Low-Bulk Fast-Eating	
Vegetables 10	Fruit 15	Starches 50	Meats 75	Sweets 150	Fats 175

TABLE 1. **Weight-Height Reference Chart (Adults)***

Height (No Shoes)		Reference Weight				
		Women		Men		
Feet, Inches	*Centimeters*	*Pounds*	*Kilograms*	*Pounds*	*Kilograms*	
4′10″	147	101	46	—	—	
4′11″	150	104	47	—	—	
5′ 0″	152	107	49	—	—	
5′ 1″	155	110	50	—	—	
5′ 2″	157	113	51	124	56	
5′ 3″	160	116	53	127	58	
5′ 4″	162	120	54	130	59	
5′ 5″	165	123	56	133	60	
5′ 6″	167	128	58	137	62	
5′ 7″	170	132	60	141	64	
5′ 8″	172	136	62	145	66	
5′ 9″	175	140	63	149	68	
5′10″	178	144	65	153	69	
5′11″	180	148	67	158	71	
6′ 0″	183	152	69	162	74	
6′ 1″	185	—	—	167	76	
6′ 2″	188	—	—	171	78	
6′ 3″	190	—	—	176	80	
6′ 4″	193	—	—	181	82	

*Data adapted from Metropolitan Life Insurance Company, Build and Blood Pressure Study, 1959.

TABLE 3. Time-Calorie Displacement Chart*

Low-Calorie High-Bulk Slow-Eating		"Lean" Left			High-Calorie Low-Bulk Fast-Eating
Vegetables	*Fruits*	*Starches*	*Dairy*	*Meat Group*	*Fats, Oils, Nuts*
Eat at LEAST 20 cal serving equiv./day	Eat at LEAST 40 cal serving equiv.	Eat 70 cal serving equiv./day	Eat 80 cal serving equiv./day	Eat at MOST 75 cal serving equiv./day	Eat at MOST 45 cal serving equiv.

Vegetables — Eat at LEAST (20 cal serving equiv./day)

Servings Listed Are for Raw Vegetables: All Cooked Vegetables Equal ½ c

Vegetable	Amount
Artichokes	½ bud
Asparagus	
Bamboo shoots	½ c
Bean sprouts	1 c
Beets	1 med
Broccoli	1 c
Brussels sprouts	
Cabbage	1 c
Carrots	1 sm
Cauliflower	⅔ c
Celery (5 inches)	6 stalks
Cucumbers	1 lg
Eggplant	1 c
Green beans	1 c
Green peppers	1 lg
Kohlrabi	½ c
Lettuce	5 lg leaves or ¼ head
Mushrooms	7 sm
Okra	
Onions (3-inch diam.)	½
Radishes	10 sm
Rutabagas	½ c
Salad, mixed	1 c
Scallions	3
Spinach	1 c
Squash, summer	1 sm
Tomatoes	½ c
Turnips	4
Water chestnut	
Zucchini	1 c

Fruits — Eat at LEAST (40 cal serving equiv.)

Fresh, Frozen, Sugar-Free

Fruit	Amount
Apples	½ med
Apricots	2
Banana	½ sm
Blackberries	½ c
Blueberries	½ c
Cantaloupe (5-inch diam.)	⅓
Cherries, red sweet	11 med
Cherries, red sour	⅓ c
Grapefruit (4-inch diam.)	½
Grapes	12 purple, 20 green
Honeydew (6-inch diam.)	¼
Mango	½ sm
Nectarine	1
Orange (2½-inch diam.)	1
Papaya	⅓ med
Peach	1 med
Pear	½ med
Pineapple	1 sl or ½ c
Plums	2 med
Raspberries	½ c
Strawberries	10 lg or ¾ c
Tangerine	2 sm
Watermelon	¾ c

Preferred Foods

Starches — Eat (70 cal serving equiv./day)

Cooked Starches Should Represent at Least ½ of Total Intake

Cooked

Beans, cooked: Lentils	⅓ c
Kidney	⅓ c
Lima	⅓ c
Pinto	⅓ c
Soy	¼ c
White	⅓ c
Cereal, cooked: Buckwheat	½ c
Millet	½ c
Oatmeal	½ c
Ralston	½ c
Seven-grain	½ c
Wheatena	½ c
Barley	½ c
Bulgar	½ c
Corn: On cob	3-inch ear
Kernels	½ c
Peas, blackeyed	⅓ c
Peas, green	⅔ c
Potato: Baked	1 med
Boiled	1 med
Mashed	½ c
Pumpkin	¾ c
Rice, brown	½ c
Squash, winter	½ c
Sweet potato	½ med

Dry

Food	Amount
Bread, whole grain	1 sl
Cereal, dry: All Bran	⅓ c
Bran Buds	⅓ c
Bran Flakes	⅔ c
Raisin Bran	½ c
Shredded wheat	½ c
Most	½ c

Dairy — Eat (80 cal serving equiv./day)

May Exchange Serving for Serving with Meat Group

Food	Amount
Skim, nonfat: Buttermilk	1 c
Evaporated diluted 1:2	1 c
Milk powder	⅓ c
Milk Low fat, 1–2%	1 c
Yogurt, plain	½ c
Whole: Buttermilk	½ c
Evaporated diluted 1:2	½ c
Milk	½ c
Yogurt, plain	½ c

Meat Group — Eat at MOST (75 cal serving equiv./day)

Weigh Portions After Cooking

Food	Amount
Fish: Bass	1 oz
Catfish	1 oz
Cod	1½ oz
Crabmeat	3 oz
Clams	10 med
Flounder	1¼ oz
Haddock	1½ oz
Lobster	2½ oz
Oysters (raw)	8 med
Perch	1½ oz
Salmon	1½ oz
Scallops	2 oz
Shrimp	20 or 2½ oz
Snapper	1½ oz
Tuna (water pack)	2 oz
Poultry: Chicken (no skin)	1½ oz
Turkey (no skin)	1½ oz
Meat: Beef	1 oz
Pork	1 oz
Lamb	1 oz
Veal	1 oz
Cheese: All hard cheese	⅔ oz
Cottage cheese (noncreamed)	½ c
Ricotta cheese (part skim)	¼ c

Fats, Oils, Nuts — Eat at MOST (45 cal serving equiv.)

Avocado (3¼ × 4 inches)	⅛
Butter: Regular	1 t
Whipped	1½ t
Cream: Half & Half	2 T
Sour	1½ T
Whipping	1 T
Non dairy	3 t
Cream cheese	1 T
Margarine: Diet	1 T
Whipped	1½ t
Regular	1 t
Mayonnaise: Regular	1½ t
Low calorie	1 T
Nuts, unsalted: Almonds	7
Brazil	2
Cashew	4
Hickory	7
Peanuts	9
Pecans (halves)	5
Walnut (halves)	5
Oil	1 t
Peanut butter	1 t
Salad dressing: Regular	2 t
Low calories	2–4 T (see label)
Seeds, unsalted: Pumpkin	1 T
Sesame	1 T
Sunflower	1 T

Crackers
Rye Crisp 4
Venus Wafers 4
Popcorn, plain 1½ c

Occasional Foods
(Up to 2 Items/wk from Each Group)

Canned vegetable	½ c	Canned fruit†	
Pickle, sour	1 lg	Applesauce	½ c
Sauerkraut	⅔ c	Fruit cocktail	½ c
Tomato juice	3 oz	Mandarin oranges	½ c
V-8 juice	4 oz	Dried fruit	
		Apricots	2
		Dates	1½
		Figs	1
		Prunes	1½
		Raisins	2 T
		Fruit juice	
		Apple	⅓ c
		Cranberry	¼ c
		Grape	¼ c
		Grapefruit	½ c
		Orange	⅓ c
		Pineapple	⅓ c
		Prune	¼ c

Angel food cake 3 × 4 × ½ inches	1 sl
Biscuit or Muffin	½
Bread, white	1 sl
Cornbread 2 × 2 × 1½ inches	1 pc‡
Cereal, dry, other, (see non-sugared label)	
Cereal, cooked white	½ c
Crackers	
Graham	2½ sq
Oyster	20
Soda	5
Pasta, cooked	½ c
Rice, cooked white	½ c
Roll, dinner	1 sm

Bologna	2 oz‡
Cured meats	1 oz
Duck	¾ oz‡
Egg	1 med
Frankfurters	1⅔ oz‡
Goose	¾ oz‡
Luncheon meat	1½ oz§
Organ meat	1 oz
Ricotta cheese	2½ T
Sausage	1¼ oz§
Bacon	1 sl
Bacon drippings	1 t
Chitterlings	¼ c
Cracklings	1 t
Gravy	2 T
Salt pork	¼ oz
Alcohol, count 2	fats
Beer	
Regular	3 oz
Lite	5 oz
Liquor	¾ oz§
Wine	
Dry	2 oz
Sweet	1 oz
Lite	4 oz

Special Occasion Foods
(Up to 200 cal/wk)
Calorie Content of Selected Items

Cakes			Ice cream ½ c, 1 scoop	150
Pound (3 × 3 × ½ inches)	125		Ice milk ½ c, 1 scoop	100
Brownies (2 × 3 × 2 inches)	145		Jello ½ c	65
Cake with icing (2 × 3 × 2 inches)	210		Jelly 1 level T	50
Candy—1 oz	150		Juice, sweetened ("drinks") ½ c	50
Cereals, dry, sugared (see label)			Pies ⅙ pie	380
Cookies			Potato chips 10	115
Ginger snaps	70		Puddings	
Vanilla wafers	20		Whole milk ½ c	130
Crackers, snack (see label)			Skim milk ½ c	70
Cranberry sauce 1 T	30		Sherbert ½ c	130
Donuts			Soda 10 oz	130
Plain 1 med	125		Soups, cream 8 oz	150
Jelly 1 med	225		Sugar 1 t	20
French fries 10 pcs	135		Yogurt, sweetened or fruited 1 c	250
Fruits, canned, sweetened, 2 halves or ½ c	80			
Honey 2 t	40			

*From Weinsier R, Johnston M, and Doleys D: Time Calorie Displacement: Approach to Weight Control. Philadelphia, George Stickley Co., 1983, pp 8–11. Used by permission.
†Unsweetened.
‡Count 1 fat.
§Count 2 fats.

TABLE 4. **Guide to the Number of Serving Equivalents to Select**
from Each Food Group Per Day for Weight Reduction

Diet	Vegetable Group	Fruit Group	Starch Group	Milk Group	Meat Group	Fat Group
A (975 cal)	3	4	4	½	4	3
B (1030 cal)	4	4	4	½	4½	3
C (1200 cal)	4	5	5	½	5	3½
D (1370 cal)	5	6	6	½	5½	3½
E (1540 cal)	5	7	7	½	6	4
F (1700 cal)	5	8	8	½	6½	4½

the diabetic "exchange" list system. No upper limit is placed on vegetable and fruit intake, and patients are encouraged to eat as much as they desire because the calorie content is low and larger intakes tend to prevent hunger and decrease the risk of binges, which occur with more restricted diets. An upper limit is set for fats, and less intake is encouraged. Foods in each group are divided into "preferred," "occasional," and "special occasion" categories (Table 3). The preferred foods require more time to consume, are the least refined, and have the highest fiber content. The special occasion foods are high-calorie snack and dessert foods. Permitting patients up to 200 kcal per week of these items allows flexibility and removes the guilt associated with using these foods on special occasions.

Most adult men are started at approximately 1200 kcal per day and women at 1000 kcal per day. The serving equivalents, or "exchanges," for each of the food groups for various calorie levels are shown in Table 4. At these calorie levels and using the types of food described in the TCD plan, vitamin and mineral intake is usually adequate without supplementation.

Adherence to this dietary approach tends to be high because of the opportunity to select from among a variety of foods within each of the food groups. Post-treatment weight maintenance is achieved in approximately 50 per cent of the patients an average of 2 years later. Detailed information about the TCD approach is described in the book *Time-Calorie Displacement: Approach to Weight Control,* published by the George Stickley Company in Philadelphia.

Physical activity may minimize the loss of lean body mass associated with weight loss. Low-impact aerobic exercise that is tailored to the individual is generally recommended. Cardiovascular conditioning is achieved by exercising 3 to 5 days a week for at least 30 minutes at 60 to 85 per cent of maximum heart rate (220 minus the age). Lifestyle changes through the use of "step-losing" activities (e.g., using stairs instead of the elevator) help to establish long-standing patterns of increased physical activity.

Behavior and psychologic therapy should in-clude the following therapeutic modalities. Daily self-monitoring of dietary intake for at least 4 months is the key to establishing improved eating habits. Because chronically restrained eaters are prone to binging, practicing controlled intake of highly desired foods (rather than total avoidance) helps to prevent the "on-off" attitude toward dieting. Finally, attention should be directed toward improving feelings of self-worth and self-control by using such strategies as assertiveness training and supportive psychotherapy.

Three components of a weight control program must be considered together and interrelated: diet, physical activity, and behavior modification with emotional support. Although any one of these components may be used to achieve weight loss in certain individuals, when such an interdisciplinary program is applied to unselected patients, it is likely to maximize the odds of achieving long-term weight control.

PELLAGRA

method of
JOSÉ ERNESTO DOS SANTOS, M.D.
Universidade de São Paulo
São Paulo, Brazil

Pellagra is a disease caused by nutritional deficiencies, frequently multiple, in which niacin and tryptophan inadequacies predominate. There is evidence for the participation of other vitamin and mineral deficiencies in the etiology of the disease. It is diagnosed mainly in alcoholic patients and less frequently in food faddists, elderly people, and persons with malabsorption syndromes or other illnesses that cause an increased requirement for niacin and its precursor, such as the malignant carcinoid syndrome. In this syndrome, 60 per cent of the dietary tryptophan is converted to serotonin (in contrast to only 1 per cent in a normal situation), with a consequent decrease in niacin coenzyme synthesis. Pellagra-like skin lesions have been reported in 7 per cent of patients with carcinoid syndrome. Another disease associated with pellagra is Hartnup's disease, a familial abnormality in monoaminomonocarboxylic amino acid absorption by the intestine and reabsorption by renal tubules.

Primary pellagra, in which diet is the only etiologic factor, is observed in underdeveloped countries where corn, millet, and jowar *(Sorghum vulgare),* cereals with low niacin and tryptophan contents, are staple foods. The disease is rare in countries where corn is treated with alkali before human consumption, probably as a consequence of the liberation of niacin bound to peptides or carbohydrates by the alkali treatment. The effect of excess leucine (as in jowar) as an inhibitor of niacin coenzyme synthesis is also considered a possible explanation.

The clinical picture of pellagra is characterized by diarrhea, symmetric scaling and sometimes ulcerating dermatitis on sun-exposed skin surfaces, irritability, anxiety, depression, and ultimately psychosis. Other frequent clinical signs are scarlet glossitis and fatigue. As a multiple deficiency state, it is frequently associated with anemia, peripheral neuropathy, and other signs related to deficiency of other nutrients.

PREVENTION

The most important preventive method is the provision of a diet with sufficient amounts of energy, protein, vitamins, and minerals. Such a diet includes vegetables, cereals, meat, dairy products, and fruits. A daily intake of 2400 to 2800 kcal, 45 to 55 grams of protein of high biologic value, and 20 niacin equivalents (NE) (1 NE is equal to 1 mg of niacin or 60 mg of dietary tryptophan) will prevent pellagra in healthy adults. For patients who cannot or should not eat, a multivitamin supplementation given orally, by tube, or parenterally must be added to the prescription. The Food and Nutrition Board of the National Academy of Sciences in the United States (1980) recommends 6 to 9 NE for healthy infants, and 11 to 19 NE for older children and adults. For lactating or pregnant women, it is advisable to supplement the normal diet with 5 or 2 NE, respectively.

TREATMENT

The acute manifestations should be treated with 150 to 300 mg of niacinamide orally. For children, the dose must be reduced to 60 to 150 mg a day. Usually this amount is prescribed for a period of 15 days. When diarrhea and anorexia are also present, the utilization of tube feeding or parenteral nutrition is indicated. In this case, commercial products should contain the recommended amounts of vitamins. With appropriate treatment, the skin signs and other symptoms disappear in 10 to 20 days.

RICKETS AND OSTEOMALACIA

method of
JOHN M. PETTIFOR, M.B., CH.B.,
PH.D. (MED.)
University of the Witwatersrand
Johannesburg, South Africa

Rickets and osteomalacia are metabolic bone diseases characterized by a failure of or delay in mineralization of preformed matrix. In the case of rickets, which by definition is a disease of children with open epiphyses, the defect occurs in cartilaginous matrix at the epiphyseal growth plate and manifests with deformity of and often delay in closure of the growth plate. Osteomalacia is associated with a mineralization defect in the osteoid at the endosteal bone surfaces (both cortical and trabecular). Children thus manifest with features of both rickets and osteomalacia, whereas in adults, only osteomalacia is found.

Biochemically, both rickets and osteomalacia are associated with disturbances in calcium or phosphorus homeostasis or both. Clinically, rickets is generally accompanied by progressive deformities of the long bones, and in young infants, craniotabes and delayed closure of the fontanelles may be found. In both adults and children, the disease is often associated with muscle weakness, especially of the proximal muscles, bone pain, and skeletal fragility. Radiologically, rickets is generally diagnosed easily by the characteristic appearances at the growth plates, especially in those of the distal radius and ulna and around the knee. Osteomalacia is often more difficult to diagnose, and a bone biopsy may be required to confirm the diagnosis. Radiographically, bone mass is generally decreased, but it may be normal or even increased, as in X-linked hypophosphatemic vitamin D–resistant osteomalacia or renal osteodystrophy.

PATHOGENESIS OF RICKETS

Table 1 lists the causes of rickets and osteomalacia. They have been divided into several groups: two larger ones, depending on whether the disease is mainly caused by a defect in calcium or phosphorus homeostasis, and a smaller third group in which the pathogenesis is caused by direct impairment of mineralization. These divisions are helpful in delineating the pathogenesis and treatment of the disease. Calciopenic rickets and osteomalacia are characterized primarily by hypocalcemia, which in the majority of cases is caused by an abnormality in the metabolism or a deficiency of vitamin D. The resultant secondary hyperparathyroidism leads to increased phosphate clearance by the kidney and variable hypophosphatemia. Hypocalciuria and a generalized increase in urinary excretion of amino acids are also manifestations of secondary hyperparathyroidism.

Phosphopenic rickets and osteomalacia, on the other hand, are associated primarily with hypophosphatemia. Serum calcium and parathyroid hormone values are generally normal. Urinary findings are variable,

TABLE 1. **Pathogenesis of Rickets and Osteomalacia**

Calciopenic
1. Inadequate formation of 1,25-dihydroxyvitamin D
   Vitamin D deficiency
     Dietary lack
     Lack of sunlight exposure
     Malabsoprtion syndromes
   Failure of hepatic hydroxylation—severe liver disease
   Increased vitamin D catabolism—? anticonvulsant therapy
   Failure of renal hydroxylation
     1-Alpha-hydroxylase deficiency
     (vitamin dependency type I)
     Renal failure
2. Peripheral resistance to 1,25-dihydroxyvitamin D
   Defects in target organ receptors (vitamin D dependency type II)
3. Inadequate calcium intake
   Dietary calcium deficiency
   High fluoride intake

Phosphopenic
1. Inadequate phosphate absorption
   Dietary lack (e.g., breast-fed, very-low-birth-weight infants)
   Binding of dietary phosphate in the gastrointestinal tract
2. Increased renal losses
   Renal phosphate leak
     Genetic or sporadic hypophosphatemic vitamin D–resistant rickets
     Hypercalciuria vitamin D–resistant rickets
     Adult-onset hypophosphatemia vitamin D–resistant osteomalacia
     Oncogenous osteomalacia
     Neurofibromatosis or polyostotic fibrous dysplasia
   Complex renal tubular abnormalities
     Proximal tubular defect
       Primary (Fanconi's syndrome)
       Secondary (multiple myeloma, outdated tetracyclines)
     Distal renal tubular acidosis

Impaired Mineralization
1. Hypophosphatasia
2. Aluminum toxicity
3. Fluoride
4. Disodium etidronate

depending on the cause of the phosphopenic bone disease, but in all these cases, the phosphate level is decreased.

DIAGNOSIS OF RICKETS AND OSTEOMALACIA

The diagnosis of rickets and osteomalacia can usually be made on the basis of the clinical history, physical examination, and radiographic and biochemical investigations. Difficulties, however, may arise in cases of suspected osteomalacia, where the radiographic and biochemical changes are not diagnostic. In such situations, histologic examination of undecalcified sections of an iliac crest bone biopsy specimen, obtained generally under local anesthesia, is of diagnostic value because impaired mineralization can be quantitated by prior labeling of the bone with tetracycline. Table 2 gives some of the biochemical investigations required for the establishment of the etiology of the bone disease, although the physician needs to be selective because the initial history, physical examination, and biochemical investigations may point to a particular diagnosis. Mistakes can be made in the diagnosis because of the lack of awareness of the changes that occur in serum phosphorus and alkaline phosphatase levels with age. Serum phosphorus levels are highest in the immediate newborn period, falling during the following couple of years to plateau until the pubertal growth spurt, when they fall slowly to adult levels. Alkaline phosphatase levels show a similar pattern, although there is often a rise in values associated with the pubertal growth spurt before they fall to adult levels.

PHYSIOLOGY OF MINERAL HOMEOSTASIS AND BONE MINERALIZATION

The physiology of the mineralization of newly formed bone or growth plate matrix is a complex process that is incompletely understood. However, the maintenance of normal serum calcium and phosphorus concentrations is an important factor in normal mineralization. The enzyme alkaline phosphatase, which is present in osteoblasts and chondrocytes, also appears to play a pivotal role in the mineralization process, as an inherited absence of the bone isoenzyme (hypophosphatasia) leads to a marked mineralization defect and to the clinical and radiologic picture of severe rickets and osteomalacia. Certain elements, such as fluoride and aluminum in excess, inhibit the mineralization process, as do drugs such as disodium etidronate (Didronel), a bisphosphonate.

The control of serum calcium levels is achieved by several factors, the most important of which are parathyroid hormone and the active metabolite of vitamin D (1,25-dihydroxyvitamin D or 1,25-$(OH)_2$D). Parathyroid hormone, which is secreted in response to a fall in the ionized calcium level, increases serum calcium values by (1) increasing osteoclastic bone resorption,

TABLE 2. **Biochemical Investigations Useful in the Diagnosis of Rickets and Osteomalacia**

Serum
  Calcium (ionized if possible)
  Phosphorus
  Alkaline phosphatase (bone isoenzymes if liver disease is considered possible)
  Magnesium
  Creatinine
  Blood gases (if renal tubular acidosis is suspected)
  25-Hydroxyvitamin D (if vitamin D deficiency suspected)
  1,25-Dihydroxyvitamin D (only of limited value; more of a research tool)
  Parathyroid hormone

Urine
  24-hr calcium excretion (or calcium/creatinine ratio)
  Tubular reabsorption of phosphorus
  Amino acid excretion
  pH and acidification test (if renal tubular acidosis is suspected)
  Glucose

(2) decreasing renal calcium loss, and (3) increasing the production of 1,25-(OH)$_2$D by the kidney. 1,25-(OH)$_2$D increases calcium absorption from the gastrointestinal tract and acts synergistically with parathyroid hormone in increasing osteoclastic bone resorption. Through its metabolite, 1,25-(OH)$_2$D, vitamin D plays a central role in the maintenance of normal mineral homeostasis.

The control of serum phosphorus levels is less well understood, and values are not as tightly controlled as are those of serum calcium. Unlike calcium, serum phosphorus levels appear to be largely controlled by alterations in the renal excretion of phosphate, which, in turn, is partially controlled by parathyroid hormone and growth hormone.

VITAMIN D AND ITS METABOLITES

Vitamin D occurs in two major forms. Vitamin D$_3$ (cholecalciferol) is formed in the skin by the conversion of 7-dehydrocholesterol under the influence of ultraviolet radiation. Vitamin D$_2$ (ergocalciferol), the form usually used for the fortification of foods and pharmaceutical preparations, is an irradiated plant sterol. Although there is some evidence in humans that the two preparations have slightly different actions, for practical purposes they may be used interchangeably.

Vitamin D is stored in muscle and fat. Thus, if toxicity caused by vitamin D overdosage develops, it may take several months before symptoms subside. Vitamin D is transported to the liver, where it is hydroxylated to 25-hydroxyvitamin D (25-OHD), the major circulating form of the vitamin. The circulating level of 25-OHD (normal range, 10 to 50 mg per ml) is a useful indicator of the vitamin D status of an individual; low levels (<4 ng per ml) indicate vitamin D deficiency, whereas values higher than 200 ng per ml suggest vitamin D toxicity. The physiologically active metabolite of vitamin D, 1,25-(OH)$_2$D, is formed in the kidney, where increased parathyroid hormone concentrations and hypophosphatemia stimulate its formation. Table 3 provides the pharmaceutical preparations of vitamin D and its metabolites and analogues that are available. 1-Alpha-hydroxyvitamin D$_3$ (One-Alpha), a synthetic analogue of vitamin D, behaves in a very similar manner to 1,25-(OH)$_2$D$_3$ (Rocaltrol), as it is rapidly hydroxylated by the liver to 1,25-(OH)$_2$D$_3$. Thus its indications for use are similar to those of the active metabolite. Dihydrotachysterol (Hytakerol), an irradiated plant sterol, is a 5,6-trans vitamin D$_3$ analogue that has a hydroxyl group in a "pseudo-one" position and thus does not require 1-alpha hydroxylation by the kidney for its biologic activity. 1,25-(OH)$_2$D$_3$ and 1-alpha-hydroxyvitamin D$_3$ have relatively short durations of action of between 3 and 7 days, whereas dihydrotachysterol's action may persist for some 2 to 8 weeks. As mentioned previously, the parent vitamin may have a duration of action of up to 6 months, depending on the amount accumulated in tissue stores before therapy is stopped.

TREATMENT

General Considerations

Accurate diagnosis of the etiology of rickets and osteomalacia is of paramount importance, as treatment regimens differ markedly, depending on the cause. This includes not only the types of drugs or the dosage used but also the duration of therapy. Further, a dose of vitamin D that may be needed to correct the bone disease in some forms of vitamin D–resistant rickets could lead to severe vitamin D toxicity in others. In those patients who require prolonged therapy, regular measurement of serum and urinary parameters helps to monitor the response to therapy and prevents under- or overtreatment (Table 4).

Calciopenic Rickets and Osteomalacia

Vitamin D Deficiency

Vitamin D deficiency was a major problem in the industrial towns of Europe and the United States at the turn of the century. Since then, the general practice of fortifying various foods, especially milk, with vitamin D has markedly reduced the prevalence of privational vitamin D deficiency. In developed countries, the problem is almost totally confined to the socioeconomically disadvantaged, the elderly, vegans, and members of certain religious groups, who either do not get sufficient exposure to sunlight because of dress or who do not drink milk and milk products. Breast-fed infants are also at risk because breast milk does not provide sufficient vitamin D to maintain the vitamin D status of the infant.

Prevention. The recommended daily dietary allowance for vitamin D is 10 micrograms (400 IU) per day. In adults it has been suggested that requirements might be even lower (2.5 micrograms, or 100 IU, per day). It is considered prudent to recommend vitamin D supplementation, either in the form of a multivitamin preparation or as vitamin D alone, in all those groups who are at risk. This is particularly true for breast-fed infants and institutionalized elderly persons, for whom adequate exposure to sunshine cannot be guaranteed. There is no evidence that vitamin D toxicity can be produced with a vitamin D intake of 400 IU per day. Health education, stressing the importance of a good diet and the need for sufficient exposure to sunlight (very little is actually required to maintain a normal vitamin D status—up to 30 minutes several times a week), is an essential part of any program designed to eradicate vitamin D deficiency.

Diagnosis of Vitamin D Deficiency Rickets. Vitamin D deficiency rickets or osteomalacia is characterized by the typical features of calciopenic rickets or osteomalacia. Vitamin D deficiency may be confirmed by measuring serum 25-OHD levels, which in vitamin D deficiency are generally less than 4 ng per ml. However, in the majority of cases, this investigation is usually unnecessary.

TABLE 3. **Pharmaceutical Preparations of Vitamin D and Its Analogues**

Form of Vitamin D	Generic Name	Trade Name	Dosage Form	Physiologic Dosage (μg/day)
Vitamin D_2	Ergocalciferol	Drisdol	Caps 625 μg* and 1.25 mg Tablets 1.25 mg Liquid 8000 U/ml	10
25-OHD$_3$	Calcifediol	Calderol	Caps 20 μg, 50 μg	5
1,25-(OH)$_2$D$_3$	Calcitriol	Rocaltrol	Caps 0.25 μg, 0.5 μg	0.5
		Calcijex	Injection 1 μg/ml, 2 μg/ml	
Dihydrotachysterol		Hytakerol DHT	Tablets 0.125 mg, 0.2 mg, 0.4 mg Solution 0.25 mg/ml	20
1-Alpha-hydroxyvitamin D$_3$		One-Alpha	Caps 0.25 μg, 1 μg	0.5–1

*1 μg vitamin D_3 = 40 IU.

It should probably be reserved for those patients in whom there is uncertainty about the diagnosis or in whom there is an inadequate response to treatment.

Vitamin D deficiency caused by a malabsorption syndrome (e.g., after gastrointestinal surgery, celiac disease, or pancreatic insufficiency) should be considered in any patient who has symptoms referable to the gastrointestinal tract. In these patients, the bone disease may be caused by a combination of calcium deficiency, malnutrition, and vitamin D malabsorption, and bone histology may reveal features of osteoporosis rather than osteomalacia.

Treatment. Privational vitamin D deficiency responds rapidly to vitamin D replacement, even in small doses. Oral vitamin D_2 (4000 to 5000 IU [100 to 125 micrograms] per day) produces biochemical and radiologic evidence of healing within a month. However, therapy should be continued for about 3 months before the dose is reduced to the recommended dietary allowance of 400 IU per day. In some countries in Europe, a single intramuscular or oral dose of 600,000 IU

TABLE 4. **Investigations Useful in Monitoring Vitamin D Therapy**

Serum
  Calcium
  Phosphorus
  Alkaline phosphatase
  25-OHD*
Urine calcium/creatinine ratio
24-hr urine calcium excretion

*Of value only if vitamin D or 25-OHD is used in therapy.

(15,000 micrograms) is given as therapy. The advantage of this form of therapy is that the problem of patient compliance is removed. A further dose may be given after 1 or 2 months. Vitamin D toxicity does not occur generally if only one or two doses are given. A biochemical response to this form of therapy may be noted after several days, and radiographic healing may be seen after several weeks. There are no reasons for the use of other vitamin D metabolites or analogues in the treatment of privational vitamin D deficiency. Calcium supplementation is generally not indicated in the majority of cases unless the diet is low in calcium. If rickets or osteomalacia is associated with signs and symptoms of hypocalcemia (e.g., convulsions or apneic spells), intravenous calcium may be given (10 per cent calcium gluconate—1 to 2 ml per kg up to maximum of 10 ml slowly while monitoring the heart rate), and a daily oral supplement of between 1 and 1.5 grams may be given during the initial stages of therapy (Table 5).

The short-term response to therapy may be determined by monitoring serum calcium and phosphorus levels, and alkaline phosphatase levels are of value for long-term monitoring. With the onset of therapy, alkaline phosphatase levels initially rise and then gradually fall over several months. Depending on the severity of the bone disease, alkaline phosphatase levels may not return to normal for up to 6 months or occasionally even longer.

The treatment of vitamin D deficiency associated with malabsorption may require a more individualized assessment of vitamin D absorp-

TABLE 5. **Calcium Preparations for the Treatment of Rickets/Osteomalacia**

Generic (Trade) Name	Preparation	Calcium Concentration	Route of Administration	Side Effects
Calcium chloride	10% solution	27 mg/ml	IV	Peripheral vasodilation; cutaneous burning sensation; do not give IM
Calcium gluceptate	22% solution	18 mg/ml	IV	Less irritating than $CaCl_2$
Calcium gluconate	10% solution Tablets 500 mg, 650 mg, 975 mg, 1000 mg,	9 mg/ml 60 mg/tablet 90 mg/tablet	IV PO	Do not give IM Does not irritate gastrointestinal tract
Calcium lactate	Tablets 325 mg, 650 mg	42 mg/tablet 84 mg/tablet	PO	Absorption improved if given with lactose
Calcium carbonate (Titralac; numerous)	Tablets 420 mg, 650 mg, 750 mg, 1250 mg, 1500 mg	168 mg/tablet 260 mg/tablet 267 mg/tablet 300 mg/tablet 500 mg/tablet 600 mg/tablet	PO	Do not use in achlorhydria
Calcium glubionate syrup (Neo-Calglucon)		115 mg/5 ml	PO	
Calcium lactate-gluconate (Calcium Sandoz forte)	Effervescent tablets*	500 mg/tablet	PO	

*Not available in the United States.

tion because the degree of malabsorption varies from patient to patient. Pharmacologic doses of vitamin D_2 are usually successful in treating the bone disease if it is caused by vitamin D deficiency, but higher doses than those used in privational vitamin D deficiency are often required (10,000 to 100,000 IU [250 micrograms to 2.5 mg] per day). The response to therapy can be monitored by measuring serum 25-OHD levels, which provide an indication of the absorption of the enterally administered vitamin D_2. Concomitant dietary supplementation with calcium (1 to 1.5 grams of elemental calcium per day) is advisable because calcium malabsorption is a frequently associated finding. Magnesium depletion may also need to be corrected in certain situations before hypocalcemia responds to therapy.

25-OHD$_3$ and 1,25-(OH)$_2$D$_3$ are more water soluble than vitamin D. Thus their absorption may be less affected by fat malabsorption. However, there is no real indication for their use because given the appropriate dose of vitamin D_2, the majority of patients respond. Furthermore, patients with gastrointestinal malabsorption should be encouraged to spend as much time as possible in the sunshine because this will eliminate the need for vitamin D absorption from the gut.

Decreased Hepatic Hydroxylation

Severe liver damage may be associated with low 25-OHD levels. However, in the majority of cases, this is not caused by a failure of hepatic hydroxylation but rather by an inadequate dietary intake of vitamin D and a lack of exposure to sunlight. Biliary cirrhosis and severe obstructive jaundice may be associated with rickets or osteomalacia caused by poor vitamin D absorption. More often, the bone disease associated with cirrhosis is osteoporotic, perhaps because of the poor nutritional status of the individual and the direct effect of alcohol abuse on bone metabolism. If impairment of hydroxylation does occur in severe liver disease, it is not usually a therapeutic problem, as an adequate intake of vitamin D ensures normal circulating levels of 25-OHD.

Impaired hydroxylation of vitamin D has also been incriminated as a factor in the bone disease of very-low-birth-weight infants. Although there is biochemical evidence of such an impairment, vitamin D_2 supplementation of the diet (800 IU

[20 micrograms] per day) ensures normal circulating 25-OHD levels. The metabolic bone disease associated with prematurity is primarily a problem of inadequate phosphate intake caused by the low phosphate content of breast milk. It can be corrected by phosphate supplementation of breast milk (20 mg per kg body weight per day). Some experts also recommend calcium supplementation.

Increased Vitamin D Metabolism

Patients receiving long-term anticonvulsant therapy have been shown to have increased metabolism of vitamin D caused by the induction of hepatic enzymes. However, in most patients, clinical vitamin D deficiency is an uncommon problem. Nevertheless, it may occur more readily in the institutionalized or severely handicapped patient, whose vitamin D intake (dietary and sunlight exposure) is suboptimal.

In those patients in whom vitamin D deficiency may be a problem, vitamin D_2 supplementation (2000 IU [50 micrograms] per day or 50,000 IU [1.25 mg] once weekly) ensures an adequate vitamin D intake and prevents the development of hypocalcemia, which might aggravate the seizure disorder.

When biochemical variables are used to monitor the evidence of vitamin D deficiency and metabolic bone disease, care should be taken in interpreting the alkaline phosphatase levels because total levels are frequently elevated in patients receiving anticonvulsant therapy as a result of the induction of hepatic alkaline phosphatase. The determination of the isoenzymes of alkaline phosphatase establishes whether the bone isoenzyme fraction is elevated.

Failure of Renal Hydroxylation

Vitamin D Dependency Type I. This rare condition is inherited as an autosomal recessive condition and usually manifests in the first year of life with severe hypocalcemia, rickets, and bone deformities. The defect is thought to be located in the renal 1-alpha-hydroxylase enzyme. Thus, the patient typically has normal 25-OHD levels but low 1-25(OH)$_2$D levels.

As the name implies, the patient does not respond to physiologic doses of vitamin D. Vitamin D_2 in a dose of 25,000 to 60,000 IU (625 to 1500 micrograms) per day is required to maintain normal bone metabolism, but the condition can be treated with physiologic doses of 1,25-(OH)$_2$D$_3$ or 1-alpha-hydroxyvitamin D$_3$. Although the latter metabolites are more expensive than vitamin D, because of their short half-life the dosage can be monitored more effectively. Lifelong therapy is required to prevent recurrence of the bone

disease, and treatment should be started early in life to prevent the development of severe bone deformities.

Renal Failure. Renal osteodystrophy is a complex metabolic bone disease that is characterized by a variable mixture of features of osteomalacia, hyperparathyroidism, and aluminum bone disease. The pathogenesis of the bone disease is not clearly understood, although several factors are known to contribute to its development:

1. Uncontrolled hyperphosphatemia developing during the gradual decline in renal function leads to hypocalcemia and secondary hyperparathyroidism.

2. A gradual decline in the production of 1,25-(OH)$_2$D by the kidney occurs, with an associated decrease in intestinal calcium absorption.

3. Aluminum accumulates at the mineralization front, which impairs mineralization of preformed osteoid. This accumulation results from the use of aluminum-containing phosphate-binding agents and from aluminum contamination of dialysate water.

A comprehensive discussion of the treatment of renal osteodystrophy is beyond the scope of this chapter. However, the principles of therapy are outlined.

Vitamin D supplementation early in the decline of renal function maintains more normal serum 1,25-(OH)$_2$D levels and reduces the rate of progression of hyperparathyroidism and renal osteodystrophy. Further, the often associated muscle weakness improves. At present, there is no uniform opinion as to when vitamin D supplementation should begin or which of the vitamin D analogues or metabolites should be used. However, it is reasonable to suggest that the 1-alpha-hydroxylated analogues are more physiologic. The recommended starting doses are as follows: vitamin D_2—20,000 to 80,000 IU (0.5 to 2.0 mg) per day; 25-OHD$_3$—50 micrograms daily; 1,25-(OH)$_2$D$_3$—0.25 microgram daily; 1-alpha-hydroxyvitamin D—0.25 to 0.5 microgram daily. Dihydrotachysterol has also been used but probably confers no advantage. Serum calcium levels need to be monitored carefully for evidence of hypercalcemia and the vitamin D dosage adjusted accordingly. As intestinal phosphate absorption is increased and secondary hyperparathyroidism is decreased with the use of these metabolites, hyperphosphatemia should be controlled before starting therapy with vitamin D or its analogues, and the dose of phosphate-binding agents during therapy should be carefully adjusted. Serum phosphate levels should be maintained at 4.0 to 5.5 mg per dl (1.3 to 1.8 mmol per liter) with the use of a low-phosphorus diet (less than 1 gram daily) and phosphate-binding agents such as calcium carbonate (Titralac), which also provides an additional source of calcium. The use of aluminum-containing antacids should be kept at a minimum because they may increase the accumulation of aluminum in the bone.

If aluminum bone disease is a problem, the use of desferoxamine (Desferal) should be considered to chelate aluminum and reduce its deposition in bone. In some patients with severe renal osteodystrophy, hyperparathyroidism cannot be controlled by conservative medical therapy, and parathyroidectomy may be necessary.

Peripheral Resistance to 1,25-(OH)₂D

Recently, several kindreds have been reported with various abnormalities in the 1,25-$(OH)_2$D receptor. These patients, usually children, present with severe rickets, hypocalcemia, and markedly elevated 1,25-$(OH)_2$D levels. Alopecia may also be an accompanying clinical feature. These patients respond poorly or not at all to high doses of vitamin D or its analogues. In some cases, as much as 50 micrograms of 1,25-$(OH)_2D_3$ daily fails to produce a clinical response. Recently, healing of the bone disease and improvement of the biochemical abnormalities have been achieved by intravenous infusions of calcium, with or without oral phosphate supplementation.

Inadequate Calcium Intake

Dietary Calcium Deficiency. Severely restricted calcium intake (less than 25 per cent of the recommended dietary allowance), especially in infants and young children, has been implicated in the pathogenesis of rickets, despite an adequate vitamin D status. The clinical and biochemical picture is that of calciopenic rickets, but the presentation can be differentiated from that of privational vitamin D deficiency by the finding of normal serum 25-OHD and elevated 1,25-$(OH)_2$D concentrations. The bone disease responds to an increased calcium intake, which may be achieved by improving the diet (increasing dairy products) or by giving calcium supplements (1000 mg per day).

High Fluoride Intake. Excessive fluoride ingestion, such as that occurring in areas of high water fluoride concentration or when fluoride is used for the treatment of osteoporosis, leads to a rise in osteoblastic activity with an increase in osteoid formation. Fluoride also directly impairs mineralization of newly formed osteoid. Thus sclerosis and features of osteomalacia may be found histologically. A low dietary calcium intake probably exacerbates the degree of osteomalacia. Endemic fluorosis can be effectively treated only by reducing the fluoride intake (e.g., changing the water supply in the area). However, increased calcium intake can reduce the osteomalacic component of the bone disease.

Phosphopenic Rickets and Osteomalacia

Inadequate Phosphate Absorption

Dietary Lack. A dietary deficiency of phosphate occurs only in exceptional circumstances because phosphate is present in most foods. Rickets and osteopenia are well-recognized complications in breast-fed, very-low-birth-weight infants during the first 3 months of life. Although the pathogenesis of the disease is probably multifactorial, phosphate deficiency caused by the low phosphate content of breast milk (approximately 150 mg per liter) is considered to be the major factor in its development. Treatment consists of maintaining an adequate vitamin D intake (800 IU [20 micrograms] per day) and increasing the dietary intake of phosphorus, and possibly calcium, by supplementing breast milk with phosphorus (20 mg per kg per day) or by using special premature infant milk formulas.

Intestinal Phosphate Binding. Hypophosphatemia, hypercalcemia, muscle weakness, and osteomalacia are uncommon complications associated with long-term ingestion of aluminum-containing antacids, which are usually taken for upper gastrointestinal tract disturbances. Other biochemical features include hypercalciuria, which leads to nephrocalcinosis, and almost absent renal phosphate excretion.

Management that consists of stopping the antacid therapy and increasing the phosphate intake (2 to 4 grams per day) (Table 6) leads to a rapid improvement in signs and symptoms.

Increased Renal Losses

X-Linked Hypophosphatemic Vitamin D–Resistant Rickets and Osteomalacia. In many developed countries, X-linked hypophosphatemic vitamin D–resistant rickets (XLH) is probably the most common form of rickets. The disease usually presents

TABLE 6. **Phosphate Supplements Available for the Treatment of Rickets and Osteomalacia**

Preparation	Phosphorus Content	Comment
Joulie's solution	30 or 48 mg/ml*	Bad taste, poor compliance
Neutra-Phos	250 mg/capsule	Dissolve in 75 ml water
K-Phos Neutral	250 mg/tablet	
K-Phos Original	110 mg/tablet	
Phosphate-Sandoz	500 mg/effervescent tablet	Dissolve in 75 ml water

*Depending on whether the dibasic sodium phosphate used is anhydrous.

in infancy with progressive leg deformities (usually bowing), short stature, and hypophosphatemia. About two-thirds of these patients have evidence of X-linked inheritence. Females with the disease may not be phenotypically abnormal but have hypophosphatemia and lowered tubular reabsorption of phosphorus. Apart from this lowered reabsorption, which is characteristic of the disease, no other renal abnormalities, except for glycosuria in an occasional child, are detected. The primary defect in the disease is thought to be an abnormality in renal phosphate reabsorption. Although there is evidence of altered control of vitamin D metabolism, this does not appear to be a major factor in the pathogenesis.

Early diagnosis and the early institution of correct management are important in preventing progressive deformities and the development of short stature. Hypophosphatemia in an infant of an affected mother should alert the physician to the diagnosis before the onset of growth retardation or clinical rickets.

Phosphate supplementation is the mainstay of therapy, the objective being to maintain serum phosphorus levels as close to the normal range as possible (keeping in mind the normal range for the age of the patient). Phosphate therapy should be given four to six times a day, spread as evenly as possible over the 24 hours, and the dosage should be increased slowly to the required amount (1 to 4 grams per day). Serum phosphorus levels should be monitored 45 to 75 minutes after an oral phosphate dose is given. Loose stools are a frequent complaint when therapy is commenced, but this problem generally resolves over the first couple of months. Although phosphate therapy alone improves the radiologic appearance of rickets, histologic osteomalacia is only minimally improved. Further, phosphate supplements alone tend to cause hypocalcemia and secondary hyperparathyroidism, which has been reported in patients with XLH. Although vitamin D in large doses was used in the past as an adjunct to therapy, more recently the 1-alpha-hydroxylated metabolites have been shown to be more efficacious and, when used with phosphate supplements, have returned the features of osteomalacia to almost normal. Treatment with $1,25\text{-}(OH)_2D_3$ should commence with a dose of 0.25 microgram twice daily and should be increased slowly to 0.5 to 1.0 microgram twice daily. 1-Alpha-hydroxyvitamin D_3 appears to work equally effectively, although the drug need be given only once daily in a dose of 1 to 2 micrograms per day. The response to therapy is monitored by serum phosphorus and alkaline phosphatase levels, the latter returning to normal during a period of 6 to 12 months. Serum calcium levels and urine calcium/creatinine ratios should be assessed at 2- to 3-month intervals once treatment has been stabilized to detect evidence of vitamin D toxicity. Calcium supplements may be beneficial during the early stages of therapy but are not necessary once radiologic and biochemical healing of the disease has been observed.

Therapy should be continued until longitudinal growth has ceased. Whether therapy should be continued in adulthood is not clear because there is no well-documented evidence to point to the clinical benefits of continued therapy, although histologically the features of osteomalacia will be prevented from recurring. If osteotomies are required to correct deformities, these should be done only if compliance with therapy is adequate and the osteomalacia is biochemically under control. If these precautions are not observed, deformities recur postoperatively. Serum calcium and urine calcium/creatinine ratios need to be monitored frequently postoperatively to detect evidence of hypercalcemia associated with immobilization. With the use of the 1-alpha-hydroxylated metabolites, a reduction in the daily dose may be required, but cessation of therapy is generally not indicated.

Hypercalciuric Hypophosphatemic Vitamin D–Resistant Rickets. This rare inherited disease is differentiated from XLH by the presence of hypercalciuria and elevated $1,25\text{-}(OH)_2D$ levels. Treatment with phosphate supplements alone leads not only to the healing of the rickets but also to a fall in $1,25\text{-}(OH)_2D$ levels and correction of the hypercalciuria.

Adult-Onset Hypophosphatemic Vitamin D–Resistant Osteomalacia. This form of osteomalacia does not appear to be inherited. The biochemical abnormalities are similar to those of XLH, except that glycinuria may also be detected. Clinically unlike XLH, the disease generally occurs between 20 and 40 years of age and is associated with severe muscle weakness. It is possible that this condition is the same as oncogenous osteomalacia, which is discussed next. Treatment is similar to that for XLH if no tumor can be found.

Oncogenous Osteomalacia. As the name implies, the hypophosphatemia and osteomalacia are secondary to an often small, benign mesenchymal tumor, which is thought to secrete a factor that not only decreases phosphate reabsorption by the kidney but also suppresses $1,25\text{-}(OH)_2D$ production. The tumors are characteristically either nonossifying fibromas, which appear as small, radiolucent areas in bone, or mesenchymal hemangiopericytomas. Removal of the tumor results in a permanent remission of the osteomalacia and the biochemical abnormalities. If the tumor cannot be found or resected, treatment with the 1-alpha-hydroxylated metabolites and phosphate supplements results in amelioration of the symptoms.

A similar form of osteomalacia and/or rickets has been described in some patients with neurofibromatosis or polyostotic fibrous dysplasia. The pathogenesis is thought to be similar to that of oncogenous osteomalacia. Resection of the lesions is often not possible. Symptomatic treatment with $1,25\text{-}(OH)_2D_3$ and phosphate supplements is generally the only form of therapy available.

Fanconi's Syndrome. Fanconi's syndrome, which has many different etiologies, is characterized by varying degrees of proximal renal tubular dysfunction. Typically, glycosuria, aminoaciduria, phosphaturia, hypokalemia, and proximal renal tubular acidosis occur. If rickets or osteomalacia is associated with the disease, therapy with $1,25\text{-}(OH)_2D_3$ and phosphate supplements leads to healing. However, potassium supplements and correction of the metabolic acidosis with bicarbonate therapy or Shohl's solution are frequently required. The underlying etiology of Fanconi's syndrome should be actively sought and treated where possible.

Distal Renal Tubular Acidosis. Distal renal tubular acidosis may lead to severe rickets and osteomalacia. It is associated with a failure of hydrogen ion excretion in the distal tubule and manifests with hypercalciuria, nephrocalcinosis, and hypophosphatemia. Correction of the acidosis with bicarbonate therapy (1 to 4 mmol per kg per day) leads to disappearance of the phosphaturia and hypercalciuria and healing of the bone disease. Occasionally, potassium supplements are also required, especially once bicarbonate therapy has commenced.

Impaired Mineralization

Hypophosphatasia. Hypophosphatasia is a genetic disease (inherited as autosomal dominant or recessive) that is characterized by low or absent serum levels of the bone isoenzyme of alkaline phosphatase. Clinically, the picture varies, but it is generally associated with a severe mineralization defect mimicking rickets and osteomalacia. There is no known treatment for the condition.

Aluminum Toxicity. Aluminum accumulation is rare in otherwise healthy individuals; it does, however, occur in uremic patients, who ingest large quantities of aluminum-containing antacids or who are receiving dialysis with water contaminated with aluminum. Treatment should be aimed at removing the aluminum from the body pool with chelating agents such as desferoxamine.

Fluoride Toxicity. The effects of fluoride excess have been discussed in the section on high fluoride intake, which deals with the calciopenic causes of rickets or osteomalacia.

Disodium Etidronate. The diphosphonates are being used increasingly in clinical medicine to treat Paget's disease and the hypercalcemia associated with malignant tumors. The use of disodium etidronate (Didronel), a diphosphonate, has been associated with the development of osteomalacia, especially when used in large doses (greater than 40 mmol per kg per day) for more than 1 month. The newer diphosphonates do not have this complication.

SCURVY AND VITAMIN C

method of
JOHN H. CRANDON, M.D.
Tufts University Medical School
Boston, Massachusetts

INCIDENCE

During the past 30 years, scurvy has virtually vanished from the American scene. Coincidentally, requests for blood ascorbic acid levels, the sine qua non for a positive diagnosis of subclinical ascorbic acid deficiency, have become so infrequent that even the larger hospitals now send these blood samples to special laboratories for analysis.

During this period, nevertheless, there has been a marked proliferation of studies, both experimental and statistical, relating to the possibly beneficial actions of ascorbic acid, particularly in megadoses, for diseases ranging from cancer to colds. Many of the conclusions drawn from these studies must remain hypothetical because ethics committees and a litigious society have reduced human experimental studies to zero.

CLINICAL FINDINGS

The clinical diagnosis of scurvy is made on the basis of the dietary history, petechiae or hyperkeratotic plugs in the hair follicles, scattered ecchymoses, bleeding gums (if teeth are present), hemarthroses, lassitude, postural hypotension, and a markedly limited ability to perform strenuous work. A tourniquet test for petechiae is of no value. In infants there may be tenderness over the tibiae, bony epiphyses, or costochondral junctions, with a characteristic x-ray picture in these areas.

The fundamental finding seen by the pathologist (generally in wound biopsy specimens) is lack of intercellular "cement substance," or collagen, between proliferating fibroblasts in the soft tissues and between endothelial cells in the small blood vessel walls. A diagnosis of scurvy on the basis of perifollicular petechiae alone is incorrect in at least one-third of the cases.

When blood determinations, wound biopsy specimens, or gum biopsy specimens are not available, a therapeutic test with oral or parenteral ascorbic acid in doses of 500 mg per day in adults and 100 to 200 mg per day in children for 10 days should be performed. It should be borne in mind that petechial hemorrhages of the extremities from whatever cause may show some improvement with bed rest alone.

ACTION

Ascorbic acid is a strong reducing agent that is easily destroyed by alkalis. Aside from its vital role in the formation of intercellular substance, ascorbic acid facilitates the absorption of heme iron and enhances the action of the immune system and leukocytes; the action of catecholamine, norepinephrine, and dopamine; and the biosynthesis of carnitine. It participates in the conversion of folic acid to folinic acid, in the metabolism of tyrosine, and in the oxidation-reduction of sulfhydryl groups. It also protects against certain toxic substances, such as the heavy metals (e.g., cadmium).

An exciting discovery was the action of ascorbic acid in preventing the formation in the stomach of cancerogenic nitrosamines produced by the ingestion of nitrate-rich foods (foods to which nitrate had been added as a preservative). Coincidental with the advent of better vitamin C nutrition, there has been, in the opinion of most surgeons, a considerable decline in the incidence of gastric carcinoma. Improved control of peptic ulcer disease could also be a factor in this decline.

In the treatment of cancer, ascorbic acid has been found to be of no value.

REQUIREMENT

The recommended daily allowance of ascorbic acid for the average adult is 60 mg, for pregnant women 80 mg, and for infants 35 mg. With disease or increased metabolism, stress, trauma (particularly severe burns), or extensive inflammatory processes, the requirement is much higher. With surgery, the blood ascorbic acid level generally falls, and among heavy smokers it is usually below average. The minimal amounts of the vitamin necessary on a surgical ward to maintain adequate blood levels in adults with various diseases and surgeries are shown in Table 1.

In recent years, megadoses of vitamin C (1000 to 3000 mg per day) have been recommended by some people for a variety of reasons ranging from promoting good health to preventing cancer and colds. Ascorbic acid is relatively inexpensive and can serve as a good placebo. However, it has now been established that overdoses cause oxaluria, with production of renal stones, and may cause iron poisoning from too much absorption of heme iron. Megadoses in pregnant women may produce a rebound phenomenon in the newborn infant. Large doses may interfere with Clinitest and Testape determinations in the urine and Hemoccult tests of the feces.

It is noteworthy that most pharmaceutical firms have reduced the amount of ascorbic acid in their multivitamin tablets from 500 to 600 mg to 100 to 200 mg. In addition, ascorbic acid is added to some canned foods and bottled drinks as a preservative and to some drugs as a buffer (parenteral Achromycin, Tofranil).

TABLE 1. **Ascorbic Acid Required to Maintain Adequate Blood Levels**

Condition	Daily Dose (mg)
Tuberculosis	100–200
Burns (severe)	200–500
Ulcerative colitis	200–400
Urinary infection	200–300
Wounds (granulating)	100–200
Postoperative benign course	100
Diarrhea (severe)	200
Hyperthyroidism	200
Pregnancy or lactation	100

Deficient Blood Ascorbic Levels
Plasma: less than 0.2 mg/dl*
Buffy coat: less than 4 mg per 100 grams†

*Roe and Kuether method.
†Butler and Cushman method.

VITAMIN K DEFICIENCY

method of
JONATHAN C. GOLDSMITH, M.D.
University of Nebraska Medical Center
Omaha, Nebraska

Vitamin K is a fat-soluble vitamin that is essential for normal human nutrition. Biologic activity indicative of vitamin K is expressed by 1,4-naphthoquinones substituted at the 3 position. Vitamin K_1, or phylloquinone, is found in green leafy vegetables; vitamin K_2 (menaquinone series) is synthesized by intestinal flora, especially *Bacteroides fragilis*. Vitamin K_3, or menadione, is a lipid-soluble provitamin. Daily requirements for vitamin K in normal humans have been estimated to be between 10 micrograms per day and 2 micrograms per kg body weight per day. Body stores are limited.

An essential role has been identified for vitamin K in blood coagulation and bone formation. Vitamin K is required for the postribosomal modification of coagulation Factors II, VII, IX, and X, proteins C and S, and calcium-binding bone proteins. Substrate specificity is provided by basic amino acid–rich propeptides between the leader sequence and the amino terminus of the mature protein. Glutamic acid residues found in the amino terminal region of coagulation factors are converted to gamma-carboxyglutamic acid residues by a hepatic membrane–bound microsomal vitamin K–dependent carboxylase. Pairs of gamma-carboxyglutamic acid residues are essential for calcium binding and for the normal interaction of coagulation factors and phospholipids. For vitamin K to participate in the carboxylase reaction, it must be present in the reduced form. Vitamin K is converted to a 2,3-epoxide form after carboxylation and must be regenerated to the reduced form. Coumarin interferes with this latter step.

CLINICAL FEATURES

The clinical manifestations of vitamin K deficiency or antagonism by coumarin are hemorrhagic. Bleeding is due to a deficiency of coagulation factor activity and is therefore similar to hemophilia rather than platelet defects. Soft tissue, cutaneous, gastrointestinal, genitourinary, and central nervous system bleeding may occur, in addition to intra-articular hemorrhage. Bleeding can be life-threatening or merely cosmetically disfiguring. Laboratory diagnosis of vitamin K deficiency is essential for proper management.

LABORATORY FEATURES

Deficiencies of Factors II, VII, IX, and X lead to a prolongation of both the prothrombin time (PT) and the partial thromboplastin time (PTT). However, vitamin K is not required for fibrinogen formation, hematopoiesis, or platelet function. Therefore, the thrombin time, fibrinogen quantitation, platelet count, and bleeding time are normal in the absence of or antagonism of vitamin K. Abnormalities in these last parameters suggest an alternative diagnosis such as liver disease or disseminated intravascular coagulation (Table 1).

To assess vitamin K deficiency, serum phylloquinone levels can be determined by high-pressure liquid chromatography. Normal levels are in the range of 1.0 to 1.5 mg per ml. It is also possible to measure inadequately gamma-carboxylated proteins induced in vitamin K's absence or antagonism (PIVKA's) as indicators of vitamin K deficiency. Radioimmunoassays and enzyme-linked immunosorbent assays have been used to measure PIVKA's of prothrombin, which have plasma disappearance times of approximately 3 days.

DEFICIENCY STATES

Hemorrhagic disease of the newborn (HDN) typically occurs 1 to 7 days post partum and is characterized by gastrointestinal, cutaneous, nasal, umbilical stump, and circumcision site bleeding. Breast-fed infants and those born to mothers taking anticonvulsants, antibiotics, or anticoagulants are at risk, although idiopathic cases are common. A severe variant of HDN occurs in the first 24 hours after delivery and is marked by life-threatening intracranial, intrathoracic, or intra-abdominal bleeding. Late HDN occurs at 1 to 3 months of age and is marked by cutaneous, gastrointestinal, or intracranial bleeding. Etiologies of these late cases include diarrhea, malabsorption, anticoagulant exposure, and breast-feeding; idiopathic cases also occur.

Malabsorption or dietary deficiency of vitamin K also leads to a hemorrhagic diathesis. Cystic fibrosis, alpha$_1$-antitrypsin deficiency, biliary atresia or obstruction, and hepatitis can produce malabsorption of fat-soluble materials such as vitamin K. Inadequate dietary intake may occur in total parenteral nutrition, debilitation, intentional omission, and infants exclusively fed breast milk. Breast milk contains 15 micrograms per liter or less of vitamin K compared with 50 micrograms per liter in commercial formula and cow milk.

Broad-spectrum antimicrobial agents cause vitamin K deficiency by elimination of ileal bacteria capable of vitamin K$_2$ synthesis. Some cephalosporin antibiotics have been postulated to interfere directly with hepatic utilization of vitamin K. Coumarin-containing drugs block vitamin K–epoxide reductase activity, which results in a depletion of reduced vitamin K and inadequate gamma-carboxylation of coagulation factors.

PREVENTION AND TREATMENT

For patients who are receiving coumarin and who have significant bleeding, immediate but temporary reversal of the effect of coumarin can be achieved by the infusion of 10 to 15 ml of fresh frozen plasma (FFP) per kg of body weight. Ten milligrams of vitamin K$_1$ (AquaMEPHYTON) subcutaneously corrects the coagulation abnormalities but only after 6 to 24 hours, and it makes subsequent anticoagulation with coumarin, if required, difficult. Life- or limb-threat-

TABLE 1. **Laboratory Findings in Acquired Hemorrhagic Disorders**

Laboratory Test	Vitamin K Deficiency	Liver Disease	Disseminated Intravascular Coagulation
PT	↑	↑	N or ↑
PTT	↑	↑	N or ↑
Thrombin time	N	N or ↑	N or ↑
Fibrinogen	N	N or ↓	↓
Platelet count	N	N or ↓	↓
Fibrin(ogen) degradation products	N	N or ↑	↑
Bleeding time	N	N or ↑	N or ↑

* ↑ = prolonged or raised; N = normal; ↓ = reduced.

ening hemorrhage should be treated with both FFP and vitamin K$_1$. Water-soluble analogues of vitamin K (Synkavite) are not effective in this clinical situation. Laboratory abnormalities such as PTs up to 2½ to 3½ times the control value in the absence of significant hemorrhage can often be managed by omission of coumarin and careful monitoring rather than by FFP and vitamin K$_1$ therapy.

Postoperative vitamin K deficiency can be avoided by weekly parenteral administration of 10 mg of vitamin K$_1$ to patients who receive nothing by mouth or who have poor oral intake. More frequent administration of vitamin K$_1$ is not necessary.

Neonates should receive 1.0 mg vitamin K$_1$ (Konakion, intramuscularly; Mephyton, subcutaneously) or 2.0 mg vitamin K$_1$ orally or 5.0 mg vitamin K$_2$ orally immediately after birth to prevent HDN. These doses should be repeated every 4 weeks if the infant has malabsorption or is exclusively breast fed. Newborns of mothers who are receiving anticoagulant or anticonvulsant agents may benefit if the mothers receive 10 mg of vitamin K$_1$ parenterally each week for 2 to 3 weeks before delivery.

Prothrombin complex concentrates (Factor IX concentrates) contain many of the vitamin K–dependent coagulation factors. However, they should not be used to reverse the effect of warfarin or to treat vitamin K deficiency. Prepared from thousands of donors, Factor IX concentrates (Konyne, Profilnine, Proplex) carry a significant risk of transmitting hepatitis. These concentrates also have additional procoagulant effects that can result in life-threatening venous and arterial thrombosis.

In general, vitamin K should be given intramuscularly or subcutaneously. Intravenous dosing may achieve a more rapid clinical response but may cause hypersensitivity or anaphylactic reactions, and fatalities have occurred. Careful monitoring and the availability of resuscitation equipment are mandatory during the intravenous administration of vitamin K. Intravenous doses are, in general, 10 to 30 per cent of the subcutaneous or intramuscular doses.

OSTEOPOROSIS

method of
IAN H. THORNEYCROFT, Ph.D., M.D.
Tulane University Medical Center
New Orleans, Louisiana

Osteoporosis is reduced bone mass per unit volume with a normal ratio of matrix to mineral. Basically, the bone is normal but reduced in quantity. Patients can be considered to have osteoporosis when their bone density is less than 80 per cent of that of young adults.

DIAGNOSIS

Clinically, osteoporosis can be suspected by kyphosis secondary to crush fractures (dowager's hump) and by a gradual loss in height. Unfortunately, by the time osteoporosis is detected clinically, the disease is well advanced. An ordinary radiograph does not detect osteoporosis until 25 per cent of bone is lost. Single-beam photon absorptiometry is an accurate and reliable technique, but it measures only cortical bone, not trabecular bone. Fifty per cent of osteoporosis involves trabecular bone. Dual-beam photon absorptiometry and computed tomography scanning are the most practical methods of measuring bone density, and both measure trabecular bone. There is debate as to which is better. I prefer photon absorptiometry. The best method of diagnosing osteoporosis is a bone biopsy, but, of course, this is not practical. The causes of osteoporosis are shown in Table 1.

Osteoporosis is more common in relatives of patients with osteoporosis. Nonblack females are most likely to develop osteoporosis.

INCIDENCE, EPIDEMIOLOGY, AND CONSEQUENCES

Women lose bone rapidly after the loss of ovarian function; 25 per cent of caucasian women over the age

TABLE 1. **Differential Diagnosis (Etiology)**

Unknown
  Senile
  Juvenile

Endocrine
  Hypogonadism
    Male
    Female
      Menopause
      Hypoestrogenic amenorrhea
  Thyrotoxicosis (includes excess thyroid replacement)
  Glucocorticoid excess
  Diabetes mellitus
  Hyperparathyroidism

Cancer
  Multiple myeloma
  Leukemia
  Lymphoma
  Mastocytosis

Drugs
  Heparin
  Ethanol
  Caffeine

Immobilization
  Confinement to bed
  Space flight

Metabolic bone diseases
  Osteogenetic diseases
  Homocystinuria
  Ehlers-Danlos syndrome

Other
  Primary biliary cirrhosis

of 60 years have radiographic evidence of osteoporosis. Fractures are more common in the presence of osteoporosis, and hip fractures are the twelfth leading cause of death in the United States. From 10 to 30 per cent of women who experience a hip fracture die within 6 months, and 50 per cent of the survivors are severely incapacitated, necessitating nursing home care. Spinal compression fracture causes severe back pain. The cost is billions of dollars per year.

TREATMENT

In the case of osteoporosis, an ounce of prevention is worth a pound of cure. Risk factors should be identified and reduced or eliminated.

There is no effective method to reverse osteoporosis. Fluoride builds spinal trabecular bone, but there is controversy as to whether it reduces cortical bone density at the same time. Fluoride is associated with severe gastrointestinal side effects in 20 per cent of patients, frequently leading to anemia. It is also associated with arthritis and fluorosis. For these reasons, fluoride should be reserved for the most severely affected individuals.

Postmenopausal women and women with hypoestrogenic amenorrhea lose bone secondary to the low estrogen level. Lost estrogen should be promptly replaced. The minimum effective dose to prevent osteoporosis is 0.625 mg of conjugated equine estrogens (Premarin). The dose-response curve is steep, and generic drugs of unknown biopotency should be avoided. In younger women, oral contraceptives are effective. If estrogens are contraindicated, depomedroxyprogesterone acetate may be effective. Women who still have a uterus should be given a progestin such as 10 mg of medroxyprogesterone acetate for 10 to 13 days per month to prevent uterine hyperplasia and carcinoma. The estrogen is usually given for the first 25 days of the month, and the progestin is given on days 13 to 16. I usually give estrogen every day and add a progestin for the first 10 to 13 days of the month. Therapy should be initiated within 5 years of menopause and continued for 10 to 15 years to prevent osteoporotic fractures.

Calcium deficiency may also play a role in osteoporosis. American women ingest an average of 500 mg of elemental calcium per day. The recommended daily minimum intake is 1000 mg in premenopausal women and 1500 mg in menopausal women. Replacement of the calcium alone is not effective. However, combining 1500 mg of elemental calcium per day with conjugated equine estrogens may reduce the minimum effective estrogen dose to 0.3 mg. Premenopausal calcium prophylaxis may increase bone density at menopause and prevent fractures afterward.

PAGET'S DISEASE OF BONE

method of
STANLEY WALLACH, M.D.
University of South Florida College of Medicine, Tampa, Florida, and the VA Medical Center Bay Pines, Florida

Paget's disease is a focal, sometimes generalized, inflammatory disease of the skeleton that is characterized by both excessive bone resorption and bone formation. The disease can be traced back to skeletal remains in England dating from 1000 A.D. The best clinical and pathologic description, although not the earliest, was that of Sir James Paget 110 years ago. He was well aware of the painful, deforming nature of the disease and gave it the name "osteitis deformans."

We know that Paget's disease is of focal occurrence both geographically and anatomically. The disease is most prevalent in England, Australia, New Zealand, France, Germany, and the United States. Approximately 3 per cent of the caucasian population older than age 40 years have the condition in either a focal or generalized anatomic distribution. In the area of England where the earliest traces of the disease have been found, the prevalence is double that of other areas: 6 to 8 per cent of the population older than age 40 years. A discrete geographic focus also exists in the area surrounding Naples, Italy, although the condition is not otherwise particularly common in southern Europe. Paget's disease is distinctly infrequent in Scandinavian countries and among the Oriental and black races. With regard to anatomic distribution, any bone in the body can be affected. Most commonly involved bones are the pelvis, skull, dorsolumbar spine, femur, and tibia.

There is a distinct hereditary component to the disease in that 15 to 50 per cent of patients, depending on the study, also have an afflicted first-order relative. Both parents and siblings are affected equally, suggesting a hereditary rather than an environmental influence. It has been estimated that the prevalence of the disease is 10 times greater among the first-order relatives of index patients than of their spouses. However, a classic hereditary transmission of the disease cannot be demonstrated, and it is generally accepted that the hereditary influence is expressed as a predisposition to a discrete etiologic factor or to the expression of that factor.

A large body of data amassed during the past decade suggests that the etiologic factor in Paget's disease is a slow virus infection. The nuclei and cytoplasm of pagetic osteoclasts invariably contain arrays of inclusion bodies that appear to be identical to the nucleocapsids of the Paramyxoviridae family of ribonucleic acid viruses. This finding is almost specific for Paget's disease, although a few cases of isolated giant cell tumor of bone, osteopetrosis, and pyknodysostosis have also been reported to have such inclusion bodies. By the use of immunofluorescence techniques, the inclusion bodies have been found to react with antibodies to approximately six different viruses. However, serum antibody titers to these viruses are not unusually

TABLE 1. **Clinical Features of Paget's Disease**

    I. Musculoskeletal
        a. Pain
        b. Deformities
        c. Fractures
        d. Neoplastic conversion
        e. Miscellaneous
            i. Resorptive-sclerotic components
            ii. Increased bone vascularity
    II. Neurologic
        a. Cranial nerve deficits and syndromes
        b. Medulla and cerebellum
        c. Spinal cord and nerves
        d. Miscellaneous
            i. Steal syndromes
            ii. Peripheral neuropathies
            iii. Carpal/tarsal tunnel syndromes
    III. Cardiovascular
        a. Increased cardiac output
        b. Generalized atherosclerosis
        c. Cardiovascular calcifications
    IV. Metabolic
        a. Increased skeletal turnover
        b. Abnormal calcium metabolism
        c. Abnormal uric acid metabolism

prominent among Paget's disease patients, nor has any of these viruses been isolated from affected osteoclasts. As a result, the slow virus etiology of Paget's disease remains conjectural until virus rescue is achieved and the discrepant data regarding the causative virus are reconciled.

Whatever the inciting cause, the initial pathophysiology is the transformation of osteoclasts in discrete skeletal locations into extremely abnormal bone-resorbing cells that proceed to digest bone rapidly and indiscriminately. These pagetic osteoclasts have an abnormal appearance and contain many more nuclei than normal osteoclasts. The extremely chaotic bone resorption evokes an equally disorganized and excessive osteoblastic response, so that the full-blown histologic picture consists of a combination, in varying proportions, of abnormal bone loss and sclerotic bone of poor structural quality. Affected bones are thickened, subject to deformation and pathologic fracture, and often painful. Pagetic bone is also vascular and contains a large capillary bed of low pressure, thereby "stealing" blood flow from other organs. To compensate for this condition, when the amount of pagetic bone is extensive, cardiac output increases. Pagetic bones near skin surfaces (e.g., an affected tibia) are often warm to the touch because of the greatly increased blood flow. The process of alternating bone resorption and formation is not only repeated several times in affected bony areas but also tends to encroach on previously unaffected adjacent bone. The rapidity of progression is variable, and most patients show very little change in their abnormal x-ray films from year to year. However, elevated serum alkaline phosphatase levels or increased radiotechnetium uptake on bone scans or both are usually present continuously, which indicates disease activity.

DIAGNOSIS

The diagnosis of Paget's disease is usually not difficult if it is considered in the differential diagnosis when suggestive symptoms are present. Appropriate x-ray appearances and an elevated serum alkaline phosphatase level are usually sufficient for diagnosis, although osteoblastic or mixed osteoblastic-osteolytic metastases from prostate, breast, and other carcinomas may rarely present a similar radiographic appearance. Bone scans define the extent of disease but should not be used in lieu of x-ray films. It is extremely important to take x-ray films of all positive areas on bone scans to define the anatomy of the bony lesions as precisely as possible. It is generally unnecessary to measure serum osteocalcin or urinary hydroxyproline levels or other parameters of skeletal turnover. An isolated elevation of the serum alkaline phosphatase level is sometimes the only clinical finding because symptoms may be absent or so mild as to be ignored. In such cases, if x-ray films and a bone scan are negative, liver disease or a skeletal condition other than Paget's disease should be considered. An elevated 5'-nucleotidase or gamma-glutamyl transpeptidase level can be used to incriminate liver disease.

CLINICAL FEATURES

The most common clinical features of Paget's disease are summarized in Table 1. Orthopedic, rheumatologic, neurologic, ophthalmologic, otolaryngologic, and even cardiologic features can sometimes dominate the clinical picture of Paget's disease and distract the physician from considering Paget's disease in the differential diagnosis. Pain is the most common presenting symptom and may be directly skeletal in origin or partially muscular if deformities are present that cause abnormal muscular relationships. Associated osteoarthritic pain is extremely common because deformities cause abnormal wear and tear of joint surfaces. There is also degeneration of articular cartilage when the underlying bone is pagetic. Headaches are frequently present with skull involvement even when there are no obvious neurologic abnormalities or head enlargement. Radicular pain occurs secondary to impingement of the pagetic bone of affected vertebral bodies on exiting spinal nerves. Deformities may take many forms, but anterior bowing of the long bones of the legs is the most common finding. Pagetic vertebrae are subject to compression and can cause kyphoscoliosis. When the pelvis is involved, the acetabular cups usually become osteoarthritic. As the underlying bone becomes structurally incompetent, pressure of the femoral heads may cause medial displacement of the acetabular cups, so-called acetabular protrusion. Chronic progressive hip pain is thus a common problem in Paget's disease of the pelvis. When the resorptive component of the Paget's disease predominates, large areas of resorption may be present in the skull, so-called osteoporosis circumscripta. Similar advancing fronts of pagetic bone resorption may be seen in long bones and produce flame-shaped areas of demineralization. Behind such fronts, lunate areas of resorption may fail to undergo subsequent sclerosis and may remain as cyst-like areas devoid of structure. In some patients, cracks occur along the lateral aspects of sclerotic bones in the lower extremities. These fissure fractures, as well as the lunate areas of bone resorption, are subject to fracture with minimal trauma. Such fractures can be catastrophic, not only because of possible nonunion but also because the subsequent immobilization causes extreme bone loss and predisposes to further fractures.

Pagetic bone lesions undergo neoplastic transformation in approximately 1 per cent of patients. The resulting lesion is sometimes a benign giant cell tumor, but even these tumors can have serious consequences if they are in a strategic location such as the spine. Malignant transformation to an osteosarcoma or other type of sarcoma is usually catastrophic and leads to death in 2 years or less.

Neurologic deficits sometimes dominate the clinical picture because of extensive Paget's disease of the skull and spine. The neurologic impairments arise from a combination of direct bony impingement on exiting cranial and spinal nerves and on the spinal cord, and from a pagetic steal of blood supply away from neurologic structures to surrounding pagetic bone sharing a common blood supply. Any cranial nerve can be impaired, but the auditory branch of the eighth cranial nerve is most commonly affected because the temporal bone encases the hearing apparatus. High-frequency sensorineural hearing loss, similar to that of presbycusis but progressing at a more rapid rate, is relatively common. Visual problems can be caused by either optic nerve or oculomotor impairment. In addition, pagetic patients are susceptible to two retinal lesions, retinal mottled degeneration and angioid streaks, that do not correlate with the degree of optic or oculomotor impairment. The lower cranial nerves and the medulla and cerebellum are particularly susceptible to damage when the posterior skull becomes so pagetic as to be flattened in the area of the foramen magnum, a condition known as "platybasia." Lower cranial nerve palsies, ataxia, and Valsalva's maneuver–induced headaches characterize this neurologic syndrome, with the headaches resulting from partial obstruction of the aqueduct. When the aqueduct is completely obstructed, a hydrocephalus-dementia syndrome may occur. In the peripheral nervous system, neuropathies and carpal tunnel or tarsal tunnel syndromes are common, but they do not correlate with anatomic impingement on spinal or peripheral nerves.

Atherosclerosis and medial calcinosis of medium-sized arteries are almost always present in older pagetic patients to a greater extent than would be expected based on age alone. Subendocardial calcification, mitral annulus calcification, and calcific aortic stenosis also occur with increased frequency. However, the major cardiovascular feature of Paget's disease is the increased cardiac output required by the greatly increased blood flow through pagetic bones. Although this may ultimately result in left ventricular hypertrophy, overt congestive heart failure is rare except in patients with associated coronary artery disease sufficient to depress myocardial contractility.

Patients with Paget's disease are particularly prone to defects in both calcium and uric acid metabolism. Approximately 5 per cent of these patients are hypercalcemic as a result of concomitant primary hyperparathyroidism. By contrast, a nonparathyroid form of hypercalcemia secondary to an imbalance between the rates of bone resorption and bone formation resulting

from immobilization is rare. Even in the absence of hypercalcemia, hypercalciuria, with or without calcium stone formation, is relatively common. Hyperuricemia, with or without gouty features or uric acid stone formation, is as common as abnormal calcium metabolism. The basis for these metabolic defects and their relation to the underlying Paget's disease are unclear.

TREATMENT

After the diagnosis of Paget's disease has been made based on clinical, radiologic, and biochemical features, it is necessary to define the extent and anatomic location of the disease because these factors determine the functional impact of the condition and the potential for future complications involving the musculoskeletal and neurologic systems. Of the approximately 3 million cases estimated to exist in the United States, approximately three-quarters can be classified as trivial on the basis of a lack of significant symptoms and a limited amount of structural involvement of nonstrategic parts of the skeleton. The remaining 750,000 patients have moderate to severe symptomatic Paget's disease in need of treatment. Table 2 outlines the features seen in these more severe cases and should be used as indications for treatment. If pain is the major symptom and cannot be relieved by simpler agents such as nonsteroidal anti-inflammatory drugs, specific treatment is indicated. Clinical evidence of a loss of skeletal integrity, radiologic evidence of extensive bone resorptive features that predispose to fracture, and neurologic deficits are the key indications for treatment. Although the research to date is inconclusive, it is reasonable to treat the patient if visual or auditory defects are progressive. However, there is no evidence that stable visual or auditory defects can be improved. Treatment is also effective in rapidly reducing bone blood flow and should be used before orthopedic surgery to reduce intra- and postoperative bleeding and thereby improve healing. Prolonged immobilization secondary to fracture or surgery causes severe, irreversible bone loss, and it is necessary to reduce this possibility by starting treatment as early as pos-

TABLE 2. **Indications for Treatment of Paget's Disease**

Pain (unrelieved by nonsteroidal anti-inflammatory drugs)
Loss of skeletal integrity
Excessive resorptive component
Neurologic deficits
Prolonged immobilization
Preparation for orthopedic surgery
Complications secondary to increased cardiac output
Extreme elevation of serum alkaline phosphatase level

sible. By reducing bone blood flow, treatment also normalizes cardiac output, which benefits patients who have abnormal cardiac function. Whether or not to treat patients with extreme elevations of the serum alkaline phosphatase level (i.e., 5 to 30 times normal) in the absence of other indications is unclear but is probably defensible.

Specific Agents

Three types of drugs are presently available in the United States for the treatment of Paget's disease (Table 3). All three operate by inhibiting osteoclastic bone resorption, although their mechanisms differ. The calcitonins inhibit bone resorption hormonally, whereas disodium etidronate inhibits all processes involved in skeletal turnover by physicochemically adsorbing to bone surfaces, rendering them inert. Plicamycin (mithramycin) causes toxic damage to osteoclasts. In all three instances, the suppression of bone resorption permits more normal bone formation and remodeling to occur. Resorptive lesions improve or disappear, and the mass of enlarged bones

TABLE 3. **Specific Drugs for Paget's Disease**

Calcitonins
 Synthetic salmon calcitonin (SCT) (Calcimar)
  Dose: 50–100 IU, SC or IM, daily to three times a week
  Duration: 18 mo, with repeat courses as needed
  Side effects: Metallic taste, anorexia, nausea, vomiting
        Nonspecific rash, urticaria
        Flushing of ears and face
        Polyuria
        Diarrhea (rare)
  Drug resistance: Primary: 15%
        Secondary: 20–40%

 Synthetic human calcitonin (HCT) (Cibacalcin)
  Dose: 0.5 mg, SC or IM, daily to three times a week
  Duration: Same as for SCT
  Side effects: Same as for SCT, but rash and urticaria
        rare
  Drug resistance: Primary: 15%
        Secondary: unknown, probably rare

Disodium etidronate (EHDP) (Didronel)
  Dose: 5–20 mg/kg daily, orally on empty stomach
  Duration: 6 mo (3 mo for 20 mg/kg dose)
  Side effects: Increased bone pain
        Diarrhea, nausea, vomiting
  Drug resistance: Primary: 15%
        Secondary: 10–20%

Plicamycin (mithramycin)
  Dose: 25 μg/kg, daily or qod, by IV infusion
  Duration: 9–10 infusions during 1½–3 wk, with repeat
        courses as needed
  Side effects: Anorexia, nausea, vomiting
        Abnormal hepatic and/or renal function
        Thrombocytopenia with gastrointestinal
        hemorrhage
  Drug resistance: None reported

decreases. As a result, and in association with a reduction in the degree of pagetic steal, neurologic deficits improve in many patients. The biochemical counterpart of these changes is a 30 per cent reduction or more in the serum alkaline phosphatase level.

Calcitonin

Synthetic salmon calcitonin (SCT) (Calcimar) was the first of the three agents to receive U.S. Food and Drug Administration (FDA) approval and has been in routine use for more than 15 years. In most patients, the initial response is similar regardless of whether 50 IU is injected subcutaneously three times a week or 100 IU daily. However, because most, if not all, secondary resistance to SCT is caused by neutralizing antibody production, higher doses of up to 200 IU daily may sometimes be needed to overcome secondary resistance. In cases of secondary resistance occurring during the initial or repeat courses of SCT, it is usually preferable to switch to synthetic human calcitonin (HCT) (Cibacalcin). The side effects of SCT shown in Table 3, except for diarrhea, occur in approximately 10 per cent of patients but are usually self-limited and ameliorate with continued treatment. Rarely, urticaria or severe nausea and vomiting may make it necessary to discontinue SCT. HCT has similar side effects, except that gastrointestinal side effects are more frequent, whereas dermatologic reactions are infrequent. In general, SCT is better tolerated than HCT and is preferred in initiating treatment. Both SCT and HCT have approximately 15 per cent rates of primary resistance, the reason for which is unknown.

The duration of calcitonin treatment in responsive cases is unsettled. Beneficial clinical and biochemical responses usually begin within 2 weeks to 2 months and are usually maximal within the first 10 to 12 months of treatment. Short courses of treatment usually result in suboptimal responses and rapid relapses, whereas prolonged courses of treatment do not increase the maximal response and may predispose to secondary resistance. For these reasons, an 18-month course of calcitonin treatment is advocated if an acceptable initial response is seen. After a course of calcitonin treatment is completed, the serum alkaline phosphatase level gradually increases to the baseline value. Despite this response, clinical features may remain improved indefinitely. In other patients, clinical phenomena return toward baseline at a variable rate. When the clinical features again become sufficiently disabling to justify treatment, a new course of calcitonin should be started. In some cases, partial or complete secondary resistance to

SCT may be seen with subsequent courses of treatment and may require a change to HCT or to disodium etidronate (EHDP).

Disodium Etidronate (Didronel)

This drug has been approved by the FDA for Paget's disease and has been in routine use for more than 10 years. It is a nondegradable analogue of sodium pyrophosphate, a naturally occurring modulator of bone metabolism that inhibits bone formation, mineralization, and bone resorption by adsorbing to bone surfaces and rendering them inert. In addition, the analogue reduces the generation of 1,25-dihydroxyvitamin D_3 in the kidney, which further contributes to inhibition of bone mineralization. The synthetic analogue is not hydrolyzed by alkaline phosphatase, which is also a potent pyrophosphatase.

The major advantages of EHDP over calcitonin are its oral route of administration and its lower cost. Although gastrointestinal side effects are infrequent, especially with the 5 mg per kg per day dose, approximately 20 per cent of patients develop increased bone pain at the site of pagetic lesions. In these patients, the inhibiting effect of the drug on mineralization appears to predominate over its antiresorptive action, and a painful osteomalacia-like lesion develops that requires discontinuation of the drug.

In the average patient with multiple sclerotic lesions, EHDP is as effective as calcitonin. Although its rate of primary resistance is similar to that of calcitonin, it has a considerably lower frequency of secondary resistance. With secondary resistance, there may be a dissociation between the clinical and biochemical responses, with a recurrence of clinical findings despite a suppressed serum alkaline phosphatase level. When this happens, the latter becomes useless in judging the response to a replacement agent.

For a limited number of indications, calcitonin is preferred to EHDP because of the tendency of the latter to inhibit bone formation and mineralization, as well as bone resorption. When there is an excessive resorptive component to the disease process or a need to heal a fracture or an operative bony defect, calcitonin is preferred to EHDP. Some physicians also prefer calcitonin for neurologic complications, although improvement in neurologic deficits has been reported with both calcitonin and EHDP.

Plicamycin (Mithramycin)

This chemotherapeutic agent causes sufficient toxic damage to osteoclasts to produce the same overall beneficial effects as the other two agents. However, because of its concurrent toxicity to the gastrointestinal tract, liver, kidneys, and bone marrow, it should be reserved for patients who have become resistant to or have serious side effects from SCT, HCT, and EHDP. The FDA has not officially approved it, although it has been in common use for Paget's disease as long as calcitonin. Most patients should be hospitalized for a course of plicamycin because of its inherent toxicity, but some physicians have been able to adapt it to outpatient administration under special conditions in selected patients. The major advantage of plicamycin is that an almost universal response can be expected.

Other Agents

Newer analogues of EHDP are currently undergoing clinical trials in the United States, and some have been in common use in Europe and other countries for several years. These newer analogues have the same beneficial effect on osteoclastic bone resorption as EHDP, but lesser inhibitory effects on bone formation and mineralization. As a result, they can be used interchangeably with calcitonin and have the additional advantage of being effective orally. Intravenous forms also exist and, like plicamycin, can achieve prolonged suppression of Paget's disease after a short course of intravenous treatment, but with very little toxicity. The analogue that will soon enter routine use in the United States is the aminohydroxypropylidene bisphosphonate analogue, also known as "APD." Ongoing clinical trials have thus far yielded promising results.

Other forms of calcitonin, such as porcine calcitonin and a modified form of eel calcitonin, are available in other countries but do not have any advantages over SCT and HCT. The latter is the preferred calcitonin in Asia because it was developed in Japan. Whether any new animal forms of calcitonin, or new modifications of the natural molecule, offer advantages over SCT or HCT is unknown. However, several manufacturers have developed noninjectable forms of calcitonin. The most promising of these is a nasal form of SCT, which has already been shown to be as effective as injectable SCT in the treatment of Paget's disease.

Nonsteroidal Anti-Inflammatory Drugs

As noted earlier, osteoarthritis is a concomitant of Paget's disease, and it is often difficult to differentiate the two on the basis of pain. It is sometimes necessary to treat both conditions simultaneously to achieve optimal benefit with regard to pain and disability. In patients treated with a specific agent alone, and in whom there is a clear-cut response, as indicated by a declining serum alkaline phosphatase level, but an inadequate alleviation of the pain, the addition of a nonsteroidal anti-inflammatory agent may make the difference between therapeutic success and failure.

PARENTERAL NUTRITION IN ADULTS

method of
J. CAMILO PALACIO, M.D.
School of Medicine
University of Pennsylvania
Philadelphia, Pennsylvania

and

JOHN L. ROMBEAU, M.D.
VA Medical Center
Philadelphia, Pennsylvania

Parenteral nutrition (PN) is defined as the intravenous administration of nutrients. There are two types of PN: (1) peripheral PN, the administration of water, electrolytes, protein, and caloric substrates through a peripheral vein to meet partial nutrient requirements; and (2) total parenteral nutrition (TPN), the provision of all daily required nutrients through the central venous system because of the tonicity of the solutions. The terms "total parenteral nutrition" and "central venous alimentation" are analogous. However, "hyperalimentation" implies excessive nutrient support; thus, this term should generally be avoided.

PHYSIOLOGIC CONSIDERATIONS

In terms of cellular nutrition, it makes little difference whether nutrients are delivered orally or intravenously. However, the administration of nutrients directly into the blood bypasses the gastrointestinal (GI) tract, which leads to intestinal atrophy, reductions in GI hormone secretions, and decreases in intestinal enzyme activity. Because of these adverse effects of TPN on the GI tract, enteral nutrition should be given if the gut can be used safely.

NUTRITIONAL ASSESSMENT

To determine the need for PN accurately, an assessment of the patient's nutritional status must be made. Nutritional assessment is the process of diagnosing malnutrition and determining nutrient requirements. Although most clinicians agree that nutritional assessment should be performed, there is less agreement as to how this is best accomplished. Recently, a subjective global assessment (SGA) of nutritional status has

been developed and validated in hospitalized patients (Table 1). The SGA is based on nutritionally relevant features of the medical history and physical examination, and it classifies the patient's nutritional status into one of three categories: (1) well nourished, (2) moderately malnourished, or (3) severely malnourished.

It is emphasized that the SGA is subjective; consequently, there are no absolute values for its measurement. Consideration of the complete clinical picture and the physician's experience and judgment determine the value of this assessment. The SGA combined with measurement of serum albumin levels is superior or equal to single objective parameters in predicting the development of nutritionally related complications in patients undergoing major operations.

INDICATIONS

As a general rule, PN is indicated when the GI tract cannot or should not be used. Careful consideration should be given to the nutritional status, clinical condition, and GI function of the patient to assess whether TPN or another type of nutritional support should be used. The indications for TPN are either absolute or relative (Table 2).

NUTRIENT REQUIREMENTS

Careful consideration should be given to the requirements and administration of all nutrients—protein, carbohydrate, fat, vitamins, electrolytes, trace elements, and water—because efficient use of one nutrient requires the presence of others. The amount of protein and calories to be administered depends on the goals of PN (either to deliver complete nutritional support [TPN] or to provide only some protein and calories for a short course of therapy [partial PN], anticipating oral intake within 5 to 7 days).

Energy Requirements

Energy requirements are based on age, sex, body build, activity level, and disease state. The formula most widely used to predict the resting metabolic expenditure (RME) is the Harris-Benedit equation:

$$\male = \text{RME (kcal/day)} = 66 + (13.7 \times W) + (5 \times H) - (6.8 \times A)$$
$$\female = \text{RME (kcal/day)} = 655 + (9.6 \times W) + (1.7 \times H) - (4.7 \times A),$$

where RME = resting metabolic expenditure;

TABLE 1. **Classification of Nutritional Status***

Criteria	Well Nourished	Moderately Malnourished	Severely Malnourished
A. Subjective Global Assessment			
I. Medical History			
a. Body weight change in the last 6 months	Loss < 5%	Loss 5–10%	Loss > 10%
b. Dietary intake	Balanced diet that meets requirements	70–90% of required	<70% of required
c. GI symptoms (vomiting, diarrhea)	No	Intermittent	Daily for >2 wk
d. Functional capacity	Full capacity	Reduced	Bedridden
II. Physical examination			
a. Subcutaneous fat	Normal	↓	↓↓
b. Muscle mass (quadriceps, deltoids)	Normal	↓	↓↓
c. Edema (ankle, sacral)	No	+	+
d. Ascites	No	+	+
B. Serum albumin level	>4.0 grams/dl	3.0–4.0 grams/dl	<3.0 grams/dl

*From Palacio JC and Rombeau JL: Nutritional support. *In* Fazio VW (ed): Current Therapy in Colon and Rectal Surgery. Philadelphia, B.C. Decker, Inc., 1989. Used by permission.

W = weight in kg; H = height in cm; and A = age in years.

After the determination of the RME, total energy requirements are adjusted according to the patient's disease or state, as indicated in Table 3.

Giving calories in excess of requirements is of questionable value because it increases lipogenesis and the deposition of fat in the liver. Excessive delivery of calories also produces a respiratory quotient greater than 1.0, which implies fat synthesis and suggests that the extra calories are not required. Therefore, there is enough evidence to support the conclusion that hyperalimentation may be dangerous.

TABLE 2. **Indications and Rationale for TPN**

Indications	Rationale
Absolute	
Abdominal sepsis	Prolonged ileus
GI fistulas	>500 ml/day of output
Short-bowel syndrome	↓ absorptive capacity
Complicated pancreatitis	Pseudocyst, hemorrhagic abscess
Postoperative severe malnutrition with unsafe use of GI tract	↑ risk of postoperative complications
Relative	
Acute tubular necrosis	↑ renal function recovery
Preoperative malnutrition	Severely malnourished patients in need of major surgery
Cancer and immune incompetence	Selected patients may benefit from TPN
GI disease	↓ nutrient absorption (e.g., regional enteritis, chemotherapy)
Anorexia nervosa	↑ nutritional status while undergoing psychiatric evaluation

Protein Requirements

To meet daily requirements, the amount of protein needed varies with the patient's clinical status and disease and ranges from 0.75 to 2 grams per kg per day; this amount is higher in the hypercatabolic patient and lower in the patient with liver disease or renal failure. Protein appears to be replaced at a finite rate and cannot be stored. When excess protein is administered, it is catabolized or excreted in the urine.

Electrolyte and Micronutrient Requirements

Requirements for sodium, potassium, bicarbonate, chloride, magnesium, calcium, and phosphate should be based on the patient's pre-TPN levels, with estimates of daily requirements and ongoing losses.

Vitamins should be administered daily in amounts recommended by the Nutritional Advisory Group of the American Medical Association. Standard amounts of commercial trace element

TABLE 3. **Correction Factors for Predicting Energy Requirements for Hospitalized Patients***

Clinical Condition	Correction Factor (× RME)
Physical activity	
Confined to bed	1.2
Out of bed	1.3
Fever	1.0 + 0.13 per °C
Elective surgery	1.0–1.2
Peritonitis	1.2–1.5
Soft tissue trauma	1.14–1.37
Major sepsis	1.4–1.8
Starvation	0.7

*Adapted from Bernard MA, Jacobs DO, and Rombeau JL: Nutritional and Metabolic Support of Hospitalized Patients. Philadelphia, W.B. Saunders Co., 1986, p. 13.

mixes are usually adequate for short-term parenteral feeding. Copper and manganese should be omitted from the TPN, as they are predominantly excreted in the bile in patients with liver disease.

COMPLICATIONS

The complications of TPN are grouped into three categories: technical, metabolic, and septic.

1. *Technical complications*: Technical complications are the result of efforts to obtain access to the central venous system. Immediate complications include pneumothorax, injury to the subclavian artery or brachial plexus, and misdirection of the catheter. Late complications include central venous thrombosis.

2. *Metabolic complications*: The metabolic complications of TPN can involve any of its components. Excessive protein administration is associated with increases in blood urea nitrogen level, oxygen consumption and resting energy expenditure, and ventilatory drive. Excessive caloric intake, particularly excessive glucose, results in hyperglycemia, increased oxygen consumption, carbon dioxide production, and resting energy expenditure. Excessive fat administration can result in hyperlipidemia with increased plasma triglyceride levels and decreased cellular immune function. Excessive water and sodium can result in salt and water overload.

3. *Septic complications*: Septic complications occur in 5 to 10 per cent of patients receiving TPN and are caused by contamination of the central venous catheter. The most common infectious organism is *Staphylococcus epidermidis*, which contaminates the catheter at its contact point with the skin. Careful monitoring of central venous catheters by an experienced nutritional support nurse reduces catheter sepsis.

PARENTERAL FLUID THERAPY IN INFANTS AND CHILDREN

method of
WILLIAM A. PRIMACK, M.D.
Fallon Clinic
University of Massachusetts Medical School
Worcester, Massachusetts

Fluid and electrolyte therapy consists of three components: (1) *maintenance therapy* replaces the daily *normal expenditure* of fluids and electrolytes; (2) *deficit therapy* replaces *pre-existing abnormal losses* of fluid, electrolytes, or both; and (3) *replacement therapy* replaces *ongoing abnormal losses* such as those caused by nasogastric drainage or persistent diarrhea. Fluid therapy may be given orally, but it is given parenterally if the infant or child is unable to meet his or her needs by the oral route.

Dehydration from gastroenteritis is the most common clinical situation where fluid therapy is required in infants and children. Since the 1930s, parenteral (i.e., intravenous) fluid therapy has been the standard route of rehydration. Recently, following the lead of health care workers in the Third World, the need in the Western World for parenteral fluid therapy in the treatment of gastroenteritis has been lessened by the use of oral rehydration solutions (ORSs) and glucose and electrolyte oral maintenance solutions.

MAINTENANCE FLUID AND ELECTROLYTE THERAPY

Maintenance therapy replaces normal metabolic losses from respiration, urine, sweat, and stool. This therapy should allow fluid and electrolyte homeostasis with minimal renal compensation and provide sufficient calories to prevent protein catabolism and ketosis. Parenteral maintenance therapy should meet all the daily needs of an adequately hydrated child with normal renal function who is temporarily unable to ingest oral fluids and who has no excessive ongoing water or electrolyte losses. An example is the preoperative or postoperative patient who is allowed no oral hydration.

In the infant, about two-thirds of *insensible water losses* are from the skin and one-third are from the lungs. These losses are evaporative and account for about 50 per cent of daily maintenance water requirements in the infant and about 30 to 35 per cent of daily needs in the older child. Urinary losses account for the remainder of maintenance fluid needs, except in infants, in whom stool water averages 10 to 20 ml per kg per day. Because daily physiologic insensible water losses are proportional to caloric expenditure, correlating the maintenance water requirement with the caloric expenditure gives a convenient estimate of fluid needs that is reliable for most infants and children. The hospitalized child requires approximately 120 ml of water for every 100 kcal metabolized. Because water of oxidation and preformed water provide about 17 ml and 3 ml per 100 kcal metabolized, respectively, approximately 100 ml of water is required for each 100 kcal metabolized. A formula to estimate caloric expenditure based on body weight is given in Table 1. Thus, a hospitalized 16-kg child should receive about 1300 kcal or about 1300 ml of water per day (1000 ml for the first 10 kg plus 50×6 = 300 ml for the remaining 6 kg). Similarly, a 38-kg child requires about 1860 kcal or 1860 ml of water daily (1000 ml for the first 10 kg, plus

TABLE 1. **Estimate of Maintenance Fluid Requirements**

Body Weight (kg)	Maintenance Fluids (ml/day)
4–10	100 ml/kg
11–20	1000 ml + 50 ml/kg over 10 kg
21–80	1500 ml + 20 ml/kg over 20 kg

$50 \times 10 = 500$ ml for the next 10 kg, plus $20 \times 18 = 360$ ml for the remainder).

Insensible losses are increased by about 12 per cent for each degree of body temperature above 38° C. An increased respiratory rate or a high ambient temperature also increases insensible fluid losses, which are decreased if the child is in a mist tent or is breathing humidified air via an endotracheal tube.

Water loss from the kidneys depends on the solute load that must be excreted. The clinician may assume that the average child who requires fluid therapy is not receiving an excessive dietary solute load, so that the estimated renal solute load can be assumed to be 10 to 40 mOsm per 100 kcal. Unless the child has significant renal abnormalities, a urinary concentration range of 150 to 600 mOsm (specific gravity 1.005 to 1.020) can be achieved. Thus, an average renal solute load of 30 mOsm per kcal can be excreted in as little as 50 ml of urine (urine osmolarity = 600 mOsm) or as much as 200 ml (urine osmolarity = 150 mOsm). Most infants and children can easily excrete their renal solute load in approximately 70 ml of water per 100 kcal.

Average daily urinary electrolyte losses are approximately 2 to 3 mEq of sodium and 1 to 2 mEq of potassium per kg of body weight. Chloride is the principal inorganic anion in urine. Water lost from the lungs is electrolyte free. Daily electrolyte losses in sweat are about 0.5 mEq per kg each of sodium and potassium. Electrolyte losses in stool are minimal in the absence of diarrhea. Thus, replacement should approximate 2 to 3 mEq of sodium and 2 mEq of potassium per 100 kcal metabolized (or per 100 ml of fluid

required). A solution containing 20 to 30 mEq per liter of sodium chloride (NaCl) and 20 mEq per liter of potassium chloride (KCl) given at a rate calculated from Table 1 will meet the maintenance fluid requirements of the average hospitalized infant or child. Glucose is added to the intravenous solution to provide sufficient calories (about 20 per cent of basal caloric needs) to prevent protein catabolism and the osmotic diuresis of starvation ketosis.

The euvolemic child with normal renal function should excrete 1 to 3 ml per kg of urine per hour. Urine output of less than 0.8 ml per kg per hour suggests oliguria. The anuric patient should receive replacement only for insensible losses, or approximately one-third of the fluid recommended in Table 1, with 0.5 to 1.0 mEq of sodium per kg daily and no potassium. An anuric child should lose about 0.5 per cent of body weight daily, or overhydration may occur.

DEFICIT THERAPY

Dehydration is caused by an acute loss of body fluids and electrolytes, with a resulting deficit of total body water and variable deficits of electrolytes. In infants and children, the most common causes of dehydration are gastrointestinal losses from diarrhea or vomiting. Less common causes include the osmotic diuresis of diabetic ketoacidosis or dehydration from vigorous activity in a warm environment.

The most accurate estimation of dehydration is the direct measurement of body weight loss. Often an accurate preillness weight is not available, and the clinician is forced to use subjective physical signs to estimate the degree of dehydration (Table 2). Estimates of the degree of dehydration assume that the observed changes are not caused by malnutrition or chronic illness. In infants and small children, estimates are usually no more accurate than 5 per cent of body weight. *Mild or 5 per cent dehydration* occurs with a history compatible with fluid and electrolyte loss, but with relatively few physical signs, except

TABLE 2. **Estimate of the Degree of Isotonic Dehydration by Physical Signs**

Physical Sign	Symptoms of Dehydration for Degree Shown*			
	< 5%	5–10%	10–15%	>15%
Turgor	Normal	Decreased	Tenting	Poor
Mucous membranes	Moist	Dry	Very dry	Parched
Eyeballs	Normal	Soft	Sunken	Very sunken
Fontanelle	Flat	Soft	Sunken	Very sunken
CNS	Consolable	Irritable	Lethargic	Comatose
Pulse	Normal	Orthostatic	Increased	Thready
BP	Normal	Normal	Orthostatic	Shock

*Hypotonic dehydration: physical signs accentuated; hypertonic dehydration: physical signs diminished, with "woody" turgor.
Abbreviations: CNS = central nervous system; BP = blood pressure.

possibly thirst and dry mucous membranes. *Moderate or 10 per cent dehydration* occurs when there are clear physical signs of fluid loss, such as loss of subcutaneous tissue turgor ("tenting") or a sunken fontanelle, but no signs of circulatory or central nervous system compromise. *Severe or 15 per cent dehydration* indicates more dramatic physical signs with impending circulatory compromise, and the patient may be near shock. In older children and young adults, similar clinical findings are used to estimate dehydration. In these children, states of mild, moderate, and severe dehydration are estimated as 3, 6, and 9 per cent of body weight loss, respectively.

Classification of dehydration depends on the quantity of electrolytes lost relative to water losses. Most fluids lost have sodium concentrations ranging from 30 to 70 mEq per liter, with the notable exception of the situation in cholera, in which the sodium concentration of stool is nearly isotonic with plasma (Table 3). *Isotonic dehydration* (sodium level 130 to 150 mEq per liter) indicates that the loss of free water and electrolytes is proportional to normal physiologic concentrations.

Hypotonic dehydration (sodium level < 130 mEq per liter) occurs when solute is lost in excess of water, causing the serum sodium level to fall. It may be seen in children with dehydration in whom free water is replaced in excess of solute, especially when sodium-containing losses persist. An example is an infant with several days of moderately severe diarrhea who is receiving replacement solely with low-sodium–containing solutions such as soda or diluted infant formula (Table 4). Because sodium is the principal extracellular cation, hypotonic dehydration indicates a disproportionate loss of electrolytes and fluid from the extracellular space, with consequent exaggerated physical signs of dehydration (see Table 2).

Hyponatremia can occur in many clinical settings other than hypotonic dehydration. As Table 5 shows, the child with hypotonic dehydration should have evidence of weight loss and clinical findings of dehydration. The urinary sodium level should be low (<10 mEq per liter) and the urine osmolarity high. Similar urinary findings are observed with congestive heart failure and nephrosis, but the patient shows weight gain and edema. Hyponatremia can also occur when free water is received in excess of solute, such as with water intoxication. The urine sodium level is low and the urine is hyposmotic to plasma. An inability to concentrate the urine, as may be seen with renal insufficiency or obstructive uropathy, produces a high urine sodium level (>50 mEq per liter) and an isotonic or mildly hypotonic urine. Similar findings associated with hyperkalemia suggest adrenal insufficiency. Inappropriate release of antidiuretic hormone (SIADH) produces hyponatremia from excessive renal reabsorption of free water, resulting in urine with a high sodium level and an osmolarity inappropriately high for the hypotonic serum. High serum concentrations of osmotically active materials can cause an artificially low serum sodium level (pseudohyponatremia). Examples include marked hyperglycemia, severe hyperlipidemia, and high serum concentrations of mannitol or radiocontrast materials.

Hypertonic dehydration (sodium level > 150 mEq per liter) occurs when too little free water is given. The classic example is replacement of the relatively low sodium losses of rotavirus diarrhea with a relatively high-sodium solution such as boiled skim milk (see Table 4). The high sodium concentration protects the extracellular space at the expense of the intracellular space. Consequently, the child often has few classic physical signs of dehydration, and the clinician tends to underestimate the degree of volume deficit (see Table 2). Hypertonicity causes the formation of intracellular osmotically active substances (idiogenic osmole) that protect intracellular volume from the high extracellular osmolarity. If hypertonicity is corrected too rapidly, the cells swell as water is osmotically drawn in before the idiogenic osmole can leave. In the brain, the swelling can cause cerebral edema, seizures, intracerebral bleeding, or all three.

TABLE 3. **Electrolyte Content of Common Body Fluids**

	Electrolyte Content (mEq/Liter) of Diarrheal Fluid			Electrolyte Content (mEq/Liter) of Body Fluid		
Electrolyte	Cholera	Rotavirus Infection	ETEC Infection	Gastric Fluid	Sweat	Ileal Fluid
Sodium	88	37	53	60	45	129
Potassium	30	38	37	10	5	11
Chloride	86	22	24	84	58	116
Bicarbonate	32	6	18	0	0	29

Abbreviation: ETEC = enterotoxic *Escherichia coli.*

TABLE 4. Electrolyte Content of ORS, Maintenance, and Commonly Used Oral Fluids

Solution	Sodium (mEq/Liter)	Potassium (mEq/Liter)	Chloride (mEq/Liter)	Base (mEq/Liter)	CHO (Grams/Liter)	Type of CHO	Storage Form*
Rehydration Solutions							
WHO ORS	90	20	80	30	20	Glucose	Powder
Rehydralyte	75	20	65	30	25	Glucose	Liquid
Maintenance Electrolyte Solutions							
Infalyte	50	20	40	30	20	Glucose	Powder
Lytren	50	25	45	30	20	Glucose	Powder
Pedialyte	45	20	35	30	25	Glucose	Liquid
Resol	50	20	50	34	20	Glucose	Liquid
Clear Fluids							
Gatorade	21	17	17	6	61	Glucose	Liquid
Kool-Aid	0–5†	0.1	0	†	88	Sucrose	Powder
Soda	0–8†	1–12†	??	0	80–120†	‡	Liquid
Apple juice	0.4	26	??	0	119	Fructose	Liquid
Chicken soup	105	2	100	0	32	??	Liquid
Cherry Jell-O	25	0.25	10	†	166	Sucrose	Powder
Milk and Infant Formula							
Skim milk	23	47	29	0	50	Lactose	Liquid
Formula	8–12†	18–28†	12–18†	0	67	Lactose	Liquid

*All values represent powders diluted according to directions.
†Range for commonly used brands.
‡High-fructose syrup, sucrose, or both.
Abbreviations: WHO = World Health Organization; CHO = carbohydrate.

ONGOING LOSSES

Replacement of ongoing losses is essential to successful fluid therapy. Common examples are persistent diarrhea and nasogastric drainage. The volume of these losses can be accurately measured and the electrolyte content measured or estimated (see Table 3), so that accurate replacement can be planned. Diarrheal losses in infants are accurately estimated by weighing dirty diapers and subtracting the weight of the empty diaper.

TREATMENT PRINCIPLES

Most mild and moderate dehydration can be safely and effectively treated by the use of ORS, to be discussed. If the oral route is unavailable,

TABLE 5. Hyponatremia

Clinical Condition	Weight	Urine Sodium (mEq/Liter)	Urine Osmolarity (mOsm/kg H₂O)
Hypotonic dehydration	Decreased	<10	>500
CHF or nephrosis	Increased	<10	>500
Water intoxication	Increased	<10	<200
Chronic renal insufficiency	No change	>50	<300
Adrenal insufficiency	Decreased	>50	<300
SIADH	Increased	>50	>500

Abbreviation: CHF = congestive heart failure.

the intravenous route is the only parenteral route usually required. In extreme situations, isotonic fluids can be administered into the intraosseous spaces of the anterior tibia or posterior iliac crest, using a large-bore spinal needle.

Fluid Resuscitation. If dehydration is moderate or severe, immediate expansion of the extracellular space is begun to preserve cardiovascular function and renal perfusion. An infusion of 0.9 per cent NaCl (normal saline) with 5 per cent dextrose or Ringer's lactate solution with 5 per cent dextrose at a rate of 10 to 20 ml per kg per hour for 1 to 2 hours usually provides adequate fluid resuscitation while awaiting the results of initial laboratory tests and planning further therapy. Plasma or albumin infusions are rarely required.

Rate of Fluid Infusion and Treatment Duration. Fluid repair usually takes about 24 hours. One-half of the deficit is replaced in the first 8 hours and the remainder over the next 14 to 16 hours. In hypertonic dehydration, treatment is usually planned over 48 hours. Maintenance fluid requirements are added to the deficit fluids. Replacement of all losses, including restoration of full nutrition, usually takes several days.

Body Fluid Spaces. Knowledge of the body fluid spaces and their principal constituents aids in the prescription of fluid and electrolyte therapy. The *total body water* of an infant is about 70 per cent of body weight, decreasing to the adult value of 60 per cent by 1 year of age. Of the total body water, approximately two-thirds is in the *intracellular fluid* (ICF), where potassium is the major cation and proteins and energy-containing phosphate compounds are the major anions. The remaining one-third of body water is in the *extracellular fluid* (ECF), which includes the interstitial space and the intravascular space. The major cation of the ECF is sodium at a concentration of about 140 mEq per liter, and the major anion is chloride at a concentration of 100 mEq per liter. The potassium concentration in the ECF is only 5 mEq per liter.

In the typical clinical situation, acute weight loss from dehydration is nearly all from the total body water space. Approximately one-half of the loss is from the ECF and one-half from the ICF. Consequently, if electrolyte loss is isosmotic to fluid loss (isotonic dehydration), each liter (kilogram) of acute body weight loss suggests an approximate deficit of sodium of $140 \times 0.50 = 70$ mEq and of potassium of $150 \times 0.50 = 75$ mEq. The more rapid the onset of dehydration, the greater the relative deficit of the ECF.

Potassium. Potassium losses vary, depending on the source of the electrolyte deficit, with relatively high losses caused by gastric or intestinal drainage (see Table 3). Extracellular (serum) potassium values are only an approximate reflection of intracellular potassium values and may be misleading. For example, metabolic acidosis raises the serum potassium level as hydrogen ions displace potassium ions within the cell. Some of the displaced potassium is rapidly excreted, so that the child with acidosis may have a normal, or even elevated, serum potassium level but a large potassium deficit. There are no clinical signs of potassium loss, unless it is extreme, with muscle weakness or electrocardiographic changes (usually the potassium level < 2 mEq per liter).

Potassium replacement should be gradual, as the total intracellular store of potassium is much greater than the extracellular store, and potassium should never be added to an intravenous solution until urine output is assured to avoid the arrhythmias associated with severe hyperkalemia. In most clinical situations potassium replacement of 20 to 30 mEq per liter of intravenous fluid is adequate because total replacement of potassium losses may take several days. A potassium concentration more than 40 mEq per liter should never be exceeded in parenteral fluids without administration into a central line, where a great deal of mixing can occur. High potassium concentrations should be given only in a patient care setting where adequate monitoring is available. Potassium is usually added as KCl or occasionally as potassium phosphate.

Hyponatremia. Treatment of hyponatremia depends on the etiology. If it is caused by water intoxication, it resolves spontaneously when the excess water is withheld. Mineralocorticoids are required in adrenal insufficiency. Water restriction is essential to treat SIADH successfully.

In hypotonic dehydration, solute (NaCl) must be replaced (see Case 2, later). The quantity of NaCl necessary to replace a solute deficit is calculated as

$$(\text{Na desired} - \text{Na measured}) \times \%\text{TBW} \times \text{body weight}$$

where %TBW is percentage of total body water. Because about one-half of the solute losses are intracellular potassium, only about one-half of the amount of the calculated sodium deficit is placed in the fluid prescription.

If hyponatremia is severe (sodium level < 120 mEq per liter) and the patient has symptoms such as seizures, hypertonic (3 or 5 per cent) saline can be infused at a maximal rate of 5 mEq per kg per hour (10 ml per kg per hour) until symptoms remit. Rapid repair of severe hyponatremia is controversial and should be done only if absolutely required.

Hypernatremia. Correction of hypernatremia must proceed slowly to minimize the risk of cerebral edema, seizures, or both. Most authorities recommend replacement of the total deficit over 48 hours or more and believe that *the serum sodium level should decrease by no more than 10 to 12 mEq per liter per day.* Hypertonicity represents a greater deficit of free water compared with solute. The water deficit equals the normal water volume minus the measured water volume, as shown:

Deficit =

$$\frac{\%\text{TBW} \times \text{body weight (kg)} \times \text{measured osmolarity}}{\text{normal plasma osmolarity}}$$

$$- \%\text{TBW} \times \text{body weight}$$

If the measured serum osmolarity value is not available, substituting two times the serum sodium value gives a usable estimation. This formula is used in Case 3. Hypotonic solutions must be given carefully to prevent a too rapid fall of the serum osmolarity. Hypocalcemia and hyperglycemia are frequent complications of hypernatremic dehydration. Severe hypernatremia (sodium level > 180 mEq per liter) may require peritoneal dialysis.

Acid-Base Disturbances. The poor tissue perfusion in severe dehydration or the loss of bicarbonate (HCO_3)-rich fluids, such as in profuse diarrhea, may result in a *metabolic acidosis.* Unless the acidosis is severe, adequate rehydration with re-establishment of tissue and renal perfusion usually causes rapid resolution of the acidosis without requiring exogenous base therapy. If the acidosis is severe (serum HCO_3 level < 10 to 12 mEq per liter) or a large anion gap is present, the initial resuscitation fluid can contain up to 40 to 60 mEq per liter of sodium bicarbonate ($NaHCO_3$). This should be mixed into a hypotonic solution such as 0.45 per cent (half-normal) saline with 5 per cent dextrose. Routine intravenous infusion of hypertonic solutions should be avoided, as should rapid infusion of undiluted $NaHCO_3$, which may result in a paradoxical intracellular acidosis in the central nervous system.

Metabolic alkalosis can be caused by loss of hydrogen ions in gastic juice, as with frequent vomiting or nasogastric suction. The classic example in infants is the persistent vomiting of pyloric stenosis (Case 4). Chloride losses are also high, usually resulting in a hypochloremic metabolic alkalosis, often associated with hypokalemia. Replacement with chloride-containing solutions such as NaCl and KCl is necessary because administration of HCl or NH_4Cl is impractical.

Re-Evaluation of the Treatment Plan. In the acute setting, the patient should be frequently re-examined, and repeated measurements of body weight, serum electrolytes, or both (e.g., every 8 to 12 hours) may be required. The fluid prescription can then be revised appropriately. This is especially true when large ongoing losses occur.

EXAMPLES OF TREATMENT PLANS

The patient in the first three cases is a 10-kg infant with a temperature of 37° C and without abnormal ongoing losses. All laboratory results are given in Table 6. From Table 1, the infant's maintenance fluid requirements would be 1000 ml per day or about 40 ml per hour. Electrolyte requirements would be about 25 mEq of NaCl and about 20 mEq of KCl daily.

This infant develops gastroenteritis and rapidly becomes 10 per cent dehydrated. This indicates that the fluid deficit is about 1 liter (0.1 × 10 kg). The infant's initial fluid resuscitation requires 0.9 per cent saline with 5 per cent dextrose at a rate of 100 ml per hour for the first

1 or 2 hours (10 ml per kg per hour). Because the degree of dehydration is a rough estimate, the resuscitation fluids are not usually included in the calculation of the fluid prescription.

Case 1: Isotonic Dehydration. Because the total estimated deficit of 1 liter is approximately evenly divided between the ECF and the ICF, the sodium and potassium deficits are 70 and 75 mEq, respectively. These are added to the maintenance requirements of 25 and 20 mEq each. Thus, 2 liters of solution containing a total of 95 mEq each of sodium and potassium is required (given as 50 mEq per liter of NaCl and 30 mEq per liter of KCl). Because one-half of the deficit is to be replaced in the first 8 hours, the initial rate of infusion would be 500 ml per 8 hours + maintenance (40 ml per hour), or about 100 ml per hour, and the remainder would be infused at a rate of 500 ml per 16 hours + 40 ml per hour, or about 70 ml per hour.

Case 2: Hypotonic Dehydration. The sodium and potassium deficits from dehydration and the rate of fluid administration are the same as in Case 1. The formula to replace the additional sodium deficit is

$$(\text{Na desired} - \text{Na measured}) \times \%\text{TBW} \times \text{body weight}$$
$$\text{or}$$
$$135 - 125 \times 0.6 \times 10 \text{ kg} = 60 \text{ mEq}$$

Thus, using the calculations from Case 1, a total of 160 mEq of sodium and 60 mEq of potassium is mixed into 2 liters of water (80 mEq per liter of NaCl and 30 mEq per liter of KCl) administered at the same rate as in Case 1.

Case 3: Hypertonic Dehydration. Correction should be planned over 48 hours once initial fluid resuscitation is complete. The formula to calculate the water deficit is:

Deficit =

$$\frac{\%\text{TBW} \times \text{body wt (kg)} \times \text{measured osmolarity}}{\text{normal plasma osmolarity}}$$
$$- \%\text{TBW} \times \text{body wt}$$
$$\text{or}$$
$$= \frac{0.6 \times 10 \text{ kg} \times 326}{280}$$
$$- 0.6 \times 10 \text{ kg} = 6.98 - 6 = 980 \text{ ml}$$

The maintenance requirements for 48 hours are 2000 ml of water, 50 mEq of sodium, and 40 mEq of potassium. The deficit of water is 1000 ml from the dehydration and 980 ml from the hypernatremia. Even though the serum sodium level is elevated, sodium must be added to the rehydra-

TABLE 6. **Case Examples**

Case No. (Dehydration Type)	Weight (kg)	mEq/Liter			
		Na	*K*	*Cl*	*CO$_2$*
1 (isotonic)	10	140	4.5	108	18
2 (hypotonic)	10	125	4.5	93	18
3 (hypertonic)	10	163	5.0	128	19
4 (pyloric stenosis)	4.2	128	3.4	75	34

tion solution, as in the other examples, because there is a total body deficit of sodium associated with the dehydration, and too rapid correction of hypernatremia must be avoided. The hypertonicity results from an excess loss of free water relative to sodium. Thus, 75 mEq of sodium and 70 mEq of potassium are added to the maintenance electrolyte requirement, giving a total of 125 mEq of sodium and 110 mEq of potassium in 3980 ml (about 35 mEq per liter of NaCl and 30 mEq per liter of KCl) to be administered over 48 hours: The volume deficit should be replaced in the first 12 hours.

Case 4: Pyloric Stenosis. A 6-week-old infant who weighed 4.2 kg 3 days before becoming ill has had projectile vomiting of all fluids for 30 hours. The weight is 3.7 kg (12 per cent dehydration), and there is an "olive" mass in the right upper abdomen. Laboratory results (see Table 6) show a hypochloremic metabolic alkalosis with hyponatremia.

Therapy must repair the dehydration because volume contraction causes the proximal tubule of the kidney to reabsorb excess HCO_3, aggravating the metabolic alkalosis. Normal saline rather than Ringer's lactate must be used as the initial resuscitation fluid. The infant's deficit from dehydration is $0.12 \times 0.7 \times 4$ kg $= 336$ ml of water and $(0.34$ liter $\times 70$ mEq per liter$) = 24$ mEq of sodium. The sodium deficit is $(135 - 128$ mEq$) \times 0.7 \times 4$ kg $= 20$ mEq. The potassium deficit is often large and takes several days to replace. The infant's maintenance needs are 400 ml of water and 10 and 8 mEq of sodium and potassium, respectively. Thus, a total of 54 mEq of sodium in about 740 ml of water is required (about 75 mEq of NaCl and 40 mEq of KCl per liter) and should be administered at a rate of 46 ml per hour for the first 8 hours and 23 ml per hour for the rest of the day. Any ongoing losses from nasogastric suction must also be replaced (see Table 3).

ORAL REHYDRATION THERAPY

The observation that the coupled transport of sodium and glucose in the small intestine persists despite infectious gastroenteritis has led to the development of glucose and electrolyte solutions for the oral treatment of patients with dehydration. Glucose facilitates the absorption of sodium. Water is absorbed osmotically after sodium absorption. Potassium is transported passively by solvent drag with absorbed water. Properly formulated glucose and electrolyte ORSs provide a net positive absorption of electrolytes and water despite persisting diarrhea. A glucose concentration of 2 per cent (111 mmol) allows maximal

sodium absorption. Much higher concentrations of glucose may not be fully absorbed from the intestine, and the osmotic effect of the remaining glucose may cause excess water to be lost in the stool.

Experience has shown success with ORS in all forms of mild and moderate dehydration both in the Third World and the West. ORS use allows rapid rehydration, with a complication rate similar to that of parenteral rehydration, at a much lower cost. The principal contraindications to ORS use are altered consciousness or seizure activity, severe hypotension or shock, persistent vomiting (as in pyloric stenosis), or absent bowel sounds. In these situations, parenteral rehydration therapy should be used until the patient stabilizes, at which time ORS may be added or substituted. Because continuing losses from the stool are often somewhat higher in patients receiving ORS than when the gut is put "to rest" (the child is receiving no oral feeding) during parenteral rehydration, the volumes recommended for rehydration with ORS are larger than those recommended for parenteral rehydration. The child's thirst and appetite assist in determining the rate, volume, and type of fluid administration with ORS.

The prototype ORS is the World Health Organization (WHO) solution (Table 7). This solution has been used successfully for more than 20 years in the treatment of cholera. It can be mixed by adding the ingredients in Table 6 to 1 liter (1.05 quarts) of clean water. Recent work has shown that glucose can be replaced by sucrose or rice powder, both of which are less expensive and easier to store. HCO_3 can be replaced by citrate, which is much more stable in solution. The ingredients should be provided in premixed packets or solutions to avoid iatrogenic errors in mixing.

In developed countries, the organisms causing gastroenteritis result in a stool sodium concentration that is much lower than that typically seen in cholera (see Table 3). Consequently, rehydration solutions developed for the West are lower in sodium content than is the WHO solution (see Table 7). Oral rehydration solutions have higher sodium concentrations than do oral maintenance electrolyte solutions. Oral maintenance solutions are formulated to prevent dehydration when an infant or child has mild gastroenteritis or another acute illness limiting the intake of food or milk (see Table 7).

TABLE 7. **WHO ORS Formula**

To 1 liter of water add	Substitutions
½ tsp NaCl	
½ tsp NaHCO₃	½ tsp sodium citrate
¼ tsp KCl	
2 Tbsp glucose	4 Tbsp sucrose

Clear fluids, such as fruit juices or soda, which are often recommended in the United States for mild gastroenteritis maintenance, are not as effective as the oral maintenance electrolyte solution. Clear fluids are low in sodium, and fructose is often the most prevalent carbohydrate, because high-fructose corn syrup has replaced sucrose as the major sweetener in many soda pops and juice drinks (see Table 7). Fructose is an ineffective substitute substrate for the glucose-sodium transporter in the small intestine. Also, if clear fluids are used alone for oral rehydration, or if they are used alone for prolonged periods as oral maintenance solutions, their low sodium content may cause hyponatremia. Clear fluids are good sources of additional fluids and calories once the recommended volumes of ORS or oral maintenance solutions have been ingested.

TREATMENT PLAN USING ORAL REHYDRATION SOLUTIONS

Clinical assessment of the degree and type of dehydration is identical to that given before parenteral therapy (see Table 2). The rehydration phase generally should last for 3 to 6 hours, with the estimated deficit being replaced with ORS. For example, replacement of 50 ml per kg over 4 hours should be planned for mild dehydration, and 100 ml per kg over 6 hours should be planned for moderately severe dehydration. If the child has hypertonic dehydration, oral rehydration should be planned over 12 to 24 hours. If the infant or child continues to vomit, as is common with rotavirus infections, small amounts (<30 ml) of ORS administered frequently are usually tolerated.

After rehydration is complete, ORS should not be used as the only fluid intake, because the high sodium content may lead to hypernatremia. ORS can be replaced with a maintenance electrolyte solution, or ORS can be ingested with extra free water in the form of breast milk in nursing infants, or as plain water, fruit juices, or other low-sodium clear liquids. The ratio of ORS to clear fluids should be approximately 1:1. Refeeding should begin as soon as the rehydration phase is complete. Breast-feeding should continue ad libitum. Generally, solids such as a BRAT diet (*B*anana, *R*ice, *A*pple sauce, *T*oast) or other carbohydrate-rich, low-lactose foods such as boiled potatoes are well tolerated. Refeeding may cause an increase in stool volume, which the infant or child usually tolerates well by increasing the appetite for fluids.

The timing of the reintroduction of lactose-containing formulas is controversial. The usual practice in the United States has been to delay the reintroduction of milk-based formula for several days, because some experienced pediatricians have observed recurrence of dehydrating diarrhea with early reintroduction of such formulas. However, breast milk, which is rich in lactose, is well tolerated. Nevertheless, delay in reintroducing milk-based formulas is probably still prudent. Infants can temporarily use a casein hydrolysate or other non–lactose-containing formula. The older infant or child should be able to tolerate the normal diet for several days before the use of cow milk.

The Endocrine System

ACROMEGALY

method of
WILLIAM F. YOUNG, JR., M.D.
Mayo Medical School
Rochester, Minnesota

Chronic growth hormone (GH) excess from a GH-producing pituitary tumor results in the clinical syndrome acromegaly. If untreated, this syndrome is associated with morbidity and mortality. Although the annual incidence is estimated to be only 3 per 1 million population, GH-secreting pituitary adenomas are the second most common hormone-secreting pituitary tumors. Ectopic neoplasms that produce GH or GH-releasing hormone (GHRH) are rare (<1 per cent) causes of acromegaly.

The mass effects of GH-producing pituitary macroadenomas (>10 mm) are similar to those of other pituitary macroadenomas. They include visual field defects, oculomotor pareses, headaches, and pituitary insufficiency. The effects of the chronic GH excess include acral and soft tissue overgrowth, progressive dental malocclusion, degenerative arthritis related to chondral and synovial tissue overgrowth within joints, low-pitched sonorous voice, excessive sweating and oily skin, perineural hypertrophy leading to nerve entrapment (e.g., carpal tunnel syndrome), eustachian tube obstruction leading to recurrent serous otitis media, proximal muscle weakness, carbohydrate intolerance, hypertension, and cardiac dysfunction.

DIAGNOSTIC EVALUATION

The patient with acromegaly has a characteristic appearance, with coarsening of facial features, prognathism, frontal bossing, spade-like hands, and wide feet. Often there is a history of progressive increase in shoe, glove, ring, or hat size. These changes may occur slowly and may go unrecognized by the patient, family, and physician. Comparison with earlier photographs of the patient is helpful in confirming the clinical suspicion of acromegaly.

High plasma GH levels are not diagnostic of acromegaly. Basal plasma GH levels are increased in patients with poorly controlled diabetes mellitus, chronic hepatic or renal failure, or conditions characterized by protein-calorie malnutrition such as anorexia nervosa. The diagnosis of acromegaly depends on two criteria: a GH level that is not suppressed to less than 2 micrograms per liter after an oral glucose load (75 to 100 grams) and an increased serum concen-

tration of somatomedin C (SmC; a GH-dependent growth factor responsible for many of the effects of GH). The laboratory assessment of acromegaly is supplemented with imaging of the pituitary by either computed tomography or magnetic resonance imaging and with visual field examination by quantitative perimetry. If imaging of the pituitary fails to detect an adenoma, computed tomography imaging of the chest and abdomen is indicated in search of an ectopic GHRH-producing tumor (e.g., pancreatic adenoma, small cell lung tumor). The plasma GHRH concentration can be measured in some research laboratories; this may be done in atypical cases (e.g., normal sella on imaging in an acromegalic patient with an uncharacterized lung nodule on a chest radiograph) but is not done for routine screening.

TREATMENT

Treatment is indicated for all patients with signs and symptoms of acromegaly and biochemical confirmation. The goals of treatment are to prevent the long-term consequences of GH excess, to remove the intrasellar mass, and to preserve normal pituitary tissue and function. Treatment options include surgery, irradiation, and medical therapy (Figure 1). In my opinion, surgery is the treatment of choice and is supplemented, if necessary, with irradiation or medical therapy or both. The criteria for cure are (1) clinical remission, (2) normal suppression of the GH level by oral administration of glucose, and (3) a normal SmC level.

Surgical Therapy

Trans-sphenoidal adenectomy by an experienced neurosurgeon is the only treatment option that has the potential for providing a permanent cure. If diagnostic imaging studies are negative, trans-sphenoidal surgery is indicated for a presumed GH-secreting microadenoma (≤10 mm). Selective adenectomy of a GH-secreting microadenoma with preservation of surrounding normal pituitary tissue is routinely possible.

Potential complications of trans-sphenoidal surgery include anterior pituitary insufficiency, transient or permanent diabetes insipidus, cerebrospinal fluid rhinorrhea, loss of vision, and hemorrhage. All patients are given glucocorti-

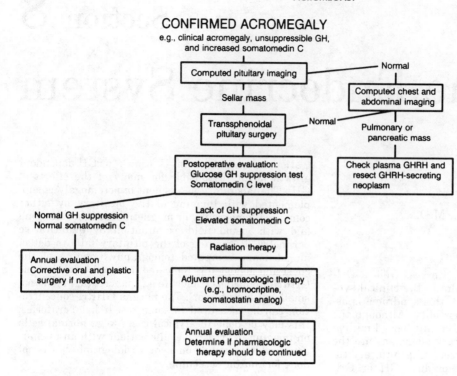

CONFIRMED ACROMEGALY
e.g., clinical acromegaly, unsuppressible GH, and increased somatomedin C

Computed pituitary imaging — Normal

Sellar mass

Computed chest and abdominal imaging

Transsphenoidal pituitary surgery — Normal

Pulmonary or pancreatic mass

Postoperative evaluation: Glucose GH suppression test Somatomedin C level

Check plasma GHRH and resect GHRH-secreting neoplasm

Normal GH suppression Normal somatomedin C

Lack of GH suppression Elevated somatomedin C

Annual evaluation Corrective oral and plastic surgery if needed

Radiation therapy

Adjuvant pharmacologic therapy (e.g., bromocriptine, somatostatin analog)

Annual evaluation Determine if pharmacologic therapy should be continued

Figure 1. Algorithm for the treatment of acromegaly. A somatostatin analogue is not currently available for routine clinical use but may be approved for this disorder by mid-1990.

coids perioperatively, and endogenous glucocorticoid production is assessed before dismissal; the typical hospital stay is 5 days. The mortality is approximately 0.4 per cent. The cure rate after trans-sphenoidal surgery is approximately 80 per cent for microadenomas and 30 per cent for macroadenomas. The recurrence rate after apparent surgical cure is less than 10 per cent.

In many patients with GH-secreting macroadenomas, trans-sphenoidal surgery is primarily a debulking procedure before radiation therapy. Radiation therapy is indicated if biochemical evidence of acromegaly persists postoperatively, and it is usually initiated 1 to 3 months postoperatively (Figure 1).

The transcranial surgical approach occasionally is necessary for debulking a massive macroadenoma with marked suprasellar extension. This approach is associated with a longer hospital stay and increased morbidity.

Surgical removal of an ectopic GHRH-producing neoplasm usually results in return of the blood GH level to normal and regression of acromegaly.

Radiation Therapy

When conventional radiation therapy, administered with a linear accelerator (4500 to 5000 cGy given over a period of 6 weeks), is used as the initial treatment, GH levels of less than 5 micrograms per liter are found in 20 per cent of patients at 2 years, in 40 per cent by 5 years,

and in 70 per cent by 10 years. Unfortunately, the irradiation affects the normal pituitary cells as well as the adenomatous tissue. Various degrees of hypopituitarism (e.g., hypogonadism, hypothyroidism, and secondary adrenal insufficiency) are present in at least 50 per cent of the patients 10 years after irradiation. Other potential side effects include damage to the optic nerves, brain necrosis, and radiation-induced neoplasia.

Use of heavy particle radiation from a cyclotron (available at only a few centers in the United States) gives results comparable to those of conventional radiation therapy, with a similar side effect profile.

Because of the temporal lag between the treatment and the return of GH and SmC levels to normal and the high incidence of hypopituitarism, radiation therapy should be considered to be adjunctive and reserved for patients with persistently high GH levels after trans-sphenoidal surgery.

Medical Therapy

Dopamine agonists have been found to be partially effective in the treatment of acromegaly. Approximately 70 per cent of patients respond to bromocriptine (Parlodel), a lysergic acid derivative of ergoline, with some decrease in the basal GH level. However, in only approximately 15 per cent of the patients does the GH level become normal with this treatment. The best responders are patients with pituitary tumors that secrete both GH and prolactin. The usual effective dose of bromocriptine, available as a 2.5-mg tablet or a 5-mg capsule, is 20 to 40 mg daily given in three or four doses. Treatment is begun with one-half of a 2.5-mg tablet taken with food at bedtime. The daily dose is increased by one-half tablet every week until the blood GH level becomes normal. Most patients develop a tolerance to the early side effects—postural lightheadedness and nausea. Less common side effects include constipation, headache, fatigue, and nasal congestion. Bromocriptine should not be taken during pregnancy. It does not decrease the size of the GH-secreting pituitary adenoma. Therefore, this form of treatment is partially effective, not curative, and should be reserved for adjunctive therapy for patients who are not cured by surgery or irradiation.

An analogue of somatostatin (SMS-201-995 [Octreotide], Sandoz) may be an addition to our armamentarium of pharmacologic agents in the near future. This drug is still investigational and not available for general use. When given subcutaneously three times per day, SMS 201-995 is effective in bringing GH and SmC levels to normal. Decreased pituitary tumor size, documented by computed tomography, during treatment with SMS 201-995, has been reported. If the results from a multicenter trial to be completed by mid-1990 show SMS 201-995 to be an effective adjunctive treatment, it will be indicated for patients who are not cured by operation and are waiting for the postoperative radiation therapy to be effective.

MONITORING OF TREATMENT RESULTS

The immediate postoperative serum GH level predicts the degree of cure. Frequently, after complete removal of a GH-secreting pituitary adenoma but before dismissal from the hospital, patients note that their fingers feel less stiff and that the hyperhidrosis has disappeared. The GH response to an oral glucose load and the SmC level 6 weeks postoperatively determine whether the patient may be considered to have a short-term cure. Screening for the status of other pituitary hormones is done at this time (e.g., blood analyses for cortisol, thyroxine, testosterone, or estradiol, and urinalysis for fasting-state osmolality). These studies and visual field examination by quantitative perimetry are repeated 3 and 12 months postoperatively. Computed imaging of the pituitary is done 12 months after the operation for microadenomas and at 3 and 12 months for macroadenomas.

If all studies give normal results 1 year post-operatively, a long-term cure is probable; an annual general medical examination, measurement of basal GH and SmC values, and a visual field examination are needed. Steroid coverage for stress is indicated for 1 year postoperatively, regardless of glucocorticoid levels.

If glucocorticoid or posterior pituitary insufficiency is identified, these patients should carry identification indicating that they need additional corticosteroids or vasopressin in the event of an accident or serious illness. A bracelet or necklace may be obtained from the Medic Alert Foundation.

After successful surgical treatment, there is a marked regression of the soft tissue excess but the bone changes are permanent. After the soft tissue changes have stabilized, combined oral and plastic surgery may be indicated (e.g., mandibular osteotomies, recessing the supraorbital ridges, rhinoplasties, and reducing the size of the tongue). Disabling hypertrophic osteoarthropathy of the hip may require total hip replacement.

The annual follow-up program for patients who have radiation therapy includes assessing the GH response to an oral glucose load, determination of the SmC level, computed tomography imaging of the sella, visual field examination, and surveillance for anterior and posterior pituitary insufficiency. If pituitary target gland deficiencies are identified, the secondary nature of these deficiencies should be confirmed and replacement therapy should be started (see Hypopituitarism chapter). In the interval before the radiation therapy affects the autonomous GH secretion, pharmacologic therapy is begun and is continued if found to be effective. The pharmacologic agent is then withdrawn for 4 weeks annually to see if the radiation therapy returned the GH and SmC values to normal; if not, the pharmacologic treatment is continued for another year.

ASSOCIATED CONDITIONS

A GH-secreting pituitary tumor may be part of multiple endocrine neoplasia type I (pituitary tumor, pancreatic tumor, and primary hyperparathyroidism). Hypertension and impaired glucose tolerance are commonly associated with acromegaly and are frequently relieved or cured with effective treatment. Acromegaly is associated with an increased incidence of neoplastic lesions (e.g., adenomatous colonic polyps and carcinoma), and these patients should have periodic general medical examinations.

ADRENOCORTICAL INSUFFICIENCY

method of
JULIUS SAGEL, M.D.

Medical University of South Carolina and
Medical Service, Veterans Administration
Medical Center
Charleston, South Carolina

Adrenal insufficiency results from either primary disease of the adrenal gland (Addison's disease) or deficiency of adrenocorticotropic hormone (ACTH) secondary to hypothalamic or pituitary disease.

Autoimmune adrenal destruction is now the most common cause of Addison's disease in the United States. This is frequently associated with one of two polyglandular autoimmune (PGA) syndromes that result in multiple endocrine deficiencies. PGA Type 1, also known as the candidiasis endocrinopathy syndrome, usually occurs before the age of 15 years. In addition to adrenal insufficiency, hypoparathyroidism and chronic mucocutaneous candidiasis occur. PGA Type 2 (Schmidt's syndrome), which is characterized by Addison's disease, autoimmune thyroid disease, and insulin-dependent diabetes mellitus, is more fequent in adults. Because failure of one endocrine gland in the PGA syndromes is often associated with or followed by deficiency of other glands, and because hormonal replacement therapy may be influenced by the function of another gland, evaluation of all endocrine glands should be considered when failure of one is recognized.

Other causes of primary adrenal failure include tuberculosis, fungal disease (in particular histoplasmosis, blastomycosis, and coccidioidomycosis), sarcoidosis, amyloidosis, hemochromatosis, adrenal hemorrhage, and bilateral adrenalectomy. Recently, the association of the acquired immunodeficiency syndrome with adrenal insufficiency has been reported. This may be the result of adrenal destruction caused by involvement of the adrenal gland by cytomegalovirus, *Mycobacterium avium-intracellulare*, or metastatic Kaposi's sarcoma. Several drugs can alter steroidogenesis or the metabolism of glucocorticoids (see later discussion).

Secondary adrenal insufficiency (ACTH deficiency) frequently follows withdrawal of glucocorticoid therapy if therapy has been continued long enough to produce sustained suppression of the hypothalamic-pituitary-adrenal axis. Other causes of secondary insufficiency include pituitary tumors, as well as infiltrating diseases and vascular events in the hypothalamus or pituitary.

CLINICAL PRESENTATION

The clinical features of both primary and secondary adrenal insufficiency may be nonspecific and in the unstressed patient tend to be subtle. These features include anorexia, nausea, vomiting, diarrhea, and abdominal pain. Hyperpigmentation accompanies Addison's disease but is not a feature of secondary insufficiency.

Any intercurrent stress, such as infection, trauma, or surgery, may precipitate an adrenal crisis if increased glucocorticoid is not administered to a patient with adrenal insufficiency. This crisis is manifested by weakness, hypotension, and fever and may be fatal if not treated promptly.

All three zones of the adrenal cortex are involved in diseases that produce primary adrenal insufficiency. As a result, there is deficiency of cortisol, aldosterone, and adrenal androgen. In contrast, secondary adrenal insufficiency spares the zona glomerulosa, which is mainly under the control of the renin-angiotensin system. Hence, aldosterone secretion is not significantly deficient, as is secretion of cortisol and adrenal androgen.

In primary adrenal failure, the laboratory findings include the features of mineralocorticoid deficiency, namely, hyponatremia, hyperkalemia (not present with severe vomiting or diarrhea), and hyperchloremic metabolic acidosis. These findings are usually not observed in secondary adrenal insufficiency. The blood urea nitrogen and serum creatinine concentrations are often elevated because of volume depletion and reduced glomerular filtration. Hypoglycemia, particularly in the setting of shock, should suggest adrenal crisis.

A screening test for adrenal insufficiency can be performed by administering 0.25 mg of synthetic ACTH (Cortrosyn: 1–24 amino acid sequence of human [1–39] ACTH) intramuscularly or intravenously and measuring the serum cortisol response at baseline and at 30 and 60 minutes. A normal response (a maximal post-ACTH cortisol value of more than 20 micrograms per dl with an increment of at least 6 micrograms per dl) excludes the diagnosis of Addison's disease (primary adrenal failure). However, a blunted or deficient response is found in either Addison's disease or secondary hypoadrenalism. Confirmation of end-organ insufficiency can be obtained by demonstrating an inadequate response after a prolonged ACTH infusion test consisting of an 8-hour infusion for 3 consecutive days.

In addition, an important part of the diagnostic work-up is the determination of the cause of Addison's disease.

TREATMENT

As with all endocrinopathies, the objective is to replace the deficient hormone in a physiologic fashion during normal phases as well as during intercurrent illnesses. The normal cortisol secretion rate under basal conditions averages 12 mg per M² of body surface area per day, or 20 to 25 mg per day.

Hormonal Replacement. The replacement glucocorticoid dose in a nonstressed patient with hypoadrenalism is 20 mg of cortisol in the morning and 10 mg in the evening. Synthetic glucocorticoids in biologically equivalent doses, such as 5 and 2.5 mg of prednisone, may be substituted. Although this replacement attempts to simulate the normal circadian pattern of cortisol secretion, it does not reproduce the continuous and pulsatile endogenous secretion. Glucocorticoids with a long half-life, such as dexamethasone, do not mimic this rhythm and should not be used.

Adjustment of the replacement glucocorticoid dose under nonstressed conditions may be necessary under the following circumstances:

1. The patient is taking drugs that increase the metabolism of glucocorticoids, thus requiring an increase in the replacement dosage. These drugs include phenobarbital, diphenylhydantoin, and rifampin; the last may be given for tuberculosis of various organ systems, including the adrenal system. Rifampin accelerates catabolism of cortisol by inducing hepatic microsomal enzymes and can precipitate adrenal crisis in patients with partial hypoadrenalism.

2. Patients with hepatic disease may need a reduced dose because the liver is important in the metabolism of glucocorticoids.

3. Although replacement doses are usually constant over a wide range of body sizes, the large individual may require a higher dose.

4. Both the production and the catabolism of several hormones, including cortisol, are reduced in the elderly. Therefore, it is appropriate to prescribe a slightly lower dose of glucocorticoid for geriatric patients.

5. The presence of associated endocrinopathies may have an impact on glucocorticoid therapy. This is particularly relevant in patients with PGA Types 1 and 2, as well as in those with hypopituitarism. Diabetes mellitus may be "brittle" and difficult to control in an addisonian patient before glucocorticoid replacement therapy is given. Thyroid and adrenal failures may also coexist in hypothalamic or pituitary disease (hypopituitarism) and when primary thyroid and adrenal failures occur in Schmidt's syndrome (PGA Type 2). These patients may present principally with features suggesting hypothyroidism. In these patients, thyroid hormone replacement may precipitate an adrenal crisis by increasing the metabolic clearance rate of the small residual cortisol secretion. In such patients, replacement glucocorticoid therapy should be instituted before initiating thyroid hormone therapy.

The adequacy of glucocorticoid replacement in adrenal insufficiency is monitored clinically. It may be associated with a decrease in pigmentation in primary adrenal insufficiency. Monitoring ACTH levels during replacement is not generally useful in Addison's disease.

Most patients with Addison's disease (as opposed to pituitary insufficiency) require mineralocorticoid replacement. A synthetic mineralocorticoid, fludrocortisone acetate (Florinef), is presecribed in a dose of 0.05 to 0.1 mg per day. The dose is adjusted according to the blood pressure response (particularly when standing), body weight, presence of edema, and maintenance of normal electrolyte levels (particularly potassium).

Dietary Adjustment. All patients with Addison's disease should have a sodium intake of at least 150 mEq per day. This amount should be supplemented in the presence of diarrhea or profuse sweating.

Patients with secondary hypoadrenalism do not usually require mineralocorticoid replacement. The minor abnormalities in aldosterone secretion in these patients are usually compensated for by sufficient dietary sodium intake.

Patient Education. It is important for patients with hypoadrenalism to carry identification indicating their diagnosis to ensure appropriate adjustment of the dose of glucocorticoid in the face of any intercurrent illness and stress. Parenteral therapy is often necessary with vomiting. Patients should also be informed that elective surgical procedures require adjustment of their steroid dosage.

Treatment of the Underlying Cause. The underlying cause of the condition, such as tuberculosis or fungal infection causing Addison's disease, or the hypothalamic or pituitary lesion in patients with secondary hypoadrenalism, needs specific treatment.

TREATMENT OF ACUTE ADRENAL INSUFFICIENCY (ADRENAL CRISIS)

The features of adrenal crisis include fatigue, weakness, fever, hypotension, and, in some cases, hypoglycemia. This medical emergency may be precipitated in a patient with hypoadrenalism under the following circumstances:

1. Acute intercurrent medical illnesses.

2. An elective surgical procedure in the presence of unexpected hypoadrenalism.

3. Treatment with ketoconazole for fungal disease (e.g., blastomycosis of the adrenal gland). This imidazole derivative, in high doses, is able to suppress steroidogenesis by inhibiting cytochrome P-450–dependent enzymes involved in steroid synthesis. Similarly, metyrapone, an in-

hibitor of 11-hydroxylase, is contraindicated in patients with suspected Addison's disease.

The diagnosis of adrenal crisis is initially clinical, requiring the immediate initiation of treatment before the result of a plasma cortisol level determination is available. If the cortisol level is inappropriately low for the level of stress (e.g., less than 10 micrograms per dl), a confirmatory test can be done at a later date when the patient is receiving maintenance therapy. At this stage, the patient is changed to dexamethasone, which is a potent synthetic steroid that does not interfere with cortisol measurements, and an ACTH stimulation test is performed.

The steps involved in the therapy of acute adrenal crisis are as follows:

1. *Glucocorticoid replacement.* It is important to emphasize that during major stress the cortisol secretion rate of the normal adrenal gland is increased by approximately fifteen- to twentyfold. Hence the maximum secretion is between 300 and 400 mg per day. Therefore, therapy consists of administering hydrocortisone parenterally as a water-soluble sodium succinate or phosphate ester preparation. The patient is given a 100-mg intravenous bolus followed by 100 mg every 8 hours as a continuous intravenous infusion. Intramuscular cortisone acetate should not be used because this form is insoluble and irregularly absorbed, particularly in hypotensive patients. It is generally not necessary, even in patients with Addison's disease (primary adrenal failure), to administer mineralocorticoid because a dose of hydrocortisone in excess of 75 mg per day provides an adequate mineralocorticoid effect. However, a parenteral mineralocorticoid, desoxycorticosterone acetate, is available if needed.

2. *Replacement of fluids and electrolytes.* Initially, intravenous normal saline should be given in an amount determined by the degree of extracellular volume depletion. In addition, intravenous glucose should be administered because of the predisposition to hypoglycemia caused by inadequate hepatic gluconeogenesis. Serum glucose concentrations should be monitored throughout therapy. The hyperkalemia accompanying addisonian crisis usually responds to volume expansion and hormonal therapy.

3. *Treatment of precipitating factors.* These factors were mentioned earlier and include the use of antibiotics for sepsis, as well as the elimination of medications that may have precipitated the crisis.

THERAPY OF STRESS (INCLUDING COVERAGE FOR SURGERY) IN ADRENAL INSUFFICIENCY

Under normal circumstances, mild stresses such as a minor surgical procedure or an influenza-like illness are accompanied by a two- to fourfold increase in cortisol secretion. Therefore, with a mild viral syndrome and fever, the physician should immediately increase the glucocorticoid dose by two- or threefold. The temperature of the patient should be monitored. A temperature above 39° C signals a need for increased glucocorticoids, whereas a normal temperature is an indication to reduce the steroid dosage. If, during the acute illness, the temperature remains between 38° and 39° C, the dose should be considered to be appropriate.

With more severe stress, such as major surgery, the cortisol secretion rate normally increases approximately fifteenfold above the basal rate, with elevated levels persisting for up to 3 days after surgery. Glucocorticoid therapy is started the day before or hours before the surgical event because there is a slight delay in the effect after administration. This may be in the form of either 100 mg cortisone acetate intramuscularly the night before or a continuous infusion of 100 mg hydrocortisone sodium succinate intravenously through the night before. After surgery the patient should receive hydrocortisone sodium succinate (100 mg) every 8 hours by continuous infusion until stable postoperatively. During the next few days there is a rapid reduction in the dose by 50 per cent on a daily basis, so that on the fourth postoperative day the patient is receiving maintenance therapy. This protocol should be modified in the face of postoperative complications such as infection or hemorrhage.

SELECTIVE OR ISOLATED HYPOALDOSTERONISM

Selective aldosterone deficiency is most commonly seen in the setting of hyporeninemic hypoaldosteronism, the clinical features of which are nonspecific. The diagnosis is generally made from laboratory features, which consist of hyperkalemia in the presence of mild renal insufficiency (a creatinine clearance rate higher than 20 ml per minute) and hyperchloremic metabolic acidosis. Further investigation reveals subnormal renin and aldosterone responses to provocative stimuli (posture or volume depletion) in the face of normal cortisol secretion.

This condition is seen most frequently in patients with renal disease caused by diabetes mellitus, gout, lead, analgesic abuse, obstructive uropathy, and pyelonephritis.

Treatment. Treatment is usually needed to control the metabolic abnormalities. Mineralocorticoid administration tends to improve both the hyperkalemia and the hyperchloremic metabolic acidosis. However, the dose of fludrocortisone acetate needed is often high, frequently 0.2 mg per day. The reason for the increased dosage compared with that required in Addison's disease is thought to be the presence of renal disease which limits the response to the mineralocorticoid. Caution should be exercised in the patient with hypertension or compromised cardiac function. Fludrocortisone acetate therapy may further elevate blood pressure or precipitate congestive cardiac failure. Similar complications may be encountered with the use of sodium bicarbonate or potassium-binding exchange resins, which might be used in selected cases. Diuretic therapy such as furosemide, which increases net acid excretion, might be used alone or in combination with fludrocortisone acetate, particularly if the latter produces excess salt and water retention.

CONGENITAL ADRENAL HYPERPLASIA

Congenital adrenal hyperplasia results from deficiency of one of several enzymes necessary for adrenal steroidogenesis. With the reduction in cortisol concentration, the ACTH level increases, stimulating synthetic pathways proximal to the enzyme defect and causing an accumulation of precursor steroids. Other pathways in the adrenal glands that are not blocked are also driven by the elevated ACTH level.

A deficiency of 21-hydroxylase, which is involved in secretion of both aldosterone and cortisol, is the most common enzyme deficiency. When it is severe, the chemical changes resemble those of Addison's disease, and acute adrenal insufficiency may occur. In another form, the simple virilizing variety, the enzyme block involves only the zona fasciculata or glucocorticoid pathway. Manifestations differ depending on the age of onset and the severity of the enzyme deficiency.

Treatment. The therapy is similar to that of primary adrenal failure, except that higher glucocorticoid doses may be needed initially to suppress ACTH and reduce the excess production of adrenal androgens. The adequacy of therapy can be monitored by measuring serum 17-hydroxyprogesterone levels. A patient with this condition should always be evaluated and treated by an endocrinologist with experience in this disorder. Inadequate treatment can result in inappropriate sexual development and early skeletal maturation with fusion of the epiphyses and stunted growth. Optimal therapy should be achieved without evidence of glucocorticoid excess.

The second most common enzyme deficiency is that of the 11-hydroxylase enzyme, which is accompanied by hypertension. This condition requires therapy with cortisol without mineralocorticoid replacement.

CUSHING'S SYNDROME

method of
PAUL C. CARPENTER, M.D.
Mayo Clinic and Mayo Medical School
Rochester, Minnesota

Cushing's syndrome is caused by prolonged exposure to excessive exogenous or endogenous glucocorticoid hormones. This can result from exogenous administration of adrenocorticotropic hormone (ACTH) or glucocorticoids, or from endogenous increased secretion of cortisol, ACTH, or corticotropin-releasing hormone (CRH).

ACTH-dependent Cushing's syndrome, which accounts for 85 per cent of endogenous cases, is caused by excessive pituitary ACTH secretion (80 per cent) and ectopic ACTH or CRH secretion (20 per cent) from nonpituitary neoplasms. The pituitary ACTH-dependent form is designated Cushing's disease. ACTH-independent Cushing's syndrome is caused by benign or malignant adrenocortical neoplasms in most instances. A minority of cases are caused by ACTH-independent micro- or macronodular adrenocortical disease in which the adrenals contain multiple small, autonomous, cortisol-secreting adenomas. This form can be a familial disease.

"Pseudo-Cushing's syndrome" is a term used to describe the mild hypercortisolism seen in alcoholic or depressed patients that resolves with elimination of depression or abstinence from alcohol.

DIAGNOSTIC STRATEGY

Appropriate treatment of Cushing's syndrome relies on accurate diagnosis. The majority of cases can be precisely diagnosed by combining clinical and laboratory assessments. However, in some cases of ACTH-dependent Cushing's syndrome, the differential diagnosis is challenging.

All forms of endogenous Cushing's syndrome have in common increased secretion of cortisol. The first step in diagnosis is the establishment of hypercortisolism. The single best laboratory test for this purpose is measurement of the urinary free cortisol level, preferably with a chromatograph-purified assay. Virtually all patients with Cushing's syndrome have increased urinary cortisol excretion. Measurement of urinary 17-ketogenic or 17-hydroxysteroid excretion, corrected for daily creatinine excretion, is useful but has more false-negative results than measurement of urine free cortisol. Plasma cortisol determinations have limited precision because of the wide normal range and the pulsatile nature of cortisol production. The highest precision is found in late afternoon measurements.

When hypercortisolism has been demonstrated, tests are done to establish the diagnosis of Cushing's syndrome and the differential diagnosis. These tests include (1) static and dynamic tests to determine the condition of the pituitary-adrenal axis and (2) imaging techniques to find pituitary neoplasms, define adrenal shape and size, and search for ectopic ACTH- or CRH-secreting neoplasms.

A diagnostic algorithm is used to establish the cause of Cushing's syndrome. The major components of biologic diagnostic testing have existed for more than 20 years and include low-dose dexamethasone, high-dose dexamethasone, and metyrapone testing. More recently, CRH stimulation testing and petrosal venous sampling for ACTH levels have been added to improve diagnostic precision. Advances in computed tomography and magnetic resonance imaging have improved the ability to detect neoplasms in adrenal and pituitary glands.

TREATMENT

Surgical Therapy

The primary definitive therapy of the various forms of Cushing's syndrome currently is surgical. Trans-sphenoidal removal of pituitary microadenomas by experienced pituitary surgeons generally produces a remission in Cushing's disease (80 to 90 per cent) and minimizes the chance of recurrent disease (4 to 8 per cent). Failure to obtain remission generally results from the presence of invasive pituitary tumors or rare instances of anterior pituitary corticotroph hyperplasia. The potential for predicting recurrent Cushing's disease, using CRH stimulation testing after trans-sphenoidal surgery, is being studied.

Complete extirpation of adrenocortical neoplasms is the preferred therapy for ACTH-independent forms of Cushing's syndrome. Unilateral adrenalectomy, preferably from a posterior approach, cures benign adrenocortical adenomas causing Cushing's syndrome. An anterior abdominal surgical approach should be used when adrenocortical carcinoma is suspected. Unfortunately, many individuals with adrenocortical carcinoma as the origin of their Cushing's syndrome have distant metastatic spread of disease at the time of the original diagnosis. Bilateral adrenalectomy, by the flank or posterior approach, is used to manage ACTH-independent bilateral nodular adrenocortical hyperplasia.

Removal of the neoplastic tissue secreting CRH or ACTH eliminates the ectopic forms of Cushing's syndrome. However, as with adrenocortical malignancy, metastatic spread of the sources of ectopic peptides can make surgical cure untenable.

Radiation Therapy

As primary therapy, conventional x-rays or proton beams can be used to treat pituitary neoplasms or corticotroph hyperplasia causing Cushing's disease. These modalities produce approximately 40 and 70 per cent success rates, respectively. Remission rates are somewhat higher if radiation therapy is used adjunctively after failed trans-sphenoidal pituitary surgery. Disease remission using conventional x-ray therapy is also higher in children. Adrenocortical malignancies are generally radiation resistant, but there is some success in the palliation of bone pain from metastases. Radiation can be used as augmentive therapy in the treatment of some forms of ectopic ACTH-producing tumors.

Medical Therapy

Pharmacologic therapy of Cushing's syndrome has had limited use, but in some instances it can become an important component in the management of hypercortisolism. The agents used are of three types: (1) drugs that modify pituitary ACTH release; (2) agents that interfere with the production of adrenocortical hormones; and (3) drugs that modify the cellular effects of glucocorticoids (cortisol) or mineralocorticoids (aldosterone, deoxycorticosterone).

The various drugs to be cited should always be used under the supervision of an experienced physician because significant toxicity can occur with each. Several of these agents are considered to be investigational and are therefore used only under established research or therapeutic protocols. Many clinicians routinely administer small doses of dexamethasone (0.25 to 0.75 mg per day) when using these drugs to avoid clinical adrenocortical insufficiency if the drug therapy is highly effective.

Table 1 lists some of the drugs, both available and investigational, that are in the adjunctive management of Cushing's syndrome. The antiserotoninergic properties of cyproheptadine and the investigational drug metergoline appear to be the origin of the effect of these agents. Both have been used in the short- and long-term management of selected cases of Cushing's disease but with minimal success; even when successful, remissions have generally been incomplete. Cyproheptadine and metergoline have generally not been effective in altering secretion of ACTH from ectopic sources. Bromocriptine* may lower ACTH production from the pituitary in a few patients with Cushing's disease. It has been suggested that the pituitary neoplasm in these patients is derived from neural elements in the pars intermedia of the pituitary, as opposed to the much more common eosinophilic corticotroph adenomas of the anterior pituitary. This group of patients represents less than 10 per cent of all patients with Cushing's disease, which explains the limited utility of bromocriptine. On an investiga-

---

*This use is not listed by the manufacturer.

TABLE 1. **Drugs for Adjunctive Management of Cushing's Syndrome**

Drug	Daily Doses	Major Complications
Inhibit Pituitary ACTH Release		
Cyproheptadine	12–24 mg	Very limited yield; drowsiness; weight gain
Inhibit Cortisol Production		
Ketoconazole*	200–800 mg†	Liver toxicity; nausea; oligospermia
Mitotane (*o,p'*-DDD)	2–10 grams	Gastrointestinal disturbances (80%); central nervous system depression, somnolence, dizziness (30%); rash (15%)
Aminoglutethimide	1–2 grams	Drowsiness (35%); rash (16%); postural hypotension, dizziness (6%); headache (5%); hypothyroidism (5%)
Metyrapone	1–4 grams†	Hypokalemia; virilization; gastrointestinal disturbances
Inhibit Steroid Receptor		
RU-458*	10–20 mg/kg	Low yield; ? effect overridden by increased ACTH production in Cushing's disease

*These drugs should be considered to be investigational and require review by institutional human investigation resources.

†Drug dosages are higher than those conventionally recommended.

tional basis, somatostatin and some of the longer-acting somatostatin analogues have also been noted to diminish ACTH production in Cushing's disease after repeated subcutaneous administration. These agents are also under investigation for the adjunctive management of ectopic ACTH production. Rare cases of Cushing's disease may respond to reserpine treatment.

There has been much experience with drugs that interfere with adrenocortical steroid production and release. Metyrapone, aminoglutethimide, and ketoconazole diminish adrenocortical steroid production by interfering with one or more of the enzymatic steps involved in adrenocortical steroid biosynthesis. Mitotane (*o,p'*-DDD) is an adrenal cytolytic agent that inhibits adrenal steroid synthesis and destroys normal and neoplastic adrenocortical cells.

The best-tolerated of these drugs is ketoconazole, which is currently the most popular one for the management of hypercortisolism, particularly because it is relatively free of side effects. Individual sensitivity to ketoconazole varies widely, necessitating close monitoring of steroid production and dose adjustment. Substantial hepatic toxicity is noted particularly when high

doses are used. This effect is generally reversible when the dosage is lowered or the drug is discontinued.

Large doses of metyrapone can cause gastrointestinal upsets. Its major effect is the inhibition of 11-beta hydroxylation in the adrenal cortex. Diminished cortisol production is achieved at the expense of accumulation of androgenic cortical products, resulting in virilization in women, and excess deoxycorticosterone, resulting in hypertension and hypokalemia. Many patients with Cushing's disease respond to the diminished cortisol levels created by metyrapone with increased ACTH production, resulting in effective override of the competitive enzymatic blockade. This phenomenon is seen less often when aminoglutethimide, mitotane, or ketoconazole is used.

The primary problems with mitotane (Lysodren) use are gastrointestinal, manifested by anorexia, nausea, and vomiting. Rashes are common. Symptoms of depression, excessive somnolence, and lightheadedness occur in one-third of patients. The drug may affect the zona glomerulosa in the adrenal cortex, leading to mineralocorticoid deficiency that may require replacement with oral fludrocortisone in doses of 50 to 150 micrograms daily. Mitotane can be used as an adjunct to pituitary x-ray therapy because clinical and biochemical improvement can be delayed for several months after radiation therapy. The drug can be used in divided doses ranging from 1 to 4 grams daily to gain more rapid control of the hypercortisolism. The dose can be diminished as the effects of pituitary irradiation become more prominent with the passage of time.

Aminoglutethimide (Cytadren) also has significant gastrointestinal side effects. For many patients, however, the most bothersome side effects are significant lethargy and sedation. Aminoglutethimide has the peculiar side effect of causing hypothyroidism in a small number of patients. A maculopapular rash is often seen during the first 2 weeks of therapy, but it generally resolves despite continuation of treatment. Similar problems were observed with the use of trilostane when it was under investigation.

There has been a long search for agents that specifically interfere with the glucocorticoid effect on target cells. The focus has been predominantly on drugs that block the cortisol receptor. Most of those developed in the past had limited success and were abandoned. Currently, RU-468 is being used in some clinical trials of hypercortisolism in children and adults, with limited success. Modification of the steroid-receptor complex interaction with nuclear protein is another area of research.

Many individuals with severe hypercortisolemia, particularly those with adrenocortical malignancy or ectopic ACTH syndrome, may have substantial hypertension and severe hypokalemia as a result of overproduction of mineralocorticoid in the form of deoxycorticosterone, aldosterone, or even cortisol. Spironolactone (Aldactone) interferes with the renal mineralocorticoid effect, and its use is often necessary and efficacious. In addition, spironolactone is known to block androgen receptors partially in various tissues. It also diminishes the skin oiliness, acne, and hirsutism that occur in Cushing's syndrome, accompanied by androgen excesses. Most individuals require 100 to 200 mg per day to achieve significant benefit, and as much as 400 mg per day in divided doses may be necessary. In severe cases, potassium supplementation may still be used, but the need for it is markedly diminished when spironolactone is used.

All of the preceding agents are used in the various forms of Cushing's syndrome predominantly as adjunctive or temporizing therapy. In some instances, the drugs that diminish steroid production, either by interfering with ACTH or by their direct adrenocortical effect, are used to try to improve the patient's condition before surgery. They are also used on a short-term basis while awaiting the effects of pituitary irradiation in Cushing's disease. In inoperable adrenocortical carcinoma with Cushing's syndrome, mitotane is the only drug shown to have relatively consistent antitumor effects, but even then it does not significantly alter the long-term prognosis of this malignancy. Its use for 6 to 12 months in all patients after resection of adrenocortical malignancy is currently being investigated, even in those with no apparent residual disease, in an attempt to alter the poor long-term prognosis in those cases that initially seem to be apparent cures. Recent reports suggest that cisplatin may offer therapeutic benefit for inoperable adrenocortical carcinoma.

In some cases of Cushing's syndrome, combined therapy using adrenolytic agents and steroidogenic enzyme inhibitors may be of benefit, but to date, no results of long-term clinical trials have been reported. Because metyrapone, mitotane, and aminoglutethimide inhibit different steroidogenic enzymes and have different side effects, combinations using low doses of these drugs may lead to effective therapy with diminished side effects as a result of the lesser doses.

Therapeutic Goals

The goal of therapy in Cushing's syndrome, similar to the goal in other therapeutic endeavors, is to treat the patient with modalities that involve minimal risk, obtain complete remission from the hypercortisolism or other steroid excesses, and ideally allow the patient to lead a medication-free life. Selective trans-sphenoidal adenomectomy for Cushing's syndrome generally yields these results. After pituitary surgery, patients are ACTH deficient, presumably because of the hypercortisolism's suppressing normal CRF production and perhaps directly inhibiting normal anterior pituitary corticotroph function. These patients require glucocorticoid but not mineralocorticoid replacement. Intraoperatively and during the first 2 or 3 postoperative days, parenteral glucocorticoid is given at a rate of approximately 100 mg per M^2 per day of hydrocortisone or an equivalent water-soluble steroid. This agent can be given by continuous intravenous infusion or by intramuscular injection every 12 hours. We routinely use prednisolone sodium phosphate (Hydeltrasol) perioperatively, giving 40 mg parenterally every 12 hours on the day of surgery. The dose is tapered rapidly over 2 or 3 days by halving the dose daily and then starting oral replacement with hydrocortisone or cortisone (12 to 15 mg per M^2 per day) or prednisone (5 mg per M^2 per day) in divided doses. This regimen is maintained for 1 month, and then tapering begins. The dose can be diminished by discontinuing the lower evening doses of glucocorticoid replacement for 1 or 2 months and then tapering the morning doses, or the daily doses can be doubled but given on an every-other-day basis for 1 or 2 months. Recovery of the pituitary-adrenal axis can be monitored by measuring the morning plasma cortisol level before administering morning steroid doses or by monitoring the response to a short ACTH stimulation test (Cortrosyn, 250 micrograms intramuscularly, with cortisol measurements at 0 and 60 minutes). If the response to stimulation is normal (doubling of plasma cortisol levels or absolute values above 20 micrograms per dl), replacement steroid therapy can be discontinued in most instances. If suboptimal plasma levels are noted or there is insufficient ACTH stimulation, steroid therapy can be continued for another 1 or 2 months and testing repeated. In our experience, the majority of patients are able to stop glucocorticoid replacement therapy in 3 or 4 months, but some require therapy for as long as 1 year. During recovery time, stress illnesses should be treated by doubling the daily dose of glucocorticoid, and severe stresses such as major trauma, substantial body burns, or surgery with general anesthesia should be covered with parenteral steroid injections at 4 to 10 times daily replacement levels. After extirpation of unilateral benign, cortisol-secreting adenomas, a similar tapering glucocorticoid schedule and testing can be used.

In cases of ectopic ACTH or CRH production causing Cushing's syndrome, complete surgical extirpation of the neoplasm is the preferred therapy. If the tumor is completely removed, the patient generally undergoes prompt remission of Cushing's syndrome or returns to good health. Again, glucocorticoid replacement therapy on a tapering schedule is necessary for several weeks to months after surgical curative therapy. Replacement mineralocorticoid therapy is not necessary. When faced with the problem of incompletely resectable tumor, one must choose from among a variety of adjunctive therapies. Pharmacologic therapy, noted earlier, can be used to control hypercortisolism, mineralocorticoid excess, or androgen excess. Embolization of residual tumor, particularly hepatic metastases, has also been used to diminish ectopic peptide production. Intraoperative focal radiation therapy and direct organ infusion chemotherapy are other options for some neoplasms. When laboratory evaluation indicates the diagnosis of ectopic ACTH syndrome and no tumor is found with imaging or localization techniques, the patient is periodically re-evaluated, with attempts to find the source of the occult tumor. If cortisol overproduction causes significant Cushing's syndrome, bilateral adrenalectomy can be considered. Adrenalectomy is also warranted when long-term survival is anticipated in unresectable malignancies causing ectopic ACTH syndrome.

DIABETES INSIPIDUS

method of
DIANE K. JORKASKY, M.D.
University of Pennsylvania School of Medicine
Philadelphia, Pennsylvania

DIAGNOSIS

Diabetes insipidus (DI) results in the formation of a dilute urine and presents clinically as polyuria. It can be categorized as either central or nephrogenic. The partial or complete failure of antidiuretic hormone (ADH) secretion from the posterior pituitary in central DI occurs in the majority of patients because of head trauma, neoplasms in the central nervous system, hypophysectomy, or hypoxic encephalopathy. Less frequent etiologies include granulomatous diseases (sarcoidosis, tuberculosis), meningitis, encephalitis, a rare inherited form of DI, and an idiopathic variety. Exogenous administration of ADH in both types of central DI results in enhanced renal concentration. Patients with partial central DI, however, maintain a modest ability to concentrate urine during water deprivation.

Although a congenital form exists, nephrogenic DI occurs most often as an acquired defect caused by a variety of renal diseases including chronic renal failure, chronic interstitial nephritis, medullary and polycystic diseases, obstructive uropathy, sickle cell disease and trait, amyloidosis, light chain nephropathy, and sarcoidosis. In nephrogenic DI, the renal tubules are unresponsive to ADH, and thus exogenous administration of ADH analogues does not result in enhanced renal concentrating ability. Certain other clinical states may temporarily impair this ability such as starvation, hypokalemia, and hypercalcemia. Drugs have also been implicated in the induction of nephrogenic DI: lithium carbonate (Lithobid), demeclocycline (Declomycin), amphotericin B, cisplatin, gentamycin (Garamycin), and methoxyflurane (Penthrane). The measurement of urine osmolality after a standard water dehydration test, followed by the subcutaneous administration of 5 units of aqueous vasopressin (Pitressin), should differentiate partial or complete central DI from nephrogenic DI.

TREATMENT

The cause and chronicity of the diabetes insipidus dictate the approach to management. Regardless of etiology, however, the patient who has a normal thirst mechanism and access to water should be able to maintain a relatively normal plasma osmolality and serum sodium concentration, albeit at the expense of polydipsia and polyuria. When chronic therapy is indicated, the options are outlined in Table 1. The actual dose of drug used for a specific patient should be tailored to the individual's urinary response because responses vary considerably among patients.

Central Diabetes Insipidus

The usual therapy of choice for acute central DI, like the therapy after hypophysectomy, is short-acting vasopressin injection given parenterally. The DI under these conditions may be transient, and the use of long-acting agents may result in water intoxication. In chronic central DI, vasopressin has no role, and the therapy of choice is intranasal desmopressin acetate (DDAVP) (see Table 1). It has virtually no vasopressor activity, is rarely allergenic, and is well tolerated. Headache, nasal congestion, and intestinal cramping occur on occasion. For patients intolerant of the intranasal formulation, DDAVP can be administered subcutaneously (or intravenously), but the equivalently effective parenteral dose is usually less than the intranasal dose. Vasopressin tannate in oil (Pitressin Tannate in Oil) has the advantage of a long duration of action (see Table 1), but it must be given as a deep intramuscular injection. The vials must be warmed and shaken vigorously before adminis-

TABLE 1. **Therapeutic Options in Chronic Diabetes Insipidus (Presented in Order of Preference)**

Indication	Agent	Usual Dose
Complete central DI	Desmopressin acetate (DDAVP)	2.5–20 μg by intranasal administration q 12–24 hr
	Vasopressin tannate in oil (Pitressin Tannate in Oil)	2–5 U intramuscularly q 24–48 hr
	Lysine-vasopressin (Diapid nasal spray)	Intranasal administration, 1 spray/nostril q 4–6 hr
Partial central DI	Chlorpropamide (Diabinese)*	250–1000 mg daily†
	Clofibrate (Atromid S)*	1–2 grams daily in 3–4 divided doses
	Carbamazepine (Tegretol)*	400–600 mg daily in 3–4 divided doses
Nephrogenic DI	Thiazide diuretics	25–100 mg daily (titrate according to diuretic response)

*Not approved for this use.
†This dose exceeds the manufacturer's recommended dose.

tration. As an alternative, lysine-vasopressin (Diapid nasal spray) can be administered intranasally, but its short duration of action requires frequent dosing. This agent has variable absorption from the nasal mucosa and may produce irritation and rhinorrhea.

Partial central DI, which accounts for more than one-half of all cases of central DI, has several therapeutic options. Small doses of DDAVP may be used intranasally, but an alternative approach to therapy is to enhance endogenous ADH release and action through the use of several pharmacologic agents: chlorpropamide* (Diabinese), clofibrate* (Atromid S), and carbamazepine* (Tegretol). A single drug may be used, although synergy has been reported with the combination of any two of these agents in low doses. The onset of antidiuretic action may take several weeks after starting the drug. Many adverse side effects, including hypoglycemia (chlorpropamide); nausea, diarrhea, and flu-like syndrome (clofibrate); and leukopenia, vertigo, and ataxia (carbamazepine), have limited the usefulness of these drugs.

Nephrogenic Diabetes Insipidus

Nephrogenic DI differs from central DI in that the kidney is unresponsive to endogenous ADH and thus to any exogenous analogue. Most patients require no intervention and can ingest water in response to an intact thirst mechanism. In acquired nephrogenic DI, electrolyte abnormalities should be corrected and offending drugs withdrawn if possible. For the patient who has excessive polyuria, a reduction in salt and protein intake may enhance proximal reabsorption of solutes and water in the kidney, reduce distal delivery, and attenuate the polyuria. By producing mild extracellular volume contraction, the

*See Table 1.

thiazide diuretics may be similarly useful as adjunctive therapy. Such management could result, however, in orthostatic hypotension and hypokalemia.

SIMPLE GOITER

method of
MARY KORYTOWSKI, M.D., and
DAVID S. COOPER, M.D.
*Johns Hopkins University School of Medicine
Baltimore, Maryland*

The term "goiter" refers to any visible or palpable enlargement of the thyroid gland. The enlargement may be diffuse or nodular (i.e., containing one or more nodules) and generally results from hyperplasia of thyroid follicular cells. Simple goiters are those goiters that have no clear etiology and are therefore justifiably also called idiopathic or sporadic goiters. Thyroid function in individuals with simple goiters is usually normal, although hyperthyroidism is occasionally seen (toxic nodular goiter or Plummer's disease).

The etiology of simple goiter (i.e., goiter occurring in a nonendemic goiter region) is far from clear. In the United States, iodine deficiency as a cause of goiter was eliminated with the introduction of iodized salt in the 1920s; however, the prevalence of goiter still varies from 0.4 to 7.2 per cent. Disorders of thyroid hormone biosynthesis account for only a very small percentage of goiters; such patients are usually identified in childhood and are often hypothyroid. As with other disorders of the thyroid gland, women are affected more frequently than men.

Numerous factors have been postulated in the etiology of simple goiter. These include genetic predisposition, an increased sensitivity of the thyroid gland to the growth-stimulating effects of thyroid-stimulating hormone (TSH), or cyclic periods of clinically undetectable thyroid hypofunction, with subsequent increases in TSH. Recently, thyroid growth-stimulating immunoglobulins have been identified in the sera from a large proportion of patients with simple goiters, suggesting that autoimmunity may be important. In some geographic areas, environmental pollutants may contribute to goiter development. Certain drugs, especially iodine-containing medications (e.g., amiodarone) and lithium, have been associated with goiter, particularly in individuals with underlying subclinical autoimmune thyroid disease. Not uncommonly, patients with a past history of head and neck irradiation will also develop the disease with a small diffuse or nodular goiter.

DIAGNOSIS

Any patient presenting with either a nodular or a diffuse goiter should have thyroid function tests performed, including serum thyroxine level determination, tri-iodothyronine (T_3) resin uptake (T_3RU), TSH level determination, and antithyroid antibodies; serum T_3 levels should be obtained if hyperthyroidism is suspected clinically. Radioisotope scanning is indicated to rule out the presence of a dominant hypofunctioning region, particularly if a nodule is enlarging or if there is a history of head and neck irradiation. Thyroid ultrasonography is not particularly useful in the evaluation of goiter.

The presence of antithyroid antibodies and/or an elevated serum TSH is evidence for autoimmune (Hashimoto's) thyroiditis. If a dominant cold area is noted on radioisotope scan, needle biopsy is indicated, especially if there is a history of rapid growth, compressive symptoms, or radiation exposure. While nodular goiters are not premalignant, malignancy can arise in a pre-existing goiter, making detection more difficult.

THERAPY

In treating the patient with a simple goiter, several factors need to be considered, including the age of the patient, the length of time the goiter has been present, the consistency of the goiter (diffuse or nodular), the patient's thyroid function, and whether there has been a recent increase in the size of the goiter.

Patients with a small diffuse goiter and normal thyroid function do not necessarily require treatment unless they find the presence of a goiter cosmetically unacceptable. If suppressive treatment with thyroid hormone is not initiated, patients are followed up initially at 6 months and then at yearly intervals to monitor the size of the thyroid gland and the potential development of nodules.

Long-term therapy with L-thyroxine (Synthroid, Levothroid) is the cornerstone of therapy for patients with simple goiters. The goal of treatment is to suppress the patient's endogenous TSH secretion and therefore to remove a potent stimulus for thyroid gland growth. In general, an L-thyroxine dose of 2 micrograms per kg is required to render circulating TSH undetectable; smaller doses should be used in the elderly. Regression of the size of the goiter occurs in about 60 per cent of patients. Some goiters, however, function independently of TSH and may continue to grow even though TSH secretion is completely inhibited. Regression in the size of the gland is dependent on (1) the size of the goiter at the initiation of treatment, with large goiters showing less response, and (2) the duration of treatment, with greater regression occurring with longer treatment. A lack of response is usually due to the presence of cysts, fibrosis, and calcifications within long-standing goiters as well as the presence of foci of autonomous function. Continued growth despite suppressive therapy is an indication for biopsy or surgery because of the concern about malignancy.

In patients with one or more autonomously functioning thyroid nodules, L-thyroxine therapy may cause iatrogenic thyrotoxicosis due to continued function of the nonsuppressible nodular tissue. Because of the possibility of autonomous function within a goiter, caution must be used in starting therapy with L-thyroxine, especially in individuals older than 60 years of age or those with a history of cardiovascular disease. Iatrogenic thyrotoxicosis can be minimized by seeing the patient 4 weeks after the initiation of treatment for repeat thyroid function studies and by starting elderly and cardiac patients on low doses of L-thyroxine. Thyroid scanning *while the patient is taking L-thyroxine* is the best way to document the presence of autonomously functioning nodules (suppression scanning). Patients with autonomous nodules can also develop hyperthyroidism when exposed to iodide-containing medications and contrast media (jodbasedow phenomenon). These compounds should be avoided in individuals with nodular goiters.

Surgical management of simple goiter becomes necessary when the goiter is unresponsive to thyroid hormone therapy and/or becomes large enough to cause local pressure symptoms, such as shortness of breath, wheezing, dysphagia, or hoarseness, or if there is concern about malignancy. Some patients with large asymptomatic goiters may choose surgical management as the initial therapy for cosmetic reasons. Postoperative thyroid hormone is then prescribed to prevent recurrence of the goiter.

HYPERPARATHYROIDISM AND HYPOPARATHYROIDISM

method of
MARK S. NANES, M.D., PH.D., and
BAYARD D. CATHERWOOD, M.D.
Emory University School of Medicine and VA Medical Center
Decatur, Georgia

CALCIUM HOMEOSTASIS

The parathyroid glands maintain a normal concentration of calcium in blood (8.5 to 10.5 mg per dl) by influencing three tissues: bone, kidney, and intestine. Because 55 per cent of blood calcium is protein bound, mostly to albumin, total serum calcium should be interpreted after adjusting the serum calcium level plus 0.85 mg per dl for each gram per dl of albumin outside the median normal value. Parathyroid hormone (PTH) increases the blood calcium concentration by stimulating bone resorption, renal calcium reabsorption, and renal production of 1,25-dihydroxyvitamin D_3 (1,25-$(OH)_2D_3$). PTH also stimulates renal phosphate excretion. PTH effects on intestinal calcium absorption are mediated by the action of 1,25-$(OH)_2D_3$ on duodenal calcium transport. A negative feedback loop formed by blood ionized calcium inhibition of PTH in the blood maintains calcium homeostasis. The consequences of excessive secretion of PTH are hypercalcemia, hypercalciuria, and associated neurologic, renal, and skeletal complications. Inadequate secretion of PTH results in hypocalcemic paresthesias, muscle cramps, cataracts, and tetany.

PRIMARY HYPERPARATHYROIDISM

Diagnosis

Primary hyperparathyroidism is a disorder of excessive production of PTH characterized by hypercalcemia. The prevalence of primary hyperparathyroidism is estimated at 100 to 250 per 100,000 population. The median age of onset is in the fifth decade. The PTH level is elevated in plasma as a normal response to hypocalcemia (secondary hyperparathyroidism) in vitamin D deficiency, vitamin D resistance, and renal failure, conditions best treated by correcting the primary defect. In some patients with renal failure, chronic stimulation of parathyroid secretion results in parathyroid hyperplasia and hypercalcemia (tertiary hyperparathyroidism).

The diagnosis of primary hyperparathyroidism is made by demonstrating elevated plasma PTH levels in the presence of hypercalcemia. In some patients, the serum calcium level may be elevated sporadically. For these patients, three sets of data collected over 1 week increase confidence in the diagnosis. Alternatively, the PTH level can be measured in plasma frozen immediately after collection and stored until the calcium value for that sample is known to be elevated. The normal range for PTH depends on the assay used because different antibodies cross-react differently with inactive PTH fragments. The prolonged half-life of mid–carboxy terminal fragments of PTH in patients with renal dysfunction falsely elevates the PTH value, making the diagnosis of hyperparathyroidism difficult. Immunoradiometric assays that are selective for intact PTH are more specific than the older radioimmunoassays and should be used if available. Measurement of the urinary cyclic adenosine monophosphate (UcAMP) level is a useful adjunct in the diagnosis of hyperparathyroidism because more than 50 per cent of UcAMP is derived from the action of PTH on proximal renal tubules. The creatinine level should be determined in the same urine sample as UcAMP, and in serum, so that UcAMP can be corrected for the glomerular filtration rate (normal range of UcAMP = 2 to 4 nM per dl of glomerular filtrate). The UcAMP level may be elevated in some forms of hypercalcemia of malignancy because PTH-related peptide, produced by these tumors, has amino terminal homology with PTH and binds to the PTH receptor. PTH levels are suppressed in patients with hypercalcemia of malignancy because PTH-related peptide does not cross-react with PTH in radioimmunoassays. False-positive elevations of PTH levels can occur in patients with malignancy because of renal dysfunction. Hyperparathyroidism also causes hypophosphatemia, phosphaturia, hyperchloremia, and a normal anion gap metabolic acidosis as a result of direct actions of PTH and calcium on proximal tubule function. These changes are not specific for hyperparathyroidism and should not be relied on to make a diagnosis.

Primary hyperparathyroidism is caused by a single adenoma in over 80 per cent of cases. Recent surveys estimate that less than 2 per cent of patients with primary hyperparathyroidism have parathyroid carcinoma. The remaining 15 to 20 per cent have parathyroid hyperplasia. All three forms of primary hyperparathyroidism can be familial, although this is rare for adenoma and carcinoma. Parathyroid hyperplasia also presents as a component of familial multiple endocrine neoplasia (FMEN) Type 1, in which hyperplasia of the parathyroids, pituitary, and pancreatic islets may occur in the same patient. Parathyroid hyperplasia is less commonly associated with medullary carcinoma of the thyroid or pheochromocytoma in MEN Type 2 and, rarely, with MEN Type 3. Modest parathyroid enlargement is also observed in familial hypocalciuric hypercalcemia (FHH), an autosomal dominant disorder characterized by mild elevation of plasma PTH and serum calcium levels. FHH is distinguished from primary hyperparathyroidism by hypocalciuria (calcium clearance to creatinine clearance < 0.01) and a benign clinical course. There is no increase in the incidence of nephrolithiasis, bone disease, or neurologic symptoms in patients with FHH compared with normal persons, and hypercalcemia almost always recurs after subtotal parathyroidectomy. It is important to rule out FHH with a 24-hour urine calcium and creatinine measurement in every patient suspected of having primary hyperparathyroidism because surgery is rarely indicated in FHH.

Treatment

Surgery

Indications for Parathyroidectomy. There have been few long-term studies on the natural history of primary hyperparathyroidism; therefore, the usual criteria for surgery differ among centers. In all cases, the expectation of cure should be tempered by the risk of surgical complications. Complications of parathyroid surgery include recurrent laryngeal nerve damage, hypoparathyroidism, bleeding, infection, and the risk associated with general anesthesia. Five per cent of parathyroid surgeries are unsuccessful. The risk of surgical complications is increased for individuals who have had previous neck surgery, a factor that should be considered when recommending a second parathyroid exploration.

In the authors' experience, parathyroid exploration should be done in patients with complications caused by hyperparathyroidism, including altered mentation, nephrolithiasis or renal parenchymal calcification, renal failure, bone disease (low bone density, fracture, elevated bone alkaline phosphatase level, brown tumors or cysts), or soft tissue calcification (chondrocalcinosis, skin calcification with pruritus). A serum calcium level consistently higher than 12 mg per dl has been considered a sufficient criterion for surgery, but there are no prospective studies comparing the rate of new fractures or renal stones in asymptomatic patients randomized to surgical treatment or medical follow-up. Untreated patients with mild primary hyperparathyroidism are unlikely to present with extremely elevated serum calcium levels. A loss of cortical bone is observed in primary hyperparathyroidism, which could increase the probability of hip fracture in untreated patients. Although there is no evidence that a delay in treatment increases the hip fracture rate in patients with mild hypercalcemia, it is prudent to recommend surgery in patients younger than age 40 years who have a serum calcium level higher than 11 mg per dl and in patients older than age 40 years whose serum calcium level is higher than 12 mg per dl.

Patients who have a serum calcium level below 12 mg per dl can be followed with careful medical observation unless complications occur. Dual-photon or computed tomography bone densitometry provides objective data on changes in bone density. New elevations of serum alkaline phosphatase or serum osteocalcin levels are also useful indices of bone disease.

Surgical Approach. Chvostek's sign, a useful monitor of postoperative hypocalcemia, should be checked preoperatively because it is present in 5 per cent of normal persons. Another preoperative concern is whether noninvasive parathyroid localization studies should be done. Preoperative localization of enlarged parathyroid glands by ultrasound, computed tomography, nuclear magnetic resonance, and thallium-technetium subtraction scans is useful for patients undergoing a second parathyroid exploration; however, noninvasive localization has not been demonstrated to improve the probability of successful surgery, shorten the operative time, or decrease the incidence of surgical complications in patients undergoing a first parathyroid exploration.

An effort should be made to identify and perform biopsy of parathyroid glands during surgical exploration to confirm their identity. The size of each gland should be noted because the pathologic distinction between adenoma and hyperplasia is not always clear and the presence of multiple enlarged glands suggests hyperplasia. Once the number of abnormal parathyroids is known, the surgeon can decide on the appropriate operative approach.

ADENOMA. Most parathyroid adenomas are found at the expected location near the upper and lower poles of the thyroid. The occurrence of "ectopic" parathyroid glands (<10 per cent) is explained by the variable length of migration of embryonic inferior parathyroid glands from the third branchial pouch and of embryonic superior glands from the fourth branchial pouch. Glands arising from the third branchial pouch migrate caudally with the developing thymus; therefore, migration beyond the lower pole of the thyroid results in a mediastinal parathyroid, often embedded in the thymus. Inferior glands have been found in the carotid sheath and the retropharyngeal area. Parathyroid glands arising from the fourth branchial pouch remain near the superior pole of the thyroid. They have been found in the tracheoesophageal groove. Parathyroid glands are also found embedded within the thyroid. If no adenoma is found in the typical locations, neck exploration should extend to the retropharyngeal area and the tracheoesophageal groove. The surgeon is frequently able to pull up the thymus and superior thymic fat from behind the sternal notch, a maneuver that may yield a parathyroid adenoma embedded in thymic tissue. If an adenoma is still not found, a hemithyroidectomy should be done on the side of the neck on which only one gland was identified. Mediastinal exploration should be reserved for the second parathyroid exploration after localization studies are done. If a single adenoma is found and the remaining glands are normal in size and on frozen section analysis, removal of the adenoma results in cure for most patients.

HYPERPLASIA. Multiple enlarged parathyroid glands and a family history of hyperparathyroidism are indications for a more aggressive surgical approach. Removal of a single enlarged parathyroid gland in patients with hyperplasia may result in temporary normalization of the serum calcium level, but hyperparathyroidism often recurs. Two surgical approaches have been used for parathyroid hyperplasia. The first is subtotal parathyroidectomy, leaving only one-half of the most normal-appearing gland in situ. The second is complete parathyroidectomy followed by transplantation of a parathyroid autograft to the forearm. Hyperparathyroid patients with FMEN Type 1 should have total parathyroidectomy and parathyroid autotransplantation because the recurrence rate of hyperparathyroidism after subtotal parathyroidectomy in this group is 50 per cent in 10 years. Patients with parathyroid hyperplasia caused by renal failure also have a high rate of recurrence of hyperparathyroidism after subtotal parathyroidectomy; therefore, total parathyroidectomy and autotransplantation are frequently done for these patients. The long-term success of subtotal parathyroidectomy in non–FMEN Type 1 familial hyperparathyroidism or sporadic parathyroid hyperplasia is not known, and subtotal parathyroidectomy is often done in these cases. Parathyroid autografts can cause recurrent hyperparathyroidism because of unregulated secretion of PTH; therefore, autografts do not always result in cure for patients with hyperplasia. The rate of recurrent hyperparathyroidism in properly selected patients with autotransplants should be low.

Parathyroid autotransplantation can be done with a fresh autograft at the time of parathyroidectomy or with a frozen autograft 2 to 3 months after parathyroidectomy. The advantage of a fresh autograft is the greater probability of successful vascularization. Parathyroid autografts usually take up to 6 months to function; there-fore, the completeness of total parathyroidectomy can be established during this period by the observation of persistent postoperative hypocalcemia. In specialized centers, intraoperative UcAMP measurement has been used to confirm that a total parathyroidectomy has been done. Frozen autografts can be placed electively, thereby allowing a longer period of observation to confirm the completeness of total parathyroidectomy.

CARCINOMA. Parathyroid carcinoma is insensitive to external radiation therapy or chemotherapy; therefore, surgery is the preferred treatment. Patients with parathyroid carcinoma benefit from removal of as much tumor tissue as possible. Debulking lowers the serum calcium level for a length of time that is more dependent on the aggressiveness of the tumor than on the aggressiveness of the surgeon.

SECOND OPERATION. The reasons for unsuccessful parathyroid surgery include distorted neck anatomy caused by prior surgery or goiter, failure to diagnose parathyroid hyperplasia or FHH, "ectopic" location of parathyroid glands, the presence of more than four parathyroid glands, and inexperience of the surgeon. Even the most experienced surgeon occasionally misses an adenoma. Ninety per cent of parathyroid adenomas found during a second operation are in expected locations near the superior and inferior poles of the thyroid. The remainder are in the tracheoesophageal groove, carotid sheath or mediastinum or are embedded in the thyroid. Parathyroid adenomas have been found in the pericardium. As many as six parathyroid glands in one individual have been reported.

Second operations are an indication for preoperative localization techniques. The sensitivity and specificity of ultrasound, technetium-thallium subtraction, computed tomography, and nuclear magnetic resonance are highly dependent on the institution where they are performed. Selective arteriography and venous sampling for PTH have been useful at specialized centers. Second operations have a greater risk of complications; therefore, every effort should be made to locate abnormal parathyroid tissue before surgery. The benefit of a second operation should outweigh the risk of recurrent laryngeal nerve damage.

PREGNANCY. Primary hyperparathyroidism rarely occurs during pregnancy. There is little danger to the fetus from maternal hypercalcemia before parturition; however, hypercalcemia in utero increases the probability of severe hypocalcemic tetany during the neonatal period. Neonates of hyperparathyroid mothers should be followed with twice daily monitoring of serum calcium levels and should receive intravenous calcium, if necessary, to prevent the onset of tetany. Once feedings are begun, calcium and vitamin D supplementation may be necessary to prevent hypocalcemia. These supplements can be tapered over a period of months. There is a theoretical risk of worsening maternal hypercalcemia during the last trimester of pregnancy because of unregulated production of 1,25-$(OH)_2D_3$ by placental and decidual tissue. Given these risks to the neonate and the mother, parathyroidectomy should be considered in pregnant women who have serum calcium levels higher than 12 mg per dl. Parathyroidectomy should be done during the second trimester, when the risk of anesthesia-induced congenital malformation is lowest.

Medical Therapy

Emergency Treatment of Hypercalcemia. Altered mentation or coma may result from severe hypercalcemia. The goal of emergency therapy in these cases is to lower the serum calcium level by expanding the intravascular volume and promoting renal calcium excretion with furosemide and forced saline diuresis. Treatment with intravenous saline (4 to 8 liters per day) and intravenous furosemide (Lasix), 20 to 40 mg per hour, promotes calcium excretion. Treatment with furosemide before or in the absence of forced saline diuresis does not lower the serum calcium level and may promote hypercalcemia by causing dehydration. Complications of furosemide include hypokalemia and hypomagnesemia. Careful attention should be directed to balancing urine output with the rate of intravenous fluid administration to prevent congestive heart failure.

If the response to diuresis is inadequate, intravenous plicamycin (Mithracin), 25 micrograms per kg per day, can be administered to inhibit osteoclastic bone resorption directly. Plicamycin is effective for up to 1 week. Complications include anorexia, nausea, bone marrow suppression, inhibition of clotting factor synthesis, hepatic and renal failure, hypophosphatemia, and hypokalemia. Plicamycin should be used as a temporary treatment in patients awaiting surgery. It is contraindicated in pregnancy. Hemodialysis against a low calcium bath has been used to lower serum calcium levels in dialysis patients.

Chronic Therapy. Medical therapy for primary hyperparathyroidism is indicated when there is an unacceptable risk of surgery, attempts to locate abnormal parathyroid tissue have been unsuccessful, or patients refuse surgery.

Patients with primary hyperparathyroidism should be instructed to maintain good hydration by drinking an extra glass of water with each meal and at bedtime. Hydration decreases the concentration of calcium in urine, thereby preventing the formation of renal stones. Thiazide diuretics should be discontinued because they decrease renal calcium clearance and worsen hypercalcemia.

Estrogen therapy can lower the serum calcium level 1 mg per dl in postmenopausal women with primary hyperparathyroidism. Estrogen decreases hypercalciuria and slows the rate of bone resorption. Conjugated estrogens (0.625 to 2.5 mg per day) should be administered for 25 days a month. Medroxyprogesterone acetate (10 mg per day) should be added on days 15 to 25 to allow endometrial shedding. The risks of estrogen therapy include thromboembolism, stroke, and uterine carcinoma. If patients do not smoke and medroxyprogesterone acetate is used to cycle the endometrium, the risks of estrogen therapy are small compared with those of hyperparathyroidism.

Oral phosphate therapy can be used to lower the serum calcium level in patients who have normal renal function. Phosphate therapy decreases the serum calcium level by complexing with dietary calcium and promoting deposition in bone. There is a danger of calcium-phosphate deposition in soft tissues, including the kidney, which could cause renal failure. Phosphate therapy also increases the secretion of PTH, which may accelerate the rate of bone resorption. Oral phosphate is available as a mixture of sodium and potassium salts or as the sodium-free potassium salt. Treatment is initiated with 2 grams per day in divided doses for the first 2 to 3 days, followed by 1 to 1.5 grams daily in divided doses.

Corticosteroids and calcitonin are not effective for chronic therapy of primary hyperparathyroidism. Treatment with etidronate disodium (Didronel), a diphosphonate that arrests bone resorption and formation, has not been effective. New diphosphonate analogues and PTH antagonist peptides are currently experimental but may be useful in the future.

HYPOPARATHYROIDISM

Diagnosis

Hypoparathyroidism results in hypocalcemia and hyperphosphatemia as a result of insufficient PTH secretion or action. Symptoms of hypocalcemia include tingling and burning periorally and in the hands and feet, muscle cramps including carpal and pedal spasm, and tetany.

Hypoparathyroidism is most often a complication of surgery. It may be congenital (DeGeorge's syndrome), caused by polyglandular autoimmune disease Type I, or idiopathic.

Pseudohypoparathyroidism, or Albright's hereditary osteodystrophy, is a disorder characterized by hypocalcemia, hyperphosphatemia, and elevated plasma PTH levels caused by resistance to PTH action. Patients with pseudohypoparathyroidism usually have a characteristic phenotype that includes short stature, short fourth metacarpals or metatarsals, mental retardation, and associated hypothyroidism and hypogonadism. The diagnosis of pseudohypoparathyroidism is established by demonstrating an absent or subnormal elevation of the UcAMP level during administration of PTH. Hypoparathyroidism has also been reported to occur in patients with hemachromatosis and other infiltrative diseases. Insufficient PTH secretion and diminished PTH action may occur in magnesium depletion.

Treatment

The goal of therapy is to increase the serum calcium level sufficiently to prevent the symptoms and signs of hypocalcemia without causing hypercalcemia or hypercalciuria. Hypocalcemia can be corrected by adequate delivery of elemental calcium and the administration of vitamin D analogues, which stimulate intestinal absorption of calcium.

Tetany

Emergency treatment of tetany should be done with intravenous infusion of calcium. Administration of 200 mg of elemental calcium (21 ml of 10 per cent calcium gluconate) intravenously in 100 ml 5 per cent dextrose over 15 minutes stops tetany. This therapy should be continued until patients are taking adequate oral calcium and vitamin D. Infusion of 5 to 10 mg per kg of elemental calcium (70 ml of 10 per cent calcium gluconate) over 24 hours in 1 liter of normal saline prevents recurrence of tetany. The dose of intravenous calcium should be reduced after 24 hours to prevent hypercalcemia. Once tetany is controlled, the infusion rate should maintain the serum calcium level in the low to low-normal range (8 to 8.5 mg per dl). Tetany after parathyroidectomy is more likely to occur in patients with bone disease. These patients are more likely to require prolonged intravenous calcium therapy than those without bone disease.

After Parathyroidectomy

Hypocalcemia usually occurs after parathyroidectomy within 12 to 24 hours but may be delayed. Therapy of mild hypocalcemia should be withheld to document the development of symptoms and the fall in the serum calcium level, both of which indicate that the surgeon has completely removed

TABLE 1. **Calcium Content of Oral Calcium Preparations**

Preparation	Elemental Calcium (%)
Calcium carbonate	40.0
Calcium citrate	21.0
Calcium lactate	12.8
Calcium gluconate	8.8
Calcium glubionate	6.5

abnormal parathyroid tissue. The serum calcium level may fall to the normal range after neck exploration even if a parathyroid adenoma is not found because of intravenous fluid volume expansion; however, hypercalcemia recurs within 48 to 72 hours. Indications for starting therapy include uncomfortable paresthesias, muscle cramps, a positive Chvostek's sign, or a serum calcium level rapidly falling below 8 mg per dl. Patients with evidence of bone disease are most likely to develop severe hypocalcemia because of accelerated deposition of calcium into "hungry" bones. A postoperative serum phosphate level higher than 6 mg per dl predicts permanent hypoparathyroidism in patients with normal renal function.

Mild hypocalcemia can be treated by increasing the dietary calcium intake. Calcium intake is more predictably controlled by administering oral elemental calcium (1 to 2 grams per day). The elemental calcium content of commonly prescribed oral calcium preparations is shown in Table 1. We recommend 1.2 grams of calcium carbonate four times a day (4.8 grams of calcium carbonate per day = 1.9 grams of elemental calcium per day). The fractional absorption of calcium is increased when calcium carbonate is taken with food. Hypoparathyroid patients who are unable to take medications by mouth because of vomiting or surgery should be treated intravenously with 1 gram of elemental calcium every 24 hours.

If hypocalcemia persists despite therapy with elemental calcium, vitamin D analogues should be administered to stimulate intestinal calcium absorption. $1,25\text{-}(OH)_2D_3$ (calcitriol) is the vitamin D analogue of choice for patients with postoperative hypoparathyroidism because it has a rapid onset of action and a short biologic half-life (1 to 2 days). Thus, hypercalcemia from overtreatment can be rapidly corrected by lowering the dose. Calcitriol (Rocaltrol) is initiated with 0.25 to 0.50 micrograms twice a day (0.03 micrograms per kg per day in children*). The dose can be increased to 1 to 2 micrograms per day if needed. Vitamin D analogues other than calcitriol may be used for chronic therapy of permanently hy-

---

*Dosage in children has not been established by the manufacturer.

poparathyroid patients; however, patients should be monitored carefully to prevent toxicity. Dihydrotachysterol (Hytakerol) is a synthetic analogue of calcitriol that has the advantage of low cost; however, its biologic half-life is 7 days. The daily dose is 400 micrograms per day (20 micrograms per kg per day in children). Ergocalciferol (vitamin D_2), the least expensive preparation, is administered as 1500 micrograms per day (50 micrograms per kg per day in children). The deposition of ergocalciferol in body fat may result in toxicity that does not resolve for months.

All patients taking vitamin D analogues should be monitored by measurement of 24-hour urine calcium levels. Nephrolithiasis or renal parenchymal calcification can be prevented by maintaining urine calcium excretion below 200 to 250 mg per 24 hours. Serum calcium levels should be maintained between 8 and 8.5 mg per dl. Correction of the serum calcium level to "normal" often results in hypercalciuria and subsequent nephrolithiasis.

Hypoparathyroidism during pregnancy is treated according to the principles outlined earlier. The vitamin D requirement for pregnant patients is decreased compared with that of nonpregnant patients because of the production of $1,25\text{-}(OH)_2D_3$ by placenta and decidual tissue. Patients with pseudohypoparathyroidism require lower doses of vitamin D when they are pregnant.

HYPOPITUITARISM

method of
ANDREW G. FRANTZ, M.D.
Columbia University College of Physicians and Surgeons
New York, New York

Hypopituitarism is defined as a deficiency of one or more anterior pituitary hormones. It is important to remember that pituitary disease of any kind can result in deficiencies that are single or multiple and that virtually any combination of deficiencies may coexist. With some hormone-secreting tumors (e.g., with prolactinomas or with adenomas causing acromegaly), excess production of one hormone may be accompanied by deficiencies of others. In practice, gonadotropin deficiency is among the most commonly encountered. Growth hormone deficiency may also be shown by stimulation tests in many patients with pituitary disease, although its diagnosis is not clinically important in the adult because no replacement therapy is currently given to adults. Somewhat less frequently encountered are clinical deficiencies of adrenocorticotropic hormone (ACTH) and thyroid-stimulating hormone (TSH), although with these disorders, the diagnosis is of clinical importance because of the necessity of insti-

tuting therapy. Prolactin deficiency occurs very rarely, and replacement therapy is not given for this condition.

Pituitary tumors are among the most common causes of hypopituitarism in adults. Treatment of the mass lesion itself by surgery, radiotherapy, or tumor-shrinking drugs (e.g., bromocriptine for prolactinomas) may infrequently correct a deficiency of a tropic hormone that was caused by compression of the gland itself or the stalk. Prolactin reduction may also correct a functional defect in gonadotropin secretion caused by hyperprolactinemia. The decision to treat hypopituitarism is made by careful assessment of each of the individual hormones. It must also be remembered that with mass lesions, hypopituitarism not present initially may develop gradually over the course of months or years either as a result of progression of the lesion itself or as a late result of treatment, especially after radiotherapy.

GONADOTROPIN DEFICIENCY

Hypogonadotropic hypogonadism could in theory be treated by giving either gonadotropins or gonadal steroids. In practice, except when fertility is desired, gonadal steroids are always chosen for reasons of convenience and expense.

Males

Testosterone administered orally is ineffective because of rapid degradation and inactivation by the liver. Derivatives have been synthesized that resist degradation; all of these oral preparations carry a small risk of causing cholestatic jaundice, which is reversible on discontinuation of the drug. The oral replacement dose for an adult male with 17α-methyltestosterone (Oreton Methyl, Metandren, Neo-Hombreol-M) is 20 to 50 mg per day (e.g., 10 to 25 mg twice daily). A buccal tablet, to be dissolved slowly in the cheek pouch and not swallowed, is said to be about twice as effective as the oral preparation and should therefore be given in half the above dose; some individuals find this route of administration annoying. Fluoxymesterone (Halotestin, Ultandren, Ora-Testryl) is another androgen about as effective as methyltestosterone and should be given orally in total doses of 10 to 20 mg per day, preferably twice daily.

In my experience the oral androgens are frequently not as effective as one could wish, and I prefer the administration of a long-acting testosterone ester intramuscularly. Testosterone enanthate (Delatestryl) and testosterone cypionate (Depo-Testosterone) are available in a sesame oil preparation of 200 and 100 mg per ml. Maximal effects are produced by administering 400 mg intramuscularly every 2 weeks, and it is probably never necessary to exceed this dose for replacement therapy. Administration of 200 mg every 2 weeks or 300 mg every 3 weeks provides an adequate replacement dose for most men.

Side effects of androgen therapy include variable degrees of fluid retention, sometimes seen as worsening of pre-existing congestive heart failure; gynecomastia, which may regress with continued therapy; and male pattern baldness in individuals genetically predisposed. With oral preparations, in addition to cholestatic jaundice, peliosis hepatis (blood-filled cysts of the liver) and hepatoma have rarely been noted.

In treating previously virilized males who have become hypogonadal, I generally start out with full doses of parenteral steroids. Therapy may then be tapered somewhat to what seems a satisfactory dose, depending on degree of libido and sexual performance. For reasons of convenience, one may experiment at this point with oral androgens if the patient so desires, but he should be advised that they may be less effective. In inducing virilization for the first time in a patient who has failed to go through a normal puberty, it is generally desirable to proceed at a slower rate because of profound and potentially unsettling psychic changes that may accompany too rapid virilization. In young men with concomitant growth hormone deficiency whose epiphyses are unfused and who are short, one may also wish to use low doses or to defer therapy pending the use of growth hormone. The object in this case is to achieve as much statural growth as possible before epiphyseal closure occurs.

Not all male hypogonadism requires treatment. Patients often make what are to them satisfactory long-term adjustments to reduced or absent libido. Disturbance of a long-established pattern by the induction of desires that the patient is ill equipped to fulfill may do him a real disservice. Such therapy should be undertaken only after careful consideration and discussion with the patient. Finally, it should be mentioned that impotence due to hypogonadism of long duration, particularly that associated with pituitary tumors, may be quite resistant to androgenic replacement therapy; sometimes there is no therapy that is entirely satisfactory for these patients.

Fertility is rarely restored in hypogonadotropic males by treatment with androgens alone, but prior use of androgens does not impair the subsequent effectiveness of gonadotropin therapy. The usual approach is therefore to use androgens until the point at which fertility is actively sought. At this time treatment is changed to parenteral hCG (human chorionic gonadotropin, a luteinizing hormone–like preparation of placental origin derived from the urine of pregnant women), which is given three times weekly for many weeks to months. In some cases this is adequate to initiate spermatogenesis, but additional parenteral therapy with a preparation having follicle-stimulating hormone activity (Pergonal, derived from the urine of postmenopausal women) is usually also required. Treatment may be necessary for as long as 6 to 12 months, is expensive, and on the whole is less successful than corresponding treatment to induce fertility in women.

In both men and women with hypogonadotropism due to hypothalamic deficiency (who constitute the majority of those with "idiopathic" hypogonadotropism), considerable success has recently been achieved in inducing fertility by means of luteinizing hormone–releasing hormone delivered subcutaneously in pulsatile fashion by means of a special pump.

Females

Young women in the premenopausal age range who are clearly hypogonadal should usually be treated, with the object of preventing premature osteoporosis, maintaining normal secondary sex characteristics and skin texture, and possibly reducing susceptibility to coronary artery disease. Low cyclic doses of estrogen should be used, as well as a progestational agent to ensure normal withdrawal bleeding. A satisfactory regimen is either 10 to 20 micrograms of ethinyl estradiol (Estinyl) or 0.625 to 1.25 mg of conjugated estrogens (Premarin) once a day for the first 25 days of each month. An oral progestin such as medroxyprogesterone acetate (Provera), 10 mg, is also given once a day for days 16 through 25 inclusive.

Side effects of estrogens that have been reported when they are used for birth control purposes include edema, a somewhat increased risk of thromboembolic disease as well as of endometrial cancer, hypertension, hepatic adenoma, and hepatocellular carcinoma. These risks are small, and it is unclear whether they even exist to a significant degree when estrogen is used in low doses as suggested for replacement in hypogonadotropic hypogonadism. Recently, a transdermal form of estrogen (Estraderm) has become available to be applied to the skin as a patch twice weekly. It may decrease some of these risks still further, as a result of bypassing the liver after absorption, but whether it has advantages over oral estrogen for the treatment of hypopituitarism is uncertain.

Libido may be depressed in women with hypopituitarism, and if so, it is usually not restored with estrogens alone. In women who complain of diminished libido, a trial of low-dose androgen therapy, e.g., 25 mg of testosterone enanthate (Delatestryl) or testosterone cypionate (Depo-Testosterone) intramuscularly every 4 to 6 weeks, may be worthwhile. There is danger, however, in the use of androgens because women who respond favorably may want to continue them indefinitely; prolonged use even at these low-dose levels may lead to irreversible deepening of the voice as well as hirsutism, clitoromegaly, and acne. The physician should be alert to these changes and should discuss the possibility of them in advance with the patient.

Fertility in women with hypopituitarism, if desired, is usually brought about with the use of exogenous gonadotropins. The length of treatment required is shorter, and the success rate is considerably higher than when these agents are used for men, as mentioned previously. Because of the risks involved, which include the ovarian hyperstimulation syndrome and multiple births, such treatment should be undertaken only by physicians familiar with this form of therapy.

ACTH DEFICIENCY

Hypoadrenocorticism, when present in patients with hypopituitarism, is seldom as severe as that seen in patients with Addison's disease or after bilateral adrenalectomy. Glucocorticoid production, although impaired, usually persists to some degree. Furthermore, since aldosterone production is not primarily under ACTH control, replacement mineralocorticoid is rarely required.

Hydrocortisone production rate in the normal adult is of the order of 15 to 20 mg per day, and this defines the usual replacement dose. I prefer to give either hydrocortisone, 10 mg twice daily, or cortisone acetate, 12.5 mg (one-half tablet) twice daily. A higher dosage than this is rarely necessary in hypopituitarism. Some argument could be made for giving more of the total dose in the morning and less in the late afternoon, to mimic more closely the normal secretory pattern, but the above regimens are usually satisfactory. Prednisone, 2.5 mg twice daily, may also be given. Occasionally, a patient with hypopituitarism may appear to be borderline with respect to the need for steroid replacement. On such occasions I sometimes give hydrocortisone, 5 mg twice a day, or 10 mg in the morning and 5 mg in the afternoon. Hypothyroidism, if present in the patient with hypopituitarism, may diminish the need for steroid replacement by slowing the degradation of circulating steroids. Under these circumstances, treatment of the hypothyroidism may necessitate the simultaneous institution of glucocorticoid therapy. In all cases, patients should be advised to increase their steroids to double or triple the usual daily dose in the event of unusual stress or minor febrile illnesses. They should be in touch with their physician at once in case of severe illness, and if any delay in securing medical help is anticipated, particularly in the event of severe vomiting, they or a family member should be provided with an injectable form of steroid such as dexamethasone sodium phosphate (Decadron), available as 4 mg in 1.0 ml in a disposable syringe, to be taken intramuscularly. This may be repeated after 6 to 8 hours if a doctor is not available. Patients with hypoadrenocorticism should also wear a medical information bracelet or necklace with information about their condition. Such devices are obtainable from the Medic Alert Foundation International, P.O. Box 1009, Turlock, CA 95381-1009 (telephone 1-800-344-3226). In the event of severe or life-threatening infections or stress, including major surgery, hospitalized patients with hypopituitarism should be treated like addisonian patients, with large total daily steroid doses of the order of 300 mg per day of hydrocortisone equivalents given intravenously or intramuscularly in divided doses. Therapy is frequently initiated with a bolus dose such as 4 mg of dexamethasone phosphate intravenously (or sometimes intramuscularly, in preparation for operation) followed by 100 mg of hydrocortisone sodium succinate (Solu-Cortef) every 6 to 8 hours by slow intravenous drip.

TSH DEFICIENCY

Sodium L-thyroxine is the drug of choice for treating hypothyroidism. The daily replacement is 50 to 200 micrograms, given as a single oral dose, with 150 micrograms being appropriate for the majority of both older children and younger adults. In these individuals, therapy may be started directly with this dose. In older patients, and particularly in those with coronary artery disease, a lower starting dose should be used, generally not more than 50 micrograms per day and sometimes as low as 25 micrograms or even 12.5 micrograms if angina is present and severe. This can be increased in 25- to 50-microgram increments every 3 to 4 weeks, depending on the clinical response and the serum thyroxine (T_4) measurements. With optimum therapy the serum T_4 will generally be at the upper end of the normal range and may even slightly exceed it in some cases. Serum tri-iodothyronine (T_3) will be normal, however, unless the patient is being overtreated. It has been shown that when L-thyroxine therapy is substituted for desiccated thyroid in a dose that is therapeutically equivalent, serum T_4 will rise by approximately 3 micrograms per dl, and serum T_3 (which may have been elevated on desiccated thyroid therapy) will fall. For practical purposes, serum T_3 measurements are usually unnecessary, particularly if the patient feels well and serum T_4 is not elevated.

As noted previously, consideration should be given to the possible need for instituting, or increasing the dose of, glucocorticoid therapy when L-thyroxine therapy is begun in hypopituitary patients, who may have defects of ACTH secretion as well as of TSH.

GROWTH HORMONE DEFICIENCY

Growth hormone deficiency in hypopituitarism is not treated unless the patient is of short stature and the long bone epiphyses are unfused. If these conditions exist, however, growth rates approximating those of a normal child may be achieved with parenteral growth hormone therapy. Growth hormone obtained from cadaver pituitaries is no longer available in the United States because of the development of Creutzfeldt-Jakob disease in a small number of patients after long-term treatment with this preparation. Two human growth hormone preparations made biosynthetically by recombinant DNA techniques (Protropin and Humatrope) are currently available. The usual dose is in the range of 0.1 to 0.2 IU per kg, given intramuscularly three times a week. Therapy is expensive and must be continued for many months to years. It is desirable to withhold sex hormone therapy and to treat concomitant ACTH deficiency, if the latter is present, with the minimum necessary dose of glucocorticoid, in order to prevent steroid antagonism of growth hormone action.

HYPERPROLACTINEMIA

method of
NICHOLAS P. CHRISTY, M.D.
*Columbia University College of Physicians
   and Surgeons*
New York, New York

Hyperprolactinemia is defined as a persistent, chronic elevation of the plasma prolactin concentration; it is fairly common in the population at large and is the most prevalent neuroendocrine disorder. Prolactinoma, that is, prolactin-secreting tumor of the pituitary gland, an important cause of hyperprolactinemia, is the most common hormone-producing tumor of the human adenohypophysis, occurring in as many as 10 per cent, and in some studies up to 25 per cent, of random autopsies.

Hyperprolactinemia is observed as a result of or in association with various clinical circumstances. Those diverse circumstances dictate the diagnostic plans and procedures and determine the need for and nature of the treatment. The consensus of most endocrinologists is that most patients with hyperprolactinemia require treatment under most circumstances. If the decision is made to withhold treatment, continuous, careful monitoring of most patients is necessary. Certain categories of patients, to be discussed, do not need treatment of the hyperprolactinemia per se, although they may require correction of the associated disorder. Proper therapy or a rational decision to withhold it demands precise diagnosis.

CLINICAL PRESENTATION

Many patients with hyperprolactinemia have no symptoms or signs ascribable to a raised plasma prolactin concentration. This is true of most patients who have drug-induced or drug-related hyperprolactinemia, which usually abates when the drug is stopped. Examples are some agents that block dopamine agonist receptors or reduce dopamine synthesis in various parts of the brain. Specific drugs include neuroleptics such as chlorpromazine, perphenazine, haloperidol, metoclopramide, and sulpiride; antidepressants like imipramine and amitryptiline; and antihypertensives like reserpine and methyldopa. Opiates, verapamil, and intravenous cimetidine may induce hyperprolactinemia, as may administered estrogens, but not in the small doses found in contraceptive agents. Asymptomatic hyperprolactinemia is observed in hypothyroidism, correction of which slowly brings down the raised plasma prolactin concentration. The same is true in patients with chronic renal failure, wherein the mechanism is completely unknown. Especially high values are seen with renal hemodialysis. Successful renal transplantation and correction of the zinc deficiency of renal failure restore the serum prolactin concentration to normal.

In some other conditions associated with hyperprolactinemia, the laboratory abnormality may have clinical significance. Abnormally high prolactin concentrations are sometimes observed in women with syndromes of hyperandrogenicity, such as polycystic ovary (Stein-Leventhal) syndrome. It is now known that hyperprolactinemia may stimulate the adrenal cortex to secrete excessive quantities of dehydroepiandrosterone sulfate. In isolated galactorrhea (i.e., galactorrhea without oligo- or amenorrhea), where one would expect to find hyperprolactinemia, the situation is complex. The incidence of this type of galactorrhea in hyperprolactinemic women is variably reported as 30 to 80 per cent, whereas, conversely, galactorrhea can occur with normal serum prolactin concentrations in many women, more than 85 per cent in one series.

The hyperprolactinemia of Addison's disease and that associated with the presumably neurogenic injuries to the chest wall are of no known clinical significance (Table 1).

Hyperprolactinemia is most often observed in the setting of gonadal dysfunction: amenorrhea or infertility in women, loss of libido or impotence in men. Reduced sexual activity is a frequent finding in both sexes, as are headache and other signs of hypothalamic or pituitary tumor, including visual disturbances and visual field defects. This group of patients most often has prolactinoma. In these patients, hyperprolactin-

TABLE 1. Causes of Hyperprolactinemia

Physiologic Causes
Sleep
Pregnancy
Suckling
   Nipple stimulation
Coitus with orgasm
Stress

Hypothalamic Diseases
Diffuse—encephalitis, radiation
Granulomatosis—sarcoid, histiocytosis
Tumors—astrocytoma, craniopharyngioma, Rathke's pouch
   cyst, germinoma, metastases
Pseudoprolactinomas
Pituitary stalk section
Head trauma

Pituitary Diseases
Prolactinomas
Pseudoprolactinomas
Acromegaly
Cushing's disease
Granulomas

Drugs
Neuroleptics—chlorpromazine, metoclopramide
Antihypertensives—methyldopa
Antidepressants—amitriptyline
Opiates
Estrogens (not anticontraceptive agents)
Cimetidine

Lesions of the Chest Wall
Chest trauma
   Burns
   Surgery
Herpes zoster virus

Miscellaneous
Primary hypothyroidism
Chronic renal insufficiency
Addison's disease
Polycystic ovary (Stein-Leventhal) syndrome
Undefined cause

emia induces hypoestrogenism, probably through inhibition by the excessive prolactin of hypothalamic gonadotropin-releasing hormone, although the mechanism is still debated. The hypoestrogenic state has been proved to cause osteopenia. In hyperprolactinemic women, there is also the theoretical possibility that hypoestrinism may predispose to a greater susceptibility to coronary artery disease (compared with normal premenopausal women).

DIAGNOSIS

Symptomatic hyperprolactinemia is strongly associated with prolactinoma. Even under ideal conditions, diagnosis is imperfect in some cases and treatment may have to be either protracted or repeated. Finally, close, continuous follow-up with laboratory and radiologic monitoring is required.

Because prolactin is secreted episodically, with a sharp rise during sleep, and because the plasma prolactin concentration is labile in the face of multiple stimuli, sustained hyperprolactinemia can be documented only by repeated measurements (on 3 different days) under basal, trauma-free conditions. The best time for this determination is in the morning, 2 hours after waking. The upper limit of the normal serum (plasma) prolactin concentration is 18 to 20 ng per ml. The importance of a large, experienced, and busy laboratory for the measurement of prolactin concentration resides in several characteristics of the prolactin radioimmunoassay; prolactin is fairly easily damaged by prolonged storage, which may result in loss of immunoactivity and cause falsely high readings on plasma specimens; an altered molecular form of either the standards or the circulating prolactin ("big" or "big-big" prolactin) may result in serial dilutions that yield curves wherein the standard and the specimen (unknown) are not parallel, which produces errors in assays done at high versus low dilutions. Small laboratories that perform only occasional prolactin assays cannot be expected to circumvent all these difficulties, so that their results are not reliable.

The many patients who have obvious symptoms or signs of disease of the sellar region or who, in the setting of gonadal insufficiency, are prime candidates for a diagnosis of prolactinoma or pseudoprolactinoma require careful radiographic study of the pituitary fossa and contiguous structures. Large supra- and intrasellar tumors and pseudoprolactinomas (large hypothalamic, pituitary, or parapituitary tumors that induce hyperprolactinemia, not by causing prolactin hypersecretion but by interfering with the hypothalamic-pituitary vascular pathway by squeezing or displacing the infundibulum or pituitary stalk, so that dopamine, the tonic prolactin-inhibiting hormone, does not reach the pituitary) can sometimes be visualized by plain skull films taken in the sagittal and coronal planes. Nevertheless, the best results are now obtained with computed tomography (CT) scanning or magnetic resonance imaging (MRI). These are particularly useful in distinguishing hypothalamic from pituitary tumors. Provocative (chlorpromazine, thyrotropin-releasing hormone) stimulation and inhibition tests are not discriminatory because both the hypothalamus and the pituitary contain dopamine agonist receptors. Such pharmacologic tests do not enable a differential diagnosis between a diencephalic and a pituitary etiology of prolactin hypersecretion. The most accurate technique for the definition of the pituitary anatomy now available is the high-resolution CT scan (with or without contrast medium enhancement), with 1.5-mm sections through the substance of the pituitary gland. Characteristic findings in prolactinoma are a hypodense area within the enhanced gland, a convex (i.e., upwardly bulging) upper surface of the pituitary, and a measurement of 9 to 10 mm for the height of the gland. These characteristics are not entirely specific for prolactinoma. Still, these findings, together with lateral displacement of the infundibulum or pituitary stalk, although not completely specific for prolactinoma, are diagnostically quite reliable in the presence of sustained hyperprolactinemia.

MRI can demonstrate prolactinomas. The pituitary is often slightly enlarged by the tumor, which produces a signal intensity slightly less than that of contiguous normal pituitary tissue in a so-called T1-weighted image.

As to the relative advantages of CT scanning and MRI, it has been found that CT is superior in about 10 per cent of studies, MRI is better in 10 per cent, and the results are equivalent in 80 per cent. MRI may yet show better resolution of the sellar region. It has the advantages that there is no need for contrast medium and there is no exposure to radiation. A potential disadvantage is that MRI often fails to demonstrate lateral spread or extension of tumor into the cavernous sinuses. More observations with MRI are needed to establish the relative or absolute value of this new technology.

One more detail must be added concerning plasma prolactin concentrations in prolactinoma. Roughly speaking, the larger the tumor, the higher the prolactin concentration. In several clinics, it has now been well established that concentrations of 200 to 250 ng per ml may have any cause; concentrations above 250 ng per ml indicate a prolactinoma; and concentrations higher than 300 ng per ml always indicate a prolactinoma.

As can be seen in Table 1, the cause of hyperprolactinemia can usually be accurately identified by the history, the clinical picture, or both. The patients who have the most important clinical consequences for treatment, namely, those with prolactinoma, require intense radiologic examination. Even in the best hands, some prolactinomas, especially small ones (1 to 2 mm in diameter), will be missed; some workers suggest that the portion escaping detection may be up to 30 per cent. Nevertheless, as CT and MRI techniques improve and become more widely used, we may expect that the number of cases of "idiopathic," "undefined," or "functional" hyperprolactinemia will grow progressively smaller.

TREATMENT

Most patients with hyperprolactinemia should be treated at large medical centers with extensive laboratory facilities, experienced endocrinologists, and neurosurgeons who have had wide experience with trans-sphenoidal pituitary adenomectomy.

Once pregnancy, postpartum lactation, other endocrine conditions (hypothyroidism, primary adrenocortical insufficiency, polycystic ovary syndrome), and drugs have been excluded, the diagnosis of prolactinoma is established by CT scan or MRI. Then, as will be seen, there are several therapeutic choices, including some that entail combining two or more treatment modalities. Several considerations enter into the best choice of therapy for the individual patient.

A few general statements can be made. If a microadenoma is suspected but cannot be rigorously proved, there is a reasonable option not to treat. In the face of a proven hypothalamic tumor or prolactinoma of the pituitary, one is obliged to treat if only because the tumor mass itself is a threat to life or to normal neuroendocrine function. In the presence of prolactinoma associated with infertility, treatment is mandatory if fertility is desired. Galactorrhea with a normal menstrual cycle and hyperprolactinemia need not be treated unless the inappropriate lactation is so voluminous as to constitute a major nuisance. Treatment of hyperprolactinemia with the aim of preventing or ameliorating the osteopenia associated with hypoestrinism and for the possible prevention of coronary artery disease in women will be discussed under "Hyperprolactinemia of Undefined Cause."

Pituitary Microadenoma

Microadenoma, defined as a tumor with radiographic (CT) dimensions less than 10 mm in diameter, is the most common assignable cause of hyperprolactinemia when no other etiology can be identified. The first step is to rule out drug-induced hyperprolactinemia; the second is to eliminate medical conditions (alcoholism and liver disease, in addition to the etiologies listed in Table 1) and neurologic disorders (epileptic seizures, electroconvulsive therapy; rarely, empty sella). Then the question of whether and how to treat rests on associated symptoms and signs, the specific needs or wishes of the patient, and knowledge of the natural history of hyperprolactinemia. This has been studied in three groups of patients with pituitary tumors, mostly microadenomas. In the first series of 43 patients, who were followed for 3 to 20 years, evidence of pituitary tumor was definite; 2 patients experienced moderate suprasellar extension within 5 years and required surgery; the remaining 41 patients showed no radiologic progression of tumor, and in 3 of them, galactorrhea, amenorrhea, and hyperprolactinemia resolved spontaneously. In a second series, 25 hyperprolactinemic patients were followed for a long period (mean, 11 years); 18 had or were assumed to have microadenoma, the remaining 7 macroadenoma. Only one of the 25 patients showed tumor progression (by x-ray film); the mean serum prolactin value declined by more than 50 per cent over time in the patients with microadenoma. In a third series of patients, studied in Italy, about 20 per cent showed some radiologic progression during 3 years. In summary, most patients with demonstrated microadenoma show no progression of growth of the pituitary tumor over time. Criteria for treatment are thus other than the tumor considered simply as an intrasellar mass lesion (e.g., infertility).

In a group of 41 hyperprolactinemic patients without evidence of pituitary tumor (by definition, idiopathic hyperprolactinemia) followed for as long as 12 years, more than 80 per cent had either no change or a fall in serum prolactin concentration; in more than one-third, it fell to the normal range; more than one-half of the patients demonstrated a decrease to less than 50 per cent of the control level. In general, the higher the initial prolactin concentration, the smaller was its fall. Pituitary tumor developed in only 1 of these 41 patients.

For hyperprolactinemic patients who are asymptomatic, a good case can be made to with-hold treatment and to observe over time. Obser-vation includes prolactin measurements about every 6 months and CT scanning of the sellar region about every 2 to 4 years. Given the like-lihood that a number (up to 30 per cent) of small (<1 to 3 mm in diameter) microadenomas will be missed by CT scan, the clinician can assume that a few patients will develop significant pituitary tumor. The data show that the number of patients will be small and the rate of progression slow.

Symptomatic Pituitary Microadenoma

The decision to treat a microadenoma is based on or at least related to the presence or absence of symptoms of disturbance in or near the sella and the status of gonadal function. The natural history of treatment by observation only has been discussed. Apart from theoretical considerations, other factors entering into the decision are the infrequency and slow rate of progression of mi-croadenomas, the high rate of recurrence of treated tumors over the long term, and, if phar-macotherapy is used, the need for indefinite treat-ment because hyperprolactinemia recurs when the therapeutic agent is stopped. The major in-dication for treatment is the need to restore relatively normal pituitary function to achieve normal gonadal activity, including normal men-ses, ovulation, and fertility in women; and to improve libido, sperm count, and potency in men. There are five therapeutic options: surgery, bro-mocriptine, radiotherapy to the sellar region, various combinations of these three therapies, and observation alone.

Surgery: Trans-Sphenoidal Adenomectomy. This procedure is most often the treatment of choice in the United States because endocrinologists and surgeons here have had the widest experience with it. It should be emphasized that the data presented here are based on results obtained by experienced neurosurgeons. It should also be added that the procedure used is an adaptation of the one revived at the turn of the twentieth century by Harvey Cushing; by the mid-1920s, Cushing had reduced the mortality rate to 5.6 per cent, a figure now decreased to less than 1

per cent in most centers. The effectiveness of this treatment is variable. In the British experience, the initial cure rate (substantial reduction of the prolactin concentration or its restoration to or near normal) is 80 to 85 per cent and mortality is 0.27 per cent, with major morbidity occurring in 0.4 per cent and cerebrospinal rhinorrhea fluid being observed in 1 to 2 per cent. The rate of recurrence of hyperprolactinemia is 20 to 50 per cent; relapse occurs within 1 to 2 years, a few becoming evident at 2 to 5 years. Most often, the recurrent tumor cannot be seen by CT scan. The inference is either that residual tumor fragments have grown back or that there is a stimulatory hypothalamic influence, new or recurrent. Other large series have reported a long-term recurrence rate of 50 per cent; still lower rates (of 0 to 30 per cent) have been described. Most workers hold that these rates, like all others, will continue to increase over the years of postoperative follow-up.

In patients who show an initial cure, there is a high rate of return of normal ovulatory menses and of achievement of pregnancy. The treatment of prolactinomas, microadenomas, or macroad-enomas is further discussed under "Pregnancy." Surgical treatment involving craniotomy (never used for microadenoma) is far more hazardous than the trans-sphenoidal approach.

Pharmacotherapy: Bromocriptine. The use of an ergot derivative, 2-bromo-alpha-ergocryptine me-sylate, or bromocriptine (Parlodel) started in 1970, chiefly in Europe and the United Kingdom. There, most endocrinologists regard this drug and its congeners as the treatment of choice. Bromo-criptine is a dopamine receptor agonist. It is the natural hypothalamic hypophysiotropic hormone that exerts the principal tonic inhibitory influ-ence on pituitary prolactin secretion; that is, it is a prolactin-inhibiting factor or hormone (PIF, PIH). Untoward effects of bromocriptine are nau-sea, vomiting, and orthostatic hypotension; psychic effects (rarely, psychosis) are uncommon, but they may persist and become more or less troublesome in about 10 per cent of patients. These disadvantages can be minimized by very gradual attainment of the therapeutic dose and by careful follow-up. A practical regimen is this: A dose of 1.25 mg (orally) is given with a bedtime feeding; after a week without side effects, this dose is moved to the time of the evening meal; after another week or so, another 1.25-mg dose is added with another meal. Thereafter, the dose is gradually increased to 2.5 mg two to three times a day until the serum prolactin concentra-tion has fallen into the normal range. This usu-ally occurs within days to a few weeks (some favorable effect on the prolactin concentration is seen within hours) and at a total dose of 7.5 mg a day, which after some weeks can sometimes be given as a single dose. Patients develop tolerance to the side effects of the drug within days to weeks. Only occasionally are larger doses, up to 30 mg per day, required. Long-term therapy is safe; untoward effects of clinical significance are not seen even after years of treatment (see also under "Pregnancy").

Bromocriptine therapy is rapid and effective. At the usual dose, 7.5 mg per day, the general experience has been that microadenomas shrink—by as much as three-quarters of their volume—in 50 to 100 per cent of cases. Menses return in 85 per cent of treated women, and documented ovulation is restored in about 60 to 100 per cent. Coexistent deficiencies of pituitary function tend to improve to or toward normal; an exception is failure of serum testosterone concentrations to rise in about one-half of the treated men. After continuous treatment for 2 years or more, it is sometimes possible to reduce the bromocriptine dose if the serum prolactin concentration has fallen and the tumor has shrunk. Prolactin concentrations rise when bromocriptine is stopped, but after prolonged drug therapy, that rise may be delayed until many months after cessation of the drug.

Bromocriptine therapy is only rarely curative. When the drug is stopped, the tumor or the hyperprolactinemia or both recrudesce. Treatment therefore must be continued indefinitely. Symptoms and signs of the pituitary adenoma as a tumor mass are relieved as the tumor shrinks. As indicated, there is a very high rate of restoration of gonadal function, especially among women, and a number of hyperprolactinemic men with hypogonadism and depression respond to bromocriptine with improvement in emotional state, libido, potency, and sperm count, whether or not there is an accompanying rise in the serum testosterone concentration.

Disadvantages of long-term treatment with bromocriptine are these: The drug is expensive; no one knows how long treatment must be continued; and, in theory, there may be untoward effects—so far not identified—of therapy over many years.

Radiation Therapy. This modality is never used as primary treatment for microadenoma. If used adjunctively, the dosage is 4500 rad to the sellar region, delivered through three portals at a rate of 200 rad per day. The serum prolactin concentration falls to normal in fewer than 25 per cent of patients, even over many years. The fall, if it occurs, is exceedingly slow, like that of growth hormone in radiation-treated acromegaly. There is also a substantial risk of hypopituitarism after

20 years or more: hypogonadism in more than one-half of the patients, hypoadrenalism in about one-third, and thyroid deficiency in 15 to 20 per cent. Therapeutic results and unwanted sequelae are about the same with alpha-particles or proton beam therapy as with conventional radiotherapy.

Combination Therapy. Various combinations have been used to treat microadenoma. Second surgical procedures after tumor recurrence with initial surgical cure carry a much higher rate of untoward effects and sequelae. Bromocriptine is safe and effective if re-treatment is needed, for example, several years after trans-sphenoidal resection. Some workers have advocated initial treatment with bromocriptine, followed by surgery. The drawback with this sequence is that the planes of dissection between the adenoma and the contiguous normal pituitary tissue may be partly or completely obliterated, which renders surgery more difficult. Surgery followed by radiotherapy (or the reverse) is more likely to effect a permanent cure, but the incidence of hypopituitarism is higher and the patient is exposed to the risks of both procedures. The most useful combination appears to be prepregnancy radiation followed by bromocriptine (see under "Pregnancy"). To date, there are not enough reported statistics on the results of combination therapies to establish a clear preference. Treatment has to be individualized.

Observation Only. "Expectant" treatment is usually safe. Microadenomas progress in very few cases (well under 4 per cent). With alert monitoring (prolactin measurements, CT scans every 6 months to 2 or more years) and following patients for signs of tumor enlargement (headache, vision and visual field changes), recurrences can be anticipated or treated promptly. The larger the original tumor, the less likely is expectant therapy to be a reasonable alternative.

Pituitary Macroadenoma

By definition, macroadenomas are tumors with a diameter of greater than 10 mm (by CT scan). They are far less common than microadenomas. They seem to be more frequent in men than in women, perhaps because they are discovered later. Without the obvious clinical sign of amenorrhea as a marker, the clinical presentation is slower and more gradual; furthermore, male patients are reluctant to complain of reduced frequency of shaving, loss of libido, or impotence. The plasma prolactin concentration correlates only roughly with the tumor size. Values range from 300 to higher than 1000 ng per ml. With these large tumors, the tumor viewed as a mass is often the primary factor in governing treatment, not the hyperprolactinemia and its consequences (e.g., infertility).

Trans-Sphenoidal Adenomectomy. Cure (normal prolactin concentration) is achieved in only 10 to 40 per cent of patients; results are far less favorable than those for microadenomas. The larger the tumor, the lower the success rate. In some series, the rate of recurrence has been 20 to 80 per cent over several years; some workers believe that this rate will approach 100 per cent after enough time has passed. The mortality is 0.9 per cent, with a major morbidity of 14 per cent, which includes a 10 per cent incidence of diabetes insipidus, sometimes transitory and sometimes permanent. Repeat trans-sphenoidal operation is far more hazardous than a first or primary procedure, as is any approach that requires craniotomy. Secondary treatment is usually done with bromocriptine.

Bromocriptine. The tumor shrinks by one-half or more in about 70 per cent of the treated patients; some shrinkage occurs in the remaining 30 per cent. The prolactin concentration always falls but does not correlate with the tumor size before or during treatment. The rate of shrinkage is rapid, with reduction occurring within 1 to 2 weeks and almost always by 6 to 12 weeks. There are no indices that enable prediction of the amount or rate of reduction. A good plan is to treat during a period of many months. Even with signs of chiasmal compression, clinical improvement occurs in more than 90 per cent of patients, so that such signs do not necessarily imply a surgical emergency. This method tends to be the treatment of choice in the United Kingdom; in the United States, most clinics favor surgery as primary therapy.

Combination Therapy. For macroadenomas, many, perhaps most, patients require the addition of radiotherapy or trans-sphenoidal resection to the bromocriptine regimen. Not enough patients have been systematically followed to enable a clear statement as to the optimal order of therapeutic methods.

Observation Only. Because of the size of the tumor mass, this method is not appropriate for macroprolactinomas.

Pseudoprolactinomas

These hypothalamic or pituitary tumors, which induce hyperprolactinemia by their pressure effects on the infundibulum or the pituitary stalk, can sometimes be effectively treated with bromocriptine. Usually the treatment of choice is trans-sphenoidal resection (if the tumor is not too large and does not extend too far outside the pituitary fossa) or radiotherapy. It is probably true that many of these tumors are what endocrinologists used to call "chromophobe" or "null cell" adenomas; many of them are now known to be prolactinomas.

Pregnancy

Probably the best method of treating microadenomas and some macroadenomas in women who desire pregnancy is by initial radiation, followed by bromocriptine therapy (the latter to achieve a more rapid fall in the serum prolactin concentration). Once several ovulatory cycles (three or more) are achieved, conception may be attempted. If the attempt is successful, the patient is closely monitored. If in the course of the normal pituitary swelling during gestation there is apparent tumor recurrence, bromocriptine can be safely reinstituted. So far, there is no evidence of bromocriptine teratogenicity; the frequency of congenital anomalies in the fetus is no higher than that in the population of pregnant women at large. The question of whether breast-feeding should be permitted has not yet been settled (compare the stimulatory influence of suckling on pituitary secretion of prolactin).

Bromocriptine treatment has been successfully carried out in more than 3000 pregnant women. In a few patients, trans-sphenoidal surgery—where strongly indicated—has been done with perfect safety during gestation.

Hyperprolactinemia of Undefined Cause

As indicated earlier, many of these patients do not need treatment. It is not possible to predict with certainty to which patients this statement applies. Still, it is certain that only a tiny minority of microadenomas, even those that can be demonstrated, progress to macroadenomas and that this evolution is slow. Arguments in favor of treating these patients include restoration of fertility (if desired), restoration of normal estrogen levels (in premenopausal women), restoration of libido and potency (in men), and prevention of possible pituitary tumor (theoretical). In one controversial class of patients who show prolactin level elevations at about the time of the preluteal estradiol peak (in association with infertility), bromocriptine therapy may permit conception. Arguments against treatment include lack of evidence that undefined hyperprolactinemia is harmful, the observation that in some patients the hyperprolactinemia disappears spontaneously, the possibility that prolonged bromocriptine treatment may induce untoward effects not yet recognized, the high cost of the drug, and the apparent need for indefinite courses of treatment.

As to prevention of osteopenia, it is clear that it occurs as a result of hyperprolactinemia, but it is not yet proved that treatment has a favorable effect on the bone loss of calcium.

HYPOTHYROIDISM

method of
MICHAEL M. KAPLAN, M.D.
Southfield, Michigan

DIAGNOSIS

Hypothyroidism is the syndrome resulting from insufficient secretion of thyroid hormone from the thyroid gland. In mild to moderate cases, there is predominant deficiency of the main circulating thyroid hormone, thyroxine (T_4). In severe cases, there is also decreased secretion of tri-iodothyronine (T_3), the main active form of thyroid hormone inside cells. However, because most T_3 is made outside of the thyroid gland from T_4, intracellular T_3 deficiency can result from T_4 deficiency, as well as from reduced thyroidal T_3 secretion. Like anemia, hypothyroidism is not a diagnosis, but rather the result of specific thyroid pathology. Thus, there are two important aspects of diagnosis: establishing the hypothyroid state and determining its cause. Most hypothyroid patients require lifelong treatment, but those with self-limited diseases should not be committed to decades of unnecessary therapy. Moreover, if no etiology can be found, the presence of hypothyroidism should be questioned and verified.

To establish hypothyroidism, the important laboratory tests are an estimate of the serum free T_4 concentration and measurement of the serum concentration of thyroid-stimulating hormone (thyrotropin; TSH). The total serum T_4 level is often obtained, but many conditions besides hypothyroidism can cause low total T_4 values (Table 1), and many mildly hypothyroid patients have normal serum T_4 levels. The serum free T_4 level can be estimated by several methods, but by any of them, subnormal values are obtained in several conditions other than hypothyroidism (see Table 1), and again, mildly hypothyroid patients often have normal serum free T_4 concentrations.

Given the limitations of T_4 tests, the most sensitive and accurate test for hypothyroidism is the serum TSH concentration, particularly by a highly sensitive TSH assay. Serum TSH concentrations are elevated in virtually all patients with hypothyroidism caused by intrinsic thyroid disease, even in the mildest cases. By contrast, patients with low total and free T_4 values caused by nonthyroidal illnesses usually have normal TSH values by highly sensitive assays. The only patients who are missed if the serum TSH test is the primary screening method for suspected hypothyroidism are the rare individuals with pituitary and hypothalamic diseases, in whom the serum TSH level is usually normal and sometimes low. To minimize the chances of missing either mild primary hypothyroidism or hypothyroidism caused by unsuspected pituitary or

TABLE 1. **Causes of Subnormal Serum Total and Free T_4 Values and Elevated Serum TSH Values**

1. Subnormal serum total T_4 values
   a. Hypothyroidism
   b. Reduced serum concentration of thyroxine-binding globulin on a genetic basis
   c. Drugs: phenytoin (diphenylhydantoin), androgens, danazol, L-asparaginase, glucocorticoids, T_3, fenoclofenac, phenylbutazone, 5-fluorouracil, high-dose salicylates, and high-dose furosemide therapy in patients with renal impairment
   d. Severe nonthyroidal illnesses of many types

2. Subnormal serum free T_4 or free T_4 index values
   a. Hypothyroidism
   b. Therapy with T_3, phenytoin, or high-dose salicylates (the free T_4 concentrations are truly low in patients taking T_3 or phenytoin and artifactually low in patients taking salicylates)
   c. Severe nonthyroidal illnesses (less common than subnormal total T_4 values)

3. Elevated serum TSH values (the upper limit of normal is 4–6 μU/ml in most current, highly sensitive assays)
   a. Hypothyroidism caused by thyroid (not pituitary or hypothalamic) disease
   b. Recovery phase of severe nonthyroidal illness (TSH values of up to 20 μU/ml)
   c. Antibodies in serum against rabbit IgG (for conventional TSH assays) or against mouse IgG (for monoclonal TSH assays); this is rare
   d. Old age (a few individuals over age 60 yr have serum TSH levels of up to about 10 μU/ml, with no other evidence of thyroid disease)

hypothalamic disease, both serum free T_4 and TSH tests are needed. Causes of elevated serum TSH concentrations other than hypothyroidism are rare (see Table 1).

Of the causes of hypothyroidism (Table 2), Hashimoto's thyroiditis is by far the most common, accounting, along with prior ablative treatment for hyperthyroidism, for perhaps 90 per cent of the cases of hypothyroidism. The hallmarks of Hashimoto's thyroiditis are goiter and elevated serum titers of antithyroid microsomal antibodies and/or antithyroglobulin antibodies. In both the painful and painless varieties of subacute thyroiditis, hypothyroidism often occurs, but it usually lasts only for a period ranging from a few weeks to 3 months, with restoration of normal thyroid function thereafter. A radioiodine uptake test helps to distinguish Hashimoto's thyroiditis (radioiodine uptake usually normal or high) from subacute painless thyroiditis (radioiodine uptake usually quite low), and the latter disease should be suspected in a woman who presents with hypothyroidism in the first 6 to 8 months post partum. A painful thyroid gland strongly suggests subacute granulomatous thyroiditis. Other causes of thyroid damage in adults should be revealed by a careful medical history, and congenital hypothyroidism should be detected by neonatal screening programs. Pituitary and hypothalamic hypothyroidism are usually accompanied by signs and symptoms of other pituitary hormone deficiencies, and sometimes by the hypersecretory syndromes amenorrhea and galactorrhea, acromegaly, and hypercortisol-

TABLE 2. Causes of Hypothyroidism

1. Chronic lymphocytic (Hashimoto's) thyroiditis
2. Primary thyroid atrophy (probably a variant of Hashimoto's thyroiditis
3. Subacute granulomatous (de Quervain's) thyroiditis
4. Subacute painless lymphocytic thyroiditis
5. [131]I therapy or thyroid surgery for hyperthyroidism; may also occur late (10–20 yr) in the natural history of Graves's disease treated only with antithyroid drugs
6. Radiation therapy for head, neck, or upper chest malignancies
7. Antithyroid drugs; propylthiouracil or methimazole in overly high doses
8. Goitrogenic drugs: lithium, inorganic iodide, sulfonylureas (probably requires underlying thyroid damage in most cases); amiodarone can cause either hypothyroidism or hyperthyroidism
9. Infiltrative diseases, such as cystinosis, amyloidosis, or leukemia (rare)
10. Iodine deficiency (virtually nonexistent in North America)
11. Congenital hypothyroidism; usually thyroid dysgenesis or agenesis, less often goitrous cretinism (intrathyroidal enzyme deficiency), rarely autoimmune
12. Syndromes of tissue resistance to thyroid hormone (rare)
13. Hypopituitarism (TSH deficiency)
14. Hypothalamic disease (thyrotropin-releasing hormone deficiency)

ism. In cases of concomitant corticotropin (ACTH) and TSH deficiency, glucocorticoid replacement should be started before thyroid hormone treatment.

TREATMENT

The optimal treatment for hypothyroidism is oral levothyroxine sodium (Levothroid), that is, synthetic L-T_4. Dextrothyroxine (Choloxin) is available for treating hyperlipidemia; its merits as a hypocholesterolemic agent are debatable, but it has no place in the treatment of hypothyroidism. Therefore, all subsequent references to T_4 denote levothyroxine. Treatment with oral T_4 concomitantly restores the serum free T_4, free T_3, and TSH concentrations to normal in most cases. It also results in only minimal fluctuations of these measurements from hour to hour, thus approximating the normal pattern of euthyroid patients. Finally, treatment with T_4 allows the normal regulatory mechanisms to determine the serum and tissue levels of T_3 by allowing deiodination of T_4 to T_3 in each organ, again as in normal persons. The small contribution of thyroidal T_3 secretion is missing and the serum ratio of T_4 to T_3 is slightly elevated, but serum T_3 and free T_3 concentrations are well within the normal range.

Levothyroxine is available under several brand names (e.g., Levothroid, Levoxine, and Synthroid) and generically from many manufactur-

ers. There are well-documented cases of differences in bioequivalence between T_4 tablets from different manufacturers. In some cases, this is a result of incorrect hormone content in the tablets, reported in one generic preparation as recently as 1987. Even when the T_4 content of tablets of different brands is the same, for some patients differences in bioavailability and therapeutic effect exist. Therefore, I advocate specifying a T_4 brand that the physician trusts and not allowing generic substitution or brand switching. At an extra cost of no more than $40 per year, this policy avoids variations in thyroid status when patients refill their prescriptions.

Levothyroxine Dosage

Levothyroxine tablets are available in a wide range of strengths: 25, 50, 75, 100, 112, 125, 150, 175, 200, and 300 micrograms (often specified in milligrams, i.e., 0.025 to 0.3 mg). Even finer adjustments of the T_4 dosage can be made by having the patient take different doses on different days of the week or skipping 1 or 2 days a week. Because the half-life of T_4 in the blood is about 7 days, such schedules do not appreciably alter the serum free T_4, free T_3, or TSH concentrations from one day to the next. The long half-life of T_4 in the blood has several other practical implications. The time of day the tablets are taken does not matter. There is no reason to divide the daily dose. Skipped doses should be made up by taking a double or even a triple dose the day the omission is discovered. When a dosage adjustment is made, it takes 5 to 6 weeks for the patient's serum hormone concentrations to reach the new steady state.

The average daily levothyroxine dose needed to maintain a normal serum TSH concentration in a patient with little or no endogenous thyroid hormone production is about 120 micrograms, or 2 micrograms per kg body weight. However, there is wide variation from one patient to another in the T_4 requirement. In the author's practice, the great majority of hypothyroid patients need daily T_4 doses between 50 and 150 micrograms.

Factors influencing the optimal T_4 replacement dose are summarized in Table 3. The endogenous T_4 production rate in normal individuals falls with age, as does the optimal T_4 dose in hypothyroid patients: 50 micrograms daily may be sufficient for some patients over age 60 years. Body weight is a determinant and may account for the higher average dose needed in men. Another important variable is the patient's endogenous thyroid function. Small doses of T_4 may suffice in patients who have had ablative treatment for hyperthyroidism or surgery for large multinodu-

TABLE 3. **Factors Influencing Optimal Levothyroxine Dosage**

1. Age. Older patients need lower average doses; children need higher doses per kg of body weight.
2. Weight. The required dose tends to increase as body weight increases, but the correlation is weak.
3. Sex. Men tend to require higher doses up to age 60 yr, perhaps because they weigh more than women.
4. Residual secretory capacity of the thyroid gland. Substantial levels of autonomous secretion can lower the required dose.
5. Drugs. Cholesterol-lowering resins and soybean-based infant formulas bind T_4 within the gut and interfere with T_4 absorption.
6. Intestinal function. Short-bowel syndromes, intestinal bypass surgery, and inflammatory bowel disease can cause T_4 malabsorption.

lar goiters and whose residual thyroid function is subnormal but nonsuppressible. Malabsorption of T_4, necessitating increased doses, can occur in patients with inflammatory bowel disease or the short-bowel syndrome after intestinal resection or bypass surgery. The cholesterol-lowering resins cholestyramine and cholestipol bind T_4 (and T_3) in the intestine and impair absorption of T_4 (and T_3) into the blood. It is best if these resins can be avoided in patients taking thyroxine. If it is necessary for a patient to take T_4 and a cholesterol-lowering resin, they should be taken as far apart in time as possible, and the timing of the doses for both drugs should be exactly the same from day to day. Soybean-based infant-feeding formulas may also contain substances that interfere with T_4 absorption.

Initial Treatment

At the time of initial diagnosis, the rapidity with which the hypothyroid state is to be corrected must be given careful consideration. The hazard of overly rapid thyroid hormone replacement is myocardial ischemia in a patient with coronary artery disease. Thyroid hormone has direct inotropic and chronotropic effects on the heart, and correction of hypothyroidism also increases oxygen consumption by many tissues. Both of these thyroid hormone effects increase the demand on the myocardium for oxygen delivery. Moreover, coronary artery disease is often asymptomatic, probably has an increased prevalence in chronically hypothyroid patients, especially those with hypertension, and increases in prevalence with age.

Guidelines for initial doses of T_4 are summarized in Table 4. At one extreme, young hypothyroid patients may be given the estimated full replacement dose. At the other extreme, in patients over age 60 years with known heart dis-

ease, it may be advisable to start with as little as 25 micrograms of T_4 every other day and monitor the cardiac status carefully before every dose increase. The guidelines in Table 4 are offered only as reference points for decision-making; if in doubt, proceed cautiously. On rare occasions, a more aggressive approach may be appropriate; for example, a pregnant, severely hypothyroid woman could be given a loading dose of 200 micrograms of T_4 daily for 1 to 2 weeks if she and her physician decide that the increased risk of spontaneous abortion caused by hypothyroidism outweighs the cardiac risks of rapid replacement.

TABLE 4. **Guidelines for Initial T_4 Dosage in Hypothyroid Adults**

Clinical Situation	Reasonable Starting T_4 Dose*
1. Otherwise healthy patient under age 45 yr with low risk of heart disease and mild to moderate hypothyroidism (serum TSH 30 μU/ml or less)	Full estimated replacement dose: 100–150 μg daily, depending on age, weight, and sex; check in 6 wk, adjust as needed
2. Patient under age 45 yr with moderate to severe hypothyroidism and possible heart disease	Subreplacement dose: 50 μg daily; increase in 4–6 wk as needed if no adverse cardiac reactions occur
3. Patient aged 45–60 yr, mild to moderate hypothyroidism, and no known or suspected heart disease	Subreplacement dose: 50 μg daily; increase in 4–6 wk as needed if no adverse cardiac reactions occur
4. Patient aged 45–60 yr with severe hypothyroidism or with mild to moderate hypothyroidism and known or suspected heart disease	Subreplacement dose: 25 μg daily; increase in 4–6 wk as needed if no adverse cardiac reactions occur
5. Patient over age 60 yr with mild hypothyroidism and no known heart disease	Subreplacement dose: 25 μg daily; increase in 4 wk as needed if no adverse cardiac reactions occur
6. Patient over age 60 yr with moderate to severe hypothyroidism or with known or suspected heart disease	Very low dose: 25 μg every other day; increase in 2–4 wk if no adverse cardiac reactions occur

*These doses are guidelines for typical patients, not hard and fast rules. Individual patients often have additional medical conditions that necessitate modification of these recommendations to suit their particular needs. The recommendations apply to patients with hypothyroidism of unknown or presumed long duration. Patients with hypothyroidism of known brief duration, such as after ^{131}I therapy for hyperthyroidism or after T_4 withdrawal in a thyroid cancer patient for diagnostic tests or ^{131}I therapy, can generally be given a full replacement T_4 dose.

Monitoring Treatment

The adequacy of each patient's T_4 dose is best monitored by using a highly sensitive serum TSH assay that can reliably distinguish subnormal from normal serum TSH concentrations. The goal is to achieve a serum TSH concentration in the normal range. There is no evidence that any serum measurement of total or free T_4 or total or free T_3 is better in assessing the patient's thyroid status than a sensitive TSH determination. Indeed, when the TSH level is normal, the T_4 and free T_4 values are often at the upper limit of normal, or even high, when blood is sampled within 2 to 8 hours after the patient's last T_4 dose. In this setting, mildly elevated total or free T_4 values are generally ignored because decreasing the T_4 dose often causes the TSH level to rise into the hypothyroid range.

If a patient treated with T_4 has a highly sensitive TSH value below normal, the T_4 dose is higher than it needs to be. Currently, there is controversy over whether mild T_4 over-replacement leads to a decrease in bone mineral density; it might. Furthermore, there can be subtle changes in cardiac dynamics caused by mild thyroid hormone over-replacement, which could potentially have deleterious consequences in elderly patients with heart disease. In patients with unmeasurably low TSH concentrations by the sensitive assays, a small dose reduction can be made (e.g., omitting one tablet a week or reducing the average daily T_4 dose by 12.5 to 25 micrograms) to allow the TSH level to rise to normal without having it overshoot into the hypothyroid range. Because this is quite easy to do, because there may be adverse effects from over-replacement, and because there are no obvious advantages to over-replacement, I advocate precise T_4 dose titration so that the patient's serum TSH level, by highly sensitive assays, is within the normal range. Once this is achieved, annual checkups are generally sufficient, and the patient's dose is usually stable from year to year. Annual dose adjustments are at most minor ones, unless one or more of the factors listed in Table 3 has changed greatly.

Adjustment of the T_4 dose based on a sensitive TSH assay is much more reliable than adjustment by clinical intuition. Patients with slightly excessive or inadequate doses usually have no attendant physical findings. Many patients taking T_4 report that they have difficulty losing weight or are tired. These symptoms are exceedingly common in patients taking correct doses of T_4 and in patients with no thyroid disease. Trying to alleviate these patients' symptoms by raising the T_4 dose higher than that dictated by their own pituitary-thyroid set point achieves, at most, a transient placebo effect, risks the possible adverse effects of excessive doses noted earlier, and fails to address the real causes and appropriate management of the symptoms.

Patients who are taking optimal T_4 doses should be specifically informed that they are euthyroid. Other than the cholesterol-lowering resins, they may take any other medication that would otherwise be appropriate, including over-the-counter cold remedies with labels that advise patients with thyroid disease to consult a physician before use. After pregnancy there is no reason that a woman taking T_4 should avoid breast-feeding her infant.

Other Thyroid Hormone Preparations

Oral thyroid hormone preparations are available that contain L-T_3 (also termed "liothyronine"), either alone or in combination with T_4. These preparations include synthetic T_3, combinations of synthetic T_3 and T_4, and thyroid tablets USP. The last, available as desiccated thyroid and thyroglobulin, are made from porcine thyroid. They require gastrointestinal hydrolysis of T_4 and T_3 from the thyroglobulin and subsequent absorption of the released hormones. When patients take any preparation containing T_3, including thyroid USP, their serum T_3 concentrations fluctuate widely during the day. This never happens in patients with normal thyroid glands. Furthermore, in states of caloric deprivation and nonthyroidal illnesses, the serum T_3 level normally falls because of inhibition of T_4 deiodination. This appears to be an adaptation to illness, possibly serving a protein-sparing function. Treatment with T_3 prevents the body from making this adaptive response. In summary, there is no reason to use any preparation containing T_3 for chronic treatment of hypothyroidism and no reason at all to use the animal-derived preparations.

In three special situations, brief treatment with synthetic T_3 alone (Cytomel and generic preparations) might be considered.

1. In a hypothyroid patient with congestive heart failure or unstable angina, in whom treatment with thyroid hormone is considered necessary while the heart disease is stabilized. Such a patient could be treated with a low dose of T_3, 5 to 10 micrograms daily, with the rationale that if the myocardial ischemia worsens, the T_3 can be stopped, and its action will dissipate sooner than if T_4 were used. However, in most cases, it is better to start vigorous treatment of the cardiac ischemia first, and then introduce T_4 cautiously.

2. In myxedema coma. This condition is discussed later.

3. In thyroid cancer patients whose thyroid hormone is being withdrawn in preparation for diagnostic imaging studies or ^{131}I therapy. The duration of symptomatic hypothyroidism can be shortened, usually without interference with the cancer management, by treating the patients for 2 to 4 weeks with T_3 during T_4 withdrawal. The usual dose is 50 to 75 micrograms daily, and the T_3 must be stopped 2 to 3 weeks before the diagnostic or therapeutic procedures.

SPECIAL TREATMENT SITUATIONS

Congenital Hypothyroidism

In congenital hypothyroidism, the optimal dose per kilogram of body weight is much higher than that in adults. In some affected children in the first months of treatment, the serum TSH level fails to drop until the T_4 dose is raised to the point where deleterious effects of hyperthyroidism occur. The T_4 dose must therefore be monitored by a combination of careful clinical assessment, especially linear and skeletal growth, and serum T_4 measurements, with serum TSH measurements as an adjunctive test. After this initial phase, the pituitary-thyroid axis normalizes. Consultation with a pediatric endocrinologist is usually advisable for children with congenital hypothyroidism.

Pregnancy and the Postpartum Period

Some hypothyroid women taking a stable T_4 dose develop elevated serum TSH levels during pregnancy. Neither the frequency of this phenomenon nor the reason for it is clear; it occurs in a minority of cases. It is advisable to check the serum TSH level in the second trimester and adjust the T_4 dose if necessary. In the postpartum period, there can be a flare-up in the activity of Hashimoto's thyroiditis and an increase in the patient's T_4 need. Thus, a check of the TSH level about 6 weeks post partum is also advisable.

Painless subacute thyroiditis occurs with unusually high frequency in the postpartum period. This disease often has a phase of hyperthyroidism preceding a phase of hypothyroidism. The hypothyroidism is usually self-limited, lasting for up to about 3 months. Nevertheless, I offer a 3-month course of T_4 treatment to women with hypothyroidism caused by postpartum painless subacute thyroiditis, with the rationale that this may be a busy and stressful time in their lives, and subtle fatigue, weakness, or mood changes caused by hypothyroidism are intuitively undesirable and preventable. When painless subacute thyroiditis occurs in the postpartum period, it progresses to permanent hypothyroidism in up to 30 per cent of cases, more often than the 5 to 10 per cent incidence of permanent hypothyroidism after painless subacute thyroiditis occurring at other times. Thus, follow-up testing is needed whether or not T_4 treatment is administered.

Hypothyroid Patients Who Need Urgent Surgery

In the past, it was thought that hypothyroid patients tolerated surgery poorly. They are indeed more sensitive to depressant drugs such as narcotics and sedatives. However, recent studies suggest that with modern anesthetic techniques and careful attention to drug dosage, hypothyroid patients tolerate procedures such as coronary artery bypass with mortality and complication rates similar to those of euthyroid patients. If surgery is elective, it makes sense to render the patient euthyroid beforehand, but if surgery is urgent, current evidence indicates that it is prudent to proceed with surgery as dictated by the disease, with individualized preoperative and perioperative T_4 treatment.

Myxedema Coma

Myxedema coma is the extreme form of hypothyroidism, characterized by abnormalities of the sensorium ranging from obtundation to coma, hypothermia, and circulatory compromise caused by bradycardia and hypotension. There is usually a precipitating event superimposed on pre-existing severe hypothyroidism. Respiratory failure is common, and gastrointestinal atony (pseudo-obstruction) may occur. General therapeutic measures include identification and vigorous treatment of the precipitating disease, gradual correction of the hypothermia, oxygen and mechanical ventilatory assistance when needed, correction of abnormalities of intravascular volume and serum electrolytes, and administration of glucocorticoids (e.g., dexamethasone, 4 mg intravenously daily) in case there is concomitant adrenal insufficiency. These measures are at least as important as thyroid hormone replacement.

The optimal thyroid hormone dose in myxedema coma is not known. Paradoxically, although it is usually advisable to replace thyroid hormone slowly in severe hypothyroidism, thyroid hormone is replaced rapidly when myxedema coma is present. The explanations of this paradox are that the untreated condition has a mortality rate of about 80 per cent, and the potentially lethal aspects of the syndrome may begin to improve as early as a few hours after initiation of thyroid hormone repletion; thus, the potential benefits of aggressive thyroid hormone treatment outweigh the risks of precipitating myocardial ischemia. Intravenous administration of thyroid hormone is more reliable than oral or nasogastric tube administration because gastrointestinal absorption may not be normal in myxedema coma. T_4 for intravenous injection is available in 200- and 500-microgram vials. An injection kit for T_3 (Cytomel) is available from the manufacturer by special request. Some authorities advocate a loading dose of 500 micrograms of T_4 intravenously. Others advocate starting with 100 micrograms of T_4 intravenously once daily for 5 days, with clinical and laboratory assessment of cardiac and metabolic status several times daily, and adjustment of the T_4 dose thereafter. Successful treatment has also been reported with T_3 in doses of 20 to 40 micrograms daily, although published experience with T_3 treatment is not extensive.

The effects of thyroid hormone therapy in myxedema coma are monitored by careful clinical assessment, and laboratory tests, including a free T_4 estimate (if T_4 is given) and serum TSH levels. If T_3 is given, serum T_3 concentrations fluctuate widely and are difficult to interpret. TSH measurements are less helpful guides than usual because with long-standing severe hypothyroidism, there may be a nonsuppressible component of TSH secretion for several weeks, and the TSH level may fall but fail to normalize despite adequate or even excessive doses of thyroid hormone. Therefore, TSH determinations can provide reassurance that the thyroid hormone treatment is having some beneficial effect, but they cannot be used for T_4 or T_3 dose titration in the initial treatment of myxedema coma.

HYPERTHYROIDISM

method of
JAMES C. SHEININ, M.D., and
ARTHUR B. SCHNEIDER, M.D., PH.D.
Michael Reese Hospital and Medical Center
Chicago, Illinois

The presence of hyperthyroidism (thyrotoxicosis) and its underlying cause can be readily detected with current diagnostic techniques. Although available therapeutic modalities satisfactorily result in the reversal and eventual correction of the metabolic abnormalities, their major shortcoming is that they are usually directed at the result (e.g., the overactive thyroid or the excess thyroid hormone) rather than the pathogenesis (e.g., thyroid-stimulating immunoglobulins in Graves' disease) of the condition. Before discussing the options for treating hyperthyroidism, it is helpful to understand how the newer "high sensitivity" thyroid-stimulating hormone (TSH) assays facilitate

diagnosis. It is also important to highlight some steps in the differential diagnosis, so that the appropriate therapeutic choices can be considered.

Measurement of total thyroxine (T_4) and free thyroxine index (FTI) remains the first step in evaluating thyroid function. TSH assays that allow for the clear distinction between normal and low TSH levels are now widely available. Hyperthyroidism is associated with immeasurably low TSH levels (the very rare TSH-producing pituitary tumors are an exception). It appears that these TSH assays obviate the need for throtropin-releasing hormone stimulation testing. A normal TSH level, as measured by one of the new assays, virtually eliminates the possibility of hyperthyroidism. This can be especially helpful in patients with changes in levels of or with abnormalities of thyroxine-binding proteins. Occasionally, an undetectable TSH level may be found in patients with autonomous functioning nodules or Graves' disease who are euthyroid. Such patients require no treatment but close follow-up for evidence of hyperthyroidism.

The physical examination often establishes the cause of hyperthyroidism. Infiltrative ophthalmopathy (exophthalmos and/or extraocular muscle weakness) is found in Graves' disease, a nodular goiter in toxic multinodular goiter, and characteristic pain and tenderness in subacute thyroiditis. In other cases the cause cannot be determined without further tests. Hyperthyroid states can be divided into those with elevated or normal uptake and those with low uptake. Of the former, Graves' disease can be treated with antithyroid drugs or ablative therapy with radioactive iodine (^{131}I) or surgery. Toxic multinodular goiter or toxic adenomas are best treated with ablative therapy. Therapy must be directed at the rare tumors that produce TSH or human chorionic gonadotropin (hCG). Causes associated with low uptake (subacute thyroiditis, painless thyroiditis, thyrotoxicosis factitia, and other rare causes) are often self-limited and require no treatment or palliative treatment. Other tests may be helpful. A high free T_4 level by equilibrium dialysis or high tri-iodothyronine (T_3) level may indicate hyperthyroidism when the total T_4 level is normal or borderline high. Conversely, a normal free T_4 level by equilibrium dialysis or normal T_3 level when the total T_4 level is elevated may identify a euthyroid state with increased or abnormal T_4-binding proteins.

GRAVES' DISEASE

Graves' hyperthyroidism is an organ-specific autoimmune disorder in which thyroid-stimulating immunoglobulins (TSIs) cause overactivity of the thyroid gland independent of normal hypothalamic-pituitary control. Hence, the thyroid in Graves' disease can be thought of as the victim and not the culprit. It is a lifetime disease that is characterized by spontaneous exacerbations and remissions. In time, up to 20 per cent of patients may spontaneously develop overt or subclinical hypothyroidism. The ophthalmopathy and dermopathy of Graves' disease appear to be separate but related organ-specific autoimmune disorders that do not occur in all patients with Graves' disease. They may occur before or after the onset of hyperthyroidism and may occur in euthyroid or hypothyroid patients with Hashimoto's thyroiditis.

Unfortunately, no treatment of Graves' hyperthyroidism now available will regularly bring about permanent cure of the disorder without causing untoward effects. Current treatments limit the response of the thyroid to the TSIs and thereby control the production of thyroid hormones. Unlike other forms of hyperthyroidism, Graves' hyperthyroidism may go into remission, so all three therapeutic alternatives may be considered. These are inhibition of thyroid hormone synthesis with thioureylene drugs, ablation of thyroid tissue with ^{131}I, and ablation with surgery. Recent surveys in the United States and in Europe show that there is no consensus among endocrinologists in the approach to Graves' hyperthyroidism. Most favor a trial of thioureylene therapy as the initial management of young adult women, a view that we share. In older patients we most frequently recommend ^{131}I therapy. A recent report suggests that children and adolescents with Graves' hyperthyroidism are less likely to go into a thioureylene-related remission than adults. For them we prefer long-term thioureylene therapy. If a remission is not achieved, we consider either subtotal thyroidectomy or ^{131}I therapy on a case by case basis. Many endocrinologists now feel comfortable giving ^{131}I to adolescents and young adults. When, as in many patients with Graves' hyperthyroidism, two or all three therapeutic alternatives would be appropriate, the patient should be an enlightened participant in the decision-making process.

Thioureylene Drugs

Since the thioureylene drugs cause no permanent damage to the thyroid gland, permanent hypothyroidism does not occur as a consequence of their use. Most recent data suggest that there is about a 50 per cent likelihood of a remission following treatment with thioureylene drugs for 2 years. It has been suggested that the likelihood of remission following thioureylene therapy is inversely related to dietary iodine intake and that more frequent remissions are being seen now because of decreased dietary iodine.

Thioureylene drugs inhibit thyroid hormone biosynthesis by inhibiting incorporation of iodide into the tyrosine residues in thyroglobulin. In addition, one of the thioureylene drugs, propylthiouracil (PTU), inhibits 5'-deiodinase activity and thereby inhibits peripheral conversion of T_4

to the more active hormone T_3. Thioureylene drugs do not block the release of performed, stored thyroid hormone into the circulation. Consequently, thyroid hormone levels may not fall, and peripheral manifestations of hyperthyroidism may not abate until stored hormone is depleted. This may take 2 to 3 weeks after initiation of treatment. Therapeutic measures that block release of stored hormone and control peripheral manifestations of circulating hormones will be discussed subsequently.

Increasing evidence indicates that thioureylene drugs may have a direct or indirect immunosuppressive effect on the autoimmune disorder underlying Graves' disease. Clearly, however, the putative immunosuppressive effect does not ensure that a sustained remission will occur in all patients treated with thioureylene drugs. Characteristics of patients that tend to be associated with sustained remission are short duration of disease, mild disease, and small goiter. Conversely, long duration of disease, large goiter, ophthalmopathy, other autoimmune disorders, and family history of autoimmune thyroid disorders are associated with a greater chance of relapse.

There is controversy involving several fundamental aspects of thioureylene therapy, including selection of drug, size and timing of dosage, and duration of therapy. The therapeutic efficacy and side effects of PTU and methimazole (Tapazole) are quite similar. The potency of methimazole is about tenfold that of PTU. The serum half-lives of methimazole and PTU are about 5 and 1 hours, respectively. In most clinical settings either drug would be appropriate. There are some situations in which the longer half-life of methimazole or the inhibition of 5'-deiodinase activity by PTU makes one or the other the preferred drug. Our preponderant experience has been with PTU, and we have found it to be remarkably effective and safe. We begin therapy with 100 to 200 mg of PTU or 10 to 20 mg of methimazole every 8 hours. To maximize compliance, we recommend taking the medication upon arising, in midafternoon, and at bedtime. We see patients every 3 weeks for the first 6 weeks until the patient is euthyroid. Because of the postulated immunosuppressive effect of thioureylene drugs and because of recent data suggesting that higher dosages of thioureylene drugs may be associated with a higher incidence of remission, it is uncertain whether the dosage of thioureylene drugs should be decreased or be kept at a relatively high level with thyroid hormone added to maintain a euthyroid state. A recent survey of European endocrinologists found that 55 per cent favored the former, and 45 per cent favored the latter. Until recently, we favored the former approach, but reassessment now seems warranted, except in pregnancy. Parenthetically, thyroid enlargement in a patient being given thioureylene therapy may be an important clue to development of hypothyroidism resulting from stimulation of the thyroid by TSH.

Another unresolved aspect of treatment is the frequency of administration of thioureylene drugs. Although there have been advocates of giving either drug as a single daily dose, methimazole clearly appears more appropriate for such a regimen because of its longer half-life. If we thought that single daily-dose therapy would enhance patient compliance, we would select methimazole but initiate therapy every 8 hours and switch to a single daily dose when the patient became euthyroid. Once a euthyroid state and a stable medical regimen are established, we monitor our patients every 3 months, reverting to 3- to 6-week intervals should the clinical state or medical regimen change.

Yet another area of uncertainty involves the optimal duration of thioureylene therapy. Reports of duration of therapy range from as little as 3 months to 4 years or more. Although remissions may occur in as little as 3 months, sustained remissions apparently are more likely to occur after 1 to 2 years of therapy and may be even more likely to occur after more prolonged therapy. Although thioureylene therapy has been given for many years without untoward effects, the bulk of thioureylene-related sustained remissions appear to occur within 2 years of initiation of therapy.

Unfortunately, none of the currently available clinical or laboratory parameters assessed before or during thioureylene therapy are reliable predictors of thioureylene-related sustained remission. Therefore, after 1 to 2 years, we withdraw patients from thioureylene therapy as a clinical trial. Such patients should be seen every 4 to 6 weeks for the first 3 months and at 3-month intervals for the remainder of the first year off therapy, since this is the period of time during which hyperthyroidism is most likely to recur. However, as patients are followed for prolonged periods, more will relapse, and some will develop overt or subclinical hypothyroidism. Hence, we recommend that patients be seen at least once a year for their lifetime.

Untoward effects of thioureylene drugs occur in 1 to 5 per cent of patients, with fever, rash, urticaria, and arthralgia or arthritis most commonly seen. More significant but less frequent reactions include a lupus-like syndrome, toxic hepatitis (with PTU), and cholestatic jaundice (with methimazole). All patients treated with thioureylene drugs must be told about the small risk of acute agranulocytosis and should be instructed to stop the drug and to contact their physician immediately if they develop fever or sore throat. Agranulocytosis occurs in less than one-half of 1 per cent of patients treated, nearly always within 3 months of starting therapy. It should be noted that although neutropenia is common in untreated Graves' hyperthyroidism and that a dose-related neutropenia is associated with thioureylene therapy, agranulocytosis is acute, idiosyncratic, and not dose related and cannot be predicted from previous blood cell counts.

Ablative Therapy

Radioactive Iodine

Optimally, ablative therapy with ^{131}I or surgery would be sufficient to damage or to remove sufficient thyroid tissue to control the hyperthyroidism but not enough to cause lifetime hypothyroidism. Unfortunately, neither form of ablative therapy reliably fulfills this expectation.

Various approaches to ^{131}I therapy have been used in Graves' hyperthyroidism. These include doses calculated to attempt to achieve the optimal goal, smaller doses that attempt to minimize the incidence of post–^{131}I hypothyroidism, and larger doses that attempt to ablate the gland totally, accepting hypothyroidism and treating it with thyroid hormone replacement. The size of the ^{131}I dose is directly related to the incidence of hypothyroidism within the first year of therapy and is inversely related to the failure of the dose to restore a euthyroid state. However, the increasing incidence of hypothyroidism with time is independent of size of the ^{131}I dose given. It should be noted that up to 28 per cent of patients may develop transient hypothyroidism soon after ^{131}I therapy and subsequently may become either euthyroid or hyperthyroid again.

We calculate the ^{131}I dose to be given using the following formula:

$$\text{Dose (mCi)} = \frac{\text{base dose (μCi per gram)} \times \text{estimated thyroid weight (grams)}}{\text{fractional 24-hour } ^{131}\text{I uptake} \times 1000}$$

In an uncomplicated case of Graves' hyperthyroidism, we use a base dose of 80 μCi per gram. With this dose, we find that about 90 per cent of patients are rendered euthyroid within 6 months, that there is an incidence of hypothyroidism of about 10 to 20 per cent in the first year after therapy, and that there is a continuing incidence of hypothyroidism of about 2 to 5 per cent per year thereafter. Consideration is given to using thioureylene drugs, iodides, or beta blockers after ^{131}I therapy if more prompt restoration to a euthyroid state or if blocking peripheral manifestations of hyperthyroidism is desired. After ^{131}I therapy, we follow our patients at 6-week intervals for the first 3 months, at 3-month intervals for the remainder of the first year, and once a year for their lifetime.

Complications of ^{131}I therapy are rare. Radiation-induced thyroiditis or sialitis and mild exacerbations of hyperthyroidism may occur. Radiation-induced thyroid storm, which tends to occur in elderly patients, patients with complicating diseases, patients with long-standing hyperthyroidism, and patients with large glands, can be prevented by thioureylene drug treatment to restore a euthyroid state and deplete the gland of stored thyroid hormone prior to ^{131}I administration. To date, there is no evidence for increased incidence of any long-term genetic or neoplastic complications of ^{131}I therapy.

Surgery

Subtotal thyroidectomy carries with it not only the benefits and risks of ^{131}I therapy but the additional risks of a surgical procedure. It does result in prompt resolution of the hyperthyroid state. We favor the standard preparation for surgery, consisting of thioureylene drugs for 6 weeks to restore a euthyroid state and deplete the gland of stored thyroid hormone and potassium iodide as Lugol's iodine, 5 to 15 drops three times a day, or a saturated solution of potassium iodide (SSKI), 1 to 3 drops three times a day, for the 10 days just prior to surgery to decrease the vascularity of the gland. We feel that preparation for thyroid surgery using beta blockers and potassium iodide is less effective because it leaves the gland with a large amount of stored thyroid hormone and therefore should be limited to situations in which surgery cannot be delayed. Even in the hands of experienced thyroid surgeons and anesthesiologists, in addition to the minimal risk of intraoperative mortality, the risks of recurrent laryngeal nerve damage and permanent hypoparathyroidism are reported to be about 3 per cent. There may also be a minimal risk of thyroid storm, even after preoperative preparation. The risks of persistent or recurrent hyperthyroidism and of short- and long-term permanent hypothyroidism are correlated with the amount of residual thyroid tissue, which is not unlike the situation with ^{131}I therapy. Studies have demonstrated a 6 to 12 per cent incidence of persistent or recurrent hyperthyroidism—unacceptably high in our perspective—and up to about a 50 per cent incidence of hypothyroidism, depending on the amount of residual thyroid tissue and duration of follow-up. As with ^{131}I therapy, transient hypothyroidism may occur in up to 20 per cent of patients in the first postoperative year.

Adjunctive Therapy and Thyroid Storm

Beta-adrenergic blocking agents have proved to be valuable adjuncts because they ameliorate the peripheral sympathomimetic effects of hyperthyroidism. Propranolol (Inderal) has the additional advantage of inhibiting peripheral conversion of T_4 to T_3. Beta blockers are particularly useful in patients with supraventricular arrhythmias. Although they have been used as the sole therapy for Graves' hyperthyroidism and as preparation for surgery, we believe that such treatment is suboptimal. They are an essential part of the treatment of thyroid storm. Representative doses of propranolol in hyperthyroidism as adjunctive therapy are 40 to 160 mg daily, and in thyroid storm they are 160 to 480 mg daily or 1 to 10 mg intravenously.

Iodides are used to block release of stored thyroid hormone in thyroid storm and in other settings in which prompt lowering of thyroid hormone levels is desirable; they are also used to decrease the vascularity of the thyroid gland preoperatively. In thyroid storm, SSKI is given as 8 drops every 6 hours and 1 to 3 drops three times a day in other settings. Because iodides are incorporated into thyroid hormone, they should not be given until hormone biosynthesis is blocked by an initial dose of thioureylene drugs. Recently, iodinated contrast agents such as ipodate* (Oragrafin) and iopanoic acid* (Telepaque) have been used in thyroid storm. They are extremely effective in blocking the conversion of T_4 to T_3, but their exact role remains to be determined.

High dosages of glucocorticoids have been used empirically to treat thyroid storm due to "relative adrenal insufficiency," but it has been shown that such dosages inhibit peripheral conversion of T_4 to T_3 and may inhibit thyroid hormone secretion. In thyroid storm, 100 mg of hydrocortisone every 8 hours is recommended.

Since thyroid storm often occurs in association with a precipitating illness, the latter should be searched for and treated vigorously. Also, the systemic manifestations of thyroid storm, including fever, fluid loss, and cardiac complications, should be treated aggressively.

---

*This use of these agents is not listed in the manufacturers' directives.

Complicating Illnesses

There are certain clinical settings that favor one therapeutic modality or contraindicate another. There are patients for whom hyperthyroidism is a more significant risk, e.g., the elderly patient, patients with antecedent or hyperthyroidism-related cardiovascular disease, or patients with related autoimmune endocrine disorders such as adrenal insufficiency or insulin-dependent diabetes mellitus. Such patients require therapy that will promptly block the peripheral effects of hyperthyroidism, will rapidly restore a euthyroid state, will prevent release of stored thyroid hormone that may adversely affect their condition or may provoke thyroid storm, and will ensure no recurrence of hyperthyroidism. We initiate treatment of such patients with higher doses of PTU, 200 mg every 8 hours, and with propranolol, 40 to 240 mg daily in single long-acting or divided doses, for 6 weeks to render the patient euthyroid and to deplete the gland of stored hormone. Propranolol is continued, PTU is stopped for 3 to 5 days, and ^{131}I therapy is administered using the formula given earlier with 120 microcuries per gram of thyroid used as the base dose.

Pregnancy

Accurate assessment of thyroid status in pregnancy, in which thyroxine-binding globulin is elevated, requires estimation or measurement of the concentration of free T_4. Free T_4 is unchanged in normal pregnancy. It is estimated by the FTI (calculated from the T_3 resin uptake, which is low or low normal, and the total T_4, which is high in normal pregnancy) or measured by equilibrium dialysis. Graves' disease tends to abate or to remit in the second and third trimesters of pregnancy, possibly owing to immunologic alterations during pregnancy, and to exacerbate post partum. Because of the risk of thioureylene-induced fetal goiter and hypothyroidism, the dose of thioureylene drugs should be minimized and the mother should be kept at a high normal or minimally elevated free T_4 level. Thyroid hormones do not effectively cross the placenta, so that giving thyroid hormone medication to the mother will not prevent fetal goiter. PTU clearly is preferred to methimazole during pregnancy and lactation because it crosses the placental barrier about one-fourth as much as methimazole and is concentrated in milk about one-tenth as well. The suggestion that methimazole may be associated with congenital skin defects recently has been challenged. No teratogenic effects have been attributed to PTU.

Clearly, ablative therapy with ^{131}I is contraindicated during pregnancy. Should thioureylene therapy not be tolerated or should high doses be required, subtotal thyroidectomy in the midtrimester of pregnancy following the usual preoperative preparation is an appropriate and safe alternative. The safety of beta blockers in pregnancy has not yet been established. Because of the natural history of the disease during and after pregnancy and because of the desirability of minimizing PTU dosage, we follow our pregnant patients with Graves' hyperthyroidism at 4- to 6-week intervals during and for 3 to 6 months after pregnancy.

Recurrent Graves' Disease

Finally, the question arises of how to treat patients with persistent or recurrent Graves' hyperthyroidism following thioureylene therapy, subtotal thyroidectomy, and ^{131}I therapy. A patient who has not become euthyroid within 6 months after ^{131}I should be given a second dose, calculated with 120 to 150 microcuries per gram of thyroid as the base dose. Second operations carry with them significantly greater risks of hypoparathyroidism and laryngeal nerve injury, so patients with recurrent hypothyroidism following subtotal thyroidectomy should be given ^{131}I. The surveys previously alluded to demonstrate a clear lack of consensus on the approach to patients with persistent or recurrent hyperthyroidism following thioureylene therapy. Since most thioureylene-related remissions will occur within the first 2 years of therapy, hyperthyroidism will be controlled, but remission will occur infrequently after additional thioureylene therapy. Although long-term thioureylene has been well tolerated, we and most others would recommend ablative therapy, and we prefer ^{131}I therapy in all but the youngest patients. Should there be an exacerbation of hyperthyroidism after a sustained remission of years, we would favor another course of thioureylene therapy.

OTHER FORMS OF HYPERTHYROIDISM

Toxic Multinodular Goiter

The considerations for treatment of this form of hyperthyroidism are very similar to those for Graves' disease. Since toxic multinodular goiters do not go into spontaneous remission, thioureylene drugs are only indicated as a preparatory measure for ablative treatment with ^{131}I or surgery. Such preparatory treatment to deplete the gland of stored hormone is often indicated because toxic multinodular goiters occur most frequently in older patients. Preparatory treatment with PTU, 100 to 200 mg every 8 hours, should be continued until thyroid hormone levels fall into the normal range. These goiters tend to be more difficult to treat with ^{131}I. It is likely that this resistance occurs because different parts of the gland have different levels of function and autonomy. Therefore, larger doses of ^{131}I are usually given using the formula noted previously, with 150 microcuries per gram of thyroid as the base dose, and repeated treatments are sometimes required. Adjunctive therapy with beta blockers, as described previously, should be used as necessary.

Solitary Toxic Adenoma

Hyperthyroidism caused by a single overactive thyroid nodule is effectively treated with ^{131}I. The "hot" nodule concentrates ^{131}I, while the remainder of the thyroid has reduced uptake, resulting from suppression of pituitary TSH secretion, and is protected. It should be remembered that a "warm" nodule does not cause hyperthyroidism. The continued function of the remaining thyroid tissue indicates that pituitary TSH secretion has not been suppressed. Further, while all "hot" nodules are functioning autonomously, not all of them cause hyperthyroidism. Surgery is an acceptable, but usually unnecessary, alternative to ^{131}I therapy. The surgical procedure is limited to removal of the nodule or lobe and therefore is relatively safe.

Thyroiditis

Two forms of thyroiditis may present as hyperthyroidism. One form (subacute, de Quervain's or giant cell thyroiditis) is associated with a painful thyroid gland. The other form (silent, painless, or lymphocytic thyroiditis) is not associated with pain and often occurs in the postpartum period. In both instances, hyperthyroidism is caused by a process that destroys the thyroid gland, resulting in leakage of hormone into the circulation. Therefore, neither thioureylene drugs nor ablative therapy has a role in treatment. Both forms of thyroiditis resolve spontaneously, although lymphocytic thyroiditis may recur after subsequent pregnancies. In the acute phase, treatment is directed at controlling the peripheral manifestations of hyperthyroidism and controlling discomfort. Silent thyroiditis may be treated with beta blockers and subacute thyroiditis with aspirin (up to twelve 325-mg tablets per day in divided doses) or other nonsteroidal anti-inflammatory agents. In unusually resistant cases, prednisone may be used, starting with 40 mg per day and rapidly tapering the dose. The hyperthyroid phase of the disease may be followed by transient and rarely permanent hypothyroidism.

THYROID CANCER

method of
BLAKE CADY, M.D.
New England Deaconess Hospital
Boston, Massachusetts

Cancer of the thyroid is an uncommon disease that provokes considerable interest and controversy in its management because of the frequency of thyroid nodules and the often puzzling clinical evaluation of patients in terms of the need for surgery or other therapy. There is enormous variability in the outcome of cancers in the old and the young, which adds to the confusion and uncertainty about how to manage this disease. There are 11,000 cases of thyroid cancer in the United States per year but only 1100 deaths. Therefore, this is a relatively uncommon cancer and deaths are very uncommon, representing only 10 per cent of cases, compared with other visceral organ cancers. Thyroid cancer is predominant in women (more than 70 per cent of cases), particularly in the younger age groups. One of the confusing aspects of thyroid cancer is the frequency of occult, microscopic foci of papillary carcinoma seen in thyroid glands removed for benign problems. The incidence of these occult papillary carcinomas in microscopic foci may be as high as 30 per cent in routine autopsies in some parts of the world and is at least 10 per cent in autopsies in this country. The frequency is related, in part, to the number of sections of the thyroid gland inspected.

The known etiologic factors of thyroid carcinoma include radiation in childhood, which has been shown to be associated with an increased frequency of thyroid nodules and thyroid cancers many years later. This susceptibility to radiation occurs only in the developing thyroid glands of infants and children, however, and is reported in patients after radiation treatments of the thymus, adenoids, and skin in the years before 1950. Few patients with radiation-associated thyroid cancer are seen currently because of the complete cessation of childhood irradiation after the 1950s. Although family histories are common in benign thyroid disorders, only a few family clusters of differentiated thyroid carcinoma have been reported. In contrast, 20 per cent of medullary carcinomas of the thyroid occur in familial clusters, particularly in association with multiple endocrine neoplasia syndromes.

There is a relationship between environmental and dietary iodine levels and the frequency and type of differentiated thyroid carcinoma. Iodine-deficient areas have a higher incidence of cancers by a factor of about three; these cancers are more commonly follicular carcinomas.

PATHOLOGY

The most frequently used pathologic classification of thyroid carcinoma is seen in Table 1.

TABLE 1. **Classification of Thyroid Cancers**

1. Differentiated (from follicular epithelium): represents more than 95% of cases
   Papillary; mixed papillary and follicular
   Follicular (Hürthle's cell)
2. Undifferentiated (from follicular epithelium)
   Anaplastic, spindle and giant cell, small cell
3. Medullary (from parafollicular C cells)
4. Lymphoma
5. Other rare forms
   Squamous, sarcoma, teratoma
6. Metastatic
   Renal, lung, melanoma, breast

Any cancer with papillary features is classified as papillary carcinoma, whether it is pure papillary, mixed papillary and follicular, or predominantly follicular with only minor papillary elements. All cancers with papillary features behave in a biologically similar fashion. In contrast, pure follicular adenocarcinomas have a distinct biologic behavior, with few if any lymph node metastases and more common distant metastases, particularly to the lungs. Follicular carcinomas must be separated into low-grade, encapsulated lesions with minimal tumor capsular invasion by cancer cells and lesions marked by significant tumor capsular invasion by malignant cells and with blood vessel invasion. These latter tumors have a more aggressive behavior and a high incidence of metastatic disease. Hürthle's cell carcinomas are considered to be a separate entity by some investigators, but we view them as a variant of follicular adenocarcinoma, with biologic behavior similar to that of other follicular carcinomas. Medullary thyroid carcinoma is not a cancer of the thyroid cells but arises within the thyroid gland from parafollicular cells that produce calcitonin. Eighty per cent of medullary carcinomas are sporadic, with a unifocal origin in one thyroid lobe. The other 20 per cent are associated with familial syndromes and are characterized by multifocal origin throughout in the thyroid gland. Calcitonin produced by the parafollicular C cells is easily detectable in the serum and can be used as an accurate tumor marker. With few exceptions, the calcitonin level is elevated in cases of either familial or sporadic medullary carcinoma, and is particularly useful in screening familial endocrine syndrome persons without apparent clinical disease so that an early curative operation can be performed.

Undifferentiated thyroid carcinomas consist of anaplastic varieties with spindle and giant cells but also include some small cell types; they are extremely aggressive, lethal, and rapidly growing cancers. Fortunately, they have occurred with far less frequency in recent years and now make up only 2 or 3 per cent of all cancers, in contrast to more than 20 per cent in the 1930s and 1940s. In some parts of the world, they are still common. Thyroid lymphoma is relatively uncommon, but it is necessary both to recognize it and to separate it from generalized lymphomas that involve the thyroid gland. Thyroid lymphoma frequently arises in the background of Hashimoto's lymphoid thyroiditis, and this must be recognized in the differential diagnosis of thyroid masses in Hashimoto's thyroiditis. Rare cases of squamous cell carcinoma of the thyroid must be separated from squamous cell carcinomas of the larynx that grow into the thyroid gland and present as a thyroid mass.

RISK GROUP ASSESSMENT

Although the pathologic features of thyroid carcinoma are important, the age of the patient with differentiated thyroid carcinoma is the most important prognostic feature. No other human cancer has such a wide disparity of outcome on the basis of age. For many years, the excellent prognosis in the young and the modest prognosis in the old have been recognized, but in recent years this age separation has been more carefully analyzed and quantified. In differentiated thyroid cancer of childhood and in adults up to the age of 40 years in men and 50 years in women, less than 1 or 2 per cent of patients die of this disease. Children and young to middle-aged adults make up two-thirds of these cases. In contrast, men over age 40 years and women over age 50 years have a recurrence rate of at least 25 per cent and a death rate of more than 20 per cent.

The reasons for this great separation in outcome based on age are obscure. However, age is such a strong determinant of the prognosis that it supersedes the effects of size, extent, pathologic type, type of surgery, use of radioactive iodine, and all other clinical and therapeutic features of the disease.

In attempts to make the risk group assessment of cases more inclusive, clinical scoring systems have been developed. They indicate that in addition to age, the size and invasiveness of the differentiated cancers in the older age group should be taken into account to produce a more inclusive low-risk group that includes almost 90 per cent of all patients. In this more inclusive low-risk group, the cancer mortality rate is less than 2 per cent and the recurrence rate is less than 5 per cent. In the residual high-risk group, which makes up about 10 per cent of patients, the mortality rate is close to 50 per cent. Simple clinical criteria can be used to separate patients into low-risk and high-risk groups for help in assessing therapeutic options and outcomes. The definition of low-risk and high-risk patients is given in Table 2.

CLINICAL ASSESSMENT OF PATIENTS

Thyroid cancer patients usually present with either thyroid nodules or lymph node metastases in the neck. Rarely is a distant metastasis from thyroid carcinoma the presenting complaint in the absence of a thyroid mass. Assessment of the likelihood of cancer in the patient with a thyroid nodule hinges on its size; a history of recent growth; firmness, hardness, or fixation of the nodule; and symptoms suggestive of invasion of surrounding tissue, such as hoarseness from vocal chord paralysis, dysphagia from compression of the esophagus, or stridor from compression of the trachea. In young patients, 25 per cent present with an enlarged lymph node in the neck, sometimes without a palpable mass in the thyroid gland itself. Older patients usually present with a thyroid nodule.

Physical examination is essential and should be

TABLE 2. **Differentiated Thyroid Carcinoma:**
Inclusive Risk Group Definition

Low Risk (90% of All Patients)
1. Men 40 years or younger and women 50 years or younger
   A. All papillary cancers, regardless of local extent
   B. All follicular cancers with minor tumor capsular invasion
   C. Without distant metastases

2. Men >40 years and women >50 years
   A. Cancers less than 5 cm in diameter
   B. Follicular cancers with minor tumor capsular invasion
   C. Papillary cancers confined within the thyroid gland capsule

High Risk (10% of All Patients)
1. Men 40 years or younger and women 50 years or younger
   A. Follicular cancers with major tumor capsular invasion
   B. With distant metastases

2. Men >40 years and women >50 years
   A. Cancers greater than 5 cm in diameter
   B. Follicular cancers with major tumor capsular invasion
   C. Papillary cancers extending outside the thyroid gland capsule
   D. With distant metastases

performed in detail from both in front of and behind the patient. A careful evaluation of all the cervical lymph nodes is necessary, as well as evaluation of the thyroid gland itself.

Because thyroid cancer is an anatomic rather than a functional disease, measurements of thyroid function are of little help in assessing the risk of thyroid carcinoma in a particular nodule.

Anatomic studies of the thyroid gland, such as ultrasonography, radioactive thyroid scans, or computed tomography scans, may be helpful but are not diagnostic. Nodules that show increased activity may also harbor thyroid carcinoma. Thus, radioactive iodine scans of the thyroid gland should not be used as the sole basis for decisions about the surgical approach. Similarly, ultrasonic examination of thyroid nodules that reveals cystic lesions does not rule out the cystic presentation of a papillary carcinoma, which is not uncommon. Thus, the laboratory evaluation of thyroid nodules offers little specificity and should be viewed with caution.

Needle Biopsy

In contrast, thyroid needle aspiration of palpable thyroid masses or cervical lymph nodes is an extremely valuable technique. Although a specific diagnosis of cancer frequently cannot be made by thyroid needle cytology or biopsy, the essential discrimination between thyroid nodules that need to be removed surgically and those that can be observed can be made. Thyroid needle aspiration cytology showing a microfollicular pattern of cells consistent with either a benign or a malignant follicular neoplasm should lead to surgical removal. The thyroid needle aspiration may give a definitive diagnosis of papillary, anaplastic, or medullary carcinoma. Needle aspiration cytology or biopsy of the thyroid is usually not accurate enough to

discriminate between Hashimoto's thyroiditis and lymphoma of the thyroid. Thus, an argument can be made for thyroid nodule needle aspiration cytology or biopsy as the first diagnostic procedure after the history and physical examination. Once thyroid needle aspiration cytology has revealed cells consistent with adenomatous goiter and the nodule does not require removal because of its size or symptoms, functional tests can be performed to assess that aspect of thyroid physiology, and scans can be obtained to confirm the diagnosis of multinodular gland or act as a baseline for the follow-up of such patients. The separation of follicular thyroid lesions into benign or malignant categories by aspiration cytology is not possible at the present time; indeed, accurate discrimination between an adenomatous nodule in a multinodular gland and a follicular adenocarcinoma cannot be made. Therefore, any thyroid aspiration cytology that reveals a microfollicular pattern should lead to surgical removal. If there is any uncertainty about the interpretation of the thyroid needle cytology, it can be repeated, if necessary, before settling on a course of management.

Studies that have compared core cutting needle biopsy with fine needle aspiration cytology of the thyroid indicate that both techniques are highly accurate and equivalent. Fine needle aspiration has fewer complications, such as bleeding, and is easier and more acceptable to patients. Thus, at present, most thyroid needle biopsies should be aspiration cytology examinations. Use of a No. 18 or No. 19 needle for the aspiration cytology is recommended because more thyroid tissue can be obtained and even clumps of cells can be produced as a microbiopsy for examination by the pathologist.

Thyroid needle aspiration cytology is a laboratory test and, like all tests, needs to be put into a clinical context. If the patient has a mass that is so large that it should be removed anyway, there is little purpose in performing thyroid needle biopsy. If the nodule has clinical characteristics of cancer, it should be operated on regardless of the thyroid needle cytology findings. Although thyroid needle cytology can be extremely helpful in separating patients into those who require surgery and those who do not, it may not supply a specific diagnosis and must be placed in the clinical context.

TREATMENT

Operative Approach

Thyroid surgery is extremely safe and uncomplicated in experienced hands. The rate of recurrent laryngeal nerve injury should be less than 1 per cent, and hypoparathyroidism should not occur unless a bilateral thyroid operation is undertaken, in which case its incidence postoperatively should be less than 1 per cent to justify bilateral thyroid surgery. Death after thyroid surgery is extraordinarily rare. The average patient can walk the night of surgery, have food by mouth the next day, and leave the hospital within 3 days, if not earlier. Thus, the simplicity, ease, safety, and lack of complications after thyroid surgery should be appreciated to place the role of thyroid surgery in the management of thyroid nodules in context. Seventy-five per cent of patients operated on for thyroid disease today are explored for the possibility of cancer. Roughly one-third of patients with solitary thyroid nodules or predominant thyroid nodules in a multinodular gland undergoing aspiration cytology do not need surgery. The incidence of carcinoma ranges between 25 and 50 per cent in patients undergoing thyroid surgery for nodules. Benign follicular adenomas should also be removed because they apparently progress and later lead to follicular adenocarcinoma. Thus, the large majority of patients operated on have pathology that should be removed. The widespread use of thyroid needle aspiration cytology has perhaps doubled the incidence of carcinoma in surgical specimens by the elimination of small, innocuous nodules, but it is better to err on the side of surgical removal of ambiguous thyroid nodules.

The surgical approach to the thyroid gland is made through a low collar incision, which heals rapidly with a thin scar and minimal disfigurement. The median diameter of thyroid cancers operated on in recent years has decreased to less than 2 cm in diameter; thus patients can be easily handled with a thyroid lobectomy, either total or subtotal, as the initial operative step. Once the pathologist has examined the specimen and made the diagnosis, benign lesions need no further surgery; cancers sometimes need additional tissue removal. Most cancers in young patients at extremely low risk of death from disease are adequately treated by a unilateral thyroid operation. The opposite thyroid lobe should be examined at surgery because multicentric cancers sometimes occur in the opposite thyroid lobe in patients with papillary thyroid carcinoma; those abnormal lobes should also be removed. Lymph node metastases in papillary carcinoma are common. When encountered in the area of the thyroid bed they can be removed by a "node-picking" operation. If lymph node metastases were palpable before surgery, the thyroid incision can be extended to perform a modified neck dissection, preserving the spinal accessory nerve and usually the sternocleidomastoid muscle and the jugular vein.

In patients with a significant risk of recurrence and death, the thyroid operation needs to be more extensive for ease in the use of radioactive iodine. This mandates a total lobectomy on the side of the primary thyroid cancer and a subtotal thyroid gland removal on the opposite side. On occasion, total thyroidectomy may be required for multifocal thyroid carcinoma, but this does not increase curability and is associated with significant increases in complications.

For patients with medullary carcinoma of the thyroid, total thyroidectomy should be performed because, at the time of surgery, the complete family history is usually not known; the patient may be the index case of a familial cluster and may have multicentric cancer. If thorough documentation of a medullary carcinoma is available before surgery, so that its sporadic nature is completely confirmed, total thyroidectomy is not required. In medullary carcinomas, ipsilateral neck dissection should be performed in a more traditional fashion, including the sacrifice of the jugular vein, sternocleidomastoid muscle, and all the lymph nodes from the superior mediastinum and lateral and upper neck, with sparing of the spinal accessory nerve. Submandibular dissections are not required. Node metastases are common and imply a poor prognosis in patients with medullary carcinoma, although the typical disease course is indolent and may extend over many years.

Patients with anaplastic thyroid carcinoma can seldom have a complete removal of the tumor because it usually invades the surrounding tissues widely and is large. The major therapeutic goal in surgery of anaplastic carcinoma is to achieve a satisfactory airway by unroofing the trachea and, if necessary, performing a tracheostomy. In thyroid lymphoma the tumor should be completely removed if possible because the prognosis is excellent if the lymphoma is confined to the thyroid gland. Frequently, complete removal is impossible because of the large size of the tumor and the extensive involvement of surrounding tissues.

Follow-up of Thyroid Cancer Patients

Postoperative management of thyroid carcinoma remains controversial. In low-risk patients, because the prognosis is so good, radioactive iodine therapy cannot add to the control of disease. In patients with high-risk, differentiated thyroid carcinoma, radioactive iodine should be routinely used postoperatively, first to ablate any normal thyroid gland and later diagnostically to seek out the presence of metastases. Metastases can be treated with therapeutic radioactive iodine if they concentrate the tracer dose, which unfortuntely occurs in a minority of cases.

Although thyroid hormone administration postoperatively to suppress thyroid-stimulating hormone is routine, there is some doubt about whether it makes a difference in the long-term prognosis. Standard therapy today includes thyroid hormone administration, but for young patients with a small carcinoma and a hemithyroidectomy with a 100 per cent chance of cure, thyroid hormone administration postoperatively should be optional if patients are euthyroid.

The use of thyroglobulin as a tumor marker postoperatively is effective only in the presence of a total thyroid ablation and thus is not widely applicable. It has little use in young patients, who have almost no risk of recurrence or death, but it can be used in high-risk patients for follow-up. Unfortunately, treatment of metastatic disease is uniformly unsuccessful in older patients. Chest x-ray films should be taken if symptoms are present or pulmonary metastases are suspected. Thyroid function tests should be performed occasionally to analyze the success of thyroid-stimulating hormone suppression if thyroid hormone is administered. Routine bone scans, radioactive iodine scans, and other tests in the low-risk group are probably of little value. They may be used in the high-risk group for follow-up when metastases are suspected.

Lymphoma of the thyroid is curable with the use of multidrug chemotherapy and radiotherapy after surgery. Multidisciplinary management of anaplastic carcinomas should include both chemotherapy and radiotherapy, but unfortunately, cures are essentially unprecedented.

PHEOCHROMOCYTOMA

method of
SHELDON G. SHEPS, M.D.
Mayo Clinic and Mayo Medical School
Rochester, Minnesota

Just over a century ago (1886), Fränkel described a young woman with symptoms of pheochromocytoma in whom, at autopsy, bilateral adrenal tumors were found. In 1922, Labbé reported a case and was the first to attribute the symptoms to the adrenal tumors. The next year, Professor Villard of Lyon operated on a patient who died in shock. In 1926, C. H. Mayo, at the Mayo Clinic, and G. Roux, in Switzerland, successfully removed adrenal tumors and dramatically reversed hypertensive episodes.

Epinephrine was isolated in crystalline form and the chemical structure was elucidated in 1897. The hormone was synthesized in 1904 and later was shown to be present in increased amounts in pheochromocytomas. Some years later, identification of norepinephrine, dopamine, other precursors, and metabolites led to rapid advances in the biochemical diagnosis of pheochromocytoma. Precision in the measurement of these compounds was further refined by high-pressure liquid chromatography (HPLC) and radioisotopic labeling techniques, which have greatly contributed to the preoperative diagnosis and follow-up in patients with catecholamine-producing tumors.

INCIDENCE

Pheochromocytoma is a rare tumor that occurs at any age, but the peak incidence is in the fourth through the sixth decades. Among the general population in Olmsted County, Minnesota, pheochromocytoma occurs in 1 or 2 adults per 100,000 per year, whereas in Sweden, occurrence is one-fourth that rate. Among hypertensive persons, the incidence of pheochromocytoma has decreased because essential hypertension has been diagnosed in an increased number of persons in recent years. From 1973 to 1975, the annual incidence of pheochromocytoma at the Mayo Clinic was estimated to be 0.4 per 1000 hypertensive persons with diastolic pressures of 95 mmHg or more.

Pheochromocytoma may be part of a polyglandular endocrine derangement or may be associated with other neuroectodermal disorders. There is an increased incidence in families, particularly those of children with pheochromocytoma and especially when pheochromocytoma is present in both adrenal glands. Autosomal dominant inheritance is seen in multiple endocrine neoplasia, Type II (MEN Type II), in association with pancreatic islet cell tumors, and in neuroectodermal disorders (neurofibromatosis and von Hippel-Lindau disease). Families with multiple adrenal and extra-adrenal pheochromocytomas unassociated with other tumors or syndromes also have been reported.

PATHOLOGIC FEATURES

Pheochromocytoma is a tumor of chromaffin cells located in the adrenal medulla. The cells are derived from the cells of the neural crest, which also contribute to the central nervous system and sympathetic ganglia. Neuroblastomas, ganglioneuromas, and pheochromocytomas may arise from these tissues. Mixtures of these cell types may be present in the tumors. These cells are part of the amine precursor uptake and decarboxylation (APUD) cell system and retain the biochemical mechanisms to synthesize, store, and secrete many biogenic amines and peptides. This development explains some of the isolated and familial polyglandular tumor relationships and the many potential secretory products.

Ninety per cent of pheochromocytomas arise in the adrenal medulla. Solitary lesions are more common on the right. About 5 per cent of occurrences are bilateral, and about 10 per cent of tumors are extra-adrenal and solitary. The location of extra-adrenal chromaffin tissue may be anywhere from the base of the brain to the testicle, including the interatrial cardiac septum. Extra-adrenal tumors account for up to 19 per cent of catecholamine-producing tumors. Most are within the abdomen, but a few are within the chest and neck. About 10 per cent of tumors recur.

Malignancy is a difficult problem because of the potential for multicentric origin of pheochromocytoma and because of the lack of specific histologic, biochemical, and electron microscopic criteria of malignancy.

For malignancy to be diagnosed, tumor cells must be found in sites where chromaffin tissue does not normally occur (for example, lymph nodes, liver, bone, muscle, and lung). The incidence of malignant disease may range from 3 to 14 per cent. Hosaka and associates performed nuclear DNA studies on ploidy by flow cytometry in 75 patients with pheochromocytomas who had a follow-up of 10 years. All patients with a normal DNA histogram had a benign course, whereas 30 to 40 per cent of those with aneuploid or tetraploid-polyploid DNA had evidence of malignant disease. The importance of these observations in the diagnosis and follow-up of patients operated on remains to be clarified.

CLINICAL FEATURES

Nearly all tumors produce symptoms or signs related to the excessive production and release of catecholamines; even manipulation of a "nonfunctioning" tumor at surgery can release catecholamines. Symptoms are not related to the size, location, or histologic appearance of the tumor. Symptoms, entirely or in part, are episodic in most patients. The episodes usually are uniform in composition, although they tend to vary in duration and increase in severity and frequency with time. The onset of each episode is characteristically sudden, and peak severity is reached within a few minutes. The duration is less than 15 minutes in half the patients and shorter than an hour in most. The paroxysms either are spontaneous or are elicited by exercise, bending over, urination, defecation, pressure on the abdomen, induction of anesthesia, or injection of histamine, guanethidine, glucagon, droperidol, tyramine, metoclopramide, cytotoxic drugs, saralasin, tricyclic antidepressants, or phenothiazines.

The clinical clues to pheochromocytoma are symptomatic paroxysms, including headache, pallor, perspiration, and palpitations; unusual lability of blood pressure; accelerated hypertension; a pressor response to induction of anesthesia or to any antihypertensive drugs; and a suprarenal or midline abdominal mass. Hypertension may appear only with a paroxysm or may be more persistent. Rarely, hypotension is a presenting feature; when it is, the patient usually has a tumor that secretes predominantly epinephrine, dopa, or dopamine.

MEN Type II consists of medullary carcinoma of the thyroid gland, pheochromocytomas, and parathyroid disease. A variant of this syndrome, MEN Type IIB, is manifested as an abnormal phenotype and rarely includes parathyroid disease. Pheochromocytomas in MEN Type II are asymptomatic in about half the patients and are diagnosed by biochemical testing, indicated by detection of abnormalities in the thyroid and parathyroid glands or by a positive family history (autosomal dominant inheritance). In this syndrome, the thyroid tumor and pheochromocytomas are preceded by hyperplasia of the appropriate cell type, and the tumors are multiple, bilateral, and potentially malignant with metastasis.

CATECHOLAMINE METABOLISM

Norepinephrine is synthesized from tyrosine by way of dopa and dopamine in the brain, chromaffin tissue, and sympathetic nerve endings (Figure 1). In mammals, epinephrine is formed from norepinephrine almost entirely in the adrenal medulla. Small amounts of epinephrine and norepinephrine are excreted unchanged or conjugated, but the rest is excreted primarily as the respective catechol O-methyl derivatives (metanephrine and normetanephrine) and, after additional oxidation of the amine group, as vanillylmandelic acid (VMA).

DIAGNOSIS

Diagnostic studies generally include measuring the urinary excretion of norepinephrine, epinephrine, dopamine, total metanephrines, and VMA and the plasma concentrations of norepinephrine and epinephrine. The urinary determinations may be done on specimens collected during 24 hours or less, and the results may be expressed as either 24-hour rates, hourly rates, or per milligram of creatinine. The determination of total metanephrines has given the fewest false-negative results, from 1 to 2 per cent, and has been our choice for a screening test because of its accuracy and the ease of processing many specimens every day. Methylglucamine, a component of many iodinated contrast media used in radiology, may cause metanephrine values to be falsely normal for as long as 72 hours after its use. Determinations of VMA are positive in about 90 per cent of patients with pheochromocytoma.

Methods that use HPLC for the determination of fractionated catecholamines (norepinephrine, less than 80 micrograms in 24 hours; epinephrine, less than 20 micrograms in 24 hours; and dopamine, less than 400 micrograms in 24 hours) in urine are highly sensitive: More than 95 per cent of tumor patients have had positive results (norepinephrine and epinephrine, greater than 100 micrograms in 24 hours). At these diagnostic decision levels, the clinical specificity of the test is relatively low. Higher decision levels (norepinephrine of greater than 170 micrograms in 24 hours or epinephrine of greater than 35 micrograms in 24 hours) provide good clinical specificity (greater than 95 per cent), even in patients receiving antihypertensive medications, while maintaining the same level of sensitivity for tumor detection. Examining both the norepinephrine and the epinephrine values and considering an increase of either catecholamine to be positive are important. From 50 to 70 per cent of patients have increased values of epinephrine, and 75 to 80 per cent have increased values of norepinephrine. When norepinephrine and epinephrine are considered together, more than 95 per cent of patients have increased concentrations of either. Dopamine adds little diagnostic information except in relatively rare situations when extraordinary amounts are secreted.

One must be aware of clinical situations and drugs that could influence the test result (Table 1). Mildly increased values for total metanephrines may be noted in 10 to 20 per cent of patients without tumor. Values above the normal range in these patients often are due to interference by drugs or unusual urine pigments. Special precautions that we have described enable these interfering substances to be differentiated from

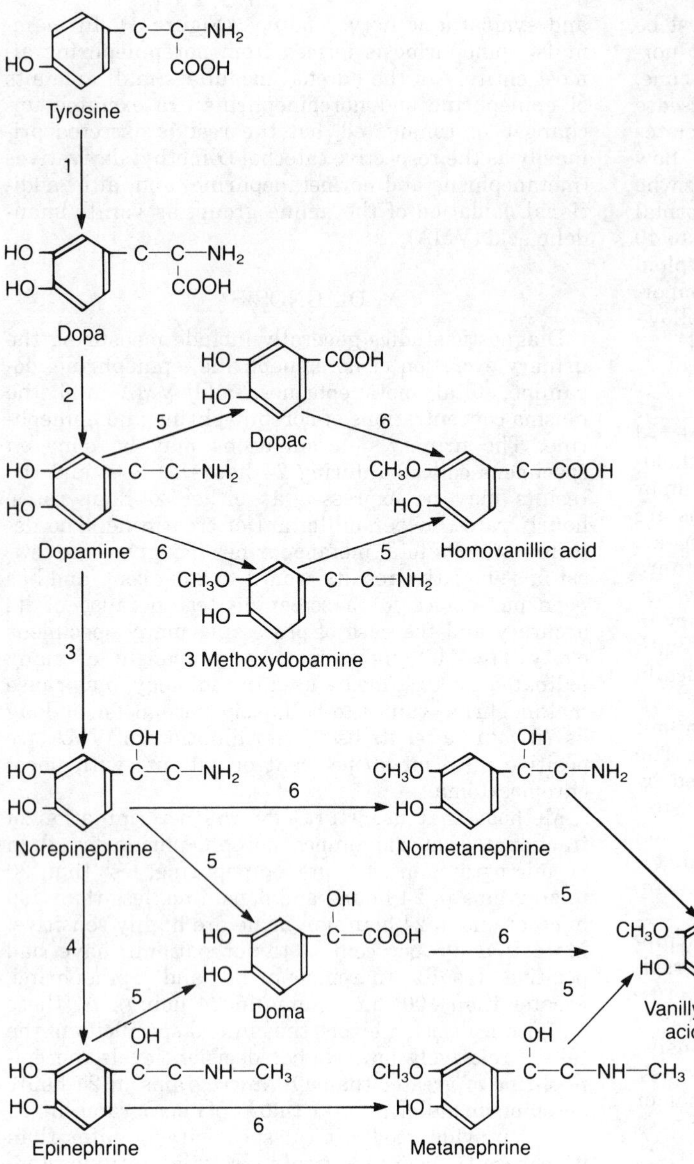

Figure 1. Pathways and enzymes of catecholamine metabolism: 1, tyrosine hydroxylase; 2, aromatic amino acid decarboxylase; 3, phenylamine beta-hydroxylase; 4, phenylethanolamine *N*-methyltransferase; 5, monoamine oxidase plus aldehyde dehydrogenase; and 6, catechol *O*-methyltransferase. (From Sheps SG: Pheochromocytoma. *In* Spittell JA Jr (ed): Clinical Medicine. Vol. 7. Philadelphia, Harper & Row, Publishers, 1984, pp 1–26. Used by permission.)

true increases in metanephrines. The combination of determination of urinary metanephrines as a screening test and confirmation by determination of urinary fractionated catecholamine excretion is a noninvasive laboratory regimen that has excellent predictive value for the identification of the patient with pheochromocytoma.

The application of much more specific methods for measuring catecholamine concentrations in plasma (radioenzymatic, HPLC) also has added to diagnostic acumen. Catecholamines in plasma are chemically labile, and the samples must be handled carefully. Many alterations in physiologic and pathologic states can profoundly affect the concentration of plasma free norepinephrine. To enhance accuracy, one must pay careful attention to blood drawing and preparation of the patient. The variability associated with age, sex, and renal failure is uncertain. Even when samples are collected properly, plasma measurements of norepi-

nephrine and epinephrine are not as sensitive as urinary measurements for the detection of pheochromocytoma. Plasma norepinephrine concentrations of greater than 750 pg per ml or epinephrine concentrations of greater than 110 pg per ml are found in 90 to 95 per cent of patients with tumors, but as with urinary measurements, the specificity of the measurements at these upper limits for normal subjects is not good for separating patients with tumors from other patients with similar symptoms. When high diagnostic decision levels are used to overcome the specificity problem, the sensitivity of the measurements for tumor detection decreases. At decision levels of 2000 pg per ml for norepinephrine or 200 pg per ml for epinephrine, the specificity is about 95 per cent, but the sensitivity for tumor detection drops to about 85 per cent.

Clonidine can be given orally to distinguish between the patient with pheochromocytoma, whose hypersecretion of plasma norepinephrine does not respond to

TABLE 1. **Situations and Drugs Interfering with Biochemical Diagnosis of Pheochromocytoma***

Stimulation of Endogenous Catecholamines

Plasma and urine catecholamines are most sensitive, but metanephrines and VMA can be abnormal as well: emotional and physical stress, surgery, acute central nervous system disturbance (stroke, hemorrhage, tumor, encephalopathy), acute coronary ischemia, angiography, hypoglycemia, caffeine, nicotine, diazoxide, theophylline, drug withdrawal (alcohol, clonidine), vasodilator therapy (nitroglycerine, sodium nitroprusside, calcium channel blockers administered acutely).

Exogenous Catecholamines

All the tests can be abnormal but HPLC and radioenzymatic assays are more specific and sensitive for catecholamines: nose drops, sinus and cough remedies, bronchodilators, appetite suppressants.

Drugs Altering Catecholamine Metabolism
1. Reduction in plasma or urine catecholamines: alpha$_2$ agonists, chronic use of calcium channel blockers, converting enzyme inhibitors, bromocriptine.
2. Decreased VMA; catecholamines and metanephrines increased: methyldopa,† monoamine oxidase inhibitors.‡
3. Variable changes in any test: phenothiazines,‡ tricyclic antidepressants,‡ L-dopa.‡
4. Increase in plasma or urine catecholamines: alpha$_1$ blockers, beta blockers, labetalol.

Specific Interference
1. ↓ Metanephrine: metanephrine assay interference by the methylglucamine§ in radiographic contrast medium.
2. ↓ Urinary catecholamines: mandelamine destroys catecholamines in bladder urine.
3. VMA ↓: clofibrate.
   VMA ↑: nalidixic acid, anileridine.
4. Labetalol: metabolite(s) interfering with all tests.

*From Sheps SG, Jiang N-S, and Klee GG: Diagnostic evaluation of pheochromocytoma. Clin Endocrinol Metab 17:397, 1988.

†HPLC assays can accurately determine catecholamines and metanephrines in presence of methyldopa.

‡Drugs with prolonged half-lives may need to be discontinued for 2–3 wk before accurate determinations can be made.

§Methylglucamine destroys a reagent in the Pisano metanephrines assay; this is most pronounced in urine collected the same day as the contrast medium is administered but may last up to 72 hours.

the drug, and the patient without tumor, whose high basal concentration is decreased to normal by the drug. Careful attention to the procedure of this test is necessary to avoid false-positive results, for example, during concomitant administration of propranolol. Provocative pharmacologic tests are rarely necessary.

LOCALIZATION

Although most pheochromocytomas arise in the adrenal glands or nearby and almost all are located within the abdomen, the tumors may exist anywhere from the base of the brain to the scrotum and may be multicentric. Localization methods help the surgeon plan the operation and reduce the chance of negative findings at laparotomy if the tumor happens to be outside the abdomen. However, the surgeon still must determine whether there are multiple and bilateral

tumors. At present, computed tomography (CT) is the most reliable method for preoperative localization: Well over 90 per cent of the tumors are visible if included in the area of examination. CT is accurate, noninvasive, and reproducible; magnetic resonance imaging (MRI) and CT are the only imaging techniques that can visualize normal adrenal glands when the diagnosis is equivocal. MRI may emerge as a desirable procedure for extra-adrenal locations and in pregnant patients. In adrenal MRI, relaxation times of pheochromocytomas are often dramatically greater than those of normal adrenal tissue. More experience is needed to evaluate this observation. CT-guided percutaneous adrenal biopsy in unsuspected pheochromocytoma has been associated with cardiovascular crises.

Scintigraphy with ^{131}I-labeled meta-iodobenzylguanidine (MIBG) is an exciting new method for localizing pheochromocytomas. MIBG concentrates in adrenergic vesicles, and where these vesicles are sufficiently numerous, an image can be produced. Catecholamine-producing tumors and metastatic lesions have been demonstrated throughout the body; the normal adrenal medulla in humans generally is not imaged. About 10 per cent of tumors are not demonstrated; false positives are rare (1 to 2 per cent). Positive studies can be used to direct CT scanning efforts to provide precise anatomic localization of the tumor or tumors. MIBG may also image other APUD tumors. At present, CT, because of general availability, should be used for initial localization attempts, first to scan the adrenals and, if results are negative, next to study the entire abdomen and pelvis. MIBG scintigraphy should be used if results of this study are negative or if metastasis or familial disease is considered likely. MRI can be directed at any extra-abdominal site for further anatomic localization.

TREATMENT

Surgical excision is the definitive therapy. Proper preparation for surgery has greatly reduced the previously high surgical morbidity. Most institutions now prepare their patients with alpha-adrenergic blocking agents (phenoxybenzamine [Dibenzyline], prazosin [Minipress], terazosin [Hytrin], phentolamine [Regitine]) until they have been normotensive and free of spells for about a week. Preoperative volume expansion is seldom necessary with this approach. Beta-adrenergic blocking drugs are added for several days before the operation, particularly if the patient has had arrhythmia. Caution should be taken with the addition of beta-adrenergic blocking agents if cardiomegaly or evidence of cardiomyopathy exists. Labetalol or other alpha- and beta-adrenergic blocking agents can be very effective, but the proportion of the alpha and beta blockade in the drug may not be applicable to all patients with pheochromocytoma. If the blocking drugs are not well tolerated, metyrosine (Demser) may be used preoperatively. Additional drugs that have been useful in some cases are calcium channel blocking agents and converting enzyme inhibitors. Preoperative preparation with glucocorticoid should be done in patients likely to have bilateral adrenalectomy, such as those with MEN Type II. Attempts to preserve the adrenal cortex have occasionally been successful.

A transabdominal approach is generally necessary to allow thorough exploration of all chromaffin tissue in the abdomen, and associated intra-abdominal disease, particularly cholelithiasis (occurring in almost 30 per cent of patients with pheochromocytoma), can be corrected at the same time. The posterior approach, although safe, usually entails excessive manipulations of the tumor. During surgery, careful attention to anesthesia, cardiovascular hemodynamics, and blood volumes contributes to greatly reduced surgical mortality. The present consensus is that enflurane is the anesthetic agent of choice because it does not sensitize the myocardium to exogenously administered catecholamines or stimulate the release of catecholamines from the tumor or sympathetic system. During the operation, the electrocardiogram, central venous pressure, and mean arterial pressure are monitored continuously. A Swan-Ganz catheter is used almost routinely to measure the filling pressures of the left ventricle. Intraoperative blood pressure crises are handled with infusions of sodium nitroprusside or nitroglycerin; phentolamine (Regitine) and labetalol (Normodyne, Trandate) can also be used. Arrhythmias can be treated by parenterally administered beta-adrenergic blocking drugs and lidocaine.

The operative mortality at the Mayo Clinic from 1980 to 1986 was 1 in 77 patients (1.3 per cent). In our previous experience, the 5-year survival rate was 96 per cent for patients with benign tumors and 44 per cent for those with malignant tumors.

After curative surgery, 10 per cent of patients have recurrence; thus, catecholamine and metabolite levels should be measured annually for at least 5 years and perhaps longer—and certainly promptly if symptoms appear or hypertension recurs. The recent findings of flow cytometry suggest that patients with abnormal DNA patterns should have closer and longer follow-up to detect malignant disease earlier.

For inoperable or metastatic tumors, consideration has been given to surgical intervention and therapeutic embolization to reduce tumor load and catecholamine production. Repeated therapeutic doses of MIBG have not produced a substantial long-lasting benefit. Radiation therapy is generally successful if doses of 40 Gy or more can be administered to the area because the tumors are relatively radioresistant. Chemotherapy trials have not had a persistent benefit on catecholamine production or tumor growth, although striking transient decreases have been reported with cyclic administration of cyclophosphamide, vincristine, and dacarbazine. The effects of excess circulating catecholamines can be controlled by the use of alpha- and beta-adrenergic blocking agents, alone or in combination with the previously mentioned drugs.

THYROIDITIS

method of
NADIR R. FARID, M.B., B.S.
Memorial University of Newfoundland
St. John's, Newfoundland, Canada

Traditionally, thyroiditis has been classified temporally as acute, subacute, and chronic, with these descriptions often superimposed upon other relevant characteristics, e.g., acute suppurative or chronic goitrous. The recent recognition of the clinical entity of painless thyroiditis (associated or unassociated with pregnancy) has further complicated this classification. Silent thyroiditis unassociated with pregnancy is subacute in duration, whereas postpartum thyroiditis may fall in the categories of subacute to chronic. In the latter event, it would be important to differentiate postpartum from chronic autoimmune thyroiditis, as the management is different. A viable alternative to the traditional classification of thyroiditis has, however, not emerged.

ACUTE (SUPPURATIVE) THYROIDITIS

Acute thyroiditis is now rarely seen in adults except in immunocompromised patients. It is usually associated with infection with gram-positive organisms. It presents as an acute inflammatory process with exquisite localized swelling and tenderness, lymphadenopathy, fever, and leukocytosis. In the event of recurrent attacks or involvement of the left lobe, pyriform sinus fistula should be suspected. Appropriate parenteral antibiotics should be instituted immediately while awaiting the results of bacteriologic culture. Aspirates of the affected area should be cultured both aerobically and anaerobically, and antibiotic therapy should be altered accordingly. Surgical intervention may be necessary if an abscess is formed.

Although they do not present acutely, tuberculosis and (even more unusually) syphilis and fungal infections can result in suppurative thyroiditis.

SUBACUTE (DE QUERVAIN'S) THYROIDITIS

Pain is generally a cardinal feature of subacute thyroiditis; unusual patients presenting with protracted malaise have been described. Subacute thyroiditis is probably due to viral and rickettsial infections of the thyroid triggering cell-mediated injury. This form of thyroiditis predominantly occurs in the summer and early fall, particularly around the Great Lakes. The pain over the thyroid area may be flitting in nature and may be transmitted. The thyroid gland is tender to touch and presents a localized or generalized "woody" texture. More severe cases are associated with marked systemic symptoms, including fever, malaise, and hyperthyroidism. The diagnosis is made on clinical grounds, corroborated by mild to moderate hyperthyroxinemia in the presence of thyroidal radioiodine uptakes greater than 5 per cent and high erythrocyte sedimentation rates; thyroid autoantibody titers are usually negative to low.

Reassurance of the patient and anti-inflammatory agents usually suffice in the case of mild attacks. Coated aspirin, 600 mg every 6 to 8 hours, for a week to 10 days is prescribed with gradual reduction of the dose thereafter. Steroids should be used in severe attacks as well as for recurrent mild bouts. Dexamethasone (Decadron) is started at a dose of 8 mg per day and is rapidly halved by 7 to 10 days and then reduced slowly thereafter, with the view to discontinuing therapy by the end of a month. In the event of recurrence of symptoms on reducing or discontinuing the drug, the lowest dose compatible with symptom control should be reinstituted. Symptoms of hyperthyroidism should be controlled with propranolol (Inderal), 20 to 40 mg every 8 hours.

With severe attacks or after several recurrences, patients may experience symptomatic hypothyroidism; this is usually short-lived and does not require replacement therapy. Permanent hypothyroidism is not a usual sequela of subacute thyroiditis.

PAINLESS THYROIDITIS

Painless thyroiditis is immunogenetically and immunologically allied to autoimmune thyroiditis. The reason these conditions are usually self-limiting, whereas chronic autoimmune thyroiditis is not, is unknown. They generally run a subacute course associated with variable degrees of thyroid dysfunction. The condition is characterized by lymphocytic infiltration of the thyroid associated with no to moderate goiter formation, and variable degrees of hyperthyroxinemia followed by no to fairly severe thyroid insufficiency;

during the acute phase the 24-hour radioactive iodine uptake is 5 per cent or less. This condition tends to occur preferentially post partum, and then it is more likely to be associated with goiter, a symptomatic acute hyperthyroid phase, and severe prolonged hypothyroidism. In some areas postpartum hypothyroidism is not usually preceded by a thyrotoxic phase; the extent to which variation in diagnostic criteria, dietary iodide intake, and disease severity contribute to this phenomenon is unclear. Mothers with elevated titers of antimicrosomal antibodies in the second/third trimester of pregnancy are at approximately 50 times the risk for postpartum thyroiditis than are antibody-negative women. The prevalence of postpartum thyroiditis is 6 per cent in these women, and they stand a 25 to 30 per cent chance of recurrence in future pregnancies. Thyroid autoantibody titers are lower in painless thyroiditis not related to pregnancy.

Painless thyroiditis unrelated to pregnancy at most requires symptomatic control of the hyperthyroid phase with beta-adrenergic blockers; rarely do these patients become symptomatically hypothyroid. The hyperthyroid phase of postpartum thyroiditis usually requires symptomatic management. Thyroid replacement therapy is necessary in about 30 per cent of patients with postpartum thyroiditis. While hormone replacement may be necessary for several months to a year, we have seen patients who required treatment, albeit at a reduced dosage, for up to 4 years after a single episode of postpartum thyroiditis. The need for continued thyroid replacement therapy should be reviewed on a 6-month basis after discontinuing the drug for 4 to 5 weeks. Circulating thyroid hormones, basal, and if necessary thyroid-releasing hormone (TRH)–stimulated thyroid-stimulating hormone (TSH) should be measured. When in doubt as to whether postpartum hypothyroidism is related to chronic or postpartum thyroiditis, I elect to manage the patient in the same fashion as I would a patient with postpartum thyroiditis. Recovery from painless thyroiditis is often associated with a decline and even a disappearance of thyroid autoantibodies.

CHRONIC AUTOIMMUNE THYROIDITIS

Chronic autoimmune thyroiditis may or may not be associated with diffuse (goitrous) goiter (Hashimoto's thyroiditis) and atrophic (idiopathic myxedema) thyroiditis, respectively. The underlying pathologic processes, lymphocytic infiltration, thyroid cell death, and attempts at regeneration and fibrosis, are common to both conditions; in goitrous thyroiditis, thyroid growth predominates over destruction. The manifold increase in the prevalence of goitrous thyroiditis over the last three decades has been attributed to the increase in iodide intake. Atrophic thyroiditis affects an older group more readily than does the goitrous variety. In Hashimoto's thyroiditis, goiter is diffuse and may reach large proportions even in iodide-sufficient areas. The vast majority of patients with autoimmune thyroiditis remain euthyroid and asymptomatic, although it remains the most important cause of noniatrogenic thyroid failure.

The diagnosis of goitrous autoimmune thyroiditis is confirmed by high titers of antimicrosomial antibodies; although a patchy pattern on thyroid scintiscan provides further confirmation, it is not necessary to establish a diagnosis. Serum (preferably serum-free) thyroxine and basal TSH should be measured; slight elevations of serum TSH are an indication for TRH stimulation tests. On the basis of this battery of tests, different degrees of thyroid failure may be established: from minimal, with normal serum thyroid hormone concentrations and increased pituitary TSH reserve, to severe, associated with marked symptoms, very high basal TSH, and low serum thyroxine concentrations. Atrophic thyroiditis is uncovered in epidemiologic or hospital surveys or in patients found to be hypothyroid in the absence of goiter.

The purpose of thyroxine treatment should be to correct symptomatic hypothyroidism and limit or suppress goiter growth. Epidemiologic data suggest that symptomatic individuals who are positive for thyroid autoantibodies and have a slight elevation of serum TSH may drift in and out of a euthyroid state. Unless they have an expanding goiter, these patients do not require therapy but should be maintained under close surveillance. Symptoms of mild thyroid failure may be subtle, and therapeutic trials may sometimes be justified. No control studies are available to date to separate the placebo effect from a physiologic effect of such a policy.

The goal of therapy of thyroid failure is to correct symptoms and to normalize serum TSH. The advent of high-sensitivity TSH assay has made it unnecessary for most patients to undergo the TRH stimulation test to ascertain suppression of pituitary TSH. Many TSH assays cannot confidently separate "undetectable" from normal serum TSH, and concomitant free-serum thyroxine measurement may be necessary. Over-replacement is particularly relevant in the older patient, as even mild hyperthyroxinemia may induce insomnia, weight loss, or cardiac symptoms. In younger patients with goiter in whom the goal is complete suppression of pituitary TSH secretion, mild hyperthyroxinemia may be well tolerated. Older recommendations concerning optimal replacement doses of L-thyroxine were recently revised as the amounts of the bioavailable hormone in older formulations (before 1985) were apparently overestimated. This phenomenon was reflected by the need to reduce the L-thyroxine dose of patients on stable chronic doses. Patients with symptomatic hypothyroidism should be advised not to expect improvement for 3 to 5 weeks after onset of therapy. Younger patients with moderate to severe hypothyroidism may be started on 0.075 to 0.1 mg of thyroxine and followed up some 6 weeks later for clinical assessment and measurement of serum-free thyroxine and high-sensitivity TSH, with dosage adjusted accordingly. Patients above the age of 55, particularly if they have symptoms or electrocardiographic evidence of ischemic heart disease, are started on 0.025 mg per day, with a stepwise increase by 0.025 mg per day every 4 to 6 weeks, and thyroid function is reassessed when a dose of 0.075 mg per day is attained. The dose of L-thyroxine may then be adjusted to bring serum TSH within the normal range. In patients with moderate to severe symptoms of ischemic heart disease, a smaller dose of thyroid and/or prior institution of beta-adrenergic blockers may be necessary. Clearly, the thyroid replacement dose should be individualized on the basis of thyroid function tests. Because in some patients the autoimmune injury is progressive, the dose of L-thyroxine may have to be adjusted depending on symptoms, goiter progression, and thyroid function tests after many months of apparent stable activity. There is no place for the use of thyroid extracts of L-tri-iodothyronine for the correction of hypothyroidism or suppression of goiter growth. The physician should stress to the patient the importance of compliance with chronic thyroid replacement.

It is good practice to monitor shrinkage of goiter in patients with goitrous thyroiditis. Unequal reduction of goiter may be due to a coincidental nodule or thyroid lymphoma and warrant further investigations. Infrequently, the goiter may continue to grow despite suppression of serum TSH, and surgery is indicated if evidence of pressure on underlying or retrosternal structure is suspected.

RIEDEL'S THYROIDITIS

Riedel's thyroiditis is a rare condition in which the thyroid and surrounding structures are involved in a progressive fibrotic process. Patients with retroperitoneal fibrosis and biliary cirrhosis are particularly prone to this disorder. The thyroid is stony hard. Surgery may be required to relieve pressure symptoms, and thyroid hormones may be necessary if hypothyroidism supervenes.

Section 9

The Urogenital Tract

BACTERIAL INFECTIONS OF THE URINARY TRACT IN MEN

method of
PHILIP M. HANNO, M.D.
Hospital of the University of Pennsylvania
Philadelphia, Pennsylvania

Asymptomatic infections of the urinary tract are rare, present in less than 0.6 per cent of men under 60 years, 1.5 per cent of men 60 to 69 years, and 3.6 per cent of men over 70 years. The incidence of symptomatic infection is 10 per cent that of women, and infections in adult males mandate urologic investigation. Cystitis is normally secondary to a primary infection of the prostate or kidney or to recent use of instrumentation or urologic surgery. In the absence of lower urinary tract obstruction, urinary stasis, a foreign body (e.g., catheter), or calculus disease, recurrent urinary infections will usually be traced to bacterial persistence in prostatic fluid. A prostatic antibacterial factor has been isolated from prostate fluid. It is a zinc salt that along with the protective length of the male urethra may be an important extrinsic defense mechanism against infection in men. Intrinsic bladder defense mechanisms include hydrokinetic clearance of bacteria through voiding (compromised in patients with outlet obstruction and residual urine), bacterial antiadherence activity of luminal mucopolysaccharides of the bladder mucosa, and possibly some bacterial growth-inhibitory characteristics of urine.

DIAGNOSIS AND LOCALIZATION OF URINARY TRACT INFECTION

Segmented bacteriologic localization cultures will differentiate cystitis from urethritis and allow determination of whether the prostate is the source of infection. Following cleansing of the glans, the patient initiates urination, and the physician collects 5 to 10 ml of urine first voided in a sterile container (VB 1). A sterile midstream urine is next obtained (VB 2). The patient is asked to stop voiding and prostatic massage is conducted, following which the expressed prostatic secretion is collected from the meatus (EPS). Finally, the patient completes voiding, and the fourth specimen is collected (VB 3). Quantitative culture and sensitivity data are collected from each of the above specimens.

If VB 1 is positive and greater than VB 3, the diagnosis is urethritis. If EPS or VB 3 is greater than VB 1, a prostatic infection is primary. If VB 2 indicates greater than 10^4 organisms of pure culture, the patient has cystitis and needs to be treated for 5 days with an appropriate antimicrobial (Table 1) that does not diffuse into the prostate (e.g., nitrofurantoin macrocrystals), following which cultures are repeated to determine the source of the infection.

BACTERIAL CYSTITIS

This presents with some combination of urinary frequency, urgency, dysuria, nocturia, suprapubic discomfort, low back pain, and hematuria. Systemic symptoms of fever, chills, and rigors are generally absent unless acute bacterial prostatitis or pyelonephritis is concomitant. Urine culture confirms the diagnosis, showing at least 10^5 colonies of pathogen. *Escherichia coli* is found in 80 per cent of infections. *Klebsiella, Enterobacter, Proteus, Pseudomonas,* and *Serratia* organisms are also found. Other pathogens include *Streptococcus faecalis* and *Staphylococcus.* Treatment requires 10 to 14 days of oral antibiotics, the choice determined by culture and sensitivity data. Urologic investigation to rule out complicating anatomic or functional pathology in the urinary tract is carried out during or after completion of therapy.

ACUTE AND CHRONIC BACTERIAL PROSTATITIS

Acute bacterial prostatitis is manifested by the sudden onset of chills, fever, pain in the lower back and perineum, and difficulty in urination. The urine sediment is positive for white cells and bacteria. On rectal examination the prostate is

TABLE 1. **Oral Antibiotics Commonly Given for Urinary Tract Infection in Men**

Antibiotic	Recommended Dose
Nitrofurantoin macrocrystals (Macrodantin)	50 mg 4 times daily
Trimethoprim-sulfamethoxazole (Septra, Bactrim)	Two tablets (160 mg trimethoprim, 800 mg sulfamethoxazole) twice daily
Carbenicillin indanyl sodium (Geocillin)	One or two tablets 4 times daily
Cephradine (Velosef)	250–500 mg 4 times daily
Norfloxacin (Noroxin)	400 mg twice daily
Ciprofloxacin (Cipro)	250–500 mg twice daily

exquisitely tender. Excessive prostatic palpation can induce septicemia. This condition is usually treated on an inpatient basis with 5 to 10 days of parenteral antibiotics, chosen according to bacterial sensitivities. Empiric therapy with a penicillin or cephalosporin in conjunction with an aminoglycoside is recommended prior to tailoring therapy after sensitivity data become available. Following parenteral treatment, outpatient treatment for another 2 weeks is the rule with oral antibiotics. As opposed to chronic bacterial prostatitis, there is good penetration of antibiotic into the acutely inflamed gland, and the choice of drug is not as critical.

Chronic bacterial prostatitis, in contrast, is insidious in onset. In most cases, the patient has no history of acute prostatitis, and there is no fever. Patients usually present with a history of recurrent bacterial cystitis but may be surprisingly asymptomatic in the intervals. They may have perineal pain and a tender, "boggy" prostate on examination. Diagnosis is made on the basis of the localization studies already described. Treatment is prolonged, as diffusion of antibiotics into the non–acutely inflamed prostate is poor, and 6 to 8 weeks of oral antibiotic therapy is not uncommon. Trimethoprim-sulfamethoxazole (Septra, Bactrim), carbenicillin indanyl sodium (Geocillin), and norfloxacin (Noroxin) reportedly give adequate prostatic levels of antibiotic in many cases. One should not confuse true bacterial prostatitis with nonbacterial prostatitis and prostatodynia, much more common conditions for which antibiotics are *not* indicated.

SPECIAL CIRCUMSTANCES

Patients with chronic indwelling catheters and asymptomatic bacterial colonization should not be treated, as sterilization of the urine is virtually impossible, and resistant organisms are likely to establish residence in the presence of long-term antibiotic suppression. Treatment should be instituted only for symptoms of acute infection. Asymptomatic bacteriuria in elderly patients, although associated with an increased mortality rate, has not been found to be the cause of the mortality. This condition is difficult to cure and probably should not be treated.

BACTERIAL INFECTIONS OF THE URINARY TRACT IN WOMEN

method of
C. DAVID CAWOOD, M.D.
St. Luke's Episcopal Hospital
Houston, Texas

Urinary tract infections in women are extremely common, yet are an urgent and vexing problem for patient and physician alike. For the most part, they are lower tract in origin (bladder), are not serious, and if left untreated are usually self-limiting. The usual presenting symptoms are frequency, dysuria, urgency, suprapubic pressure, and a feeling of incomplete emptying. If untreated, these symptoms may progress to gross hematuria with the passage of blood clots as a result of rapid proliferation of organisms and local severe bladder mucosal inflammation (hemorrhagic cystitis). Subsequent ascent into the upper urinary tract occurs in a small proportion of these patients, with the development of flank pain, malaise, and fever, indicating renal infection (pyelonephritis). Recurrent urinary tract infections in women do not lead inevitably to renal damage and renal loss of function, although this is possible in women who have reflux or who are pregnant.

Unlike the man, who has no natural portal for the entry of bacteria into the intact urinary tract, the women has a very short (3 cm) urethra, which has been shown to be the origin of entry in the overwhelming majority of infections. The classic example is that of "honeymoon cystitis" experienced by the newlywed woman, who develops frequency, urgency, and dysuria, often with hematuria. This initial episode of cystitis marks many an adult woman's entry into the pattern of recurrent cystitis or urinary tract infections; the vast majority of such infections are temporally related to coitus. It has been shown unequivocally that the organisms responsible for such infections are almost always indentifiable by serotype in the colon and on the perineum hours or days before the cystitis develops.

DIAGNOSIS

The benchmark for diagnosing a urinary tract infection is a properly collected mistream urine specimen for urinalysis and culture. However, urethritis may be present without a positive urine culture because the midstream urine may have washed the bacteria and white blood cell–rich initial urethral washings into the toilet, replacing them with relatively innocuous-looking urine and low-colony-count culture results. Also, a colony count of 10^5 organisms per ml is no longer generally considered to be the sine qua non of a significant urinary tract infection; a patient with a proven colony count of 10^6 organisms at 7 a.m. can easily have a colony count of 10^1 or 10^2 organisms in a midstream or catheterized specimen by 2 p.m. as a result of normal fluid intake, so that dilution of the urine is more rapid than the doubling rate of the organism. In the initial stages of infection, a woman may have fairly intense symptoms, yet the urinalysis may show only a few white blood cells or a few bacteria; a culture, if performed, is generally positive, although the colony count may be low.

Urine specimens sent to the laboratory are subject to many changes during transport, storage, handling, and interpretation. If possible, the physician should centrifuge and examine the urine personally (a simple 2-minute test), which often yields far more meaningful results. If an adult woman presents with only lower urinary tract irritative symptoms, she is presumed to have cystitis or urethritis and should be treated, irrespective of the paucity of the results of urinalysis, culture, or both. The woman who experiences cystitis only after becoming sexually active rarely has associated upper urinary tract symptoms or pathology.

TREATMENT

Asymptomatic Bacilluria

Chronic asymptomatic bacilluria is present in 2 to 10 per cent of all women. It is significant only in the pregnant woman. If the bacilluria is untreated, one-fourth of these women develop acute pyelonephritis at some point in their pregnancy. Two-thirds of such pyelonephritic episodes can be prevented by treating the bacilluria. Treatment of the infection also seems to lower the incidence of hypertension during pregnancy.

In addition, there seems to be an increased incidence of premature delivery in patients who have bacilluria during pregnancy. Treatment should be guided by the results of the culture.

Cystitis

Virtually all infections that are localized completely to the lower urinary tract (no localizing flank pain, fever, or systemic symptoms) can be eliminated with any broad-spectrum antibiotic given orally for 5 to 10 days. Indeed, many such episodes of cystitis clear spontaneously in 5 to 7 days by forcing fluids alone. In treating simple cystitis, the more common drugs, such as amoxicillin (Amoxil), 250 mg three times daily; a cephalosporin (cephalexin [Keflex]), 250 mg four times daily; a sulfonamide (Gantrisin) 1 gram four times daily; trimethoprim-sulfamethoxazole (Bactrim DS), one tablet twice daily; or nitrofurantoin (Macrodantin), 50 mg four times daily, are effective when given for 1 to 10 days. I prefer

to treat the patient for 7 days because symptoms seem to persist longer if they are treated for a shorter period. Some of the sulfonamides have fallen out of favor because of the rare but potentially serious and sometimes fatal reactions to them, such as Stevens-Johnson syndrome, hepatic necrosis, toxic dermal necrolysis, and blood dyscrasias.

If the infection is uncomplicated by upper urinary tract or systemic symptoms, a culture is an unnecessary expense (Table 1). A follow-up urinalysis in 3 weeks to ensure clearance of the urine (and to discover chronic or unresponsive infections) is recommended. If the urinalysis is still positive or there are persistent symptoms, a culture should be obtained, therapy instituted according to the culture results, and intravenous pyelography (IVP) and cystoscopy performed.

For women who have repeated episodes of cystitis, particularly those associated with coitus, the simple expedient of drinking two glasses of water before and voiding promptly after intercourse mechanically flushes the bacteria from the lower urinary tract and prevents the majority of these infections.

If infections are a recurrent problem despite this procedure, a single dose of nitrofurantoin (50 mg), tetracycline (Achromycin V, 250 mg), or penicillin (Penn•Vee K, 250 mg) within an hour of coitus often prevents recurrence.

For women who have a chronic lower urinary tract infection that does not clear despite 7 to 10 days of appropriate therapy as determined by culture, who have no anatomic abnormality by IVP or cystoscopy, and who do not have significant residual urine, a single nightly dose of the same drug (after full-dose therapy) for 30 days often eliminates the problem.

Other causes should be sought for urinary ir-

TABLE 1. **Management of Cystitis and Pyelonephritis**

Cystitis	Pyelonephritis
No culture needed	Culture blood and urine
Colony counts may be low	Begin therapy IV pending results of culture;
UA may be near normal	acquired as:
Treat with common drugs	Outpatient—cephalosporin or aminoglycoside
Follow-up UA in 3 wk	In hospital—cephalosporin and aminoglycoside
No studies if no symptoms and	Follow BUN and creatinine levels
negative UA at 3 wk	Hydrate; obtain IVP; BUN and creatinine levels first
Study if symptoms occur or if	Give pre-IVP mannitol if patient is diabetic
positive UA	Perform renal ultrasound if patient has iodine allergy or is
Suppress infection with drugs	pregnant; IVP contraindicated with myeloma
after coitus if related	Treat per culture results for 10 days
	Treat for 14 days if blood culture(s) positive
	Suppress infection for 30 days more with PO therapy
	Do cystoscopy when infection is controlled, retrograde pyelo-
	gram if iodine allergy exists, voiding cystogram if renal
	atropy exists (rule out reflux) or ureteral tunnels abnormal

Abbreviations: UA = urinalysis; BUN = blood urea nitrogen.

ritative symptoms that mimic those of cystitis (frequency, dysuria, urgency, nocturia), if the urinalysis is persistently normal (Table 2). These causes include atrophic vaginitis, urethral stenosis, large cystocele, and detrussor hyper-reflexia or uninhibited bladder; the latter is commonly seen in younger women with multiple sclerosis or amyotrophic lateral sclerosis. In older women, interstitial cystitis, carcinoma in situ of the bladder, parkinsonism, brain tumors, and stroke are frequent causes. Some women lose the fine cortical integrating function over bladder control as a result of cerebral atrophy or subclinical stroke. Atrophic vaginitis is best treated with topical estrogen, urethral stenosis by periodic dilation, cystocele by surgical repair, and hyperreflexia (once carcinoma in situ and underlying neurologic disease have been ruled out) by anticholinergic drugs such as propantheline (Pro-Banthine), 15 mg four times daily.

Pyelonephritis

Upper urinary tract infections (pyelonephritis) occur when intervening factors are present that allow the ascent of organisms to the kidney(s), as in reflux, or when there is a septic blood-borne process that localizes in the kidney. Lower urinary tract infections in women rarely lead to pyelonephritis unless a complicating factor is present. Such factors that are commonly seen are anatomic urinary tract abnormalities (reflux, stones, upper urinary tract obstructions, colonic fistulas, radiation cystitis, high bladder residual from neurogenic or anatomic causes), general debilitation (from diabetes or malignancy), or the presence of an indwelling Foley's catheter or other foreign body (stone, balloon fragment, iatrogenic objects) in the bladder.

In all cases of upper urinary tract infection, the kidneys must be visualized as soon as possible to detect the presence of obstruction or stone. The method of choice is the IVP. The long-held opinion of waiting a few days before performing an IVP to prevent contrast allergy, renal failure, or both is incorrect. Contraindications to this test include allergy to iodine, fish, or shrimp and pregnancy. If there is any question about the adequacy of renal function, a serum creatinine assay should be performed first because the administration of contrast material to a patient with impaired renal function may result in acute renal failure. Iodine contrast should be given with caution in diabetics who should not be dehydrated, preferably administering mannitol, 12.5 grams, intravenously as a bolus before the dye is given in an attempt to protect the renal tubules. Similarly, contrast should not be given in those patients who have known myeloma to prevent precipitation of acute renal failure.

If there is a contraindication to using contrast material, a renal ultrasound test should be performed. Further imaging (if needed) can be obtained with a renal scan or retrograde pyelogram performed at the time of cystoscopy.

In upper urinary tract infections, cultures of urine (midstream or catheterized) and blood are mandatory before initiating therapy. Ten per cent of patients with pyelonephritis have positive blood cultures. Depending on the severity of the illness, the patient may either be treated as an outpatient or be hospitalized and given antibiotics intravenously if quite ill. As soon as cultures have been obtained, empiric antibiotic therapy should be started. For nonhospitalized patients, an oral cephalosporin, 250 to 500 mg every 6 hours, is a reasonable first choice until the culture results are known. For patients ill enough to require hospitalization, intravenous fluids are begun and a cephalosporin (cefazolin [Ancef]), 500 mg to 1 gram every 8 hours, or gentamicin or tobramycin (Garamycin or Nebcin), 1 mg per kg every 8 hours, is given until the results of the culture are known. If the patient has a hospital-acquired infection, a beta-lactam ceftazidime (Fortaz), 500 mg every 8 to 12 hours, and amikacin (Amikin), 5 mg per kg every 8 hours, should be started for broadest coverage. Once sensitivities are available, these drugs should be changed to a single drug that is the least toxic and least expensive one available. If nephrotoxic drugs such as an aminoglycoside are used, blood urea nitrogen and creatinine levels should be obtained and the dosage decreased or interval changed if these are elevated. The blood urea nitrogen and creatinine levels are monitored throughout treatment, along with serum peak and trough levels. Therapy is continued for 10 days. If positive blood cultures are obtained, 14 days of parenteral therapy are required, followed by 30 days of oral treatment with suppressive doses of a drug indicated by the culture.

TABLE 2. **Causes of Urinary Irritative Symptoms That Mimic Cystitis**

Atrophic vaginitis
Urethral stenosis
Ureteral stones (lower one-third)
Carcinoma in situ
Radiation cystitis
Interstitial cystitis
Large cystocele
Detrussor instability caused by
Multiple sclerosis
Amyotrophic lateral sclerosis
Stroke
Brain tumor
Parkinsonism
Incomplete emptying (overflow)

Pyelonephritis that does not respond within a few days to culture-specific antibiotics should prompt a search for other factors, such as renal abscess, inappropriate dose or choice of antibiotics, or underlying debilitating disease. A computed tomography scan of the kidneys may be indicated under such circumstances to ensure the absence of a small abscess that may require surgical drainage.

Indications for Investigational Studies of the Urinary Tract

All patients with pyelonephritis should undergo IVP unless there is diminished renal function, iodine allergy, or pregnancy; in these cases, a renal ultrasound study should be done instead. If bladder drainage is not adequate, either on IVP or clinically, a postvoid catheterized residual urine determination should be obtained.

Once the infection and fever are controlled, cystoscopy should be performed, either during hospitalization or on a subsequent visit to the urologist's office. If upper urinary tract changes of pyelonephritis are seen on the IVP, or if abnormal ureteral orifices are seen at cystoscopy, a voiding cinecystourethrogram should be done. If an ultrasound study was performed during the acute episode, retrograde pyelography can be done at the time of cystoscopy to delineate upper urinary tract anatomy.

Cystometric studies help identify the presence of neurogenic disease, incomplete bladder emptying, and mechanical outlet obstruction (rare in women). Women who have (1) frequent (two or more a year) recurrences of cystitis, (2) infections unrelated to coitus, or (3) irritative symptoms without positive urine findings should have at least a postvoid residual urine determination, cystoscopy, and, most likely, an IVP to rule out such underlying problems as interstitial cystitis, carcinoma in situ, radiation cystitis, tuberculosis, urethral diverticulum, lower ureteral stones, neurogenic disease, or upper urinary tract sources of infection.

BACTERIAL INFECTIONS OF THE URINARY TRACT IN GIRLS

method of
DAVID A. DIAMOND, M.D.
University of Massachusetts Medical Center
Worcester, Massachusetts

Urinary tract infection (UTI) is defined as the persistent presence within the urinary tract of actively multiplying organisms. During childhood, 5 per cent of girls develop a UTI and approximately 80 per cent develop a recurrence, which makes this a most common pediatric problem. In most children, these infections do not compromise immediate or long-term health. In a small percentage of patients, however, a UTI is the first sign of significant underlying pathology such as obstructive uropathy or vesicoureteric reflux and renal scarring, which together are a major cause of end-stage renal disease in the child. Thus, evaluation and management of UTI in the female child are of the utmost importance.

DIAGNOSIS

The diagnosis of UTI must be made on the basis of a positive urine culture, and the technique of urine collection and the clinical presentation of the child must be considered. Statistically, a properly done midstream urine culture that grows more than 10^5 colonies is 80 per cent accurate in diagnosing a UTI. An identical result for a repeat midstream urine specimen increases the accuracy to 95 per cent. Obtaining a properly collected midstream specimen may present a challenge. The older girl may be instructed to wash her perineum with an iodophore preparation and to separate the labia to maintain a midstream clean catch specimen. For the infant and younger child, an adhesive U-bag must be applied. The incidence of skin contamination of such specimens is high. Thus, although a negative U-bag urine culture is meaningful, often a positive result requires confirmation by a sterile catheterized specimen using a No. 5 French feeding tube or a carefully done suprapubic aspiration of the bladder. *Any* significant bacterial growth in such specimens is indicative of a UTI. In some situations urinary frequency may result in lower bacterial colony counts. Thus, the child with a pure bacterial growth of 10^3 to 10^4 colonies of a single organism and with symptoms consistent with a UTI should be presumed to have an infection.

Virtually all urinary pathogens are bowel commensals, and *Escherichia coli* is responsible for approximately 80 per cent of bacterial UTIs in girls. Under normal circumstances, the urinary tract has various defense mechanisms that prevent UTI. These mechanisms include dilution of bacteria entering the bladder by urine production, regular emptying of the bladder, resistance of bladder mucosa to adherence of bacteria, and the immunologic response of the bladder to bacteria. The diagnosis of UTI suggests a breakdown in these defense mechanisms.

The clinical presentation of UTI in the female child is variable and quite dependent on age. Infants have notoriously nonspecific signs and symptoms referable to UTI, including failure to thrive, jaundice, colic, vomiting, and fever. Thus, any severely ill infant should have a urine culture as part of a routine evaluation. Older girls present with histories more classic for urinary pathology, which include enuresis, frequency of urination, hematuria, abdominal and loin pain, and fever.

The first clearly documented UTI in the female child warrants radiologic evaluation to rule out an anatomic

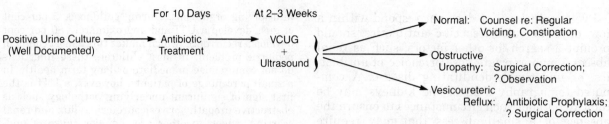

Figure 1. Algorithm for management of UTIs in girls.

abnormality that predisposes the child to recurrent UTI or progressive renal damage. Routine imaging should include a complete ultrasound scan of the urinary tract from the upper pole of the kidneys to the bladder neck, as well as a properly done voiding cystourethrogram (VCUG). The VCUG is particularly useful in screening for vesicoureteric reflux, whereas the ultrasound scan is most valuable in diagnosing hydronephrosis associated with an obstructive lesion or quite severe reflux. The intravenous pyelogram remains a valuable functional and anatomic study of the upper and lower urinary tracts, particularly in situations of more complex anatomy suggested by the ultrasound scan, such as in delineating duplex collecting systems. The yield of these diagnostic studies is high. Vesicoureteric reflux is noted on approximately one of three VCUGs in girls with UTI, and although obstructive lesions are far less common, they are particularly important to diagnose early, before renal deterioration occurs.

Although the diagnosis of an anatomic abnormality is critical in these children, it is equally important to diagnose a functional voiding problem, which a majority of girls with UTI have. By far the most common abnormality is infrequent voiding. Constipation is also commonly associated with recurrent UTI and should be pursued in any thorough history. Often the most effective management of anatomically normal girls with bacterial UTI includes voiding every 3 to 4 hours by the clock during the day and effective control of constipation.

TREATMENT

After the initial diagnosis of UTI, the child should be treated with a 10-day course of oral

TABLE 1. **Oral Antimicrobials for Urinary Infections in Girls**

Drug	Dosage
Trimethoprim-sulfamethoxazole (Bactrim, Septra)*	Suspension: 0.5 ml/kg bid Tablets: 10–20 kg, one tablet bid; over 20 kg, two tablets bid
Nitrofurantoin (Furadantin)†	2 mg/kg qid (8 mg/kg/day)
Sulfisoxazole (Gantrisin)*	40 mg/kg qid (160 mg/kg/day)
Amoxicillin (Amoxil)	12 mg/kg tid (36 mg/kg/day)
Cefaclor (Ceclor)	10 mg/kg tid (30 mg/kg/day)

*Contraindicated in children younger than 2 months old (jaundice).

†Contraindicated in children younger than 1 month old (hemolytic anemia).

antibiotic. Any of the medications shown in Table 1 are appropriate, although nitrofurantoin (Furadantin) and trimethoprim-sulfamethoxazole (Bactrim, Septra) are preferable. Nitrofurantoin is absorbed entirely by the small bowel so that resistant colonic bacteria do not develop. Trimethoprim-sulfamethoxazole achieves high concentrations in the vaginal secretions, which makes it a particularly effective genitourinary antibiotic for the female. The particularly ill child who has vomiting and dehydration should be admitted to the hospital for intravenous antibiotic treatment. After completion of the 10-day course of oral antibiotic, it is reasonable to continue with prophylaxis with nitrofurantoin or trimethoprim-sulfamethoxazole until diagnostic studies have ruled out an anatomic lesion. A reasonable time frame for scheduling imaging studies is 2 to 3 weeks after the initiation of antibiotic treatment.

After the child has undergone ultrasonography and a VCUG has been done, she should be seen by a pediatric urologist who can interpret the studies and perform a thorough history and physical examination to rule out a functional voiding disorder (Figure 1). In this way, the likelihood of recurrent infection or progressive renal damage is minimized.

CHILDHOOD ENURESIS

method of
H. GIL RUSHTON, M.D.
*Children's Hospital National Medical Center
Washington, D.C.*

Enuresis is the involuntary voiding of urine beyond the age by which normal control is expected. Nocturnal enuresis refers to persistent wetting during sleep past the age of 5. Primary enuresis is defined as bed wetting in patients who have never been dry for extended periods of time. In contrast, secondary enuresis is the onset of wetting following a continuous dry period greater than 6 months.

Nocturnal enuresis is prevalent in as many as 15 to 20 per cent of 5-year-old children. Approximately 15 per cent of bed wetters will achieve nocturnal control each year, so that by age 15 only 1 to 2 per cent of adolescents remain enuretic. Approximately 15 per cent of bed wetters also have diurnal enuresis (wetting while awake).

ETIOLOGY

Although many etiologic theories for enuresis have been proposed, the bulk of data supports a biologic basis in most patients. Cystometrogram evaluation in up to 85 per cent of enuretic children reveals a persistent pattern of infantile-type detrusor instability, with uninhibited bladder contractions and a small capacity. Enuresis is considered by most to represent a "maturational lag" of normal inhibitory control by the central nervous system. Genetic factors clearly appear to contribute to enuresis. In one survey, when both parents had a history of enuresis, 77 per cent of the children were enuretic. When only one parent had a history of enuresis, 44 per cent of the children were enuretic. When neither parent had a history of enuresis, only 15 per cent of the children were enuretic. Sleep and arousal disorders have also been implicated in some enuretics. This relationship is poorly understood, and supporting data are both equivocal and conflicting. Although most enuretics do not suffer from underlying psychopathology, emotional stress can at times manifest as secondary or "onset" enuresis. In a recent retrospective study of 1265 children, the factors most predictive of the age of attainment of bladder control were a family history of enuresis, the child's developmental level at 1 and 3 years of age, and the child's early sleeping patterns.

TREATMENT

Evaluation and treatment are contingent upon the pattern of enuresis, physical examination, and urinalysis and culture. Physical examination should include abdominal and genital examination, observation of the child while voiding, and neurologic evaluation. Neurologic evaluation should include checking peripheral reflexes, evaluation of perineal sensation and anal sphincter tone, and inspection of the lower back for evidence of sacral dimpling or cutaneous anomalies suggestive of spina bifida occulta.

Uncomplicated Enuresis

The incidence of organic uropathology in children with nocturnal enuresis, normal physical examination, and negative urine culture does not appear to be significantly higher than in the normal population. Frequently, these children will have associated mild daytime frequency or enuresis with a normal urinary stream, a positive family history of enuresis, and perhaps slightly delayed developmental milestones. No further

urologic evaluation is indicated in most of these patients.

Numerous therapeutic programs for uncomplicated nocturnal enuresis have been recommended. These include psychotherapy, hypnotherapy, diet therapy, motivational therapy, drug therapy, and behavioral modification (conditioning) therapy. Although no single therapeutic plan is ideal for all patients, the last two approaches are the most effective and practical. There is no objective evidence that withholding fluids in the evening, random awakening of the child to void, or punitive measures result in significant cessation of enuresis.

Drug Therapy. A number of pharmacologic agents have been used to treat enuresis. Tricyclic antidepressants, particularly imipramine (Tofranil), have been used with the best results. The exact pharmacologic mechanism of action on the bladder is not well understood. However, it does appear to result in a measurable increase in functional bladder capacity when it is effective. Imipramine should not be used to treat enuresis in children under age 6 to 7 years and should be kept out of the reach of small children, owing to its extreme toxicity in excessive doses. Success rates are best in older children, with complete cessation of enuresis reported in up to 40 per cent and improvement in 10 to 20 per cent. However, the relapse rate following discontinuation is high, particularly when the drug is stopped abruptly or prematurely, and many children escape control and require an increasingly higher dosage for effectiveness. The dose of imipramine is 25 mg taken 1 to 2 hours prior to bedtime for patients 6 to 8 years old and 50 to 75 mg in older children and adolescents (not to exceed 2.5 mg per kg per day). A sustained-release form (Tofranil PM) may be most effective. Therapy should be continued for at least 2 weeks prior to assessing efficacy and possibly adjusting the dosage. The optimal duration of therapy in patients who respond favorably is uncertain. Generally, I recommend treatment for 3 to 6 months, at which time the patient is "weaned" by gradually reducing the dose and/or frequency, i.e., every other night over 3 to 4 weeks. Should relapse occur, a repeat course of treatment can be started. Often, imipramine will work on an as needed basis, and use may be reserved for times when staying dry is particularly important to the child (sleepovers, camp).

Side effects from treatment with imipramine are uncommon but include anxiety, insomnia, and adverse personality changes. Overdoses have been reported secondary to excessive ingestion and can cause potentially fatal toxicity with cardiac arrhythmias and conduction blocks, hypotension, and convulsions. Physostigmine therapy is used to manage life-threatening imipramine toxicity.

Anticholinergic drugs, specifically oxybutynin* (Ditropan), reduce or abolish uninhibited bladder contractions and may be particularly beneficial in patients who also have daytime frequency or enuresis. The dose in children over 6 years old is usually 5 mg two or three times daily. Common side effects include dryness of the mouth and facial flushing. Excessive dosage may result in blurring of vision.

Recent studies have reported promising results from treatment with desmopressin, an analogue of the antidiuretic hormone vasopressin. The proposed mechanism of action is a reduction in nocturnal urine output to a volume less than the functional bladder capacity of the enuretic child. This explanation assumes that when a child wets at night, he or she exceeds his or her bladder capacity. A significant improvement in enuresis has been consistently reported with doses of 10 to 40 micrograms administered intranasally. Significant side effects have not been reported; however, relapse rates after discontinuation of short-term therapy are high.

Behavioral Modification (Conditioning) Therapy. Behavioral modification therapy revolves around use of a signal alarm device that is electrolytically triggered when the child voids, awakening the patient. Initially, the child wakens after or during voiding. A conditioned response is gradually evoked by the association of awakening and inhibition of micturition. Long-term success rates of 75 per cent have been reported following 4 to 6 months of treatment. Essential to the success of such a program are strong patient compliance and motivation.

Numerous systems are available at reasonable cost. Occasional complications have been reported with pad and buzzer systems such as "buzzer ulcers" of the skin or alarm failure if the child is not positioned properly on the pad. A modification of the alarm system, known as the "Wet-Stop" (Palco Labs, 1595 Soquel Dr., Santa Cruz, Calif. 95065), uses a small sensor that is placed into a cotton pocket in the child's underwear and an alarm that is attached to the child's pajama collar. These units are compact, safe, and effective and avoid many of the problems associated with a pad and buzzer.

As success depends on a cooperative and motivated child, behavioral modification therapy is generally used in patients over 7 years old. In some children who fail to awaken to the alarm or who awaken in a confused state, a low dose of

imipramine in conjunction with the alarm system may be beneficial. Adjunctive measures that will increase the effectiveness of the alarm system include positive reinforcement programs in which the child receives a "reward" following a predetermined number of successive dry nights. The child is encouraged to keep a record of progress, such as using a calendar with stars for each dry night. Parental support, empathy, and patience are key elements in successful management of the child with enuresis. Likewise, reassurance, periodic feedback, and encouragement of the parents and child by the physician are necessary for optimal results.

Complicated Enuresis

Patients with a positive urine culture or history of urinary tract infection, abnormal neurologic examination, or significant voiding dysfunction characterized by either infrequent voiding or severe frequency associated with incontinence, poor urinary stream, and/or encopresis have complicated enuresis. These patients should be further evaluated with a renal/bladder sonogram and voiding cystogram (with spine films) to exclude vesicoureteral reflux and/or hydroureteronephrosis associated with a thickened, unstable bladder. The latter findings indicate the need for further urologic and/or urodynamic evaluation. Neurosurgical evaluation may also be indicated in some of these patients to exclude spina bifida occulta or a tethered cord.

In those patients with secondary-onset enuresis associated with severe voiding dysfunction, including infrequent voiding and encopresis, a careful family and social history may reveal underlying psychosocial stresses. Treatment of these children is initially directed toward emotional support. Those patients with bladder or upper urinary tract damage secondary to severe voiding dysfunction who do not have an organic obstructive or neurologic lesion may also benefit from timed voidings, anticholinergic therapy, and/or biofeedback therapy. Occasionally, renal damage may be so severe as to necessitate a program of intermittent catheterization if bladder emptying cannot be achieved by other means. In some cases psychotherapy or professional counseling may also be warranted.

URINARY INCONTINENCE
method of
EDWARD J. McGUIRE, M.D.
University of Michigan
Ann Arbor, Michigan

Incontinence may be due to abnormalities of urethral or bladder function. Bladder abnormalities include

---

*Safety and efficacy of this drug in children under 5 years of age have not been established.

poor reservoir function manifested by decreased compliance or an increase in pressure with increasing volume. These abnormalities are relatively subtle and often poorly diagnosed and poorly managed. Abnormalities of the control of bladder reflex activity are probably the most common reason for incontinence, although the etiology of this kind of abnormality is multiple. In addition, "paradoxic" or overflow incontinence results from lack of reflex bladder contractility.

TREATMENT

Bladder-Related Incontinence

Disorders of Compliance. An abnormal increase in intravesical pressure with filling, indicating loss of bladder reservoir function, occurs after radical pelvic surgery, in cases of peripheral neuropathy, in patients with myelodysplasia, and in those with sacral cord or sacral root injuries or disease. These disorders are frequently associated with lack of reflex bladder contractility, but the major abnormality is a loss of low-pressure volume accommodation. The increased pressure volume relationship has a direct hydraulic effect on ureteral delivery of urine to the bladder and induces leakage across a fixed continence mechanism at low to moderate vesical volumes. The intent of treatment is to empty the bladder periodically and to preserve and to protect low-pressure storage of urine. This can usually be accomplished by intermittent catheterization and anticholinergic drugs. If vesical pressures cannot be kept below 35 cmH$_2$O at the volumes obtained at the time of intermittent catheterization, some method to improve reservoir function is essential to preserve upper urinary tract function. This can be done by augmentation cystoplasty using bowel tissue or by reducing the outlet resistance and lowering the pressure at which leakage occurs (with the acceptance of more incontinence). Increasing urethral resistance to improve continence is directly prejudicial to upper urinary tract function if vesical compliance (volume tolerance at pressures under 35 cmH$_2$O) is indicated.

Disorders of Control of Reflex Vesical Activity. These disorders may be associated with spinal cord injury or disease and multiple sclerosis, in which case control of reflex bladder activity is poor or absent and both the storage and voiding phases of bladder activity are disordered. Approximately 70 per cent of the patients can be managed by anticholinergic medication and intermittent catheterization. Because the major effect of such lesions in men is related to upper urinary tract changes related to high bladder pressure, sphincter obviation procedures and condom catheter drainage are frequently used—these sacrifice

continence. In women, bladder pressures are lower, and continence is of major importance. Interruption of reflex pathways at the trigone, sacral root, or cord levels or partial cystectomy and augmentation cytoplasty can be used to achieve good vesical storage function, with intermittent catheterization used for periodic bladder emptying. Quadriplegic women are a special problem; provision for a continent stoma to allow self-catheterization permits avoidance of treatment by Foley's catheter drainage or ileal loop diversion; both methods have a dismal long-term outlook. Treatment of male spinal cord–injured patients by ileal loop diversion, cutaneous ureterostomy, suprapubic tube, or Foley's catheter drainage is associated with equally dismal long-term complications.

"Idiopathic" Detrusor Contractile Incontinence. Poor control of reflex vesical activity without high-pressure bladder dysfunction is a fairly common problem that is frequently encountered in the elderly, those with cerebrovascular disease or lesions of the basal ganglia, adult men and women without neurologic disease, and children. The urodynamic finding is basically a sudden bladder contraction that occurs unwillingly.

Warning of detrusor events is poor, and reflex contractility is provoked by volume. Treatment is directed at delay of the reflex bladder response with anticholinergic agents such as oxybutynin chloride (Ditropan), 5 mg three times daily; propantheline bromide (Pro-Banthine), 15 to 30 mg three times daily; dicyclomine (Bentyl), 20 mg four times daily; or imipramine (Tofranil), 10 to 25 mg three times daily or 50 mg at bedtime. These should be coupled with a regular program of timed voiding, which tends to short-circuit the uninhibited response of the bladder to filling. Urodynamically, no qualitative differences distinguish hyperactive bladder activity in one group from that in another. Poor response to one agent often can be circumvented by using two agents that act differently—e.g., imipramine, 10 mg three times daily, and oxybutynin, 5 mg three times daily.

Obstructive Uropathy. Poor control of reflex vesical activity is also associated with obstructive uropathy, most commonly, benign prostatic hyperplasia. Residual urine or symptoms suggesting obstruction, e.g., hesitancy or a slow stream, should prompt investigation and initially contraindicate anticholinergic therapy.

Stress Incontinence

Stress incontinence related to poor urethral support in women, associated with visible urethral hypermobility, responds most predictably to surgical repair. Alternative methods include tampon use to achieve urethral support, and temporary treatment with drugs with alpha-stimulating properties (e.g., phenylpropanolamine, 25 mg three times daily, or imipramine, 25 mg three times daily). These agents have not been approved by the U.S. Food and Drug Administration for this usage and have somewhat limited value.

Weakness of urethral sphincter function in elderly women, not associated with urethral hypermobility with an increase in intra-abdominal pressure, responds reasonably well to intravaginal Premarin (one-third of an applicator at night) and imipramine (10 mg three times daily). Men with very mild postprostatectomy incontinence *may* respond to alpha-stimulating agents, but this does not happen often.

When internal sphincter function is absent in patients with myelodysplasia and following radical prostatectomy, and occasionally following radical surgery for uterine or rectal malignant disease, medication is of no benefit, and usually complicated surgical procedures are required for relief.

EPIDIDYMITIS

method of
PETER T. NIEH, M.D.
Lahey Clinic Medical Center
Burlington, Massachusetts

Inflammation of the epididymis is characterized by scrotal pain and by enlargement and induration of the posterior-lying epididymis, with eventual scrotal edema, testicular involvement, and hydrocele formation. Epididymitis usually is caused by infection of the urinary tract but may be associated with trauma, tuberculosis, or even syphilis or gonorrhea. Reflux of sterile urine down the vas deferens after prostatectomy may produce a chemical epididymitis.

In males younger than age 35 years, chlamydia is the common pathogen, usually presenting with expressible urethral discharge. In older men, the typical coliform bacteria predominate, often associated with distal urinary tract obstruction. Tuberculosis should be considered in the older patient with sterile pyuria and nodularity of the vas deferens.

In prepubertal boys, the rare instances of epididymitis are usually caused by bacteria, and careful evaluation for congenital urinary anomalies, such as vesicoureteral reflux or ectopic ureter, should be undertaken. In adolescents and young adults, acute epididymitis must be differentiated from testicular torsion, which is a surgical emergency. Radionuclide scan or Doppler ultrasonography may be useful in this situation.

Urinalysis may reveal pyuria and sometimes bacteriuria. A smear of any urethral discharge should be made and stained for *Neisseria gonorrhoeae*. A urine culture should be obtained before any antibiotic therapy is instituted. If tuberculosis is suspected, a sample for acid-fast bacilli should also be submitted.

TREATMENT

Immobilization

In mild cases, scrotal support is adequate. However, in more severe cases, the testis may need to be elevated on several soft folded towels or even strapped to the pubic symphysis by using cloth tape after the scrotum is shaved.

Strict bed rest for the first 24 to 48 hours minimizes further irritation and pain. The patient should be permitted to leave the bed only to use the bathroom.

Analgesia

Application of an ice pack limits edema and provides appreciable relief. Codeine with acetaminophen or aspirin, combined with nonsteroidal anti-inflammatory drugs such as ibuprofen, usually suffices to control pain. In particularly severe cases, a local anesthetic block provides further relief and permits better examination of the enlarged scrotal contents. Local anesthesia is performed after appropriate preparation of the skin with iodine, by using 10 ml of 0.5 per cent lidocaine (Xylocaine) or bupivacaine (Marcaine) injected carefully through a 21-gauge needle into the spermatic cord at the level of the pubic tubercle.

Broad-Spectrum Antibiotics

The therapy for gonorrhea is described elsewhere. For the patient younger than age 35 years with nongonococcal epididymitis, chlamydia is most effectively treated with tetracycline, 500 mg orally every 6 hours for 10 days, or doxycycline, 100 mg orally twice daily for 10 days. If bacteria are seen on urinalysis, either ciprofloxacin (Cipro), 250 mg, or trimethoprim-sulfamethoxazole (Septra or Bactrim), one tablet orally twice daily for 10 days, is advisable. If the patient appears to be in a toxic condition with a high fever and leukocytosis, use of a third-generation cephalosporin or parenteral aminoglycoside is preferable.

Surgery

Aspiration of an acute hydrocele under local anesthesia allows a more careful examination of the underlying structures and often permits more rapid resolution of scrotal discomfort. If there is any doubt whether epididymitis or testicular torsion is the problem, early surgical exploration is recommended. If a area of fluctuance develops, which suggests abscess formation, surgical drainage or excision may be necessary. If pain and fever persist in an older man, an epididymoorchiectomy must be considered. If a mass persists after treatment, the possibility of an underlying testicular tumor should be considered, and ultrasonography and inguinal exploration may be required.

COMPLICATIONS

Most patients with acute epididymitis respond to proper treatment with relatively rapid resolution of pain, although induration may take several weeks to resolve completely. In some instances, chronic epididymitis may persist, with recurrent episodes of scrotal pain and induration. In these patients, fibrosis and ductal obstruction are usually present, with resultant sterility if involvement is bilateral. In patients who are immunocompromised, epididymitis may progress to produce Fournier's gangrene, a necrotizing, synergistic infection of the scrotal wall. This condition requires radical excision of all infected tissue and epididymo-orchiectomy in selected patients.

GLOMERULAR DISORDERS

method of
GERALD C. GROGGEL, M.D.
University of Utah Health Sciences Center
Salt Lake City, Utah

Glomerular disorders may result from a variety of pathologic processes, the primary one being immunologic. The principal clinical manifestations of glomerular disorders are hematuria, proteinuria, hypertension, edema, and reduction of the glomerular filtration rate.

Glomerular disorders can be divided into four major clinical syndromes: acute glomerulonephritis, rapidly progressive glomerulonephritis (RPGN), the nephrotic syndrome, and asymptomatic urinary abnormalities (proteinuria and hematuria). They can also be divided into primary disorders, in which only the kidney is involved in the disease process and all clinical manifestations arise from alterations in glomerular structure or function, and secondary or systemic disorders, in which the kidney is part of a disorder affecting multiple organs, such as diabetes mellitus.

ACUTE GLOMERULONEPHRITIS

Most patients with acute glomerulonephritis have had a recent infection of the pharynx or skin with a group A beta-hemolytic *Streptococcus*. Acute glomerulonephritis similar to poststreptococcal glomerulonephritis may occur after many bacterial, viral, or parasitic infections. Certain systemic diseases such as systemic lupus erythematosus, infective endocarditis, and vasculitis may also cause acute glomerulonephritis.

Poststreptococcal Glomerulonephritis

This form of acute glomerulonephritis is secondary to an infection with certain strains of group A beta-hemolytic *Streptococcus*. The hallmark of this disorder is depression of the levels of the third and fourth components of complement. These levels return to normal after 6 to 8 weeks. If the component levels remain persistently low, another diagnosis should be sought. Treatment of the streptococcal infection does not prevent the occurrence of glomerulonephritis, but it may suppress the development of streptococcal antibodies. Treatment of the infection is recommended with a 10-day course of either penicillin or erythromycin. Treatment with antibiotics probably does not affect the course of acute glomerulonephritis. Thus only conservative management is used to treat the symptoms of the glomerulonephritis, including the management of hypertension and edema. There is no evidence that corticosteroid therapy is of value in acute glomerulonephritis. An occasional patient with acute poststreptococcal glomerulonephritis presents with crescentic glomerulonephritis and rapid loss of renal function. In these instances, it is appropriate to treat the patient's RPGN just as any other patient with this condition would be treated (see the section on RPGN). The prognosis for this disorder is in general very good.

Infectious Endocarditis

Glomerulonephritis may be associated with subacute bacterial endocarditis, infected ventriculoatrial shunts, or visceral abscesses. In each situation, the primary purpose of therapy should be to eradicate the infection as rapidly as possible. The glomerulonephritis usually resolves with appropriate antibiotic or surgical treatment of the underlying process.

In the rare patient who develops diffuse crescentic glomerulonephritis with rapid loss of renal function, the use of high-dose steroid therapy may be considered. However, the benefits of steroid therapy need to be weighed against the detrimental and potentially life-threatening effects of such therapy on the course of the underlying infection. I consider the administration of high-dose steroids only if the infection has been adequately treated. In that case, the physician could consider using intravenous methylprednisolone, 15 to 30 mg per kg, given over several hours every other day for three doses, followed by a short course of oral prednisone, 60 mg per day, for 4 weeks.

Systemic Lupus Erythematosus

The therapeutic approaches to the management of lupus nephritis are controversial. All patients with active lupus have some form of renal involvement, but only those with significant glomerular involvement require treatment. When there is no evidence of clinical renal disease, the physician can assume that the patient does not have significant glomerulonephritis. But if the patient has proteinuria, hematuria, an active urinary sediment, or an elevated serum creatinine level, treatment should be considered. Before treatment is instituted in this setting, it is appropriate to perform a renal biopsy to classify the patient according to the microscopic appearance of the kidney. The major forms of lupus nephritis, according to the World Health Organization's classification, are minimal, mesangial, focal proliferative, diffuse proliferative, and membranous glomerulonephritis.

Minimal and Mesangial Lupus Nephritis

Minimal lupus nephritis is characterized by rare mesangial immune deposits in otherwise normal-appearing glomeruli. In mesangial nephritis there are more mesangial deposits, and these are associated with mild mesangial expansion and proliferation. Usually these patients have normal renal function and minimal proteinuria. The goal of therapy is to control the extrarenal manifestations of the lupus. No specific therapy is required for this form of glomerular disease. If the serum creatinine level rises or heavy proteinuria develops, the clinician should suspect the development of a more severe form of lupus nephritis.

Focal and Diffuse Proliferative Lupus Nephritis

Focal lupus nephritis is characterized by focal and segmental glomerular lesions that are often associated with necrosis and intercapillary thrombi. The immune deposits are extensive, involving both the mesangium and the glomerular capillary wall, primarily in a subendothelial location. Diffuse proliferative lupus nephritis involves almost all the glomeruli and is characterized by extensive glomerular hypercellularity, necrosis, capillary wall thickening, and fibrinoid changes. Crescent formation may be present in both of these diseases. In diffuse proliferative lupus nephritis, immune deposits may be found in the mesangium, the subendothelium, and even the subepithelial space. These patients typically have heavy proteinuria, an active urinary sediment, frequent hypertension, and a reduced glomerular filtration rate.

Present evidence indicates that steroid therapy alone is probably not effective. These patients also require some form of cytotoxic therapy. They can be initially treated with high-dose oral prednisone, 60 to 80 mg per day, with tapering after 1 month of therapy. After the prednisone has been tapered, they should be treated with either cyclophosphamide or azathioprine. Regimens that have proved to be successful in treating lupus nephritis include cyclophosphamide, 1 to 3 mg per kg per day; azathioprine, 1 to 3 mg per kg per day; a combination of cyclophosphamide, 1 mg per kg per day, and azathioprine, 1 mg per kg per day; or cyclophosphamide, 500 to 1000 mg per M^2 of body surface intravenously. There is some preliminary evidence that the intravenous form of cyclophosphamide is associated with fewer adverse reactions than the other regimens and may provide better preservation of renal function.

Thus, presently I recommend treating proliferative lupus nephritis with intravenous cyclophosphamide, beginning with a dose of 500 mg per M^2 of body surface. This is given in 250 ml of normal saline and is followed by a minimum of 1 liter of normal saline. The white blood cell count is followed carefully, with a goal of reaching a nadir of approximately 2000 to 3000 cells per mm^3. If this dose is tolerated, it is increased the next month to 750 mg per M^2 and again to a maximal dose of 1000 mg per M^2. This dose is given monthly for a total of 6 months.

It should be emphasized that extensive scarring seen on renal biopsy, particularly with interstitial fibrosis and tubular atrophy, suggests that the lupus nephritis is less amenable to therapy. In this situation, the risks of continuing immunosuppressive therapy probably do not outweigh the potential benefits.

Membranous Lupus Nephritis

In this form of lupus nephritis there is diffuse capillary wall thickening, with immune deposits located in the subepithelial space. In contrast to idiopathic membranous nephropathy, there can also be mild mesangial changes with mesangial immune deposits. The clinical course of this form of lupus nephritis is usually more indolent than that of the proliferative forms. Although there are no controlled therapeutic trials of this form of lupus nephritis, I would recommend treating these patients just as patients with idiopathic membranous nephropathy are treated. They should receive 120 mg of prednisone orally every other day for 8 weeks, with the dose tapered over a 4-week period. These patients may require lower doses of prednisone to control their extrarenal lupus.

Necrotizing Vasculitis

Systemic necrotizing vasculitis is a heterogeneous disorder in which blood vessels of various sizes in many different organs may be involved with inflammatory necrotizing lesions. Polyarteritis nodosa, hypersensitivity vasculitis, and Wegener's granulomatosis may all involve the kidney.

As initial therapy, it is appropriate to treat these patients with a combination of high-dose prednisone, 60 to 80 mg per day, and oral cyclophosphamide, 1 to 3 mg per kg per day. The prednisone can be tapered over 1 to 3 months. The cyclophosphamide is continued for at least 3 months or until the disease becomes quiescent.

For Wegener's granulomatosis, therapy consists of cyclophosphamide, 1 to 3 mg per kg per day, and prednisone, 40 to 60 mg a day. After 1 year of therapy, the cyclophosphamide can be slowly discontinued. In all forms of vasculitis, it is important that treatment be initiated early to maximize the preservation of renal function.

Henoch-Schönlein Purpura

Henoch-Schönlein purpura is a syndrome consisting of dermal, articular, abdominal, and renal manifestations. It is a leukoclastic vasculitis with deposits of IgA in both the skin and the kidney. The glomerulonephritis can vary in severity from mild to severe. In general, this is a benign, self-limited disease, with less than 10 per cent of patients progressing to renal failure. Treatment does not appear to alter the course of the renal disease. An occasional patient may have crescentic glomerulonephritis on renal biopsy. These patients should be treated just as other patients with crescentic glomerulonephritis are treated, as described in the next section.

RAPIDLY PROGRESSIVE (CRESCENTIC) GLOMERULONEPHRITIS

RPGN is a form of glomerulonephritis associated with progressive renal insufficiency that develops over weeks to months. The morphologic hallmark of this disorder is extensive glomerular crescent formation. If it remains untreated, end-stage renal disease always develops. Thus early diagnosis and treatment are essential.

Any type of acute glomerulonephritis can result in crescentic glomerulonephritis. The term "idiopathic rapidly progressive glomerulonephritis" is reserved for patients who do not have evidence of another type of glomerulonephritis and do not have evidence of a systemic disease. In the presence of pulmonary involvement, this disorder is called Goodpasture's syndrome. This disorder has been divided into three types. Type I is characterized by linear deposits of IgG along the glomerular capillary membrane and is associated with circulating antiglomerular basement membrane antibodies. Approximately 20 per cent of the patients have this form. Type II is characterized by granular immune deposits of IgG and complement. Approximately 40 per cent of the patients have this form. Type III is characterized by no glomerular immune deposits on immunofluorescence. Approximately 40 per cent of the patients have this form. There are few studies of the treatment for this disorder, and none of them have been well controlled.

The initial treatment for the antiglomerular basement membrane antibody–mediated disease should be plasma exchange (plasmapheresis) combined with oral prednisone, 60 mg per day, and cyclophosphamide, 1 to 3 mg per kg per day. Plasmapheresis should consist of 2- to 4-liter exchanges daily for the first 2 to 5 days. The frequency of plasmapheresis can then be gradually reduced over 2 to 4 weeks until the serum antiglomerular antibody level decreases and a good clinical response is obtained. The cyclophosphamide can be discontinued after 2 to 3 months, and then the prednisone can be slowly tapered. These patients are monitored by following serum levels of antiglomerular basement membrane antibody. This therapy is most effective in nonoliguric patients with an initial serum creatinine level of less than 6 to 7 mg per dl. Patients who have oliguria and severe renal failure should be treated conservatively with dialysis and transplantation. Plasmapheresis should not be instituted without simultaneous immune suppression because there is often a clinical relapse caused by a rebound in circulating antibody levels after the plasmapheresis is stopped.

The treatment of patients with Type II RPGN or granular immune deposits is pulse methylprednisolone. Methylprednisolone, 30 mg per kg per day, is given intravenously over 30 minutes three times on alternate days, followed by oral prednisone, 1 mg per kg per day, tapered over several months. In contrast to Type I RPGN, the benefit of treatment has been seen even in patients who are oliguric and receiving dialysis, but the best results occur in patients treated early. There is no evidence that plasmapheresis is superior to pulse steroids in Type II RPGN. If there is evidence of an underlying vasculitis based on clinical features and focal necrotizing glomerular lesions, a cytotoxic agent should be added, usually cyclophosphamide, in a dose of 1 to 3 mg per kg per day for 3 to 6 months.

The treatment of Type III RPGN or no immune deposits disease is identical to the treatment of Type II. Again, if there is evidence of an underlying vasculitis, patients should be treated with cytotoxic therapy, usually cyclophosphamide, as noted earlier. Although there have been anecdotal reports of the use of anticoagulants (heparin, warfarin) and antithrombotics (dipyridamole) in this disorder, the risk of life-threatening complications clearly outweighs any potential benefit.

Goodpasture's Syndrome

Goodpasture's syndrome is an antiglomerular basement membrane antibody–mediated disease with systemic involvement manifested primarily by pulmonary hemorrhage. The therapeutic approach to these patients is similar to that used for patients with idiopathic antiglomerular basement membrane antibody–mediated disease. The pulmonary manifestations should respond to plasmapheresis in the vast majority of patients. In patients with advanced renal disease, that is, with a serum creatinine level greater than 7 mg per dl and/or oliguria, the response of the renal disease to plasmapheresis will probably be poor. In these patients, the renal disease should be treated conservatively with dialysis and transplantation. Patients who are to undergo transplantation should have low or undetectable serum antibody levels for at least 3 to 6 months to minimize the risk of disease recurrence in the transplanted kidney.

IDIOPATHIC IgA NEPHROPATHY

IgA nephropathy is one of the most frequent forms of glomerulonephritis. Its clinical features are variable. Many patients have recurrent episodes of gross (macroscopic) hematuria, particularly after virus-like syndromes. On examination of the renal biopsy specimen, the hallmark of this disorder is deposits of IgA in the mesangium by immunofluorescence. A subset of patients with IgA nephropathy may have the nephrotic syndrome. Patients with heavy proteinuria, hypertension, and abnormal renal function at the time of presentation probably have a worse prognosis.

Approximately 20 to 25 per cent of patients with IgA nephropathy develop end-stage renal disease during a period of 20 years. Henoch-Schönlein purpura is the systemic form of this disease.

Presently, the treatment for IgA nephropathy is entirely supportive. There is no evidence that any therapeutic measures are effective in this disorder. Therapies that have been tried include corticosteroids, cytotoxic agents, antibiotics, and phenytoin.

ASYMPTOMATIC PROTEINURIA

Patients with low-grade proteinuria (less than 1 gram per 24 hours) and a normal urinary sediment are said to have asymptomatic proteinuria. The vast majority of these patients have postural proteinuria, which occurs only when they are in the upright position. This can be documented by collecting a split 24-hour urine sample consisting of the urine produced both while the patient is recumbent and while the patient is upright. If protein appears only in urine collected in the upright posture, the patient can be identified as having postural proteinuria. These patients can be reassured that the prognosis is good, and they do not need further evaluation or treatment. If the proteinuria is not postural, these patients should be followed closely. If they develop evidence of severe proteinuria (more than 2 grams per 24 hours), an abnormal urinary sediment, or loss of renal function, they should undergo a renal biopsy. Based on the biopsy findings, specific therapy can then be instituted.

NEPHROTIC SYNDROME

The nephrotic syndrome is a clinical syndrome manifested by heavy proteinuria (usually more than 3.5 grams per day per 1.72 M² body surface area), hypoalbuminemia, hyperlipidemia, lipiduria, and edema. The hallmark of this syndrome is hypoalbuminemia. This, rather than the degree of proteinuria, defines the syndrome.

There are many causes of the nephrotic syndrome, idiopathic as well as systemic. In children the vast majority have the idiopathic form, whereas in adults approximately one-third are associated with a systemic disease, drug, or toxin. The most common systemic diseases causing the nephrotic syndrome are diabetes mellitus, systemic lupus erythematosus, amyloidosis, drugs, and neoplasms. Diabetic nephropathy is always accompanied by other manifestations of microangiopathy, particularly retinopathy. There is no known specific therapy for the renal disease. Rigorous control of blood pressure and blood glucose level may delay the development of end-stage renal failure. There are some anecdotal reports that converting enzyme inhibitors are effective in reducing the proteinuria in this disorder and possibly in slowing the progression to end-stage renal disease. Further studies are needed before the therapeutic benefits of converting enzyme inhibition are established.

Amyloidosis may be primary or associated with a variety of systemic diseases. If the underlying disease can be identified, it should be treated if possible. Unfortunately, no specific therapy is of proven benefit. In patients with familial Mediterranean fever, colchicine diminishes the frequency of attacks and prevents the development of amyloidosis. Many drugs have been associated with the nephrotic syndrome, including the nonsteroidal anti-inflammatory agents, gold, captopril, and penicillamine. The nephrotic syndrome usually resolves when the offending agent is discontinued. Many neoplasms have also been associated with the nephrotic syndrome. If the neoplasm can be effectively treated, the nephrotic syndrome usually remits.

Causes of the Idiopathic Nephrotic Syndrome

Minimal Change Disease

This disease accounts for 85 to 90 per cent of children with the nephrotic syndrome and 15 to 20 per cent of adults. Generally the urine sediment is benign, blood pressure is normal, and there is little tendency toward loss of renal function. Thus the indications for treatment are primarily symptomatic.

These patients, both adults and children, should be treated initially with oral prednisone, 2 mg per kg (up to 80 mg per day), given as a single daily dose for 4 weeks, and then on an alternate-day basis for an additional 4 weeks. As soon as the nephrotic syndrome completely remits (urine protein level less than 200 mg per day), one should switch to alternate-day steroid therapy. Prednisone should then be slowly tapered over the remainder of the 8-week treatment period. If alternate-day treatment is used as initial therapy, it usually takes longer to induce a remission.

With this approach, more than 90 per cent of patients achieve a remission. However, 60 per cent of these patients have subsequent relapses. For patients with infrequent relapses (one to two per year), repeating the initial therapy is usually effective. Patients who have frequent relapses may benefit from either oral cyclophosphamide, 1 to 2 mg per kg per day, or chlorambucil, 0.15 mg per kg given for 6 to 8 weeks, plus prednisone. Patients who relapse as the prednisone is being

tapered or immediately after it is discontinued are considered to be steroid dependent. In these patients the benefits of long-term, low-dose steroid therapy are probably outweighed by the side effects. Therefore, treatment with cyclophosphamide or chlorambucil to induce a long-lasting remission would be appropriate. These patients may require slightly higher doses of chlorambucil (0.15 to 0.2 mg per kg per day). All adult patients should have a renal biopsy before being treated. For children, who are usually assumed to have minimal change disease and are treated without a renal biopsy, it is appropriate to perform a renal biopsy before instituting cyclophosphamide or chlorambucil therapy.

There are significant side effects associated with both of these alkylating agents, and they should be used with caution. The white blood cell count, hematocrit, and platelet count need to be measured weekly. If signs of bone marrow toxicity develop, the dose of the alkylating agent should be reduced or discontinued. To avoid gonadal dysfunction, the patient should be treated with cyclophosphamide for 6 weeks or less, and the total cumulative dose of chlorambucil should be kept below 7 mg per kg. A urinalysis should be performed at regular intervals to detect hemorrhagic cystitis from the cyclophosphamide. The use of these agents has also been associated with a high risk of malignancies, particularly leukemia and lymphoma, in later life. Given the natural history of this disease and the risk of side effects with the use of alkylating agents, the majority of patients should not be so treated. These drugs should be reserved for the patient who frequently relapses and is debilitated from both the consequences of the nephrotic syndrome and the long-term side effects of steroid therapy.

Mesangial Proliferative Glomerulonephritis

Mesangial proliferative glomerulonephritis is characterized by increased cellularity in the mesangial region in a patient without systemic illness. There are usually immune deposits of IgM in the mesangium. Treatment of mesangial proliferative glomerulonephritis is similar to that of minimal change disease. The drug of choice is prednisone. Patients should be treated to the point of remission or for up to 8 weeks. With this treatment, approximately 50 per cent of the patients can be expected to achieve a complete remission of the nephrotic syndrome. However, the majority of patients relapse as soon as the steroid dose is tapered or discontinued. If prednisone is ineffective or if the patient is steroid dependent and the nephrotic syndrome is significant, cyclophosphamide can be used at a dose of 1 to 2 mg per kg per day for 8 weeks. Adding prednisone to the cyclophosphamide does not improve the outcome. The cyclophosphamide does not need to be tapered. Some of these patients develop focal glomerulosclerosis.

Focal Segmental Glomerulosclerosis

Focal glomerulosclerosis accounts for approximately 10 to 15 per cent of the adults with idiopathic nephrotic syndrome. The majority of these patients have progressive renal failure and hypertension and develop end-stage disease after 5 years. Patients who achieve a partial remission of the nephrotic syndrome tend to have a better prognosis than those with persistent, heavy proteinuria. There have been no controlled clinical trials, but certain patients have had a remission of proteinuria associated with steroid therapy. Patients who respond to therapy appear to have a better prognosis than nonresponders or patients who have not been treated. Thus, if there are no contraindications to steroid therapy and renal function is well preserved, I recommend a trial of corticosteroids. Patients should be treated with 100 to 120 mg of prednisone on alternate days until a complete remission occurs or for a maximum of 8 weeks. The prednisone can then be tapered over the next 4 weeks. Although there is no proven benefit at this time, the risks and side effects from a short course of alternate-day prednisone therapy are low and the potential benefits may be great. If there are contraindications to steroid therapy or the patient has advanced renal failure, conservative management with control of blood pressure is indicated. There is no evidence that alkylating agents are of benefit. Recent preliminary work suggests that cyclosporine may be effective in inducing a remission, but patients appear to relapse as soon as the drug is discontinued. Thus, at this time, cyclosporine cannot be recommended for these patients. In patients who respond to steroids but who have frequent relapses or are steroid dependent, a prolonged remission in proteinuria may be induced with the use of cyclophosphamide, 1 to 2 mg per kg per day, or chlorambucil, 0.1 to 0.2 mg per kg per day, in addition to the prednisone for an 8-week course. But this therapy should be reserved for patients with significant side effects from the nephrotic syndrome and the steroid treatment. Patients with focal sclerosis who have non-nephrotic proteinuria should be treated conservatively because they generally do not progress to end-stage renal disease.

Membranous Nephropathy

Idiopathic membranous nephropathy is the most frequent cause of the nephrotic syndrome in adults, accounting for about 50 per cent of these cases. The outcome is highly variable. Spontaneous remission can occur. The treatment of membranous nephropathy remains highly controversial. However, a number of well-done prospective studies have demonstrated the benefits of therapy in slowing the progression of the renal disease.

Initial treatment of membranous nephropathy is 120 mg of prednisone orally given on alternate days for 8 weeks. The drug is then tapered and discontinued over the next 4 to 8 weeks. The patient who relapses later should be treated in a similar manner. This treatment has been shown to preserve renal function and slow the progression to end-stage renal disease. These benefits have been achieved even without remission of the proteinuria. A second form of treatment that has been shown to be effective is methylprednisolone, 1 gram intravenously for 3 days, followed by oral prednisone, 0.5 mg per kg per day for a month, alternated with chlorambucil, 0.2 mg per kg per day for a month, for a total of 6 months. The dose of chlorambucil is reduced if the white blood cell count falls below 5000 per mm^3. This therapy has also been shown to be beneficial in preserving renal function.

Recently it has been shown that cyclophosphamide in a dose of 1.5 mg per kg per day for 12 to 24 months slows the progression to end-stage renal disease. This treatment is particularly effective in patients with serum creatinine levels higher than 1.8 mg per dl. In patients with membranous nephropathy and non-nephrotic, asymptomatic proteinuria (less than 2 grams per day), the prognosis is good and treatment is not recommended.

Membranoproliferative Glomerulonephritis

Membranoproliferative glomerulonephritis is an uncommon cause of the idiopathic nephrotic syndrome, accounting for less than 5 per cent of adults with this syndrome. These patients usually present with the nephrotic syndrome or with acute glomerulonephritis manifested by hematuria and low-grade proteinuria. Many patients have a decreased serum complement level at some stage of their disease. Most patients with membranoproliferative glomerulonephritis progress to end-stage renal disease. Occasional spontaneous remission may occur. There are two histologic subtypes of membranoproliferative glomerulonephritis. Type I is characterized by prominent C3 deposits along the glomerular capillary and in the mesangium, and by electron-dense deposits in subendothelial and mesangial locations. In Type II membranoproliferative glomerulonephritis (intramembranous deposit disease), C3 deposits are present in the capillary walls and mesangium, but immunoglobulin is absent. The glomerular basement membrane is usually thickened with electron-dense deposits. I recommend treating patients with both Type I and Type II membranoproliferative glomerulonephritis with dipyridamole, 75 mg three times per day, and aspirin, 325 mg three times per day. In Type I membranoproliferative glomerulonephritis, this regimen has been shown to delay the progression to end-stage renal disease.

A number of other therapeutic regimens have been tried in patients with membranoproliferative glomerulonephritis. Particularly in children, uncontrolled trials of alternate-day prednisone have been shown to be of benefit in slowing the progression of the renal disease. But until controlled trials show a benefit of this form of therapy, I cannot recommend it. The combination of cyclophosphamide, dipyridamole, and warfarin (Coumadin) has been shown to be ineffective in the treatment of membranoproliferative glomerulonephritis.

GENERAL MANAGEMENT OF GLOMERULAR DISEASE

In addition to the treatment of the underlying disorder, management of patients with glomerular disease, particularly the nephrotic syndrome, includes therapy directed at relief of symptoms, correction of deficiencies resulting from urinary losses, and preservation of renal function.

Edema

Edema may occur in patients with glomerular diseases for various reasons. First, hypoalbuminemia resulting from the nephrotic syndrome reduces plasma oncotic pressure, leading to a disturbance in Starling forces in the peripheral capillary. Intravascular fluid is redistributed into the interstitial compartment, producing edema. The decreased intravascular volume then leads to increased resorption of sodium chloride and water by the kidney. Second, avid sodium chloride resorption can be found in the absence of hypoalbuminemia in glomerular disorders marked by intense glomerular inflammation. Third, a decrease in the glomerular filtration rate may limit urinary sodium chloride and water excretion, which leads to intravascular volume expansion. The consequences of the fluid retention in addition to edema can include hypertension and pulmonary congestion. Patients with mild to moderate edema do not need treatment except for moderate salt restriction (dietary sodium limit of 2 grams per day). Ony severe symptomatic edema should be treated. Diuretics can be used to treat this condition. Hydrochlorothiazide, be-

ginning at a dose of 25 mg per day, can be used in patients with a glomerular filtration rate exceeding 50 ml per minute. For patients with more compromised renal function, the loop diuretics furosemide or ethacrynic acid should be used in doses of 40 to 160 mg per day. If the hydrochlorothiazide or loop diuretics alone are not effective, a potassium-sparing agent such as amiloride, spironolactone, or triamterene can be added. These agents must be used with great caution in patients with compromised renal function because the risk of hyperkalemia is considerable. These patients must be monitored carefully for overdiuresis and the development of volume depletion. The goal of therapy should not be the eradication of edema but the control of the symptoms of edema. All of these patients have edema to some extent at all times.

Hypertension

Hypertension associated with glomerular disorders may be secondary to volume expansion or excessive systemic vasoconstriction. Clearly sustained hypertension accelerates the progression and irreversible loss of renal function, whatever the underlying disorder. Thus hypertension must be aggressively treated in these patients because it is an important factor in the progression of the renal disease. Generally a diuretic should be the initial therapy. The thiazide diuretics can be used in patients with serum creatinine levels less than 2.5 mg per dl. In those with serum creatinine levels higher than 2.5 mg per dl, the loop diuretics should be used. If the blood pressure is not controlled with a diuretic alone, a second agent, either a converting enzyme inhibitor, captopril and enalapril, or a beta blocker such as propranolol should be used. Captopril should be instituted at a dose of 25 mg twice per day and increased to a total of 150 mg per day. Enalapril should be initiated at a dose of 5 mg once per day and increased to a total dose of 20 or 30 mg per day. Propranolol should be started at a dose of 40 mg twice per day and increased to a total dose of 160 to 240 mg per day. Other agents that can be used include a calcium channel blocker such as nifedipine or diltiazem. For resistant hypertension, minoxidil can be effective, beginning at a dose of 2.5 to 5 mg per day and increasing to 20 to 30 mg per day.

A few words of caution about the use of drugs in patients with glomerular disease must be kept in mind. Because many drugs circulate bound to albumin, the hypoalbuminemia present in these patients may lead to high levels of free drug and increased toxicity. Certain agents, particularly the sulfonamide diuretics, can cause acute interstitial nephritis and lead to deterioration of renal function. Certain agents, such as the beta blockers nadolol and atenolol, are excreted primarily by the kidney, and their dosage needs to be adjusted for the level of renal function. The angiotensin-converting enzyme inhibitor captopril has been associated with the development of membranous nephropathy in a small number of patients. Doses greater than 150 mg per day should not be used in patients with impaired renal function or in those with systemic lupus erythematosus.

Thrombosis

Patients with the nephrotic syndrome have an increased prevalence of thromboembolic disease, which may be related in part to loss of inhibitors of coagulation, particularly antithrombin III, and to increased platelet aggregation. Renal vein thrombosis is particularly common in patients with the nephrotic syndrome secondary to membranous nephropathy. Pulmonary emboli can complicate renal vein thrombosis. Patients who present with evidence of either pulmonary emboli or an acute worsening of proteinuria or renal function that cannot be explained by other means should undergo venography. Patients with documented renal vein thrombosis or thromboembolic events need to be treated with oral anticoagulants. This therapy should be continued for as long as they remain nephrotic and hypoalbuminemic. There is no evidence that prophylactic anticoagulation is of benefit.

Hyperlipidemia

One of the hallmarks of the nephrotic syndrome is hyperlipidemia, manifested primarily by elevation of the serum cholesterol level but also, in patients who are severely nephrotic, with elevation of serum triglyceride levels as well. The etiology of the hyperlipidemia is multifactorial in these patients. Clearly, patients with persistent, long-term proteinuria and long-term elevations of serum lipid levels are at risk for premature atherosclerosis. Until recently there has been no safe, effective treatment for this disorder. Now, however, the fibric acid congener gemfibrozil has been found to be safe and effective at a dose of 600 mg twice per day. A combination of gemfibrozil plus the bile acid–binding resin colestipol, at a dose of 10 grams twice per day, was particularly effective in these patients. Unfortunately, many patients are unable to tolerate the gastrointestinal side effects of the bile acid–binding resins. Recent studies also suggest that the new lipid-lowering agents, the hydroxymethyl-

glutaryl coenzyme A reductase inhibitors, particularly lovastatin, may also be effective in this disorder. Further studies of this agent are needed before its use can be recommended.

Nutritional Therapy

In patients with the nephrotic syndrome, deficiencies of a variety of plasma proteins may occur. Significant hypogammaglobulinemia may be present and may be associated with increased susceptibility to infections. Hyperimmune gamma globulin may be beneficial in patients with recurrent infections. The loss of vitamin D–binding globulin may lead to vitamin D deficiency, hypocalcemia, and bone disease. These patients may require therapy with oral vitamin D preparations. There may be urinary losses of trace metals such as iron, zinc, and copper.

The optimal dietary intake for patients with the nephrotic syndrome and renal insufficiency remains to be established. There is some clinical evidence that moderate dietary protein restriction may retard the progression of renal disease in patients with chronic renal failure. There is also evidence that moderate protein restriction, rather than increased protein intake, may be more effective in maintaining serum albumin levels in patients with the nephrotic syndrome. However, the long-term safety and efficacy of protein-restricted diets in patients with heavy proteinuria, diabetes, and systemic diseases have not been demonstrated. In selected patients, moderate protein restriction may be appropriate. Initial therapy should include dietary counseling and a diet containing 0.7 to 0.8 gram per kg of protein per day. These patients need to be monitored closely for maintenance of body weight and serum albumin concentrations. Frequent visits with a nutritionist are probably required to ensure dietary compliance.

PYELONEPHRITIS

method of
STEVEN M. OPAL, M.D.
Brown University
Providence, Rhode Island

Pyelonephritis is defined as acute or chronic inflammation of the kidney resulting from the presence of microorganisms within the renal pelvis and interstitium. The disease generally presents as a clinically apparent, toxic illness with symptoms referrable to the urinary tract. However, it is important to note that infection of the upper urinary tract may occur in the absence of localizing symptoms. This condition is referred to as subclinical pyelonephritis and is observed primarily in children or the elderly. Pyelonephritis is the most common recognized source of bacteremia in hospitalized patients with gram-negative sepsis, and urinary tract infections remain the most common cause of nosocomially acquired infection. Although the optimal therapy for pyelonephritis is yet to be defined, general guidelines for this clinical entity have been developed. The recent introduction of various new antimicrobial agents has improved and widened the therapeutic options available to clinicians who treat pyelonephritis.

ACUTE PYELONEPHRITIS

The diagnosis of acute pyelonephritis is based on clinical findings of urinary frequency, dysuria, pyuria, and bacteriuria accompanied by fever, flank pain, and systemic toxicity. Despite the development of various techniques to localize infection in the upper urinary tract (antibody-coated bacteria, ureteral catheterization, Fairley's bladder washout, and imaging techniques), no method is sufficiently safe and reliable to be used routinely.

Pyelonephritis generally occurs as a result of ascending urinary tract infection from the urethra and urinary bladder. Infection of the kidney via the hematogenous route occurs infrequently (less than 5 per cent of cases) after disseminated infection with invasive microbial pathogens such as *Staphylococcus aureus, Candida* species, and *Salmonella* species. The Enterobacteriaceae and *Enterococcus faecalis* account for more than 95 per cent of the microorganisms causing pyelonephritis. Infection of the upper urinary tract is abetted by functional or mechanical obstruction of urinary flow and vesicoureteral reflux. Urinary calculi may contribute to pyelonephritis by producing urinary obstruction. Certain organisms (*Proteus* species, some *Klebsiella* species, *Staphylococcus saprophyticus*) may promote urolithiasis by producing urease, which alkalinizes the urine by releasing ammonia. The change in urinary pH results in precipitation of magnesium-ammonium-phosphate (struvite) stones. These stones may encase viable bacteria, which results in recalcitrant urinary tract infections.

Acute pyelonephritis is generally caused by a single strain of bacteria. Polymicrobial urinary tract infections are uncommon and should prompt a search for enterovesical fistulas or other structural abnormalities of the urinary tract. Polymicrobial infection is occasionally associated with urinary tract instrumentation or urolithiasis.

A Gram's stain of urine provides a rapid and reliable technique for diagnosis of pyelonephritis. The finding of one or more organism per oil immersion field on Gram's stain of uncentrifuged urine indicates at least 10^5 organisms per ml. Gram's stain also distinguishes gram-negative bacilli from gram-positive cocci (enterococci or staphylococci), which permits an early guide to empiric therapy. Urinary culture and susceptibility studies, when available, can be used to direct antimicrobial therapy. Blood cultures are generally warranted in patients with acute pyelonephritis. White blood cell casts in the urinary sediment are specific for renal medullary infection and are often found in urinary tract infections that are complicated by obstruction or papillary necrosis. Pyelonephritis in the absence of significant bacteriuria may occur under the following circumstances: pyelonephritis with complete urinary obstruction, prior antimicrobial therapy, or suppurative complications (intrarenal or perinephric abscess).

Treatment

The toxic-appearing patient with acute pyelonephritis should be hospitalized for intravenous antimicrobial therapy. A rapid assessment of fluid and electrolyte status should be conducted, in addition to a review of potential complicating factors such as recent use of urinary tract instrumentation, prior antimicrobial therapy, pregnancy, diabetes mellitus, prior urinary tract infections, or functional or mechanical abnormalities of urinary flow. Intravenous fluids are indicated to promote an adequate urinary output and to treat volume depletion, which may develop secondary to fever and loss of urinary concentrating ability. After urine and blood cultures have been obtained and urinalysis and Gram's stain have been reviewed, empiric therapy is warranted based on an assessment of the most likely pathogen.

Uncomplicated pyelonephritis may be treated with a variety of acceptable antimicrobial regimens. Parenteral ampicillin, cefazolin (Ancef), or trimethoprim-sulfamethoxazole (Septra, Bactrim) are acceptable empiric agents. Combination therapy with aminoglycosides in addition to beta-lactam drugs is generally reserved for severely ill patients with presumed gram-negative sepsis, or for nosocomially acquired infections in which resistant gram-negative bacilli (*Pseudomonas, Providencia*) are more likely to occur. Antimicrobial therapy should be modified once the susceptibility pattern of the offending pathogen is known. Directed therapy should make use of the simplest and least expensive effective agent.

A number of second- and third-generation cephalosporins and newer antimicrobial agents such as aztreonam (Azactam), imipenem (Primaxin), and beta-lactamase inhibitor combinations such as ticarcillin plus clavulanic acid (Timentin) are well suited for treatment of acute pyelonephritis. These agents have the advantage of being active against a wide variety of resistant gram-negative bacilli (including *Pseudomonas* species) while avoiding the potential nephrotoxicity associated with aminoglycoside antibiotics. They are particularly useful in treating nosocomially acquired pyelonephritis. The fluoroquinolones norfloxacin (Noroxin) and ciprofloxacin (Cipro) have an excellent spectrum of activity and pharmacokinetic properties for use in the treatment of urinary tract infections. Intravenous preparations of fluoroquinolones will soon be available and will provide a useful alternative for the treatment of acute pyelonephritis. Enterococcal urinary tract infections are successfully treated with ampicillin alone unless the patient is septic, which indicates the need for the addition of an aminoglycoside. *S. saprophyticus* is susceptible to trimethoprim-sulfamethoxazole, ampicillin, or vancomycin.

Intravenous therapy should continue until 48 hours after the patient becomes afebrile. At that time, the patient may be switched to an effective oral antimicrobial agent for a total duration of therapy of at least 2 weeks. Therapy should continue for a total of 4 to 6 weeks in patients who have frequent relapsing infections or complicated structural abnormalities of the urinary tract. Most patients are rendered afebrile within 72 hours of initiation of appropriate antimicrobial therapy. Lack of clinical response by this time should prompt an investigation to rule out local suppurative complications (intrarenal or perinephric abscess, papillary necrosis) or urinary obstruction. Computed tomography and renal ultrasonography are useful in providing diagnostic information as well as a means of directing therapeutic percutaneous drainage if an abscess is identified.

A follow-up urinary culture 1 week after completion of therapy should be obtained in patients with documented pyelonephritis. Evidence of relapsing infection should be treated with a prolonged course (4 to 6 weeks) of an appropriate antimicrobial agent. Frequent relapsing infections in women and any urinary tract infection in men should prompt urologic evaluation to exclude potentially correctable structural abnormalities.

CHRONIC PYELONEPHRITIS

Chronic pyelonephritis connotes chronic interstitial nephritis with scarring associated with recurrent urinary tract infections. This entity is seen almost exclusively in patients who have structural abnormalities of the genitourinary tract with evidence of recurrent infection since childhood. Recurrent urinary tract infections in adults without structural anomalies of the genitourinary tract rarely, if ever, result in chronic renal insufficiency. Chronic pyelonephritis is associated with small contracted kidneys that have uneven scarring and thinning of the renal cortex. The clinical presentation is one of chronic renal insufficiency associated with hypertension, urinary concentrating defects, metabolic acidosis, hyperkalemia, and renal salt wasting.

Treatment

The optimal therapy of chronic pyelonephritis is prevention of its occurrence before irreversible loss of renal function occurs. Prevention is accomplished by careful evaluation and treatment of patients with structural abnormalities of the urinary tract. Urinary tract infections in children, in males, in women with recurrent relapsing infections, and in patients with abnormal renal function deserve a urologic investigation to exclude potentially correctable obstructive lesions.

Prolonged suppressive antimicrobial therapy may occasionally be useful in patients with recurrent urinary tract infections associated with renal scarring. A 6- to 12-week course of an oral antimicrobial agent such as trimethoprim-sulfamethoxazole, trimethoprim alone, a fluoroquinolone, or urinary acidification with methenamine mandelate (Mandelamine) is often effective.

Complete sterilization of the urine in patients with multiple genitourinary tract abnormalities is often impossible. It is recommended that patients be treated during acute symptomatic infections with a 10- to 14-day course of antimicrobial agents in an attempt to alleviate symptoms and prevent systemic infection. Continuous antimicrobial suppression is ill advised in such patients because this treatment creates selection pressures favoring the development of an antibiotic-resistant bacterial population.

TRAUMA TO THE GENITOURINARY TRACT

method of
JOSEPH N. CORRIERE, Jr., M.D.
*The University of Texas Medical School
at Houston
Houston, Texas*

Trauma to the genitourinary tract is present in about 10 per cent of all patients with abdominal trauma seen in emergency centers. With a high index of suspicion and the use of excretory urography, cystography, retrograde urography, and computed tomography (CT), a rapid, accurate diagnosis of these lesions can be made and appropriate therapy provided in a timely fashion.

RENAL INJURIES

Everyone agrees that minor renal injuries need conservative management and major renal parenchymal and vascular lesions need immediate surgical repair. However, controversy surrounds the proper treatment of renal injuries of an intermediate nature. With the advent of CT assessment of these lesions, there has been more agreement, but the debate still is not settled.

Although the kidneys are well protected by the ribs, vertebral bodies, and heavy lumbar muscles, injuries are very common. Rapid deceleration causing excessive movement of the kidneys may lead to major vessel trauma resulting from stretching of the vessels with arterial intimal tearing and thrombosis. Approximately 80 per cent of renal injuries are caused by blunt trauma and are usually secondary to motor vehicle accidents, falls, sports, or fights. The most common penetrating injuries are caused by gunshot or stab wounds and comprise the other 20 per cent of renal injuries. Eight per cent of abdominal penetrating injuries involve the kidneys, and associated visceral injuries are present in 80 per cent of these patients.

Patients with upper abdominal trauma who have a high probability of renal injury have hematuria 90 per cent of the time, abdominal and/or flank tenderness, and occasionally contusions or abrasions over the flank area.

An excretory urogram (intravenous pyelogram [IVP]) should always be obtained in patients who have sustained significant upper abdominal or flank trauma, have significant hematuria, or have a fracture of the eleventh or twelfth rib or the transverse processes of the lumbar vertebrae. If the IVP is normal, no additional studies are necessary. If there is nonfunction of a kidney on the IVP, a renal vascular injury should be suspected and the patient should have an arteriogram. If function is seen but the architecture of the kidney is unclear or extravasation is present, a CT scan is indicated to define fully the extent of the injury.

Renal Contusion

When there is decreased perfusion on the IVP but the renal outline is complete and intact, with no evidence of contrast extravasation, the patient is said to have a renal contusion. Bed rest and conservative therapy are all that is necessary in these patients. Frequent urinalysis until there is no more hematuria can be used as a guide to ambulation. Contact sports should be prohibited for a few weeks, and blood pressure should be checked for up to 1 year to be sure that hypertension caused by a "Page" kidney does not develop.

Renal Laceration

When insufficient information is obtained on the IVP, because of an indistinct renal outline, an area of decreased perfusion, contrast extravasation, or the presence of a retroperitoneal mass, a CT scan must be obtained to evaluate the extent of renal parenchymal injury as well as the presence of an intrarenal or perirenal hematoma. Most of these lesions can be treated with bed rest and observation. The indications for renal exploration in blunt injuries are an expanding or uncontained hematoma, the presence of nonviable renal parenchyma, and, in some cases, major contrast extravasation. Less than 10 per cent of all renal injuries fall into this category. All penetrating wounds should be explored.

A midline transabdominal incision should be used. Associated injuries of the liver, spleen, and bowel should be corrected before opening a retroperitoneal hematoma unless heavy bleeding demands that this be done. A vertical incision over the aorta should be made to isolate the renal vessels where they leave the aorta and enter the vena cava. Vessel loops should be used to secure the renal artery and vein before the peritoneum lateral to the colon is incised. The colon is then mobilized, the hematoma entered, and the kidney explored.

Intrarenal hematomas should be evacuated, the wound débrided by guillotine excision, and individual arteries and veins suture ligated with 5-0 absorbable suture. The calices should be closed with a running 5-0 suture and should be made as watertight as possible. If sufficient capsule is present to cover the defect, it should be closed to tamponade persistent vessel oozing. If the capsule has been destroyed, pedicle grafts of omentum or free peritoneal patch grafts may be used. Polypropylene mesh can also be employed and sewn into a pocket for the organ. Retroperitoneal drains should be placed near the injured kidney and brought out by a separate stab wound.

If renal artery thrombosis is present, the injured segment must be removed and circulation re-established. Vein or artery grafts may be needed. Autotransplantation should be considered before nephrectomy is used. Small vessel occlusions can be left alone without fear of complications. Venous injuries should be sutured with 5-0 vascular suture. Segmental veins may be ligated safely. The venous system has many intrarenal anastomoses, unlike the arterial system, which has end arteries.

URETERAL INJURIES

The ureter transports urine from the kidney to the bladder. When it is injured by external violence, a fistula may occur and lead to urinary extravasation into the retroperitoneum or the peritoneal cavity. If injury to another structure has occurred at the time of the ureteral injury, a fistula may develop to the vagina, skin, or bowel. If the urine is infected, life-threatening sepsis may occur.

Gunshot wounds account for over 95 per cent of ureteral injuries. Knife wounds are the next most common etiology. Rarely, patients fall and become impaled on a spike.

The IVP is the best way to diagnose a ureteral injury. Urinary extravasation is seen on the study, as well as some decrease in visualization of the collecting system.

If the injury is first seen at surgical exploration, the ureter should be dissected from its bed and examined where it lies in proximity to the missile tract. If it cannot be positively determined whether an injury is present, one vial (5 ml) of indigo carmine should be injected intravenously. Within 7 to 10 minutes, the dye will leak into the periureteral tissues if the ureter has been lacerated.

If the patient is not undergoing exploration, and if after the IVP there is still a question about the presence of an injury, the most definitive study is a retrograde ureterogram. Most of the time, this study is not feasible. In this case, a CT scan of the area best demonstrates the presence of extravasation.

Contusion

This injury is discovered during exploration of a patient who has had a missile pass close to the ureter but in whom the structure has remained intact. No therapy is necessary in these patients. If a high-velocity bullet (traveling at a rate of more than 2500 feet per second) has caused the wound, there is always the danger of late necrosis of the ureter. In this instance, placement of an internal stent and a drain in the area of the injury should be considered.

Laceration

If a partial laceration is present and the ureter that is still in continuity is viable, placement of an indwelling "double-pigtail" stent and closure of the wound with interrupted 4-0 or 5-0 absorbable sutures give the best results.

If the remaining intact ureter is of questionable viability or if there is a complete laceration of the ureter, all devitalized tissue must be excised and a suitable repair selected.

The ureteroneocystostomy has the lowest complication rate but can be performed only in the patient with an injury below the level of the iliac vessels. The kidney can usually be mobilized and lowered so that the gap between the ureter and bladder can be decreased by an additional few centimeters. A bladder flap can also be used to bring the bladder closer to the ureter. Sometimes merely suturing the bladder to the psoas fascia (psoas hitch) can avoid tension on the repair. A nonrefluxing reimplantation is most desirable but cannot always be performed.

If the injury is too high to perform a ureteroneocystostomy, a ureteroureterostomy should be done.

If a major length of ureter is lost, consideration should be given to a transureteroureterostomy or merely to bring the cut end of the ureter to the skin as a cutaneous ureterostomy for later definitive repair. Autotransplantation of the kidney to the hypogastric vessels plus ureteroneocystostomy should also be considered. This adds major operative time and risk to the patient, but in the patient with a solitary kidney it can be lifesaving.

BLADDER INJURIES

When the bladder is distended or the pelvis is fractured, the normal protective influence of the intact pelvic ring is lost and the shearing force of a pelvic fracture tears the bladder at its moorings. A spicule of bone may lacerate the organ, or it may rupture at the dome by a direct blow to the abdomen without causing bony injury. Missiles, on the other hand, may find the bladder despite its level of distention.

Penetrating trauma to the bladder from external violence is most commonly caused by gunshot wounds. The most common etiology of blunt bladder injuries is from motor vehicle accidents, but it can also be caused by falls, crushing injuries to the bony pelvis, or blows to the abdomen.

Hematuria is a hallmark finding with bladder injuries; gross hematuria occurs more than 95 per cent of the time, and microscopic hematuria is present in the remaining cases.

The static cystogram is the only study that can definitely diagnose a ruptured bladder. In the male, if a urethral injury is suspected because of a pelvic fracture, the presence of blood at the urethral meatus, a high-riding prostate on rectal examination, or marked ecchymosis and edema of the perineum, scrotum, and/or penis, a retrograde urethrogram must be done before urethral catheterization is attempted.

Penetrating Injuries

All patients with penetrating injuries from external violence should undergo exploration of the abdomen and of the tract the missile followed from its entrance wound to its exit wound. The peritoneal cavity should be opened even if the injury is felt to be entirely extraperitoneal, and the intra-abdominal viscera and major vasculature should be examined for damage. All devitalized tissue and debris (e.g., bullets, bone spicules, clothing) should be removed from the bladder and abdomen.

After débridement, any extraperitoneal vesical defects should be closed with a one-layer running suture of 3-0 chromic or polyglycolic suture through the interior of the bladder. Extensive mobilization of the bladder to ensure a watertight closure or to place the knots on the outside of the bladder usually only increases bleeding. If it is impossible to close the extraperitoneal defects, they should not be disturbed. With adequate bladder drainage, they eventually heal without difficulty. A suprapubic cystotomy tube is then inserted in the bladder.

The intraperitoneal bladder incision is closed with a double layer of 3-0 chromic or polyglycolic suture in a running watertight fashion, as are any intraperitoneal defects.

Bladder Contusions

An injury of the bladder mucosa or muscularis without loss of bladder wall continuity secondary to blunt trauma is a bladder contusion. Extravasation of contrast is not seen. These injuries need Foley's catheter drainage for a few days or, if minor, no therapy at all.

Intraperitoneal Rupture

Intraperitoneal rupture of the bladder occurs when there is a sudden rise in intravesical pressure secondary to a blow to the pelvis or lower abdomen. This increased pressure results in rupture of the dome, the weakest and most mobile part of the bladder. Contrast material fills the cul-de-sac, outlines loops of bowel, and eventually extends into the paracolic gutter.

All intraperitoneal bladder ruptures caused by blunt abdominal trauma should undergo formal repair. The bladder usually has a rent at the dome measuring 5 cm or more. Devitalized tissue should be excised and, after a suprapubic tube has been placed as previously described, the dome wound should be closed with absorbable suture material.

Extraperitoneal Rupture

Extraperitoneal bladder ruptures are almost exclusively seen with pelvic fractures. Most of the time, the bladder is sheared on the anterior lateral wall near the bladder base by the distortion of the pelvic ring disruption. Occasionally, the bladder is lacerated by a sharp, bony spicule. On cystography, flame-shaped areas of extravasation that are usually confined to the perivesical soft tissues are visualized.

Isolated extraperitoneal bladder ruptures can be easily handled by 10 days of Foley's catheter drainage. One cannot decide, as some authors state, to treat small extraperitoneal ruptures with catheter drainage and to formally close large ruptures because it is difficult to relate the amount of contrast extravasation to the extent of the injury.

If the patient with an extraperitoneal bladder rupture is to be explored for associated injuries and is not gravely ill, it is best to open the dome of the bladder, not disturb the pelvic hematoma, repair the rupture intravesically, close the bladder, and insert a suprapubic tube, as previously described.

URETHRAL INJURIES

When considering injuries to the male urethra, a classification that helps to determine appropriate therapy is (1) posterior urethral injuries (those of the prostatic and membranous urethra, above and including the urogenital diaphragm) and (2) anterior urethral injuries (those of the bulbous and penile, or pendulous, urethra below the urogenital diaphragm).

The female urethra is rarely injured. When it is damaged, however, the injury is usually accompanied by a severe bony pelvic disruption with concomitant injury to the bladder neck and vagina. Urethral injury is more common in female children than in adults.

Almost all injuries of the posterior urethra in the male occur in conjunction with fracture of the bony pelvis. Ninety per cent of these injuries are caused by motor vehicle accidents involving passengers in automobiles, persons on motorcycles, or pedestrians. Falls from a height, industrial crushing injuries, and sporting accidents result in the other 10 per cent of pelvic fractures.

This injury is most commonly caused by the shearing force of the bone disruption. The prostate, attached by the puboprostatic ligaments, is pulled in one direction, while the membranous urethra, attached to the urogenital diaphragm, is pulled in another direction.

Penetrating wounds of the posterior urethra from external violence are uncommon but do occur.

Most injuries to the anterior urethra caused by external violence result from blunt trauma to the perineum. The bulbous urethra is usually crushed against the pelvic arch, generally when the patient falls astride an object. This may happen while falling from a height, straddling a fence, or having a foot slip from the rung of a ladder. It is sometimes caused by a kick to the perineum or by hitting a bump in the road while riding a bicycle and coming down hard on the seat or the crossbar.

Patients with a history of trauma to the perineum or a fracture of the bony pelvis should be suspected of having a urethral injury. The majority of patients with a ruptured urethra have blood at the urethral meatus, and many of them have swelling and ecchymosis of the penis, scrotum, and/or perineum. This is caused by urine, blood, or both leaking into these structures.

In the patient with a fractured pelvis, rectal examination may reveal the prostate to be in a higher position than usual. This "high-riding" prostate is caused by disruption of the urethra, with the prostate elevated from its normal position by a large pelvic hematoma. The soft, boggy hematoma is felt where the prostate is normally found.

Any patient with a suspected urethral injury must have a retrograde urethrogram performed. Under no circumstances should an attempt be made to catheterize the urethra until this study delineates the anatomy and any damage done to that organ. Injudicious catheterization of the injured urethra carries the risk of converting a partial urethral rupture into a complete urethral rupture, as well as possibly infecting a sterile periurethral or pelvic hematoma.

Type I Posterior Urethral Injury

The patient with a pelvic hematoma compressing the urethra often has difficulty voiding, so a urethral catheter should be left in place for a few days. This urethral compression is classified as a Type I injury.

Partial Posterior Urethral Rupture, Types II and III

A Type II posterior urethral injury has extravasation of contrast only above the urogenital diaphragm into the true pelvis, whereas in a Type III injury the urogenital diaphragm is ruptured and contrast extravasates both above and below this structure. The injuries can be either partial or complete. The patient with a minimal partial urethral rupture may be treated with urethral catheter drainage for 14 to 21 days, followed by a voiding cystourethrogram to ensure that the injury has healed. If the catheter does not pass easily into the bladder or if the injury is extensive, urethral catheterization should not be done for fear that the partial rupture may be converted to a complete rupture. The patient should undergo suprapubic cystotomy. A cystogram must then be done to rule out a concomitant bladder rupture.

The most conservative way to handle all of these injuries is to place a suprapubic cystotomy and not attempt urethral instrumentation. A voiding cystourethrogram through the cystotomy tube should be performed 14 to 21 days after the injury. If extravasation is no longer present and the urethra is of normal caliber or there is only a minimal stricture at the site of the injury, the tube should be removed and the patient allowed to void. If urethral occlusion is present, suprapubic drainage should be continued for 4 to 6 months and delayed open repair performed.

Complete Posterior Urethral Rupture, Types II and III

There are two ways to treat the patient with a complete rupture of the posterior urethra: immediate surgical realignment or suprapubic cystotomy and delayed surgical repair. Immediate surgical realignment is the procedure of choice in the stable patient who is going to have immediate pelvic exploration for a concomitant vascular or rectal injury or, as is frequently seen in children, has major bladder neck lacerations or prostatic fragmentation.

The procedure is performed through a lower abdominal midline incision. A catheter is passed per urethra through the urogenital diaphragm into the perivesical space. Another catheter is passed via the bladder out of the bladder neck, through the prostatic urethra, and brought into the surgical field by sight. The catheters are tied together, and the bladder catheter is used to guide the urethral catheter into the bladder and is tied by a lock stitch to the abdominal wall to fix the catheter in place.

The prostate and bladder should now be repositioned easily and without tension against the urogenital diaphragm. A suprapubic tube should be placed in the bladder and a drain in the perivesical space.

Delayed surgical repair is the procedure of choice if (1) the patient is medically unstable or (2) the surgeon is unskilled in performing major urethral reconstructive surgery. The delayed repair is my procedure of choice.

Once the diagnosis of a complete posterior urethral disruption has been made, a suprapubic tube is placed in the bladder either by trochar or by formal cystotomy. A cystogram is then performed to ensure that there is no bladder rupture, and nothing more is done about the urethral injury at that time. Approximately 6 months later, a definitive repair is performed.

Anterior Urethral Contusions

No special therapy is necessary for patients with this injury. It is seen in straddle injuries when the urethrogram is normal but initial or terminal hematuria exists. Patients usually are able to void normally, and their hematuria promptly clears.

Partial Anterior Urethral Rupture

If the extravasation on the urethrogram is minimal, contained by Buck's fascia, and there is good urethral continuity, these patients may be allowed to void or a urethral catheter can be placed in the bladder for a few days. If the injury is extensive and extends outside Buck's fascia, a suprapubic tube should be placed in the bladder and a voiding cystourethrogram repeated in 10 to 14 days.

Complete Anterior Urethral Rupture

In this injury there is extensive extravasation and loss of urethral continuity. These patients should have a suprapubic tube placed in the bladder and followed closely. If the urine is infected, they should receive antibiotics.

When the skin of the genitalia and perineum is intact and at least 14 days have elapsed from the time of the injury, a voiding cystourethrogram and possibly a combined voiding cystourethrogram and retrograde urethrogram should be done to delineate the injury. If urethral continuity is intact but a minimal stricture is present, a visual urethrotomy may be needed to incise the stricture.

Most of these patients usually develop complete occlusion of the urethra caused by a very short stricture. They should continue to receive suprapubic drainage for 4 to 6 months until the perineum is well healed before reconstruction. A delayed one- or two-stage repair is then necessary.

Penetrating Anterior Urethral Injury

These wounds need prompt attention. Clean knife wounds merely need minimal débridement, closure of the defect with absorbable sutures, and suprapubic catheter drainage for 2 to 3 weeks.

Dirty wounds with extensive tissue destruction and embedded foreign material (e.g., metal pellets, oil, grease, hair, clothing) need to be thoroughly cleansed with antiseptic solution and copious irrigation. Although débridement of devitalized tissue is important, it must be stressed that contused corpus spongiosum tissue is hemorrhagic and ecchymotic and may appear necrotic when it is only badly bruised. If débridement is vigorous, more urethra than is necessary may be removed and discarded, making eventual repair a formidable task. In this instance, suprapubic diversion should be done until the perineum has healed. This may take weeks to months. Radiographic studies usually demonstrate a residual stricture, which can be handled by formal urethroplasty.

PENILE INJURIES

The penis contains both urinary tract and reproductive tract structures. Therapy of wounds of the penis should be directed at preservation of these organ system functions. When the penile urethra is lacerated, the treatment choices are (1) primary repair (spatulated reanastomosis over a Foley's catheter) if the injury is minimal and the wound is clean or (2) delayed repair (requiring a perineal urethrostomy) if major tissue destruction is present.

When injuries to the penile skin are trivial, they can be treated the same way as skin wounds anywhere on the body; however, if a circumferential injury has occurred to the penile shaft skin, the skin distal to this injury must be removed because the lymphatics are disrupted and this distal penile skin becomes permanently edematous. After removal of the distal shaft skin, the penis can be buried in a scrotal flap, to be matured at a second operation or a split-thickness skin graft applied to the denuded penile shaft.

Penetrating injuries of the penis and penile fractures caused by blunt trauma to the erect penis require closure of the corporal defect after assessment of the continuity of the urethra. This closure should be performed with absorbable suture because corporal defects closed with permanent suture may leave behind palpable subcutaneous knots that may be annoying or painful to the patient. Early surgical treatment of penile fracture is superior to nonoperative treatment.

Treatment of extensive penile injuries should be conservative and staged in an attempt to rescue marginally viable tissue. All but frankly necrotic and dysfunctional tissue should be left behind during débridement of the penis. Frequent débridement of small amounts of tissue, rather than an aggressive session of débridement, results in a greater amount of functioning tissue being saved in patients with massive penile injury.

Rarely, one is faced with the management of a patient who has had an amputation of the penis, either self-induced or as a result of external violence. Reimplantation of the amputated penis using microscopic assistance should be attempted.

TESTICULAR INJURIES

When the diagnosis of testicular rupture is made or suspected, exploration of the scrotum is required. Evacuation of the overlying hematoma, débridement of the testicular tubules, and closure of the tunica albuginea, when performed early, lead to a high rate of testicular salvage. Similarly, exploration of the scrotum for penetrating injuries should be performed early because bleeding vessels within the scrotum do not tamponade because the scrotum expands to accommodate large amounts of blood.

SCROTAL INJURIES

Trivial scrotal injuries can be débrided and closed with absorbable suture under local anesthesia. When the tunica vaginalis has been lacerated, the scrotal contents should be inspected and a drain placed in the wound. Many scrotal injuries can be closed primarily, even when there is a large loss of scrotal skin, because of the elastic nature of the remaining scrotum. When there is a major loss of scrotal skin, especially if an avulsion has exposed the testes, management should consist of staged closure of the scrotal skin, with or without skin grafting. During the time when the testes have no scrotal covering, they are covered by moist saline dressings. Some urologists advocate the creation of thigh pouches or immediate skin grafting; however, this approach is not necessary.

BENIGN PROSTATIC HYPERPLASIA

method of
MICHAEL E. MAYO, M.B., B.S.
University of Washington
Seattle, Washington

In benign prostatic hyperplasia (BPH) there is an enlargement of a small volume (5 per cent) of tissue surrounding the central third of the urethra. The urethra is usually elongated and both lateral and middle lobes may enlarge and distort the neck and trigone of the bladder. This prevents the normal funneling of the bladder neck, obstructing voiding. BPH is an age-related condition rarely found before age 40 but is present in 80 per cent of men over 80 years of age. Today, there is a 29 per cent probability that a 40-year-old man will have a prostatectomy during his lifetime.

The history of prostatism typically encompasses two sets of symptoms: obstructive and irritative. Hesitancy, poor stream, intermittency, terminal dribbling, double voiding, and incomplete emptying are the most common obstructive symptoms. Men with BPH rarely strain to void unless chronic retention has developed. The irritative symptoms of frequency and urgency are present in most patients, and these are often more troublesome than the obstructive ones, especially when sleep is disturbed by nocturia. Incontinence (urge and overflow), retention (acute and chronic with azotemia), infection (producing pain on urination), and hematuria are all less common forms of presentation. Physical examination should include an assessment of the size and consistency of the prostate. Although size does not always correlate with the degree of obstruction, a very large gland may need a different surgical approach and any suspicion of malignancy will usually require a tissue diagnosis before treatment can be planned. Physical signs of retention of urine or neuropathy should also be sought.

Initial investigations should be noninvasive, and a flow rate determination is the most useful screening test. Urinalysis, and culture if indicated, a hemogram, and blood chemistry are standard investigations in all cases. Although upper urinary tract imaging is not essential, except when there is a history of stones or hematuria, an ultrasonogram and/or excretory urogram will allow for an estimate of trabeculation and residual urine without the necessity for urethral instrumentation. Cystoscopy will be indicated if a decision on the management of prostatism cannot be made or if there is any suspicion of other bladder pathology, especially a tumor. A simple cystometrogram (CMG) may demonstrate detrusor muscle instability, which is present in 60 to 70 per cent of men with prostatism but is rarely helpful in deciding on treatment. The CMG may document a large capacity bladder with reduced sensation in men with chronic retention; however, to determine the contractility of the detrusor muscle, a complex multichannel urodynamic study with voiding pressure is required. Any man with a neuropathy and possible obstruction should also have a urodynamic evaluation to determine the significance of each component. The most common indications for intervention in BPH are the symptoms of prostatism. Men with moderate symptoms (nocturia of twice or less) have a good chance of remaining the same or improving over time, and, indeed, a large placebo effect has been found in controlled trials of drug treatment for BPH. Therefore, in men with mild to moderate symptoms a period of observation is advisable. Retention (acute or chronic with azotemia), recurrent infection, and persistent hematuria are much less common but more urgent reasons for intervention.

TREATMENT

Nonsurgical

Surgical removal of the obstructing tissue is still the most effective treatment but there are nonsurgical therapies that should be discussed with the patient and recommended if there is a high surgical risk.

Alpha-Adrenergic Antagonists. The prostate and bladder neck contain a large number of alpha-adrenergic receptors, and inhibition of these has been shown to improve both the obstructive and irritative symptoms in many well-controlled trials. The drug most often used is phenoxybenzamine* (Dibenzyline), 10 mg per day orally, increasing as tolerated over a period of 1 week to 30 mg per day. Prazosin* (Minipress), 1 to 2 mg orally, increasing as tolerated to 4 to 8 mg per day, is also effective and may be associated with fewer side effects (dizziness, lack of concentration, stuffy nose). A reduction in circulating testosterone by using estrogens or performing orchiectomy will often allow atrophy of a benign gland but is not generally acceptable in men without disseminated cancer of the prostate. However, the intracellular conversion of testosterone to dihydrotestosterone can be blocked by inhibiting the enzyme 5α-reductase, which is responsible for this conversion; therapeutic trials of a 5α-reductase inhibitor are now in progress. Balloon dilation of the prostatic urethra is also under therapeutic trial.

Surgical

Transurethral Surgery. Transurethral resection of the prostate (TURP) has become the surgical treatment of choice in most cases. Resection of relatively small glands (less than 20 grams) seems to be associated with a higher incidence of bladder neck contracture, and the early results of incising the bladder neck and prostate (transurethral incision of the prostate [TUIP]) are excellent. It remains to be seen if a TURP will be

---

*This use of these agents is not listed in the manufacturers' directives.

required more often in the TUIP patients at a later date.

Open Surgery. Only 10 per cent of prostatectomies are performed by open procedure, the indications being very large glands, inadequate urethral size for the resectoscope, and the presence of certain bladder pathologies. In a *suprapubic* prostatectomy the gland is approached through the bladder, and in the *retropubic* prostatectomy the anterior prostate capsule is incised directly just below the bladder neck. In the *perineal* prostatectomy the posterior prostatic capsule is incised in the perineum, but the latter procedure is rarely indicated because of significant impotence and incontinence problems that ensue.

In all resection procedures the objective is to remove the adenoma, leaving the surgical capsule. Clearly, the open procedure is more complete but is usually associated with a higher morbidity.

Anesthesia. Spinal or epidural anesthesia is excellent for a transurethral approach and may be adequate for open surgery if high enough to give adequate relaxation of the abdominal muscles. General anesthetic is required if there are contraindications to spinal or epidural anesthesia. It is also possible to do the procedure under local anesthetic, infiltrating the prostate from both the perineal and urethral aspects.

Antibiotics. Appropriate antibiotic therapy should be started parenterally at least 12 hours prior to surgery and continued for 5 days after catheter removal in patients with bacteriuria and in those with indwelling urethral catheters. Even if the urine from Foley's catheter is sterile, there is an increase in urethral colonization around it. Prophylactic antibiotics given to patients with sterile urine and no preoperative catheters appear to reduce postoperative bacteriuria but do not show any benefit in reducing the rare but serious complications of septicemia. Also, in the majority of patients, this postoperative bacteriuria is asymptomatic and transient. Prophylactic antibiotics should, however, be given to high-risk patients with diabetes, neurogenic bladder, and immunosuppression and to those with cardiac and other prostheses.

Blood Transfusion. It is rare to need blood transfusion in transurethral surgery, and cross-matching is not performed routinely unless the preoperative hematocrit is borderline. In open prostatectomy blood is more often required and should be cross-matched beforehand.

Postoperative Care. Bleeding with obstruction of the drainage catheters is probably the most troublesome problem. It is not important which type of catheter and method of irrigation are used as long as the nursing staff caring for the patient is thoroughly familiar with their management. There is a real advantage to having all postoperative prostatectomy patients on a designated urology nursing unit. The catheter is removed usually in 1 to 3 days after a TURP when the urine has cleared to a light pink or brown if there are no other factors such as fever, a large perforation, or other active medical problem that would compromise a voiding trial. The patient should be warned to expect some increased frequency, urgency, and even urge incontinence. Unless the voided volumes are very small, the stream should be noticeably better than before operation. Bleeding should be monitored by saving the three most recent urine samples. The postvoid residual should be determined if there is any clinical suspicion of incomplete emptying.

COMPLICATIONS

Early Complications

Mortality. Traditionally, the operative mortality (death within 30 days of surgery) for open prostatectomy and TURP was thought to be less than 2 per cent and less than 1 per cent, respectively. However, recent figures based on health care claims data have revealed the mortality (occurring in or out of hospital within 91 days of prostatectomy) is 3.1 per cent for open prostatectomy, and 2.8 per cent for TURP in teaching hospitals. This compares with a high figure of 6.1 per cent for open prostatectomy and 9.0 per cent for TURP for small nonteaching hospitals (less than 150 beds). Within 1 year of TURP 9 per cent of men age 55 to 69 years of age die as compared with a predicted rate of 3.5 per cent in age-matched men not undergoing surgery. If these figures are confirmed, it is clear that in high-risk patients, with poor life expectancy, alternative management of prostatic enlargement should be carefully considered.

TURP Syndrome. An average of 1 liter of irrigation fluid is absorbed in a TURP and this causes little clinical or biochemical disturbance. However, if large venous sinuses are opened or if large perforations in the prostate capsule or bladder neck are made and large amounts of irrigating fluid are extravasated, considerable amounts of fluid may enter the patient's circulation. The irrigating fluid used is usually a slightly hypotonic solution of glycine or sorbitol, which causes a dilutional hyponatremia that is responsible for most of the clinical manifestations (nausea, vomiting, confusion, coma, bradycardia, hypertension, and muscle paralysis). Many patients will correct the clinical and metabolic problem of the TURP syndrome with diuresis, which may, if necessary, be induced by diuretics. Attempting to correct the hyponatremia with hypertonic saline may be indicated in patients with coma, but cardiac failure is likely to be precipitated.

Hemorrhage. Venous bleeding at the end of the procedure can usually be controlled with gentle catheter traction and tamponade of the bladder neck and prostatic fossa for a few hours. Heavy arterial bleeding restarting after the procedure will usually require a recystoscopy under anesthetic with evacuation of clots and coagulation of the bleeding point.

Secondary venous hemorrhage is often brought on by straining, and readmission to hospital with cystoscopy is occasionally required. Patients should be advised not to be too active and to try to avoid straining for defecation, and they should not allow the bladder to become overdistended.

Urinary Tract Infection. The use of preoperative antibiotics, whether for treatment or prophylaxis, has been discussed. If antibiotics are not used, it is advisable to check a urine culture before discharge and at 3 to 4 weeks, as asymptomatic bacteriuria that does not clear may be associated with delayed healing of the prostatic fossa and increased scarring. Urinalysis will usually reveal pyuria and microhematuria for 6 weeks until the prostatic fossa has re-epithelized, and urine culture is needed to confirm bacteriuria and to check sensitivities. Epididymitis occurs in 2 per cent of patients after TURP, and vasectomy does not appear to prevent it.

Wound Infection. The incidence of wound infection may be as high as 20 per cent even in patients with uninfected urine. The source of these organisms is probably the distal urethra, and prophylactic antibiotics are advisable in open procedures and will usually halve the risk. The condition of osteitis pubis is rarely seen now that most urinary tract infections can be adequately treated prior to surgery.

Incontinence. Detrusor muscle instability present in 60 to 70 per cent of men prior to surgery may cause urgency incontinence for several months after operation; however, 60 per cent of these patients will lose their instability within 6 months. Sphincter weakness incontinence is seen in less than 1 per cent of patients in the long run, although it may be present for a few days after removal of the catheter. Sphincter incontinence after prostatectomy is usually due to damage to the passive component of the distal sphincter. The patient may be able to prevent leakage by active pelvic floor contraction, but when this voluntary muscle fatigues, a slow drip will occur when the patient is upright. Improvement in sphincter function will occur over time and with pelvic floor exercises. Surgical correction with an artificial sphincter is not usually considered for 6 to 12 months, which will allow spontaneous improvement to occur.

Impotence and Retrograde Ejaculation. Potency may decrease in a number of men after suprapubic and retropubic prostatectomy, TURP, or TUIP but rarely can an organic cause be found for this. Sexual activity often decreases at this time of life, and the prostatectomy, with the associated local discomfort, adds a further psychologic factor. Ejaculation is nearly always partly or largely retrograde after surgery except in patients who have had a TUIP. Preoperative counseling should include a generally positive outlook with regard to change in potency but should contain a warning about the problem of retrograde ejaculation, especially if the patient is relatively young and may want to father more children.

Inadequate Emptying. This may be due to persistent adenoma or hypocontractility of the detrusor muscle. It is important to determine which of these is present before undertaking further surgery, and this evaluation may require at least a CMG, or preferably multichannel urodynamics to determine detrusor contractility during attempted voiding. If obstructing tissue is still present, further resection is generally indicated. Hypocontractility should be treated with a further period of catheter drainage, preferably by a self-intermittent catheterization program, or if this cannot be performed, a Foley's catheter may be inserted for a few weeks. The patient may have to learn to void by straining or Credé's method. The addition of parasympathetic agents (bethanechol [Urecholine] orally 25 mg three times per day) may be tried but is usually ineffective unless much larger doses are taken, in which case unacceptable side effects will occur.

Late Complications

Urethral Strictures. These occur in approximately 6 per cent of patients after TURP and are most common in the submeatal area. Attempting to use instruments and catheters that are too large for the urethra may predispose to stricture, and the meatal and submeatal areas may be damaged by allowing dried blood and secretions to build up on the catheter. Treatment consists of dilation and occasionally internal urethrotomy, but if the stricture is in the membranous urethra, gentle and repeated dilations only should be performed, otherwise the passive sphincter may be damaged.

Bladder Neck Contracture. This is a scarring of the bladder neck that constricts in ring-like fashion and prevents adequate funneling. It seems to be more common after small TURPs or if the bladder neck is resected too deeply. The condition presents with obstructive and irritative symptoms, often with infection. Endoscopic incision rather than resection is the treatment of choice, and this may have to be done more than once. Occasionally, an open Y-V plasty is necessary to resolve the problem.

Regrowth of Prostatic Tissue. Health care claims data have revealed a much higher incidence of repeat prostatectomy than the 10 per cent quoted from traditional retrospective studies. For patients surviving 8 years, the cumulative probability for a second operation is 20 per cent for TURP and 10 per cent for open operation.

PROSTATITIS

method of
EDWIN M. MEARES, Jr., M.D.
Tufts University School of Medicine
Boston, Massachusetts

ACUTE BACTERIAL PROSTATITIS

Acute bacterial prostatitis generally is recognized easily because its clinical presentation is typical: sudden chills and fever, perineal and low back pain, both irritative and obstructive voiding dysfunction, generalized malaise, and occasional arthralgia and myalgia. On rectal examination, the prostate is usually tender and is partially or totally swollen, indurated, and warm to the touch. The prostatic expressate is purulent and readily grows large numbers of the bacterial pathogen (usually coliforms) on culture plates. However, because massage of an acutely inflamed prostate is painful and may lead to bacteremia, this procedure should be avoided. Bacteriuria usually accompanies acute prostatitis; therefore, the pathogen may generally be identified by culture of the voided urine.

General Therapy

Hospitalization often is warranted, especially when significant urinary retention develops. The administration of analgesics, antipyretics, stool softeners, and adequate hydration is indicated. Cystoscopy and urethral catheterization should be avoided. Patients who develop significant urinary retention as a result of acute bladder outlet obstruction are managed best by the insertion of a temporary punch suprapubic tube and a drainage system under local anesthesia. A variety of punch suprapubic tubes and drainage systems are available for use in this setting.

Antibacterial Therapy

Many antibacterial drugs are effective in the treatment of acute bacterial prostatitis, even agents that fail to cure chronic bacterial prostatitis. The intense inflammatory reaction that develops in acute prostatitis apparently alters the pharmacokinetics sufficiently so that drugs that normally are excluded diffuse in therapeutic concentrations into prostatic fluid. I prefer to initiate therapy with trimethoprim-sulfamethoxazole (TMP-SMX) (Bactrim, Septra), one double-strength tablet (160 mg TMP, 800 mg SMX each) twice daily, until the results of the culture and sensitivity tests are known. If the patient is allergic to sulfonamides but not to TMP, I begin therapy with TMP (Proloprim, Trimpex) alone, 200 mg orally twice daily. Other new agents that usually are highly effective include norfloxacin (Noroxin), 400 mg by mouth twice daily, and ciprofloxacin (Cipro), 500 mg by mouth twice daily. If the results of susceptibility tests of the pathogen and the clinical response are favorable, I continue therapy in full dosage for at least 30 days to cure the infection and prevent the development of chronic bacterial prostatitis.

If initial therapy with an oral antimicrobial agent is undesirable, I administer gentamicin sulfate (Garamycin), 3 to 5 mg per kg of body weight per day, divided into three intravenous doses, *plus* ampicillin, 1 gram, administered intravenously every 6 hours, until the results of the culture and sensitivity tests are known. If the patient responds favorably to this therapy, after about 1 week a suitable oral antimicrobial agent is substituted and given in full dosage for at least 30 days.

Operative Therapy

Surgical therapy generally is not required in the management of acute bacterial prostatitis. Occasionally, however, a prostatic abscess evolves. The clinician should suspect an abscess in patients who respond poorly or incompletely to what should be appropriate antimicrobial therapy. Presumptive diagnosis of a prostatic abscess is made by palpation of a localized, tender, fluctuant mass within the prostate during rectal examination. Definitive diagnosis is made by means of transrectal prostatic ultrasonography or computed tomography. Overt prostatic abscesses usually require surgical drainage.

CHRONIC BACTERIAL PROSTATITIS

Chronic bacterial prostatitis (CBP) is a common cause of relapsing recurrent urinary tract infection (UTI) in men because the bacterial pathogen often persists unaltered in the prostatic secretions during antibacterial therapy and eventually reinfects the urine after medication is withdrawn. The most common causative pathogens are various strains of *Escherichia coli,* although infections caused by species of *Klebsiella, Enterobacter, Proteus, Pseudomonas,* and other less common gram-negative organisms occasionally are found. *Enterococcus (Streptococcus faecalis)* is a definite cause of some cases of chronic prostatitis; however, prostatitis caused by other gram-positive organisms is confirmed infrequently and rarely leads to relapsing bacteriuria. Prostatic infection caused by two or more pathogens occurs occasionally.

The clinical manifestations of chronic bacterial prostatitis vary considerably; however, most patients complain of irritative voiding dysfunction and pain perceived in various sites (penile, perineal, scrotal, suprapubic, low back, and even inner thighs). The hallmark of CBP is relapsing UTI caused by the same pathogen. Men with CBP typically have prostatic expressates that show leukocytosis (more than 10 white blood cells per high-power field) and increased numbers of macrophages containing fat. The most accurate method of diagnosing bacterial prostatitis is to perform essentially simultaneous quantitative cultures of the urethra, midstream urine, and expressed prostatic secretions.

General Therapy

Men with CBP seldom have symptoms that warrant hospitalization. Chills, fever, and acute urinary retention are unusual and generally reflect an acute exacerbation of a chronic infection. Although appropriate antibacterial therapy usually quickly controls the symptoms of CBP, adjunctive therapy is sometimes indicated. The liberal use of hot sitz baths is especially soothing. Some patients also benefit from the temporary use of anti-inflammatory agents (e.g., ibuprofen [Advil, Motrin], 600 mg orally four times daily) and anticholinergics (e.g., oxybutynin chloride [Ditropan], 5 mg orally three times daily).

Antibacterial Therapy

Pharmacokinetic studies using dogs confirm the clinical experience in men: Few antimicrobial agents achieve therapeutic levels in prostatic secretions. TMP does diffuse into prostatic fluid and has the best-documented success in curing chronic bacterial prostatitis caused by susceptible pathogens. Long-term therapy (12 weeks) has proved to be more successful than short-term therapy (2 weeks) in achieving cures. Norfloxacin and ciprofloxacin, new fluoroquinolone agents, are still under investigation for use in CBP but already have shown excellent efficacy in curing many cases of CBP caused by coliforms. Based on my experience and that of others, I recommend the following therapeutic regimens for treating nonazotemic men with culture-proven susceptible pathogens infecting the prostate:

1. TMP-SMX, one double-strength tablet (160 mg TMP, 800 mg SMX) orally twice daily for 12 weeks *or*

2. TMP, two tablets (100 mg each) orally twice daily for 12 weeks *or*

3. Ciprofloxacin, 500 mg orally twice daily for at least 4 weeks *or*

4. Norfloxacin, 400 mg orally four times daily for at least 4 weeks *or*

5. Carbenicillin indanyl sodium (Geocillin), two tablets (382 mg each) orally four times daily for at least 4 weeks

Specific therapy must always be tailored to meet the individual patient's needs and drug tolerance. (See also the manufacturer's directions regarding the use of these agents.)

Most men with CBP who are not cured by medical therapy can be kept relatively comfortable with sterile bladder urine by the use of continuous low-dose suppressive daily therapy with an appropriate oral antibacterial agent, such as a single 100-mg capsule of nitrofurantoin or a single regular-strength tablet of TMP-SMX per day. Typically, however, cessation of drug therapy eventually results in reinfection of the bladder urine and a return of symptoms.

Operative Therapy

For patients with CBP who are not cured or adequately controlled by medical therapy, treatment by surgical means may prove to be necessary. Men with CBP and prostatic calculi often are candidates for surgical therapy, especially because infected prostatic calculi cannot be sterilized by antimicrobial therapy alone. Total prostatovesiculectomy cures CBP but is seldom recommended because of its sequelae. Provided that the resectionist successfully removes all foci of infected stones and tissue, transurethral prostatectomy can cure CBP. Unfortunately, this goal is difficult to achieve, especially because the peripheral zone of the prostate contains the largest foci of infection.

NONBACTERIAL PROSTATITIS

Although its specific cause remains obscure, nonbacterial prostatitis (NBP) is the most common form of prostatitis syndrome. Many of the clinical symptoms and features of NBP and CBP are indistinguishable, except that patients with NBP characteristically do not have relapsing UTI. Despite having prostatic fluid leukocytosis, men with NBP have negative cultures localizing a causative pathogen to the prostate. Studies of an infectious cause of NBP have generally eliminated as pathogens aerobic bacteria, obligate anaerobes, mycoplasmas, ureaplasmas, chlamydia, trichomonads or other parasites, and viruses. Some investigators believe that NBP is an autoimmune disease. The diagnosis is confirmed only by excluding other forms of prostatitis.

General Therapy

When bacteriologic localization cultures demonstrate no bacterial pathogen in a patient who has symptoms of chronic prostatitis and inflamed prostatic secretions, a clinical diagnosis of nonbacterial prostatitis is made. Because mycoplasmas, ureaplasmas, and *Chlamydia trachomatis* have not been completely excluded as causative agents in cases of NBP, I recommend a clinical trial of antimicrobial therapy directed toward these agents. The tetracyclines and erythromycin are the most effective drugs against these organisms; therefore, a trial using either minocycline or erythromycin is recommended. I administer minocycline (Minocin), 100 mg orally twice daily for 4 weeks, or erythromycin, 500 mg orally four times daily for 4 weeks.

Because most patients who have NBP respond poorly to antimicrobial therapy, the clinician should not persist in using antimicrobial agents in management. Instead, efforts should be made to assist the patient in coping with his disease. I tell the patient that he has a noninfectious inflammation of the prostate that is similar to noninfectious arthritis. The condition tends to be chronic and causes annoying symptoms but will not lead to serious complications or shorten his life. The use of alcoholic beverages, coffee, and spicy foods should be restricted if the patient notices that these substances aggravate his symptoms. Normal sexual activity should usually be encouraged. Indeed, the patient should try to lead as normal a life as possible. For symptomatic flare-ups, I recommend hot sitz baths, short courses of anti-inflammatory agents (e.g., ibuprofen, 600 mg orally four times daily), and an anticholinergic agent (e.g., oxybutynin chloride, 5 mg orally three times daily).

Antibacterial Therapy

Antimicrobial therapy is seldom warranted in managing NBP, especially in men who respond poorly to empiric therapy with minocycline or erythromycin.

Operative Therapy

Unless the patient with NBP also has obstructive voiding dysfunction associated with bladder outlet obstruction, surgical therapy is seldom indicated in the management of NBP. Indeed, irritative voiding symptoms may grow worse after transurethral prostatectomy.

PROSTATODYNIA

Some patients with symptoms of prostatitis, especially prostatic pain, have a normal urinalysis and culture and prostatic expressates that are normal by microscopy and culture. These men suffer from prostatodynia, a syndrome usually associated with an acquired voiding dysfunction. In most patients with prostatodynia, urodynamic testing discloses a voiding dysfunction associated with apparent spastic obstruction of the bladder neck and prostatic urethra. These patients often respond to therapy using alpha blockers, such as prazosin (Minipress), 1 or 2 mg orally twice daily in gradually increasing doses. Other patients have pelvic floor tension myalgia and respond best to treatment using hot sitz baths, muscle relaxants such as diazepam (Valium), 5 mg orally three times daily, and special exercises. In still other patients, emotional problems seem primary and psychiatric consultation is warranted.

ACUTE RENAL FAILURE

method of
JOHN T. HARRINGTON, M.D.
Tufts University School of Medicine
Newton-Wellesley Hospital
Newton, Massachusetts

Acute renal failure (ARF) is the origin of clinical nephrology. In 1941 Bywaters and Beall reported their experience with patients with ARF from crush injuries after the bombing of London. A few years later in the Netherlands, Kolff used the artificial kidney for the first time on a patient with uremia from malignant hypertension. Kolff made eight artificial kidneys during World War II; after the war, three were dispatched abroad—one to London, one to New York, and one to Montreal. Merrill's group at the Brigham Hospital in Boston built its own machine, using Kolff's blueprints, and, according to Kolff, "probably did more for the further propagation of dialysis than any other group." ARF was the major indication for the early use of the artificial kidney. Chronic hemodialysis did not become feasible until the early 1960s, after the invention of the Quinton-Scribner shunt.

In the nearly 45 years since the end of World War II, an enormous amount has been learned about ARF at the cellular, nephronal, whole-kidney, and whole-body levels. Nevertheless, survival of ARF patients still hovers around 50 per cent, a figure not dissimilar to that seen in the first decade after the end of World War II. Thus, ARF remains a challenging clinical entity. The fact that a patient can survive for a prolonged period with total loss of a vital organ system and then recover virtually complete function highlights the unique aspect of ARF.

Acute renal failure remains a generic term, encompassing a variety of clinical situations. I restrict the use of this term to patients in whom renal function deteriorates over a period of 2 weeks or less. At a macroscopic level, ARF, like Gaul, can be divided into three parts: prerenal azotemia, postrenal azotemia, and intrinsic renal failure. It is important to rule out both prerenal and postrenal azotemia before deciding that intrinsic renal failure is present. The reason for this is obvious: Rapid correction of prerenal azotemia (e.g., dehydration) or relief of postrenal azotemia (e.g., benign prostatic hypertrophy with obstruction) can rapidly return renal function to normal. In both of these circumstances, the kidney is intrinsically normal, at least during the early phases. Historically, ARF was almost always associated with oliguria (<400 ml per day). The last decade has demonstrated that intrinsic renal failure caused by acute tubular necrosis (see later) is associated with urine output of approximately 1000 ml per day in at least 20 to 30 per cent of cases.

Prerenal azotemia is caused by inadequate renal perfusion. Inadequate renal perfusion results either from salt and water depletion (e.g., severe diarrhea or "third space" accumulations from acute pancreatitis) or from volume overload (e.g., congestive heart failure, where renal function deteriorates because of the impaired cardiac output). In either case, prerenal azotemia is manifested by a reduction in urine output, a benign urine sediment, excretion of concentrated urine (specific gravity > 1.015 to 1.020), and urine sodium excretion of less than 5 to 10 mEq per liter (in the absence of diuretic administration).

Given that prerenal azotemia can be caused by either volume depletion or volume overload, determination of the volume status of the ARF patient is essential. This determination requires careful attention to the patient's immediate history, accurate knowledge of fluid intake and ouput, analysis of daily weight (still all too often lacking in hospitalized patients in the United States), and a careful physical examination. Physical examination of a patient in whom one is attempting to determine the intravascular volume should stress (1) measurement of orthostatic blood pressure and pulse; (2) skin turgor, particularly over the anterior thigh, where the presence of "tenting" is an excellent sign of intravascular volume depletion even in elderly patients; and (3) a careful search for edema, either pretibially or in the sacral region. All too often, I see "dehydrated" patients (a diagnosis erroneously made on the basis of a dry tongue—simply a function of mouth breathing) who have 4 + pitting sacral edema—edema that has been missed by attending physicians and house staff alike. The presence of edema establishes the fact that total body sodium overload exists. Although in unusual circumstances edema can be present with a decrease in effective intravascular volume, statistically it is much more likely to be accompanied by increased intravascular volume. If doubt remains regarding the status of the intravascular volume after the history and physical examination, a recent chest x-ray film may be helpful; findings consistent with congestive heart failure establish the presence of volume excess. Finally, invasive hemodynamic measurements, using either a central venous pressure line or a Swan-Ganz line, can be made. Volume challenges, if used in the patient with prerenal azotemia who is thought to be volume depleted, should consist of 250 ml isotonic saline or lactated Ringer's solution (no difference between these two replacement solutions has ever been shown), given over 15 minutes, with repeated clinical observations or hemodynamic measurements made. In patients with severe third space accumulations (e.g., acute pancreatitis), 10 liters or more may be required in extreme circumstances before intravascular volume, blood pressure, and renal perfusion are restored.

Postrenal failure, defined as obstruction to urine flow, is seen most typically in elderly men with prostatic hypertrophy. The presence of total anuria or alternating swings between high and low urine output strongly suggests the possibility of obstruction and the need for appropriate urologic investigation. Abdominal percussion and palpation, rectal examination, and an estimate of postvoid residual urine (by Foley's catheter or by ultrasonography) should be done in all oliguric patients. A pelvic examination is mandatory in any woman with oliguria or ARF to eliminate the possibility of bilateral ureteral obstruction secondary to widespread pelvic cancer. Detection of obstructive uropathy was once difficult, frequently requiring cystoscopy and retrograde catherization; the advent of ultrasonography has virtually eliminated their use. Renal ultrasound provides not only evidence regarding the possibility of obstruction, but also information on postvoid residual urine and renal size (see later).

Recalling that the kidney has only four main structures (i.e., glomeruli, blood vessels, renal tubules, and interstitium) is helpful in focusing on the precise cause of *intrinsic renal failure.* Globally, ARF may be caused by acute glomerulonephritis, renovascular disease, acute tubular necrosis (ATN), or acute interstitial nephritis (AIN). In patients with *hospital-acquired ARF,* the vast majority of instances are caused either by prerenal azotemia or by ATN. In patients who *enter* the hospital with ARF, the likelihood of finding entities other than ATN is considerably higher, and more attention must be paid to the differential diagnosis in these patients.

DIAGNOSIS

My approach to the differential diagnosis of intrinsic renal failure relies heavily on a recent history; a careful physical examination establishing the patient's volume status; measurement of urine specific gravity (or osmolality) and urine sodium level (the latter only in the patient who is not receiving furosemide, a rare finding in today's hospitalized oliguric patient); and, most importantly, a careful examination of the spun urine sediment. A plethora of urinary diagnostic indices has been promulgated during the last two decades. In my experience, they rarely add anything beyond what can be obtained by the methods just noted. As mentioned earlier, the patient with prerenal azotemia has a benign urine sediment, concentrated urine, and a low urinary sodium concentration. The patient with postrenal azotemia has a benign urine sediment and, occasionally, red blood cells (caused by previous urologic investigation or the disease causing the obstruction); urine specific gravity and urinary sodium concentration are not helpful in making the diagnosis of postrenal azotemia.

In the patient with ARF caused by intrinsic renal disease, urinary sediment examination by the experienced clinician-uroscopist is particularly helpful. Classically, one finds proteinuria, hematuria, and red blood cell casts in the patient with acute glomerulonephritis; white blood cells, perhaps eosinophils, and, rarely, white blood cell casts in the patient with AIN; and renal tubular cells, muddy brown pigmented casts, and occasionally renal tubular cell casts in the patient with ATN. In my experience, diagnostic urine sediment abnormalities are found in more than 95 per cent of patients with acute glomerulonephritis, in a comparable percentage in patients with AIN, and in approximately 75 to 85 per cent of patients with ATN. Jaundiced patients have a urine sediment typical of that seen in patients with ATN, with the obvious addition of bilirubinuria.

Urinary specific gravity is elevated and urinary sodium excretion is decreased in patients with acute glomerulonephritis (of any sort), whereas in ATN, urinary specific gravity is usually in the 1.010 to 1.012 range and urinary sodium concentration is more than 30 to 40 mEq per liter. Urinary specific gravity and sodium concentration are not helpful in the diagnosis of AIN. The remainder of this discussion focuses on the patient with ATN because that is the likely cause of ARF in hospitalized patients. Renal biopsy may be required in instances where there is little clinical evidence of ATN, in helping to distinguish cortical necrosis from ATN, and in diagnosing suspected acute glomerulonephritis or AIN.

ACUTE TUBULAR NECROSIS

Epidemiology, Risk Factors, and Prognosis

Two recent, major reports have defined the epidemiology of hospital-acquired ARF, its risk factors, and its prognosis. ARF, variably defined by a rise in the serum creatinine concentration, occurred in 2 to 5 per cent of hospitalized patients in these studies. In one study, 80 per cent of the episodes of hospital-acquired renal insufficiency were caused by decreased renal perfusion, postoperative renal insufficiency, radiographic contrast media, or aminoglycoside administration. In the second study, volume depletion, aminoglycoside use, congestive heart failure, radiographic contrast media, and septic shock were the major risk factors identified. Poor prognostic factors include the presence of oliguria (nonoliguric patients seem to have both less severe ATN and a smaller likelihood of dying), urinary sediment abnormalities, and severe renal insufficiency. The adverse effect of volume depletion was increased in diabetics; the risk of aminoglycoside use increased with increasing age. In one study, an increase in the serum creatinine level of 3 mg per dl or more was associated with a mortality rate of 64 per cent! In most instances, however, patients did not die of renal failure per se but rather of the diseases that precipitated it.

Prevention

Knowledge of the limited number of risk factors associated with hospital-acquired ARF should provide the clinician with all the ammunition needed to reduce its incidence dramatically. To prevent ARF, attention should be directed at avoiding nephrotoxic aminoglycoside antibiotics, avoiding radiocontrast media, and moderating the use of diuretics to prevent too rapid diuresis, particularly in a diabetic patient. All clinicians have the tools to monitor their own patients efficiently and cheaply. The requirements are simple: (1) *mandatory* daily weight determinations in all patients admitted to medical and surgical units; (2) avoidance of nephrotoxic agents when possible; (3) measurements of peak and trough serum levels of aminoglycosides at appropriate intervals, coupled with measurement of the serum creatinine concentration every other day; and (4) infection surveillance and control programs. In this regard, careful attention must be directed especially at the use of Foley's catheters and indwelling arterial and venous lines.

Treatment

Treatment of ARF encompasses both conservative (nondialytic) therapy and various dialytic modalities. At present, treatment of established ATN is primarily supportive in that no demonstrated, effective method of hastening recovery from ATN exists. A number of innovative treatment protocols, including the intravenous administration of adenosine triphosphate–magnesium chloride are being examined experimentally, but information on their use in clinical ARF is scanty. High-dose furosemide (200 to 400 mg intravenously) and mannitol (12.5 to 25 grams intravenously) have been shown to convert early oliguric

renal insufficiency into nonoliguric renal failure. No effect on overall mortality rates has been demonstrated, however.

Conservative Therapy

Conservative therapy of the oliguric patient, based on principles established in the 1950s, is still applicable to ARF patients as we approach the 1990s. The physician must be attuned to abnormalities in all organ systems, not simply to those of the kidneys. Normal volume status must be maintained. Fluid (water) should be administered only to replace urine output and nonrenal losses, and to provide an additional 400 to 500 ml per day. If the serum sodium level falls below 130 mEq per liter, more rigid water restriction must be used; the input may need to be reduced to as little as 400 ml per day. Sodium should be given to the oliguric patient only to the extent that it is lost by nonrenal routes or to replace third space losses. The oliguric patient should have a sodium chloride intake of 2 grams per day or less orally and no sodium chloride in intravenous fluids. The administration of 0.5 N sodium chloride to the edematous, oliguric patient, inexplicably still a common practice in U.S. hospitals, results only in further edema and more profound hyponatremia. Potassium administration should be forbidden in the oliguric patient unless hypokalemia and potassium depletion from a nonrenal route are present. The daily diet should consist of an adequate protein intake (40 to 60 grams) and large amounts of carbohydrates (at least 100 grams). In fact, the introduction of a low-sodium, low-potassium diet that contained adequate protein, coupled with 100 grams of glucose, resulted in a decline in the mortality of ARF from approximately 90 per cent in the 1940s to its current level of approximately 50 per cent even by the early 1950s. Although these conservative maneuvers are in a sense old-fashioned, they remain the bedrock of modern treatment of the patient with ARF.

Dietary Treatment

Dietary treatment has been a major area of investigation in ARF in the past 20 years. No one dietary prescription can be given to all patients with ARF, but some general guidelines can be provided for patients with ARF of varying severity. First, in the patient with mild ARF who is in mild negative nitrogen balance, a diet that includes 20 to 30 grams per day of high-biologic-value protein or its equivalent as essential amino acids is indicated (along with sodium and potassium restriction, as just noted). At least 100 grams of carbohydrate per day should be given; increased calories should be supplied if renal failure lasts for more than 5 to 7 days. In patients with moderately severe ARF (e.g., secondary to sepsis), intravenous nutritional support is often required. One should give sufficient calories to maintain the nitrogen balance (clinically estimated by a stable weight in the edema-free patient); carbohydrates should comprise 60 to 70 per cent of the total calories, with the remaining calories being given as a 20 per cent fat emulsion. Essential amino acids given intravenously may be required; a variety of commercial preparations are available. Concentrated dextrose is the major caloric source in most of these feeding solutions, along with 10 to 20 per cent fat emulsions. In the severely catabolic patient (e.g., the patient with ARF after trauma and rhabdomyolysis), 3000 calories per day or more is required. From 20 to 30 grams per day of essential amino acids may be needed, along with large amounts of glucose and 10 to 20 per cent fat emulsions.

In the patient who cannot be fed, parenteral nutrition is required. Hypertonic nutrient solutions must be infused centrally through a subclavian vein catheter. Knowledge of a number of technical details is required to provide total parenteral nutrition safely; the clinician is referred to specialized textbooks on ARF for such details. Finally, it should be pointed out that although maintenance of nitrogen balance is a reasonable goal of therapy, it has not been demonstrated that advances in nutritional therapy have improved survival rates in ARF patients.

Conservative management of the patient with ARF must also focus on prevention of infection, prevention and treatment of gastrointestinal bleeding, and maintenance of normal cardiac and pulmonary functions. Foley's catheters should not be used unless urologically indicated; urine volumes can be obtained by intermittent bladder catheterization, with less risk of infection in the oliguric patient. Although not proved effective in reducing uremic gastrointestinal bleeding, my approach is to use aluminum hydroxide (antacids) and an H_2 receptor antagonist (e.g., cimetidine, 300 mg orally twice daily). In patients in whom bleeding continues, particularly those in whom any surgical procedure is required, administration of 1-deamino-8-D-arginine-vasopressin (DDAVP), 0.3 microgram per kg over 20 minutes intravenously, or intranasally at 3.0 micrograms per kg; cryoprecipitate, 7 to 10 bags; or conjugated estrogens, 0.6 mg per kg per day for 4 to 5 days, helps to correct the platelet dysfunction that causes the bleeding in these patients. I prefer to use DDAVP. Adequate dialysis (daily in the bleeding patient with a prolonged bleeding time) is the initial treatment of choice in uremic bleeding.

Finally, *any drug* that is being given to a patient with renal failure should be carefully scrutinized both for its absolute necessity and for the appropriateness of its dosage and of the intervals between doses. A number of tables are available to guide the clinician on the dosage and time intervals of the most commonly used drugs. These tables also provide information on the dialysis of drugs, either by hemodialysis or by peritoneal dialysis.

Dialytic Therapy

Dialysis is required in patients with ARF for the same indications as in chronic renal failure. Absolute indications include volume overload, severe acidosis, hyperkalemia, and gross manifestations of uremia, such as seizures or pericarditis. Dialysis may be required daily to keep the blood urea nitrogen level below 100 mg per dl and the serum creatinine level below 10 mg per dl. Three techniques of dialytic therapy are currently available: hemodialysis, peritoneal dialysis, and continuous arteriovenous hemofiltration (CAVH). Peritoneal dialysis, although still an excellent therapeutic modality, is not used as often as in the past, having been superseded by hemodialysis, with its greater ease, convenience, and rapidity. Peritoneal dialysis suffers from the problem of slow clearance and frequently cannot be used in patients who have undergone major abdominal surgical procedures. Because of the ability to dialyze hemodynamically unstable patients and to use small amounts of anticoagulants (without causing clotting in the external device), as well as the ease of insertion of double-lumen dialysis catheters, hemodialysis is now relied on heavily for management of ARF patients.

I do not wait for the absolute indications for hemodialysis noted earlier. My approach is to use hemodialysis on a prophylactic basis, starting before the major uremic complications appear. Dialysis should be done for 4 hours per treatment for a minimum of three times per week until the onset of the postoliguric phase and stability or a decline in blood urea nitrogen and serum creatinine levels are observed. Bicarbonate, not acetate, should be used as the source of alkali in dialysis in ARF patients. In my experience, subclavian venous access provides a better alternative than femoral vein catheterization because the subclavian route allows the patient to move about, thereby reducing the likelihood of deep venous thrombosis and other complications of strict bed rest.

The last decade has seen the introduction of several nondialytic techniques for the treatment of ARF, including CAVH and slow continuous arteriovenous ultrafiltration (SCUF). Both techniques, which are essentially the same, consist of continuous removal of a large volume of uremic ultrafiltrate via a dialyzer. When the ultrafiltrate removed is replaced by a nearly equal volume of an appropriate electrolyte solution, the technique is considered CAVH; when the fluid is not replaced, it is considered SCUF. Proponents of CAVH argue that it is particularly useful in ARF patients who cannot be peritoneally dialyzed or in those who are hemodynamically unstable and therefore not suitable for acute hemodialysis. The hemofiltration device, in essence a high-flux dialyzer, operates without the use of a blood pump, requiring the patient's systolic blood pressure to be higher than 70 mmHg. Blood flow rates of approximately 100 ml per minute can be obtained by cannulation of the femoral artery, with return of blood to any peripheral vein. Large amounts of fluid can be removed by ultrafiltration with these devices; 10 liters or more per day of ultrafiltrate is not unusual. It is thus obvious that unless the patient is grossly volume overloaded, physiologic solutions must be infused to match the fluid lost. In contrast to hemodialysis, which removes fluids and waste products by ultrafiltration and diffusion, convective forces account for removal of uremic molecules in CAVH. Many complications of hemodialysis, peritoneal dialysis, and CAVH exist. Accordingly, these techniques should be used only by a nephrologist who has experience with them.

CHRONIC RENAL FAILURE

method of
K. SHASHI KANT, M.D.

University of Cincinnati College of Medicine
Cincinnati, Ohio

Chronic renal failure (CRF) can be said to be present when the kidneys are affected by irreversible and usually progressive conditions. Various common causes of chronic renal failure are given in Table 1. The current incidence of new cases is between 100 and 250 persons per 1 million, depending on the racial mixture of the population, there being a higher proportion of hypertensive renal disease among black persons.

CLINICAL FEATURES AND DIAGNOSIS

The single most frequent laboratory datum indicating renal failure is the serum creatinine level or creatinine clearance (CCr). When muscle mass (the source of creatinine) is constant, the CCr is a good index of the glomerular filtration rate (GFR), except in far advanced renal failure, when CCr overestimates GFR. The blood urea nitrogen (BUN) concentration is not as accurate an estimate of renal function because

TABLE 1. Causes of CRF

Cause	Prevalence (%)
Diabetic nephropathy	40–50
Other primary and systemic glomerular diseases	20–30
Hypertension	15–20
Stones, obstruction, interstitial nephritis, polycystic kidneys	10

it is affected by other considerations, such as dietary protein intake and the state of the patient's hydration.

The physician faced with a patient with renal failure must first make the distinction between acute renal failure (ARF) and CRF because ARF is generally associated with recovery of renal function and demands a different form of diagnosis and treatment. Table 2 provides the common means of differentiating ARF from CRF.

The clinical features of established CRF with a GFR level higher than 50 ml per minute are subtle and are often not detected by patients. This is also true because the serum creatinine may not rise above the normal range until the GFR falls below 40 to 50 ml per minute because of hypertrophy in the remnant nephrons. Patients with known mild CRF therefore must be followed with accurate CCr measurements. When GFR falls below 40 ml per minute, various general features such as easy fatigability, hypertension, and mild anemia become evident. With further decline in function (GFR

TABLE 2. Features That Help to Distinguish ARF from CRF

Distinguishing Feature	ARF	CRF
History and examination	Previously known normal renal function Distinct episode of hypotension, exposure to nephrotoxin, or features of acute glomerulonephritis or interstitial nephritis	Previously established renal disease with documented progressive deterioration of function
	Patient tolerates azotemia poorly; usually does not have neuropathy	Patient appears to be well adapted despite azotemia; clinically detectable neuropathy present
Laboratory features	Anemia is mild, and serum phosphate level may not be elevated	Moderate to severe normocytic and normochromic anemia; phosphate level elevated
Radiologic features	Kidney size normal by ultrasound; bones normal	Kidneys small; radiologic features of osteodystrophy present

TABLE 3. Systemic Manifestations of CRF

Fluid and Electrolyte Imbalance

Sodium and H_2O retention leading to hypertension and congestive heart failure; obligate sodium wasting when intake severely decreased, leading to extracellular fluid decreases and reversible acute decrease in GFR

Metabolic acidosis with increased anion gap and a tendency toward hyperkalemia

Hematologic or Immunologic Problems

Anemia, bleeding diathesis, decreased T cell immunity, and decreased neutrophil chemotaxis and killing capacity

Calcium, Phosphate, PTH

Phosphate retention, decreased vitamin D metabolites leading to increased parathyroid hormone, bone disease, vascular calcifications, pruritus; skeletal and cardiac muscle dysfunction

Metabolic

Hyperlipemia, sexual dysfunction

Others

Nausea, vomiting, gastritis

Pericarditis, peripheral neuropathy, intellectual dysfunction

---

15 to 30 ml per minute) there is progressive anemia, metabolic acidosis with an increasing anion gap, increasing hypertension, itching, declining performance at work and at home, and rising serum phosphorus levels. CRF can be said to be end-stage renal disease (ESRD) when GFR values are at or about 10 ml per minute. The patient may still be able to function, but fluid and electrolyte balance is tenuous and azotemic complications such as nausea, vomiting, pericarditis, and peripheral neuropathy are likely to be present. Ideally, a strategy to manage the ESRD by dialysis, transplantation, or both should be worked out before this condition occurs.

TREATMENT

CRF is a syndrome of protean manifestations. Management requires a knowledge of derangements in various systems. Regardless of the specific cause of CRF, certain features are seen in all cases. These features are present in all patients to varying degrees (depending on the severity of CRF). Table 3 shows these manifestations of CRF and general principles of management. In all patients with CRF, the aim should be to optimize the renal function and prevent further deterioration. The principles of management discussed in the following sections apply to all patients, even when ESRD supervenes.

Conservative Management of the Patient with Chronic Renal Failure

The various factors requiring attention in a patient with known CRF are listed in Table 4.

Reversible Factors

Although CRF implies irreversible disease, various factors may be responsible for deterioration at a rate more rapid than that ascribable to the primary underlying renal disease itself. For some years, it has been believed that the relationship between serum creatinine level and time is linear. Any increase in the slope for an individual patient suggests a superimposed and possibly reversible factor. Commonly encountered factors that may lead to a reversible deterioration in function are given in Table 5.

Extracellular Volume Depletion. Subtle volume depletion may be the most common cause of reversible renal functional deterioration in CRF. For reasons to be discussed, there is an obligate sodium loss in the patient with CRF. Extracellular fluid (ECF) depletion decreases renal blood flow and thereby diminishes GFR further. Causes of ECF depletion include overzealous use of diuretics, intercurrent illness with decreased oral intake, and inappropriate dietary sodium restriction. Data to support these factors should be sought vigorously, including historical facts and documentation of rapid weight loss. Clinical features such as postural hypotension or dry mucosal surfaces may be seen only in advanced stages. Even in the absence of hard data, *slow* and *careful* intravenous hydration with half-normal saline could be used to test this hypothesis. It goes without saying that the patient must be carefully observed for central signs of fluid overload. Another prerenal factor is cardiac failure. This is often difficult to correct, but improved pump function could be associated with improving GFR.

Urinary Tract Obstruction and Infection. Obstruction is commonly seen in men with prostatic hypertrophy. Ultrasonographic demonstration of

TABLE 4. Factors Requiring Attention in Managing CRF

1. Primary disease (evaluate, treat)
2. Reversible factors (search for)
3. Sodium, potassium, H_2O balance
4. Acid-base balance
5. Calcium, phosphate, vitamin D abnormalities
6. Anemia
7. Hypertension
8. Diet
9. Drug therapy and usage

TABLE 5. Factors Commonly Leading to Reversible Decline in GFR in CRF Patients

1. Hemodynamic—extracellular fluid volume depletion, hypertension, congestive heart failure
2. Urinary tract obstruction, infection, or both
3. Nephrotoxins—aminoglycosides, diuretics, antibiotics leading to interstitial nephritis, nonsteroidal anti-inflammatory drugs, radiocontrast dye, angiotensin-converting enzyme inhibitors
4. Renal vein thrombosis
5. Hypercalcemia, hypokalemia

hydronephrosis indicates a need for surgical correction of this problem. Infection may be associated with obstruction or may occur by itself. Even though infection alone may not cause long-term damage, it makes sense to treat all urinary tract infections expeditiously. Antibiotics should be used judiciously, with avoidance of all nephrotoxins. Broad-spectrum penicillins or cephalosporins are good choices for most patients.

Hypertension. Hypertension (HTN) is the result of expanded ECF volume in 90 per cent of patients with CRF. Strict attention to dietary sodium intake, and hence control of ECF volume, controls blood pressure in most instances. Patients with underlying hypertensive disease also respond to these measures. Control of high blood pressure (especially in the patient with accelerated HTN) may transiently worsen renal function. In many of these cases, function may improve if HTN is adequately controlled in the long run. The damaged renal vasculature in these patients loses the capacity to maintain blood flow as perfusion pressure falls (loss of autoregulation). Nevertheless, HTN control decreases mortality from cardiovascular and cerebrovascular accidents. In addition, control of HTN may be important in slowing the progression of CRF in the patient with diabetic nephropathy. There is now sufficient evidence to indicate that angiotensin-converting enzyme (ACE) inhibitors significantly retard the progression of diabetic nephropathy when used early in the course of that disease (i.e., in the stage when no proteinuria is detectable by routine laboratory methods).

Drug therapy for HTN in CRF should include ECF volume control by the use of dietary sodium restriction and diuretics. Thiazides are ineffective at a GFR of less than 40 ml per minute, and loop diuretics may be used. Potassium-sparing diuretics (spironolactone, triamterene, amiloride) should not be used in patients with a GFR of less than 50 ml per minute, as hyperkalemia will result. If diuretics are ineffective, vasodilators, calcium channel blockers, or centrally acting agents can be used. ACE inhibitors should be used with caution in the CRF patient, as they may produce an increase in proteinuria, a decrease in kidney function, and bone marrow toxicity. In hypertensive patients with an element of renovascular disease, ACE inhibitors may precipitate acute renal failure.

Nephrotoxic Agents. These agents are the second most common cause of acute worsening in a patient with CRF. Major nephrotoxins causing renal damage include antibiotics, nonsteroidal anti-inflammatory drugs (NSAIDs), sulfonamide diuretics, and iodinated contrast media. Risk from these agents is increased with advancing age, underlying diseases such as diabetes, and plasma cell dyscrasias. In addition, various states (cirrhosis, congestive heart failure, aging, and impaired renal function) in which renal blood flow is maintained by increased local production of vasodilatory prostaglandins are particularly susceptible to decreased blood flow produced by prostaglandin antagonists such as NSAIDs. These agents should be avoided if possible.

Antibiotics may produce direct tubular toxicity (aminoglycosides) or damage by causing acute interstitial nephritis. Aminoglycosides may produce damage even when used in appropriate doses. Sulfonamides (antibiotics), diuretics, and penicillins are more likely to produce acute interstitial nephritis when previous damage exists and must be suspected when acute worsening of function in CRF occurs. Iodinated contrast media cause tubular damage that worsens kidney function in patients with the following risk factors: decreased GFR, diabetes mellitus, and plasma cell dyscrasias. Intravenous contrast media can cause a serious and often irreversible decrease in GFR in these cases. If a contrast medium must be used, the patient should be hydrated overnight and receive 12.5 to 25 grams of mannitol immediately after dye injection to maintain urine flow and decrease tubular toxicity. There is no conclusive proof that renal toxicity can be avoided by newer nonionic contrast media.

Other Reversible Factors. Electrolyte disturbances such as hypercalcemia and hypokalemia may cause deterioration in function that is reversible on correction. Patients with established nephrotic syndrome may develop superimposed renal vein thrombosis. This condition is the result of hypercoagulability and may be clinically silent or become manifest by a sudden increase in proteinuria, pulmonary embolism, or vague abdominal and flank pains. Renal vein thrombosis should be treated with full-dose heparin intravenously for 10 to 14 days, followed by long-term use of coumarin derivatives.

Sodium, Potassium, and Water Balance

With progressively decreasing GFR, fractional sodium excretion in the remnant nephrons must increase progressively, as dietary intake of sodium does not decrease. Sodium and other osmotically active solutes must thus be excreted at a higher fraction of the filtered load by the remnant nephrons to maintain homeostasis. This increased osmotic load per nephron, along with features such as mild ECF volume expansion and structural anatomic defects in the distal nephron, results in an obligate sodium loss. As dietary sodium intake falls, the normal kidney is able to increase reabsorption to conserve sodium and thus defend the ECF volume. The kidney of the CRF patient is unable to reabsorb sodium to the same extent or with the same alacrity as the kidney of the normal person for the reasons previously discussed. As a consequence, it is easy for the CRF patient to develop a negative sodium and ECF balance when intake is decreased for any reason. As the kidney is less able to conserve sodium, it is also unable to excrete large loads because of the decreased GFR. Moderate sodium restriction (100 to 120 mEq per day) may become necessary when the GFR falls below 20 ml per minute, especially in the volume-expanded, hypertensive patient. The possibility of an ECF volume decrease and an associated decrease in GFR must, however, be watched for. Similarly, water conservation (i.e., urine concentration) is harder to achieve in CRF; the obligate osmotic diuresis, as well as the structural nephron damage, diminishes the ability to concentrate urine and causes excretion of urine with low, fixed osmolality. Restriction of water intake then leads to dehydration (and azotemia). In the conscious individual, the normal thirst mechanism is able to regulate water intake, and it is not necessary to consider water restriction even when GFR values approach 10 to 15 ml per minute.

Potassium is normally excreted largely by secretion in the distal nephron. Factors affecting its handling in CRF include urine flow rate and aldosterone level. There may also be some potassium secretion into the gastrointestinal tract. Serum potassium levels do not rise above 5.5 mEq per liter until the GFR falls below 10 ml per minute. The homeostatic mechanisms, however, are unable to compensate when there is a sudden large increase in intake or load, when urine flow falls (dehydration), or when mineralocorticoid antagonists are used. Drugs such as NSAIDs and ACE inhibitors may also cause hyperkalemia.

Acid-Base Balance

With progressive decline in the GFR, there is decreasing excretion of the daily hydrogen ion load of 60 to 80 mmol per liter. Decreased ammonia production is the major cause of this defect. With progressive hydrogen ion retention, ECF and bone buffers maintain blood pH and ECF bicarbonate concentrations at levels higher than 15 mmol per liter. Decreased hydrogen ion excretion in the absence of decreased GFR can occur when there are tubular defects in hydrogen ion excretion (bicarbonate reclamation) in renal tubular acidosis. In general, mild acidosis is well tolerated. Bicarbonate supplements are usually not needed and have the adverse effect of increasing sodium loads and associated ECF expansion

and HTN. From 20 to 40 mEq per day of sodium bicarbonate or sodium Shohl's solution can be used when needed. Potassium Shohl's solution must obviously be avoided.

Phosphate, Calcium, Vitamin D, and Osteodystrophy

Phosphate retention and decreased 1,25-dihydroxyvitamin D production by the kidney lead to a decrease in ionized calcium in CRF. This stimulates parathyroid hormone (PTH) secretion, as does skeletal resistance to the calcemic action of PTH. Prolonged elevation of the PTH level leads to bone resorption and other manifestations, including anemia, pruritus, and soft tissue and vascular calcification. The last is especially likely to happen if the serum calcium level rises (as a result of calcium or vitamin D supplementation or autonomous hyperparathyroidism) while phosphate levels are still elevated. Serum phosphorus levels may not rise until the GFR is less than 30 ml per minute as a result of an adaptive PTH increase. Treatment should be directed at controlling serum phosphate levels by restricting the intake of protein and dairy products. Phosphate binders such as calcium carbonate or citrate may be used. Patients who are likely to be long-term dialysis candidates should not receive aluminum hydroxide or carbonate as phosphate binders. The latter can be used to control phosphate elevations only in the short term. Calcium and vitamin D products should not be used as long as phosphate levels are high.

Renal osteodystrophy results from the interplay of elevated PTH levels, altered vitamin D and collagen metabolism, elevated levels of calcification inhibitors (such as magnesium), chronic acidosis, and excessive intake of aluminum antacids. Conservative management should be directed at normalizing the calcium and phosphate levels and avoiding aluminum products.

Anemia and the Hematopoietic and Immune Systems

In the undialyzed uremic patient, anemia is usually the result of a decrease in erythropoietin synthesis. Other causes, such as blood loss and nutritional deficiencies, must be excluded. Aluminum excess may also contribute to anemia. The general availability of recombinant erythropoietin in the near future should help to alleviate this problem.

Uremia is an immunosuppressed state. Deficient T lymphocyte immunity, neutrophil function, and mild deficits of humoral immunity have all been described. Platelet function is depressed because of accumulation of dialyzable products of guanidine metabolites, as well as increased production of prostacyclin by the endothelium in uremia. The prolonged bleeding time caused by the preceding abnormalities usually responds to adequate dialysis.

Diet

Many of the symptoms and signs of advancing uremia are caused by retention of nitrogenous waste products that result from protein breakdown. Before the widespread availability of dialytic treatment, severe protein restriction (20 to 30 grams per day) was the only alternative. Negative nitrogen balance leading to severe muscle wasting, osteopenia, and anemia was noted. The aims of dietary therapy in CRF today are to (1) provide adequate energy and protein to prevent malnutrition, (2) ensure adequate control of minerals such as phosphate, calcium, and trace minerals, and (3) prevent deterioration of existing renal function. Animal experiments in various types of experimental renal disease have clearly shown that protein restriction (to 8 to 10 per cent of total caloric intake) and possibly phosphate restriction significantly slow the progress of CRF. Associated slowing of progressive glomerular and tubular lesions has been shown by several authors. In chronic renal disease, progressive nephron destruction may be the result of glomerular hyperfiltration in the remnant nephrons. Factors responsible for this include increased glomerular capillary flow and pressures in these remnant nephrons. Dietary protein restriction reverses these pathogenetic mechanisms in the experimental animal. In human CRF, proof for this hypothesis is not yet available.

I therefore suggest that patients with known CRF and a GFR less than 40 ml per minute be placed on a diet that restricts dietary protein to 0.5 to 0.6 gram per kg of high biologic value protein. Phosphate can, therefore, be restricted to 600 to 800 mg per day, especially by avoiding dairy products. Energy needs of about 30 to 35 kcal per kg per day should be met from carbohydrate and fat sources. Fat should be predominantly from sources high in polyunsaturated fatty acids. Once the GFR falls below 20 ml per minute, sodium and potassium restriction of 100 mEq per day should be instituted and adjusted. If chronic dialysis or transplantation is not being contemplated, the dietary protein level can be lowered further to 20 grams per day and supplemented with essential amino acids. This diet is unpalatable and hard to enforce. Because of the possible ill effects of a negative nitrogen balance, such diets should be prescribed and monitored by experts.

Drug Therapy

Prescribing drugs in CRF requires a knowledge of the metabolism and excretion of the drug, as well as the mechanisms by which the drug may cause a further decline in GFR. Drugs that are eliminated by the kidney should have dosage adjustments based on CCr values rather than serum creatinine concentrations. A simple bedside formula to use in calculating the CCr is

$$\frac{(140 - age) \times wt\ in\ kg}{Serum\ creatinine \times 72}$$

This value should be multiplied by 0.85 in women. Nephrotoxicity may also be caused by tubulointerstitial disease of the allergic (e.g., sulfonamides, penicillins) or vasomotor (e.g., NSAIDs) varieties. A good source of information is *Drug Prescribing in Renal Failure* by William M. Bennett et al. This booklet is published by the American College of Physicians and is available from them.

Specific Therapy

Definitive therapy for CRF is necessary when kidney function is no longer able to support life. The alternatives are to map out a program of dialysis, kidney transplantation, or both, or to use palliative treatment with dietary restriction of sodium, potassium, fluid, and protein. The onset of ESRD is associated with many changes in the life of the patient. These include changes in physical and emotional well-being, the threat of disability leading to loss of employment and self-esteem, and the fear of various treatment regimens. When ESRD is imminent, the treatment alternatives should be discussed with the patient and the family. These discussions will probably have to be held repeatedly, and the input of other professionals such as dietitians, social workers, and nurses should be actively sought. An informed patient is more likely to make appropriate treatment choices and to comply with difficult and unpalatable therapeutic regimens. Finally, successful treatment of ESRD involves planning ahead to select a treatment option. This is necessary because definitive vascular or peritoneal access must exist several weeks before commencing chronic dialysis.

Determining the start of definitive therapy is based on documentation of ESRD with BUN and creatinine values above 80 to 100 mg per dl and 8 to 10 mg per dl, respectively. Dialysis must be started earlier in diabetics and, not infrequently, when the patient is clinically uremic even though BUN and creatinine values are not inordinately high.

Choice of Therapy

Dialysis and transplantation are complementary modes of therapy. In patients under the age of 55 years, transplantation should be considered the definitive mode, with dialysis being used to improve the patient's condition while arrangements for a transplant are made. With the advent of cyclosporine and other potent nonsteroidal immunosuppressives, patients up to the age of 60 years can be considered transplant candidates, especially if a live donor is available. Transplantation from a living donor source can be planned electively and is less likely to be associated with severe rejection episodes and hence fewer infective complications.

Dialysis and associated technology have improved steadily over the past two to three decades. This is exemplified by a steady improvement in the survival of these chronically ill patients. However, unlike a functioning transplant, neither hemodialysis nor peritoneal dialysis can correct the metabolic effects of CRF, such as anemia, osteodystrophy, cardiovascular disease, and sexual and intellectual dysfunction.

Hemodialysis involves passage of blood through a hemodialysis filter, where the blood path is separated from a countercurrently flowing dialysate by a semipermeable membrane. Average predialysis BUN values should be maintained at about 80 mg per dl. Depending on the patient's size and dietary compliance, azotemia and ECF volume can be controlled with 3 to 4 hours of dialysis three times a week. With dialyzers made from newer, more permeable membranes, satisfactory control may be achieved with 2 to 3 hours of dialysis three times a week. Patients can be trained to perform hemodialysis at home. This requires a trainable partner and a satisfactory water supply. It has the advantage of being less intrusive into the patient's normal lifestyle.

In *peritoneal dialysis* the peritoneal membrane functions as the semipermeable membrane, and dialysate is instilled into and drained out of the peritoneal cavity via a catheter implanted surgically into the abdominal wall. The latter process is minor and can often be accomplished under local anesthesia. The most common form of peritoneal dialysis is called continuous ambulatory peritoneal dialysis (CAPD). It involves exchanging the peritoneal dialysate (available in plastic bags) four times a day. Patients can be trained to do this at home. Other forms of peritoneal dialysis include the use of a mechanical cycler to exchange fluid automatically during sleep at night and leave 2 liters of dialysate in the peritoneal space during the day. This method is particularly useful for patients who cannot perform exchanges during the day (e.g., because of work space limitations). Peritoneal dialysis has the advantage of being better tolerated by older patients with cardiovascular problems. CAPD is easy to learn and is a form of self-dialysis that allows easy travel. It does require scrupulous attention to aseptic technique; breakdowns lead to bacterial peritonitis. The latter is the major disadvantage of CAPD but can usually be managed by the addition of intraperitoneal antibiotics on an outpatient basis.

Survival of patients on dialysis has steadily improved, with average 5-year survival now being in the 50 to 60 per cent range. Risk factors that increase mortality include age, diabetes, and cardiac, cerebral, and pulmonary disease. For instance, 5-year survival in an otherwise healthy 45-year-old man may be 85 to 90 per cent, whereas a teenage diabetic may have a survival at 5 years of 40 to 50 per cent. These figures should continue to improve in the future.

GENITOURINARY TUBERCULOSIS

method of
ARNOLD C. CINMAN, M.D.
University of California School of Medicine
Los Angeles, California

The introduction of effective chemotherapeutic agents has dramatically reduced the incidence of pulmonary tuberculosis. However, the occurrence of genitourinary (GU) tuberculosis has not paralleled this decline. This may be due to the long latent period preceding the appearance of tuberculosis in extrapulmonary sites; moreover, in Western Europe and the United States it may be due to the massive influx of people from developing countries where the incidence of tuberculosis is higher.

TREATMENT

The primary therapy for GU tuberculosis is medical. Surgical intervention is reserved for the treatment of complications or for the correction of postchemotherapeutic sequelae. The principles of chemotherapy include the simultaneous use of multiple antituberculous drugs, prolonged therapy, regular follow-up, and diligent monitoring to ensure adequate disease control, drug compliance, and early return to a normal lifestyle. Ideally, the drugs should be bactericidal, taken orally, free of serious side effects, and reasonably inexpensive. Except for preventive treatment of persons in contact with patients recently diagnosed as having tuberculosis and with recent tuberculin skin converters, the use of single-drug treatment is condemned, since it rapidly causes the development of resistant organisms. Adult converters should be closely monitored, and chest radiographs should be obtained every 3 to 6 months. Child converters should be treated with isoniazid, 10 to 15 mg per kg body weight, in two divided daily doses for 1 year.

Commitment to a sanatorium or isolation is unnecessary for renal tuberculosis. However, proper precautions should be taken when disposing of urine. Ideally, a male patient with positive urine cultures should use his own toilet and avoid any urinary spillage. Men are instructed to void in the sitting position. A nourishing diet, adequate rest, and minimal, nonfatiguing activity represent integral parts of the general management of patients with urinary tuberculosis.

Chemotherapy

Treatment is not commenced until the diagnosis is firmly established. Although short-term therapy of 6 to 9 months is recommended in treating pulmonary tuberculosis, it has been customary to treat patients with GU tuberculosis for 2 years. For the first 8 to 12 weeks triple-drug therapy, namely isoniazid, rifampin, and ethambutol, is used. A double-drug regimen is then instituted for the remaining treatment period based on the results of sensitivity testing. The recommended regimen consists of isoniazid, 300 mg; rifampin, 600 mg; and ethambutol, 15 mg per kg body weight in a single daily oral dose. The most effective double-drug therapy to be continued for 2 years is isoniazid, 300 mg, and rifampin, 600 mg, in single daily doses. Substitution of ethambutol for rifampin, 1000 to 1200 mg in a single daily dose, in conjunction with isoniazid is effective but is not as desirable because ethambutol is bacteriostatic and has a higher incidence of side effects. To prevent isoniazid-induced polyneuritis, 100 mg of pyridoxine (vitamin B_6) is given as a daily supplement.

In children the recommended regimen is isoniazid, 10 mg per kg (up to 300 mg), and rifampin, 10 to 20 mg per kg, not to exceed 600 mg per day in single or divided doses. Ethambutol is not recommended for children younger than 13 years of age.

No incidence of relapse has been observed with the above treatment regimens. In most instances urine cultures become negative within 1 month after initiation of treatment, which is a positive indication of the effectiveness of therapy. Patients are followed with urine cultures at 1 month, 3 months, and every 6 months thereafter for the first 2 years. If the culture taken at 1 month is negative, the 3-month study is not performed. A final culture is obtained 1 year after cessation of treatment. An intravenous pyelo-gram or nuclear renogram is obtained twice a year for the first 3 years. Periodic follow-up once a year and radiographic studies once every 2 to 3 years are necessary to ascertain the long-term arrest of the disease.

More recent data suggest that double-drug therapy using two bactericidal drugs, namely isoniazid and rifampin, for 6 to 9 months is as effective as the previously recommended regimen (Table 1). The rationale for using a triple-drug regimen for the first 8 to 12 weeks is that ethambutol is a bacteriostatic drug (affects both intra- and extracellular organisms) and therefore, at least on theoretical grounds, inhibits development of resistant mutants.

Other antituberculous agents are available, although they are used to a lesser extent and are defined as second and third line drugs.

First Line Drugs

Isoniazid. Isoniazid is the least toxic of currently used antituberculous drugs and is bactericidal to both intra- and extracellular organisms. Peripheral neuropathy occurs more often in malnourished patients and is largely prevented by the administration of 100 mg of pyridoxine daily. Hypersensitivity reactions such as fever, skin eruptions, lymphadenopathy, vasculitis, and occasionally fatal hepatitis are rarely encountered. Central nervous system reactions, including seizures, toxic encephalopathy, and psychosis, have been reported. Caffeine and amphetamine derivatives, both central nervous system stimulants, must be avoided while taking isoniazid. The usual oral dosage is 5 mg per kg per day for adults (up to 300 mg) and 10 to 15 mg per kg per day for infants and children (up to 300 mg per day).

Rifampin. Rifampin (Rifadin, Rimactane) inhibits DNA-dependent RNA polymerase activity and is a bactericidal drug. Because it occasionally causes liver dysfunction, concomitant administration of hepatotoxic agents must be avoided. It crosses the placental barrier, and therefore neonates of rifampin-treated mothers should be carefully observed. While undergoing treatment with rifampin, patients should be given liver function tests every 4 to 6 months. Renal impairment is not a contraindication, since the drug is excreted by the liver. It causes orange-colored urine. The usual dosage is 600 mg per day for adults and 10 to 20 mg per kg per day for children, not to exceed 600 mg per day.

Ethambutol. Ethambutol (Myambutol) is a bacteriostatic drug affecting intra- as well as extracellular organisms. It induces reversible optic neuritis, although this is rarely encountered with

TABLE 1. **First Line Drugs in Short-Course Chemotherapy of Tuberculosis**

Drug	Dosage		Activity
	Daily	*Twice Weekly*	
Bactericidal Drugs			
Isoniazid*	5–10 mg/kg, usually 300 mg PO	15 mg/kg, usually 900 mg	Active in both extracellular and intracellular bacilli
Rifampin*	10 mg/kg, usually 450–600 mg PO	10 mg/kg, usually 450–600 mg	As above, particularly on closed lesion "persistors"
Streptomycin	20–40 mg/kg, 5 days/wk IM	25–30 mg/kg	Active in neutral or slightly alkaline pH against extracellular bacilli in cavities
Pyrazinamide†	30–35 mg/kg, usually 1.5–2 grams PO	50–60 mg/kg, usually 1.5–2 grams	Active in acid pH medium on intracellular bacilli
Capreomycin†	0.75–1 gram, 5 days/wk IM	1.5 grams	Same as streptomycin
Bacteriostatic Drug			
Ethambutol‡	15–25 mg/kg, usually 1200–1600 mg PO	50 mg/kg	Acts both on intracellular and extracellular bacilli to inhibit development of resistant mutants

*A combination capsule containing 150 mg of isoniazid and 300 mg of rifampin is available.
†Safety and efficacy of these drugs in children have not been established.
‡Not recommended for children under 13 years of age.

doses of 15 mg per kg daily. Patients should therefore be tested for visual acuity and red-green color discrimination prior to commencing therapy and every 3 months thereafter, unless visual acuity diminishes in the interim. If this happens, an ophthalmologic examination should be carried out immediately, and the drug should be temporarily discontinued. Rashes may also occur. The usual daily dose is 15 to 25 mg per kg. In patients with reduced renal function, the dosage should be smaller because the drug is excreted mainly by the kidneys.

Second Line Drugs

These drugs are always used in combination with first line drugs and are only used when treatment failure occurs with primary drugs or when retreatment is required. Although these drugs are effective, their side effects are greater than those encountered with first line drugs.

Streptomycin. Streptomycin is bacteriostatic to extracellular organisms but causes eighth nerve toxicity, with auditory and vestibular impairment. It should be used cautiously in older patients or in those with renal impairment because of its nephrotoxicity. Vestibular function studies and audiograms in conjunction with blood urea nitrogen and serum creatinine should be obtained prior to treatment. Patients should be carefully monitored during treatment. The peak serum concentration should not exceed 20 to 25 micrograms per ml in persons with decreased renal function. During initial treatment, streptomycin is given intramuscularly in doses of 15 to 25 mg per kg (up to 1 gram) on a daily basis. After 6 to 8 weeks, a twice weekly regimen is instituted using doses of 25 to 30 mg per kg.

Pyrazinamide. Pyrazinamide is the synthetic analogue of nicotinamide and is bacteriostatic to intracellular organisms. Hepatotoxicity is the most common serious side effect. It may induce hyperuricemia because it inhibits excretion of urate, and acute episodes of gout have been described in patients taking the drug. Elevation of plasma glutamic-oxaloacetic acid as well as glutamic-pyruvic transaminase is the earliest abnormality induced by the drug. Close monitoring of serum glutamic-oxaloacetic transaminase (SGOT), serum glutamic-pyruvic transaminase (SGPT), and serum uric acid is mandatory during its administration. The usual dosage is 15 to 30 mg per kg, up to 2 grams, given orally in three or four divided doses. When administered on a twice weekly basis, the dosage is 50 to 70 mg per kg.

Cycloserine. Cycloserine* (Seromycin) is a broad-spectrum antibiotic that is bacteriostatic to both intra- and extracellular organisms. Its untoward effects commonly involve the central nervous system; psychotic states, paranoid reactions, personality changes, and convulsions have been described. Alcohol use during the administration of the drug aggravates the psychiatric problems. The usual dosage is 10 to 20 mg per kg or 250 mg orally twice a day. At this dosage the risk of adverse reactions is small. In order to minimize toxicity, plasma levels should not exceed 30 micrograms per ml. Side effects may be prevented with 100 mg of pyridoxine given daily.

---

*Safety and dosage of this drug have not been established for pediatric use.

Third Line Drugs

These drugs are less commonly used and include the following.

Capreomycin. Capreomycin* (Capastat) is bactericidal to extracellular organisms in cavities. It is nephrotoxic and causes eighth nerve damage. Vestibular function studies, audiograms, and blood urea nitrogen and serum creatinine should be obtained at frequent intervals during drug administration. The usual daily dose is 15 to 20 mg per kg intramuscularly up to 1 gram. The drug should be used cautiously in older patients, and its use should be avoided in those with decreased renal function.

Kanamycin. Kanamycin (Kantrex) is bactericidal to extracellular organisms. Side effects and dosage are the same as those for capreomycin.

Ethionamide. Ethionamide (Trecator S.C.) is bacteriostatic to both intracellular and extracellular organisms. It induces gastrointestinal disturbances and is hepatotoxic, thus requiring close monitoring of SGOT and SGPT. It has a metallic taste. Divided doses may minimize gastrointestinal side effects. Use of the drug should be avoided during pregnancy. The usual dosage is 15 to 30 mg per kg up to 1 gram daily.

Para-aminosalicylic Acid. Para-aminosalicylic acid (PAS) is bacteriostatic to extracellular organisms only. The importance of this drug in the management of tuberculosis has decreased markedly since more active agents have been developed. It induces irritation of the gastrointestinal tract and, at times, severe diarrhea. Patients with peptic ulcers tolerate the drug poorly. Hypersensitivity reactions are common. Because it may cause hepatic damage of varying degrees, SGOT and SGPT levels should be monitored. This drug may induce acidosis, especially in children, because it is a relatively strong organic acid. When the sodium salt is used, excessive sodium loading may result. The usual dose is 150 mg per kg up to 12 grams daily in three or four divided doses.

Several general principles should be followed in the chemotherapeutic management of GU tuberculosis: (1) selection of drug regimen should be based on susceptibility testing, (2) the regimen should contain two bactericidal drugs, and (3) the concomitant use of drugs with the same type of side effects should be avoided whenever possible.

Hypoadrenalism (Addison's syndrome) caused by tuberculosis is rare today but should be looked for and treated appropriately.

---

*Safety and efficacy of this drug in children have not been established.

Surgical Therapy

Whereas surgical management of GU tuberculosis was widely used in the 1950s and 1960s, today operative therapy has become the exception rather than the rule. The indications for surgical intervention in GU tuberculosis are (1) obstruction, (2) destruction, and (3) reconstruction. Occasionally, diagnostic surgery may be indicated to confirm the presence of tuberculosis prior to instituting chemotherapy. Tuberculotic patients should be on antitubercular chemotherapy for at least 3 weeks prior to undergoing surgery.

Obstruction. The most common sites of urinary tract obstruction in tuberculosis occur in areas of anatomic narrowing. The process may be silent, causing unrecognized loss of a kidney, and may be accelerated during the healing phase, while the patient is on chemotherapy. Partial nephrectomy or cavernotomy may be necessary to treat intrarenal obstruction, whereas strictures at the ureteropelvic junction are amenable to standard pyeloplasty techniques. Ureteric strictures have been successfully treated with transcystoscopic dilations, with or without steroids. Transluminal balloon dilation of ureteric strictures has been reported and can be performed via a percutaneous nephrostomy if difficulty is encountered with ureteric instrumentation. Internal double-J stents are of great value in keeping ureteric strictures patent. Surgical resection followed by ureteroureterostomy, ureteroneocystostomy, or ileal interposition is reserved for the management of cases that cannot be managed with the preceding more simple treatments.

Destruction. A unilateral nonfunctioning kidney, especially associated with calcification, pain, hematuria, or hypertension, should be removed after adequate antituberculotic coverage. The poorly vascularized kidney may be a reservoir for viable mycobacteria, which may reactivate the disease when the patient's immunity is weakened as the result of old age or debilitating diseases. Epididymectomy is performed only rarely in patients with enlarged, fistulizing lesions or for diagnostic purposes in the differential diagnosis of an intrascrotal mass lesion.

Reconstruction. Augmentation enterocystoplasty or ileocecocystoplasty is advised for managing the contracted bladder of "burnt-out" tuberculosis. The bowel-to-bladder anastomosis should be made as wide as possible to prevent the development of stenosis. Vasovasostomies or vasoepididymostomies may be the only method of restoring fertility to males with tuberculotic vasal strictures.

MALIGNANT TUMORS OF THE UROGENITAL TRACT

method of
KENNETH B. CUMMINGS, M.D.
Robert Wood Johnson Medical School
New Brunswick, New Jersey

ADRENAL CARCINOMA

Carcinoma of the adrenal cortex is a rare, although highly lethal, malignancy, accounting for less than 0.2 per cent of deaths from all cancers. The predominant age distribution is between 20 and 50 years, but this cancer may occur at any age. In reported series, approximately two-thirds of the patients are female. Adrenal carcinomas are classified as functional or nonfunctional, depending on the presence or absence of clinical endocrinologic manifestations or abnormal laboratory determinations. From 50 to 80 per cent of these tumors are functional and predominate in females. The most common clinical manifestations are virilization and Cushing's syndrome, which are more easily recognized in females. By contrast, from reported series, it appears that nonfunctional adrenal carcinomas predominate in males. Less common manifestations of functional tumors are feminization and hyperaldosteronism.

Apart from the endocrinologic manifestations, common presenting symptoms and signs are nonspecific. Weight loss, weakness, fever, and abdominal masses have been recorded.

The widespread use of computed tomography (CT) scans has led to the incidental diagnosis of adrenal masses. This is consistent with the acknowledged 10 to 20 per cent incidence of adrenocortical adenomas from autopsy series. Measurements of the plasma and urinary steroids complement the CT scan and provide the key to diagnosis. An important finding is the size of the lesion because most adrenocortical carcinomas are larger than 6 cm when initially discovered. The pathologic stage of the tumor is the best prognostic indicator.

Staging

Stage	Characteristics
I	Localized tumor less than 5 cm in size
II	Localized tumor more than 5 cm in size
III	Tumor with local invasion or lymphatic metastases
IV	Distant metastases

Treatment

The primary treatment for adrenal carcinoma is surgical extirpation. Because local disease extension is frequently present when the diagnosis is made, wide operative exposure is necessary for successful removal. This can be achieved by a generous subcostal incision or, as I prefer, an ipsilateral thoraco-abdominal incision with the patient in the modified flank position. Ipsilateral renal involvement necessitates en bloc nephrectomy with the tumor mass. Large left-sided lesions may require concomitant splenectomy. Systematic lymphadenectomy of all regional lymph nodes is performed.

Metastatic disease is treated with o,p'-DDD (mitotane), currently the only active agent. The duration of response is not long, and toxicities (anorexia, nausea, vomiting, and diarrhea) are dose limiting. Mitotane produces objective responses in most patients and reduces steroid production. The recommended initial dose of mitotane (Lysodren) is 9 to 10 grams orally per day in three or four divided doses. It is increased every 48 hours to the maximum tolerated dose (up to 20 grams per day). Aminoglutethimide (Cytadren) and metyrapone,* used to achieve medical adrenalectomy, may aid in alleviating the symptoms produced by tumor steroid production.

Follow-up is rigorous and includes imaging studies (CT scan and chest x-ray film) at 3-month intervals. Periodic steroid excretion studies are obtained and may be the first evidence of tumor recurrence.

Five-year survival rates are 80 per cent for Stage I tumors, 50 per cent for Stage II, 15 per cent for Stage III, and 0 to 5 per cent for Stage IV.

RENAL CELL CARCINOMA

Renal cell carcinoma (hypernephroma) is the most common primary renal neoplasm, with approximately 20,000 new cases per year. The etiology is unknown, but the incidence is reported to be more common in industrial areas and predominates in males with a ratio of 2:1. A predisposition to this malignancy is observed in patients with von Hippel–Lindau disease and in patients with polycystic kidney disease. The peak incidence occurs between the fifth and seventh decades of life.

The most common presenting symptom is hematuria (gross or microscopic). Not infrequently, mass lesions of the kidney are noted on routine imaging studies: intravenous pyelography (IVP), CT, or ultrasonography. The last study usually distinguishes benign cysts from neoplasms. Renal arteriography may be appropriate to establish

---

*This use is not listed by the manufacturer.

the diagnosis (80 per cent of renal cell cancers are hypervascular) or to define preoperatively the vascular supply to large tumors.

Paraneoplastic syndromes are common with this tumor and are believed to be related to hormones or hormone-like substances (erythropoietin, parathyroid hormone, renin, and prostaglandins). The most common paraneoplastic syndrome is hepatic dysfunction, which is reported in approximately 20 per cent of patients in the absence of hepatic metastases.

CT scan with contrast is the most cost-effective staging study. Bone metastases may be evaluated with bone scans.

Staging

Stage	Characteristics
I	Tumor confined to the renal capsule
II	Tumor confined to Gerota's fascia but invading perinephric fat
III	Tumor extension to the renal vein or metastatic to regional lymph nodes
IV	Tumor extension to adjacent organs or distant metastases

Inferior vena cava involvement occurs in approximately 15 per cent of patients. However, even a finding as ominous as this should not deter therapeutic intervention, even if the cephalad extension is supradiaphragmatic. Magnetic resonance imaging and ultrasonography are appropriate to diagnose the amount of caval extension. However, for surgical planning, inferior venacavography defines the magnitude of collateral venous drainage, and catheterization of the right side of the heart may be required to define this cephalad extent when retrohepatic or supradiaphragmatic tumor extension is present.

Treatment

The only treatment with curative intent is surgical extirpation of all tumor. At present, radical nephrectomy (perifascial) is rarely indicated when biopsy-confirmed distant metastases exist. The goal of operative therapy of localized renal cell carcinoma is complete removal of Gerota's fascia and its contents, including the ipsilateral adrenal gland and the regional lymph nodes. Resection of adjacent structures (liver, tail of the pancreas, mesocolon, and bowel) may be appropriate in selected cases. Surgical extirpation of intraluminal extension of tumor in the vena cava should be performed in the absence of pathologically confirmed metastases. This procedure can be performed safely by trained urologic oncologists. It may require circulatory arrest of the lower torso, depending on the cephalad extent of the tumor and the magnitude of the collateral

venous return needed to support cardiac output. Alternatively, the procedure can be safely performed with cardiac bypass. Survival in such cases is more dependent on the primary (T) tumor stage and the (N) nodal involvement.

The surgical approach must be tailored to the patient and the magnitude of the anticipated extirpation. A subcostal extraperitoneal approach, although ideal in the elderly patient with a small tumor, may be inadequate for more complicated presentations. I prefer a transabdominal approach or a thoraco-abdominal incision in selected cases.

Preoperative and postoperative adjuvant radiation therapy has not proved to be effective. Radiation therapy does have a role in palliation of bone metastases. Angioinfarction is appropriate to palliate symptoms related to the primary renal tumor in patients with metastatic disease. There is no effective chemotherapy for renal cell carcinoma. Recent experiences with biologic response modifiers—interferons, interleukins, and tumor necrosis factor—have shown promise. Complete remissions of long duration have not been achieved, and current treatment-related toxicities may be significant.

Appropriate postsurgery follow-up should occur at 3-month intervals for the first 3 years and, if the patient remains disease free, at 6-month intervals thereafter. Follow-up should include a baseline CT scan, chest x-ray film, and liver function tests (LFTs). Chest x-ray films and LFTs are routinely performed, as well as repeat CT scanning at 6 months and thereafter as appropriate.

The 5-year survival rate for Stage I disease is 70 per cent. Extension to the renal capsule and the perinephric fat decreases this rate to 50 per cent. Renal vein or inferior vena cava involvement is associated with a 5-year survival rate of 40 to 50 per cent. Five-year survival is dramatically reduced to 0 to 30 per cent when regional lymph node involvement is defined. The prognosis for patients with distant metastases is poor, with fewer than 10 per cent surviving for 1 year. Chemotherapy regimens are changing, but combination therapy with dacarbazine, vincristine, and cyclophosphamide has activity.

WILMS'S TUMOR (NEPHROBLASTOMA)

Wilms's tumor is the most common genitourinary malignancy in children. It is a rare tumor in the neonate but commonly presents as an abdominal mass before the age of 6 years. Interestingly, the tumor has been associated with congenital anomalies including aniridia and hemihypertrophy. IVP is usually sufficient to make the diagnosis. Real-time ultrasonography helps to differentiate the diagnosis of Wilms's tumor and may provide information regarding disease extension as well as venous extension. CT scans and arteriography, although performed with difficulty in this age group, may occasionally be warranted.

Staging

Stage	Characteristics
I	Tumor limited to the kidney and completely excised
II	Tumor extending beyond the kidney but completely excised
III	Residual nonhematogenous tumor confined to the abdomen
IV	Hematogenous metastases
V	Bilateral renal involvement

The tumors are also classified with respect to histology as favorable or unfavorable.

Treatment

Surgical extirpation is the cornerstone of therapy but is no longer regarded as the emergency it once was. The transrectus subcostal abdominal incision (chevron) is preferred.

Abdominal exploration is initially performed to determine the extent of disease and resectability. The contralateral kidney is mobilized from within Gerota's fascia to permit complete visual inspection. Suspicious areas require biopsy. It is not unusual for this tumor to invade through the renal capsule or to invade contiguous organs or structures (adrenal, duodenum, liver, pancreas, spleen, diaphragm, colon, or musculature of the abdominal wall). It may be appropriate to do limited resection of these structures at the time of radical (perifascial) nephrectomy. In contrast to renal cell carcinoma, this tumor is both responsive to radiation and sensitive to combination chemotherapy.

Initial heroic surgery is unwarranted, and in the case of bilateral renal involvement, it is appropriate to perform surgical extirpation only if two-thirds of the functional renal mass can be preserved. Unilateral nephrectomy should be avoided under these circumstances, and the child should be treated with combination chemotherapy. Re-exploration after objective tumor shrinkage can be performed as early as 6 weeks.

Successful multimodality therapy has been developed under the aegis of the National Wilms' Tumor Study. Actinomycin D and vincristine given to patients with Stage I disease for 6 months achieve a 2-year disease-free state in 95 per cent. The addition of doxorubicin (Adriamycin) to this combination has produced improved 2-year disease-free survival in Stage II and III patients with favorable histologies of 90 and 84 per cent, respectively. Patients with Stage III or IV disease and those with unfavorable histologies continue to recieve radiation therapy to the tumor bed. Survival in Stage IV disease is 54 per cent, and in Stage V with favorable histology it is as high as 80 per cent.

The prognosis depends primarily on the tumor stage, the patient's age, and the degree of tumor differentiation. Survival for Stages I and IV-S is greater than 90 per cent. Stage II patients less than 1 year of age have a 91 per cent cure rate, compared with 48 per cent for patients over the age of 2 years. Stage III patients less than 1 year of age have a 77 per cent survival, in contrast to 28 per cent for patients aged more than 2 years. With Stage IV patients less than 1 year of age, the cure rate is 27 per cent compared with less than 5 per cent for older patients.

PRIMARY RETROPERITONEAL TUMORS

Primary retroperitoneal tumors are rare. Approximately 40 per cent of patients present with primary lymphoreticular tumors. The remainder of the primary retroperitoneal tumors are derived from mesenchyme (liposarcoma, fibrosarcoma, and leiomyosarcoma).

The predominant presenting symptom is increasing abdominal girth, occasionally associated with abdominal or back pain.

Diagnostic evaluation may be difficult and must rule out retroperitoneal malignancy of lymphoid origin. The CT scan with contrast is the fundamental imaging study. CT-guided needle aspiration biopsy is of unique value. Lymphoproliferative diseases cannot be managed with extirpative surgery. The management of all other retroperitoneal primary malignancies is surgical. Because these tumors usually involve contiguous structures and have a variable magnitude of vascular involvement, detailed imaging studies (arteriography and venacavography, gastrointestinal series, barium enema) may be appropriate.

Treatment

The choice of surgical exposure depends somewhat on the size and location of the lesion. In general, I prefer a thoraco-abdominal approach for tumors extending into the epigastrium or located high in the retroperitoneum. The patient is placed in the modified flank position and approached through an eighth or ninth rib incision extended paramedian on the ipsilateral side. The right colon and root of the mesentery are mobilized, exposing the great vessels. All disease must be resected, as in the fashion of postchemotherapy salvage operations for nonseminomatous germ cell tumors. This may include kidney, bowel, pancreas, spleen, inferior vena cava, and occasional aortic replacement.

Radiation has not been shown to have a role, except possibly postoperatively. The role of chemotherapy as an adjuvant, particularly with doxorubicin, suggests activity. Brachytherapy after loading techniques using ^{125}I or ^{192}Ir can provide high-dose radiation to a limited volume.

The prognosis depends on the completeness of resection and on differentiation of the malignancy. Because of the rarity of this entity, a uniform staging system has not been developed. The 5-year survival for patients with completely excised low-grade tumors has been reported to be as high as 80 per cent. Poorly differentiated tumors, with all visible disease resected, are associated with a 5-year survival of less than 10 per cent.

NEUROBLASTOMA

Neuroblastoma is the most common malignant tumor of infancy, with 50 per cent of cases reported before the age of 2 years. The tumors arise from cells of the neural crest, and in the abdomen the adrenal medulla and sympathetic ganglia are the most common sites.

The most common clinical presentation is an abdominal mass that extends under the costal margin and may cross the midline; it is hard and fixed. On a plain film of the abdomen, the mass commonly exhibits stippled calcification. IVP is appropriate and frequently reveals downward displacement of the kidney without distortion of the renal collecting system. A CT scan may be helpful. Catecholamines are frequently produced by these tumors and may be detected by the measurement of vanillylmandelic acid and homovanillic acid excreted in the urine.

Staging

Stage	Characteristics
I	Tumor confined to the organ or structure of origin
II	Tumor extending beyond the organ or structure of origin but not crossing the midline, with or without regional lymph node involvement
III	Tumor extension across the midline
IV	Distant metastases
IV-S	Patients less than 1 year of age at diagnosis who would be Stage I or II, but who have metastatic disease confined to the liver, skin, or bone marrow

Treatment

Surgical extirpation is the primary therapy and usually consists of complete surgical removal in Stages I and II. When the disease has crossed the midline (Stage III), involvement of the aorta and

vena cava is common. En bloc removal of the tumor with adjacent organs is not justified, with the exception of the ipsilateral kidney.

In children more than 1 year of age with Stage II to IV disease, chemotherapy and radiation therapy are used. Chemotherapy regimens are changing, but combination therapy with dacarbazine, vincristine, and cyclophosphamide has activity.

The prognosis depends primarily on the tumor stage, the patient's age, and the degree of tumor differentiation. Survival for Stages I and IV-S is greater than 90 per cent. Stage II patients less than 1 year of age have a 91 per cent cure rate compared with 48 per cent for older patients. Stage III patients less than 1 year of age have a 77 per cent survival rate, in contrast to 28 per cent for those more than 2 years old. With Stage IV patients less than 1 year of age, the reported cure rate is 27 per cent compared with less than 5 per cent for older patients.

UROEPITHELIAL TUMORS

Carcinoma of the Urinary Bladder

Approximately 45,000 new cases of bladder carcinoma are diagnosed each year, and 12,000 of these patients die annually. This cancer has a male/female ratio of 3:1. Tobacco use has a strong association, as does industrial exposure (particularly in the analine dye and rubber industries). The peak incidence occurs in the fifth and sixth decades of life, but the disease may occur at any age.

The most common presentation is hematuria (either gross or microscopic). Irritative symptoms may be present and are indicative of an associated inflammatory disease, carcinoma in situ (CIS), or both.

The diagnostic evaluation should include IVP, which precedes endoscopic extirpation. Abnormalities in the renal pelvis or ureters may require retrograde pyelographic definition at the time of endoscopy. The goal of endoscopy is evaluation as well as therapy. The patient with bladder cancer should be considered to have a poly (multiple), chrono (time), topic (place), malignant diathesis that may become lethal. A diagram of the endoscopic evaluation should map the location of the tumor(s) and should describe the tumor configuration (flat, papillary, or sessile) and the measured size. As part of the evaluation, select mucosal biopsies (SMBs) are obtained from endoscopically normal sites. In addition, bladder washings by barbotage with saline are obtained for cytology or flow cytometry. A bimanual examination under anesthesia reveals evidence of a mass or induration associated with large and/or invasive tumors. CT scans or ultrasound studies performed before pertubation by endoscopic resection in selected cases may define the depth of tumor invasion and dictate the endoscopic goal (staging biopsy versus resection for cure).

Comparative Clinical Staging

See unnumbered table at bottom of page.

Treatment

Endoscopic resection is the cornerstone of therapy for bladder carcinoma. The tumors are resected, with care taken to provide sufficient tissue deep to the tumors to allow the pathologist to comment on the presence or absence of muscle invasion. The pathologist is expected to give a consistent statement with respect to the following: (1) tumor grade; (2) evidence of CIS or mucosal atypia from selected endoscopically normal biopsy sites; (3) the presence or absence of muscle in the specimen; and (4) the presence or absence of tumor invasion of the muscle.

The tumor characteristics described previously, as seen endoscopically, and the grade and stage of the tumor(s), when pathologically assessed, determine if the initial diagnostic treatment was adequate or if additional therapeutic intervention is indicated. Eighty per cent of initial bladder tumors are superficial (not invading muscle).

The predominant goal of the urologist is to cure the patient. To this end, the urologist should attempt to reduce the number and frequency of subsequent tumor occurrences. Factors associated with increased risk of recurrence, progression, or both include (1) CIS or dysplasia in SMBs; (2) multiplicity of tumors; (3) tumors larger than 3 cm; and (4) any invasion. The probability of recurrence in superficial bladder cancer is 50 to 70 per cent.

Intravesical therapy is appropriate for patients with recurrence within 1 year, or for patients with tumor multiplicity or CIS, when resection is deemed to be incomplete. In the former instance, intravesical treatment is considered to be prophylactic, whereas in the latter it is adjuvant. The choice of agent depends on the tumor grade and the presence of CIS. Thiotepa is given at a dose of 30 to 60 mg with 30 to 60 ml of distilled water weekly for 4 to 6 weeks and retained for 2 hours. It may be appropriate to give responders monthly maintenance instillations.

Patients who have associated positive cytology, documented CIS, or lamina propria invasion have a significant probability of therapeutic failure with thiotepa. For such patients, I use intravesical bacille Calmette-Guérin (BCG).* The usual dose is an ampule containing 5×10^8 colony-forming units in 60 ml of solution. A treatment course consists of weekly instillations for 6 to 8 weeks, with follow-up and endoscopic evaluation at 3 months.

Therapeutic failure in these patients, as manifested by visible recurrent tumor or positive cytology, requires restaging. If the tumor remains superficial or the CIS does not invade the prostatic ducts, as defined by transurethral prostatic biopsy, a further course of BCG is appropriate. In patients who then fail, I use mitomycin C, delivered at a dose of 40 mg in 40 ml of solution weekly for 8 weeks. Occasionally patients so treated develop a palmar, genital, or diffuse rash, which is considered to be a contact dermatitis. Another drug that has activity is doxorubicin, given at a dose of 40 mg in 40 ml weekly for 6 to 8 weeks. Irritative symptoms with this drug are a treatment-limiting toxicity.

Tumors invading muscle of Stage T2 or higher require more aggressive management. Surgical extirpation (radical cystectomy and pelvic lymphadenectomy) can be expected to achieve a 5-year cure of 40 to 50 per cent in patients with Stage pT2 and T3 disease. Megavoltage radiation therapy with curative intent has achieved only 35 per cent 5-year cures and is associated with a high local failure rate in patients who have a history of polychronotopic malignant diathesis. It is of interest that muscle-infiltrating bladder car-

---

*This use is not listed by the manufacturer.

Jewett-Marshall Classification	International Union Against Cancer Classification	Characteristics
Stage 0	Ta	Papillary tumor involving only mucosa
	TIS	Grade III flat intraepithelial carcinoma
A	T1	Lamina propria invasion
B$_1$	T2	Superficial muscle invasion
B$_2$C	T3a, T3b	Deep muscle or perivesical fat invasion
	T4	Invasion of contiguous structures
D$_1$	N1–3	Regional lymph node involvement
D$_2$	N4	Juxtaregional lymph node involvement
	M1	Distant metastases

cinoma, based on patterns of failure after treatment with curative intent, suggests that systemic disease was present at the time treatment was given.

The availability of active combination agent chemotherapy marks a new era in the management of deeply invasive and metastatic bladder carcinoma. M-VAC (monthly cycles of intravenous methotrexate, 30 mg per M^2, followed 24 hours later by vinblastine, 3 mg per M^2, Adriamycin, 30 mg per M^2, and cisplatin, 70 mg per M^2, with vinblastine and methotrexate repeated on days 15 and 22) has been reported to produce complete remissions in 30 to 50 per cent of patients with metastatic disease which is durable (median duration of response > 12 months). This regimen, although active, is toxic, with myelosuppression and poor patient tolerance being the dose-limiting toxicities.

There is theoretical benefit in using this therapy as an adjuvant to surgery or radiation therapy. A number of pilot studies have been done, but no controlled Phase III trial has yet defined an actual advantage for any particular combination.

Urinary diversions using continent reservoirs (e.g., Koch and Indiana procedures) and orthotopic bladder replacement using reconfigured, detubularized bowel, are significant surgical advances. However, patient selection is important in the elderly, as the ileal conduit still represents the standard against which other forms of diversion are compared.

I prefer to stage the patient clinically with deeply invasive bladder cancer by using CT scanning. Patients clinically considered to be Stage T3 or above or node positive are initially given two cycles of (neoadjuvant) M-VAC, re-evaluated, and considered for radical cystectomy. If they have been shown to be down-staged based on pathologic evaluation of the surgical specimen, consideration is given to use of M-VAC as an adjuvant after cystectomy. I prefer to divert the upper tracks into a continent reservoir or orthotopic bladder substitution if the patient is a suitable candidate. Patients who are Stage T2 or below and node negative are initially treated with radical cystectomy. If pathologic staging indicates that the stage is T3 or above or node positive, at least two cycles of adjuvant M-VAC are given. Patients medically unsuitable for surgical extirpation are treated with high-dose, small-field radiation therapy (65 Gy to the bladder volume) and given concomitant cisplatin (70 mg per M^2 intravenously initiated just before radiation therapy and every 3 weeks thereafter for a total of eight courses). The response rate and the disease-free survival in pilot studies have been encouraging.

Patients with superficial bladder cancer require surveillance endoscopy and cytology, usually every 3 months for the first 2 years; then every 4 months for 2 years; then every 6 months for 1 year; and finally, if disease free, annually. Follow-up in patients treated for deeply invasive disease is at 3-month intervals and includes imaging studies (CT scan and chest x-ray film) as appropriate.

Renal Pelvic Carcinoma

Transitional cell carcinoma accounts for 7 per cent of all renal tumors. The peak incidence is in the sixth and seventh decades of life and implies a 30 to 50 per cent likelihood of the development of malignant bladder cancer. The most consistent clinical findings are hematuria (gross or microscopic) and pain, which is usually caused by ureteral obstruction.

The diagnosis is established with imaging studies (IVP and retrograde pyelography). Tissue to establish the diagnosis may be obtained by retrograde brushing with fluoroscopic control and selective washings for cytology or by ureteroscopy.

Staging

Stage	Postsurgical Class	Characteristics
I	pTa	Papillary but noninvasive
II	pT1	Lamina propria invasion
III	pT2, pT3a	Muscularis or renal parenchymal invasion but confined to the renal capsule
IV	pT3b, pT4, N⁺	Peripelvic or renal capsule extension and/or regional lymph node involvement

Treatment

The preferred treatment is radical nephroureterectomy including a bladder cuff. In rare instances (solitary kidney or compromised renal function), conservative endourologic surgery may be appropriate for solitary low-grade (I) and low-stage (≤cT1) tumors. The risk of such surgery is significant in patients with positive cytology from the upper urogenital tract because of unrecognized CIS. Survival for low-stage (I and II) patients is 80 per cent at 5 years compared with 30 per cent for Stage III patients and 0 per cent for Stage IV patients. It would seem appropriate to employ M-VAC adjuvant chemotherapy for patients with Stage III or IV disease.

Carcinoma of the Ureter

These tumors are less common than renal pelvic tumors, and approximately 75 per cent occur in the distal one-third of the ureter. The presentation is similar to that of renal pelvic tumors, as is the diagnostic evaluation. Current ureteroscopic techniques represent a significant diagnostic and possibly therapeutic advance.

Staging

Stage	Postsurgical Class	Characteristics
I	pTa, pTIS	Noninvasive
II	pT1	Lamina propria invasion
III	pT3, pT3a	Muscularis invasion
IV	pT3b, pT4, N⁺	Periureteral extension or regional lymph node involvement

Treatment

The treatment depends on the grade, stage, and location of the tumor. A low-grade, low-stage tumor in the lower one-third of the ureter with negative cytology may best be managed ureteroscopically or by resection of the distal ureter and reimplantation of the ureter. Prognosis is as for renal pelvic tumors and depends on the stage.

Female Urethral Carcinoma

This rare tumor presents most frequently with urethral bleeding. The most common histologic type is squamous cell carinoma, followed by adenocarcinoma and then transitional carcinoma. The diagnosis is made on urethroscopy and confirmed by biopsy. The relative rarity of this tumor has precluded staging other than for (1) the distal one-third of the urethra and (2) the proximal two-thirds of the urethra. The management depends on tumor location rather than histologic type or degree of cellular differentiation.

Treatment

Tumors of the distal one-third of the urethra are best treated by surgical resection followed by external beam radiation therapy. Tumors involving the proximal two-thirds of the urethra demand aggressive management. Preoperative radiation therapy with 50 Gy delivered over 4 to 6 weeks, followed by anterior exenteration with removal of the anterior vagina and limited pubectomy, is appropriate. Pelvic lymphadenectomy should be performed, but it is not likely to be curative. The ilioinguinal lymph nodes are followed clinically.

The prognosis is reasonably good, with survival of patients with tumors of the distal one-third of the urethra reported to be 50 per cent at 5 years. Five-year survival of patients with tumors of the proximal two-thirds, in contrast, is 10 to 20 per cent.

Male Urethral Carcinoma

This neoplasm is less common than female urethral carcinoma. The common presentation includes symptoms related to stricture, as this is frequently part of the history. The most common histologic type is squamous cell carcinoma. The most common location is the bulbomembranous urethra. Diagnosis is made by transurethral biopsy.

Staging

Stage	Characteristics
0	Confined to mucosa
A	Lamina propria invasion only
B	Invasion into but not beyond the corpus spongiosum or substance of the prostate
C	Direct extension into tissue beyond the corpus spongiosum (corpora cavernosa, muscle, fat, fascia, skin, direct skeletal involvement) or beyond the prostate capsule
D₁	Regional metastases, including inguinal and/or pelvic lymph nodes
D₂	Distant metastases

Treatment

For therapeutic purposes, it is appropriate to classify these tumors as anterior and posterior urethral in location. Endoscopic resection suffices for tumors of Stages 0 and A with routine follow-up endoscopy. The diagnosis, unfortunately, is seldom made before invasion into the corpus spongiosum or beyond has occurred (Stages B and C). Lesions of these stages involving the anterior urethra are appropriately managed by partial penectomy with a 2- to 3-cm disease-free margin.

Posterior urethral carcinomas are, unfortunately, most common and may have significant bulk when diagnosed. The disease mass may best be appreciated on magnetic resonance imaging with coronal and sagittal views. There is usually significant extension into the musculature of the urogenital diaphragm with bulbomembranous tumors. The corporal bodies in this location are lateral and may not be involved. I believe that these patients should be initially treated with external beam radiation (50 Gy) over 4 to 6 weeks. Total urethrectomy, limited pubectomy, and anterior exenteration with pelvic lymphadenectomy should be performed. Total penectomy and even emasculation may be required for large, bulky tumors. However, although local recurrence is the most common site of failure, not all patients require total penectomy. The prognosis is similar to that of the urethral carcinomas in the female. There is reasonable 5-year survival for patients with anterior urethral tumors but only 20 per cent 5-year survival for those with posterior urethral tumors.

Prostate Cancer

Approximately 100,000 new cases of prostate cancer are reported each year. The annual death rate from this disease is more than 25,000. It is the second most common cancer in males and the third most common cause of male deaths from cancer. The peak incidence is in the seventh decade of life; however, it is not uncommon in the fifth decade. Unfortunately, localized prostate cancer is not characteristically symptomatic. Fewer than 20 per cent of these cancers are confined to the prostate when first diagnosed. It is presumed that annual digital rectal examination after age 40 years suffices to suspect the presence of localized prostate cancer. This suspicion could then be confirmed by transperineal or transrectal needle biopsy. The availability of ultrasonography-guided biopsy of palpably suspicious prostates has likely improved the ease and accuracy of biopsy. However, ultrasonography should not be considered a screening tool for prostate cancer. Although this modality is useful, it only complements the "educated finger." Prostate-specific antigen (PSA) has been a significant advance in following patients with prostate cancer. In general, I believe that its sensitivity is greater than that of acid phosphatase, but it has not replaced this study. Neither PSA nor acid phosphatase determination should be considered a screening test for localized prostate cancer.

Imaging studies to evaluate the extent of disease in patients with prostate cancer include bone scans and CT scans, as well as IVP.

Staging

Stage	Characteristics
A	Occult carcinoma usually discovered after transurethral resection for clinically benign disease: Stage A_1 (focal), less than 5 per cent and well differentiated; Stage A_2 (diffuse), more than 5 per cent and other than well differentiated
B	Palpably confined to the prostate: B_1, tumor occupying less than one entire lobe of the prostate; B_2, tumor occupying one lobe or more
C	Locally advanced carcinoma invading the prostatic capsule or seminal vesicles
D_1	Pelvic nodal metastases
D_2	Distant disease, most commonly detected in bone

Treatment

Few cancers have caused as much controversy and diversity of expert clinical opinion regarding optimal management strategies and rationale. The views presented for management, stage for stage, reflect my own bias.

Localized prostate cancer should be curable (Stages A and B) and the best curative procedure considered. I believe that radical prostatectomy offers the best prospect of 15-year disease-free survival for cancer confined to the prostate. Patients should have a life expectancy of 10 years and be good surgical candidates. A pelvic lymphadenectomy is performed, and if the nodes are found to be disease free, I proceed with a radical nerve-sparing (potency-sparing), retropubic prostatoseminal vesiculectomy. Up to 80 per cent of patients who are potent preoperatively have a return of erectile function during the ensuing 6 to 8 months postsurgery. Continence is recovered in the first 3 months, and incontinence requiring corrective measures should occur in fewer than 2 per cent of patients. Patients found at surgery to have positive lymph nodes are closed and treated 6 weeks postsurgery with external beam radiation therapy for local regional disease control.

Patients judged clinically to have Stage C disease have a 50 per cent probability of having positive lymph node involvement. In young, vigorous patients, it may be appropriate to consider radical prostatectomy for "small C" disease if the lymph nodes are free of disease. Alternatively, external beam radiation therapy achieves comparable results and is currently my preference.

Patients with Stage D_1 disease must be considered to have systemic disease. Eighty per cent of such patients have positive bone scans within 5 years. It is not known at present whether primary hormonal manipulation or delayed therapy will alter the end results. Symptomatic patients with Stage D_2 disease have a significant probability of becoming symptom free with hormonal manipulations, possibly for 2 years.

The methods used for hormonal manipulation include bilateral orchiectomy, diethylstilbestrol (DES), luteinizing hormone–releasing hormone (LH-RH) agonists, and experimental antiandrogens (flutamide). Orchiectomy is a simple surgical procedure and has the advantage of complete patient compliance. DES given orally (1 mg three times daily) suppresses plasma testosterone to castration levels in all patients. The dosage may be reduced later to an average of 1 mg per day. However, such patients are at greater risk for cardiovascular complications and develop significant gynecomastia if the breasts are not irradiated before the initiation of treatment. Leuprolide and LH-RH agonists are as effective as DES without the toxicities. It is now available as a depo-injection but may not be cost effective for all patients. Antiandrogens, although not yet available in this country, may have significant clinical activity and preserve libido, which is frequently lost with the previously described methods of hormonal manipulation.

My current preference is to use bilateral orchiectomy when the patient is symptomatic or has chemical and/or bone scan evidence of rapid progression. In patients who refuse removal of the testicles and are not at increased risk of cardiovascular complications, I use DES (1 mg three times daily). Alternatively, if toxicities develop with DES or if the patient is at increased risk for cardiovascular complication, I use leuprolide.

Carcinoma of the prostate refractory to hormonal therapy is clinically a management challenge. Treatment is largely palliative, and both objective responses (reduction in acid phosphatase and PSA levels with stabilization on bone scan) and subjective responses (reduction in pain and improved performance status) are relatively short. Agents such as aminoglutethimide and high-dose (7800 mg per day) ketoconazole* block adrenal androgen production but have significant dose-related toxicities. Spinal cord compression from metastases of the dorsal spine must be anticipated. This must be treated emergently with radiation therapy, decompression laminectomy, or both.

Demonstration of the efficacy of therapy for organ-confined disease requires long-term tumor-free survival without adjunctive hormonal therapy. Radical prostatectomy for Stage B_1 disease has been reported to be 51 per cent curative at 15 years. Recently the value of radiotherapy for local control has been challenged because the incidence of positive postirradiation biopsies in patients with Stage B disease has been reported to be as high as 50 per cent. However, symptom-free survival for patients with Stage B disease has been reported to be comparable to that of surgery in the first 10 years after treatment. An abiding problem is that radiation therapy given at a dose of 70 Gy to small-volume tumors should eradicate the disease but is not expected to eliminate the factors that cause occurrence or recurrence of disease.

Stage C carcinoma patients may expect a 30 per cent overall survival of 10 years. Patients with metastatic disease have an overall 5-year survival of 29 per cent. The average survival after endocrine therapy for metastatic prostate cancer is 3 to 4 years. No effective chemotherapy for prostate cancer is yet available.

Sarcoma of the Prostate and Bladder

Rhabdomyosarcoma is a significant malignant tumor of the distal genitourinary tract in children and adolescents. Seventy-five per cent of these tumors present before the age of 4 years. Tumors

of the prostate are most common, with bladder tumors second, and are distributed equally between males and females. Vaginal tumors are less common, and occasionally rhabdomyosarcoma arises from the body of the uterus.

The most common clinical presentation is a palpable mass. Symptomatic bladder outlet obstruction occurs in 30 per cent of patients. The diagnosis is usually made by endoscopic biopsy or needle biopsy. The disease is rarely disseminated at presentation, but it may have significant regional extension.

Intergroup Rhabdomyosarcoma Study Staging

Group	Characteristics
I	Localized disease completely resected
II	Local regional disease incompletely resected
III	Incomplete resection or biopsy with gross residual disease
IV	Distant metastases

Treatment

Advances in management with the advent of effective chemotherapy have preserved survival without causing attendant loss of bladder or bowel function. Appropriate local excision is performed without the sacrifice of pelvic organs. If primary chemotherapy and radiotherapy are used, they are initiated after biopsy and appropriate imaging studies to define the extent of disease. Chemotherapy usually consists of pulse VAC (vincristine, actinomycin D, and cyclophosphamide) at monthly intervals. Tumor regression is followed by appropriate imaging studies. When maximum tumor reduction is judged to have been achieved (after two or three cycles of therapy), appropriate organ-sparing surgery is performed. If all tumor cannot be resected, radiotherapy should be administered and chemotherapy continued for a total of 2 years. Approximately 20 per cent of these tumors are nonresponsive to chemotherapy and relatively resistant to radiotherapy. Such patients require more extensive surgery. Overall survival in patients without distant metastases is 75 per cent.

Sarcomas of the prostate and bladder in adults are rare. The presentation is variable and relates to the location and size of tumor. Leiomyosarcomas are most common, followed by carcinosarcomas and rhabdomyosarcomas.

Surgical extirpation provides the basis for cure, either with preoperative radiation therapy or with adjuvant radiation therapy. The prognosis is related to the degree of tumor differentiation. In patients with well-differentiated tumors, appropriate surgery alone has produce durable, disease-free survival.

---

*Ketoconazole is an approved drug but this use is not listed by the manufacturer.

Malignant Scrotal Tumors (Excluding Testes)

The most common tumor is squamous cell carcinoma of the scrotal wall. Once an occupational disease in chimney sweeps, it is now rare. The disease presents with inflammation and ulceration of the scrotum.

Treatment

Wide local excision of the scrotal wall, as considered appropriate, is the treatment of choice. Ilioinguinal lymphadenectomy is performed only when metastases are documented.

Malignant intrascrotal tumors (excluding those of the testes) are rare. Sarcomas originating from the spermatic cord are the most common and present as a mass. Treatment is with radical orchiectomy accompanied by wide local excision. Five-year survival with this therapy alone is 60 to 80 per cent. Rhabdomyosarcoma is the most common paratesticular tumor in childhood and presents as a mass. Treatment includes radical orchiectomy and retroperitoneal lymphadenectomy. Chemotherapy is given postoperatively, with VAC. Radiotherapy is also used in node-positive patients. Five-year survival with negative nodes is more than 80 per cent, but it is less than 60 per cent when the retroperitoneal lymph nodes are positive.

Cancer of the Testes

Germinal tumors constitute approximately 97 per cent of all primary testicular cancers. The incidence is 6 per 100,000 males. There is a significantly increased incidence in individuals with cryptorchidism, which is not eliminated by orchiopexy.

The most common presentation is a palpable mass. Pain is not a common symptom, but it may be associated with hemorrhage into the tumor.

The diagnosis is made by inguinal node exploration and radical orchiectomy. Scrotal exploration should never be performed because of the potential for tumor dissemination.

Preoperative blood studies should include alpha-fetoprotein (AFP) and the beta subunit of human chorionic gonadotropin (beta-HCG). The incidence of elevated beta-HCG levels in patients with nonseminomatous germ cell tumors (NSGCT) has been found to be 40 to 60 per cent. Approximately 10 per cent of patients with pure seminoma have been found to have elevated levels. AFP levels are elevated in 70 per cent of patients with teratocarcinoma and embryonal carcinoma. The metabolic half-life of these markers is 5 days for AFP and 45 minutes for beta-HCG. Therapeutic considerations have divided testicular tumors into seminomas and NSGCT.

CT scanning of the abdomen, pelvis, and chest is the preferred imaging modality. In addition, a routine chest x-ray film is obtained.

Staging (TNM Classification)

Stage	Characteristics
T	Primary tumor
T1	Tumor limited to the testes, including rete testes
T2	Tumor invading beyond the tunica albuginea or into the epididymis
T3	Tumor invasion of the spermatic cord
T4	Scrotal invasion
N	Regional lymph node involvement
N0	No regional lymph node involvement
N1	Metastases to a single lymph node, 2 cm or less in the greatest dimension
N2	Metastases to lymph node(s) more than 2 cm but not more than 5 cm in the greatest dimension
N3	Metastases to lymph node(s) more than 5 cm in the greatest dimension
M	Distant metastases
M0	No distant metastases
M1	Distant metastases

Treatment

Radical inguinal orchiectomy is the primary treatment. If the tumor is pure seminoma, radiation therapy is given to the periaortic lymph nodes and ipsilateral iliac area at a dose of 25 Gy. Bulky retroperitoneal involvement (Stage N3) is treated as an NSGCT.

Because of the remarkably complete remission achieved currently with cisplatin-based combination regimens, efforts are now being made to reduce the toxicities or side effects of these treatments. This is particularly germane for clinical staging of any T, N0 patients in whom preoperative levels of serum markers were elevated but returned to normal postorchiectomy. Traditionally, patients with NSGCT underwent retroperitoneal lymphadenectomy with curative intent. An attendant consequence of the traditional lymphadenectomy was infertility secondary to retrograde ejaculation or failure of emission.

A response to this problem was the introduction of a surveillance program for clinical Stage N0, M0 patients with normal postorchiectomy serum markers. It is now acknowledged that 20 per cent of these patients have a relapse, and 80 per cent of the relapses occur within a year of diagnosis. A major criticism of this surveillance policy is its potential lack of safety, particularly if follow-up compliance is compromised. I prefer to offer such patients a modification of the standard bilateral lymph node dissection, which preserves fertility in more than 80 per cent of patients without compromising control of disease in the retroperitoneum.

Clinical stage patients (any T, N2, M0) are

most appropriately treated with radiational lymphadenectomy. Patients whose serum marker levels normalized postlymphadenectomy and in whom all visible disease was resected are followed without adjuvant chemotherapy. In patients whose marker levels remain elevated or who fail in follow-up, standard chemotherapy is given. This currently consists of intravenous cisplatin, 20 mg per M^2 for five daily courses every 3 weeks for three or four courses; bleomycin, 30 units per week for 13 weeks; and etoposide (VP-16), 100 mg per M^2 for five daily courses every 3 weeks for three or four courses.

Advanced NSGCT patients (clinical stage any T, N3, M0, M1) are treated with this chemotherapy regimen for cytoreduction, preferably with return of elevated serum markers (AFP and beta-HCG) to normal before surgical extirpation of residual disease. This is advocated for either residual retroperitoneal or pulmonary disease seen on imaging studies. In patients treated surgically for residual disease, it is our practice to accompany this regimen routinely with a classic retroperitoneal lymph node dissection. In the 30 per cent of patients who have residual carcinoma in the resected specimen, we have used further chemotherapy with high-dose cisplatin in combination with VP-16 for at least two cycles.

Follow-up evaluation, including serum marker (AFP and beta-HCG) levels and a chest x-ray film, is performed monthly for 18 months, then every 2 months for 12 months, then every 3 months for 12 months, and finally every 6 months until the fifth year.

Virtually complete cure should be achievable in patients with limited disease burden, such as Stage T1, N0, M0 and Stage any T, N2, M0.

For patients with Stage N3, M1 disease, a cure is achieved in approximately 70 to 80 per cent.

Penile Carcinoma

Epidermoid cancer of the penis is a rare condition in the United States, affecting only 0.2 per 100,000 males. The peak incidence is in the sixth and seventh decades of life. Neonatal circumcision almost entirely eliminates this disease. The most common presentation is a visible lesion associated with a purulent discharge in an uncircumcised patient. The predominant location (80 per cent) of the lesions is on the glans penis or prepuce. Most tumors are locally infiltrating, and 50 per cent of patients have inguinal lymph node metastases. Systemic disease is a late manifestation.

The staging parameters used, in addition to pathologic confirmation of the diagnosis and physical examination, include IVP, CT scan, and chest x-ray film.

Staging

Stage	Characteristics
I (A)	Tumor confined to the glans or prepuce or both
II (B)	Tumor extending into the shaft of the penis
III (C)	Tumors with inguinal node metastases that are operable
IV (D)	Tumors involving adjacent structures or tumors associated with inoperable inguinal node metastases or distant metastases

Treatment

Surgical extirpation is the only effective treatment, and depends on tumor location and depth of penetration. Circumcision alone may suffice for carcinoma limited to the prepuce. Selected patients with tumors involving the glans or distal one-third of the penile shaft may be candidates for Moh's chemosurgery if such therapy is available. More commonly, these lesions are treated with partial penectomy with a 2-cm disease-free margin, which allows the patient to preserve the ability both to stand while urinating and to have sexual intercourse. More extensive tumors require penectomy and perineal urethrostomy.

Because reactive lymphadenopathy is usually present, evaluation of the inguinal lymph nodes is deferred and the patient is treated with appropriate antibiotics for 3 to 4 weeks. Patients who become clinically node negative may be observed. Twenty per cent of these patients have clinically evident metastases in 2 to 3 years and are managed by delayed lymphadenectomy. Alternatively, if follow-up is unlikely because of poor patient compliance, it is appropriate to consider biopsy of the sentinel node(s) of Cabanas and, if they are positive, to proceed with formal ilioinguinal lymphadenectomy.

Patients who have persistent adenopathy at 6 weeks should undergo superficial and deep inguinal lymphadenectomy. Based on the pathologic documentation of lymph node metastases, the decision to perform bilateral ilioinguinal node dissection and pelvic lymphadenectomy is made. I prefer to stage the procedure and to perform pelvic lymphadenectomy at the time of the contralateral ilioinguinal node dissection.

Radiation therapy may be used in patients with advanced regional disease but should be considered palliative. Metastatic disease has shown a limited response to chemotherapy employing bleomycin, methotrexate, and cisplatin. Multiagent therapy may be appropriate.

Survival at 5 years in patients with positive lymph nodes is 50 to 70 per cent. Patients with systemic metastases rarely survive for 12 months.

URETHRAL STRICTURE

method of
GUY W. LEADBETTER, JR., M.D.
University of Vermont
Burlington, Vermont

In the past, most strictures of the urethra developed because of gonococcal urethritis. Today, because of the use of antibiotics, most strictures are iatrogenic, traumatic, or accidental. Strictures cause obstruction, but because their development may be gradual, the symptoms of decreasing size and force of the urinary stream may not be recognized by the patient until the urethral lumen is almost occluded.

If not treated, urinary retention or infection (i.e., periurethral abscess, cystitis, pyelonephritis, or possibly gram-negative sepsis) may occur.

The diagnosis is first suspected from the history, difficult voiding, loss of pressure, and recurrent urinary tract infections. It is confirmed by endoscopy and urethrography. When a voiding cystourethrogram is performed, the distal penis should be partially occluded during voiding. This procedure shows the extent of the stricture by dilating the distal urethra beyond the stricture. A retrograde urethrogram helps to visualize the position of the stricture's distal limit. Endoscopy allows visualization of the stricture. In most strictures a pediatric endoscope, because of its small size, is used and the entire stricture may be visualized. To complete the evaluation, a renal ultrasound scan or intravenous pyelogram is done to evaluate any damage of the upper urinary tract. In addition, urinalysis, culture, and blood studies for blood urea nitrogen and serum creatinine levels are obtained.

TREATMENT

Treatment methods include urethral dilation, urethrotomy, and open surgical repair. The choice depends on the associated problems and the severity of the stricture. It may be necessary to perform temporary urinary diversion, usually by suprapubic catheter drainage.

Urethral Dilation

A local anesthetic of 2 per cent Xylocaine jelly is used. Patients who have short strictures without a periurethral scar may be cured by a series of dilations with Van Buren sounds or filiforms and followers. However, it must be recognized that if the stricture is hard and the mucosa tears during dilation, the stricture may worsen.

If the stricture is small in caliber, filiforms and followers are used. These may be passed blindly or under vision through the endoscope. Use of Van Buren sounds under these circumstances may result in false passage and further damage.

If dilation is used as a treatment, three or four dilations at weekly intervals may be necessary. If the stricture recurs or needs to be dilated more than twice a year, an alternative therapy should be chosen. Patients should be given a broad-spectrum antibiotic before and after dilation (i.e., norfloxacin* or ciprofloxacin, 500 mg twice daily the evening before and for the next 48 hours if the urine is uninfected). If the urine is infected, the medication should be continued for 7 to 10 days. Gram-negative sepsis after dilation may occur whether the urine is infected or not.

Urethrotomy

A direct-view urethrotome is available to incise strictures. Strictures resistant to dilation and those with no periurethral scar may be incised with the urethrotome. The stricture must be incised at the 6 o'clock position through the thickness of the scar. This allows the lumen to open and heal open. A urethral catheter placed after the incision is made tamponades any bleeding that may result. The catheter may be removed in 2 to 3 days. If the catheter is left in for long periods, it may cause more inflammation and scarring. If it is selected properly, the success rate should be about 85 per cent. If there is a periurethral scar, the stricture will recur. In case of failure, urethrotomy may be attempted a second time with a deeper cut. However, repeated failure is an indication for open surgery.

Open Surgery

The procedure is as follows:

1. Resection of the stricture and reanastomosis
2. Free skin grafts
3. Pedicle grafts from scrotum or penile skin
4. Two-stage procedure
   a. Incision and marsupialization
   b. Three to 6 months later: tubularized closure using skin previously sutured to the opened stricture

---

*Usual dose is 400 mg twice daily.

Resection and reanastomosis are the least successful methods and cannot be used if the defect is too long.

Free full-thickness skin grafts are successful but should be used only by experienced surgeons.

Pedicle grafts from the scrotum or penile skin are vascularized and used as an overlay of the incised stricture. These are simple to do and are successful.

The two-stage procedure may be inconvenient for the patient but has the highest success rate, particularly for difficult strictures. A urethral catheter may be left in place for 6 to 7 days after all procedures have been completed.

RENAL CALCULI

method of
DEAN G. ASSIMOS, M.D.
The Bowman Gray School of Medicine
of Wake Forest University
Winston-Salem, North Carolina

During the past 10 years, the surgical management of patients with renal calculous disease has dramatically changed. The development of less invasive treatment techniques such as extracorporeal shock wave lithotripsy, ureteroscopic stone removal, and percutaneous stone removal has made open surgical lithotomy an uncommon event. Despite these advances, patients with renal calculous disease are still at risk for stone recurrence; therefore, preventive measures should be considered.

The major goals of prevention are to eliminate or reduce recurrent nephrolithiasis and to limit the growth of calculi already present without subjecting the patient to undue treatment-related morbidity. This can be accomplished by identifying and correcting certain pathophysiologic abnormalities that predispose individuals to stone formation. Stone prevention is based on decreasing the urinary concentration of constituent ions, lowering the saturation of stone-forming salts, correcting deficits in urinary inhibitors of crystallization, and modulating such factors as urinary pH.

Calcium oxalate calculi occur in 70 to 80 per cent of patients with renal stones. Other types of calculi include those consisting of calcium phosphate, calcium oxalate mixed with uric acid, cystine, struvite (magnesium ammonium phosphate), uric acid, 2,8-dihydroxyadenine, xanthine, and triamterene.

PATIENTS WHO WARRANT THERAPY AND METABOLIC EVALUATION

Approximately 50 per cent of first-time calcium stone formers form another stone within 10 years. The interval to recurrence tends to decrease with each new stone formed. Therefore, it is certainly justifiable to evaluate and recommend medical therapy for patients with recurrences, especially those with short stone-free intervals (less than 2 years). Patients with a solitary kidney or renal insufficiency are at greater risk of stone-related morbidity and may benefit from such therapy after the formation of only one stone, whereas others may require it because of their vocation (e.g., airline pilots).

PATIENT EVALUATION

The minimum work-up of a first-time stone former includes stone analysis by x-ray diffraction, polarization microscopy, or infrared spectroscopy; urine culture; and a serum chemistry panel. A serum parathyroid hormone (PTH) level is obtained in patients with hypercalcemia. If this level is elevated, parathyroid surgery is indicated. While on their regular diet, recurrent stone formers collect two 24-hour urine specimens, which are analyzed for calcium, creatinine, uric acid, oxalate, magnesium, phosphorus, sodium, and citrate levels. In addition, a cystine screen (cyanide-nitroprusside test) is done. If it is positive, a quantitative urinary amino acid analysis is performed. A fasting urinary pH level is also obtained. If it is above 6, an ammonium chloride acid load test is done to assess for renal tubular acidosis. Individuals with hypercalciuria (greater than 250 mg per 24 hours for adults) undergo further testing. After 1 week of a low-calcium (400 mg) and restricted-sodium diet (100 mEq), they collect another 24-hour urine specimen for similar testing. At the end of this week, calcium load testing is performed. Urine is collected after a 12-hour fast and after a 1-gram oral calcium gluconate load. PTH activity is indirectly assessed by monitoring nephrogenous cyclic adenosine monophosphate (NcAMP) levels. Patients with renal leak hypercalciuria have a form of secondary hyperparathyroidism and remain hypercalciuric during low-calcium intake, fasting, and calcium loading. NcAMP levels remain elevated during fasting and after calcium loading. Individuals with Type I absorptive hypercalciuria remain hypercalciuric while on a low-calcium diet but revert to a normal calciuric state during fasting. In contrast, patients with Type II absorptive hypercalciuria have normal urinary calcium levels while on the low-calcium diet and during fasting. In both types of absorptive hypercalciuria, there is a marked increase in calcium excretion after the calcium load associated with suppression of NcAMP activity.

GENERAL TREATMENT

Hydration is one of the most effective and morbidity-free treatments that benefits all stone-forming patients. Adults are urged to increase their urine output to 2 to 3 liters daily, with special emphasis given to increased hydration before bedtime. Patients are instructed to drink at least 8 to 10 ounces of fluid hourly while awake. Despite the simplicity of this therapy, many individuals are noncompliant. Having such individuals monitor their urinary specific gravity by dipstick testing may involve them more actively in their therapy. Patients are instructed to check their specific gravity early and later in the day and to drink enough fluid to keep it below 1.015.

SPECIFIC TREATMENT

Calcium Stones

Renal Leak Hypercalciuria

Thiazide diuretic therapy is the treatment of choice for patients with renal leak hypercalciuria. Thiazides decrease urinary calcium excretion by increasing calcium reabsorption in the early portion of the distal convoluted tubule and by promoting calcium reabsorption in the proximal tubule. Various types can be used, including hydrochlorothiazide (25 to 50 mg twice daily), trichlormethiazide (1 to 2 mg twice daily), and chlorthalidone (25 mg twice daily). Thiazide preparations that contain triamterene should not be used because triamterene can crystallize and form renal stones. Sodium intake should be limited to increase the hypocalciuric action of the thiazide. Adverse side effects of thiazides include hypokalemia, hyperglycemia, hyperuricemia, hypercalcemia, hypercholesterolemia, hypertriglyceridemia, rash, and interstitial nephritis. Thiazide therapy is contraindicated in untreated primary hyperparathyroidism. Periodic serum chemistry panels and 24-hour urinary calcium levels are monitored to detect electrolyte disturbances and to ensure that calcium excretion is decreasing. Hypokalemia requires correction because it results in lower renal excretion of citrate, an inhibitor of crystallization of stone-forming calcium salts. Potassium supplementation with potassium chloride or potassium citrate can be used. Potassium citrate is preferred because it also increases the urinary citrate level.

Type I Absorptive Hypercalciuria

There are two therapeutic options for these patients: thiazide diuretics and cellulose sodium phosphate. A disadvantage of thiazide diuretics is that with time patients become refractory to their hypocalciuric action. Bone density may also increase with thiazide treatment in these patients, but this increase probably causes no serious long-term problems. This approach might be the best for children or individuals with osteoporosis. When taken with meals cellulose sodium phosphate (5 grams two or three times per day for adults) binds both calcium and magnesium, which decreases their gastrointestinal absorption and limits urinary excretion of these ions. This agent may also promote an increased urinary

excretion of oxalate and phosphorus. Magnesium (1 to 1.5 grams twice daily between meals) prevents hypomagnesemia. Moderate dietary restriction of calcium, oxalate, and sodium is also recommended. Cellulose sodium phosphate is contraindicated in patients with primary or secondary hyperparathyroidism, hypomagnesemia, bone disease, hypocalcemia, and hyperoxaluria. It is not recommended for pediatric patients. Every 6 months during therapy, a complete blood count should be performed and the levels of urinary calcium, magnesium, sodium, and oxalate and serum PTH, calcium, magnesium, alkaline phosphatase, copper, zinc, and iron should be assessed.

Type II Absorptive Hypercalciuria

Moderate dietary calcium restriction (400 to 600 mg per day) combined with limited sodium intake (100 mEq per day) may control hypercalciuria in these patients. This diet provides less calcium to complex with oxalate in the gut. Therefore, dietary oxalate restriction should also be imposed to prevent absorptive hyperoxaluria.

Renal Phosphate Leak

In these individuals, the renal phosphate leak causes hypophosphatemia, which stimulates the synthesis of calcitriol. This promotes calcium absorption from the gut and mobilization of calcium from bone, which results in hypercalciuria. These patients are treated with neutral orthophosphates (500 mg three times daily). Orthophosphates are contraindicated in patients with an active urinary tract infection or struvite calculi. Diarrhea is the most common side effect of orthophosphate therapy.

Hyperuricosuria

Hyperuricosuria promotes calcium oxalate stone formation through a variety of mechanisms including epitaxy, heterogeneous nucleation, and binding of crystallization inhibitors. Decreasing the urinary uric acid level helps to retard calcium oxalate stone formation in such individuals. This can sometimes be accomplished by limiting purine intake. If dietary restriction is unsuccessful, allopurinol (Zyloprim), 200 to 300 mg per day, is recommended. Adverse side effects of allopurinol include fever, rash, acute gouty arthritis, xanthine stone formation, and Stevens-Johnson syndrome.

Hypocitraturia

Low urinary citrate levels are encountered in a variety of calcium stone–forming patients, including those with distal renal tubular acidosis and chronic diarrhea. Citrate lowers the urinary saturation of calcium oxalate by complexing calcium. Citrate also inhibits nucleation and crystallization of stone-forming calcium salts. Hypocitraturia can be corrected with oral potassium citrate, 10 to 20 mEq three times daily, either as a liquid or as a tablet. The liquid preparation is preferable for patients with rapid gastrointestinal transit, such as those with diarrhea. Potassium citrate is contraindicated in patients with hyperkalemia, peptic ulcer disease, decreased gastrointestinal transit time, renal insufficiency, active urinary tract infection, or struvite stones. Adverse side effects are mainly gastrointestinal.

Enteric Hyperoxaluria

Enteric hyperoxaluria may occur in individuals with inflammatory bowel disease, short bowel syndrome, or a jejunoileal bypass. It occurs when calcium in the gut complexes with unabsorbed fat, which facilitates free oxalate absorption and increased delivery of bile salts to the large colon, further promoting oxalate transport. Most patients are treated with supplemental oral calcium, 0.25 to 1 gram four times daily with meals, and restriction of dietary fat and oxalate. Some of these individuals have concomitant metabolic acidosis and hypocitraturia, which are correctable with administration of oral potassium citrate. Treatment-associated hypercalciuria is best managed with oral thiazides.

Infectious Stones

These stones form as a result of urinary tract infection with certain organisms, including *Proteus, Klebsiella, Pseudomonas,* and staphylococcal species. These urease-producing bacteria hydrolyze urea and generate high levels of bicarbonate and ammonia, which promotes formation of struvite and carbonate apatite stones. Total stone removal and prevention of recurrent infection are the two most important therapeutic goals. Individuals with residual postoperative stone fragments and patients who are prone to stone recurrence, such as those with neurogenic bladder or urinary diversion, may benefit from treatment with acetohydroxamic acid, a urease inhibitor, 10 to 15 mg per kg per day in three or four divided doses. Acetohydroxamic acid is contraindicated

in patients with moderate to severe renal insufficiency or anemia, as well as during pregnancy. Adverse reactions include hemolytic anemia, bone marrow suppression, and gastrointestinal problems.

Uric Acid Stones

Treatment is based on hydration, diet, urinary pH manipulation, and allopurinol therapy. The solubility of uric acid is markedly increased at urinary pH values of 6.5 to 7.0, which can be achieved with sodium bicarbonate or potassium citrate therapy. Patients should monitor their urinary pH levels to ensure adequate alkalinization. Overalkalinization (pH 7.5 or higher) is discouraged because this might promote formation of calcium phosphate stones. Allopurinol, 100 mg three times per day, decreases urinary uric acid excretion. The preceding measures should prevent recurrent uric acid lithiasis and may cause dissolution of existing calculi.

Cystine Stones

Conventional treatment attempts to lower the concentration of cystine below the solubility limit of 300 mg per liter and to increase its solubility by urinary alkalinization to a pH greater than 7.0. Good oral hydration during the day and night is imperative. Sodium bicarbonate or potassium citrate therapy should achieve appropriate urinary alkalinization. Unresponsive patients can be treated with sulfhydryl medications such as D-penicillamine (Cuprimine), 1 to 2 grams per day in four divided doses, and alpha-mercaptopropionylglycine (Thiola), 1 to 2 grams per day in three divided doses. These agents may induce dissolution of cystine stones. The mechanism is based on a thiol-disulfide exchange reaction in which cystine reacts with the sulfhydryl groups of these medications to form a disulfide compound and cysteine, which are both highly soluble. Many patients do not comply with D-penicillamine therapy because of its many side effects, which include epidermolysis, rash, loss of taste and smell, fever, nephrotic syndrome, arthralgia, and pancytopenia. The side effects of alpha-mercaptopropionylglycine are less severe which makes it a better treatment choice.

The Sexually Transmitted Diseases

CHANCROID

method of
WILLIAM L. ALBRITTON, M.D., PH.D.
University of Saskatchewan
Saskatoon, Canada

Chancroid, or soft chancre, was differentiated clinically from syphilis, or hard chancre, in the middle 1800s, but the etiologic agent of chancroid, *Haemophilus ducreyi*, was not recognized until the late 1800s. The chancre usually begins as a tender papule that becomes ulcerated during a 24- to 48-hour period. An associated painful unilateral inguinal adenitis is a characteristic feature in about one-half of the cases. Painful ulcer and inguinal adenitis are useful clinically in differentiating chancroid from syphilis. Autoinoculation ulcers and the absence of vesicular lesions are also useful clinical indicators.

Chancroid is endemic in many tropical areas of Asia and Africa where its prevalence is exceeded only by that of gonorrhea. Recently a number of urban outbreaks have been reported in the United States and Canada. Epidemiologic studies of these outbreaks have shown symptomatic infections to occur more commonly in uncircumcised males, in lower socioeconomic groups, and often in association with prostitution. Asymptomatic carriage of *H. ducreyi* does not appear to contribute significantly as a source of infection, but asymptomatic ulcers in females and atypical syndromes such as urethritis in males may contribute to unrecognized reservoirs of disease. Increased awareness of chancroid and improved methods of isolation of *H. ducreyi* have demonstrated the endemic nature of the disease in North America, with more than 5000 cases reported in the United States and Canada in 1987.

DIAGNOSIS

The laboratory diagnosis of chancroid depends on the isolation of *H. ducreyi*. Primary isolation from genital ulcers has been reported with varying success. Best results have been reported with nutritionally rich, selective media containing antibiotics. No reliable serologic or antigen detection test is currently available. A clinical diagnosis can usually be made by exclusion of other etiologies with similar clinical findings such as herpes simplex virus infection, syphilis, and lymphogranuloma venereum.

TREATMENT

Plasmid-mediated antibiotic resistance in *H. ducreyi* has been described for ampicillin, sulfonamides, chloramphenicol, tetracycline, streptomycin, and kanamycin. In vitro testing of clinical isolates from diverse geographic areas indicates a wide range in the prevalence of selected resistance determinants and the need for local susceptibility testing, especially if treatment failures with standard regimens are seen.

Current recommended regimens include oral erythromycin, 500 mg four times per day, or 160 mg of trimethoprim–800 mg of sulfamethoxazole (Bactrim, Septra) (one double-strength tablet) twice a day for 7 days, although therapeutic failures have been observed with the second regimen. Acceptable alternative regimens may include a long-acting third-generation cephalosporin, such as intramuscular ceftriaxone (Rocephin), 250 mg; oral amoxicillin, 500 mg, plus clavulanic acid, 125 mg (Augmentin), three times per day for 7 days; and certain of the newer fluroquinolones, such as oral ciprofloxacin (Cipro), 500 mg twice daily for 3 days. Alternative regimens, however, have usually had only limited trials in North America.

Clinical response is usually noted within 48 to 72 hours; persistent positive cultures at 72 hours is predictive of clinical failure. Local cleansing of the ulcer is usually all that is required. Fluctuant buboes should be aspirated rather than incised and drained. Systemic disease related to *H. ducreyi* has not been reported, but local relapse is not uncommon. Re-treatment with the same regimen is usually sufficient.

Treatment of sexual contacts with the same regimen as the index case is essential to prevent reinfection. Dual infection with another sexually transmitted disease is common. Syphilis serology as well as empiric therapy with long-acting benzathine penicillin, 2.4 million units intramuscularly, may be important in some clinical settings because the usual regimens for chancroid are not adequate for syphilis.

GONORRHEA

method of
SUMNER E. THOMPSON, III, M.D., M.P.H.
Emory University School of Medicine
Atlanta, Georgia

The major issue in the therapy of gonococcal infections is antibiotic resistance. Highly penicillin-resistant penicillinase-producing *Neisseria gonorrhoeae* (PPNG) strains were first described in 1975 and are endemic in the United States, particularly in New York, Florida, and California. In the past 3 years, high-level resistance to tetracycline has been described, as well as more widespread lower-level but clinically significant resistance to penicillin, tetracycline, and occasionally cefoxitin. Sporadic spectinomycin resistance has also been seen.

Sexually transmitted diseases, particularly those that are ulcerative or produce inflammation, and hence disruption of mucosal integrity, are thought to increase the risk of co-transmission of the human immunodeficiency virus, the cause of acquired immunodeficiency syndrome. Therefore, the prompt and adequate treatment of gonorrhea has an important, even urgent, implication for the control of this disease.

GENERAL PRINCIPLES OF ANTIBIOTIC USE

Whenever ceftriaxone is indicated, other third-generation cephalosporins, such as ceftizoxime, cefotaxime, or cefoperazone, may be substituted in the appropriate dose if the clinician is more familiar with their use. Doxycycline and tetracycline may be used interchangeably. In pregnant women and in individuals intolerant of tetracycline, erythromycin in the same dose may be substituted.

DIAGNOSIS AND FOLLOW-UP

A gram-stained urethral smear is adequate for diagnosis of symptomatic urethritis in men. For all other situations, the impression gained from a gram-stained smear should be confirmed by culture. Treatment, particularly of women exposed to gonorrhea, should be given immediately, without waiting for the culture result.

TREATMENT

Uncomplicated Gonorrhea (Symptomatic and Asymptomatic Urethritis in Both Sexes and Cervicitis)

If PPNG is uncommon (estimated at less than 1 to 2 per cent of cases), the drugs of choice, in order of preference, are

1. Ceftriaxone (Rocephin), 250 mg intramuscularly, or ceftizoxime (Cefizox), 500 mg intramuscularly
2. Amoxicillin, 3 grams orally with 1 gram of probenecid
3. Ampicillin, 3.5 grams orally with 1 gram of probenecid
4. Spectinomycin hydrochloride (Trobicin), 2 grams intramuscularly
5. Penicillin G procaine, 4.8 million units intramuscularly in two injections, plus probenecid, 1 gram orally

Note: All regimens should be followed by tetracycline, 500 mg orally four times a day, or doxycycline (Vibramycin), 100 mg twice a day for 7 days.

The injectable regimens have the advantage of ensuring that full therapy has been completed at the first visit. The injectable cephalosporins and spectinomycin do not require probenecid. However, spectinomycin and ceftriaxone are the two most expensive regimens (costs about equal).

Tetracycline alone was formerly a recommended regimen, but because of the rise of tetracycline resistance in gonococci, it should be avoided for primary therapy. However, up to one-third of patients with gonorrhea may have urethral or endocervical co-infection with *Chlamydia trachomatis*, a sexually transmitted pathogen that is not sensitive to the penicillins, cephalosporins, or spectinomycin. If cultures or chlamydia antigen detection tests are not done to rule out infection, the 7-day tetracycline regimen should be instituted. Failure to treat this organism results in a high proportion of male patients developing postgonococcal urethritis and female patients developing pelvic inflammatory disease.

The penicillins, and probably ceftriaxone, appear to treat incubating syphilis acquired at the time of gonorrhea infection. It is not clear whether this is true for spectinomycin. All patients should have a test for syphilis at the time of initial treatment, and again 8 weeks later.

Sexual partners of patients with confirmed gonorrhea should be examined and treated with one of the preceding regimens, even if they are asymptomatic or have no signs of gonorrhea. Patients with early disease, who may have no signs of infection, or with asymptomatic infections can transmit the disease.

Because individuals with one sexually transmitted disease tend to have others, consideration must be given to obtaining informed consent and testing for human immunodeficiency virus. This is most important in persons with a history of repeated infections.

Penicillinase-Producing *Neisseria gonorrhoeae*

Like endemic areas of the United States, many parts of the world now have high levels of infection with this organism. The clinician should suspect infection with PPNG and institute appropriate therapy in

1. Patients with a history of exposure in the Far East or Africa, or individuals from these areas who have recently moved to the United States
2. Prostitutes in one of the endemic areas: southern California, New York City, or southern Florida
3. Individuals who have failed treatment with one of the penicillin regimens given previously

The treatment of choice is an injectable third-generation cephalosporin or spectinomycin, as detailed earlier. Failure of either of these regimens should prompt a call to the local health department for further investigation. To treat patients who have failed with one of these regimens, I use the other recommended antibiotic.

Gonorrhea During Pregnancy

Any regimen mentioned earlier is safe to use in pregnancy except tetracycline. Erythromycin of either base, stearate or estolate, may be substituted.

Nongenital, Uncomplicated Gonorrhea in Both Sexes

Pharyngeal Infection. There is debate about whether the gonococcus causes pharyngitis or is merely a colonizer, like another *Neisseria*, the meningococcus.

The oral regimens listed earlier do not seem to eradicate the gonococcus consistently from the pharynx. If there is a need to treat at all, other than symptomatically, the recommended regimens are (1) penicillin G procaine with probenecid or (2) ceftriaxone. Doses are the same as those for genital gonococcal infection.

Rectal Infection. Rectal cultures should be taken routinely in homosexual men but are not necessary in women who do not give a history of rectal intercourse, provided that an endocervical culture is taken.

Ceftriaxone is now the drug of choice in homosexual men because it appears to eradicate gonococcal infections of the urethra, pharynx, and rectum at the same dose. Penicillin G procaine with probenecid, as described earlier, is the other regimen of choice. Either regimen can be used effectively in women.

Conjunctivitis. Although traditionally a disease of the newborn, this is seen occasionally in adults. I would hospitalize this patient and give ceftriaxone, 1 gram intravenously in two divided doses for 5 days, or aqueous penicillin G, 2 million units every 4 hours (12 million units a day) for 5 days. This infection should be considered to be an emergency, and treatment should be begun promptly after a presumptive diagnosis from a gram-stained smear of eye exudate has been obtained.

Complicated Gonococcal Infections

Salpingitis (Pelvic Inflammatory Disease). Women with a first or second episode of pelvic inflammatory disease (PID) or who have partners recently treated for sexually transmitted diseases usually have infections caused by either the gonococcus or *C. trachomatis*. In this setting, if an antigen detection assay for chlamydia cannot be done, it is important to treat for both organisms. Women who are ambulatory, who do not have high fever, and who are not vomiting may be treated as outpatients.

Women with multiple episodes of PID are more likely to have infection with their own endogenous vaginal flora. This includes anaerobic and enteric organisms. PID in this setting is often a mixed infection. Women who have high fever or prostration, or who are pregnant or do not respond to outpatient regimens, should be hospitalized for parenteral therapy (Table 1).

TABLE 1. **Antibiotic Therapy of PID**

Type	Severity	Therapy
First or second episode	Mild	Ceftriaxone* (Rocephin), 500 mg IM, days 1 and 5, plus doxycycline† (Vibramycin), 100 mg bid for 14 days
	Severe	Ceftriaxone, 1 gram qd IV × 5 days, plus doxycycline, 100 mg bid for 14 days
More than 2 episodes	Mild	Ceftriaxone, 500 mg qd IM on days 1 and 5, and doxycycline, 100 mg bid for 14 days, plus metronidazole (Flagyl), 250 mg qid, both PO, for 14 days
	Severe	Ceftriaxone, 1 gram IV qd for 5 days, plus doxycycline, 100 mg bid, and metronidazole, 250 mg qid PO for 14 days

*Other third-generation cephalosporins can be used with appropriate dosing schedules.
†Tetracycline, 500 mg qid, can be used in place of doxycycline.

Epididymitis. In patients under 50 years of age, the gonococcus and *C. trachomatis* are the most important infectious causes of epididymitis. Outpatient therapy with antibiotics plus scrotal elevation, bed rest, warm sitz baths, and analgesia are also important components of therapy. Antibiotic therapy consists of (1) ceftriaxone, 250 mg intramuscularly, on days 1 and 4, plus doxycycline, 100 mg orally twice a day for 10 days or (2) aqueous penicillin G procaine, 4.8 million units intramuscularly, in two divided doses given together with 1 gram of probenecid orally. These drugs are followed by ampicillin, 500 mg orally four times daily for 7 days, and then tetracycline, 500 mg orally four times daily for 7 days.

Disseminated Gonococcal Infection. Two major syndrome complexes cause the majority of disease, a tenosynovitis with a petechial or pustular rash and a true septic arthritis that is usually monarticular. Occasionally, hematogenously circulating organisms may cause endocarditis or meningitis; hence it is best to hospitalize all patients for treatment and observation. The antibiotic regimens are the same for both syndromes, but joint aspiration is important diagnostically and therapeutically for septic arthritis. It is neither necessary nor advisable to inject antibiotics intra-articularly. Open drainage of joints is also contraindicated, except in the rare case of hip joint infection. Adequate treatment consists of aqueous crystalline penicillin G, 2 million units intravenously every 6 hours for 3 or 4 days, followed by 5 days of ampicillin, 500 mg orally four times daily.

For the penicillin-allergic patient, or the patient with disseminated gonococcal infection caused by PPNG or other resistant strains, treatment consists of ceftriaxone, 1 gram intravenously once daily for 3 or 4 days, followed by cefaclor, 500 mg orally four times a day for 5 days.

Pediatric Gonococcal Infections

Infants born to women with gonorrhea should receive 50,000 units of aqueous crystalline penicillin G either intramuscularly or intravenously. Low-birth-weight babies should receive 20,000 units. An alternative is ceftriaxone, 125 mg intramuscularly in one dose. Clinical gonococcal syndromes require extra treatment.

Ophthalmia Neonatorum. Infants should be hospitalized and isolated for 24 hours after therapy is started. Treatment consists of aqueous crystalline penicillin G, 100,000 units per kg of body weight per day in four divided doses for 7 days. Ophthalmia caused by PPNG may be treated with ceftriaxone, 25 to 50 mg per kg of body weight intravenously or intramuscularly every 12 hours for 7 days.

Gonococcal Infections in Children (Vulvovaginitis, Urethritis, Proctitis, or Pharyngeal Infection). Children weighing 100 pounds (45 kg) or more should receive adult doses of antibiotics. Others should receive amoxicillin, 50 mg per kg orally, plus probenecid, 15 mg per kg orally (to a dose limit of 1 gram), or penicillin G procaine, 100,000 units per kg intramuscularly plus the oral probenecid. An alternative is ceftriaxone, 125 mg intramuscularly without probenecid.

Complicated Infections (Disseminated Gonococcal Infections, Meningitis, Peritonitis). Children weighing more than 100 pounds (45 kg) should be hospitalized and treated with adult doses of antibiotics. Smaller children should be hospitalized and treated with aqueous crystalline penicillin G, 100,000 to 150,000 units per kg per day intravenously for 7 to 10 days. Ceftriaxone, 25 mg per kg intravenously for 7 to 10 days, may be substituted in penicillin-allergic children.

NONGONOCOCCAL URETHRITIS

method of
JACKSON E. FOWLER, JR., M.D.
University of Illinois College of Medicine
Chicago, Illinois

Urethritis in men is manifested by a urethral discharge, dysuria, or both. More than four polymorphonuclear leukocytes per high-power field in the urethral exudate or secretions, or five leukocytes per high-power field in the sediment of a first-voided urine specimen, provide objective evidence of urethral inflammation. The diagnosis of nongonococcal urethritis is not entertained until gonorrhea is ruled out by Gram's stain or culture.

Chlamydia trachomatis, Ureaplasma urealyticum, and *Trichomonas vaginalis* are responsible for about 50, 25, and 5 per cent of nongonococcal infections, respectively. In 20 per cent of patients there is no identifiable microbial etiology for the syndrome. Definitive diagnosis of chlamydial urethritis is made by immunofluorescent or enzyme-linked immunosorbent assay of urethral specimens. *U. urealyticum* can be identified by culture, but the organism may also colonize the urethras of normal men. Isolation studies, therefore, do not prove a causal role. Infection by *T. vaginalis* is established by microscopic visualization of the parasite in the first voided urine specimen.

TREATMENT

The treatments of choice for both chlamydial and suspected ureaplasma urethritis are tetracycline hydrochloride, 500 mg by mouth four times daily, or doxycycline, 100 mg by mouth twice daily. Erythromycin stearate, 500 mg by mouth four times daily, is also effective and is recommended if the tetracyclines are contraindicated or not well tolerated. Regardless of the agent administered, 7 days of treatment is necessary. Most patients with urethritis of uncertain etiology also respond to the tetracycline or erythromycin regimens.

Metronidazole (Flagyl), 250 mg by mouth three times daily for 7 days, is the treatment of choice for trichomonal infections.

Persistent or recurrent symptoms usually result from reinfection and should be investigated as described for an initial episode of urethritis. However, about 20 per cent of men with chlamydial urethritis, 25 per cent with ureaplasma urethritis, and 50 per cent with urethritis of unknown etiology experience recurrent symptomatic inflammation that is not caused by identifiable infection. The erythromycin or metronidazole regimens may prove to be useful in these circumstances.

A small proportion of individuals have prolonged, intermittent symptoms. Urethroscopy is advisable to rule out a stricture, diverticulum, or condyloma acuminatum, which may simulate urethral infection. However, the examination is usually unrevealing. A 3- to 5-day course of tetracycline or erythromycin at the onset of symptoms is recommended for the management of these troublesome cases.

GRANULOMA INGUINALE
(Donovanosis)

method of
MARGARET C. DOUGLASS, M.D.
Henry Ford Hospital
Detroit, Michigan

Granuloma inguinale, which is caused by *Calymmatobacterium granulomatis,* is characterized by granulomatous lesions of the genital region. Pseudobuboes rather than true lymphadenopathy are produced by direct granulomatous involvement of subcutaneous tissue of the groin. Diagnosis is made histologically by demonstration of Donovan's bodies in macrophages by using a Wright's or Giemsa's stain. Concurrent infection with gonorrhea or syphilis is not unusual and must be excluded before treatment.

Tetracycline, 500 mg orally four times daily, is recommended as the first line therapy, although resistance to this drug has been encountered.

Chloramphenicol, 500 mg every 8 hours orally, and gentamicin, 1 mg per kg twice daily, although probably the most effective drugs, are reserved for resistant cases because of concerns about toxicity. Chloramphenicol may be the first line drug in developing countries because it is inexpensive, highly effective, and associated with higher patient compliance rates than tetracycline. Trimethoprim-sulfamethoxazole, one double-strength tablet orally twice daily, is also effective. Erythromycin, 500 mg every 6 hours, can be used during pregnancy. Results with ampicillin are variable; penicillin is not effective. Streptomycin and lincomycin have also been used. Therapy should be continued until lesions are completely healed. If an antibiotic is effective, a clinical response should be evident in 7 days. Healing usually occurs in 3 to 5 weeks.

LYMPHOGRANULOMA VENEREUM

method of
MARGARET C. DOUGLASS, M.D.
Henry Ford Hospital
Detroit, Michigan

The characteristic lymphadenopathy of lymphogranuloma venereum (LGV) is frequently unilateral and evolves over several weeks into large, painful masses associated with systemic symptoms. Spontaneous rupture and suppuration may occur, with the formation of draining sinus tracts. Diagnosis can be confirmed by identification of the causative organism, *Chlamydia trachomatis,* by a rapid diagnostic test—either an enzyme-linked immunosorbent assay or a direct fluorescent antibody method—using a specimen from a primary lesion or from an aspirate from a bubo.

Various antibiotics have been used for LGV, but there is no singularly effective drug that guarantees a cure. Evaluation of drug regimens is complicated by the highly variable natural history of LGV. Tetracycline, 500 mg four times daily, or doxycycline, 100 mg twice daily for 2 to 6 weeks, is the drug of choice. Erythromycin, 500 mg orally four times daily, is preferred during pregnancy. A sulfonamide such as sulfisoxazole, 1 gram four times daily, is another alternative therapy. Chloramphenicol, minocycline, and rifampin are also effective. Dual infections with other sexually transmitted diseases are common and require appropriate therapy. Surgical treatment of the acute inguinal syndrome may be indicated. Aspiration of large fluctuant lymph nodes can be performed with a large-bore needle and syringe through healthy adjacent normal skin. Incision and drainage should be performed only under antibiotic coverage to minimize the risk of subsequent sinus formation. Sexual contacts should be treated with a 2-week course of one of the recommended antibiotics.

SYPHILIS

method of
NICHOLAS J. FIUMARA, M.D., M.P.H.
Tufts University School of Medicine
Boston, Massachusetts

Syphilis is an infectious disease caused by *Treponema pallidum*. Except for congenital syphilis, it is acquired principally through sexual exposure and sex play during the infectious period. In acquired syphilis, the disease passes through the primary stage, which is manifested by a chancre, an ulceration at the point of inoculation; a secondary stage, with systemic symptoms, adenopathy, and rash; a latent stage, which is an asymptomatic period of variable duration with reactive serologic tests; and finally, a late stage with mucocutaneous, osseous, visceral, cardiovascular, and neural involvement. Infectious syphilis, however, consists of the primary and secondary stages and the early latent phase of less than 1 year's duration. During these stages syphilis may be spread sexually. During pregnancy, however, syphilis in all stages, particularly early syphilis, is potentially infectious to the developing fetus.

The average incubation period of primary syphilis is 3 weeks, and the lesion appears at the point of inoculation. By the time the chancre is 7 days old, the reagin blood test—the rapid plasma reagin (RPR) test—is reactive. The diagnosis of primary syphilis is established by finding *T. pallidum* on dark-field microscopic examination, a positive RPR test plus a reactive treponemal test such as the microhemagglutination (MHA) test, the fluorescent treponemal antibody absorption (FTA-ABS) test, the fluorescent treponemal absorption double staining (FTA-ABS [DS]) test, or the hemagglutination treponemal test for syphilis (HATTS). Most laboratories perform the MHA treponemal test. If this test is nonreactive in a patient with a persistently positive RPR, the laboratory then performs the more sensitive FTA-ABS or its modification, the FTA-ABS (DS).

The secondary stage follows the onset of the chancre by 9 to 90 days, with an average of 3 weeks. The chancre is frequently present at the beginning of the secondary stage but is usually healing. The secondary stage appears within 6 months and usually 6 to 8 weeks after exposure to infection. The signs and symptoms of secondary syphilis are protean but may be conveniently grouped within three syndromes.

Early in this stage, the patient complains of an influenza or grippe-like syndrome consisting of headaches, lacrimation, nasal discharge, sore throat, and generalized arthralgia. There is a slight rise in temperature, in addition to a severe loss of weight. There may be secondary anemia, an increase in the white blood cell count with an absolute lymphocytosis, and an increase in the erythrocyte sedimentation rate. With these constitutional symptoms, the patient has enlargement of the lymph nodes. A generalized lymphadenopathy is one of the most common findings of secondary syphilis. The lymph nodes are enlarged but not painful and have a hard, rubbery feel. This adenopathy usually precedes the cutaneous eruption. At about this time, palpation of the abdomen may reveal an enlarged spleen and, less commonly, an enlarged liver.

The generalized eruption completes the picture of secondary syphilis. It is often positive by dark-field microscopy. The evolution of the eruption is macular, maculopapular, papular, and, lastly, pustular. Relapsing secondary syphilis is manifested by annular lesions.

Both the reagin and treponemal blood tests are reactive in secondary syphilis.

Patients with primary and secondary syphilis are infectious sexually.

RECOMMENDED TREATMENT SCHEDULE FOR SYPHILIS

Early Syphilis: Primary, Secondary, and Early Latent Disease of Less Than 1 Year's Duration

1. *Benzathine penicillin G,* 2.4 million units intramuscularly immediately, repeated in 7 days for a total of 4.8 million units.
2. *Patients allergic to penicillin*
   a. *Tetracycline,* 500 mg orally four times daily for 15 days.
   b. *Doxycycline,* 100 mg orally two times daily for 15 days.
   c. *Minocycline,* 100 mg orally two times daily for 15 days. *Erythromycin* is not recommended because of a cure rate of only 70 per cent.
   d. *Ceftriaxone* (Rocephin), 250 mg intramuscularly daily for 10 days, has not been fully evaluated but should be effective.

Patients with their first attack of primary syphilis who are treated effectively have a nonreactive RPR circle card (RPR-CT) test within 1 year; patients with secondary syphilis have a nonreactive RPR-CT test within 2 years; and patients with early latent syphilis of less than 1 year's duration are seronegative within 4 years.

Syphilis of More Than 1 Year's Duration (Except Neurosyphilis)

This category includes early latent syphilis of 1 to 4 years' duration, late latent (syphilis of 4 years' duration or longer), and late (tertiary) stages, including mucocutaneous, osseous, visceral, and cardiovascular manifestations.

1. *Benzathine penicillin G,* 2.4 million units intramuscularly immediately to be repeated at weekly intervals for a total of 4.8 to 7.2 million units.
2. *Procaine penicillin G in aqueous suspension,* 600,000 units intramuscularly daily or every other day for a total of 10 doses.
3. *Patients allergic to penicillin*
   a. *Tetracycline,* 500 mg orally four times daily for 15 days.
   b. *Doxycycline,* 100 mg orally two times daily for 15 days.
   c. *Minocycline,* 100 mg orally two times daily for 15 days.

Patients with a first attack of early latent syphilis of 1 to 4 years' duration treated with the preceding regimens have a nonreactive RPR-CT in 5 years. This has been found in 75 per cent of the patients so studied.

In patients with late latent syphilis, 45 per cent are seronegative in 5 years and the remainder are Wassermann or reagin fast.

Cerebrospinal fluid examination is not performed unless the patient has neurologic or psychiatric signs and symptoms.

Neurosyphilis

1. *Benzathine penicillin G,* 2.4 million units intramuscularly at weekly intervals for not less than 3 weeks for a total of 7.2 million units.
2. *Crystalline penicillin G aqueous,* 10 to 20 million units intravenously daily for 10 days followed by benzathine penicillin G, 2.4 million units daily for 5 days.
3. Patients allergic to penicillin
   a. *Tetracycline,* 500 mg orally four times daily for at least 20 days.
   b. *Doxycycline,* 100 mg orally two times daily for at least 20 days.
   c. *Minocycline,* 100 mg orally two times daily for at least 20 days.

Syphilis in Pregnancy

1. *Benzathine penicillin G,* 2.4 million units intramuscularly immediately, repeated in 7 days for a total of 4.8 million units.
2. Patients allergic to penicillin
   a. *Doxycycline,* 100 mg orally two times daily for 15 days.
   b. *Oral or intravenous desensitization.* Any pregnant woman with a positive blood test for syphilis and with no previous history of

treatment should be treated prophylactically pending the results of a diagnostic work-up.
Note: Erythromycin is not recommended in pregnancy. Although it is 70 per cent effective for the mother, it does not pass the placenta in sufficient concentration to protect the fetus. Thus, congenital syphilis has occurred in spite of administration of 30 grams of erythromycin over 15 days. The U.S. Public Health Service discourages the use of erythromycin for the treatment of syphilis in pregnancy.
   c. *Ceftriaxone,* 250 mg intramuscularly daily for 10 days except in patients who have had an immediate hypersensitivity reaction to penicillin such as anaphylaxis, angioedema, urticaria, or bronchospasm.

Early Congenital Syphilis in Patients Younger Than 2 Years of Age

1. *Procaine penicillin G in aqueous suspension,* intramuscularly for a total of 100,000 to 250,000 units per kg (2.2 pounds) of body weight divided into 10 doses; for practical purposes, 100,000 units of procaine penicillin G in aqueous suspension, intramuscularly daily for 10 days for a total of 1 million units.
2. *Crystalline penicillin G aqueous,* 50,000 units per kg intravenously daily for 10 days.
3. *Benzathine penicillin G,* 100,000 units per kg (2.2 pounds) of body weight, either as a single intramuscular injection or divided into two doses a week apart. *Note:* A cerebrospinal fluid examination is not required before treatment.
4. Patients allergic to penicillin, *erythromycin,* half the adult dose.

Reinfection Syphilis

Treatment schedules are the same as for the initial infection.

Contacts of Patients with Early Syphilis

1. *Benzathine penicillin G,* 2.4 million units intramuscularly if the RPR-CT test is nonreactive.
2. Patients allergic to penicillin
   a. *Tetracycline,* 500 mg orally four times daily for at least 7 days.
   b. *Doxycycline,* 100 mg orally every 12 hours for 7 days.
   c. *Minocycline,* 100 mg orally every 12 hours for 7 days.

Section 11

Diseases of Allergy

ANAPHYLAXIS AND SERUM SICKNESS

method of
RENEE LANTNER, M.D.,
MARK BALLOW, M.D.
*State University of New York at Buffalo and
The Children's Hospital of Buffalo*
Buffalo, New York

and

RICHARD D. deSHAZO, M.D.
*University of South Alabama School of Medicine
Mobile, Alabama*

EPIDEMIOLOGY

Anaphylaxis is a potentially life-threatening symptom complex resulting from the sudden release of mast cell or basophil-derived mediators into the circulatory system. Anaphylaxis is a major medical problem because 1 in every 2700 hospitalized patients experiences drug-induced anaphylaxis and between 400 and 800 patients die each year from allergic reactions to beta-lactam antibiotics alone. Serum sickness results in a different symptom complex whereby immune complexes activate the complement system, resulting in localized inflammatory tissue damage. Serum sickness reactions are much less common than they were several decades ago, when animal-derived antitoxins were used for passive immunizations.

ANAPHYLAXIS

Pathophysiology

Classic anaphylaxis results from the bridging of IgE molecules on the surface of mast cells or basophils by an antigen-causing mediator release (Figure 1). Mediators released from mast cells and basophils include histamine, arachidonic acid metabolites (leukotrienes and prostaglandins), platelet-activating factor, and chemotactic factors that contribute to smooth muscle contraction, increased vascular permeability, secretion of mucus, and inflammatory responses characteristic of anaphylaxis.

Anaphylactoid reactions are reactions that mimic the symptoms of classic anaphylaxis but

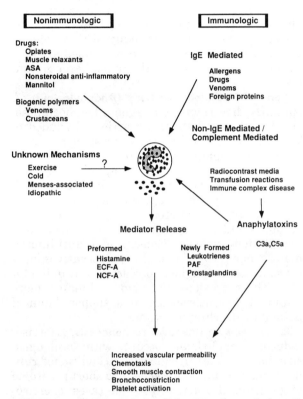

Figure 1. Diagram of anaphylactic and anaphylactoid mechanisms. ASA = acetylsalicylic acid; ECF-A = eosinophilic chemotactic factor of anaphylaxis; NCF-A = neutrophil chemotactic factor of anaphylaxis; PAF = platelet-activating factor.

are produced by non–IgE-mediated mechanisms, such as direct mast cell degranulation, modulation of arachidonic acid metabolism, or activation of the complement cascade by immune complexes. Anaphylatoxins derived from complement component fragments (e.g., C3a, C5a) cause increased vascular permeability, smooth muscle contractility, and inflammatory cell mobilization, as well as release of additional mediators from mast cells. The distinction between anaphylaxis and anaphylactoid reactions has little clinical meaning because the symptom complex and the treatment are the same for each.

Etiology

IgE-Mediated Reactions (Anaphylaxis). Hundreds of agents are known to cause anaphylaxis. Some examples of these are shown in Table 1. Recent additions include anaphylaxis associated with murine monoclonal antibodies used for diagnostic purposes or in transplantation rejection therapy, reactions to chymopapain used for chemonucleolysis, anaphylaxis to the venom of the imported fire ant (a growing problem in the southern United States), reactions occurring during dialysis to ethylene oxide gas used in the sterilization of dialysis tubing, and anaphylaxis to natural rubber, which is found in latex surgical gloves, balloons, and ileostomy bags. IgE-mediated hypersensitivity to many of these agents can be demonstrated in vivo by immediate-type skin testing or in vitro by the radioallergosorbent test.

Non–IgE-Mediated Reactions (Anaphylactoid). A similarly diverse group of agents has been associated with anaphylactoid reactions. Included in Table 2 are agents that cause the same symptom complex as anaphylaxis but are mediated by nonimmunologic mechanisms. Anaphylactoid reactions to iodinated contrast media have been studied extensively. These agents not only cause direct release of mediators from mast cells and basophils but also activate the complement and coagulation systems. Nonsteroidal anti-inflammatory agents and bisulfite preservatives may cause acute anaphylactoid reactions in individuals with no previous history of asthma or, more commonly, bronchospasm in a subpopulaton of patients with chronic asthma.

Reactions with Unknown Pathogenesis. Exercise-induced anaphylaxis occurs with prolonged, strenuous exercise, frequently in conditioned runners, and is usually preceded by a short prodrome of generalized pruritus. In some cases, exercise-induced anaphylaxis occurs only after the inges-

TABLE 1. Classes and Examples of Agents That Cause Anaphylaxis

Hormones: adrenocorticotropic hormone, insulin, hydrocortisone, estradiol, synthetic luteinizing hormone–releasing hormone, parathormone

Animal or human proteins: horse serum (snake antivenin, antilymphocyte globulin), seminal fluid, Factor VIII, protamine sulfate, monoclonal antibodies, human serum albumin

Enzymes: chymotrypsin, chymopapain, streptokinase, asparaginase

Venoms: fire ants, wasps, yellow jackets, snakes

Animal danders: cat, horse, dog, and others

Foods: eggs, milk, shellfish, nuts, and others

Drugs: penicillin, cephalosporin, and others

Polysaccharides: dextran, iron dextran

Miscellaneous: ethylene oxide gas on dialysis tubing, hyatid cyst rupture, natural rubber (latex)

TABLE 2. Representative Agents That Cause Anaphylactoid Reactions

Nonsteroidal anti-inflammatory agents: acetylsalicylic acid, indomethacin, ibuprofen, and others

Diagnostic agents: iodinated contrast media*

Muscle relaxants†: *d*-curare, succinylcholine

Preservatives: bisulfites, metabisulfites

Opiates: codeine, morphine, and others

Mannitol

Blood products: intravenous gamma globulin, blood, plasma, cryoprecipitate

*Incidence of repeat reactions decreased to <5% by pretreatment with prednisone, 50 mg PO, at 6-hr intervals for three doses, with the last dose 1 hr before the procedure, plus diphenhydramine, 50 mg PO or IM, and ephedrine, 25 mg PO, 1 hr before administration (the latter not to be used in the presence of cardiac disease).
†Some of these reactions may be IgE mediated.

tion of certain foods, such as shellfish or celery. Recently a group of women who experienced attacks of anaphylaxis associated with menses have been successfully treated with a luteinizing hormone–releasing hormone analogue and/or oophorectomy, implying a role for sex hormones in the pathogenesis of this condition. The mechanism of cold urticaria, which can lead to severe hypotension with total body exposure, is not totally understood; however, cryoglobulins may be involved causing mast cell mediator release. A syndrome of repeated episodes of anaphylaxis for which no etiology can be determined despite extensive evaluation is idiopathic anaphylaxis.

Clinical Manifestations

The signs and symptoms of anaphylaxis reflect the effects of the released mediators on target organs, involving either a single organ, such as the skin, or multiple organ systems in more severe cases (Table 3). These reactions usually occur within seconds to minutes after exposure

TABLE 3. Signs of Anaphylaxis

Organ System	Signs and Symptoms
General	Sense of impending doom, malaise, weakness
Cutaneous	Erythema, urticaria, angioedema, pruritus, warmth
Respiratory	Sneezing, rhinorrhea, nasal congestion, dysphagia, laryngospasm, bronchospasm
Cardiovascular	Tachycardia, hypotension, arrhythmias, faintness, palpitations
Gastrointestinal	Vomiting, diarrhea, abdominal cramps, tenesmus
Genitourinary	Uterine contractions, bladder urgency

to the responsible agent but may be delayed for hours with some agents, especially foods. Anaphylactic reactions are commonly preceded by a short prodrome of nasal, eye, and genital itching or burning and then by urticaria and angioedema. In cases of massive mediator release, laryngospasm, bronchospasm, hypotension, arrhythmias, syncope, diarrhea, and uterine cramping may ensue. Some patients experience recurrence of symptoms up to 8 hours after the initial reaction, termed "biphasic anaphylactic reactions." These recurrences may be caused by partial therapy of the initial reaction or a secondary response similar to the late-phase response in asthma. Persistent anaphylaxis is a form of anaphylaxis that may last for 5 to 32 hours and occurs in up to 28 per cent of patients.

Differential Diagnosis

Vasovagal reactions that occur under stress—for example, during dental surgery—must be distinguished from anaphylactic reactions. In vasovagal reactions (compared with anaphylaxis), the pulse is slow rather than rapid, the blood pressure is normal or elevated rather than decreased, and the skin is cool rather than warm from vasodilation. Patients with systemic mastocytosis have recurrent episodes of flushing, tachycardia, pruritus, headache, abdominal pain, diarrhea, or syncope. Pseudoanaphylactic reactions have been described after intramuscular injection of procaine penicillin and are thought to be caused by the release of free procaine. Symptoms include visual hallucinations, unusual tastes, fright, combativeness, twitching, and seizures. Factitious anaphylaxis is defined as repeated, self-induced episodes of anaphylaxis. Patients with hereditary angioedema have episodes of laryngeal edema and painless, nonpruritic swelling of the extremities, frequently associated with abdominal pain and often occurring after trauma, such as dental surgery. Globus hystericus should be considered when the major complaint is a chronic "lump in the throat" and no anatomic abnormalities are found.

Treatment

The treatment of anaphylaxis depends on the severity of the reaction. The use of aqueous epinephrine is key because it inhibits mediator release, restores vasomotor tone, and relaxes bronchial smooth muscle. The early use of antihistamines blocks histamine effects such as cardiac arrhythmias and peripheral vasodilation. Establishing an airway, as in any critical situation, is imperative. A step-by-step approach to

the management of anaphylaxis is outlined in Table 4. If the agent causing anaphylaxis has been injected into an extremity, continued absorption of the agent can be decreased by the use of tourniquets and the local injection of epinephrine. If the patient is cyanotic, oxygen should be administered. If bronchospasm is present, administration of an inhaled beta agonist or intravenous aminophylline should be added, keeping in mind that aminophylline may cause hypotension if infused too rapidly. If the patient is hypotensive, rapid infusion of intravenous fluid is indicated. If peripheral administration of epinephrine is unsuccessful, cautious intravenous administration of epinephrine, preferably with cardiac monitoring, should be considered. If hypotension persists, the use of vasopressors and the monitoring of pulmonary wedge pressure should be under-

TABLE 4. **Treatment of Anaphylaxis**

1. Establish secure airway with oropharyngeal or endotracheal tube or, if necessary, by cricothyroidotomy. Administer oxygen if appropriate.

2. Inject aqueous epinephrine 1:1000, 0.01 ml/kg, up to 0.3 ml SC; repeat every 15–20 min as needed.

3. If anaphylaxis followed an injection, apply tourniquet proximal to injection site, removing briefly every 10–15 min, and give additional epinephrine 1:1000, 0.01 ml/kg, up to 0.2 ml, into injection site.

4. Give diphenhydramine, 1–2 mg/kg, up to 50 mg IV or IM; repeat every 4–6 hr as needed for urticaria and angioedema.

5. Monitor vital signs frequently.

6. Place patient in recumbent position and elevate legs.

7. If patient is hypotensive, begin IV infusion with isotonic crystalloid or colloid solutions, using large-bore catheter.

8. If hypotension persists, consider slow administration of IV epinephrine 1:10,000, 0.1 ml/kg, up to 10 ml (1 mg), over 5–10 min; this may be administered as a continuous infusion of 0.5–5 μg/min (0.1–1 μg/kg/min in children).

9. If preceding regimen fails, administer dopamine, 2–50 μg/kg/min, titrating to blood pressure.

10. For resistant hypotension caused by beta blockade, glucagon, 1–5 mg IV over 1 min may be beneficial; because of short-term effects, a continuous infusion, 1–5 mg/hr, may be required. Side effects may include nausea, vomiting, and hypoglycemia. Bronchospasm may not be affected.

11. For bronchospasm, infuse aminophylline, 6 mg/kg IV over 20 min, followed by a continous drip of 0.5–0.8 mg/kg/hr (base on pre-existing plasma theophylline level, if applicable) and administer inhaled beta adrenergics (metaproterenol, albuterol, terbutaline) every 1–2 hr as needed.

12. Corticosteroids should be administered to prevent late phase reactions as hydrocortisone, 250–500 mg IV every 4–6 hr (4–8 mg/kg for children); or methylprednisolone, 40–120 mg IV every 4–6 hr (1 mg/kg/dose for children); or prednisone, 30–40 mg PO every 12 hr (1–2 mg/kg/day for children) if less severe. Taper doses appropriately, if necessary.

13. For resistant or prolonged anaphylaxis, cimetidine, 300 mg IV or IM, may be beneficial in some cases.

taken. Individuals who experience anaphylaxis while taking beta-adrenergic blockers are at risk for severe reactions that may be difficult to reverse. These individuals require much larger volumes of fluid replacement and vasopressor drug treatment than does the usual patient with anaphylaxis. Glucagon may reverse the hypotension in these patients. However, effects may be short-lived (less than 30 minutes unless a continuous infusion is used), and side effects include hypoglycemia with prolonged use resulting from depletion of glycogen stores, nausea, and vomiting, which can be hazardous in a patient with altered consciousness. Further studies are required to determine optimal dose regimens. The administration of corticosteroids does not help in the early stages but may prevent late or prolonged reactions and should be given in all severe cases of anaphylaxis. All patients should be observed for several hours after anaphylaxis has resolved because symptoms may occur up to 8 hours later in 20 per cent of the patients.

SERUM SICKNESS

Serum sickness develops when antigen-antibody complexes form in the presence of slight antigen excess, have a critical size, and are present in sufficient amounts to be deposited in the blood vessels of various tissues. Symptoms are not present when the inciting antigen is first introduced. The appearance of host antibody 1 to 2 weeks later results in immune complex formation. These immune complexes lodge in the vascular walls, where complement activation occurs. Activated complement components, particularly C3a and C5a anaphylatoxins, increase vascular permeability and are chemotactic to neutrophils, which cause tissue damage by releasing proteolytic enzymes. As the immune response continues and antibody excess develops, these larger complexes are taken up by the mononuclear phagocytic system, and symptoms eventually resolve.

The causative antigens may be exogenous, from infecting organisms or drugs, or endogenous (organ specific or nonspecific), from damaged tissues. Drugs are the most common cause of these reactions and include heterologous sera (antilymphocyte globulin, antivenins), antibiotics (penicillin, sulfonamides), nonsteroidal anti-inflammatory drugs (phenylbutazone, naproxen), hydantoins, and thiazides. Serum sickness can also occur in association with infections such as hepatitis B,

rickettsial disease, and subacute bacterial endocarditis.

Patients with serum sickness experience fever, urticarial or morbilliform eruptions, lymphadenopathy, arthralgia or arthritis, and vasculitis with palpable purpuric lesions on the skin of the extremities (Table 5). Patients may also have a purpuric or erythematous band at the junctions of plantar and palmar skin. In severe cases, neuritis, glomerulonephritis, and hypertension may occur and, rarely, a Guillain-Barré–type picture is seen. The diagnosis of serum sickness is made on the basis of the typical symptom complex, although certain laboratory findings are helpful. Total hemolytic complement (CH_{50}) and the specific complement components C3 and C4 may be decreased, suggesting complement consumption. The erythrocyte sedimentation rate may be elevated. Circulating immune complexes are often detected by C1q binding or Raji cell assay, as well as by immunofluorescence of skin or kidney biopsy specimens.

If the agent causing serum sickness can be identified, exposure to it should be stopped and subsequently avoided. Most commonly, symptoms resolve within 2 to 3 weeks after exposure to the causative agents ceases, and recovery is generally complete. If exposure is chronic, a syndrome of systemic vasculitis may result.

During the acute phase of serum sickness, the patient should be treated with antihistamines such as hydroxyzine (Atarax, Vistaril), 25 to 50 mg at bedtime or every 4 to 6 hours if needed. If arthralgia or arthritis is present, nonsteroidal anti-inflammatory agents may be helpful. More commonly, prednisone, 1 to 2 mg per kg per day (maximum, 60 mg), is administered as two divided doses for 5 to 7 days, followed by a single daily dose for several days. This dosage is then tapered over an additional 7 to 10 days. In severe cases, prednisone may be required for longer periods.

TABLE 5. **Features of Serum Sickness**

Signs and Symptoms	Frequency (%)
Fever, malaise	100
Cutaneous eruptions (urticarial, morbilliform)	90–95
Arthralgia	50–77
Generalized vasculitis	Rare
Peripheral neuritis	Rare
Glomerulonephritis	Rare
Guillain-Barré syndrome	Rare

ASTHMA IN THE ADOLESCENT AND THE ADULT

method of
MARTA M. LITTLE, M.D., and
THOMAS B. CASALE, M.D.
*VA Medical Center and University of Iowa
College of Medicine
Iowa City, Iowa*

Asthma symptoms most frequently develop during childhood and often diminish or resolve completely during adolescence. Nevertheless, symptomatic asthma frequently recurs or develops de novo in adults. Among adults, asthma remains a relatively common disease and is estimated to affect approximately 7 per cent of the general population.

DIAGNOSIS

Currently, there is no universally accepted definition of asthma. Nevertheless, *airway hyper-responsiveness* to various stimuli and *reversible airway obstruction* are clinical features that have become the cornerstones of asthma diagnosis. Although the exact mechanisms underlying airway hyper-responsiveness in asthma are not known, factors that potentially contribute include abnormalities in airway geometry, airway epithelium, airway smooth muscle, and autonomic nervous system regulation of airway tone. Potential imbalances in autonomic neural control of airway tone, specifically beta-adrenergic hyporesponsiveness and cholinergic hyper-responsiveness, have particular clinical relevance because current diagnostic and therapeutic maneuvers commonly involve the use of agonists and antagonists of these nervous systems.

The degree of airway hyper-responsiveness, the frequency and severity of airway obstruction, and the large variety of stimuli that may trigger acute episodes make asthma a heterogeneous disease clinically. Asthma has traditionally been classified as *extrinsic* when allergic sensitivity is involved in triggering asthmatic episodes and as *intrinsic* when no allergic cause is readily apparent. It may also be classified in terms of severity and chronicity as *intermittent* asthma when acute obstructive episodes are separated in time by relatively long symptom-free periods without airway obstruction, and as *chronic* asthma when obstruction is more frequent and prolonged and does not completely resolve between episodes, perhaps as a result of airway inflammation. Classification of asthma by both its triggers and its chronicity has important therapeutic implications for individual patients.

Although many patients with asthma present with a characteristic clinical history of episodic wheezing and dyspnea, it is important to remember that not all patients with asthma have these symptoms. Instead, they complain of vague tightness in the chest or of recurrent cough without overt wheezing. It is also important to remember the old adage "not all that wheezes is asthma," because a number of disease processes may similarly present with wheezing. Thorough consideration of alternative diagnoses is partic-

ularly important in the adult patient at risk for cardiovascular disease or chronic lung disease related to smoking. In addition to a thorough history and physical examination, a plain chest roentgenogram, pulmonary function testing, and sputum analysis may be particularly helpful in assessing the diagnostic possibilities. In uncomplicated asthma, the chest roentgenogram may show hyperinflation but is otherwise normal. During an asymptomatic period, spirometric (forced vital capacity [FVC], forced expiratory volume in 1 second [FEV_1]), and peak flow measurements may be totally normal, but residual volume and total lung capacity are frequently increased because of air trapping. Diffusion capacity is normal to increased. During a period of acute asthma, there is a significant reduction in FEV_1, peak expiratory flow rate, and FEV_1/FVC ratio. Sputum from asthmatics is remarkable for the presence of eosinophils. Characteristic Charcot-Leyden crystals and Curschmann's spirals may also be noted.

To establish a diagnosis of asthma definitively, it is essential to demonstrate reversible airway obstruction or airway hyper-reactivity, which are the hallmarks of this disease. Airway reversibility and hyper-reactivity can often be easily demonstrated by monitoring changes in pulmonary functions before and after inhalation of therapeutic or provocative agents. When initial spirometric measurements are abnormal, administration of an inhaled beta$_2$ agonist followed by repeat spirometry 15 minutes later is useful in assessing reversibility. Traditionally, an increase in FEV_1 or flow rates by 20 per cent or more has been considered diagnostic. A few patients with chronic airway obstruction do not respond to inhaled beta agonist medication but have significant reversal of airway obstruction after a trial of oral prednisone, 40 to 60 mg daily for 1 to 2 weeks. Such a corticosteroid trial may be critical in distinguishing asthma from nonreversible chronic obstructive lung disease.

When initial spirometric measurements are normal, hyper-reactivity of the airways can be confirmed by bronchoprovocation challenges with methacholine (cholinergic agonist), histamine, or exercise testing. In a patient with a suggestive clinical history, a decline in FEV_1 or flow rates by 20 per cent or more during the provocative test is strongly supportive of a diagnosis of asthma, especially if the decline occurs in response to low concentrations of the provocative agent or during minimal exercise. Alternatively, the patient with a suggestive history but normal spirometry may be given a portable peak flow meter with which to monitor peak flows during a baseline, asymptomatic period and during any recurrence of symptoms. In a reliable patient, the finding of a significant decline in peak flows associated with symptoms may verify a suspected diagnosis of asthma. Ambulatory peak flow monitoring is also a useful means of monitoring the adequacy of maintenance therapy in a known asthmatic.

TREATMENT

Treatment of asthma can be divided into chronic maintenance therapy and management of the acute attack.

Chronic Maintenance Therapy

The goal of maintenance therapy should be to provide long-term, symptom-free existence with minimal side effects from the medications used. Greatest success is achieved when the therapeutic approach includes both *avoidance* of provoking stimuli and a carefully individualized therapeutic regimen. The first step is a comprehensive history and physical examination, particularly aimed at identifying the triggers of acute attacks and gauging the intensity of the therapy required. A history of the degree of symptom control achieved with previous therapeutic regimens is also useful. To identify triggers that may precipitate asthma in an individual patient, it is particularly important to note the following:

Exposures to potential provocative agents found in the home and work place (e.g., pets, dust, mold, irritants, and industrial chemicals such as isocyanates)

Smoking (active or passive exposure)

Seasonal pattern of symptoms suggesting sensitivity to aeroallergens

Relationship of asthma symptoms to exercise

Relationship of asthma symptoms to ingestion of foods, preservatives, and medications, especially metabisulfites, aspirin, and beta blockers

Relationship of asthma symptoms to upper and lower respiratory tract infections

Skin testing for allergic sensitivity to inhalant allergens is a useful adjunct to a thorough history in identifying triggers of asthma. Once identified, these provocative agents should be removed or avoided as much as possible. Avoidance measures may involve counseling the patient in ways to minimize exposure to dust, molds, or animal danders in the home environment or to irritants and sensitizing chemicals in the work place. It may involve instructions to stop smoking or to discontinue the use of prescription and nonprescription drugs believed to be exacerbating factors.

Pharmacologic therapy of asthma begins with an aerosolized beta$_2$ agonist as the first line medication. Every adult asthmatic should have ready access to and know how to use an aerosolized beta$_2$ agonist. Whether or not this and other medications will be required on a regular basis for maintenance therapy can be predicted largely from the chronicity of symptoms (intermittent versus chronic) and previous medication needs. Thus, a previously untreated patient who experiences only mild, intermittent asthma may require a beta$_2$-agonist inhaler only for acute symptoms. A patient with chronic asthma, however, would benefit from regular use of an aerosolized beta$_2$ agonist every 4 to 6 hours plus stepwise addition of other agents as needed. The aim of therapy is to provide long-term, symptom-free periods. In severe asthma, however, this may mean weighing residual asthmatic symptoms against the side effects caused by further increases in therapy, especially with corticosteroids. The medications currently available for pharmacologic therapy in asthma will now be described.

Beta$_2$-Adrenergic Agonists

Most of the beta-adrenergic agonist medications currently used in asthma are beta$_2$ selective. However, this selectivity is relative and varies with the dosage and route of administration. Thus, although the predominant action of these medications is to stimulate lung beta$_2$ receptors, beta$_1$ and peripheral beta$_2$ receptors may also be stimulated, thereby resulting in side effects of palpitations and tremor, respectively. These medications are thought to be therapeutic in asthma by increasing cyclic adenosine monophosphate levels in airway smooth muscle and in mast cells, causing bronchodilation and inhibiting mast cell mediator release, respectively. Beta-adrenergic agonists are available in three forms: (1) aerosol formulations, including metered-dose inhalers (MDIs) and solutions for delivery by a compressor-driven jet nebulizer; (2) oral tablets; and (3) preparations for parenteral (subcutaneous) administration. Parenteral therapy is most appropriate for emergency room management and is discussed under therapy for the acute attack. Table 1 shows the aerosol and oral beta$_2$-agonist medications currently available and their recommended dosages. In general, the beta$_2$-agonist aerosols are preferred over the oral tablets because the oral preparations may not be as effective as aerosols, and they cause more side effects. The aerosol medications are administered directly to the airway by inhalation and result in more rapid onset of bronchodilation at relatively small doses.

Maximal deposition of aerosolized drug in the airways and maximal therapeutic effect are achieved only when proper inhalation technique is followed. For optimal use of an MDI, the patient should hold the inhaler 2 inches in front of the open mouth, inhale slowly from end-tidal volume to total lung capacity, trigger the inhaler to deliver medication at the beginning of the inhalation, and hold the breath for 10 seconds before exhaling. Patients should be thoroughly instructed and made to demonstrate proper MDI use during future clinic visits. Patients who find it difficult to coordinate inhalation and actuation of the inhaler precisely may benefit from the use

TABLE 1. Beta$_2$-Adrenergic Agonists

Drug	Dosage Per Treatment (mg)			Duration of Action (hr)
	MDI	Nebulizer	Oral	
Albuterol (Proventil, Ventolin)	0.18 (two puffs)	2.5	2–4	4–6
Bitolterol (Tornalate)	0.74–1.11 (two puffs)			4–6
Metaproterenol (Alupent, Metaprel)	1.3–1.95 (two or three puffs)	10–15	10–20	3–4
Terbutaline (Brethaire, Brethine)	0.40 (two puffs)		2.5–5	4–6
Pirbuterol (Maxair)	0.2–0.4 (one or two puffs)			4–6

of a volume reservoir or spacer. When attached to the MDI, these spacers act as a holding chamber from which the aerosolized medication can be inhaled without the need for coordination of activation and inhalation. Administration of aerosolized beta$_2$ agonists via a powered nebulizer unit also obviates the need for coordinated ventilatory maneuvers, but this is typically reserved for treatment of acute asthma attacks. Nebulizers are less suited for chronic maintenance therapy, as they are not portable and are much more expensive.

When administered as aerosols in the recommended dosage, the selective beta$_2$ agonists noted in Table 1 (albuterol, bitolterol, metaproterenol, terbutaline, and pirbuterol) differ from each other only slightly in potency and length of action. For many patients, these medications are equally effective, and individual patient preference and cost may be the best determinants in selecting one for chronic use.

Theophylline

Theophylline has a proven record of effectiveness in asthma and has been used in the treatment of asthma for more than 50 years. Despite this long history of use, precisely how theophylline mediates its therapeutic effect remains unclear. Today, theophylline's most important role is as oral maintenance therapy in the management of patients with chronic asthma. Intravenous administration of theophylline for acute attacks of asthma is discussed later.

An important guide to optimal therapy with theophylline is measurement of the serum theophylline level. Theophylline is most effective when serum levels are in the range of 10 to 20 micrograms per ml, although some patients achieve benefit at lower levels. Serum theophylline levels above 20 micrograms per ml should be avoided because of frequent side effects and potentially serious toxicity. Although these serum levels are reliable therapeutic standards, the theophylline dosage regimen that maintains them varies considerably among patients and among different formulations of theophylline. A typical maintenance dosage of oral theophylline for a generally healthy, nonsmoking adult is 10 to 12 mg per kg per day, usually administered in divided dosage. Multiple factors may, however, alter the pharmacokinetics of the drug. Factors that decrease theophylline metabolism and result in a lower dosage requirement include advanced age, liver disease, congestive heart failure, and concurrent use of macrolide antibiotics (erythromycin) or cimetidine. Factors that increase theophylline metabolism and result in higher dosage requirements include younger age, smoking, and concurrent use of certain other medications such as phenytoin.

Theophylline is available in rapidly absorbed, short-acting formulations and in slow-release, sustained-action formulations. The slow-release compounds are preferred for maintenance therapy because of the longer dosing intervals (resulting in better patient compliance) and less variation in serum concentrations. A large number of slow-release theophyllines (either bead-filled capsules or tablets) are currently available (Table 2). The manufacturers recommend 12-hour dosing intervals for most of these medications. However, some patients with rapid elimination of the drug may require 8-hour dosing intervals. In addition to the 8- to 12-hour slow-release theophyllines, two 24-hour ultra-slow-release

TABLE 2. Slow-Release Theophylline Compounds

Brand Name	Doses (mg)	
	Capsules	Tablets
Elixophyllin SR	125, 250	
Slo-bid Gyrocaps	50, 100, 200, 300	
Slo-Phyllin Gyrocaps	60, 125, 250	
Somophyllin-CRT	100, 200, 250, 300	
Theobid Duracaps	130, 260	
Theo-Dur Sprinkle	50, 75, 125, 200	
Theovent Long-Acting	125, 250	
Theo-24*	100, 200, 300	
Theo-Dur		100, 200, 300
Theolair-SR		200, 250, 300, 500
Uniphyl*		400

*Once-a-day preparations.

theophyllines are now on the U.S. market. These once-a-day preparations have been associated with variable absorption and greater fluctuation in serum concentrations. They may not be optimal for use in patients who require tight maintenance of therapeutic serum theophylline concentrations to avoid breakthrough asthma, but they may be used to treat selected patients with milder disease. Maintenance theophylline therapy should be initiated gradually by incremental increases in dosage over 1 to 2 weeks. This avoids many of the minor adverse side effects (nervousness, tremor, gastrointestinal symptoms) associated with rapid initiation of therapy. After the anticipated maintenance dosage has been reached, serum theophylline measurements should be used to make any final dose adjustments.

Cromolyn Sodium

Cromolyn is a prophylactic agent for asthma that may act in part by stabilizing mast cell membranes. Cromolyn has no bronchodilator action of its own and is thus of no benefit in acute asthma. In fact, because of its irritating effects on the airway, it should be avoided during acute attacks. Cromolyn is potentially useful as a substitute for theophylline in chronic maintenance therapy, especially in children, for whom it has been shown to be most effective. Although cromolyn has generally been disappointing in the management of asthma in adults, there are a few situations in which it may be the drug of choice. In particular, if the patient can identify a certain event or exposure that precipitates asthma attacks, the prophylactic use of cromolyn can be highly effective. For example, cromolyn can be effectively used just before exercise or before anticipated exposure to a pet or laboratory animal known to trigger asthmatic symptoms.

Cromolyn is poorly absorbed when given orally and must be given by inhalation. It is available as a powdered capsule for use in a spinhaler, but this has largely been superseded by the introduction of a cromolyn MDI (Intal). The dose for the MDI is two puffs four times daily, and a 6-week trial is necessary before efficacy can be adequately assessed in chronic asthma.

Corticosteroids

Rational use of corticosteroids in asthma takes into account two variables. Corticosteroids are the most potent agents in the asthma pharmacopeia, but their use for long periods is associated with severe side effects, such as weight gain, cataracts, osteoporosis, glucose intolerance, hypertension, poor wound healing, and immunosuppression. Fortunately, short (1- to 2-week) courses of high-dose corticosteroids (such as oral

prednisone, 40 to 60 mg per day) followed by a rapid taper are both well tolerated and extremely effective in managing exacerbations of asthma. In patients with frequent exacerbations requiring frequent short courses of prednisone, chronic inhaled steroid therapy for maintenance should be tried. Inhaled steroid therapy can be administered chronically, without the severe side effects associated with chronic systemic corticosteroid use. The major side effects of inhaled steroids are dysphonia and oral candidiasis. The risks of these side effects can be minimized by using a spacer and by rinsing the mouth after inhaler use.

The steroid inhalers currently available in the United States and their recommended dosages are shown in Table 3. The recommended dosage can be doubled if necessary to suppress disease activity, but systemic steroid side effects may become evident with chronic administration of higher doses. The patient who is well maintained on inhaled steroids may occasionally need a short burst and taper of oral prednisone for asthma exacerbations. It should be noted that inhaled steroids, although useful in maintenance therapy, are not as useful in the treatment of acute exacerbations of asthma. We generally recommend that inhaled steroids be preceded by inhaled beta agonists.

For a minority of steroid-dependent patients, inhaled steroids are not sufficient; chronic oral prednisone is necessary for adequate symptom control. If possible, such patients should be maintained on alternate-day prednisone therapy to decrease adrenal suppression and side effects. Patients with the most severe steroid-dependent asthma may, however, notice significant diminution of lung function on the alternate days when they do not take steroids. These patients often require daily prednisone, usually 10 to 15 mg per day, for maintenance therapy. Overall, the goal should be to determine the minimum dose of prednisone necessary to control asthma adequately while being careful not to withhold steroids when they are needed. Indeed, inappropriate withholding and too rapid withdrawal of steroids have been repeatedly cited as contributing factors in cases of fatal asthma.

TABLE 3. **Corticosteroid Inhalers**

Drug	Recommended Dosage
Beclomethasone dipropionate (Vanceril, Beclovent)	Two puffs (84 μg) tid or qid
Flunisolide (AeroBid)	Two puffs (500 μg) bid
Triamcinolone acetonide (Azmacort)	Two puffs (200 μg) tid or qid

New therapies aimed at reducing the need for daily steroid use and decreasing the side effects in severe asthmatic patients are currently being investigated. Troleandomycin, a derivative of the macrolide antibiotics, slows elimination of methylprednisolone and, when used in combination with methylprednisolone in clinic trials, improves clinical control of asthma and allows significant reductions in steroid dosage (usually from a daily to an alternate-day dosage). Adverse effects associated with this regimen, including enhancement of steroid side effects, elevated liver transaminase levels, and the risk of disseminated varicella infection, limited its usefulness in the past. The theophylline dosage should be decreased by about 25 per cent and blood levels frequently monitored during troleandomycin therapy. New protocols that appear to decrease the incidence of many of these adverse effects while maintaining clinical efficacy may make this a more useful therapeutic intervention in the future.

With accumulating evidence that airway inflammation is an important feature of chronic asthma, there has been increasing interest in the use of anti-inflammatory drugs as steroid-sparing agents in severe steroid-dependent asthma. The most promising of these is the folate antagonist methotrexate, which is already being used in place of high doses of corticosteroids in the treatment of rheumatoid arthritis and psoriasis. In a recent clinical trial, methotrexate in low dosage reduced the corticosteroid requirements of patients with severe asthma without causing deterioration of pulmonary functions. Because of methotrexate's potential toxicity and teratogenicity, patients must be carefully selected and closely followed by a physician familiar with its use. Future trials should be helpful in determining the proper use of methotrexate in asthma. However, until these studies are completed, routine use is not recommended. Nevertheless, it is hoped that methotrexate, and perhaps other anti-inflammatory agents, will provide new avenues for effective treatment of severe asthma with minimal corticosteroid morbidity.

Anticholinergic Agents

Because the cholinergic nervous system is the most important regulator of airway tone, and because asthmatics have cholinergic hyper-responsiveness, anticholinergic agents should theoretically be effective in the treatment of asthma. Anticholinergic agents in the form of datura leaves and stramonium were among the earliest bronchodilators used. Nevertheless, administration of atropine and related tertiary ammonium compounds is associated with troublesome side effects that limit their usefulness in asthma. The recent introduction of ipratropium bromide, a quaternary ammonium compound that is poorly absorbed and is associated with negligible systemic side effects, has allowed further analysis of the efficacy of anticholinergic agents in asthma. The amount of bronchodilation produced by ipratropium inhalation varies from person to person. In general, older asthmatics and those with intrinsic asthma seem to have the most favorable response. For most patients, anticholinergic agents are less potent than beta$_2$-adrenergic agents, but the combination may have an additive bronchodilatory effect. A particular situation in which anticholinergic agents may be significantly more effective than beta$_2$-adrenergic agents is in bronchospasm occurring in a patient taking beta blockers.

In general, inclusion of ipratropium in maintenance therapy should be considered for patients who have not had a full bronchodilatory response to beta$_2$ agonists and theophylline. It is important, however, to evaluate its efficacy in the individual patient before making a commitment to long-term therapy. Efficacy can be estimated by measuring the bronchodilatory response 30 to 60 minutes (the time to peak effect) after inhalation of ipratropium. The recommended dose for ipratropium administered via an MDI (Atrovent) is two puffs (36 micrograms) four times daily.

Other Therapies

Desensitization to allergens, which has been shown to be effective in the treatment of allergic rhinitis, may also benefit selected patients whose asthma is exacerbated by common aeroallergens. Other therapeutic considerations that should not be overlooked are the importance of physical conditioning and attention to recommended vaccination schedules. With proper instruction to avoid cold air and to use a beta$_2$-agonist or cromolyn inhaler before exercise, even patients with chronic asthma can tolerate some form of regular exercise, particularly swimming. This regular exercise program is rewarded by improved functional capacity. Patients with chronic asthma and other chronic pulmonary diseases should receive the polyvalent pneumococcal vaccine and annual influenza vaccinations. New therapies being investigated for potential efficacy in chronic management of asthma include calcium channel blockers and antiallergic agents (azelastine, ketotifen).

Emergency Room and Hospital Management of Acute Asthma

Initial rapid assessment of the patient with acute asthma should include a pertinent history and physical examination aimed at ruling out other causes of wheezing and dyspnea (pneumonia, pulmonary embolism, congestive heart failure) and at assessing the severity of the asthma attack. Historical details that are helpful in assessing severity and in predicting how well the asthmatic obstruction will respond to bronchodilator therapy include the duration of symptoms, precipitating factors, current medications, and severity of previous attacks.

Of the physical examination findings, the most ominous is a disturbance of consciousness, as this suggests respiratory failure and the need for immediate aggressive therapy, possibly including mechanical ventilation. Other physical findings and observations that are indicative of relatively severe obstruction include tachycardia (>120 beats per minute), use of accessory muscles of respiration, diaphoresis, inability to lie flat, and severe breathlessness during speech. Generalized wheezing is typically present, and the absence of wheezing may be an ominous sign indicative of very severe obstruction.

These clinical findings are useful guides, but they are not by themselves completely reliable. Severe physiologic impairment can be present in the absence of many of the clinical findings suggesting severity. Objective measurement of lung function with spirometry is therefore imperative. FEV_1 measurements of 30 per cent or less of the predicted value and peak expiratory flow rates of 130 liters per minute or less are evidence of severe asthma requiring immediate intensive therapy. Arterial blood gas determinations to assess gas exchange are essential in patients with severe obstruction (including those too ill to perform spirometric maneuvers) but are of limited value in patients with mild to moderate attacks. In severe asthma, these determinations provide an important clue to impending respiratory failure (rising Pco_2 in a tiring patient) and a means to check for adequacy of supplemental oxygen therapy.

Many of these clinical parameters have been used to develop an index or formula for determining which emergency room patients need to be hospitalized. Nevertheless, the decision to hospitalize a patient for acute asthma is ultimately made when, in the physician's clinical judgment, outpatient management is unlikely to be successful or when an initial attempt at outpatient management has already failed.

As in chronic maintenance therapy, the first line medications in emergency treatment of asthma are sympathomimetics, including beta-adrenergic agonists. Patients may be treated with epinephrine (1:1000), 0.3 ml, or with terbutaline (1 mg per ml), 0.25 ml subcutaneously at 20-

TABLE 4. Adult Dosages of Intravenous Aminophylline and Theophylline

	Aminophylline	Theophylline (in 5% Dextrose)
Loading dose (mg/kg)	5–7	4–6
Maintenance dose (mg/kg/hr)		
Nonsmoker	0.5–0.7	0.4–0.6
Smoker	0.9	0.75
Elderly	0.4	0.3
Heart failure or liver dysfunction	0.2–0.3	0.2

minute intervals for a maximum of three doses. Alternatively, 0.5 ml of isoproterenol (0.5 per cent) or 0.3 ml of metaproterenol or albuterol (see Table 1) can be administered via a wet nebulizer every 20 minutes for three doses. The patient should be re-evaluated clinically and by spirometry after each treatment. Although theophylline's role in the emergency treatment of asthma is secondary to that of the beta-adrenergic agonists, additional bronchodilation may be achieved by theophylline loading in the emergency room in a patient not previously taking theophylline. Theophylline loading may be accomplished with an oral loading dose of a rapid-release preparation or, more rapidly, by intravenous administration of aminophylline, 5 to 7 mg per kg, or theophylline, 4 to 6 mg per kg (Table 4). A loading dose should not be given to a patient already taking theophylline unless a serum theophylline concentration is used as a guide to adjust the loading dose appropriately. In some patients with a limited response to sympathomimetics and theophylline, an anticholinergic medication such as atropine, 0.025 to 0.035 mg per kg, via a nebulizer may be of benefit. Recommendations for the treatment of acute asthma in the emergency room usually emphasize the use of corticosteroids only when the response to conventional bronchodilator therapy has been inadequate. Nevertheless, earlier use of corticosteroids as part of *initial* therapy in the emergency room (such as methylprednisolone, 125 mg intravenously) is sometimes indicated. For example, an asthmatic patient who presents to an emergency room with a several-day history of a viral upper respiratory tract infection and asthmatic symptoms that have worsened despite frequent use of a beta-agonist inhaler at home is unlikely to have an immediate and full response to bronchodilator therapy in the emergency room. The maximum bronchodilation possible from relaxation of bronchial smooth muscle may already have been achieved. The remaining obstruction is predominantly the result of inflammation, mucosal edema, and mucous plugging, and successful management requires the use of corticosteroids.

If there has been a good response to treatment in the emergency room, the management may continue on an outpatient basis after release from the emergency room on an intensified maintenance program and with close medical follow-up. In most cases, the medications given on release from the emergency room include a burst and taper of prednisone. If the response to treatment in the emergency room has been poor, with either little clinical improvement or failure of FEV_1 to improve to above the 40 to 50 per cent predicted, the patient should be hospitalized for further intensive bronchodilator therapy and intravenous corticosteroids. In the hospital, maintenance theophylline or aminophylline may be given by continuous intravenous infusion. Guidelines to the adult dosage of aminophylline and theophylline, including suggested alterations in special clinical situations, are shown in Table 4. Because of considerable interpatient variability in theophylline metabolism, serum theophylline levels must be monitored and therapy adjusted to maintain equilibrium levels between 10 and 20 micrograms per ml. The physician should be cognizant of the signs of theophylline toxicity, including nausea, vomiting, restlessness, arrhythmias, and convulsions, and know how to treat them. The response to corticosteroids may take several hours, and steroid therapy should be instituted without undue delay. Intravenous corticosteroid doses are empiric, but moderate to high doses of methylprednisolone (40 to 125 mg every 6 hours) or of hydrocortisone (200 to 1000 mg every 6 hours) have been effective. Whether there is any significant advantage for high versus moderate doses is controversial. The response to this intensive therapy can be followed by spirometry and arterial blood gas determinations. Once steady improvement is demonstrated, the therapy can be gradually converted to a regimen of inhaled and oral medications that can be continued on an outpatient basis with close follow-up after discharge.

ASTHMA IN CHILDREN

method of
NANCY P. CUMMINGS, M.D.
Stanford University Hospital
Menlo Park, California

Asthma is a common disorder affecting millions of children. It appears to be increasing in Western countries, with an incidence of approximately 5 per cent in

1974 and 8 per cent in 1980. Black persons are more commonly affected than caucasians, with an incidence of 9 per cent compared with 6 per cent. Asthma is the leading cause of morbidity in childhood, with an estimated 2.8 million restricted activity days per year attributed to asthma in 1983. Asthma and wheezing were the tenth most frequent causes of visits to the pediatrician's office in 1980–1981, accounting for 2.2 million visits. Most children with asthma have the first episode by their third birthday. Ninety per cent improve during adolescence. However, mild persistent wheezing is relatively common, and it is estimated that only 20 per cent of those with childhood asthma become totally asymptomatic in adult life. Children who have persistent symptoms at age 14 and abnormalities in spirometric measurements often have persistent and severe symptoms in young adulthood.

The spectrum of the disorder ranges from a very mild, intermittent course to severe, life-threatening disease. Until recently, mortality caused by asthma had been stable or declining slowly. However, during the past 5 years, it has been increasing in a number of Western countries, including the United States. The reasons for this increase are not yet clear. However, considerations have included increased prevalence, increased severity of the disease, drug toxicity, and management deficiencies such as inadequate long-term treatment, discontinuity of medical care, poor patient compliance, and inadequate monitoring of lung function, especially between acute exacerbations.

The key feature of asthma is airway hyper-reactivity, an exaggerated bronchoconstrictor response to a variety of stimuli. Airway hyper-responsiveness is associated with inflammation of the airways. Postmortem lungs show marked inflammation of the airways with infiltration of inflammatory cells (particularly eosinophils), disruption of airway epithelium, and plugging of the airway lumen by viscous mucus. Mast cells have been assumed to play a role in the pathogenesis of asthma, with mast cell–released mediators such as histamine, prostaglandins, and leukotrienes causing bronchial smooth muscle contraction, microvascular leakage, and airway mucous secretion and acting as chemotactic agents for other inflammatory cells. Eosinophilic infiltration, a characteristic feature of asthmatic airways, differentiates asthma from other inflammatory conditions of the airways. Eosinophils release a variety of mediators including leukotriene C_4, platelet-activating factor, major basic protein, and eosinophilic cationic protein. These mediators are toxic to airway epithelium, and this epithelial damage may be a critical feature of airway hyper-responsiveness. In addition, the cholinergic and adrenergic autonomic nervous systems are involved in control of the airways. Recently, neuropeptides such as vasoactive intestinal peptide and substance P have been identified as having effects on airway function.

When a child presents with asthma or symptoms suggestive of asthma, a careful history and physical examination should precede therapy. Important points in the history include the precipitants of symptoms, the duration of symptoms, and current and past medications. If symptoms or attacks have occurred, the details of, as well as the response to, therapy are important. Usually the diagnosis is easy, especially when the asthma is severe. The diagnosis may be more difficult when the asthma is mild or if it presents in an atypical manner. Children who present six to eight times each winter with a diagnosis of "bronchitis" are unusual unless they have an underlying immunodeficiency disorder or chest problem. The common diagnosis is asthma. Chronic cough without wheezing or shortness of breath has been well described as a primary manifestation of asthma. In children who can perform the spirometry test, the most appropriate evidence is the demonstration of reversible obstructive airways disease. In older children in whom baseline pulmonary functions are normal and asthma is suspected, a provocative challenge either with exercise or by inhalation of methacholine or histamine may be needed to make the diagnosis of asthma apparent. Methacholine challenge has been safely performed in children as young as 2 years of age by experienced investigators. A therapeutic trial of oral or inhaled bronchodilators may also be diagnostic for asthma.

TREATMENT

There are four basic approaches to the outpatient management of the child with asthma: (1) identifying the precipitants of the asthma and manipulating the environment to control the child's exposure to them; (2) controlling bronchospasm and the inflammatory component of asthma with medication; (3) altering the immune response to environmental allergens with immunotherapy; and (4) educating the patient and family to improve their ability to manage this chronic illness adequately.

The goals of asthma therapy are to obtain maximum control of symptoms with a minimal number of the safest medications. Ideally, children should be able to participate in normal daily activities and sports with few or no restrictions. School absenteeism should be minimized. Decreasing the number of acute episodes of wheezing that require emergency treatment and reducing the number and frequency of hospitalizations are desirable. Normal growth and development should occur. Ideally, there should be complete relief of airway obstruction and normalization of pulmonary function. The patient and family should be able to understand, accept, and manage the asthma within the context of the family's lifestyle.

Identifying Precipitants of Asthma and Instituting Environmental Controls

Asthmatic children have a higher prevalence of allergies than the normal population. Approximately one-half of the children with asthma demonstrate allergen skin test reactivity compared with approximately 20 per cent of nonasthmatics. Pollens and molds, house dust, dust mites, and animal danders may all induce wheezing in asthmatic children. Allergen-induced asthma generally occurs within minutes after exposure to an allergen, peaks 10 to 15 minutes later, and lasts for 1 to 2 hours. Symptoms develop rapidly and are readily apparent. In some children, often those with severe asthma, a late asthmatic response may occur 2 to 4 hours after allergen exposure, peaking 5 to 12 hours later and lasting for 1 to several days. Both immediate and late responses are precipitated by exposure to various allergens to which the patient has antigen-specific IgE, as demonstrated by skin test or in vitro measures of specific IgE. Dust mites, animal danders, pollens, and molds may be associated with both early and late asthmatic reactions. Avoidance of allergens can lead to a decrease in IgE-mediated reactions and may also decrease nonspecific airway hyper-reactivity. Avoidance of dust and dust mites requires special attention to the child's bedroom. Pillows, mattresses, and box springs should be encased in plastic covers and wiped weekly. Bedding should be washed weekly in hot water. Furniture and wall hangings should be limited. Bare floors are preferred, and if carpeting is present, a low pile is best. Carpeting should be vacuumed several times a week. Room air vents should be closed and covered with cheesecloth. Closets should contain only the current season's clothes. The bedroom should be dusted frequently. Animal allergens that may precipitate both early and late asthmatic reactions should be removed from the home. Allergy to air-borne fungi is an especially difficult problem, and a search for possible mold growth should be made in the home. Use of a dehumidifier may be considered to keep the general area as dry as possible.

Nonallergic precipitants of asthma include inhaled irritants, both particulate and gaseous. The most important of these irritants is cigarette smoke. Maternal cigarette smoking correlates most closely with the frequency and severity of acute asthmatic attacks in the child. Both parents, however, should be encouraged to stop smoking, and smoking should be prohibited in the home of an asthmatic child. Asthmatic teenagers should be strongly discouraged from smoking. Other pulmonary irritants include sulfur dioxide, nitrogen dioxide, and ozone; thus, smog exposure should also be avoided if possible. Irritants from wood-burning stoves, fireplaces, assorted oil-based heaters, and various chemicals (e.g., formaldehyde, cleaning products) may also cause bronchoconstriction.

Air purification systems may be useful for both

allergen- and irritant-induced symptoms. Room units can be purchased for the bedroom (see *Consumer Reports,* January 1985). Central air purification systems can also be purchased; however, they are often expensive (between $500 and $1,000). A Humidist (Honeywell) can be installed in homes with central air conditioning and heating systems as an aid in controlling indoor humidity. Relative humidity of 40 to 50 per cent is ideal because higher humidity (70 to 80 per cent relative humidity) encourages the presence of dust mites and molds.

A major precipitant of asthma in children is viral respiratory infection, especially in young children. Viral infections can also increase nonspecific airway hyper-reactivity, which may persist for weeks after resolution of the viral infection. Major pathogens implicated in triggering asthma in children include *Mycoplasma,* parainfluenza virus, rhinovirus, respiratory syncytial virus, adenovirus, and influenza virus. Except for the use of erythromycin for *Mycoplasma* infections and possibly ribavirin (Virazole) for respiratory syncytial virus, no effective treatment is available once the infection begins. Consideration can be given to removing children from high-exposure environments such as day care centers. Careful handwashing should be emphasized for all persons who care for children.

Exercise, hyperventilation, and cold air trigger bronchospasm, possibly by shared mechanisms of heat and/or water loss from the bronchial mucosa. At least 90 per cent of asthmatic children have exercise-induced bronchospasm. Despite this, most asthmatic children should be encouraged to exercise, with appropriate pharmacologic pretreatment beforehand. Swimming tends to cause the least bronchoconstriction and long periods of running the most bronchoconstriction.

Emotions can occasionally be involved in triggering asthma. However, parents should be assured that asthma is not a psychosomatic disease.

Asthma may also be aggravated by changes in weather, such as an increase in relative humidity or a sudden change in barometric pressure. Smog, storms, and air turbulence may contribute to an asthmatic episode. The reasons for these changes are largely unknown.

Pharmacotherapy

The major drugs employed for the treatment of asthma are (1) adrenergic or sympathomimetic drugs, (2) theophylline, (3) sodium cromoglycate (cromolyn), and (4) corticosteroids. Other less often used medications include atropine and its derivatives, antihistamines, antibiotics, anti-inflammatory medications, and antimetabolites.

Adrenergic or Sympathomimetic Drugs

A major advance in recent years has been the development of adrenergic compounds, which are predominantly beta$_2$ agonists that produce more prolonged bronchodilation and fewer cardiovascular side effects than previously available medications. In the early part of this century, both ephedrine and epinephrine, nonselective adrenergic agents, were used. With the identification of the beta$_1$ and beta$_2$ receptors, more specific beta$_2$ agonists were developed for wide use. The beta$_2$ receptor is the primary adrenergic receptor that stimulates relaxation of bronchial smooth muscle. The most widely used beta$_2$ agonists include metaproterenol (Alupent and Metaprel), terbutaline (Brethine, Bricanyl), albuterol (Ventolin, Proventil), and bitolterol (Tornalate). These medications are available in liquid preparations, tablet form, metered-dose inhalers (MDI), and liquid solutions for inhalation. The usual doses of these agents are shown in Table 1.

These drugs are generally well tolerated, although increased heart rate, tremor, and irritability can occur. Side effects often decrease with time. Liquid and tablet preparations are rapidly absorbed from the gastrointestinal tract and often produce more hyperactivity and tremor than inhalants. Inhaled forms of medications are particularly useful, with rapid onset of action and minimal side effects. Their use is limited primarily by the child's ability to coordinate activation of a MDI or to use a nebulizer.

Theophylline

Theophylline has been used as a bronchodilator since the 1940s. It is probably the most commonly prescribed drug for asthma in this country. The mechanism of action remains unclear. Although it was previously assumed that it acted as a phosphodiesterase inhibitor, it now appears that other mechanisms are responsible for theophylline's action. Theophylline effectively prevents symptoms of asthma but has a low therapeutic index. Serum levels thought to produce the maximal bronchodilating effect are between 10 and 20 micrograms per ml, although some children have relief of symptoms and improved pulmonary function with lower doses. Many children have difficulty tolerating theophylline. Side effects include irritability, restlessness, nightmares, decreased attention span, sleepwalking, misbehavior, enuresis, and poor school performance. Adverse effects can be noted with doses that produce serum levels within or below the therapeutic range.

There is significant intersubject variation in theophylline metabolism, and individualizing therapy is critical. Generally, if a child is initially

TABLE 1. **Dosing Guidelines for Adrenergic Drugs**

Drug	Subcutaneous Administration	Oral Administration	Aerosol Administration	Metered-Dose Inhaler
Epinephrine	0.01 ml/kg up to 0.30 ml (1:1000 solution)	—	—	—
Isoetharine	—	—	0.02 ml/kg/dose up to 0.05 ml diluted with 1.5–2 ml normal saline (1% solution)	Two inhalations q 2–3 hr (340 μg/inhalation)
Metaproterenol	—	0.3—0.6 mg/kg/dose 4 times/day (10- and 20-mg tablets; 10 mg/5 ml syrup)	0.01 ml/kg/dose up to 0.30 ml diluted with 1.5–2 ml normal saline (5% solution) or 1-unit dose (0.6% solution)	Two inhalations q 4 hr (65 μg/inhalation)
Albuterol	—	0.1–0.15 mg/kg/dose 3–4 times/day (2- and 4-mg tablets; 2 mg/5 ml syrup)	0.01–0.03 ml/kg/dose up to 0.5 ml diluted with 1.5–2 ml normal saline (0.5% solution)	Two inhalations q 4 hr (90 μg/inhalation)
Terbutaline	0.01 ml/kg up to 0.30 ml (1% solution)	0.075–0.10 mg/kg 3–4 times/day (2.5- and 5.0-mg tablets)	0.1 mg/kg diluted up to 2 ml with normal saline (marketed for subcutaneous use)	Two inhalations q 4 hr (200 μg/inhalation)
Bitolterol	—	—	—	Two inhalations q 6 hr (370 μg/inhalation)

given a low dose of theophylline and is gradually increased to therapeutic doses based on body weight (Table 2), side effects can be avoided or decreased. For young children, theophylline capsules may be used that are opened and the contents sprinkled in food. Most young children must take the drug three times a day. In older children and adolescents, a new longer-acting theophylline preparation that maintains blood levels for 24 hours may be beneficial when asthma has significant diurnal variation and nocturnal exacerbations.

Theophylline levels should be determined and should be a guide for therapy. Peak (2 to 4 hours after a dose) and trough (before the preceding dose) levels have been recommended; however, long-acting theophylline preparations may be variable in their peak and trough times.

TABLE 2. **Dosing Guidelines for Oral Theophylline***

Age	Total Daily Dose (mg/kg/24 hr)
6–51 wk	(0.30) × (age in weeks) + 8
1–9 yr	24
9–12 yr	20
12–16 yr	18
More than 16 yr	13 (or 900 mg/day, whichever is less)

*Data From Weinberger M, Hendeles L, and Ahrens R: Clinical pharmacology of drugs used for asthma. Pediatr Clin North Am *28*:47–75, 1981.

Cromolyn

Cromolyn has been thought to inhibit IgE-dependent release of mediators from human lung mast cells. However, recent evidence has shown this property to be surprisingly weak. Cromolyn may inhibit secretory properties of other inflammatory cells, thereby modulating mechanisms that contribute to the inflammatory component of asthma. Cromolyn has minimal side effects and appears to be as effective as theophylline in the first line treatment of asthma. It is especially useful in children who tolerate theophylline and beta-adrenergic agents poorly. It must be used prophylactically, and most children require it at least three times a day. As the asthma improves over months of routine use, many children can be adequately maintained with lower doses of cromolyn.

Cromolyn is available for administration in three forms. The oldest is a 20-mg capsule using lactose as a carrier, which is opened using a Spinhaler device. Because lactose is present inside the capsule and can be swallowed, gastrointestinal symptoms can occur in the lactose-intolerant patient. Cromolyn available as an MDI is generally chosen by older children and adolescents. A solution containing 20 mg per ml of cromolyn solution in 2-ml ampules is available for use with nebulizers.

Atropine and Ipratropium Bromide (Atrovent)

Atropine has been used in the treatment of asthma for almost 2 centuries. It inhibits bronchoconstriction by its action as an anticholinergic agent. Atropine is rarely used in children. The pharmacist can prepare it by dissolving atropine tablets, 0.6 mg in normal saline (without preservatives) to a concentration of 1 mg per ml and sterile filtered. From 1 to 2 ml (0.05 mg per kg, maximum 2 mg) of this solution may be placed in a nebulizer and used either alone as a bronchodilator or with a beta-adrenergic drug or cromolyn. Atropine solution may also be used; however, it is more expensive. Atropine can be absorbed into the systemic circulation and is associated with anticholinergic side effects such as dry mouth, blurred vision, and altered heart rate.

Ipratropium bromide is a quaternary isopropyl derivative of atropine. It is poorly absorbed and has few systemic side effects. It has only recently been approved for use in the United States and can be used only with adults. However, a number of studies have shown its efficacy in childhood asthma. It is active as a bronchodilator, with a peak onset at 10 minutes and a duration of 4 to 6 hours. When it is used in combination with an inhaled beta agonist, prolonged bronchodilation occurs. The dose is generally two inhalations three or four times a day. Atropine and ipratropium bromide are drugs of choice in patients who have asthma induced by beta-blocking agents.

Corticosteroids

Corticosteroids are very effective drugs in the treatment of both acute and chronic asthma. They do not produce immediate bronchodilation but instead act at many sites to help reverse the pathologic process of asthma. Some of the actions of corticosteroids include enhancement of the beta-adrenergic response to relieve bronchospasm, reversal of mucosal edema, decrease in vascular permeability by vasoconstriction, inhibition of the release of leukotrienes, reduction of mucous secretion, and interference with chemotaxis (this action may be caused by leukotriene B_4). Corticosteroids also produce an eosinopenic effect, which may help prevent the cytotoxic effects of major basic protein and other inflammatory mediators released from the eosinophil. Corticosteroids have no direct effect on immediate hypersensitivity. They block the late asthmatic reaction and the increased airway hyper-reactivity observed after the late asthmatic reaction.

Toxicity of corticosteroids is related primarily to the duration rather than to the dose and includes a cushingoid appearance, growth suppression, striae and purpura, cataracts, osteoporosis, and muscle weakness. Because of their side effects, corticosteroids have traditionally been reserved for highly intractable disease in children who respond poorly to other medications. However, early intervention with corticosteroids in children who become unresponsive to bronchodilators may, with minimal risk, abort a severe impending asthma attack and prevent hospitalization. A dose of 2 mg per kg per day to a maximum of 60 to 80 mg in two divided doses may be administered for 4 to 7 days and discontinued abruptly or tapered. Although it would be ideal to target intervention with corticosteroids at patients who will not improve spontaneously, it is difficult to distinguish those in whom spontaneous resolution will not occur.

Aerosolized corticosteroids have been of considerable value in the management of patients with moderate to severe asthma. These preparations allow effective control of symptoms and improve pulmonary function in the majority of patients, with minimal risk of the systemic side effects associated with long-term oral steroid therapy. Preparations available for use by inhalation include beclomethasone (Beclovent, Vanceril), flunisolide (AeroBid), and triamcinolone (Azmacort). Therapy with aerosolized steroids is generally initiated after asthma is under maximal control with aggressive bronchodilator therapy and, if necessary, a short course of oral steroids. A starting dose for beclomethasone is generally 84 micrograms four times a day. A twice-a-day schedule may be equally effective. In patients who respond poorly to conventional doses of inhaled corticosteroids, the use of high-dose inhaled beclomethasone (up to 1600 micrograms per day) may improve asthma control and reduce systemic steroid requirements. Serious systemic side effects such as iatrogenic Cushing's syndrome and growth suppression have not yet been noted with the usual doses of inhaled corticosteroids. Abnormal pituitary and adrenal function has been reported with high-dose therapy. All patients should rinse their mouths after using these agents to avoid both nonspecific throat irritation and the development of oral candidiasis. Oral candidiasis may also be prevented by using spacer devices.

Other Medications

Antihistamines carry a warning that they should not be used in asthma patients. However, a number of studies have shown that not only are they safe in patients with severe asthma, they may have a bronchodilator effect. Newer antihistamines and antihistamines available in Europe have been shown to give dose-dependent protection against histamine-induced bronchoconstriction.

Antibiotics have not been shown to be beneficial in the treatment of asthma. However, an exception is the presence of sinusitis, which should be aggressively treated in patients with asthma because it has been demonstrated that treatment of sinusitis may improve the asthma. Erythromycin is often necessary to treat *Mycoplasma* infections that may precipitate an episode of wheezing. Erythromycin and troleandomycin (TAO) are two antibiotics that are steroid sparing. TAO has been well studied, and when used with methylprednisolone but not prednisone, it decreases the clearance of methylprednisolone, allowing the steroid dose to be decreased. These drugs also reduce the clearance of theophylline. Thus, the theophylline dose should be decreased at least 25 to 33 per cent when initiating therapy with erythromycin or TAO. TAO has been associated with significant liver abnormalities, which can necessitate discontinuation of the drug.

Expectorants have not been demonstrated to benefit the child with asthma. Their use cannot be recommended.

Medications for anxiety and sedation are generally contraindicated in patients with asthma.

In a small number of adult patients, pulmonary functions have been shown to improve after ingestion of nonsteroidal anti-inflammatory agents such as aspirin. However, a larger number of asthmatic patients may develop bronchoconstriction after taking aspirin, so it is recommended that aspirin not be given to asthmatic children. Aspirin allergy is rare in childhood asthma and more common in adult-onset asthma.

Gold salt preparations have been used for the management of asthma in Japan. Although their mode of action is uncertain, they are thought to be effective through their anti-inflammatory mechanisms.

Methotrexate has been used in severe steroid-dependent asthma in adults. Use of this antimetabolite has allowed a decrease in the daily dose of steroids.

Use of Aerosols

Therapeutic aerosols used in the treatment of asthma include MDIs, dry powder inhalers, and nebulizer solutions. Beta agonists, cromolyn, ipratropium bromide, and inhaled corticosteroids are available in aerosol form for the management of patients with asthma. MDIs are compact and portable and are ideal for children older than 6 to 7 years of age. Approximately 10 per cent of the drug reaches the airways, even with perfect inhalation technique. Because many studies have shown that these medications are improperly used, proper inhalation technique should be reviewed at each visit to the physician. MDIs

should be shaken well before inhalation. The head is tilted back to straighten the airway. Children should be instructed to breathe out fully (but not forcibly). The MDI is held between the index finger and thumb, and the mouthpiece is placed just outside a wide-open mouth and directed toward the back of the throat. Inhalation should be slow and even, and the canister should simultaneously be firmly pressed. Deposition of aerosol particles in the lung can be enhanced by low inspiratory flow rates and breath holding for 10 seconds after inhalation. A second dose may be given immediately.

To increase the efficiency of the MDI, various extension tubes (spacer devices) can be placed between the MDI and the mouth. Activation of the MDI releases the aerosol into the spacer, from which the patient slowly inhales. Inhal-Aid, InspirEase, and the Monahan aerochamber have all been useful for children who are unable to use an MDI properly. Spacers do not confer any advantage in children who use an MDI correctly.

Several beta agonists, cromolyn, and pharmacist-made atropine solutions are available as solutions that can be delivered by nebulization with either a face mask or mouthpiece. They are delivered by using a compressor (Pulmo-Aide, DeVilbiss, Somerset, Pa., 15501) or powered by wall oxygen. Many types of nebulizers are available. The main advantage of the nebulizer is that little patient coordination is required, and it can be used in crying and dyspneic children and in those too young to coordinate an MDI. The addition of intermittent positive pressure breathing does not improve the efficacy of nebulized solutions.

Approaches to Treatment

Mild Asthma. More than one-half of children with asthma have mild asthma that occurs infrequently. Often their symptoms are precipitated only by viral respiratory infections, and they may be completely symptom free, with normal or near-normal pulmonary functions, between episodes. This group includes patients who have primarily exercise-induced bronchospasm, who present only with cough, and who have fewer than two or three mild non–life-threatening acute asthmatic episodes a year. These children generally require only intermittent medications and rarely need corticosteroids.

Exercise-induced bronchospasm is best managed with either an inhaled beta-adrenergic bronchodilator or cromolyn before exercise. Albuterol has the longest duration of effect and is generally considered to be the beta agonist of choice. Cromolyn, either one capsule by Spinhaler or two inhalations of an MDI, also effectively blocks exercise-induced bronchospasm. In children in whom a beta agonist and cromolyn only partially block exercise-induced bronchospasm, the combination of albuterol followed by cromolyn is recommended. An adequate warm-up period also improves children's response to exercise.

Mild acute exacerbations of asthma can generally be treated with inhaled beta-adrenergic agents. These can be given by MDI, two inhalations every 4 to 6 hours, or as solution delivered by nebulization. An oral agent, either theophylline or an oral beta agonist, may also be beneficial. The doses given in Table 1 are provided only as guidelines. Treatment usually begins with a smaller dose and, if needed and tolerated, is increased to a larger dose. Therapy should be continued for 5 to 7 days after the child is asymptomatic and then discontinued.

Moderate Asthma. Approximately 20 per cent of asthmatic children have moderate asthma. They have frequent acute exacerbations that significantly affect their ability to function normally at their age level. Generally, these children have acute symptoms at least every 4 to 6 weeks (if not properly managed). Pulmonary functions may remain abnormal until proper control is achieved. These children generally require continuous use of medications. The initial medication may include either an inhaled or oral beta agonist, inhaled cromolyn, theophylline, or a combination. Because of the importance of inflammation in asthma, the second drug added to a beta agonist is often cromolyn, which decreases the inflammatory response, decreases bronchial hyper-reactivity, and inhibits both immediate IgE-mediated bronchoconstriction and the late asthmatic response. Occasionally, a short course of steroid therapy is required for acute exacerbations of asthma. If there is a seasonal pattern to the asthma, there may be times when less intensive therapy is adequate to control symptoms.

Severe Asthma. From 1 to 5 per cent of asthmatic children have daily symptoms, limitation of physical activity and exercise, abnormal pulmonary functions at initial evaluation, and evidence of chronic hyperinflation on physical examination. These patients require aggressive management to control their disease, including an inhaled beta agonist, cromolyn, and theophylline. If this therapy proves to be inadequate, corticosteroids are indicated. Inhaled corticosteroids should be initiated after a course of oral steroids to maximize pulmonary functions. In children who continue to experience difficulty, even with optimal doses of inhaled bronchodilators and inhaled anti-inflammatory agents such as cromolyn and/or corticosteroids, and who require large doses of oral corticosteroids to treat acute episodes, consideration should be given to alternate-day corticosteroid therapy. The use of alternate-day corticosteroids often provides optimal control of the asthma and may result in the use of lower total doses of corticosteroids. Control of the asthma should be achieved with larger doses of prednisone initially, then tapering to 20 to 40 mg every other day, using the minimal dose that controls symptoms. If the child remains well for 6 to 8 weeks, the dose should be slowly tapered.

Severe Acute Asthma (Status Asthmaticus). Treatment of severe acute asthma ideally requires an understanding of the child's history, the treatment given before presentation, and the duration and symptoms of the present episode. This information should be elicited as briefly as possible while preparations for the child's care are undertaken. Once treatment has begun, the remainder of the child's history can be obtained.

The physical examination should also be brief and should be directed at assessing the severity of the respiratory distress and detecting the complications of the attack. Signs associated with severe obstruction include intercostal and suprasternal retractions, sternocleidomastoid contractions, pulsus paradoxus greater than 20 mmHg, cyanosis, agitation or lethargy, and poor air movement with a quiet chest. With a few exceptions, there is no clear benefit to obtaining various laboratory or radiologic tests. Complete blood tests are frequently ordered, but because of various medications the child may be taking, they seldom provide useful information. Electrolyte evaluations are useful if dehydration is suspected. Chest x-ray examinations are rarely necessary unless the presence of pneumothorax or pneumonia is considered likely. Arterial blood gas levels should be obtained if there is any question as to how the child is responding and certainly if the development of ventilatory failure is suspected. A theophylline level may be useful, especially to assess compliance or to rule out toxicity. However, care should be taken if long-acting oral theophyllines have been administered because the peak level can vary from patient to patient.

Oxygen should be administered but may be discontinued as the patient condition improves. Administration of adrenergic drugs by aerosol has been shown to be as effective as administration of injected epinephrine or terbutaline. Effective bronchodilation is achieved with a much smaller inhaled than parenteral dose, and side effects are reduced. The onset and duration of action are similar. Nebulizers should be powered by wall oxygen in the emergency room and, if available, in the office, although compressors may be used. Older children may use nebulized solutions through a T tube, and infants may sit on their mothers' laps with a mask attached to the nebulizer. Doses for nebulized beta agonists are listed in Table 1. Nebulized treatments can be repeated every 20 minutes as long as the heart rate remains less than 80 per cent of the predicted maximum. If there is no satisfactory response after two or three treatments, or sooner if the patient's condition deteriorates, hospitalization and observation are probably necessary. Alternatively, treatment may begin with aqueous epinephrine (0.01 ml per kg subcutaneously) or terbutaline (0.01 ml per kg subcutaneously). If there is a good response, epinephrine crystalline suspension (Sus-Phrine, 0.005 ml per kg subcutaneously) may provide longer clinical effects; however, tachycardia and tremor are significant. Intravenous theophylline does not appear to add significantly to the bronchodilator effects of inhaled beta-adrenergic agents and should be administered cautiously if a long-acting theophylline preparation is present.

The decision to hospitalize should be made if there is severe obstruction with little response to the medications just mentioned, if improvement is not complete within 3 to 4 hours after therapy, or if an infant has symptoms with less than a complete response. Most children with an attack that has recurred within 48 hours should be hospitalized. Careful observation is the most important goal of hospitalization, and vital signs should be recorded frequently every 30 minutes to 1 hour for the first 8 hours of hospitalization. The basic laboratory studies include a chest x-ray film, arterial blood gas analysis, and peak expiratory flow measurements. A complete blood count is generally done; however, it may reveal information that is difficult to interpret. Urinalysis may demonstrate the presence of ketones and elevated specific gravity. Treatment consists of aerosolized beta agonists given every 30 minutes to 1 hour, with decreasing frequency as the child improves. Aminophylline can be administered as a bolus dose of 7 mg per kg if theophylline has not previously been given, followed by a constant infusion of 1.2 mg per kg per hour. Corticosteroids should be administered to all patients who are already using oral or inhaled corticosteroids. Corticosteroids appear to decrease the subsequent need for hospitalization. However, studies have not confirmed whether children who receive corticosteroids acutely improve faster than those who are not given corticosteroids. Most hospitalized children should receive either hydrocortisone, 5 to 7 mg per kg bolus, followed by approximately 15 mg per kg per day,*

or methylprednisolone, 1 to 2 mg per kg bolus, followed by 1 to 2 mg per kg every 4 to 6 hours.

Whether the patient is discharged from the hospital or the office, a treatment plan for the next 10 to 14 days should be carefully considered and reviewed with the patient and parents. Oral theophylline is begun at a dose extrapolated from the intravenous requirement (24-hour aminophylline dose $\times$ 0.85 divided by the dosing interval of the oral preparation). Inhaled adrenergic agonists are continued using an MDI or nebulizer. An outpatient return visit should be scheduled for less than 1 week.

Immunotherapy

Although there is no absolutely convincing evidence from controlled double-blind studies that immunotherapy is effective for children with allergic asthma, there is strongly suggestive published evidence and respectable anecdotal evidence that immunotherapy may be helpful. Experimental evidence shows that airway hyperreactivity to inhaled allergens is reduced after high-dose appropriate immunotherapy. Immunotherapy is indicated for children who have a history of allergen-induced asthma and who demonstrate IgE-mediated sensitivity to the suspected allergen by properly performed epicutaneous prick skin tests or in vitro measures of specific IgE. Immunotherapy is not indicated if there is an adequate response to environmental control and appropriate pharmacotherapy without side effects. It is important to determine the appropriate allergens to be used in patients with allergic asthma. These should include unavoidable allergens such as pollens, house dust mites, and possibly certain molds, especially *Alternaria,* which is prevalent in many parts of the United States. There is no place for immunotherapy with bacterial vaccines, tobacco, histamine, or food allergens. It is essential that reliable and potent extracts be used for both diagnosis and therapy, and that the administration of allergen extracts be started with appropriately low doses and increased progressively during a period of weeks and months at a rate that the patient can tolerate without risk of systemic anaphylactic reactions. Injections should always be administered in the office under the guidance of a physician. The child should be observed carefully for 20 minutes after each injection.

Education

To many patients and families, asthma remains a mystery. They are angry that they have the problem, confused about what triggers

---

*Usual dose is 4 mg per kg, then 2 to 10 mg per kg per day, but dose varies with disease.

asthma, and frustrated in their attempts to deal with it. The goal of an educational program is to acknowledge these issues and to convince the family that they are able, with help and support, to control the problem. The physician's attitude in this regard is critical. There is no substitute for spending enough time with the child and family to deal with these issues.

Excellent materials can be obtained from the Asthma and Allergy Foundation of America (1717 Massachusetts Ave. N.W., Suite 305, Washington, D.C., 20036, 202–265–0265); and the American Lung Association (1740 Broadway, New York, N.Y., 10019, 212–315–8770). A number of self-management programs (Air Power, Open Air, Air Wise, Living with Asthma, Family Asthma Program) have been developed and are frequently sponsored by local chapters of the Asthma and Allergy Foundation and the American Lung Association. Most asthma self-management programs deal with the following four principles: (1) asthma is a common disease, and having asthma is annoying but not disgraceful; (2) people with asthma can lead full and active lives; (3) it is much easier to prevent than to treat an asthmatic attack; and (4) people do not become addicted to asthma medications.

Armed with knowledge from the physician, and perhaps self-management programs, the patient and family can deal more easily with the stress that accompanies an acute episode of asthma, as well as the stress associated with chronic disease.

ALLERGIC RHINITIS CAUSED BY INHALANT FACTORS

method of
HOWARD M. DRUCE, M.D.
St. Louis University School of Medicine
St. Louis, Missouri

The symptoms of seasonal allergic rhinitis (hay fever) include paroxysms of sneezing, nasal pruritus and congestion, clear rhinorrhea, and palatal itching. In severe cases, especially in the peak pollen season, the mucous membranes of the eyes, middle ear, and paranasal sinuses may also be involved. This involvement may lead to conjunctival irritation, redness, and tearing; ear fullness and popping; and pressure in the cheeks and forehead. There may also be systemic symptoms of malaise, weakness, and fatigue. Classically, the symptoms appear during a defined season in which specific inhalant allergens are abundant outdoors. With this presentation, the syndrome is relatively easy to diagnose, provided that the physician is familiar with the pollinating season of the major trees, grasses, and weeds of the locale. Perennial allergic

rhinitis is caused by allergens present in the environment throughout the year. Examples include house dust mite and cockroach and animal proteins.

When the symptom complex is partially expressed, diagnosis is more difficult. Isolated chronic nasal obstruction may be a manifestation of perennial rhinitis. The nasal obstruction, in turn, may lead to sinus ostial occlusion and consequent sinusitis. Thus, although allergy is not thought to be a direct cause of sinusitis, the latter may result from obstruction of sinus drainage.

Other types of exposure may lead to special patterns of symptom production. For instance, exposure to airborne allergens in the work place may lead to symptoms occurring only during work, with a symptom-free period on weekends. Some patients who are sensitive to animal proteins may display such exquisite sensitivity that they develop symptoms of rhinitis and asthma merely by entering a house where an animal had been several hours earlier.

Ingested food allergens rarely produce rhinitis without involving other organ systems as well. Clearly, symptoms closely related in time to eating a given food may suggest a cause-and-effect relationship, but this may not be IgE mediated. Manifestations that include hives, facial swelling, or bronchospasm strongly suggest an allergic reaction, but rhinitis alone is unlikely to be mediated in this fashion. Certain medications, such as aspirin and reserpine, may induce nasal congestion and rhinorrhea, respectively. Pregnancy or the use of oral contraceptives may also produce rhinitis. Many persons develop rhinorrhea or nasal congestion when exposed to cold air or drafts, during periods of high humidity, when exposed to fumes or strong odors, after drinking wine or beer, and during emotional stress. This syndrome, known as "vasomotor rhinitis," can be differentiated from allergic rhinitis by the lack of associated nasal, palatal, or conjunctival pruritus, by symptoms displayed out of season, by negative skin tests, and by an absence of eosinophils on nasal smear.

About 10 to 12 per cent of the U.S. population suffers from allergic rhinitis, the onset of which occurs before 30 years of age in two-thirds of the patients. The peak incidence occurs in the early teens, but new cases are identifiable at any age. There is no predilection for either sex. In evaluating a case of possible allergic rhinitis, the patient's history is paramount in establishing the diagnosis. Thus, the seasonal nature of the disease and conditions that exacerbate or relieve the symptoms should be discussed. Nonspecific precipitants such as noxious fumes, smoke, odors, environmental conditions, bright lights, and alcohol should be identified because they may aggravate a hyperirritable airway.

PHYSICAL EXAMINATION

Nasal examination using a speculum is generally sufficient and should be supplemented by repeated examination after the use of a topical decongestant (such as 1 per cent phenylephrine) to reveal the posterior structures. Attention should be paid to structural abnormalities that may impede nasal airflow, such as a deviated nasal septum, septal spurs, nasal polyps, or hypertrophied turbinates. Decongestion also permits an estimate of the reversibility of mucosal swelling.

Stigmata of other atopic diseases, such as atopic eczema, conjunctivitis, or asthma support a diagnosis of allergic rhinitis, as does a family history of similar conditions. Children with allergic rhinitis often have dark patches under the eyes termed "allergic shiners" and may wipe their nose in a characteristic manner—the "allergic salute."

DIAGNOSTIC TESTS

To confirm IgE-mediated sensitivity to suspected allergens, skin tests with appropriate antigen extracts are useful. Skin testing gives a rapid result (within 15 minutes) at the time of initial consultation and is specific and sensitive. Epicutaneous (prick) skin tests are now the method of choice. Intradermal testing is used less frequently as an initial test because of its greater incidence of false-positive results. In highly suspicious cases, an intradermal test can support the results from epicutaneous testing.

Nasal smears to detect eosinophils may be used to differentiate infectious rhinitis (increased numbers of neutrophils) from allergic rhinitis (eosinophilia). However, absence of eosinophilia on the smear does not rule out an allergic etiology. Presence of eosinophilia, although suggestive of allergy, is not diagnostic, as it is also found in nonallergic rhinitis with eosinophilia (NARES syndrome). Eosinophilia does, however, suggest the likelihood of a good therapeutic response to topical nasal steroids.

In recent years, advances in technology have produced several in vitro blood tests for allergy diagnosis. These tests (such as the radioallergosorbent test or RAST) measure either the total serum IgE or specific IgE antibodies directed at defined allergens. Because of the wide variation in normal values and their overlap with patient values, total IgE levels are of limited use in the diagnosis of allergic rhinitis. Similarly, the in vitro tests for specific IgE antibodies are not required when competent skin testing can be performed. These tests are of use when dermographism and severe dermatitis preclude skin testing or in certain cases of anaphylactic sensitivity.

If there is suspicion of an anatomic abnormality that is not clearly seen through use of the speculum, posterior rhinoscopy is indicated. This procedure may be performed using the intraoral mirror; however, it may be poorly tolerated by many patients. Fiberoptic rhinoscopy with a flexible endoscope permits convenient assessment of the entire upper respiratory tract, including the nasopharynx, the openings of the eustachian tubes, and the vocal cords.

In cases with airflow obstruction possibly caused by a deviated nasal septum, an estimate of the aerodynamic flow can be obtained by measuring nasal airway resistance by rhinomanometry in each nostril before and after topical decongestion. In many cases, normal airflow values are restored after decongestion. This response suggests blockage secondary to mucosal swelling and may reduce the indications for surgery.

If there is any suspicion of chronic sinusitis (i.e., postnasal drainage, headaches, facial pain and fullness, or halitosis), sinus radiographs should be obtained.

PATHOPHYSIOLOGY

To cause allergic rhinitis, an air-borne allergen must make contact with the respiratory mucosa. Particles of the size of pollens, molds, and animal allergens (2 to 60 micrometers) are efficiently trapped and deposited on the nasal mucosa. It has been observed recently that pollen allergens can be detected in particle-free fractions of air, which suggests that microfragmentation occurs. Allergens are water-soluble proteins of 10,000 to 60,000 daltons, which on contact with either the lower or upper respiratory tract mucosa diffuse into the epithelium and stimulate the formation of specific IgE antibody in susceptible hosts.

The capacity to make increased quantities of IgE is genetically determined and requires prolonged, low-dose exposure to allergens. Exposure of atopic individuals to new allergens is usually without consequence for several years. However, after two or three allergy seasons, allergic rhinitis or asthma may develop.

Mast cells, found either in the mucosa or free in the nasal cavity, bear specific IgE directed against allergens. Contact by allergens with these cells leads to degranulation, a noncytotoxic exocytosis and release of cytoplasmic granules containing a variety of enzymes and chemical mediators into the immediate vicinity of the mast cells. The mediators released from mast cells may be preformed and thus rapidly acting (e.g., histamine), preformed and slowly eluted from the granule matrix (e.g., heparin and trypsin), or newly synthesized (e.g., the leukotrienes). Thus, an immediate, rapidly apparent reaction may lead to a prolonged inflammatory reaction as the various mediators exert their specific effects. The released mast cell mediators cause all the signs and symptoms associated with allergic rhinitis (Table 1). Many of the responses are attributable to histamine acting through its H_1 receptor, which explains why antihistamines are generally effective in treating allergic rhinitis.

Several mediators initiate reactions that do not appear until 4 to 24 hours after mast cell degranulation. These "late phase" mast cell–mediated reactions appear mainly as nasal obstruction and are caused by cellular infiltration. They are thus more difficult to treat and, not surprisingly, are poorly responsive to antihistamines and decongestants. It is thought that the late phase may be the underlying reaction in chronic rhinitis.

The amount of antigen required to elicit symptoms varies in a given individual at different times of the year. Thus, for a person who is sensitive to ragweed pollen, a greater amount of antigen is required to elicit symptoms out of season than in the height of the season. The development of nasal hyper-reactivity during allergen exposure is caused by the accumulation of neutrophils in the nasal mucosa as part of the late phase allergic reaction.

TABLE 1. **Allergic Rhinitis: Major Symptoms and Responsible Mediators***

Pathologic Event	Symptoms Elicited	Mediator(s) Responsible
Pruritus	Tickling, palatal "clicking"	Histamine (H_1 receptor), prostaglandins
Mucosal edema	Nasal obstruction	Histamine (H_1), eicosanoids, kinins
Sneezing	Sneezing and the irrepressible feeling of the need to sneeze	Histamine (H_1), eicosanoids
Secretion of mucus	Runny nose, postnasal drip	Histamine ($H_1 \pm H_2$), eicosanoids, muscarinic discharge
Late phase allergic reactions	Congestion, nasal hyperirritability	Inflammatory factors, eicosanoids, chemotactic factors

*From Druce HM and Kaliner MA: Allergic rhinitis. *In* Cherniak RM (ed): Current Therapy of Respiratory Disease–2. Toronto, B.C. Decker, 1986, p 5. Used by permission.

TREATMENT

Environmental Control

If it is practical, the patient should minimize exposure to antigens known to exacerbate the disease. This is more feasible for antigens within the home than for outdoor pollens. Exposure to the latter may be reduced by keeping windows closed and using air conditioning in the house and in automobiles. It is thus important that the physician and patient be aware of the pollinating season of allergenic species in their area, as well as in regions in which vacations might be spent.

There are a number of ways to reduce indoor air-borne allergens. Whenever possible, pets should be kept outdoors and should not be admitted to bedrooms. A significant reduction in airborne dust is possible. Patients may use zippered plastic covers over mattresses, box springs, and pillows; move books and toys to closets; dust with damp rather than dry cloths; and remove carpeting, venetian blinds, and other dust collectors. High-efficiency filter units may be helpful but should be tested before purchase. Electrostatic dust precipitators are not recommended because the ozone generated by the electrical discharge may irritate the airway mucosa.

Symptomatic Therapy for Allergic Rhinitis

Antihistamines are usually prescribed as first line therapy in allergic rhinitis, but many patients are disturbed by the soporific side effects of these drugs. Newer nonsedating antihistamines (such as terfenadine) are well accepted by patients previously unable to use antihistamines. Terfenadine (Seldane), 60 mg twice daily as needed, is currently the antihistamine of choice, despite its high cost. Other commonly prescribed antihistamines are given in Table 2.

Antihistamines are effective against sneezing, itching, and rhinorrhea; however, they are not as effective in reversing nasal congestion. For this reason, as well as to counter the soporific effects of antihistamines, decongestants, which are alpha-adrenergic agonists, have been prescribed in combination with antihistamines.

The principal side effects of oral decongestants are insomnia and irritability. Administration of these agents may interfere with urinary flow in males. Their use is contraindicated in patients who have hypertension or glaucoma, and during concomitant monoamine oxidase inhibitor therapy. Examples of combination products include clemastine fumarate and phenylpropanolamine hydrochloride (Tavist-D) and azatadine maleate and pseudoephedrine sulfate (Trinalin), prescribed as one tablet twice daily. A number of other similar drugs are available. If the side effects of one drug are unacceptable, a product

TABLE 2. **Some Commonly Used Antihistamines***

Class	Generic Name	Trade Name
Ethylenediamine	Pyrilamine	Poly-Histine†
	Tripelennamine	PBZ
Ethanolamine	Diphenhydramine	Benadryl
	Clemastine	Tavist
Alkylamine	Chlorpheniramine	Chlor-Trimeton
	Brompheniramine	Bromfed
	Triprolidine	Actifed†
Phenothiazine	Promethazine	Phenergan
Piperazine	Hydroxyzine	Vistaril
Piperidine	Azatadine	Optimine
		Trinalin†
	Cyproheptadine	Periactin
Miscellaneous	Terfenadine	Seldane

*Because so many combination and compound formulations are available, the author suggests that the physician consult the latest edition of the *Physicians' Desk Reference* for dosing details.

†Combination product with a decongestant.

containing an antihistamine from a different pharmacologic class should be selected.

Sodium cromolyn (Nasalcrom), acts by stabilizing mast cells and preventing mediator release. It has been marketed for several years as a nasal spray for treatment of allergic rhinitis. For effective topical nasal use, the medication has to be used at least four times daily. One advantage of topical nasal cromolyn therapy is that virtually no significant side effects have been reported.

Topical nasal steroids have made a major impact on the treatment of both allergic and nonallergic rhinitis. Corticosteroids have a variety of pharmacologic actions that are useful in treating allergic disease. They reduce inflammation, suppress neutrophil chemotaxis, are mildly vasoconstrictive, reduce intercellular edema, and suppress mast cell–mediated late phase reactions. Three preparations of topical nasal steroids are currently available in the United States: flunisolide (Nasalide), beclomethasone (Beconase, Vancenase), and dexamethasone (Decadron Turbinaire). At the prescribed doses, the former two may be given for a prolonged period without fear of adrenal suppression. Studies have demonstrated no evidence of mucosal atrophy, even after several years of continuous use. Dexamethasone may be given in short courses and, for treating exacerbations of chronic sinusitis, should be used in combination with antibiotics and oral decongestants. However, dexamethasone can suppress adrenal function and should be used cautiously.

Nasal steroids are relatively long-acting and can be administered twice daily. They do, however, have to be taken regularly because they are more effective in preventing symptoms than in counteracting them. The side effects of nasal steroids include nasal irritation, burning, drying, epistaxis, and, rarely, perforation. They can be minimized by the use of a saline nasal spray at intervals between the use of the steroids. Aqueous suspensions of beclamethasone are now available and are marketed as Beconase AQ and Vancenase AQ. At an initial dose of two sprays in each nostril twice daily, these preparations are currently the intranasal steroids of choice. The use of oral or intramuscular steroids is generally not indicated for treatment of allergic rhinitis. In patients receiving chronic nasal steroid therapy, a careful examination should be performed to rule out nasal septal perforation, both before commencing therapy and periodically thereafter.

Immunotherapy

Immunotherapy refers to the subcutaneous introduction of increasing doses of allergens to which the patient is sensitive. There are many putative actions of immunotherapy. Possibly the most important one is the generation of specific IgG-blocking antibody to the antigen in question. Immunotherapy also reduces IgE antibody levels, blunts the usual seasonal increase in IgE levels, reduces mast cell and basophil degranulation in response to allergen challenge, and stimulates T lymphocyte suppression of IgE production.

Immunotherapy has been demonstrated to be effective in improving rhinitis symptoms caused by grass, ragweed, birch and mountain cedar pollens, and cat allergen. Its efficacy in combatting dust and mold sensitivity is still under investigation. Immunotherapy is antigen specific; thus, the specific allergic sensitivity of the patient must be known before extracts for therapy are formulated. Allergen skin testing and a careful history are the accepted means of determining specific sensitivities. The concept of formulating an immunotherapy prescription at a laboratory remote from the patient on the basis of results of in vitro tests is strongly condemned. Allergy immunotherapy is exacting and complicated and should be administered only by an expert in this field.

The limitations of immunotherapy should be explained to the patient. Although this therapy is not a cure for allergies, 80 to 85 per cent of patients derive substantial, long-lasting symptomatic relief. If no response has occurred after 1 to 2 years at the highest tolerated maintenance dose, the patient's sensitivities should be reviewed and the prescription reformulated before proceeding. Patients given immunotherapy should be reminded of the importance of maintaining environmental control; in addition, they may have to use such concomitant medications as antihistamines.

ADVERSE REACTIONS TO DRUGS

method of
DENNIS R. OWNBY, M.D.
Henry Ford Hospital
Detroit, Michigan

Adverse reactions to drugs are common medical problems. Some estimates suggest as many as 1 in 20 pharmacotherapeutic courses results in an adverse reaction. As listed in Table 1, allergic reactions are only one form of adverse reaction accounting for 6 to 10 per cent of all adverse drug reactions. Allergic drug reactions should be differentiated from other adverse reactions because allergic reactions are likely to recur and because they are potentially more serious. Death has been reported in 1 in 10,000 allergic reactions.

TABLE 1. **Classification of Adverse Drug Reactions**

A. Immunologic or allergic reactions
 1. IgE-mediated sensitivity
 2. Antibody-mediated cytotoxicity
 3. Antigen-antibody complex disease (serum sickness)
 4. T cell–mediated immunity
B. Pseudoallergic reactions
 1. Anaphylactoid reactions from radiocontrast media
 2. Direct mediator release
 3. Sensitivity to nonsteroidal anti-inflammatory drugs
 4. Exacerbation of asthma by beta blockers
C. Probable immunologic reactions
 1. Skin eruptions
 2. Febrile mucocutaneous syndrome (Stevens-Johnson, Lyell's syndromes)
 3. Löffler's syndrome
 4. Pulmonary infiltrative disease with eosinophils
D. Nonimmunologic reactions
 1. Toxicity
 2. Side effects
 3. Drug-drug interactions
 4. Reactions related to host factors
  a. Impaired drug excretion or metabolism
  b. Enzyme deficiency
  c. Intolerance or idiosyncrasy
 5. Superinfections

ALLERGIC REACTIONS

Allergic drug reactions occur as the result of the immune recognition and response to a drug or its metabolites. Once immunologic sensitization has occurred, continued exposure or re-exposure to the drug can result in activation of the immune system and can produce a variety of clinical pictures depending on the particular portion of the immune system activated. Allergic drug reactions can usually be distinguished from other adverse reactions by using several criteria: (1) Allergic reactions to drugs usually resemble other known allergic reactions, such as urticaria, asthma, and anaphylaxis. (2) Because allergic reactions require immunologic sensitization, they do not occur on the first exposure to a drug. Symptoms of an allergic drug reaction rarely occur until at least 7 days of therapy have been completed during the initial exposure. More often, a person is sensitized to a drug during one course of treatment and reacts at the onset of a subsequent course of treatment. (3) Even though prior immunologic sensitization is required, the sensitization may not be specific for a single drug but may extend to structurally similar drugs; for example, sensitization to penicillin may result in sensitivity to other beta-lactam antibiotics. (4) The manifestations of allergic drug reactions are unlike the known pharmacologic effects of the drug (see later section on pseudoallergic reactions). (5) Reactions occur in only a small proportion of the individuals who are treated with the drug. (6) Allergic reactions can be elicited by contact with small quantities of the drug. (7) Because allergic reactions are the result of immunologic sensitization, evidence of sensitization, such as the presence of antibodies to the drug, should be present in individuals thought to have had an allergic reaction. (8) Eosinophilia is often present.

PSEUDOALLERGIC REACTIONS

Pseudoallergic reactions are difficult to differentiate from true allergic reactions because the symptoms of both result from the release of immune mediators. In contrast to true allergic reactions, pseudoallergic reactions occur as the result of direct mediator release by the drug. Immune recognition of the drug is not involved. An example of a pseudoallergic reaction is the wheal and flare response induced by the intracutaneous injection of an opiate. Although this wheal and flare response is identical to that produced by injecting allergen into allergic subjects, the wheal and flare reaction produced by opiates is classified as a pseudoallergic response because opiates are known to release histamine and other mediators directly from human mast cells. Similarly, therapeutic doses of opiates may produce generalized urticaria and pruritus that simulate an allergic reaction.

A more serious form of pseudoallergic reaction can be caused by the intravascular injection of radiocontrast agents. These agents can produce all of the signs of anaphylaxis, but because the release of chemical mediators is nonimmunologic the reactions are termed "anaphylactoid." The treatment remains the same as that for anaphylaxis.

Several other agents produce clinical symptoms that are difficult to separate from allergic reactions. Aspirin and other nonsteroidal anti-inflammatory drugs can aggravate asthma and in some individuals provoke severe asthmatic attacks within minutes of exposure. A controlled, graded aspirin challenge with repeated spirometry is the only conclusive diagnostic test, but the diagnosis should be suspected from the patient's history. A recognized syndrome is the triad of asthma, nasal polyps, and aspirin sensitivity. Individuals with aspirin-induced asthma usually cannot tolerate other nonsteroidal anti-inflammatory agents. Current options for aspirin-sensitive individuals who require therapy with a nonsteroidal agent are salsalate (Disalcid), which is usually tolerated, or desensitization by oral challenge.

Beta-adrenergic blocking drugs, including those that are relatively cardioselective, can aggravate symptoms in asthmatic patients. Even topical beta-blocking drugs such as timolol (Timoptic) have been reported to produce severe asthma attacks. These agents must therefore be used cautiously in patients with asthma.

DIAGNOSIS OF DRUG ALLERGY

The diagnosis of drug allergy is difficult because few tests are available to confirm the clinical history. Attempts can be made to detect drug-specific IgE antibodies either by skin tests or by in vitro tests such as the radioallergosorbent test or enzyme-linked immunosorbent assay. Skin tests are usually more sensitive than in vitro tests for detecting drug-specific IgE antibodies. Tests for IgE antibodies are feasible for only a limited number of drugs including beta-lactam antibiotics, insulin, heteroantisera, and some toxoids and vaccines.

Skin testing for penicillin has been extensively investigated and has been found to be safe and reliable when properly performed. Skin tests should include reagents designed to detect sensitivity to both the major and minor penicillin determinants. Benzylpenicilloyl polylysine (Pre-Pen) is a commercially available major antigen preparation. There is no commercial preparation of the minor antigenic determinants. An aqueous solution of penicillin G is often used to test for minor determinants but may not adequately represent all minor determinants and therefore a small percentage of sensitive individuals may be missed.

A common question concerning penicillin skin testing is whether negative skin tests for penicillin exclude the possibility of allergy to other beta-lactam antibiotics. The probability of an individual with a negative penicillin skin test having an allergic reaction to another beta-lactam antibiotic seems small, but there is little firm information on this issue. Studies have found positive skin tests to penicillin derivatives and cephalosporins in some individuals, but the precise value of these tests for predicting allergic reactions has not been determined.

Another issue concerning penicillin testing is the question of when to test. Most authorities have suggested that penicillin skin tests should be performed only when penicillin is the antibiotic of choice to treat an individual with a history of penicillin allergy. The practice of skin testing individuals with prior histories of possible allergic reactions to penicillin has been discouraged because of the concern that some of these individuals will be falsely reassured that they are not allergic to penicillin. In some cases the skin tests may be falsely negative; in others a previously allergic individual may have a negative test result, but with re-exposure to penicillin allergic sensitivity may return. On the other hand, many children have been labeled as allergic to penicillin because of maculopapular skin eruptions during a febrile illness that was treated with ampicillin or amoxicillin. Because of the label of penicillin allergy, these children may be treated with less effective antibiotics or antibiotics with other side effects. In this circumstance the risk of skin testing and then allowing skin test–negative children to again receive penicillin appears to be low.

The only universally applicable test for drug allergy is to rechallenge the patient with the drug in question. Before this is undertaken the relative risks and benefits must be carefully considered.

TREATMENT

The first signs suggestive of an adverse reaction in a patient taking a medication should prompt the physician to (1) attempt to define the features and severity of the reaction, (2) identify the drug most likely to have caused the reaction, (3) decide to withdraw or if necessary continue the medication, and (4) decide if therapy is needed to reduce the severity of the reaction. When a drug reaction occurs in a patient who is taking multiple medications, it may be difficult to identify the responsible drug. The first step is to attempt to relate the onset of the reaction to a change in medications, especially the addition of any medication. The second step is to consider how likely each drug is to produce a reaction. Next, each drug should be evaluated as to its necessity for the patient's care. Finally, a decision must be made to stop one or more of the patient's drugs based on the information gathered. The withdrawal of the offending drug usually results in the prompt resolution of the reaction, and no additional treatment is necessary. Whenever possible it is preferable to allow enough time for the reaction to resolve or at least begin to resolve before initiating a substitute medication.

Anaphylaxis

Anaphylaxis is the most severe form of allergic drug reaction, often starting within minutes of administration of a drug. Care must then be directed at the four life-threatening manifestations of anaphylaxis: (1) upper airway obstruction, (2) hypotension, (3) cardiac dysfunction, and (4) bronchospasm. Each of these must be repeatedly evaluated until the reaction is completely resolved.

The initial drug of choice is epinephrine, 300 micrograms (0.3 ml of a 1:1000 aqueous solution) for adults or 10 micrograms per kg up to 300 micrograms for infants and children. In most situations the epinephrine should initially be given subcutaneously. The marked peripheral vasodilatation during anaphylaxis provides rapid absorption, and the subcutaneous injection can be given with a minimum of delay. If the symptoms are severe or rapidly progressive, the dose of epinephrine can be repeated in 10 minutes. When the symptoms are profound, epinephrine can be administered intravenously, but this must be done cautiously because of the significant potential for cardiac arrhythmia. For intravenous use the epinephrine should be diluted to 1 to 2 micrograms per ml (1 mg of epinephrine equals 1 ml of a 1:1000 solution in 500 or 1000 ml of D5W). The infusion is started at 1 to 2 micrograms per minute and is then adjusted depending on the clinical response.

The patient's blood pressure must be monitored frequently. Mild hypotension often responds to the administration of epinephrine, but if this is inadequate or if marked hypotension is found, large quantities of intravenous fluids should be given rapidly. The rate of fluid delivery should be governed by the degree of hypotension, the patient's age, cardiac history, and urine output. If fluid replacement does not adequately restore blood pressure, a pressor agent such as norepinephrine or isoproterenol should be added.

The status of the patient's upper airway must

be continually assessed because obstruction can develop rapidly. The patient often first notices a sensation of swelling in the throat or pharynx followed by hoarseness or dyspnea. The airway obstruction should respond to epinephrine administration, but if severe obstruction develops rapidly intubation should be considered. Because of edema it is usually not possible to insert a full-sized endotracheal tube, and a smaller tube should be used. If total obstruction develops, cricothyroid membrane puncture should be performed to maintain ventilation.

Although they are not effective immediately, antihistamines may help control some of the manifestations of anaphylaxis, especially the cutaneous changes and the hypotension. Optimal treatment requires both an H_1 antagonist such as diphenhydramine (Benadryl) (50 to 100 mg given slowly intravenously in an adult, 1 to 2 mg per kg in children) and an H_2 antagonist such as cimetidine (Tagamet) (300 mg intravenously in an adult over 5 minutes or 5 to 8 mg per kg in children).

Cardiac dysfunction may be manifested in several ways, most commonly as low cardiac output. This condition may be caused by hypovolemia or by depression of myocardial function by anaphylactic mediators. Treatment is with epinephrine as just described or possibly with intravenous isoproterenol. A second form of cardiac dysfunction is a rhythm disturbance. Conventional treatment for the rhythm disturbance should be used along with treatment for the anaphylaxis. Oxygen should also be given to help reduce hypoxia. Refractory cardiac dysfunction may indicate that myocardial infarction occurred as a complication of the anaphylactic episode.

Bronchial obstruction may be a minor or major problem during anaphylaxis. If bronchospasm is significant and does not respond to the use of epinephrine, aminophylline should be administered. For individuals who are not currently taking oral theophylline, an initial dose of 6 mg per kg should be given intravenously during 20 to 30 minutes, followed by an infusion of 0.9 mg per kg per hour. If a patient is already taking theophylline, the dose should be reduced by at least 50 per cent and therapy is best guided by the serum levels. If the bronchospasm is not too severe, inhalation of a beta agonist may also be beneficial; in severe cases aggressive management with intubation and assisted ventilation must be considered.

With prompt treatment most episodes of anaphylaxis respond quickly to medical management; however, a second phase of anaphylaxis may occur 4 to 10 hours later. In an effort to prevent this recurrence of symptoms, corticosteroids are initially administered intravenously and then orally if possible: methylprednisolone (60 to 80 mg for adults or 1 mg per kg for children) intravenously and then an equal dose of oral prednisone 6 and 12 hours later. Because of this risk for recurrent symptoms, patients should be observed for 18 hours after an episode of anaphylaxis.

Pruritic Rashes

Pruritic rashes, including urticaria, are among the most common drug-induced reactions. Most rashes resolve within 24 to 48 hours after discontinuance of the medication. If the patient is bothered by the pruritus, antihistamines can be given either orally or intramuscularly. Among the most effective antihistamines are diphenhydramine, 25 to 50 mg every 6 hours, hydroxyzine (Atarax or Vistaril), 25 to 50 mg every 6 hours, and cyproheptadine (Periactin), 4 to 8 mg. If the pruritus is not severe or after it is initially controlled by one of these agents, a milder and less sedating antihistamine may be sufficient to control symptoms: chlorpheniramine (Chlor-Trimeton), 2 to 4 mg every 6 hours, or terfenadine (Seldane), 60 mg every 12 hours. Patients should always be warned about the sedating potential of antihistamines. Severe urticaria or urticaria combined with marked angioedema may require oral corticosteroids as for serum sickness.

Serum Sickness

Serum sickness is characterized by urticaria, angioedema, and arthralgias. Edema of the hands and feet can be severe and painful and can limit function. Fever and adenopathy may also be present. In mild cases the symptoms resolve in 1 or 2 days with only oral antihistamines. In more severe cases oral prednisone may be used to hasten resolution (prednisone, 60 mg per day tapered during 5 to 10 days for adults, 1 mg per kg per day tapered during 5 to 10 days for children).

PROPHYLAXIS AND DESENSITIZATION

Premedication has been found to be useful for preventing or reducing adverse reactions from radiocontrast medium in individuals with histories of previous reactions. Adults are given three 50-mg doses of prednisone at 6-hour intervals with the last dose 1 hour before the procedure. Also 1 hour before the procedure, diphenhydramine, 50 mg, is given orally. Ephedrine, 25 mg orally 1 hour before the procedure, has been suggested by some authorities but caution should be exercised in patients suspected of having cardiac disease. Cimetidine and aspirin have also been suggested as additional agents likely to be helpful in suppressing adverse reactions, but conclusive information is not yet available for these agents. The same pretreatment regimen might be useful to prevent allergic reactions resulting from other drugs; however, no prospective evaluations have been reported.

On rare occasions a person who is allergic to a drug must be treated with the drug because of inadequate alternatives. On these occasions desensitization may be attempted. The process of desensitization consists of administering a quantity of drug insufficient to cause a reaction and then gradually increasing the quantity of the drug until a full therapeutic dose is reached. Depending on the particular drug, the oral, subcutaneous, intramuscular, or intravenous route may be used. Desensitization should be undertaken only by experienced physicians in a hospital setting. Successful desensitization has been reported for beta-lactam antibiotics, insulin, sulfonamide antibiotics, and various antisera.

Penicillin is the drug for which desensitization is most frequently required. Although subcutaneous or intravenous routes may be used, oral desensitization is probably the safest. Penicillin is diluted in a suitable vehicle so that an initial oral dose of 100 units can be given. The dose of penicillin is then doubled every 15 minutes until a dose of 640,000 units is given, which results in a total cumulative dose of 1.4 million units. If signs or symptoms of anaphylaxis occur, treatment is given and once the symptoms are controlled the desensitization is continued. If treatment is interrupted or if the patient requires treatment again in the future, the desensitization must be repeated.

Prevention

Prevention is the ideal treatment of drug reactions. Allergic reactions can sometimes be prevented by carefully questioning patients about previous treatments and adverse effects, including potentially cross-reacting drugs. The use of drugs, especially those that more frequently produce sensitization, should be limited to essential indications. The process of starting and stopping a drug also increases the risk of allergic sensitization. Finally, a history of allergy to common environmental agents does not increase the risk of drug allergy, nor is there a relationship between allergy to seafoods and reactions to iodinated radiocontrast agents.

ALLERGIC REACTIONS TO INSECT STINGS

method of
HOWARD J. SCHWARTZ, M.D.
Case Western Reserve University,
  University Hospitals, and
    University Suburban Health Center
Cleveland, Ohio

Although insect stings usually cause only local redness, pain, itching, and swelling, which are confined to the area in which the sting has occurred and which generally subside within hours, a substantial number of persons develop systemic allergic reactions to insect stings. These allergic reactions are closely related immunologically to allergic respiratory disease in that they occur in sensitized persons, in whom these reactions are mediated by immunoglobulins of the IgE type. However, there is an equal frequency of insect sting allergy in atopic and nonatopic persons, which indicates that sensitization can occur in any person regardless of whether or not this person is otherwise allergic or comes from an allergic family.

Insect venoms contain amines and peptides, which have inflammatory and vascular effects that are responsible for the normal local, transient reactions just described. The systemic allergic reactions with which we are concerned are immunologic reactions to protein allergens in the venoms of hymenopteran insects (honeybees, yellow jackets, wasps, and hornets). These venoms contain allergens that have similar enzyme activities but different immunochemical characteristics. Therefore, testing has to be more specific than has been appreciated in the past.

The signs and symptoms of an allergic reaction are classic in that the patient first experiences local pain and other discomfort, followed in several minutes by several systemic symptoms. The symptoms may include a feeling of being ill or apprehensive, with diffuse warmth, flushing, or heat. Lightheadedness or dizziness may occur, possibly associated with observable diffuse redness, hives, and swelling of the face or lips.

The anaphylactic syndromes caused by an insect sting allergy are no different from anaphylaxis of other causes and may be manifested as cutaneous, respiratory, cardiovascular, or gastrointestinal symptoms, or a combination of these organ-specific symptoms. Most reactions begin within 15 minutes of the sting but may not reach peak intensity for 1 hour or longer. Symptoms may vary from flushing, hives, and angioedema to nausea, abdominal cramps, symptoms of upper airway edema, chest tightness, lightheadedness, hypotension, collapse, and shock. Most fatalities occur in older adults. In the United States, 50 or more deaths per year are caused by or related to insect stings. However, the true fatality rate may be higher, and postmortem analysis of serum for venom IgE antibodies may be helpful in analyzing cases of sudden death of unknown etiology.

The history usually indicates that the patient has

had many previous bee stings without incident. Often there is no history of other allergic diseases.

For the purposes of treatment, we often classify these reactions according to their pattern of severity. Large local reactions, with intense swelling at the site of the sting that may be greatly exaggerated in size and duration compared with a normal reaction, are of considerable morbidity and can frighten the patient, but they do not carry the same risk of systemic anaphylaxis or death that the other systemic reactions carry. Successive systemic reactions usually follow the same pattern in any individual but can become progressively more severe. Surveys have suggested that perhaps 3 per cent of the general population have had systemic reactions to an insect sting.

To devise a proper treatment plan, the physician must go beyond obtaining historic evidence of the reaction to look for objective evidence of venom-specific IgE antibodies. These can be demonstrated by skin testing or serologic means. If in vitro testing is chosen, it most commonly involves the radioallergosorbent test. Skin tests are performed with each of the available venom extracts (honeybee, yellow jacket, yellow hornet, bald-faced hornet, or wasp venoms) and are most safely begun with scratch or prick tests in patients in whom reactions have been very severe or nearly fatal. If these tests are negative, one proceeds to intradermal skin testing with venom concentrations of 0.001 microgram per ml and increased in tenfold increments until a clearly positive wheal and flare reaction is obtained. We do not exceed concentrations of 1.0 microgram per ml because higher concentrations may cause misleading, false-positive, nonspecific irritant reactions. The skin test responss are obtained 15 minutes after the dose is given.

If there are reasons against doing skin testing in an individual patient, venom-specific IgE antibodies can be measured in blood samples by serologic tests such as the radioallergosorbent test. These tests should be performed only by laboratories that have substantial experience and a reputation for proper standardization of controls and clinical validation of their test methods. Currently skin testing is the "gold standard." It is more frequently positive than serologic testing. Therefore, a negative blood test will not exclude venom sensitivity as frequently as a negative skin test will.

Venom skin tests are positive in more than 90 per cent of patients who have had systemic reactions. Patients who have had large local reactions often have a positive skin test as well. Therefore, a positive skin test alone should not be relied on to make a clinical decision. No one laboratory test can distinguish patients with systemic reactions from those who have had large local reactions or clinically insignificant reactions. Because the severity of the clinical reaction is not consistently correlated with the degree of test reactivity, such tests without a clinical history should not be used as the basis for clinical treatment. Asymptomatic sensitivity (i.e., a positive test with a negative history) can occur in a substantial number of patients and, again, should not be considered a reason for desensitization.

In adult patients with a history of reactions and positivity to appropriate venom antigens, the risk of a systemic reaction to another sting is as high as 60 per cent. This risk may drop many years after a sting because of a spontaneous decline in sensitivity, and it has been seen in other examples of anaphylaxis such as drug hypersensitivity. However, many individuals remain at risk for decades. Therefore, the time elapsed from the clinical sting reaction cannot reliably be used as a reason for nontreatment in any patient. Appropriate venom immunotherapy reduces the risk of a serious systemic reaction to less than 3 per cent.

The natural history of venom reactivity in children is different than in adults. The majority of children up to age 16 years who have had reactions confined to the skin (urticaria and angioedema), without respiratory or cardiovascular involvement, suffer a similar systemic reaction in up to 10 per cent of cases, but the risk of progressing to more serious anaphylaxis is less than 1 per cent.

Nonsystemic child reactors with positive skin tests also have a low risk of systemic reaction to subsequent stings compared with adults. Patients who have had only large local reactions have a 5 to 10 per cent risk of a subsequent reaction. These risk exposure rates are generally not considered high enough to warrant the use of venom immunotherapy. In children who have had systemic reactions that do involve respiratory or cardiovascular symptoms, it is thought that venom immunotherapy should be used.

PREVENTION AND THERAPY

Principles

The management of persons with a history of allergic reactions to an insect sting and with objective evidence of specific antivenom IgE is based on the substantially increased risk these persons have of suffering a severe reaction to a subsequent sting, especially if the patient is an adult. Therapeutic considerations include (1) measures to reduce exposure (i.e., avoidance), (2) making certain that the patient always possesses and knows how to use emergency medications in the event of a subsequent sting, and (3) specific venom immunotherapy.

Patients at high risk should be counseled to use special precautions. Insect repellents may not prevent hymenopteran stings. Insect nesting areas should be avoided or eliminated. Patients should avoid using trash receptacles, eating outdoors, mowing the lawn, and going barefoot. If they cannot avoid such activities, proper clothing including shoes, long-sleeved shirts, long-legged pants, and gloves should be worn and highly scented or brightly colored materials should be eschewed. Smooth-textured, snug-fitting clothing of subdued color is preferred. Food and strong odors attract insects, so great care should be taken when picnicking outdoors.

For patients with a known allergy to stinging insects, epinephrine in prefilled syringes (EpiPen,

TABLE 1. **Evaluation and Treatment of Insect Sting Allergy**

Clinical History	Conduct Test	Venom Immunotherapy
Systemic adult	Yes	Yes if test is positive
Systemic, noncutaneous in children	Yes	Yes if test is positive
Systemic, cutaneous in children only	Optional	No (risk ≤10%)
Large local	Optional	No (risk <10%)
Normal	No	No

Ana-Kit) should always be available, and the patient must be instructed in its proper use. The EpiPen has several distinct advantages. It is operated automatically and is available in a junior strength as well as the single full dose of 0.3 mg. Patients must be cautioned that this kit is not a substitute for medical attention and that after its use medical attention should be sought immediately because additional observation and treatment are often required. Antihistamines are helpful for relief of cutaneous symptoms but not for more severe anaphylactic reactions. Corticosteroids take several hours to begin working and are not important in the acute phase of the reaction. They are not a substitute for the proper use of epinephrine. Careful observation is important because symptoms may recur when the effect of the aqueous epinephrine wears off. Large local reactions are best treated with ice, antihistamines, and analgesics. A brief tapering course of oral steroids for several days may speed the resolution of a severe, large local reaction. There is a pressing need for public education by physicians and emergency room staff in short- and long-term treatment of these patients, because surveys have revealed that most individuals with systemic reactions are not informed of the risk of future reactions and frequently fail to seek proper medical consultation with an allergist after the acute reaction for proper long-term care.

Preventive Therapy: Immunotherapy

Whether or not any patient is a candidate for venom immunotherapy is determined by criteria outlined in Table 1. Whole-body extracts of stinging insects are ineffective and should not be used in treating patients with insect sting anaphylaxis. Patients who have had systemic reactions and who demonstrate clear-cut skin test reactions to tests with 1 microgram per ml of venom or less should be treated with each venom that shows a positive reaction. When maintenance immunotherapy is achieved, the same dose is repeated at intervals of up to 4 weeks. At the end of the first year of therapy, intervals can be extended to 6 weeks. Intervals beyond 6 weeks have not definitely been shown to be reliable for immunotherapy. Responses to therapy may be measured by obtaining serial determination of venom-specific IgG antibodies and by sequential measurement of IgE antibody levels. Although adverse reactions to venom immunotherapy are possible, the frequency of their occurrence is no different from that of reactions occurring in patients receiving high-dose immunotherapy for inhalant allergies. There has been no evidence of any increased risk for women receiving *maintenance* venom immunotherapy during pregnancy.

It is not clear how long venom immunotherapy must be continued. The standard recommendation is that treatment should be continued until venom sensitivity disappears. Almost 50 per cent of patients retested after receiving venom immunotherapy for 8 years are skin test negative. Although it may be safe to discontinue therapy 5 to 8 years after the institution of therapy, there is still some uncertainty in this area and further research data are needed to prove this point. Patients who stop receiving immunotherapy and are restung should be re-evaluated for the possible recurrence of systemic reactivity because the venom challenge from the new sting can represent a booster dose for the patient who has had IgE hypersensitivity.

Diseases of the Skin

ACNE VULGARIS AND ROSACEA

method of
MICHAEL T. GOLDFARB, M.D., and
CHARLES N. ELLIS, M.D.
University of Michigan Medical Center
Ann Arbor, Michigan

ACNE VULGARIS

Acne vulgaris is a disorder of the pilosebaceous unit affecting more than 80 per cent of teenagers and young adults. Comedones, pustules, papules, nodules, and cysts are found primarily on the face, chest, and back. This condition is often distressing to the patient and may lead to a poor image of the personal appearance and low self-esteem. Therefore, therapy for this benign but potentially disfiguring disease is frequently sought by the patient.

To understand how to treat acne vulgaris adequately, it is important to know its pathogenesis. An active sebaceous gland is necessary for the development of acne. Activation first occurs at puberty, when androgens stimulate the gland to produce sebum. People with acne tend to produce more sebum than those without the problem. Also, for an unknown reason, the acne patient has hyperkeratinization of the epithelium of the sebaceous follicle. This leads to a mass of keratinized cells that plug the follicle and create the first lesion of acne, the microcomedo.

Although the microcomedo is not visible, trapped sebum and keratin accumulate behind the plug, and the lesion grows into a closed comedone or whitehead. The pore may widen slowly and the lesion becomes an open comedone, or blackhead. The dark pigment seen in blackheads is not "dirt," but probably melanin from melanocytes at the follicular orifice.

Open comedones, having a wide pore, are able to discharge accumulated debris into the outside environment; in rare cases, they rupture or become inflamed. The closed comedo cannot discharge its contents and creates the perfect environment for the overgrowth of a normal bacterial inhabitant of the sebaceous follicle, *Propionibacterium acnes*. This anaerobic bacterium produces chemotactic substances that diffuse across the abnormal epithelium and attract neutrophils. The neutrophils, in turn, ingest *P. acnes* and release hydrolytic enzymes that rupture the follicular wall. The entire content of the follicle, including keratin, hair, bacteria, and sebum, may be discharged into the dermis, producing inflammation.

P. acnes produces lipases that break the sebum triglycerides into free fatty acids. Free fatty acids are especially irritating when they enter the dermis and promote inflammation. Thus, ruptured microcomedones and closed comedones become the pustules, papules, nodules, and cysts of inflammatory acne.

Treatment

With therapy, acne vulgaris can usually be brought under control. However, most acne treatments do not offer a cure, and the problem recurs if therapy is discontinued. Therefore, the patient and physician may have a long relationship until the acne slowly abates, usually but not always in the early twenties.

During early visits, patients should be carefully educated about the pathogenesis of acne and the rationale for treatment. There are numerous myths about acne that must be dispelled. First, acne is not caused by poor hygiene, so excessive washing and scrubbing of the skin are not only unnecessary but may even stimulate the disease. Second, picking and popping pimples can lead to increased inflammation and scarring of the skin and must be avoided. Third, the notion that a high-fat diet (e.g., chocolate, fried foods) worsens acne has been disproved by clinical studies. Only if a patient complains that a certain food consistently flares the skin should any dietary restrictions be imposed.

A careful history concentrating on current skin care is essential. Many patients have used various over-the-counter (OTC) preparations for acne before their first visit. They may also be applying an oil-based moisturizing cream or cosmetic that is comedogenic and causes the disease to flare. An occasional patient may be taking a systemic medication that is inducing or exacerbating the acne. Certain occupations, including short-order cook and mechanic, expose the skin to excessive external greases and can cause acne to flare. Finally, emotional stress worsens the condition.

Patients should be instructed to wash the involved areas of the skin gently with a mild soap twice a day. They must be warned never to manipulate or aggressively scrub the acne lesions. Also, only water-based or oil-free products should be used on the skin.

Topical Therapy

The mainstay of acne treatment is topical medications. These agents are extremely safe, with local irritation being the only common side effect. Most cases of comedonal or papular acne can be brought under control without systemic therapy. In general, topical treatments work primarily by preventing the formation of acne and are less effective at clearing lesions already present. Therefore, the patient should apply the medication to the entire area that is involved, not only to individual lesions. Improvement usually takes a minimum of several weeks. Currently, a wide variety of effective topical medications is available for the treatment of acne.

Tretinoin. The best agent for comedonal acne is topical tretinoin (Retin-A), which is also efficacious for papular and pustular disease. Tretinoin is available as a cream (0.025, 0.05, 0.1 per cent), gel (0.01, 0.025 per cent), or liquid (0.05 per cent). It works by reducing the cohesiveness of the keratinocytes at the follicular orifice, which leads to a decrease in comedo formation and the expulsion of existing comedones.

Tretinoin should be applied to the involved area once or twice a day. Initially, the patient may complain of irritation and inflammation of the skin, but these usually resolve in 1 to 2 months. Of the three different preparations, tretinoin cream is the least irritating and easiest to tolerate. Therefore, we frequently begin therapy with tretinoin 0.025 per cent cream daily. Improvement takes approximately 4 to 6 weeks, and there may even be an exacerbation of the acne during the first weeks of therapy. As the skin becomes more tolerant of the tretinoin therapy, the strength of the cream can be increased to 0.05 per cent. Alternatively, medication may be changed to the more penetrating but also more irritating gel preparation.

Benzoyl Peroxide. Topical benzoyl peroxide is available as both a prescription and OTC medication for acne vulgaris. It is currently the most frequently used therapy for acne. There are numerous different preparations available, including gels, creams, lotions, washes, and even a facial mask in concentrations of 2.5, 5, and 10 per cent. The primary effect of benzoyl peroxide is antibacterial, greatly reducing the concentration of *P. acnes* on the skin. It also has some mild comedolytic properties. Therefore, comedonal and papular acne respond well to this therapy.

Benzoyl peroxide can be irritating and drying at the initiation of therapy. Approximately 1 to 2 per cent of patients develop an allergic contact dermatitis, and therapy must be discontinued. The vehicle plays an important role in the delivery of benzoyl peroxide. Prescription gel formulations (Desquam-X, PanOxyl, Persa-Gel) are the most effective but also the most irritating. We frequently begin patients with the 5 per cent gel on a daily basis. The benzoyl peroxide washes are convenient for treating large areas of involved skin, especially the chest and back.

Topical Antibiotics. The use of topical antibiotics for acne vulgaris has become popular during the past decade. Clindamycin (Cleocin T), erythromycin (T-Stat, A/T/S, Erycette, Erygel), tetracycline (Topicycline), and meclocycline (Meclan) are currently available in a variety of vehicles (solutions, pads, gels, creams) at concentrations ranging from 0.22 to 2 per cent. These antibacterial agents inhibit the growth of *P. acnes* but have no comedolytic effect. They are most effective in patients with papular and pustular disease.

Currently, topical clindamycin and erythromycin solutions are the most widely used. They are applied to the involved areas twice daily. Topical antibiotics are well tolerated, and patients have less irritation and dryness than with benzoyl peroxide or tretinoin. A rare patient has developed diarrhea and even pseudomembranous colitis while using topical clindamycin. Therefore, all patients should be warned to stop applying clindamycin if persistent diarrhea occurs.

Other Agents. Numerous OTC exfoliating medications are currently available for the treatment of acne, including salicylic acid, resorcinol, and sulfur. By drying and peeling the skin, they hasten the resolution of comedones, papules, and pustules. In general, they are not comedolytic and are unable to prevent the formation of new lesions. For patients who are unable to tolerate tretinoin or benzoyl peroxide, these agents may be a viable alternative. Salicylic acne pads are convenient and effective.

Topical Therapy for Black Patients. Many black patients are accustomed to applying various emollients and ointments to their skin to keep it moist. It is important to discourage this practice to avoid additional comedo formation. Also, the dryness and scaling associated with the use of topical tretinoin and benzoyl peroxide can give skin of black patients an ashy appearance. This may be cosmetically unacceptable to the patient. Therefore, we tend to use more topical antibiotics and avoid the higher concentrations of tretinoin or benzoyl peroxide when treating the black patient.

Combination Therapy. Often two topical agents are prescribed concurrently, with excellent results. Successful combinations include tretinoin and benzoyl peroxide, tretinoin and a topical antibiotic, or benzoyl peroxide and a topical antibiotic. The rationale for combination therapy is to attack different aspects of the pathogenic pathway simultaneously. Also, tretinoin, with its comedolytic effect, can enhance the penetration of benzoyl peroxide or a topical antibiotic into the sebaceous follicle.

If two topical medications are applied at exactly the same time, they may inactivate each other. Therefore, we recommend that the patient use one agent in the morning and the other in the evening. However, there is currently one product available that contains both erythromycin and benzoyl peroxide in a stable form (Benzamycin Topical Gel). This medication remains active for up to 3 months if kept refrigerated and is quite effective, partly because it provides dual therapy in a single convenient application.

Systemic Therapy

Although topical medications are usually sufficient, some patients require systemic therapy. Oral medications should be considered when the acne has proved to be recalcitrant to topical therapy, when large areas of the body are involved, or when cystic lesions are present.

Systemic Antibiotics. For more than 30 years, oral antibiotics have played an important part in acne management. By suppressing the growth of *P. acnes*, they can markedly improve inflammatory acne. However, systemic antibiotics are ineffective for noninflammatory comedonal disease. When antibiotics are used orally instead of topically, improvement is frequently greater and occurs in less time. Also, oral antibiotics are far more convenient for the treatment of widespread disease and for treating areas not easily reached by the patient.

Tetracycline (Sumycin, Achromycin V) is the most commonly prescribed systemic antibiotic for the treatment of acne. It is effective, generally free of serious side effects, and inexpensive. The usual dose is 500 to 1000 mg per day orally, depending on the size of the patient and the severity of the disease. As the acne clears, the dose can be slowly tapered. The absorption of tetracycline is greatly hindered by food, especially dairy products. Therefore, it must be taken on an empty stomach 1 hour before or 2 hours after meals. Also, tetracycline is phototoxic, and patients are more susceptible to a severe sunburn. The most common side effects reported are gastrointestinal upset and candida vaginitis. Tetracycline can permanently stain developing teeth, so it should not be used in pregnant or lactating patients or in children under 9 years of age.

The second most commonly used oral antibiotic for acne is erythromycin (E-Mycin, ERYC). It is effective at a dose of 250 to 1000 mg per day orally. Erythromycin is well tolerated. An occasional patient may experience significant gastrointestinal discomfort and may have to discontinue therapy.

Many other antibiotics have been used systemically to treat acne with excellent results. Minocycline (Minocin), a derivative of tetracycline, is extremely efficacious at a dose of 100 to 200 mg per day orally. Unfortunately, it is expensive, and some patients may experience headaches and dizziness. Cefadroxil (Duricef), at 500 mg orally per day, is safe and effective, but quite expensive. Oral clindamycin (Cleocin) is an effective therapy for acne, but the risk of pseudomembranous colitis has limited its use. For severe cases of cystic acne, sulfone (Dapsone) has been a successful treatment. However, the risk of hemolytic anemia makes it difficult to use. Finally, trimethoprim-sulfamethoxazole (Bactrim) has been used with positive results.

Many systemic antibiotics have been said to reduce the effectiveness of oral contraceptives; patients should be appropriately advised.

The addition of topical agents (e.g., benzoyl peroxide or tretinoin) to systemic antibiotic therapy provides improved results.

Systemic Retinoids. In the past, vitamin A (retinol) was used systemically for the treatment of acne. However, high doses were required to achieve even minimal improvement. Therefore, patients had only slight clearing of their acne and experienced many of the side effects of hypervitaminosis A.

The development of the retinoid isotretinoin (Accutane), a synthetic derivative of vitamin A, has revolutionized the treatment of severe, recalcitrant nodulocystic acne. It is currently the most efficacious therapy for acne and can reduce the number of inflammatory lesions by 90 per cent in almost all cases. Isotretinoin is the only treatment that can lead to prolonged remissions of acne even after therapy is discontinued.

The exact mechanism of action of isotretinoin is unknown, but it does have many different effects that are clearly of benefit for the treatment of acne. During therapy, isotretinoin decreases sebum production, reduces the concentration of

P. acnes, reverses the abnormal follicular keratinization, and even has a direct anti-inflammatory effect on the skin. None of these effects appear to be permanent after treatment is discontinued, and the reason for the long-term remission of disease remains obscure.

There are many side effects associated with isotretinoin therapy, and it is reserved for severe cases of cystic acne resistant to other treatments. Patients should be treated with 1 to 2 mg per kg per day orally for approximately 20 weeks. We tend to use the higher doses for disease involving the chest and back. Some patients have a flare of their acne during the first month of therapy. Most show significant improvement after 2 months of treatment. Even if patients are not clear at the end of the course of isotretinoin, they may continue to improve afterward. A second course is rarely needed, and a minimum of 8 weeks should be allowed before it is considered.

The side effects of isotretinoin are the same as those of hypervitaminosis A. Almost all patients complain of dryness of the mucous membranes. Chapped lips (cheilitis), dry nose, and dry eyes are extremely common. We recommend that patients use an ointment on the lips and apply natural tears to the eyes during therapy. Other problems less commonly experienced during therapy include myalgias and arthralgias, hair loss, and headaches. Laboratory tests should be monitored before and monthly during therapy. Up to 25 per cent of patients have elevated serum lipid levels, especially triglycerides. Also, abnormal liver function tests are occasionally noted during treatment. Fortunately, these side effects and laboratory abnormalities resolve 1 month after therapy has been discontinued.

Isotretinoin is a potent teratogen, and this has become the most serious problem with its use. If any isotretinoin is taken during pregnancy, there is a significant risk of serious birth defects. No woman who is pregnant or trying to conceive should ever be given isotretinoin. Women with childbearing potential should have a negative serum pregnancy test before and monthly during therapy. Also, only the highly effective oral contraceptive pills are adequate protection for birth control while taking isotretinoin. After the patient has had one normal menstrual cycle without therapy, she can conceive without any increased risk of birth defects.

Systemic antibiotics, especially tetracyclines, should be stopped during isotretinoin therapy to reduce the risk of pseudotumor cerebri.

Estrogen Therapy. Systemic estrogens have been helpful in the management of acne in women who fail to respond to topical agents and systemic antibiotics. They work by suppressing androgen production, which results in a decrease in sebaceous gland activity. Treatment usually consists of using an oral contraceptive pill in a 3-week cycle. At least 0.05 mg orally of ethinyl estradiol or mestranol (Ovulen) daily is required to suppress sebum production. It usually takes 3 to 4 months to achieve significant sebum suppression and improvement of the acne. Also, during the first 2 months of therapy, many patients experience a flare of their disease. Estrogen therapy has numerous side effects, including nausea, weight gain, hypertension, and even the serious risk of thromboembolism.

Corticosteroid Therapy. Oral corticosteroids, with their anti-inflammatory action, are sometimes necessary to treat an explosive episode of inflammatory acne. This severe acne flare may occur spontaneously or may be caused by the initiation of therapy. Oral prednisone (Deltasone), at a dose of 20 to 40 mg daily for approximately 7 to 10 days, is usually efficacious. Prolonged therapy with corticosteroids may lead to serious side effects as well as steroid acne.

Low-dose corticosteroids can be a successful therapy for women with acne caused by overproduction of adrenal androgens. This can be demonstrated by an elevated blood level of dehydroepiandrosterone sulfate. Oral dexamethasone (Decadron), 0.25 to 0.5 mg nightly, suppresses the activity of these androgens and helps to clear the acne. Unfortunately, it frequently takes months to achieve any substantial improvement.

Other Systemic Therapies. The nonsteroidal antiinflammatory medication ibuprofen (Motrin) enhances the efficacy of oral tetracycline. Spironolactone (Aldactone), with its antiandrogen effect, has been helpful for some women with treatment-resistant acne. Oral zinc, which was initially found to be an excellent therapy for acne by a clinical study, has not proved to be effective in general use.

Office Therapy

Minor Office Surgery. Open comedones or blackheads are unsightly and easily expressed with a comedo extractor. Closed comedones, or whiteheads, which have the potential to become inflammatory lesions, can be expressed only after the pore has been widened with, for example, a No. 11 Bard-Parker scalpel blade or needle. Acne "cysts" are not true, walled cysts. They should not be lanced, as increased scarring is likely to occur; instead, it is preferable to instill corticosteroids.

Intralesional Corticosteroid Injections. Intralesional corticosteroids are useful to clear nodular or cystic acne lesions rapidly. Less than 0.1 ml of short-acting triamcinolone (Kenalog), 2.5 mg per ml, injected into the center of the lesion with a 30-gauge needle, usually causes the acne cyst or nodule to resolve in only a few days. Care must be taken not to inject an area with a large amount of corticosteroids to avoid the possibility of skin atrophy. Also, a persistent lesion should not be reinjected for at least 2 to 3 weeks.

Cryosurgery. The resolution of cystic acne lesions can be hastened by a superficial freeze with liquid nitrogen. With either a cotton swab or spray apparatus, liquid nitrogen is applied to the involved skin for two 15-second freeze cycles. It is believed to work by superficially desquamating the skin.

Ultraviolet Light. The use of artificial ultraviolet light in the physician's office has greatly decreased during the past decade. It has been found to be only minimally effective and may even increase the comedo count. Many patients report improvement of their acne with natural sunlight. This is probably the result of a tan, which makes the lesions less evident.

Treatment of Acne Scars. Deep inflammatory acne lesions may leave a scar after they resolve. This scar can be a sharply punched-out pit, an atrophic macule, or a keloid. Keloids are more commonly found on the chest and back. These scars are permanent but may become less prominent with time.

Numerous surgical procedures have been developed to correct acne scarring. Patients with multiple depressed scars of even depth may have a 50 per cent improvement with dermabrasion. Sharply punched-out pits can be removed with punch excision. Keloid scars of the chest and back often flatten with the intralesional injection of triamcinolone, 10 to 40 mg per ml. Depressed scars can be improved by injecting purified bovine dermal collagen (Zyderm).

ROSACEA

Rosacea, or acne rosacea, is a chronic skin disorder that occurs primarily in middle age. it is characterized by erythema, telangiectasias, papules, and pustules without any comedones. The face is primarily involved, especially the nose, cheeks, forehead, and chin. Rosacea involves the eyes in approximately 50 per cent of patients. Ocular rosacea is characterized by blepharitis, conjunctival hyperemia, chalazia, and even keratitis and iritis. Some rosacea patients, usually men, develop a lobulated enlargement of their nose called rhinophyma. This is caused by hypertrophy of both the sebaceous glands and connective tissue of the nose. The nasal tip and ala are most commonly involved. The etiology of rosacea is unknown. Many theories have been proposed, including an increased propensity to flushing, overexposure to sun and heat, and even infestation with the mite *Demodex folliculorum.*

Treatment

Patients should avoid stimuli that provoke facial vasodilation and may aggravate their condition. This includes excessive exposure to extreme heat, cold, and sunlight, as well as ingestion of hot liquids, spicy foods, and alcohol.

Systemic Therapy

Tetracycline is the treatment of choice for rosacea. It can effectively clear the papules, pustules, and ocular lesions. However, the telangiectasias and rhinophyma do not respond well to tetracycline. The mechanism of action of tetracycline in rosacea is unclear. It may work by suppressing the inflammation of the disease rather than as an antibacterial agent.

An effective dose for oral tetracycline therapy is 500 mg daily. The patient usually begins to respond in 1 to 2 months. Once the rosacea has sufficiently cleared, the tetracycline can frequently be tapered to 500 mg three times a week. Because of the chronic nature of the disease, therapy may have to be continued for years.

Many other systemic antibiotics, including metronidazole (Flagyl), erythromycin, minocycline, and ampicillin, have been used with some success for the treatment of rosacea. In general, they are not as effective as tetracycline therapy. Therefore, we use these agents only for patients who are unable to tolerate or have failed to improve with tetracycline.

For severe, recalcitrant rosacea, isotretinoin has been tried with some success. However, isotretinoin does not induce the same dramatic clearing and long-term remission with rosacea as it does with nodulocystic acne. It should be used only if all other therapeutic attempts have failed.

Topical Therapy

Topical corticosteroids may help to reduce the erythema and inflammation of rosacea. They should be used for only short periods to avoid accentuating the telangiectasias. Also, it is best to use only a weak corticosteroid, such as hydrocortisone 1 per cent cream (Hytone) once daily.

In the past, topical antibiotics have not been effective for rosacea. Recently, topical metronidazole 0.75 per cent gel (MetroGel) became available. It works primarily by producing an anti-inflammatory effect. When this agent is applied twice daily, there is a significant reduction of the papules and pustules of rosacea.

Creams containing 2 to 10 per cent precipitated sulfur have been used for the treatment of rosacea for many years. They are well tolerated and can be quite helpful for some patients. However, results of this therapy vary greatly, and it does not stand up to rigorous clinical testing. A combination of sodium sulfacetamide and sulfur in a flesh-tinted lotion (Sulfacet-R) can effectively camouflage as well as help clear the papules and pustules of rosacea.

Surgical Therapy

The fine telangiectasias can be removed by electrodesiccating the vessels with a fine epilating needle. Because of the multiple connections of these vessels, the telangiectasias frequently recur and require retreatment.

A variety of surgical techniques have been developed to treat rhinophyma. The excess tissue can be removed with scalpel excision, electrodesiccation, liquid nitrogen cryosurgery, dermabrasion, and argon or carbon dioxide laser surgery. Therapy can greatly reduce the size of the nose and improve the patient's overall appearance.

HAIR DISORDERS

method of
ROBERT B. SKINNER JR., M.D., and
E. WILLIAM ROSENBERG, M.D.
University of Tennessee
Memphis, Tennessee

There are many hair disorders, both inherited and acquired. However, most fall into one of a few common categories.

PATTERN HAIR LOSS

Pattern (androgenic) hair loss is common in men (25 per cent of men by age 30; 60 per cent by age 60) and, to a lesser degree, in women. it is a result of an inherited tendency whose expression is modified by androgen and estrogen. A diagnostic hallmark of pattern hair loss is its familiar location at the man's frontal hairline and vertex and the woman's crown. A further diagnostic aid is the fact that the patient is usually not aware that an increased amount of hair is coming out but finds unexpectedly that the hair on the scalp is becoming sparse.

Men who wish to treat their pattern hair loss should be reminded that it is not considered to be a disease, that the costs of treating it are not ordinarily reimbursable, and that most women don't mind it. Those who wish to treat it can be offered the choice of surgical procedures (e.g., punch graft transfers, scalp reductions, flaps), which are expensive but permanent, or medical treatment, which is less expensive but is expected to last only for the duration of treatment.

The only proven medical therapy for male pattern hair loss is 2 per cent minoxidil solution (Rogaine) applied twice daily. It works best in preventing further hair loss at the male vertex. Those men most likely to be helped by minoxidil are younger than 40 years old, have fewer than 10 years of balding, and have less than a 10 cm² bald area at the vertex. The concomitant use of a 0.025 per cent retinoic acid preparation once a day appears to enhance the effectiveness of minoxidil treatment. We think that, once started, the treatment should be continued for at least 12 months before failure is determined. There appear to be no important side effects.

Although minoxidil is not officially approved for the woman with pattern hair loss, we prescribe it and retinoic acid for these patients. A different approach to the treatment of pattern hair loss in women is to try to modify the hormonal effect on scalp hair bulbs with the use of either estrogen replacement or spironolactone. We do not use this treatment.

TELOGEN HAIR LOSS

Human hairs grow for about 4½ years at a rate of about 0.1 mm per day. They then stop growing, loosen their connection to the root, and fall out at the rate of about 100 per day. Some 4 to 6 months later, a new hair begins to grow from the same root.

A variety of medical conditions stop some, many, most, or almost all hairs from growing. When that happens, there is pronounced shedding after a delay of 3 to 8 months. By far the most common event causing telogen hair loss is childbirth. Usually the baby is 4 to 5 months old when the hair loss is discovered and is walking and talking by the time it has spontaneously resolved. No treatment except reassurance is required or helpful.

Other causes of telogen hair loss need to be looked for and sometimes corrected. These include sudden or pronounced weight loss (especially if great enough to interfere with the menstrual cycle), withdrawal of birth control pills, iron deficiency anemia, hypo- or hyperthyroidism, or a reaction to any severe illness or trauma such as high fever, general anesthesia, or automobile accidents.

We do not think that mental stress induces this condition.

ALOPECIA AREATA

Usually the diagnosis of alopecia areata is straightforward: the sudden, almost overnight, appearance of smooth, circular patches of total hair loss on the scalp and body. Rarely, the diagnosis is difficult. In such cases, a biopsy from the edge of a bald spot may be helpful. The finding of associated nail pitting may be an additional diagnostic aid. Most cases of alopecia areata remain confined to a limited number of spots, and most resolve spontaneously in 6 to 12 months. When treatment is desired, we use the following, in order:

1. Localized areas are injected intralesionally with 10 mg per ml triamcinolone through a 30-gauge needle, giving up to 20 mg per monthly session.

2. More extensive areas, and alopecia areata in small children, are treated by nonspecific irritation, using 1 per cent anthralin cream applied often enough (usually two or three times per week) to keep the bald areas pink and mildly irritated.

3. A more effective but more difficult treatment is the induction of allergic contact dermatitis on the bald sites. This is effective up to 85 per cent of the time on spots and 35 to 50 per cent of the time on totally bald scalps. We induce a contact sensitivity to squaric acid dibutyl ester (SADBE) by painting a small spot on the forearm with a 2 per cent alcohol solution and covering the area with an adhesive bandage for 2 weeks. Most persons become allergic to this apparently harmless chemical after about 10 days and develop a red, oozing blister at the application site. Depending on the appearance of the test reaction, a prescription is then written for a 1:1000, 1:10,000, or 1:100,000 dilution in acetone to be applied sparingly to bald areas once or twice a week. Hair growth is usually seen by the end of 4 or 5 months of treatment. SADBE is not an approved medication and is not available except through chemical supply houses. Its use requires the help of a competent pharmacist and is probably not feasible in most practices.

4. Two per cent minoxidil is easier to use and is readily available. We have had less experience with it in alopecia areata than with SADBE. It is probably a better initial choice.

TRICHOTILLOMANIA

Irregular, patchy hair loss is the result of conscious or unconscious pulling, tugging, twirling, or other manipulation of scalp hair. It is most common in young people and children and can be difficult to diagnose and communicate to the patient. Biopsy of an affected area is useful. The nightly application of petrolatum makes the hairs harder to manipulate and reminds the patient of what he or she is doing. Behavioral therapy affords the best hope for treatment of resistant cases, and the advice of a psychiatrist is sometimes advisable.

TRACTION ALOPECIA

Excessive traction exerted along the hair shaft can damage the growing root and result in hair loss. It is most commonly seen in young black women who exert traction in the process of braiding, platting, cornrowing, or trying to straighten their hair. It is not unknown in caucasians, however, and was seen as a consequence of the use of brush rollers during the bouffant era and of tightly applied rubber bands on ponytails. Characteristically, the edge of the scalp is spared (the last few hairs being impossible to grasp). The only treatment is further avoidance of trauma. Continued traction can cause permanent hair loss.

FUNGUS INFECTION

The formerly common fluorescent patchy ringworm seen only in children and easily diagnosed with a Wood's light has now virtually disappeared. In its place is a hard-to-diagnose, nonfluorescent ringworm that affects persons of all ages and varies in appearance from a mild case of dandruff to a widespread, purulent, boggy kerion. The classic lesion is a circular area of hair loss with small black dots visible when infected hairs have broken off at the scalp line.

Diagnosis is best made by gently removing a tiny black dot fragment of hair and examining it with a potassium hydroxide microscopic preparation. The appearance of small, translucent spores within the hair shaft remnant is diagnostic. A wetted Culturette (Marion Laboratories) swab inoculated on Sabouraud's medium is the next best diagnostic measure, and a biopsy specimen stained with periodic acid–Schiff reagent is third best. The usual potassium hydroxide examination of scale is not reliable. The only effective treatment is systemic griseofulvin continued for at least 3 months. Family members also deserve close scrutiny.

OTHER CAUSES

There are many other causes of hair loss. The recent onset of patchy hair loss deserves a serologic test for syphilis. Other patients with unexplained hair loss require consultation with a specialist.

CANCER OF THE SKIN

method of
JAIME A. TSCHEN, M.D.
Baylor College of Medicine
Houston, Texas

Skin cancer accounts for 30 to 40 per cent of all new cancers each year. Malignant melanoma, the most aggressive skin cancer, has shown a rapidly climbing occurrence rate: almost 22,000 new cases in a year, with about 6000 deaths per year in the United States. No other malignancy—except for lung cancer in women—has shown such an alarming increase in mortality (currently 10 to 20 per cent).

The prognosis for all skin cancers is better now than ever before because of public education and earlier detection. In most cases, pathologic confirmation of the clinical diagnosis should precede treatment.

Some of the most important facts about skin cancer are summarized here (from the American Cancer Society: Cancer Facts and Figures. New York, American Cancer Society, 1985, p. 10, with permission):

INCIDENCE: Over 400,000 cases a year, the vast majority of which are highly curable basal or squamous cell cancers. They are more common among individuals with lightly pigmented skin, living at latitudes near the equator. The most serious skin cancer is malignant melanoma, which strikes about 22,000 men and women each year.

MORTALITY: An estimated 7400 deaths a year, 5500 from malignant melanoma, and 1900 due to other skin cancers.

WARNING SIGNALS: Any unusual skin condition, especially a change in the size or color of a mole or other darkly pigmented growth or spot.

RISK FACTORS: Excessive exposure to the sun; fair complexion; occupational exposure to coal tar, pitch, creosote, arsenic compounds, and radium. Among blacks, because of heavy skin pigmentation, skin cancer is negligible.

PREVENTION: Avoid the sun between 10:00 AM and 3 PM when ultraviolet rays are strongest, and by using protective clothing. Use 1 of the growing number of sunscreen preparations, especially those containing such ingredients as PABA (paraaminobenzoic acid). They come in varying strengths, ranging from those that permit gradual tanning to those allowing practically no tanning at all.

EARLY DETECTION: Recognition of changes in scales or the appearance of new skin growths is the best way to find early skin cancer. Basal and squamous cell skin cancers often take the form of a pale, waxlike, pearly nodule, or a red, scaly, sharply outlined patch.

Melanomas are usually distinguished by a dark brown or black pigmentation. They start as small, mole-like growths that increase in size, change color, become ulcerated, and bleed easily from a slight injury.

TREATMENT: There are 4 methods of treatment—surgery, radiotherapy, electrodesiccation (tissue destruction by heat), or cryosurgery (tissue destruction by freezing).

For malignant melanoma, adequate surgical excision of the primary growth is indicated. Nearby lymph nodes may be removed. The microscopic examination of all suspicious moles is essential.

SURVIVAL: For basal cell and squamous cell cancers, cure is virtually assured with early detection and treatment. Malignant melanoma, however, can spread to other parts of the body quickly. The 5-year survival rate for white patients with malignant melanoma is 82 percent compared with 95 percent for patients with other kinds of skin cancer.

TREATMENT OF BASAL CELL CARCINOMA

Most basal cell carcinomas are treated by curettage and desiccation under local anesthesia. Cure rates are higher than 90 per cent, and cosmetic results are usually good. Recurrent lesions or tumors located in strategic areas, for example, around the eyes, ears, nose, mouth, or fingers, frequently require Mohs' micrographic surgery. X-ray therapy is usually reserved for older individuals with tumors in areas that are difficult to reconstruct (eyelids, nose). Cryosurgery is sometimes used; however, it requires specialized equipment (thermocouples) and expertise. New treatments on the horizon include the use of retinoids and interferons.

TREATMENT OF SQUAMOUS CELL CARCINOMA

Most squamous cell carcinomas can be treated by curettage and desiccation or surgical excision with a high cure rate. Lesions arising in mucocutaneous junctions or in previously damaged tissues, such as burned areas, osteomyelitic areas with sinus tracts, or tissue affected by radiodermatitis, behave more aggressively and have a higher incidence (up to 30 per cent) of regional metastasis; therefore, complete excision should be attempted initially.

TREATMENT OF MALIGNANT MELANOMA

Early or thin melanomas (less than 1 mm thick) can be treated with complete excision with adequate margins (usually 1 to 2 cm and down to fascia). Thicker tumors usually require wider margins; in some studies, a selected group of tumors benefited from regional node dissection. No uniformly good results are obtained with any therapy for advanced disease.

As a rule, no destructive methods (curettage

and desiccation, cryosurgery) should be used for melanomas because they do not provide adequate pathologic information most often required for determination of appropriate therapy. Adequate sampling (by punch or incisional biopsies) can often be done on melanomas without compromising the final treatment.

Remember the danger signs of pigmented lesions (modified mnemonic of the American Academy of Dermatology):

A: Asymmetry—one-half of the lesion unlike the other half
B: Border irregular—scalloped or poorly circumscribed border
C: Color—varied from one area to another; shades of tan, white, brown, black, red, or blue
D: Diameter—larger than 6 mm (diameter of pencil eraser) as a rule
E. Elevation—recent change in thickness of the lesion

TREATMENT OF OTHER CUTANEOUS MALIGNANCIES

Mammary and extramammary Paget's disease, Kaposi's sarcoma, dermatofibrosarcoma protuberans, angiosarcoma, mycosis fungoides, cutaneous lymphomas, adnexal carcinomas, and other less common malignancies require specialized treatment most of the time.

PAPULOSQUAMOUS ERUPTIONS

method of
WALTER H. C. BURGDORF, M.D.
University of New Mexico School of Medicine
Albuquerque, New Mexico

Papulosquamous eruptions are as much a diagnostic as a therapeutic problem. In addition to the conditions covered in this section, drug eruptions and secondary syphilis frequently enter into the list of possible diagnoses.

SEBORRHEIC DERMATITIS

Seborrheic dermatitis is a common rash affecting everyone at some stage of their life. The eruption is erythematous and scaly and may often acquire a waxy crust if severe or untreated. Common areas of involvement include the scalp (e.g., cradle cap in infants and dandruff in adults) and face (e.g., scaling and redness of the eyelids, nasolabial folds, and retroauricular areas and along the hairline). The disease may be widespread, and typically the sternal and intertriginous regions are involved; this type of seborrheic dermatitis is a possible precursor of erythroderma in the elderly.

Except in rare cases with unusual distribution, secondary infection, or inappropriate prior therapy, the diagnosis is usually obvious on inspection.

Management

The mainstay of management of seborrheic dermatitis is frequent shampooing. The daily use is more important than the type or brand of shampoo; however, there are at least four major shampoo types with the following different active ingredients:

1. Zinc pyrithione (Head and Shoulders, DHS Zinc, Sebulon, Zincon)
2. Selenium sulfide (Selsun, Exsel)
3. Salicylic acid (Ionil, Sebulex, Vanseb)
4. Tar. The tar shampoos range from old-fashioned, smelly but effective products (Polytar, Zetar, Ionil, Sebutone) to newer, more cosmetically elegant preparations (T/Gel, Ionil T Plus, DHS Tar Gel). In addition to enjoying better patient acceptance, products in the latter group are less likely to stain blond or grey hair.

Patients should be instructed to wash their hair, rinse, reapply the shampoo, wait 2 to 3 minutes, and rinse again. It is perfectly appropriate to use rinse and/or conditioner; some are made especially for such patients (Ionil Rinse, DHS Conditioning Rinse). A minimum interval is shampooing every other day; for most patients daily shampoos are necessary. Patients with hair styles that do not allow such frequent shampooing may have to choose between their style and their scalp disease. In addition, many patients find that they do better if they alternate different types of shampoos.

Recalcitrant scalp disease, especially that with thick crusts, may require presoaking. Generations of young mothers have discovered the application of baby oil to the scalp for an hour or overnight, followed by shampooing and use of a scrub brush, will loosen most scales. Baker P&S Liquid is a more sophisticated solution for the same purpose.

Finally, topical corticosteroids may be needed, with particular attention to vehicle and strength. On the scalp itself, a relatively mid- to high-potency steroid in either a spray (Kenalog Spray), gel (Lidex Gel or Topicort Gel), lotion (Maxivate Lotion), or solution (Synalar or Halog) should be applied once a day to thickened or itchy areas. The patient should be cautioned not to use the expensive corticosteroid as a hair-dressing alternative, but to apply it sparingly to "bad" areas.

A milder corticosteroid in a less drying vehicle must be used on the hairline, face, and other areas. Seborrheic dermatitis does not respond well to high-potency steroids. Have the patient start with 1 per cent hydrocortisone cream (Hytone), applying it two or three times daily. If this does not work, usually the explanation is noncompliance or failure to shampoo. However, slightly more potent steroids such as desonide cream 0.05 per cent (DesOwen, Tridesilon) or 0.025 per cent triamcinolone cream (Kenalog, Artistocort) may be tried.

PSORIASIS

Psoriasis is a common skin disease; 1 to 3 per cent of the population are estimated to suffer from the "heartbreak" disease. The diagnosis may be made on physical examination. Lesions are usually erythematous with a thick, silvery scale; they are most commonly seen over the knees, elbows, and scalp. On the scalp, severe seborrheic dermatitis and psoriasis merge imperceptibly; the old term sebopsoriasis is useful. There may be other clues: nail changes (pitting, oil spots, subungual debris) and gluteal cleft redness are helpful. Treated lesions notoriously lose the above features and become harder to diagnose.

A type of psoriasis rarely identified by patients or nondermatologists is the guttate variant. Usually seen in children and young adults and often triggered by a streptococcal infection, guttate psoriasis is characterized by many small erythematous papules that appear suddenly, primarily on the trunk, without other stigmata.

Patients with psoriasis show a wide spectrum of disease. Those with localized disease are easily managed by any physician. As they develop more widespread disease, simple topical therapy becomes less helpful and affordable, and other approaches must be developed. In a small subset, the disease becomes so widespread as to involve the entire body (erythroderma), may have an acute pustular component with widespread sterile pustules, or may be associated with arthritis.

Management

Most psoriatics need a friendly doctor. Taking the time to explain their disease to them and promising to work with them to control but not cure the disorder are more important contributions than any prescription. Possible triggering factors occasionally can be eliminated; these include drugs (lithium and the beta blockers are notorious for causing psoriasis to flare up) and trauma (psoriasis tends to appear in areas of trauma, such as on the hands of manual laborers).

The mainstays of management of localized psoriasis, adaptable to almost any practice setting, are topical corticosteroids, tar, and anathralin (Table 1). Topical corticosteroids are cosmetically elegant and preferred by patients. One can start with the most cost-effective product, 0.025 per cent triamcinolone cream; however, stronger, far more expensive products are usually needed. In any event, one can then move up through the therapeutic range; I usually employ Lidex because it is quite potent and available in many forms (cream, emollient cream, ointment, gel, lotion). Many patients will want to use a cream or emollient cream in the morning but prefer a messier but less drying ointment at night. Patients should be encouraged to apply their medication twice daily or at most three times daily.

Several tricks are available to increase the potent effect of topical corticosteroids. Cheapest to use is Saran Wrap occlusion; some areas of the body are more amenable to this than others. Intralesional triamcinolone, 2.2 to 5 mg per ml can be used for localized plaques, injected with either a needle and Luer-Lok syringe or an air-powered injection device (Derma-jet, Mada-jet). Finally, a number of extremely potent topical corticosteroids are now available in the United States for short-term pulse treatment, often on a once daily basis. They include 0.05 per cent clobetasol propionate (Temovate Cream or Ointment), 0.05 per cent diflorasone diacetate (Psorcon Ointment), and 0.05 per cent betamethasone dipropionate (Diprolene AF Cream). None should be used for more than 2 weeks without special indications, because in addition to the well-known topical side effects such as atrophy, telangiectasia, striae, and infections, these new agents increase the possibility of adverse systemic reactions.

Two clinically relevant phenomena have been described with topical corticosteroid therapy. First, tachyphylaxis occurs (that is, patients or their disease becomes tolerant to a given compound with time); thus, it is appropriate to alternate products. Second, when high-potency corticosteroid therapy is stopped, often there is a rebound flare-up of psoriasis. For these reasons most physicians employ either tars or anthralin as adjunctive therapy, even in localized disease. While both products were messy and difficult to use in the not too distant past, major advances in their formulations have been made, and patient compliance is now much higher because of the more cosmetically elegant forms.

Tars are now available in alcoholic bases (Psorigel, Estar Gel) and creams (Fotocar Cream).

TABLE 1. **Management of Psoriasis***

	Localized Plaque-Type Psoriasis (<30% Body Surface)	Widespread Plaque-Type Psoriasis, Eruptive Guttate Type	Generalized Pustular Psoriasis	Erythrodermic Psoriasis
Treatment (in order of preference)	Tar plus topical corticosteroids *or* Anthralin plus topical cortico-steroids	(1) Anthralin plus ultraviolet light *or* Goeckerman's regimen (2) PUVA	Methotrexate *or* Oral retinoids	Methotrexate *or* Oral retinoids
Ideal setting of treatment	Outpatient	Day care center or inpatient unit	Inpatient unit	Inpatient unit

*Courtesy of Chung-Hong Hu, M.D.

Thus, it is rarely necessary to struggle to find a pharmacist who can mix one of the old crude coal tar "recipes." Tars can be applied directly to the patches of psoriasis; I typically have a patient use a topical steroid in the morning and then in the evening apply tar, let it dry, and then cover with the steroid. The choice between gel and cream is dependent on patient tolerance. Tar can also be used for simple home phototherapy. Before exposing their lesions to sunlight, patients can either bathe in a tar bath (3 capfuls Balnetar in a half-filled tub) or apply a tar product to the lesions.

Anthralin is also available in varying percentages as creams (0.1, 0.2, 0.4, 1.0 per cent Lasan Cream; 0.1, 0.25, 0.5, 1.0 per cent Dritho-cream or ointments; 0.1, 0.25, 0.5, 1.0 per cent Anthra-Derm Ointment). It can be applied, as described earlier for the tar products, in the evening. The patient should start with the lowest concentration and work up to 0.5 per cent. Alternatively, short contact use of 1 per cent anthralin can be made; the patient applies the product to the psoriatic lesions, waits 30 to 60 minutes, and removes it with a bath or mineral oil. Both anthralin and tar stain bedclothes and sheets.

Psoriasis presents unique problems in certain areas:

1. Scalp: Manage just as seborrheic dermatitis.
2. Flexural areas: Inverse psoriasis, involving the axillae and groin, is also similar to seborrheic dermatitis and does better with low-potency corticosteroids. Tar and anthralin should be avoided in these areas.
3. Palmar and plantar lesions: Treatment with topical corticosteroids, tars, and short-contact anthralin therapy should be tried.

Management of More Extensive Cases

Patients who fail to respond to the above measures generally require more complicated therapy; it may be troublesome because of expense, need for special equipment, or use of dangerous medications. Such approaches should probably be left to physicians with a special interest in psoriasis who have both the experience to choose between competing regimens and the facilities to provide most cost-effective care. Several approaches are possible (see Table 1).

Goeckerman's Regimen. Patients receive tar and ultraviolet light, in either a day care or an inpatient setting. This represents the safest, most time-tested approach to severe psoriasis but has the least patient acceptance because it requires so much of the patient's time.

Antimetabolites. Because psoriasis is a hyperproliferative disorder, it is not surprising that a variety of antimetabolites will help control the disease. Methotrexate has been best studied; a single daily weekly dose of 10 to 30 mg has proved very effective. The success of the relatively lower dosages in rheumatoid and psoriatic arthritis has encouraged me to use a weekly regimen of 7.5 to 15 mg. I currently give no patients the larger doses. The role of liver biopsies in methotrexate patients remains controversial; if more than 15 mg per week is used, there is a general consensus that a pretreatment biopsy and biopsies every 2 years are appropriate while the patient is on therapy. With lower dosages, the recommendations vary, but one should keep a log of total methotrexate dosage and at least get a biopsy after ingestion of total dosage of 1 to 1.5 grams. Patients cannot be allowed to conceive or father children while on methotrexate therapy; the safe washout period is felt to be 2 to 3 months. Other antimetabolites such as 5-fluorouracil and hydroxyurea may also be employed but are much less widely used than is methotrexate.

PUVA Photochemotherapy. Patients take the photosensitizing drug psoralen *(P)* and are exposed to high-intensity ultraviolet A *(UVA)* light in a special light box. PUVA is very effective but causes skin aging and cataracts and increases the risk of skin cancers.

Retinoids. Oral retinoids are now available in

this country in the form of etretinate (Tegison), which is approved for psoriatic erythroderma and pustular psoriasis as well as for severe psoriasis not responsive to standard measures. It may also be used as adjunctive therapy with PUVA to reduce the UVA dose and speed the response. Etretinate has a very long half-life and is a potent teratogen. I am reluctant to treat female patients with it. The lengthy package insert should be followed in detail should this drug be required for its potential lifesaving role in erythroderma or a pustular flare-up.

PITYRIASIS ROSEA

Pityriasis rosea is an idiopathic acute papulo-squamous eruption, which is diagnosed on clinical examination. Patients typically describe a single initial scaly patch, often misdiagnosed as tinea corporis. Multiple oval-shaped macules then develop, often in a Christmas-tree pattern following skin lines on the trunk. In caucasians, the arms, legs, and head are usually spared, although in black persons these areas may be involved (inverse variant). Since secondary syphilis can exactly mimic pityriasis rosea, a Venereal Disease Research Laboratory (VDRL) test should be considered.

Management

If the patient with pityriasis rosea is not itching, management consists of lubrication and reassurance. Generally, a mild soap (e.g., Dove) and bathing or showering (e.g., Alpha-Keri Bath Oil, Cetaphil) suffice. When pruritus occurs, antihistamines and distractors can be used. I typically prescribe hydroxyzine, 25 mg twice daily and 50 mg at bedtime, but other regimens and drugs are acceptable. I mix 0.025 per cent menthol with Cetaphil as an effective, inexpensive distractor; Sarna may also be used. Topical steroids can also be employed but are disappointing; they are an expensive way to lubricate and a poor way to control itch. When extreme pruritus occurs or in black patients with facial involvement or pigmentary changes, a short burst of systemic corticosteroids may be needed. I employ prednisone, 60 mg daily for 3 days, 40 mg daily for 3 days, and 20 mg daily for 3 days, taken all at once in the morning; any comparable regimen will do.

PITYRIASIS LICHENOIDES ET VARIOLIFORMIS ACUTA (PLEVA)

This tongue twister is actually an identifiable papulosquamous eruption in teenagers and young adults. It looks like "bad chronic chickenpox" with necrotic (varioliform) papules and macules with scale; the patient looks terrible but feels fine. The main differential considerations are guttate psoriasis and pityriasis rosea. Since PLEVA is characterized by lymphocytic vasculitis and hemorrhage, it can usually be identified by skin biopsy.

Management

PLEVA is generally a self-limited disease and requires no therapy. However, most patients desire something for such a severe-looking disease. Topical lubricants and distractors can be employed, as for pityriasis rosea. In addition, oral antibiotics may be helpful. Either tetracycline, 1 gram daily, or minocycline (Minocin), 100 mg daily, may be tried. Extremely low-dose methotrexate* (5 to 10 mg per week) is amazingly effective; unfortunately, PLEVA occurs in an age group where a teratogen such as methotrexate can rarely be justified for a benign disease.

LICHEN PLANUS

Lichen planus is another acute idiopathic dermatosis, characterized by violaceous, polygonal, flat-topped papules. Typical areas of involvement are the wrists, ankles, and genitalia. The oral mucosa may also be involved, either with lacy white streaks or with ulcerations. Similarly, the palms and soles may be either hyperkeratotic or ulcerated. In addition, atrophic and bullous lesions can occur. Because of the widespread and varied clinical appearance, a biopsy is often necessary; the typical band-like infiltrate of lymphocytes at the epidermal-dermal junction usually resolves the diagnostic dilemma. The disease usually persists for 3 to 6 months; almost all cases resolve by 12 months except for oral, genital, and plantar variants, which are more chronic.

Management

Treatment of the pruritus is the goal of therapy. Topically, for limited disease, high-potency topical corticosteroids such as 0.05 per cent fluocinonide cream (Lidex) may be useful for limited areas; on the genitalia, a milder form such as 0.05 per cent desonide cream (Tridesilon, Des-Owen) should be used. Application is two or three times daily. In addition, distractors such as 0.025 per cent menthol in Cetaphil can be used.

Antihistamines are used as for any other pru-

---

*This use of methotrexate is not listed in the manufacturer's directive.

ritus. Hydroxyzine has traditionally been favored, in a dosage of 25 mg two or three times daily and 50 mg at night, but newer nonsoporific agents such as terfenadine (Seldane), 60 mg, or combination blockers such as doxepin (Sinequan, Adapin), 50 to 75 mg at night and 25 mg in the morning, may be useful.

Finally, systemic corticosteroids are often needed for relief from itching. I usually prescribe 60 mg per day of prednisone in the morning tapered over a 3-week period, with consideration of alternate-day steroids if this regimen helps but the disease recurs. Griseofulvin, 500 mg twice a day, may also be tried, especially in the presence of a dermatophyte infection, but also in patients with no other indications. For the oral disease, either topical Kenalog in Orabase or 0.025 per cent isotretinoin gel (Retin-A) may be used.

CONNECTIVE TISSUE DISORDERS: LUPUS ERYTHEMATOSUS, DERMATOMYOSITIS, AND SCLERODERMA

method of
CODY WASNER, M.D.
Oregon Health Sciences University
Eugene, Oregon

and

JOSEPH L. JORIZZO, M.D.
Bowman Gray School of Medicine of Wake Forest
University
Winston-Salem, North Carolina

LUPUS ERYTHEMATOSUS

Systemic lupus erythematosus (SLE) is an inflammatory disease of unknown etiology that is characterized by the production of autoantibodies and by inflammatory involvement of several organ systems. It is unrivaled in its varying modes of presentation and spectrum of disease. Appropriate treatment depends on accurate classification of the symptom constellation into an appropriate clinical subset. SLE can mimic most other diseases, and before beginning therapy other explanations for the symptoms, especially infectious etiologies, must be ruled out.

Cutaneous Lupus Erythematosus

Skin manifestations can be subdivided into three relatively distinct subsets: chronic cutaneous (discoid) lupus erythematosus (DLE), subacute cutaneous lupus erythematosus (SCLE), and the acute cutaneous lesions that occur with systemic lupus. A complete history, physical examination, and laboratory investigation are necessary in all patients to separate cutaneous from systemic involvement. Laboratory evaluation should include a complete blood cell count, chemistry screening profile, urinalysis, and tests for antinuclear antibody (ANA) and anti-Ro (SS-A) antibody. In those patients with positive tests for autoantibodies, additional testing for anti-DNA antibodies and serum complement studies are indicated.

Discoid Lupus Erythematosus

DLE starts as erythematous patches that lead to the development of elevated edematous plaques with fine adherent scales. If left untreated, atrophy, depigmentation, and scarring result. DLE is usually confined to the skin. Fewer than 5 per cent of patients develop systemic symptoms, and most of these patients have positive ANA tests when their skin lesions develop. A negative ANA test is additional reassurance to patients of the benign nature of their illness. Because of scarring, hair loss, and depigmentation, make-up, wigs, and other cosmetic devices are an important treatment modality. Most patients are photosensitive, and thus excess sunlight and tanning booths must be avoided. For patients who are in the sun, sunscreens with a sun protection factor (SPF) of 15 or higher should be used daily to prevent exacerbation of skin lesions.

Topical corticosteroids are beneficial in mild and limited disease but require regular application for success. Care must be taken when strong topical corticosteroids are used, especially in the facial area, because they can cause skin atrophy and telangiectasia. Intralesional corticosteroids such as triamcinolone acetonide (2 to 4 mg per ml) can be useful for persistent lesions. Systemic corticosteroids may help temporarily but are rarely effective long term and have substantial toxicity. They have no place in the long-term management of DLE. Antimalarial compounds are most frequently used when the severity and extent of disease warrant systemic therapy. Hydroxychloroquine sulfate (Plaquenil), 200 to 400 mg per day, is the therapy of choice and seems to have a preventive as well as therapeutic effect. Toxicity is infrequent but includes pleomorphic drug eruptions, occasional gastrointestinal symptoms, mainly diarrhea, and rarely visual disturbances. A rare, silent retinopathy can occur after 1 to 2 years of treatment. A specialized ophthalmologic examination is recommended at the initiation of hydroxychloroquine therapy and every 6 months thereafter. Chloroquine phosphate (Aralen), 250 mg per day, and quinacrine hydrochloride, 100 mg daily, are alternative antimalarial compounds but have drawbacks. Chloroquine may have greater retinal toxicity and be less effective. Quinacrine can cause an orange-yellow discoloration of the skin and can have central nervous system and bone marrow toxicity.

Many other systemic medications have been recommended for use in DLE, but controlled studies of these compounds are lacking. These drugs include Isotretinoin (Accutane), 40 mg twice daily; auranofin (Ridaura, an oral gold product), 3 to 9 mg daily; dapsone, 100 to 150 mg per day; and immunosuppressive agents such as azathioprine (Imuran), 100 to 150 mg per day. All of these agents require elaborate monitoring precautions and should be considered only if other conventional therapy fails.

Cosmetic surgery is used infrequently in DLE because new lesions may occur at the surgical site.

Subacute Cutaneous Lupus Erythematosus

SCLE is a syndrome of intermediate severity between benign DLE and SLE. It is characterized by nonscarring erythematous annular and papulosquamous lesions, usually of the head, neck, or upper trunk. Skin biopsy is diagnostic. Frequently mild musculoskeletal symptoms also occur. Autoantibodies, especially ANA and anti-Ro (SS-A) antibodies, are present in at least one-half of patients. Occasional mild involvement of other organ systems has been reported, including leukopenia, mild proteinuria, and Raynaud's phenomenon.

Treatment modalities are similar to those used for DLE. Scarring is much less likely, but mild musculoskeletal symptoms, which can be distressing to the patient, may respond well to hydroxychloroquine sulfate. Noncutaneous disease, which usually has a benign course, rarely requires the use of strong medications such as prednisone. Lupus profundus, a recurrent, nonsuppurative panniculitis producing subcutaneous nodules that may ulcerate, is usually treated with systemic corticosteroids.

Systemic Lupus Erythematosus

SLE can attack virtually any organ system. Treatment is based on the nature and severity of the organ involvement. The diagnosis of SLE depends on more than the presence of autoantibodies. Care must be taken to avoid overlooking a curable illness, especially of infectious etiology. Drug-induced lupus must be considered, especially when the patient is taking procainamide or hydralazine. Removal of the offending drug invariably results in resolution of the patient's symptoms within 6 months. Antihistone antibodies have been associated with drug-induced lupus but are not reliably present.

Even when the diagnosis of lupus has been made, it may not be necessary to treat the patient. In the absence of clinically demonstrable organ involvement, serologic abnormalities should not be treated. Elevated erythrocyte sedimentation rates, high titers of anti-DNA antibodies or ANA, and low serum complement levels may exist for years without any clinically significant harm to the patient. The temptation to treat these laboratory abnormalities with corticosteroids must be avoided.

Treatment

Skin

Skin manifestations of systemic disease can include DLE or SCLE and are treated as discussed in the preceding sections. Skin vasculitis, most frequently leukocytoclastic vasculitis, may indicate more serious organ involvement. Vasculitis should be searched for in the lungs, kidneys, and peripheral nervous system and if found may warrant corticosteroid treatment in doses as high as 1 mg per kg per day of prednisone until resolution of the vasculitic signs.

Joints

Most patients develop a symmetric, nonerosive arthritis with frequently peripheral interphalangeal joint involvement and ligamentous laxity. Salicylates in doses of 3 to 4 grams per day or other nonsteroidal anti-inflammatory drugs are frequently all that are necessary for pain control and maintenance of joint function. Especially severe cases may require the use of hydroxychloroquine sulfate in doses of 200 to 400 mg per day or occasionally the use of oral or injectable gold salts. Intra-articular corticosteroids are particularly helpful when one joint is persistently involved. Systemic corticosteroids are rarely indicated for articular disease alone.

Serositis

Pleurisy and pericarditis are frequently seen and respond well to indomethacin (Indocin) at doses of 100 to 150 mg per day. Refractory cases may need prednisone at doses of 0.5 to 1 mg per kg per day, with a rapidly tapering dose over 2 weeks.

Hematologic

Leukopenia is a frequent manifestation of systemic lupus but rarely needs treatment. Thrombocytopenia, however, can be life-threatening, and treatment should be considered if the platelet count drops below 15,000 per mm^3. Prednisone is most frequently used at doses of 1 mg per kg per day, with a rapid tapering to 0.1 to 0.3 mg per kg given on alternate days. The goal should be to maintain a platelet count higher than 20,000 per mm^3. Splenectomy is rarely necessary. Cyclophosphamide (Cytoxan) (1 to 2 mg per kg per day) has been used when the side effects of prednisone necessitate alternative treatment. Some patients with lupus develop a thrombotic tendency, which has been associated with the presence of anticardiolipin antibody (responsible for the false-positive serologic test for syphilis). This syndrome, which can result in pulmonary emboli, cerebral thrombosis, and other serious manifestations including death, is still poorly understood. Corticosteroids appear to be of little benefit, but anticoagulants are probably indicated in patients with thromboses and high cardiolipin antibody titers.

Renal

Renal disease continues to be the leading cause of morbidity and mortality in SLE. Proteinuria, glomerulonephritis, and nephrotic syndrome as well as renal insufficiency are commonly seen clinical sequelae. Urinary sediment analysis, creatinine clearance changes, blood pressure, and occasionally renal biopsy all can give prognostic information. Corticosteroids, at a dose of 1 mg per kg per day orally, are used for the more aggressive forms of renal disease. Doses may be tapered to 0.5 mg per kg per day by 4 months of therapy. Toxicity from high-dose long-term corticosteroid use may be substantial. Frequently, immunosuppressive or cytotoxic agents such as azathioprine, 1 to 2.5 mg per kg per day, or cyclophosphamide, 1.5 to 2.5 mg per kg per day, have been used in combination with corticosteroids to lower the necessary steroid dose. Bone marrow suppression and infectious complications can occur with these agents, and there is a possible increased risk of malignancy. High-dose intravenous cyclophosphamide, given at monthly intervals in doses of 500 to 1000 mg per M^2, may be less toxic than daily oral cyclophosphamide and equally effective.

Central Nervous System

SLE can affect all levels of the central nervous system, but psychiatric illness and seizures are the most frequent presentations. Organic brain syndrome, aseptic meningitis, and cerebritis and myelopathy are also frequently seen. It is difficult to prove that treatment affects the course of central nervous system disease, but prednisone at 1 mg per kg per day and cyclophosphamide in treatment regimens similar to those used for severe nephritis have been advocated. Pulse methylprednisolone (Solu-Medrol), 1 gram intravenously per day for 3 days, is used in severe cases, but its efficacy is unproved.

Miscellaneous

Myositis, interstitial lung disease, and severe systemic symptoms (high fevers, lymphadenopathy, and serositis) are often treated like nephritis. Prednisone is begun initially followed by a steroid-sparing immunosuppressive or cytotoxic agent if the treatment course is prolonged.

In refractory cases of organ system involvement, several experimental and as yet unproven treatments have been used. Lymphapheresis, plasmapheresis, or photopheresis, cyclosporine A, and total lymphoid irradiation have been tried, but their benefit has not yet been substantiated.

DERMATOMYOSITIS

Dermatomyositis is an idiopathic inflammatory disorder that primarily affects the skin and muscle. The cutaneous eruption may precede all other disease manifestations by months to even years. Poikiloderma occurs in dermatomyositis; however, in contrast to acute SLE, the color in dermatomyositis is violaceous. The name given to the violaceous poikiloderma of dermatomyositis occurring with periorbital edema is the "heliotrope sign"; when it occurs over the knuckles it is called Gottron's sign. Periungual telangiectasia and cuticular dystrophy are other typical features.

Dermatomyositis occurs in a biphasic age distribution. The childhood form is more likely to be associated with vasculitis; the adult form may occur in association with occult malignancy. Current practice suggests a directed malignancy evaluation (i.e., pursue leads from history, physical examination, and screening laboratory studies) rather than a routine "million dollar workup" for affected adults.

The following diagnostic criteria are used for dermatomyositis:

1. Clinical signs and symptoms of proximal muscle weakness
2. Elevation of muscle enzymes (e.g., aldolase, creatine phosphokinase
3. Electromyographic changes of myositis
4. Typical histologic changes of myositis from muscle biopsy
5. Typical cutaneous eruption

Treatment

General Treatment Measures

Initial hospitalization allows for the diagnosis to be confirmed and for the necessary bed rest. A program of gradually increasing activity from full bed rest to passive range-of-motion exercises and then to increasing exercise is best coordinated by physical and occupational therapy consultants. A high-protein diet may also be beneficial during the acute stage of the disorder.

Topical Therapy

Dermatomyositis, like lupus erythematosus, is characterized by a cutaneous eruption with a photosensitivity component. Sunscreens should be used as described for lupus erythematosus.

The poikilodermatous eruption, by definition, is characterized by epidermal atrophy. Potent topical corticosteroid therapy should be avoided due to the potential to exacerbate this atrophy. Emollients and mild topical corticosteroids (1 per cent hydrocortisone) may be of benefit in alleviating pruritus.

Cosmetics such as Cover Mark, which are compounded to the patient's specific skin color, may be beneficial. The cutaneous eruption does not follow the course of the muscle disease. Many patients have cutaneous morbidity that persists long after they are asymptomatic from their muscle disease. These patients no longer perceive themselves as being acutely ill; however, physician support and understanding must continue through this period.

Systemic Therapy

Corticosteroids. Systemic corticosteroid therapy is the treatment of choice for the myositis of dermatomyositis. The usual precautions should be taken both prior to initiating therapy and during the course of long-term systemic corticosteroid therapy. Physicians should be familiar with the significant and varied complications of therapy with this agent.

Therapy is initiated with prednisone, approximately 1 mg per kg per day in a single morning dose. Extensor muscle strength and laboratory assessment of muscle enzymes should be monitored carefully. Aggressive therapy should be maintained at least until a steady plateau of improvement is reached. Response is variable; some patients improve dramatically within 2 weeks and others show very little change after 3 to 6 months. Divided daily-dose prednisone therapy, or single-dose therapy of up to 100 mg per day, in some cases with the addition of immunosuppressive agents, can be used for patients with refractory disease. Pulse therapy, with massive doses of 1 gram equivalent of prednisone per day* for 3 to 5 days, has also been described as treatment for dermatomyositis, with subsequent requirement of lower maintenance doses of prednisone. Hospital monitoring is usually required for this still experimental therapy.

As improvement occurs, the prednisone dose can be reduced slowly; with careful monitoring of muscle strength and serum enzymes on each clinic visit. An initial dosage reduction of 10 to 25 per cent can be used, followed by a 5-mg reduction every 2 to 4 weeks. If relapse occurs, a prompt substantial increase in dosage is required with a slower subsequent taper. Dermatomyositis responds well to a single-dose, every-other-day regimen. This can often be accomplished after 6 months of daily-dose therapy when prednisone dosage is in the range of 20 to 30 mg per day. Since 60 mg of prednisone on alternate days represents a significant taper from 30 mg per day, several weeks of intermediate therapy are often helpful—for example, 50 mg alternating with 10 mg; other published guidelines are available for changing to alternate-day therapy.

Maintenance prednisone therapy is usually required for a minimum of 2 years. Most patients can eventually stop therapy, but as many as 25 per cent may require therapy for more than 5 years.

Methotrexate. Methotrexate† can be added to the regimen of prednisone and supportive care if control of disease activity is not achieved with prednisone alone after 2 to 4 months or if prednisone-sparing effects are required. The dosage regimen popularized by dermatologists in the treatment of psoriasis is appropriate, and 10 to 25 mg can be given in a single weekly oral dose. Full benefit may not be derived for 3 to 4 months. Pre-existing liver disease and chronic alcohol use are contraindications to therapy, as are pregnancy, severe renal disease, and blood dyscrasias. With decreased disease activity, methotrexate can be tapered by lowering the weekly dose. The usual precautions with methotrexate therapy should be followed.

Azathioprine. Azathioprine† can be used instead of methotrexate. A dosage of 2 to 3 mg per kg per day in divided doses is usual. Again, several months of therapy may be required to assess full benefit. Hematologic toxicity, in particular, requires close monitoring. The rare but potential risk of development of malignancy exists with therapy with any immunosuppressive agent.

Antimalarials. As the cutaneous eruption does

---

*Exceeds normal dosage range.

†This use of these agents is not listed in the manufacturers' official directives.

not always respond to the aforementioned therapies, adjunctive therapy for the poikiloderma may be required. Therapy for patients with refractory cutaneous lesions of dermatomyositis is initiated as described for patients with lupus erythematosus.

Other Drugs. Cyclophosphamide, chlorambucil, and 6-mercaptopurine have been used in the management of dermatomyositis but are not standard therapies.

Plasmapheresis. Plasmapheresis may have a role in the treatment of resistant cases of dermatomyositis. Maintenance corticosteroid therapy is still necessary.

SCLERODERMA

Scleroderma is a chronic disease with the potential for significant cutaneous as well as systemic morbidity. The pathogenesis remains unknown, and therapies that are as dramatically effective as systemic corticosteroid therapy for lupus erythematosus or dermatomyositis are unavailable for scleroderma. The disease is characterized by dermal sclerosis, fibrosis of other organs, inflammation and autoantibody formation, and obliterative, proliferative, and vasospastic vascular abnormalities.

Scleroderma has a localized, primarily cutaneous subset called morphea. Plaque, guttate, generalized, and linear (includes the "en coup de sabre" variant on the face) forms of morphea occur. The linear form, especially in children, may be associated with autoantibody formation and mild systemic rheumatologic features; however, in general the primary effect of these localized variants is to produce dermal sclerosis. The linear variants are the least likely to resolve spontaneously and are more likely to involve deep underlying structures, producing hemiatrophy on the face or joint contractures on the extremities.

Eosinophilic fasciitis is a variant of scleroderma characterized by dramatic proximal extremity or truncal cutaneous induration without the acral changes of scleroderma, which will be discussed. Lesions often occur after localized trauma. Histologically, inflammation and thickening of the fascia with eosinophilia are seen. Systemic features do occur but are generally mild. These patients usually respond well to systemic corticosteroid therapy.

Systemic scleroderma occurs in two general forms: the CREST form (*C*alcinosis, *R*aynaud's phenomenon, *E*sophageal dysmotility, *S*clerodactyly, and *T*elangiectasia) (often used synonymously with acrosclerosis) and diffuse, or progressive, systemic sclerosis. Although patients with both forms can suffer from severe vaso-

spasm, gastrointestinal involvement, hypertension, scleroderma kidney, cardiac conduction abnormalities, and pulmonary hypertension and fibrosis, patients with the CREST form generally do not have significant shortening of their lives (patients are often elderly women), whereas patients with diffuse systemic sclerosis (younger men and women) may have a 5-year survival rate of only 50 per cent.

Although systemic therapies are sometimes used for the treatment of the subset morphea (described earlier), general therapy (e.g., emollients, physical therapy for linear variants) and intralesional corticosteroid therapy are the most frequently used approaches.

Overlap syndromes of scleroderma with lupus erythematosus, dermatomyositis, and rheumatoid arthritis exist. One overlap syndrome, mixed connective tissue disease, is characterized by autoantibody to ribonucleoprotein. Although these overlap syndromes are described as corticosteroid responsive, long-term follow-up has shown that many of these patients have pulmonary fibrosis and hypertension as seen in scleroderma. The following discussion relates to therapy of the patient with systemic scleroderma.

Treatment

General

Patients with scleroderma are often frustrated by the lack of a single dramatically effective therapy for this disease; therefore, emotional support is critical. Patients may benefit greatly from membership in the United Scleroderma Foundation, Inc. Emollients are important in making the "hidebound" skin more tolerable for the patient. Avoidance of smoking is crucial, as the local digital vasospasm associated with smoking may be synergistic with the vasospasm of Raynaud's phenomenon and may result in digital necrosis. Not only exposure of the hands to cold but also generalized cooling should be minimized by protective clothing and by other appropriate measures.

Areas of cutaneous calcinosis or acral erosions are particularly predisposed to secondary infection. Topical clindamycin or erythromycin or Silvadene cream can be useful in preventing recurrent infection after treatment of acute tissue infection with the appropriate systemic antibiotic.

Physical therapists can be vitally important in helping the patient maintain range of motion and in preventing contractures. Occupational therapists work with the patient's hands to maintain maximal function. Both these health professionals are invaluable partners in the total management of the scleroderma patient.

The typical "crow's beak" esophagus of scleroderma results in large part from esophageal reflux, which follows esophageal dysmotility. Scleroderma patients should be treated with an antireflux program, which might include elevation of the head of the bed, antacid and H_2 antihistamine therapy.

Systemic Therapy—Vasoactive Agents

Vasoactive agents have been used primarily to treat Raynaud's phenomenon and its sequelae. It is believed that some of these therapies may also modify basic disease mechanisms.

Topical Nitroglycerin. These vasodilating agents were originally developed to treat Raynaud's phenomenon, but their use diminished because of the rebound cardiac vessel spasm that followed the use of excessive amounts. If dosage is carefully restricted, these agents can improve signs and symptoms of Raynaud's phenomenon and promote healing of digital ulcers.

Arteriolar Dilators. Methyldopa (Aldomet), and more recently prazosin (Minipress), has been beneficial, as described with the topical nitroglycerins.

Alpha Blockers. Phenoxybenzamine (Dibenzyline) and tolazoline (Priscoline) have been used.

Beta Agonists. Terbutaline (Brethine) has been used to treat Raynaud's phenomenon.

Angiotensin-Converting Enzyme Inhibitor. Captopril (Capoten) has been used for the hypertensive crisis associated with scleroderma, but with increasing frequency it is being reported to benefit Raynaud's phenomenon and its sequelae. Some investigators believe that cutaneous sclerosis is also ameliorated.

Calcium Channel Blockers. Nifedipine (Procardia) and verapamil (Calan) have also been successfully used to treat Raynaud's phenomenon and digital ulceration.

Other Vasoactive Agents. Ketanserin, a selective Type II serotonin antagonist, has been used with success. Intra-arterial therapy with reserpine and methyldopa, and more recently with prostacyclin infusions, is of benefit and may be used when oral systemic therapies are no longer beneficial and when digital gangrene is imminent.

Hematologic Therapy

Therapy with stanozolol (Winstrol), a fibrinolytic agent, corrects laboratory fibrinolytic abnormalities and may be associated with clinical improvement in digital ulceration. Antiplatelet therapy with dipyridamole (Persantine) and aspirin may also be beneficial. Pentoxifylline (Tren-

tal), an agent that affects blood viscosity, has also been claimed to benefit digital ulceration.

Lathyrogens

D-Penicillamine alters aldehyde cross-links of Type I collagen. In addition to effects on collagen, D-penicillamine also has immunomodulating effects. Therapy with this agent (250 to 750 mg per day) may be associated with reduced dermal sclerosis and possibly with improvement in organ involvement and with increased survival. Significant side effects of D-penicillamine therapy include leukopenia; thrombocytopenia; induction of autoimmune disorders such as lupus erythematosus, pemphigus, and myasthenia gravis; renal toxicity such as the nephrotic syndrome; and cutaneous eruptions.

Immunosuppressive Therapy

Azathioprine and cyclophosphamide have been used alone in dosages like those described earlier (see SLE) or in combination with plasmapheresis for the treatment of life-threatening or potentially crippling scleroderma. Results have been equivocal, but many patients may have had significant improvement in visceral organ function. Meticulous monitoring of the patient for acute and chronic toxicity is mandatory. Experience by the prescribing physician with the use of these therapies is important.

Other Therapies

Lymphapheresis is currently an investigational therapy. Phenytoin (Dilantin) has been claimed to benefit dermal sclerosis. Antimalarials, potassium aminobenzoate, colchicine, and dimethyl sulfoxide each have their advocates, although experimental evidence of benefit in patients with dermal sclerosis and other manifestations of scleroderma is lacking.

CUTANEOUS VASCULITIS

method of
PEARON G. LANG, JR., M.D.
Medical University of South Carolina
Charleston, South Carolina

Although cutaneous blood vessels of all sizes may be affected by a vasculitic process, the most common vessel involved is the venule. Clinically, this venulitis results in palpable purpura, and the term "leukocytoclastic vasculitis" is often used to describe this cutaneous form of vasculitis. Palpable purpura, the hallmark of leukocytoclastic vasculitis, occurs most often on the lower extremities and other dependent areas or over areas of pressure. Leukocytoclastic vasculitis often is confined to the skin, but systemic involvement may occur. An etiology for leukocytoclastic vasculitis often cannot be found; however, it may be associated with infection (hepatitis B virus, *Mycobacterium leprae,* group A *Streptococcus,* and *Staphylococcus aureus*), drugs, chemicals, foreign proteins, complement deficiency (C2), underlying malignancy, cryoglobulinemia, and collagen-vascular disease. When a set of distinct clinical findings is present, the leukocytoclastic vasculitis may be given a name, for example, Henoch-Schönlein purpura or erythema elevatum diutinum.

The vasculitides are usually classified on the basis of histopathology. However, because many of the vasculitides share a common pathologic picture, they are further subdivided on the basis of clinical findings and characteristic variations in the histopathology; for example, allergic granulomatous angiitis and Wegener's granulomatosis, are both granulomatous vasculitides, but eosinophils are more prominent in the inflammatory infiltrate in the former and renal disease is more prevalent in the latter. Table 1 gives the various types of necrotizing vasculitis.

Although palpable purpura is the most common presentation of cutaneous vasculitis, depending on the disease process and the size of the vessels involved, other cutaneous presentations are possible, for example, nodules, ulcers, plaques, vesicles, pustules, gangrene infarcts, livedo reticularis, and urticaria/angioedema. The lesions may be asymptomatic or associated with pruritus, burning, or pain. The presence of nodules and large areas of necrosis usually implies larger vessel involvement typical of polyarteritis nodosa and the granulomatous vasculitides.

Vasculitis may present as a multisystem disease. Again, depending on the size of the vessels affected and the disease process, a number of organ systems may be involved, including the lungs, heart, gastrointestinal tract, joints, muscles, kidneys, eye, and central and peripheral nervous systems. Even when systemic involvement is limited, cutaneous lesions may be accompanied by fever, malaise, arthralgias, myalgias, and edema.

PATHOGENESIS

The vasculitides are considered to represent hypersensitivity reactions to a known or unknown antigen. The events involved in causing the vascular damage

TABLE 1. **Classification of the Vasculitides**

Leukocytoclastic vasculitis
Polyarteritis nodosa
  Classic
  Cutaneous
  Infantile (? Kawasaki's disease)
Granulomatous vasculitis
  Allergic granulomatous angiitis (Churg-Strauss syndrome)
  Wegener's granulomatosis
  Lymphomatoid granulomatosis
Giant cell arteritis
  Temporal arteritis
  Takayasu's arteritis

have been demonstrated best for leukocytoclastic vasculitis. In this vasculitic variant, immune complexes are deposited in the vessel walls. This deposition leads to the activation of the complement cascade, which, in turn, attracts polymorphonuclear leukocytes that via their lysosomal enzymes damage the vessel wall. This explanation, however, is probably an oversimplification because platelets, lymphocytes, mast cells, and various mediators of inflammation may also be involved. It has been postulated that the other vasculitides are mediated by a similar process.

EVALUATION

Although the diagnosis of vasculitis may be suspected clinically, this suspicion should be confirmed by biopsy. If on cutaneous biopsy both large and small vessels are involved, the vasculitis is most likely related to an underlying collagen-vascular disease; a polyarteritis nodosa–like syndrome related to use of amphetamines or to hepatitis B infection; or to one of the granulomatous vasculitides. If a leukocytoclastic vasculitis is suspected, the lesion that is selected for biopsy should be at least 24 hours old because the typical pathologic changes may not be present in younger lesions. If direct immunofluorescence is desired, however, the lesion should be less than 12 hours old because the immune deposits are rapidly removed by phagocytosis. In general, direct immunofluorescence is of limited value in the management of leukocytoclastic vasculitis. Exceptions to this are (1) a confirmation is desired of the diagnosis of Henoch-Schönlein purpura where in contrast to most leukocytoclastic vasculitides the immune deposits consist of IgA and not IgG or IgM; (2) the vasculitis appears to be associated with systemic lupus erythematosus and immune deposits in the basement membrane zone are being sought; (3) or a search is being made for the antigen that precipitated the vasculitis.

Once the diagnosis of vasculitis is made, the patient should have a complete history and physical examination to determine the presence of extracutaneous disease or other underlying disease or precipitating events. This procedure allows the clinician to select the appropriate laboratory tests. The physical examination may also give a clue about the type of vasculitis, even before the biopsy results are available: for example, if in chronic urticaria the lesions persist for more than 24 hours and are associated with purpura or hyperpigmentation, urticarial vasculitis is the most likely diagnosis; nodules following the course of a vessel probably indicate polyarteritis nodosa; and an ulceration confined to the temple is typical of temporal arteritis.

Even in the absence of signs or symptoms of extracutaneous involvement, the patient should have at the minimum a complete blood count with differential count, a platelet count, a chemistry profile that includes assessment of hepatic and renal function, a urinalysis, a stool guaiac test for occult blood, and a chest x-ray. If clinical data warrant or if the vasculitis is not short-lived, additional assays including tests for hepatitis-associated antigen, coagulation studies, cryoglobulin determination, serum protein electrophoresis, antinuclear antibody determination, complement studies, and an antistreptolysin O titer or throat culture should be obtained. If polyarteritis nodosa is suspected, angiography can be used to evaluate systemic disease and confirm the diagnosis because 80 per cent of patients have arterial aneurysms. In temporal arteritis there is a marked elevation of the erythrocyte sedimentation rate, which can be used as a guide to therapy. In patients with chronic urticaria related to urticarial vasculitis, the erythrocyte sedimentation rate is often elevated and thus serves as a useful screening test in patients with chronic urticaria who are suspected of having vasculitis.

TREATMENT

Treatment should be tailored to the severity and extent of the vasculitis. If an underlying disease is thought to be causally related, treatment should be directed at that disease; if a drug is suspected, it should be discontinued. If a leukocytoclastic vasculitis is mild, confined to the skin, and self-limited, minimal treatment in the form of leg elevation, support stockings, antihistamines, or nonsteroidal anti-inflammatory agents may be all that is required. These latter agents may also alleviate any accompanying myalgias or arthralgias.

For severe, extensive leukocytoclastic vasculitis, with or without systemic involvement, corticosteroids, in doses of 40 to 60 mg per day (prednisone), are the mainstay of treatment. However, if the dosage cannot be significantly reduced after initial control is achieved or if long-term treatment is required, it is best to add an immunosuppressive agent to spare the patient the long-term side effects of high-dose corticosteroid administration. The immunosuppressive agents most commonly used are azathioprine* (Imuran) and cyclophosphamide* (Cytoxan), usually in doses of 1 to 2 mg per kg per day. Of these, cyclophosphamide appears to be the most effective. The side effects of the immunosuppressive agents include bone marrow toxicity, hepatitis, hemorrhagic cystitis, infertility, and the possibility of therapy-associated malignancies. Close monitoring of a patient who is given these agents is essential.

In severe, rapidly progressive vasculitis with systemic involvement, cyclophosphamide may be given initially in doses of 3 to 4 mg per kg per day intravenously. After 3 days the patient is switched to oral administration, with doses of 2 mg per kg per day. Patients taking cyclophosphamide and corticosteroids who respond poorly to therapy or who develop hemorrhagic cystitis may respond to pulse therapy with cyclophosphamide in doses of 0.5 to 1 gram per M^2 given intrave-

nously at intervals that vary from once a month to every 3 months.

Pulse therapy with methylprednisolone (Solu-Medrol), 1 gram per day intravenously for 3 to 5 days, has also been used to induce a more rapid remission, to induce a remission in patients who are unresponsive to immunosupressive agents and/or oral corticosteroids, or to maintain a remission. This therapy should not be undertaken lightly, however, because cardiac arrythmias and arrest caused by rapid electrolyte shifts may occur.

Although experience with colchicine is limited, doses of 0.6 mg two or three times a day sometimes control leukocytoclastic vasculitis, and the drug deserves a trial in patients who do not have severe, rapidly progressive disease.

Plasmapheresis has been reported to be of benefit in some patients with vasculitis. It has been used to induce a remission or to facilitate the induction of a remission, as well as to maintain a remission. Unless plasmapheresis is combined with the use of immunosuppressive agents, however, the patient usually suffers a relapse. It has been proposed that plasmapheresis mediates its benefit via the removal of circulating immune complexes and the promotion of the removal of these complexes by the reticuloendothelial system; however, other mechanisms may also be involved.

Antimalarial agents such as hydroxychloroquine (Plaquenil) have on occasion been reported to be of benefit in the management of leukocytoclastic vasculitis, but there have been no controlled studies of the use of these agents, and in general the drugs mentioned previously are more effective.

Diaminodiphenylsulfone (DDS, dapsone), in doses of 100 to 300 mg per day, has been reported to control leukocytoclastic vasculitis, but again there are no large studies of its usefulness. Of the leukocytoclastic vasculitides, the one that seems to respond most consistently is erythema elevatum diutinum. This chronic vasculitis is unusual, low grade, and usually confined to the skin, which is characterized by purple or red-brown or occasionally yellow papules and plaques occurring over joints and extensor surfaces.

There is no universally effective treatment for urticarial vasculitis. H_1 antihistamines alone or in combination with H_2 antihistamines alleviate the pruritus, and indomethacin (Indocin) may control the skin lesions and joint symptoms. In some patients, oral corticosteroids, 40 to 60 mg per day (prednisone), are required to control the skin lesions and associated systemic disease. Favorable responses to cyclophophamide, hydroxychloroquine, and colchicine have also been reported.

---

*This use not listed in manufacturers' directives.

Nodular vasculitis, a chronic low-grade vasculitis that is usually confined to the skin and consists of subcutaneous plaques and nodules that ulcerate and usually occur on the lower legs of women, has shown a variable response to a number of therapeutic modalities including colchicine, diaminodiphenylsulfone, saturated solution of potassium iodide (SSKI), oral and intralesional corticosteroids, indomethacin, and dipyridamole (Persantine).

Livedoid vasculitis (atrophie blanche; segmented hyalinizing vasculitis) is another low-grade chronic vasculitis that is seen primarily in women and presents as extremely painful ulcers around the ankles and over the dorsum of the feet, which heal leaving depressed white scars (atrophie blanche). This entity again shows no uniform response to any one therapy. Responses to anticoagulants, corticosteroids, nicotinic acid (Nicobid), low-molecular-weight dextran, colchicine, aspirin, dipyridamole, phenformin* (DBI), and ethylestrenol (Maxibolin) have been reported.

In managing polyarteritis nodosa and the granulomatous vasculitides, a combination of corticosteroids and immunosuppressive agents (cyclophosphamide, azathioprine) offers the most effective therapy. Cyclophosphamide is the treatment of choice for Wegener's granulomatosis and is also preferred in the treatment of polyarteritis nodosa and the other granulomatous vasculitides.

Oral corticosteroids (prednisone, 40 to 60 mg per day) are the treatment of choice for temporal arteritis. The erythrocyte sedimentation rate can be used as a guide to taper the corticosteroid dosage.

Local measures for managing areas of cutaneous necrosis include soaks, whirlpool baths, gentle débridement, topical antibiotics, and nonadherent dressings.

---

*Withdrawn from the U.S. market.

DISEASES OF THE NAILS

method of
ROBERT BARAN, M.D.
Centre Hospitalier
Cannes, France

The nail is a convex, hard, horny plate covering the dorsal aspect of the tip of the digits. Its appearance is determined by the integrity of the terminal bony phalanx, periungual tissues, nail bed, and matrix.

The nail plate, produced by the matrix, grows from a pocket-like invagination of the epidermis and adheres firmly to both the nail bed and the undersurface of the proximal nail fold, which, at its free border, forms the cuticle and seals the nail pocket.

The most distal part of the matrix, the whitish semicircular lunula, is not covered by the proximal nail fold. Distal to the lunula, the pink nail bed epithelium presents with parallel longitudinal rete ridges and subepithelial capillaries running longitudinally at different depths.

Distally adjacent to the nail bed, the hyponychium, an extension of the epidermis under the nail plate, marks the point at which the nail separates from the underlying tissue.

There is little space between the nail and the bone of the distal phalanx. This space is occupied by nonkeratinizing nail epidermis and highly vascular dermis containing glomus organs.

The following should be borne in mind: (1) The proximal matrix forms the surface of the nail plate, and the distal matrix forms its inferior part. It is therefore possible to locate the initiating pathology by a thorough examination of the nail. (2) Fingernails grow at a rate of 0.1 mm a day; toenails grow much more slowly (it takes 12 to 18 months to replace a large toenail).

FUNGAL INFECTIONS OF THE NAILS

Fungi gain initial entry into a nail by three main routes: (1) via the lateral nail groove and the distal subungual area; (2) via the dorsal aspect of the nail; and (3) via the undersurface of the proximal nail folds, which remain normal in dermatophytic invasion or become swollen (chronic paronychia), as, for example, in *Candida* infection.

Before initiating treatment, potassium hydroxide examination and mycologic culture are essential. Sometimes, however, isolation of fungi is difficult (in proximal white subungual onychomycosis) or the problem is compounded if the patient has already received topical or systemic treatment. Pieces of nail (from simple trimming, including a bit of hyponychium, or 4-mm punch biopsy) should be sent to the pathologist, the hyphae being stained by the periodic acid–Schiff reaction.

The large number of therapeutic regimens available appears to indicate a wide range of effective treatments, but cure rates are uneven.

The current treatment of onychomycosis is still unsatisfactory because:

1. It is seldom possible to achieve a cure using topical antifungal therapy alone, except in superficial white onychomycosis (where simple scraping may be sufficient), *Candida* paronychia, and *Candida* onycholysis.

2. Drug-related toxicity may limit the use of oral therapy.

3. Oral antifungal therapy is necessarily prolonged and, particularly in the case of toenails,

may be unsuccessful because of inadequate dosage or inadequate assessment of drug effectiveness.

To improve the results, an adjunct to antifungal chemotherapy should be used to remove as much nail material bearing fungi as possible. The following techniques can be used to shorten the duration of treatment:

1. Forty per cent urea paste can be applied under an occlusive dressing after thorough protection of the surrounding skin. Softening of the diseased portion of the nail permits its atraumatic separation from adjacent tissue after 1 week.

2. Partial surgical nail avulsion is suitable for onychomycosis of limited extent. Like the previous technique, it results in reasonable remission rates and reduces the time needed for systemic therapy by 50 per cent.

Partial surgical avulsion is also advisable in *Candida* paronychia with secondary nail plate invasion.

Dermatophytes. Dermatophytes are best treated with micronized griseofulvin, 500 mg twice daily at mealtimes. The dosage may be doubled to treat resistant infections.* Oral ketoconazole (one tablet, 200 mg daily) is an alternative because it is effective in treating dermatophytes and *Candida albicans*. However, side effects, including an antiandrogen effect and hepatotoxicity, limit the use of this drug. Liver function tests should be carried out before therapy, at 2 and 4 weeks during therapy, and once a month thereafter. A topical antifungal preparation should be applied daily until full nail growth is obtained, subject to the patient's willingness to persevere with therapy on the treated areas and toewebs.

Candida Species. Oral ketoconazole use should be limited to chronic mucocutaneous candidiasis and distolateral subungual onychomycosis despite its effectiveness in treating milder diseases such as *Candida* paronychia or *Candida* onycholysis.

Nondermatophyte Molds. These are resistant to the available oral antifungal drugs. Topical 28 per cent tioconazole or cyclopiroxolamine may be effective in *Hendersonula toruloidea* infection. Nail avulsion is recommended when feasible. Finally, despite correct management, all nails do not respond equally; some may remain unaffected by treatment. Therefore, in many patients, particularly the elderly or those with only toenail involvement, simple grinding down of the mycotic nail plates may be the best therapy.

---

*This dosage may be higher than that recommended by the manufacturer.

INGROWN NAIL

Regardless of the initial cause, an ingrowing nail ultimately has a nail bed that is too narrow for its nail plate. Treatment depends on the degree, duration, and type of the deformity.

Distal Nail Embedding. Avulsion of the nail or even spontaneous nail shedding may produce this condition. Sculptured artificial nails can be used to override the distal nail wall. When this procedure fails, a crescent wedge tissue excision is carried out around the entire distal phalanx, and the defect is closed with 5-0 monofilament suture.

Juvenile Ingrown Toenail. Treatment of the early stage (pain and erythema) of this disorder is conservative. The nail spicule is removed under local anesthesia, and a wisp of cotton wool kept moist with a disinfectant is placed beneath the nail and between it and the lateral groove. The nails should always be cut square along the top, and sharp corners should be smoothed away with an emery board.

In advanced-stage juvenile ingrown toenail (edema, granulation tissue, purulent drainage), after removal of the lateral strip of the offending nail, hemostasis is achieved with a tourniquet and the blood is carefully cleared from the nail pocket. The surrounding skin is protected with petroleum jelly, and a saturated solution of phenol is applied to the lateral matrix horn on a small cotton pack for 3 minutes, followed by neutralization with alcohol. Two major drawbacks to this procedure are (1) the long time required for healing and (2) the prolonged drainage caused by the chemical burn from the phenol's caustic effects, with possible secondary infections (treated by soaking the foot twice daily in a quart of warm water containing three capsules of povidone-iodine [Betadine]).

Hypertrophic Lateral Nail Lip. A thick, hypertrophic lateral nail fold results from long-standing ingrown nails. An elliptic wedge of tissue, taken from the lateral nail wall of the toe to the bone, pulls away the lateral nail fold from the offending lateral nail margin.

Pincer Nail. The nail brace technique, using a stainless steel wire fitted to the nail, is useful for correcting the inward distortion of the nail in this condition. Haneke's technique is suitable for a definitive cure. The nail is narrowed with bilateral cautery of the matrix horn, using phenol. The distal half of the nail is removed, and a longitudinal median incision of the nail bed is carried down to the bone. The nail bed is undermined, and the dorsal tuft is cut with a rongeur. The nail bed is sutured with 6-0 polyglactin (Vicryl), and reversed tie-over sutures are put in the folds and tied over the plantar aspect of the toe.

Ingrown Toenail in Infancy. Ingrown toenails in infancy fall into three groups: (1) congenital hypertrophic lip of the hallux, a condition that disappears spontaneously; (2) distal embedding with a normally oriented nail, in which conservative treatment should be undertaken at all costs because proper growth recurs at the age of 6 months; and (3) congenital malalignment of the big toenail. Management here depends on accurate assessment of the degree of the malalignment and its associated changes. If the deviation is mild and without complications, the nail, as it hardens, may overcome the initial slight distal embedding, and sufficient normal nail may grow to the tip of the digit to prevent further secondary traumatic changes.

If the deviation is marked and the nail is buried in the distolateral tissues, disabling changes may occur in childhood and in adult life. Surgical rotation of the misdirected matrix is essential to prevent permanent nail dystrophy, despite the possibly spontaneous favorable course of some cases.

INFECTION OF THE NAIL FOLDS

This disorder is characterized by inflammation, swelling, and abscess formation. It can be either acute or chronic.

Acute Paronychia. If this disorder does not respond to penicillinase-fast antibiotics within 48 hours, it should be treated surgically by removing the base of the nail plate, whose proximal third is transversally cut with a nail splitter. In distal subungual infection, probing determines the most painful area and provides an indication for the site of fenestration of the nail plate.

Chronic Paronychia. This condition may result from maceration or from *C. albicans* perpetuating the inflammatory process. Keeping the lesion dry is essential. Nystatin-triamcinolone acetonide ointment (Mycolog) should be applied two or three times daily until the cuticle has regrown. Monthly injections of triamcinolone acetonide suspension (2.5 mg per ml) into affected nail folds facilitate resolution of the paronychia.

Conditions that do not respond to medical therapy (e.g., a foreign body) should be treated by the excision of a crescent-shaped, full-thickness piece of the proximal nail fold, including its swollen portion. Complete healing by granulation takes about 6 to 8 weeks.

TRAUMAS

Acute Subungual Hematoma. As soon as the hematoma is visible, it should be drained with a sharp, pointed scalpel or hot paper clip cautery.

This treatment relieves the pain produced by pressure resulting from the trapped blood. A hematoma involving more than 25 per cent of the visible aspect of the nail is a warning sign of nail bed injury, and x-ray films are mandatory to rule out fracture. The nail is then removed and the hematoma evacuated. The nail bed is sutured with 6-0 polyglycolic acid (Dexon). The nail plate is cleaned, shortened, narrowed, and replaced. Sutures maintain the nail to the lateral nail folds.

Repeated Minor Trauma. Chronic hematomas from ill-fitting footwear or sporting activities are painless and often associated with onycholysis of the large toenail. They sometimes grow out longitudinally and may occasionally persist, which makes partial nail avulsion necessary.

Self-Induced Trauma (Factitial Nail Alterations). Onychophagia (nail biting) and onychotillomania (neurotic picking or tearing of the nails) are nervous habits. Periungual warts are common in nail biters.

Hangnails that may become infected should be removed with sharp-pointed scissors.

The longitudinal split known as median nail dystrophy is probably caused by repeated pressure on the base of the nail, the proximal nail fold of which is intact. It usually affects the thumbs and must be differentiated from the washboard nail, which results from pushing back the cuticle. Micropore tape, changed daily and kept on for 6 months, may deter the patient's habit.

MISCELLANEOUS CONDITIONS

Curative and prophylactic treatment of the following four conditions necessitates maintenance of a state of dryness, requiring the use of cotton gloves under rubber gloves: paronychia (see earlier), onycholysis, brittle nails, and dermatitis.

Onycholysis. In this condition, separation of the nail plate starts distally and spreads toward the proximal edge. Whatever the cause, some rules are mandatory.

Thorough clipping away of as much detached nail as possible, repeated at 2-week intervals.

Gentle brushing with plain soap and water once daily, followed by careful rinsing and drying.

Depending on the cause of the complaint (e.g., fungal organisms, psoriasis, impaired peripheral circulation), appropriate local treatment, systemic treatment or both, is prescribed; in all cases, dryness of the onycholytic areas should be maintained.

Brittle Nails. Nails may split lengthwise or laterally into layers. This occurs mostly in persons who have an occupation involving exposure to moisture.

Avoid repeated immersions in soap and water.

Follow each hydration by application of an ointment to retain the moisture in the nail plate.

Use Cetaphil as an alternative to excessive exposure to water.

Keep the nails short.

Oral iron for 6 months, even in the absence of overt anemia, may be helpful.

Nail polish is protective, but only oily removers should be used.

Nail wrapping limited to the distal portion of the nail may afford protection and camouflage in recalcitrant fragility of the nail keratin.

Dermatitis. Allergic or irritant contact dermatitis involving the digits may interfere with nail plate formation, produce onycholysis, or both. Paraben-free topical corticosteroids, applied three or four times daily to surrounding soft tissues, are effective, and provide thorough protection of hands.

DERMATOSIS

Psoriasis. Treatment of nail changes in psoriasis is tedious and sometimes unsatisfactory. Nail polish should be used to hide discrete nail changes. Some patients get better spontaneously, and others improve when the associated skin lesions are treated.

Potent topical corticosteroids are helpful for treating the dorsal aspect of the proximal nail. Although the efficacy of topical corticosteroids can be enhanced by overnight occlusion, this technique should be used only for limited periods.

An intralesional long-acting steroid is injected into the proximal nail fold or into the subungual affected area, using triamcinolone acetonide (Kenalog-10), diluted to 2.5 mg per ml, at a dose of 0.2 to 0.5 ml per nail. Injections should be repeated monthly for 6 months, then every 6 weeks for the next 6 months, and finally every 2 months for 6 to 12 months.

A digital block is useful to make the treatment less painful, but when several digits are involved, a wrist block may be the appropriate anesthesia.

With the exception of acropustulosis, in which the treatment is consistently effective, variable responses to etretinate are found in nail psoriasis.

Lichen Planus. With the exception of mild disorders such as "20-nail-dystrophy" (which may pertain to lichen planus), treating the nail dystrophy resulting from lichen planus to prevent severe and sometimes permanent lesions such as pterygium and onychatrophy is highly recommended. An intralesional long-acting steroid should be used in the same manner as for treating

psoriatic nails. If more than one or two digits are affected and there is no medical contraindication, triamcinolone acetonide is injected intramuscularly (80 mg the first month, then 40 mg monthly for 6 months). The frequency of the injections should be adjusted to the patient's response. Treatment may last for 18 months to 2 years.

Onychogryphosis. The nail is thickened and distorted in this disorder, often resembling a ram's horn in the elderly. Conservative treatment is indicated, especially in high-risk patients. The nail should be trimmed at regular intervals with rotating grinders. Should radical treatment be needed, phenol cautery is superior to cold steel surgery for matricectomy.

TUMORS

Longitudinal Melanonychia. Longitudinal linear pigmentation of the nail in persons with fair complexion may be perplexing to the physician and distressing for the patient. Complete excisional biopsy is recommended for both diagnosis and treatment. The appropriate technique depends on three factors: (1) the width of the band; (2) the matrix melanin production site; and (3) the anatomic location of the band on the nail plate. Longitudinal melanonychia with periungual pigmentation, nail dystrophy ulceration, or a mass that bleeds easily should be treated a priori as a malignant melanoma.

Subungual Epidermoid Carcinoma. This disease is not as rare as it might appear from the medical literature. It should be regarded as a low-grade malignancy. The microscopically controlled excision of fresh tissue results in complete removal of the lesion (even when cortical bone is involved), with maximum preservation of normal tissue and function.

Pyogenic Granuloma. This vascular post-traumatic tumor is easily removed by surgical shaving (for the pathologist to examine) under local anesthesia. Hemostasis is achieved with aluminum chloride.

Warts. Recurrences of warts are frequent and are not related to treatment. A spontaneous or "magic" cure is by no means unusual. Chemical ablation with monochloroacetic acid, Cantharone, and podophyllin, as well as electrodesiccation and curettage, is still in use.

Liquid nitrogen is more convenient. To minimize the throbbing pain produced by the frozen lesion, pretreatment application of clobetasol propionate under a Blenderm reduces the inflammatory response to the freeze. Massages with this steroid may be continued twice daily for 3 days. Oral aspirin, 600 mg three times daily, beginning

2 hours before and for 3 days after treatment, is also helpful.

Intralesional injection of bleomycin is unquestionably effective. The powder should be diluted to a concentration of 1.0 ml with saline. Part of this solution should be further diluted to 0.1 ml according to the region under treatment (nail matrix is highly susceptible). Patients with vascular impairment should not be treated with bleomycin, and it is also contraindicated in pregnancy.

Warts respond well to carbon dioxide laser treatment under local anesthesia.

Mucoid Cysts. The injection of a sclerosing agent, such as 1 per cent sodium tetradecyl sulfate (Sotradecol), into mucoid cysts has superseded cryosurgery, surgery, radiotherapy, steroid injections, and other treatments. After the cyst has been pierced and its jelly-like material expressed, 0.20 ml is injected painlessly. One procedure may be enough. A second can be performed after 1 month.

Subungual Glomus Tumor. Characteristic radiating pain, either spontaneous or provoked by minor trauma, is associated with glomus tumor. Small tumors of the central nail bed may be removed after punching a 6-mm hole, restricted to the nail plate, and incising the subungual tissue. For tumors in a lateral situation, an L-shaped incision, permitting dissection of the nail bed dermis from the bone, is made until the tumor is reached.

KELOIDS

method of
O. G. RODMAN, M.D.
Henry Ford Hospital
Detroit, Michigan

Keloids are benign proliferative cutaneous lesions composed of excessive collagenous tissue. Trauma is the triggering factor in the vast majority of patients with spontaneously arising keloids most commonly noted on the anterior chest. Common areas of keloid formation include the ears, jawline, chest, shoulders, and upper back. There is a higher incidence in black patients. By definition, keloids extend beyond the original trauma site in a crab-like configuration, whereas hypertrophic scars are confined within the border of the initial site of trauma.

PREVENTION

Unnecessary surgery should be avoided in known keloid formers. If surgery is essential, incisions should be parallel to skin tension lines with the final closure under minimal tension. Midchest incisions should be minimized and the crossing of joint spaces should be avoided. Pressure garments or devices worn postoperatively further hinder keloid regrowth.

TREATMENT

There is no single best treatment for keloids. In virtually all patients, combination therapeutic modalities are indicated, including intralesional steroids, surgical excision, pressure dressings, laser therapy, and radiotherapy. My treatment for such patients invariably includes the triad of intralesional steroids, excisional surgery, and pressure devices. Regardless of the therapeutic modality used, the physician should periodically monitor all patients over a period of 18 to 24 months for potential keloid recurrence.

Intralesional Steroids

Intralesional steroid therapy plays a definite role in the improvement of all keloid patients, since it promotes collagen breakdown and overall size shrinkage. Triamcinolone acetonide suspension (Kenalog) is employed in concentrations ranging from 2 to 40 mg per ml. A 27-gauge or larger-bore needle should be used to prevent suspension clogging. The use of a Luer-Lok syringe will prevent leakage, thereby significantly enhancing drug delivery.

Most patients will accept a 10- to 15-second freeze with liquid nitrogen prior to steroid injection, because of local anesthetic effects from the cryotherapy. The resultant tissue edema allows for further ease in subsequent steroid injections. All injections should be placed within the substance of the keloid and not sublesionally, to avoid unnecessary cutaneous atrophy. Repeated higher concentrations of triamcinolone acetonide are more likely to produce hypopigmentation that may last 6 to 12 months before resolution.

Earlobe keloids are much more amenable to predictable and successful improvement than are keloids located presternally. Nevertheless, I prefer to treat initially all larger keloids with a steroid injection of 40 mg per ml injection, diluting with 1 to 2 per cent lidocaine to achieve my final desired concentration. After injections for two to four visits spaced approximately 3 to 4 weeks apart, Kenalog-10 (triamcinolone acetonide) may be used full strength or diluted with lidocaine to a minimum strength of 2 mg per ml. Surgery is virtually never performed on a patient who has not first received a minimum of three steroid injections without benefit.

Surgery

The surgical approach to removal of keloids varies depending on the size, location, and configuration of the lesions. In all instances, atraumatic and sterile techniques are of paramount importance. It is best to use 6-0 or 5-0 interrupted nylon sutures, carefully avoiding tension and unnecessary trauma to all tissue.

Small, simple posterior pedunculated earlobe keloids may be shaved, followed by postoperative steroid therapy and pressure hemostasis. Keloids with narrow bases may be excised with careful undermining and injected at the base. Larger, dumbbell-shaped keloids may be meticulously cored out, with low-tension interrupted sutures for closure. Sutures generally are removed in 10 to 14 days with subsequent injections of Kenalog-10 two weeks later. Within 2 months, steroid injections may be stopped; however, the patient should return for follow-up at the first sign of recurrence.

Chest or presternal keloids tend to be more painful and much more recalcitrant. However, combining maximum intralesional steroid injections with fine electrocoagulation and postradiation therapy, good to excellent results can be obtained. A dose of 250 rad is given postoperatively, followed by four similar treatments every 2 weeks. A youthful patient and the lack of an experienced radiotherapist are relative contraindications to this latter modality because of potential carcinogenesis.

Other Therapeutic Measures

Carbon dioxide laser excision has now been used for treatment of keloids in all anatomic sites. As with other modalities, facial lesions respond best to the carbon dioxide laser. The cutting mode of the laser is controlled to yield minimal thermal damage to uninvolved skin, and the resultant wound is left to heal via secondary intention. Standard wound care and postoperative follow-up with pressure dressings and/or intralesional steroids are recommended.

In the face of failures with the aforementioned treatments, other regimens include methotrexate, colchicine, nitrogen mustard, thiotepa, and beta-aminopropionitrile fumarate. Asiatic acid, topical tretinoin, and zinc therapy have also yielded variable degrees of success.

VERRUCA VULGARIS
(Warts)

method of
DAVID P. CLARK, M.D.
University of Missouri Health Science Center
Columbia, Missouri

Despite all efforts, no effective antiviral chemotherapy for verruca has been discovered. All current therapy to eliminate warts is dependent upon tissue destruction and induction of the host's immune system. Some warts are difficult to eradicate; periungual, perirectal, and plantar warts are most resistant to therapy. Immunosuppressed patients are frequently plagued by multiple verrucae and respond poorly to any therapy. Warts are epithelial growths caused by human papillomaviruses (HPV). Over 45 different types of HPV have been isolated from human infections. HPV DNA is incorporated into human DNA. Viral DNA can be recovered in normal-appearing cells up to 15 mm from the base of a clinical wart.

INITIAL THERAPY

Simple destructive chemical or cryosurgical methods will eliminate most verrucae and were the first therapeutic measures used to treat warts. Fifty to 60 per cent of common warts will disappear without therapy over a 12- to 18-month period. In evaluating all therapeutic intervention, the risk of scar, pain, infection, and drug side effects must be balanced against the known natural history of warts.

Chemical Destruction

Salicylic acid preparations are an effective first line therapy. After softening and paring of the wart with a blade or pumice stone, 17 per cent salicylic acid in a collodion base is applied daily. Alternatively, 40 per cent salicylic acid plasters are applied to the treatment area for 48 hours followed by 48 hours of rest and gentle débridement. Daily therapy for 2 to 3 months is needed for elimination of most warts. However, morbidity and cost are low and results are equal to all other methods.

Caustic acids, such as bichloroacetic acid or trichloroacetic acid, may be applied with or without tape occlusion weekly by the physician. An extract from the blister beetle, cantharidin, is used alone or in combination with salicylic acid to cause vesiculation and slough of wart tissue. Although initial application of cantharidin is usually painless, blisters develop over 4 to 8 hours that can be painful or secondarily infected.

Flat Warts. Flat warts are multiple, flat-topped,

flesh-colored papules found on the face, arms, and legs. These warts may spread rapidly and are difficult to treat. Retinoic acid (Retin-A)* and 5-fluorouracil* have been used successfully to treat flat warts, but chemical treatments for facial flat warts cause considerable skin irritation. Shaving encourages dissemination and must be stopped.

Condylomata Acuminata. These are HPV infections found on mucous membranes and spread primarily through sexual contact. Therapy must start with a complete evaluation of both partners. Podophyllin, an extract of the May apple, is applied as a 25 per cent solution in tincture of benzoin every 5 to 14 days. The surrounding tissue is protected with Vaseline and the medication washed off in 2 to 6 hours. Patients vary greatly in response to podophyllin; some patients have little reaction while others have a dramatic inflammatory response. Podophyllin is systemically absorbed after application to mucous membranes. Considerable morbidity and even death have resulted from applications of large amounts of the drug (i.e., greater than 1.4 ml of 25 per cent). Gross visual inspection is insufficient to determine adequacy of therapy. After the wart is not visible on gross inspection, compresses saturated with 3 per cent acetic acid are placed over the treatment site for 10 minutes. Inspection with a hand lens will often demonstrate areas of white scale indicating residual wart tissue.

Cryosurgery

Application of liquid nitrogen ($-320°$ C) by a cotton swab or spray device is effective. The area is usually treated until a 1 to 2 ml halo of frost surrounds the wart. A blister develops, causing the slough of wart tissue and adjacent skin. Local pain is usually minimal and rarely requires local anesthesia. Scarring is minimal but cases of hypertrophic scar following cryosurgery have been reported. Due to a high number of nonhealing ulcers, cryosurgery is to be avoided on the lower extremities and over bony prominences. Cryosurgery over the lateral aspects of digits may result in sensory loss. Frequently a wart will require two or three sessions of cryotherapy.

TREATMENT MODALITIES FOR DIFFICULT TO TREAT WARTS

Chemical Destruction

Dinitrochlorobenzene (DNCB) has been used successfully to treat recalcitrant warts—particularly the difficult to treat periungual warts. Al-

though a large experience with physician-applied DNCB has demonstrated few side effects, DNCB is a contact sensitizer and can induce a variety of immune responses. DNCB, in high concentration, has been associated with a positive Ames test for mutagenicity; however, this agent has never been found to be a carcinogen. Currently the drug must be compounded locally because no medical-grade DNCB is marketed in the United States.

Bleomycin, a chemotherapeutic agent, has been injected into verrucae with excellent results. However, the procedure can be associated with considerable pain. Necrosis of digits and induction of Raynaud's phenomenon have been reported after injection of periungual warts with bleomycin.

Use of DNCB and bleomycin for treatment of verrucae is investigational and both drugs have considerably more side effects than any of the initial chemical therapies. Expertise and caution are required.

Surgical Destruction

Surgical methods to treat warts are rapid and often effective but have the potential to scar, require local anesthesia for pain control, and do not have superior cure rates. Cold-steel surgery, electrosurgery, and laser therapy are all used to treat difficult verrucae. Because these nonspecific surgical methods involve considerable destruction of normal tissue and have definite morbidity, they should be reserved for recalcitrant warts.

Carbon Dioxide Laser. The carbon dioxide laser generates high temperatures, $150°$ C, with a column of infrared light. The laser beam is focused in a very small area and causes vaporization and destruction of the wart. Due to limited heat transfer to normal tissue and improved accuracy, there is less risk of scarring with laser destruction than with electrosurgical methods. Recent success with treating condyloma acuminata with carbon dioxide laser therapy may be due to the treatment of an entire "field" rather than isolated lesions. Laser surgery seals nerve endings and lymphatics, which minimizes postoperative discomfort. Laser surgery is not universally available and the technology remains expensive.

Cold-Steel Surgery. Removing wart tissue with a curette or scalpel has been used for many years. However, scalpel excision has been almost wholly abandoned due to unacceptable recurrence rates. The curette is most effectively used following light desiccation with an electrosurgery unit. Cold-steel surgical methods are best used to "debulk" large, exophytic warts prior to chemical or laser therapy.

---

*This use of these agents is not listed in the manufacturers' directives.

Electrosurgery. Electrosurgery units destroy tissue with heat produced when current passing through tissue encounters electrical resistance. Electrosurgery involves considerable heat transfer to adjacent normal tissue. If extensive treatment of the wart is necessary, scarring will occur. The amount of scarring is unpredictable due to variable heat transfer. If electrosurgery is performed in the periungual region, permanent nail distortion may occur.

Multiple unsafe or useless therapies are used too often because no one definitive cure for warts is accepted. Patients and families are often less knowledgeable about the long-term consequences of therapy and insist that "something be done." Physicians should persist in conservative treatment and avoid multiple, painful office visits. Fortunately, the large majority of all warts will disappear with simple therapy.

MOLES AND MELANOMA

method of
THOMAS REA, M.D., and
VINCENT C. HUNG, M.D.
University of Southern California
 School of Medicine
Los Angeles, California

Moles and pigmented lesions of all sorts are one area of increasing concern for both the public and the physician at a time when there is a general increased awareness of skin cancers and the deleterious effects of excessive sun exposure. Nevocellular nevi, more commonly known as moles, are the most common tumor of humans. Moles themselves undergo a natural, predictable change in clinical and histologic appearance that spans the normal human life. The rising incidence of melanoma and the fact that approximately 60 per cent of melanomas arise from pre-existing moles make it necessary for physicians to be able to recognize the appearance of benign moles during all stages of their normal metamorphosis, as well as the characteristics of malignant transformation.

One per cent of all newborns have moles at birth or shortly thereafter. The incidence of moles increases throughout childhood and early adolescence. Moles are most prevalent in young caucasian adults, who may have from 20 to 40. Darker-skinned individuals in general have fewer moles. In all individuals, the majority of moles gradually involute, and by the time the patient is in the seventies, few moles are present. From onset to later involution, these moles possess typical clinically and histologically distinct features that allow them to be separated into three categories: junctional, compound, and intradermal.

CLASSIFICATION OF MOLES

Junctional Nevi

Junctional moles initially appear in children. They are generally hairless, light to dark brown, flat surfaced, and from 1 to 5 mm in size. Skin markings are preserved, and most lesions are ovoid or elliptic. The borders and pigmentation of junctional nevi should have only slight irregularities. Junctional nevi are so named because histopathologically nevus cells are found at the junction of the epidermis and dermis. These nevi are commonly seen in children. In later life, they progress to compound and intradermal nevi. Only on the distal extremities, palms, and soles may moles routinely maintain their junctional qualities.

Compound Nevi

Although compound nevi may be present from birth, they are generally seen in older children and adults. They differ from junctional nevi in that they tend to be more elevated and somewhat irregular in texture. Pigmentation varies from flesh colored to dark brown. Histopathologically, nevus cells can be found at the junction of the epidermis and dermis but also within the dermis itself.

Intradermal Nevi

The most common variety of moles in adults, intradermal nevi are fleshy, raised growths that are either broad based or pedunculated. Pigmentation ranges from flesh colored to dark. When found on the head and neck, coarse hairs, often cosmetically annoying, are also present. Histopathologically, the original nevus cells may largely be replaced with adipose and fibrotic tissues.

TREATMENT OF CLINICALLY BENIGN-APPEARING MOLES

The majority of moles are easily identified as benign and need to be removed only if they are cosmetically bothersome or symptomatic to the patient. Facial moles are often troublesome, especially to women, as they become fleshy with increasing age or because coarse hairs grow from within them. Intradermal nevi on the faces of men are often annoying because of repeated nicking while shaving. Other moles, particularly pedunculated ones, frequently become irritated as they catch on clothing or jewelry, particularly when located on the neck, axilla, or brassiere line. Raised compound or intradermal nevi can generally be removed by shave excision level to the surface of the surrounding skin. Deeper shave excision is likely to leave a permanent depressed scar. In raised moles where pigment or hairs are still growing, the patient should be cautioned that shave excision may leave residual pigment or hair. Excision of moles is the definitive method of removing deep-seated pigment, hairs, or flat junctional nevi. The patient should be advised that surgical fusiform excision leaves a scar that is generally at least two and one-half to three times the width of the mole. Surgical experience and skill, the location of the mole, and the age of the patient all influence the ultimate cosmetic result. Excisions in older patients that fall in existing creases and wrinkle lines generally have a good outcome. Excisions in younger patients, who have more reactive wound healing, in darker-complexioned patients, or in anatomic areas without definite creases and wrinkle lines generally have a poorer cosmetic outcome. Treated moles should always be submitted for pathologic examination, therefore precluding such destructive techniques as cryotherapy, curettage, or electrodesiccation.

SUSPICION OF MELANOMA

Patients may seek medical attention because of a change in their moles, the development of new pigmented lesions, or general concern about skin cancer and melanoma. Usually the cardinal features observed in skin lesions that prove to be melanoma are changes that develop over a period of months. Lesions that have changed over several years or a few weeks generally do not turn out to be melanoma. Changes noted by patients include an alteration in color, an increase in the width or height of the lesions, bleeding, ulceration, or itching. Of interest is the fact that the first lesion noted by the patient may not be the factor that causes the patient to seek medical attention. In one series, more than one-third of the patients with proven melanoma sought consultation at the urging of a spouse or other family member. This is often the case with lesions in areas such as the back, which are difficult for the patient to observe. In about 20 per cent of patients with melanoma, a history of trauma precipitating a change in an otherwise stable mole can be elicited. Sometimes patients request an examination of their nevi after another family member has recently been diagnosed as having melanoma. This history may alert the clinician to a possible familial tendency toward melanoma. A personal history of previous melanoma also increases the likelihood of developing another melanoma. Moles can darken or change color in response to sun exposure, steroid therapy, puberty, or pregnancy. However, these changes are wholesale and affect most or all of the moles.

Approximately 60 per cent of melanomas develop from pre-existing moles. When the clinician evaluates changing moles or de novo pigmented lesions, the following ABCD guidelines are helpful: A—*asymmetry* of the lesion is a hallmark of melanoma; imaginary bisection of benign lesions generally gives mirror images, whereas melanomas are generally asymmetric. B—*borders*: benign lesions have regular, smooth borders, but melanomas, because of irregular malignant growth, have uneven, scalloped, or notched borers. C—*color*: benign lesions vary from flesh colored to light to medium brown and are relatively uniform in color. Malignant lesions are irregular in color, ranging from black to dark brown, red, or blue. Blue coloration is said to be the result of Tyndall's effect of deep pigment and therefore portends the development of thicker, more advanced lesions. D—*diameter*: benign lesions are generally less than 6 mm. Malignant lesions are generally larger.

Any lesion suspected of being melanoma requires biopsy. Based on the assumption that a totally excised lesion is better sampled histopathologically than a partially removed lesion, an excisional biopsy of a suspicious lesion produces the highest number of diagnoses of malignant melanoma. With an increase in the size of lesions, both complete excision and complete histologic examination become increasingly difficult, necessitating other approaches. One approach is to perform multiple biopsies to be sure of achieving an adequate sample. Another approach is the biopsy of exactly the area of suspicion, such as the black macula in the midst of an otherwise lightly colored, melanotic freckle. Shave biopsies of suspected melanomas are not advised. If a punch biopsy is performed, using a large trephine (4 mm or greater) is advisable. In large lesions or lesions with ulceration or necrosis, multiple biopsies may be more likely to give an accurate diagnosis and estimation of thickness. Lymph node examination should be performed in any patient with a suspected melanoma to look for evidence of metastasis. The pathologic diagnosis of melanoma, particularly early melanoma, can be difficult. The tissue should be reviewed by a pathologist with experience in these lesions. In cases where the pathologic diagnosis is unclear, it is prudent to seek a second opinion.

PREDISPOSING FACTORS IN THE DEVELOPMENT OF MELANOMA

The incidence of melanoma has risen dramatically, doubling every decade for the past 50 years. It is therefore important to identify bearers of precursor lesions and other patients at increased risk so that they can be carefully followed and prophylactically treated if indicated. The prototypic patient at increased risk of melanoma is of northern European origin; has blue or green eyes;

has red, blond, or light brown hair; and tends to freckle or burn instead of tan. The highest incidence of melanoma is in Sunbelt areas such as Tucson, Arizona, and Queensland, Australia, but melanoma is by no means restricted to areas of year-round sunny weather. In fact, rather than having a history of chronic heavy sun exposure, many melanoma patients have a history of episodic sun exposure and sunburns as children and young adults. Patients at increased risk for the development of melanoma need to be advised to avoid excessive sun exposure, to use sunscreens routinely, and to be alert to suspicious changes in their moles or the development of new lesions.

PIGMENTED LESIONS AT RISK FOR THE DEVELOPMENT OF MELANOMA

The familial dysplastic nevus syndrome is a relatively recently described constellation of (1) numerous clinically atypical nevi, (2) characteristic atypical histologic features of moles, and (3) one or more family members with a history of melanoma. Family members may have up to a 500-fold increased risk of melanoma compared with the general population. These patients have many, sometimes hundreds, of atypical moles with clinical features ranging from those of ordinary benign nevi to those of frank melanoma. They have variegated color, are larger than 5 mm in diameter, and may have irregular borders. Differentiation from melanoma may be difficult. These patients must be followed carefully, probably every 3 to 4 months. Follow-up is probably best done by those who deal with the entity on a regular basis. These patients must be instructed in careful self-examination and avoidance of sun. Any suspicious lesion that has changed on serial examination is best removed. Serial photographs can be useful in determining changes from one examination to the next.

To add to the confusion, the term "dysplastic nevus" has also been liberally applied to atypical-appearing nevi in individuals without a family history of melanoma. These lesions may be solitary or multiple. In some cases, the patients have a history of melanoma. When biopsy is done, these nevi show a variable degree of the histologic atypia seen in full-bloom familial dysplastic nevus syndrome. No statistics are available on what percentage of these patients with nonfamilial, atypical nevi later develop melanoma. Again, careful follow-up, excision, and histologic examination of any suspicious lesion are warranted.

Congenital nevi are found in approximately 1 per cent of newborns. Giant nevi, defined as lesions greater than 20 cm in diameter, make up only a small fraction of these congenital nevi.

Small congenital nevi have been defined as lesions less than 1.5 cm in diameter. Intermediate congenital nevi are defined as those measuring 1.5 to 20 cm in diameter. It is difficult to ascertain the true incidence of melanoma in congenital nevi. The strongest data are derived from individuals with giant congenital nevi; it is estimated that approximately 6 per cent will develop melanoma. The overall incidence of melanoma is extremely low in childhood and rises with the onset of puberty. In contrast, the incidence of melanoma arising in giant congenital nevi is highest during the first 5 years of life, with nearly 60 per cent of these melanomas developing during the first decade. Giant congenital nevi are problematic. Ideally, total excision is desired. Often, however, they are so large or extend so deeply that total removal is not possible. Leptomeningeal involvement is not uncommon, and the leptomeninges may also be a site of later melanoma development. Even after subtotal excision, melanomas have been reported to develop under skin grafts. It is hoped that new technologic advances, such as tissue expanders, will offer better treatment of giant congenital nevi.

Most congenital nevi are small or medium sized. They too appear to have an increased risk of developing into melanomas; however, it is more difficult to be definitive on specific rates of malignancy. This is an area of some controversy. However, it is generally recommended that small and medium-sized congenital nevi be excised as prophylaxis against future melanoma development. Unlike giant congenital nevi, small and medium-sized congenital nevi generally do not give rise to melanomas before puberty. Therefore, they do not necessarily have to be removed in the first few years of life. In advising parents of children with these moles, it is explained that there is probably a small but increased risk of melanoma transformation. Complete removal of these lesions totally eradicates this potential danger. The ultimate cosmetic result of excision depends on the location and size of the lesion. Excision of larger lesions that require split-thickness skin grafting, or of lesions on the trunk and extremities where scars tend to stretch, leaves more noticeable cosmetic results. In general, however, even these results are less apparent than the original congenital nevus. It should be emphasized that the major purpose of excision of small and medium-sized congenital nevi is melanoma prevention, not cosmetic appearance. The risk of general anesthesia can be avoided in most cases by performing excision under local anesthesia when the patient is either manageable or cooperative (i.e., either during the first few weeks of life or before puberty). If the parents elect not to have excision, or to wait for the child to come of age so that he or she will cooperate with a local procedure, they should be educated to look periodically for changes in the child's congenital nevus and to have the mole re-evaluted by the physician on an annual basis. Prudent avoidance of sunburn or excessive sun exposure is also advisable.

PREMALIGNANT LESIONS

method of
JAMES B. BRIDENSTINE, M.D.
New Orleans, Louisiana

Premalignant conditions may be classified as primary lesions, which occur spontaneously; secondary lesions, which occur in association with other conditions; and hereditary conditions. Of all the precancerous skin lesions encountered by the practitioner, at least 99 per cent are actinic keratosis, leukoplakia, lentigo maligna, dysplastic nevus, or congenital nevocellular nevus. Of these, actinic keratosis accounts for the overwhelming majority.

Patients inquire about precancerous conditions because of their cosmetic disfigurement and malignant potential. Although the malignant potential varies, most precancerous conditions have a low rate of conversion to the malignant state. Therefore the practitioner must consider the cosmetic result when treating these lesions.

Because it is important to establish a definitive diagnosis in premalignant conditions, it is advisable that punch biopsies be performed to provide microscopic identification. Because precancerous conditions may degenerate into frank malignancy at any time, practitioners must ensure themselves and the patients that malignancy has not already occurred. With the exception of actinic keratoses without an inflammatory response or hyperkeratosis, typical keratoacanthomas, and congenital nevocellular nevi, we recommend that all conditions receive biopsy preoperatively. Because of their frequency and our ability to identify actinic keratosis clinically, it is not cost effective to perform biopsy before definitive treatment. When hyperkeratosis or an inflammatory response suggests possible malignant change in an actinic keratosis, a biopsy to rule out squamous cell carcinoma is imperative. Keratoacanthoma and congenital nevocellular nevus do not require a preoperative biopsy for identification, but microscopic evaluation for malignant degeneration should be performed at the time of excision. This is best done with serial sectioning to be certain that no nidus of malignancy is present.

PRIMARY LESIONS

Actinic Keratoses

These scaling, erythematous or hyperpigmented plaques found on sun-exposed areas are the most common premalignant conditions. They often cause concern because of their cosmetic disfigurement. Their malignant potential is low; therefore treatment should provide excellent cosmetic results. Because these lesions are superficial, I prefer to remove them under local anesthesia by thin, tangential shave excision, with the scalpel or razor blade slicing through the papillary dermis. A few millimeters of margin of epidermis surrounding the treatment site is then lightly electrodesiccated at such a low-power setting that a slow blanching (without bubbling or charring) of the surface is seen. Many practitioners overtreat these relatively benign lesions by overzealous electrodesiccation or cryotherapy, with resultant permanent hypopigmented scarring. Another acceptable treatment is superficial curettage. Bleeding after shave excision or curettage is rarely a problem and is controlled by pressure or a chemical cauterant such as 35 per cent aluminum chloride. Any lesion that recurs after treatment or one that initially has a thick surface scale should be considered for total excision, if feasible.

Multiple actinic keratoses involving major portions of the head and neck, trunk, and upper extremities can be treated with topical 5-fluorouracil (5-FU). The 5 per cent cream is usually applied twice daily. Treatment should be continued for 3 to 4 weeks on the face and neck and for 4 to 6 weeks on the scalp, trunk, and upper extremities. Patients must be forewarned that after several days of treatment and long before treatment is complete, the skin will become inflamed and will have a burning pain. For these reasons, I discourage 5-FU treatment. Once my patients have gone through one such treatment, they rarely elect it again. The end of 5-FU treatment occurs when most of the lesions that initially became inflamed have become eroded and exudative. Lesions on the scalp, trunk, and upper extremities usually need 2 weeks of pretreatment and/or concomitant treatment with tretinoin 0.05 per cent cream (Retin-A) to remove or soften thick surface scales. After treatment, any residual lesions require biopsy to rule out squamous cell carcinoma.

Three surgical procedures that effectively remove multiple actinic keratoses are facial dermabrasion, phenol chemical peel, and trichloroacetic acid (TCA) peel. These are considerably more effective than topical 5-FU and should be used when numerous lesions are present or in patients who have a poor response to 5-FU or who have multiple basal cell carcinomas. A procedure used extensively in my practice, mainly on the head and neck, is peeling with 35 per cent TCA. Higher concentrations of TCA can be used but are much more likely to cause scarring and therefore are not recommended. The TCA peel can be enhanced by pretreatment with Jessner's solution or 50 to 70 per cent lactic acid. After these surgical procedures, the skin is rejuvenated. In addition to providing marked therapeutic effects, these treatments provide excellent cosmetic improvement.

Although cryosurgery with liquid nitrogen is used by many physicians, I prefer to avoid it because it can result in permanent hypopigmentation. Because actinic keratoses are directly related to sun damage and are found most commonly in light-complexioned individuals, patients should be advised to regularly apply sunscreens with a sun protection factor of 10 or higher.

Leukoplakia

This condition may be seen on the vermilion border of the lips and the mucous membranes of the oral, anal, and genital regions. The white, hyperkeratotic changes of leukoplakia on the lips can be best defined clinically by grasping the lip at the angles of the mouth and placing it under stretch pressure. I perform biopsy of the most suspicious area, using a 2- or 3-mm punch, followed by primary closure with a braided suture, which is more comfortable than the stiff monofilament suture materials. Leukoplakia in this area most commonly results from chronic sun exposure, irritation from smoking, or chronic biting of the lip. Ill-fitting dentures, poor oral hygiene, excessive use of tobacco, and sharp or chipped teeth may create intraoral changes of leukoplakia.

Definitive treatment consists of infiltration of the affected area with local anesthesia, followed by cautery using a flat, spatula-shaped electrode capable of evenly distributing the destructive force. The affected area and some normal-appearing adjacent tissue are cauterized until a white hue is attained. A curette is used to loosen the treated tissue. Repeat cautery may be necessary to eliminate the deeper, more stubborn areas. Antibiotic ointments such as gentamicin (Garamycin), erythromycin (Ilotycin), or polymyxin B–bacitracin (Polysporin), which do not contain the sensitizing substance neomycin, should be applied every 1 to 2 hours to keep the surgical site soft. Re-epithelialization generally is complete between 7 and 15 days, postoperative pain is mild, and healing is usually complete, without any visible scar formation. Initial evaluation and follow-up examination performed on a semiannual basis should include examination of the regional lymph nodes in the cervical chain and those that are palpable while performing an intraoral bimanual examination using a gloved hand. Laser surgery accomplishes the same results as electrodesiccation cautery.

In severe cases of leukoplakic changes involving a major portion of the lower lip, vermilionectomy and resurfacing of the lip, using an advancement flap from the labial mucosa, is a satisfactory procedure but is more formidable and may cause some deformity of the lower lip.

Red lesions of the oral cavity, known as erythroleukoplakia, have a much higher rate of degeneration into malignancy and should be excised in toto. Genital lesions may be excised or cauterized and curetted.

Lentigo Maligna (Melanotic Freckle of Hutchinson)

These hyperpigmented and often irregularly colored macular lesions, commonly found on sun-exposed areas in the elderly, should be adequately evaluated by punch biopsy, particularly in areas that demonstrate nodularity or changes of depigmentation. Because degeneration of these lesions leads to malignant melanoma, I prefer to treat them early. Punch biopsy shows dysplastic melanocytes, in comparison with the increased number of normal melanocytes seen in lentigo senilis, better known as a liver spot.

Because the abnormal melanocytes extend deep into the hair follicles, complete excision is indicated. Curettage and cautery, liquid nitrogen, and chemical peel using full-strength phenol have been recommended but do not adequately treat the deeper portions of the lesion and usually result in a disfiguring, hypopigmented scar. Dermabrasion, when carried below the hair follicles, cures the lesion but produces permanent scarring. Radiation therapy is not recommended.

Complete surgical excision with serial microscopic evaluation of the tissue is the treatment of choice. The lesion may be so large that it requires several surgical sessions of simple excision for complete removal. In more complex lesions, resurfacing with skin flaps is superior to grafting.

Bowen's Disease

This condition is a particular type of squamous cell carcinoma in situ and usually presents on sun-exposed areas as a well-defined, erythematous, scaling plaque. It is often mistaken for an actinic keratosis; however, its malignant potential is considerably greater. When found in areas not normally exposed to sunlight, it may result from earlier exposure to arsenic ingestion and can be associated with internal malignancy.

When nodularity or erosion is present, biopsy should encompass these areas.

Complete excision of Bowen's disease is imperative, and the specimen should be sent for serial sectioning to determine definitively tumor-free borders. Most lesions are small and can be closed by using primary closure. Margins must be adequate to encompass areas of involvement that are not clinically perceptible. Although cautery and curettage, radiation therapy, chemotherapy using 5-FU, and cryotherapy with liquid nitrogen are used by many physicians, I do not rely on these methods because they do not provide a surgical specimen for microscopic evaluation.

Erythroplasia of Queyrat

This condition represents Bowen's disease of the mucous membranes, usually of the penis. It is a potentially dangerous condition because it can invade the distal urethra or rapidly degenerate into squamous cell carcinoma with regional lymph node metastases. Because of these two complicating factors I do not use topical chemotherapy with 5-FU, cryotherapy using liquid nitrogen, or cautery and curettage, which have been recommended by some. Surgical excision with serial evaluation of the entire specimen is obligatory to identify positively tumor-free borders. Although cold knife surgery can be used, special microscopic techniques are necessary for evaluating the surgical specimen. Mohs's micrographic surgery is the treatment of choice and should be used even if patients must be sent to distant centers using this technique. Initial treatment must be effective and complete to prevent penectomy in the event of recurrence. Circumcision should be performed as a preventive measure.

Keratoacanthoma

This lesion is typical in appearance, with its rapid onset and characteristic dome shape with a central crater containing a keratotic plug. The clinical difficulty arises in distinguishing this tumor from a squamous cell carcinoma. Although some physicians have suggested that a wedge resection be removed from the central portion of a keratoacanthoma to induce spontaneous resolution, I believe that this is ill-advised because rapid extension of the tumor may continue and adequate microscopic identification may be impossible. It is well known that these lesions frequently resolve spontaneously, but the result is always a noticeable, hypopigmented, atrophic scar. A rapidly enlarging squamous cell carcinoma that has been clinically misdiagnosed as keratoacanthoma is another reason for permanent and complete excision of the keratoacanthoma.

In cases in which multiple keratoacanthomas are found, complete surgical excision may not be necessary. After several lesions have been adequately evaluated microscopically to rule out squamous cell carcinoma, the remaining lesions may be treated by using cautery and curettage, cryotherapy with liquid nitrogen, intralesional infiltration of full-strength 5-FU, or intralesional triamcinolone (Kenalog), 20 to 40 mg per ml. Other reported treatment methods for multiple keratoacanthomas are oral methotrexate, 2.5 mg per day for 3 months, and a compounded 3.5 per cent ointment of bleomycin. Multiple keratoacanthomas of the eruptive type are resistant to most forms of therapy.

Cutaneous Horn

These exophytic lesions may develop into squamous cell carcinoma. Treatment consists of excision with primary closure and subsequent microscopic examination of the base of the lesion. Cautery and curettage and other modalities do not provide a surgical specimen for microscopic evaluation and are not recommended.

Miscellaneous Primary Lesions

Arsenical Keratoses, Tar Keratoses, Paget's Disease, and Verrucous Carcinoma. These conditions are mentioned here for completeness. They are rare. If they are found, the patient should be referred to a dermatologist who has experience in their treatment.

SECONDARY LESIONS

Congenital Nevocellular Nevus

These nevi come in two varieties: the giant, hairy, pigmented nevus, often referred to as bathing trunk nevus, and the smaller, nonhairy, congenital, pigmented nevus. Studies have shown that malignant degeneration into melanoma is much greater for congenital nevi compared with acquired nevi. Some studies indicate that pigmented nevocellular nevi that develop before the age of 2 are also at increased risk of malignant degeneration. Most physicians now believe that all congenital nevi should be surgically excised as soon as possible because deaths have been reported as early as the first decade of life. Most smaller lesions can be excised in toto with one operation. Larger lesions may be removed in serial excisions, allowing 8 to 12 weeks to elapse between surgical sessions. When feasible, advancement flaps should be used rather than skin grafting for obvious cosmetic reasons. Recently, dermabrasion has been recommended for large lesions. When used during the first 8 weeks of life, this method is effective in permanently removing pigmentation and destroys most of the melanocytes before they migrate to the deeper portions of the dermis. The procedure must be performed by a dermatologic surgeon who is well trained in the technique of dermabrasion.

Nevus Sebaceus of Jadassohn

This congenital tumor, also known as organoid nevus, can develop into a basal cell carcinoma, apocrine carcinoma, adnexal carcinoma, or squamous cell carcinoma. Because malignant degeneration usually occurs in adulthood, it is advisable to excise these lesions surgically during adolescence. Superficial cautery and curettage do not destroy the deeper portions of this tumor and, in addition, produce an alopecic scar.

Chronic Conditions

Malignant degeneration in chronic irritant conditions is well known. It is often associated with chronic discharge or pruritus. These conditions include but are not limited to thermal burn scars, radiation dermatitis, cutaneous ulcers, ill-fitting appliances, cheilitis, lichen sclerosus et atrophicus, lichen planus, and lupus vulgaris. The practitioner must be aware that these conditions predispose to malignant degeneration. Periodic follow-up is indicated, and any suspicious change should prompt a skin biopsy.

HEREDITARY CONDITIONS

The genodermatoses that are associated with malignant change are xeroderma pigmentosum, pachyonychia congenita, dyskeratosis congenita, epidermodysplasia verruciformis, basal cell nevus syndrome, and dysplastic nevus syndrome with B-K mole. Little can be done to prevent malignant changes. Therefore, careful monitoring of these patients is necessary to correct the malignant and premalignant changes as early as possible.

Dysplastic Nevus (B-K Mole) Syndrome

The dysplastic nevus syndrome is growing rapidly in importance. Studies have shown that 10 per cent or more of the U.S. caucasian population carries the gene for this syndrome. Patients with this condition have a propensity to develop many pigmented lesions with irregular, indistinct (fuzzy) borders and multiple shades of color. Although most common on the trunk, lesions can appear in any location. Evolution to malignant melanoma occurs with disturbing frequency. Therefore, any suspicious lesion should be excised with a margin of 2 to 5 mm of normal tissue. Photographic documentation every 6 months is helpful, and family members should be screened for the condition.

BACTERIAL DISEASES OF THE SKIN

method of
ROBERT ZANE, M.D.,
ARNOLD W. GUREVITCH, M.D., and
SAMUEL E. WILSON, M.D.
Harbor-UCLA Medical Center
Torrance, California

The skin is the largest organ of the body. The normal stratum corneum layer is the major barrier against infection, being virtually impermeable to bacteria. Important factors that limit bacterial colonization include the presence of inhibiting normal flora, primarily species of *Corynebacterium* and *Staphylococcus epidermidis;* a dry, cool surface with a poor nutrient supply; and a lipid-rich, acidic environment. Most infections of the skin result from traumatic disruption of these barriers. Common inoculates are *Staphylococcus aureus,* which forms bullae or pustules, and group A beta-hemolytic streptococci, which produce a spreading, erythematous character, lymphocytosis, and central necrosis.

IMPETIGO

This bacterial infection, seen in all age groups but most commonly in children, occurs in two forms: the more common thick, golden-crusted, nonbullous lesions and a bullous form. In the past, most cases of nonbullous impetigo (impetigo contagiosa) were caused by group A beta-hemolytic streptococci, although *S. aureus* was often isolated from cultures as well. In most recent studies, however, *S. aureus* was the most frequent isolate. The initial lesion of nonbullous impetigo is an erythematous papule that progresses to a transient, superficial vesicle or pustule. The vesiculopustular lesion ruptures, resulting in a thick, yellow crust surrounded by a slightly edematous, red border. Bullous impetigo is characterized by large, superficial bullae that rupture easily, leaving a thin, varnish-like crust. Bullous impetigo is caused almost exclusively by phage group II *S. aureus.* Both forms of impetigo are highly contagious, especially to children.

Treatment of nonbullous impetigo begins with topical cleansing of the area and application of warm compresses. Mupirocin, a topical antibiotic, has recently been reported to provide good results for localized lesions. Widespread impetigo should be treated with a systemic antibiotic. Currently, oral erythromycin (E-Mycin), 250 mg four times a day (30 to 50 mg per kg per day in divided doses for children) for 7 to 10 days is recommended. Alternative but more expensive choices are dicloxacillin (Dynopen) (250 to 500 mg every 6 hours), amoxicillin-clavulanic acid (Augmentin) (250 mg every 8 hours), or a cephalosporin. Recent studies indicate a 25 to 50 per cent failure rate with penicillin V. Bullous impetigo should be treated similarly. If the impetigo progresses to cellulitis, an intravenous antibiotic may be required.

STAPHYLOCOCCAL SCALDED SKIN SYNDROME

The staphylococcal scalded skin syndrome, characterized by widespread erythema, bullae, and exfoliation, is seen predominantly in newborns or young infants and rarely in adults who are immunocompromised or who have renal failure. The disease is caused by the exfoliative exotoxin exfoliatin, which is produced by the phage group II strain of *S. aureus*. In children the most common site of primary staphylococcal infection is the conjunctiva. The exotoxin causes cleavage and blister formation high in the epidermis within the granular layer, without damage to the lower epidermis. These clinical features grossly resemble a scald produced by boiling water. However, the staphylococcal scalded skin syndrome is manifested by sudden onset of fever, erythema, edema, and exquisite tenderness of the skin. The skin lesions commonly affect the neck, face, groin, and axillae but can become generalized, including the palms and soles (mucous membranes are usually spared). Within 1 to 2 days the upper layers of the epidermis become separated, causing flaccid bullae and the peeling off of large sheets of skin. The skin is extremely sensitive to a light touch and peels off easily (Nikolsky's sign), leaving a moist, red surface.

Treatment consists of local care and systemic antibiotics. Supportive measures, such as burn cradles, blankets, and intravenous fluid and electrolyte management, are critical in severe cases. Beta-lactamase–resistant antistaphylococcal antibiotics, such as those used to treat bullous impetigo, are recommended. Mortality in untreated cases is greatest in neonates, and death usually results from sepsis and electrolyte imbalance. With early treatment the prognosis is excellent, and healing occurs without scarring.

TOXIC EPIDERMAL NECROLYSIS

Toxic epidermal necrolysis is usually related to hypersensitivity to drugs such as sulfonamides, barbiturates, hydantoins, penicillin-related antibiotics, vaccines, and salicylates. In contrast to the scalded skin syndrome, toxic epidermal necrolysis involves necrosis of the entire epidermal layer, with cleavage at the dermal-epidermal border. Accurate diagnosis, which is accomplished by skin biopsy, is mandatory because of the severity of this disease. Patients are best managed at burn centers with full resuscitation using balanced electrolyte solutions. Skin loss may reach 100 per cent of the total body surface. Topical antibacterials are recommended; however, sulfa-containing creams should be avoided because of the high incidence of allergy in these patients. Systemic corticosteroids are probably not useful and may even be harmful. There is a 25 to 70 per cent mortality, even with appropriate treatment. In general hospitals, however, a reduction in mortality may be achieved by early referral to a burn center, use of biologic dressings such as porcine grafts, and intensive support.

FOLLICULITIS, FURUNCLES, AND CARBUNCLES

Bacterial folliculitis often occurs as a superficial infection within a hair follicle and is usually caused by *S. aureus*. Found most commonly on the scalp, beard, and extremities, folliculitis is characterized by small, red papules that progress to pustules that spontaneously rupture. The hair follicle is relatively isolated from host defenses. Treatment includes topical cleansing with antibacterial soap such as hexaclorophene (pHisoHex) and chlorhexidine (Hibiclens) twice daily, followed by application of topical antibiotics such as erythromycin topical solution (T-Stat), 1 per cent clindamycin solution (Cleocin T), or mupirocin ointment (Bactroban). Daily application of 6.25 per cent aluminum chloride hexahydrate in ethanol (Xerac AC) has also been reported to be effective. Systemic antibiotic therapy may be needed for widespread chronic folliculitis. Erythromycin, 250 to 500 mg orally every 6 hours, is recommended.

In contrast to superficial folliculitis, a furuncle (boil) is a deep follicular abscess caused almost exclusively by *S. aureus* and found most commonly in areas where the skin is moist, occluded, and subject to friction, such as the buttocks, groin, thighs, axillae, and waist. The face, neck, and extremities may also be involved. A furuncle begins as a small, red, follicular papule or nodule that progresses to a pustular and then a necrotic stage. The follicle is then destroyed, and healing occurs with scar formation.

A carbuncle is a multiloculated abscess resulting from coalescence of contiguously infected hair follicles. These uncommon infections usually occur in areas of thick skin such as the back of the neck, shoulders, hips, or thighs. The presenting lesion is a smooth, red, firm, painful lump that may reach a diameter of up to 10 cm. Eventually, pus drains from several follicular orifices. If untreated, the central area becomes necrotic and sloughs. Cultures or Gram's stain of purulent fluid, revealing *S. aureus,* may aid in the diagnosis.

Furuncles commonly become fluctuant and drain spontaneously with application of warm compresses. When further treatment is indicated, simple incision and drainage are especially helpful. Both furuncles and carbuncles should always be treated with systemic antibiotics in addition to incision and drainage. Dicloxacillin (Dynapen), 250 mg every 6 hours, cephalexin (Keflex), 250 mg every 6 hours, cefadroxil (Duricef), 500 mg every 12 hours, or erythromycin (E-Mycin), 500 mg every 6 hours (in penicillin-allergic patients), is useful in preventing further spread and sepsis. In recurrent cases, prophylaxis may be obtained with good hygiene and routine bathing with antibacterial cleansers such as chlorhexidine (Hibiclens). A search for underlying conditions such as diabetes, immune deficits, and nasal carriage is important. In some cases, the use of long-term, low-dose systemic antibiotics such as erythromycin, 250 mg, or clindamycin, 150 mg orally once a day, may be required. Nasal carriage may be suppressed by a topical antibacterial ointment.

ERYSIPELAS AND CELLULITIS

Erysipelas is a superficial form of cellulitis involving chiefly the dermis and upper subcutaneous layers of the skin. Cellulitis is a deeper infection involving primarily subcutaneous tissue. Erysipelas is caused by group A beta-hemolytic streptococci, whereas cellulitis is caused by streptococci, *S. aureus, Haemophilus influenzae,* and, occasionally, a variety of other bacteria. Clinically, erysipelas, also known as St. Anthony's fire, is characterized by a sharply circumscribed area of erythema and edema, most commonly involving the face and neck. Cellulitis presents as a warm, erythematous, edematous, tender lesion with less distinct margins and an advancing border. Both forms may be accompanied by fever, malaise, lymphangitis, and lymphadenitis. The most common predisposing conditions include trauma, diabetes, venous stasis, immunosuppression, or an underlying cutaneous disease. Diagnosis is based on the clinical presentation because it is quite difficult to culture bacteria from these lesions.

Early limited erysipelas in an uncompromised patient can usually be treated with penicillin V, 250 to 500 mg orally every 6 hours for 10 days. Erythromycin, 250 to 500 mg every 6 hours, may be substituted in the penicillin-allergic patient. The patient must remain well hydrated, and the affected limb should be elevated to promote lymphatic drainage. Warm compresses should be applied three times daily. In more extensive cases or when significant systemic signs are present, parenteral penicillin G is recommended, 2 million units every 4 to 6 hours. If evidence of previous damage to the skin is present, combination antibiotic coverage is recommended. Erysipelas frequently shows little improvement until the fifth day of therapy.

In cellulitis, penicillinase-resistant antibiotics are recommended to cover *S. aureus.* Vancomycin, 500 mg every 6 hours, should be used in the penicillin-allergic patient. Gram-negative anaerobic organisms must be suspected when chronic ulcers are present, especially in the diabetic or immunosuppressed patient. In general, incision and drainage are contraindicated in the absence of local necrosis. However, failure to achieve a reasonable response to antibiotics may indicate abscess formation or necrosis. Failure to drain necrotic areas can be fatal.

HAEMOPHILUS INFLUENZAE CELLULITIS

H. influenzae cellulitis, most commonly seen in children under 5 years of age, causes a reddish-blue to purple, warm, raised, tender area on the face, neck, or upper extremities. This usually is preceded by several days of fever and coryza and often occurs in conjunction with otitis media, epiglottitis, sinusitis, or pneumonia. The cellulitis is caused by hematogenous spread from a primary focus, and it may precede meningitis. Therefore, a spinal tap is an important part of the work-up.

Current treatment recommendations are hospitalization for hydration and parenteral antibiotics such as ampicillin, 200 to 400 mg per kg per day,* and chloramphenicol, 75 to 100 mg per kg per day,* each divided into four doses. Cultures from blood, cerebrospinal fluid, pleural effusions, and so on should be done before therapy. Because of major problems of resistance of *H. influenzae,* the treatment should be re-evaluated in 48 hours and the most appropriate therapy chosen.

HIDRADENITIS SUPPURATIVA

Hidradenitis suppurativa is not a primary infectious process but rather a chronic, suppurative,

---

*May exceed manufacturer's recommended dose.

inflammatory disease of the pilosebaceous apparatus and apocrine sweat glands. It probably results from occlusion of the follicular pore and leads to the formation of tender, red, subcutaneous nodules, abscesses, sinus tracts, and scarring. Hidradenitis is often seen together with severe cystic acne. It is most commonly found in the axillae, groin, perineum, and perirectal areas. Any abscess in the apocrine gland region should be suspected to be hidradenitis, and multiple abscesses with sinus tract formation are diagnostic. Secondary bacterial infection occurs rather commonly, and cultures often reveal *S. aureus*. However, a variety of other pathogens occasionally occur, and in many cases only normal skin flora grow. Appropriate treatment depends on the stage and severity of the disease. If a specific pathogen is found, an appropriate antibiotic should be used until the secondary infection has resolved. If no pathogen is present, erythromycin or tetracycline, 250 mg four times daily given orally, is usually helpful. Long-term maintenance therapy is almost always required to prevent recurrences. The antibiotic dose should be gradually reduced to the lowest amount that controls the disease. This therapy must be continued for months to years. In the acute setting, incision and drainage of abscesses are appropriate for symptomatic relief; however, this treatment may cause sinus formation. Intralesional injection of nonfluctuant nodules, using a long-acting corticosteroid (triamcinolone acetonide, 2.5 to 3.0 mg per ml), is quite helpful. In addition, some patients with early hidradenitis respond to isotretinoin (Accutane), 1 to 1.5 mg per kg per day. In severe cases that are not controlled by medical therapy, wide local excision of the apocrine gland–bearing tissue has remained an essential form of treatment. After complete excision, the defect can be managed by primary closure, delayed healing by granulation, split-thickness skin grafting, or rotation flaps. Another surgical approach involves probing and unroofing, by scalpel or electrocoagulation, all interconnecting sinus tracts. The areas are thoroughly curetted to remove necrotic tissue and epithelial linings. Complete healing, by secondary intention, occurs in 1 to 2 months.

VIRAL DISEASES OF THE SKIN

method of
BRENT G. PETTY, M.D.
The Johns Hopkins University School of Medicine
Baltimore, Maryland

This chapter deals with the treatment of viral infections that are usually limited to the skin (Table 1).

TABLE 1. **Viral Infections of the Skin**

Herpesviruses
  Herpes simplex virus, type 1
    Orolabial
    Cutaneous
    Whitlow
  Herpes simplex virus, type 2
    Genital herpes
    Herpetic proctitis
  Varicella-zoster virus
    Localized
    Disseminated

Poxviruses
  Molluscum contagiosum
  Orf (ecthyma contagiosum)
  Milker's nodules

Papillomavirus
  Warts

Drug therapy specific for viral inhibition is available for treatment of the herpesviruses, but to date, no specific antiviral chemotherapy has been found for the other viral diseases discussed.

HERPES SIMPLEX VIRUS, TYPE 1

Clinical Manifestations

Orolabial Herpes. Painful ulcerative pharyngitis and stomatitis caused by herpes simplex virus type 1 (HSV-1) are usually seen in children and resolve within 2 weeks without complications. When the disease is severe and extensive, however, the patient may become dehydrated because of inability to maintain adequate fluid intake.

The most common manifestation of HSV-1 is herpes labialis, the typical cold sore. It usually emerges at the vermilion border of the lip, frequently recurring in the same location in association with an illness, exposure to sunlight, after surgery, or after other physiologic stress. Herpes labialis is usually self-limited and is problematic primarily because of pain and cosmetic concerns.

Cutaneous Herpes. A patch of vesicular lesions with surrounding erythema, the appearance typical of herpetic lesions, may develop anywhere on the skin. Like herpes labialis, the eruption may recur in the same location. These lesions are usually less extensive than the dermatomal distribution of herpes zoster (see later). Although cutaneous herpes is generally self-limited, in some patients it causes extensive erythema multiforme as a nonspecific response, often extending well beyond the area where the cutaneous viral infection was localized.

Herpetic Whitlow. The term "whitlow" refers to an infection localized to a finger tip after direct inoculation of virus through a break in the skin. It is usually seen in dentists or medical personnel or occurs as a result of self-inoculation by a patient with herpes elsewhere. Although the majority of cases are caused by HSV-1, many are caused by herpes simplex virus type 2 (HSV-2). Pain and swelling associated with vesicular lesions, pustular lesions, or both are typical at presentation.

Diagnosis

The diagnosis of HSV-1 infection is largely clinical, and treatment is often initiated on the basis of clinical suspicion alone. Additional diagnostic aids are Tzanck's smear, viral culture, and antigen detection methods. Tzanck's smear is a toluidine blue stain of the material scraped from the base of a punctured, fresh vesicle. The presence of multinucleated giant cells supports the diagnosis of herpetic infection. Viral culture is perhaps the most specific and reliable method for confirming the presence of infectious virus, but it requires 2 to 3 days for the characteristic cytopathic effect to appear. The time needed to confirm the diagnosis can be shortened to 16 hours by detecting HSV antigens from cultured specimens, using monoclonal antibodies or biotinylated DNA probes. The monoclonal antibodies have the slight advantage of providing type-specific identification (either HSV-1 or HSV-2), whereas the biotinylated DNA probes react with both serotypes.

Serologic assays are available to identify individuals who were previously infected with HSV and who, by presumption, still have latent viral infection in ganglia. Identifying such individuals from among those who are to undergo organ transplantation is important in the prophylaxis of reactivated disease.

Treatment

The development of the nucleoside analogue acyclovir allows specific treatment for HSV infections. This substantial step forward was part of the reason for awarding the 1988 Nobel Prize in Medicine and Physiology to Dr. Gertrude Elion, the developer of acyclovir. Acyclovir selectively inhibits viral replication because the virus contains an enzyme (thymidine kinase) that converts acyclovir to its active form (acyclovir triphosphate) in infected cells; uninfected human cells do not have this enzyme and so cannot produce the active triphosphate in a significant amount. This property allows acyclovir to act as a "magic bullet," affecting virus-infected cells and having no effect on uninfected cells.

Acyclovir is marketed in topical, oral, and intravenous formulations, with increasing degrees of efficacy, respectively. Topical therapy is no more or only slightly more beneficial clinically than placebo; the oral formulation is so well tolerated that, in my opinion, the topical preparation is not worth the mess and inconvenience. For either primary or recurrent HSV-1 infections, oral acyclovir, 200 mg five times per day for 5 days, is recommended. This dose is effective for orolabial or cutaneous disease and herpetic whitlow. When orolabial herpes is severe or is associated with herpes esophagitis, thereby preventing oral therapy, or if the patient is immunosuppressed, intravenous acyclovir, 5 mg per kg every 8 hours, should be administered. Because acyclovir is eliminated primarily by the kidneys, the dosage, whether given orally or intravenously, should be reduced in patients with renal insufficiency.

Inasmuch as herpes tends to be a recurrent disease, often with known precipitating factors (e.g., ultraviolet light exposure or surgery for trigeminal neuralgia), smaller doses of acyclovir have been found to decrease the incidence of recurrences. Doses of 200 mg of oral acyclovir twice daily* may provide protection from recurrent disease. This prophylactic therapy can be given continuously in patients who have severe recurrent disease or who are prone to develop serious complications with recurrences, such as erythema multiforme. On the other hand, many patients fare well if they simply take the prophylactic therapy in anticipation of an exposure likely to initiate a recurrence, such as extended exposure to sunlight. In patients with serologic evidence of past infection who are to undergo bone marrow, renal, or cardiac transplantation, intravenous acyclovir, 5 mg per kg every 8 hours, is highly effective in preventing the morbidity of recurrent herpes infection in such immunocompromised hosts.

HERPES SIMPLEX VIRUS, TYPE 2
Clinical Manifestations

Genital Herpes. Genital herpes presents as multiple bilateral lesions on the external genitalia. The lesions may be vesicular, pustular, or ulcerative. With time the lesions crust over and heal. In women there may be associated vaginal and cervical involvement. The symptoms include pain, dysuria, and vaginal and urethral discharge. Although some cases of genital herpes are caused by HSV-1, the majority are caused by HSV-2. The painful lesions usually remit spontaneously, but there is a propensity for recurrence, particularly with HSV-2, and, less frequently, with HSV-1.

Herpetic Proctitis. Pain, discharge, tenesmus, and ulcerative rectal lesions on proctoscopy are

---

*This dose may be lower than that recommended by the manufacturer.

the hallmarks of rectal herpes infection. Like genital herpes, this condition is more often caused by HSV-2 than by HSV-1. It has become increasingly recognized in homosexual men and in heterosexual women who practice anal receptive intercourse.

Diagnosis

The diagnostic considerations for HSV-2 were mentioned in the discussion of HSV-1.

Treatment

Again, acyclovir provides specific antiviral treatment. Given in doses of 200 mg orally five times a day for 5 days, acyclovir causes initial or recurrent episodes of HSV-2 to remit more quickly than the resolution observed in patients treated with placebo. An alternative regimen of 800 mg twice daily for 5 days* may be equally effective, but it has been studied far less extensively. Because recurrence remains a major problem, prophylaxis with low-dose oral acyclovir is indicated in patients who have frequent and/or extensive recurrences. Doses as low as 200 mg orally twice daily have been shown to have a significant effect in reducing the frequency of the painful, debilitating episodes in predisposed patients. If 200 mg twice daily proves to be inadequate to reduce the incidence of recurrence, the dose can be increased to 200 mg three times daily or 400 mg twice daily. A single oral dose of 800 mg of acyclovir also appears to be superior to placebo in preventing recurrences, but it has not been compared with the lower-dose regimens.

VARICELLA-ZOSTER VIRUS

Clinical Manifestations

Varicella (chickenpox), usually contracted in childhood, invariably leads to latent viral infection of dorsal root ganglia. Reactivation of latent virus, with migration along sensory nerves to the skin, leads to the syndrome known as herpes zoster. Clinically, there may be a brief (3- to 5-day) period of pain, hyperesthesia, or both, in a dermatomal distribution before the eruption of typical grouped vesicles with surrounding erythema in a patchy distribution along the dermatome. Generally, herpes zoster is a self-limited disease with spontaneous remission. Nevertheless, there may be occasions, most commonly in immunosuppressed patients, when the involvement extends beyond single or contiguous dermatomes and affects distant dermatomes, visceral organs, or both, particularly the lungs and liver. Such "disseminated zoster" constitutes a

serious disease. Even in the absence of dissemination, about 30 per cent of patients have persistent pain after resolution of the cutaneous lesions, a condition known as postherpetic neuralgia. Postherpetic neuralgia increases in incidence with increasing age.

Diagnosis

Herpes zoster is commonly a clinical diagnosis, based on the characteristic combination of clusters of vesicular lesions with surrounding erythema associated with pain in a dermatomal distribution. Tzanck's smear should be positive, just as with HSV, and viral culture can confirm the diagnosis but is rarely used outside of rigorous clinical trials or epidemiologic investigations.

Treatment

Acyclovir has activity against varicella-zoster virus. Given orally or intravenously, it significantly reduces the duration of viral shedding, new lesion formation, and acute pain. Nevertheless, because the majority of immunocompetent patients with herpes zoster experience a self-limited illness, it is not clear that acyclovir should be used, except when the disease affects the ophthalmic branch of the trigeminal nerve, thereby threatening the eye. In spite of its antiviral effect, acyclovir has been disappointing in preventing postherpetic neuralgia, either alone or in combination with corticosteroids. If oral acyclovir is used to treat herpes zoster,* it should be used as early as possible in the illness, and because varicella-zoster virus is less sensitive to acyclovir than is HSV, larger doses must be used, namely, 800 mg five times a day for 5 to 7 days.† Prodrugs of acyclovir and sustained-release preparations of oral acyclovir have been under investigation, but none have yet been marketed.

Because immunosuppressed patients are at special risk to develop disseminated disease, oral therapy must be monitored carefully to detect the earliest evidence of dissemination; alternatively, intravenous acyclovir, 10 mg per kg every 8 hours,‡ should be given instead of oral therapy. If dissemination occurs, even in an immunocompetent patient, intravenous acyclovir treatment with this dose should be started promptly and continued for 7 to 10 days, or longer if there is no positive clinical response. Human leukocyte interferon-alpha appears to be just as effective as intravenous acyclovir but has more adverse side effects, such as fever and nausea.

The treatment recommendations for herpesvirus infections are summarized in Table 2.

---

*This dosage regimen is not listed by the manufacturer.

*This use is not listed by the manufacturer.
†This dosage regimen is not listed by the manufacturer.
‡May exceed manufacturer's recommended dose.

TABLE 2. **Acyclovir Treatment of Herpesvirus Infections**

Infection	Treatment	Prophylaxis
HSV-1	200 mg PO 5 times a day*	200 mg PO bid†
HSV-2	200 mg PO 5 times a day*	200–400 mg PO bid
Herpes zoster		
Localized disease in slightly immunosuppressed patients	800 mg PO 5 times a day‡	
Localized disease in severely immunosuppressed patients	10 mg/kg IV q 8 hr‡	
Disseminated disease	10 mg/kg IV q 8 hr‡	

*For extensive disease, when oral therapy is not possible, or in immunosuppressed patients, 5 mg/kg IV q 8 hr is recommended.
†May be lower than manufacturer's recommended dose.
‡May exceed manufacturer's recommended dose.

POXVIRUSES

Clinical Manifestations

Molluscum Contagiosum. This illness is characterized by small, papular lesions with a central depression. It occurs primarily in children, in whom the lesions are located on the face, trunk, and limbs. In adults, the lesions most commonly occur in the genital and inner thigh areas, probably related to sexual contact. In both children and adults, the lesions are present without systemic symptoms. Molluscum contagiosum is usually a self-limited illness, requiring no treatment. The lesions clear in 6 months to 3 years after their appearance.

Orf. Also known as ecthyma contagiosum, orf is an endemic viral illness among sheep and is transmitted to humans by contact with the animals' secretions by those responsible for handling them (e.g., sheepherders, veterinarians). The virus causes the development of nodules on exposed areas, which are self-limited but may become secondarily infected; this is the main concern in this disease.

Milker's Nodules. This poxviral illness is spread from infected cattle to handlers and causes a self-limited nodular eruption that lasts for 4 to 6 weeks. No therapy is recommended.

Treatment

If treatment for molluscum contagiosum is contemplated because of the extent of the lesions, one can consider removal with a curette or liquid nitrogen, use of a keratolytic agent such as Duofilm (combination salicylic acid and lactic acid),

or stimulation of a local inflammatory reaction in the dermis by puncturing the lesions and applying iodine. Orf nodules may be resected if they are extensive or necrotic. Secondary infections can be treated if they develop.

PAPILLOMAVIRUS

Clinical Manifestation

Warts. Warts are caused by as many as 42 different types of human papillomavirus. Each type is largely specific for warts erupting at a particular body site. Warts are generally spread by direct contact, including self-inoculation, but may also be spread by fomites, particularly with plantar warts, which can be acquired through contact with shower floors. Although they may be persistent or long-standing, most warts spontaneously regress. Venereal warts (condyloma accuminata) may be especially extensive, persistent, and resistant to treatment.

Treatment

Removal by electrodesiccation, curettage, or blistering agents such as liquid nitrogen or cantharidin has been used. Keratolytic agents, such as salicylic acid paint, and formalin soaks have been used particularly for plantar warts. A 25 to 50 per cent podophyllin solution is used, with or without surgical excision or liquid nitrogen application, in the treatment of genital warts. Intralesional interferon injections have been successful in the treatment of some patients with vulvar warts.

PARASITIC INFESTATIONS

method of
HOBART K. RICHEY, M.D.,
PHILIP D. SHENEFELT, M.D., and
NEIL A. FENSKE, M.D.
University of South Florida
Tampa, Florida

SCABIES

Scabies is an infestation by the mite *Sarcoptes scabiei hominis*. It is characterized by marked pruritus, which is usually worse at night, excoriations, and secondary infection. The itching is caused by sensitization to the mite; thus, close contacts may be affected despite the absence of symptoms.

Infestation occurs when a female mite burrows through the epidermal stratum corneum and creates tiny tunnels in which fecal debris and eggs can be found. After contact with the mite, a previously sensitized patient may develop symptoms within 24 hours. Patients who have not had prior contact with the mite may remain asymptomatic for 6 to 8 weeks, after which sensitization usually develops and the clinical symptoms become apparent. The characteristic lesion is a burrow, a subtle violation of the integrity of the epidermis. It is generally several millimeters in length and serpiginous in nature. Burrows are usually present in the interdigital finger-web spaces, as well as in other intertriginous locations. In males, the glans penis is also a frequent site of involvement. In addition to burrows, numerous papules and pustules may be found.

Infestation in adults rarely involves the face or scalp. However, infants and young children with scabies often have widespread involvement including the neck, face, and scalp.

A variant referred to as crusted or Norwegian scabies occurs in physically debilitated, mentally retarded, or immunocompromised patients. It is characterized by infestation with thousands of mites and results in a diffuse, hyperkeratotic, crusted eruption involving predominantly the hands, feet, and nails. Despite the myriad mites, pruritus is minimal.

The diagnosis of scabies can be confirmed by obtaining a scraping, using a No. 15 scalpel blade with a drop of mineral oil adherent, from a burrow or nonexcoriated papule. This material is placed on a glass slide and examined under the light microscope. The yield for identification of the scabies mite, eggs, or fecal debris is increased by scraping multiple burrows and papules.

Treatment

The most common agent used for the treatment of scabies is lindane 1 per cent (Kwell) in a lotion or cream. The patient should be instructed to apply the Kwell from the neck down, with special attention to the axilla, umbilicus, interdigital webs, groin, and intergluteal cleft. The Kwell should be left on overnight for 6 to 12 hours and washed off in the morning. This procedure should be repeated in 3 days.

In studies, lindane 1 per cent has been shown to be 90 per cent curative at 6 hours and 98 per cent curative at 12 hours. It is a cosmetically acceptable product that is not malodorous and does not sting when applied to the skin. There have been isolated case reports of resistance to the product, especially in areas where scabies infestation is endemic and treatment with lindane has been liberal.

Neurotoxicity associated with lindane use has generally been reported in infants and usually is caused by either inappropriate topical use or accidental ingestion of the lindane. We do not recommend lindane for the treatment of scabies in infants and modify its use in young children, preferring a half-strength solution that is left on for only 3 to 4 hours. Although lindane is not a known teratogen, we avoid its use in pregnant or lactating women. Irritant dermatitis may result from excessive use; therefore, we limit the amount prescribed to that sufficient to treat the individuals involved.

Another agent that has been used in the treatment of scabies is 6 per cent precipitated sulfur in hydrophilic petrolatum. The agent is applied once a day for 3 consecutive days without removal of the agent or bathing during the intervening time period. Twenty-four hours after the last application, the patient may bathe and remove the medication. Treatment for infants and young children should include application of the antiscabetic agent to the face and scalp, with particular attention to the postauricular folds. Reported success rates for the eradication of the mite are variable, and patient acceptance is lower because the treatment is messy. This treatment is safer in small children, infants, and pregnant and lactating women.

Crotamiton (Eurax) and 25 per cent benzyl benzoate creams are of limited efficacy and are not considered to be the treatment of choice.

Malathion 0.5 per cent aqueous emulsion (Prioderm) is effective as a single dose, which should be repeated after 7 days for maximal efficacy. It reportedly has a low mammalian toxicity with low dermal penetration.

The use of permethrin 5 per cent in dermal cream is reportedly an excellent scabicide when used in a single-dose schedule. It is cosmetically elegant, has no odor, and does not stain clothing. It reportedly has a low mammalian toxicity and is broken down by esterases in the skin. Systemic absorption is thus of minimal concern.

Norwegian scabies may be treated with any of the previously mentioned products. However, the mite is often sequestered in the subungual debris, which is characteristic of the infestation, and cases refractory to treatment are common. Dissolution of the nail with 40 per cent urea, with subsequent application of the scabicide, may help to eradicate this nidus of infection.

Treatment of scabies should include the patient and all close contacts. In addition, at the time of treatment, linens including bedclothes, towels, and recently worn clothing should be laundered. Kwell shampoo can be added to the laundry wash cycle for complete mite eradication.

Postscabetic dermatitis, nodular scabies, and scabetic granulomas are sensitization phenomena that may remain for days or weeks after eradication of the mite. They can be treated with mild- to moderate-potency topical corticosteroids or with oral antihistamines.

CUTANEOUS LARVA MIGRANS

Cutaneous larva migrans, also known as creeping eruption, is seen quite frequently in the southeastern United States and, less often, in the northern states. In this era of worldwide travel, this diagnosis should be kept in mind especially for vacationers who have recently returned from the Caribbean or subtropics. The infestation is with a nematode larva that has been contracted through contact with warm, moist, sandy areas such as those found at the beach, in a sandbox, or under houses. In the United States, the infestation is most commonly caused by *Ancylostoma braziliense,* the dog and cat hookworm. Animal droppings containing the ova are deposited on the soil, and within 1 to 2 days the rhabditiform larva hatches. In a few days it matures into the filariform larva, which has the ability to penetrate skin after direct contact. The larva can reportedly penetrate through clothing. Persons at high risk for this eruption include sunbathers, gardeners, plumbers, and electricians.

The clinical condition develops within a few hours of contact and presents as a pruritic, erythematous papule. Within 1 to 2 days erythematous, urticarial-appearing, serpiginous tracks 2 to 4 mm wide develop; they are extremely pruritic. The track is an inflammatory response to the larva migrating throughout the epidermis. The larva may die within a 2- to 8-week period, or it may persist as an infestation for up to 1 year, characterized by cycles of remission and exacerbation. Certain varieties have been reported to enter the dermis and migrate to the lungs, where mild cough, eosinophilia, and a transient pulmonary infiltrate develop. This hypersensitivity reaction is known as Löffler's syndrome or pulmonary infiltration with eosinophilia (PIE syndrome).

Diagnosis is made clinically, based on a slowly migrating, serpiginous track that moves 1 to 2 cm per day and is extremely pruritic. Biopsy is of little use, as the larva is seldom found. Stool examination for ova and parasites is also of no benefit.

Treatment

Treatment of extensive involvement is with thiabendazole (Mintezol), 500-mg chewable tablets, two tablets administered twice daily for 2 days. The pruritus usually abates within 2 to 4 days, and the track resolves within 7 to 10 days of initiation of therapy. Side effects include nausea, vomiting, diarrhea, headaches, anorexia, dizziness, and hematuria and are often sufficiently severe to compromise patient compliance.

Milder infestations respond well to the topical application of thiabendazole pediatric suspension, 500 mg per 5 ml, four times daily for 10 days. The pruritus resolves within 48 hours, and the tracks generally resolve within 5 to 7 days. The treatment should be continued for 1 to 2 days after resolution of the last track. Side effects of topical therapy include mild burning, erythema, and edema at the site of application. Cryosurgery with ethyl chloride or liquid nitrogen has also been used, but treatment failures are more common than successes.

Instruction in preventive measures is important. If work must be performed in an area that may be used by domestic animals, the ground should be draped with plastic. In addition, it is recommended that sandboxes be covered when not in use to limit the risk to children.

Larva currens infestation is caused by the autoinoculation of the intestinal filariform larva of *Strongyloides stercoralis.* It usually starts in the perianal region and is characterized by a rapid rate of migration, which may reach up to 10 cm per day. Migration of this larva is through the dermis. Diagnosis is made on examination of stool for larvae, and treatment is with oral thiabendazole, 25 mg per kg per day,* twice a day for 2 days. This eradicates both the cutaneous and intestinal infestations.

PEDICULOSIS

Pediculosis Capitis. This infestation is caused by the head louse *Pediculus humanus capitis.* Pruritus and secondary infection confined primarily to the occipital region of the scalp and neck are the main symptoms, and lymphadenopathy is frequently present. Neither *P. humanus capitis* nor *Phthirus pubis* (the crab louse) has been implicated in the transmission of disease.

The adult female *P. capitis* louse lays her eggs near the scalp in concretions that are adherent at an angle to the base of the hair shaft. These eggs hatch in 4 to 14 days, leaving empty nits on the hair shaft. The louse has a life span of approximately 30 days. There are an average of 12 to 24 mites per infested host. If the louse is separated from its human host, it dies within 2 to 10 days. Therefore, spread may occur from close contact with an infested human or with fomites carrying the louse.

---

*May be lower than the manufacturer's recommended dose.

Diagnosis is made on examination and identification of the characteristic nits. The adult head louse is elongated and moves rapidly; thus, it is seldom seen. By contrast, the pubic louse is more squat and sluggish and is easily visible.

Pediculosis Pubis. The majority of patients infested with *P. pubis* have involvement limited to the pubic area, but the infestation can also involve the eyelashes, axillae, and hair of the chest and abdomen. Pruritus is a prominent feature.

The majority of patients have minimal inflammation at the site of the louse bite. However, gray-blue macules termed "maculae ceruleae" can be seen.

Pediculosis Corporis. Pediculosis corporis is an uncommon infestation and has been implicated in the spread of typhus, relapsing fever, and trench fever. The body lice live and reproduce in the seams of clothing and return to the surface of the skin only to feed. For this reason, the body louse is rarely identified on routine examination of the skin. The diagnostic nits attached to fibers in the seams of the clothing can be identified.

Treatment

Pyrethrins, naturally derived from chrysanthemums, have been a mainstay of therapy. However, their photoinstability, which results in a loss of potency 12 to 24 hours after exposure to light, limits their usefulness.

Pyrethrins have been combined with piperonyl butoxide for use as a nonprescription pediculocide (RID). The piperonyl butoxide potentiates the effect of the pyrethrins by decreasing their rate of metabolism within the louse.

A synthetic pyrethrin, permethrin (Nix), has been developed that is photostable and has a residual activity on the scalp and hair for 10 days after application. It has been demonstrated to have a low mammalian toxicity, especially in its trans isomer form. In addition, there is low dermal absorption when it is topically applied.

Pyrethrin piperonyl butoxide liquid and permethrin in 1 per cent solution, when applied as recommended by the manufacturer, have recently been found to be equally effective in reducing live louse populations. The pyrethrin piperonyl butoxide is applied to dry hair, allowed to stand for 10 minutes, and then washed out with shampoo. This is followed by combing of the hair with a fine-tooth comb to remove the nits. Its ovicidal properties are not 100 per cent effective. For this reason, the manufacturer recommends reapplication 1 week later.

Permethrin is applied in a slightly different manner. The patient is instructed to shampoo the hair, towel it dry, and then apply the preparation and massage it evenly into the scalp. The preparation is allowed to remain in contact with the scalp for 10 minutes and then rinsed out with water. The permethrin appears to have excellent pediculocidal as well ovicidal activities and is effective in a single-dose regimen.

Adverse reactions noted with the pyrethrins and permethrin include pruritus, erythema, tingling, and stinging, all of which are usually mild.

Malathion, an organophosphate, is a potent cholinesterase inhibitor, acting on the nervous system of the louse. It has been shown to be an effective pediculocide, as well as an ovicide. It should be applied to a moistened scalp, allowed to dry, and then washed out in 8 to 12 hours, with subsequent combing of the hair with a fine-tooth comb to remove the nits. Side effects include mild stinging of the scalp.

Lindane is a good pediculocide but has poor ovicidal activity. It is applied to the hair and allowed to remain in contact with the scalp for 4 minutes before being washed out with shampoo, followed by combing of the hair with a fine-tooth comb. Acute side effects include erythema, pruritus, and irritation. Neurotoxicity, which has been previously described, must also be considered when treating pregnant women and infants with pediculosis capitis.

For any of the three forms of louse infestation—pediculosis capitis, corporis, or pubis—the home environment should be addressed for control of reinfestation. All clothing and linen should be washed in hot water and dried mechanically for a minimum of 20 minutes. Articles that cannot be washed in this manner should be either stored in sealed plastic for at least 10 days or dry cleaned. Combs and other hair care instruments should be soaked in a pediculocidal shampoo and rinsed in hot water.

FUNGAL DISEASES OF THE SKIN

method of
NARDO ZAIAS, M.D.
Mt. Sinai Medical Center
Miami Beach, Florida

There are two very effective, orally administered antimycotics available, and soon there may be more.

Griseofulvin (Fulvicin, Grisactin) is a fungistatic drug that is used only in the treatment of dermatomycosis. It has been available for 30 years and is, by and large, a safe drug whose side effects are well known. Side effects commonly include headaches, soft stools, abdominal gas, and photosensitivity. Griseofulvin interferes with Coumadin (warfarin-like) drugs.

Barbiturates decrease the effect of griseofulvin. Griseofulvin increases the effect of alcohol.

Ketoconazole (Nizoral), an imidazole derivative, is an effective antifungal agent that is also fungistatic. It is a broad-spectrum agent and therefore is active against fungi that cause dermatomycosis, *Candida albicans* and other yeasts, and various fungi that produce subcutaneous and deep mycoses. Ketoconazole has side effects related to alterations of liver function and treatment with this drug should be carefully monitored. Patients who have active hepatitis or abnormal liver function should not be given ketoconazole. This drug is antiandrogenic and can affect the function of the adrenal cortex.

SUPERFICIAL MYCOSES

Tinea Versicolor

Tinea versicolor (caused by *Malassezia furfur*) is probably the most common superficial mycosis. The fungus is found in the sebum-rich areas of the skin surface, including the scalp, face, and midline chest, and may occur elsewhere on the body. The condition starts as a perifollicular lesion that coalesces to form typical macular, hypopigmented, or hyperpigmented lesions.

Treatment

The skin should be scrubbed well from face to abdomen with selenium disulfide, 2.5 per cent (Selsun shampoo), avoiding the eyes. Suds should remain for 20 to 30 minutes and then should be washed off. Selsun should not be left on skin overnight because irritation may result. Treatment should not be limited to involved sites; instead, all areas previously mentioned should be treated.

Oral ketoconazole,* one 200-mg tablet once a day, should be administered for 5 consecutive days.

Repigmentation of the hypo- or hyperpigmented spots is enhanced by exposure to sunlight, and the rapidity of this reaction may be used as an index of cure. Relapses are common.

Cutaneous Candidiasis

Cutaneous candidiasis commonly involves the intertriginous areas of skin, especially the underside of breasts, groin, intergluteal cleft, scrotum, interdigital spaces (fingers and toes), and the oral mucosa.

Topical Treatment

There are many topical anticandidal creams that are effective in the treatment of this condi-

---

*Ketoconazole is an approved drug but this use is not listed by the manufacturer.

tion. Pruritus is a very pronounced symptom; therefore, for the initial 2 to 3 days, the anticandidal agent should be used in combination with a mild or moderate-strength topical corticosteroid. The patient must make sure that the topical preparation covers all involved skin areas and that the medication is applied frequently and directly to the lesion.

Effective topical agents include nystatin, ciclopirox, miconazole, clotrimazole, bifonazole, ketoconazole, econazole, nystatin plus corticosteroid, clotrimazole plus corticosteroid, and naftifine creams.

Candidiasis of the Oral Mucosa

Candidal lesions of the oral mucosa can be treated with nystatin troches (Mycostatin Pastilles), in a dose of 200,000 units, that are slowly dissolved in the mouth. In younger patients, 2 to 4 ounces of nystatin oral suspension, in a dose of 100,000 units per ml, can be given four to six times a day. Patients should be instructed to delay swallowing the solution to give the nystatin a chance to interact with the yeast in the mouth.

Recurrent Cutaneous Candidiasis

C. albicans occurs in the bowel of approximately 40 to 50 per cent of individuals. In some patients whose physical or chemical makeup favors easier reinfection from the bowel, a course of oral nystatin, 500,000 units four times daily for 1 to 2 weeks, controls the candidal population in the gastrointestinal tract. Naturally, topical treatment should be applied at the same time.

In patients with chronic mucocutaneous candidiasis, a special syndrome in childhood, the use of systemic ketoconazole is effective. Contact Janssen Pharmaceuticals (40 Kingsbridge Rd., Piscataway, NJ 08854) for the most recent regimen.

Tinea Capitis (Scalp)

Tinea of the scalp (ringworm) is a childhood disease except in rare instances. Two types of scalp ringworm are common: fluorescent and nonfluorescent. Griseofulvin, 11 mg per kg per day of microsize oral suspension, is the specific treatment for both. If the patient can swallow, crush ultramicrosized griseofulvin-polyethylene glycol (PEG), at 7.3 mg per kg per day, giving one tablet with ice cream once a day for 4 to 6 weeks.

In the United States, nonfluorescent scalp ringworm, caused by *Trichophyton tonsurans*, is the most prevalent type.

Tinea Barbae

Tinea barbae (Majocchi's granuloma), or ringworm involving the hair follicle in the bearded area, is usually caused by *Trichophyton rubrum*. Treatment is 330 to 375 mg twice daily of ultramicrosized PEG, taken with meals, for 4 to 6 weeks.

If griseofulvin is not clinically effective, ketoconazole, 200 mg daily, may be effective.

CUTANEOUS DERMATOPHYTOSIS

Tinea Corporis

There are numerous effective topically antifungal creams. However, whenever there is extensive involvement, or if noncompliance with the regimen is suspected, a systemic antifungal is indicated. In acquired immunodeficiency syndrome (AIDS) and AIDS-related complex (ARC) patients, systemic treatment is indicated.

Superficial Dermatophytosis

Two systemic drugs are effective for dermatophytosis: griseofulvin and ketoconazole. Oral griseofulvin (PEG or ultramicrosized), 500 mg daily, is given in divided doses for 4 to 6 weeks. Ketoconazole, 200 mg daily, is given for 4 to 6 weeks. Liver, androgenic, and adrenal functions should be monitored. For localized areas of involvement, one of the following broad-spectrum topical antifungals may be used:

1. Ciclopirox (Loprox)
2. Miconazole (cream)
3. Clotrimazole (Lotrimin, Mycelex)
4. Econazole (Spectazole)
5. Ketoconazole (Nizoral)
6. Naftifine (Naftin)

Tinea Pedis (Athlete's Foot)

Three clinical types of tinea pedis occur: (1): interdigital dermatomycosis, (2) a vesicular type involving the arch of the foot, and (3) a scaling type involving the plantar surface. The interdigital type and the vesicular type are easily controlled by any of the topical preparations mentioned earlier.

The plantar scaling type of tinea pedis, which when severe is termed the "mocassin" type, can be controlled by oral medications because no topical cream has appeared that is able to control the disease. Treatment is by oral griseofulvin, 750 to 1000 mg daily of microsized or 660 to 750 mg daily of ultramicrosized PEG or ultramicrocrystalline, for 8 to 12 weeks. Topical application of creams may decrease the symptoms. Treatment is given for 3 months or more.

Onychomycosis

No topical antifungal is effective against onychomycosis. Systemic griseofulvin should be started at 500 mg daily and increased if the patient does not show progressive improvement. Fingernails usually require 10 to 12 months of therapy.

Ketoconazole, although effective, is not recommended for toenail infection because of the long treatment time required, and great care should be taken if it is used in fingernail disease.

TRUE FUNGAL INFECTIONS

Cryptococcosis, coccidioidomycosis, generalized histoplasmosis, visceral candidiasis, aspergillosis, North American blastomycosis and paracoccidioidomycosis (South American blastomycosis), and some forms of eumycetomas are caused by true fungi, not actinomycetes. In patients with human immunodeficiency virus infection and either ARC or AIDS, the clinical picture is atypical, usually being severe, and the treatment response is never the same as that in normal patients. The physician must use all available treatments to control such infection.

Treatment

The treatment of choice is ketoconazole, 200 mg daily. Higher doses should be used if the disease is life-threatening. Each disease has its own treatment schedule. Hepatic, androgenic, and adrenal functions should be monitored closely.

Amphotericin B is given intravenously, packaged as a sterile powder, 50 mg per vial. It should be dissolved in 1000 ml of 5 per cent dextrose and water (never with saline solution because it precipitates). It is given by slow intravenous drip for 4 to 8 hours, using an intravenous catheter (Intracath).* The dose is 1 mg per kg per day. The initial dose should be one-fifth to one-half of the maintenance dose, with daily increases of 5 to 10 mg as tolerated.

Impairment of kidney function is common with amphotericin B therapy, and an increase of the nonprotein nitrogen or blood urea nitrogen level demands temporary discontinuance. A total dose of more than 5 grams may result in permanent kidney damage. Fever, chills, nausea, vomiting,

---

*The manufacturer recommends a 1-mg test dose infused slowly.

headache, and anorexia are usually encountered with daily administration of the drug. These symptoms can be treated with conventional supportive therapy (e.g., aspirin, chlorpromazine, steroids) and with pretreatment before the next daily dose of amphotericin is given. The drug can be given intrathecally* or intracisternally in doses of not more than 1 mg every 48 hours.

Treatment of Fungal Infections Not Responsive to Ketoconazole, Griseofulvin, or Amphotericin B

Actinomycosis (Actinomyces israelii)

Give penicillin (procaine or aqueous), 1 million units or more daily, until all traces of the disease have disappeared, and then continue this regimen for another 2 weeks. Use conservative surgical intervention whenever possible to promote drainage, and excise bone cysts. Give erythromycin, 250 mg four times daily, to patients allergic to penicillin.

Nocardiosis (Nocardia asteroides, Nocardia brasiliensis, and Streptomyces)

The treatment of choice is the combination of trimethroprim and sufamethoxazole (Bactrim). This drug may produce severe side effects. The patient should be monitored carefully and the drug discontinued at the first sign of rash. The initial dosage should be increased to accomplish a clinical cure if the patient does not show ill effects. In some of these diseases, treatment may have to be given for several months.

Chromomycosis

No effective treatment is available. Early lesions may respond to thiabendazole or ketoconazole.

Sporotrichosis

Localized sporotrichosis can be treated with a saturated solution of potassium iodide (1 gram per ml), 20 drops (1 ml) orally three times daily initially and then increased by 0.5 ml daily to 9 to 12 ml daily. Drug use should be continued for 2 weeks after all lesions heal. Side effects such as acneiform skin eruptions, lacrimation, nausea, and parotid gland swelling are often encountered. These usually subside on discontinuance of the drug; the acneiform skin eruption may take weeks to disappear. Ketoconazole, 200 mg daily, is also effective.

---

*This use is not listed by the manufacturer.

DISEASES OF THE MOUTH

method of
WILLIAM J. MORAN, D.M.D., M.D.
University of Chicago
Chicago, Illinois

LIP LESIONS

Cleft Lip and Palate

This congenital anomaly may vary from a small notching of the lip or hard palate to extensive deformity of the lip, premaxilla, and palate. It may occur in isolation or in association with other anomalies. The frequency of occurrence is about 1 in 1000 births. A multidisciplinary team approach is necessary in caring for these children. Pediatricians, surgeons experienced in dealing with these defects, dental specialists, otologists, speech therapists, geneticists, and psychologists should work in concert in counseling the family and planning and carrying out treatment.

Cheilitis

Contact cheilitis is manifested by erythema and vesiculation of the lips. It is usually caused by sensitization to lipstick, lip balms, or food and is seen more often in women than in men. Treatment is elimination of the causative agent. Triamcinolone acetonide (Aristocort) ointment is helpful.

Angular cheilitis refers to a condition in which painful fissures develop at the corners of the mouth. This is found most commonly in children and the elderly. It is thought to be related to lip sucking, edentulism, or ill-fitting dentures. Saliva bathes the fissures, producing maceration. Candidiasis may be present. Treatment with an ointment containing nystatin (Mycostatin) is helpful, along with elimination of the causative factors.

In solar cheilitis, keratinization with areas of erosion develops on the lower lip and is due to excessive exposure to the elements, especially the actinic rays of the sun. It occurs more commonly in fair-skinned individuals. Treatment consists of excision with either the carbon dioxide laser or standard lip shave technique. Patients should avoid sun exposure and use a sunscreen lip balm. Because the lesion may progress to carcinoma, patients must be followed carefully, and any suspicious lesion should be biopsied to rule out carcinoma.

Cheilitis glandularis apostematosa is a condition in which the mucous glands of the lip become inflamed, enlarged, and nodular. The ductal ostia appear as small red papules on the lip, and mucus may seep from these inflamed orifices. Exposure to the elements or other irritants such as tobacco seems to be the cause. Treatment consists of eliminating irritants such as tobacco, careful cleansing of the lips, and use of a sunscreen lip balm. Carbon dioxide laser vaporization of affected areas or lip shaving may be helpful.

Mucous Retention Cyst

Mucous retention cysts usually occur in the lower labial mucosa. They are due to trauma to mucous glands with or without secondary infection, which produces ductal obstruction and results in an expanding collection of mucoid material within the tissues. Treatment is unroofing or excision; incision or aspiration usually results in recurrence.

GINGIVAL AND PERIODONTAL LESIONS

Simple Gingivitis

Inflammation of the gingival tissues surrounding the teeth is known as simple gingivitis. The inflammation is manifested by redness and swelling and is due to irritation from bacterial plaque and calculus, which build up as a result of poor oral hygiene. Treatment should consist of dental referral for complete removal of plaque and calculus, along with patient education regarding oral hygiene.

Acute Necrotizing Ulcerative Gingivitis

Intense erythema and edema of the gingiva with necrosis of the interdental papillae are the hallmarks of acute necrotizing ulcerative gingivitis. The patient may have considerable pain, fever, and cervical lymphadenopathy. A mixed fusiform/spirochete etiology has long been proposed; more recently, viral infection and secondary bacterial infection are suspected. Treatment consists of fluids, analgesics, rest, and gentle oral rinses and débridement. Antibiotic therapy may be added.

Desquamative Gingivitis (Gingivosis)

Gingivosis is characterized by vesiculation and desquamation of the gingiva. It occurs most frequently in middle-aged women. The etiology is not known. It may be a manifestation of various disorders such as bullous pemphigoid and pemphigus vulgaris. A biopsy should be obtained for histologic as well as direct immunofluorescent examination. A topical steroid such as fluocino-

nide (Lidex) gel, 0.05 per cent applied six times a day, may be helpful.

Gingival Enlargement

Generalized gingival enlargement and inflammation that occurs during puberty and pregnancy may arise in response to hormonal changes. A presumed hereditary generalized enlargement known as hereditary gingival fibromatosis may occur at the time of tooth eruption; the gingiva may become quite large and fibrotic. Treatment consists of gingivoplasty and maintenance of excellent hygiene to retard regrowth. A similar type of enlargement that occurs in individuals on phenytoin (Dilantin) therapy may require gingivoplasty if enlargement results in trauma during mastication. Rarely, generalized gingival enlargement is caused by leukemic infiltration. Focal gingival enlargement may be inflammatory or neoplastic in origin; pyogenic granuloma and fibroma are frequently encountered examples. Biopsy, in an excisional manner when possible, is indicated for diagnosis and is often therapeutic.

Eruption Cyst

An eruption cyst is a bluish, translucent, dome-shaped lesion overlying the crown of an erupting tooth. It may be incised to relieve pressure and discomfort. A topical anesthetic ointment may also be of help, especially in young children.

Pericoronitis

In pericoronitis, inflammation surrounds the crown of a partially erupted tooth, due to trapping of plaque and debris beneath a flap of soft tissue overlying the crown. Treatment consists of removal of plaque and debris from under the soft tissue flap and maintenance of good oral hygiene. Antibiotic therapy should be instituted. Occasionally, removal of the overlying soft tissue flap or tooth extraction is necessary to prevent recurrent infection. Deep space abscess may complicate pericoronitis.

Dental Sinus

A sinus tract may be found in the gingiva. It usually extends from an apical periodontal infection. A panoramic or periapical radiograph may reveal a periapical radiolucency. Dental referral should be made for evaluation and treatment.

TONGUE LESIONS

Median Rhomboid Glossitis

Median rhomboid glossitis is characterized by an irregularly shaped, smooth red patch located on the mid-dorsum of the tongue; it is usually slightly depressed. Histologically one sees stratified squamous epithelium with absence of lingual papillae. This condition may be developmental or perhaps related to chronic low-grade candidiasis. It is usually asymptomatic, but if symptoms are present an antifungal agent may be tried. If symptoms persist, surgical excision is indicated.

Benign Migratory Glossitis

As its name implies, this is a harmless condition characterized by migratory, smooth red patches on the tongue. It is rare and of unknown etiology, although associated occasionally with psoriasis or Reiter's disease. Although this disorder is often asymptomatic, a burning discomfort may occur; this is generally mild and self-limiting. A mild hydrogen peroxide mouth rinse and bland diet may help.

Fissured Tongue

This congenital anomaly may be an isolated finding or associated with Down's, Melkersson-Rosenthal, or Sjögren's syndromes. The tongue is deeply fissured, predisposing to food trapping, inflammation, and infection. Good oral hygiene, including brushing the tongue with a soft toothbrush and a mild hydrogen peroxide oral rinse after meals and at bedtime, is the only treatment required.

Macroglossia

Enlargement of the tongue may be due to a variety of conditions, including neoplasms, developmental anomalies such as hemangioma and lymphangioma, and metabolic derangements such as amyloidosis. Infection, angioedema, and superior vena cava syndrome may also produce tongue enlargement.

Black Hairy Tongue

In this condition, the filiform papillae of the tongue undergo hyperplasia and elongation and become discolored because of overgrowth of pigment-producing oral flora. The etiology is unknown, although it is associated with prolonged antibiotic therapy; chronic irritation also may play a role. Treatment includes brushing of the tongue with a soft toothbrush and using a mild hydrogen peroxide mouthwash. Use of tobacco and other oral irritants should be avoided. Extremely elongated papillae may be snipped with scissors.

WHITE MUCOSAL LESIONS

Candidiasis (Thrush)

Candida albicans produces infection mainly in immunosuppressed patients. Patients receiving steroid or prolonged antibiotic therapy are also at risk. White, cheesy patches on the mucosa can be wiped off, leaving an eroded and bleeding surface. Treatment includes determining and correction of underlying factors and the use of antifungal agents such as nystatin (Mycostatin) (solution or oral tablets). Ketoconazole (Nizoral) appears to be more effective for cases of *Candida* laryngitis or esophagitis related to radiotherapy.

Nicotinic Stomatitis

The lesions of nicotinic stomatitis occur on the palate and appear to be related to smoking, especially pipe smoking. The palatal mucosa is thickened and gray-white in color, with multiple small red dots that are the inflamed ostia of minor salivary gland ducts. Histologically, hyperkeratosis and inflammation with mild dysplasia are seen. The lesion usually regresses slowly upon cessation of smoking and is not considered premalignant. Atypical lesions should be biopsied.

Oral Burns

Any caustic agent may injure the oral epithelium, leaving a sloughing white membrane; placement of an aspirin in the oral vestibule to relieve toothache is perhaps the most well-known example of this. Healing is usually uneventful and treatment is symptomatic.

Lichen Planus

Lichen planus can affect the mouth or skin, or both. The typical appearance in the mouth is a white reticular network on the buccal mucosa; however, there are many variations, including annular patterns and erosive and bullous lesions. Histologic confirmation is often required. Associated skin lesions most commonly occur on the flexor aspects of the wrists and lower legs bilaterally. Painful lesions may be palliated with topical or intralesional steroids. Fluocinonide gel, 0.05 per cent, may be applied six times daily. Triamcinolone acetonide, 5 mg per ml, may be injected 0.1 ml per cm^2 using a 30-gauge needle. In more severe cases, oral prednisone in daily doses of 40 to 60 mg may be given for 14 days and then tapered over a week. The etiology is unknown.

Leukoedema

This is a variation from normal seen mostly in black persons. The buccal mucosa appears opalescent white. There are no inflammation or symptoms. Histologically, the epithelium is thickened with edema of the spinous layer; dysplasia is absent.

Leukoplakia

Leukoplakia literally means "white patch." The term usually refers to a keratotic plaque that may be premalignant or malignant. If examination suggests an obvious etiology such as infection or trauma from dentition, every effort should be made to resolve these. If the lesion regresses after 2 to 4 weeks, it may be followed up. All other lesions should be examined histologically. Any lesion demonstrating erosion or induration should be considered to be carcinoma until proved otherwise.

Papilloma

Papillomas of the oral cavity, caused by the human papilloma virus, are most frequently seen on the palate, uvula, tongue, and lips. The typical appearance is warty and keratotic. Excisional biopsy is diagnostic and therapeutic.

Squamous Carcinoma

Squamous carcinoma is the most common carcinoma of the upper aerodigestive tract. It may present as a white keratotic lesion or as a red, ulcerated lesion. The most important etiology is heavy tobacco use, including "smokeless" tobacco (snuff); heavy alcohol use seems to have a synergistic effect. A positive family history even in the absence of tobacco use appears to increase risk. While the typical patient is traditionally described as male and in the sixth decade, more women and younger patients are being diagnosed, probably because of changing social habits. Early stage (I and II) carcinomas have a good to fair prognosis. Treatment consists of wide excision or radiotherapy. Advanced stage (III and IV) carcinomas have a poor prognosis (overall 30 per cent 5-year survival) but vary by site. Advanced lesions are usually treated with combination therapy consisting of surgery and radiotherapy, with or without chemotherapy. A multidisciplinary team, including surgical, radiation, and medical oncologists, speech and swallowing therapists, and dental specialists, is required to care for patients with advanced stage lesions.

RED AND PIGMENTED MUCOSAL LESIONS

Denture Stomatitis

Poor oral hygiene in the denture wearer can lead to inflammation beneath the denture, and secondary candidiasis may occur. The mucosa beneath the denture is red and painful. This mucositis occurs most often in the maxilla and corresponds exactly to the area beneath the denture. Treatment consists of thorough daily cleansing of the denture and removal of the denture at night. If secondary candidiasis is present, nystatin or ketoconazole should be prescribed.

Hemangioma

Hemangiomas appear to be hamartomas and may vary greatly in size and resultant deformity. Most congenital lesions regress during childhood; small lesions may be completely excised. Large, deforming lesions that infiltrate structures (e.g., the tongue) can be debulked using carbon dioxide laser therapy.

Hereditary Hemorrhagic Telangiectasia

This condition has an autosomal dominant pattern of inheritance. Multiple, small telangiectasias may affect the oral cavity, pharynx, and/or nose, producing recurrent bleeding. Cryotherapy, laser therapy, and steroid therapy have been used for treatment.

Amalgam Tattoo

This is an exogenous pigmentation produced when silver amalgam filling material becomes implanted in soft tissue during dental restoration procedures. The tattoo is blue-black in color and asymptomatic. Its nature may be confirmed by a radiograph, revealing radiopaque metallic flecks. If confirmed radiographically further treatment is unnecessary; otherwise, excisional biopsy is indicated. The differential diagnosis includes pigmented nevus and malignant melanoma.

Pigmented Nevus

Benign pigmented nevi of all types may occur in the oral cavity. This includes lentigos and junctional, compound, and blue nevi. Except for the blue nevus, they are generally brown in color. They may be raised or flat and are relatively unchanging. These lesions should be excised to exclude the possibility of melanoma. A radiograph may be obtained to exclude amalgam tattoo.

EROSIVE, ULCERATIVE, AND VESICULOBULLOUS LESIONS

Recurrent Aphthous Stomatitis

This condition consists of recurring, painful ulcerations that can occur on any area of the oral mucosa except the gingiva and anterior hard palate. The shallow ulcerations may be single or multiple and can range from less than 2 mm to greater than 10 mm in size. They have a yellowish-gray pseudomembranous base and are surrounded by an erythematous halo. There may be associated fever and lymphadenopathy. The lesions are self-limiting and usually resolve in 7 to 14 days.

The etiology of this condition is unknown. It occurs mainly in adults, more commonly in women than in men.

Only symptomatic treatment is possible. Avoidance of spicy, acidic, and salty foods as well as sharp, hard foods such as crackers promotes comfort. A mixture of diphenhydramine (Benadryl) elixir and Kaopectate in equal parts used as a mouth rinse six times a day may be helpful. Tetracycline, 250 mg in 30 ml of water, used as a mouth rinse and then swallowed four times a day, has been of benefit in some patients.

Behçet's Syndrome

Behçet's syndrome is composed of the triad of recurrent oropharyngeal ulcerations, genital ulcerations, and uveitis. Other manifestations include gastrointestinal lesions, vasculitis, synovitis, and neurologic abnormalities. Patients are generally in their second or third decade, and men are affected more often than women. Treatment consists of symptomatic measures and systemic steroids. Cyclophosphamide (Cytoxan) and other cytotoxic drugs have also been used.

Herpetic Stomatitis

Herpetic stomatitis is due to infection of the oral mucosa with herpes simplex virus, either type 1 or type 2. Primary herpetic stomatitis generally occurs in the pediatric age group, although it may also occur in adults. Vesicular lesions may involve the entire oral mucosa; these then rupture, producing painful ulcerations. Patients usually suffer from fever, lymphadenopathy, malaise, and headache. They may be unable to swallow, with resultant drooling and dehydration. Treatment includes analgesics and antipyretics. Parenteral fluids may be necessary. The course usually lasts from 7 to 14 days.

In secondary herpetic stomatitis, recurring lesions most often involve the lips, hard palate, and attached gingiva. Factors that may precipitate these lesions include upper respiratory infection, trauma, and psychologic stress. Healing usually occurs in 7 to 10 days.

Erythema Multiforme

Erythema multiforme is a disease of the skin and mucous membranes and occurs in two forms. The minor form lasts 2 to 3 weeks; the major form, known as Stevens-Johnson syndrome, may last up to 6 weeks. The disease occurs in young adults and appears to be more common in men. The etiology is unknown, but precipitating factors include infections, such as herpes simplex and mycoplasma, and drugs, especially sulfonamides. The lesions begin as vesicles or bullae and then slough, leaving large, painful ulcerations with whitish pseudomembranous bases. The lips, buccal mucosa, and tongue are the most frequently involved sites in the oral cavity. In Stevens-Johnson syndrome, there is severe skin, oral, conjunctival, and genital involvement. When oral lesions are the only manifestation, establishing the diagnosis is difficult. Differentiation from bullous pemphigoid and pemphigus vulgaris may require biopsy. Severe lesions may be treated with prednisone, 40 to 60 mg daily for several weeks.

Herpangina

Herpangina is an infection of the oropharynx caused by coxsackievirus (groups A and B) and encountered in children. Small vesicles are seen on the soft palate, uvula, and tonsillar pillars symmetrically. They quickly rupture, leaving small painful ulcerations. Fever, lymphadenopathy, headache, and malaise are associated. This disease is distinctive enough to allow clinical diagnosis. Treatment is symptomatic, and healing occurs rapidly.

Pemphigus and Pemphigoid

Pemphigus and pemphigoid appear to be autoimmune diseases and present as oral bullae of varying size that slough, leaving painful ulcerations with a whitish pseudomembranous base. The buccal mucosa, palate, and gingiva are most frequently involved. Patients are usually in the fifth and sixth decades. An important differentiating feature is that pemphigus also affects the skin. However, the oral lesions may precede the skin lesions by years. Conjunctival lesions may occur in pemphigoid. The histologic appearance of the bullae is similar in both disorders; however, in pemphigus, round desquamated epithelial cells

(Tzanck's cells) may be seen within bullae. Immunofluorescent examination reveals IgG antibodies to intercellular substance in pemphigus, whereas IgG is seen within the basement membrane in pemphigoid.

Systemic steroids are used to treat both diseases. In pemphigus high doses are often necessary and patients may develop steroid complications. Cyclophosphamide has been added in severe cases in order to reduce steroid levels. Steroids are not always effective in pemphigoid, and dapsone has been used with some success. Ophthalmologic examination should be done to rule out ocular involvement in pemphigoid.

OTHER LESIONS

Tori

Tori are benign hyperostoses that occur in the midline of the hard palate (torus palatinus) or lingual aspect of the mandible (torus mandibularis). They generally require no treatment.

Fordyce's Spots

Fordyce's spots are small, discrete, light yellow papules found in the buccal and labial mucosa of approximately 80 per cent of the general population. They are ectopic sebaceous glands and require no treatment other than patient reassurance.

Orolingual Paresthesia

Orolingual paresthesia most often affects the tongue (glossodynia), but other oral mucosal surfaces may be affected. It is usually encountered in older women. Patients complain of a burning discomfort, yet the mucosa appears normal. Possible causes of this symptom include vitamin deficiency anemia, referred pain from dental or periodontal disease, and mild candidiasis. It may also be a manifestation of stress. Often no cause can be pinpointed. Treatment includes reassurance, along with counseling regarding good oral hygiene and nutrition. Dental evaluation may be helpful if the patient does not receive regular dental care. Any mucosal changes should be biopsied.

Xerostomia

Xerostomia, or dry mouth, is a bothersome symptom and often causes halitosis. It may have many causes. Virtually all patients who have had radiotherapy to the head and neck have some degree of xerostomia. Systemic illnesses including lymphoproliferative disorders (Mikulicz's disease, Sjögren's syndrome), rheumatoid arthritis, lupus erythematosus, scleroderma, and sarcoid may involve the salivary glands and cause xerostomia. Exogenous substances such as anticholinergics, antihypertensives, antihistamines, and antimotion drugs frequently produce xerostomia. Finally, xerostomia may be related to stress or may be idiopathic. If a patient has a history of radiotherapy or is taking a drug that causes xerostomia, symptomatic relief may be obtained by frequent intake of fluids and use of artificial saliva such as XERO-LUBE. Otherwise, systemic causes should be ruled out. Dental referral should be made, because patients with xerostomia may have an increased incidence of caries and require good oral hygiene and regular dental follow-up.

VENOUS STASIS ULCERS

method of
P. J. OSMUNDSON, M.D.
Mayo Clinic
Rochester, Minnesota

Venous stasis ulcers are a major cause of morbidity and disruption of normal lifestyles because of the frequency of venous diseases and the ensuing chronic venous insufficiency of the lower extremities.

PATHOPHYSIOLOGY

For proper management, it is essential to understand the fundamental problem underlying the development of venous stasis ulcers. Abnormally high leg venous pressures occur in patients with venous disease when they are standing or sitting with their legs in dependent positions. The elevated venous pressure is transmitted to the subcutaneous tissues and skin. Venous pressure elevation with leg dependency is usually caused by chronic deep venous insufficiency with incompetent valves in the deep veins that occurs as a late consequence of deep venous thrombosis. Rarely, chronic venous insufficiency develops because of an absence of valves in the deep veins. Varicose veins involving the superficial venous system, with perforating veins connecting the superficial and deep venous systems, may contribute to the venous stasis.

DIAGNOSIS

Accurate diagnosis underlies correct management. Venous stasis ulcers must be differentiated from a wide variety of other vascular and nonvascular diseases causing leg ulcers (Table 1). Characteristics of venous stasis ulcers are edema, pigmentation, dermatitis, cellulitis, induration, and ulceration. Venous stasis ulcers have a predilection for the lower third of

TABLE 1. **Etiology of Commonly Occurring Leg Ulcers**

Venous stasis ulcers
  Unusual types
    Combined stasis and ischemic ulcer
    Complicating arteriovenous malformations
Ischemic ulcers
  Arteriosclerosis obliterans
  Thromboangiitis obliterans
  Arteriolar ischemic ulcers
    Hypertensive ischemic ulcer
    Inflammatory arteritides and collagen vascular
      diseases
Infections
Neoplastic diseases
Neurotrophic diseases
Hemoglobinopathies

the leg and ankle, more often on the medial than the lateral side.

Laboratory aids in the diagnosis of venous stasis ulcers are usually unnecessary, although noninvasive studies to document the venous pathophysiology and to exclude arterial diseases and ischemia are sometimes helpful. Venography may be necessary in the rare instances where venous reconstructive surgery is being considered as therapy for recurrent stasis ulcers resistant to standard therapy.

TREATMENT

Physicians and patients alike need to understand the two-phase approach to management: (1) healing the ulcer and (2) preventing recurrence.

The size of the ulcer and its chronicity determine the initial therapy. Many small ulcers in the early stages heal rapidly with bed rest and elevation of the legs to a height greater than right atrial pressure. Wet-to-dry dressings with a 0.25 per cent aqueous solution of aluminum subacetate or a 0.9 per cent solution of sodium chloride are used to clean the ulcer bed. For larger, recurrent, deeper ulcers, additional measures may be necessary, including whirlpool baths and enzymatic debridement with chemical agents such as a combination of fibrinolysin and desoxyribonuclease (Elase) ointment. Additional mechanical débridement may also be necessary. Locally applied or systemically administered antibiotics are necessary only if there is a significant infectious component. When the ulcer base is clean, with healthy granulation tissue, an occlusive dressing with hydroactive granules (Duoderm) may hasten healing. The dressings are applied for 1 to 7 days, and the ulcer is redressed until final healing occurs.

Therapy on an ambulatory basis often permits healing of small ulcers with clean bases. External elastic support is provided by sponge rubber pads lined with gauze, which are placed over the ulcer and supported with two heavy-duty, 4-inch elastic wraps. An alternative pressure dressing for ambulatory treatment is the Unna boot.

Surgical treatment is necessary for large, recurrent venous stasis ulcers. Skin grafts applied after the ulcer bed is clean often shorten the healing time. Ligation and stripping of varicose veins, combined with ligation of incompetent perforating veins in the leg, may also help to heal the ulcer and prevent recurrence. Venous reconstructive surgery is reserved for recalcitrant, recurring ulcers.

Once the venous stasis ulcer has healed, it is essential to instruct the patient in the need for adequate support with elastic stockings or elastic wraps, which are worn whenever the leg is in a dependent position. Lastly, elevation of the legs at night while in bed minimizes recurrence of the ulcer.

DECUBITUS ULCERS
method of
GEORGE C. XAKELLIS, M.D.
University of Iowa
Iowa City, Iowa

Decubitus ulcers have been present since antiquity and have been identified by many different names. In the past, they were termed "bed sores." More recently, research has suggested that they are caused by pressure, and they are becoming known as "pressure ulcers" or "pressure sores."

The increase in the elderly population has resulted in increased numbers of patients at risk for this problem. Any physician who is actively engaged in the care of elderly patients is likely to be confronted with a decubitus ulcer.

ETIOLOGY

It has become clear over the past 30 years that the main causative factor in the development of decubitus ulcers is pressure. Decubitus ulcers occur in areas where the skin is compressed between a firm surface (e.g., a hospital mattress) and a bony prominence.

Research has demonstrated that a compressive pressure of 70 mmHg applied for 2 hours results in irreversible tissue necrosis. It has also been demonstrated that the pressure required to occlude capillary blood flow is approximately 32 mmHg. Currently it is believed that the compressive pressure results in occlusion of blood flow to the skin and subcutaneous tissue overlying the bony prominence, resulting in ischemia and cell death. However, it has also been demonstrated that reducing pressure to a value below this level does not uniformly prevent decubitus ulcers. Consequently, it appears that the physiologic changes resulting from compressive pressure are not yet totally understood.

Normal people do not develop decubitus ulcers. In a normal person, compressive pressure over a bony prominence results in pain, which causes the person to shift position, thus alleviating the pressure. This protective mechanism must be damaged for compressive pressure to cause tissue damage. The patient may have decreased sensation or mobility, so that he or she is unable to feel pain or move to relieve the pressure. In addition, a number of medical conditions may contribute to the development of decubitus ulcers. For instance, poor nutrition, as documented by a low serum albumin level, may predispose to decubitus ulcer formation.

GRADING

Decubitus ulcers have been classified in many different ways. One method that I have found to be useful is Shea's grading system. The ulcer is graded from I to IV based on the depth the wound has penetrated into the skin, subcutaneous tissues, and deep tissues overlying the bony prominence. The definition of the four grades in presented in Table 1.

GENERAL TREATMENT CONCEPTS

Physicians frequently ask, "Is there anything I can do to treat this patient's decubitus ulcer besides turning the patient every 2 hours?" General treatment of decubitus ulcers can be divided into two general areas: systemic and local treatment.

Systemic Treatment

Systemic tratment can be classified into three broad categories: nutrition, infection control, and other general medical interventions.

Nutrition. Protein and calorie intake must be adequate for optimal wound healing. In addition, wound healing is hampered by vitamin and mineral deficiencies. Vitamin C, vitamin A, and zinc

TABLE 1. **Shea's Classification System***

Grade I: Irregular, ill-defined area of soft tissue swelling and induration, with associated heat and erythema. There may be superficial breakdown that is limited to the epidermis.

Grade II: Shallow ulcer extending to but not involving the subcutaneous fat. Ulcer edges are distinct, with early fibrosis and pigment changes blending into a broad, indistinct area of heat, erythema, and induration.

Grade III: Irregular, full-thickness skin wound extending into the subcutaneous fat. Usually, it has undermined the skin for a variable distance. The anatomic limit is the deep fascia.

Grade IV: The deep fascia has been penetrated. Muscle or bone is usually exposed in the ulcer base. Fistulas to the bowel or the bladder may exist.

*From Shea JD: Pressure sores: classification and management. Clin Orthop *112*:89–100, 1975. Used by permission.

deficiencies all may result in retarded wound healing. A diet history, serum albumin level, and total lymphocyte count help to establish the patient's nutritional status. If evidence of malnutrition or inadequate diet exists, nutritional supplementation should be instituted.

Infection Control. In the absence of systemic infection, systemic antibiotics are not helpful in healing decubitus ulcers. However, decubitus ulcers complicated by systemic infection require antibiotic treatment. Systemic infection as a complication of decubitus ulcers is usually manifested as bacteremia and sepsis, osteomyelitis, or spreading cellulitis. Signs of infection include fever, elevated white blood cell count, changing mental status, or spreading cellulitis around the wound. Because decubitus ulcers are typically colonized with multiple organisms, a combination of agents that treat anaerobes, gram-positive cocci, and gram-negative rods needs to be given until blood cultures identify the causative agent. Clindamycin (Cleocin), 600 mg every 8 hours intravenously, and gentamicin (Garamycin), 3 mg per kg per day in divided doses intravenously (adjusted downward if renal failure exists), is one acceptable regimen for initial empiric therapy. Wound cultures often grow multiple organisms and are of questionable value in determining correct antibiotic therapy. The diagnosis of osteomyelitis is particularly difficult. In general, one should consider the possibility of osteomyelitis if bone is visible in the base of the ulcer. The best method of diagnosing osteomyelitis is by bone biopsy. Noninvasive testing, including an x-ray film and a bone scan, is helpful if negative. However, the bone scan is often difficult to interpret. If noninvasive tests are inconclusive, treatment can be initiated as if osteomyelitis is not present, and the progress of wound healing can be monitored. If healing does not occur, bone biopsy should be performed for diagnosis.

General Medical Interventions. Systemic treatment also includes measures such as optimizing treatment of other medical conditions that may decrease tissue perfusion, worsen urinary or fecal incontinence, or limit mobility. These measures include optimizing the treatment of conditions such as congestive heart failure or Parkinson's disease.

Local Interventions

The single most important intervention is motivation of the nursing staff. Increasing the nursing attention that patients with decubitus ulcers receive can be accomplished in a number of ways. First, a skin care program should be established in the institution. One person should be identified as the skin care coordinator, and all skin break-downs are to be reported to this individual. The skin care coordinator should keep records of the wound size, the grade, and the treatment plan instituted by the attending physician. A schedule of regular skin care rounds should be initiated at the institution. Finally, one should avoid assigning guilt for decubitus ulcer occurrence.

Local therapy consists of four steps. First, all pressure must be removed from the wound. With continued pressure, the wound will not heal.

Second, all necrotic tissue must be débrided. Healing does not occur while necrotic tissue is present in the wound bed. This débridement can take one of three forms: surgical débridement, enzymatic débridement, or mechanical débridement. For thick eschar or extensive necrotic tissue, surgical débridement is the most expedient method. For smaller amounts of necrotic tissue, either mechanical or enzymatic débridement can be used. Mechanical débridement uses saline wet-to-dry dressings. A wet saline dressing is placed in the wound and allowed to dry. It adheres to the wound bed. When it is removed, the adherent tissue is removed at the same time, thereby débriding the wound. Enzymatic débridement uses enzymes such as collagenase, which attack the devitalized tissue and spare the healthy tissue in the wound bed. Theoretically, normal tissue is not affected, but in clinical practice, no clear advantage over the other methods of débridement has been demonstrated.

Third, the bacterial count in the wound needs to be kept low. It has been demonstrated that unless wound bacterial counts are lowered below 10^6 bacteria per ml of exudate, wound healing does not occur. Also, the surgical literature suggests that unless wound bacterial counts are reduced below a critical level, skin-grafting procedures are less likely to succeed. Although the critical level of bacteria may vary, the important principle is that wound bacterial counts must be decreased for healing to occur.

Last, a moist wound-healing environment needs to be maintained. Not long ago, it was common practice to dry the decubitus ulcer using heat lamps. Today a large body of literature suggests that re-epithelialization occurs more quickly across a moist wound surface. On the basis of this finding, it is recommended that the decubitus ulcer be kept moist during the wound-healing process. This can be done in a number of ways, which will be addressed.

Topical Agents

Since the time of Hippocrates, numerous topical remedies have been used to treat decubitus ulcers. Examples of topical agents that have been available for many years include sugar paste, gold leaf, antacids, and various topical antibiotics. Unfortunately, most of these agents have not been tested in a controlled fashion, and their benefit compared with placebo is not known.

More recently, topical agents have been developed that attempt to address the principles of local intervention noted earlier. Some are designed to débride necrotic tissue, some to decrease wound bacterial counts, and some to maintain a moist wound environment. The agents designed to débride devitalized tissue, such as collagenase, appear to be effective. However, when compared with surgical débridement or mechanical saline wet-to-dry débridement, they appear to offer no significant advantages. Many agents, such as topical antibiotics, attempt to decrease wound bacterial counts. However, it appears that saline gauze dressings changed every 4 hours are effective for this purpose and that topical antibiotics, which have the potential to cause a hypersensitivity reaction, are unnecessary. One exception is silver sulfadiazine cream (Silvadene), which, if applied every 8 hours, lowers bacterial counts more quickly than saline for the first 3 days of use. After 3 days the effectiveness of these two agents becomes similar. Consequently, in a situation where rapid lowering of the wound bacterial count is essential, such as during in-hospital preparation for skin grafting, silver sulfadiazine cream for 3 days may be valuable; otherwise, saline-wetted gauze dressings are adequate.

A number of topical agents work to maintain a moist wound-healing environment. The traditional example of this type of dressing is the saline-saturated gauze dressing, which is changed every 4 to 6 hours and wetted once between dressing changes. An entire class of new dressing materials termed "occlusive dressings" have been developed that also work on this principle. In experimental animal studies, re-epithelialization of shallow skin wounds occurred more quickly with the occlusive dressing. Randomized trials are currently under way to compare these dressings with saline-saturated gauze in the treatment of decubitus ulcers. These dressings are particularly popular with the nursing staff, as they must be changed an average of once every 3 days rather than every 4 to 6 hours.

Last, another class of topical agents, "growth factors," is currently under development. There is a lot of interest in these agents, as they have the potential to speed the natural rate of healing rather than simply optimizing the healing environment.

Topical Treatment by Ulcer Grade

Grade I—Remove pressure.

TABLE 2. **Norton's Risk Assessment Scale***

Physical Condition		Mental Condition		Activity		Mobility		Incontinence	
Good	= 4	Alert	= 4	Ambulant	= 4	Full	= 4	None	= 4
Fair	= 3	Apathetic	= 3	Walks with help	= 3	Slightly limited	= 3	Occasional	= 3
Poor	= 2	Confused	= 2	Wheelchair bound	= 2	Very limited	= 2	Usually/urinary	= 2
Very bad	= 1	Stuporous	= 1	Bedfast	= 1	Immobile	= 1	Urinary and fecal	= 1

*From Norton D, McLaren R, and Exton-Smith AN: An Investigation of Geriatric Nursing Problems in Hospital. London: National Corporation for the Care of Old People, 1962 (reprinted by Churchill Livingstone, Edinburgh, 1975). Reproduced by permission of NCCOP (now known as the Centre for Policy on Aging).

Grade II—Remove pressure, débride necrotic tissue, and cover ulcer with saline-moisture gauze. Change the dressing every 4 to 6 hours and remoisten it once between changes. If the dressing is dry at the time of removal, remoisten it before removal. Occlusive dressings may be a useful alternative. Several weeks are usually required for healing to occur.

Grade III—Remove pressure, débride necrotic tissue (this may require surgical débridement), and evaluate the ulcer for sepsis. The preferred dressing is saline-saturated gauze, changed every 4 to 6 hours and remoistened once between changes. Several months are usually required for healing to occur.

Grade IV—Remove pressure, initiate extensive surgical débridement, and evaluate the ulcer for osteomyelitis and sepsis. Use saline-saturated dressings, as described previously. Major surgical reconstruction may be required.

Surgical Reconstruction

For Grade IV wounds and some large Grade III wounds, formal surgical débridement may be necessary. Numerous types of skin grafts, skin flaps, and myocutaneous flaps have been advocated over the years. These alternatives are particularly appealing for young paraplegics, whose immobility can be lessened by teaching them repositioning techniques. These interventions are probably less useful for older, more debilitated patients, for whom the problems of immobility will, at best, remain unchanged over time.

Specialized Beds

During the last few years, numerous specialized beds have been developed for the treatment of decubitus ulcer. These range from inexpensive air, water, or foam mattresses, to viscoelastic gel pads, to motorized low-air-loss and air-fluidized beds. The simpler devices are designed to place a layer of air, fluid, or gel between the patient and the hospital mattress. The more sophisticated devices actually replace the hospital bed with an air- or fluid-filled surface. These mattresses and beds conform to the patient's body contours and support the body over a larger surface area, thus decreasing the compressive pressure generated at any given point. The cost of these mattresses and beds ranges from $30 to $50 for an air mattress to $50 to $80 a day for rental of an air-fluidized bed. It seems reasonable to use an inexpensive mattress as an adjunct to, but not instead of, the intensive nursing care required to treat these patients. The air-fluidized bed has been shown to be more effective than the simpler mattresses in healing large wounds, but because of its high cost, its cost effectiveness remains in doubt.

PREVENTION

Currently, there is increasing emphasis on the prevention of decubitus ulcers. These wounds are being used as a quality assurance measure for nursing home care, and their presence is being construed as a failure to provide adequate care. Although it is unlikely that all of these wounds can be prevented, it appears that their incidence could be reduced by instituting a risk assessment protocol in the institution. Patients at high risk could be placed on more rigorous nursing care schedules and/or on an inexpensive soft mattress rather than on a regular hospital bed. One such risk assessment scale was developed by Norton more than 20 years ago and is illustrated in Table 2. The patient receives a score from 1 to 4 in each of five categories. The scores for each category are then totaled. The total possible score for any individual patient is 20. A total score of less than 12 puts a patient at high risk for developing a decubitus ulcer.

With this increased emphasis on prevention, it is hoped that treatment modalities outlined previously will be required much less frequently during the next few years.

ATOPIC DERMATITIS

method of
J. B. KOPSTEIN, M.D.
Windsor, Ontario, Canada

Atopic dermatitis may be defined as a chronic cutaneous disease occurring primarily but not exclusively in individuals from families in which asthma and hay fever are prevalent. The clinical appearance and location of skin involvement are fairly characteristic. Certain fungal, bacterial, and viral infections are particularly common in these patients.

RECOGNITION

Atopic dermatitis occurs in all racial groups, but caucasians and Orientals are most frequently affected. The disease appears to have an unusually high prevalence in Asians emigrating to temperate areas of North America. Approximately 90 per cent of cases appear to occur by the age of 2 years. Approximately 70 per cent of patients have family members with atopic diseases. Adult-onset atopic dermatitis occurs rarely. Most of the new cases seen in adults are recurrences of childhood atopic dermatitis that may not be recalled. Itching is a paramount symptom. The classic presentation is in an infant with an eczematous eruption on the cheeks, anterior aspect of the legs, and dorsa of the arms. An associated diaper dermatitis is not infrequent. Scalp involvement also occurs and must be distinguished from the yellowish, greasy scales seen in seborrheic dermatitis. Nummular, or coin-like, patches, especially on extensor surfaces, may occur. These patches frequently form crusts, and a seropurulent discharge from their surfaces may occur. This variety also occurs in adults and is not always atopic in origin.

The Dennie-Morgan atopic fold is a pleat of skin around the eyes that may be an early cutaneous marker of atopic dermatitis. In black skin, the eczema tends to be more papular and may leave areas of hyper- or hypopigmentation on clearing. The infantile phase of the disease may subside or progress to the childhood variety, in which flexural eczematous patches appear, especially in the antecubital and popliteal areas. Infraorbital darkening with facial pallor also is frequently seen in children and adults with the disease. Excoriation and rubbing may lead to thickening or lichenification of the skin. The adult variety is similar, with additional involvement around the eyes and neck, although this may also be seen in the childhood variety. Accentuation of the palmar lines, with or without ichthyosis, frequently coexists with atopic dermatitis. The ichthyosis is of the dominant type (ichthyosis vulgaris).

Juvenile plantar dermatitis is a dry, scaly form of eczema that is almost always atopic in origin. It may be the only manifestation of the disease. This condition is especially prevalent in older children and teenagers, particularly males. Keratosis pilaris often coexists with atopic dermatitis and is characterized by large numbers of keratotic papules on the upper arms, the anterior thighs, and occasionally the face. Pityriasis alba is a disorder that is also likely atopic in origin and is characterized by whitish, scaly patches, especially on the face and arms. It may persist for long periods, often into the twenties or even the thirties. Chronic hand eczema, especially in young adult women, is often seen, and a history of atopic disease is frequently obtained in this group. Primary household irritants are etiologically important in these patients. Similarly, much industrial contact dermatitis of the primary irritant variety occurs in atopic individuals, which accounts for its frequent intractability.

PRECIPITATING FACTORS

It is well known that atopic dermatitis is seasonal, with worsening especially at seasonal changes. Most atopics appear to do better during the warmer months in temperate climates if excessive humidity and high temperatures are avoided. Some appear to do better during the winter. Atopic skin appears to cope with sudden temperature changes poorly, and flare-ups may occur with prolonged exposure to cold, windy weather. Emotional factors may be operative in older children and adults and may be associated with exacerbations of the disease. The role of diet is controversial, but many believe that in infancy some foods do play a role in flare-ups of the disease (see later).

COMPLICATIONS

Atopic patients appear to have diminished T cell numbers and functions, as well as defects in chemotaxis. IgE levels are often but not always increased. These abnormalities may account for the unusual susceptibility of these patients to herpes simplex and molluscum contagiosum infections. These infections may be quite widespread in the case of herpes simplex, causing serious, widespread inoculation lesions within the patches of eczema. This is known as Kaposi's varicelliform eruption. Systemic or oral acyclovir may be required in these patients if they have severe, widespread involvement. Fungal infections with dermatophyte pathogens also appear to have an increased frequency and are responsive to oral or topical miconazole (Micatin) or clotrimazole (Lotrimin). Atopic patients are also highly susceptible to cutaneous infection with coagulase-positive staphylococci. Boils, carbuncles, folliculitis, and impetigo are seen with high frequency in patients with atopic dermatitis. However, colonization of lesions with these organisms without obvious infection is extremely frequent and may be important in causing persistence of the lesions. Scabies may coexist in patients with atopic dermatitis and may produce a clinical picture that may be unrecognizable. Nevertheless, a careful search with a hand lens may reveal burrows around the wrists, axillary folds, breasts, or penis. Scrapings suspended in mineral oil may reveal the acari under low-power microscopy. The use of lindane in coexistent scabies and widespread atopic dermatitis may result in potentially toxic levels of the drug. Careful monitoring of such patients is required, as convulsions may occur, especially in young children. If there is any doubt about the use of lindane, physicians are advised to apply 6 per cent sulfur in petrolatum twice daily for 3 days as an alternative therapy.

NATURAL HISTORY AND PROGNOSIS

Atopic dermatitis tends to decrease with age, with fewer relapses during adult life. In perhaps 60 to 70 per cent of infants and children with atopic dermatitis, the disease resolves before adulthood. However, recurrences in the form of adult hand eczema or industrial dermatitis are frequently seen after earlier remissions. It is best not to prognosticate to parents about the future in childhood atopic dermatitis. Furthermore, at least one-third of infant and childhood patients will develop bronchial asthma, and another one-third will develop hay fever.

MANAGEMENT

There seems little doubt that infantile atopic dermatitis may be aggravated by certain foods, especially cow milk, eggs, and wheat products. It is probably better to avoid these foods when they appear to be a factor. Prolonged, restrictive diets with little or no rationale may interfere with nutrition and should not be prescribed. Anaphylactic reactions to peanuts, chocolate, and eggs are relatively rare but can be fatal. Allergy to penicillin is also more frequent in atopic individuals. Tomatoes and citrus products may produce a characteristic circumoral erythema in some of these patients. The use of a straw may be helpful in young children in whom this occurs. Wool, dust, feathers, cats, dogs, horses, and guinea pigs should be avoided. Atopic infants and children should not be allowed to play directly on household carpets, whether these are wool or synthetics. Cotton garments and socks should be worn, if possible, although smooth synthetic fabrics may be tolerated. The use of regular alkaline soap is contraindicated. Cleansing can be achieved with Cetaphil Lotion, Aveenobar, Lowila Cake, and numerous other soapless cleansers. In my opinion, bleaches, fabric softeners, and antistatic pads should be avoided in washing clothing. Double rinsing may sometimes be required to rid the clothing completely of detergents.

Topical corticosteroids are the single most important modality in the management of this disease. Most importantly in children, the least potent steroid that is effective should be used. One per cent hydrocortisone cream or ointment may be quite effective, especially in children, and there is little, if any, absorption. If it is ineffective, desonide cream (Tridesilon) or ointment and 0.2 per cent hydrocortisone valerate (Westcort) are slightly more potent alternatives. Sometimes a diluted form of a more potent steroid may be useful. In this regard, triamcinolone 0.1 per cent cream, 15 grams diluted to 120 or 240 grams with one of the commercial cream or ointment bases, is often effective and is quite economical. The high-potency topical steroids such as betamethasone dipropionate (Diprosone) and valerate (Valisone) or clobetasol propionate (Temovate) may have a place in localized, intractable atopic dermatitis. Widespread use for prolonged periods should be avoided because of the risk of absorption and adrenal suppression. There is also evidence that in childhood, widespread use of intermediate or strong topical steroids may delay or reduce the adolescent growth spurt. On the scalp, the alcohol–propylene glycol steroid lotions may burn and may not be tolerated. There are several light steroid creams and lotions available for use in this location. Nothing stronger than 1 per cent hydrocortisone should be used in intertriginous sites because of the risk of atrophy and striae formation. Ichthyosis frequently coexists with atopic dermatitis. Emollients such as petrolatum, Eucerin, Nivea, or Aquaphor should be applied after a bath. Urea 5 to 20 per cent ointments often are used in ichthyosis but may burn if applied to hot, wet skin. Similarly, lactic acid and some of the newer hydroxy acid creams may be useful in ichthyosis. Burning and stinging may also be occasional problems here as well. Tar preparations are rarely indicated in the modern management of this disease, although they are occasionally helpful in nummular eczema.

Bath oils may be helpful in either the bath or the shower. If applied to the entire skin in the shower, they should be partially rinsed off. These oils should be unscented. Lubath and Aveeno Oilated are two bath oils that are often used. Natural sunlight or professionally supervised shortwave ultraviolet light therapy may be helpful in some cases of atopic dermatitis. Home sun lamps and tanning facilities are best avoided.

Systemic corticosteroids may be indicated for severe flare-ups that cannot be controlled by topical therapy alone. They should be withdrawn as soon as possible after clearing occurs. Their use in children is difficult to justify unless an emergency situation exists. Hospitalization may provide great benefit in cases where the disease has become intractable. Here intensive nursing care with ultraviolet light, baths, and supervised administration of ointments and oral sedation results in rapid resolution in many cases.

Antihistamines such as hydroxyzine (Atarax) or diphenhydramine (Benadryl) may be useful for their sedative and antipruritic properties. The newer nonsedative antihistamines have no antipruritic or sedative properties and are not indicated in atopic dermatitis. As previously indicated, staphylococcal infection or colonization often occurs in these patients. Erythromycin and cloxacillin or its derivatives may be used for frank infections. In addition, in some cases of recalcitrant atopic dermatitis, empiric use for 7 to 10 days may result in clearing of the disease, presumably because of removal of staphylococcal colonization.

ERYTHEMAS

method of
ALAN E. LASSER, M.D.
Northwestern University Medical School
Skokie, Illinois

Erythema is a nonspecific reaction pattern in the skin to a multitude of stimuli, including drugs, physical agents, infections, autoimmune diseases, and malignancy. Erythema is also a component of most dermatologic diseases. However, when we think of "the erythemas," certain disease entities come to mind.

ERYTHEMA MULTIFORME

Erythema multiforme is an acute, often recurrent eruption of the skin and mucous membranes. The hallmark of the disease is the presence of distinctive skin lesions consisting of rings of color, the "target lesion." As in most dermatologic conditions, only a few of the typical lesions need be present to focus thinking toward the correct diagnosis. Minor to major expressions of disease can occur and are labeled as such. Erythema multiforme major has skin involvement along with extensive erosions of two or more mucosal surfaces. The most severe expression is called Stevens-Johnson syndrome, which is truly a medical emergency. If this syndrome is suspected, an emergency ophthalmologic consultation should be obtained. A prodrome of fever, malaise, and myalgias is often present and is especially valuable for the patient with recurrent disease to appreciate its significance.

Almost anything can trigger erythema multiforme. The most frequently identified precipitating factors are recurrent herpes simplex infections, *Mycoplasma* infections, and drug reactions, especially to sulfonamides, penicillin, phenytoin, and phenylbutazone.

The eruption is symmetric and usually self-limiting; minor forms resolve in 1 to 4 weeks. The primary lesion is an erythematous papule. The lesion enlarges for a few days and may coalesce. The typical iris or target lesion develops as the individual lesion enlarges, with the most severe damage being in the center. The center of the lesion may become gray, white, or deep purple. Outside the center there may be a dusky red inflammatory zone surrounded at the periphery by a lighter edematous zone. Fluid may accumulate beneath the epidermis and bullae may form. Scarring in the minor variant is uncommon but postinflammatory hyperpigmentation, hypopigmentation, or both are common.

All symptoms and manifestations are more severe in the major variant. Involvement of the mucous membranes of the eye and oral and genital areas can be a difficult management problem. Fluid and electrolyte imbalances, extensive denudation of the skin, blindness, esophageal stricture, secondary infection, and death can occur.

Treatment

Therapy is conservative symptomatic for the minor variant. Tepid wet compresses with tap water or Burow's solution diluted 1:40 for bullae and denuded areas and antihistamines for itching and urticarial erythema are the mainstays of therapy. Vigilon's dressings are often beneficial for intertriginous erosions. Oral lesions can be helped with half-strength hydrogen peroxide rinses and/or an anesthetic cocktail of equal parts of elixir of diphenydramine (Benadryl) and Kaopectate. Xylocaine Viscous may also be of benefit. Extremes of temperature and the trauma of sharp-edged foods should be avoided. A liquid diet may be necessary. Cultures for bacteria and cultures and serologic studies for *Mycoplasma* should be obtained. If secondary infection is suspected, use of antibiotics is advised. Any drugs suspected of causing erythema should be discontinued. Herpes simplex may be the etiologic agent; however, the use of acyclovir (Zovirax) has not been effective once erythema multiforme is present. In recurrent disease, starting acyclovir at the earliest prodromal sign, before the appearance of erythema multiforme or at the onset of the lesions of herpes simplex, may be of benefit. If this treatment is successful, these patients should have acyclovir on or near their person at all times.

The use of systemic steroids is controversial at this time. There is evidence that systemic steroids do not alter the course of established disease and may even increase morbidity. A case can be made for steroid use early, before the disease is fully expressed, because of the potential seriousness of the illness. For example, prednisone so used should be started in a dosage of 1 to 2 mg per kg per day and tapered slowly according to the response.

ERYTHEMA NODOSUM

Erythema nodosum is characterized by the sudden appearance of erythematous, tender nodules in the skin, usually of the pretibial area. The lesions are usually symmetric and oval. Pain is variable and may be severe. A few days after onset of disease in the typical case, redness begins to subside. A prodrome is often present. Females are affeted more often than males, and there seems to be some seasonal clustering in the spring and fall. Erythema nodosum is a reaction pattern in the skin that can be triggered by a whole litany of conditions. Infections (often streptococcal), collagen disease, inflammatory bowel disease (ulcerative colitis or Crohn's disease), sarcoidosis, and drugs (especially oral contraceptives, estrogens, and sulfonamides) are the most frequent etiologic triggers. However, in most cases no etiology is identified.

The work-up includes a complete history and physical examination. Laboratory studies should include throat culture, antistreptolysin O titer, antinuclear antibody, erythrocyte sedimentation rate, and chest x-ray. If there is any doubt about the diagnosis, a deep cutaneous biopsy should be obtained.

Treatment

Therapy includes limitation of activity to bed rest, elevation of legs, wrapping with elastic bandage, elimination of any drug suspected of causing disease, and treatment of any specific etiology found on evaluation. Aspirin or nonsteroidal anti-inflammatory agents (Motrin) are usually given. Because of the relatively frequent association of a recent streptococcal infection, many practitioners give a course of empiric penicillin therapy, if the drug is not contraindicated. In severe or long-lasting cases, prednisone, if it is not contraindicated, 40 to 60 mg per day tapering over 15 to 30 days, is recommended.

ERYTHEMA CHRONICUM MIGRANS
(See also Lyme Disease in Section on Infectious Diseases)

Lyme disease is caused by the spirochete *Borrelia burgdoferi* that resides in the adult tick *Ixodes dammini*. The first stage of this disease consists of the eruption erythema chronicum migrans, which begins within days of a tick bite as an erythema around the area of the bite. The erythema gradually expands with a flat or elevated border and partial clearing of the center; it is usually nontender and nonpruritic. Several days after the primary lesion, more than 50 per cent of patients develop multiple annular secondary lesions, which are usually smaller, migrate less, and typically spare the palms and soles. Without treatment this eruption subsides during 3 to 4 weeks.

If this disease is suspected, therapy should be started early to modify signs and symptoms, prevent recurrences, and prevent late complications. Antibiotic therapy is often begun before laboratory studies are complete. Tetracycline HCl, 250 to 500 mg every 6 hours, is recommended. In children younger than age 8 years, penicillin, 250 mg every 6 hours, or erythromycin, 250 mg every 6 hours, can be used. Erythromycin is also used in patients who are allergic to penicillin.

BULLOUS DISEASES
method of
DONALD P. KADUNCE, M.D., and
JOHN J. ZONE, M.D.
University of Utah Medical Center
Salt Lake City, Utah

The most severe bullous diseases appear to be humorally mediated by cutaneous immunoglobulin deposition. The remainder of the bullous diseases, which are not discussed here, are of genetic (e.g., hereditary epidermolysis bullosa), infectious (e.g., bullous impetigo, toxic shock syndrome), physical (e.g., friction blisters), or idiopathic (e.g., erythema multiforme) etiology.

Immune-mediated bullous diseases may be pathogenetically grouped into those mediated by IgG—pemphigus vulgaris, bullous pemphigoid, and epidermolysis bullosa acquisita—and those mediated by IgA—dermatitis herpetiformis and linear IgA bullous dermatosis. There is a large amount of clinical and histologic overlap among these diseases, which necessitates the use of direct and indirect immunofluorescence for confirmation. Care should be exercised to include routine histology of the blisters, as well as direct immunofluorescence of normal-appearing perilesional skin.

DERMATITIS HERPETIFORMIS AND LINEAR IgA BULLOUS DERMATOSIS

Dermatitis herpetiformis (DH) is an extremely pruritic papulovesicular disease that occurs on extensor surfaces and is characterized pathologically by an accumulation of neutrophils in the dermal papillary tips, a vesicle occurring in the basement membrane zone, and the granular deposition of IgA in the dermal papillary tips. There is a strong association between DH, gluten-sensitive enteropathy, and the human leukocyte antigen B8/DR3/DQw2 haplotype. Linear IgA bullous dermatosis has an identical histologic picture but is characterized by linear deposition of IgA in the basement membrane zone, a somewhat more variable clinical picture, and no association with gluten-sensitive enteropathy or the human leukocyte antigen phenotype.

Treatment

Optimal therapy of DH includes two major interventions: (1) dapsone or sulfapyridine and (2) a gluten-free diet. These therapies are complementary and should not be thought of as alternative approaches to treatment. Although patients with linear IgA bullous dermatosis are generally unresponsive to gluten-free diets, the other therapies to be described pertain to both diseases.

Although pharmacologic therapy is the cornerstone of DH treatment, a gluten-free diet may allow a reduction in the dose of suppressive medication and, in some cases, may provide clinical remission. Gluten (a dietary protein present in rye, barley, wheat, and oats) is prevalent in the diet of Western cultures, making compliance difficult. Dietary counseling is necessary for this therapy to succeed, but even modest reductions in gluten intake may moderate the activity of the disease. The drug dose can generally be reduced during an average of 8 months of dietary restriction and the drug eliminated at an average of 29 months.

Dapsone is the drug of choice for DH. Once the suppressive threshold has been reached, disease activity generally subsides within 24 to 72 hours. We generally begin with doses of 25 to 50 mg per day and increase them in 25-mg increments every 3 days until suppression is achieved; in most patients, suppression is complete with doses of 75 to 150 mg per day. The dose is increased gradually to avoid severe acute hemolysis, which may otherwise limit tolerance. After suppression, the dose of dapsone may be tapered to the lowest level, allowing two or three new lesions per week. The maximal long-term suppressive dose recommended is 400 mg per day.* Doses greater than 200 mg per day may be associated with peripheral neuropathy, cholestatic jaundice, and psychosis. Despite these precautions, the patient's skin may develop a bluish tinge secondary to methemoglobinemia. All patients should have a complete blood count at baseline and weekly for 1 month, once per month for 6 months, and then semiannually. A chemistry profile should be done at baseline, at 6 months, and annually. Patients at

risk for glucose-6-phosphate dehydrogenase deficiency should have the initial level checked.

Sulfapyridine is an alternative suppressive therapy, although some patients do not respond to any dose. Initial dose of sulfapyridine are 500 mg three times daily to 1000 mg twice daily, with the same response time as that for dapsone. Doses of up to 4 grams per day may be required for suppression and should be given in divided daily doses.* Side effects are generally limited to those of other sulfa drugs, including nephrolithiasis. The neuropathy and psychosis of dapsone are avoided, and hemolysis, if it occurs, is much less severe.

Localized relief, without an increase in the dose of dapsone, may be obtained by the use of topical steroids such as fluocinonide gel (Lidex). This form of therapy is most effective if the vesicles are broken. Other therapies, including colchicine, cholestyramine, pyribenzamine, indomethacin, nicotinic acid, and cromolyn sodium, have been minimally effective in our hands.

PEMPHIGUS VULGARIS AND BULLOUS PEMPHIGOID

Pemphigus vulgaris (PV) is characterized by acantholytic, intraepidermal blisters induced by IgG directed against an epidermal cell surface antigen. These blisters, which are often on the face, trunk, and oral mucosa, are fragile and demonstrate a positive Nikolsky's sign. Before the advent of steroids, this disease was usually fatal. Successful therapy is directed at eliminating the circulating antibody, the titer of which closely parallels disease activity.

Bullous pemphigoid (BP) appears to be mediated by the deposition of IgG and C3 in the basement membrane zone. The blister, which forms at the dermal-epidermal junction, is tense, and Nikolsky's sign is usually negative. Mucous membrane involvement is less frequent than in pemphigus. Therapy leads to clinical remissions for the majority of BP patients and parallels the disappearance of circulating anti–basement membrane antibody levels.

Treatment

The drugs of choice for BP and PV are systemic steroids and/or immunosuppressive agents. The vast majority of patients respond to oral prednisone in doses of 0.5 to 1.0 mg per kg per day. The response is initially characterized by a decrease in the number of new lesions and by healing of old lesions during 2 to 3 weeks. Doses of prednisone of up to 2.0 to 2.5 mg per kg per day* may

---

*May exceed manufacturer's recommended dose.

*May exceed manufacturer's recommended dose.

be necessary in recalcitrant PV but are rarely required in BP. When PV proves to be unresponsive to this regimen, we have occasionally used pulse-dosed steroids: intravenous methylprednisolone (Solu-Medrol), 1 gram per day for 5 days, followed by the previously mentioned oral regimen. Once a response has been obtained, the steroids may be tapered at a rate of 10 mg per week until a daily dose of 20 mg per day is reached. At that point, the prednisone should be tapered at a rate of 2.5 mg per week. If at any point new lesions occur, we return to the next highest dose. Numerous acute and chronic side effects accompany the use of steroids and are dose dependent. Acutely, patients may suffer from glucose intolerance, hypokalemia, metabolic alkalosis, opportunistic infections, exacerbation of hypertension, and psychosis. Chronic steroid use also produces osteoporosis, cataracts, and cutaneous fragility.

Immunosuppressive agents are steroid-sparing *adjuncts* that allow steroids to be tapered more rapidly. The immunosuppressive agents most commonly used in the therapy of BP and PV are cyclophosphamide (Cytoxan) and azathioprine (Imuran).* Azathioprine is our drug of choice in the long-term management of BP. It is given orally in doses of 2 to 3 mg per kg per day; should this regimen fail, we replace azathioprine with cyclophosphamide, 2 to 3 mg per kg orally per day. Methotrexate, 25 mg intramuscularly per week, has been used by others.† Complete blood counts should be done weekly for the first month and then monthly until the medications can be tapered. In general, steroids are tapered first, followed by tapering of the immunosuppressive agents. These agents are tapered at a rate of 50 mg of each daily dose per month once the patient is clear of lesions, is no longer receiving steroids, and has negative antibody titers. Side effect profiles are similar for cyclophosphamide and azathioprine, including depression of both primary and secondary immune responses, cell-mediated immunity, hepatic damage, and bone marrow suppression. Cyclophosphamide causes sterility and cystitis; the latter may be avoided by generous fluid intake and morning administration of the drug. Hepatic and renal damage impair excretion of these agents and exacerbate toxicity. Finally, when any of the agents mentioned earlier are used, the patient must be skin tested for tuberculosis. Patients who have positive test results should receive isoniazid, 300 mg per day,

while receiving steroid or immunosuppressive therapy.

For patients who fail the previously discussed therapies, gold is a reasonable alternative.* After a test dose of 5 mg intramuscularly, we begin administering 25 mg intramuscularly each week and advancing to 50 mg per week as tolerated. Typically, a total dose of 500 to 1500 mg must be achieved for a therapeutic response, and once the disease is under control, monthly maintenance therapy can be instituted. Baseline complete blood cell counts and urinalysis must be performed before each injection because of the relatively high frequency of glomerulonephritis, thrombocytopenia, and neutropenia. Dermatitis may complicate this form of therapy.

We reserve plasmapheresis for patients who fail to respond to an adequate trial (each trial lasts for about 6 months) of all the previously discussed regimens (nearly all of our patients are receiving steroids and immunosuppressives at this point). Three to five plasmapheresis procedures are performed during 2 weeks, each with an exchange of 60 ml per kg.

A brief word should be said about cyclosporine A. This potent immunosuppressive drug has theoretical benefits for patients who fail all of the preceding therapies, but none of our patients have required this agent. Because of the risk of irreversible nephrotoxicity, one should be cautious in using it.

If disease activity is localized to the lower extremities, local therapy with saline or aluminum subacetate wet dressings and potent topical steroids (we favor fluocinonide cream) can avoid parenteral therapy.

EPIDERMOLYSIS BULLOSA ACQUISITA

Epidermolysis bullosa acquisita (EBA) is an acquired immunobullous disorder mediated by an IgG class immune response directed against Type VII collagen (a component of the normal basement membrane zone). EBA may be differentiated from BP by immunoelectron microscopy or indirect immunofluorescence using saline split skin, which shows adherence of IgG to the dermal side of the basement membrane zone in EBA and to the epidermal side in BP. Blisters are most commonly present over joint surfaces but, because of skin fragility, may be present at any site of minor trauma. The therapy of EBA is similar to those mentioned previously. It is nearly always long-term and, at best, suppressive.

---

*Cyclophosphamide and azathioprine are approved drugs but this use is not listed by the manufacturer.

†Methotrexate is an approved drug but this use is not listed by the manufacturer.

---

*Gold is an approved drug but this use is not listed by the manufacturer.

Treatment

As with BP and PV, steroids are the mainstay of therapy for EBA. Doses of up to 2 mg per kg are often required for suppression. Unlike patients with BP and PV, most patients with EBA do not achieve a complete cure, although skin fragility does appear to be decreased, pruritus often improves, and the rate of blister formation slows. There is a poor correlation between antibody titers and response to therapy.

Because patients with EBA require long-term steroid therapy, with all the attendant side effects noted earlier, the use of steroid-sparing agents is preferred. These include dapsone, azathioprine, and cyclophosphamide and are used as discussed earlier. The response to these modalities is usually poor.

Two methods that appear more promising are cyclosporin A* therapy and plasmapheresis. Cyclosporin A is begun at 1 to 2 mg per kg per day and cautiously increased to a maximum of 5 to 6 mg per kg per day. Urinalysis, blood urea nitrogen, creatinine, cyclosporin A levels, and the complete blood cell count must be followed at least twice weekly during initiation and dosage changes and biweekly to monthly only after maintenance is reached. Irreversible nephrotoxicity is the most serious side effect of cyclosporin A. Plasmapheresis is approached in the same manner as described earlier for PV and has been effective in the hands of several investigators. We favor a trial of plasmapheresis before committing the patient to cyclosporin A.

---

*Cyclosporine A is an approved drug but this use is not listed by the manufacturer.

CONTACT DERMATITIS

method of
JOHN E. WOLF, Jr., M.D.
Baylor College of Medicine
Houston, Texas

The skin is, among many other things, a barrier—an interface between a person's internal and external environments. It is generally an effective barrier, but one often achieved at a price—contact dermatitis.

There are two general types of contact dermatitis—irritant and allergic—and these, in turn, like any other form of dermatitis (e.g., eczema), may be acute, subacute, or chronic. The management of contact dermatitis must account for these variations and must be prefaced by careful description and accurate diagnosis.

Irritant contact dermatitis results from exposure of the skin to inherently injurious chemicals or toxins and does not require allergic sensitization. Examples include dermatitis caused by detergents, household or industrial cleansers, or the sting of the Portuguese man-of-war, *Physalia physalis*. On the other hand, allergic contact dermatitis follows exposure to a substance capable of sensitizing the skin; subsequent reexposure may elicit a contact dermatitis. The classic illustration is *Rhus* contact dermatitis (poison ivy).

AVOIDANCE AND PHYSICAL PROTECTION

With either form of contact dermatitis, a critical component of proper management is identification of the inciting agent followed by careful avoidance of that substance. In the case of irritant contact dermatitis, this information is generally obtained by a probing patient history, sometimes combined with a careful examination of the home or work place. Evaluation of allergic contact dermatitis may also include open or closed patch testing.

Once an inciting or provocative agent has been identified, the patient must make every effort to avoid further contact with that substance, which may be difficult. A bricklayer with a contact allergy to chromates may be unable to avoid contact with chromate-containing cement. Seemingly ubiquitous substances like nickel may also be difficult to avoid. Short of outright avoidance, the use of protective clothing such as gloves, boots, masks, and long-sleeved shirts may be helpful. The use of barrier creams, especially in an industrial setting, may also be useful, but in my experience their utility is minimal.

TREATMENT OF ACUTE CONTACT DERMATITIS

Acute contact dermatitis, irritant or allergic, is usually a weeping, oozing, exudative process, which is often accompanied by vesicles or bullae and sometimes complicated by secondary bacterial infection. The application of cool or tepid soaks or compresses may be both soothing and drying; tap water or Burow's solution (Domeboro) may be used. Colloidal oatmeal (Aveeno) baths may also be quite comforting. Itching is often intense and may be controlled by antihistamines such as diphenhydramine (Benadryl), trimeprazine (Temaril), hydroxyzine (Atarax), or the nonsedating terfenadine (Seldane).

Most cases of acute contact dermatitis require the use of topical or systemic corticosteroids for effective management. Systemic steroids, used for the more severe cases, may be administered either orally (as prednisone, 40 to 60 mg daily for 10 to 14 days) or intramuscularly (as triamcinolone acetonide [Kenalog] or betamethasone acetate [Celestone]). Oral steroids are generally tapered over a 1- to 2-week period, whereas intramuscular preparations may persist for 1 (betamethasone) to 3 (triamcinolone) weeks. The well-known contraindications for the use of systemic corticosteroids must, of course, be considered when deciding whether to use them in the treatment of acute contact dermatitis.

For an acute contact dermatitis, topical corticosteroids are most often prescribed in the form of a lotion, cream, or solution. Solutions are particularly useful for hair-bearing areas or for sites such as the ears or interdigital spaces, whereas lotions may be spread easily over larger areas of affected skin; creams may be ideal for hands, feet, or smaller patches of contact dermatitis. In any format, topical corticosteroid preparations may be mild (hydrocortisone), moderate (Westcort, Tridesilon, Locoid), potent (Topicort, Lidex, Cyclocort), or super potent (Diprolene, Psorcon, Temovate) formulations. Milder preparations should be used on the face, breasts, groin and axillae. With the potent or super potent preparations, local (atrophy, telangiectasia, striae) or even systemic (adrenal axis suppression) side effects are potential problems. The super potent steroids must be used with special caution.

TREATMENT OF CHRONIC CONTACT DERMATITIS

In the chronic form, allergic or irritant contact dermatitis generally produces thickening, lichenification, and fissuring, often intermixed with acute or subacute manifestations of the eczematous process. As with acute contact dermatitis, secondary infection may be a problem and necessitate the use of topical (bacitracin, Bactroban) or oral (erythromycin, tetracycline, cephalosporins, dicloxacillin) antibiotics.

The dry, cracked, thickened skin of chronic contact dermatitis is generally treated with the application of moisturizing or emollient lotions, creams, and ointments, rather than with the baths, soaks, and compresses that are most helpful in acute forms of the disorder. Likewise, when topical corticosteroid preparations are used, creams or ointments are generally favored over the less emollient lotions and solutions. Because a chronic disease process predicts a prolonged therapeutic course, the physician must be especially vigilant when using the more potent topical corticoid preparations. Certainly the same caveat applies to systemic corticosteroids, which should be used carefully and infrequently to control severe flare-ups of chronic contact dermatitis. Pruritus is, indeed, a problem here, as with the acute process, and oral antihistamines may provide at least temporary relief.

SKIN DISEASES OF PREGNANCY

method of
ROBERT A. SWERLICK, M.D.
Emory University
Atlanta, Georgia

Pregnancy is marked by profound physiologic changes that can result in a number of cutaneous changes, some of which are considered to be pathologic. Pregnancy is almost invariably associated with various pigmentary changes, such as darkening of the areolae or genitalia, linea nigra, or development of melasma. Often, pregnancy is associated with the growth of skin tags or the development of pyogenic granulomas, both of which tend to involute after parturition. Certain inflammatory skin conditions not specific for pregnancy, such as acne or eczema, have been noted to worsen or to improve dramatically during pregnancy.

A group of disorders are thought to be relatively specific for pregnancy, two of which are discussed here: herpes gestationis (HG) and pruritic urticarial papules and plaques of pregnancy (PUPPP).

HERPES GESTATIONIS

HG is a rare disorder that is characterized by urticarial wheals, bullae, and marked pruritus. It may begin as early as the first trimester, or it may not become apparent until after delivery. The severity of symptoms is variable, with some patients having spontaneous resolution during pregnancy and others having severe, widespread vesiculation. The histologic findings are similar to those seen with bullous pemphigoid: a subepidermal blister associated with variable infiltration with neutrophils and eosinophils. The diagnosis of HG is best made by using direct immunofluorescence microscopy of perilesional skin. All patients with HG have linear deposits of C3 at the basement membrane zone of the dermal-epidermal junction. About one-quarter of patients have IgG deposits that are detectable by direct immunofluorescence.

The disease resolves after pregnancy, although an immediate postpartum flare is extremely common. Some patients have periodic eruptions after delivery, particularly after menstruation begins, and some have exacerbations of HG after ingestion of oral contraceptives. Rarely, a transient cutaneous eruption has been noted in children born to mothers with HG, but this eruption requires no therapy. A much more controversial point is whether children born to mothers with HG are at higher risk for fetal morbidity or mortality. Widely disparate results have come from different studies, but at least one study suggests a somewhat high incidence of fetal problems, especially prematurity, in these infants.

Therapy

The therapy of HG should be directed at control of symptoms. A few patients can be treated with topical medications, thus obviating any potential problems with ingestion of oral medications during pregnancy. Topical steroids, such as triamcinolone 0.1 per cent in a cream base applied as often as four or five times daily, may control disease activity. Open areas can be soaked in tap water or alluminum acetate soaks before steroid application. Diphenhydramine, 25 to 50 mg three or four times daily, may be used to control pruritus.

Many patients with severe, widespread disease do not have the disease controlled with topical medications and require the use of systemic corticosteroids. Control is usually obtained with 20 to 40 mg of prednisone daily as a single morning dose. This regimen should be tapered to the lowest possible dose needed to control activity or to alternate-day doses, but it should be expected that higher doses may be required post partum, when disease in many patients flares. The use of immunosuppressive agents such as azathioprine is contraindicated during pregnancy and in nursing mothers. The use of corticosteroids during pregnancy is also controversial, but experience with pregnancy in steroid-dependent asthmatics suggests that the risks are not significant.

PRURITIC URTICARIAL PAPULES AND PLAQUES OF PREGNANCY

PUPPP is an extremely pruritic eruption that usually occurs late in pregnancy. It characteristically begins in the striae distensae and then spreads to the thighs and abdomen. The primary lesions are edematous papules, which unlike HG, rarely vesiculate. Histologic examination demonstrates a lymphohistiocytic infiltrate with variable numbers of eosinophils. Differentiation from HG can be made with certainty by direct immunofluorescence, which does not demonstrate C3 at the epidermal basement membrane zone.

There is no known association with PUPPP and maternal or fetal morbidity. The eruption promptly improves and clears after delivery. Treatment before that time consists of the use of high-potency topical corticosteroids such as fluocinonide cream 0.05 per cent, applied three or four times daily, and the use of diphenhydramine, 25 to 50 mg three or four times daily, to control itching. Patients with PUPPP only rarely require oral steroids to control the eruption.

PRURITUS ANI AND VULVAE

method of
EUGENE LEIBSOHN, M.D.
St. Joseph Hospital
Phoenix, Arizona

Pruritus ani and vulvae is a condition in these areas characterized by severe chronic itching, usually with some lichenification without a specific etiology.

Before this diagnosis is made, it is essential to rule out both dermatologic and internal diseases, which frequently produce itching in these areas. Dermatologic conditions include atopic dermatitis, seborrheic dermatitis, lichen planus, urticaria, contact dermatitis, lichen sclerosus et atrophicus, leukoplakia, Paget's disease, Bowen's disease, parasitoses, dermatitis herpetiformis, and drug allergies. Internal disorders that are frequently associated with pruritus are diabetes, hepatic and biliary diseases, blood lymphomas, chronic renal failure, and thyroid disease. Local factors that are associated with pruritus ani and vulvae are hemorrhoids, cryptitis, fissures, cervicitis, and hyperhidroses.

Once these factors are eliminated, it can be assumed that the condition results from various combinations of heat, dryness, and local irritation, including overmedication.

GENERAL TREATMENT

All types of soap should be avoided. Room-temperature showers or baths are recommended not more often than once daily. After the shower or bath, a moisturizing lotion such as Cetaphil may be used. Toilet paper should be avoided and the area cleansed with cotton and mineral oil, with a careful attempt to eliminate fecal matter in the folds of the anal canal. Any type of occlusion should be eliminated, and nylon undergarments and pantyhose should not be used. Increasing the bulk of the stool is helpful, and a tablespoonful of psyllium (Metamucil) daily can frequently achieve this purpose. Spicy foods should be eliminated from the diet.

TOPICAL MEDICATIONS

In acute cases with oozing, wet Domeboro compresses (one packet or tablet to a pint of cool water) should be used three times a day for 15 minutes. The area is allowed to dry by evaporation, and a lotion containing 1 per cent clindamycin hydrochloride (Cleocin) in a nonfluorinated steroid such as 1 per cent Cetacort is applied. In resistant cases, half-strength carbol-fuchsin (Castellani's Paint) is used and allowed to dry before the lotion is applied. This solution stains, and the patient should be so advised.

In the more chronic cases with dry lichenified mucosa and skin, a keratoplastic antibacterial, anti-inflammatory cream may be used, such as 3 per cent iodochlorhydroxyquin with hydrocortisone cream (Vioform Hydrocortisone), 0.5 per cent salicylic acid, 0.5 per cent sulfur in 1 per cent hydrocortisone (Hytone cream) applied three times a day.

In more resistant cases with increased lichenification, capsaicin (0.025 per cent) (Zostrix cream) diluted four times with 1 per cent Cetacort cream may be tried. Frequently, intradermal injections of diluted triamcinolone, 2 mg per ml in 1 per cent lidocaine, are helpful. Ultraviolet light and grenz ray therapy used in conjunction with the preceding medications frequently break the itch-scratch reflex.

SYSTEMIC THERAPY

Antipruritics such as cyproheptadine (Periactin), 2 mg three times a day and 4 mg at bedtime, are frequently helpful. In older patients, doxepin (Sinequan), 10 to 25 mg twice daily, is often antipruritic as well. Oral prednisone, 20 mg in daily individual doses, may be used for short periods if no contraindications such as ulcers or tuberculosis are present.

URTICARIA AND ANGIOEDEMA

method of
ROBERT B. SKINNER, JR., M.D., and
DENISE M. BUNTIN, M.D.
University of Tennessee
Memphis, Tennessee

Urticaria is a common cutaneous disorder often referred to as hives or wheals. Lesions consist of raised, well-circumscribed, erythematous pruritic plaques. These are transient and resolve in a few hours. Urticarial lesions range in size from a few millimeters to several inches (giant urticaria). Most urticaria results from an IgE-mediated immune response to a variety of antigens, producing areas of localized cutaneous edema. Urticarial lesions are characterized by edema in the superficial dermis; edema in the deep dermis and subcutaneous tissue produces the condition called angioedema. Evaluation and treatment of urticaria are based on classification into one of the following categories: acute, chronic, physical, or contact urticaria; urticarial vasculitis or angioedema.

ACUTE URTICARIA

Acute urticaria is defined as eruptions lasting less than 6 weeks; it usually responds to oral antihistamines. Work-up consists of a history with particular emphasis on medications and a physical examination. Laboratory tests are not usually necessary unless the urticaria persists for more than 6 weeks. The history should particularly explore drugs, especially aspirin, aspirin-containing products, and penicillin. Aspirin-allergic patients can have cross-sensitivity to nonsteroidal anti-inflammatory agents, azo dyes (tartrazine), and benzoic acid. Over-the-counter medications must be explored, including headache relievers, cold preparations, laxatives, and vitamin supplements.

Foods are a common cause of urticaria. Most commonly associated foods are shellfish, nuts, eggs, chocolate, cheese, peanut butter, tomatoes, and strawberries. Questions should concentrate on food eaten immediately prior to the eruption and foods possibly associated with previous episodes of urticaria.

Treatment

Treatment of acute urticaria usually requires full adult doses of oral antihistamines to control symptoms. Adult doses of oral antihistamines include diphenhydramine (Benadryl), 50 mg; hydroxyzine (Atarax, Vistaril), 50 mg; cyproheptadine (Periactin), 4 mg; chlorpheniramine (Chlortrimeton), 4 mg; trimeprazine (Temaril), 2.5 mg. All should be taken four times daily. The main side effect of oral antihistamines is drowsiness. This can sometimes be avoided by using the nonsedating antihistamines astemizole (Hismanal), 10 mg once daily, or terfenadine (Seldane), 60 mg twice daily. Doxepin* (Sinequan), 10 mg three times daily, can be effective when antihistamines fail.

The goal of treatment in acute urticaria is to control symptoms until the antigen inducing the urticarial eruption is eliminated from the system. Antihistamines should be taken around the clock until symptoms are eliminated. They can then be slowly tapered, with resumption of full dosage if the urticaria recurs. When one antihistamine fails to control symptoms, a second or even a third antihistamine from another pharmacologic class can be added—for example, the combination of diphenhydramine and hydroxyzine.

Topical modalities such as cool compresses or an antipruritic lotion (Sarna) will help to control itching. For severe urticaria or laryngeal edema, subcutaneous or intramuscular administration of 1:1000 epinephrine (0.2 to 0.5 ml) is sometimes required.

---

*This use is not listed by the manufacturer.

CHRONIC URTICARIA

Chronic urticaria is defined as an urticarial eruption lasting longer than 6 weeks. Studies show that laboratory work-up for chronic urticaria is not cost effective; however, the studies that seem most productive are complete blood count, multichannel chemistry profile, erythrocyte sedimentation rate, and urinalysis. Thyroid function tests and chest x-ray or sinus films are rarely of benefit. A search for infection should pursue infected teeth, sinuses, gallbladder, and kidney as well as signs and symptoms of viral infections. A food diary may sometimes be helpful; since the urticarial eruption frequently begins within several hours after ingestion of the offending food, the diary may reveal the same food eaten prior to other urticarial attacks. Special diets such as lamb and rice or the food-additive elimination diet may clear the urticaria, and then gradual addition of foods to the diet may reveal the triggering substance.

Treatment

Treatment is with the same agents mentioned earlier for acute urticaria. General treatment measures include avoidance of aspirin and aspirin-containing products, nonsteroidal anti-inflammatory agents, alcohol, exertion, and excessive heat, all of which increase cutaneous vasodilation and exacerbate urticaria.

THE PHYSICAL URTICARIAS

The physical urticarias can be diagnosed by history and mechanical tests. *Pressure urticaria* is manifested by development of urticaria several hours after local pressure has been applied to the skin. Common areas are the buttocks after sitting, the feet after walking, and areas subjected to pressure from tight clothes or belts. *Cold urticaria* can be diagnosed by a history of an urticarial eruption of hands and face during rewarming after cold contact. An ice cube placed on the patient's arm for several minutes will produce urticaria after removal of the ice cube and rewarming. *Cholinergic urticaria* is characterized by tiny, highly pruritic, punctate wheals or papules occurring on any part of the skin and lasting from 30 to 90 minutes. Precipitating factors include exercise, increased environment temperature, fever, and emotional stress. Physical urticarias are also reported to occur in association with light, vibration, heat, and water. *Dermographism* is the eruption of a linear wheal when the skin is stroked with a firm object. This differs from *contact urticaria*, which is the production of wheals when the skin is touched by any of a variety of substances. Avoidance of contactants relieves contact urticaria.

Treatment

Treatment of physical urticarias consists of oral antihistamines and avoidance of triggering factors. Dermographism is treated with low-dose antihistamines and avoidance of unnecessary trauma.

URTICARIAL VASCULITIS

Urticarial vasculitis can be suspected when individual urticarial lesions are present in one location for several days instead of several hours and there are associated complaints of fever, abdominal pain, arthralgias, and myalgias. The lesions sometimes hurt rather than itch. A skin biopsy of an urticarial lesion will reveal leukocytoclastic vasculitis. Urticarial vasculitis is frequently associated with medications, hepatitis B, mononucleosis, and systemic lupus erythematosus.

Treatment

Oral antihistamines are ineffective in urticarial vasculitis. Reported treatments include oral prednisone, 40 to 60 mg daily and tapering off in 10 to 14 days; oral colchicine,* 0.6 mg twice daily; dapsone,* 100 mg daily; and indomethacin* (Indocin), 75 to 200 mg daily in divided doses.

ANGIOEDEMA

Angioedema is a severe form of urticaria involving the deep dermis or subcutaneous tissue and manifested by severe swelling. Usually affected are the more distensible tissues such as the eyelid, lips, ear lobes, external genitalia, oral mucous membranes, tongue, and larynx. The hands and feet can develop severe edema. Urticaria frequently precedes angioedema, and the etiology and treatment of angioedema are the same as for urticaria. In hereditary angioedema, which consists of sudden attacks of gastrointestinal, laryngeal, and pharyngeal edema, there is a functional deficiency of the inhibitor of the activated first component of the complement system. Treatment is with the oral anabolic steroid danazol (Danocrine), 200 mg twice or three times daily.

---

*This use is not listed by the manufacturers.

PIGMENTARY DISORDERS

method of
CHRISTY A. LORTON, M.D., and
JAMES J. NORDLUND, M.D.
University of Cincinnati College of Medicine
Cincinnati, Ohio

The four pigments that are primarily responsible for normal skin color are oxygenated and reduced hemoglobins, carotenoids, and melanin. Of these, melanin is the major determinant of skin color. Disorders of pigmentation can be caused by at least three mechanisms: (1) an enhanced or diminished production of melanin by the melanocyte, (2) an increase or decrease in the number of melanocytes, or (3) an abnormal location of melanin and/or melanocytes within the dermis. The clinical result is either decreased pigment (hypopigmentation) or increased pigment (hyperpigmentation).

HYPERPIGMENTATION

Ultraviolet Light—Induced Hyperpigmentation (Suntan)

The constitutive or baseline skin color is genetically determined. It is independent of extrinsic factors such as exposure to sunlight. Facultative skin color is the inducible darkening of the skin that most often follows exposure to ultraviolet radiation. Suntan results from two different mechanisms. Longwave ultraviolet light (type A [UVA], 320 to 400 nm or "black light") causes immediate darkening of pigment. This occurs within 15 to 30 minutes after exposure and disappears within hours. It is probably caused by an oxidative change in the pre-existing melanin molecules. Immediate tanning is responsible for the attractive bronzing of the skin that most individuals observe after intense exposure to summer sunlight.

Shortwave ultraviolet light (type B [UVB], 290 to 320 nm) produces sunburn as well as delayed tanning. Delayed tanning is often much darker than the immediate type and is caused by proliferation of melanocytes as well as enhanced production of melanin. It takes 3 to 4 days to develop and lasts for many weeks.

Both longwave ultraviolet light and shortwave ultraviolet light contribute to photoaging, and both increase the risk of developing skin cancers. Both types of ultraviolet light are responsible for the mottled hyperpigmentation and wrinkling that are observed on heavily exposed areas of the skin such as the face, neck, and dorsum of the hands. Exposure to ultraviolet radiation in tanning parlors also hastens the processes of photoaging and wrinkling and possibly increases the risk of developing skin cancers.

Treatment

The patient must recognize that sun-induced pigmentation can be reversed only by avoiding exposure of the skin to all forms of ultraviolet light. There are many physical sun blocks that reflect ultraviolet light and protect the skin well. Clothing such as beachwear or hats, which can be very elegant, are excellent protectants. Other chemical sun blocks such as zinc oxide, calamine, talc, titanium dioxide, and kaolin are opaque and are effective sun shields. These products must be applied in a thick coat. Some preparations, which are available commercially in numerous spectacular colors, are now cosmetically and socially acceptable. For individuals who are unusually sensitive to sunlight and who desire to enjoy outdoor activities, these sun blocks are essential.

Chemical sunscreens function in a different way. They absorb ultraviolet light, especially in the shortwave range (UVB, 290 to 320 nm). The most common chemical sunscreens contain para-aminobenzoic acid (PABA), the esters of PABA, and salicylates. Other chemicals, like the benzophenone derivatives, anthranilates, and cinnamates, absorb UVB and offer additional absorption in the UVA (320 to 350 nm) range.

Two factors should be considered when choosing a sunscreen: the sun protection factor (SPF) and the substantivity. The SPF is the ratio of the minimal sunburn (UVB) dose of sunlight on chemically protected skin compared with that on unprotected skin. In midsummer (June 21) the average unprotected person burns after 15 to 20 minutes of direct exposure to the sun at noontime. A sunscreen with SPF 2 absorbs one-half of the UVB striking the skin. Therefore it takes twice

TABLE 1. **A Partial List of Combination Sunscreens with an SPF Equal to or Greater Than 15 That Have Good to Excellent Substantivity**

Brand Name Sunscreens (SPF)	Active Ingredients
Total Eclipse (15)	2.5% glyceryl PABA, 2.5% octyldimethyl PABA, 2.5% oxybenzone
SuperShade (15)	7% octyldimethyl PABA (padimate O), 3% oxybenzone
PreSun-15 (water resistant)	8% padimate O, 3% oxybenzone
Elizabeth Arden Suncare Creme (15)	Padimate O, oxybenzone
MMM-What-A-Tan! (15)	3% octyldimethyl PABA, 2.5%
Sundown (15) (sunblock)	7% padimate O, 5% octyl salicylate, 4% oxybenzone
Photoplex (15)	7% padimate O

as long to burn the treated skin (30 to 40 minutes of exposure on June 21). An SPF of 15 to 20 (which requires 15 to 20 times more UVB to burn the skin) is considered to be adequate protection against UVB radiation.

The substantivity of the sunscreen is its ability to withstand sweating and water immersion. Table 1 gives examples of current commercially available sunscreens with SPFs equal to or greater than 15 that also have good to excellent water and sweat resistance. Ideally, all sunscreens should be reapplied after prolonged swimming or heavy sweating.

Postinflammatory Hyperpigmentation

A variety of inflammatory conditions and infections (Table 2) cause hyperpigmentation of the skin, usually called "postinflammatory hyperpigmentation." The dyschromia follows the pattern and distribution of the original disease, but its intensity is not necessarily related to the degree of the previous inflammation. Postinflammatory hyperpigmentation is common and rather persistent in darkly pigmented people. It is caused by stimulation of melanocytes to produce excessive amounts of melanin. If the melanin remains in the epidermis, the color of the skin appears to be deep tan to dark brown. Often the inflammation is associated with disruption of the dermal-epidermal barrier. Melanin is then deposited in the upper dermis. When brown melanin is located in the dermis, its color appears to be slate gray or bluish.

Treatment

Epidermal forms of hyperpigmentation may respond to treatment with bleaching agents. Dermal hyperpigmentation does not respond to any medical treatments and usually is permanent. It is important, therefore, to determine whether the pigmentation has mainly an epidermal or a dermal component. Examination of the patient with a Wood's lamp (black light) in a totally dark room can facilitate this evaluation. Epidermal melanin turns almost black when viewed with the Wood's lamp. In contrast, dermal pigmentation, when observed with a Wood's lamp, is not visible to the

TABLE 2. **Some Common Causes of Postinflammatory Hyperpigmentation**

Exanthems	Acne
Drug eruptions	Tinea versicolor
Lichen planus	Cutaneous lupus
Atopic dermatitis	Psoriasis
Trauma, burns	Lichen simplex chronicus
Herpes zoster	Pityriasis rosea
Ashy dermatosis	Fixed drug eruption

TABLE 3. **Some Bleaching Agents for Hyperpigmentation (Applied Twice or Three Times Daily)**

Over-the-Counter Preparations
Eldopaque cream with opaque base (2% hydroquinone)
Eldoquin (2% hydroquinone)
Esoterica Cream (2% hydroquinone)
Atra (2% hydroquinone)

Prescription Preparations
Eldopaque Forte with opaque base (4% hydroquinone)
Solaquin Forte (4% hydroquinone, PABA ester, benzophenone)
HCQ Kit (4% hydroquinone, 1% hydrocortisone)
Ambi (2% hydroquinone, PABA ester)
Melanex (3% hydroquinone)

Combination of Medications (to be prescribed as separate medications)
Hydroquinone 4% and salicylic acid 2% cream
Hydroquinone 2% or 4%, hydrocortisone 2%, and tretinoin cream 0.05% applied sequentially
Hydroquinone 4%, tretinoin 0.1%, and dexamethasone 0.1% applied sequentially

examiner, and the blemishes on the patient's skin disappear.

There are several topical therapies for hyperpigmentation (Table 3). Prevention of further hyperpigmentation is paramount. Optimal management of the primary skin problem is essential.

Melasma (Chloasma)

Melasma ("mask of pregnancy") is a common patchy, irregular, tan to brown pigmentation that is usually located on the face of women. It occurs in women who are taking oral contraceptives or who are pregnant. It usually fades slowly after the termination of either event and is exacerbated by exposure to sunlight. It also occurs in women who are not taking birth control pills or whose last pregnancy occurred many years earlier. Occasionally, it occurs in men. Melasma is caused by increased epidermal melanization, although in some patients there is a moderate amount of dermal pigment as well. In these latter individuals, treatment can never return the skin entirely to its normal appearance.

Freckles (Ephelides)

Freckles first appear in childhood in individuals who have fair complexions and who are genetically of Celtic or Northern European ancestry. Freckles fade in the winter and become more prominent after exposure to sunlight. Middle-aged and older adults usually lose some or all of their freckles.

Solar Lentigines

Solar or senile lentigines are dark brown macules, usually 1 to 3 cm in diameter, that occur on the chronically sun-exposed surfaces of elderly individuals, especially on the dorsum of the hands or on the face. They are commonly misnamed "liver spots." In contrast to freckles and melasma, they do not fade in the winter but persist throughout the calendar year. They must be distinguished from lentigo maligna (Hutchinson's freckle) or seborrheic keratoses.

Treatment

Patients with these sun-induced pigmentary disorders must avoid further exposure to sunlight. Sunscreens or sunblocks help to prevent further pigmentary abnormalities.

Various bleaching medications are available, either as single agents or in combinations (Table 3). There is considerable individual variation in the response to treatment, but in general, most patients respond to one of the combination preparations. Most bleaching medications must be applied conscientiously, often for 6 to 12 months, to achieve optimal results.

Hydroquinone suppresses pigmentation, probably by blocking the activity of tyrosinase, the enzyme that is primarily involved in melanin synthesis. Side effects from hydroquinone are rare but include mild skin irritation. At higher concentrations, colloid milia, dermal pigmentation, or both have been reported. The addition of a corticosteroid cream increases the effectiveness of the hydroquinone and possibly reduces the frequency of skin irritation. Caution must be exercised when prescribing corticosteroids for prolonged periods. On the face, steroids can cause telangiectasia, atrophy, or acneiform lesions. The more potent fluorinated corticosteroids should not be used on the face except under special circumstances. On the arms and trunk, potent topical steroids can cause striae. These are irreversible.

Tretinoin cream (Retin-A) can also be used in conjunction with hydroquinone and/or mild corticosteroids to decrease epidermal hyperpigmentation. Recently, there has been a great deal of interest in the use of tretinoin alone to remove pigmentation associated specifically with photoaging. Tretinoin can be very irritating to the skin and can cause erythema, desquamation, and soreness. To minimize the side effects, the following approach is suggested. Therapy should be initiated with 0.025 or 0.05 per cent tretinoin applied at bedtime twice weekly for 1 month, then three times weekly for the second month, followed by nightly applications. Thereafter the concentration of the cream can be increased to 0.1 per cent if tolerated by the patient.

Monobenzyl ether of hydroquinone (monobenzone) (Benoquin) should *never* be used to treat disorders of hyperpigmentation. It is always contraindicated because in some individuals it causes destruction of melanocytes and leaves permanent disfiguring white spots. It is used only for complete depigmentation of patients with extensive vitiligo.

There are other modalities for treating localized pigmented spots like freckles or solar lentigines. Gentle freezing with liquid nitrogen can decrease the amount of color. Melanocytes are particularly susceptible to destruction by this treatment. One must avoid causing necrosis of the skin or blistering. Dark-skinned patients should not have lesions frozen except in special circumstances because of the risk of permanent depigmentation.

Trichloroacetic acid (TCA) is another agent that is effective in removing freckles and solar lentigines or other localized patches of pigmentation but is generally not useful in dark-skinned individuals. It must be used with extreme caution because it is highly reactive chemically and can cause instantaneous necrosis of the epidermis, which can produce severe scarring. Patients with solar freckles, lentigines, or localized pigment can be treated by applications of TCA by the physician. One cautious approach is to begin with a single application of 25 per cent TCA on one or two test areas in cosmetically less critical locations. If the patient notes a burning sensation, the area is washed with soap and water. Generally, 25 per cent TCA produces little effect or results. Subsequently areas are tested with 35, 50, or, if necessary, 75 per cent TCA. The concentration of TCA that produces desquamation and loss of the lesion without excessive injury is used as the treatment of choice. The physician should be well acquainted with and thoroughly trained in the use of these preparations to avoid severe complications.

Systemic Causes of Hyperpigmentation

Generalized hyperpigmentation is associated with many systemic disorders. Usually the color is due to melanin, for example, in Addison's disease. Metabolic, nutritional, or endocrine disorders should be considered in patients with widespread or diffuse hyperpigmentation. Generalized hyperpigmentation can also be caused by drugs or heavy metals. A partial list of these disorders and drugs is given in Table 4.

Treatment

Treatment for hyperpigmentation caused by systemic disorders is directed at correcting the

TABLE 4. **Some Systemic Causes**
of Hyperpigmentation

Metabolic Conditions	Drugs and Heavy Metals
Hemochromatosis	Mercury
Porphyria cutanea tarda	Silver
Addison's disease	Arsenic
Vitamin B_{12} deficiency	Gold
Pellagra	Antimalarial agents
Scleroderma	Minocycline
Acanthosis nigricans	Phenothiazines
Pregnancy	Carotenemia

underlying disease or discontinuing the medication.

HYPOPIGMENTATION

Vitiligo

Vitiligo is a common acquired depigmenting disorder that occurs in about 1 per cent of the general population. It is characterized by white (depigmented) patches on the skin. Only about 5 per cent of affected individuals have a positive (primary family) history of vitiligo. About 15 per cent of patients with vitiligo have thyroid disease, and 5 per cent have diabetes mellitus. Rarely, the patient with vitiligo has Addison's disease, pernicious anemia, or other endocrine disorders.

There are two types of vitiligo. In the generalized form, the white patches are spread symmetrically over the body. In the second form, segmental vitiligo, the patches are limited to localized areas (e.g., one-half of the face, an entire arm, or one leg). Segmental vitiligo usually does not follow dermatomes. In either type of vitiligo, the white patches generally appear spontaneously without a pre-existing rash. The depigmented areas are completely devoid of epidermal melanin and melanocytes. The cause of vitiligo is not known. Although it is commonly assumed to be an autoimmune disease, depigmentary disorders in several animal models that resemble human vitiligo suggest that the disorder may have a biochemical basis.

Treatment

The physician should be aware of the strong psychosocial impact that vitiligo has on the patient and should be prepared to provide reassurance, explanation, and appropriate referral to support groups, consultants, or psychiatrists as needed. For most people, vitiligo is a devastating disfigurement.

For certain individuals, the use of cosmetics or stains to conceal the more apparent vitiligo is all that is desired. Cover Mark and Dermablend are two opaque types of makeup that some patients find helpful. Vita Dye and Dy-o-Derm are quick-tan preparations. Both are stains that contain dihydroxyacetone. They are less acceptable because they tint the skin an orange-brown hue. Patients may need assistance from trained personnel in developing the skill to apply cosmetics or dyes.

Judicious use of broad-spectrum sunscreens is recommended for three reasons. First, the areas of vitiligo burn more easily than normal skin when exposed to sunlight. Second, injury like sunburn extends the depigmentation, a process called "Koebner's phenomenon." Third, exposure to sunlight induces darkening of the surrounding normal-appearing skin and causes accentuation of the cosmetic disfigurement.

Repigmentation requires regrowth of melanocytes into the white epidermis. Unfortunately, melanocytes do not migrate more than a few millimeters from the edge of a lesion. Thus successful repigmentation requires the presence of hair bulbs from which melanocytes can be stimulated to migrate into the surrounding white skin. Skin on the dorsa of the hands or distal to the ankles cannot repigment because this skin lacks sufficient numbers of hair bulbs.

The most effective method of treatment for vitiligo is photochemotherapy. It requires a motivated patient who is committed to prolonged therapy. It is intended for patients older than 10 years of age who are neither pregnant nor lactating. There must be no history of a photosensitivity disorder. If a collagen vascular disorder is suspected, an antinuclear antibody level and other evaluations should be obtained before starting photochemotherapy.

Psoralen (available as Oxsoralen-ultra or Trisoralen) is a potent photosensitizer in combination with UVA (PUVA). PUVA therapy for vitiligo takes 6 to 24 months and must be given optimally (i.e., three times a week in correct dosages). The patient must be given careful instruction in the proper use of protective glasses that block out UVA, which might damage the eyes. Physicians prescribing PUVA should have special training in the correct use of this medication.

Topical PUVA is intended for treatment of limited areas of vitiligo. Skin treated with topical psoralen is extremely sensitive to sunlight and UVA. Even inadvertent exposure of the treated skin to sunlight through car windows for a few minutes can cause painful second-degree burns. Topical psoralen should be used only by physicians thoroughly acquainted with its safe use.

Topical steroid creams like hydrocortisone 2.5 per cent or triamcinolone acetonide 0.1 per cent, applied once daily, often successfully treat vitiligo. The medication must be applied for 6 to 12 months. The patient should be observed carefully to prevent damage to the skin from the steroids. Caution must be used when applying steroids around the eyes. Patients with vitiligo probably should have a baseline eye examination that is repeated yearly if they are receiving PUVA or applying steroids near the eyes.

For patients with extensive (more than 50 per cent) vitiligo, careful consideration should be given to total depigmentation of the remaining pigmented skin. This is accomplished by application of 20 per cent monobenzyl ether of hydroquinone twice daily. The medication is applied until depigmentation is complete. This medication causes irreversible destruction of melanocytes. This procedure should be done only after the patient gives informed consent. Patients need to understand that the depigmentation is permanent and makes them ineligible for repigmentation. They will always be sensitive to sunlight. However, the cosmetic result is outstanding. This type of therapy probably should be undertaken only by physicians with appropriate training.

Postinflammatory Hypopigmentation

Many of the same inflammatory disorders or infections that cause postinflammatory hyperpigmentation can also cause hypopigmentation. The most common of these are eczema, atopic dermatitis, tinea versicolor, secondary syphilis, chickenpox, and psoriasis. Pityriasis alba is a mild form of dermatitis that is common in children. It is characterized by hypopigmented patches with fine scales. Although most commonly noted on the face, it can also affect the arms, thighs, or trunk.

Treatment

Unlike postinflammatory hyperpigmentation, most instances of postinflammatory hypopigmentation resolve slowly over time. Hydrocortisone 2.5 per cent in a cream or lotion applied twice daily may accelerate repigmentation.

Idiopathic Guttate Hypomelanosis

This common condition is characterized by hypopigmented, confetti-like macules on the extremities. These macules also can occur on the trunk and, rarely, on the face. The condition occurs in all races but is more noticeable in dark-skinned people. It must be distinguished from vitiligo. The cause of idiopathic guttate hypomelanosis is not known, although sunlight is thought to be a contributing factor. The lesion is caused by a reduction in the number of the melanocytes in the white patch. There is no satisfactory treatment for this condition.

OCCUPATIONAL DERMATITIS

method of
HAROLD PLOTNICK, M.D.
Wayne State University School of Medicine
Detroit, Michigan

Occupational dermatoses include a large assortment of cutaneous abnormalities that are primarily caused or aggravated by components in the work place. Chemical agents by far are the leading cause of occupational skin disease. These agents include an array of primary irritants, allergic sensitizers, photosensitizers, and systemic intoxicants absorbed through the skin.

Despite the introduction of many protective devices, breakthroughs in controls occur. Chemicals that are used and well harnessed in one industry can become unleashed and hazardous in another. The industries with the greatest number of work-related dermatoses are machine tool production, plastic manufacturing, rubber production, food processing, leather tanning and finishing, and metal plating and cleaning.

Most work-related skin diseases affect the exposed areas of the body. The clinical picture of an acute contact eruption is characterized by the appearance of erythema, edema, vesiculation, and weeping. This reaction is the same whether the cause is a primary irritant or an allergic sensitizer.

A primary irritant source produces a direct physical change in the skin. The allergic patient must initially undergo an incubation period to develop antibodies against the specific antigen. Once antibodies are formed, subsequent exposure to the recognized antigen will elicit an eczematous response within 24 hours in the target skin area. Unlike the primary contact dermatitis that is localized to the areas of exposure, the allergic response may appear over other areas of the body besides the locus of contact.

MANAGEMENT

The Physician's Role in Industry

The physician's role in industry is not limited to the diagnosis and treatment of work-related skin injuries, but also includes identifying the cause and recommending protective measures to prevent future recurrences. Medical treatment must be prompt and comprehensive to lessen the degree of morbidity and hasten the recovery of the skin to its preinjury state. When possible, the worker is kept on the job while receiving treatment. If this approach is impractical, the worker should be moved to another area of the work place or given time off until the skin is clear. A worker who has developed an allergic reaction to a recognized chemical may experience a recurrence of the dermatitis even on minimal re-exposure despite the employment of protective safeguards. In these selected cases, a change in job assignment is mandatory.

Patch Testing

The patch test is not a perfect bioassay but it does possess unique and valuable features since it serves as a miniature model of the disease under investigation. The patch test is recommended for suspected allergens, not for evaluating known or suspected primary irritants. The latter would only contribute to a false-positive reaction and confuse the purpose of the test.

The majority of patch testing is performed under a closed system with the exact materials to which the worker is exposed. Dry materials can be utilized as is, but liquids should be diluted with equal parts of a compatible vehicle prior to testing. This cautionary procedure is necessary to avoid a potential primary irritation that could result in a false-positive reaction.

The test materials should be covered by a nonallergenic material and fixed in place by an allergy-free adhesive-treated paper tape (3M Micropore, Scanpor) for a period of 48 hours. The patch is then removed and a 45-minute rest period is observed prior to the reading. A positive test is recognized either as erythema and edema (2+), a weak reaction; or as erythema, edema, and vesiculation (3+), a stronger allergic reaction. A negative response indicates the absence of an allergic reaction.

Hand Protection

Hands are the most common site of contact dermatitis. The use of protective gloves or a barrier cream is a necessary part of the working uniform in industries in which corrosive chemicals are encountered. These agents include low-pH acids, high-pH alkalis, chromates, coolants, cutting oils, some greases, free or uncombined monomers of epoxy and polyester systems, organic solvents, and rust preventatives.

Protection is the key to the avoidance of primary irritants and allergic-sensitizing contact dermatitis in industry. Where hand protection is a must, the choice is the right type of glove for the specific job (e.g., canvas, leather, rubber, or vinyl).

Canvas gloves are suitable for dry work. They do protect the hands from the rough edges on stock and from stains when handling various chemically coated materials. Leather gloves can be used in dry work as well, but their real advantage is in types of work in which there is a need for gripping objects, such as in the buffing and polishing industry.

Wet jobs require the use of rubber or vinyl gloves. Rubber gloves are pliable and supple and are composed of either natural latex or synthetic materials. In some industries in which contact is with organic solvents or uncured plastic monomers, rubber gloves may allow minuscule amounts of chemicals to enter. In these situations, a vinyl glove is preferred because of its alleged nonpermeable nature. The prolonged wearing of rubber or vinyl gloves prevents evaporation of sweat, and retention of sweat within the interior of the glove may cause maceration of the epidermal surface. It is advisable that vinyl gloves contain an inner fleece cotton lining to absorb the sweat. Unlined rubber gloves can be worn over absorbent, light-weight cotton gloves. Excessive sweat production within the interior of rubber gloves can sometimes leach out uncombined rubber accelerators and antioxidants that may cause allergic contact dermatitis in susceptible individuals. Workers who develop this problem should wear synthetic rubber (Neoprene) or vinyl gloves.

Protective gloves can be hazardous to workers engaged in machine tool production; the gloves may be grabbed by the machine and cause injury to the worker. In this type of industry in which manual dexterity is essential, a suitable barrier cream (Kerodex 71) can be used as a protective agent. Kerodex 71 has been used effectively in industries in which coolants and cutting oils are the primary contactants. The barrier cream must be removed every 2 hours and the hands must be washed to free any retained residue and dried. A fresh application of the barrier cream is then applied to all contact areas.

The Problem of Sweaty Hands

Hyperhidrosis (excessive sweat production) with its frequently accompanying pompholyx (dyshidrosis) may precede or become symptomatic from the prolonged use of protective rubber or vinyl gloves. A worker with an active pompholyx may develop a hand dermatitis from materials that normally do not call for gloved protection. The reason for this is that open blisters may provide an easy access for potential irritants and sensitizers to invade the skin and initiate an inflammatory response.

Workers with dyshidrosis or its aggravated form (dyshidrotic eczematous dermatitis) respond favorably to appropriate local care. This includes soaking the hands in Burow's aluminum acetate 1:30 solution (Domeboro), one tablet per quart of water, for 15 minutes twice a day. Following the soaks, a midpotency glucocorticoid cream (e.g., fluocinolone acetonide 0.025 per cent [Synalar], desonide 0.05 per cent [Tridesilon], or betamethasone valerate 0.1 per cent [Valisone]) can be helpful in clearing the dyshidrotic reaction. Workers with active pompholyx who cannot tolerate cotton-lined protective gloves or whose reaction is unresponsive to local medication must be assigned to a dry job.

Physical and Climatologic Influences in Contact Dermatitis

The intact epidermis is provided with a natural lipid-wax protective mantle that can ward off the majority of irritants encountered by the skin. When lipid solvents bathe the skin's surface, the protective layer is washed away. The unprotected keratin layer is free to lose its water content to the atmosphere, a factor that results in a dry stratum corneum and a potential opening for primary irritants to enter the skin.

Climatologic conditions that influence the water content of the skin are recognized as the dew point and humidity. During the colder months of the year, when the ambient water content is low, there is an increase in the loss of water from the skin to the atmosphere. The physical change in the skin is recognized as chapping or dehydration secondary to a low dew point and humidity.

Skin dryness resulting from the coupling of the two examples just noted can evolve into an eczematous process, a problem often seen in the machine tool industry during the cold winter months. The worker's bare hands are in and out of various lipid solvents (coolants, cutting oils, degreasing agents) many times a day. This sequence of repeated exposure to lipid solvents followed by evaporation of solvent and epidermal water loss to the low water content of the ambient work atmosphere may account for the measurable increase in symptomatic hand eczema during the colder months of the year. The same exposure and work methods usually present little problem during the other seasons of the year.

Treatment

The basic treatment for dehydration-induced eczematoid dermatitis is restoration of water to the thirsty epidermis. This phenomenon can be corrected by avoiding soaps and utilizing a water-miscible oil (Alpha-Keri) as a hand cleaner and by the after-work use of hygroscopic creams or lotions. These agents restore water to the epidermis and decrease its evaporation to the ambient water-deficient atmosphere. The following proprietary medications are suggested: a water-in-oil emollient (Eucerin), and lactic acid derivatives of azelaic acid (LactiCare Cream, Lac-Hydrin Lotion). These water-holding agents are best applied to a moist skin after work hours and at bedtime.

SUNBURN AND PHOTOSENSITIVITY

method of
VINCENT A. DELEO, M.D.
Columbia University
New York, New York

"Sunburn" is the term used to describe a normal but painful acute response to excessive solar exposure. Repeated, chronic exposure to solar radiation over several years results in changes of aging and skin cancer development. The term "photosensitivity" is usually reserved for an abnormal response to the sun's rays. These responses are the result of absorption of electromagnetic radiation in the ultraviolet (UV) spectrum by skin cells. The UV spectrum has been arbitrarily divided into the shortwave, middle range, and longwave segments, known respectively as UVC (2 to 290 nm), UVB (290 to 320 nm), and UVA (320 to 400 nm). UVC rays are totally absorbed by the ozone layer, so this radiation is not of clinical significance. UVB radiation is also referred to as "sunburn" radiation because radiation in this spectrum is most efficient at inducing inflammation in the skin. UVA radiation can also produce inflammation in normal skin, but not as effectively as UVB. UVA radiation, however, is responsible for most photosensitivity responses. This response is of growing importance because tanning salons use UVA sources, which are capable of delivering huge quantities of radiation in this range.

SUNBURN

Sunburn is a classic wounding response. The skin begins to become red and edematous 3 to 6 hours after being damaged. The reaction peaks 24 hours after exposure and may include blisters (second-degree burns). In severe cases, systemic symptoms including weakness, chills, fever, and dehydration may require hospitalization and treatment, as for thermal burns. In mild and moderate cases, the individual should be instructed to use cool compresses and take aspirin (for its anti-inflammatory effects, not just for pain relief). Topical steroid agents are also beneficial. The use of systemic steroids is controversial and not recommended.

The most important service physicians can provide their patients in relation to sun exposure is to instruct patients in prevention of sunburn and

TABLE 1. **Recommended Sunscreens for Various Skin Types**

Reaction to Sun	Example	Skin Type	Recommended Sunscreen SPF
Always burns easily, never tans	Red-haired, freckled	I	≥15
Always burns easily, tans minimally	Fair-skinned, blue-eyed	II	≥15
Burns moderately, tans gradually	Darker caucasian	III	≥15
Burns minimally, tans always	Mediterranean	IV	8–15
Burns rarely, tans profusely	Middle Eastern, Latin American, light-skinned negroid	V	8
Never burns	Dark-skinned negroid	VI	4–8

the delayed effects of sun exposure. This includes stressing that *all sun exposure is damaging* and that *there is no safe tanning.* Effective chemical sunscreens are now available to protect skin from sun damage. The effectiveness of this protection is indicated by the product's sun protective factor (SPF). This value is required labeling on all marketed sunscreen products and is determined by standardized testing procedures in human volunteers. The SPF represents the ratio of the amount of radiation necessary to produce redness in skin with the sunscreen to the amount necessary to produce redness in skin without the sunscreen. Therefore, the higher the SPF, the greater the protection. Products are also labeled to indicate the substantivity of the product on skin after immersion in water—water resistant or waterproof. Table 1 lists recommendations for sunscreen usage determined by skin type. These sunscreens prevent not only sunburn but also actinic carcinogenesis and photoaging of the skin.

Photoaging and Carcinogenesis

The chronic exposure of human skin to sunshine leads to the development of well-documented changes in the skin. UV radiation is known to be the primary carcinogen in more than 90 per cent of all *basal cell and squamous cell carcinomas.* UV radiation also appears to play a causative role in melanoma development. In addition, chronic UV radiation exposure induces most of the changes previously thought to represent *normal aging.* These changes include thickening, wrinkling, hypo- and hyperpigmentation, and the development of benign and premalignant lesions, actinic keratoses, and solar lentigos.

The dose of radiation required to induce these changes varies directly with the skin type, so that darker individuals (Skin Types III to VI) can tolerate larger doses of radiation without the ravages seen in individuals with Skin Types I and II. Proper sunscreen use and sun avoidance can prevent these changes. There is early evidence that tretinoin cream (Retin-A) 0.05 per cent applied twice daily can induce repair or reversal of some of these changes, or both. The

medication is irritating and should be started slowly (twice a week), with a gradual increase to the twice daily regimen. Patients must use sunscreens because tretinoin is photosensitizing. The agent should not be used during pregnancy.

Actinic keratoses should be treated because they represent precancerous lesions. Common methods include cryosurgery with liquid nitrogen and electrodesiccation. For extensive actinic damage with many keratoses, topical 5-fluorouracil (Efudex Cream 2 per cent) can be used. The agent is applied twice daily and produces a severe irritant reaction. The drug is discontinued when lesions become minimally eroded. The treatment requires careful monitoring by the physician and a well-informed patient who is willing to tolerate the physical and cosmetic trauma involved. Efudex also causes photosensitivity and should not be used during pregnancy.

PHOTOSENSITIVITY

A classification of common types of photosensitivity is presented in Table 2 and includes idiopathic, exogenous chemical, genetic-meta-

TABLE 2. **Classification of Photosensitivity Disorders**

Genetic and Metabolic	Degenerative and Neoplastic
Xeroderma pigmentosum	Actinic keratosis
Rothmund-Thomson syndrome	Squamous cell carcinoma
Cockayne's syndrome	Malignant melanoma
Bloom's syndrome	Basal cell epithelioma
Porphyrias	Photoaging
Albinism	
Pellagra	**Photoaggravated**
Kwashiorkor	Discoid lupus erythematosus
Hartnup's disease	Systemic lupus erythematosus
	Dermatomyositis
Idiopathic	Herpes simplex virus
Polymorphous light eruption	Darier's disease
Hydroa vacciniforme	Acne rosacea
Actinic prurigo	Atopic dermatitis
Chronic photosensitivity	Disseminated superficial actinic porokeratosis
Solar urticaria	Lichen planus actinicus
	Pemphigus foliaceus
Exogenous Chemicals	Transient acantholytic dermatosis
Photoallergic reactions	
Phototoxic reactions	

TABLE 3. Causes of Photochemical Sensitivity

Photoallergy	Phototoxicity
Topical	*Topical*
Antibacterials	Tars
Halogenated salicylani-	Therapeutics
lides	Pitch
Bithionol	Furocoumarins
Jadit	Therapeutics
Multifungin	Fragrance materials*
Fenticlor	Plant products†
Phenothiazines	Lime
Chlorpromazine	Celery
Promethazine	Parsnip
Fragrances	Fig
Musk ambrette	Dyes
6-Methylcoumarin	Eosin, methylene blue,
Sunscreens	and others
Para-aminobenzoic acid	*Systemic*
esters	Antibiotics
Benzophenones	Griseofulvin
Digalloyl trioleate	Nalidixic acid
Miscellaneous	Sulfanilamide
Stilbenes	Tetracyclines
Sandalwood	Chemotherapeutic agents
Diphenhydramine	Dacarbazine
Psoralens	5-Fluorouracil
Thiazides	Vinblastine
Sulfonylureas	Chlorpromazine
Plants of the Compositae	Amiodarone
family	Diuretics
Systemic	Furosemide
Sulfanilamide	Hydrochlorothiazide
Chlorpromazine	Hematoporphyrin
Piroxicam	Nonsteroidal anti-inflam-
	matory drugs
	Benoxaprofen‡
	Piroxicam
	Naproxen
	Psoralen
	Tolbutamide

*Berlock dermatitis.
†Phytophotodermatitis (not all-inclusive).
‡Withdrawn from the U.S. market.

bolic, and light-aggravated conditions. Metabolic abnormalities like the porphyrias are discussed elsewhere, as is the light-aggravated disease lupus erythematosus.

Exogenous chemical photosensitivity reactions can occur to chemicals taken systemically or applied topically, and the reactions can be phototoxic or photoallergic (Table 3). In all cases, however, both chemicals and light energy are necessary for induction of the response. Whereas allergic reactions are usually eczematous, toxic reactions can assume a large array of morphologic patterns including exaggerated sunburn, bullous, eczematous, papular, lichenoid, pigmented, and that seen in pseudoporphyria. Phototoxic and systemic photoallergic reactions are diagnosed by the history. Suspected contact photoallergy is confirmed by photopatch testing. Treatment consists of avoidance of the chemical and short-term avoidance of light exposure until the drug has completely cleared the body. Treatment with topical steroids is usually sufficient once the chemical is avoided.

By far the most common type of photosensitivity seen in the United States is the idiopathic condition *polymorphous light eruption*. It is estimated to affect about 15 per cent of the population at some point during their lives. It occurs predominantly in young adults (in females more than males). After intense exposure (usually on vacation), the individual develops an itchy rash on scattered areas of sun-exposed skin, but not usually on all exposed areas. The eruption is either of a small papular or papulovesicular type or a large papular or plaque type and persists for days. It is important to rule out lupus erythematosus in these patients by skin biopsy for histology and direct immunofluorescence and serologic tests (antinuclear antibody and anti-Ro, anti-La antibodies). Photochemical reactions must be ruled out by the history, photopatch testing, or both. Therapy includes sunscreens and sun avoidance for mild cases. More severe cases have been treated with beta-carotene (Solatene), 180 mg per day, or psoralen photochemotherapy.

Solar urticaria is a rare but debilitating photosensitivity. Patients are usually young individuals who describe the development of hives on all (or most) areas of skin exposed to sunshine. The reaction appears with minimal exposure, may occur to narrow- or broad-spectrum UV radiation, and disappears within 24 hours. Patients who are sensitive to radiation in the UVA range react to light filtered through window glass, as in a car. The diagnosis is confirmed by phototesting, and treatment with antihistamines, especially terfenadine (Seldane), 60 mg two or three times a day, is usually sufficient to allow a normal lifestyle. Large exposures (sun tanning) must still be avoided.

The Nervous System

BRAIN ABSCESS

method of
SYDNEY M. FINEGOLD, M.D.
VA Wadsworth Medical Center
University of California School of Medicine
Los Angeles, California

Brain abscess begins as a cerebritis, then becomes an abscess, and ultimately becomes encapsulated. The first two stages may often be managed medically.

ETIOLOGY

The etiologic agents of intracranial suppuration vary primarily with the site and kind of antecedent infection and also with predisposing host factors. The common isolates are anaerobic bacteria (including anaerobic cocci, *Bacteroides, Porphyromonas, Fusobacterium, Actinomyces,* and, less often, *Clostridium*) and aerobic or microaerophilic gram-positive cocci (*Staphylococcus aureus, Streptococcus pneumoniae, Streptococcus pyogenes,* and viridans group streptococci such as *S. anginosus*). Fastidious bacteria such as *Haemophilus (Actinobacillus) actinomycetemcomitans* and *Haemophilus aphrophilus* may also be found. Although certain organisms such as *S. aureus* are usually found in pure culture, polymicrobial infections are common when other pathogens, such as the anaerobes or Enterobacteriaceae, are involved.

Brain abscesses that arise as a direct extension of infection from the middle ear, mastoids, sinuses, or oropharynx frequently yield anaerobes and microaerophilic streptococci, although other aerobes, such as·*S. aureus, Haemophilus influenzae,* and Enterobacteriaceae (e.g., *Proteus*), may be encountered. In the compromised host, however, unusual pathogens must be considered. For example, in rhinocerebral zygomycosis, direct extension of fungal infection of the nasopharynx may lead to intracranial abscess. In patients with acquired immunodeficiency syndrome, *Toxoplasma gondii* must be considered the most likely cause of focal central nervous system infection.

Brain abscesses after hematogenous spread from a preceding lung abscess or other pleuropulmonary infection are commonly caused by anaerobic pathogens and various streptococci. *Nocardia, Aspergillus,* and the zygomycetes may also be found in this setting, especially in the compromised host.

S. aureus may cause brain abscess in association with endocarditis and is the most likely pathogen in brain abscess that follows accidental or surgical trauma to the head. Gram-negative rods are also found in this setting. In patients with congenital heart disease, brain abscesses are most often caused by aerobic or microaerophilic streptococci and anaerobic cocci, less often by *Haemophilus*. Additional, uncommon causes of brain abscess include various Enterobacteriaceae such as *Klebsiella* and *Enterobacter,* which may originate from primary genitourinary or intra-abdominal infections; *Neisseria meningitidis* and *Listeria monocytogenes,* which are usually associated with meningitis; *Mycobacterium* and protozoa, including *Entamoeba histolytica.*

TREATMENT

Medical Therapy

In the stage of acute suppurative encephalitis or cerebritis before the formation of an encapsulated abscess, prolonged high-dose antimicrobial therapy may be curative without surgical intervention. When the etiology is known because of a positive culture from a primary source, therapy can be directed specifically. In the case of positive blood cultures, however, it should be remembered that not all organisms in the brain abscess may appear in the blood culture. Given the diversity of organisms that may cause brain abscess, particularly in immunocompromised subjects, surgery (burr hole with aspiration) is desirable to make a specific bacteriologic diagnosis. It is important that a good anaerobic transport setup be used in sending the specimen to the laboratory. In certain patients with fully formed abscesses, especially those for whom the risk of surgery is prohibitive, treatment with antimicrobial therapy alone may be attempted. Close observation of such patients is obligatory, using serial imaging procedures with monitoring for signs of a decreasing level of consciousness and developing focal neurologic deficits.

Table 1 lists the antimicrobial agents useful in the management of brain abscess, their spectrum of activity, and information concerning dosage and administration. In most situations when the etiology is not known, metronidazole plus penicillin G represents the initial treatment of choice.

Anticoagulation is contraindicated in the presence of brain abscess because of the danger of intracranial hemorrhage. Measures to decrease

TABLE 1. **Antimicrobial Agents Useful in the Treatment of Brain Abscess**

Drug	Susceptible Organisms	Dosage
Penicillin G	Streptococci, many anaerobes	200,000–300,000 U/kg/day (given IV every 2–4 hr)
Metronidazole (Flagyl)	Anaerobes except *Actinomyces* and other gram-positive non-sporing rods	30 mg/kg/day (given IV every 6 hr)*
Chloramphenicol (Chloromycetin)	Gram-negative bacilli, anaerobes	50–60 mg/kg/day initially, then 30 mg/kg/day (given IV every 6 hr)
Nafcillin (Nafcil, Unipen)	*S. aureus*	100–200 mg/kg/day (given IV every 4 hr)
Trimethoprim-sulfamethoxazole (Bactrim, Septra)	*Nocardia,* gram-negative bacilli, methicillin-resistant *S. aureus*	20 mg/kg/day trimethoprim plus 100 mg/kg/day sulfamethoxazole (given IV or PO every 6 hr)
Cefotaxime (Claforan)†	Gram-negative bacilli	120–175 mg/kg/day (given IV every 4–6 hr)
Vancomycin (Vancocin)	Methicillin-resistant *S. aureus,* streptococci	30 mg/kg/day (given IV every 6 or every 12 hr)
Rifampin (Rimactane) (use only in combination)	*S. aureus,* anaerobes	15 mg/kg/day (given PO every 12 hr)
Amphotericin B (Fungizone)	Fungi	1-mg test dose IV; then gradually build up to 0.5 mg/kg/day by the fifth day

*Usual loading dose is 15 mg/kg followed by 7.5 mg/kg every 6 hr; dosage should be reduced if there is severe liver disease.
†Other agents such as ceftazidime and piperacillin may be used for gram-negative bacillary infection.

intracranial pressure may be necessary. Anticonvulsants such as phenytoin (Dilantin), 100 mg intravenously or orally every 8 hours, or phenobarbital, 30 to 60 mg intravenously every 6 to 8 hours, should be used. Blood levels of anticonvulsants should be monitored. Anticonvulsants should be continued until the abscess has definitely resolved. At that point, they may be stopped if the patient has been free of seizures.

Surgical Therapy

Operation is mandatory when neurologic deficits are severe or progressive, particularly when signs of brain stem compression (herniation) are present. The situation is especially urgent when the abscess is in the posterior fossa. Abscess drainage is by far the most rapid and effective method of reduction of intracranial pressure in the setting of a severe deficit.

When the abscess abuts the ventricular wall, rupture of the abscess into the ventricle is a threat. Drainage is indicated to prevent this possibility, which would lead to disseminated meningeal infection. Operation is also indicated when serial computed tomography (CT) scans or magnetic resonance imaging (MRI) shows progression of an abscess during antibiotic treatment.

Corticosteroids are useful for reduction of edema caused by the operative procedure. Dexamethasone (Decadron), 10 mg intravenously, then 4 mg every 4 to 6 hours, is given. Immunosuppressive effects are minor and temporary with short-term use. Steroids may be tapered rapidly as the patient's neurologic condition improves. They will not usually be required for more than a week after drainage.

Most abscesses can be drained via a needle through a burr hole under local anesthesia. Needle drainage may be repeated as necessary. When the abscess is located in a deep or neurologically sensitive site, CT-guided stereotactic equipment may be used to perform drainage.

If the abscess is large or multiloculated, craniotomy with abscess drainage under direct vision may be needed. A drainage catheter may be left in the cavity and hooked up to a closed-suction system. Significant drainage does not usually continue beyond 48 hours, and the catheter may then be removed.

Craniotomies should be performed, if possible, through an osteoplastic (vascularized) bone flap to minimize the risk of osteomyelitis. Excision of an abscess or of a postabscess scar occasionally may benefit the patient who has seizures that have resisted ordinary treatment.

Antibiotics should be continued for at least 6 to 8 weeks after drainage. CT scans or MRI must be performed to confirm that progressive resolution of the abscess is taking place. Antibiotics may be discontinued even though there is a small residual nonenhancing abnormality on the enhanced CT scan or MRI. Such an abnormality should be re-examined by CT or MRI, about a month after the antibiotics are stopped, to rule out re-emergence of the abscess.

ALZHEIMER'S DISEASE
method of
J. THOMAS HUTTON, M.D., PH.D.
Texas Tech Health Sciences Center
and the Lubbock VA Outpatient Clinic
Lubbock, Texas

Therapy for Alzheimer's disease is limited because its causes and pathophysiology remain unclear. Symptomatic treatment and supportive care benefit selective aspects of Alzheimer's disease and reduce the family's great burden.

Alzheimer's disease accounts for 50 to 60 per cent of patients with dementia. Another 10 to 20 per cent have underlying causative or complicating medical disorders for which effective treatment exists. Most of these disorders result from hepatic, renal, or endocrine abnormalities, hypoxia, toxic states, infectious diseases, hydrocephalus, depression, or space-occupying lesions. Among the remaining 30 per cent, diagnosis, prognosis, and supportive care can assist patients with disorders such as multi-infarct dementia, Creutzfeldt-Jakob disease, and Pick's disease. Making a correct diagnosis provides the best opportunity for specific and effective therapeutic intervention.

Initial evaluation for dementia should include a careful history, general physical examination, and neurologic examination. Basic diagnostic tests uncover most of the readily reversible disorders. Although modifications should be made according to individual circumstances, a reasonable initial screen includes a complete blood count, electrolyte levels, metabolic panel, thyroid function, vitamin B_{12} level, serum folate level, serologic tests for syphilis and, if appropriate, for acquired immunodeficiency syndrome, urinalysis, electrocardiogram, and chest x-ray film. In certain instances, other tests may prove to be useful. The principal purpose of brain imaging is to identify space-occupying lesions and evidence of strokes. One should not overinterpret cerebral atrophy in patients beyond the age of 65 years as disease. The magnetic resonance imaging scan may demonstrate periventricular changes and unidentified bright objects that may be misidentified as lacunar strokes. The significance of these magnetic resonance imaging findings remains controversial. Electroencephalography, lumbar puncture, carotid and vertebral ultrasound scans, and cisternography are not routinely needed and are best used after neurologic consultation. Psychiatric consultation may be helpful in differentiating depression as a cause or a complicating factor. Neuropsychologic studies may identify depression, establish a baseline, and assess impairment resulting from focal brain disorders.

Before discussing the treatment of various aspects of Alzheimer's disease, the following overarching clinical concepts should be considered:

1. The physician's major impact may result from periodic follow-up of the patient and family to assist with problem-solving and decision-making and to be available when the inevitable crises occur.

2. Sudden worsening almost always results from superimposed metabolic, infectious, toxic, depressive, or cerebrovascular insults. Acute changes should be viewed as potentially reversible and warrant medical evaluation.

3. Support for the family caregiver is as important as treatment of the patient.

4. Dosages of medications for elderly, demented persons often need to be reduced by one-half compared with those for younger persons.

5. Tranquilizing medications should not become substitutes for caregivers trained in basic behavioral management and communication skills.

THERAPY FOR ASSOCIATED ASPECTS OF ALZHEIMER'S DISEASE

Cognitive and Memory Impairment

At present, no medications exist that reliably improve cognitive and memory impairment. The most widely used and tested agent is a combination of ergoloid mesylates (Hydergine). Although this agent is not clinically impressive, many research studies suggest that it benefits some symptoms of dementia. A realistic issue is whether this combination favorably alters the rate of behavioral decline, a question now being addressed through research. Also, an evaluation is being conducted to determine whether doses of up to 9 mg per day are more useful than the currently recommended 1 mg three times a day. This agent is classified as a metabolic enhancer, but its effect may derive from its reduction of concomitant depression. Papaverine (Pavabid) and cyclandelate (Cyclospasmol) are vasodilators. Their therapeutic rationale was compromised when senile dementia was shown to be associated with primary neuronal changes rather than increased cerebral arteriosclerosis.

The brain acetylcholine level is reduced with Alzheimer's disease. Therapeutic strategies consist of precursor loading with lecithin or choline, or of preventing the rapid lowering of the acetylcholine level by centrally acting anticholinesterase agents. Results of lecithin and choline clinical studies were disappointing. Centrally acting anticholinesterase agents such as tetrahydroaminoacridine (THA) and physostigmine are being tested, often in combination with precursor loading. An enthusiastic report on THA prompted a multicenter, large-scale clinical study. Hepatotoxicity required lowering of the THA dose. Results of this study should soon be available.

Aggressive Outbursts, Delusions, and Hallucinations

Aggressive outbursts may reflect misperceived threats and mounting frustration. Such reactions can often be avoided if the family maintains flexibility in scheduling care for the patient and does not signal impatience or anger. At times, emotional outbursts cannot be related to external causes, and patients require tranquilization for safety reasons. Patients with delusions and visual hallucinations respond well to tranquilizers. Thioridazine (Mellaril), haloperidol (Haldol), chlorpromazine (Thorazine), and thiothixene (Navane) should be tried on an as needed basis rather than on a fixed dosage schedule. Thioridazine has the least severe extrapyramidal side effects, minimizing bradykinesia, muscular rigidity, and falls.

TABLE 1. **Functional Rating Scale for Symptoms of Dementia**

Instructions:

1. The scale must be administered to the most knowledgeable informant available. This usually is a spouse or close relative.
2. The scale should be read to the informant one category at a time. The informant is presented the description for behavior in each category. The informant is read each of the responses, beginning with zero response. All responses should be read before the informant endorses the highest number response that best describes the behavior of the patient.
3. Responses obtained for each category are summed to give an overall score.

Circle the highest number in each category that best describes behavior during the last 3 months.

Eating:
   0 Eats neatly, using appropriate utensils
   1 Eats messily, has some difficulty with utensils
   2 Able to eat solid foods (e.g., fruits, crackers, cookies) with hands only
   3 Has to be fed

Dressing:
   0 Able to dress appropriately without help
   1 Able to dress self with occasional mismatched socks, disarranged buttons or laces
   2 Dresses out of sequence, forgets items, or wears sleeping garments with street clothes—needs supervision
   3 Unable to dress alone, appears undressed in inappropriate situations

Continence:
   0 Complete sphincter control
   1 Occasional bed-wetting
   2 Frequent bed-wetting or daytime urinary incontinence
   3 Incontinent of both bladder and bowel

Verbal Communication:
   0 Speaks normally
   1 Minor difficulties with speech or word-finding difficulties
   2 Able to carry out only simple, uncomplicated conversations
   3 Unable to speak coherently

Memory for Names:
   0 Usually remembers names of meaningful acquaintances
   1 Cannot recall names of acquaintances or distant relatives
   2 Cannot recall names of close friends or relatives
   3 Cannot recall name of spouse or other living partner

Memory for Events:
   0 Cannot recall details and sequences of recent experiences
   1 Cannot recall details or sequences of recent events
   2 Cannot recall entire events (e.g., recent outings, visits of relatives or friends) without prompting
   3 Cannot recall entire events even with prompting

Mental Alertness:
   0 Usually alert, attentive to environment
   1 Easily distractible, mind wanders
   2 Frequently asks the same questions over and over
   3 Cannot maintain attention while watching television

Global Confusion:
   0 Appropriately responsive to environment
   1 Nocturnal confusion or confusion upon awakening
   2 Periodic confusion during daytime
   3 Nearly always quite confused

Spatial Confusion:
   0 Oriented, able to find his/her bearings
   1 Spatial confusion when driving or riding in local community
   2 Gets lost when walking in neighborhood
   3 Gets lost in own home or in hospital ward

Facial Recognition:
   0 Can recognize faces of recent acquaintances
   1 Cannot recognize faces of recent acquaintances
   2 Cannot recognize faces of relatives or close friends
   3 Cannot recognize spouse or constant living companion

Hygiene and Grooming:
   0 Generally neat and clean
   1 Ignores grooming (e.g., does not brush teeth and hair, shave)
   2 Does not bathe regularly
   3 Has to be bathed and groomed

Emotionality:
   0 Unchanged from normal
   1 Mild change in emotional responsiveness—slightly more irritable or more passive, diminished sense of humor, mild depression
   2 Moderate change in emotional responsiveness—growing apathy, increased rigidity, despondent, angry outbursts, cries easily
   3 Impaired emotional control—unstable, rapid cycling or laughing in inappropriate situations, violent outbursts

Social Responsiveness:
   0 Unchanged
   1 Tendency to dwell in the past, lack of proper association for present situation
   2 Lack of regard for feelings of others, quarrelsome, irritable
   3 Inappropriate sexual acting out or antisocial behavior

Sleep Patterns:
   0 Unchanged from previous, "normal"
   1 Sleeps, noticeably more or less than normal
   2 Restless, nightmares, disturbed sleep, increased wakefulness
   3 Up wandering for all or most of the night, inability to sleep

If anxiety is prominent, a benzodiazepine agent may help.

Depression

Depression occurs in about one-third of Alzheimer's patients, usually in the early stages of the disease. Also, pseudodementia caused by depression can mimic Alzheimer's disease. The tricyclic antidepressants may reduce depression and whatever portion of the cognitive decline that results from the depression. Doxepin (Sinequan), nortriptyline (Pamelor), and amitriptyline (Elavil, Endep) are used in doses of 25 to 100 mg per day; if given at bedtime, they may obviate the need for a hypnotic.

Sleeplessness

Sleep is often fragmented, with frequent nocturnal arousals and reduced rapid eye movement sleep. Patients tend to awaken and wander and disrupt the sleep of the caregiver. Sleep maintenance for the patient is usually a larger problem than sleep induction. Temazepam (Restoril) has a half-life of 10 hours (clinical effect of about 6 hours), with little or no residual medication effects the next day. Triazolam (Halcion), with a half-life of 2 hours, does little for sleep maintenance. Levels of longer-acting flurazepam (Dalmane) may build up with regular usage and cause unacceptable daytime sedation. Chloral hydrate, with a half-life of 8 hours, continues to be a good hypnotic agent in doses ranging from 250 to 500 mg.

Physician as Advisor

The physician often must advise the family on practical management hints. Table 1 is a functional rating scale for symptoms of dementia that quickly identifies major problem areas and can be administered by a nurse at each appointment. The sum of the scores from the forced-choice format is graphed on a time scale. Scores above 30 predict imminent nursing home placement. Items with strong individual predictive value include "unable to speak coherently," "has to be bathed and groomed," and "incontinent of both bowel and bladder." The decision to institutionalize is a family one, but the doctor may mitigate the inevitable family guilt by providing assurance that the burden is equal to or greater than that of other affected families who have been forced to seek placement.

Families should speak to the demented family member in short, unambiguous sentences. The Alzheimer patient understands nonverbal gestures, touching, and affect long after complicated sentences become incomprehensible. Assistance with bathing and grooming may be needed; in-home and institutional respite care extend the duration of family caregiving. If urinary tract infections and other medical disorders are excluded as a cause of urinary incontinence, practical assistance is derived from establishing regular opportunities for elimination and, if necessary, using adult diapers. Indwelling catheters are to be avoided, and external catheters are generally poorly tolerated. A home assessment may discover sources of potential danger or unnecessary environmental confusion. Television, radios, and mirrors are frequent sources of anxiety because of faulty perception. Shadows are incorrectly identified as holes, flowered wallpaper as flowers in need of picking, pebbled linoleum as in need of being picked up. Alzheimer patients functionally have a limited gaze to the central field, making low-lying tables, chairs, and throw rugs dangerous and placing high objects out of view. Interior key locks or locks involving several steps befuddle the patient and usually prevent escapes. A tailored exercise program for the patient and the caregiver fosters general health, reduces anxiety and depression, and promotes sleep.

The physician is often the source of helpful referrals. Assistance may be derived from visiting nurses; counselors; social workers; physical, occupational, and speech therapists; lawyers; support groups and chapters of the Alzheimer Association; area agencies on aging; and Alzheimer's special care units and day programs. Practical information on caring for the Alzheimer's patient is now available in books, videos, and pamphlets; their use should be encouraged.

INTRACEREBRAL HEMORRHAGE

method of
ANGELA M. O'NEAL, M.D., and
CARLOS S. KASE, M.D.
Boston University School of Medicine
Boston, Massachusetts

Intracerebral hemorrhage (ICH) results from arterial bleeding directly into the brain parenchyma. These hemorrhages account for only 10 per cent of stroke subtypes, but they contribute substantially to stroke mortality; their 30-day mortality rate is about 30 per cent.

PATHOPHYSIOLOGY

The location of ICH favors the deep portions of the cerebral hemispheres, especially the basal ganglia and thalamus, followed in frequency by the subcortical white matter. Infratentorially, the pons and the cerebellum are most commonly affected. These areas are supplied by small, perforating arteries 50 to 200 micrometers in size, including the lenticulostriate branches of the middle cerebral artery, the thalamoperforant branches of the posterior cerebral artery, and the paramedian basilar perforators. The rupture of these arteries results in the predominantly deep hemispheric and brain stem locations of ICH.

A strong association of systemic hypertension with ICH has long been recognized. Efforts to elucidate the vascular pathology underlying this disorder have been made since the beginning of this century. Charcot and Bouchard described the association of ICH with "miliary aneurysms" or pseudoaneurysms of the deep, penetrating arteries. It was believed that hypertension led to "weakening" of the vessel wall at sites of microaneurysm formation, ultimately resulting in rupture and hemorrhage. C.M. Fisher pointed out the common sites of predilection for lacunar infarction and ICH, and showed that the underlying pathologic substrate for both entities corresponded to "lipohyalinosis." This process represents the deposition of a hyaline, eosinophilic material in the media of small, perforating arteries as the result of long-standing hypertension. This can cause either occlusion of the vessel, leading to a lacunar infarct, or vessel rupture, causing ICH.

ICH is usually a monophasic event. The period of active bleeding is generally thought to be less than 1 hour. The clinical deterioration that at times occurs over the course of several hours is generally the result of cerebral edema rather than continuing bleeding, but there are occasional exceptions to this rule, that is, instances in which slow progression of the neurologic deficits and deterioration in the level of consciousness can be correlated with computed tomography (CT) documentation of hematoma enlargement. Hypertensive ICH is usually a nonrecurrent event, unlike other causes of ICH, in which repeated episodes of bleeding are characteristic (see later).

CLINICAL SYNDROMES

Putaminal hemorrhage accounts for the majority (35 to 50 per cent) of ICHs. The clinical syndrome is quite variable, reflecting both the different patterns of extension of the hemorrhages and their variability in size. Classically, patients with a massive putaminal hemorrhage present with sudden onset of hemiparesis, hemisensory loss, a field cut, and disturbance in the level of consciousness. On examination, patients have a contralateral hemiparesis combined with a sensory deficit, a gaze palsy of the supranuclear type (with conjugate ocular deviation at rest toward the affected hemisphere), and a homonymous hemianopsia. In addition, aphasia may be present in patients with dominant hemisphere hemorrhages, whereas elements of hemineglect are present in nondominant hemisphere hemorrhage patients. The language disturbances are best categorized as either global aphasia or fluent paraphasic speech with relatively preserved repetition. Patients commonly follow an initial progressive, deteriorating course in both focal deficits and level of consciousness. Headache and vomiting frequently occur at onset but are not reliable in distinguishing putaminal hemorrhage from other sites or causes of ICH. Signs of a relatively good clinical outcome include alert mental status, full visual fields, full extraocular movements, and only partial motor deficit at the onset of ICH. In contrast, massive hemorrhages with progression to coma have mortality rates in the 65 to 75 per cent range.

Caudate hemorrhage represents only about 5 to 7 per cent of ICHs. The caudate nucleus is supplied by the same group of perforating arteries as the putamen, and the more frequent involvement of the putamen possibly reflects a more severe involvement of distal middle cerebral artery perforators by lipohyalinosis.

Symptoms of primary caudate hemorrhage are similar to those of subarachnoid hemorrhage and reflect the ventricular proximity of the caudate nucleus, leading to early ventricular extension of the hemorrhage. Patients generally present with headache and vomiting, followed by loss of consciousness. On examination they usually have a stiff neck and an acute confusional state. In a series of 12 patients with caudate hemorrhage, the following characteristics were found: the onset was acute, with maximal deficits present within minutes; headache occurred in 11 of the 12 patients before loss of consciousness; disturbances in level of alertness (ranging from drowsiness to coma) were usually transient and resolved within 48 to 72 hours; confusional states were present in three-fourths of the patients. Language disturbances or nondominant behavioral syndromes are an infrequent finding in caudate hemorrhage.

Because of the location of the hemorrhage, ventricular extension, frequently associated with acute hydrocephalus, is a common feature in this condition. A CT scan can generally distinguish caudate hemorrhage from subarachnoid hemorrhage and ruptured anterior communicating artery aneurysm because the last commonly bleeds into either the basal frontal lobes or the interhemispheric fissure, whereas primary caudate hemorrhage does not extend so far inferiorly.

In general, caudate hemorrhage has a more benign outcome than other types of ICH. This may reflect its rapid decompression into the ventricular system or the smaller amount of blood collected in the substance of the brain.

Thalamic hemorrhage accounts for 10 to 15 per cent of ICHs. Characteristically, these patients develop the abrupt onset of a dense contralateral hemiparesis associated with a severe hemisensory loss. The motor deficit usually involves the face, arm, and leg to a comparable degree. The sensory syndrome includes a dense loss of all sensory modalities over the contralateral half of the body. However, these findings do not reliably distinguish thalamic from putaminal hemorrhage because the combined sensory-motor deficits are a feature of both.

The most distinctive features of thalamic hemorrhage are the associated oculomotor abnormalities. These include vertical gaze palsy, loss of convergence, and miotic, unreactive pupils (Parinaud's syndrome). Other ocular abnormalities may be present, including skew deviation, down-gaze palsy, nystagmus retractorius, and Horner's syndrome. Aphasic or neglect syndromes may be present, depending on the side of the hemorrhage, but are not usually prominent.

Thalamic hemorrhages frequently show ventricular extension because of the proximity of the thalamus to the third ventricle. This is associated with a significant (25 per cent) incidence of hydrocephalus. The prognosis of thalamic hemorrhage relates to the level of consciousness on admission, the presence of hydrocephalus, and the size of the hemorrhage. Hemorrhages with a diameter of 4 cm or more are generally fatal, but some patients with larger hemorrhages survive. Occasionally, emergency ventriculostomy in the presence of acute hydrocephalus is associated with dramatic improvement in the patient's condition.

Subcortical white matter or *lobar hemorrhages* make up 30 per cent of ICHs. They tend to cause bleeding, which dissects along the white matter tracts parallel to the cortical surface, leading to the so-called slit hemorrhages. The mortality from these hemorrhages (11 to 32 per cent) is substantially lower than that from hemorrhages at other sites. Lobar hemorrhages tend to predominate in the posterior aspects of the hemispheres (occipital and parietal areas), and their peripheral location explains the majority of the presenting features and their differences from deep ganglionic ICHs. These patients usually complain of headache and vomiting, are less often comatose, have milder degrees of hemiparesis, and frequently have visual field defects. Seizures at onset are more common than in other forms of ICH.

Hypertension still accounts for the majority of cases, but nonhypertensive causes of ICH are more common than in the deep locations. More than 50 per cent of lobar hemorrhages are caused by cerebral aneurysms, arteriovenous malformations, or primary or metastatic brain tumors. Warfarin sodium (Coumadin) anticoagulation, other bleeding diatheses, and amyloid angiopathy are responsible for the remainder.

Cerebellar hemorrhage accounts for 5 to 17 per cent of ICHs. Hypertension is the most frequent causative factor, being present in approximately 60 per cent of patients. Cerebellar hemorrhages usually occur deep in the hemisphere, in the area of the dentate nucleus. The cardinal symptoms include acute onset of dizziness, headache, nausea, vomiting, and inability to walk. On examination, the findings of ataxia, appendicular or axial, ipsilateral horizontal gaze palsy, and ipsilateral peripheral facial weakness are a useful diagnostic triad in cerebellar hemorrhage. The finding of hemiplegia is exceedingly rare, to the point of virtually ruling out the diagnosis of hemorrhage in this location. Other less common or specific signs include a decrease in the level of alertness, pinpoint reactive pupils, dysarthria, and head tilt. The constellation of physical findings in cerebellar hemorrhage represents a combination of unilateral cerebellar deficits and those resulting from compression of the tegmentum of the pons ipsilaterally.

The need to make an early diagnosis is critical because these patients may quickly deteriorate into coma from brain stem compression. Surgical evacuation of the clot can be lifesaving.

Pontine hemorrhages comprise 5 to 15 per cent of all ICHs. Almost all of these hemorrhages are secondary to hypertension. Hemorrhage occurs from rupture of midpontine perforating arteries off the basilar trunk.

Patients can present with a variety of symptoms. Classically, patients are comatose, with a flaccid quadriparesis or decerebrate posturing, and pinpoint but reactive pupils. Hyperthermia and abnormal respiratory patterns complete the picture. Hemorrhages that are less massive and primarily lateral tegmental may produce a number of eye movement abnormalities, including paresis of horizontal gaze and the "one-and-a-half" syndrome, internuclear ophthalmoplegia, ocular bobbing, sixth nerve palsy, and skew deviation. The incidence of seizures is markedly lower than in supratentorial hemorrhages. The vital prognosis is poor, as there is no effective medical or surgical treatment.

NONHYPERTENSIVE MECHANISMS OF INTRACEREBRAL HEMORRHAGE

Although hypertension is the etiologic factor in the majority of ICHs, some 20 to 30 per cent result from other causes. These should be considered in patients whose hemorrhage is atypical because of lack of a history of hypertension, recurrent episodes of bleeding, young age of the patients, or unusual locations of the hemorrhage. *Vascular malformations* probably account for 4 to 8 per cent of ICHs. The most frequent malformation responsible for hemorrhage is arteriovenous or venous angioma. These malformations are more often located superficially in the cerebral hemispheres. Malformations most often present with rupture in the young adult, and the clinical syndrome depends on the location of the hemorrhage. The diagnosis is usually made by arteriography. However, a contrast CT scan may demonstrate the abnormal serpiginous vascular channels. Currently, magnetic resonance imaging offers another possible method for noninvasive diagnosis of small arteriovenous malformations, as T_2-weighted images of the malformation can be visualized as a high signal containing multiple flow voids.

Hemorrhage may occur into a *brain tumor*. This a rare event, occurring in only 1 per cent of all brain tumors. Malignant tumors, either primary or metastatic, are more commonly associated with ICH. This probably relates to their tendency to undergo central necrosis, to have a rich blood supply, and occasionally, as in choriocarcinoma, to invade blood vessels directly. The tumors most frequently associated with hemorrhage include glioblastoma multiforme and metastases from bronchogenic carcinoma, melanoma, renal cell carcinoma, and choriocarcinoma. A number of clinical features typify these hemorrhages: patients may have chronic headache or focal neurologic deficits preceding the hemorrhage; the finding of papilledema on initial funduscopic examination may indicate a mass lesion with increased intracranial pressure preceding the ICH; a CT scan may show multiple areas of hemorrhage; and the hemorrhage may affect areas atypical for hypertensive hemorrhages, such as the corpus callosum or the medial frontal lobe area.

Amyloid angiopathy is a significant contributor to ICH in the elderly. This angiopathy is caused by deposits of amyloid in the media and adventitia of small and medium-sized arteries located primarily in the superficial cortical layers and the subarachnoid space. Cerebral amyloid angiopathy is not associated with systemic amyloidosis. The condition is usually sporadic, with a striking increase with age; its frequency at autopsy is 8 per cent for individuals in their seventies and rises to 60 per cent for patients over the age of 90. A familial autosomal dominant form of the disorder has been identified in certain families from Iceland and the Netherlands. The sporadic form has a striking association with the changes of Alzheimer's disease on histopathologic studies. Clinical dementia is present in approximately 30 per cent of the cases. These hemorrhages usually occur in a lobar location, with a predilection for the posterior aspects of the hemispheres. Because of the superficial location of the intraparenchymal hemorrhages, a subdural or subarachnoid extension may also be present. In addition, these hemorrhages have a remarkable tendency to recur. The diagnosis is established by cerebral biopsy, which shows cortical and leptomeningeal arteries with deposits of Congo red–positive amyloid in the media and adventitia, deposits that are birefringent under polarized light.

Anticoagulant-related ICH is another important cause of nonhypertensive hemorrhage. ICH represents approximately 1.5 per cent of the bleeding complications of anticoagulant use. There is an increase in this complication of anticoagulant treatment in patients over the age of 65 years. Clinically, these patients have a relatively slow course at onset in comparison to those with hypertensive ICH, reflecting a bleeding process that evolves over longer periods. The patients most at risk for this complication are those whose prothrombin time is excessively prolonged, greater than the usual therapeutic range of one and one-half to two times control values. The mortality rate of these anticoagulant-related ICHs is high, on the order of 65 per cent.

ICH can occur after the use of *amphetamines and related sympathomimetic drugs,* such as cocaine, ephedrine, pseudoephedrine, and phenylpropanolamine. Hemorrhage usually occurs in chronic users, but it may happen after the first use of amphetamines and over-the-counter decongestants such as ephedrine or phenylpropanolamine. Transient hypertension has been documented after the use of these drugs. On arteriography, some patients have a beading pattern resulting from alternating constriction and dilatation of intracranial arteries. It is possible that the combination of this direct vascular effect and the hypertension resulting from the sympathomimetic action of the drug is the cause of bleeding in these patients.

TREATMENT

Medical treatment of ICH is aimed at preservation of neurologic function and prevention of further deterioration secondary to elevated intracranial pressure. The history and physical examination should be promptly followed by a noncontrast CT scan of the head to make a rapid anatomic diagnosis, including the presence of a mass effect, hydrocephalus, or signs of herniation. A lumbar puncture is probably no longer necessary in the work-up of ICH and is contraindicated in the presence of a mass effect. Angiography should be restricted to the diagnosis of atypical cases of ICH. This can help to decide whether arteritis, arteriovenous malformation, or tumor is the underlying pathology. Laboratory studies should always include a platelet count and coagulation parameters.

Patients with ICH should be managed in an intensive care setting. The head should be elevated 30 degrees to decrease intracranial pressure by facilitating venous drainage. Careful attention to pulmonary toilet can avoid the common complications of atelectasis and pneumonia. Passive range-of-motion exercises and elastic stockings should be used to decrease the risk of venous thrombosis. Once the patient has stabilized, oral or nasogastric feedings can be instituted. Physical therapy can be initiated in alert patients after approximately 1 week. Issues of tracheostomy and gastrostomy must be addressed in persistently comatose patients.

Patients who present in coma require intubation and hyperventilation to maintain a PCO_2 in the range of 25 to 30 mmHg. After placement of Foley's catheter, mannitol is given intravenously in a dose of 0.5 to 1 gram per kg over 20 minutes, is continued every 6 hours for the first 24 hours, and then is gradually tapered. Furosemide (Lasix) and other diuretics can be used initially in conjunction with mannitol to achieve a rapid hyperosmolar state. Serum osmolality should be maintained in the range of 300 to 310 mOsm. Serum and urine electrolyte levels must be closely followed to monitor hyperosmolar therapy, as well as to check for the potential development of the syndrome of inappropriate antidiuretic hormone secretion. All patients should have an intravenous catheter placed. Isotonic saline solutions should be infused slowly. Hypotonic solutions such as 5 per cent glucose should be avoided because of the possibility of increasing edema surrounding the ICH. Intravenous fluids should be maintained for the first several days to ensure adequate urine output.

The routine use of steroids in ICH has not been shown to be beneficial. In fact, patients treated with steroids have fared worse than untreated control subjects because of an increased rate of complications, including infections and decompensation of diabetes. This emphasizes the fact that the increase in intracranial pressure from ICH results primarily from the mass of the hemorrhage itself rather than from the surrounding edema.

Patients with ICH caused by abnormal clotting factors should receive fresh-frozen plasma. Those with liver disease or those who have received warfarin should also be given vitamin K_1 (phytonadione), 10 mg subcutaneously. Intravenous vitamin K should be avoided because of the danger of precipitating hypotension. Heparin anticoagulation can be quickly reversed by using intravenous protamine sulfate.

Blood pressure management is extremely important in patients with ICH. Many of these patients have uncontrolled hypertension, and others may have a reflexly increased blood pressure caused by the effect of increased intracranial pressure. As cerebral perfusion is determined by the difference between mean arterial blood pressure and intracranial pressure, caution must be used initially in lowering the blood pressure aggressively. In the absence of cardiac ischemia, normotensive blood pressure should not be the goal, as this may result in diminished cerebral perfusion pressure, leading to cerebral ischemia.

Seizures occur in approximately 17 per cent of patients with nontraumatic supratentorial ICH. In a recent study of seizures with ICH, it was found that seizures tended to occur at the time of ICH onset, without new seizures in the later stages of ICH. Patients with ICH involving the cerebral cortex have an increased risk of seizures. These data indicate that anticonvulsants should not be used routinely in ICH unless the patient has had seizures at onset or has a hemorrhage that is closely related to the cerebral cortex.

Surgery is of benefit in several instances. In patients with large cerebellar hemorrhages (greater than 3 cm in diameter) or in those with signs of brain stem compression, surgical evacuation of the clot can be lifesaving. The other major role of surgery is in the treatment of hydrocephalus, particularly in cases of thalamic hemorrhage. Surgery may be beneficial in large lobar hemorrhages with progression of symptoms despite maximal medical therapy. Other types of ICH are not clearly benefited by surgical intervention.

ISCHEMIC CEREBROVASCULAR DISEASE

method of
JOHN W. NORRIS, M.D.
University of Toronto
Toronto, Ontario, Canada

About 60 per cent of ischemic cerebral events (transient ischemic attacks [TIAs] and stroke) are due to cerebral embolism or decreased flow from atherosclerosis of the internal carotid artery. Emboli from the heart (mural thrombosis after myocardial infarction, or valvular heart disease) account for at least another 20 per cent. Lacunar infarctions, small infarctions in the fine penetrating arterioles of the white matter in the internal capsule or brain stem, cause another 10 per cent of events. The remaining 10 per cent of TIAs are accounted for by rarer causes, such as carotid dissection and arteritis.

Treatment depends on both the cause of the ischemic event and whether the goal is to prevent further stroke or to treat the current episode.

Management of stroke has changed radically in the last decade because of the advent of effective imaging techniques for the brain and cerebral circulation. Computed tomography (CT) allows an accurate diagnosis of the location and, in most cases, the pathology of the lesion. For instance, many minor stroke deficits that were diagnosed as ischemic lesions and treated with anticoagulants were probably hemorrhagic. This error affects the effectiveness of treatment as well as the complication rate. About 25 per cent of TIA patients have areas of cerebral infarction seen on a CT scan.

Magnetic resonance imaging (MRI) has advanced the speed and accuracy of stroke diagnosis because although CT is often negative for the first day after infarction, MRI detects ischemic lesions within hours.

Carotid Doppler, both continuous wave and pulsed wave techniques, has proved to be an accurate method of estimating the degree of stenosis in the carotid vessels in the neck. The sensitivity and specificity of this method compared with those of angiography are more than 95 per cent. Real-time imaging (B-mode or Duplex scanning) visualizes ulceration, intraluminal clot, and intraplaque hemorrhage, which may relate to plaque activity and are clinically important. Transcranial Doppler techniques with low-frequency ultrasound beams that penetrate the skull allow evaluation of the circle of Willis and its branches. Recent developments of this relatively new technique suggest that it may be useful in determining the pathogenesis of acute ischemic stroke and prognosis of these patients.

RISK FACTORS

Whether the event is transient (TIA) or permanent (completed ischemic stroke), risk factors for vascular disease should be investigated unless the patient is terminally ill or in a neurovegetative state.

The major risk factor for stroke is hypertension,

and the recent decline in the incidence of stroke reflects the control of high blood pressure in the community. The diagnosis of hypertension should not be based on blood pressure recordings taken during the acute stage of stroke because blood pressure is commonly elevated in the early weeks after an ischemic event. Blood pressure should be reduced gradually if the patient is hypertensive because infarcted brain loses the capacity to autoregulate, and perfusion becomes dependent on systemic blood pressure. Sudden drops in pressure may worsen the area of infarction or induce it in patients with recent TIAs and critical carotid stenosis.

Ischemic heart disease occurs in 60 per cent of stroke patients and is the most common cause of death in patients with TIAs, ischemic stroke, or asymptomatic carotid stenosis. Cardiac causes should be sought in patients with ischemic cerebral events and normal carotid Doppler or carotid angiograms.

Cardiac arrhythmias, especially atrial fibrillation, also cause ischemic cerebral events, and cardiac monitoring is needed in patients in whom cardiac causes are suspected because the use of anticoagulants may be indicated.

Serum cholesterol, low-density lipoprotein, and high-density lipoprotein levels should be corrected if they are abnormal. The role of smoking as a risk factor for stroke is uncertain, but in younger patients smoking is best avoided for cardiac and peripheral vascular reasons, as well as for prevention of further strokes.

TRANSIENT ISCHEMIC ATTACKS

TIAs last less than 24 hours (usually 1 to 3 hours), and the most common type is transient monocular blindness or amaurosis fugax. Although harmless, these TIAs carry an annual stroke risk of 5 to 8 per cent and an annual mortality (mainly myocardial) of 5 per cent.

Stroke prophylaxis 25 years ago was based primarily on the use of anticoagulants such as warfarin (Coumadin) or heparin, but no randomized study of these agents was ever conducted so their role cannot be evaluated. Also, they carry at least a 1 to 2 per cent chance of serious bleeding, often into the brain. There is thus no justification for their use unless a cardioembolic source is identified, preferably by two-dimensional echocardiogram.

Numerous antiplatelet drugs are claimed to be effective in stroke prophylaxis for TIAs, but so far only aspirin has a documented prophylactic effect. Dipyridamole (Persantine) and sulfinpyrazone (Anturane) have not been shown to be beneficial. The results of a large multicenter trial

of a new drug for stroke prevention, ticlopidine, are not yet available, but preliminary communications indicate that the drug is a more effective prophylactic for stroke than aspirin. At present, the drug of choice is aspirin, which is probably of no value in women but which reduces the risk of stroke by 50 per cent in men with TIAs. The initial dose of 1300 mg daily is no more effective therapeutically than low-dose aspirin of 325 mg daily. The low-dose format has significantly fewer side effects, most notably gastrointestinal bleeding, which is often fatal in patients in the stroke-prone age group. Aspirin is best given in the enteric-coated form.

In patients with carotid occlusion or with carotid stenosis inaccessible to surgery, anastomosis of a scalp artery to a brain artery through a craniotomy (extracranial-intracranial bypass) was practiced until recent years. Unfortunately, a large multicenter study of this technique showed that it was ineffective, and its use has now been largely abandoned, at least for cerebral ischemia.

Carotid endarterectomy probably remains the best method of stroke prophylaxis in symptomatic patients with carotid stenosis and TIAs or minor stroke. Because the severity of carotid stenosis with or without ulceration relates directly to the risk of stroke, carotid endarterectomy is more justified in patients with carotid stenosis of more than 75 per cent. In patients with nonstenosing but severely ulcerated lesions, carotid surgery is also performed but there is less evidence to justify its use. B-mode carotid Doppler techniques can image these lesions and even demonstrate a fresh clot in the lumen or in the arterial wall and are proving of to be increased value in surgical assessment. Although at present there are several multicenter studies in progress in North America and Europe, this procedure is now the most widely practiced vascular surgery in North America. In 1971, 15,000 of these procedures were performed in the United States, and by 1985 this number had climbed to 107,000. The projection for 1986 was 124,000, but in fact, it was only 83,000; by 1987, the number was 81,000.

One reason for this sudden decline is that doubts were raised regarding its efficacy in patients with asymptomatic carotid stenosis, in whom the annual stroke risk is only 2 to 3 per cent. The combined stroke and death rate from carotid surgery differs widely, and although it is reported as only 1 to 2 per cent in some centers, in others it is more than 20 per cent. At this level, the operation is more hazardous than the disease. Misgivings about its use have spread to symptomatic patients with carotid stenosis, although the annual stroke risk for these patients is two to three times higher than that for asymptomatic patients.

The problem complicating all neurovascular procedures is the threat of death or severe disability from myocardial ischemia because surgical benefits are negated if the patient's survival is short-lived.

COMPLETED STROKE

Recovery from cerebral infarction depends on a number of factors, including the type of infarct, the pathogenesis of the ischemia, and the site of the lesion. For instance, small lacunae usually produce transient hemiparesis. They are rarely more than 1 cm in diameter and are often too small to be visualized by CT or even MRI scanning. Cardioembolic strokes, even if small, may undergo hemorrhagic transformation and produce devastating effects. However, they may resolve rapidly if the embolus lyses and disintegrates. Recovery from cerebral infarction depends partly on the size of the surrounding halo of partially ischemic brain, the ischemic penumbra. Drug therapy is unlikely to affect the necrotic core; however, it may reverse the metabolic damage of the inert but viable neurons in the penumbra.

In all ischemic strokes, the primary disturbance is reduced cerebral perfusion, which causes a loss of high-energy phosphates and loss of homeostasis of cellular ionic pumps with electrolyte imbalance and cellular edema. Partial ischemia is more dangerous than total ischemia because metabolism with inadequate oxygenation generates lactic acidosis and destroys astrocytes and later neurons.

Vasodilator therapy such as carbon dioxide is useless because it shunts blood to normally reacting cerebral vessels from the hyperemic area of infarction (intracerebral steal). Hyperventilation should produce the opposite, but in clinical trials it has proved to be of no value. Similarly, no drug has been effective in reducing ischemic cerebral edema, which is the most common cause of death in the first week after cerebral infarction.

Anticoagulants may prevent further embolism in cardioembolic stroke, when an embolic source is demonstrated or is strongly suspected. However, because embolic strokes are more likely to be hemorrhagic than other types of ischemic stroke, devastating cerebral hemorrhage may result. Anticoagulants have no place in treatment of cerebral infarction from carotid stenosis, and in the few randomized studies in which they were used for treatment of partial completed strokes, they were no more effective than placebo in preventing further severe neurologic deficits.

In stroke in evolution (progressing stroke), where the neurologic deficit continues to increase within a few hours of onset, anticoagulants are often given on the rationale that the causal process is progressing thrombosis. There is no evidence that progressing stroke represents progressing thrombosis. It may simply represent spreading cerebral edema.

In one double-blind randomized study, calcium channel blockers apparently reduced the neurologic deficits in patients with cerebral infarction. The result awaits confirmation by additional studies. Other therapies such as hemodilution and drugs such as prostacyclin, pentoxifylline (Trental), and naloxone (Narcan) have all proved to be disappointing. At present, there are several studies in progress to test thrombolysis in treatment of acute ischemic stroke by using tissue plasminogen activator (Activase) or Ancrod (Malayan pit viper venom). The results are awaited with interest.

The most effective treatment of completed ischemic stroke may be the use of a cocktail that incorporates calcium blockers and vasodilators, possibly starting with a thrombolytic agent to allow access of these drugs to ischemic brain. At present, no effective regimen has been developed for completed ischemic stroke, although the subject is under intense scrutiny by investigators throughout the world.

REHABILITATION OF THE PATIENT WITH HEMIPLEGIA

method of
JOSEPH GOODGOLD, M.D.
New York University School of Medicine
New York, New York

Strokes are heterogeneous in their etiology, clinical manifestations, and therapeutic specificity (embolic occlusion versus intracerebral hemorrhage), so that accurate diagnosis should be established before beginning treatment. It is generally estimated that approximately 500,000 new cases of stroke occur annually, of which 40 per cent are fatal; thus, the problem is indeed important in our society. As a matter of relative reference, there are approximately 10,000 new cases of spinal cord injury and about 500,000 cases of head injury each year in the United States.

Rehabilitative treatment of stroke embodies the essential philosophy and methodology of rehabilitation medicine. It is a holistic approach to care and adds to medical and physical treatment a full complement of humanistic and social dimensions, including behavioral considerations and educational and vocational issues, as well as social service, family, societal, and environmental factors. The basic physical examination and history are supplemented in rehabilitation medicine by addressing all of these issues and by assessing the level of residual functional capacity and the possibility of recovery of function. The prevention of some complications that occur quickly and insidiously, such as joint contracture and decubiti, is also an important aspect of the therapeutic regimen.

The efficacy of rehabilitative intervention in stroke is difficult to state accurately because of the multifaceted nature of the medical problem, the possibility of spontaneous recovery of at least some functions, and the difficulty of evaluating the psychosocial and economic factors. But the overwhelming practical observation is that the number of stroke victims who are almost vegetative and bedridden is markedly reduced. At the same time, the increased ability to locomote, to manipulate impaired and unimpaired limbs, and to participate socially and economically increases the individual's quality of life while reducing the level of support required from family and social services.

TREATMENT DURING THE ACUTE STAGE OF STROKE

Rehabilitative measures must be integrated with medical care and should be instituted immediately. Some of the complications that occur during the period when life support systems may be required increase the problems of care when and if the patient survives. For example, flexion contractures of the elbow, wrist, and fingers; abduction of the arm and interval rotation of the limb; external rotation of the hip; and flexion of the knee and equinovarus of the foot all contribute to later difficulties in ambulation, limb manipulation, and body balance. Therefore, early positioning and passive and active joint exercises, within tolerance and safety limits, are essential. As another example, the development of decubiti in the paralytic and often comatose patient can be notoriously rapid and is responsible for many additional hospital days or weeks of subsequent care of this complication. The rehabilitation team is acutely aware of these problems and the means of implementing the appropriate preventive regimens. A more energetic program of mobilization can usually be commenced within 48 hours after onset of stroke, and the patient can be transferred to a rehabilitation section, if available, when medical stability is attained.

CHRONIC CARE

Patient selection is a serious and difficult matter when long-term therapy is to be initiated. Patients who are overwhelmingly affected physically fare poorly, and individuals who have become demented by stroke are not appropriate candidates. The major group of patients who cannot participate in a program are those whose cognitive deficiency is so severe that comprehension of instructions and memory retention are seriously impaired. Full, comprehensive rehabilitative treatment for these patients should be deferred until recovery of sufficient mental capacity has been demonstrated.

The most effective approach to the rehabilitative care of the stroke patient is the multidisciplinary team, which usually consists of a physical therapist, occupational therapist, speech pathologist, social worker, psychologist, and rehabilitation nurse. The team is led by a physician who integrates all activities as a case manager—a function that is now becoming recognized as essential to all aspects of medical care. In most instances, the most effective leader is the physician who is trained in rehabilitation medicine, the physiatrist. The contributions of some members of the rehabilitation team are summarized in the following sections.

Physical Therapy

Physical therapy has evolved in two directions. The old and still time-honored approach uses stretching exercises and joint range-of-motion maneuvers in an attempt to prevent muscle-tendon shortening and loss of joint mobility. Muscles are exercised by passive range of motion; later, with recovery of movement, active exercises are commenced. The patient is rapidly progressed to balancing exercises and training and is started on a program designed to restore some degree of locomotion via careful, progressive gait training. The orthotic and prosthetic divisions are frequently enlisted to produce bracing to control the loss of movement and distortion of the foot and leg. These services are also used to produce static and dynamic devices to support and substitute for deficiencies involving the upper extremity.

During the past 10 to 15 years, newer methods of physical therapy have been introduced that are based on neurophysiologic information and reflexology. It is an appealing and seemingly scientific approach, but regrettably, the results of this approach to central nervous system disease have not been proved by critical methodologic and statistical analysis. The most popular of these methods are identified by the names of their proponents (e.g., Brunstrom, Kabat, Bobath, Rood, Knott). For a time, all share a popularity and in-vogue status sometimes bordering on theological fervor. More recently, functional electrical stimulation has become popular again. Theoretically, it improves strength and coordination and enhances proprioceptive sense about joints by virtue of the muscle contractions that occur. Biofeedback techniques are also popular and seem to be of some value in retraining function of the lower extremity and attaining better control of the proximal upper extremity. The persistently paralyzed hand is not affected.

Occupational Therapy

The most important purpose of the occupational therapist is to retrain the upper extremities. The goal is to attain maximal functional use and recovery of the finer motor skills. The therapist has major responsibility for training the patient in the various elements of the activities of daily living so as to attain maximal independence. When necessary, various devices are introduced, ranging from specially made eating utensils to a completely planned home environment—ramps for wheelchair access, bathroom and shower or bathtub rails, and specially designed kitchens with a variety of substituting mechanical and electrical devices.

Speech Pathology

The treatment of residual speech problems in the stroke patient is not a simple, routine matter. In the dysarthric patient, standard methods of retraining in sound formation and control of the muscles involved may be of considerable help, but the aphasic patient poses a different problem. Many proposed methods of treatment have proved to be problematic. Indoctrination by nonverbal means of communication and, recently, by using adaptive approaches provided by computer technology seem to have potential for improving the patient's skills.

Other Components

Rehabilitation Nursing

In most rehabilitation settings, the schedule of treatment sessions averages 3 to 6 hours per day, so that the role of the rehabilitation nurse as an integrator and coordinator of various aspects of treatment during the remaining 18 to 21 hours is easily understood. The nurse functions in all areas (e.g., medical, physical, psychosocial). It is important to involve the patient and family in all aspects of preparation for home care. The family is recruited and actively participates in the care system from the onset of the program. Detailed information and instructions on care and coping are given to them daily by the staff and in regularly scheduled family-patient-staff conferences.

Social Services

In these days of government oversight, rules, and regulations, coupled with the zealous cost accounting and cost-effective concerns of the insurance industry, the intervention of the social workers is of critical importance. These persons are important in handling the myriad details of fiscal entitlement from government and private sources and are crucial in patient placement—whether it be from an acute medical facility to a rehabilitation center or from the center to an intermediary facility, a long-term chronic nursing institution, or the home-family environment. Their constant presence and practical knowledge are an important stabilizing force.

Psychologic Services

The patient who requires rehabilitative services must be able to learn and relearn basic information and motor-sensory skills. Therefore, poststroke dementia must be clearly identified, as well as other behavioral aberrations with bizarre and irrational emotional content. Essentially, then, we must respond to the following questions: Is there a psychosis? Can the patient remember information and apply it? Is there a significant component of depression? This problem is common in the poststroke patient. Behavioral scientists have developed methods of cognitive treatment that are widely used but not universally accepted as making a significant impact. Clearly, however, as a simple example, helping the patient to remember information by taking notes in a readily accessible booklet carried on the patient's person is of practical help. The significant incidence of visual perception and left-sided defects is rapidly identified during the behavioral work-up. Psychologists have developed therapeutic interventions centered on retraining in basic visual scanning, with stress on augmented head movement to compensate for field deficiency. There is emphasis on anticipation of the loss caused by impaired perception, so that compensatory head movement becomes routine in enlarging the scanning zone.

Psychologic support is important not only to the patient but also to the immediate family, including siblings, who are often in dire need of supportive care. Sometimes small conferences with all concerned persons are sufficient; in other instances, a series of therapeutic consultations are required. In my experience, most patients have a negative behavioral reaction to the catastrophe of a stroke, although the compensatory demeanor may make it difficult to detect the underlying turmoil and stress.

Other problems are also encountered in caring for the stroke patient. Included are shoulder subluxation of the paralyzed arm, as well as brachial plexus and peripheral nerve injuries usually caused by abnormal compression and body habit.

Occasionally, ectopic ossification occurs around the elbow or shoulder and may be the cause of considerable distress during the stage of early inflammatory changes. In some patients, there is severe reflex sympathetic dystrophy affecting the involved hand. As always, treatment of this autonomic nervous system dysfunction is difficult, running the gamut from psychotherapy, courses of steroids, analgesics, therapeutic stellate ganglion blocks, and sometimes cervical sympathectomy. The response to treatment is as difficult to predict as the severity of the patient's symptoms.

Approximately 10 per cent of stroke victims begin to have seizures and should be treated with phenytoin (Dilantin) or carbamazepine.

Care of the stroke patient has some aspects of a continuum because complications of the process itself are recurrent and because the patient may also have other illnesses. For example, underlying diseases such as hypertension, diabetes mellitus, and other metabolic disorders and biochemical aberrations that foster vascular lesions will continue to take their toll. It is thus imperative that the future care of the patient be structured around a regularly scheduled follow-up system that is prophylactically oriented and marked by cooperation between the medical clinician and the physiatrist.

EPILEPSY IN ADOLESCENTS AND ADULTS

method of
ROGER J. PORTER, M.D.
*National Institute of Neurological Disorders
and Stroke
Bethesda, Maryland*

Approximately 1 per cent of the U.S. population has active epilepsy. Although reports of its worldwide incidence vary, there is no proof of geographic variation. Differences in terminology and inclusion criteria may be largely responsible for the apparent discrepancies. If a 1 per cent incidence rate and a global population of 4.8 billion are assumed, 48 million people worldwide suffer from epilepsy. A sizable minority of them, perhaps 20 to 25 per cent, respond poorly and are chronically refractory to currently available therapies.

DIAGNOSIS

There are multiple levels of diagnosis in every patient with epileptic seizures. At a fundamental clinical level, the *etiologic diagnosis* involves identification of the cause of the epileptic seizures. At a more superficial yet therapeutically important level, the *seizure diagnosis* is based on the nature of the seizure. These two diagnostic levels are often combined with other criteria (Table 1) to provide the *epilepsy syndrome diagnosis*; an epileptic syndrome may be defined as a disorder characterized by a cluster of signs and symptoms customarily occurring together.

The search for all three levels of diagnosis is necessary for the proper care of the patient with epilepsy. Failure to establish the etiologic diagnosis means that some patients continue to have seizures because of undiagnosed brain lesions, such as a brain tumor. Failure to establish the seizure diagnosis means that some patients continue to have seizures because the therapy is incorrect; for example, absence seizures are mistaken for complex partial seizures, and the incorrect medication is prescribed. Failure to establish the syndrome diagnosis prevents the physician from understanding the prognosis and duration of therapy, such as mistaking juvenile myoclonic epilepsy (benign course) for progressive myoclonic epilepsy (malignant course). There is a clear relationship among the etiologic, seizure, and syndrome diagnoses; the first two are subsets of the last, as noted in Table 1. Also, the etiologic diagnosis may contribute to the seizure diagnosis, and vice versa. Although the etiologic diagnosis often cannot be established with certainty, the seizure diagnosis can almost always be determined. It is from the base of knowledge outlined in Table 1 that the physician establishes the syndrome diagnosis.

ETIOLOGY

Epilepsy can be caused by virtually any major category of serious disease or disorder in humans. It can result from congenital malformations, infections, tumors, vascular diseases, degenerative diseases, or injury. In more than three-fourths of patients with epilepsy, the seizures begin before the age of 18 years.

TABLE 1. **Data Needed to Provide a Syndrome Diagnosis***

I. Information on Etiology
  A. Etiologic diagnosis is either definitively known or definitively unobtainable (idiopathic)
          or
  B. Etiologic diagnosis is suggested by some of the following:
    1. Neurologic history, including age of onset and family history
    2. Neurologic examination
    3. Electroencephalogram
    4. Radiologic (and related) examinations
    5. Other tests, including psychologic examination

II. Information on Seizure Type
  A. Seizure type is definitively known
          or
  B. Seizure type is suggested by some of the following:
    1. Neurologic history, including age of onset
    2. Neurologic examination
    3. Direct or indirect (e.g., videotape) observation of a seizure
    4. Electroencephalogram, ictal and interictal
    5. Other tests, as above

*From Porter RJ: Epilepsy: 100 Elementary Principles, 2nd ed. London, Bailliere Tindall, 1989.

The reason for this age of onset is not clear, but the increased vulnerability of the young nervous system to seizure development is known clinically and documented experimentally. In a substantial proportion of patients, the etiology of the seizures remains undetermined. Future scientific advances are likely to identify inherited susceptibility as a principal cause of epilepsy. Although there is considerable evidence that absence seizures, for example, are an expression of an autosomal dominant gene, the role of genetic factors in epilepsy has been almost wholly unexplored. Likewise, it is tempting to hold a "genetic predisposition" responsible when one patient has epilepsy after a head injury and another equally injured patient has no seizures; however, this implication is, at the moment, almost pure speculation.

SYNDROMES

There is a fundamental difference between seizures and epilepsy. A seizure is a finite event; it has a beginning and an end. Hughlings Jackson, in 1870, stated that a seizure is "a symptom . . . an occasional, an excessive and a disorderly discharge of nerve tissue." Epilepsy, on the other hand, is a chronic disorder. The World Health Organization has stated that epilepsy is "a chronic brain disorder of various etiologies characterized by recurrent seizures due to excessive discharge of cerebral neurons." Epilepsy is a group of syndromes rather than a disease; the "epilepsies" or "epileptic syndromes" have arisen to classify patients and to emphasize the heterogeneity of these symptom complexes. The classification of epileptic syndromes is now becoming useful to the practitioner, even though it has proved to be much more difficult to devise than the classification of epileptic seizures.

The classification of the epilepsies depends on the ability to determine a framework of similarity in patient characteristics—including seizures and many other factors. The earliest and most persistent subdivision is between epilepsy with a recognizable cause (symptomatic) and epilepsy without a recognizable cause (cryptogenic or idiopathic). The terms "primary epilepsy" (meaning that the etiology is unknown) and "secondary epilepsy" (meaning that the etiology is clinically identifiable) have also been used in a similar way to differentiate the epilepsies even though these terms present special semantic difficulties. Secondary epilepsy is a quite different concept from secondary generalization of seizures, with which it may be confused.

In 1985, the International League Against Epilepsy published a proposal for syndrome classification. The fundamental observations reflect the earlier success of the classification of epileptic seizures by beginning first with the partial, generalized concept followed by the etiology concept:

1. Partial (localization-related) epilepsies
   a. Idiopathic
   b. Symptomatic
2. Generalized epilepsies
   a. Idiopathic
   b. Idiopathic, symptomatic, or both
   c. Symptomatic

3. Epilepsies undetermined whether partial or generalized
4. Special syndromes

The next subdivision below partial-generalized and idiopathic-symptomatic, especially for the generalized epilepsies, is the *relationship of age to onset,* one of the most important variables underlying the classification. Whenever possible, it is desirable to categorize a patient into an epileptic syndrome; a syndrome classification provides prognostic information for the patient that neither the seizure diagnosis nor the etiologic diagnosis can provide. Unfortunately, it is not always possible to classify a patient into an epilepsy syndrome, just as the etiology of the epilepsy may remain elusive. It is almost always possible, however, to classify the patient's seizures.

SEIZURES

Although interest in modifying and improving the classification of epileptic syndromes continues, the classification of *epileptic seizures* has been a more successful effort. Even though the seizure diagnosis is a highly empiric method of determining therapy, for the foreseeable future the seizure type is the best information on which to base a therapeutic decision for the symptomatic treatment of epilepsy.

Seizures are fundamentally divided into two groups—partial and generalized. Partial seizures have clinical or electroencephalographic (EEG) evidence of a local onset, but the word "partial" does not imply a highly discrete focus; such a focus often does not exist. The abnormal discharge usually arises in a portion of one hemisphere and may spread to other parts of the brain during a seizure. Generalized seizures, however, have no evidence of localized onset. The clinical manifestations and abnormal electrical discharge give no clue to the locus of onset of the abnormality, if indeed such a locus exists.

Partial Seizures

There are three types of partial seizures, determined to some extent by the degree of brain involvement by the abnormal discharge.

The least complicated partial seizure is the elementary or *simple partial seizure,* characterized by minimal spread of the abnormal discharge such that normal consciousness and awareness are preserved. For example, the patient may have a sudden onset of clonic jerking of an extremity lasting for 60 to 90 seconds; residual weakness may last for 15 to 30 minutes after the attack. The patient is completely aware of the attack and can describe it in detail. The EEG may show an abnormal discharge highly localized to the involved portion of the brain.

The *complex partial seizure* also has a localized onset, but the discharge becomes more widespread (usually bilateral) and almost always involves the limbic system. Most (not all) complex partial seizures arise from one of the temporal lobes, possibly because of the susceptibility of this area of the brain to insults such as hypoxia or infection. Clinically, there may be a brief warning followed by an alteration of consciousness during which some patients may stare and others may stagger or even fall. Most, however, demonstrate fragments of integrated motor behavior termed "automatisms," for which the patient has no memory. Typical automatisms are lip smacking, swallowing, fumbling, scratching, or even walking about. After 30 to 120 seconds, the patient gradually returns to normal consciousness but may feel tired or ill for several hours after the attack.

The last type of partial seizure is the *secondarily generalized seizure,* in which a partial seizure immediately precedes a generalized tonic-clonic (grand mal) seizure. This seizure type is described with the generalized seizures.

Generalized Seizures

Generalized seizures are those in which there is no evidence of localized onset. The group is quite heterogeneous.

Generalized tonic-clonic (grand mal) seizures are the most dramatic of all epileptic seizures and are characterized by tonic rigidity of all extremities, followed in 15 to 30 seconds by a tremor that is actually an interruption of the tonus by relaxation. As the relaxation phases become longer, the attack enters the clonic phase, with massive jerking of the body. The clonic jerking slows over 60 to 120 seconds, and the patient is usually left in a stuporous state. The tongue or cheek may be bitten, and urinary incontinence is common. Primary generalized tonic-clonic seizures begin without evidence of localized onset, whereas secondary generalized tonic-clonic seizures are preceded by another seizure type, usually a partial seizure.

The petit mal or *absence seizure* is characterized by both sudden onset and abrupt cessation. Its duration is usually less than 10 seconds and is rarely more than 45 seconds. Consciousness is altered; the attack may also be associated with mild clonic jerking of the eyelids or extremities, with postural tone changes, autonomic phenomena, and automatisms. The occurrence of automatisms can complicate the clinical differentiation from complex partial seizures in some patients. Absence attacks begin in childhood or adolescence and may occur up to hundreds of times a day. The EEG during the seizure shows a highly characteristic 2.5- to 3.5-Hz spike-and-wave pattern. Atypical absence patients have seizures with postural changes that are more abrupt, and the patients are often mentally retarded; the EEG may show a slower spike-and-wave discharge, and the seizures may be more refractory to therapy.

Myoclonic jerking is seen, to a greater or lesser extent, in a wide variety of seizures, including generalized tonic-clonic seizures, partial seizures, absence seizures, and infantile spasms. Treatment of seizures that include myoclonic jerking should usually be directed at the primary seizure type rather than at the myoclonus. Some patients, however, have myoclonic jerking as a major seizure type.

Atonic seizures are those in which the patient has sudden loss of postural tone. If standing, the patient falls suddenly to the floor and may be injured. If seated, the head and torso may suddenly drop forward; the patient's face typically falls directly into a plate of food set on the table. Although most often seen in children, this seizure type is not unusual in adults. Many patients with atonic seizures wear helmets to prevent severe injury.

TREATMENT

Antiepileptic drugs are often quite specific for various types of epileptic seizures, and proper seizure classification is crucial to appropriate therapy. The clinical evidence for specificity of antiepileptic drugs against various seizure types is impressive:

1. Some drugs, such as phenytoin or carbamazepine, are virtually ineffective against absence seizures or myoclonic seizures but control most partial seizures and generalized tonic-clonic seizures.
2. Some drugs, such as ethosuximide or trimethadione, have no effect against partial seizures, generalized tonic-clonic seizures, or myoclonic seizures but are useful in treating absence seizures.
3. Valproic acid is effective against both absence seizures and myoclonic seizures, as well as primarily generalized tonic-clonic seizures.
4. Corticotropin may stop infantile spasms but has little effect on other seizure types.

Monotherapy

Much has been written in the past few years regarding the merits of monotherapy compared with polytherapy. The latter, which merely means the use of more than one drug at a time in a single patient, has been declared unnecessary and inappropriate, without adequate and reasoned consideration that multiple drugs may, in fact, be useful in some patients. The following statements consider the arguments both for and against monotherapy.

The best state of health is the medication-free state. Although this statement is, on its own, self-evident, it points out that any therapy—including monotherapy—is inferior to a drug-free state when such a state is possible. Some patients with epilepsy prefer to risk an occasional seizure than risk toxicity from drug therapy. Others benefit so little from therapy that they may be better off without medication. Such patients are uncommon, but clearly monotherapy is less desirable than the absence of therapy when none is needed or indicated. Finally, and perhaps most importantly, some patients who once required medical therapy may no longer need it and deserve a trial of drug withdrawal.

The advantages of limiting the total antiepileptic drug intake (either in number or in quantity) are well documented. When a single drug is taken to excess, both physician and patient become aware of the consequences; dose-related adverse effects are obvious, and the patient becomes ill. Less obvious is the advantage of taking fewer medications. Most physicians and patients agree, however, that the administration of fewer antiepileptic drugs has certain advantages:

1. Adverse drug-drug interactions are much less likely; they obviously do not occur with monotherapy.
2. Side effects in general may be fewer.
3. Compliance by the patient may be better. However, compliance problems may also relate to inadequate attention by the physician to this issue.
4. The cost may be lower. However, it may be higher if more expensive drugs are chosen.
5. Seizure control is better in some patients. But improvement in seizure control may not relate to a fundamental alteration in the propensity to have seizures. It may, rather, relate to increased compliance because of few adverse side effects.

A multidrug regimen may occasionally be superior to monotherapy. In certain patients, almost always with severe, difficult to control epilepsy, multiple drugs appear to be more effective than single medications. Although only a minority of patients may respond, the physician should not automatically reject a multidrug regimen as having no potential benefit for the patient.

A nonsedative regimen may be more important than monotherapy. In the past decade, an increasing number of studies have suggested that certain antiepileptic drugs, notably those with sedative-hypnotic effects, may cause drowsiness and cognitive dysfunction in many patients with epilepsy. If one accepts that barbiturates and benzodiazepines are, with certain limited exceptions, second line antiepileptic drugs because of their sedating properties, one is limited, in most cases, to four primary antiepileptic drugs. These are phenytoin, carbamazepine, valproic acid, and ethosuximide. Logically, one should begin therapy with one of these four drugs as monotherapy. When a multidrug regimen is indicated, combinations of nonsedative medications are preferable to combinations including barbiturates or benzodiazepines. Whether monotherapy with barbiturates or benzodiazepines is worth the effort before embarking on a multidrug regimen has not been adequately investigated by clinical trials. Only scant data are available to support a regimen of monotherapy with sedative-hypnotic antiepileptic drugs except for (1) certain specific seizure types, such as the myoclonias, which may respond to chronic benzodiazepine therapy and (2) patients who are intolerant of the usual first line drugs.

In summary, when treatment is needed for epileptic seizures, all patients should first be tried on a single medication. This medication, before being abandoned as ineffective, should be "pushed" gently to the point of producing dose-related side effects. Should the first medication fail, a second trial of another single agent should probably be attempted before considering a multidrug regimen. A few patients, however, have their epilepsy optimally controlled with multiple drugs.

Pharmacokinetics

The pharmacokinetics of antiepileptic drugs, like those of other drugs, follow certain rules that must be learned and understood by the prescribing physician if optimal therapy is to be achieved. These rules are as follows.

The key to drug intake intervals is the drug's half-life. The spacing of antiepileptic drugs throughout the day should be scientifically based. If maximum therapeutic effectiveness of the short–half-life drugs is desired, they must be delivered frequently—often four times a day. Two antiepileptic drugs, valproic acid and carbamazepine, have short half-lives. When valproic acid is given only every 12 hours, its plasma level fluctuates widely. It is most important, therefore, to space out the administration of these drugs during the day, especially in patients whose attacks are not completely controlled and who require maximum effectiveness from the limited antiepileptic armamentarium. The observation may be of even greater importance for carbamazepine. These same recommendations apply—to a lesser extent—to primidone, whose antiepileptic action is complicated by its long–half-life metabolite, phenobarbital. Multiple daily doses are also important for drugs with gastrointestinal toxicity. Some drugs can be administered infrequently and with little attention to the time of day or the relation to meals. The most widely publicized of these antiepileptic drugs is phenytoin, in which once-a-day administration has become popular. Some patients find such a regimen convenient and entirely satisfactory, but others are bothered by toxic effects and find that twice-a-day administration eliminates these unpleasant side effects.

The key to determining intervals between changes in drug dose is the drug's half-life. The disadvantage of drugs with short half-lives is the necessity of frequent administration. The advantage of drugs with short half-lives is the ability to change from one steady-state level to another in a relatively short time. The pharmacokinetic rule is simple: after every dose change, it takes five half-lives to reach 97 per cent of a new steady-state plasma drug level. Only after the new steady-state level is reached can drug efficacy be evaluated. Although dose-related toxicity can occur at any time in the course of drug administration, like efficacy it cannot be fully evaluated until the new steady-state level is achieved. The fact that a patient tolerates a 400-mg daily dose of phenytoin for the first 3 days of administration does not mean that toxicity will not occur after 1 or 2 weeks at that dose. Occasionally, toxicity occurs before a steady-state level is reached, and a dosage decrease is indicated.

The time needed to reach a steady-state plasma drug level is not determined by the amount of the dose change. Whether the dose of an antiepileptic drug is increased by 15 or 150 mg daily, the time necessary to achieve a new steady-state level is the same. Although this assumption is based on linear kinetics, only phenytoin deviates from this model. Explained in another way, the eventual height of the new steady-state plasma drug level is a function of the daily dose of the drug, whereas the time needed to reach this steady-state level is related not to the total dose or to the amount of the dose change but to the half-life of the drug. The longer the half-life, the longer the time needed to reach a steady state, regardless of the dose. When altering the dose of a drug, especially at higher plasma levels, changes should be made infrequently and in small increments. Dose-related toxicity, when encountered, is thus relatively mild. The time required to reach a steady state for the major antiepileptic drugs is shown in Table 2.

Use the therapeutic plasma drug level only as a guide. Table 3 demonstrates optimal therapeutic plasma drug levels. The usual therapeutic level

TABLE 3. Effective Plasma Levels of Six Antiepileptic Drugs*

Drug	Effective Level (μg/ml)	High Effective Level† (μg/ml)	Toxic Level (μg/ml)
Carbamazepine	4–12	7	8
Primidone	5–15	10	12
Phenytoin	10–20	18	20
Phenobarbital	10–40	35	40
Ethosuximide	50–100	80	100
Valproic acid	50–100	80	100

*From Porter RJ: Epilepsy: 100 Elementary Principles, 2nd ed. London, Bailliere Tindall, 1989.

†Level that should be achieved, if possible, in patients with refractory seizures, assuming that the blood samples are taken before administration of the morning medication. Higher levels are often possible—without toxicity—when the drugs are used alone (i.e., as monotherapy).

of phenytoin, for example, is 10 to 20 micrograms per ml, which suggests that most patients experience optimal seizure control with minimal toxicity if their plasma phenytoin level is within this range. Unfortunately, there are many exceptions to this guideline, and many patients are well controlled at higher or lower levels. For example, some patients tolerate phenytoin levels exceeding 20 micrograms per ml and require these high levels for seizure control. The main considerations in the use of plasma drug levels are as follows:

1. Antiepileptic drug monitoring is useful only as a guide to changes in therapy; it is not a substitute for clinical judgment.

2. Expected therapeutic plasma drug levels are average values; each patient has an individually optimal value.

3. The determinations help to achieve maximal effects of each medication. The use of gradually increasing doses to establish the maximally tolerated dose is a valid concept in patients with seizures refractory to therapy.

4. The determinations are invaluable in the presence of toxic side effects, especially in patients taking multiple drugs and when using phenytoin, which has nonlinear kinetics.

5. Noncompliance, malabsorption, and altered (idiosyncratic) metabolism can be identified, but only noncompliance is a common problem.

6. A reliable laboratory is critical to proper interpretation of the results.

Except in special metabolic circumstances, the need for free levels of antiepileptic drugs remains in doubt. Many studies have emphasized that the free fraction (i.e., the portion not bound to plasma proteins) of antiepileptic drugs is the only portion of the circulating drug that can diffuse through plasma membranes. Until recently, however, the

TABLE 2. Plasma Half-Life of Six Antiepileptic Drugs*

Drug	Half-Life	Time to Reach Steady State
Carbamazepine	12 hr	3 days
Valproic acid	12 hr	3 days
Primidone†	12 hr	3 days
Phenytoin	1 day	5 days‡
Ethosuximide	2 days	10 days
Phenobarbital	4 days	3 wk

*From Porter RJ: Epilepsy: 100 Elementary Principles, 2nd ed. London, Bailliere Tindall, 1989.

†Primidone is converted rapidly to phenobarbital.

‡Phenytoin obeys saturation kinetics.

question of clinical relevance has been largely ignored. The fundamental argument is not whether the free fraction is the fraction that is diffusible; the argument is whether changes in the free fraction are relevant in clinical practice. Only in special circumstances, and only with phenytoin and valproic acid, is there any probability of clinical relevance.

Monitor the plasma drug level first thing in the morning. Monitoring of plasma levels of antiepileptic drugs is confusing because determinations are made on blood samples obtained randomly at various times during the day. Especially with short–half-life drugs such as valproic acid, it is important to establish a fixed relationship between drug intake and blood sampling. The only rational time to take routine samples is in the morning, before the first dose of medication is administered. Such samples reflect the baseline (trough) level and are directly comparable. To detect the toxic offender in a multidrug regimen, it is sometimes necessary to take blood samples at times other than in the morning. This is only occasionally required, however, because the levels determined from the morning samples usually indicate which drug is present in the blood at a high level.

A reliable clinical laboratory is critical for accurate monitoring of plasma drug levels. Each physician must be certain that the laboratory used is competent (i.e., the reported values are close to the correct or true values) and reliable (i.e., the laboratory consistently gives accurate results). The laboratory should subscribe to a proficiency testing program. Two such programs are available in the United States.

Watch for saturation kinetics with phenytoin. The problem with phenytoin, a problem not shared by other antiepileptic drugs, is the relationship between the dose and plasma level of the drug. With phenytoin, this relationship becomes more and more nonlinear as higher doses are given. In practical terms, it means that the half-life of the drug may be much longer at higher doses than at lower doses. To avoid problems with phenytoin, note the following:

1. At higher doses, the increases should be spread over long intervals to avoid the occurrence of toxicity many days later; even weeks may be necessary between dose changes.
2. The plasma phenytoin level may not change immediately after a dose change; the level may plateau for up to a week before further increases or decreases occur spontaneously. This apparent steady state may be of varying duration and may be followed by a prominent increase or decrease in the phenytoin plasma level during a period of constant dosage.

3. Evaluation of seizure control must be delayed until a steady-state level is achieved.
4. Drug interactions may be exaggerated.

Drugs Useful for Simple Partial, Complex Partial, and Generalized Tonic-Clonic Seizures

Carbamazepine (Tegretol)

Seizure Type. Carbamazepine is considered by many to be the drug of choice for partial seizures, and many physicians also use it first for generalized tonic-clonic seizures. It is used with phenytoin in many patients who are difficult to control. Carbamazepine is nonsedative in its usual therapeutic range.

Pharmacokinetics. The rate of absorption of carbamazepine varies widely among different patients, although almost complete absorption apparently occurs in all. Peak levels are usually achieved 6 to 8 hours after administration. Slowing the absorption by giving the drug after meals helps the patient tolerate larger total daily doses.

Carbamazepine has an initial half-life of 36 hours, which decreases to less than 20 hours with continuous therapy. Thus, considerable dosage adjustments are to be expected during the first weeks of therapy.

Carbamazepine is metabolized in part to the stable epoxide carbamazepine-10,11-epoxide, which has been shown to have anticonvulsant activity. The contribution of this and other metabolites to the clinical activity of carbamazepine is unknown.

Some generic forms of carbamazepine have significantly different bioavailability and should be used with great caution.

Therapeutic Levels and Dose. Carbamazepine is available only in oral form. The initial dose is typically 200 mg twice daily, increased at weekly intervals by an additional 200 mg per day. In adults, doses of 1 gram or even 2 grams are tolerated. Higher doses are achieved by giving multiple doses daily. In patients receiving three or four daily doses, in whom the blood is taken just before the morning dose is given (trough level), the therapeutic level is usually 4 to 8 micrograms per ml; although many patients complain of diplopia above 7 micrograms per ml, others can tolerate levels above 10 micrograms per ml.

Toxicity. The most common dose-related side effects of carbamazepine are diplopia and ataxia. The diplopia often occurs first and may last for less than an hour during a particular time of day. Rearrangement of the divided daily dose can often remedy this complaint. Other dose-related complaints include mild gastrointestinal upsets, unsteadiness, and, at much higher doses, drowsiness. Hyponatremia and water intoxication have occasionally occurred and may be dose related.

Some concern exists regarding the occurrence of idiosyncratic blood dyscrasias with carbamazepine, including fatal cases of aplastic anemia and agranulocytosis. Most of these have involved elderly patients, and most have occurred within the first 4 months of treatment. The occurrence of blood dyscrasias is similar to that of other commonly used drugs. A mild, persistent leukopenia is also seen in some patients; this is not necessarily an indication to stop treatment, but it obviously requires careful monitoring. The most common idiosyncratic reaction is an erythematous rash; other responses, such as hepatic dysfunction, are unusual.

Drug Interactions. Drug interactions involving carbamazepine are almost exclusively related to the enzyme-inducing properties of this drug. The increased metabolic capacity of the hepatic enzymes may cause a reduction in the steady-state carbamazepine concentration and an increased rate of metabolism of primidone, phenytoin, ethosuximide, valproic acid, and clonazepam. Other drugs, such as propoxyphene, troleandomycin, and valproic acid, may inhibit carbamazepine clearance and increase the steady-state carbamazepine blood level. Other anticonvulsants, however, such as phenytoin and phenobarbital, may decrease the steady-state concentrations of carbamazepine through enzyme induction. No clinically significant protein-binding interactions have been reported.

Phenytoin (Dilantin)

Seizure Type. Phenytoin is one of the most effective drugs against partial seizures and generalized tonic-clonic seizures. In the latter, it appears to be effective against attacks that are either primary or secondary to another seizure type.

Pharmacokinetics. Absorption of phenytoin is highly dependent on the formulation of the dosage form. Particle size and pharmaceutical additives affect both the rate and the extent of absorption. Some generic forms do not have the same bioavailability as Dilantin, the most commonly prescribed formulation. Oral absorption of phenytoin sodium is nearly complete in most patients, although the time to peak effect may range from 3 to 12 hours. Absorption after intramuscular injection is unpredictable, and some drug precipitation in the muscle occurs; this route of administration is not recommended.

Phenytoin has no active metabolites. It has dose-dependent (saturation) kinetics. Increases in dose may produce large changes in concentrations. In such cases, patients may quickly develop symptoms of toxicity.

The half-life of phenytoin varies from 12 to 36 hours, with an average of 24 hours for most patients in the low to middle therapeutic range. Much longer half-lives are observed at higher concentrations. At low blood levels, it takes 5 to 7 days to reach steady-state blood levels after every dosage change; at higher levels, it may be 4 to 6 weeks before blood levels are stable.

Therapeutic Levels and Dose. The therapeutic plasma level of phenytoin for most patients is between 10 and 20 micrograms per ml. A loading dose can be given either orally or intravenously; the latter is the method of choice for convulsive status epilepticus. When oral therapy is started, it is common to begin adults at a dosage of 300 mg per day regardless of body weight. Although this may be acceptable in some patients, it frequently yields steady-state blood levels below 10 micrograms per ml, the minimum therapeutic level for most patients. If seizures continue, higher doses are usually necessary to achieve plasma levels in the upper therapeutic range. Because of its dose-dependent kinetics, the phenytoin dosage should be increased each time by only 25 to 30 mg in adults, and ample time should be allowed for the new steady state to be achieved before further increasing the dose. A common clinical error is to increase the dose directly from 300 to 400 mg per day; toxicity frequently occurs at a variable time thereafter.

Toxicity. Dose-related side effects caused by phenytoin are, unfortunately, similar to those of other antiepileptic drugs in this group, making differentiation difficult in patients receiving multiple drugs. Nystagmus occurs early, as does loss of smooth extraocular pursuit movements, but neither is an indication for decreasing the dose. Diplopia and ataxia are the most common dose-related side effects requiring dose adjustment; sedation usually occurs only at considerably higher levels. Gingival hyperplasia and hirsutism occur to some degree in most patients; the latter can be especially unpleasant in females. In some patients, long-term chronic use is associated with coarsening of facial features and mild peripheral neuropathy, the latter usually manifested by diminished deep tendon reflexes in the lower extremities. Reports of decreased cognitive function with phenytoin are suggestive but inconclusive.

Idiosyncratic reactions to phenytoin are relatively rare. Most commonly, a typical rash reveals the hypersensitivity of the patient to the drug, which is then appropriately discontinued. Fever may also occur, and in rare cases the skin lesions may be severe and exfoliative. Lymphadenopathy may be difficult to distinguish from malignant lymphoma, and although some studies suggest a causal relationship between phenytoin and Hodgkin's disease, the data are far from conclusive. Hematologic complications are exceedingly rare, although agranulocytosis has been reported in combination with fever and rash.

Drug Interactions. Drug interactions involving phenytoin are related primarily either to protein binding or to metabolism. Because phenytoin is highly bound, other highly bound drugs, such as phenylbutazone, sulfonamides, benzodiazepines, or anticoagulants, can displace phenytoin from its binding site, causing an increase in free drug levels. The protein binding of phenytoin is markedly decreased in the presence of renal disease. The drug has an affinity for thyroid-binding globulin, which confuses some tests of thyroid function; the most reliable screening test of thyroid function in patients on phenytoin appears to be the measurement of thyroid-stimulating hormone levels.

Phenytoin has been shown to induce the production of microsomal enzymes responsible for the metabolism of a number of drugs. Other drugs, notably phenobarbital and carbamazepine, cause decreases in phenytoin steady-state concentrations.

Phenobarbital

Seizure Type. Phenobarbital is useful in the treatment of partial seizures and generalized tonic-clonic seizures, although the drug is often tried for virtually every seizure type, especially when attacks are difficult to control. There is little evidence for its effectiveness in generalized seizures such as absence seizures, atonic attacks, or infantile spasms; it may worsen the condition of certain patients with these seizure types.

Some physicians prefer either metharbital (Gemonil) or mephobarbital (Mebaral)—especially the latter—to phenobarbital because of their supposedly decreased side effects. Only anecdotal data are available for such comparisons.

Pharmacokinetics. Phenobarbital is completely absorbed over 6 to 18 hours. Plasma protein binding is clinically unimportant. No active metabolites are formed.

Therapeutic Levels and Dose. The usual dose is 3 to 5 mg per kg per day. The drug can be given once per day because of its long half-life; typically, it is given at bedtime. The therapeutic level of phenobarbital in most patients is approximately 10 to 40 micrograms per ml. The upper end of the therapeutic range is more difficult to define, as many patients appear to tolerate chronic levels above 40 micrograms per ml.

Toxicity. The most common dose-related side effect is sedation. Phenobarbital (and other barbiturates and benzodiazepines) have been impli-

cated in long-term cognitive impairment and are used much less frequently for this important reason. Ataxia occurs at high levels. Idiosyncratic reactions are rare; the most common one is a typical drug-induced dermatitis.

Drug Interactions. Valproic acid can elevate plasma phenobarbital levels dramatically. Patients taking phenobarbital may need a dose reduction if valproic acid is added. Phenobarbital also has interactions with phenytoin and other commonly used drugs such as warfarin and digoxin.

Primidone (Mysoline)

Seizure Type. Primidone is metabolized to phenobarbital and phenylethylmalonamide. All three compounds are active anticonvulsants. The drug, like its metabolites, is effective against partial seizures and generalized tonic-clonic seizures and may be more effective than phenobarbital. It was previously considered to be the drug of choice for complex partial seizures, but recent studies of partial seizures in adults strongly suggest that carbamazepine and phenytoin are superior to primidone. Overall, the clinical use of primidone is similar to that of phenobarbital.

Pharmacokinetics. Primidone is absorbed slowly but completely. The time required to reach the peak concentration after oral administration is about 3 hours, but considerable variation has been reported.

The appearance of phenobarbital corresponds to the disappearance of primidone. Phenobarbital accumulates slowly but eventually reaches therapeutic concentrations in most patients when therapeutic doses of primidone are administered. Phenobarbital levels derived from primidone are usually two to three times higher than primidone levels. Phenylethylmalonamide, which probably makes a minimal contribution to the efficacy of primidone, has a half-life of 8 to 12 hours and therefore reaches a steady state more rapidly than phenobarbital.

Therapeutic Levels and Dose. Primidone is most efficacious when plasma levels are in the range of 8 to 12 micrograms per ml. Concomitant levels of its metabolite, phenobarbital, at steady state usually vary from 15 to 30 micrograms per ml. Doses of 10 to 20 mg per kg per day are necessary to obtain these levels. It is important, however, to start primidone at low doses and gradually increase it over a few days to a few weeks to avoid prominent sedation and gastrointestinal complaints. Primidone rapidly reaches a steady state (30 to 40 hours), but the active metabolite, phenobarbital, does so much more slowly (20 days).

Toxicity. The toxic side effects of primidone are

similar to those of its metabolite, phenobarbital, except that drowsiness occurs early in treatment and may be prominent if the initial dose is too large; gradual increments are indicated when starting the drug.

Drug Interactions. Primidone interactions are similar to those of phenobarbital.

Drugs Useful for Absence Seizures

Ethosuximide (Zarontin)

Seizure Type. Ethosuximide's spectrum is quite narrow, even though it is quite effective for absence seizures.

Pharmacokinetics. Absorption is complete after administration of the oral dosage forms. Peak levels are observed 3 to 7 hours after oral administration of the capsules. Ethosuximide is not protein bound. It is completely metabolized, principally by hydroxylation to inactive metabolites. The drug has a half-life of approximately 40 hours, although values from 18 to 72 hours have been reported.

Therapeutic Levels and Dose. Therapeutic levels of 60 to 100 micrograms per ml can be achieved in adults with doses of 750 to 1500 mg per day, although lower or higher doses may be necessary. Some authors report that higher levels (up to 125 micrograms per ml) are needed in certain patients to achieve efficacy; such patients may tolerate the drug without apparent toxicity at these levels. The drug might be administered as a single daily dose were it not for its gastrointestinal side effects; twice-a-day dosage is common. The time of day at which the level is measured is not particularly important for ethosuximide, as its half-life is relatively long. No parenteral dosage form is available.

Toxicity. The most common dose-related side effect of ethosuximide is gastric distress, including pain, nausea, and vomiting. This can often be avoided by starting therapy at a low dose, with gradual increases to the therapeutic range. When the side effect does occur, temporary dosage reductions may allow adaptation. Other dose-related side effects include transient lethargy or fatigue and, much less commonly, headache, dizziness, and hiccups. Non–dose-related side effects of ethosuximide are extremely uncommon.

Drug Interactions. Administration of ethosuximide with valproic acid results in higher steady-state concentrations caused by inhibition of metabolism. No other important drug interactions have been reported.

Valproic Acid (Depakene)

Seizure Type. Valproic acid (valproate) is effective against absence seizures and might be con-

sidered the drug of choice in this seizure type were it not for its hepatotoxicity. Because of this toxicity, ethosuximide is preferred. Valproic acid is unique in its ability to control certain types of myoclonic seizures; in some cases, the effect is dramatic. The drug is effective against generalized tonic-clonic seizures, and a few patients with atonic attacks may also respond. There is no evidence from controlled clinical trials that the drug is effective in partial seizures or infantile spasms.

Pharmacokinetics. Valproic acid is well absorbed after an oral dose, with bioavailability greater than 80 per cent. Peak blood levels are observed within 2 hours. Food may delay absorption, and decreased toxicity may result if the drug is given after meals. The drug is also 90 per cent bound to plasma proteins. No active metabolites have been clearly documented.

The enteric-coated tablet (Depakote) is the preferred foundation. This product, a 1:1 mixture of valproic acid and sodium valproate, is absorbed much more slowly. Peak concentrations after administration of the enteric-coated tablets are seen in 3 to 4 hours. The sodium salt is also used, in syrup, primarily for pediatric use.

Therapeutic Levels and Dose. Doses of 25 to 30 mg per kg per day may be adequate in some patients, but others may require 60 mg per kg or even more. Therapeutic levels of valproic acid range from 50 to 100 micrograms per ml. The drug should not be abandoned until morning trough levels of at least 80 micrograms per ml have been attained; some patients may require and may tolerate levels in excess of 100 micrograms per ml.

Toxicity. The most common dose-related side effects of valproic acid are nausea, vomiting, and other gastrointestinal complaints such as abdominal pain and heartburn. The drug should be started gradually to avoid these symptoms; a temporary reduction in dose can usually alleviate the problems. Sedation is uncommon with valproic acid alone but may be striking when valproic acid is added to phenobarbital. A fine tremor is frequently seen at higher levels. Other reversible side effects, seen in a small number of patients, include weight gain, increased appetite, and hair loss.

The idiosyncratic toxicity of valproic acid is largely limited to hepatotoxicity, but this may be severe. In most cases, the patients are also taking other antiepileptic drugs. Initial serum glutamic-oxaloacetic transaminase values may not be elevated in susceptible patients, although these levels eventually become abnormal. Most fatalities have occurred within 4 months after initiation of therapy. Careful monitoring of liver function is obviously mandatory when starting the drug; the hepatotoxicity is reversible in some cases if the drug is withdrawn. The incidence of hepatotoxic deaths related to valproic acid (Figure 1) is fortunately decreasing, for reasons that are unclear. The other observed idiosyncratic response with valproic acid is thrombocytopenia, although documented cases of abnormal bleeding are lacking. Reports suggest an increased incidence of spina bifida in the offspring of women who take the drug during pregnancy.

Drug Interactions. Because of its avid binding, valproic acid displaces phenytoin from plasma proteins. In addition to binding interactions, valproic acid inhibits the metabolism of several drugs, including phenobarbital, phenytoin, and carbamazepine, leading to higher steady-state concentrations.

Other Antiepileptic Drugs

The following antiepileptic drugs have occasional specialized uses, but most are second line drugs whose utility in therapy is quite limited. The exceptions are those benzodiazepines used in the acute treatment of status epilepticus.

Succinimides

Phensuximide (Milontin) and methsuximide (Celontin) were developed and marketed before ethosuximide. They are used primarily as anti–absence seizure drugs. Methsuximide is generally considered to be more toxic—and phensuximide much less effective—than ethosuximide. Methsuximide has been used for partial seizures by

some investigators. The desmethyl metabolite of methsuximide has a half-life of 25 hours or more and exerts the major antiepileptic effect.

Oxazolidinediones

Trimethadione (Tridione), the first oxazolidinedione, was introduced as an antiepileptic drug in 1945 and remained the drug of choice for absence seizures until the introduction of succinimides in the 1950s. The use of the oxazolidinediones (trimethadione, paramethadione, and dimethadione) is now limited, primarily because of their toxic side effects.

Hydantoins Other Than Phenytoin

Three congeners of phenytoin are marketed in the United States and are used to a limited extent. These are mephenytoin (Mesantoin), ethotoin (Peganone), and phenacemide (Phenurone).

Mephenytoin and ethotoin, like phenytoin, appear to be most effective against generalized tonic-clonic seizures and partial seizures. The incidence of severe reactions such as dermatitis, agranulocytosis, or hepatitis is higher for mephenytoin than for phenytoin. Ethotoin may be recommended for patients who are hypersensitive to phenytoin, but larger doses are required. Therapeutic levels of mephenytoin range from 5 to 16 micrograms per ml, and levels above 20 micrograms per ml are considered toxic. Therapeutic blood levels of its active metabolite, nirvanol, are between 25 and 40 micrograms per ml. A therapeutic range for ethotoin has not been established.

Phenacemide, the straight-chain analogue of

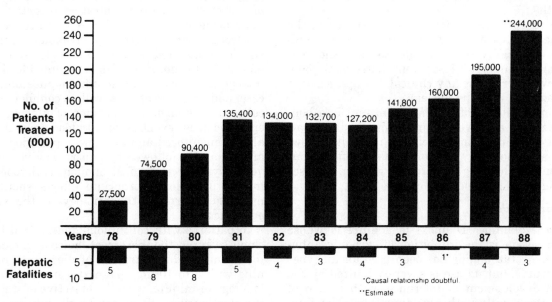

Figure 1. Increasing use of valproic acid in the United States versus the decline in reported hepatic fatalities, 1978–1988. Data from 1988 are estimated. (From Porter RJ: Epilepsy: 100 Elementary Principles, 2nd ed. London, Bailliere Tindall, 1989.)

phenytoin, is a toxic drug of last resort for refractory partial seizures. It is well absorbed and completely metabolized. The relationship between blood levels and effect has not been established. Serious and sometimes fatal side effects have been reported in association with the use of phenacemide.

Benzodiazepines

Diazepam (Valium) used intravenously is the drug of choice for stopping continuous seizure activity, especially generalized tonic-clonic status epilepticus. The drug is marketed as an adjunct to therapy and is occasionally given orally on a chronic basis, although it is not considered to be effective in this application, probably because of the rapid development of tolerance.

Lorazepam (Ativan) is a newer benzodiazepine that, when given intravenously, is an alternative to diazepam in the treatment of status epilepticus.

Clonazepam (Klonopin) is a long-acting drug with documented efficacy against absence seizures and one of the most potent antiepileptic agents known. It is also effective in some cases of myoclonic seizures. Sedation is prominent, especially on initiation of therapy; starting doses should be small. Maximal tolerated doses are usually in the range of 0.1 to 0.2 mg per kg, but many weeks of a gradually increasing daily dosage may be needed to achieve these doses in some patients. Therapeutic blood levels are usually less than 0.1 microgram per ml and are not routinely measured in most laboratories. As with other benzodiazepines that are chronically administered, tolerance often develops within a few months.

Nitrazepam (Mogadon) is not marketed in the United States but is used in many other countries, especially for infantile spasms and myoclonic seizures. It is less potent than clonazepam, and whether it has any clinical advantages over clonazepam remains unclear.

Clorazepate dipotassium (Tranxene) is a benzodiazepine approved as an adjunct in the treatment of complex partial seizures in adults. Drowsiness and lethargy are common side effects, but as long as the drug is increased gradually, doses as high as 45 mg per day can be given.

Acetazolamide

Acetazolamide (Diamox) is a diuretic whose main action is the inhibition of carbonic anhydrase. Acetazolamide has been used for all types of seizures, but its use is severely limited by the rapid development of tolerance, with return of seizures usually within a few weeks. The drug may have a special role in epileptic women who experience seizure exacerbations at the time of menses; seizure control may be improved and tolerance may not develop because the drug is not administered continuously. The usual dose is approximately 10 mg per kg up to a maximum of 1000 mg per day.

Bromide

Although largely discarded, bromide is still occasionally useful, such as in management of epilepsy in patients with porphyria, in whom other drugs may be contraindicated. Its half-life is approximately 12 days, and it is given in doses of 3 to 6 grams per day in adults to obtain plasma levels of 10 to 20 mEq per liter. Major toxic problems are unfortunately frequent, including rashes, sedation, and behavioral changes.

Generalized Tonic-Clonic Status Epilepticus

The treatment of generalized tonic-clonic (grand mal) status epilepticus depends on the severity of the presentation. Occasionally, patients present with persistent, or nearly persistent, tonic-clonic activity that is bilateral and severe. Control of such seizure activity demands minute-to-minute emergency efforts. More commonly, patients present with a short history of a series of tonic-clonic seizures; perhaps one attack has been observed by the emergency room physician. The seizures are separated by prolonged stuporous periods. These periods may be the predominant clinical presentation when the seizures are separated by intervals of 20 to 40 minutes or more. In either case, certain life support measures are necessary. These include maintenance of satisfactory cardiorespiratory function and monitoring of respiration, blood pressure, and the electrocardiogram. An intravenous catheter should be inserted, and blood samples should be obtained for chemistry tests, including blood urea nitrogen, electrolytes, calcium, magnesium, glucose, and drug screens, as well as complete blood cell counts and determinations of plasma antiepileptic drug levels. Arterial blood gases should also be monitored and an airway provided. Usually, thiamine followed by glucose is given intravenously, especially if alcoholism or hypoglycemia is possible. Appropriate efforts should be made to determine the etiology of the status epilepticus.

In patients with continuous generalized tonic-clonic seizures, the therapy of choice is immediate intravenous administration of diazepam, beginning with 5 to 10 mg, given at a maximum rate of 5 mg per minute, with the objective of stopping the attacks; up to 20 mg can be given to an adult. Alternatively, lorazepam can be given, up to a total of 8 mg. As soon as the tonic-clonic activity has momentarily ceased, loading should begin with an intravenous injection of phenytoin (see later discussion of precautions). The anticonvulsant effect of intravenously administered diazepam is relatively short—usually only 20 to 30 minutes—but highly effective in most cases. The drug does have a sedative effect, like other benzodiazepines, and this effect long outlasts the anticonvulsant activity. Respiratory depression occurs, especially in the presence of barbiturates. Bradycardia and hypotension also complicate therapy.

If the attacks cease temporarily or if the patient has status epilepticus with prolonged stuporous periods between attacks, intravenous injection of phenytoin should be started immediately. In patients who experience status epilepticus with prolonged periods between attacks (sometimes called "serial seizures"), benzodiazepines may be avoided entirely. Thus, the patient's already depressed consciousness is not further depressed by a sedative antiepileptic drug. Phenytoin has the outstanding advantage of being nonsedative in a setting where depression of consciousness may greatly decrease the opportunity to obtain information from the neurologic examination. If the patient does not respond to diazepam and phenytoin, phenobarbital should be given intravenously. Doses as high as 18 mg per kg—1000 to 1500 mg in adults—may be required. Respiratory depression and hypotension are common, especially at high doses, and especially if benzodiazepines have recently been administered; endotracheal intubation should usually be done at or before this step in therapy. Some patients simply do not respond to intravenous doses of diazepam, phenytoin, or phenobarbital, and other drugs such as paraldehyde may be tried. Paraldehyde can be given intravenously in a dose of 5 to 10 ml diluted in 50 ml of normal saline. Paraldehyde can cause metabolic acidosis, pulmonary hemorrhage, and cardiovascular depression. Other drugs such as intravenous lidocaine, rectal valproic acid, or carbamazepine are not recommended; they are rarely effective. When intravenous phenytoin and phenobarbital fail to control the status, most neurologists now prefer to move directly to general anesthesia. General anesthesia stops brain function, and treatment of status epilepticus may occasionally require its use. Pentobarbital is generally used, and pharmacologic support of blood pressure is routine.

Although the intravenous use of phenytoin is now standard, either to achieve a loading dose (when oral intake is not possible) or to treat status epilepticus, precautions are required.

1. Do not exceed a 50 mg per minute infusion rate. Administration at 25 mg per minute is an excellent way to decrease the likelihood of acute toxicity even further. The risk is generally much higher in older patients and patients with a history of cardiac arrhythmias, hypotension, or compromised pulmonary function.

2. Use a cardiac monitor. Because cardiac arrhythmias from either phenytoin or the vehicle propylene glycol are the most likely form of acute toxicity, monitoring of the cardiac rhythm is indicated and helps to provide an early warning of cardiotoxicity.

3. Take the blood pressure every 2 to 4 minutes during the infusion. Acute hypotension is an indication to slow or discontinue the infusion.

4. Direct intravenous injection is preferable to slower infusion by intravenous drip. When mixed with intravenous solutions, phenytoin precipitates as the pH is lowered during the dilution process. Never mix phenytoin with glucose-containing solutions, as precipitation is much more rapid and extensive. When phenytoin is to be given by intravenous drip, 1 gram of phenytoin should be mixed with 200 ml of physiologic saline.

5. Aim for a total dose of approximately 20 mg per kg. One of the most important errors is to give an inadequate dose and then to conclude prematurely that the drug is ineffective. In status epilepticus, the chief concerns with intravenously administered phenytoin are the cardiotoxic symptoms during the acute period of administration, rather than the toxicity that results from giving an excessive total dose. The latter can be alleviated by a reduction in dose after the acute period, and in most patients in whom intravenous administration of phenytoin is indicated, temporary dose-related ataxia is not a problem because they are likely to be confined to bed. Monitoring plasma phenytoin levels can be extremely useful throughout the entire treatment process and can help to indicate when maintenance therapy should be instituted. Usually such therapy should begin about 12 hours after the loading dose has been given.

Finally, for patients who are awake and can take medication by mouth, oral administration of phenytoin is an effective way to give a loading dose. With oral administration, therapeutic levels can be reached within a few hours—not fast enough for the treatment of status epilepticus, but sufficient for many nonurgent problems.

Pregnancy and Epilepsy

One of the most controversial subjects related to epilepsy is the proper management of pregnant epileptic patients and their offspring. The complex issues are summarized in a few statements:

1. Pregnancy virtually never causes epilepsy, except as a complication of other neurologic insults, such as cerebral sinus thrombosis.

2. Epilepsy occasionally worsens with pregnancy. About one-half of the patients with epilepsy who become pregnant have no change in seizure frequency, but the remaining patients are more likely to have worsening than improvement. The chief factors in increased seizure frequency during pregnancy seem to be poor compliance with medication schedules and altered absorption or metabolism of drugs.

3. Eclampsia does not cause epilepsy, although seizures may occur during severe eclampsia. The seizures do not persist after delivery and recovery from the metabolic disturbances.

4. Status epilepticus does not occur more frequently during pregnancy.

5. Pregnancy may change the pharmacologic action of antiepileptic drugs and involve alterations in absorption, plasma protein binding, metabolism, and volume of distribution. If a change occurs, it usually consists of a fall in plasma drug levels, which return to normal after delivery. The only sure way to maintain seizure control is to monitor the plasma drug levels more frequently during pregnancy and immediately after delivery.

6. Fetal abnormalities are slightly more frequent if the mother has epilepsy. Overall, a twofold or threefold increase in the risk of fetal abnormalities is the current consensus. If the usual rate of abnormalities is considered to be 2 per cent, the likelihood may be 4 to 6 per cent in such children.

Compliance

Noncompliance is the principal cause of uncontrolled seizures. Poor compliance with the physician's instructions regarding medication is not a problem unique to epilepsy; it is a difficulty encountered in any chronic disease for which daily therapy is indicated. The typical patient with infrequent seizures forgets, for many reasons, to take the medications and thereby continues to have seizures. The frustrated physician prescribes higher and higher doses of drugs, observing neither toxic effects nor seizure control. Then, if the patient suddenly becomes compliant, toxicity occurs swiftly; the physician is dumbfounded and the patient disillusioned. A concerted effort by the physician may be required to control this problem.

Drug Cessation

Drug cessation is controversial and not always successful. The discontinuation of medication in patients who have been seizure free for some time is a complex medical issue, as the heterogeneity of epilepsy renders decisions about drug discontinuation difficult. After 3 or 4 years without a seizure, most patients—especially if they are taking more than one antiepileptic drug—deserve an attempt at gradual discontinuation of medications. However, the matter remains complex for the individual patient. The patient may have drugs withdrawn at the most conservative rate, with the most frequent, benign EEG follow-up, and with meticulous documentation of the seizure-free state during the process of withdrawal, only to crash with a flurry of seizures as the ultimate goal seems within the grasp of patient and physician. How is the physician to know when drugs are no longer needed and what process should be used for their withdrawal? First, the physician must be candid with the patient and admit the uncertainty of the prognosis. Second, as remission is clearly possible in some patients, a trial of gradual drug removal is reasonable after some seizure-free years. Possibly important variables include EEG findings, seizure types (and their combinations), age at onset of seizures, duration of epilepsy, and presence of neurologic dysfunction. The impetus for decreasing and stopping antiepileptic drugs is their chronic long-term toxicity; the anxiety of withdrawal is caused by the patient's fear of seizure recurrence. At this time, individualization of the decision is the best that can be offered the patient.

EPILEPSY IN INFANTS AND CHILDREN

method of
EILEEN P. G. VINING, M.D.
Johns Hopkins Hospital
Baltimore, Maryland

A seizure is a sudden, paroxysmal electrical discharge of neurons in the brain. For us to make the clinical diagnosis of a seizure, this electrical discharge must recruit sufficient surrounding neurons to alter the child's function or behavior. Epilepsy is generally defined as recurring, unprovoked seizures. In recent years, careful attention has been paid to classification of seizures (Table 1) and more recently to classification of the epilepsy syndromes (Table 2). Since etiology, therapy, and prognosis depend upon proper recognition of the disorder, this classification scheme is of great importance.

TABLE 1. Seizure Classification

International Classification	"Old Terms"
I. Partial Seizures	Focal or local seizures
A. Simple partial seizures (consciousness not impaired)	Focal motor seizures
1. With motor symptoms	Jacksonian seizures
2. With somatosensory or special sensory symptoms	Focal sensory seizures
3. With autonomic symptoms	
4. With psychic symptoms	
B. Complex partial seizures (with impairment of consciousness)	Psychomotor seizures
1. Simple partial onset	Temporal lobe seizures
2. With impairment of consciousness at onset	Petit mal seizures
C. Partial seizures that secondarily generalize	
II. Generalized Seizures (Convulsive or Nonconvulsive)	
A. Absence seizures	
1. Absence	
2. Atypical	
B. Myoclonic seizures	Minor motor seizures
C. Clonic seizures	Grand mal seizures
D. Tonic seizures	Grand mal seizures
E. Tonic-clonic seizures	Grand mal seizures
F. Atonic seizures (astatic)	Akinetic, drop attacks

TREATMENT

Why Seizures Are Treated

Prophylactic medication is prescribed because of fear of the consequences of seizure recurrence, including the fear of neurologic and physical injury. There are no data to support the concept that a few seizures are linked to intellectual deterioration or any other form of neurologic damage, nor is there convincing evidence in humans of seizures begetting seizures. Although

TABLE 2. Classification of the Epilepsy Syndromes

1. Localization-related epilepsies
   Benign rolandic
   Benign occipital
2. Generalized epilepsies
   Age related (benign neonatal convulsion, West's syndrome, childhood absence, benign juvenile myoclonic epilepsy)
3. Undetermined (? focal or generalized)
4. Special syndromes
   Chronic progressive epilepsia partialis continua in children

sudden, unexplained death is somewhat more frequent in persons with epilepsy, there are no data to suggest that therapy reduces this occurrence. Obviously there is a risk of physical injury if a seizure should occur in a dangerous or unsupervised setting. The greatest motivation to treat is because of the fear of the psychosocial consequences of recurrence. These risks are best managed by appropriate counseling concerning the nature of seizures, by minimizing the risk of physical or neurologic consequences, and by avoiding overprotection of the child.

A seizure should be treated when the risk of recurrence and the consequences of that recurrence are clearly greater than the risk of treatment and the consequences of daily prophylactic therapy.

Recent data suggest that an individual with a first seizure, on average, has a 30 per cent chance of having a second seizure. Children with absence seizures, myoclonic seizures, or atonic seizures routinely have had multiple seizures prior to consultation with the physician and will continue to do so unless treated. There is increasing evidence that in children who have had a generalized idiopathic tonic-clonic seizure with a normal electroencephalogram (EEG), the recurrence rate is as low as 15 per cent. However, recurrence rate after a second seizure is closer to 75 per cent.

The Treatment Plan

The decision to treat should be made *after* a discussion of the risk/benefit ratio with the patient and family. This includes the risks of seizure recurrence, the benefit of prophylaxis, and the risks and possible side effects of the medications. The treatment plan must be described to the patient and family to ensure their understanding and knowledgeable participation (Table 3). The diagnosis must be certain, since the choice of anticonvulsant is based primarily on the type of seizure (Table 4). This choice also is influenced by possible side effects. In some children, the possible cosmetic side effects of phenytoin (Dilantin) would not be a concern, whereas in others it would be very undesirable. Many medications (carbamazepine* [Tegretol], primidone [Mysoline], valproic acid [Depakene, Depakote]) must be started at suboptimal doses to avoid immediate side effects. The amount of drug is then increased until the desired goal is achieved. That goal is control of seizures without toxicity. Toxicity means evidence of clinical dysfunction and not

---

*Safety and efficacy for use in children under 6 years of age have not been established.

TABLE 3. Treatment

1. Discuss plan with patient and/or parent.
2. Be sure of diagnosis and classification
3. Choose the most appropriate drug; consider seizure type and possible side effects.
4. Increase the drug dose until control of seizures is achieved or there is clinical toxicity (not just high serum levels).
5. If the drug is not effective (i.e., if there is not control of seizures without side effects), add a second drug. When it is in therapeutic range, slowly discontinue first drug. ACHIEVE MONOTHERAPY.
6. MONITOR THOROUGHLY.
7. Provide support, counseling, and education.
8. If seizures are controlled for 2 years, consider tapering off drug.

simply high serum levels. If the drug is not effective, the drug of second choice should be added. When the second drug is in therapeutic range, the first drug should be tapered and discontinued. This will lead to the use of monotherapy. Increasing data indicate that monotherapy has many advantages including equal efficacy, fewer side effects, and easier monitoring. Also it frequently allows less costly treatment of seizures.

Once the medication regimen has been established, monitoring of the patient is essential, not only to be certain that the seizures are controlled but, more important, to ascertain that there are no unwanted side effects. This requires going beyond the traditional monitoring of hematologic and hepatic side effects to ensure that physical appearance, motor coordination, learning, and behavior are not being adversely affected. Frequently, the physician will have to rely on more than his or her own observation of the patient, and it may be necessary to carefully question both parents and school regarding any changes they may perceive in the child.

The therapeutic plan must include an awareness that seizures may not occur forever. Probably 70 to 75 per cent of children will ultimately have their seizures completely controlled. Once the seizures have been controlled for 2 or more years, it is reasonable to consider discontinuation of medication. Recent studies show that children who have been seizure free for 2 or more years have a 75 per cent chance of remaining seizure free when medication is discontinued. The children who appear to have the greatest likelihood of nonrecurrence are those who have a recent normal EEG.

A therapeutic plan is not complete without

TABLE 4. Antiepileptic Drug Therapy for Children

Drug	Indications	Usual Dose (mg/kg/day)	Usual Dosage Schedule	Half-life (hr)	Therapeutic Range (μg/ml)	Side Effects
Carbamazepine* (Tegretol)	F, C, G	10–40	bid–qid	10–30	5–14	Headache, drowsiness, dizziness, diplopia, blood dyscrasia, hepatotoxicity, arrhythmia
Clonazepam (Klonopin)	M, A	0.05–0.10	bid–qid	24–36		Drowsiness, ataxia, secretions, hypotonia, behavioral problems
Ethosuximide (Zarontin)	A (? C, M)	20–40	bid	24–42	40–100	GI distress, rash, drowsiness, dizziness, SLE, blood dyscrasia
Phenobarbital	F, C, G, S	2–8	qd–bid	48–100	10–25	Drowsiness, rash, ataxia, behavioral and cognitive problems
Phenytoin (Dilantin)	F, C, G, S	4–8	qd–bid	6–30	10–20	Drowsiness, gum hyperplasia, rash, anemia, ataxia, hirsutism, folate deficiency, teratogenicity
Primidone (Mysoline)	F, C, G	12–25	bid–qid	6–12	6–12	Drowsiness, dizziness, rash, anemia, ataxia, diplopia
Valproic acid (Depakene, Depakote)	F, C, G, M, A	10–60	bid–qid	6–18	50–100	GI distress, hepatitis, alopecia, drowsiness, ataxia, tremors, pancreatitis, thrombocytopenia

*Safety and efficacy for use in children have not been established.

Abbreviations: F = focal (partial-simple); G = generalized (tonic-clonic); C = partial-complex; A = absence; M = minor motor (akinetic, atonic, myoclonic); S = status; GI = gastrointestinal; SLE = systemic lupus erythematosus.

dealing with the informational, psychosocial, and emotional needs of the patient and family. This may require considerable counseling that can be augmented by the Epilepsy Foundation of America; the family may request information by calling 800–EFA–1000.

Seizure Types and Epilepsies

Generalized Tonic-Clonic Seizures

The standard anticonvulsants are phenobarbital, phenytoin, carbamazepine,* and valproic acid. Phenobarbital is inexpensive and well known to pediatricians. Its major disadvantages are hyperactivity, behavioral disorders, cognitive difficulties, and sleep disorders in at least 30 to 40 per cent of children. Data indicate that many patients experience more subtle alterations in learning and behavior. If phenobarbital is used, it is mandatory that the physician pay careful attention to any adverse changes in the child. Phenytoin is also an effective anticonvulsant, but changes in appearance and gingival hyperplasia may occur in up to 90 per cent of children. One must also recall that phenytoin has nonlinear kinetics. As the therapeutic range is approached, small increases in dosage may cause dramatic increases in serum drug levels. Carbamazepine appears to have fewer adverse effects on neuropsychologic function than other drugs. This drug has a fairly short half-life and may need to be given as frequently as four times a day in order to smooth the peak and trough levels. Aplastic anemia associated with carbamazepine use is extremely rare and apparently cannot be predicted by routine hematologic monitoring. On the other hand, neutropenia is more frequent but rarely produces clinical problems. Valproic acid is useful in generalized seizures and also appears to have minimal effects on neuropsychologic function or behavior. It also has a short half-life. The hepatic side effects of sodium valproate are quite rare but are more frequent in children less than 2 years of age who are receiving polytherapy. Children over 11 years of age and on monotherapy have had no hepatic failures reported.

Partial Seizures

Both simple and complex partial seizures can be effectively treated by phenobarbital, phenytoin, carbamazepine,* and primidone. Primidone is readily converted to phenobarbital. Prior to conversion, primidone and another active metabolite (phenylethylmalonamide) are also active anticonvulsants. Primidone has many of the side effects of phenobarbital and in addition has significant initial toxicity, requiring that it be introduced at very low doses and increased in small increments. Valproic acid may be helpful in treating partial complex seizures, especially when there is a significant element of absence. In addition, if the partial seizures secondarily generalize, valproic acid is a useful medication.

Absence Seizures

Absence seizures are best treated with either succinamides or sodium valproate. Valproate is probably more effective in atypical absence seizures and would certainly be preferred when a patient has both absence and tonic-clonic seizures. Ethosuximide (Zarontin) is effective in classic absence seizures; side effects include headaches and nausea. Benzodiazepines are frequently used as adjunctive drugs. These drugs include clonazepam (Klonopin), clorazepate (Tranxene), and lorazepam (Ativan).* It is discouraging that the benzodiazepines are effective initially but decrease in efficacy over time. Side effects may be quite intolerable and include sedation, behavior changes, and at times difficulty handling secretions.

Myoclonic and Atonic Seizures

Valproic acid is the drug of choice for these seizures. The benzodiazepines also may be effective. The ketogenic diet can play an important role in controlling these seizures. The diet involves fasting the child into ketosis and maintaining this ketosis chronically by using a diet containing a high portion of ketogenic foods (fats). The diet usually consists of a ratio of 4 grams of fat to 1 gram of protein plus carbohydrate, making a 40-calorie unit. Children require 60 to 75 calories per kg per day and at least 1 gram per kg per day of protein. Fluids are restricted to 600 to 1200 ml per day. The diet is deficient in calcium and fat-soluble vitamins and requires supplementation with 1 gram, twice daily, of calcium carbonate and multivitamins with minerals and iron. The child is monitored by examining urinary ketones; the level should be high, especially late in the afternoon.

Febrile Seizures

Febrile seizures occur in 3 to 4 per cent of all children, most commonly between 9 and 20 months of age; 30 to 40 per cent will experience a recurrence. Even with recurrence, there is no increased risk of mental retardation, cerebral palsy, or other significant neurologic sequelae. Only children with two or more risk factors are

---

*Safety and efficacy for use in children under 6 years of age have not been established.

*This use is not listed in the manufacturer's directive.

at a significantly increased risk for epilepsy. These factors include atypical febrile seizure (i.e., lasting longer than 15 minutes, recurring within 24 hours, or focal in nature), a first-degree relative with a history of epilepsy, and abnormal neurodevelopmental status prior to the first febrile seizure. Even with two or more of these risk factors, the risk of afebrile seizures does not exceed 13 per cent.

Therefore, the use of prophylactic therapy should be considered only in the face of these risk factors or multiple recurrences. Daily phenobarbital, at a dosage that maintains blood levels of greater than 15 micrograms per ml, will reduce recurrence. However, this therapy frequently produces the previously mentioned behavioral changes. Valproic acid is apparently effective but potentially too toxic to consider for use. For temperatures greater than 38.5° C, rectal diazepam (Valium) (not available in the United States), 0.5 mg per kg every 8 hours, is also reported to be effective, producing only mild sedation. The intravenous preparation of diazepam can be substituted. *Normally we do not recommend prophylactic therapy for children with febrile seizures.*

Neonatal Seizures

Neonatal seizures are the most reliable predictor of later neurologic deficit. However, the majority of infants with neonatal seizures who survive do well. The most important therapy is the search for the cause and the appropriate treatment. If the neonatal seizures are recurrent or appear to significantly threaten or interfere with the child's well-being, therapy with anticonvulsants is utilized.

Phenobarbital is the drug of choice, with a loading dose of 20 mg per kg intravenously as a slow bolus or in divided doses over a short period of time. Phenytoin can also be used, again with a loading dose of 20 mg per kg. Diazepam is a useful agent in its rapidity of action; however, it has a short half-life. It can be used at a dose of 0.2 to 0.5 mg per kg. Concern regarding its diluent does not appear to be warranted any longer. Frequently, we will treat an infant with a loading dose of phenobarbital. If this is effective and ongoing insult to the brain does not appear to be occurring, we will not place the child on maintenance phenobarbital. The long half-life (approximately 100 hours) can be expected to protect the infant over the period of recovery from asphyxia.

Infantile Spasms

These seizures classically consist of sudden flexion of the head, abduction and extension of the arms, and simultaneous flexion of the knees. These are the only type of seizures that occur in series or clusters. Frequently the EEG pattern will be that of hypsarrhythmia. Prognosis is generally poor for this group, especially in the two-thirds who are considered symptomatic and who are experiencing these seizures owing to a definable underlying pathology.

Treatment should begin promptly since there is some indication that earlier therapy leads to better outcome. ACTH gel, given 10 to 40 units intramuscularly twice daily, is the treatment of choice, although variations, including higher doses and alternate-day therapy, have been reported to be successful. Prednisone, 2 mg per kg or 75 mg per M², may be equally effective, but is not used as the first therapy in our center. Duration of treatment varies from 2 weeks to many months. We treat for 4 to 6 weeks and then begin to taper. Side effects of ACTH or prednisone are almost universal and include hypertension and susceptibility to infection. Behavioral disturbances, including severe irritability and transient decrease in psychomotor performance, are not uncommon. Valproic acid and benzodiazepines may also be effective.

Lennox-Gastaut Syndrome

The Lennox-Gastaut syndrome consists of an EEG pattern of slow spike waves and rapid spikes, two or more types of seizures (one of which is usually myoclonic or atonic), and mental retardation. Onset is usually between 1 and 6 years of age and may frequently be seen as part of an evolution from infantile spasms. Valproic acid is the treatment of choice but often must be used with additional anticonvulsants. We find the ketogenic diet particularly helpful in this seizure disorder.

Benign Rolandic Epilepsy

This benign form of epilepsy generally begins between 3 and 13 years of age and consists of seizures characterized by facial movements, grimacing, and vocalization, followed by a tonic-clonic component. The EEG frequently shows characteristic repetitive spikes in the midtemporal or parietal area. It is generally much worse in non–rapid eye movement sleep. Seizures are quite benign and often occur only at night. Often anticonvulsant medication is not necessary. When necessary, carbamazepine appears to be the drug of choice.

Juvenile Myoclonic Epilepsy of Janz

This disorder begins in late childhood or early adulthood with mild myoclonic seizures, often on awakening. These may then lead to tonic-clonic or absence seizures. This seizure disorder is particularly sensitive to valproic acid.

Status Epilepticus

While brief tonic-clonic seizures almost certainly do not cause brain damage, there is fear that status epilepticus, or seizures lasting more than 30 minutes, may be a threat to the integrity of the central nervous system, as well as to life itself. In treating status epilepticus, there is a fine line between aggressive therapy to stop the seizures and the production of iatrogenic problems requiring intubation and ventilation and the potential morbidity associated with these complications. Before medications are given, maintenance of vital functions should be established, including adequate aeration and monitoring of vital signs. An intravenous line should be placed to obtain blood for appropriate studies and to administer glucose (as necessary) as well as anticonvulsant drugs. Diazepam is usually the initial drug of choice because of low toxicity and rapid onset of action. It is given as 0.2 to 0.5 mg per kg over a 2-minute period with a maximum single dose of 10 mg. The dose may be repeated in 10 minutes if the seizure persists. This can also be done using rectal diazepam.* Lorazepam,† 0.05 to 0.10 mg per kg (4 mg maximum), is increasingly being utilized as an alternative because of its longer duration of action. Because diazepam is effective for only a short time, the child should also be treated with an intravenous loading dose of phenytoin or phenobarbital. A loading dose of 15 to 20 mg per kg of phenytoin is infused at a rate not to exceed 50 mg per minute, or phenobarbital can be given in a loading dose of 15 to 20 mg per kg. Simultaneous electrocardiographic and blood pressure monitoring is mandatory. Maintenance dosages should be begun within 6 to 8 hours.

Surgical Therapy

Medical therapy is effective in perhaps 75 per cent of children. However, in those individuals whose seizures are intractable and/or who are experiencing life-altering side effects, the search for identifiably abnormal tissue and the potential for surgical remediation should be considered. This frequently requires intensive monitoring to determine the exact focus of the seizure activity. Sometimes a subdural electrode grid is necessary, enabling the clinician to identify the source of the seizure as well as areas that should be spared to preserve important neurologic functions (e.g.,

movement and speech). In addition, some youngsters have progressive disease of a single hemisphere due to developmental abnormalities, trauma, or Rasmussen's encephalitis. These children should be considered for hemispherectomy.

HEADACHES

method of
JOEL R. SAPER, M.D.
Michigan Headache and Neurological Institute
Ann Arbor, Michigan

Headache is a pervasive and widespread illness, estimated to affect more than 70 per cent of American households. Over 300 medical illnesses can produce headache. The most troubling and chronic of the headache conditions are those referred to as primary headaches, which are characterized by the absence of structural pathology or systemic disease.

PRIMARY HEADACHE DISORDERS

As the perspectives on chronic headache change, the "headache villains" of the past hundred years—the blood vessels and muscles—are coming to be seen more as accomplices. The central hypothesis, which is supported by the current understanding of brain mechanisms, advances the premise that chronic recurring headaches (primary headache disorders) arise in part, if not exclusively, from fundamental disturbances in neuronal, neurotransmitter, receptor, or nerve function. The peripheral muscular or vascular activity is secondary to the central and primary disturbances; as a result, changing attitudes to headache treatment have evolved.

Treatment

The treatment of patients with chronic recurring headache is enhanced by conveying a sincere interest in their distress and by establishing worthwhile and frank communication. Although emotional factors are at times important, psychologic and stress-related factors have been overemphasized as the etiologic basis for headache. Presumptive and premature emphasis on psychologic elements is counterproductive and may prevent recognition of the important physiologic changes, usually inherited, that most experts now believe predispose patients to this disorder.

Nonmedical Management

Nonmedical management of headache requires the identification and, if possible, the elimination

---

*Rectal diazepam is not available in the United States.
†This use is not listed in the manufacturer's directive.

TABLE 1. Migraine-Provoking Influences

Psychologic	Localized or generalized in-
Stress/anxiety	fection
Anger	
Let-down	Dietary
Exhilaration	
	Medicines
Dazzling light	Reserpine
	Hydralazine
Hormonal	MAOIs*
Menarche	Nonsteroidal anti-inflam-
Menstruation	matory agents*
Menopause	Vasodilators*
Pregnancy (first trimester)	Antiasthmatic agents
Delivery	Thiazide derivatives
Birth control pills	Propranolol*
Exogenous estrogens	Amphetamines, diet pills
	Ephedrine
Sleep	
Too much	Marked weather changes
Too little	
Napping	Head/neck trauma
	Mild
Toxins	Severe
	Smoking

*May also be of benefit.

of provoking influences (Tables 1 and 2). Often, interventions such as biofeedback and stress management are very important in treatment of patients. Stopping smoking has proved valuable in the treatment of many apparently refractory headache cases; discontinuance of smoking reduces nicotine and carbon monoxide effects, both of which may produce headache. Perhaps the most important of all nonmedical approaches is the elimination of daily or almost daily use of symptomatic medicines such as analgesics or ergotamine tartrate. It is now apparent that too frequent use of ergotamine tartrate or analgesics (more often than 2 days per week) may accentuate headache frequency. Discontinuance of excessively used symptomatic medications may be basic to control and prevention.

Simultaneously present medical conditions, particularly those along the distribution of the trigeminal nerve, can aggravate pre-existing pri-

mary headache disorders. Therefore, careful evaluation of dental pathology and treatment of disorders such as microabscesses, moderate to severe temporomandibular joint dysfunction, and cracked teeth, as well as treatment of sinus disease or other disturbances about the head and neck, can have a marked beneficial effect on primary headache control.

MIGRAINE HEADACHES

Although traditionally classified into common and classic forms, differences of opinion exist as to whether classic migraine (with a preheadache neurologic aura) and common migraine (without a distinct, identifiable neurologic aura) are different entities. Moreover, it is now apparent that in many individuals, the intermittent migraine during the early course of their headache years "transforms" or evolves from the intermittent pattern to a daily or almost daily nonmigraine headache pattern, with superimposed acute exacerbations of typical migraine events. This latter entity, referred to variously as transformed migraine, daily chronic headache, or combined headache, may well represent a progressive disturbance in the pathophysiology of intermittent migraine. Currently, however, migraine is still classified as an intermittent entity, characterized by the absence of headache between acute events.

Treatment

Symptomatic (Rescue) Treatment

Table 3 describes criteria for symptomatic versus preventive treatment of migraine. The basis for symptomatic treatment is established by frequency. Acute attacks of migraine occurring less than once a week and in the absence of any contraindication to the use of symptomatic therapies warrants this form of treatment. The route of administration for symptomatic therapy may

TABLE 2. Some Foods That May Trigger Headaches

Tyramine-containing foods	Onions
Chocolate	Alcohol products
Aged cheeses	Wine/champagne, liquor,
Vinegar	beer
Relishes, dressings,	Fatty foods
sauces, catsup	Nitrite-containing foods
Liver, kidney, other	Hotdogs, sandwich meats,
organ meats	others
Alcohol	MSG-containing foods
Sour cream	Caffeine
Yogurt	Too much
Yeast extracts	"Rebound" effect
Citrus fruits	Seafood
Milk and milk products	

TABLE 3. Guidelines for Symptomatic Versus Preventive Therapy

Symptomatic Guidelines
Frequency less than 1 or 2 headaches/wk
No medical contraindications
For ergot derivatives: No coronary artery disease, severe hypertension, peripheral or cerebrovascular disease
For analgesics containing aspirin: No peptic ulcer disease, anticoagulant use, aspirin-sensitive asthma

Preventive Guidelines
Frequency greater than 1 or 2 headaches/wk
Medical contraindications for symptomatic therapies
Failure of symptomatic therapies
Reliable, predictable regularity of attacks (e.g., at or around menstrual period)
Known substance abuse tendencies

be as critical as the choice of medication. Delay of gastric absorption has been demonstrated in patients during both the preheadache and headache phases and occurs even in the absence of nausea and vomiting. The following interventions are of greatest value.

Ergotamine Alkaloids. Ergotamine alkaloids are estimated to be effective within the first 1 to 2 hours in up to 90 per cent of cases when administered parenterally, in 80 per cent of patients given the rectal form, and up to 50 per cent of patients given the oral form. Recent reports propose that central (brain) effects may be equally or more important than peripheral vasoconstrictive influences. The ergotamine alkaloids ergotamine tartrate and dihydroergotamine (DHE-45) are available in parenteral (intravenous, intramuscular, and subcutaneous), oral, rectal, inhalant, and sublingual forms. The oral and sublingual forms are less effective than those administered by the parenteral or rectal routes. The oral forms (Cafergot, Cafergot P-B, and Wigraine) each contain 1 mg of ergotamine tartrate. They are administered as two tablets at the onset of an attack, followed by one tablet every half hour until relief is obtained or until 5 mg have been taken. Sublingual tablets (Ergomar, Ergostat, Wigrettes) contain 2 mg of ergotamine tartrate and are given as one tablet sublingually at the onset of a headache and may be repeated once.

In rectal form, a suppository containing 2 mg of ergotamine tartrate (Cafergot, Cafergot P-B, Wigraine, Wigraine P-B) can be administered initially with a repeat dose in 1 hour, up to a maximum daily dose of 4 mg. I recommend beginning at a dose of one-third to one-half of a suppository in order to avoid the known adverse effects of ergotamine tartrate when excessive or too rapid absorption occurs. Cafergot P-B (tablets and suppositories) and Wigraine P-B suppositories contain the added ingredients butalbitol and belladonna, considered to enhance efficacy and reduce the gastrointestinal (GI) and other untoward effects of ergotamine tartrate. All preparations of Cafergot and Wigraine also contain caffeine, but sublingual, inhalant, and intravenous preparations do not.

Parenteral treatment with DHE-45 (1 to 2 ml intramuscularly or 0.5 to 1 ml intravenously) is effective in most instances and can be combined with parenterally or rectally administered antinauseants. (Treatment regimens using intravenous DHE-45 are described later.)

Well-known contraindications and untoward reactions are described in easily obtained reference sources. Less widely known, however, is the potential for physical dependence on ergotamine tartrate, reported in patients taking ergotamine as infrequently as three times per week, and resulting in "rebound" or "ergotamine headache," a self-sustaining headache/medication cycle in which the next headache represents the withdrawal symptom from the last dose of drug. Therefore, ergotamine tartrate should be used no more than 2 days per week, since greater frequency of usage leads to dependency and increasing headaches.

Isometheptene Mucate. Isometheptene mucate (Midrin) is a sympathomimetic agent combined with acetaminophen and dichloralphenazone (a tranquilizer). It produces less GI distress than ergotamine tartrate and occasionally is more effective.

Midrin is recommended for the symptomatic relief of mild to moderate migraine. Dosage is two capsules at the onset of an attack, followed by one or two capsules 1 hour later, to a maximum of five capsules per attack. Usage more than 2 days per week should be avoided.

Nonsteroidal Anti-Inflammatory Drugs. Nonsteroidal anti-inflammatory drugs (NSAIDs) have symptomatic as well as preventive properties in migraine therapy. A large number of agents are available, but naproxen sodium (Anaprox) has been most widely evaluated. The dose of naproxen is 275 mg, one or two tablets, to be taken at the onset of headache. Other agents include meclofenamate sodium (Meclomen), 100 to 200 mg, which can be repeated in 1 to 2 hours.

Other Agents

Although analgesics (narcotic and non-narcotic) may benefit some patients during an acute migraine attack, overuse risks make these agents unacceptable for routine usage except when proper limits can be established and when other therapies are of little value. Injectable narcotics are more effective than oral medication. Some patients with migraine benefit only from analgesic therapy, given alone or in conjunction with the symptomatic therapies noted earlier. While physicians must be cautious and alert for the somatic expression of psychologic despair and drug-seeking behavior, patients should not be deprived of necessary and available therapy as a result of professional timidity or unfounded prejudice. In selected cases, narcotics may represent the most appropriate and safest treatment.

Other Adjunctive Agents. Antinauseants are administered in conjunction with symptomatic drugs and are most effective by parenteral and suppository routes. The dose of chlorpromazine (Thorazine) is 25 to 50 mg intramuscularly, rectally, or in tablet form. Promethazine (Phenergan) is administered at a dose of 25 mg intramuscularly or rectally or 50 mg orally. Prochlorperazine (Compazine), 25 mg rectally or intramuscularly, should be used with particular caution because of the higher incidence of acute dystonic reactions associated with its use when compared with other agents such as chlorpromazine. Metoclopramide hydrochloride (Reglan), 10 mg orally three times a day or in intravenous form (same dose), can have antiemetic effects and may also enhance oral absorption.

Steroids may also be useful for symptomatic treatment of migraine. Patients with prolonged attacks may benefit from prednisone, 40 to 60 mg orally for 3 to 5 days, or dexamethasone, 8 to 16 mg intramuscularly.

Recently, a treatment protocol has been recommended that uses intravenous DHE-45 for refractory migraine. The starting dose is 0.5 to 1 mg every 8 hours over a period of 3 to 5 days, after an initial test dose of 0.1 to 0.3 mg. This therapy is best carried out in an inpatient setting and should be reserved for patients in whom standard interventions have been ineffective. Intravenous antinauseant therapy can be given simultaneously for accompanying GI distress.

Similarly, a 4-day protocol of intravenously administered hydrocortisone can be used for severely acute and refractory cases. This regimen consists of 100 mg of hydrocortisone added to 100 ml of an intravenous preparation of dextrose and water, given over 20 to 30 minutes. It is given four times a day during the first day; three times on the second day; twice on the third day; and once on the fourth day.

Preventive Treatment

The Beta-Adrenergic Blockers. The most important drugs for the prevention of migraine are the beta-adrenergic blocking agents. Their value in chronic daily headache and mixed forms is also recognized. Nadolol* (Corgard) and propranolol (Inderal) are the most widely administered and tested agents, but others may be of similar value. Individual dose determination is required. Nadolol is started at 20 mg per day and increased to tolerance, often to a range 80 to 160 mg per day. Twice daily dosing may be of added benefit in some patients. The short-acting form of propranolol is used in a range of 20 to 40 mg three or four times per day, whereas the long-acting form (Inderal LA) is best employed in a twice daily regimen, beginning at 80 mg once or twice a day and increasing to 160 mg twice daily as tolerated.

Methysergide. Methysergide (Sansert), the old-

est of the migraine prophylactic agents, is marred by a history of adverse consequences, but most authorities believe that selective and carefully monitored usage is both appropriate and necessary in difficult to manage cases. The drug is given as 2 mg three or four times a day in equally divided dosages. Treatment should be continued for no more than 6 months. A "drug holiday" of at least 1 month should separate periods of treatment. A chest x-ray, electrocardiography, and intravenous pyelography or magnetic resonance imaging of the abdomen is recommended to evaluate for the presence of retroperitoneal, cardiac valvular, and pulmonary changes.

Calcium Antagonists. Of the three available calcium antagonists (verapamil* [Isoptin, Calan], diltiazem* [Cardizem], and nifedipine* [Procardial]), verapamil and diltiazem seem to have the greatest effectiveness for treatment of headache. Calcium antagonists do not appear to be as effective as the beta blockers for prophylaxis of migraine but may be very effective in certain instances. They are agents of choice in patients who cannot take beta-adrenergic blockers, such as patients with asthma. Verapamil* is given in a dose range of 40 to 160 mg, two to four times per day, and diltiazem* is administered in a dose range of 30 to 90 mg, two or three times per day. Many patients administered nifedipine report increased headache, at least initially, although successful results are occasionally evident.

Nonsteroidal Anti-Inflammatory Drugs. The NSAIDs are used for both the symptomatic and preventive treatment of migraine. Naproxen sodium has been successfully established as an effective preventive agent in dose ranges of 275 mg, one or two tablets twice daily. Other NSAIDs may also be effective. Appropriate monitoring for untoward reactions, including aggravation of hypertension, is necessary.

Antidepressants. *Tricyclic antidepressants* (TCAs), particularly amitriptyline (Endep, Elavil) and nortriptyline (Aventyl, Pamelor), can be of dramatic benefit in patients with frequently occurring headache. In addition to reducing pain, these agents can ameliorate the frequently present sleep disturbances. Amitriptyline is administered in a dose of 25 to 150 mg per day, often in a single bedtime regimen. Nortriptyline dosages range from 25 to 75 mg at bedtime.

The *monoamine oxidase–inhibiting antidepressants* (MAOIs), particularly phenelzine (Nardil), can dramatically reduce the frequency of migraine and mixed headache forms. The traditional taboo against the simultaneous adminis-

---

*This use of this agent is not listed in the manufacturer's directives.

*This use of these agents is not listed in the manufacturers' directives.

tration of MAOIs and TCAs has diminished somewhat, and MAOI and amitriptyline treatment programs are employed for refractory depression and/or headache. Phenelzine, 15 mg one to three times daily, is usually given before midafternoon.

When simultaneously administering TCAs (amitriptyline, nortriptyline) and MAOIs, both drugs should be started on the same day, gradually increasing dosages to tolerance. Imipramine-related TCAs should not be used in conjunction with MAOIs to avoid hypertensive reactions. Severe orthostatic hypotension can occur in patients taking MAOIs alone or in conjunction with other antidepressants.

Other Preventive Agents. Clonidine hydrochloride* (Catapres), carbamazepine* (Tegretol), and methylphenidate* (Ritalin) are occasionally useful in intractable cases of migraine. Cyproheptadine* (Periactin) may be effective in adults with migraine; it is of considerable importance in the treatment of childhood migraine, and many consider it to be the drug of first choice. Dosages range from 4 to 8 mg, three or four times a day, in adults and 4 mg, two or three times a day, in children.

MIXED HEADACHE FORMS (TRANSFORMATIONAL MIGRAINE, DAILY CHRONIC HEADACHE, SO-CALLED TENSION HEADACHE)

Although the term "chronic tension headache" is still used, many experts consider it a variation of migraine or other mixed headache forms. Many authorities doubt that muscular pain is the primary basis for headaches in patients with frequent head and neck pain syndromes. It is possible that *acute* tension headache may be a separate and distinctive entity from that of the chronic form. Distinguishing mild to moderate migraine with muscle components from acute tension headache is not possible clinically and contributes to the disagreement as to whether acute muscular headache actually exists. Many believe that central mechanisms are responsible for the co-called muscular elements seen in the primary headache conditions.

Preventive Treatment

Frequent, recurring headache patterns in which migrainous and nonmigrainous features coexist are best treated with the pharmacologic and nonpharmacologic programs already described for migraine. Acute tension headache, if such actually exists, can be treated with mild analgesia (e.g., aspirin, acetaminophen) or NSAIDs. Simple muscle relaxants may also be helpful. For acute migrainous elements, symptomatic treatments are appropriate. For the more frequent or daily component, combinations of beta-adrenergic blockers and TCAs are most effective. One such regimen includes nadolol,* 60 to 160 mg daily, or propranolol (Inderal LA), 80 to 360 mg, and amitriptyline,* 50 to 150 mg at bedtime. The NSAIDs may be added if necessary.

The population of patients suffering frequent mixed element headaches (e.g., daily chronic headache) is a complex and challenging group of headache sufferers. In these patients, even the most appropriate pharmacotherapeutic intervention may be ineffective because of analgesic overuse, psychologic distress, and family and other complicating problems. It is the opinion of many authorities that the symptoms in these individuals reflect an endogenous pain syndrome that manifests as pain and other physiologic and psychologic distresses, including periodic depression, sleep disturbance, and substance overuse. Effective treatment often requires multidisciplinary interventions and sometimes hospitalization (see later). Biofeedback, psychotherapy, family involvement, lifestyle regulation, and other nonmedical and medical therapies are often necessary.

CLUSTER HEADACHE

Perhaps the most sinister of the well-recognized headache disorders is cluster headache. Few headaches are a greater challenge to the clinician's knowledge, compassion, and pharmacotherapeutic skills. Cluster headache can be divided into three major forms: episodic, chronic, and variants.

Episodic cluster headache is well known and most commonly characterized by recurring bouts of intensely painful attacks of cephalalgia. The pain is usually centered around an eye or the temple area and accompanied by nasal drainage, lacrimation, and other autonomic disturbances. Each headache lasts between 1 and 2 hours, and cycles of headache occur an average of every 2 to 4 months.

Chronic cluster headache is divided into primary and secondary forms. The term "chronic" is applied when the headache continues day after day, year after year, without remission or an interim period. *Primary chronic cluster headache* occurs without an interim period or remission

---

*This use of these agents is not listed in the manufacturers' directives.

*This use of these agents is not listed in the manufacturers' directives.

from the time the first cycle begins; the *secondary chronic cluster headache* is characterized by a pattern of typical, episodic cycles that eventually evolve to a chronic (without an interim period of remission) pattern.

Many variant forms of cluster headache exist, including *chronic paroxysmal hemicrania* (CPH). This disorder, first reported in 1974, is in many ways similar to cluster headache but often affects young women (cluster headache generally strikes adult men). The variant forms of cluster headache, including CPH, may be shorter-lasting than those of a typical cluster headache (less than 1 hour) and generally occur with greater frequency—up to 10 to 12 attacks compared to 2 to 4 cluster attacks per day. These variant forms rarely awaken patients from sleep, which is more typical of cluster headache.

Treatment

The treatment of cluster headache requires persistence, diligence, and innovation. Patients with cluster headache must discontinue all alcoholic products and avoid daytime napping. Discontinuance of smoking may be extremely important, although this is very difficult to achieve in the cluster headache population.

Symptomatic Treatment

Inhalation of 100 per cent oxygen is an effective means of symptomatically relieving the pain in many patients. Patients are administered 100 per cent oxygen at 7 liters per minute for a period of 15 minutes or more.

Symptomatic medications include rectal ergotamine tartrate and chlorpromazine. Injectable narcotics are discouraged because of the risks of overuse in patients with the daily headache patterns. Risk of overuse of ergotamine is also a concern.

Preventive Treatment

Preventive therapies are most appropriate for cluster headache.

Prednisone. Prednisone is the most reliable and effective drug for the prevention of cluster headache and can dramatically reduce both chronic and episodic varieties within hours of first administration. Several regimens are available, including that listed in Table 4. Although some headache cycles can be terminated with steroids, re-emergence of headaches may occur as dosages decrease to 15 to 20 mg per day.

Lithium Carbonate. Lithium carbonate* (Eskal-

---

*This use of this agent is not listed in the manufacturer's directives.

TABLE 4. Ten-Day Protocol for Prednisone Treatment of Cluster Headache*

	Drug Dose (mg)			
Day	8:00 a.m.	4:00 p.m.	Bedtime	Total (per day)
1	20	20	20	60
2	20	20	20	60
3	20	20	20	60
4	20	20	20	60
5	20	15	15	50
6	15	15	10	40
7	10	10	10	30
8	5	5	5	15
9	5	0	5	10
10	5	Finished		5

*A total of seventy-six 5-mg tablets are needed for this protocol.

ith, Lithobid, Lithane) is effective in more than 60 per cent of cases. The usual starting dose is 300 mg administered two to four times daily. Therapeutic response does not necessarily correlate with blood levels, and serum levels exceeding 0.7 mEq per liter are rarely necessary for good results.

Calcium Antagonists. Verapamil* (Isoptin, Calan) can be particularly valuable in dosages ranging from 80 to 160 mg three or four times per day.

Methysergide. Methysergide can be useful in cluster headache, since many cycles of the episodic form last less than the 6-month limit on continued usage of methysergide. Dosages are the same as those used in migraine treatment.

Nonsteroidal Anti-Inflammatory Agents. NSAIDs can be effective for cluster headache but appear to be most useful for the variant forms. Indomethacin (Indocin) at dosages of 25 to 50 mg three or four times per day is often effective.

Chlorpromazine. Chlorpromazine in dosages ranging from 75 to several hundred mg per day has been reported as useful in cluster headaches, but most authorities have not found this treatment to be acceptable, except rarely. Chlorpromazine can be used as an adjunctive therapy, however.

Other Therapies. Intravenous DHE-45 or hydrocortisone, as described for symptomatic (rescue) treatment of migraine, can be markedly beneficial to alter cluster headache (reduce the attacks for several days), but its value beyond the actual days of usage cannot be predicted. Nonetheless, the termination, for at least several days, of a severe and disabling pain syndrome can in itself be worthwhile, while allowing other treatments to be started.

Histamine desensitization to alleviate cluster headache is considered by most authorities to be of little value. However, in severely intractable cases, this intervention can be considered.

Surgery and other ablative procedures on the sphenopalatine ganglion, the nervus intermedius, or the branches or ganglion of the trigeminal nerve may be effective and appropriate in some absolutely intractable cases. Surgical treatment is recommended only in the most severe and extreme circumstances.

HEADACHES IN CHILDREN

Children, like adults, suffer headaches. The treatment regimens are generally similar, although greater reliance on nonmedicinal interventions is appropriate. Biofeedback, dietary regulation (e.g., not missing meals and avoidance of headache-provoking foodstuffs), and limiting other provoking factors can be helpful. Cyproheptadine, beta-blocker therapy, TCAs, calcium antagonists, and NSAIDs are useful for prophylaxis. Symptomatic treatment can be accomplished in a manner similar to that for adults with migraine.

POST-TRAUMATIC CEPHALGIA

The incidence of headache following closed-head injury varies from 33 to 80 per cent and can take one of several forms. Often the headache is a component of the *post-traumatic* or *postconcussion syndrome,* which represents a constellation of symptoms that can follow even mild head or flexion-extension neck injury. Among the headache symptoms are generalized throbbing or non-throbbing cephalgia; unilateral, intermittent, or continuous throbbing (similar to migraine); localized occipital/cervical pain with neuralgic qualities; and unilateral, intense, intermittent cephalgia in the anterior triangle of the neck or in the orbital area, resembling episodic cluster headache. Other mixed forms exist as well.

Treatment

The treatment of these conditions is similar to that of other headache types, emphasizing non-pharmacologic as well as pharmacologic therapies. Transneural stimulation, physical therapy, and nerve-blocking procedures may be additionally helpful. Local tenderness may respond to local anesthetics and/or to neuralgic medication, such as carbamazepine, 100 to 200 mg three times daily, or baclofen (Lioresal), 10 to 20 mg two or three times daily.

Hospital Treatment

Since 1979, when the first inpatient specialty unit for headache was developed in Ann Arbor, patients with severe and refractory headaches have been admitted to the few similar units around the country. The inpatient headache programs provide a comprehensive and intense intervention and include drug detoxification programs, aggressive pharmacotherapy, milieu treatment, dietary manipulation, identification and reduction of provoking influences, and psychologic and family intervention. Admission to such a unit is appropriate for patients with refractory daily or almost daily headache.

EPISODIC VERTIGO

method of
LINDA M. LUXON, B.Sc.
*The National Hospital for Nervous Diseases
Queen Square, London, England*

Humans have developed a sophisticated mechanism for maintaining perfect balance that depends on the integration and modulation in the brain stem of visual, proprioceptive, and vestibular sensory information. A deficiency of one or more of these sensory inputs may result in episodic vertigo, as may integrating abnormalities caused by central nervous system disease. Such disorientation is generally described by patients as "dizziness": a nonspecific symptom that may result from pathology in various body systems. In contrast, vertigo is defined as "a hallucination of movement" and is a cardinal manifestation of a disordered vestibular system. However, such semantic differences are rarely volunteered by the patient, who is frightened and confused by new and unfamiliar sensations of movement.

For diagnostic and management purposes (Figure 1), episodic vertigo and dizziness should be considered to be synonymous terms requiring a full history and physical examination, with special reference to the cardiovascular, neurologic, ophthalmologic, and otologic systems to identify treatable causes of nonotologic vertigo such as occult cardiac dysrhythmias, temporal lobe epilepsy, and transient ischemic attacks in the vertebrobasilar territory. In addition, there is a small proportion of patients with episodic vertigo of central vestibular origin in whom visuovestibular oculomotor abnormalities indicate the need for specific neurologic investigation.

Having excluded general medical and neurologic causes of episodic vertigo, the physician must then consider otologic causes. In particular, it is essential to exclude the presence of chronic middle-ear disease with occult labyrinthine erosion.

However, the majority of patients with episodic vertigo may be identified as suffering from a peripheral (i.e., labyrinthine or, rarely, eighth cranial nerve) pathology. In certain cases, specific pathology, for example, syphilitic labyrinthitis, Meniere's disease, or an acoustic neurinoma, may be identified. Definitive treatment may then be instituted. However, in many cases the pathophysiology of isolated vertigo of periph-

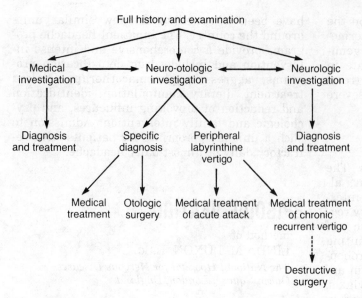

Figure 1. Management of episodic vertigo.

eral labyrinthine origin is poorly understood, and it is impossible to consider specific drug therapy for most patients. The symptomatic treatment of such cases may be divided into medical and surgical aspects.

MEDICAL TREATMENT

Counseling

Recurrent vertigo frequently gives rise to acute anxiety, in part because of the fear of an underlying fatal pathology and in part because of the embarrassment of suffering an attack in public.

A full history and physical examination, together with appropriate investigations and followed by a simple and clear explanation of the problem and of the therapeutic measures available, are invaluable to reassure the patient of the benign nature of the condition despite the severity and unpleasantness of the symptoms.

Cawthorne-Cooksey Head and Balance Exercises
(Table 1)

Resting neural activity in the labyrinth of a normal subject is equal but opposite in each ear. When injury results in asymmetry of neural activity in the two ears, vertigo is experienced.

TABLE 1. **Cawthorne-Cooksey Exercises**

Sitting

Eyes Movements at first slow, then fast
1. Up and down, side to side
2. Focus on finger moving from 3 ft to 1 ft from face

Head Movement at first slow, then fast (also with eyes closed)
1. Bend forward and backward
2. Turn from side to side

Trunk
1. Bend forward to pick up objects from the floor
2. Bend forward to pick up ball from the floor, return to sitting and twist body to put ball behind, first to left, then right
3. Drop shoulder and head sideways to left and right
4. Throw and catch ball to the side and above head

Standing

As Above, Plus
1. Change from sitting to standing with eyes open and closed; also turning around in between
2. Turn on the spot to left and right, eyes open and closed (will require supervision)
3. Walk with another person, throwing and catching ball, in a circle and straight line
4. With another person's help, walk with eyes open and closed, backward and forward, sideways, turning head, looking in all directions to avoid fixating with eyes
5. Walk in a circle forward and backward with head turned to left and right, eyes open and closed

Lying Down

1. Roll head from side to side, also over edge of bed
2. Roll whole body from side to side
3. Sit up straight, forward and from side lying down

For relaxation, practice shoulder shrugging and circling

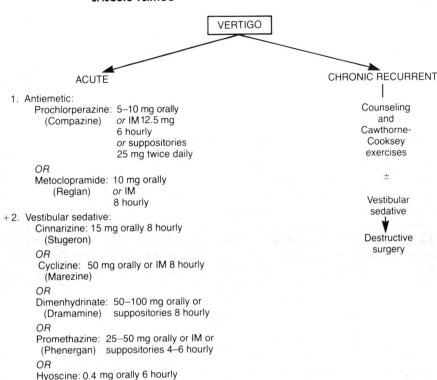

Figure 2. Treatment of episodic vertigo.

Elegant experiments in cats and baboons have shown clearly that stimulation of visual input and the promotion of movement, after a unilateral vestibular neurectomy, result in more rapid recovery of balance. Thus, the basis of head and balance exercises in vestibular disorders is to deliberately and systematically provoke episodes of vertigo such that compensation may develop more rapidly. These exercises are of particular value in patients with peripheral vestibular lesions but are of no value in the treatment of central causes of vertigo because the mechanisms subserving compensation are deranged. The exercise regimen that is used at The National Hospital for Nervous Diseases is outlined in Table 1.

The patient is encouraged to perform one exercise at a time for 3 minutes three times a day and to progress gradually from one exercise to another as the patient can accomplish more without undue symptoms of vertigo. It is emphasized that the exercise regimen is not an endurance test and that a gentle, systematic, consistent approach is more efficacious than infrequent bursts of aggressive exercises, which merely precipitate troublesome vertigo associated with vegetative symptoms. Antivertiginous drugs are given only in association with acute symptoms because such drugs may suppress vestibular activity, which is required for compensation.

Drug Therapy (Figure 2)

The so-called vestibular sedative drugs provide the mainstay of symptomatic treatment, but because no rationale exists for their use, the response to treatment is, not surprisingly, often disappointing. It must be emphasised that the use of drugs in acute vertigo should be advocated only after full investigation and consideration of other therapeutic maneuvers. In addition, any benefit must be weighed against potential side effects.

Antihistamines. These drugs have been widely used in the treatment of dizziness because they lower the threshold of vestibular reactivity, but in elderly persons, anticholinergic (blurred vision, urinary retention) and sedative side effects may be troublesome. Cinnarizine (Stugeron*) is probably the most effective antivertiginous agent currently available. The standard oral dose is 15 mg three times daily and, although it is well tolerated, drowsiness is a common side effect in the elderly person, and it may be necessary to titrate the dose.

Psychotropic Drugs. Psychotropic drugs including sedatives, antidepressants, and tranquilizers have frequently been prescribed for the treatment of dizziness, partly in an attempt to alleviate the

---

*Not available in the United States.

psychologic sequelae of vestibular pathology and partly on the false assumption that symptoms are nonorganic in origin. Such drugs act directly on the central nervous system and may prevent the normal compensatory mechanisms that facilitate recovery from peripheral vestibular dysfunction. It is therefore my view that such drugs should not be prescribed, except for specific psychiatric indications. Moreover, it should be emphasized that chronic use of these drugs may result in dizziness, particularly in the elderly patient. Furthermore, dizziness is a withdrawal symptom after long-term administration of both antidepressants and minor tranquilizers.

Antiemetics. In this category, prochlorperazine (Compazine), a phenothiazine derivative, deserves special mention in view of its widespread use. It has minor antihistaminic activity and is thought to act directly on the brain stem. It is of particular value in the control of nausea and vomiting associated with vertigo, by intramuscular injection of 25 mg or by use of suppositories of 25 mg given twice during the first 24 hours. There is little evidence of efficacy in ameliorating vertigo itself. Metoclopramide (Reglan) may also be of value in the treatment of vomiting with vertigo in adults but may cause extrapyramidal side effects.

Anticholinergics. Anticholinergics diminish the excitability of the vestibular nuclei neurons, which may be the action by which antihistamines exert an antivertiginous effect. Both atropine, 0.4 to 0.6 mg, and hyoscine, 0.32 to 0.65 mg, given intramuscularly produce symptomatic relief in acute vertigo of labyrinthine origin, but care should be taken if there is evidence of prostatic enlargement, constipation, glaucoma, or cardiac insufficiency, particularly in elderly persons.

Vasodilators. These drugs have been proposed as the treatment of choice in vertigo of vascular etiology, for example, endolymphatic hydrops, sudden vestibular failure, whiplash injury, and head trauma. The aim of such treatment is to reestablish adequate blood flow in ischemic areas. The histamine analogue betahistine* has been demonstrated experimentally to increase capillary blood flow in the stria vascularis of the inner ear. Side effects occur rarely but include headaches, rash, and gastric discomfort. It should be recalled that histamine may exacerbate asthma, rhinitis, and pheochromocytoma, and in these conditions betahistine is contraindicated.

Diuretics. Diuretics have no place in the treatment of episodic vertigo, with the exception of the specific management of Meniere's disease.

Anticoagulants. These agents have been pre-

*Not available in the United States.

scribed frequently to elderly patients with episodic vertigo on the false assumption that these episodes are related to vertebrobasilar insufficiency. Prolonged recurrent vertigo, in isolation, is rarely a manifestation of this diagnosis. Hence, the known risks of anticoagulation, particularly in elderly persons, must be balanced against careful and precise diagnosis.

SURGICAL TREATMENT

Surgical intervention in the treatment of episodic vertigo is indicated in three situations:

1. The treatment of complications of chronic middle-ear disease
2. To improve the quality of life of a patient suffering from severe, recurrent vertigo in whom medical measures have failed
3. To exclude the presence of a perilymph fistula

It cannot be overemphasised that before destructive surgery is undertaken, there must be no doubt as to the exact site and side of the lesion. Moreover, particularly in the elderly person, vestibular compensation may be prolonged or indeed incomplete as a consequence of an age-related deterioration in the ability to integrate information within the central nervous system. The risk of persisting imbalance must therefore be carefully weighed against any possible advantage.

MENIERE'S DISEASE

method of
GALE GARDNER, M.D.
University of Tennessee–Memphis
Memphis, Tennessee

Meniere's disease is not simply an instance of dizziness or vertigo. It is a specific disorder of the labyrinth (inner ear) that produces a combination of complaints including vertigo (sensation of spinning), hearing loss (of a particular type), tinnitus (ear noise, usually roaring), and frequently a sensation of fullness in the ear. To qualify as true Meniere's disease, all these symptoms must occur, followed by varying periods with no attacks. During the attacks, the patient is frequently nauseated, may vomit, and is clearly ill and probably apprehensive.

Meniere's disease is *not* any of these symptoms occurring singly. It is not dizziness alone, although many patients have this symptom, nor is it hearing loss or tinnitus alone. These isolated symptoms must be evaluated separately.

ETIOLOGY

A number of disease processes may produce the combination of vertigo, hearing loss, and tinnitus. The most important is an acoustic neuroma, usually arising in the internal auditory canal and apparently producing symptoms by causing pressure on the neurovascular contents of the canal. It is crucial for the physician to think of this possibility whenever treating a patient with the symptoms of Meniere's disease. Primary care physicians should think of the possibility of a tumor when dealing with a patient who has unilateral hearing loss or tinnitus, with or without dizziness or vertigo. In the presence of these symptoms, and if the hearing loss is of the sensorineural type (nerve dysfunction rather than conductive or mechanical dysfunction), an imaging study is indicated.

Other disorders that may produce this combination of symptoms are syphilis (usually localized in the inner ear and central nervous system), hyperlipidemia, food allergy, hypothyroidism, and others.

The condition that we refer to as "true" Meniere's disease is believed to be caused by an increase in the amount of inner ear fluid (endolymph), producing hydrops of the labyrinth. We do not yet know the cause of this condition or the mechanism whereby it occurs, which, of course, makes treatment difficult.

DIAGNOSIS

True Meniere's disease is diagnosed by the history of attacks of vertigo, with associated hearing loss (that usually fluctuates in severity) and tinnitus, with initial involvement of usually only one ear. The severity of the attack is helpful in differentiating true Meniere's disease from other labyrinthine disorders. A hearing test (audiogram) is needed to show that the hearing loss involves nerve dysfunction (sensorineural hearing loss). If the hearing loss is caused by mechanical factors such as dysfunction of the eardrum, ear bones (ossicles), or ear canal, it is referred to as conductive, and Meniere's disease may be ruled out. Tuning fork tests, if performed properly, can also help in making this determination, but the diagnosis should be confirmed with audiometry. A caloric test, or more desirably an electronystagmographic examination, may also help to make the diagnosis. These tests are likely to show spontaneous or positional nystagmus during attacks, and perhaps a reduction in caloric response on the involved side. At some point, I obtain a computed tomography scan or a magnetic resonance imaging scan with gadolinium of every patient who I believe has Meniere's disease because some of them will be found to have an acoustic tumor instead.

TREATMENT OF THE ACUTE ATTACK

Those who have never had Meniere's disease frequently underestimate the impact of the attack on a patient. Lacking medical knowledge, the patient is at the mercy of imagination and suspects everything from a stroke to a heart attack. Reassurance and support are therefore essential in managing the acute attack. Fortunately, the patient can be told that attacks rarely last longer than 2 or 3 hours. Supportive treatment during this time is all that is required.

For a mild attack without nausea or vomiting, meclizine (Antivert or Bonine), 25-mg tablets, or cyclizine lactate (Marezine), 50-mg tablets, may be given every 4 to 6 hours for dizziness.

For a more severe attack with nausea and vomiting, one may use cyclizine lactate, 50 mg (1 ml) intramuscularly, immediately and every 4 to 6 hours thereafter. Prochlorperazine (Compazine) may be given as a 25-mg suppository immediately and then used twice daily. For emergency room settings with severe attacks, I use atropine sulfate, 0.0125 mg per kg intravenously or intramuscularly; it can be repeated in 2 hours. Atropine should be used with caution in patients with a history of cardiac disease, particularly in the presence of supraventricular tachycardia. Diazepam (Valium) may also be given intravenously or intramuscularly, at a dosage of 5 to 10 mg, and may be repeated in 3 to 4 hours.

In an unusually severe attack or in the presence of complicating factors, it may be necessary to admit a patient to the hospital and to provide fluid replacement.

PREVENTION OF ATTACKS

To list the medications and treatment programs that have been used and advocated in the past for Meniere's disease would exceed the space limitations of this section. Suffice it to say that the following general types of treatment may be considered: tranquilizers, vagal blockers (such as atropine), antihistamines, vasodilators, diuretics, vitamins, histamine, steroids, low-salt diet, special head exercises, and avoidance of alcohol, caffeine, and tobacco, to name only a few.

My own medical maintenance regimen is fairly simple. Primarily, the patient is repeatedly reassured that if worse comes to worse the disease can be controlled surgically, but that 80 to 90 per cent of individuals can be controlled successfully with nonsurgical measures. For individuals less than 60 years of age, I use a combination of (1) belladonna-ergotamine-phenobarbital (Bellergal), one tablet given twice daily, (2) meclizine, one 25-mg tablet given at bedtime, and (3) diazepam, one 2-mg tablet (or even less if necessary) three times a day, unless contraindications to any of these regimens exist.

For patients over the age of 60 years, I generally use a combination of (1) meclizine and (2) diazepam, as indicated previously, as well as (3) nicotinic acid, 50-mg tablets, in a flushing dose before breakfast and at bedtime.

Certain qualifications are necessary. In my office, we spend a great deal of time counseling patients on reducing the amount of these medications to below the point at which sedation or other side effects occur. We also spend time determining any contraindications to their use, either because of other conditions that may be present (e.g., glaucoma in the case of belladonna-ergotamine-phenobarbital) or because of incompatibility of these medications with other medications the patient may be taking.

SURGERY

Surgery should be considered when medical treatment has failed; when there are no medical, age-related, or other contraindications; and when the condition is significantly affecting the patient's life.

Types of Surgery

Generally, surgery takes two forms. In situations in which hearing remains relatively good, conservative surgery that does not sacrifice hearing function is preferred. If the hearing has gradually deteriorated with the passage of time, which is not uncommon, a destructive procedure is indicated. The rationale is that this type of surgery is generally more effective than the conservative type, and there is no valid reason to preserve hearing that is no longer useful.

Without discussing surgical details that are of little interest to the primary care physician, here are the procedures I prefer to offer these patients. These procedures are performed by approaching the labyrinth either from behind the auricle (postauricular), from above, or directly through the ear canal. The conservative procedure I prefer to use initially is to place a shunt tube between the endolymphatic sac of the labyrinth and the adjacent subarachnoid space (endolymphatic sac–subarachnoid shunt) through a postauricular incision. A variation is to place the shunt tube between the endolymphatic sac and the mastoid space. Should these operations fail, I prefer to cut the balance (vestibular) nerve while preserving the hearing nerve, using either a posterior fossa approach (retrolabyrinthine vestibular nerve section) or a middle fossa approach (middle fossa vestibular nerve section).

When hearing in the involved ear is not considered useful to the patient, but the balance problem is incapacitating and medication has not controlled the problem, I prefer to destroy the balance end organ with nerve endings, with sacrifice of hearing (labyrinthectomy). In a younger patient I do this through a postauricular incision, drill away the three balance canals, open the vestibule of the labyrinth, and remove the membranous end organs for balance (transmastoid labyrinthectomy). In an elderly patient I do the operation through the ear canal, open the vestibule, connect the oval and round windows in the middle-ear space, and remove the membranous end organs (transcanal labyrinthectomy).

Effectiveness of These Procedures in Relieving the Effects of Meniere's Disease

Nothing in life is perfect, but as surgical procedures go, labyrinthectomy is highly effective, eliminating balance problems or significantly alleviating them 95 per cent of the time, but with sacrifice of hearing. The conservative sac procedures allow preservation of hearing and improve the patient's balance function (in my experience, in approximately 80 per cent of cases) but do little, if anything, to improve the hearing, which usually continues to deteriorate slowly.

The retrolabyrinthine and middle fossa nerve section procedures appear to offer the best of both worlds, controlling vertigo as effectively (95 per cent or better) as labyrinthectomy but preserving hearing as well. Yet these are both intracranial procedures and carry greater risks than the other procedures, which are all relatively low-risk operations.

None of these procedures have a high or even a predictable rate of success in stabilizing or improving hearing or in controlling tinnitus; however, in some cases, dramatic improvement in these areas occurs. Because of the tendency for this disease to fluctuate in severity, it is difficult, if not impossible, to know with certainty whether to attribute postoperative improvement to the effects of surgery or to the fluctuating nature of the disease.

Bilateral Involvement

Unfortunately, 20 to 40 per cent of patients may ultimately develop bilateral Meniere's disease. In this situation, conservative surgery may be indicated, but the use of streptomycin may also be considered to reduce balance dysfunction nonsurgically. This must be done with care to avoid undue injury to the labyrinth by following the hearing and balance function with testing during the course of treatment.

VIRAL MENINGOENCEPHALITIS

method of
HARLEY A. ROTBART, M.D., and
MYRON J. LEVIN, M.D.
*University of Colorado School of Medicine
Denver, Colorado*

Many viruses are capable of infecting the central nervous system (CNS) and causing symptomatic disease (Table 1). Several distinct syndromes are recognized, although there is significant overlap in etiologic agents, laboratory findings, and clinical manifestations. *Aseptic meningitis* is the most common CNS viral syndrome, characterized by headache, stiff neck, photophobia, and nonspecific constitutional signs such as fever, vomiting, and lethargy. *Encephalitis* is the result of parenchymal brain infection and is often associated with a change in level of consciousness and/or affect, frequently with accompanying focal neurologic deficits and seizures. *Myelitis* is a relatively rare syndrome (in the postpolio era) that results from infection of spinal cord neurons, with attendant motor signs and symptoms. Each of these entities is best diagnosed by a combination of clinical findings and cerebrospinal fluid (CSF) analysis. The CSF typically contains leukocytes, usually with a lymphocyte predominance, although polymorphonuclear cells may be in excess early in infection. Glucose levels are usually normal or slightly low, and protein is often modestly elevated (more so in herpes simplex and other necrotizing viral infections).

Most CNS viral disease is acute in onset and of short duration. Chronic (or "slow") infections occur with

TABLE 1. **Etiologic Agents of Viral Meningoencephalitis**

Agent/Disease	Most Common Clinical Syndrome*		Comment
	Aseptic Meningitis	Encephalitis	
Acute Infection			
Arenaviruses			
Lymphocytic choriomeningitis	X		Rodent handlers at risk
Lassa, Junin, Machupo		X	Hemorrhagic fevers
Bunyavirus			
California encephalitis		X	Arthropod borne; regional, seasonal
Cytomegalovirus		X	Neonates, immunocompromised patients at risk
Enterovirus	X		Most common cause of aseptic meningitis
coxsackie, echo, polio			
Epstein-Barr virus	X	X	Association still poorly defined
Herpes simplex		X	Type 1 more common
Human immunodeficiency virus		X	Cause of various CNS syndromes
Influenza A	X	X	
Measles		X	
Mumps	X	X	
Orbivirus	X		Colorado tick fever; seasonal
Togaviruses			
Eastern, western, St. Louis encephalitis		X	Regional, seasonal; arthropod borne
Rubella		X	Part of congenital rubella syndrome
Varicella-zoster		X	Immunocompromised patients at greatest risk; primary infection or reactivation (herpes zoster)
Subacute, Chronic, or Persistent Infections			
Creutzfeldt-Jakob disease		X	Transmitted by direct inoculation of infected nervous tissue; perhaps by other routes
Enterovirus	X		Hypogammaglobulinemic and agammaglobulinemic patients at risk
Kuru		X	Associated with cannibalism of infected brains
JC and BK viruses		X	Progressive multifocal leukoencephalopathy
Measles		X	Subacute sclerosing panencephalitis
Rabies		X	
Rubella		X	

*The most common syndrome is indicated for each virus, but significant overlap exists, with many agents capable of causing both meningitis and encephalitis. When there is an X in both columns, the syndromes are equally common.

certain viruses (e.g., Creutzfeldt-Jakob disease, sub-acute sclerosing panencephalitis) or in certain hosts (e.g., chronic enteroviral infection in hypogammaglob-ulinemic patients). A postinfectious CNS inflammatory disease has also been described following several viral diseases, including varicella-zoster, measles, and ru-bella.

TREATMENT

Approach to therapy is three-pronged: (1) rule out other treatable causes of infection (empiric therapy for nonviral agents may be required while awaiting results of laboratory studies); (2) provide supportive care; and (3) administer spe-cific antiviral therapy when appropriate.

Implicit in the diagnosis of viral CNS infection is the exclusion of other treatable disease. Since that may require hours to days, empiric initiation of antibiotics (for acute bacterial, mycobacterial, or rickettsial infection) or, rarely, antifungal drugs may be indicated. Empiric therapy may also be warranted when parameningeal infec-tions (sinusitis, abscess, epidural and subdural collections) are suspected, as they may be ini-tially indistinguishable from acute viral infec-tion. Noninfectious CNS diseases that may mimic viral infection and require specific therapy in-clude malignancy, collagen-vascular diseases, Reye's syndrome, and lead poisoning. Occasion-ally antibiotic therapy itself, usually with sulfa compounds, causes an aseptic meningitis-like syndrome.

TABLE 2. **Specific Therapies for CNS Viral Infections**

	Pathogen/Disease	Drug and Dosing	Comment
Established Therapy	Herpes simplex	Acyclovir (Zovirax),* 10 mg/kg q 8 hr IV × 10 days†	Brain biopsy recommended prior to start of therapy; give acyclovir as 1-hr infusion; adjust dose for renal impairment
	Varicella-zoster	Acyclovir (Zovirax), as above	One-hr infusion; adjust dose for renal impairment
	Human immunodeficiency virus	Azidothymidine (Retrovir), 200 mg q 4 hr PO; *or* 2.5–5 mg/kg q 4 hr IV‡	Important to exclude other concomi-tant CNS infection/malignancy; monitor blood counts
	Rabies	Human diploid cell vaccine, 1 ml IM on days 1, 3, 7, 14, 28; *and* human rabies immune globulin, 20 IU per kg (½ given into wound, ½ given IM)	Begin immediately postexposure; local wound cleansing also recommended
Experimental Therapy	Cytomegalovirus	Ganciclovir, 2.5–7.5 mg/kg q 8 hr IV; *or* 5 mg/kg q 12 hr IV, for duration of symptoms	Available on compassionate use basis from Syntex Corp.; biopsy diagnosis required; adjust dose for renal im-pairment or neutropenia
	Epstein-Barr virus	Ganciclovir or acyclovir, as above	Duration of therapy uncertain
	Influenza A	Amantidine, 200 mg/day PO (for >10 years old) × 7–10 days	Adjust dose for renal impairment
	Arenaviruses	Ribavirin,§ 2 grams IV load, then 1 gram q 6 hr IV × 4 days, followed by 0.5 gram q 6 hr IV × 6 days	Only Lassa fever trials report; hemol-ysis may complicate therapy; tera-togenic
	Measles		
	Acute encephalitis	Ribavirin,§ 2.5 mg/kg qid PO × 7 days	This dosing reported for acute mea-sles; higher dose may be considered for encephalitis; teratogenic
	Subacute sclerosing panencephalitis	Ribavirin,§ 10 mg/kg tid PO × 3 days followed by 10 mg/kg bid × 6 wk	
	Enteroviruses		
	Chronic infection	Human immunoglobulin, 200–400 mg/kg q 2–4 wk IV†; duration based on response	Intrathecal therapy may be more ef-fective; gammaglobulin lots may be screened for specific antibody titers to infecting serotype
	Neonatal (high risk)	Human immunoglobulin, 400 mg/kg IV as single dose	High-risk factors include concurrent maternal illness, age at onset <1 wk, prematurity

*This use is not listed by the manufacturer.
†This dose may exceed the manufacturer's recommended dose.
‡The IV formulation of azidothymidine is investigational.
§The currently marketed formulation of ribavirin is for aerosol administration only.

Supportive therapy, which is directed at the sequelae of severe viral CNS infections, is applicable regardless of the specific pathogen. *Respiratory failure* may result from depression of central pathways, concomitant tracheobronchopulmonary infection, or airway obstruction with or without seizures. An artificial airway, assisted ventilation, and tracheal toilet all may be necessary. *Fluid/electrolyte imbalance* due to dehydration, dilutional hyponatremia, or inappropriate secretion of antidiuretic hormone is common with any CNS infection. Electrolytes and urine/serum osmolality should be monitored and fluid input adjusted regularly. *Brain edema* secondary to the inflammatory response to viral infection should be suspected with the occurrence of new neurologic deficits or changes in pupil size. A computed tomography or magnetic resonance imaging scan may help in this diagnosis, and an intracranial pressure monitor will confirm and quantitate the elevated pressure and facilitate management. Fluid input should be adjusted to avoid overhydration. Mannitol (0.5 gram per kg of 20 per cent solution given over 20 minutes intravenously) osmotically removes excess CNS fluid and should be given in repeat doses every 4 to 6 hours as needed. Hyperventilation to constrict CNS blood vessel caliber is generally used after other modalities have failed. The response is usually brisk, but may wane after 24 hours. The use of glucocorticoids is controversial, and in some settings may be harmful.

Seizures may result from direct viral or inflammatory damage of neurons, increased intracranial pressure, or fluid and electrolyte imbalance. Phenytoin (Dilantin), 15 mg per kg given intravenously as a loading dose at a rate not to exceed 50 mg per minute, while monitoring blood pressure and electrocardiogram, is the drug of choice, as it does not cloud the sensorium. Maintenance dosing is with 3 to 5 mg per kg daily for adults and 4 to 8 mg per kg for children. Phenobarbital, 5 mg per kg intravenously every 30 minutes, at a rate not to exceed 100 mg per minute, until seizures cease or blood pressure falls (total loading dose not more than 20 mg per kg), is an alternative. Maintenance dosing of phenobarbital is 2 to 3 mg per kg daily for adults and 3 to 5 mg per kg for children. Refractory seizures may require additional antiepileptics or paralysis (to prevent hyperthermia and increased metabolic requirements). We do not recommend prophylaxis against seizures in hospitalized patients with viral CNS infection.

Bladder atony/hypotony secondary to myelitis or severe encephalitis requires catheterization. Patients with protracted courses may develop malnutrition and require hyperalimentation.

Specific established antiviral therapy is available only for herpes simplex, varicella-zoster, human immunodeficiency virus, and rabies (Table 2). Experimental treatments, however, have shown promise in a number of serious viral CNS diseases (see Table 2) and may be considered on a compassionate basis in certain appropriate settings.

REYE'S SYNDROME

method of
DORIS A. TRAUNER, M.D.
University of California, San Diego School of Medicine
La Jolla, California

Reye's syndrome is an acute metabolic encephalopathy with hepatic dysfunction that occurs almost exclusively in children, although rare cases have been reported in adults of all ages. It is a biphasic illness with characteristic clinical features. In the initial phase, the child has a viral syndrome, most often a flu-like illness, with gastrointestinal tract or upper respiratory tract symptoms. While influenza B virus is associated with the majority of cases, varicella is the prodromal illness in approximately 10 per cent. The child typically is recovering from this viral ailment when the second phase begins with repeated vomiting, followed by changes in sensorium. These may include lethargy, hyperexcitability, or combativeness; symptoms may progress to obtundation or coma. Hyperventilation is a prominent feature on examination. Seizures may occur at any time during the course of the second phase.

Infants under 1 year of age have a more subtle presentation. Although the prodromal illness is usually present, vomiting may be minimal or absent; respiratory distress is present early, and the initial sign of the second phase may be sudden apnea or seizure activity.

Laboratory abnormalities include evidence of hepatocellular dysfunction with elevated serum transaminase and creatine phosphokinase levels, hyperammonemia, and prolonged prothrombin time. Serum bilirubin concentrations are not significantly elevated. Hypoglycemia occurs in about 40 per cent of children. A mixed metabolic acidosis and respiratory alkalosis is typical, with alkalosis predominating. Abnormalities of fatty acid, glucose, and urea cycle metabolism have been demonstrated during the acute illness. All of the metabolic abnormalities are reversible once the acute phase of the illness is over.

Pathologic changes include microvesicular fatty accumulation in the liver, depletion of hepatic glycogen stores, decreased hepatic activity of the succinic acid dehydrogenase enzyme, and mitochondrial swelling and pleomorphism. Massive brain swelling is a potentially fatal complication.

Reye's syndrome affects 0.3 to 3.5 per 100,000 children under the age of 18 years in the United States.

The cause of this disorder is unknown. There is evidence of a potential association between salicylate ingestion during the prodromal illness and subsequent development of Reye's syndrome. No causal relationship has been established.

A number of metabolic disorders can mimic Reye's syndrome and need to be considered in the differential diagnosis. These disorders include urea cycle defects, organic acid disorders, systemic carnitine deficiency, and medium-chain acyl coenzyme A dehydrogenase deficiency.

TREATMENT

Treatment of the acute illness is limited by a lack of knowledge about causation. Most approaches to therapy are based on intensive supportive care, correction of metabolic abnormalities, treatment of seizures, and reduction of intracranial pressure. In addition, because of experimental evidence of a possible carnitine deficiency state in these patients, we use carnitine as an adjunct to therapy.

A uniform staging system for Reye's syndrome has been proposed by the National Institutes of Health Consensus Development Conference on the Diagnosis and Treatment of Reye's Syndrome. This consists of five stages:

Stage I: Vomiting; lethargy or sleepiness; responds appropriately to verbal stimuli.

Stage II: Stupor, disorientation, delirium, combativeness; may not respond to verbal stimuli but responds appropriately to painful stimuli.

Stage III: Obtundation or coma; decorticate posturing to painful stimuli; intact brain stem reflexes.

Stage IV: Coma; decerebrate posturing spontaneously or in response to painful stimuli; brain stem reflexes may be impaired, with sluggish pupillary response to light and incomplete oculocephalic (doll's eyes) reflexes.

Stage V: Coma; flaccid quadriparesis; no response to painful stimuli; sluggish or absent oculocephalic and pupillary responses.

General Considerations

Any infant or child with suspected Reye's syndrome should be hospitalized in a pediatric intensive care unit, even if the child is awake and responsive. The clinical condition can deteriorate very quickly, and a child may pass from Stage I to Stage III or IV in a matter of minutes. Continuous cardiac and respiratory monitoring should be instituted immediately. Blood should be drawn for serum glucose, ammonia, bilirubin, transaminase and creatine phosphokinase determinations, and electrolytes and prothrombin time.

Stages I and II

The child should not be given any oral feedings initially. An intravenous line should be inserted and hypertonic glucose solution (10 to 15 per cent) with appropriate electrolyte concentrations should be administered at low maintenance fluid levels. Serum glucose determinations should be monitored every 8 hours, and the rate of infusion adjusted to maintain serum glucose concentrations between 125 and 175 mg per dl. Treatment should be continued until the child has been clinically stable for 36 to 48 hours and until laboratory confirmation has been obtained that serum ammonia concentrations are stable or decreasing and liver function tests are normalizing. If deterioration in the clinical state occurs, more vigorous therapy as outlined later should be instituted.

Stages III and V

For children in the more advanced stages of Reye's syndrome, the mortality rate is significant, and aggressive therapy is required, including insertion of arterial and central venous lines, elective endotracheal intubation, and mechanical ventilation. Since hyperthermia is a common occurrence, the child should be placed on a cooling blanket to regulate body temperature within the normal range. A nasogastric tube and a Foley's catheter should be inserted, and intake and output precisely recorded. Intravenous solutions containing hypertonic (15 per cent) glucose with appropriate electrolyte concentrations should be administered at 75 per cent of maintenance levels. Intravenous fluid administration rates should be adjusted as needed to maintain serum osmolality below 320 mOsm. Serum glucose concentrations should be monitored every 4 to 6 hours and kept between 125 and 175 mg per dl. Careful fluid and electrolyte balance should be maintained.

If serum ammonia concentrations exceed 150 micrograms per dl, lactulose and neomycin (25 to 50 mg per kg every 6 hours*) can be administered by nasogastric tube, or neomycin by enema. When serum ammonia concentrations exceed 350 micrograms per dl, more aggressive measures such as exchange blood transfusion or peritoneal dialysis may be warranted, since ammonia levels of this magnitude have been correlated with higher mortality rates. Transfusions with fresh-frozen plasma are helpful in correcting clotting abnormalities if prothrombin time is markedly prolonged, especially if intraventricular catheter

---

*May exceed the manufacturer's recommended dose.

placement is to be considered. We also use L-carnitine, 100 mg per kg every 12 hours intravenously, as an adjunct to therapy.

Seizures can be treated using intravenous phenytoin, with an initial loading dose of 15 mg per kg followed by a daily dose of 5 to 8 mg per kg in two divided doses. If the child is to be paralyzed for a prolonged period, it is helpful to use continuous electroencephalogram (EEG) monitoring to identify seizure activity. Alternatively, prophylactic phenytoin may be administered.

Brain swelling and increased intracranial pressure (ICP) may account for significant morbidity and mortality; for this reason, aggressive measures to control ICP appear warranted. An ICP monitoring device should be inserted. We prefer an intraventricular catheter, but many centers use surface recording devices. ICP should be kept within the normal range (under 15 torr). However, perfusion pressure (PP) of the brain is more important than the absolute ICP value. PP is the difference between mean arterial blood pressure (MABP) and ICP. In order to protect the brain from ischemia, PP should be kept above 50 torr. Thus, if MABP is 60, ICP must be 10 or less to ensure adequate PP.

Reduction in ICP may be achieved in several ways. Paralysis with a neuromuscular blocking agent such as pancuronium bromide at a dose of 0.1 to 0.2 mg per kg is useful, not only to reduce ICP but also to prevent the child from fighting the respirator. The child's head should be elevated 30 degrees. Controlled hyperventilation to maintain a PCO_2 of 25 to 30 torr will also help to reduce ICP. Administration of an osmotic diuretic such as mannitol, at a dose of 0.25 gram per kg, is also effective. The dose may be repeated or increased to as high as 2 grams per kg per dose every 4 hours as needed to control ICP. Serum osmolality should be monitored and kept below 320 mOsm in order to maintain the effectiveness of mannitol and prevent complications of hyperosmolar states.

The use of high-dose barbiturates to control ICP should be reserved for the most refractory cases, since this mode of therapy is associated with additional complications, including decreased cardiac output and systemic hypotension. The usual method for barbiturate treatment is to administer a loading dose of 3 to 5 mg per kg pentobarbital intravenously, and then 1 to 3 mg per kg per hour to maintain a blood level of 3 to 4 mg per dl and a burst-suppression pattern on EEG. When ICP has remained normal for 24 to 48 hours, the pentobarbital is gradually reduced over 36 to 48 hours.

OUTCOME

The mortality rate for all cases of Reye's syndrome remains about 30 per cent. There is evidence that the disease is less likely to progress in children who are diagnosed in Stage I and who receive hypertonic glucose therapy. Survivors of Reye's syndrome over the age of 1 year are likely to return to normal levels of function, even in severe cases. Sequelae include mild cognitive dysfunction, seizure disorders, and, rarely, more severe impairment such as psychomotor retardation. Infants less than 1 year of age are more likely to suffer long-term, significant neurologic sequelae such as psychomotor retardation and spastic quadriplegia.

MULTIPLE SCLEROSIS

method of
GARY BIRNBAUM, M.D.
University of Minnesota
Minneapolis, Minnesota

DIAGNOSTIC CONSIDERATIONS

Multiple sclerosis (MS) is a chronic demyelinating disease of the central nervous system (CNS). Its course is variable, ranging from illness so mild as to be detected only at autopsy to severe disability and death within several years. Most individuals with MS have a mild to moderate form of the disease. Neurologic symptoms usually appear between the ages of 18 and 50, although instances of earlier or later onset are not rare. Women are affected more often, with female/male ratios approaching 2:1. The incidence of the disease varies with geographic location, being more common in northern and southern temperate zones and less common as one approaches the equator. In high-risk areas, incidences of more than 150 per 100,000 have been reported.

Because no single diagnostic parameter, either on history, physical examination, or laboratory test, is pathognomonic of MS, the diagnosis rests on a combination of clinical and laboratory findings. The most important information comes from the history and physical examination, which should reveal objective evidence of multifocal involvement of CNS white matter not attributable to other causes (e.g., emboli, vasculitis, diabetes mellitus, neoplasm, vitamin B_{12} or vitamin E deficiency). Any CNS function can be affected, although sensory, visual, motor, and bowel and bladder difficulties are most common. The disease often has an exacerbating and remitting course, with various degrees of recovery between attacks. In some individuals the disease is chronically progressive from onset, whereas in others the illness is characterized by a combination of chronic progression with superimposed attacks. The pattern of disease can change with time;

exacerbations and remissions early in the course can become chronic progressive symptoms later in the illness.

Two categories of laboratory tests corroborate the clinical diagnosis: those that demonstrate multiple areas of CNS white matter dysfunction and those that demonstrate evidence of an in situ immune response within the CNS. The former types of tests are particularly important early in the illness when multifocal CNS involvement may be subclinical. Such tests include visual, brain stem, and somatosensory evoked responses; magnetic resonance imaging of the brain and spinal cord; and computed tomography of the brain. The best test for determining the presence of an immune response in the CNS is the analysis of cerebrospinal fluid. In cases of active MS, there are typically a lymphocytic pleocytosis, an increased percentage of immunoglobulin, an increase in synthesis of immunoglobulin in the CNS, and the presence of three or more bands of gamma globulin on cerebrospinal fluid protein electrophoresis. Bands are usually not present in serum, which should be electrophoresed concurrently. Early in the course of the disease, any or all of the above laboratory tests may be normal, and repeat evaluations may be necessary.

The cause of MS is not known but it appears that multiple factors are important in pathogenesis. Evidence from family studies, population studies, and studies of monozygotic twins indicates that there is a strong genetic component involved in determining susceptibility to disease. In addition, there is strong evidence for an immunologic response in the CNS that contributes to the demyelinating process. Finally, studies of both humans and animals suggest that an exogenous agent such as a virus may be responsible for either initiating or perpetuating the disease process. The nature of either the immune abnormality or the exogenous agent (or agents) involved is not known.

TREATMENT

There is no cure for MS at this time. However, a nihilistic approach to treatment is not warranted. A large number of therapies may significantly relieve symptoms of the disease, and various experimental treatments now under investigation may alter the duration of an exacerbation and perhaps the short-term course of the disease.

Treatments may be divided into two general categories: those aimed at alleviating symptoms and those directed against the presumed underlying disease process.

Symptomatic Treatments

Spasticity

Corticospinal tract dysfunction occurs frequently in patients with MS. The associated spasticity results in painful flexor and extensor spasms, nocturnal cramping and myoclonus, and extremity tightness with decreased ability to ambulate and perform fine motor movements. Many paraparetic MS patients rely on lower extremity extensor spasticity for support, and care should be taken in reducing spasticity in such individuals.

There is no entirely satisfactory treatment for spasticity in MS, but a number of drugs are useful. One of the safest and most commonly used is baclofen (Lioresal). The mechanism of its action is not known, but it inhibits poly- and monosynaptic spinal reflexes. At the start of treatment, baclofen may have depressant effects on the CNS, with increased weakness and fatigue. Thus, it must be administered slowly. The usual starting dose is 5 mg one to three times per day. Doses are gradually increased as tolerated to levels as high as 20 mg four or five times per day. If nocturnal spasms, painful cramping, and myoclonus are the predominant symptoms of spasticity, baclofen can be administered in the evening and at bedtime. Because weakness and fatigue are not as apparent at night, a higher starting dose (e.g., 10 mg at bedtime) may be tolerated. Benzodiazepines such as diazepam (Valium) have been used with some success in MS patients. Dosages vary with the drug, but because all drugs can cause sedation and increased fatigue, low dosages should be used initially. With diazepam an initial dose of 2 mg at night is usually well tolerated. Because of its long half-life, diazepam can be given in single daily doses. Clonazepam (Klonopin), another benzodiazepine, can be used in the treatment of nocturnal myoclonus and restless legs syndrome. The usual starting dose is 0.5 mg at bedtime. Another useful antispasticity drug is dantrolene (Dantrium). Initial doses are 25 mg two or three times per day. Timing of doses can be tailored to the specific needs of the MS patient. Because this drug may cause significant hepatic dysfunction, particularly at dosages above 400 mg per day, liver functions should be monitored while this medicine is given. In the severely disabled patient with intractable flexor or extensor spasms and pain, tenotomy or rhizotomy can be considered.

Bladder Dysfunction

MS patients with spinal cord dysfunction frequently have difficulties in controlling urination. The most common bladder symptoms are urgency, urge incontinence, and frequency. Less often, patients experience difficulties in initiation of urination, lack of an urge to urinate, and constant dribbling without feelings of urgency. Treatment can reduce and may alleviate entirely many of these bladder difficulties.

Symptoms of urgency and frequency are caused

by bladder and detrusor spasticity and dysynergia. Anticholinergic drugs such as propantheline (ProBanthine) are effective treatments for this condition. Initial doses are 7.5 mg every 3 to 4 hours. If the drug is well tolerated, doses can be increased to 15 mg three or four times daily, with an additional 15 to 30 mg at night to prevent nocturnal incontinence. Because anticholinergic effects last only 3 to 4 hours, timing of dosages can be tailored to an individual's needs (such as before a car journey or social engagement). Other drugs of benefit are oxybutynin chloride (Ditropan), 5 mg three or four times per day, and amitriptyline (Elavil), 10 mg at night, gradually increasing to 50 to 100 mg at night.

The presence of urinary hesitancy, difficulty with initiation of voiding, constant, low-volume incontinence, and frequent urinary tract infections suggests bladder atony, sphincter spasticity, or both. In either case, such patients cannot empty their bladders completely, which results in large, atonic bladders. The use of anticholinergics in such cases only compounds this difficulty. To determine if incomplete bladder emptying occurs, postvoiding residual urine volume is measured. Patients are asked to void and are then immediately catheterized. The presence of urine volumes of more than 100 ml indicates inadequate bladder emptying. If structural urinary tract abnormalities are excluded (with cystoscopy and ureteroscopy), it is best to treat this condition with intermittent bladder catheterization one to four times per day. Some patients may benefit from the use of a parasympathomimetic agent such as bethanechol (Urecholine), but often this treatment only increases the frequency of incontinence without inducing complete bladder emptying. If incontinence persists between catheterizations, anticholinergics, as noted earlier, can be added. Many patients initially resist the concept of self-catheterization. However, when properly taught and supervised, this technique becomes quite acceptable. Proper techique is also important in preventing urinary tract infections. If upper extremity disability or the unavailability of a care giver precludes intermittent straight catheterization, an indwelling catheter can be used. This is less desirable because of the increased incidence of urinary tract infections, local perineal irritation, and the encumbrances of tubes and bags. If patients continue to have recurrent infections, bladder calculi, or other complications of indwelling catheters, significant benefit may accrue from construction of a ureteroileal conduit.

Some patients experience frequent urinary tract infections despite proper bladder care. In such patients the use of prophylactic antibiotic therapy is warranted. Drugs that have been successfully used are trimethoprim-sulfamethoxazole (Septra DS and Bactrim DS), one tablet per day; nitrofurantoin (Macrodantin), 50 to 100 mg at bedtime; and methenamine mandelate (Mandelamine), 1 gram four times per day. An acidic urine is required for the antibacterial activity of the last drug.

Bowel Dysfunction

Constipation is the most frequent bowel symptom in patients with MS. Diarrhea is relatively uncommon. Constipation may be worsened by voluntary fluid restriction that some patients utilize to decrease bladder urgency and incontinence. Constipation is best managed by adequate fluid intake and the consumption of fiber-rich foods such as salads and bran. In addition, bulk-producing agents such as psyllium hydrophilic mucilloid (Metamucil or Fibercon) are effective, as are stool softeners such as docusate (Colace), 50 mg one to four times daily. In refractory constipation, the use of stimulant laxative suppositories, such as bisacodyl (Dulcolax) or glycerine, may be necessary. Some patients manage chronic constipation by stimulating the anus (manually or with hot water) and by manual disimpaction.

Less often, patients with MS experience bowel urgency and urge incontinence. Anticholinergics, as described earlier for bladder symptoms, are of benefit. Diarrhea is uncommon in MS, and other causes for this condition should be sought. Short-term use of antidiarrheal agents such as tincture of opium, diphenoxylate plus atropine (Lomotil), or bismuth subsalicylate (Pepto-Bismol) may be helpful.

Sexual Dysfunction

Many MS patients experience decreased genital sensation with decreased ability to achieve orgasm. In males, impotence is common. Any of these symptoms can result from an exacerbation of the disease and can be managed as such (see later discussion). If impotence persists, there are several therapeutic options. Intracavernous injections of the smooth muscle relaxant papaverine hydrochloride (30 mg per ml) in volumes of 0.25 to 1 ml are effective in inducing erections lasting 30 to 45 minutes. Alternatively, papaverine (25 mg per ml) can be mixed with phentolamine mesylate (Regitine), 5 mg per ml, and injected intracavernously in similar volumes. Orgasm and ejaculation are not affected by these medications. These treatments should be carried out after urologic evaluation and under supervision of the physician because orthostatic hypotension, injection site fibrosis, and sustained erections (>4 hours) may occur, especially with long-term use. Surgical implantation of either an inflatable or a semirigid penile prosthesis is an effective alternative treatment of impotence.

Fatigue

Overwhelming fatigue can be a disabling symptom of MS. It may not be relieved with rest and often does not correlate with motor weakness or psychologic dysfunction. There are no completely satisfactory treatments, but amantadine (Symmetrel), 100 mg twice per day, or pemoline (Cylert), 18.75 to 75 mg in the morning, can be of benefit to some patients.

Incoordination and Tremors

These symptoms cause major disability and are among the most difficult to treat. Patients respond to antitremor medications in different ways, and an empiric approach is warranted. Several drugs, either alone or in combination, can be tried.

If these drugs are not medically contraindicated, a beta-adrenergic blocker such as propranolol (Inderal) can be useful. Starting doses are 10 to 20 mg three or four times daily. These doses can be increased gradually as tolerated if salutary effects are noted. Low-dose primidone (Mysoline), 25 to 50 mg one to four times per day, can also be administered. Finally, clonazepam, 0.5 mg one to four times daily, may benefit some patients.

Psychologic and Cognitive Dysfunction

Although the stresses and disabilities imposed by MS can cause psychologic dysfunction, alterations in mood and cognitive function can be a direct result of the underlying disease process. Such changes may occur at any time in the course of MS and can cause major disability. Alterations in mood can range from psychotic-like symptoms of depression and paranoia to euphoria and emotional lability, with inappropriate crying or laughing. Mood changes are often associated with cognitive dysfunction, such as difficulties with memory, concentration, and judgment. There is little correlation of these affective changes with motor, visual, or sensory disabilities.

If mood or cognitive changes result from an acute disease exacerbation, they can be treated as such, by using corticosteroids (see later discussion). The psychologic dysfunction is often insidious in onset or persists after treatment of an acute exacerbation of disease. When this occurs, psychotropic drug therapy is appropriate. In cases of depression, and especially in individuals with emotional lability, amitriptyline can be of great value. Its potent anticholinergic effects are of additional benefit to the patient with symptoms of bladder and detrusor spasticity. Because of its sedating action, amitriptyline should be given in low doses (10 to 25 mg) at bedtime. Doses are increased as tolerated. In patients with paranoia or mania, haloperidol (Haldol) and lithium carbonate (Eskalith, Lithane, and others), respectively, can be used. Mood changes are especially frequent during steroid treatments of acute disease exacerbations. If such changes have been previously observed, they can be anticipated with future steroid administration and can be treated prophylactically by concurrent administration of lithium carbonate, 300 mg orally twice daily. Renal function and lithium levels should be monitored.

Cognitive impairment can be severe in patients with MS and again can represent a symptom of exacerbation of disease. It may persist and require extensive changes in work and family duties. If impairment is sufficiently severe, custodial care may be necessary.

Cognitive impairment may result from pseudodementia, an apparent cognitive deficit related to severe underlying depression. Pseudodementia can be differentiated from true dementia by psychiatric evaluation and neuropsychometric testing. Its treatment is the treatment of the underlying depression.

Pain and Sensory Symptoms

Pain and uncomfortable sensory symptoms are common in MS, the most common being musculoskeletal discomforts. These symptoms usually occur in the joints of paretic limbs, such as hips or knees, particularly if there is associated hyperextension of the joint because of limb weakness. Joint symptoms are also frequent during tapering and cessation of steroid therapy. Physical therapy and nonsteroidal anti-inflammatory drugs benefit such patients. Some patients receive help from orthotic appliances that prevent joint hyperextension.

A large number of MS patients experience burning, drawing, and tight, band-like dysesthesias in the limbs, chest, or abdomen, presumably because of involvement of spinal cord sensory tracts. A smaller number of MS patients develop the sudden onset of sharp, shooting, hemifacial pains, or deep facial aching, presumably associated with an area of demyelination in the outflow tract of the trigeminal nerve. Both the tic-like hemifacial pains and the dysesthesias can respond to carbamazepine (Tegretol). Initial doses are 100 or 200 mg once or twice per day. This amount is gradually increased to a total daily dosage of between 600 and 1600 mg given three or four times daily. Careful monitoring of trough drug levels and blood counts is necessary. If symptoms are most prominent at night, amitriptyline, with its associated sedating actions, can be useful. Initial dosages are 10 to 25 mg at night. Amounts are gradually increased as tolerated until therapeutic levels are achieved. This drug's analgesic actions may not be noted for 7 to 14 days, and patients should be so advised. Additional drugs that may be effective are phenytoin (Dilantin) and baclofen.

Limb spasticity may be associated with painful nocturnal cramps, which can be eased considerably with night-time doses of baclofen.

Physical Therapy

Careful stretching, conditioning, and mild aerobic exercises can increase an MS patient's feeling of well-being and can reduce limb spasticity and fatigability. The only limits to be imposed are those dictated by the patient's physical condition. Overexertion and exposure to warm temperatures (such as in heated swimming pools, whirlpool baths, or saunas) should generally be avoided because many patients with MS note an increase in neurologic symptoms with elevations of body temperature.

Treatments Aimed at the Disease Process

Immunotherapy

The presence of inflammation at sites of demyelination, the abnormalities of cerebrospinal fluid in MS patients, and the alterations in blood and cerebrospinal fluid lymphocytes suggest that an immunologic abnormality is an important component of the MS disease process. Various immunomodulating drugs thus have been used to treat the disease. Although most neurologists treat MS patients with such drugs, there is no conclusive evidence that this treatment alters the overall course of the illness.

Corticosteroids. This class of drugs is the most widely used to treat acute MS exacerbations. They are usually prescribed for short periods (i.e., weeks). Long-term administration of corticosteroids has no effect on the course of MS and often results in increased disability because of the many side effects that are associated with chronic steroid administration.

The drug most often used to treat an MS exacerbation is adrenocorticotropic hormone, or ACTH (Acthar, Cortrophin, and others). Dosages are 40 units intravenously, intramuscularly, or subcutaneously, twice per day for 1 to 2 weeks, followed by a gradual taper over an additional 7 to 10 days. Recently, high doses of intravenous methylprednisolone (Solu-Medrol, A-Methapred,

and others) have been used with success in acute attacks. Uncomfortable side effects from this drug may also be less than those noted with ACTH. The usual dose of methylprednisolone is 500 to 1000 mg per day for 7 to 10 days. The drug is administered in volumes of 100 to 200 ml of 5 per cent dextrose, infused during 90 to 120 minutes. As with all intravenous preparations, patients should be monitored for acute allergic reactions to the medication. After a 7- to 10-day course of intravenous therapy, the dose can be rapidly tapered by administering methylprednisolone orally. A total of 48 mg in divided doses is given on the first day after intravenous therapy. The dose is reduced by 8 mg per day on subsequent days until no more medication is given. Some patients experience increased fatigue after the taper, but this usually subsides within 1 to 2 weeks. Exacerbations of MS can also be treated with intravenous and oral dexamethasone (Decadron, Hexadrol), and with oral prednisone. Oral steroids may be sufficient for milder exacerbations, and it is reasonable to reserve high-dose intravenous therapy for more severe attacks. As a rule, steroids are not recommended for mild or short (<48 hours) attacks and should not be administered chronically.

Any additional body stresses, such as intercurrent infections, can result in significant increases in MS symptoms. Therefore, all patients with a presumed exacerbation of MS should be evaluated for the presence of infection, fever, or other confounding variables.

During steroid therapy, particularly with oral administration, the use of antiulcer medications is recommended. These include ranitidine (Zantac), cimetidine (Tagamet), or antacids such as aluminum hydroxide (Alterna Gel, Amphojel, Dialume, and others). Such drugs can prevent the abdominal discomfort often associated with this treatment regimen.

Azathioprine (Imuran). Azathioprine has been used as treatment for various presumed autoimmune disorders. Its benefit to patients with MS is uncertain. The drug has been used to reduce the number of disease exacerbations and/or to halt or reduce the rate of chronic progression of symptoms. It is not used to treat an acute attack. Azathioprine is administered daily, in single or divided doses after meals, at 1.5 to 2 mg per kg per day. At least 1 year of treatment may be necessary for beneficial effects to accrue. Recent evidence suggests that any beneficial effects of azathioprine may be enhanced by the periodic administration (e.g., every 4 to 6 weeks) of single high doses of intravenous methylprednisolone.

Patients receiving azathioprine should be monitored for evidence of suppression of bone marrow and for liver dysfunction, and dosages should be reduced or drugs discontinued accordingly. The incidence of malignancy in MS patients, at low dosages of this drug, appears to be small.

Cyclophosphamide (Cytoxan and Neosar). Cyclophosphamide is a potent DNA-alkylating agent that has profound immunosuppressing effects by virtue of its actions on rapidly dividing cells in bone marrow. It has been used to treat severe cases of MS in the hope of reducing the numbers and severity of disease exacerbations and halting or reducing the progression of chronic symptoms. Its efficacy is not proved, but in some series up to two-thirds of patients with chronically progressive disease stabilize for several years. The drug can be administered orally at dosages of 2 to 2.5 mg per kg per day for several months. It can also be administered intravenously, and various dosage regimens have been used. In one clinical trial, cyclophosphamide was administered at 600 mg per M^2 for five doses given over 8 days. Additional single monthly doses have been used in some protocols to continue the immunosuppressant effects of the drug. Several large, multicenter trials of cyclophosphamide are now in progress.

Use of cyclophosphamide is associated with a large number of side effects, including nausea and vomiting; bladder urgency, frequency, and hematuria; alopecia; sterility; an increased risk of infection; and an increased risk of bladder and hematologic malignancy. The last effect may be more likely with prolonged, lower-dose oral administration.

Interferons. Interferons are biologically active substances that are produced by various cells including macrophages, fibroblasts, and lymphocytes. There are at least three kinds of interferons: alpha, beta, and gamma. Administration of interferon-gamma has been associated with an increased number of MS exacerbations and is no longer used. Several preliminary trials of interferon-beta administration to patients with exacerbating-remitting MS have suggested a salutary effect in reducing the numbers of attacks. Large, multicenter clinical trials are now in progress to confirm these results and determine the best routes of administration and dosages.

Total Lymphoid Irradiation. A preliminary study of patients with chronic progressive MS suggested that total lymphoid irradiation may decrease the rate of disease progression. Additional, larger trials are in progress.

Cyclosporine (Sandimmune). Several large, multicenter trials of cyclosporine as a treatment of chronic progressive MS have recently been completed. Preliminary evidence suggests that this drug may have a mild beneficial effect, but its use is associated with a high incidence of side effects, which may preclude use of this drug for a large number of patients.

Miscellaneous Therapy

Great caution must be exercised in evaluating any therapeutic claim in MS because a hallmark of the disease is the spontaneous remission of symptoms and signs in a large number of patients. Indeed, the corridors of neurologic care are littered with the remains of "effective" treatments or cures for MS. Some of the more recent casualties are hyperbaric oxygen, colostrum, megavitamin therapy, acupuncture, special diets (such as gluten-free, saturated fat–free, lactose-free, or "allergen"-free diets), intravenous organic calcium administration, use of colchicine, and use of antifungal (anticandidal) drugs.

MS is a disease that can affect all aspects of an individual's life. Its treatment is truly a therapeutic challenge. Although no cure is yet available, many of the symptoms and signs of the illness can be significantly ameliorated and, in some instances, even eliminated.

MYASTHENIA GRAVIS

method of
CHRISTIAN HERRMANN, JR., M.D.
University of California
Los Angeles, California

Present findings indicate that autoimmune myasthenia gravis is an acquired immune complex disorder of neuromuscular transmission in voluntary striated muscle. Elevated titer of antibody to acetylcholine receptor is detectable in the serum of most patients. There is a break in immunologic tolerance with blocking and degradation of acetylcholine receptors; widening of the synaptic cleft; and partial destruction, simplification, and shortening of the postjunctional membrane. Thymic hyperplasia and/or thymoma may be associated.

Clinically, myasthenia gravis is characterized by variable weakness and easy fatigability. After a short rest of the muscles, there is partial to total recovery of strength. Extraocular, facial, and oropharyngeal muscles are usually affected early, but any of the voluntary striated muscles of the body may be involved. Commonly, its onset in women occurs before the age of 40 years and in men after the age of 40. Either sex may be affected at any time. About 12 per cent of infants born to myasthenic mothers have a transient transmitted form of neonatal myasthenia gravis that remits permanently in days or weeks. Pregnancy is not generally contraindicated in myasthenia gravis.

TREATMENT

Anticholinesterase Therapy

Anticholinesterase drugs are the usual first line of treatment for myasthenia gravis. Their action is attributed to inhibition of cholinesterase at the neuromuscular junction, allowing acetylcholine to accumulate and facilitate remaining neuromuscular transmission. The three most frequently used are (1) neostigmine bromide (Prostigmin), (2) pyridostigmine bromide (Mestinon), and (3) ambenonium chloride (Mytelase). These partially reduce the defect in neuromuscular transmission and improve strength but are not a cure.

A fourth, very short-acting anticholinesterase agent, edrophonium chloride (Tensilon), is used to aid in the diagnosis of myasthenia gravis and to assess the effectiveness of the dosage of anticholinesterase drugs noted before. It is not useful for ongoing treatment. The diagnostic edrophonium test is best done when the patient has stopped taking all anticholinesterase drugs for 8 to 12 hours. A detailed test of muscle strength is done throughout the body, with areas of weakness noted, including cranial, oropharyngeal, and respiratory muscles. This is followed by a control injection or protective placebo injection of atropine sulfate, 0.4 mg intravenously. This acts to protect the patient from muscarinic side effects of the edrophonium to be given subsequently, as well as to assess psychologic effects of an intravenous injection. A detailed test of muscle strength of the areas previously noted to be weak is done again. This is followed by edrophonium, 2 mg intravenously, with repeated muscle testing in 30 seconds to 2 minutes, as after the atropine injection. Not all areas of weakness may respond equally to the edrophonium. A second injection of edrophonium, 4 to 8 mg intravenously, may be given in 3 to 5 minutes after the first if the first was not definitive and detailed muscle testing of weak areas is done again. In most myasthenics there is a clear-cut, although transient, improvement in strength that may not be uniform in all areas of weakness. This lasts usually 2 to 5 minutes and occasionally longer.

A list of commonly used anticholinesterase drugs and comparable dosage forms and routes of administration is given in Table 1. Anticholinesterases do not occur naturally in humans. Excessive anticholinesterase therapy may have adverse effects, increasing weakness and provoking other unpleasant and potentially dangerous side effects. These are listed under the column "Cholinergic Crisis" in Table 2.

Oral anticholinesterase therapy may be started gradually with one-half of a 15-mg tablet of neostigmine (7.5 mg) or one-half of a 60-mg tablet of pyridostigmine (30 mg) at 4-hour intervals or two or three times daily. Patients with weakness in chewing and swallowing will find it helpful to take the drug 30 to 60 minutes before meals and refrain from talking while eating. Gastrointestinal effects will be fewer if a small amount of milk, bread, crackers, or other bland food is eaten before the anticholinesterase. Foods such as coffee, fruit, tomato juice, or carbonated or alcoholic beverages tend to increase the parasympathetic side effects on the gut, bladder, bronchi, and mucous glands. They are best avoided or taken at the end of a meal.

The dosage of anticholinesterase drug may be increased gradually at about 2-day intervals and the dose intervals shortened to 3 hours only if these changes are followed by objective improvement in symptoms and signs. Increases of one-fourth to one-half tablet per dose are recommended. Both the physician and patient must realize that anticholinesterase drugs seldom restore muscle strength to more than 80 per cent of normal strength with optimal dosage. Weakness of extraocular, oropharyngeal, respiratory, and other muscles at times selectively or together may show little improvement with anticholinesterase drugs.

Neostigmine and pyridostigmine are quite similar in their action and effectiveness. Some patients note more muscarinic side effects such as abdominal cramps, diarrhea, nausea, salivation, tearing, and sweating with neostigmine than with pyridostigmine. The action of neostigmine is about 30 to 45 minutes shorter than that of pyridostigmine. A few patients find that neostigmine gives more prompt and slightly greater improvement in muscle strength than pyridostigmine.

There are additional helpful forms of pyridostigmine. The syrup contains 60 mg in 5 ml (approximately 1 teaspoonful). This is palatable and easily administered and adjusted for young myasthenic children. Patients with swallowing difficulty may handle this form more easily and with greater safety than the tablets. It is also easily given by nasogastric tube. The other useful form of pyridostigmine is Mestinon Timespan tablets. Each contains 180 mg of pyridostigmine. About one-third of the dosage is released promptly, and the remainder is released over the next 6 to 12 hours. When a tablet is given at bedtime, it allows the moderate to severe myasthenic to sleep through the night without awakening to take regular anticholinesterase medication. Usually, only patients with moderate to severe myasthenia require medication during sleeping hours and the dosage may be reduced to

TABLE 1. **Anticholinesterase Drugs Used in Diagnosis and Management of Myasthenia Gravis**

Drug	Form	Adult Single Dose and Route	Usual Effective Duration and Range
Tensilon (edrophonium chloride)	10 mg/ml	2–10 mg IV	10 min (2 min to 2 hr)
Prostigmin (neostigmine methylsulfate)	0.25, 0.5, and 1 mg/ml	1 mg IM	2 hr (2–4 hr)
Prostigmin (neostigmine bromide)	15-mg tablet	15 mg PO	3 hr (2–5 hr)
Mestinon (pyridostigmine bromide)	10 mg/2 ml	2 mg IM	2 hr (2–4 hr)
Mestinon (pyridostigmine bromide)	60-mg tablet	60 mg PO	4 hr (3–7 hr)
Mestinon Timespan (pyridostigmine bromide)	180-mg tablet (slow release)	90–180 mg PO	8 hr (6–12 hr)
Mestinon Syrup (pyridostigmine bromide)	60 mg/5 ml syrup	60 mg/5 ml (1 tsp PO)	4 hr (3–7 hr)
Mytelase (ambenonium chloride)	10-mg tablet	5–10 mg PO	6 hr (4–8 hr)

one-half or two-thirds of that taken during waking hours. Since the regular forms of pyridostigmine give more prompt and dependable release and absorption, Mestinon Timespan is not recommended for daytime use.

When patients are temporarily unable to take anticholinesterase drugs by mouth or are unable to swallow, parenteral forms of neostigmine methylsulfate or pyridostigmine bromide may be substituted. The equivalent of a 15-mg tablet of neostigmine is 1 to 1.5 mg of neostigmine methylsulfate intramuscularly. The equivalent of a 60-mg tablet of pyridostigmine bromide is 2 mg of pyridostigmine bromide intramuscularly. Parenteral anticholinesterase therapy is seldom more effective than oral therapy. It is not practical for long-term care.

Ambenonium chloride is the third available oral anticholinesterase drug. It is used much less frequently than neostigmine and pyridostigmine. It may be more effective against weakness of the extremities than of the cranial muscles. Duration of action is a bit longer than that of pyridostig-

mine. Patients not responding well to neostigmine or pyridostigmine may be tried carefully on ambenonium. Muscarinic toxic effects are less prominent, but nicotinic and central nervous system symptoms and signs of toxicity may appear. The nicotinic manifestations include muscle twitching and weakness. The central nervous system manifestations include headache, restlessness, and anxiety. Between 5 and 7.5 mg of ambenonium chloride is equivalent to 15 mg of neostigmine or 60 mg of pyridostigmine (tablets) given orally. One may start with 5 mg of ambenonium every 4 to 6 hours and increase by 2.5 mg per dose if there is objective improvement and no undesirable side effects.

To assess effects of anticholinesterase drugs, it is useful to examine patients just before the next dose of drug and 45 to 75 minutes after it. Helpful areas to test include the following:

1. The patient's inability to sustain upward gaze can reveal fatigue of the lid levators or extraocular muscles.

2. Continuous counting on a single breath

TABLE 2. **Symptoms and Signs of Myasthenic and Cholinergic Crises**

Myasthenic Crisis		Cholinergic Crisis	
Ocular ptosis	*Muscarinic Symptoms and Signs:*		*Nicotinic Symptoms and Signs:*
Dysarthria or anarthria			
Dysphagia or aphagia	Sweating		Muscle fasciculations
Dyspnea or apnea	Salivation		Dysarthric speech
Facial weakness	Lacrimation		Dysphagia
Masticatory weakness	Abdominal cramping		Trismus
Difficulty handling secretions	Nausea		Muscle cramps and spasms
General weakness	Vomiting		General weakness
	Diarrhea		
	Urinary frequency		*CNS Symptoms and Signs:*
	Incontinence of bowel and bladder		
	Miosis		Restlessness
	Blurred vision		Anxiety
	Bradycardia		Vertigo
	Bronchorrhea		Headache
	Substernal pressure		Confusion and stupor
	Dyspnea and wheezing		Coma
	Bronchospasm		Convulsions
	Pulmonary edema		

gives a rough estimate of respiratory muscle strength and vital capacity.

3. The time the patient is able to keep the arms or legs elevated is an indication of the fatigability of these muscles.

4. The number of times the patient is able to cross and uncross one thigh over the other, squat, and arise or repeatedly compress a partially inflated blood pressure cuff or hand dynamometer is a simple test of strength and fatigability of neuromuscular transmission in these areas.

5. The patient's abilities to close the jaw tightly against resistance, to protrude the tongue into each cheek against resistance, to elevate the soft palate, to cough, to swallow, and to speak are useful signs that aid in assessing oropharyngeal strength.

Measurement of the vital capacity is a simple test of respiratory muscle function and reserve. It is weakness in oropharyngeal and/or respiratory muscle strength that constitutes the greatest threat to the myasthenic's life. Treatment should be directed to achieve optimal improvement in these areas.

The edrophonium chloride test may also be used in an attempt to determine how adequate ongoing anticholinesterase therapy is. One hour after the oral dose of the drug, the patient's strength is tested. The patient is then given 2 mg (0.2 ml) of edrophonium chloride intravenously, and strength is retested in 30 seconds to 2 minutes. If strength is significantly improved, the dosage of oral anticholinesterase may be increased. If strength is unchanged or declines, the oral anticholinesterase dosage is not changed. If muscarinic and nicotinic effects appear after 2 mg of edrophonium chloride, along with increased weakness, the oral anticholinesterase dosage should be lowered.

Although some differences are noted among the effects of neostigmine, pyridostigmine, and ambenonium, overall results are quite similar. Of the three, currently pyridostigmine is the most frequently used oral anticholinesterase drug.

Crisis

Muscle weakness leading to inability to maintain a patent airway free of secretions and/or adequate respiratory exchange constitutes crisis in the myasthenic. It may be caused by increase in the myasthenia gravis itself, too much anticholinesterase drug, or both. Rapid distinction among myasthenic, cholinergic, or mixed or insensitive crises may be difficult in the acute situation, if not impossible. Promptly providing an adequate airway with tracheal intubation, if

necessary, suctioning of excessive tracheobronchial secretions to clear the airway, and positive-pressure assisted or controlled respiration may be lifesaving. Bilateral weakness of the abductors of the vocal cords may obstruct the airway, thus limiting exchange. Factors often associated with myasthenic crisis are infections, especially upper respiratory tract infections, menses, omitting anticholinesterase medication, vigorous physical activity, certain drugs, and emotional upsets.

Drugs having an adverse effect on neuromuscular transmission include most hypnotics, tranquilizers, and antihistaminics, as well as thiazides, quinine, quinidine, procainamide, calcium channel blockers, beta-blockers, ether, d-tubocurarine, pancuronium, succinylcholine, magnesium sulfate, D-penicillamine, adrenocorticotropic hormone (ACTH), adrenocorticosteroids, and aminoglycoside antibiotics. The latter include colistimethate, colistin, dihydrostreptomycin, kanamycin, neomycin, novobiocin, polymyxin B, gentamicin, streptomycin, and tobramycin.

Cholinergic crisis may be caused by too much anticholinesterase medication. It may develop in the course of a spontaneous remission, or following thymectomy or an overenthusiastic use of anticholinesterase drugs by the physician or patient. Some patients become unresponsive, insensitive, or resistant to anticholinesterase drugs. This happens particularly when the dosage is gradually increased to high levels over a long period of time. It must be remembered that both the antibody to acetylcholine receptor and anticholinesterase drugs are attacking and acting on the postjunctional membrane of the neuromuscular junction. Each may adversely affect neuromuscular transmission. The symptoms and signs of myasthenic and cholinergic crisis are listed in Table 2.

In the presence of cholinergic crisis or an unresponsive, resistant, or insensitive state, the anticholinesterase drug is stopped for 3 days or more. This is best done in a hospital, since the patient frequently initially becomes still weaker and may require an airway and mechanical ventilation for a time before strength spontaneously improves. This allows junctions that may be damaged and depolarized by excessive prolonged administration of an anticholinesterase drug to recover. Fluid balance and nutrition are maintained parenterally or by nasogastric tube.

If endotracheal intubation is required for more than 3 to 4 days, tracheostomy will be more comfortable for the patient, provide better tracheobronchial toilet, and reduce risk of damage to the larynx. A short, low-pressure cuffed tube is used. At times, patients withdrawn from anticholinesterase drugs and supported improve to the point that they may function for days or weeks without anticholinesterase medication.

Atropine is best used only sporadically or in an emergency to counteract muscarinic side effects of anticholinesterase drugs. Regular use may obscure the signs of cholinergic intoxication. Oral and tracheobronchial secretions are reduced and become thick, tenacious, inspissated, and difficult to aspirate. Bronchial plugging with atelectasis may result. Sedative and tranquilizing drugs are best avoided in the anxious apprehensive myasthenic. These symptoms and signs may be those of failing respiratory function rather than a psychologic reaction to illness. Such drugs may aggravate hypoxia and hypercapnia, setting up a vicious circle of more respiratory depression with vagal activity already increased by the anticholinesterase drug, leading to arrhythmia and asystole.

The patient in crisis should be turned frequently and given postural drainage, percussion to the chest, and meticulous tracheobronchial toilet. Auscultation of the chest, chest x-rays, and fiberoptic bronchoscopy may help to remove mucous plugs. Smears, cultures, and sensitivities of tracheobronchial secretions, along with appropriate antibiotics, aid in recovery and reduce mortality. Periodic determination of arterial blood gases aids evaluation of adequacy of mechanical ventilation, need for supplemental oxygen, and adjustment of depth and rate of respiration. Automatic periodic sighing, available on some respirators, may help prevent atelectasis and contractures of the chest wall from lack of full range of movement because of weakness. The lung in most myasthenics is normal and compliant once infection and atelectasis are overcome. For this reason, compressed air is best used for long-term operation of the positive pressure respirator.

Thymectomy

Improvement or remission of autoimmune myasthenia gravis following thymectomy has been reported in up to 80 per cent from several centers dealing with large numbers of myasthenic patients. It is most apt to occur in patients without thymoma. However, thymoma, which may occur in 15 per cent of patients with myasthenia gravis, is also an indication for thymectomy, since about 35 per cent of thymomas may become invasive or malignant. Exactly why improvement or remission occurs is not known. Results cannot be predicted in advance in the individual patient. Thymectomy is not helpful in congenital myasthenia. It may be less effective in patients older than 60 years of age, in whom the thymus is usually atrophic. It is not recom-

mended for debilitated patients or those showing malignant spread of thymoma. It is not done as an emergency procedure or in the presence of active pulmonary infection, pregnancy, or rapidly worsening myasthenia. Improvement following thymectomy may not occur for weeks or months. Operative risk is small in the hands of a competent thoracic surgeon in a facility where neurologic and medical staff are familiar with the disorder and have intensive care facilities including respiratory support available. The transcervical or suprasternal approach to the thymus has been used at a few centers, but this is not usually satisfactory for removal of thymomas and may not allow removal of all thymic tissue, since the surgeon's operative field is restricted. Most centers continue to use a median sternotomy, which avoids these problems.

Treatment with alternate-day corticosteroid therapy for a few weeks or months before thymectomy is helpful in myasthenic patients with moderate to severe oropharyngeal and/or respiratory muscle weakness. It is not recommended for all patients having thymectomy.

Preoperatively, the patient is allowed to take usual doses of anticholinesterase medication with small sips of water up to the time of surgery. Postoperatively, anticholinesterase medication is resumed in 12 to 24 hours as weakness occurs, and dosage requirements are usually less. About one-half to three-quarters of the preoperative dose is given to start with. Close cooperation with postoperative follow-up by the neurologist is essential. Meperidine (Demerol) rather than morphine is used to relieve pain.

Corticosteroid Therapy

Although some physicians have used alternate-day prednisone as the first choice of treatment even in essentially limited ocular myasthenia gravis, we have generally reserved its use for patients with more generalized weakness not responding favorably to anticholinesterases or thymectomy or both. This regimen may be considered in older patients who are not suitable candidates for thymectomy. However, both the patient and physician should be aware of the long-term commitment, side effects, risks, and complications of chronic use of corticosteroids, since fewer than 10 per cent of patients are able to discontinue them completely in most cases. Strength may greatly improve, but the majority of patients remain dependent upon the corticosteroids for their improvement. Withdrawal is usually followed by recurrent weakness in weeks or months and by the need for even higher doses to reverse the weakness. In some, the improvement may be maintained on a relatively low dose, compared with amounts required to initiate the improvement. Improvement takes place over weeks or months.

Since there may be some paradoxical worsening of the myasthenia gravis when corticosteroids are first begun, they are best started in a hospital setting with staff familiar with this form of treatment in myasthenia gravis and with facilities for mechanical respiratory support and intensive care, should these be needed.

Patients with obesity, hypertension, and/or diabetes mellitus are best not treated with steroids. Patients who are anergic or who have positive skin tests for tuberculosis are best given simultaneously prophylactic isoniazid and pyridoxine with the corticosteroids.

We recommend that patients taking corticosteroids maintain a diet high in protein, potassium, and calcium; moderate in complex carbohydrates; and low in fat with no added free sugars. Supplemental 10 per cent potassium chloride may be needed to keep the serum potassium in the upper normal levels. We recommend that patients receiving corticosteroids take antacid or nonfat milk 1 to 2 hours after each meal and at bedtime. We prefer to avoid chronic cimetidine or ranitidine therapy.

The blood count, serum potassium, and blood glucose are determined at office visits. Liver function tests are recommended for those on isoniazid; progress chest films are recommended at 6- to 12-month intervals.

We prefer to start alternate-day prednisone at 20 to 25 mg and increase this by 5 mg every second or third dose cycle. When strength begins to improve (which is usually not immediately), the dosage may be maintained at that level. We have seldom needed to exceed 100 mg on alternate days. If the patient already requires mechanical respiratory support, a higher initial starting dose, up to 100 mg, may be used in attempt to reverse severe weakness sooner. This seldom happens before the second or third week. Methylprednisolone, 60 mg intramuscularly, or dexamethasone, 12 mg orally, in divided doses daily, has also been used in such states.

Nonsteroidal Immunosuppressive Therapy

Azathioprine (Imuran),* cyclophosphamide (Cytoxan),* and methotrexate* have been used for long-term treatment in some patients. Those not responding to thymectomy or corticosteroids or those in whom corticosteroids are unacceptable because of side effects or contraindications may

*This use of these agents is not listed by the manufacturers.

find these drugs helpful. These agents may also be used to reduce the dosage of corticosteroids required when side effects of these are troublesome. They are useful to provide ongoing immunosuppression in conjunction with plasmapheresis. The major long-term experience with them has been abroad rather than in the United States. Azathioprine, 2 to 3 mg per kg daily, is given in single or divided oral doses. Significant response may not be noted for 2 months to 1 year. Maximal improvement may not occur for up to 24 months, but once it is achieved it is quite even, with little fluctuation from day to day. When the patient is stable, dosage may be tapered slowly. Side effects and complications include nausea, vomiting, leukopenia, thrombocytopenia, anemia (often megaloblastic), and hepatotoxicity. Patients receiving this are best followed initially with weekly blood counts and a monthly blood chemistry panel, with particular attention to liver function tests. Lowering or discontinuing the drug usually reverses these effects. A comparable dose of cyclophosphamide is used. Results and side effects are the same except for the added risks of hemorrhagic cystitis and alopecia. Azathioprine and cyclophosphamide are not recommended for women in childbearing years because of possible developmental defects in the fetus. A risk of malignancy, as well as increased susceptibility to infection, is another consideration.

Plasmapheresis Therapy

Exchange of 2 liters of plasma for equal amounts of human albumin and saline every other day three times a week may relieve weakness temporarily. Long-term benefit from this regimen usually requires combining it with corticosteroids, other immunosuppressants, and/or thymectomy. It may be helpful in preparing moderately to severely weak patients for thymectomy or to shorten the time of crisis. Since plasmapheresis requires special facilities and skills and entails other risks, it is best done at centers familiar with both myasthenia gravis and pheresis.

Adjuvant Therapy

Ephedrine sulfate, 25 mg orally two or three times daily, is helpful to some patients. It may make patients wakeful if given late in the day or evening. It should be avoided in men with prostatism, since it inhibits micturition. Potassium chloride, 1 to 2 grams given orally in 10 per cent solution two or three times daily with meals, is helpful to other patients who function better with serum potassium levels at high normal. A few patients appear to benefit from calcium gluconate or lactate, 1 to 2 grams taken orally two to four times daily.

Care for Surgery

Myasthenics may require surgery apart from thymectomy. Preoperative cathartics and enemas are avoided. The patient may take usual anticholinesterase drugs with small sips of water up to the time of surgery. If necessary, this may be converted to a parenteral dose of neostigmine or pyridostigmine. Muscle relaxants and sedatives are best avoided. Spinal, local, or regional anesthesia is preferable. When general anesthesia is necessary, ether is avoided—although it is seldom used for patients at present. Sodium pentothal and inhalation agents, such as nitrous oxide, cyclopropane, or halothane, may be used. In those with significant oropharyngeal and/or respiratory weakness preoperatively, the endotracheal tube may be left in place postoperatively until the patient is well awake and demonstrates stable respiratory function by adequate measured vital capacity. Meperidine is given to relieve pain. Meticulous care should be given to the respiratory tract to promote full expansion of the lungs using intermittent positive-pressure breathing (IPPB), assisted coughing, and careful tracheobronchial toilet to prevent atelectasis and pulmonary infection. Since patients with myasthenia gravis tend to fatigue with repeated voluntary effort, incentive spirometry is usually counterproductive as compared with IPPB to expand the lungs in someone with pre-existing respiratory muscle weakness. If antibiotics are needed, those listed earlier that are known to interfere with neuromuscular transmission are avoided. Dosage requirements for anticholinesterase are often lower postoperatively. Therapy may be started parenterally as weakness develops. When the patient is able to swallow and is no longer nauseated and bowel sounds are normal, medication may be given by nasogastric tube or orally.

Associated Disorders

The presence of one autoimmune disease increases the likelihood of another in the same patient. As a consequence, one may see such conditions as Graves's disease, Hashimoto's thyroiditis, rheumatoid arthritis, polymyositis, dermatomyositis, scleroderma, vitiligo, pernicious anemia, lupus erythematosus, pemphigus, idiopathic thrombocytopenic purpura, red cell aplasia, autoimmune hemolytic anemia, autoimmune secondary amenorrhea, and multiple sclerosis.

The most common are disorders of the thyroid, especially hyperthyroidism. Periodically, tests of thyroid function as well as determinations of creatine phosphokinase levels are desirable.

OUTLOOK

Better and newer forms of treatment, including improved mechanical respiratory support, antibiotics to combat infection, corticosteroids, other immunosuppressants and current discoveries, and understanding of the immunopathophysiology of neuromuscular transmission have all helped to reduce mortality and morbidity as well as increase longevity. It is important for patients to learn to pace their physical activities. Patients and their families benefit from learning the nature of myasthenia gravis and general principles of management to reduce unnecessary anxiety, to allow them more control of their care, and to promote a smoother course. Most patients with myasthenia gravis are able to lead gainful, productive, satisfying lives.

TRIGEMINAL NEURALGIA

method of
G. ROBERT NUGENT, M.D.
West Virginia University
Morgantown, West Virginia

Trigeminal neuralgia (tic douloureux) is probably the worst pain afflicting human beings, but fortunately the lightning-like attacks are of brief duration, spontaneous remissions are frequent, and the condition is treatable. As the process progresses, however, one attack follows another, the remissions are shorter, and sometimes the response to medication is less satisfactory.

Trigeminal neuralgia is a stereotyped clinical entity that is easily diagnosed by the history alone. The pain usually affects the older patient, is limited to the distribution of the trigeminal nerve, and is set off by touching a trigger area, which is usually in the snout region (side of the nose, nasolabial fold area, upper or lower lip, or chin). The trigger may also be in the gum or, if the first division is involved, in the eyebrow or hairline. It is extremely rare for pain to begin in and remain localized to the first division. The pain is also set off by talking, eating, washing the face, shaving, and especially brushing the teeth.

There are no abnormal neurologic findings except in those rare cases in which an identical pain may result from a cerebellopontine angle neoplasm or other posterior fossa lesion. Two to 3 per cent of patients with trigeminal neuralgia have multiple sclerosis. An enhanced computed tomography scan of the head should be performed to rule out other lesions causing the pain if the patient is young, the history is atypical, there are abnormal neurologic findings, or the pain has been present for only a short period of time. Rarely there may be clinical confusion with glossopharyngeal neuralgia, cluster headache, or pain of dental or sinus pathology.

For many years the cause of trigeminal neuralgia was unknown; however, there is evidence now that the pain results from cross-compression of the trigeminal nerve, at the point where it enters the pons, by an aberrant blood vessel, usually a branch of the superior cerebellar artery. This artery can often be found compressing, indenting, or otherwise physically injuring the nerve when visualized during surgical approach to the nerve in the posterior fossa.

MEDICAL TREATMENT

Carbamazepine (Tegetrol) is the treatment of choice and the mainstay of early treatment. This is almost universally successful in stopping the pain, provided side effects do not limit its use. The usual side effects are ataxia, dizziness, drowsiness, nausea, and, in some patients, mental confusion; rarely it may cause a rash. Treatment is started at 200 mg per day and is increased an additional 200 mg in divided doses until relief of the pain is obtained. Frequently one or two 200-mg tablets per day are adequate to manage the pain. Some patients require 1200 to 1600 mg per day, but side effects may be a limiting factor at this dosage. Rarely carbamazepine may cause aplastic anemia or a fall in the white blood cell or platelet count. Therefore, a complete blood count should be obtained prior to starting therapy and monitored periodically thereafter. Liver function studies should also be monitored and treatment discontinued if there is any alteration in the above studies.

Phenytoin (Dilantin) has been used for many years but is much less effective than carbamazepine. Its use in combination with carbamazepine may prove beneficial; 300 to 400 mg per day is the usual dose.

A better drug than phenytoin is baclofen (Lioresal), which can be used alone or in combination with carbamazepine. The suggested regimen is a starting dose of 10 mg three times daily for 3 days, then increasing the dose by 5 mg for 3-day increments to a total of 20 mg three times daily. The dosage should not exceed that which provides relief of pain.

In my opinion and experience, acupuncture, treatment for temporomandibular joint dysfunction, vitamin B_{12}, and surgery for gum and bone pathology have no place in the treatment of this disorder.

NERVE BLOCKS

A traditional therapeutic approach has been to make the trigger area insensitive; to achieve this, various techniques have been in vogue over the years. Second-division pain can be treated by an alcohol or radiofrequency (RF) block of the infraorbital nerve in the cheek; if the gum is a trigger site, the maxillary nerve can be blocked in the pterygomaxillary fissure. Open avulsion of the infraorbital nerve can also be used. For third-division pain, the mandibular nerve may be blocked at the foramen ovale; first-division pain may be treated by open avulsion of the nerves in the supraorbital ridge. These techniques may provide 1 to 2 years of pain relief; however, as the nerve regenerates, the pain recurs.

SURGERY

For more permanent pain relief, it is necessary to treat the trigeminal nerve proximal to the gasserian ganglion. Two therapeutic approaches are popular at this time.

The first approach, vascular decompression (popularized by Jannetta), involves a major intracranial procedure to separate the nerve from the blood vessel, usually a branch of the superior cerebellar artery, that is compressing the trigeminal nerve at the root entry zone. An implantable sponge is inserted between the compressed nerve and the artery; this often stops the pain without facial numbness. With this procedure, there is some risk of deafness in the ear on the side of the surgery. Also, the mortality is 1 per cent, the recurrence rate is more than 20 per cent, and in approximately 10 per cent of cases, the offending vessel is not found and the nerve is cut, producing facial numbness.

The second currently popular treatment is RF thermocoagulation of the retrogasserian rootlets, which stops the pain by producing permanent numbness in the trigger area of the face. About 5 per cent of patients experience annoying paresthesias and dysesthesias in the numb area; this is a major problem with any procedure that relieves pain by creation of facial numbness. Most patients, however, are grateful for the numbness, which stops not only the pain but also the necessity for medication. The patient is able to leave the hospital on the day of the RF thermocoagulation procedure. The recurrence rate is about 23 per cent, but this minor procedure can be repeated.

Those patients who are unhappy with the numbness produced by a nerve block should consider the vascular decompression procedure despite the greater risks, greater expense, and extended hospitalization.

GLOSSOPHARYNGEAL NEURALGIA

The pain in glossopharyngeal neuralgia is as severe as that of trigeminal neuralgia but is centered in the area of the tonsil and radiates deeply into the ear. The triggering mechanism is swallowing. It is much less common than trigeminal neuralgia. Carbamazepine should be used in the same dosage as for trigeminal neuralgia. Temporary relief can be obtained by anesthetizing the posterior oropharynx with 2 per cent lidocaine (Xylocaine) jelly. If topical anesthesia of this area stops the pain, it is also diagnostic. If medication is not helpful, the pain can be eliminated by sectioning the ninth cranial nerve and upper two rootlets of the tenth nerve in the posterior fossa.

OPTIC NEURITIS

method of
JAMES R. KEANE, M.D.
*University of Southern California School of
   Medicine*
Los Angeles, California

There is no proven treatment for demyelinative optic neuritis. As the prognosis is good and the condition is commonly overdiagnosed, it is imperative not to overlook more treatable causes of visual loss. These include the following:

1. *Anterior chiasmal compression* may present as monocular visual loss with a central scotoma. Careful evaluation of the visual field in the apparently normal eye should reveal a subtle upper temporal defect.
2. *Optic nerve compression* usually has a more indolent course, but as damage to one optic nerve often goes unnoticed until the patient inadvertently covers the other eye, the course of the visual loss may be obscure. Surprisingly, a dramatic response to steroid therapy is more common with compression than with neuritis.
3. *Ischemic optic neuropathy* is nearly always associated with a pale, swollen optic disk and is frequently accompanied by an altitudinal visual field defect. Four varieties have been described:
   a. A not uncommon condition in late middle age, associated with a "crowded" optic disk, generally unresponsive to steroid therapy.
   b. A condition associated with temporal arteritis in the elderly, requiring emergency, high-dose steroid treatment.
   c. A less common variety, found with lupus and other types of vasculitis in younger patients, and probably responsive to steroid therapy.
   d. Superficial disk ischemia in juvenile diabetics associated with mild visual loss and a good prognosis.
4. *Nutritional-toxic amblyopia* is painless and bilaterally symmetric.
5. *Increased intracranial pressure* should be considered in patients with bilateral disk swelling, especially in those with normal vision.
6. *Macular disease* may present with acuity loss accompanied by visual distortions, positive scotoma, minor involvement of color vision, and no afferent pupillary defect.

PRESENTATION

Optic neuritis is termed "papillitis" if the optic disk is swollen and "retrobulbar neuritis" if it is not. It typically presents as painful (particularly with eye movement) visual loss in one eye, progressing over hours to several days in younger adults (ages 15 to 50 years). Optic neuritis in children is less common, more often bilateral with disk swelling, and less likely to presage multiple sclerosis (MS).

Visual acuity loss is variable, and abnormal color vision and a sense of decreased brightness are almost always present. The usual visual field loss is a central scotoma; involvement of the lower, or less commonly the upper, half of the field suggests ischemic optic neuropathy; a vertical midline edge to the field defect indicates chiasmal compression. Optic atrophy represents nerve damage more than 6 weeks old rather than acute neuritis.

Continued worsening of vision beyond 2 weeks or failure to show improvement by 2 months suggests an alternative diagnosis. Ultimate recovery of function is good, with about 75 per cent of patients achieving an acuity of 20/30 or better.

EVALUATION

The basic evaluation of typical optic neuritis includes a complete history and general physical examination, a careful ocular and neurologic examination, serum syphilitic serologic tests (preferably one more sensitive and specific than that of the Venereal Disease Research Laboratory, such as the microhemagglutination–*Treponema pallidum* or fluorescent treponemal antibody absorption test), and a complete blood count, as well as an erythrocyte sedimentation rate and an antinuclear antibody test. Patients with bilateral optic neuritis should review the possibility of exposure to potentially toxic medicines or chemicals. Diligent follow-up of visual acuity is necessary until recovery takes place.

Any atypical features in the presentation, initial evaluation, or course require prompt further work-up. Possible optic nerve or chiasmal compression should be investigated by outlining the entire anterior visual pathway with magnetic resonance imaging (MRI) (or computed tomographic scanning if high-quality MRI results are not available locally). Lumbar puncture may be indicated to rule out subacute meningitis or tumor infiltration of the meninges. Local epidemiologic patterns may suggest additional tests for such conditions as sarcoidosis, Lyme disease, or acquired immunodeficiency syndrome.

The desire to search for evidence of MS should be resisted until further symptoms develop or until an effective treatment for that condition is found. About 50 per cent of patients with isolated optic neuritis eventually develop MS. Concurrent findings of multiple white matter lesions on MRI or minor cerebrospinal fluid changes at lumbar puncture do not necessarily predict future clinical problems, however, and discussing such results or even broaching the subject of MS with the patient who has isolated optic neuritis seems unwarranted.

TREATMENT

Disciplined inaction appears to be the best therapeutic approach. As in MS, an occasional patient improves more rapidly when given steroids. Present evidence indicates, however, that the end results of steroid treatment are no better than those achieved with no treatment. A cooperative trial of optic neuritis treatment, currently in progress, may define the role, if any, of steroid therapy.

Patients whose color or stereoscopic vision is critical for their livelihood, those involved binocularly or in their only good eye, those in severe pain, and those with severe visual loss can be given a trial of steroids in the hope of speeding recovery.

Fashions in steroid preparations change, but there is no compelling evidence that more expensive regimens using adrenocorticotropic hormone or intravenous methylprednisolone are more effective than oral prednisone. If steroid treatment is believed to be indicated, it should consist of a *short* course, such as 50 mg of prednisone orally per day for 10 days.

GLAUCOMA

method of
ROBERT N. WEINREB, M.D.
University of California, San Diego
San Diego, California

The glaucomas are a diverse group of progressive optic neuropathies with characteristic topographic changes in the optic nerve head and loss of retinal sensitivity to light. Many, but not all, glaucomatous eyes have a high intraocular pressure. Glaucoma is diagnosed by clinical examination and ancillary visual field testing. There are two major classes of glaucoma: open-angle (common) and closed-angle (uncommon) (Table 1). Glaucoma may be also categorized as either primary, in which the direct cause is not known, or secondary, in which there is a known cause. Management depends on the diagnosis and the associated signs and symptoms.

Intraocular pressure is determined by the balance between aqueous humor flow into and out of the eye. In the normal eye, aqueous humor is secreted by the ciliary body into the posterior chamber. It passes between the iris and the lens and enters the anterior chamber, from where it drains through the trabecular meshwork, a minute tissue located in the angle be-

tween the cornea and the iris. In open-angle glaucoma, the aqueous humor has direct access to the trabecular meshwork; however, the function of this tissue is impaired at the cellular level, and resistance to fluid flow from the eye is increased. In angle-closure glaucoma, access to the iris is blocked physically, frequently by the apposed peripheral iris, with consequent impairment of outflow.

Intraocular pressure is among the leading risk factors associated with glaucoma. Although there is no definition of intraocular pressure that is related reliably to glaucomatous damage, it is high in most, but not all, glaucomatous eyes. In population studies, intraocular pressure resembles a Gaussian curve, skewed toward higher intraocular pressure, with a mean value of approximately 15.5 ± 2.6 mmHg. There is considerable variability in the degree to which intraocular pressure leads to impairment of optic nerve function and structural optic nerve fiber atrophy. Some eyes may tolerate for long periods an intraocular pressure that would rapidly damage others. Factors regulating fluid flow through the trabecular meshwork and those determining the resistance of the optic nerve to damage from intraocular pressure have not been delineated clearly.

PRIMARY OPEN-ANGLE GLAUCOMA

Diagnosis

Primary open-angle glaucoma is among the leading causes of blindness in the United States and worldwide; more than 2 million Americans have been diagnosed with this condition. It is generally asymptomatic. Although it is a bilateral condition, it often presents in only one eye initially. Blurring of vision and pain do not occur unless there has been a sudden increase in intraocular pressure. Because the peripheral visual field is affected first, visual acuity usually remains good until late in the course of the disease. Most often, it is recognized in association with high intraocular pressure (exceeding 24 mmHg) and abnormal cupping of the optic nerve head. However, as many as one-third of eyes with glaucoma do not have high intraocular pressure when first examined. Further, many eyes with high intraocular pressure, so-called ocular hypertensive eyes, do not have glaucoma. Hence, measurement of intraocular pressure is not sufficient to diagnose or exclude primary open-angle glaucoma. In addition, the value of intraocular pressure screening by primary care physicians has not been established. Primary open-angle glaucoma is usually diagnosed after the age of 35 years. Besides high intraocular pressure, risk factors include black race, high myopia (nearsightedness), diabetes, retinal detachment, and a family history of glaucoma.

When considering the diagnosis, ophthalmoscopic examination of the optic nerve head is

TABLE 1. **Comparison of Primary Open-Angle Glaucoma and Primary Angle-Closure Glaucoma**

Parameter	Primary Open-Angle Glaucoma	Primary Angle-Closure Glaucoma
Onset	Insidious	Sudden
Course	Progressive	Intermittent
Symptoms	None	Pain, halos around lights, decreased vision
Signs	Increased intraocular pressure, nerve fiber bundle defects in visual field, and excavation of optic nerve head	Cloudy cornea with conjunctival hyperemia
Pupil size	Normal	Mid-dilated with poor response to light
Course	Slowly progressing visual loss	Function maintained if aqueous dynamics restored
Side illumination	Flat iris (completely illuminated)	Convex iris (only the proximal side illuminated)

essential. The optic cup may extend to the upper or lower temporal rim of the optic nerve head, changes known as notches. In some cases, the pink color of the rim is lost; instead, there is general pallor. There may also be generalized enlargement of the optic cup. With stereoscopic views, the cup/disk ratio shows a Gaussian distribution, with a mean of 0.4 and with only 5 per cent greater than 0.7. Physiologic cups tend to be symmetric between the two eyes of the same individual, with a cup/disk ratio of greater than 0.2 between fellow eyes occurring in only 1 per cent of normal individuals. Visual field examination is performed to confirm the diagnosis and monitor its progression over time.

Treatment

The goal of therapy of primary open-angle glaucoma is to prevent further optic nerve damage and to stabilize the visual field by lowering intraocular pressure. Treatment is initiated with an eyedrop to lower intraocular pressure. Medical treatment either decreases the secretion of aqueous humor or decreases the resistance of the trabecular meshwork to fluid flow from the eye. Because primary open-angle glaucoma is a chronic disease, eyedrops are rarely discontinued once prescribed.

The most widely prescribed eyedrops are the beta-adrenergic blocking agents. Two nonselective agents (timolol maleate 0.25 or 0.5 per cent and levobunolol hydrochloride 0.5 per cent) and a cardioselective agent (betaxolol hydrochloride 0.5 per cent) are available. Each of these agents reduces the flow of aqueous humor into the eye. They are well tolerated and have few ocular side effects when prescribed twice daily. Like other topically administered medications, these drops may flow through the nasolacrimal duct and be absorbed by the nasal mucosa into the blood, leading to systemic side effects. The nonselective agents are contraindicated in patients with congestive heart failure and chronic obstructive pulmonary disease. Betaxolol has been used in patients with chronic obstructive pulmonary disease who do not have serious impairment of pulmonary function. Other side effects associated with the use of these agents include bradycardia, systemic hypotension, depression, and impotence.

Adrenergic agonists (epinephrine hydrochloride 1 or 2 per cent and the epinephrine prodrug dipivefrin 0.1 per cent) also can be used twice daily to lower intraocular pressure. They appear to increase aqueous humor flow through the ciliary muscle, a nonconventional path for fluid outflow from the eye. Use of these drugs is associated with conjunctival hyperemia, dilated pupil, and sometimes adrenochrome (black pigment) deposit in the conjunctiva. They may also cause tachycardia and cardiac arrhythmia.

Parasympathomimetic agents are also extremely effective in lowering intraocular pressure. They decrease the resistance of the trabecular meshwork to aqueous humor flow. Included in this group are the cholinergic agents (pilocarpine 1, 2, 4, or 6 per cent and carbachol 0.75, 1.5, or 3 per cent) and the cholinesterase inhibitors (echothiophate iodide 0.125 or 0.25 per cent). Because they constrict the pupil, their use is associated with decreased vision, particularly at night, and ciliary muscle spasm may cause aching or pain. These agents should be used with caution in highly myopic eyes because of their association with retinal detachment. Pilocarpine is inconvenient to use because it is administered four times daily. Use of these drugs is associated with few systemic side effects. Sustained-release formulations of pilocarpine (Ocusert and Pilopine HS Gel) are available and may have fewer side effects.

Oral carbonic anhydrase inhibitors (acetazolamide or methazolamide) are prescribed if eyedrops alone do not reduce intraocular pressure sufficiently. These agents reduce the flow of aqueous humor and lower intraocular pressure considerably. Their use is associated with many systemic side effects, including frequency of urination, metabolic acidosis, nausea, gastrointestinal distress, metallic taste, depression, renal stones, and aplastic anemia. For long-term use, they are tolerated by less than 50 per cent of individuals.

In general, treatment is initiated with a beta-adrenergic blocking or adrenergic agent. If intraocular pressure is not lowered adequately or the selected drug is not tolerated, either an additional drug or a different drug is prescribed. These drugs have variable additive effects when used together. In some cases, it may be necessary to use a drug from each class to lower intraocular pressure maximally. Use of eyedrops in conjunction with a carbonic anhydrase inhibitor constitutes the maximal tolerated medical therapy.

To minimize systemic side effects with eyedrops, patients should be instructed to block their nasolacrimal ducts, a method known as punctal occlusion. Pressing against the nasolacrimal ducts near the corner of the eyes for 2 minutes minimizes systemic absorption of eyedrops. Gentle closure of the eyelids for 2 to 3 minutes after eyedrop administration is also effective in preventing systemic absorption.

If additional lowering of intraocular pressure is indicated, the argon laser can be used to perform a trabeculoplasty or photocoagulation of the trabecular meshwork. Two-thirds of eyes have decreased trabecular meshwork resistance and lower intraocular pressure with this procedure. However, 50 per cent of eyes that respond favorably return to their pretreatment intraocular pressure level within 5 years. If intraocular pressure is still not lowered adequately, incisional glaucoma filtering surgery is indicated. With this procedure, a minute fistula is created, allowing aqueous humor to drain from the eye. In most circumstances, this operation can be performed on an outpatient basis under local anesthesia. Because of the increased risks, laser or incisional surgery is performed only after a trial of medical treatment. Most other open-angle glaucoma syndromes are managed in a similar fashion.

PRIMARY ANGLE-CLOSURE GLAUCOMA

Primary angle-closure glaucoma can lead rapidly to blindness if not managed appropriately. In contrast to primary open-angle glaucoma, which is a chronic condition, immediate management of an episode of primary angle-closure glaucoma is essential. An attack is characterized by the acute onset of ocular pain, decreased vision, redness, and photophobia. Often it occurs after intentional (e.g., iatrogenic) or unintentional (e.g., in a movie theater) pupil dilation. Particularly when the pupil is mid-dilated, the flow of aqueous humor from the posterior to the anterior chamber is impeded, leading to a convex (or bowed anteriorly) iris configuration. The peripheral iris is apposed to the trabecular meshwork and blocks aqueous humor outflow.

Diagnosis

The diagnosis is confirmed by clinical examination. The intraocular pressure is high (often exceeding 50 mmHg) and the globe is firm. The pupil is mid-dilated and poorly reactive to light. Visual acuity may be decreased, the cornea is edematous with loss of clarity, and there is conjunctival hyperemia. Hyperopic (farsighted) eyes are more susceptible than myopic eyes.

Treatment

The goal of treatment is to lower intraocular pressure and to restore aqueous flow through the trabecular meshwork. One drop each of a topical beta-adrenergic blocking agent and a parasympathomimetic agent (pilocarpine 2 per cent) should be administered. A carbonic anhydrase inhibitor (e.g., acetazolamide, 500 mg) should be given orally or intravenously. An additional drop of the parasympathomimetic agent can be given again in 20 minutes. If intraocular pressure is not lowered within a brief period, a laser iridectomy should be performed. If the cornea is cloudy or the patient is uncooperative, an excisional iridectomy should be performed. Creating a hole in the iris with either a laser or surgical excision equalizes the pressure within the anterior and posterior chambers and flattens the iris, often opening the angle and allowing the aqueous humor direct access to the trabecular meshwork. An eye that has had an episode of angle-closure glaucoma and has been medically treated should undergo a prophylactic iridectomy because it is likely to have a repeat episode. The contralateral eye and eyes with extremely narrow angles often are predisposed to angle-closure glaucoma, and an iridectomy should be performed prophylactically. The treatment of secondary angle-closure glaucoma depends on both allowing access to the trabecular meshwork and restoring the normal flow of fluid.

ACUTE PERIPHERAL FACIAL PARALYSIS
(Bell's Palsy)

method of
PIETER P. DEVRIESE, PH.D., M.D.
Academic Medical Centre
Amsterdam, The Netherlands

The diagnosis of Bell's palsy is made only after exclusion of other causes of peripheral facial paralysis, which require a different medical or surgical treatment: for example, viral and bacterial infections (herpes zoster, otitis media), tumors of the ear and related structures (parotid gland), and traumas or neurologic diseases.

The cause of the disease is unknown. The paralysis is often preceded by chilling, emotional stress, and disturbance of taste. Seventy per cent of patients recover completely without treatment. Age and complete spontaneous recovery are inversely related. Of patients who are less than age 15 years, 90 per cent recover completely, whereas only 37 per cent of those older than 59 years recover. About 30 per cent of patients develop sequelae such as diminished motor function, associated movements (e.g., involuntary movements on closure of the eyelids, closure of the eyelids on speaking), spasm, and crocodile tearing. These sequelae can be very disabling because they disturb social contacts. In patients who develop complete paralysis (no voluntary motor function at all) the prognosis is definitely worse. Because the paralysis can go from slight to severe within 7 days of onset of symptoms, careful examination should be performed repeatedly during the first week so that appropriate treatment may be started as early as possible in patients with impending degeneration of the nerve. There is no electrical test to *predict* nerve degeneration.

It should be mentioned that in Bell's palsy, motor function always starts to return 3 to 4 months after onset of the paralysis, at the latest.

TREATMENT

Reassurance

Reassurance is the mainstay of treatment. Many patients believe that they are suffering from a life-endangering disease, such as a stroke or a brain tumor. It must be explained to the patient that Bell's palsy is not life-threatening.

Prednisone

Although there is no absolute proof that steroids prevent nerve degeneration, treatment with prednisone is strongly recommended as soon as *complete or almost complete loss of function* (residual function in one area of the face) is noted, *within the first week of onset*. Because the decision to treat is based on clinical assessment of motor function, this evaluation should be done very carefully. Passive movements around the eye caused by rotation of the eye (Bell's phenomenon) and movements of the face by contraction of the muscles of the healthy side (forehead, nose, mouth) should not be considered residual motor function. Table 1 provides a schedule for administration of prednisone.

Absolute contraindications for prednisone treatment are active peptic ulcer, first trimester of pregnancy, tuberculosis, Cushing's syndrome, herpes simplex virus infection of the eye, and viral infections (herpes zoster).

Relative contraindications for prednisone treatment are bacterial infections, hypertension, diabetes, previous peptic ulcer or tuberculosis, hyperkalemia, psychosis, chronic glomerulonephritis, congestive heart failure, myocardial infarction, arteriosclerosis, and thrombosis. If the physician decides to treat these patients, treatment should be done in the hospital, with frequent checks of blood pressure, glycemia, electrolyte levels, and so forth. When serious complications can be expected, it may be wise to abstain from treatment. In this respect the age of the patient is important. Severe Bell's palsy in the last trimester of pregnancy is treated in consultation with the obstetrician.

Care of the Eye

Keratitis and other complications are possible when the cornea is no longer protected by the eyelids because of loss of blinking. At night the eye can be covered by an eye bandage and sterile petrolatum can be applied, or a so-called watchglass bandage can be used. During the day, 0.5 per cent methylcellulose eyedrops can be used (a few drops five times per day); if necessary, an eye

TABLE 1. **Scheme of Prednisone Treatment (5-mg Tablets)***

Day	No. of Tablets	Dose (mg)
1	4–4–4	60
2	4–4–4	60
3	4–4–4	60
4	4–4–4	60
5	4–4–3	55
6	4–3–3	50
7	3–3–3	45
8	3–3–2	40
9	3–2–2	35
10	2–2–2	30
11	2–2–1	25
12	2–1–1	20
13	1–1–1	15
14	1–1	10
15	1	5

*Altogether, 114 tablets (570 mg) are given.

bandage can also be applied. The cornea should be checked regularly for keratitis. A blepharorrhaphy is rarely necessary. In elderly patients, the lagophthalmos and the cosmetic deformity can be dealt with by use of adhesive tape approximately 0.5 cm wide and 5 cm long (e.g., Blenderm Surgical Tape No. 1525, 3M Company). The tape is first fixed as high as possible in the middle of the lower eyelid. The skin at the lateral corner of the eye is then folded, and the lower eyelid is pulled upward and sideways by fixation of the tape temporally. The same method can be used to pull up the angle of the mouth for cosmetic reasons.

Rest

A period of rest of at least 2 weeks is prescribed. The patients are instructed to avoid drafts and chilling, which frequently precede Bell's palsy.

Surgery

The benefit of surgical treatment—partial or total decompression of the nerve—has not been established by valid statistical studies.

Electrotherapy

This therapy is not recommended. A positive effect on recovery has not been proved. On the contrary, electrotherapy may enhance contractures and spasm during the recovery phase.

Exercises

Exercises of the facial musculature in the paralytic phase are to be discouraged because they result in overactivation of the healthy side of the face and hence in more asymmetry. The musculature is sufficiently activated in a passive way by movements of the mandible and by movements of the other side of the face. Distinct muscular atrophy rarely occurs. In the recovery phase after regeneration of the nerve (3 to 12 months after onset), keeping the face relaxed is important to avoid sequelae. Patients are instructed to keep a poker face. When tension builds up in the face, opening the mouth a few millimeters can help.

Eventual recovery of function in patients with nerve degeneration can be judged 12 months after onset. In the worst cases (about 15 per cent), the sequelae are troublesome. These sequelae are clearly influenced by emotional stress; no surgical treatment is available for this trouble. Social rehabilitation may be attempted by mime therapy. The patients are taught to relax both physically and psychologically by means of exercises that are guided by respiration, and a new pattern of facial muscular activity is learned to regain control of facial expression as much as possible.

PARKINSONISM

method of
HEIDI SHALE, M.D., and
STANLEY FAHN, M.D.
Neurological Institute
Columbia University College of Physicians
　and Surgeons
New York, New York

Parkinsonism is a neurologic disorder diagnosed by the presence of at least two of the following cardinal signs: tremor at rest (in hands, legs, tongue, and lower face), rigidity, bradykinesia, and loss of postural reflexes. In addition, various other signs are present, such as decreased facial expression (hypomimia) with lid retraction and decreased blink rate, abnormal speech (either hypophonia and slow, monotone voice or palilalia with abnormally rapid speech), and loss of automatic movements (decreased arm swing, reduced swallowing with sialorrhea).

The most common cause of parkinsonism is Parkinson's disease, a neurodegenerative disorder of unknown etiology. Pathologically, there is a loss of pigmented neurons in multiple areas of the brain, most importantly the dopaminergic neurons in the substania nigra. Noradrenergic and serotoninergic neurons are also affected. The loss of cholinergic neurons in the forebrain may explain the frequent association of cognitive impairment with Parkinson's disease.

There are multiple other etiologies of parkinsonism (Table 1). The most frequent cause is the use of dopamine receptor–blocking agents, mainly neuroleptics that are used as antipsychotic medication (haloperidol [Haldol], thioridazine [Mellaril]), for gastrointestinal

TABLE 1. **Major Types of Parkinsonism**

1. Primary (Parkinson's disease)
2. Secondary
   a. Drugs: neuroleptics, reserpine, lithium
   b. Toxins: manganese, carbon monoxide, cyanide, methanol, carbon disulfide, 1-methyl-4-phenyl-1,2,3,6-tetrahydropyridine (MPTP)
   c. Infections and parainfections: postencephalitic Parkinson's disease, acquired immunodeficiency syndrome, Jakob-Creutzfeldt disease
   d. Vascular infarcts
   e. Metabolic: hypoparathyroidism with basal ganglia calcification, chronic hepatocerebral degeneration
3. Parkinson's plus syndromes
   a. Sporadic: progressive supranuclear palsy, Shy-Drager syndrome, striatonigral degeneration, Parkinson's disease–amyotrophic lateral sclerosis, cortical-basal ganglionic degeneration, olivopontocerebellar atrophy
   b. Inherited: Huntington's disease, olivopontocerebellar atrophy, Hallervorden-Spatz disease, neuroacanthocytosis, Wilson's disease

disorders (prochlorperazine [Compazine], metoclopramide [Reglan]), and as antidepressants (amoxapine [Asendin]). The parkinsonism that is induced by these agents is reversible, although this reversal may take months.

Other neurodegenerative diseases often have parkinsonian features. These diseases include progressive supranuclear palsy, Wilson's disease, juvenile Huntington's disease, Shy-Drager disease, olivopontocerebellar atrophy, neuroacanthocytosis, Hallervorden-Spatz disease, and cortical-basal ganglionic degeneration. These are referred to as Parkinson's plus syndromes. Features that suggest that a patient does not have idiopathic Parkinson's disease and that further work-up is needed include

1. Corticospinal tract signs
2. Amyotrophy (muscle atrophy, fasciculations, loss of tendon reflexes)
3. Postural hypotension (unless drug induced) and other autonomic features
4. Cerebellar signs
5. Ocular palsies (except limited up-gaze)
6. Profound dementia, particularly early in disease course
7. Early, prominent loss of postural reflexes
8. Poor or no response to levodopa

TREATMENT

Because there is currently no cure for Parkinson's disease, treatment consists of medications to alleviate its symptoms. The aim is to keep an individual functional and independent for as long as possible. This includes recommendations for regular exercise, although there is no evidence that formalized physical or occupational therapy is beneficial. Treatment should be individualized and depends on the patient's age and familial, social, and employment situation. If symptoms are only a minor annoyance, no treatment is necessary. Tremor is rarely debilitating, but it may be a source of embarrassment to some patients. Evaluation of a patient with Parkinson's disease includes measurements of blood pressure and pulse rate in both supine and standing positions because orthostatic hypotension is a common side effect of some antiparkinsonian medications. Another common side effect is anorexia, and patients should be weighed at each visit. Patients should be questioned about possible cognitive symptoms (depression, memory impairment, vivid dreams, hallucinations) and about their ability to perform various activities of daily living, including washing, dressing, and eating. The physical examination should assess speech, tremor at rest and with action, bradykinesia, ability to perform rapid alternating movements, gait, and postural stability.

The frequency of patient follow-up depends on the severity of the illness and how often changes

in medication are made. However, as the disease progresses, the patient's response to medications can become extremely variable throughout the day, and observation during a 1-hour office visit may be inadequate to decide what medication adjustments are needed. In this case, it is useful to have the patients or their families maintain a diary documenting the response to medications throughout the day for at least 1 week, to see if a pattern of response emerges. The patients should record whether they are "on," "on with dyskinesias," or "off" for every hour of the day. If the patient cannot do this, hospitalization may be required for evaluation many times during the course of the day.

It is important to be aware of the high incidence of depression in patients with Parkinson's disease (one-third to one-half). This may antedate the clinical appearance of Parkinson's disease or may occur concomitantly. The depression does not always correlate with the severity of the Parkinson's disease, and successful treatment of the motor symptoms does not necessarily alleviate the depression. The signs of the two may overlap (bradykinesia, masked facies), and unless depression is treated, it may be difficult to tell whether the parkinsonian symptoms are adequately treated.

Some depressed patients with Parkinson's disease have low levels of 5-hydroxyindoleacetic acid, a serotonin metabolite, in the cerebrospinal fluid, and their depression has been successfully treated with 5-hydroxytryptophan, a precursor of serotonin. When this agent is not available, commercially available antidepressants should be used. Although tricyclic antidepressants with high anticholinergic activity might improve some of the parkinsonian symptoms, the central cognitive and psychiatric side effects as well as the hypotensive effects might be detrimental. The monoamine oxidase (MAO) inhibitors that are available in the United States block the type A MAO, which deaminates serotonin and norepinephrine, as well as the type B enzyme, which deaminates dopamine. Blocking MAO-A in a patient receiving levodopa causes marked swings in blood pressure. Therefore, nonselective MAO inhibitors are contraindicated in patients taking levodopa. In Canada and Europe, selegiline (Deprenyl, Eldepryl, Jumex), a selective MAO-B inhibitor, is available and may be safely used with levodopa.

In refractory cases of depression, electroconvulsive shock therapy can be given, which might temporarily improve the signs of Parkinson's disease as well as treat the depression. If medication is necessary to control parkinsonian symptoms, first line therapy usually consists of anticholinergics and/or amantadine in the patient who is only mildly impaired.

Anticholinergics

With loss of dopaminergic activity in the striatum, there is a relative increase in activity of cholinergic interneurons secondary to disinhibition. Anticholinergics counter this. They are useful primarily for treatment of tremor and less so for the other features of Parkinson's disease. They may also benefit such autonomic features as sialorrhea and excess sweating. Their main drawback is cognitive side effects, particularly impairment of short-term memory; hallucinations and confusion can also occur. These effects are more likely in elderly patients, particularly if there is already impairment of cognitive ability because of the primary disease. Anticholinergics should be avoided or used with caution in anyone older than 70 years of age.

Other side effects, related to peripheral parasympathetic blockade, are dry mouth, blurring of near vision because of decreased pupillary accommodation, constipation, urinary retention, and aggravation of narrow angle glaucoma.

The most commonly used anticholinergics are

1. Trihexyphenidyl (Artane), 2- and 5-mg tablets; usual maintenance dose 6 to 15 mg daily

2. Ethopropazine (Parsidol), 50-mg tablets; usual maintenance dose 200 mg daily

3. Benztropine mesylate (Cogentin), 0.5-, 1-, and 2-mg tablets; maintenance dose 2 to 6 mg daily

Other anticholinergics that are used less often are procyclidine (Kemadrin) and biperiden (Akineton). The antihistamines diphenhydramine (Benadryl) and orphenadrine (Disipal) have anticholinergic activities and are also useful.

All anticholinergics should be started with the smallest possible dose (one-half tablet) and increased gradually every 4 to 7 days. They are given three or four times a day.

Amantadine (Symmetrel)

Amantadine is an antiviral agent that has a combination of anticholinergic activity and enhancement of release of dopamine and inhibition of dopamine reuptake at striatal nerve terminals. The onset of benefit is relatively rapid (approximately 2 days to 1 week), although the benefit may be lost after several months. However, reintroduction later may result in renewed benefit. Amantadine is often used in conjunction with other antiparkinsonian agents, although it might be tried alone in mild cases.

Amantadine is available in 100-mg capsules.

The starting dose is 100 mg twice daily. The maintenance dose is 200 to 300 mg daily.

The main side effects of amantadine use are cognitive (confusion, hallucinations, delerium). Other side effects are edema of the lower extremities and livedo reticularis, a purple-red mesh-like pattern on the legs.

Levodopa

Levodopa ameliorates the symptoms of Parkinson's disease by replacement of dopamine that is lost when nigrostriatal dopaminergic neurons degenerate. Dopamine itself does not cross the blood-brain barrier, but its precursor levodopa does. Levodopa is converted to dopamine by the enzyme aromatic acid decarboxylase. When used without a decarboxylase inhibitor, most of the drug is metabolized to dopamine peripherally, which increases the peripheral side effects of levodopa (anorexia, nausea, vomiting, postural hypotension, and, occasionally, cardiac arrhythmias). To minimize these side effects, levodopa is commonly combined with a peripheral decarboxylase inhibitor. This combination allows for an 80 per cent reduction in dose of levodopa needed.

The two inhibitors available are carbidopa combined with levodopa in Sinemet in a 1:10 (10/100 or 25/250 [carbidopa, 10 or 25 mg; levodopa, 100 or 250 mg, respectively]) ratio or 1:4 ratio (25/100 [carbidopa, 25 mg; levodopa, 100 mg]) or benserazide combined in a 1:4 ratio with levodopa in Madopar or Prolopa. Only Sinemet is available in the United States. The onset of action of levodopa is 20 to 30 minutes and the effect usually lasts long enough (6 to 8 hours) to produce a smooth response between doses, at least in the first few years of treatment.

When anticholinergics or amantadine is inadequate to control parkinsonism, Sinemet should be added, usually one-half of a 25/100 tablet three times a day. Increases in dose are made by one-half to one tablet every 4 to 7 days (the rate of increase depending on the patient's disability), both to minimize side effects and to establish the lowest possible dose that effectively improves symptoms. A total daily dose of 75 to 80 mg of carbidopa is usually adequate to block most peripheral side effects. Once this level is reached, further dose increases can be made with 10/100 tablets.

The most common side effects of levodopa are orthostatic hypotension, gastrointestinal symptoms, and cognitive disturbances. The hypotension is a dose-related phenomenon related to impairment of baroreceptor reflexes by dopamine. If increasing the dose of carbidopa is inadequate, use of thigh-high elastic stockings, elevation of the head of the bed at night to increase plasma renin and decrease nocturnal diuresis, increasing dietary salt intake, and fludrocortisone, a mineralocorticoid (0.1 to 0.3 mg), may be tried. Severe, refractory hypotension, particularly if it predates drug treatment and is accompanied by other signs of autonomic dysfunction (pupillary abnormalities, incontinence, laryngeal stridor), suggests Shy-Drager syndrome or striatonigral degeneration.

Anorexia, nausea, and vomiting occur early in treatment with levodopa, when the dose of carbidopa is still low, and are usually alleviated as the Sinemet dose is increased. If they persist and further increases in levodopa are not required, additional carbidopa (Lodosyn) alone can be administered, although this drug must be obtained directly from the manufacturer (Merck Sharp & Dohme). Domperidone (Motilium), an experimental medication that blocks dopamine receptors in the gut as well as those in the brain stem chemoreceptor trigger zone for vomiting (the area postrema), has been used successfully to treat levodopa-induced nausea. Although administration of levodopa with meals might delay its onset of action or decrease the degree of benefit, this timing may also help to alleviate the nausea.

Any type of psychiatric disturbance may occur with use of levodopa and is more common in patients who are elderly and/or demented. These disturbances can include vivid dreams, nightmares, hallucinations, mania, and hypersexuality. If the patient is taking other medications with potential psychoactive side effects, such as amantadine or anticholinergics, use of these drugs should be stopped first. If the symptoms persist, the levodopa dose should be slowly lowered. (Levodopa should never be discontinued abruptly because a condition resembling the neuroleptic malignant syndrome has been reported.) Some patients develop psychiatric side effects when they take doses of levodopa that are adequate to produce an "on" state but have debilitating "offs" when the medication is reduced. Use of antipsychotic agents might improve the psychosis but worsen the parkinsonism because of dopamine receptor blockade. An experimental agent, clozapine, which primarily blocks mesolimbic and mesocortical dopamine receptors but has only weak effects on striatal dopamine receptors, is being investigated in patients with Parkinson's disease who have psychotic symptoms when treated with antiparkinsonian medications.

Other side effects caused by levodopa are insomnia, myoclonus, episodic excess sweating and hot flashes, rash (with the 25/100 pill, presumably because of the yellow dye), and darkening of urine, sweat, and saliva. Levodopa is also a pre-cursor to skin melanin, and there has been some concern about whether it may produce a recurrence in patients with melanoma. To date no causal relationship has been established, but in patients with melanomas, it might be wise to avoid using levodopa.

Dopamine Receptor Agonists

These agents act by stimulating dopamine receptors directly; they are not dependent on surviving dopaminergic neurons for conversion to dopamine or storage, as is levodopa. Theoretically, they would therefore be more useful in patients with Parkinson's disease of longer duration. There are two known dopamine receptors: D_1, which when stimulated increase cyclic adenosine monophosphate, and D_2, which do not affect cyclic adenosine monophosphate. The D_2 receptor is the more important in alleviating the motor symptoms of parkinsonism, but stimulation of the D_1 receptor may produce additional benefit. Two dopamine receptor agonists are available in the United States. Bromocriptine (Parlodel) activates only the D_2 receptor, and pergolide (Permax) activates both D_1 and D_2 receptors. The latter may be a more powerful antiparkinsonian agent and have a longer duration of action than bromocriptine.

The agonists by themselves have only mild antiparkinsonian effects, and most patients can be maintained with it alone for no longer than 1 year. However, when these drugs are used in combination with levodopa, the effects are additive. Moreover, the combination may prevent some of the long-term complications of levodopa therapy (see later section).

Bromocriptine is available in 2.5-mg tablets and 5.0-mg capsules, and pergolide in 0.05-, 0.25-, and 1.0-mg tablets. Because postural hypotension may occur early in the treatment with the agonists, patients are instructed to begin with the lowest possible dose, taken immediately before retiring at night, for several days. After this time, doses can be taken during the day and can be increased by 2.5 mg of bromocriptine or 0.25 mg of pergolide every 5 to 7 days. The maintenance dose is 10 to 40 mg of bromocriptine or 1 to 4 mg of pergolide daily, in three or four divided doses (but in more advanced cases, a dose may be taken each time the patient takes levodopa).

In addition to orthostatic hypotension, other side effects of the agonists are psychiatric disturbances (which occur more frequently than with levodopa) and, less frequently, hypersexuality, pulmonary infiltrates and pleural effusions, nasal stuffiness, and elevated liver function tests. These effects resolve with discontinuation of the medication.

Pharmacokinetic Problems Occurring with Levodopa Therapy

When levodopa treatment is begun, patients often experience a "honeymoon" period during which they are relatively free of symptoms. However, by 5 years of treatment, at least 50 per cent of patients will experience troublesome fluctuations in their response to medications and by 10 years, the figure may be as high as 85 per cent.

Initially, a patient has a predictably smooth response to each dose of medication and functions at the same high level throughout the day. However, after several years of treatment, the patient begins to experience a return of parkinsonian symptoms (the off phase) some time before taking the next dose. This deterioration occurs gradually (over many minutes) and the on state does not resume until levodopa is taken again.

"Wearing-off" correlates with falling plasma levels of levodopa. Patients with early Parkinson's disease have sufficient endogenous reserves of dopamine to sustain them until the next dose of medication, even while plasma levels of levodopa are dropping. This reserve is lost as the disease progresses, with increasing death of cells in the substantia nigra, as well as loss of storage capacity of dopamine in nerve terminals.

Various therapeutic options exist to treat wearing-off. The time between doses of levodopa can be shortened. This provides only temporary benefit, however, and if the total daily dose is increased, the likelihood of other dopa-related side effects (dyskinesias, orthostatic hypotension, and psychiatric manifestations) will increase. Each individual dose of levodopa can then be reduced, but in patients with advanced disease, this may produce an inadequate on state.

Another approach is to add a dopamine agonist because its duration of action is longer than that of levodopa. Agonists also allow for some reduction (approximately 25 per cent) in the amount of levodopa given. Dopamine agonists may be more effective in the later stages of disease because they do not depend on intact dopaminergic terminals to synthesize and store dopamine.

Selegiline (Deprenyl), the MAO-B inhibitor that decreases the rate of dopamine breakdown, may also prolong the duration of action of levodopa.

With progression of Parkinson's disease and longer levodopa treatment, patients may note a lesser degree of improvement of symptoms after taking the medication. A dose that formerly provided them with a normal or near-normal level of functioning may no longer do so. In addition, the onset of action may be prolonged, and instead of an on state's occurring within 30 minutes, the drug may take 1 hour or longer to produce an effect. Finally, some doses will not produce any beneficial response at all.

There are several reasons for this diminishing response to medication. There are dopamine receptors in the stomach, and levodopa is known to delay gastric emptying. In this case, the tablets remain in the stomach. Because levodopa is absorbed only from the small intestine, levodopa may be catabolized before it can be absorbed. The patient may find that the pills taken at mealtimes fail to have the desired effect. High-protein meals containing neutral amino acids compete with levodopa for transportation across the duodenal mucosa into the plasma and also across the blood-brain barrier. A possible solution is to dissolve the tablets in water and take them on an empty stomach, 15 to 30 minutes before meals. However, in some patients this procedure causes intolerably high peak plasma levels of levodopa. Some patients try to restrict their protein intake to the end of the day, at dinner.

Initially, as the level of dopamine decreases with the death of nigral cells, dopamine turnover increases and postsynaptic receptors become hypersensitive as a compensatory mechanism to respond maximally to the limited amount of dopamine present. This may actually mask symptoms of Parkinson's disease for a time, until dopamine falls below a critical level. Continuous bombardment of the hypersensitive receptors with exogenous dopamine, however, causes a down-regulation of the receptors and undermines the brain's attempts to compensate for decreasing dopamine levels. Drug holidays have been used to try to counter this problem. These holidays consist of 1 to several weeks during which levodopa is withheld, in the hope that this will resensitize receptors and that when levodopa is resumed, lower dosages will be required with a better response and less severe side effects. However, drug holidays have not been proved to have a long-term benefit on response to levodopa or reduction of drug-related side effects. The risks of medical complications (deep venous thrombosis, pulmonary embolism, myocardial infarction, pneumonia, and malnutrition) related to increased parkinsonism during a drug holiday makes it a risky method of treatment in view of the lack of sustained benefit obtained.

Abnormal choreic movements (dyskinesias) related to levodopa can involve any body part. The movements may be severe enough to be ballistic or can be sustained (dystonic). The dyskinesias can be seen at rest but are exacerbated by action, as well as by emotional stress. Initially, dyskinesias occur as a peak-dose phenomenon correlated with high plasma levels of dopa and presumably too much dopamine in the striatum in the presence of a hypersensitive receptor. As time passes, the patient may go directly from an off state into a dyskinetic one and then go off again, without ever having a functional on period. Also, a poorly explained pattern of diphasic dyskinesias (D-I-D = dyskinesia-improvement-dyskinesia) is seen in some patients. This pattern consists of dyskinesias as the plasma levels are rising, best motor performance without abnormal movement at peak drug levels, and reappearance of dyskinesias as the effects of the drug wear off, before the patient enters the off state.

If dyskinesias are troublesome because of pain or impairment of motor control, an attempt should be made to reduce the total dose of levodopa. Some patients find that taking the medication on an empty stomach results in dyskinesias but that dyskinesias do not occur if the drug is taken with food. If an unacceptable increase in parkinsonism results, a dopamine agonist should be added to the regimen.

Freezing, consisting of inability to initiate a movement (usually walking), is a feature of advanced Parkinson's disease. It may begin as start-hesitation, when a patient has to start walking, and also when an "obstacle" (stairs, doorway, elevator) is reached. If severe, it can preclude walking because of a frequent, intermittent inability to move, as well as because of frequent falls. Freezing can be seen in both the on and off phases. Certain methods may be used to overcome freezing. Walking should be started by marching in place before moving forward and when reaching an obstacle. A turn should be made by making a wide arc. Visual cues, such as stepping on a row of markers, can also help to overcome freezing. In some patients, auditory cues (such as listening to marching music on a portable cassette tape) help. The cause of freezing is unknown. Although levodopa may help with off state freezing, excessive levodopa sometimes exacerbates the problem.

It is still debated whether the fluctuations seen in Parkinson's disease are due to progression of the disease itself or to prolonged and early treatment with levodopa. A recent study compared patients treated with levodopa alone or in combination with bromocriptine. The patients on a combined regimen received a significantly lower dose of levodopa. After 5 years, the group taking both drugs had fewer peak-dose dyskinesias and wearing-off than the group receiving levodopa alone.

We currently recommend forestalling treatment with levodopa for as long as possible by first using anticholinergics, amantadine, and dopamine agonists. If these agents are inadequate for treating the parkinsonian symptoms, levodopa is added. Once started, the dose of levodopa should be kept as low as possible. It is preferable to keep the patient mildly parkinsonian on a lower dose of levodopa than aim for a totally normal state and risk the occurrence of fluctuations, which once begun are difficult to treat. Obviously, the course of treatment depends on the patient's needs and lifestyle.

TRENDS IN MANAGEMENT

There are three new approaches to treating patients with Parkinson's disease, particularly those with intractable drug-related fluctuations. The first approach involves experimental medications with unique modes of delivery such as transcutaneous 4-propyl-9-hydroxynaphthoxazine, a D_2 receptor agonist, or subcutaneous lisuride (another D_2 agonist) delivered via an infusion pump. The aim is to avoid fluctuations by maintaining steady plasma and brain levels of medication. A sustained-release form of Sinemet has been developed. Levodopa has also been administered via the intraduodenal route to bypass the problem of delayed gastric emptying.

The second approach is surgical treatment. Thalamotomy had been developed before the availability of antiparkinsonian drugs. Current use of computed tomography–assisted stereotaxic techniques enables more precise localization of the ventrolateral thalamus. This surgical procedure is reserved for patients whose main problem is rigidity and/or tremor that is insufficiently controlled with medicines or who are unable to tolerate medications in adequate doses because of side effects.

Recently, multiple centers in the United States, Mexico, Latin America, China, and Europe have performed transplants of autologous adrenal medullary tissues into the striatum. Thus far, the patients who improved after surgery have shown an increase in on state time, with fewer dyskinesias. Most patients have not shown marked improvement. More recently, transplants of fetal mesencephalon to the striatum are being carried out. More time is needed to determine the role of this technique.

The third recent development in the treatment of Parkinson's disease involves a hypothesis of the etiology of the condition and what might be done to prevent its progression. The theory under investigation is that metabolism of dopamine by oxidation produces build-up of toxic free radicals, which in susceptible individuals (e.g., those who have already sustained damage to the substantia nigra, perhaps from an environmental toxin) causes destruction of dopaminergic neurons. When 80 per cent of the neurons are lost, parkinsonian symptoms appear. Two antioxidants, selegiline (Deprenyl) and tocopherol (vitamin E), are being administered in a multicenter trial to patients with early Parkinson's disease to see whether the disease will progress more slowly than that of patients who receive placebos.

PERIPHERAL NEUROPATHIES

method of
DAVID A. CHAD, M.D., and
LAWRENCE D. RECHT, M.D.
University of Massachusetts Medical Center
Worcester, Massachusetts

Neuropathies fall into two main groups: *inherited* and *acquired*. The pathogenesis of the inherited forms is not yet fully understood and with few exceptions specific treatments are not yet available. On the other hand, in many cases the pathogenesis of the acquired neuropathies is well understood and specific treatments are available to arrest progression and enhance recovery. Some of these neuropathies are associated with systemic diseases and may be the sole or presenting manifestations of an underlying disorder. Prompt recognition of a neuropathy may therefore allow early diagnosis of a more generalized disorder.

We would like to provide a framework for our discussion of the treatment of peripheral neuropathy by reviewing some of the basic anatomic, physiologic, and pathologic aspects of peripheral neurology.

ANATOMY AND CLASSIFICATION

Peripheral nerves are composed of a variety of fiber types: motor, sensory, and autonomic. Motor fibers are extensions of motoneurons that reside in the anterior horn of the spinal cord. The motor fibers are myelinated and innervate muscle fibers. The motoneuron, its myelinated axon, and the muscle fibers it supplies are known collectively as the motor unit. The sensory fibers are derived from neurons in the dorsal root ganglia. Large-diameter myelinated fibers subserve the modalities of touch and pressure; thinly myelinated and unmyelinated sensory fibers are responsible for sensations of temperature and pain. The autonomic fibers are unmyelinated and are derived from neurons in sympathetic ganglia; they are concerned with autonomic functions such as control of blood vessel caliber and sweating.

The classification of peripheral neuropathies can be based on a number of criteria. We favor classification schemes based on nerve fiber pathology and on clinical features.

Wallerian degeneration describes the sequence of events that occurs distal to the site of nerve fiber transection. If a fiber is cut, crushed, or rendered ischemic, its axon and myelin sheath degenerate distal to the site of the lesion. Nerve fiber regeneration will occur, but recovery of function may take a long time and may be incomplete. *Axonal atrophy and degeneration* are usually consequences of disturbed metabolism of the cell body and axon. A host of endogenous and exogenous toxins are capable of producing this pathologic pattern, which represents the most commonly encountered pathologic basis of polyneuropathy. *Segmental demyelination* refers to myelin sheath damage. Although the axon remains intact, loss of function occurs because of conduction block. When the inciting pathogenetic factors are removed, remyelination and restoration of function can occur. For example, in some instances of compression-induced mononeuropathy the underlying pathology is focal segmental demyelination without axonal injury; when pressure on the nerve is released, recovery takes place. When demyelination occurs as a consequence of axonal atrophy, it is referred to as secondary demyelination; this pathologic appearance is noted in some toxic-metabolic polyneuropathies. Last, *neuronopathy* is another pathologic subtype of neuropathy, which refers to degeneration of either motor or sensory cell bodies.

Besides this pathologic classification, one can subdivide peripheral neuropathy into mononeuropathy, mononeuropathy multiplex, polyneuropathy, radiculopathy, and plexopathy. This subdivision is often useful clinically and our treatment discussion will focus primarily on the first three subtypes.

Mononeuropathy (disturbances in motor, sensory, and autonomic functions of a single nerve) most commonly results from acute or chronic nerve injury, and ranges in severity from a mild, reversible condition to a severe, irreversible one (nerve transection). *Mononeuritis multiplex* (multiple mononeuropathies) is usually caused by nerve fiber ischemia and is encountered most often as a form of diabetic or vasculitic neuropathy; it may also be a consequence of immunologically mediated demyelination. Other etiologies include neoplastic infiltration of nerve (usually leukemia or lymphoma; see later discussion), sarcoidosis, and leprosy. Mononeuritis multiplex tends to be painful and to have an abrupt onset, asymmetric distribution, and motor function affected to a greater extent than sensory function. By contrast, *polyneuropathy* denotes disturbed function of many nerves and has a multitude of causes, including exposure to toxins, metabolic disturbances, dysimmune states, direct and indirect effects of neoplasia, and inherited factors. The clinical hallmarks of polyneuropathy are symmetric motor weakness, sensory loss, and reduction in reflex activity. *Radiculopathy,* a disorder of the motor and sensory functions of a nerve root, is a result of many of the same conditions that produce polyneuropathy. Pain is often a prominent feature; sensory loss and weakness conform to specific dermatomes and myotomes, respectively. Because roots lie freely in the subarachnoid space, radiculopathies are often associated with abnormalities of cerebrospinal fluid. *Plexopathies* (brachial and lumbar) result from many of the disorders that affect other components of the peripheral nervous system.

Given the clinical and pathologic heterogeneity of peripheral neuropathy, how is the physician to reach the correct diagnosis? In many cases the history and physical examination are helpful, but most neurologists confirm their clinical suspicion or gain useful information about the peripheral neuropathy by the use of electromyography. Electromyography allows (1) separation of patients with peripheral neuropathy into the five clinical categories we have discussed; (2) determination of peripheral nerve pathology, i.e., whether a neuropathy is characterized by axonal degeneration, demyelination, or features of both processes; and (3) assessment of severity of the pathologic process and the likelihood of recovery.

TREATMENT

Vasculitic Neuropathies

The vasculitic syndromes associated with peripheral neuropathy are polyarteritis nodosa and related disorders, hypersensitivity vasculitis (including cryoglobulinemia), Wegener's granulomatosis, and lymphomatoid granulomatosis.

The peripheral neuropathy most often associated with vasculitis is mononeuritis multiplex. It usually occurs in a patient who has an active systemic vasculitis or collagen-vascular disorder, but it can also be a presenting manifestation of these conditions. Untreated, the disorder can progress to involve multiple nerves so that overlapping mononeuritis multiplex evolves into a pattern of a severe polyneuropathy. Vasculitis is not unfailingly associated with mononeuritis multiplex: a sizable number of patients with vasculitis *present* with a sensorimotor polyneuropathy. Other, less commonly encountered forms of vasculitic neuropathy include radiculopathy, plexopathy, and cranial neuropathies. In some patients, intensive evaluation fails to disclose a definable systemic vasculitis or collagen-vascular disorder; such patients are considered to have an isolated vasculitic peripheral neuropathy. We recommend a sural nerve biopsy for the patient with mononeuritis multiplex who is not known to have vasculitis and for the patient with a rapidly developing polyneuropathy of uncertain etiology, especially if laboratory studies suggest vasculitis.

In vasculitic neuropathy, we recommend aggressive immunosuppressive treatment with prednisone and cyclophosphamide. The diagnosis should be made as quickly as possible because treatment can prevent progression and lead to clinical improvement in most patients. Patients are started with prednisone, 60 to 80 mg per day, and cyclophosphamide (Cytoxan), 1 to 2.5 mg per kg per day, which usually results in effective relief of pain and return of function. The well-known side effects of prednisone include diabetes,

cataracts, osteoporosis, aseptic necrosis of the femoral head, exacerbation of hypertension, and predisposition to infection. Cyclophosphamide may depress the white blood cell count and increase the risk of infection. To counteract these anticipated side effects, we prescribe vitamin D and calcium supplementation, antacids or H_2 histamine antagonists, and a low-salt diet. We carefully follow the serum glucose level and blood pressure and monitor the white blood cell and neutrophil counts, which should not fall to less than 3000 cells and 1500 cells per mm^3, respectively. These drugs are continued for at least 6 weeks and then tapered slowly, using either the erythrocyte sedimentation rate or clinical findings as a guide.

Inflammatory Neuropathies

Guillain-Barré Syndrome

The Guillain-Barré syndrome (GBS) is an acute inflammatory-demyelinating polyneuropathy, the most common neuropathic cause of rapidly progressive weakness. In most patients, a careful history discloses an antecedent event (viral illness, mycoplasma infection, recent inoculation, surgical procedure) or associated condition (Hodgkin's disease, lupus erythematosus, renal transplantation) that has led to an immunologically mediated attack on peripheral myelin. The pathophysiology of GBS is unclear, but antimyelin antibodies have been demonstrated and cell-mediated immunity plays an important role in the animal model of GBS.

GBS is characterized by progressive, symmetric motor weakness and areflexia. About 15 to 20 per cent of patients require respiratory assistance. Weakness develops rapidly but ceases to progress by 4 weeks into the illness; if weakness progresses for more than 1 month, consideration should be given to another diagnosis such as chronic inflammatory neuropathy. Sensory symptoms and pain may be prominent, but there is usually minimal sensory loss. Autonomic nervous system disturbances are common and potentially lethal. Recovery usually begins 4 to 6 weeks after progression stops, but it may be delayed for months. Although 80 per cent of patients make a satisfactory recovery, a significant number are left with moderate or severe disability and a small but significant percentage (perhaps as high as 5 per cent) die.

When the cerebrospinal fluid is examined, the typical findings include an elevated protein level and few cells (albuminocytologic dissociation). Recently, however, otherwise typical GBS has been observed in patients with acquired immunodeficiency syndrome (AIDS) who demonstrate cerebrospinal fluid pleocytosis. Electromyography helps to confirm the diagnosis, but in the earliest stages of the illness the study may be normal or show only slowing of nerve conduction velocity in proximal nerve segments.

The mainstay of therapy is good general medical care. Patients who are admitted to the hospital must be observed carefully for respiratory muscle weakness, preferably in an intermediate care unit. The patient should be examined two or three times a day and vital capacity measurements should be made three or four times a day. There is probably little risk of progression of disease if the patient has maintained a plateau for 3 to 4 days. If, however, weakness is noted to be increasing or vital capacity falling, arrangements should be made to move the patient to an intensive care unit. If the vital capacity falls to 20 ml per kg, we recommend elective intubation to provide the patient with positive pressure ventilation and to help re-expand atelectatic areas of lung. Expert airway management is mandatory, and any evidence of infection requires immediate treatment with antibiotics.

The nursing and medical team must be aware of the many autonomic disturbances that can occur. Careful and continuous monitoring of blood pressure, cardiac rhythm, and fluid status is essential. Manifestations of sympathetic nervous system overactivity include transient hypertensive episodes, sudden diaphoresis, general vasoconstriction, and sinus tachycardia. Marked postural hypotension and heightened sensitivity to dehydration and to sedative-hypnotic agents indicate underactive sympathetic functioning. Insufficient parasympathetic activity is associated with adynamic ileus. Postural hypotension is best treated by use of elastic stockings and fluids; pressor agents should be avoided or used judiciously because of a heightened response to these agents, which is probably related to denervation hypersensitivity. Hypertension may be managed with short-acting alpha-adrenergic blocking agents. Hyponatremia related to inappropriate secretion of antidiuretic hormone should be treated by restriction of fluids.

The bedridden patient should be turned frequently to avoid the development of pressure sores. Paralyzed limbs require physiotherapy so that passive limb movements can be carried out and contractures prevented. Compression neuropathies (most commonly involving the ulnar and peroneal nerves) can be prevented by the use of insulating pads placed over susceptible sites (the elbow and head of the fibula, respectively). Subcutaneous heparin, 5000 units twice daily, should be used to prevent venous thrombosis and pulmonary embolism.

The natural history of the disease in the moderately to severely affected patient (a patient who is unable to walk or who has severe respiratory muscle weakness requiring a ventilator) is one of gradual improvement so that the ability to walk unassisted returns in an average of about 3 months. In the subset of respirator-dependent patients, the average time to recovery is 6 months. Four factors correlate with poor outcome: a mean motor amplitude of less than 20 per cent of normal; older age; the need for ventilatory support; and rapidly progressive disease (7 days or less).

A number of multicenter studies have shown that plasmapheresis is the only variable the physician has that can influence outcome and that it has a beneficial effect on the course of the illness, even in patients with several poor prognostic signs. Patients treated with plasmapheresis are able to walk on average 1 month earlier than untreated patients; the subset of respirator-dependent patients walks 3 months sooner than those who do not receive plasma exchange. Our practice is to use plasma exchange for patients who reach or are approaching inability to walk unaided, patients who either require intubation or demonstrate a falling vital capacity, and patients who have weakness of the bulbar musculature leading to dysphagia and aspiration. We follow the GBS study group guidelines and exchange 200 to 250 ml of plasma per kg of body weight during 7 to 14 days. We use Plasmanate or 5 per cent salt-poor albumin as replacement fluid but not fresh frozen plasma. We do not use plasmapheresis in mildly affected, ambulatory patients or in patients who are more than 21 days after onset of neuropathy. At present we do not use corticosteroids in the management of GBS, although ongoing studies may establish some role for these agents in the future.

Chronic Inflammatory Neuropathy

Chronic inflammatory-demyelinating neuropathy (CIDP) is sometimes viewed as a chronic form of GBS. Indeed, in some patients the GBS resolves but weeks to months later a second episode occurs, which is then followed by a chronic neuropathy. However, most CIDP patients have not had a previous episode of GBS; their neuropathy is characterized by either a relapsing or a slowly progressive course. Motor weakness is usually more prominent than sensory loss. Reflexes are absent or severely reduced. The cerebrospinal fluid protein level is elevated. Electromyography and sural nerve biopsy indicate features of axonal degeneration and segmental demyelination. The disorder is thought to have an immune-mediated pathogenesis. In contrast to the relatively good prognosis for GBS, patients with CIDP are less likely to recover, and many are left with mild to moderate neurologic disability. The use of corticosteroids, plasmapheresis, and immunosuppressive agents has improved the outcome somewhat. Prednisone and plasmapheresis have each been shown in controlled trials to enhance recovery, although benefits may be small. Our practice is to institute high-dose daily prednisone (60 mg per day) for 4 to 6 weeks and then convert to an alternate-day regimen, with a plan to taper corticosteroid use gradually by 5 mg per month if tolerated. We add plasmapheresis if there is no response to prednisone after 6 weeks. We have encountered patients who are exquisitely dependent on plasmapheresis, requiring exchanges every few weeks to months to maintain adequate neurologic function. In some patients who are unresponsive to these modalities, we have added azathioprine (Imuran) (1 to 3 mg per kg of body weight). Patients receiving this drug must be monitored carefully for bone marrow depression and hepatotoxicity. There remains a small group of CIDP patients who are refractory to any form of treatment.

CIDP may also present with mononeuropathy multiplex, which evolves more slowly than the vasculitic form. The course of the disease is variable, but if it is untreated there may be progression with severe disability. Treatment is the same as that described for CIDP, beginning with prednisone and using plasmapheresis if there is no response. Patients not responding to prednisone or plasmapheresis may improve with other immunosuppressive agents such as azathioprine. Experience in the use of these agents for this form of CIDP is limited, however, and the value of treatment remains unproved.

Multifocal Motor Neuropathy

This neuropathy resembles the mononeuritis multiplex form of CIDP except that in its early phases the hands and arms are more affected than the legs and it evolves to closely resemble an anterior horn cell disorder. Electromyography discloses multifocal conduction block along motor fibers, and immunologic studies reveal the presence of antibodies to ganglioside antigens in high titer. In contrast to patients with CIDP, there is no response to prednisone or plasmapheresis, but there is a substantial clinical improvement after high-dose cyclophosphamide therapy if the titer can be reduced by more than 70 per cent.

Paraproteinemic Neuropathy

A chronic neuropathy resembling CIDP also occurs in association with an IgM paraprotein-

emia. In contrast to CIDP, however, it tends to affect sensory more than motor function, and patients are often most troubled by a sensory ataxia. The pathogenesis may involve IgM-mediated demyelination; in some patients, IgM is directed toward a myelin-associated glycoprotein. Untreated, the neuropathy produces severe disability. Although controlled studies are not available, it appears that this course can be altered by vigorous immunosuppressive treatment that reduces the level of IgM by more than 50 per cent. We have therefore used a combination of oral prednisone and cyclophosphamide to attempt reduction of the level of IgM and have noted improvement in a number of patients. Repeated long-term plasmapheresis may also be beneficial.

Metabolic Neuropathies

Diabetes

Diabetes commonly produces a peripheral neuropathy. It is present at diagnosis in 8 per cent of diabetics, and its frequency increases to 50 per cent after diabetes has been present for 25 years. How this disorder produces neuropathy is uncertain, but metabolic abnormalities and nerve ischemia probably play important roles. The most commonly encountered neuropathy is a subacute or chronic distal, symmetric polyneuropathy with mixed sensory, motor, and autonomic abnormalities. A smaller number of patients have a purely sensory neuropathy, which can be intensely painful. Less commonly encountered is a proximal, symmetric motor neuropathy, which at one time was termed "diabetic amyotrophy." Diabetes also produces the clinical syndrome of mononeuritis multiplex.

Proximal diabetic motor neuropathy usually evolves slowly; diabetic mononeuritis multiplex presents in a more acute fashion. In both, pain is often severe.

A pathogenesis that may explain diabetic polyneuropathy is increased activity of the polyol pathway leading to increased peripheral nerve sorbitol levels and nerve dysfunction. Therefore, attempts have been made to reduce polyol pathway activity with an inhibitor of aldose reductase, the enzyme that converts glucose to sorbitol. Some studies have suggested improvements in neurologic function and nerve conduction velocity. However, until further studies have better defined the role of these inhibitors, we do not believe that they are indicated for routine clinical use.

The mainstay of treatment is therefore still control of diabetes, although there is no evidence to support the concept that rigorous control is superior to conventional treatment. Finger stick blood sugar monitoring and assessment of glycosylated hemoglobin level are probably the most adequate guides to good control.

The physician caring for the diabetic patient with neuropathy must also provide symptomatic and preventive treatments so that complications are minimized. Because of distal sensory loss and poor circulation, diabetics are at risk for the development of trophic skin ulcers resulting from repeated painless trauma. Skin care is therefore of utmost importance. Autonomic neuropathy may cause impaired gastric motility, orthostatic hypotension, and sexual dysfunction, which may be difficult to treat. Diarrhea and disorders of gastrointestinal motility may respond to metoclopramide. Orthostatic hypotension may respond to simple measures such as avoiding volume depletion and vasodilating agents, sleeping in the head-up position, and use of elastic stockings. Fludrocortisone is sometimes helpful if these measures fail and acts by producing volume expansion. Indomethacin may act by inhibiting prostaglandin synthesis and preventing the formation of vasodilatory substances. Sexual dysfunction in men may be helped by use of a penile prosthesis.

The management of pain in diabetic neuropathy is discussed in a later section.

Other Endocrine Disorders

Hypothyroidism can be associated with mononeuropathy (usually bilateral carpal tunnel syndromes) or a mild sensorimotor polyneuropathy. Untreated, the neuropathy demonstrates an inexorable, relentless course, but it responds well to hormone replacement therapy.

Acromegaly is also associated with either a mononeuropathy (again, most likely carpal tunnel syndrome) or a mild polyneuropathy, which appears late in the clinical course of the illness. Although carpal tunnel syndrome resolves with removal of the adenoma, it is unclear whether normalization of growth hormone levels alters the course of the polyneuropathy.

Uremia

Although a number of diseases that produce renal failure are associated with peripheral nerve damage, uremia itself produces a characteristic sensorimotor axonal polyneuropathy with secondary demyelination. It is present to some degree in approximately 65 per cent of patients who are undergoing dialysis. Several potential uremic toxins have been proposed as the etiology of the neuropathy, but none has been proved to be the critical one; to date, the best correlate of uremic neuropathy is the glomerular filtration rate, which suggests that the nerve damage is a cu-mulative result of exposure to a number of toxins. The neuropathy stabilizes or improves with regular dialysis. Renal transplantation, the most effective therapy, is associated with an initially rapid improvement and then a more gradual one.

Porphyria

This manifestation of an autosomal dominant inborn error of hepatic heme biosynthesis results in increased levels of delta-aminolevulinic acid and is characterized by attacks of abdominal pain, mental symptoms, and a subacute, predominantly motor, axonal polyneuropathy that can simulate GBS. The neuropathy is the most dangerous porphyric complication and most frequent cause of death. The natural history is one of spontaneous but slow improvement.

The principles of treatment lie first in prevention; therefore, careful attention must be given to minimizing exposure to the numerous known inciting agents such as barbiturates and birth control pills. In the acute attack, propranolol is safe to use for control of anxiety and tachycardia and may cause a general improvement in clinical state, perhaps by partially repressing delta-aminolevulinate synthase induction. Chlorpromazine is effective for treatment of accompanying psychotic symptoms and associated musculoskeletal or abdominal pain. Finally, although there exists a poor correlation between porphyrin precursor levels and severity of neurologic involvement, anecdotal reports exist suggesting a beneficial effect on neuropathy by repressing induction of delta-aminolevulinate synthase with hematin.

Neoplasm-Related Neuropathies

Neoplasms lead to peripheral nerve disorders by direct spread, metastases, paraneoplastic effects, and complications of treatment.

Direct effects occur as a result of compression and infiltration of nerves by adjacent tumor. This condition is usually painful and results in a variety of clinical patterns including mononeuropathy, mononeuritis multiplex, and plexopathy. Local radiation therapy may reduce pain and halt the progress of the compressive or infiltrative process.

A variety of paraneoplastic neuropathies are associated with malignancies, including subacute sensory polyneuropathy, sensorimotor polyneuropathy, CIDP, GBS, and a small-fiber sensory-autonomic polyneuropathy.

A *subacute sensory neuropathy* that develops in a middle-aged adult should immediately raise the possibility of an underlying neoplasm (including small cell carcinoma of the lung and tumors of the breast, ovaries, and gastrointestinal tract).

The neuropathy develops subacutely during a period of weeks to months and is marked by pain, paresthesias, dysesthesias, and limb numbness. Severe unsteadiness of gait and impaired limb coordination in the face of relatively normal muscle strength are characteristic findings. The underlying pathology is a sensory neuronopathy, and the pathogenesis most likely involves antibodies directed against a nucleoprotein antigen in sensory neurons. Despite the probable immunologic pathogenesis, immunosuppressive therapy has not been successful, and the neuropathy does not respond to treatment of the underlying neoplasm, although patients generally reach a plateau after several months of deterioration.

A *sensorimotor polyneuropathy* is perhaps the most commonly encountered malignancy-associated neuropathy. The underlying pathology is axonal degeneration, and the pathogenesis is unknown, although the severity of the neuropathy is directly proportional to the amount of weight loss. We attempt to maintain good nutritional status in these patients, but unfortunately this treatment is often ineffective. No other specific therapy is available; control of the underlying malignancy does not affect the polyneuropathy.

CIDP is most often associated with the osteosclerotic form of myeloma, which it accompanies in 50 per cent of cases, frequently antedating the diagnosis. It can also be seen concurrently with lymphoma. The course is one of steady progression leading to severe disability. Treatment of the underlying malignancy is sometimes associated with improvement of the neuropathy. Plasmapheresis may also arrest progression of CIDP and may result in improvement.

A predominantly *motor neuropathy* occurs as a rare complication of Hodgkin's disease or lymphoma. The cause is a motor neuronopathy. The disorder may produce severe degrees of weakness but over time tends to improve and stabilize independent of the activity of the underlying malignancy.

A small-fiber, painful sensory and autonomic polyneuropathy is associated with amyloidosis. Pain may be difficult to treat. Unfortunately, the neuropathy does not respond to even vigorous treatment of the amyloidosis.

Perhaps the most important neuropathies associated with neoplasia are those encountered with the administration of antineoplastic agents, most often vincristine (VCR) (Oncovin) and cis-diamminedichloroplatinum (II) (DDP). Neurotoxicity is often the dose-limiting factor in their administration, but on the other hand the potential exists to administer agents prophylactically.

VCR is used in a number of standard oncologic protocols, and the dosage that is tolerated by patients is clearly limited by neurotoxicity. The drug's effects are cumulative, although symptoms can occur after one dose. An axonal sensorimotor neuropathy is most commonly encountered; complaints of constipation and colicky abdominal pain are frequent and represent autonomic involvement. Although minor paresthesias disappear in a few weeks if VCR is discontinued at the onset of symptoms, more severe paresthesias resulting from repeated dosing require months to resolve, and resolution of motor weakness may be incomplete.

The neuropathy encountered after administration of DDP is primarily sensory; the underlying pathology is a sensory neuronopathy. DDP neuropathy is uncommon when low dosages are used but occurs more often with higher doses and clearly correlates most closely with cumulative dosage. Therefore, approximately 50 per cent of patients who receive 900 mg of DDP and virtually all in whom the dosage exceeds 1300 mg will have sensory symptoms. Symptoms and signs of DDP-induced neuropathy are reversible even after high-dose administration, although it may take many months for complete resolution of symptoms.

Although early attempts at modifying VCR-induced neuropathies with folinic acid met with little success, recent experimental evidence suggests that a ganglioside mixture and glutamic acid may ameliorate VCR-induced neuropathy. In preliminary clinical trials, gangliosides have been shown to be of some benefit in modulating VCR-induced neurotoxicity, but further studies are necessary before gangliosides can be recommended for clinical use. Glutamic acid has been studied more extensively in the clinical setting, and doses of 500 mg three times daily have proved to be efficacious in preventing neuropathy. There appears to exist an adequate rationale for using glutamic acid as a preventive measure; whether it can reverse pre-existing VCR-induced toxicity remains unclear.

DDP's toxicity is probably also ameliorable. In animal studies, use of melanocortins (peptides derived from adrenocorticotropic hormone and melanocyte-stimulating hormone that have neurotrophic effects on the central and peripheral nervous systems) such as the adrenocorticotropic hormone analogue Org 2766 results in prevention of neurotoxicity without altering antitumor effects. More significant from a clinical standpoint are recent data showing a lower incidence of neuropathy and the ability of patients to tolerate higher doses of DDP when WR 2721, a cysteamine derivative that was initially developed as a radioprotective agent, is administered concurrently. Further studies are necessary before this agent becomes available for general use.

Nutritional Deficiency Neuropathies

The major nutrients whose deficiencies may result in a neuropathy are the B vitamins: thiamine (B_1), nicotinic acid (B_3), pyridoxine (B_6), pantothenic acid, and cyanocobalamin (B_{12}). A neuropathy attributable to the essential nutrient folate has also been described. It is important to recognize both that these deficiency states are the result of dietary imbalance (such as that occurring in the alcoholic patient) rather than starvation and that often more than one of these deficiencies are present in one patient.

The most frequently encountered deficiency-induced neuropathy results from a lack of thiamine, which is the underlying etiology of the neuropathic syndrome associated with alcoholism. Lack of thiamine can also result in beriberi, whose dry form has neuropathy as a prominent sign (which is clinically similar to the neuropathy seen in alcoholics). This sensorimotor axonal polyneuropathy may be very painful.

Vitamin B_{12} deficiency is usually secondary to vitamin malabsorption, a result of intrinsic factor deficiency and not dietary imbalance. A predominantly sensory axonal polyneuropathy is a fairly common manifestation of this deficiency. Although there are usually accompanying hematologic abnormalities, neurologic symptoms of vitamin B_{12} deficiency may occur in their absence and may even occur when serum cobalamin levels are normal. A more sensitive urinary methylmalonic acid determination should be performed to assess the condition more definitively. Treatment with monthly vitamin B_{12} injections usually results in gradual improvement of neurologic symptoms and signs. A condition similar to this deficiency syndrome may also be encountered in patients after complete or near-complete gastrectomies and as a result of folate deficiency.

Because lack of a specific vitamin cannot be established in most cases, if a neuropathy is determined to be a possible manifestation of a nutritional deficiency, the general therapeutic principle is to ensure adequate nutrition in the form of a balanced diet and all the B vitamins. Pain manifestations should be treated with measures outlined later.

Toxic Neuropathies

The bacteriostatic nitrofurantoin tends to produce an axonal sensorimotor polyneuropathy most often in patients with renal impairment. The neuropathy usually arises after weeks to months of drug use and can have a rapid onset, sometimes simulating the presentation of GBS. Treatment consists of supportive measures and withdrawal of the drug; patients tend to exhibit a slow recovery after withdrawal.

The most common toxic effect of isoniazid is an axonal sensorimotor polyneuropathy that is dose related; in patients who receive usual recommended doses, its frequency is approximately 2 per cent. Neuropathy tends to occur more often in malnourished individuals and in those who acetylate the drug slowly. The neuropathy is clearly related to interference with pyridoxine utilization. However, the use of pyridoxine does not seem to speed recovery once peripheral neuropathy is encountered. Withdrawal of the drug is associated with a slow recovery. Daily administration of 100 mg of pyridoxine prophylactically prevents the neuropathy in most cases. A similar neuropathy, also probably mediated by pyridoxine, is seen with the administration of hydralazine.

Misonidazole, a drug with hypoxic radiosensitizing properties, can produce a polyneuropathy dominated by painful sensory symptoms. Dexamethasone and phenytoin have been used with some success in treatment and prevention of the neuropathy. Nitrous oxide produces a mild distal symmetric polyneuropathy with prolonged (usually illicit) use that, combined with its central effects, may simulate vitamin B_{12} deficiency. Ingestion of high doses of pyridoxine produces a severe sensory neuropathy without weakness. The pathologic change is neuronopathy; treatment is normalization of pyridoxine intake.

Lead produces a motor neuropathy, sometimes with distinct patterns of involvement such as selective wrist or foot drop. It usually occurs after prolonged exposure and is associated with constitutional symptoms and a mild anemia. A blood level higher than 0.2 mg per liter is considered to be significant. Because lead is cleared so rapidly from the body, measurement of urinary excretion of lead after pretreatment with a chelating agent is sometimes necessary to make the diagnosis. Treatment consists of removing the source of lead and administering a chelating agent, either penicillamine if the syndrome is mild or calcium disodium EDTA if more severe symptoms are present.

Arsenic is also associated with a prominent and distinctive neuropathy that follows excessive exposure, which may occur either as an occupational exposure (smelting industries) or as a result of its use as a suicide or homicide vehicle. After a subacute exposure, neuropathy develops within 1 to 3 weeks and is characterized by primarily sensory symptoms, including intensely unpleasant paresthesias and varying degrees of weakness. In the more insidious form, a chronologic triad occurs characterized first by generalized constitutional symptoms, followed by Mees's lines and mucous membrane irritation and last by the appearance of an overt neuropathy. Supportive measures include treatment of the painful paresthesias. Specific treatment consists of administering penicillamine; if the neuropathy is treated early in its course, recovery is excellent.

Hexacarbon-induced neuropathy is encountered either as a result of occupational exposure or in persons who self-administer these agents for recreational purposes ("glue sniffers"). The neuropathy is insidious and predominantly sensory in industrial exposures, but it may be more severe in glue sniffers, in whom exposures can result in a subacute development of progressive weakness that simulates GBS. Even with cessation of exposure, the neuropathy can progress for months. Recovery correlates with the amount of dysfunction at time of diagnosis; however, even patients with mild to moderate symptoms may take a year to recover.

Thallium neurotoxicity now occurs rarely because its use as a rodenticide and insecticide has been discouraged. The more severe acute neuropathy is characterized by prominent gastrointestinal symptoms and a burning, progressive sensorimotor neuropathy. Hair loss, a distinctive feature of thallium intoxication, may be delayed and not present when neuropathic symptoms develop in acute cases. The subacute form produces a primarily but not exclusively sensory syndrome characterized by pain; alopecia is usually present and is a useful clue. Recovery from the subacute form is usually excellent. Diagnosis is established by analysis of urine for thallium. Use of combinations of potassium chloride and chelating agents is currently favored as treatment.

Infectious Neuropathies

The infectious neuropathies are important to recognize because they represent a largely treatable group of nerve disorders. The most important infectious agents are the spirochetes *Treponema pallidum* (neurosyphilis) and *Borrelia burgdorferi* (Lyme disease); *Mycobacterium leprae* (leprosy); varicella-zoster viruses (shingles); and the assorted disorders associated with human immunodeficiency virus (HIV).

Syphilis can lead to severe and extensive damage of dorsal roots and give rise to tabes dorsalis, the most common form of neurosyphilis. There is a characteristic set of signs and symptoms including lightning pain, impaired sensation, ataxia, and bladder disturbances. Analysis of the cerebrospinal fluid discloses a mononuclear pleocytosis, elevated protein level, and positive serology; in all cases of tabes dorsalis antibodies spe-

cific for *T. pallidum* are found. The treatment of choice is aqueous penicillin G, 4 million units intravenously every 4 hours for 2 weeks, with careful follow-up of cerebrospinal fluid measures to ensure eradication of the active infection (the aim is for a normal cell count and the protein concentration's falling into the normal range).

Lyme disease is transmitted by the tic *Ixodes dammini*. It is associated with a variety of peripheral neuropathies including limb and cranial mononeuropathies (especially facial palsy simulating Bell's palsy), mononeuritis multiplex, polyradiculopathy, and brachial plexopathy. Facial palsy may be the sole neurologic manifestation of Lyme disease. Polyradiculopathy may simulate GBS in its progression and distribution. Most often, peripheral nerve involvement, along with lymphocytic meningitis, occurs 4 weeks after the characteristic skin lesion of Lyme disease—erythema chronicum migrans. Serologic testing may be helpful to demonstrate elevated titers against the spirochete. The neurologic signs respond to intravenous pencillin G, 20 million units per day in divided doses for 10 days. Penicillin-allergic patients should be given high doses of tetracycline.

Leprosy, a chronic granulomatous infection, has a propensity to affect peripheral nerves. Neurologic involvement is more frequent and occurs earlier in the tuberculoid form; the ulnar, great auricular, and facial nerves seem preferentially affected. A progressive sensorimotor neuropathy that is characterized by repeated attacks of neuralgic pains often precedes weakness or sensory loss. Dapsone, a drug of the sulfone class, combined with rifampin is the most effective available treatment.

Reactivated *herpes zoster* or shingles is a common, painful, vesicular eruption that occurs in a dermatomal distribution, especially in the thoracic area, less frequently in the cervical area, and least frequently in the lumbosacral area. Most herpetic lesions resolve in 2 to 3 weeks, so specific antiviral therapy is usually not indicated. Nevertheless, we recommend acyclovir administration when the disease occurs in immunosuppressed hosts, when the ophthalmic division is severely affected, or when there is disseminated disease (more than three dermatomes affected or visceral involvement). A common sequela of uncomplicated shingles is postherpetic neuralgia, which occurs in about 10 per cent of patients 1 month after herpes zoster. Its incidence is related to age; it is more likely to occur when the onset of disease is after age 60 years. Sixty to 70 per cent of patients benefit from the use of tricyclic antidepressants, but troublesome anticholinergic effects limit their use. Topical capsaicin has been shown to reduce pain effectively in some patients, but double-blind control trials will be needed to confirm its efficacy.

HIV has been associated with a variety of peripheral neuropathies: GBS, CIDP, a sensorimotor primary axonal neuropathy, a sensory neuropathy, and mononeuropathy multiplex. GBS and CIDP occur with increased incidence in the early stages of HIV infection and are sometimes the earliest manifestations of AIDS. Plasmapheresis is the treatment of choice for both conditions. A sensorimotor, painful, primarily axonal polyneuropathy is usually associated with overt AIDS or AIDS-related complex and is probably the most commonly encountered HIV-associated neuropathy. This form of neuropathy does not respond to plasmapheresis, and a specific treatment is not available except for modalities to relieve pain. A primarily sensory neuropathy has also been identified and occurs in patients with well-established AIDS who have lost weight and in some who are demented. A mononeuropathy multiplex can also occur as a presenting manifestation, early in the course of HIV infection, or can occur in patients who are known to have AIDS. In some cases the underlying pathology may be vasculitis and in others, inflammation-demyelination. Patients with a demyelinating component may have a good response to plasmapheresis.

Entrapment Neuropathies

Median Nerve

Carpal tunnel syndrome arises because of chronic compression of the median nerve as it passes through the fibro-osseous carpal tunnel. Predisposing factors include excessive flexion and extension activity at the wrist, prior wrist fracture, rheumatoid arthritis, hypothyroidism, acromegaly, and amyloidosis. Presenting symptoms include paresthesias and weakness in the territory of the median nerve.

In mild cases, we recommend a course of an anti-inflammatory agent such as aspirin or one of the nonsteroidal agents, and a wrist splint to be worn at night. If the history suggests overuse of the fingers and hands, we recommend rest and if possible some form of job modification. These conservative measures are often successful in easing discomfort. If these measures fail, if it is impossible to modify an occupation, or if the electromyogram discloses a severe degree of injury, we recommend surgical decompression of the median nerve at the wrist. In most cases, surgery relieves pain and paresthesias; return of strength to atrophic muscles of the thenar eminence is less likely to occur.

Ulnar Nerve

The cubital tunnel syndrome occurs when the ulnar nerve is compressed by a tight aponeurotic band that bridges the two heads of the flexor carpi ulnaris. The syndrome presents with paresthesias along the medial aspect of the hand; as the compression increases, weakness develops in ulnar-supplied muscles. Predisposing factors include previous elbow fracture, osteoarthritis, and occupations that involve habitually leaning on the elbow or manual work with an excessive carrying angle.

If injury is mild, simple measures are used such as protecting the elbow with a soft insulating pad and administration of anti-inflammatory agents. However, if the mononeuropathy is more severe and weakness and muscle atrophy occur, little is to be gained by a conservative approach and we recommend surgery. One can either decompress the ulnar nerve by splitting the aponeurosis or transpose the ulnar nerve to a less mechanically vulnerable position over the anterior surface of the forearm.

Inherited Neuropathies

No specific treatment of the more common inherited polyneuropathies (Charcot-Marie-Tooth disease) is available. Fortunately, their course is gradual with apparent arrest of progression (clinical plateau) for many years. Most patients are not seriously handicapped because preservation of power in limb girdle groups, even in the most severely affected patients, allows for continued walking and use of the arms. In some patients, light braces can overcome foot drop and aid in ambulation. Sometimes, if foot drop is severe, stabilizing the ankle by arthrodeses is indicated.

Two rare inherited conditions in which specific treatment is indicated are Refsum's disease and abetalipoproteinemia.

Refsum's disease is characterized by deafness, retinitis pigmentosa, scaly skin, and demyelinating polyneuropathy. The serum phytanic acid level is elevated; patients should therefore be maintained on a low–phytanic acid diet. Plasma exchange may sometimes be helpful. *Bassen-Kornzweig disease,* or abetalipoproteinemia, is marked by ataxia, areflexia, retinitis pigmentosa, and marked impairment of proprioceptive sensation. All apoprotein B–containing lipoproteins are absent from the serum, and acanthocytes are present in peripheral blood. Large doses of oral or parenteral vitamin E have shown promise in arresting progression of the condition.

MANAGEMENT OF PAINFUL NEUROPATHIES

The pain resulting from peripheral neuropathy is neuropathic, that is, it results from damage to the nervous system. Neuropathic pains are differentiated from other types of pain by, among other features, their occurrence in the absence of detectable ongoing tissue-damaging processes, by the frequent presence of dysesthesia or burning sensation, by the presence of a sensory deficit in the region of the pain, and by allodynia (perceiving pain when a mild stimulus is applied). From what is known at present, neuropathic pains are sustained by some combination of (1) hyperactivity in nociceptive neurons, (2) loss of central inhibitory connections, and (3) increased activity in sympathetic efferents. In peripheral neuropathy where large myelinated nonpain fibers may be preferentially affected, the loss of inhibitory influences on secondary neurons in the dorsal horn may result in exaggerated pain responses and neuropathic pain. In addition, ectopic impulse generation in damaged afferents may also contribute to neuropathic pains, especially pains described as lightning-like sensations. Sympathetic autonomic fiber activation or facilitation of primary sensory afferent fibers may also contribute to neuropathic pain.

Of all the symptoms of peripheral neuropathy, pain can be the most disabling and is often the most difficult to treat. Therefore, an effective strategy is essential when treating the patient with neuropathic pain. The goal should be to minimize pain and maximize function. Although the use of opiates is sometimes helpful, chronic administration should be discouraged except when absolutely necessary because it can lead to tolerance and dependence as well as relative inefficacy over the long term.

The administration of certain agents that are used principally for other neurologic or psychiatric problems may provide marked relief. The anticonvulsants carbamazepine, phenytoin, and clonazepam may relieve neuropathic pains, probably by reducing discharge from sites of ectopic impulse generation in damaged nerve. Anticonvulsants have been especially effective in the control of trigeminal neuralgia. They can be beneficial in situations where lancinating pain is prominent. There may be a sharp threshold in the serum anticonvulsant levels below which a particular drug is ineffective; therefore, the dose should be increased to the limits of the therapeutic range before the drug is deemed ineffective.

Antidepressants are sometimes effective when treating neuropathic pain and act possibly by enhancing the inhibitory action of serotonin and norepinephrine on spinal transmission neurons. They have been most efficacious in postherpetic neuralgia and painful diabetic neuropathy. Because the analgesic effects are independent of antidepressant action, the usual effective dose required for tricyclic efficacy in pain is at the lower range required for treatment of depression, and daily doses of 75 mg of amitriptyline (Elavil) are often adequate for pain relief. The physician should start with a low dose of either amitriptyline or desipramine (Norpramin) (it is unclear whether other antidepressants are as effective as these agents) and gradually build up the serum level; it is probably worthwhile to continue use of the drug for at least 1 month at a dose of 75 to 100 mg per day before deciding that it is not effective.

The major tranquilizers are also used in treating neuropathic pain, mostly in combination with tricyclic agents. However, because of phenothiazine-induced tardive dyskinesia and marginal efficacy, we have abandoned their use.

The best approach to treating painful neuropathy is a systematic one. First, the physician should ensure by a careful history and physical examination that the pain is indeed neuropathic and not related to actual tissue damage (i.e., as in a diabetic with neuropathy and pain secondary to osteomyelitis). Neuropathic pains, as mentioned, are characterized by their burning and lancinating qualities and are also typically worse at night. In formulating the treatment plan, the physician should first consider using either a tricyclic antidepressant or an anticonvulsant agent. A full trial of the chosen drug—meaning that the patient either obtains relief or is at the ceiling therapeutic level of the drug—should be administered before it is considered ineffective. At that point, the physician should add an agent of the other class (rather than switching to another drug of the same class) and see if relief can be obtained. Sometimes, the use of a nonsteroidal anti-inflammatory agent may provide effective relief. In addition, data from preliminary studies suggest that topical capsaicin may reduce the pain of certain neuropathic conditions, such as those secondary to diabetes or postherpetic neuralgia. When these measures are ineffective, cautious use of opiates should be considered, especially in situations where the neuropathic condition is self-limited (such as after exposure to a toxin or in vasculitis-mediated neuropathies in which treatment of the underlying disease is likely to result in remission).

ACUTE HEAD INJURIES IN ADULTS

method of
DOUGLAS GENTLEMAN, M.B., CH.B
Institute of Neurological Sciences
Southern General Hospital
Glasgow, Scotland

Most head injuries are mild and self-limiting, but the more severe ones may threaten life or the quality of survival. Prompt assessment and effective treatment are essential for optimal care after a severe head injury and can prevent death and disability from secondary brain damage. There are two main preventable causes of secondary brain damage: delay in the treatment of intracranial hematomas and failure to correct the systemic complications of injury (especially hypoxia and hypotension). Management of a patient with a severe head injury is therefore directed toward (1) initial assessment of the severity of the head injury and of any associated injuries and (2) identification and correction of any risk factors for secondary brain damage.

ASSESSING THE INITIAL INJURY

Conscious Level

The patient's conscious level is the most important index of the initial severity of a head injury, and it is also the most sensitive guide to later progress. The Glasgow Coma Scale has been widely adopted throughout the world because it allows the rapid and reliable assessment of conscious level by a physician or nurse.

There are three components of the scale: the eye-opening response, the best motor response in the upper limbs, and the best verbal response (Table 1). Each component of the scale is assessed independently in response to graded stimuli, and the results are charted at the bedside to give both a point reading of conscious level and a trend over time. Numbers can be assigned to the levels of responsiveness and summed to yield a Glasgow Coma Score, but this score is more valuable when comparing the severity of head injury in a series of patients than when managing the individual patient.

The conscious level should be assessed by a competent observer as soon as possible after injury. In the United Kingdom, this assessment usually takes place when the patient reaches the first hospital, but in the United States and some other countries, paramedic teams often begin assessment at the accident site. Assessment of conscious level should be repeated frequently to aid evaluation of the patient's progress.

By convention, a severe head injury is one that renders the patient unconscious—unable to obey commands, speak, or open the eyes to any stimulus—for at least 6 hours. However, less profound or less prolonged alteration of consciousness can also be followed by complications. *Any* level of impaired consciousness after head injury must therefore be regarded as significant.

Focal Neurologic Signs

Altered consciousness reflects the degree of diffuse injury to the brain. Other neurologic signs reflect focal brain injury, and these should be sought at an early stage. The two most useful signs in the acute phase are (1) the size of the pupils and their reactivity to light and (2) whether the limb responsiveness to command or painful stimuli is symmetric. This information is valuable both in the initial assessment of the severity of injury and in the detection of secondary lesions such as compressive intracranial hematomas.

More subtle signs of focal brain dysfunction, such as altered limb reflexes, can be hard to elicit in the unconscious patient in the emergency room, and they add little to practical management in the "golden hour" after injury.

Respiratory Function

The fundamental principles of respiratory and cardiovascular resuscitation must be carefully applied to all patients with a severe head injury to protect the brain from further damage.

Altered consciousness, whatever the exact etiology, carries a high risk of airway obstruction and hence of blood gas disturbance (hypoxia and hypercarbia). Posttraumatic seizures or ventilatory insufficiency can also cause hypoxia and hypercarbia. It is therefore imperative to assess the airway and breathing of the patient with severe head injury at the earliest possible moment; to measure arterial blood gas levels and take effective action to correct hypoxia and hypercarbia; and to protect the airway from later compromise.

Opinion varies on how best to protect the brain from hypoxia and hypercarbia. In North America, an aggressive approach to airway protection is usual, and endotracheal intubation and ventilation are routinely

TABLE 1. **The Glasgow Coma Scale and Score**

Response	Score
Eye-opening response	
Spontaneously	4
To speech	3
To pain	2
None	1
Best motor response (in upper limbs)	
Obeys commands	6
Localizes to pain	5
Flexes to pain (withdrawal)	4
Flexes to pain (abnormal or spastic)	3
Extends to pain	2
No response	1
Best verbal response	
Oriented	5
Confused	4
Inappropriate words	3
Incomprehensible sounds	2
None	1

Glasgow Coma Score: 3–15

Definition of coma: (score 8 or less)	No eye opening to any stimulus Does not obey commands Does not speak

used in the management of traumatic coma. In the United Kingdom, endotracheal intubation and ventilation are more commonly reserved for certain categories of head-injured patient: those who are deeply unconscious, those who on arrival at the hospital already have significant blood gas disturbances from airway obstruction or pulmonary hypoventilation, and those who are to be transported from the initial hospital to a special unit. Airway protection for other patients with an altered consciousness level is based on simpler and less invasive measures: placing the patient in the lateral or semiprone ("coma") position, inserting an oral airway, oral and pharyngeal suction of debris and secretions, and emptying the stomach contents by a nasogastric tube. What matters most is probably not the precise details of technique but that any blood gas disturbances are rapidly recognized and corrected and that the patient is assessed at an early stage by a physician who has the necessary experience to decide how best to protect that particular patient from episodes of hypoxia and hypercarbia. There should be no hesitation in using short-acting muscle relaxant drugs to facilitate intubation and ventilation; their masking of neurologic signs is not an issue in a patient who is to undergo scanning, and their action can be rapidly reversed to allow neurologic reassessment.

After a severe head injury, the goal is to keep arterial oxygen tension (Pa_{O_2}) above 100 torr and the arterial carbon dioxide tension (Pa_{CO_2}) below 40 torr. Frequent measurements of Pa_{O_2} and Pa_{CO_2} by arterial blood sampling are essential. Many centers routinely hyperventilate patients with a severe head injury to keep the Pa_{CO_2} in the range of 25 to 30 torr (see the later section on medical management of raised intracranial pressure).

Cardiovascular Function

About one-half of all unconscious victims of high-velocity injuries (such as those from traffic accidents and falls from a height) have multiple injuries. These injuries can cause such severe blood loss as to threaten the perfusion of the brain and other vital organs. It is therefore a priority to assess the patient's circulatory state, to replace blood loss, and to identify and stabilize all major extracranial injuries.

Perfusion in the unconscious patient should be monitored frequently by using the pulse rate and peripheral capillary filling as sensitive guides to the adequacy of perfusion. The systolic blood pressure should be kept in the range of 120 to 170 mmHg. The central venous pressure and pulmonary artery wedge pressure are useful indices of cardiovascular function in the critically ill patient with severe multiple injuries. Incipient or actual shock should be treated aggressively with infusions of plasma or other colloid, followed as soon as possible by compatible blood. It is easy to underestimate the volume of fluid required to make good losses from hemorrhage, and the physician should err on the side of generosity when prescribing transfusions.

Continuing perfusion failure in the head-injured adult is usually the result of a failure to recognize and treat occult hemorrhage elsewhere in the body. Blood loss from the head injury itself (either intracranial or from the scalp) is almost never the cause. The diagnosis of certain extracranial injuries can be difficult in the unconscious patient, and without a thorough clinical and radiologic assessment important injuries can be easily overlooked or underestimated. A careful clinical history from witnesses and physical examination of the patient must be supplemented by good-quality radiographs of the chest, cervical spine, pelvis, and any other body areas that appear to have been injured. Abdominal paracentesis is the best way to identify intraperitoneal hemorrhage in the unconscious patient. To save life, it is sometimes necessary to give priority to the definitive treatment of major thoracic or abdominal injuries over neurosurgical investigations.

PREVENTING THE SECONDARY INSULT

Studies of mortality after head injury have shown that some deaths are due not to the severity of the initial injury but to factors that become important later and that cause secondary brain damage. The principal avoidable factors are delay in the evacuation of intracranial hematomas and failure to recognize and treat systemic hypoxia and hypotension. Less common factors are the failure to prevent or treat secondary intracranial infection and post-traumatic seizures. The management of the patient with a serious head injury after initial assessment and stabilization is therefore directed toward preventing secondary damage from these complications.

Intracranial Hematoma

A head-injured adult with no skull fracture and a normal conscious level has a low risk of developing an intracranial hematoma—about 1 in 6000. By contrast, an adult who has both a skull fracture and an altered conscious level has a one in four chance of having an intracranial hematoma significant enough to merit surgical treatment. Patients with one or the other feature have an intermediate risk of hematoma. Data like these can guide the physician who has to decide which head-injured patients should be admitted to the hospital for assessment, and which patients require urgent neurosurgical investigation. Local practice varies, but everywhere the trend is toward the pre-emptive investigation of patients at high risk of hematoma rather than merely awaiting clinical deterioration with inevitably poorer results.

The demonstration or exclusion of a skull fracture rests on good-quality skull radiographs in at least two planes (frontal and lateral). Clinical rather than economic or medicolegal considerations should determine the indications for skull radiography after a recent head injury, and Table 2 suggests what these indications are. It should be remembered that skull base fractures are usually invisible on plain radiographs and must be diagnosed on clinical grounds (see the later section on intracranial infection).

Computed tomographic (CT) scanning revolutionized the acute management of head-injured patients in the 1970s, and despite the advent of magnetic resonance imaging it remains the definitive investigation in the 1980s and 1990s. CT scanning can demonstrate collections of blood within or outside the brain, structural damage to the brain tissue, general or focal brain swelling, damage to the skull, and intracranial foreign bodies. The precise indications for CT scanning of the adult with an acute head injury vary from place to place; they are affected by the local arrangements for head injury care and by the number of scanners available. However, it is now generally agreed that patients at high risk of hematoma should undergo scanning early, before they deteriorate. Table 3 shows the indications for CT scanning after an acute head injury that have been widely adopted in the United Kingdom.

When a hematoma has been demonstrated, there are three possible courses of action. The hematoma may be evacuated by craniotomy; this approach will be usual where the hematoma is large or extradural or when the patient's condition has deteriorated. It may be left alone, especially when it is small and therefore judged to be unlikely to cause delayed deterioration. In a third group of patients, the decision about operating is finely balanced. It is here that intracranial pres-

TABLE 2. Indications for Skull Radiography in the Recently Head-Injured Adult

A history of loss of consciousness or amnesia at any time

Neurologic symptoms or signs, e.g.,
  severe headache
  vomiting
  hemiparesis
  pupil asymmetry

Suspected penetrating injury, e.g.,
  gunshot wound
  assault with blunt instrument
  palpable skull depression
  leak of cerebrospinal fluid from nose or ear

Significant scalp injury, e.g.,
  large or irregular laceration
  laceration involving galea
  contusion or swelling

Difficulty in assessing patient, e.g.,
  deaf or demented elderly patient
  patient intoxicated by alcohol or drugs
  postictal patient

CLINICAL JUDGMENT IS REQUIRED IN ALL CASES

TABLE 3. Indications for an Emergency CT Scan in the Adult with a Recent Head Injury

Fractured skull, with *any* impairment of conscious level, or
  focal neurologic signs, or
  seizures, or
  any other neurologic symptoms or signs

Deterioration in conscious level or other neurologic signs

Coma that persists after resuscitation, even if no skull fracture

Confusion or other neurologic disturbance that persists for more than 6 hours, even if no skull fracture

Suspected penetrating missile injury of brain

sure (ICP) monitoring has a part to play because there is clear evidence that a high or rising ICP is a warning of incipient clinical deterioration, which can be prevented by prompt surgery. The methods available for ICP monitoring are discussed later in the section on the medical management of intracranial hypertension.

The technical details of evacuation of intracranial hematomas are beyond the scope of this article. However, the aim of operation is simple: to decompress the brain, to prevent cerebral ischemia, and to restore a more normal internal environment to the injured neurons. The sooner a compressive hematoma is evacuated, the more likely is the patient to make a worthwhile recovery. Conversely, delayed evacuation is associated with high mortality and morbidity.

Intracranial Infection

Any compound head injury may be followed by meningitis, abscess, or empyema, especially when the dura mater is breached. The risk is highest with fractures of the skull base, compound depressed fractures of the skull vault, and missile wounds of the brain. Applying basic surgical principles of wound debridement and antibiotic prophylaxis is vital to minimize this risk.

Fracture of the skull base is a clinical diagnosis and can only rarely be confirmed radiologically, by demonstrating intracranial gas on a skull radiograph or CT scan. Basal fractures of the anterior fossa cause periorbital hematomas (often bilaterally), whereas those of the middle and posterior fossae may cause a mastoid hematoma 1 or 2 days after injury. A leak of clear cerebrospinal fluid (CSF) is uncommon in the first few days after injury, but there may be a blood-stained discharge from the nostril or ear. An obvious CSF leak may start only when the soft tissue swelling resolves a few days after injury, by which time the patient has often been discharged from the hospital. Many, if not most, patients with a basal skull fracture never develop a CSF leak, and in most of those who do the fistula closes spontaneously. A few patients eventually need a surgical repair of the torn dura because of persistent CSF leakage, but this repair is best delayed until at least 10 to 14 days after injury.

Every patient with a compound depressed skull fracture should be referred to a neurosurgeon and the wound explored, ideally within 24 hours of injury. Devitalized tissue and foreign bodies in the scalp or brain should be carefully sought and removed, the wound should be irrigated with a solution of 10 per cent hydrogen peroxide, and the dura and scalp should be closed. The larger bone fragments may be cleaned and repositioned without fear of sepsis unless the wound is heavily contaminated or surgery has been delayed. Delayed wound débridement is associated with an increased incidence of meningitis, brain abscess, and empyema. Patients with noncompound depressed fractures are best managed without operation, except for the rare case in which the cosmetic deformity is deemed to be unacceptable.

Penetrating missile injuries of the brain are more common in the United States than in Britain, where they are usually caused by low-velocity weapons like air rifles. Patients should be referred early to a neurosurgeon, and the principles of management are the same as those for compound depressed skull fractures: to carry out early débridement of the entry wound and missile track, to remove bone fragments and devitalized tissue, and to close the dura and scalp. Missiles in inaccessible sites deep within the brain are best left alone.

Pneumococcus is the most common pathogen causing intracranial infection after a penetrating brain injury. Penicillin is therefore the drug of choice for prophylaxis: an intramuscular dose of benzylpenicillin (Crystapen), 600 mg every 6 hours for the first 1 or 2 days, then an oral preparation such as phenoxymethyl penicillin, 500 mg every 6 hours for a further 5 to 7 days. The patient allergic to penicillin may be given erythromycin, 250 mg every 6 hours. Where there is a CSF leak, the antibiotic should be given for a week after the leak has ceased. The most important way to prevent post-traumatic intracranial infection is early and adequate wound débridement.

Post-Traumatic Seizures

Any head injury may be followed by a generalized or focal seizure, but the injuries that are most strongly associated with this complication are penetrating missile injuries, compound depressed skull fractures (especially where the dura is torn), intracranial hematomas (whether or not evacuated), and injuries causing altered consciousness for more than 6 hours (regardless of the CT scan findings). By convention, seizures that occur within 7 days of injury are "early," and those that occur subsequently are "late," a classification that is relevant to the long-term prognosis of the seizures.

In addition to disturbing the function of cerebral neurons, a generalized seizure raises intracranial pressure, reduces cerebral perfusion pressure, and may place the airway at risk by rendering the patient unconscious. All of these effects can cause or aggravate brain damage, so prompt treatment and prophylaxis of seizures are important in the acute phase after head injury.

A generalized seizure that does not stop spontaneously within 1 to 2 minutes should be aborted by a cautiously administered intravenous dose of diazepam (Valium); most seizures stop with less than 10 mg, and higher doses carry a risk of respiratory depression. For focal seizures, clonazepam (Klonopin), 0.5 to 1 mg, may be given intravenously. Failure to abort a seizure may lead to status epilepticus, an emergency that often requires therapy with multiple anticonvulsant drugs and ventilatory support in the intensive care unit.

Prophylaxis against further seizures is important, and indeed many physicians give anticonvulsant drugs routinely to patients who are judged to be at high risk of seizures even if none have occurred. The drug of choice in the acute stage is phenytoin (Dilantin) because it can be administered intravenously and its plasma levels are monitored easily. An adult of average build is given 1 gram in divided doses during 12 to 24 hours by slow intravenous injection or infusion, followed by 300 mg per day. A discussion of the indications for long-term prophylaxis of seizures and the drugs available is beyond the scope of this article.

Intracranial Hypertension

Severe head injury is commonly followed by a rise in ICP, whether from a focal mass lesion, such as a hematoma or burst lobe, or from generalized swelling of the injured brain. If the rise in ICP is untreated, a chain reaction results: reduced cerebral perfusion pressure, cerebral ischemia, and neuron dysfunction. It is therefore important to monitor ICP and to prevent or treat intracranial hypertension. Table 4 shows the indications for monitoring post-traumatic ICP that are widely used in the United Kingdom.

TABLE 4. **Indications for Monitoring ICP in the Adult with a Recent Head Injury**

A patient in traumatic coma who is to undergo ventilation

A patient with an intracranial hematoma when there is doubt on clinical or radiologic grounds about the need for evacuation

A patient with a diffuse brain injury in whom consciousness is impaired *and* the third ventricle or basal cisterns are indistinct or invisible

A patient who has undergone craniotomy for an intradural hematoma or who was in a coma before evacuation of an extradural hematoma

The "gold standard" for measuring ICP in clinical practice is intraventricular pressure monitoring by using a fluid-filled catheter that is inserted into the ventricle via a burr hole and connected to a fluid phase transducer. This process gives the most reliable measurements and has the bonus of allowing CSF removal for the relief of high ICP, but it is relatively invasive and carries an appreciable risk of infection if the catheter is left in position for more than 3 days. A similar catheter can be inserted subdurally but gives less accurate measurements of ICP. Alternatively, a solid-state transducer can be implanted epidurally or subdurally; subdural recordings appear to reflect ICP accurately, but there is growing doubt about the reliability of epidural recordings, and they are best avoided. Solid-state transducers are less invasive and carry a lower risk of infection than fluid phase catheters but are vulnerable to electronic malfunction and do not allow CSF drainage.

Normal ICP is generally said to be less than 15 torr. There is no doubt that pressures higher than 30 torr are associated with impaired cerebral perfusion and clinical deterioration. It is now recognized that lesser elevations of ICP can also be harmful and may respond better to therapy. Most neurosurgeons would now take active steps to reduce ICP when it is higher than 20 torr. When ICP is high or rising, a focal lesion such as a hematoma or cerebral contusion must be excluded by CT scanning; the following comments assume that this has been done.

There are several methods in clinical use to control ICP and treat intracranial hypertension. Some are very simple: for example, the patient's head may be raised by 20 to 30 degrees and held in a neutral position to help venous drainage from the brain. Overinfusion of fluids (especially hypotonic solutions) causes cerebral engorgement and should be avoided. The systolic blood pressure should be kept in the range of 120 to 170 mmHg; lower pressures reduce cerebral perfusion pressure (which is the difference between mean arterial blood pressure and ICP), whereas higher pressures can promote vasogenic cerebral edema after head injury.

In controlling ICP it is important to detect and if possible prevent episodes of hypoxia and hypercarbia, which are common in the patient with a severe head injury and are often due to the complex interaction of factors: airway obstruction from pharyngeal secretions or inhalation of gastric contents, pulmonary hypoventilation of central origin, associated chest injury, and pre-existing pulmonary disease. The chest must be kept clear of secretions by suction, physiotherapy, and frequent changes of position in the bed; chest radiographs must be taken regularly. The importance of arterial blood gas analysis in initial assessment has already been emphasized; it is equally important to monitor Pa_{O_2} and Pa_{CO_2} as long as the patient's conscious level is altered, and prompt action must be taken to correct disturbances. To supplement arterial blood gas sampling, pulse oximetry offers a noninvasive (albeit indirect) way of continuously monitoring the adequacy of oxygenation.

There is no argument that to maintain adequate arterial gases (and thus to control ICP) in some patients requires pulmonary ventilation by using sedative or paralyzing drugs. These drugs can be used without fear of masking important neurologic signs, as long as the ICP is being monitored, access to immediate CT scanning is available, and the drugs used have a relatively short half-life or their action can be easily reversed by pharmacologic antagonists. Sedative or paralyzing drugs may have a direct beneficial effect on ICP by abolishing the hypertensive response to pain and stimulation. For the same reason, control of pain by nonopiate analgesics helps to lower ICP.

More controversial is the use of hyperventilation to lower ICP by reducing the Pa_{CO_2} to the range of 25 to 30 torr. Hyperventilation is used routinely to treat traumatic coma in many centers, but in others (including Glasgow) it is reserved for the diffuse post-traumatic brain swelling occasionally seen in children. Also controversial is the use of hyperosmolar agents such as mannitol to draw water from the cerebral interstitium into the circulation to reduce vasogenic edema. As much as 200 to 300 grams of mannitol per day, given as boluses or infusion, may be needed to control ICP, and such doses can derange renal and cardiovascular function. However, there is no doubt about the value of smaller single doses of mannitol to control ICP temporarily in the acute situation, while a desperately ill patient is being prepared for a CT scan or a craniotomy.

Steroids and barbiturates have been used to control ICP after head injury, but neither has been shown convincingly to have a desirable effect on outcome, and their routine use is not recommended.

ACUTE HEAD INJURIES IN CHILDREN

method of
J. PARKER MICKLE, M.D.
University of Florida
Gainesville, Florida

Head injury is a common occurrence in our pediatric population, and of the 5 million or so that occur in this country annually, most are minor. However, 10 to 15 per cent of this number are serious and demand an aggressive, multidisciplinary approach for optimal outcome. The most common cause of death in children in this country is trauma. Most children who die of this disease category have associated head injuries, and this often is the primary cause of demise. Head injury in the pediatric patient is age dependent, ranging from the slow deformational forces experienced at birth and early in childhood, to the high-velocity impact with acceleration, deceleration injury experienced in the older child and the young adult.

TREATMENT

General Concepts and Pathophysiology

The first concept in the treatment of pediatric head injury is that the clinical outcome is a result of the initial traumatic event and certain secondary events occurring as complications of that primary event. As physicians, we have only a preventive control over the initial event. Certain injuries are not compatible with survival and no amount of intervention can retrieve a patient from the inevitable demise in this situation. However, most head injuries, especially in children, are compatible with survival and if the secondary processes listed in Table 1 are prevented and treated, then a good outcome can be expected in a very high percentage of these children. The concept here is to begin treatment as early as possible after the initiating event, and this necessitates trained personnel at the accident scene with treatment beginning prior to transport to the acute trauma hospital.

The second concept of importance in attending children with head injuries is that neurologic deterioration or improvement is a continuum, and no one single examination can make an accurate prediction of the need for therapeutic intervention or of outcome. This aspect requires frequent and sometimes virtually continuous neurologic assessment. This goal necessitates an accurate and rapid evaluation of the patient's neurologic status at any given time.

The Glasgow Coma Scale (GCS) is the most commonly used quantitative clinical assessment system in defining points along this neurologic continuum to guide the therapeutic decision-making of the clinician; it can also provide highly accurate outcome determination. This system, without relying on detailed neurologic examination, gives an excellent idea of the level of neurologic function in the head-injured patient and also gives a good estimate of the prognosis. Using three variables—eye opening, best verbal response, and best motor response—this point system can be used in patients of all ages.

It is extremely important, however, no matter which system is used, that frequent neurologic assessment be done in head-injured patients, since rapid changes can occur and a salvageable individual can rapidly deteriorate to a state with high morbidity and high mortality as expected outcome.

The third concept is that children have a better prognosis than the adult head-injured patient with the same degree of apparent injury at the time of initial evaluation. This fact demands an aggressive approach to the treatment of the head-injured child.

The fourth concept important in managing head injury in children involves the fact that the volume of the intracranial contents is fixed (except in very small children) and any mass occurring intracranially must be accommodated by the normal contents of the intracranial cavity; otherwise the intracranial pressure (ICP) will increase. If the process is general and results in swelling or edema of the brain, then a general rise in ICP will occur. If there is a focal swelling or accumulation of blood, ICP will rise, and various herniation syndromes can occur after the normal compensatory mechanisms have been exhausted. The aggressive multidisciplinary approach to the treatment of head injuries, both at the accident scene and in the emergency ward, is

TABLE 1. **Secondary Insults After Head Injury**

Shock
Anoxia/hypoxia
Diffuse axonal injury
Intracranial hemorrhage
Increased intracranial pressure
Hydrocephalus
Seizures
Infections (central nervous system, urinary, pulmonary)
Metabolic (inappropriate antidiuretic hormone, nutritional)

directed toward minimizing these effects as secondary insults on an already injured brain. All of our efforts initially are directed to protecting the injured and vulnerable brain from secondary insults that can change the outlook from excellent to terrible.

A fifth concept is more philosophical and involves prevention. Only recently, with the advent of data collection systems, is society becoming aware of the extent of this problem. We must do everything that we can as physicians and advocates of our patients to identify those activities in society that are highly dangerous and frequently result in serious head injury, such as child abuse.

Minor Versus Serious Head Injury

Most children will sustain a head injury during life. By and large, these are minor events and require no special care. However, especially in children, it is often difficult to decide when an injury should be classified as minor and when it should be classified as serious. Any injury of questionable etiology should be classified as serious, and in the case of the younger child such an occurrence dictates early report and intervention to prevent subsequent serious injury as a result of abuse or neglect. The incidence of child abuse as a cause of head injury is not known, but it appears to be much more frequent than was estimated in the past. Children with minor head injury and no loss of consciousness or significant blood loss, and with a good social situation, can be managed as outpatients. Most children with minor head injuries should have plain skull x-rays if there is deformity of the skull, significant scalp hematoma, or point tenderness of the skull or if the injury is of questionable etiology (Table 2).

Minor head injury can have delayed sequelae detrimental to the patient. This necessitates careful evaluation on initial contact as well as adequate follow-up. Often the degree of injury cannot be adequately assessed by the history taken from the family or attending personnel, and only later will the patient continue to complain of headache, memory loss, and difficulty with concentration, all of which signal a more serious injury than initially diagnosed. Minor injuries usually have an excellent outlook, and the family and patient can be assured that most of the minor complaints following these injuries will subside.

Concussive injuries in children—that is, head injuries that cause unconsciousness for a variable period of time—without obvious neurologic deficit on initial evaluation are very important injuries. Clearly these injuries can cause permanent deficit and subsequent injuries are additive. These so-called minor injuries demand thorough radiologic evaluation and careful, regular follow-up. These children should be admitted to the hospital for observation, and the family should be educated about possible problems on discharge. If complaints of headache, memory deficit, or inattention persist, a computed tomography (CT) scan of the cranium, as well as a thorough neuropsychologic evaluation, should be made.

This group of patients is by far the most common group that we see as physicians and we are often asked to re-evaluate these individuals because of persistent complaints. Only recently has the magnitude of this problem been realized.

Serious head injuries in children range from scalp lacerations with major blood loss, often seen in the young child, to the devastating high-velocity diffuse injury to the brain more common in the older child. Important aspects in the early evaluation and treatment of the comatose child include physical examination, laboratory and x-ray evaluations, resuscitation, pharmacologic treatment, monitoring, and triage.

Serious Head Injury

The team approach is essential in caring for the severely head-injured child (Table 3).

At the accident scene or in the emergency room, the child is treated for shock, the airway is secured, and further injury to the head or spine is prevented by adequate immobilization. Careful, frequent assessment of the general neurologic

TABLE 2. **Radiologic Assessment of Minor Head Injury**

Type	When
None	Minor head injury—good social situation
Skull x-rays	Deformity, point tenderness, scalp hematoma
Long-bone x-rays	Head injury of questionable etiology
CT scan of cranium	Persistent complaints

TABLE 3. **Sequence of Events in the Care of the Seriously Head-Injured Child**

Event	How
1. Evaluate	General physical examination Examination of central nervous system Radiology (CT scans)
2. Resuscitate	Secure airway, intubate Treat shock Stabilize
3. Triage	Continue resuscitation To operating room To intensive care unit

TABLE 4. **Indications for Emergency/Urgent Surgery of the Head-Injured Child**

Condition	Comment
Refractory shock	Usually due to intra-abdominal injury and hemorrhage
Depressed skull fracture	Evaluate with CT scan
Significant intracranial hemorrhage	Rare under 2 years of age

status of the patient is made and recorded. Intravenous access should be central and the fluids administered isotonic. An arterial line is helpful in monitoring the response to resuscitation. The blood pressure must be kept as normal as possible to optimize cerebral perfusion. All patients with serious head injury are assumed to have an unstable cervical spine until proved otherwise. The indications for emergency surgery on the head-injured child are listed in Table 4. This triage is made early and rapidly. The vast majority of patients with serious head injury can be stabilized before being transferred either to the radiology suite for CT scan of the head, chest, and abdomen, or to the operating room for exploratory surgery. No patient should be sent to the radiology suite in an unstable condition without adequate monitoring by trained personnel.

Medications that we routinely give to comatose children are listed in Table 5. Seizures, if present, should be treated aggressively; broad-spectrum antibiotics are administered intravenously if grossly contaminated wounds are part of the picture. Mannitol as a dehydrating agent should not be given unless the patient is clearly herniating and needs temporary decompression on the way to the operating room. The loop diuretics and pentobarbital are medications reserved for the treatment of increasing ICP of a general nature in the intensive care unit.

TABLE 5. **Medical Treatment of the Seriously Head-Injured Child**

What	How
Dilantin	15 mg/kg loading dose; 5 mg/kg maintenance
Phenobarbital	Same as Dilantin
Valium	1–5 mg IV to stop seizure
Antibiotics	IV; broad-spectrum in contaminated wounds
Mannitol*	1 gram/kg for rapid decompression
Diuretics	1 mg/kg furosemide
Pentobarbital	15 mg/kg loading dose; titrate as needed to control ICP
Dexamethasone	10 mg IV push; 16 mg/day for 3–5 days

*Can push serum osmolarity as high as 310.

TABLE 6. **Intensive Care Unit Monitoring of the Seriously Head-Injured Child**

1. Monitor vital signs—serial central nervous system examination (Glasgow Coma Score)
2. Input/output
3. Central venous pressure
4. Arterial blood gases
5. Serum electrolytes
6. Hemogram
7. ICP
8. Multimodality somatosensory evoked potentials and brain stem auditory potentials
9. Serial CT scans

The most significant improvement in the care of severely head-injured children has been the development of specialized intensive care units with sophisticated monitoring capability. We utilize routinely the monitoring technologies listed in Table 6. The flow sheet available to the attending staff makes possible a continuous and instantaneous picture of the patient's status. This entire effort is directed toward discovering early and subtle changes in neurologic status, so that early intervention can prevent secondary injury to the brain.

A very important aspect of this monitoring is the accurate measurement of ICP. Various monitors can be used for this procedure and the information obtained is invaluable in making therapeutic decisions concerning the patient's status. We monitor all children with a GCS score of 7 or lower. The ICP must be maintained below 20 torr; this is accomplished utilizing the stepwise decision-making therapeutic regimen outlined in Table 7. Clearly, early detection of increased ICP and its successful treatment are most important aspects of the treatment of the seriously head-injured child.

Multimodality somatosensory evoked potentials and brain stem auditory evoked potentials are very helpful in detecting early deterioration in a seemingly stable child. Of major importance is the utilization of serial CT scans of the head when a child is experiencing deterioration before a therapeutic plan is decided upon. Delayed intracranial hemorrhage, increased ICP from hydrocephalus, and other causes of increased ICP

TABLE 7. **Stepwise Events in the Control of Increased Intracranial Pressure***

1. Hyperventilate to P_{CO_2} of 25 torr
2. Head elevated 30 degrees
3. Sedation/paralysis
4. Keep normothermic
5. Diuresis—loop diuretics vs. mannitol
6. Cerebrospinal fluid drainage
7. Pentobarbital coma
8. Surgery—decompression

*Higher than 20 mmHg.

can be detected and treated by this radiologic technique. ICP monitoring should be continued for as long as the child is in the comatose state and not improving. We usually leave a monitor in for a week before changing it to the opposite side or removing it. We have had no incidences of infection from these transcranially placed monitors in over 100 cases.

BRAIN TUMORS

method of
DAVID R. MACDONALD, M.D.
University of Western Ontario and London Regional Cancer Centre
London, Ontario, Canada

Brain tumors may be primary (arising from the skull, meninges, intracranial blood vessels, cranial nerves, or brain) or metastatic (arising from an extracranial systemic cancer). Primary brain tumors are classified histologically according to the presumed cell of origin (Table 1). Almost two-thirds of primary brain tumors are gliomas, and most of these (almost one-half of all primary brain tumors) are histologically malignant (glioblastoma multiforme, gliosarcoma, anaplastic astrocytoma, anaplastic oligodendroglioma, anaplastic ependymoma, mixed malignant glioma). Gliomas are classified as well differentiated, anaplastic (malignant), or glioblastoma multiforme, by using the criteria of Burger and Vogel, on the basis of the degree

TABLE 1. **Histologic Classification of Primary Brain Tumors**

Gliomas
  Glioblastoma multiforme
  Gliosarcoma
  Astrocytoma
  Oligodendroglioma
  Ependymoma
  Mixed gliomas
  Optic nerve glioma
  Brain stem glioma
  Cystic cerebellar astrocytoma
Meningioma
Pituitary adenoma
Pineal tumors
  Pinealomas (pineocytoma, pineoblastoma)
  Germ cell (e.g., germinoma)
Primitive neuroectodermal tumors
  Medulloblastoma
  Cerebral neuroblastoma
Primary cerebral lymphoma (microglioma)
Choroid plexus papilloma
Craniopharyngioma
Dermoid and epidermoid tumors
Colloid cyst
Sarcoma
Nerve sheath tumors
  Neurofibroma
  Schwannoma (acoustic neuroma)

of cellularity, pleomorphism, anaplasia, and the presence or absence of mitotic figures, vascular endothelial proliferation, and necrosis.

In North America the incidence of primary brain tumors is approximately 8 to 10 per 100,000 persons per year. There is a bimodal distribution, with an early peak in childhood (ages 5 to 10 years) and a subsequent peak in adulthood (ages 55 to 65 years). In children, two-thirds of primary brain tumors arise in the posterior fossa (cystic cerebellar astrocytomas, medulloblastomas, brain stem gliomas, ependymomas) and one-third arise supratentorally (e.g., astrocytomas, ependymomas, pineal tumors, and craniopharyngiomas). In adults the overwhelming majority of primary brain tumors arise supratentorally.

The cause of most primary brain tumors is unknown. Primary brain tumors may occur as part of a well-recognized hereditary disorder such as neurofibromatosis, tuberous sclerosis, or von Hippel–Lindau disease. Rarely, several members in one family may have primary brain tumors in the absence of one of these disorders, which raises the suspicion of a hereditary factor. In most cases, however, primary brain tumors occur sporadically, and the relatives of patients with brain tumors do not seem to be at increased risk of developing a tumor. Environmental factors, especially exposure to chemicals such as vinyl chloride, have been postulated to increase the risk for primary brain tumor, but the evidence is weak and most patients do not have a history of chemical exposure. Long-term survivors of childhood cancer who have been treated with radiotherapy or chemotherapy and children who have been treated with cranial radiation for benign disorders such as tinea capitis may also have a slightly increased risk for primary brain tumor in later life.

The incidence of most primary brain tumors is slightly higher in male than in female individuals and may be slightly higher in white than in black persons (although unequal access to health care may make apparent racial differences inaccurate). Meningiomas and pituitary adenomas occur more frequently in women than men.

Most gliomas present subacutely, over several weeks, with signs and symptoms of increased intracranial pressure (ICP) (headaches, nausea and vomiting, confusion, altered consciousness, and papilledema) and focal neurologic deficits (e.g., seizures, aphasia, and hemiparesis) depending on the location of the tumor. Tumors may occasionally present acutely, with seizures, hemorrhage, or stroke-like events. Rarely, subfrontal, temporal lobe, or midline tumors may present insidiously, with personality change, confusion, and memory loss, and may mimic a dementing process. In children, posterior fossa tumors may present with increased ICP, obstructive hydrocephalus, cerebellar ataxia, or multiple cranial nerve palsies from brain stem dysfunction. Occasionally, a child with morning headaches, vomiting, and impaired school performance is labeled as having "school phobia" and is referred for psychologic therapy until more specific signs or symptoms develop.

Pituitary adenomas and other parasellar tumors (e.g., craniopharyngioma) may present insidiously with endocrine dysfunction (e.g., amenorrhea, galactorrhea, hypothyroidism, growth delay, acromegaly, and altered thirst) and only later produce visual impairment, cranial nerve palsies, or obstructive hydrocephalus from suprasellar extension of tumor. Pineal region tumors may present either with obstructive hydrocephalus or a dorsal midbrain syndrome (large, poorly reactive pupils and abnormal vertical gaze). Cerebellar-pontine angle tumors (acoustic neuromas, meningiomas) may present with hearing loss long before ipsilateral cerebellar ataxia, other cranial nerve palsies, or increased ICP develops.

TREATMENT

The optimal conventional treatment for malignant gliomas is summarized in Table 2. An accurate diagnosis is vital. Patients with appropriate signs and symptoms should have a computed tomography (CT) scan of the head with and without intravenous contrast. Almost all patients who have symptomatic primary brain tumors have readily visible lesions on contrast-enhanced CT scans. Small tumors that present early with seizures and tumors in the temporal lobe tip or low in the posterior fossa may be difficult to visualize on CT scan. The diagnostic yield can sometimes be increased by using fine cuts through the appropriate area or direct coronal cuts. A magnetic resonance imaging (MRI) scan is likely more sensitive than the CT scan but may be less specific. Sagittal T_1-weighted, axial T_1-weighted, and axial T_2-weighted images may be required to adequately visualize tumors on the MRI scan. It may be difficult to differentiate the tumor from peritumoral edema without the use of a paramagnetic contrast agent (gadolinium-DTPA). Plain skull x-ray films, pneumoencephalography, and radionuclide brain scanning seldom provide useful additional information; in addition, lumbar puncture may be hazardous in the presence of intracranial mass lesions. Cerebral angiography is seldom required, although it may be needed to exclude vascular malformations or to determine the vascular supply of tumors before experimental therapies such as intra-arterial chemotherapy.

Corticosteroids are used to control cerebral edema and increased ICP that are associated with brain tumors. Dexamethasone (Decadron), 4 mg four times daily, is the standard initial dose. Oral

TABLE 2. **Optimal Conventional Treatment for Malignant Glioma**

Accurate localization (CT scan, MRI scan)
Corticosteroids
Anticonvulsants, anticoagulants (as needed)
Maximum feasible surgical resection
Radiotherapy (6000 cGy to tumor)
Chemotherapy (BCNU)

and intravenous doses are equivalent. The dose should be adjusted as required to control symptoms and the lowest possible dose should be used to minimize side effects. The side effects are related to total dose, duration of therapy, and individual susceptibility. Common side effects include cushingoid face and body habitus, weight gain, fluid retention, hypertension, hyperglycemia, hypokalemia, proximal muscle weakness, oral candidiasis, osteoporosis, and aseptic bone necrosis. Acute neurologic deterioration from cerebral edema or from increased ICP may require higher doses of corticosteroids (up to 100 mg* dexamethasone intravenously) as well as intravenous mannitol (0.5 to 2 grams per kg, repeated every 6 hours) or intubation with hyperventilation. Mannitol is used only in acute situations because long-term use is precluded by loss of effectiveness and fluid and electrolyte disturbances. A ventriculoperitoneal shunt may be needed to control obstructive hydrocephalus.

Anticonvulsants are used to control seizures. Approximately 25 per cent of patients with gliomas have seizures as part of the initial presentation, and up to 50 per cent have seizures at some time. The use of prophylactic anticonvulsants is controversial. Phenytoin (Dilantin) is the most commonly used anticonvulsant because it is inexpensive, effective, and available in oral and intravenous preparations, and can be given in a large initial loading dose. The initial loading dose is 18 mg per kg (orally or intravenously), usually about 1000 mg for an average adult, given no faster than 50 mg per minute intravenously. Most patients can be maintained on 300 to 400 mg daily, given either as a single daily dose at bedtime or as divided doses in the morning and evening. The blood level of phenytoin should be monitored and maintained in the suggested therapeutic range (10 to 20 micrograms per ml; 40 to 80 micromoles per liter). Side effects include rash, gum hypertrophy, liver dysfunction, and intoxication (dysarthria, ataxia, and diplopia). Carbamazepine (Tegretol) is as effective as phenytoin and may have somewhat fewer side effects, but it is not available in a parenteral form, cannot be loaded, must be given in three or four divided doses, and is more expensive. The usual maintenance dose is 600 to 1200 mg daily. The therapeutic level is 4 to 12 micrograms per ml (17 to 40 micromoles per liter). Myelosuppression and hepatotoxicity are rare but potentially serious complications. Phenobarbital is effective and inexpensive but is not usually used as a first line anticonvulsant because of its sedative properties. The usual dose is 60 to 200 mg daily, as a single

---

*This dose may exceed manufacturer's recommended dose.

bedtime dose. The therapeutic blood level is 15 to 40 micrograms per ml (65 to 170 micromoles per liter). Primidone (Mysoline), clonazepam (Rivotril), and valproic acid (Depakene) may be useful if the above-mentioned drugs are ineffective or cannot be tolerated.

Patients with primary brain tumor are at high risk for deep vein thrombosis and pulmonary embolism, especially in the perioperative period. Prolonged bed rest should be avoided. Antiembolic stockings, intermittent pneumatic compression leggings, or subcutaneous heparin (5000 units twice daily) may help prevent deep vein thrombosis postoperatively. Most neurosurgeons are reluctant to use anticoagulants during the immediate perioperative period. Patients with deep vein thrombosis or pulmonary embolism require anticoagulation, initially continuous intravenous heparin and then warfarin (Coumadin). Excessive anticoagulation should be avoided. Optimal anticoagulation (partial thromboplastin time twice control; prothrombin time 1.5 times control) is safe in primary brain tumor patients and does not seem to increase the risk of hemorrhage in tumors.

Surgery

The goals of surgery for primary brain tumor include determination of a histologic diagnosis to guide further therapy; maximal tumor removal; improvement of symptoms by tumor debulking and reduction of increased ICP; and provision of additional time for other treatments such as radiotherapy or chemotherapy. Some benign tumors such as meningioma, acoustic neuroma, or pituitary adenoma may be completely resectable and cured surgically. Surgery may be curative for cystic cerebellar astrocytomas, but most intraaxial tumors cannot be completely removed. In these cases the goal is to remove as much of the tumor as possible without increasing the patient's neurologic deficit. Gross total tumor resection may be possible in polar tumors that arise in the tips of the frontal, temporal, or occipital lobes; lobectomy may be appropriate in some patients. Major resections are often possible in tumors occurring centrally in the frontal, temporal, and parietal lobes. Major resections may not be possible in deep-seated tumors; however, almost any tumor can be biopsied by using stereotactic techniques. Accessible tumors should be resected rather than biopsied because survival is increased by increasing completeness of resection.

Radiation Therapy

After surgery, radiation therapy is the primary mode of treatment for most intraparenchymal brain tumors. Although most primary brain tumors are not curable by radiotherapy alone, this treatment increases the total and tumor-free survival for most patients with incompletely resected brain tumors. Standard treatment for malignant glioma is external beam radiotherapy, 6000 cGy (rad) in 6 weeks to the tumor plus an adequate margin. Whole-brain radiotherapy for malignant glioma has generally fallen out of favor because of concerns about long-term side effects. Stereotactic radiation implants (brachytherapy) and radiosurgery (using either a linear accelerator or the Gamma-Knife) are new experimental radiotherapy techniques that are designed to deliver highly focused radiation to small brain tumors or vascular malformations. The aim is to deliver a high dose to a small area while sparing the surrounding normal brain.

The role of radiotherapy in the treatment of well-differentiated astrocytomas (low-grade gliomas) is controversial. Some retrospective studies suggest that survival is increased with focal radiotherapy (usually 5000 to 5500 cGy in 5 to 6 weeks). Radiotherapy may also prolong tumor control and increase survival in incompletely resected, recurrent, or malignant meningiomas. Focal radiotherapy is also recommended for incompletely resected pituitary adenomas or craniopharyngiomas. Radiotherapy may be curative treatment for pineal germinomas, although it is controversial whether focal or craniospinal treatment is required.

Radiotherapy prolongs survival and may be curative in patients with medulloblastoma, after surgical removal of the tumor. Standard treatment is craniospinal radiation with 5500 cGy to the posterior fossa, 3500 to 4500 cGy to the whole brain, and 3500 to 4500 cGy to the spinal neuraxis. These doses are reduced for young children. In good-risk patients (complete resection of the primary tumor and no evidence of systemic or leptomeningeal metastases), the 5-year survival is 50 to 70 per cent.

Chemotherapy

Chemotherapy may be given as part of the treatment for some malignant primary brain tumors, especially malignant glioma or medulloblastoma. Chemotherapy can be given as an adjuvant at the time of initial treatment or later at the time of tumor recurrence. Many chemotherapeutic agents have been tried, either singly or in combination. The standard chemotherapeutic agents for malignant glioma are the nitrosoureas, either BCNU (carmustine) or CCNU (lomustine). BCNU is given intravenously, 200 mg per M^2, every 6 to 8 weeks, often starting at the beginning of radiotherapy. A cumulative dose of 1500 mg per M^2 should not be exceeded. Common side effects include local vein irritation during infusion, transient nausea and vomiting on the days of treatment, myelosuppression (which may be delayed 4 to 6 weeks after treatment and which tends to be cumulative with increasing total dose), and pulmonary fibrosis (risk increases with increasing total cumulative dose, especially more than 1500 mg per M^2). CCNU is given orally at a dose of 130 mg per M^2 every 6 weeks. The toxicity is similar to that of BCNU. Several other agents have shown some effectiveness including AZQ (diaziquone), PCNU, procarbazine (Matulane), cisplatin (Platinol), and carboplatin (Paraplatin). We have found the combination of procarbazine, CCNU, and vincristine (Oncovin), termed PCV-3, effective. In PCV-3, CCNU is given at 110 mg per M^2 orally on day 1, procarbazine is given at 60 mg per M^2 orally daily for 14 days beginning on day 8 (days 8 to 21), and vincristine is given at 1.4 mg per M^2 (maximum 2.5 mg) intravenously on days 8 and 29. Cycles are repeated every 6 to 8 weeks according to blood cell counts. Gliomas vary in their chemosensitivity; anaplastic oligodendroglioma is a particularly chemosensitive tumor, especially to PCV-3.

Chemotherapy is being increasingly used in combination with radiotherapy in the treatment of children with brain tumors, especially high-risk medulloblastoma or malignant glioma, and in very young children (younger than 3 years of age) instead of cranial radiotherapy. Effective combinations include PCV-3; cisplatin plus etoposide (VP-16); CCNU, vincristine, and cisplatin; and the "8 in 1" (eight drugs in 1 day) regimen.

Experimental chemotherapy includes intra-arterial chemotherapy (usually BCNU or cisplatin), high-dose chemotherapy (sometimes with autologous bone marrow transplantation), osmotic opening of the blood-brain barrier with mannitol followed by chemotherapy, intralesional infusion chemotherapy, and the use of new agents. Biologic response modifiers, such as interferon (especially interferon-alpha), interleukin-2, lymphokine-activated killer cells, and monoclonal antibodies, are under study. None of these new approaches has yet proved to be more effective than standard systemic chemotherapy.

PROGNOSIS

Malignant glioma is almost always fatal. Data from published multicenter clinical trials (which may be more optimistic than "real life" because of selection bias that favors good-risk patients in many clinical trials) indicate that the median survival after surgery alone is 3 to 4 months and that few patients survive more than 6 months. The median survival for surgery followed by radiotherapy is 8 to 10 months, but only 5 to 10 per cent of patients survive 18 months. The addition of BCNU chemotherapy to surgery and radiotherapy increases the median survival modestly, to approximately 12 months, but increases the 18-month survival to 25 to 30 per cent. The survival is better for anaplastic astrocytoma than for glioblastoma. Favorable prognostic features include young age (under 45 years) at diagnosis, anaplastic astrocytoma (versus glioblastoma), major or complete surgical resection (versus biopsy alone), good functional status after surgery (Karnofsky's performance status 80 or better), presentation with seizures, and a history of prior low-grade glioma.

In most patients, the tumor eventually recurs. Possible treatments at the time of recurrence include repeat resection (especially if the functional status is good), brachytherapy, and alternate chemotherapy. Radiation necrosis of brain may mimic recurrence of malignant glioma both clinically and radiologically. Neither the CT nor the MRI scan can reliably differentiate radiation necrosis from recurrent tumor; positron-emission tomography may be able to make this distinction. Surgical resection or corticosteroids may be effective therapy for radiation necrosis.

BRAIN METASTASES

Brain metastases may occur in up to 15 to 20 per cent of all patients with systemic cancer. As the treatment for systemic cancer has improved and survival has increased, the incidence of metastatic brain tumor has also increased. The most common sites of primary cancer that are metastatic to brain are lung, breast, skin (melanoma), kidney, and colon. Up to 40 per cent of patients with small cell carcinoma of lung (oat cell carcinoma) develop brain metastases and up to 70 per cent of patients dying of metastatic melanoma have at least autopsy evidence of brain metastases. Brain metastasis is usually a late manifestation of systemic cancer but may occasionally produce the initial presenting symptoms of cancer.

Metastatic tumors present as any other intracranial mass, with signs and symptoms of increased ICP or focal neurologic disturbances, or both. Seizures are common. Metastatic brain tumors are single in one-half of patients affected; approximately 80 per cent occur supratentorially, 15 per cent in the cerebellum and 5 per cent in the brain stem. The initial treatment is dexamethasone to control cerebral edema and increased ICP. Patients with a single accessible brain metastasis who are stable or have no systemic disease often benefit from surgical resection followed by postoperative whole-brain radiation. Patients with multiple brain metastases or patients in whom surgical resection is inappropriate are treated with whole-brain radiotherapy. Standard treatment regimens include 2000 cGy in 5 fractions or 3000 cGy in 10 fractions. Most patients respond to corticosteroids and cranial radiation; however, the survival is poor because most patients die of progressive systemic cancer. The median survival is 3 months after radiation therapy for patients with nonresected tumors (1-year survival is 15 per cent). Rarely, brain metastases can be cured after radiotherapy. The median survival for patients with a resected single metastasis followed by radiotherapy is approximately 12 months.

Systemic chemotherapy has been attempted in some patients with brain metastases, especially those from carcinoma of the breast or small cell carcinoma of the lung. The response and survival rates are similar to those for cranial radiation therapy. No prospective randomized trials comparing radiotherapy with chemotherapy or radiotherapy plus chemotherapy have been reported. Chemotherapy would be feasible only for tumors for which effective systemic chemotherapy is available.

CENTRAL NERVOUS SYSTEM LYMPHOMA

Systemic lymphomas seldom spread to the parenchyma of the brain. Non-Hodgkin's lymphoma may involve the leptomeninges or the spinal or intracranial epidural space. Hodgkin's disease rarely involves the central nervous system.

Primary central nervous system lymphomas (microglioma, reticulum cell sarcoma) were once considered to be extremely rare. These tumors present with clinical and radiologic features similar to those of malignant gliomas. They often involve the deep periventricular regions, may be multifocal, and may occur with ocular lymphomas. The incidence is increased in patients with chronic immunosuppression (such as after renal transplantation), and most are B cell in origin. Primary central nervous system lymphomas develop in 2 to 3 per cent of all patients with acquired immunodeficiency syndrome (AIDS). The incidence of these primary lymphomas seems to be increasing in both the AIDS and non-AIDS populations. These tumors are often responsive to corticosteroids, and prolonged remissions may occur after use of steroids only, although the tumors eventually recur despite steroid therapy. Surgery is diagnostic but not curative. Cranial radiation therapy, usually 5000 to 6000 cGy in 6 weeks, is standard. Patients with clinical or cerebrospinal fluid evidence of leptomeningeal seeding are treated with craniospinal radiation. These tumors may be chemosensitive. A variety of chemotherapeutic regimens, usually similar to those used for systemic lymphoma (e.g., MOPP, CHOP), have been reported to have at least some effectiveness. The average survival after radiotherapy for non-AIDS patients with central nervous system lymphoma is 1 to 2 years but is less than 6 months in AIDS patients, usually because of concurrent systemic illnesses.

The Locomotor System

RHEUMATOID ARTHRITIS

method of
BLAKE J. ROESSLER, M.D., and
THOMAS D. PALELLA, M.D.
University of Michigan
Ann Arbor, Michigan

Rheumatoid arthritis is a chronic systemic inflammatory disease of unknown etiology. Although no cure for rheumatoid arthritis is known at the present time, various treatment modalities applied in a progressive manner are available to control its inflammatory articular and extra-articular manifestations and to retard or prevent progressive joint destruction. Thus, the approach to the patient with rheumatoid arthritis is multifaceted. The therapeutic plan includes medication, education, rest, patterned exercise and physical therapy techniques, joint protection, and orthotheses and surgery as necessary. Our ability to manage patients with rheumatoid arthritis has improved substantially in recent years. Therefore, virtually every patient who has rheumatoid disease will benefit from institution of appropriate therapy at the earliest possible time.

PRINCIPLES OF MANAGEMENT

The treatment of patients with rheumatoid arthritis requires a comprehensive approach that includes education, rest, exercise, and medication. It is important to recognize early those patients at risk for developing progressive, destructive, disabling disease. Once identified, these patients should be aggressively treated with a combination of medications designed to prevent the development of destructive sequelae.

Because of the waxing and waning nature of rheumatoid arthritis, the objective assessment of a therapeutic course in an individual patient is often difficult. Radiographs may help to assess the lack of progression or even recortication of marginal erosions, but they are not quantitative. The titer of rheumatoid factor does not correlate well with the degree of clinical disease activity. Improvement in erythrocyte sedimentation rate generally correlates with clinical improvement and may be the best laboratory indicator of disease activity. Probably the best indicator of improvement remains the patient's and physician's assessments of the therapeutic program. For example, the duration of morning stiffness reported by the patient is one of the most sensitive clinical parameters of disease activity. Administration of standardized instruments to measure improvement in joint function such as the AIMS (Arthritis Impact Measurement Scale) is often useful in evaluating the therapeutic response in patients with rheumatoid arthritis.

PHARMACOLOGIC MANAGEMENT

Many aspects of the immune system contribute to the local and systemic manifestations of rheumatoid arthritis. Locally, lymphocytes release lymphokines, which mediate activation and recruitment of inflammatory cells to the synovium and joint space. Inflammatory mediators such as prostaglandins and leukotrienes are produced at these sites and amplify the phlogistic response. Polymorphonuclear neutrophils (PMNs) infiltrate the synovium and, when activated, release proteinases, collagenases, and superoxide radicals that contribute to inflammation and result in tissue destruction. Because the inflammatory process in rheumatoid arthritis involves diverse biologic and biochemical mediators of inflammation and tissue destruction, no single medication controls all of the disease manifestations. Therefore, a multiple-drug regimen is often most effective in suppressing the inflammatory response and possibly altering the natural history of rheumatoid arthritis. With such an approach, medications that appear to have different mechanisms of action in altering the inflammatory and immune responses are combined in a manner to minimize additive toxicity and side effects. These medications can be grouped into three categories: nonsteroidal anti-inflammatory drugs (NSAIDs), glucocorticosteroids, and disease-modifying antirheumatic drugs (DMARDs) (Table 1).

Salicylates and NSAIDs are often the initial pharmacologic agents used in the treatment of rheumatoid arthritis. As a class, these drugs have been shown to inhibit the production of prostaglandins by PMNs in vitro. They probably exert this effect within the joint space as well and may

TABLE 1. **Drug Therapy for Rheumatoid Arthritis**

Drug	Total Dose (mg)	Recommended Frequency of Administration
NSAIDs		
Acetylsalicylic acid and other salicylates	3000–4000/day	q 4–6 hr
Propionic acid derivatives		
Ibuprofen (Motrin, Rufen)	1200–2400/day	q 3–6 hr
Naproxen (Naprosyn)	500–1000/day	q 8–12 hr
Fenoprofen (Nalfon)	1200–3200/day	q 6–8 hr
Ketoprofen (Orudis)	100–200/day	q 12 hr
Indoles		
Indomethacin (Indocin)	50–200/day	q 3–6 hr
Sulindac (Clinoril)	300–400/day	q 12 hr
Tolmetin (Tolectin)	600–1200/day	q 3–6 hr
Oxicams		
Piroxicam (Feldene)	10–20/day	q 24 hr
Meclofenamate sodium (Meclomen)	200–400/day	q 4–6 hr
DMARDs		
Gold (Myochrysine, Solganal)	25–50 (indefinite)	weekly
Auranofin (Ridaura)	6–12/day*	q 24 hr
D-Penicillamine (Depen)	250–750/day	q 24 hr
Hydroxychloroquine (Plaquenil)	200–400/day	q 12 hr
Sulfasalazine (Azulfidine)	1–3/day	q 12 hr
Methotrexate (Rheumatrex)	7.5–15/week	weekly
Azathioprine (Imuran)	75–200/day	q 24 hr
Cyclophosphamide (Cytoxan)	75–150/day	q 24 hr
Chlorambucil (Leukeran)	4–8/day	q 24 hr
Glucocorticoids		
Prednisone	2.5–7.5/day	

*See text for details.

also reduce blood flow and hence reduce delivery of PMNs and other inflammatory mediators to these areas. NSAIDs may reduce the rate of tissue destruction by suppressing some of the aspects of ongoing inflammation and thus limit disability.

Most of the NSAIDs that inhibit prostaglandin production are also ulcerogenic in the gastrointestinal tract. Gastrointestinal side effects including abdominal pain, nausea, vomiting, diarrhea, and bleeding are the most common chronic problems associated with the use of NSAIDs. These side effects may be minimized by using preparations with enteric coatings or administration with meals. The concomitant use of antacids, H_2 antagonists (e.g., cimetidine [Tagamet], 400 mg three times a day, or ranitidine [Zantac], 150 mg twice a day) or sucralfate (Carafate; 1 gram four times a day) may diminish these side effects. The chemically modified nonacetylated salicylates may have the fewest gastrointestinal side effects.

NSAIDs also inhibit renal prostaglandin production and may induce azotemia. This condition is especially important in patients with pre-existing renal disease or cardiovascular disease and in patients older than 65 years. Sulindac (Clinoril) may have fewer renal side effects, but azotemia may still be associated with the use of this medication. In addition, central nervous system side effects including confusion and instability of gait may occur, especially in older patients.

Low doses of corticosteroids can significantly reduce inflammation in patients with rheumatoid arthritis. The ability of treatment with low-dose corticosteroids to alter the natural history of the disease is less clear. Corticosteroids have been shown to ameliorate many of the effects of inflammatory mediators on end-organ systems. They also reduce the release of arachidonic acid from membrane phospholipids and are lymphocytolytic. The use of corticosteroids is severely limited by the incidence of serious side effects, including adrenal suppression, infection, osteoporosis, hypertension, and accelerated atherosclerosis. Therefore, low doses of corticosteroids should be used concomitantly with a DMARD and only as a temporizing measure. The form of corticosteroid most commonly used is prednisone in doses of less than 7.5 mg per day.

Corticosteroids can also be administered intraarticularly in patients with severe acute involvement of one or a few joints, or in those with persistent disease in one or more large joints despite a program that includes NSAIDs and DMARDs. The theoretical advantages are a more localized effect and possibly fewer systemic side effects, although almost all preparations of intraarticular corticosteroids have some degree of systemic absorption. Intra-articular administration is also associated with the risk of iatrogenic joint infection.

DMARDs are medications that have been shown to have some beneficial effect on the invasive and destructive aspects of rheumatoid synovium and the accompanying inflammation. As such, they have the potential to alter the joint destruction and tissue damage that are typical of rheumatoid arthritis. However, the ability of any individual DMARD to halt the progression of erosive destructive disease has yet to be conclusively determined by controlled clinical trials. Patients taking DMARDs require close monitoring for toxicity; DMARDs should be used only by experienced physicians.

Intramuscular gold preparations (aurothioglucose [Solganal] and gold sodium thiomalate [Myochrysine]) are the most commonly used DMARDs. They are typically administered at doses of 50 mg per week. The antirheumatic effects of gold salts are usually not manifest until a cumulative dose of 1000 mg is reached. Thus, efficacy of therapy cannot be judged for several months. Gold salt therapy is limited by the relatively common occurrence of side effects. Less serious side effects are rashes and mucosal ulcerations. More serious side effects involve the kidneys and bone marrow. The renal side effects most commonly observed are proteinuria, pyuria, and azotemia; hematologic side effects include leukopenia, thrombocytopenia, and, rarely, aplastic anemia. Therefore, monitoring of patients must include a weekly complete blood count, platelet count, and urinalysis.

Auranofin (Ridaura) is an orally administered gold preparation given in doses of 3 mg twice a day and increasing to 6 mg twice a day as necessary during a 3- to 6-month period. The disease-modifying activity of auranofin may be less than that of intramuscular gold, and this agent should be reserved for treating patients with mild to moderate disease. Diarrhea is the most common side effect. Rashes, leukopenia, thrombocytopenia, pyuria, and proteinuria may also occur, so laboratory monitoring is necessary.

Methotrexate (Rheumatrex) has been recently approved for the treatment of rheumatoid arthritis. Methotrexate is administered orally once *weekly* in doses of 7.5 to 15 mg. In these doses, it is well tolerated, has few side effects, and is often remarkably effective in suppressing the signs and symptoms of the disease. Laboratory monitoring of methotrexate therapy requires a complete blood count and platelet count on at least a monthly basis, and the determination of liver enzyme levels every 3 months. The use of routine liver biopsy for monitoring purposes is no longer advocated.

Hydroxychloroquine (Plaquenil) is administered orally at a maximum dose of 200 mg twice a day. The major side effect is retinal toxicity, and therefore patients require a thorough examination by an ophthalmologist every 6 to 12 months. Gastrointestinal side effects, most commonly nausea and diarrhea, may be minimized by increasing the dose gradually over a period of a week from a starting dose of 100 mg daily. Because of the limited number of side effects, hydroxychloroquine can often be used concomitantly with another DMARD, most commonly intramuscular gold, without serious additive toxicity.

Sulfasalazine (Azulfidine) continues to show promise as a useful DMARD in patients with rheumatoid arthritis. Recent studies have shown efficacy comparable to that of intramuscular gold preparations. The drug is given orally in a beginning dose of 0.5 gram twice a day and is increased to 1 gram twice a day. Several months of treatment are required before disease-modifying activity may become apparent. Side effects are primarily gastrointestinal and include abdominal pain, nausea, and vomiting. These effects may be minimized by the use of enteric-coated preparations. Because of the possibility of leukopenia and thrombocytopenia, monthly monitoring with complete blood count and platelet count is required.

Other DMARDs include D-penicillamine, azathioprine, chlorambucil, and cyclophosphamide. These medications are also effective antirheumatic agents. However, the use of these medications is often limited by the development of potentially serious side effects. The use of these agents requires frequent laboratory monitoring, and they should be administered only by physicians who have substantial experience with them.

ADJUNCTIVE MANAGEMENT

The adjunctive management of rheumatoid arthritis begins with educating the patient with regard to the natural history of the disease process itself. This information is followed by instruction in a balanced program of rest and exercise, including methods of joint protection and alternative methods for performing activities of daily living. Consultation with physical and occupational therapists is helpful in designing more individualized or specialized regimens. Educational information regarding the benefits and side effects of NSAIDs and DMARDs is also important. The goals of a combined adjunctive and pharmacologic treatment plan include decreased disability and improved function, especially with regard to the personal, occupational, and social activities of the patient. Various helpful educational pamphlets concerning rheumatoid arthritis and its treatment are available through the Arthritis Foundation.

SURGICAL MANAGEMENT

The application of arthroscopy to rheumatologic problems provides a minimally invasive and effective therapy for selective joint disease in patients with otherwise well-controlled rheumatoid arthritis. Early removal of proliferative synovium via arthroscopic synovectomy may have beneficial effects in terms of modifying the destructive results of active synovitis. Other procedures possible with rheumatologic arthroscopy include joint inspection, drainage and irrigation in cases of infection, foreign body removal, and meniscectomy. The procedure is associated with minimal morbidity and a high degree of technical accuracy. Indications for rheumatologic arthroscopy include mechanical symptoms suggestive of internal derangement or persistent monoarticular inflammatory disease despite aggressive pharmacologic management. Although most often performed on the knee, rheumatologic arthroscopy is also possible for the shoulder, ankle, and elbow.

In patients with advanced stages of joint destruction caused by symptomatic rheumatoid arthritis, replacement of the total joint may be the treatment of choice. At present, results of total knee replacement are comparable to those of total hip replacement. The role of total joint replacement in other locations (e.g., shoulder) is less clearly defined.

JUVENILE RHEUMATOID ARTHRITIS

method of
ROBERT W. WARREN, M.D., PH.D.
Baylor College of Medicine
Houston, Texas

Juvenile rheumatoid arthritis (JRA) is a chronic disease of joints and other tissues that affects approximately 250,000 children in the United States. JRA is subdivided into three major subgroups, based upon the clinical course in the first 6 months of illness. These subgroups are (1) systemic, characterized by spiking fevers, evanescent rash, and other extra-articular disease; (2) pauciarticular, with four or fewer affected joints; and (3) polyarticular, with five or more affected joints. Only a small minority of JRA patients have an illness like adult rheumatoid arthritis (RA); unlike adults with RA, 70 to 90 per cent of children who are treated appropriately recover from JRA without significant disability. The mortality rate in the United States is less than 1 per cent.

JRA must be differentiated from other causes of arthritis. Indeed, more likely etiologies of childhood arthritis include trauma and infectious and postinfectious etiologies. Whereas these processes usually resolve over days to weeks, JRA persists in at least one joint for a minimum of 6 weeks. The formal diagnosis of JRA also requires age at onset under 16 years and exclusion of other inflammatory joint diseases.

GENERAL MANAGEMENT

There is no specific cure for JRA. Anti-inflammatory medications reduce joint swelling and pain, fever, iritis, and pericarditis, but no medication safely, totally, and instantly quells the inflammation of JRA. Continuing or recurrent inflammation produces secondary phenomena, including joint destruction, soft tissue contractures, and growth abnormalities, with accompanying psychologic trauma.

Medical Follow-up

Excellent home and community-based care is critical for the child with JRA, but every child with active JRA should also be evaluated periodically by a health care team that specializes in the care of children with arthritis. The frequency of such visits depends on the diagnosis and the problems of specific patients but should be no less frequent than annually. A systemic JRA flare or acute increased joint symptoms in any JRA patient should command immediate medical attention.

Education and Counseling of Family and Patient

The family's understanding and commitment to the care of the child with JRA is the most critical element in management. Common family concerns are physical deformity and the possible dangers of physical therapy and aspirin. The physician's role in patient and family education should be supplemented by literature on diseases and medication, family support groups (such as those sponsored by the parent-run American Juvenile Arthritis Organization), and professional assistance by rheumatology nurses, social workers, and child psychologists.

Family anxieties and concerns are normal. On the other hand, the JRA-provoked psychosocial dysfunction in the patient and family may far outstrip and outlast active or even residual joint disease. The need for psychosocial intervention must be periodically assessed.

DRUG THERAPY

Nonsteroidal Anti-Inflammatory Drugs (NSAIDs)

These agents are the mainstay of medical therapy for all forms of JRA. Responses to NSAID therapy generally occur in days to weeks. Despite the fact that no one NSAID has proved to be more efficacious than the others, there are differences in chemical structure and unpredictable differences in patient response; thus, changing to another NSAID is reasonable in therapeutic failures. On the other hand, the rare child with aspirin allergy should not be given any other NSAID. Although anecdotally successful, the simultaneous use of two NSAIDs has not been carefully studied in JRA, nor is the practice approved by the U.S. Food and Drug Administration, because of the risk of significant additive side effects.

Aspirin. Aspirin is the principal chemotherapeutic agent for all forms of JRA. Used for decades, aspirin is inexpensive and efficacious; no other NSAID is clearly superior. Compliance with aspirin therapy is much easier to measure than with other drugs, although likely more difficult to obtain because of the frequency of administration, and family worries about aspirin's efficacy and about Reye's syndrome. Aspirin is often begun in doses as low as 80 mg per kg per day to decrease the chance of toxicity, but 90 to 100 mg per kg per day (to a maximum dose of 4 grams per day) divided three or four times daily is usually required for a therapeutic serum salicylate level of 20 to 30 mg per dl. Illnesses affecting gastrointestinal absorption, low serum albumin levels, other medications, and aspirin coating can influence the obtained level. Levels should be obtained 7 to 10 days after the initiation or any change of therapy, including the institution or withdrawal of other drugs, or with the advent of any signs of salicylate toxicity (e.g., tinnitus, hyperpnea). Salicylates should be temporarily discontinued with increased risk for Reye's syndrome (e.g., following exposure to influenza or chickenpox).

A number of prescription salicylate-derivative drugs are now marketed, including choline magnesium trisalicylate (Trilisate), which is approved for use in children. Potential advantages include twice daily dosing, a liquid form (500 mg per 5 ml), less gastrointestinal intolerance, and the lack of effect on platelet function. Disadvantages include higher cost and the lack of a chewable, small children's tablet. Dose ranges are identical to those for aspirin.

Potential adverse effects of aspirin therapy include gastrointestinal symptoms, such as vomiting, abdominal pain, gastritis, ulcer disease, and constipation. Although children seem less likely to develop these problems than adults, they are not exempt and should take NSAIDs with meals or snacks. Buffered aspirin products offer little additional protection. Antacids and certainly sucralfate (Carafate) are far more efficacious. Parents should report complaints of abdominal pain, vomiting, and hematochezia. A hemoglobin or hematocrit and red cell indices should be performed at least every 4 months to assess occult blood loss. Mild liver function abnormalities are common in children on NSAIDs (transaminases < 100 IU); however, rarely children develop significant hepatitis or even liver failure on aspirin, which rapidly resolves with discontinuance of the drug. Liver function studies should be obtained 2 to 4 weeks after beginning or changing therapy, and thereafter, if values are normal, as indicated by careful physical examination. Liver function should be more closely monitored and NSAID therapy changed (e.g., dose decreased) if serum glutamic-oxaloacetic transaminase and serum glutamic-pyruvic transaminase values consistently exceed 100 IU. Aspirin therapy should be temporarily discontinued when values exceed 300 IU and then restarted at a lower dose after recovery.

Renal effects of aspirin and other NSAIDs include hematuria and decreased creatinine clearance. Urinalysis should be performed every 3 to 4 months, and blood urea nitrogen and serum creatinine every 6 months. Some nephrologists recommend that creatinine clearance be checked yearly. Finally, significant central nervous system effects (e.g., hallucinations) are rare adverse effects of aspirin and other NSAIDs that necessitate discontinuance of the drug.

Other NSAIDs. Only two NSAIDs are currently approved for use in children from 2 to 14 years of age: tolmetin (Tolectin) and naproxen (Naprosyn). Tolmetin is available in 200-mg tablets and 400-mg capsules and should be initiated at 20 mg per kg per day divided into three doses, and increased to 30 mg per kg per day (maximum 1.6 grams per day) if well tolerated. Tolmetin bioavailability is decreased by food and milk. Naproxen is available in 250-, 375-, and 500-mg tablets as well as a 125 mg per 5 ml suspension. Naproxen may be given on a twice daily schedule, with doses of 10 to 15 mg per kg per day (maximum 1 gram per day).

Other NSAIDs can be used in the treatment of older children with JRA, including ibuprofen (Motrin), 35 to 40 mg per kg per day in three or four divided doses (maximum 2.4 grams per day), sulindac (Clinoril),* 150 to 200 mg twice daily, piroxicam (Feldene),* 20 mg daily, and indomethacin (Indocin), 1.5 to 3 mg per kg per day, in two to four divided doses depending on form (maximum 150 mg daily).

Each of these drugs may be useful in specific

---

*Safety and efficacy in children have not been established.

circumstances. Ibuprofen is relatively less expensive and is available without a prescription. Sulindac may have few renal side effects. Piroxicam's single daily dosing may improve compliance. Finally, indomethacin is likely to be most effective in treating HLA B27–positive pauciarticular JRA; nevertheless, the development of side effects, particularly those affecting the central nervous system, may limit its usefulness.

Slow-Acting Anti-Rheumatic Agents

In some patients, NSAIDs alone do not control the polyarticular arthritis of systemic or polyarticular JRA, as judged by the clinical examination and evidence of progressive, erosive joint disease on x-ray films. Therapy with slow-acting agents is then indicated, and NSAIDs are continued.

After years of use in JRA, gold remains the supplemental treatment of choice. Gold is available in injectable form as gold sodium thiomalate (Myochrysine) or gold thioglucose (Solganal). Auranofin (Ridaura), an oral form of gold, has recently been shown to be ineffective in JRA. Intramuscular injections of gold are begun weekly, with a test dose of 0.25 mg per kg, followed by 0.5 mg per kg, and then 1 mg per kg per week thereafter (maximum 50 mg per dose). Since improvement can be slow, treatment is generally continued for 20 weeks. If a positive response is observed, treatment is continued at 1- to 3-week intervals until there is at least 6 months of disease inactivity. Unfortunately, adverse effects limit the use of gold. Significant, relatively common problems include bone marrow suppression, nephrotoxicity, severe rash, and mouth ulcers. Nitritoid reactions are rarely seen in children on thiomalate therapy.

Because the adverse effects are common, a brief history, review of systems, physical examination, and panel of laboratory studies must precede each injection. Laboratory studies should include a complete blood count and urinalysis. The injection should be held at least temporarily and consultation sought if there is significant hematuria, proteinuria, associated rashes and mucosal lesions, an absolute white blood count below 3000 per mm^3 or a decrease of 5000, an absolute neutrophil count below 1500 per mm^3 or a decrease of 50 per cent, or a platelet count less than 150,000 per mm^3.

Other slow-acting agents used in JRA include penicillamine* (Cuprimine, Depen) and hydroxychloroquine* (Plaquenil); however, neither drug

was shown to be more efficacious than NSAIDs in a recent double-blind study done by the Pediatric Rheumatology Collaborative Study Group. Since penicillamine has many of the same side effects as gold, most practitioners are averse to treating a child who could not tolerate gold with the drug.

Hydroxychloroquine is administered in a single JRA have not been established.

Hydroxychloroquine is administered in a single oral dose of 200 mg per M^2 per day,* and is generally well tolerated by children. Eye disease is the most serious potential side effect; thus, children taking hydroxychloroquine should be examined by an ophthalmologist before beginning therapy, and then at least every 6 months.

Corticosteroids

Systemic steroids are rarely used in the treatment of JRA. Intravenous steroids are indicated in the therapy of acutely decreased cardiac function (and other life-threatening complications) in systemic JRA. Methylprednisolone should be given intravenously, 0.25 to 0.5 mg per kg every 6 hours. In addition, systemic oral steroids are occasionally needed to control chronic symptoms in systemic JRA, such as severe anemia and rheumatoid lung disease. They may also be rarely necessary to control extremely active, severe, polyarticular arthritis unresponsive to other medications. In these circumstances, oral prednisone is given daily or preferably every other day, in as low a dose as possible for therapeutic effect. Systemic steroids have no place in the therapy of pauciarticular JRA, except for severe uveitis. Possible benefits of systemic steroids must always be balanced against the well-described major short- and long-term risks, and these should be discussed in detail with the family.

Intra-articular steroid injections of triamcinolone hexacetonide (Aristospan) are sometimes used in the therapy of JRA. Although published data are sparse, intra-articular steroid injections have a role in pauciarticular JRA, as well as in single and few joint flares of polyarticular disease. The recommended dosage is 5 to 40 mg of triamcinolone (depending upon the age of the child and on the particular joint), which can be mixed with preservative-free lidocaine; this should be injected no more than twice a year per joint. Activity of the joint should be limited for 2 to 3 days thereafter. Although most patients respond well, there are potential problems associated with intra-articular injections. These in-

---

*Manufacturer's warnings: Efficacy of penicillamine and safe use of hydroxychloroquine in treatment of JRA have not been established.

---

*May exceed manufacturer's recommended dose.

clude minimal or brief overall response, postinjection arthritis flare, and the psychologic trauma of intra-articular injection. Risks of bleeding, damage to joint cartilage, and infection should be minimal. Secondary poor bone growth and weakness of surrounding structures near the injected joint have not been confirmed.

Topical steroids are used in the eye for the treatment of uveitis (discussed later).

Experimental Agents

Immunosuppressive agents, such as methotrexate, cyclophosphamide (Cytoxan), azathioprine (Imuran), and chlorambucil (Leukeran), are not approved for the treatment of JRA, although methotrexate and azathioprine are used for severe adult RA. The first controlled trial using one of these agents, methotrexate, in children is currently concluding, and results are quite encouraging. Other modalities, including high-dose pulse-dose steroids, sulfasalazine (Azulfidine), plasmapheresis, and immunoglobulin therapy, are also being studied. Use of any of these agents in JRA is strictly experimental.

PHYSICAL AND OCCUPATIONAL THERAPY

Physical therapy and occupational therapy are essential elements in the treatment of JRA. The goals of therapy are to maintain and improve range of motion, strength, and function. Specific guidelines and components for physical therapy of JRA include the following:

1. A home/school/community-based exercise program should be planned and supervised by a licensed physical and/or occupational therapist. Normal activities that accomplish the desired joint motions should be strongly encouraged. Swimming and bicycle and tricycle riding are excellent activities for the child with JRA.

2. Splinting is used for many purposes in JRA, including pain reduction, joint protection, improving contracture and muscle strength, and increasing function. Night splinting is a highly successful and standard technique for reducing peripheral joint contractures, particularly at the wrist and knees. On the other hand, daytime use of immobilizing splints should at most be only a temporizing measure while other therapies are being instituted. Dynamic splints, which hold joint position and yet encourage specific joint motions against resistance to increase strength, are sometimes used in JRA patients. Shoe inserts and other orthotic devices such as metatarsal bars and pads, as well as comfortable, well-supported shoes, reduce pain. Cervical collars may protect the unstable cervical spine that is sometimes a complication of polyarticular and systemic JRA. Serial casting is a technique occasionally used to reduce joint contractures unresponsive to physical therapy and splinting.

3. Localized therapy, and sometimes mild pain relievers such as acetaminophen, can be extremely useful in decreasing joint stiffness and discomfort. Warm baths, local application of moist heat, and frequent changes of position can combat joint stiffness. "Icing" a joint can temporarily decrease discomfort and is used as an adjunct in serial casting.

PREVENTION AND TREATMENT OF EYE DISEASE

JRA is a major cause of blindness in children. Chronic, occult iridocyclitis is most common in antinuclear antibody (ANA)–positive pauciarticular JRA, and less common in systemic and polyarticular JRA. Risk for eye disease does not correlate with the activity of arthritis. Eye pain and photophobia are uncommon complaints, and ophthalmoscopic examination rarely suggests uveitis until significant eye damage has occurred. Thus, slit-lamp examination must be done as frequently as every 6 weeks in the young, female, ANA-positive, pauciarticular JRA patient; in the patient with systemic or polyarticular JRA, the examination should be performed every 6 months. The consulting ophthalmologist should direct any needed therapy for iritis, which generally includes topical steroids and a mydriatic agent.

SURGERY

Orthopedists should see children with severe leg length discrepancy, cervical spine disease, and subluxed and/or extremely restricted joint movement or severe pain. However, surgery is not a cure for JRA; in fact, synovectomy may worsen the disease. On the other hand, surgery can be extraordinarily valuable as a reconstructive modality. Unilateral epiphyseal stapling can improve leg length discrepancy in the growing child with asymmetric, pauciarticular arthritis. Specific operations to be considered in the child with severe deforming polyarticular arthritis include soft tissue releases, metatarsal head resection, pin traction for joint subluxation, and cervical spine stabilization. Selective joint replacement may be considered for the older adolescent and young adult patient.

ANKYLOSING SPONDYLITIS

method of
A. S. RUSSELL, M.B., B.Chir., and
D. MATHERS, M.B., B.S.
University of Alberta
Edmonton, Alberta, Canada

Although not clearly recognized as a clinical entity until the 1890s by Bechterew, Strumpell, and Marie, there are skeletal remains from France, and others from Egypt dating from 5000 years ago, that show changes compatible with ankylosing spondylitis (AS). Whether these skeletal remains were correctly interpreted or whether they might have represented a different bone disease, known as hyperostosis, is now being argued.

In the United States, AS was known as rheumatoid spondylitis and was thought of as a rheumatoid variant until the past 20 years, when its clinical, genetic, and immunologic distinction from rheumatoid arthritis became recognized. It is an arthritis primarily of the axial skeleton, although peripheral joints may be involved, and it is associated, especially in the vertebrae, with a tendency to bony ankylosis.

The disease usually begins between 15 and 30 years of age with an insidious onset of pain in the low back and/or buttocks, sometimes radiating down the leg as far as the knee. A cardinal clinical feature is stiffness after resting, which is most evident when getting out of bed. Characteristically, unless modified by treatment, this stiffness may last for 1 or 2 hours and is relieved by moderate exercise. In contrast, although patients with mechanical back dysfunction may feel some temporary stiffness in the morning, their symptoms are generally aggravated by exercise. In about 10 per cent of patients, the onset is abrupt and may more closely mimic sciatica; if the onset is associated with trauma, the diagnosis can easily be missed. Other patients present with a peripheral, that is, nonaxial, arthritis, and the diagnosis of AS is made because of the characteristic distribution of joint disease (large joints predominating), with either an associated history of back problems or physical or radiologic signs of AS.

AS is more frequent in males and although at one time the relative male-to-female prevalence was thought to be 5:1 or more, it is now 2:1 or 3:1. Even this ratio may represent under-recognition in women: a ratio of 2:1 or 3:1 is seen in clinical studies, whereas in epidemiologic studies the sex ratio is nearly equal.

Physical examination, even in the early stages, often reveals a stiff back, which is most obvious by assessing lumbar flexion using the relatively standardized Schober's test in which a measured 10-cm segment up from the L_5/S_1 junction should expand to at least 14 cm on full forward flexion. Restriction of movement, however, occurs in all directions. Restricted movement is especially impressive in the absence of acute symptoms, as severe pain, such as that caused by a mechanical back derangement, also decreases range of movement. It is important not to use only the ability to touch the toes as a measure of back flexion because mobile hips can often mask a marked decrease in lumbar spine flexion. Schober's test is used to follow the course of disease in a patient. A loss of the lumbar lordosis is often seen at an early stage but is not a necessary feature. Although the first radiologic manifestations are usually in the sacroiliac joints, there is no clinical test of sacroiliac joint function that is reliable or generally accepted. Also, because the joint is so deeply buried, tenderness over the sacroiliac joints is *not* a feature of AS. The decreased lumbar flexion and the early loss of lumbar lordosis are probably due to involvement of the facetal joints of the lumbar spine. The disease may spread proximally to involve the joints of the dorsal spine; stiffness there is manifested as reduced rotation and reduced chest expansion (less than 1 inch at the nipple line). Involvement of the dorsal spine is often associated with referred pain anteriorly of a deep, gripping quality on one or both sides. We have seen several patients admitted to the hospital with a suspected myocardial infarction based on this manifestation. As the disease progresses, a more obvious stoop may be noted with a progressive dorsal kyphosis. This stoop can be best assessed by the distance from occiput to wall: the individual stands erect with heels and buttocks against the wall and attempts to have the occiput also in contact with the wall, as it should be, when looking straight ahead.

The most important peripheral joint involved is the hip because involvement here significantly decreases function and because flexion contractures increase the tendency of the patient to lean forward when erect. AS beginning in childhood presents typically as an oligoarticular disease, and hip joint involvement is more frequent in such individuals, which contributes to their worse prognosis.

AS has been described as an enthesopathy, that is, inflammation at sites of tendinous insertions. Thus, other joints that may be involved are the manubriosternal, sternoclavicular, and symphysis pubis (although the last is usually associated with radiologic features only). In addition, plantar fasciitis is common, and symptoms may be seen at other sites, such as insertion of tendo Achillis or hamstrings.

Acute, nongranulomatous, unilateral anterior uveitis may be the presenting feature and occurs at some time in about 25 per cent of patients. Its activity does not correlate clinically with that of the arthritis. Both eyes may be involved but usually at different times.

RADIOLOGY

The cardinal radiologic feature is sacroiliitis, which is manifested by sclerosis, erosions, and, eventually, fusion of the sacroiliac joints. Although it clearly takes time for radiologic changes to develop, paradoxically most patients show these by the time they present with symptoms. This situation would support the idea that the symptoms as well as the physical signs may reflect lumbar spine involvement, that is, a stage later than sacroiliac disease. Other features are erosions of the anterior vertebral margin ("shining corners"), leading to squaring of the anterior surface of lumbar vertebrae; syndesmophytes, initially best seen at the thoracolumbar junction; and apophyseal fusion. These changes normally progress from below upward but may skip areas completely. Some patients have a typical history but have a normal radiologic appearance of the sacroiliac joints. How can they be characterized? Some have a forme fruste of AS, which can be most easily recognized if they have relatives with the full-blown disease. Bone scans have been used to try to detect inflammation of the sacroiliac joints but with variable success. Tomograms may show some changes but use too high a dose of radiation. Insufficient experience with computed tomography scans is available, and there is a tendency to over-read abnormalities here. A diagnosis of "possible AS" is, however, quite permissible, and treatment can be instituted on this basis. If after 1 or 2 years there is no radiologic progression, the physician can be confident that although inflammation may be present radiologic change is unlikely to occur.

LABORATORY TESTS

These tests are of little value in the diagnosis or management of the disease except to exclude other disorders. The erythrocyte sedimentation rate is often normal. Ninety per cent of patients carry the human leukocyte antigen (HLA) B27 but because this is found in 5 to 15 per cent of most caucasian populations, it is of no value in making the diagnosis. Indeed, it has been calculated on theoretical grounds, and has now been shown by observation, that the overwhelming majority of individuals with HLA-B27 (i.e., more than 90 per cent) do *not* have AS.

THERAPY

The mainstay of therapy is exercise to achieve and retain normal spinal mobility. Along with this goes advice regarding posture, sleeping positions, and so forth. The Arthritis Foundation in the United States, the Arthritis Society in Canada, and the British Society of Rheumatology all produce useful pamphlets that describe the clinical features and treatment programs for AS. Almost any exercise is good exercise, and patients should be encouraged to lead as normal a lifestyle as possible, including participation in sporting activities. On the other hand, once spinal fusion has occurred, that is, after many years of disease, the spine becomes more susceptible to fracture with sudden stresses and contact sports should be excluded. Swimming is perhaps the ideal exercise.

Anti-inflammatory medication, usually one of the nonsteroidal anti-inflammatory drugs (NSAIDs), is effective in most patients for relieving pain and stiffness and thereby improving mobility and allowing effective exercise. Some patients, once they achieve an active exercise program, may require only minimal drug treatment. In others, the disease remains steadily active; in still others, it fluctuates year to year. Whether these medications retard radiologic progression is unproved, although many physicians believe this to be the case. That they improve function is clear. AS remains one of the few illnesses for approved phenylbutazone use in North America, but in most patients the other NSAIDs are sufficient and are roughly equivalent to each other, although many physicians use indomethacin as the drug of first choice.

Some patients are resistant to a program of NSAIDs and physiotherapy, sometimes because of a superimposed mechanical back disorder or because of psychosocial factors. Others have persistent disease or cannot tolerate the oral medications. Radiotherapy still provides a useful alternative approach in such individuals. The risks of this modality remain, but with lower doses and therapy carefully focused on only those areas with demonstrable activity (via a bone scan), it has a helpful role.

Remittive agents such as gold treatment (especially intramuscular) have been used, particularly for patients with peripheral arthritis, with apparent benefit, and although it is unproved this approach is now generally accepted even for axial disease. Salazopyrin (sulfasalazine) has recently been shown in placebo-controlled studies to have a significant effect in patients with AS whether or not they have peripheral arthritis. It may be appropriate to consider introducing this drug at a relatively early stage, especially in patients who have an apparently poor prognosis, that is, in the presence of hip disease or serious disease in the family.

If hip disease becomes a major problem, total hip replacement may be indicated as in other forms of hip disease. There is an increased risk of ectopic bone formation around the replacement, but the results of this treatment are still generally good.

COMPLICATIONS

AS, especially after many years, may be associated with dilatation of the aortic ring and aortic regurgitation. Previous studies have found this complication in 5 per cent of patients. It is now a rare complication, perhaps because the disease is less severe than in the past. Conduction disturbances, which may be intermittent, can also be seen independently of aortic ring involvement. Apical pulmonary fibrosis has been described, but this too is rare, and, indeed, apical shadows in AS are still probably more likely to be due to tuberculosis than to the AS itself. As restriction of chest wall movement occurs, some reduction in vital capacity is seen, but a compensatory increase in diaphragmatic excursion prevents any serious problems from this restriction. On the other hand, if a severe kyphosis—or even worse, a kyphoscoliosis leading to ventilation-perfusion imbalance—develops, progressive pulmonary dysfunction may occur. Amyloidosis and cauda equina syndrome both occur. Some recent echocardiographic studies have suggested that minor involvement of the myocardial wall may actually be more common (after aortic ring involvement) than had been realized.

PREVALENCE

At a clinical level the diagnosis of AS requires relevant symptoms, that is, back pain with morning stiffness, and, usually, associated radiologic evidence of sacroiliitis. However, in epidemiologic studies, the most objective feature is that of radiologic change, although even here there can be disagreement among different observers.

The prevalence for caucasians is about 0.1 per cent, but it is much lower in black and Oriental persons. It is a familial disease: First-degree relatives of a patient with AS have a risk of spondylitis of about 10 per cent. Because AS is seen only in relatives who carry the susceptibility antigen HLA-B27, in these special circumstances within the family the risk to those individuals is approximately 20 per cent.

The mechanism whereby HLA-B27 confers increased susceptibility to AS is unknown. In the general population, it provides a relative risk factor of about 200 compared with individuals without this antigen. To date, none of the available theories have been proved, although it is now known that some bacteria have antigens that are structurally similar to areas of the HLA-B27 antigen.

AS is often described as primary or secondary, the latter designation meaning associated with another disease, such as Reiter's disease; inflammatory bowel disease, usually Crohn's disease or ulcerative colitis; psoriasis, especially psoriatic arthritis; and familial Mediterranean fever. It seems that at least in some patients the relationship is genetic: thus, not only do patients with Crohn's disease have a higher prevalence of AS but so do their relatives. The relationship to another disease is clearly not cause and effect: In most patients, for example, the AS precedes the bowel disease but in some the reverse may occur. Thus, the disease is not secondary to inflammatory bowel disease but is associated with it.

PROGNOSIS

Once the diagnosis is made in a young patient, in the absence of complicating features such as active inflammatory bowel disease, the prognosis should be good. The therapeutic emphasis should be on an active exercise program to maintain the erect posture and, although less critical, to maintain, if possible, flexibility in the spine. If a patient is diagnosed at an early enough stage and faithfully follows an exercise program and, if necessary, an anti-inflammatory regimen, effective disease control should be possible in most subjects. In patients with severe hip disease, remittive therapy would be commenced earlier because hip disease is a sign of poor prognosis. In addition, spondylitis associated with inflammatory bowel disease tends to be more severe and more difficult to control than is uncomplicated spondylitis. The emphasis again must be on exercise. Taking anti-inflammatory agents to relieve discomfort is by itself insufficient.

TEMPOROMANDIBULAR DISORDERS
method of
JEFFREY P. OKESON, D.M.D.
University of Kentucky
Lexington, Kentucky

In 1983 the American Dental Association adopted the term "temporomandibular (TM) disorders" to include all functional problems associated with the masticatory structures. Structures considered to be masticatory are the teeth, the periodontal ligaments, the bones that support the teeth (the maxillae and mandible), the TM joints, and the muscles that mobilize the mandible (muscles of mastication). Other terms that are commonly used to describe masticatory problems are "temporomandibular joint dysfunction," "craniomandibular disorders," and "myofascial pain dysfunction syndrome."

It is estimated that between 5 and 20 per cent of the population suffer from TM disorders. Epidemiologic studies reveal even a greater percentage of signs related to masticatory dysfunction. For example, the prevalence of TM joint sounds is reported to be between 25 and 50 per cent of the general population. At this time, there is controversy regarding the clinical significance of some of these signs.

Approximately 5 per cent of the population actively seek treatment for TM disorders. The majority of this group are female (80 to 85 per cent), although epidemiologic studies reveal a more equal male/female ratio for signs and symptoms.

ANATOMY

The area where craniomandibular articulation occurs, called the TM joint, is one of the most complex joints in the body. It provides for hinging movement in one plane and therefore can be considered a ginglymoid joint. However, at the same time, it provides for gliding movements, which classifies it as an arthrodial joint. Thus, it is technically considered a ginglymoarthrodial joint.

The TM joint is formed by the mandibular condyle fitting into the mandibular fossa of the temporal bone. Separating these two bones from direct articulation is the articular disk (sometimes called the "meniscus"). The disk is attached to the condyle both medially and laterally by collateral ligaments. These ligaments permit rotational movement of the disk on the condyle during opening and closing of the mouth. This so-called condyle-disk complex translates out of the mandibular fossa during mouth opening.

Unlike other synovial joints, the articulator surfaces of the TM joints are lined with dense fibrous connective tissue (not hyaline cartilage). This is an important feature in the management of many TM disorders. Dense fibrous connective tissue has a greater ability to repair itself than does hyaline cartilage. This implies that management of arthritic conditions of the TM joint may be different from that of other synovial joints. The TM joint has a fair ability to adapt or remodel when proper joint conditions are introduced (see the treatment sections).

Although there are many types of TM disorders, the two most common categories are masticatory muscle disorders and disk-interference (internal derangement) disorders. Because the majority of TM disorders fall into one of these two categories, they will be discussed in more detail.

MASTICATORY MUSCLE DISORDERS

Masticatory muscle disorders are a group of disorders associated with functional problems of the muscles that move the mandible. They present as a group of symptoms that arise from an extracapsular source (outside of the TM joint). Muscle spasms and pain are the most common complaints.

Etiology. It is thought that both malocclusion and emotional stress can play a significant role in masticatory muscle disorders. Muscle hyperactivity such as bruxism and clenching of the teeth greatly contributes to muscle spasms and pain. It is presently believed that nocturnal bruxism is more closely associated with increased emotional stress than with occlusal factors. Dental malocclusion or a poor dental prosthesis may contribute to these muscle pain disorders, especially when there is a history of pain beginning with dental therapy.

Clinical Findings. The most common complaint reported by patients with masticatory muscle disorders is myalgia. The muscles of mastication (temporalis, masseter, and medial pterygoid) are often tender to palpation. The patient's ability to open the mouth widely is frequently restricted. The normal range of jaw opening is approximately 4 cm, or about the width of three fingers.) Many of the symptoms are similar to those re-

ported by patients suffering from fibrositis or fibromyalgia. Functions of the jaw such as chewing and talking usually increase the symptoms. Symptoms are most commonly bilateral and are relatively diffuse over several muscles, although this may not always be true.

Because muscle pain is deep, it can produce referred pain. A common secondary complaint of patients who experience constant muscle pain is muscle tension headache. This type of headache is frequently produced by cervical and masticatory muscle involvement. Palpation of these muscle groups is indicated to determine whether the source of the headache pain is masticatory or cervical.

Treatment. The initial therapy for masticatory muscle disorders should be conservative and reversible. Mild analgesics (ibuprofen [Motrin], 600 mg three or four times a day) are helpful in decreasing pain and lessening the likelihood of cyclic muscle spasms. The patient should be instructed to begin a soft diet and to limit jaw movement to painless motions. The patient should be encouraged to keep the jaw muscles relaxed and not to allow the teeth to contact unless chewing (avoid clenching the teeth). If nocturnal bruxism is suspected, an occlusal appliance can be fabricated and worn during sleep to decrease this muscle activity. If a change in the dental condition created the symptoms, dental correction may be indicated. When increased emotional stress is suspected, various behavioral modification therapies such as relaxation techniques assisted with biofeedback may be helpful. When muscle pain is present, physical therapy can also be useful (e.g., moist heat, ultrasound, electrogalvanic stimulation). Muscle relaxants are not generally effective, although they can be used on a short-term basis for acute conditions (e.g., cyclobenzaprine [Flexeril], 10 mg two or three times a day).

DISK-INTERFERENCE (INTERNAL DERANGEMENT) DISORDERS

Disk-interference disorders are a group of TM disorders that result from functional problems between the mandibular condyle and the articular disk. These problems are considered to be intercapsular disorders (within the TM joint). Mechanical alteration of joint movement and joint pain are common disk-interference complaints.

Etiology. Disk-interference disorders result from a mechanical disruption of normal condyle-disk function during opening and closing of the mouth. The most common cause of this disorder is trauma. Trauma, especially gross macrotrauma, can quickly elongate ligaments that support the condyle-disk complex, causing disruption in normal biomechanical relationships. Microtrauma received over time as a result of muscle hyperactivity (bruxism) or an unstable dental condition can also contribute to this disorder.

Clinical Findings. The most common reported clinical symptom of disk-interference disorders is clicking or popping of the TM joint during jaw movement. These joint sounds are created by abnormal movement between the condyle and the disk during opening and closing. On occasion, multiple grating sounds or crepitation can be heard. Crepitation is often closely associated with degenerative joint disease. On occasion, the articular disk can be dislocated anteromedially to the condyle, inhibiting normal translation of the involved joint. This condition is clinically referred to as a "closed lock" because the patient cannot open the jaw wider than 25 to 30 mm interincisally (width of one to two fingers). Joint pain may or may not be present. When pain is present, it is arthralgic and associated with joint movement. Symptoms are usually unilateral (although not always), and the patient locates the discomfort specifically to the involved TM joint. Ear pain on the same side as the involved TM joint is a common complaint.

Treatment. Treatment of disk-interference disorders is directed toward re-establishing normal condyle-disk function. In some instances, a dental appliance can be used to re-establish a normal condyle-disk relationship and therefore eliminate the joint symptoms. This appliance is generally worn 24 hours a day for at least 8 weeks to allow adaptation or healing of the intracapsular structures. The appliance is then slowly eliminated in an attempt to return the joint to its normal position and function.

If painful symptoms return, alteration of the dental condition may be indicated. When pain is present, the patient is instructed to minimize joint sounds by decreasing jaw function. Analgesics such as ibuprofen, 600 mg as needed for pain, may be helpful. If inflammation of the joint structures is suspected, an anti-inflammatory medication such as ibuprofen, 600 to 800 mg three times a day for 3 weeks, is indicated. Sometimes physical therapy is helpful in decreasing pain and increasing joint mobility.

On occasion, occlusal appliance therapy, physical therapy, and medications may not be successful in reducing symptoms. When pain persists, surgical therapy may be considered. Surgery is directed toward re-establishing normal condyle-disk function. In most cases, conservative therapy is relatively successful; therefore, surgery is indicated only in about 5 per cent of patients with intercapsular disorders.

Asymptomatic clicking of the TM joint is a relatively common finding (25 to 50 per cent of the general population). Presently, therapy to eliminate it is relatively unsuccessful and therefore is not indicated. Only joints with painful clicking or with signs of progressing intercapsular problems should be considered for treatment.

FIBROSITIS, BURSITIS, AND TENDINITIS

method of
CHARLES L. DERUS, M.D.
Dreyer Medical Clinic
Aurora, Illinois

FIBROSITIS

Clinical Features

Fibrositis is a distinct clinical entity that is characterized by chronic diffuse aching, pain, and stiffness. Women are overwhelmingly affected, and the usual age of diagnosis is 30 to 40 years. Patients frequently "hurt all over" and usually complain of deep aching neck, shoulder, and back pain. Referred pain to the limbs may be described as myalgias, burning, coolness, numbness, or swelling.

A disturbance of Stage 4 sleep is common and results in unrefreshing sleep. Patients wake up "tired" and complain of fatigue that can last all day. A history of headaches or irritable bowel syndrome is also common. Symptoms may be exacerbated by heat, cold, stress, and exercise. The etiology of this syndrome is unknown. No test is diagnostic of fibrositis.

Diagnosis of fibrositis is based on a characteristic history, exclusion of systemic diseases that produce arthralgias and myalgias (e.g., rheumatoid arthritis, lupus, polymyositis, polymyalgia rheumatica, and hypothyroidism), a normal standard rheumatologic joint examination, normal laboratory tests (complete blood count, erythrocyte sedimentation rate, and thyroid functions), and the finding of tender points.

Tender points are the diagnostic clincher. Pressure over these areas produces severe pain. Nearby control areas are painless. The most common tender point locations are bilateral and include the midposterior trapezius muscles, second costochondral junctions, lateral epicondyles, and medial fat pads of the knees.

Treatment

Symptoms are usually chronic but can be lessened by treatment. Treatment consists of reassurance, education, and pain control. The patient should be reassured that fibrositis is usually not disabling and that damage to muscles or joints does not occur. A brief explanation of the disease combined with written educational material, which is available from the Arthritis Foundation, gives the patient a good start in coping with the disease.

Pain control includes both drug and physical therapy. Drug treatment is directed at correcting the sleep abnormality. Fibrositis patients are unusually sensitive to medications, and the lowest possible doses should be prescribed. Either amitriptyline (Elavil), 10 mg, or cyclobenzaprine (Flexeril), 10 mg, at bedtime, is useful to restore normal sleep and to ameliorate symptoms. The amitriptyline dose may be increased slowly if necessary. Results are usually seen at doses below 50 mg. Cyclobenzaprine may be prescribed in split doses up to a maximum of 40 mg per day. The role of these drugs in restoring normal sleep should be emphasized to the patient.

Analgesics, such as naproxen (Naprosyn), 250 to 500 mg twice daily with meals, may have an additive effect when used with amitriptyline. Any nonsteroidal anti-inflammatory drug (NSAID) may be useful for cervical or lumbar symptoms. Injections in tender points with corticosteroids or lidocaine, or both, are useful adjuncts in some patients.

Physical therapy consists of heat, cold, ultrasound, or massage. Therapy is especially helpful to relieve local areas of pain and spasm. Aerobic exercises that result in cardiovascular conditioning are also beneficial. Walking, swimming, bicycling, or low-impact aerobics should be started slowly and gradually increased. Encourage patients to exercise 30 to 40 minutes three or four times per week. The role that patients must play in their own improvement should be emphasized.

BURSITIS

Bursa are synovium-lined fluid-filled sacs that facilitate the motion of tendons and muscles over bone. Various factors, including excessive friction, trauma, infection (especially with staphylococcus), crystal disease (gout, pseudogout, and calcium apatite), and connective tissue diseases, can result in bursitis. Symptoms include local pain, swelling, erythema, and warmth.

There are more than 80 bursa in the human body; only a few are clinically significant. The most common site of bursitis is the subdeltoid bursa of the shoulder, which separates the deltoid muscle from the rotator cuff. Subdeltoid bursitis produces lateral shoulder pain with abduction of the arm. The olecranon bursa is located over the olecranon process. Olecranon bursitis can produce dramatic swelling and can occasionally be infected or gouty. Always obtain a culture for this site and check for crystals. Trochanteric bursitis is often confused with true hip pain or low back pain. Pain is located laterally over the greater trochanter and may radiate to the knee. Pes anserinus bursitis is often confused with true knee pain. The pes bursa is located on the medial aspect of the tibia, just distal to the medial joint line where the sartorius, gracilis, and semitendinous tendons insert on the tibia. Prepatellar bursitis ("housemaid's knee") is anterior to the patella and causes swelling and sometimes pain. Again, rule out septic bursitis. Calcaneal bursitis is a common cause of heel pain.

TENDINITIS

Tendinitis occurs most commonly where tendons pass over bony prominences or through narrow openings. However, the physician should be alert for crystal diseases, infection (especially with *Neisseria gonorrhoeae*), and connective tissue diseases. Bicipital tendinitis involves the long head of the biceps in the bicipital groove and produces anterior shoulder pain. Rotator cuff tendinitis produces lateral shoulder pain with abduction of the arm. Lateral epicondylitis ("tennis elbow") results from inflammation of the origin of the extensors of the wrist and hand and produces pain over the lateral epicondyle. Similarly, medial epicondylitis ("golfer's elbow") produces pain at the origin of the flexor muscles of the wrist and hand over the medial epicondyle.

Radial wrist and thumb pain is caused by tendinitis of the abductor pollicis longus and brevis tendons (de Quervain's disease). Stenosing tenosynovitis ("trigger finger") of the flexor tendons in the palm produces snapping and locking fingers. Posterior tibial tendinitis is a common cause of medial ankle and calf pain that is often seen in association with pes planus.

Treatment

Treatment consists initially of rest. Elbow and wrist splints are particularly helpful for epicondylitis and de Quervain's disease. Ice during the acute phase and heat during the chronic phase are beneficial. NSAIDs are indicated if conservative measures fail. Aspirin, 650 mg every 4 to 6 hours with meals, ibuprofen (Motrin), 600 to 800 mg every 6 to 8 hours with meals, naproxen (Naprosyn), 375 to 500 mg twice daily with meals, and piroxicam (Feldene), 20 mg daily with food, are representative examples. Physical therapy referral for ultrasound with or without use of topical steroids may also be useful. All patients with shoulder symptoms or frozen shoulder require instruction in range of motion exercises.

If patients have severe symptoms or fail to respond to therapy, local corticosteroid injection is indicated. The area is cleaned with alcohol and then sprayed with ethyl chloride for topical anesthesia. The affected area should be injected or infiltrated by using a 22-gauge or smaller needle. A medium-potency corticosteroid, such as prednisolone tebutate (Hydeltra-T.B.A.), should be used in superficial structures to avoid potential skin atrophy. A high-potency corticosteroid, such as triamcinolone (Aristospan), can be used for deep structures where leakage to the skin is unlikely. A dose of 20 to 40 mg of corticosteroids with 1 to 2 ml of 1 per cent lidocaine should be used.* The patient should be informed of potential risks and benefits. Advise the patient to rest the injected area for several days after injection. Surgical repair is indicated in tendon ruptures. Surgical excision or repair of bursae and tendons that fail to respond to therapy is occasionally required.

Patients with persistent or recurrent symptoms should be instructed in preventive measures. Identification and modification of activities that cause problems are essential. Patients should be instructed in warm-up and stretching exercises. Physical or occupational therapy evaluations of the work place, hobbies, or sports may be indicated. Splints or braces may be useful. Elbow bands or wrist splints can be helpful in epicondylitis. Thumb splints for de Quervain's disease are also available. Orthotics can prevent recurrent posterior tibial tendinitis and calcaneal bursitis.

An occasional patient may require chronic NSAID therapy. Frequent corticosteroid injections should be avoided because of the potential deleterious effects on connective tissues.

---

*The average intra-articular dose is 2 to 20 mg of triamcinolone hexacetonide and 4 to 10 mg of prednisolone tebutate into the tendon sheath.

OSTEOARTHRITIS

method of
GERSON C. BERNHARD, M.D.
Medical College of Wisconsin
Milwaukee, Wisconsin

The most common arthritic disease—osteoarthritis—begins as early as the second or third decade of life, and its frequency increases until it is found almost universally in octogenarians, at least by radiography.

Sixteen to 17 million Americans have clinically important osteoarthritis. It can be primary (diffuse or localized) or secondary to trauma, infection, metabolic disorders, developmental defects, or chronic inflammation, such as rheumatoid disease. The earliest change is decreased production of proteoglycans in hyaline cartilage. There is associated a decreased cartilage compliance in response to stress and increased density of subchondral bone. After this, flaking and fissuring of cartilage, bone sclerosis and cysts, osteophytosis from osteoblastic stimulation, and a mild, nonspecific synovitis are seen. Pain, the cardinal clinical feature, can result from early inflammation of synovium or inflammation at joint margins where osteophytes form, and also from capsular or tendon sheath distention, or from muscle spasm. Pain arises from the periosteum, joint capsule, synovium, or muscle where pain receptors are found—not from the cartilage. Lost or decreased motion occurs as a result of pain, muscle contracture, and scarring of joint capsule, but rarely as a result of osteophyte formation. Pain in osteoarthritis is sometimes neurologic because of peripheral nerve entrapment or radiculopathy from osteophyte formation. The degree of functional impairment depends on the strategic position of the involved joints in relation to locomotion or other major daily activities and on the severity of involvement in the affected joints.

GENERAL PRINCIPLES

Patients should be informed about the nature, origins, and probable benign course of this disease. They should distinguish osteoarthritis from the destructive inflammatory arthritides and be reassured that diffuse deformities with crippling or fatal complications are not likely to ensue. Only certain severely involved joints are destroyed. The responsibility for the most effective treatment program should be shared by the patient and managing physician. Two good patient education resources are *Osteoarthritis*, which may be obtained from the Arthritis Foundation, and *Learning to Live with Osteoarthritis,* which is published by Medicine in the Public Interest. Periods of daily rest and avoidance of joint abuse are basic. This should be viewed by the patient not as a restriction or deprivation, but as a rational positive approach to continued function and a safe way to modify pain. Many patients need to be disabused of the notion that more work or physical activity will keep them limber or "work the arthritis out." Excess weight is mechanically hindering to function of the large joints and to back care. Hence, weight reduction for the obese patient is desirable and should be both a goal for and a responsibility of the patient, with a dietitian's guidance. Sport activities in moderation should not be interdicted but should be altered or modified for the specific patient.

Many patients with osteoarthritis of the hip or knee can continue to play golf but should use a motorized cart. Similarly, the jogger should change to swimming. Other activities, such as crocheting or knitting, should be done in moderation, with periods for joint rest.

PHYSICAL AND OCCUPATIONAL THERAPY

One goal of treatment should be to keep the motion of each affected joint as close to normal as possible. A physical therapist should instruct the patient in a range-of-motion exercise program to be done at home, as well as in techniques of joint protection and pain management with heat, rest, and massage. A cane used properly in the contralateral hand of a patient who has knee or hip arthritis can reduce needless weight bearing, reduce pain, provide stability, and thus enhance independence. Isometric exercises of large muscles (such as quadriceps) done regularly help maintain function and joint stability. Isotonic exercise programs should be avoided because the repetitive action, especially against resistance, is irritating and can exacerbate local synovitis. Moist heat offers some analgesia, aids mobility, and reduces muscle spasm. A therapist should instruct patients in safe techniques for using heat in the home, including a bathtub whirlpool. Patients should also know the principles of back care, posture, and positions of rest because both the lumbar spine and cervical spine are so frequently affected by osteoarthritis and degenerative disk disease.

DRUGS

There are three reasons for use of drugs in treating osteoarthritis: analgesia, suppression of inflammation, and relief of muscle spasm. In a given patient it may be possible to avoid the use of drugs or to use them intermittently.

Analgesics and Anti-Inflammatory Agents

All of the nonsteroidal anti-inflammatory drugs (NSAIDs), including aspirin, enteric-coated aspirin, and nonacetylated salicylates (e.g., salsalate [Disalcid], magnesium salicylate [Trilisate, Magan]), as well as zero-order-release aspirin (Zorprin), are effective non-narcotic analgesics. In general, the analgesic dose of these drugs is lower than the anti-inflammatory dose. Acetaminophen or propoxyphene hydrochloride can be substituted for NSAIDs but do not have an anti-inflammatory effect. Combining nonpharmacologic techniques taught by the physical or occupational therapist with occasional acetaminophen use may be sufficient in some patients. Other patients who have inflammatory periods or who have a more consistent inflammatory component to the osteoarthritis need anti-inflammatory doses of an NSAID. The choice of drug depends on convenience to the patient, absence of toxic effect, age of the patient, concomitant diseases or drugs, and patient preference. Only salicylates can cause salicylism, but other unwanted effects on the central nervous system, gastrointestinal tract, or integument can occur in an unpredictable pattern with any of the nonsalicylate NSAIDs. Therefore, random therapeutic trials are often necessary to find the most effective and least toxic agent for a specific patient. Table 1 gives the drugs currently available in the United States and their usual dose schedules.

Gastritis and gastric ulcer are the most frequent complications from the chronic use of cyclo-oxygenase–inhibiting NSAIDs (including all but the nonacetylated salicylates). Gastritis or ulcer with bleeding is more frequent and more serious in elderly patients. Renal insufficiency is the next most serious and subtle complication of long-term use of cyclo-oxygenase–inhibiting NSAIDs. It occurs primarily in patients with hypertension, chronic renal disease, or congestive heart failure, and the elderly patient whose creatinine clearance is often reduced. Therefore, drugs with a short half-life are preferable in older patients. This requirement may necessitate dose schedules of three or four times daily, which are less convenient and reduce patient compliance.

Adrenal Corticosteroids

Systemic use (oral or parenteral) of these agents is rarely of any value in the treatment of osteoarthritis. The serious side effects caused by their prolonged use make them contraindicated.

Intra-articular injection of anti-inflammatory corticosteroids can suppress severe, superimposed inflammation in a specific joint. Aspiration of the excess fluid, as well as resting the joint, may be equally effective. Furthermore, the inhibitory effect of corticosteroids on cartilage proteoglycan synthesis tends to promote the fundamental lesion of osteoarthritis. Repeated intra-articular injections of steroids may augment cartilage damage and cause the development of a severe, disorganized form of pseudo-Charcot's joint destruction. Hence, intra-articular administration of steroids should rarely be used for osteoarthritis, and after such an injection the joint should be rested for 2 to 4 weeks to allow proteoglycan synthesis to recover.

TABLE 1. **Nonsteroidal Anti-Inflammatory Drugs**

Drug	Tablet Strength (mg)	Usual Daily Dose (mg)
Salicylates		
Acetylsalicylic acid (aspirin)	325	650–1300 qid
Enteric-coated aspirin		
Ecotrin	325 or 500	650–1300 qid
Easprin or Dasprin	975	975 qid
Zero-order-release aspirin		
Zorprin	800	800–1600 bid
Nonacetylated salicylates		
Salsalate (Disalcid)	500 or 750	750–1500 bid
Choline magnesium salicylate (Trilisate)	500, 750, 1000	750–1500 bid
Magnesium salicylate (Magan)	545	545–1190 tid
Sodium salicylate (Pabalate)	325	650–1300 qid
Indole Derivatives		
Indomethacin (Indocin)	25 or 50	25–50 tid, qid
Slow-release (Indocin SR)	75	75 bid
Tolmetin (Tolectin)	200 or 400	200–400 tid, qid
Sulindac (Clinoril)	150 or 200	150–200 bid
Oxicam		
Piroxicam (Feldene)	20	20 daily
Phenamic Acids		
Meclofenamate (Meclomen)	50 or 100	50–100 tid, qid
Propionic Acids		
Ibuprofen (Motrin, Rufen)	400, 600, 800	400–800 tid, qid
Fenoprofen (Nalfon)	300 or 600	300–600 tid, qid
Naproxen (Naprosyn)	250, 375, 500	250–500 bid
Flurbiprofen (Ansaid)	100	100 bid, tid
Acetic Acids		
Ketoprofen (Orudis)	50 or 75	50–75 tid, qid
Diflunisal (Dolobid)	250 or 500	250–500 bid
Diclofenac (Voltaren)	25, 50, 75	25–75 bid, tid

Muscle Relaxants

Relief of muscle spasm is important for pain control and maintenance of joint motion. Rest, heat, splints, gentle massage, and passive-motion exercises may accomplish this goal. Muscle-relaxing agents may augment this effort. Several drugs can be tried, including diazepam (Valium), 2 to 5 mg three or four times a day, or meprobamate (Equanil, Miltown), 400 mg three or four times a day, or methocarbamol (Robaxin), 0.5 to 1 gram four times per day. These drugs should be prescribed for only a short time and infrequently because the patient may become habituated to them.

SURGERY

Various surgical procedures may relieve pain, realign joints, or remove irritating, worn cartilage. Removal of torn menisci or loose cartilage bodies may slow the degenerative process by eliminating the mechanically irritating factors. Redistribution of weight bearing onto less worn cartilage can be accomplished by osteotomy of a hip or knee, but this measure may be only temporarily effective. Total joint replacement or resurfacing has become popular with the advent of new adhesive materials and uncemented prostheses with porous coating for bone ingrowth. However, this reconstructive surgery does not restore the degenerated joint to the normal state and is not without complications or failure and infection. It should be reserved for the patient with advanced disease who has severe pain on only mild activity and/or disabling deformity with loss of motion. It should not be offered to patients as a means of returning to previously vigorous physical activity. Techniques and hardware are still being developed and are now available for ankles, knees, hips, shoulders, elbows, and wrists.

MEASURES FOR OSTEOARTHRITIS OF THE SPINE

Rest in the supine position is best for painful osteoarthritis of the lumbar spine, as well as for back sprain. The cervical spine is best rested by use of a small pillow rolled under the neck or a semisoft cervical collar. Traction of either the cervical or the lumbar spine may have its major effect by putting the affected part at complete rest. This conservative therapy, coupled with analgesics and muscle relaxants, may require many days to a few weeks for maximal benefit. It should be followed by rehabilitation of motion and muscles, with careful attention to principles of protection of the back or cervical spine. Surgical procedures are indicated infrequently. Some indications include cord compression with slowly advancing quadriparesis, and lumbar spinal stenosis.

POLYMYALGIA RHEUMATICA AND GIANT CELL ARTERITIS

method of
EDWIN A. SMITH, M.D.
Medical University of South Carolina
Charleston, South Carolina

Polymyalgia rheumatica and giant cell arteritis are syndromes related by their common coincidence in the same patient, usually a caucasian older than 50 years of age. Approximately one-half of patients with giant cell arteritis have symptoms of polymyalgia rheumatica. The percentage of patients with polymyalgia rheumatica who have giant cell arteritis is more difficult to determine but is approximately 15 per cent. The association of these two conditions has led to a supposition of a common etiology and pathogenesis, although this has not been proved. Polymyalgia rheumatica is characterized by aching and stiffness (particularly prominent in the morning) in the shoulder and pelvic girdles and the neck, without actual weakness of these muscle groups. Malaise, low-grade fevers, and weight loss are often present. The most common manifestation of giant cell arteritis is headache, which is often accompanied by jaw claudication, fever (at times spiking), temporal artery tenderness, and visual disturbances. Because the visual disturbances can include sudden blindness (resulting from ophthalmic artery involvement), prompt diagnosis and treatment of this disorder are imperative.

Most patients with either polymyalgia rheumatica or giant cell arteritis have an elevated Westergren's erythrocyte sedimentation rate (ESR), which is often higher than 100 mm per hour.

THERAPY

Polymyalgia Rheumatica

The response of the pain and stiffness of polymyalgia rheumatica to low doses of prednisone (10 to 20 mg per day, orally) is often prompt (within 12 to 48 hours of the first dose) and dramatic. This rapid, complete resolution of symptoms has been thought to have diagnostic significance in situations in which the diagnosis is in doubt. This dose of prednisone is maintained for several weeks to 1 month and then is tapered gradually. The improvement of symptoms is usually accompanied by a fall in the ESR. However, the level of the patient's symptoms should be the prime indicator for lowering the dose of glucocorticoid. A requirement for constant normalization of the ESR is associated with excessive treatment and with a risk of side effects from glucocorticoid use, particularly accelerated osteoporosis with vertebral collapse, a complication for which individuals in this age group are at increased risk.

The duration of therapy for polymyalgia rheumatica varies but is often as long as several years at dosage of 5 to 7.5 mg per day, orally. The dosage can be judged only by the individual's symptoms as the glucocorticoid taper is executed. Rapid lowering of the dose almost always results in an exacerbation of symptoms; and alternate-day therapy, in increased symptoms on the "off" day. Some patients are known to require therapy for longer than 5 years, which indicates that, although the lowest dose of prednisone should be used, there is no urgency to discontinue the therapy.

If a temporal artery biopsy has been undertaken in a patient with polymyalgia rheumatica and giant cell arteritis has been found, treatment should be that for giant cell arteritis (see later section).

All patients with polymyalgia rheumatica must be questioned for symptoms of giant cell arteritis when they are seen for follow-up. If these symptoms occur, biopsy of the artery for confirmation and adjusting the prednisone dose to the higher levels necessary to treat this more serious condition are required. The physician must take time to educate the patient with polymyalgia rheumatica about the symptoms of giant cell arteritis. The patient should be instructed to increase the glucocorticoid dose if these symptoms occur and to contact the physician at the same time.

Giant Cell Arteritis

Because of the concern for the possibility of sudden and irreversible blindness (even though this occurrence is uncommon), patients in whom giant cell arteritis is suspected are initially treated aggressively with high doses of oral glucocorticoids (prednisone, 60 mg per day), even before a biopsy is made. The biopsy should be done within a few days of the initiation of therapy to avoid possible alteration of the histology. This high-dose glucocorticoid treatment should be maintained until all symptoms are gone and the ESR has been reduced, which usually requires 4 to 8 weeks of high-dose therapy. After this initial therapy, the symptoms become more important than the ESR to guide therapy. Initial decreases in glucocorticoid therapy can be relatively larger, such as 5 mg per week until a dose of 20 mg per day is reached. At that point, tapering by 1 mg per day each week is instituted. The dose is reduced to the lowest daily dose that controls symptoms. The ESR may rise into the slightly abnormal range (40 to 50 mm per hour) but, in the absence of a recurrence of symptoms of giant cell arteritis, this level should be tolerated. The patient should be informed about the symptoms that may recur during glucocorticoid tapering so that an exacerbation of symptoms can be promptly treated.

Patients with giant cell arteritis require various durations of therapy. Most patients require therapy for at least 1 year once a stable, low dose of the glucocorticoid is reached. Some patients may require therapy for 5 years or longer.

OSTEOMYELITIS

method of
RICHARD N. GREENBERG, M.D.
Saint Louis University School of Medicine
Saint Louis, Missouri

The treatment of osteomyelitis should be scientific (not empiric). Clues to the cause of the infection and guidelines for therapy may be found by noting whether the infection is hematogenous or nonhematogenous in origin, the age of the patient, the location of the infection, the patient's signs and symptoms, and the results of certain laboratory tests and cultures. Recent advances have dramatically improved therapy for some patients.

PATHOPHYSIOLOGY

In the *neonatal* period (up to 18 months), there are numerous transphyseal vessels in bone. In this type of circulation, infection can occur on both sides of the metaphysis and can lead to destruction of the epiphysis and the metaphysis. Neonatal osteomyelitis can be subtle but very destructive, involving numerous bones. The three most common pathogens at this time are *Staphylococcus aureus*, group B beta-hemolytic *Streptococcus*, and aerobic, gram-negative rods (Enterobacteriaceae).

In *children*, infection caused by hematogenous spread of organisms most often involves rapidly growing bone (long bones) and tends to start just beneath the metaphysis, where the nutrient arterioles bend. Infection tends to spread through the cortex. It may collect under a sturdy periosteum where a fibrous capsule confines the infection (Brodie's abscess). Any significant collection of purulent material can eventu-

ally lead to an ineffective blood supply and avascular bone. Hence, early treatment of children with osteomyelitis has better long-term results than treatment after the development of purulent material in the periosteum, with subsequent sequestrum (devitalized bone) or involucrum (new periosteal bone).

In *adults* the periosteum is firmly attached to bone, so that there is less likely to be a subperiosteal abscess and more likely to be suppurative and necrotic lesions with sequestrum and avascular bone.

SPECIAL CONSIDERATIONS

In addition to age, other important predispositions include the presence of diabetes mellitus, sickle cell disease, or severe peripheral vascular disease; the presence of a prosthesis or metal device; immunologic status, a long illness, and a history of fracture, surgery, or trauma; the specific location (e.g., spine, hip, foot); and hematogenous or nonhematogenous origin.

Diabetics often have foot infections that require a combination of antibiotics because of the presence of multiple organisms. These infections do heal with adequate debridement and appropriate antibiotics *as long as there is adequate circulation*. Amputation rather than antimicrobial treatment is indicated when circulation to the infected bone is compromised and inadequate. Diabetics also often "hide" infection, as they seem to have an increased threshold for pain. Hence, a detailed examination (especially in paraplegics) and perhaps a scanning procedure (see later) may be required to find the occult osteomyelitis. Any cellulitis or draining skin lesions should be considered to involve the underlying bone until proved otherwise.

Osteomyelitis in a patient with *sickle cell disease* is frequently associated with hematogenous spread of the organisms. The infection usually occurs in the diaphysis of long bones and is caused by *Salmonella* species), other aerobic, gram-negative rods, or *S. aureus*. A major problem in these patients is to distinguish between infection and infarction. A negative bone scan suggests the presence of infarction. Osteomyelitis is more likely to cause an elevation in temperature, white blood cell count, and erythrocyte sedimentation rate and a positive bone scan. Blood, stool (e.g., *Salmonella* species), and bone cultures are needed. Once cultures have been taken, presumptive treatment should include coverage for *Salmonella* species (ampicillin, chloramphenicol, ciprofloxacin, or another effective quinolone antibiotic).

Patients with significant *peripheral vascular disease* can present with a clinical picture suggestive of osteomyelitis but actually have bone infarction caused by significant vascular trauma and interruption of the arterial blood supply. This occurs especially after vascular surgery. Cultures of affected bone (and bone biopsy whenever possible) are needed to rule out infection. Patients who have osteomyelitis must be evaluated for adequate circulation to the infected bone. Patients with a metal apparatus or prosthesis at the infection site cannot be considered curable unless treatment eventually includes removal of the foreign object and sterilization of the site (culture proven) before reintroduction of the prosthesis. Often these patients are unable to have the foreign object removed; treatment in these patients is then directed toward suppression of the infection. Regardless of whether treatment is for cure or suppression, cultures to identify the pathogen(s) are necessary for successful therapy. Suppressive treatment always includes the inherent risk of bacteremia, and patients should be instructed to seek attention if symptoms such as fever, dizziness, and nausea occur. Bacteremia in the presence of an infected appliance demands removal of the foreign object.

Immunologically compromised patients can have unusual pathogens. Culturing must be extensive, with consideration given to the presence of fungal organisms. One such fungal pathogen, *Sporothrix schenckii*, often infects joints or may appear as a cellulitis but actually has invaded the underlying bone. Sporotrichosis is associated with gardening or soil contamination of wounds. Other fungal pathogens include *Blastomyces dermatitidis, Histoplasma capsulatum, Cryptococcus neoformans, Candida* species, *Mucor* species, and *Coccidioides immitis*.

Location of the lesion often suggests a pathogen and influences the presumptive treatment. Osteomyelitis of the spine is occasionally seen after hematogenous dissemination of uropathogens (*Escherichia coli, Klebsiella* species), *S. aureus*, or *Mycobacterium tuberculosis*. The spine is the most frequent site of tuberculous osteomyelitis in adults, whereas the metaphysis of long bones is the most frequent site in children (followed by the hip and the knee). *M. tuberculosis* is the most common pathogen involving the ribs. Infection of the foot after a nail puncture is frequently caused by *Pseudomonas aeruginosa* (presumably introduced from the host's own skin flora).

Bone infections related to *trauma (open fractures)* can be caused by pathogens from the host's own flora or by those introduced by the contaminating elements. Human bites can lead to osteomyelitis involving mouth flora, including anaerobic organisms. Cat bites can introduce *Pasteurella multocida* (a common organism in the oral secretions of cats). Dog bites may introduce aerobic, gram-negative rods including DF-2 organisms (dysogonic fermenters; they are slow-growing, gram-negative rods commonly found in the oral secretions of dogs), as well as anaerobic organisms.

Hematogenous osteomyelitis in children is nearly always caused by *S. aureus*. This organism also is common in bone infections related to indwelling catheters (i.e., hemodialysis patients) or intravenous infections (i.e., drug addicts). Drug addicts have been reported with osteomyelitis caused by gram-negative rods (especially *P. aeruginosa*) and *Candida* species.

Nonhematogenous osteomyelitis is a result of contiguous spread of pathogens from nearby infected soft tissue (i.e., decubital ulcers) or is related to trauma. These patients may not have systemic signs unless the infection becomes bacteremic as well.

HISTORY

Clues to the pathogens found in the history include nail puncture (*P. aeruginosa*), exposure to plants (*S. schenckii*), or sea water (atypical mycobacteria, *Vibrio*

species, and *Aeromonas* species), recent skin infection (*S. aureus*), human bite (anaerobes), hemodialysis (*S. aureus*), drug addiction (*Staphylococcus* species, *Pseudomonas* species), dental work or periodontal disease (mouth flora), animal bite or exposure (*P. multocida*, DF-2 organisms, and *Brucella* species), and exposure to tuberculosis.

The duration of the infection is particularly important in children. It seems that if it is treated early (within 1 week of the onset of symptoms), shorter courses of antibiotics (3 to 4 weeks instead of 6 weeks) without surgical débridement may be effective. Thus, the duration of chills, sweating, fever, malaise, and pain; inability to flex or move the involved area; joint pain; redness or erythema of skin; swelling of soft tissue; or muscle spasms should be assessed.

Chronic infections are often characterized by drainage or open sinus tracts, and prior pathogens tend to be current ones. A foul odor from sinus tract drainage is highly suggestive of the presence of anaerobes. Unusual pathogens may be present in immunologically compromised patients or in those who recently traveled to tropical areas. Any metal or prosthetic devices should be identified.

Identification of a history of drug allergies is essential. Any recent surgery or joint aspirations (or injections) should be noted. Lastly, it is important to realize that neonates may have no signs or symptoms except fever, vomiting, diarrhea, or all three.

PHYSICAL EXAMINATION

Physical examination should identify the area involved (tenderness to palpation, swelling, redness, warmth over the infected bone). A draining sinus with a feculent odor indicates the presence of anaerobic pathogens. In children especially, there may be only an inability to move the adjacent joint. Systemic signs include not only fever, chills, and malaise, but also evidence of an underlying disease (periodontal disease, sinusitis, signs of diabetes mellitus, or signs of decreased peripheral circulation such as decreased pulses and nail bed filling).

LABORATORY EVALUATION

Laboratory evaluation includes a white blood cell count with differential count and an erythrocyte sedimentation rate. These are followed during treatment and should return to normal or preinfection values if the osteomyelitis is cured or suppressed. Other blood tests depend on the particular patient and may include a sickle cell preparation or a blood glucose level determination. A skin test for tuberculosis is indicated in any patient with a spine or rib osteomyelitis or an infection that does not appear to have an easily identified bacterial pathogen as a cause.

IMAGING

X-ray films, radionuclide scans, computed tomography, and *magnetic resonance imaging* are used (1) to locate the infection and (2) to observe for spread of infection. As these procedures can be extremely expensive, judgment is required to order only those that are indicated. One should take x-ray films of the area identified by the history and the physical examination. The first sign of osteomyelitis on the film is soft tissue swelling (there may be no such evidence for up to 14 days). Later there is bone destruction and periosteal elevation.

A ^{99m}Tc bone scan is specific for increased osteoblastic activity or bone formation (it is not diagnostic for infected bone, as it can be positive in areas of trauma, tumor, synovitis, arthritis, or noninfected inflammatory processes). It is positive as early as 3 days after the onset of symptoms and is helpful in locating the osteomyelitis. The scan can miss infected avascular areas.

Although the ^{67}Ga citrate scan may be more diagnostic of infection, it is less sensitive than the ^{99m}Tc scan, and its resolution is not as good in small bones. A large amount of purulent material and active phagocytosis at the infected site are required to give a positive scan. It is not necessary to obtain this scan if the involved area has been identified.

It is not necessary to obtain the ^{111}In-labeled leukocyte scan. This scan uses the labeling of the host's own leukocytes, which are then reinjected into the patient. It is more sensitive and diagnostic than gallium scanning but is not better in localizing the involved area than the ^{99m}Tc scan.

When infection is extensive or near vital organs, computed tomography or magnetic resonance imaging is helpful. These expensive studies are of value in following vertebral osteomyelitis and infection involving the skull, pelvic area, or hips. Each can delineate the depth and extent of bone involvement.

It is not possible at this time to claim with certainty that an infection requires continued treatment based on positive scans. Treatment should end at 6 weeks (when the course of therapy is complete), provided that the patient's condition has returned to baseline, with no further evidence of bony destruction by x-ray film. Scans at this time can be misleading and should not be obtained. It is preferable to follow the patient clinically and to re-treat if symptoms recur.

ISOLATION OF THE PATHOGEN

Blood cultures (up to three sets, each drawn at a different time) grow the pathogen in most cases of acute hematogenous osteomyelitis but rarely in cases of chronic osteomyelitis (<5 per cent). Bone cultures identify the pathogen in nearly all cases of acute osteomyelitis and in at least 60 per cent of chronic infections.

Treatment should never start until after at least one set of blood cultures is taken. Furthermore, an *aspiration from the infected bone* using a 16- or 18-gauge needle (with an inner stylet if possible) should be obtained before starting treatment. As acute hematogenous osteomyelitis can be associated with potential life-threatening complications, every effort should be made to obtain blood and bone material for culture quickly so that presumptive treatment with antibiotics can begin. By contrast, patients with chronic osteomyelitis need not be treated until surgical débridement

with bone cultures has been performed. Treatment in these patients can begin in the operating room once material for cultures has been obtained.

If one attempts a bone aspiration, the needle should enter through an uninvolved area of skin that has been prepared with an iodine-containing disinfectant (iodine disinfectants work quickly, whereas alcohol requires several minutes to sterilize). Lidocaine can be used only to anesthetize the skin; it should not be injected along the periosteum because it can retard bacterial growth in culture. Specimens from infected bone should be sent for Gram's stain and for aerobic, anaerobic, mycobacterial, and fungal cultures. Even if only a few drops of serous-sanguineous material are obtained, they should at least be sent for culture and Gram's stain.

Transport of the material to the laboratory is critical, and one should consult the laboratory personnel for the best transport method available in the hospital. If transport medium is not available, one should leave the material in the syringe, remove the used needle, replace it with a sterile needle still in its cap, and send this to the laboratory as quickly as possible.

Deep wound cultures or cultures taken from sinus tracts are misleading and a waste of money. Skin-colonizing organisms may mislead the physician, and the true pathogens may not be recovered.

Again, stool cultures for *Salmonella* species are indicated for patients with sickle cell disease.

BASIC TREATMENT CONCEPTS

Treatment of osteomyelitis requires removal of necrotic, avascular, infected bone and relatively long-term antibiotic treatment. Surgery is not necessary for every patient, as children and neonates treated early for acute hematogenous osteomyelitis often are cured with appropriate antibiotic treatment only. Chronic osteomyelitis requires surgical débridement for cure. The type of surgery, whether to remove a metal appliance or prosthesis, and immobilization of bone are surgical decisions based on the extent of the infection. If a foreign object must remain in place to stabilize a fracture or maintain a joint, antimicrobial treatment should be designed to suppress the infection and allow discharge of the patient from the hospital. Suppressive treatment is usually provided by an oral antibiotic given for several months and restarted if symptoms recur. An occasional patient requires nearly lifelong daily administration of antibiotics to suppress infection in a prosthetic joint. If all objects can be removed from the bone, a cure is attempted.

INITIAL TREATMENT

Choice of the antibiotics depends on the pathogen. Empiric treatment does not exist. Once cultures have been taken, it is important to select appropriate treatment based on the history and physical findings. If the patient is acutely ill (possibly bacteremic), an initial combination of antimicrobials such as vancomycin, amikacin, and metronidazole in an adult or cefotaxime and amikacin in a child can be used. This coverage is quite extensive (and potentially toxic) but may be necessary when one is faced with acute hematogenous osteomyelitis in a severely ill individual. The regimen is changed to appropriate (cost-effective) and safer drugs as soon as the culture reports are available.

TREATMENT GUIDELINES

It is preferable to give parenteral or oral antibiotics, or both, rather than only local application of antibiotics. One can determine whether the choice is appropriate by obtaining serumcidal levels against isolated pathogens. Serumcidal activity is the only true laboratory measure of an antibiotic's effectiveness in osteomyelitis. In adults, trough (just before the next dose) serumcidal (i.e., not serumstatic) levels should exist at 1:2 dilutions or higher of serum for acute bone disease and at 1:4 dilutions or higher of serum for chronic bone disease. In children, peak (30 minutes after dosing) serumcidal levels should exist at 1:8 dilutions or higher except for streptococci, which should be 1:32 dilutions or higher.

Children who respond after only 2 weeks of intravenous treatment may be switched to an effective oral antibiotic for an additional 3 to 4 weeks. Treatment for cure requires a total of 6 weeks of antibiotic therapy, except in cases of vertebral osteomyelitis, mycobacterial disease, or fungal disease. Vertebral osteomyelitis therapy continues for up to 6 months and is stopped only when x-ray films and computed tomography scans show no further disease and the erythrocyte sedimentation rate has returned to baseline. Mycobacterial disease is usually treated with isoniazid and rifampin daily for at least 9 months. (The therapy is initiated with a third drug such as pyrazinamide but is changed once sensitivities are established. Two effective drugs should always be used to treat active tuberculosis.) Fungal therapy requires amphotericin B or perhaps a new imidazole derivative (ketoconazole, fluconazole, or itraconazole) and should be discussed with an infectious disease specialist.

ANTIBIOTICS FOR SPECIFIC ORGANISMS

For osteomyelitis caused by *Staphylococcus* species, an appropriate initial choice is oxacillin or nafcillin (vancomycin for methicillin-resistant staphylococci or for the patient with penicillin allergy) (Table 1). There is no oral agent that can be relied on for consistently adequate serumcidal levels against staphylococci. Once the patient has shown clinical improvement and has been treated with parenteral antimicrobials for several weeks, oral regimens may be tried. Patients treated with oral agents must be carefully observed for signs of treatment failure and must have adequate serumcidal levels. Oral agents with antistaphylococcal activity include cloxacillin, dicloxacillin, trimethoprim-sulfamethoxazole, new quinolone derivatives (e.g., ciprofloxacin, enoxacin, fleroxacin), and clindamycin. These agents could be combined with rifampin. Rifampin should not be used alone because of the rapid development of resistance. Children seem to respond well to oral agents, whereas adults fare less favorably.

Osteomyelitis caused by *Streptococcus* species is treated with penicillin. Penicillin-allergic patients may receive vancomycin, a first-generation cephalosporin, a long-acting cephalosporin (ceftriaxone, cefonicid), or clindamycin.

Osteomyelitis caused by *Haemophilus* species (a consideration in children) is treated with ampicillin, cefotaxime, trimethoprim-sulfamethoxazole (co-trimoxazole), cefuroxime, or ceftriaxone.

Bone infections caused by Enterobacteriaceae (e.g., *E. coli*, *Klebsiella* species, *Proteus* species) are treated with ampicillin (if the pathogen is sensitive), a third-generation cephalosporin (cefotaxime), a monobactam (aztreonam), an aminoglycoside (gentamicin), or a new quinolone (e.g., ciprofloxacin, enoxacin, fleroxacin).

Pseudomonas infections of bone require an aminoglycoside (gentamicin), ceftazidime, aztreonam, or ciprofloxacin. The best antibiotic is the least toxic agent with adequate serumcidal activity. If ciprofloxacin is appropriate, it is favored, as it can be given orally.

Anaerobic osteomyelitis is treated with metronidazole; this agent can be given orally. Other choices include clindamycin, piperacillin, cefoxitin, or cefotetan.

TREATMENT WITH ORAL AGENTS

The combination of the oral agents ciprofloxacin and metronidazole should be excellent for osteomyelitis caused by Enterobacteriaceae and anaerobes. This combination may also be effective against *P. aeruginosa* and some staphylococci. After adequate débridement, these drugs might be reasonable for a foot infection. However, such coverage is inadequate for elimination of streptococci. At this time, oral therapy is possible if the patient can receive oral medication, is able to absorb drugs via the gastrointestinal tract, and has an anaerobic pathogen (metronidazole)

TABLE 1. **Antibiotic Preferences for Osteomyelitis***

Organism	Drug	Daily Dose Children (mg/kg)	Daily Dose Adults	Hours Between Doses	Route of Administration
Methicillin-sensitive *Staphylococcus aureus*	Nafcillin (oxacillin)	50–100	8 grams	6	IV
	Cefazolin	40–100	6 grams	8	IV
	Ciprofloxacin†	—	750 mg	12	PO
Methicillin-resistant *S. aureus* and other staphylococci	Vancomycin	15–40	2 grams	12	IV
	Ciprofloxacin†	—	750 mg	12	PO
Streptococcus species	Penicillin	50,000–100,000 U	12 million U	4–6	IV
Enterobacteriaceae (*Escherichia coli, Proteus* species, *Klebsiella* species)	Ciprofloxacin†	—	750 mg	12	PO
	Ampicillin	100–300	8 grams	6	IV
	Aztreonam	—	6 grams	8	IV
	Cefotaxime	50–200	6 grams	8	IV
	Aminoglycosides‡				
Pseudomonas species	Aminoglycoside with aztreonam§	—	8 grams	6	IV
	Ciprofloxacin†	—	750 mg	12	PO
	Ceftazidime‖	30–100	6 grams	8	IV
Salmonella species (ampicillin sensitive, ampicillin resistant)	Ampicillin	100–300	8 grams	6	IV
	Co-trimoxazole (trimethoprim-sulfamethoxazole)	10/50	480/2400–640/3200 mg	6–12	IV
	Ciprofloxacin†	—	750 mg	12	PO
Haemophilus species (ampicillin sensitive, ampicillin resistant)	Ampicillin	100–300	8 grams	6	IV
	Cefotaxime	50–200	6 grams	8	IV
	Co-trimoxazole (trimethoprim-sulfamethoxazole)	10/50	480/2400–640/3200 mg	6–12	IV
	Aztreonam	—	6 grams	9	IV
Anaerobes	Metronidazole¶	15–35	1.5–2 grams	8–6	PO or IV
	Clindamycin	25–40**	2.7 grams	8	IV

*The drug listed first is the first choice. Other drugs listed are options if reason exists to choose an alternative agent.

**May exceed manufacturer's recommended dose.

†Ciprofloxacin may be effective against *Staphylococcus* species but is not a first choice. If it is used, serumcidal titers should be adequate, metal should be removed from the lesion, and the minimum inhibitory concentration should be 1 μg/ml or less. Other quinolone derivatives may be as effective as ciprofloxacin.

‡The most cost-effective aminoglycoside is gentamicin, followed by netilmicin. Tobramycin and amikacin are least cost effective. Aminoglycosides could be used initially until sensitivities are available but should be discontinued if the Enterobacteriaceae species are sensitive to less toxic agents.

§In severe *Pseudomonas* infections (potential for bacteremia is present), the combination of an aminoglycoside and a beta-lactam agent should be used. Aztreonam, the most specific beta-lactam for *Pseudomonas* species, is preferred.

‖Ceftazidime is an expensive antipseudomonal cephalosporin and should be used only if the organism is resistant to aztreonam and ciprofloxacin.

¶Safety and efficacy in children have not been established.

and/or an Enterobacteriaceae organism (ciprofloxacin or a comparable quinolone). Oral treatment for *P. aeruginosa* infection with oral ciprofloxacin may be effective if serumcidal levels are adequate. Oral treatment for *S. aureus* is more problematic.

LOCAL TREATMENT

Local administration of antibiotics to bone is currently being studied. Antibiotic-impregnated polymethyl methacrylate beads placed in open bone cavities after débridement have shown good results in animal models. In vitro studies also suggest that local delivery of an appropriate antibiotic is possible. If beads are to be used, the antibiotic must remain active against the pathogen once prepared with the polymethyl methacrylate. Aminoglycosides have been studied most thoroughly as antibiotic-impregnated beads; these agents are stable and active against sensitive aerobic, gram-negative rods and staphylococci. Aminoglycosides cannot be used for streptococci or anaerobic infections. Beads need to be removed or replaced after 2 to 3 weeks, as a dense fibrous tissue starts to surround them. There is also the theoretical concern that these beads could act as foreign bodies and could harbor pathogens (resistant to antibiotics in the beads) and prolong the infection. At this time, there are not enough data to recommend treatment with beads alone; however, beads plus systemic antibiotics help to deliver antibiotic to both vascular and avascular areas of infection. Use of antibiotic-impregnated cement cannot be recommended if its purpose is to deliver antibiotic to an infected area. In theory, the cement could be used as prophylaxis in sterile areas. The use of such cement to prevent infection (rather than systemic antibiotic prophylaxis) is debatable. In uncontrolled trials, the use of antibiotic-impregnated cement has been reported to contribute to successful revision of infected arthroplasties. The major advantage of antibiotic-impregnated beads and cement is that high local concentrations of antibiotics in bone can be achieved for a short period; serum levels remain nearly negligible, and systemic toxicity is unusual. Local administration to bone of appropriate antibiotics via a *drug pump* is investigational. Its use would seem to be appropriate only for those patients who have chronic osteomyelitis with significantly devitalized, avascular bone and who have failed prior débridement and systemic antibiotic treatment.

In certain patients (i.e., those with long bone infections), microvascular *muscle grafting* may assist in clearing the infection. Bone grafting should be avoided in infected areas, as the dead bone may sequester bacteria. *Hyperbaric oxygen treatment* of osteomyelitis has not been shown to assist in the resolution of osteomyelitis.

COMMON SPORTS INJURIES

method of
BRIAN C. HALPERN, M.D.
Marlboro, New Jersey

Sports injuries occur basically in two settings, organized and recreational. Organized sports at the high school level alone account for more than 1 million injuries per year. All of these result from either

1. Chronic trauma (overuse), which develops from repetitive forces on anatomic structures, causing inflammation, pain, and disability or

2. Acute trauma (contact and noncontact), which signifies immediate failure of a bone, ligament, musculotendinous unit, or other body system, with resulting impairment of function

Overuse syndromes comprise the greatest number of sports injuries seen clinically. Accurate diagnosis, followed by activity modification with appropriate rehabilitation, is essential to their treatment. A functional classification helps to stage the overuse injury (Table 1), and sports specificity better defines the biomechanical cause.

SHOULDER

Sports requiring overhead use of the upper extremity, such as throwing sports, racket sports, and swimming, commonly cause overuse injuries of the shoulder, followed in frequency by overuse injuries of the elbow. In the shoulder, the posterior rotator cuff muscles suffer chronic inflammation when impinged against the coracoacromial ligament and the anterior part of the acromion in overhead motion. Physical examination often reveals a positive supraspinatus test (pain, weakness, or both elicited by applying downward force to the shoulder at 90 degrees of abduction, 30 degrees of forward flexion, and full internal rotation; see Figure 1), a positive impingement test (pain elicited by internal rotation of the humerus in the forward flexed position; see Figure 2), or both. As this syndrome progresses, refractory tendinitis, wearing of the supraspinatus muscle and the biceps tendon, and partial or complete thickness rotator cuff tears can occur.

Treatment. Early treatment consists of rest, strengthening and flexibility exercises, and anti-inflammatory medications. This can be followed by physical therapeutic modalities such as ultrasound and electric stimulation. An injection of a corticosteroid can be used after failure of the initial therapeutic regimen, but it should be reserved for the seasoned athlete and not used in the very young participant.

TABLE 1. **Classification of Overuse Syndromes**

Grade I
  Postactivity pain
  Symptoms of less than 2 wk duration
  Generalized soreness

Grade II
  Pain during late activity and immediately afterward
  Symptoms of 2–3 wk duration
  Localized pain

Grade III
  Pain during early activity
  Symptoms of 3–4 wk duration
  Point tenderness with evidence of inflammation
    (erythema, swelling, crepitus)

Grade IV
  Pain with activities other than training that prevent
    or affect performance
  Symptoms of more than 4 wk duration
  Grade III signs plus disturbance in function, decreased range of motion, muscle atrophy

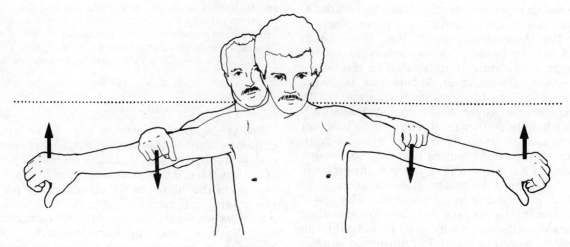

Figure 1. Supraspinatus test.

ELBOW

Elbow pain commonly evolves from tension overload on the medial aspect, compression overload on the lateral aspect, or irritation and weakness of the wrist extensors or flexors.

Treatment. Treatment is the same as that for the shoulder, plus correction of any biomechanical fault in the throwing mechanism or arm stroke.

KNEE

Sports requiring increased lower extremity loading, as in running, jumping, and biking, commonly result in overuse injuries of the knee, followed in frequency by overuse injuries of the lower leg. In the knee, patellofemoral pain predominates, with such problems as patellar ten-

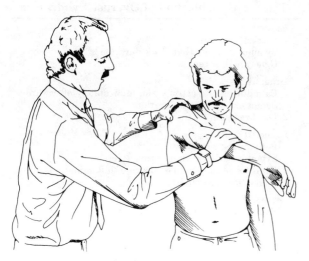

Figure 2. Impingement test.

dinitis and synovial plica irritation. Other possible diagnoses include pes anserine bursitis, iliotibial band syndrome, popliteal or biceps femoris tendinitis, meniscal tear, subluxated patella, and osteochondral damage. Physical examination usually reveals tenderness over the affected structures, and radiographs are usually normal. When evaluating the knee, a history of effusion within 2 hours of injury indicates a hemarthrosis, whereas effusion occurring 12 or more hours after injury indicates fluid of synovial origin. A hemarthrosis suggests an anterior cruciate tear, osteochondral fracture, peripheral meniscal tear, incomplete ligament tear, or subluxated or dislocated patella. The physical examination, at a minimum, should include range of motion with palpation for areas of tenderness, anterior and posterior drawer, pivot shift or jerk test, valgus and varus stress tests, external rotation recurvatum test, Lachman's test, and attempted patellar subluxation test.

Treatment. Immediate treatment should include rest, ice and immobilization, compression, and elevation. Rehabilitation should begin as early as possible. Treatment is the same as that for the upper extremity but does not include corticosteroid injection into the patellar tendon, because this can result in local atrophy and increased risk of subsequent rupture. The same risks of corticosteroid injection are seen with tendinous injections at other sites in the body as well.

LOWER LEG

In the lower leg (exclusive of the ankle and foot), the majority of syndromes are tibial periostitis (shin splints), stress fractures, and compartment syndromes. It is sometimes difficult to dis-

TABLE 2. **Classification of Sprains and Strains**

Grade I
  Microtear with some fiber tear

Grade II
  Greater fiber tear

Grade III
  Complete tear

tinguish among these conditions without the use of radiographs, bone scans, and compartment pressure measurements. Treatment consists of rest, immobilization as needed, flexibility exercises, and correction of any biomechanical fault with orthotics.

ANKLE

Lateral ankle sprains remain ubiquitous and occur biomechanically during inversion and plan-tar flexion. They often result in immediate swelling and disability to the extent of inability to bear weight.

Treatment. Ankle sprains are treated with ice immobilization, rest, elevation, compression, and rapid rehabilitation to restore normal ankle motion and strength. Return to participation hinges on the athlete's ability to run and cut without pain or instability. Some type of external support, such as taping or bracing, should be used for early return to sport participation. As in every injury, rehabilitation is the key.

Acute traumatic injuries are classified, in decreasing order of frequency, as sprains or strains, contusions, and fractures or dislocations. A grading system for sprains (injury to ligaments) and strains (injury to muscles or tendons) is presented in Table 2. Most injuries resulting from acute trauma are to the knee, followed by the ankle or foot; wrist, hand, or fingers; and shoulder.

Obstetrics and Gynecology

ANTEPARTUM CARE

method of
STEVEN D. BIGLER, M.D., and
STEVEN L. CLARK, M.D.
Utah Valley Regional Medical Center
Provo, Utah

Good prenatal care should ideally begin before pregnancy. Unfortunately, this requirement is often unrealistic. However, if the physician has the opportunity to see a woman who is anticipating pregnancy, he or she should at least encourage her to keep an accurate record of menstrual periods. This simple assignment often prevents later challenges in calculating a reliable due date. Women using oral contraceptives should be counseled to continue some reasonably effective means of birth control for one or two cycles after stopping the pill. Ovulation (and therefore conception) is often delayed for 2 weeks or more during the first cycle after the final "pill period." This delay often makes the customary menstrual estimated date of confinement inaccurate. In general, efforts to secure a firm, reliable date of last menstrual period will pay dividends during subsequent prenatal care.

THE FIRST VISIT

We usually see the normal pregnant patient at 10 menstrual weeks for her first prenatal visit. We have chosen this time because at 10 weeks the fetal heart tones can regularly be heard with the standard office Doppler instrument. If the patient is seen much before this time, little information is gained regarding the well-being of the patient and fetus, whereas at 10 weeks most patients can be reassured that the fetus is alive. We use a Doppler instrument with an audible speaker accessory so that the patient can hear the heartbeat. It has been our experience that once fetal heart tones are heard, the incidence of miscarriage is small. Mentioning this to the patient is usually quite comforting.

History

Past obstetric history is first reviewed, including gravidity, parity, abortions, ectopic pregnancies, method of delivery, duration of pregnancy, length of labor, and sex and birth weights of the infants. The patient is also questioned regarding any obstetric or general medical complications during previous pregnancies. She is asked to fill out written questionnaires dealing with risk factors for gestational diabetes and potential genetic disorders (Figures 1 and 2). General medical history, consisting of childhood diseases, operations, medical illnesses, trauma, exposures to drugs (including alcohol and tobacco), and allergies, is then explored. Previous medical records are obtained as needed, particularly for patients delivered by previous cesarean section to document the reason for the cesarean and the type of uterine incision. Family history is then reviewed as well as any history of multiple gestations. We believe that it is often advantageous for the physician to personally obtain the patient's history rather than delegating this assignment to the office receptionist or nurse.

General Physical Examination

With few exceptions, physical findings in the pregnant woman during the first trimester are identical to those in the nonpregnant woman. The patient is weighed without shoes, and blood pressure is taken, usually with the patient in the sitting position. The blood pressure is often quite normal in the first trimester and lower than usual in the second trimester; it will normally rise again somewhat during the third trimester. Dependent edema is common as pregnancy advances. Because of increased intravascular volume during pregnancy, a systolic ejection murmur may be heard. Varicosities of the lower extremities are often more prominent, even in early gestation, than in the nonpregnant woman, and they may be worse in one leg than the other. If so, the right leg is usually affected owing to compression of the right common iliac vein by the right iliac artery as it crosses superficially.

Gestational Diabetes Screening Form

A.   Name: _____ Age: _____ Date of Birth: _____

DO ANY OF THE FOLLOWING APPLY TO YOU?

Yes   No

_____   _____   1. I have delivered a baby weighing 9 lb or more at birth.
_____   _____   2. I have a family member with diabetes.
                              Relationship to you _____
_____   _____   3. I have had diabetes in a previous pregnancy.
_____   _____   4. I am diabetic now.
_____   _____   5. I have delivered a stillborn child.
_____   _____   6. I have delivered a child with a physical abnormality.
_____   _____   7. I have had 3 or more consecutive miscarriages.

Figure 1. Screening form for gestational diabetes.

Pelvic Examination

External genitalia appear as they do in the nonpregnant state, with the exception of vulvar varicosities, which may be quite common in the multipara. If these varicosities are the source of significant discomfort, some relief can be afforded by having the patient use one or two maternity pads secured by the standard belt to provide compression of the area. The vagina as well as the cervix may have a somewhat bluish hue (Chadwick's sign) because of the increased vascularity of the pelvis. The cervix is also quite friable. For this reason we use two cotton-tipped applicators, moistened with normal saline, to obtain Papanicolaou's smears in pregnant women. One applicator is inserted and rotated gently within the cervical canal, and the other is swabbed over the exocervix. This technique usually prevents the cervical bleeding often seen from the use of wooden or plastic scrapers or nylon brushes in the pregnant woman and has proved to be reliable in our experience. Monilial vaginitis is common in pregnancy and is treated with the standard antifungal agents. Examination of a vaginal wet mount under the office microscope is used to confirm this diagnosis. Branching pseudohyphae or small budding yeast cells are seen.

Bimanual pelvic examination is then done to assess the adequacy of the bony pelvis, to check for pelvic masses or other pathology, and to determine the size of the uterus. We manually check the interspinous diameter, the angle of the pubic arch, and the relationship of the pelvic side walls to each other. We do not measure the obstetric conjugate because the examination is quite painful to the patient and the dimension tends to have little bearing on her subsequent management in labor. In fact, the entire assessment of "clinical pelvimetry" is, in our opinion, of somewhat limited usefulness. We have never performed cesarean delivery based on clinical pelvimetry impressions alone without a trial of labor. Its performance merely gives a general idea of the pelvic capacity. It may, in cases where there is a strong impression of a small pelvis, modify the length of time a patient is allowed to continue in labor in the face of minimal progress.

The adnexa can be manually palpated until about 12 to 14 weeks of gestation, at which time they are carried high in the pelvis by the enlarging uterus. A palpable adnexal mass is handled in a manner similar to that in the nonpregnant patient. If the mass is cystic, unilocular, mobile, and asymptomatic, it is followed conservatively until around 16 weeks. If it persists beyond 16 weeks, increases in size, has solid components, or is multilocular, consideration of removal is appropriate. Clinical torsion is an indication for removal at any stage of gestation.

The uterine size at 10 weeks of gestation is comparable to that of a baseball. At 12 weeks, it is the size of a softball. At 10 weeks, the fundus of an anteverted uterus can just be felt at the symphysis pubis abdominally. At 12 weeks, the fundus is perhaps 3 to 4 cm above the pubis. A retroverted uterus is usually palpable abdominally by 12 weeks. The fundus of a 14-week uterus is usually found one-fourth of the way between the pubis and umbilicus. At 16 to 17 weeks, the fundus is halfway between the pubis and umbilicus, and at 20 weeks it has usually reached the umbilicus and also measures 20 cm above the symphysis. Thereafter, growth of the fundus averages 1 cm per week. Therefore, fundal height measurements in centimeters should equal gestational age in weeks (with an error factor of plus or minus perhaps 2 cm) from 20 weeks until around 32 weeks. In the later part of

The Intermountain Fetal Diagnostic and Treatment Center

Greggory R. De Vore, M.D.
LDS Hospital
Eighth Avenue and C Street
Salt Lake City, UT 84143
(801) 321-3447

Steven L. Clark, M.D.
Utah Valley Regional Medical Center
1034 North 500 West
Provo, UT 84604
(801) 373-7850, extension 2961

Prenatal Genetics Screening

Last name _____ First name _____ Date _____

Maternal Age

1. Will you be 35 years or older when the baby is due?　　　Yes _____ No _____

Genetic Diseases Common to Certain Ethnic Groups

1. Are you or the baby's father of African descent?　　　Yes _____ No _____
    If YES, have either of you been screened for sickel cell trait?　　　Yes _____ No _____

2. Are you or the baby's father of Eastern European Jewish descent (Ashkenazi)?　　　Yes _____ No _____
    If YES, have either of you been screened for Tay-Sachs disease?　　　Yes _____ No _____

3. Do you or your partner have any close relatives from Italy,
    Greece, or other Mediterranean countries?　　　Yes _____ No _____
    If YES, have either of you been screened for beta-thalassemia?　　　Yes _____ No _____

4. Do you or your partner have any close relatives from The Philippines or Southeast Asia?　　　Yes _____ No _____
    If YES, have either of you been screened for alpha-thalassemia?　　　Yes _____ No _____

Personal and Family Genetic History

1. Have you, the baby's father, or any member of your respective families ever had any of the following disorders:

    Congenital heart defects (blue baby, hole in the heart)?　　　Yes _____ No _____
    Hemophilia (bleeding disorder in which blood clots slowly)?　　　Yes _____ No _____
    Down's Syndrome (Mongolism)?　　　Yes _____ No _____
    Other Chromosomal abnormalities?　　　Yes _____ No _____
    Muscular Dystrophy (disease causing muscle weakness)?　　　Yes _____ No _____
    Cystic Fibrosis (disease involving the lungs)?　　　Yes _____ No _____
    Spina bifida (open spine), hydrocephaly (water on the brain),
        or anencephaly (absent brain)?　　　Yes _____ No _____
    A genetic disorder or birth defect not listed above?　　　Yes _____ No _____
        If YES, please list _____
        _____

    If YES to any of the above, please indicate the relationship _____

2. Do you or the baby's father have a birth defect?　　　Yes _____ No _____
    If YES, please describe _____
    _____

3. Have you had a previous stillbirth with a birth defect?　　　Yes _____ No _____

4. Have you had three or more first trimester (first 12 weeks of pregnancy) losses?　　　Yes _____ No _____

5. Do you or the father of your baby have any relatives with mental retardation?　　　Yes _____ No _____

6. Excluding iron or vitamins, have you taken any medications or recreational drugs
    (alcohol, cocaine, speed, LSD, etc.) during the pregnancy?　　　Yes _____ No _____
    If YES, please list _____

Figure 2. Prenatal screening form for genetic diseases and family history.

the third trimester, near term, it is not unusual for fundal height measurements to stabilize and remain at a constant number for 2 or 3 weeks. Occasionally, as the fetus descends into the pelvis at this time, fundal height may even appear to decrease slightly. We believe that consistent measurement of fundal height each visit is an important part of prenatal care and should not be neglected. It is a valuable screening tool for discovering intrauterine growth retardation, multiple gestation, polyhydramnios, oligohydramnios, macrosomia, inaccurate dates, and other potential problems.

Laboratory Studies

Venipuncture is performed at the first visit and the blood sample is sent for a complete blood count with indices and platelet count, blood type and Rh, antibody screen, rubella screen, and VDRL. We have found the platelet count to be useful for discovering the occasional case of immunologic thrombocytopenic purpura as well as for serving as a baseline to monitor later platelet changes in patients who become pre-eclamptic. The antibody screen (indirect Coombs's test) is important even in the Rh-positive patient to rule out the presence of irregular antibodies, some of which can cause significant fetal hemolysis. We perform a simple dipstick urinalysis to check for the presence of sugar, protein, nitrites, and leukocytes. Finally, a Papanicolaou's smear is obtained if the patient has not had one within a year. Additional testing may be appropriate depending on the patient population. For example, in our private population we have found it unproductive to do cervical cultures for gonorrhea. In other populations this would be an important test. Black patients should have a sickle cell screen. Any patient who has a positive risk factor for diabetes (see Figure 1) undergoes blood sugar screening early in the second trimester after morning sickness has subsided. This test consists of drinking a 50-gram glucose load (such as Glucola) and then in 1 hour measuring the blood sugar level. The patient need not fast and can have this screen done anytime during the day. Anyone with a blood sugar value higher than 140 mg per dl is further evaluated by a full 100-gram, 3-hour glucose tolerance test. In some patients who are at especially high risk for developing diabetes, including those with obesity, polyhydramnios, or persistent glucosuria, the simple 1-hour screen, if initially negative, is repeated at 28 weeks.

Miscellaneous

At the completion of her first prenatal visit, the patient is given a prescription for vitamins. Any brand that provides at least 60 mg of elemental iron and 1 mg of folic acid is acceptable. We have also published our own patient information booklet, which each woman receives at her first visit. This has proved to be useful in answering questions in a more detailed fashion than is usually possible during an office visit.

SUBSEQUENT VISITS

Follow-up visits are scheduled every 4 weeks until 30 weeks, then every 2 weeks until 36 weeks, and finally weekly until delivery. At each visit, weight and blood pressure are checked and the urine is assayed for the presence of protein, sugar, nitrites, and leukocytes. Fundal height is measured and fetal heart tones are auscultated either with a Doppler instrument or, beginning at 18 weeks, with a fetoscope if desired. Leopold's maneuvers are performed starting at about 30 weeks to determine fetal lie. The patient is questioned at each visit regarding fetal movement, and any perception of significantly decreased movement is checked by sending her to the hospital antepartum testing center for a fetal nonstress test (NST) and/or biophysical profile (depending on gestational age at the time). This evaluation is performed without delay immediately on completion of her office visit. A simple finger stick hematocrit may be performed, if indicated, in the office. Patients who are Rh negative receive prophylactic antenatal RhoGAM at 28 weeks. It is also important to remember to use RhoGAM in Rh-negative women who miscarry or have other antepartum episodes of bleeding. Patients with risk factors for genetic disease as determined by their answers to our questionnaire (see Figure 2) are screened and counseled as appropriate. Manual pelvic examinations are repeated at 38 and 40 weeks to confirm fetal lie and station, to determine the condition of the cervix, and to review the capacity of the bony pelvis.

ROUTINE QUESTIONS

Nausea and Vomiting. Patients quite often experience nausea and vomiting during the first trimester. This problem usually clears spontaneously by 14 weeks. In the common milder cases, relief can be found in conservative measures. Some women do better the less they eat, whereas others require frequent small snacks to "keep something in the stomach." Even in more severe cases, most women can find a few types of food that they can tolerate. During this phase of nausea and vomiting, they are encouraged to eat whatever "stays down" instead of insisting on perfectly balanced meals that promptly "come back up"! An adequate fluid intake is also important, and many women find they can best tolerate carbonated beverages or Popsicles during this time. In severe cases we have had good results with promethazine (Phenergan) rectal suppositories. The benefits of bed rest in the management of hyperemesis are also often noteworthy. Patients who do not respond to these measures may require hospitalization and intravenous infusion of fluid and electrolytes as well as the use of parenteral antiemetics. Although we acknowledge a potential risk of some antiemetic drugs in the first trimester, this must be balanced by the known deleterious effects of weight loss, dehydration, ketone production, and electrolyte imbalance on the mother and fetus in severe cases of hyperemesis.

Diet. Total pregnancy weight gain should average between 20 and 30 pounds. We have not found it practical to expect patient adherence to detailed dietary plans containing specific numbers of calories, grams of protein or sodium, and so forth. Patients are simply allowed to eat as they normally do. However, some commonsense guidelines are offered. A diet that is low in fats and sweets while emphasizing complex carbohydrates, vegetables, and lean protein sources such as fish and poultry is encouraged. Salt intake should be neither augmented nor restricted. Women are cautioned against "eating for two." Such a practice often results in an impressive weight gain. Some obese patients ask about dieting during pregnancy. Although severe caloric restriction should be avoided, we have experienced good results with obese patients who enlist in a high-quality, well-supervised weight control program such as those offered either by our hospital or by other reputable plans (e.g., Weight Watchers). Such patients have maintained good weight control while still providing for normal fetal growth.

Exercise. During pregnancy, patients are allowed to continue essentially any type of exercise they regularly enjoy. Patients who do not already exercise are allowed and encouraged to begin a program of moderate exertion such as brisk walking, swimming, or bicycling. However, such patients are cautioned to avoid exertion to the point of breathlessness. Later in pregnancy, when increased weight and a shift in one's center of gravity affect coordination and balance, the patient is counseled to avoid sports that require these skills, particularly where injury is possible. Such sports might include skiing on snow or water, gymnastics, or basketball. Patients with pregnancy-induced hypertension, more than one fetus, fetal growth retardation, or certain other additional complications are advised not to exercise and are often kept at bed rest in the left lateral recumbent position.

Drugs. Use of any type of drug should be avoided if possible throughout pregnancy and especially during the first trimester. After the first trimester, we are somewhat more liberal in allowing patients to use mild therapeutic agents. For example, in our experience, moderate use of acetaminophen (Tylenol, Datril) has proved to be safe for relief of headaches and other mild pain. We prefer to avoid aspirin for simple pain relief at all stages of pregnancy because of its effect on the clotting mechanism. Various penicillins, nitrofurantoin (Macrodantin), and cephalosporins are thought to be safe and have caused no problems in our practice when used to treat urinary tract infections or respiratory illnesses. We avoid sulfa antibiotics during the third trimester when these drugs may compete with bilirubin for binding sites in the blood, which results in elevation of bilirubin levels in the newborn. Vaginal antimonilial agents are frequently prescribed with no complications. Our experience has also been good with mild over-the-counter antihistamines and decongestants. All recreational and addictive drugs, including marijuana and cocaine, should be strictly avoided. We do not use any form of progestogen in cases of threatened abortion.

Tobacco. Smoking is actively discouraged at all times but particularly so during pregnancy. Smoking is clearly associated with low-birthweight infants related to prematurity as well as to intrauterine growth retardation. Disadvantages to the offspring of smokers also persist into childhood in areas of development and performance. Health problems can also result during childhood from the secondhand smoke of the parent, and finally, children of smokers are more likely to smoke themselves. Patients should not be satisfied with merely reducing the number of cigarettes smoked because no amount of tobacco consumption is thought to be safe.

Alcohol. Our beliefs about alcohol consumption are similar to those about smoking. Rather than allow patients to use alcohol "in moderation" (which is open to anyone's interpretation and is often under-reported), we encourage women to abstain completely from the use of alcohol during their pregnancy. Heavy use of alcohol can result in fetal alcohol syndrome, including craniofacial abnormalities, prenatal and postnatal growth retardation, cardiovascular and limb defects, impaired motor function, and speech impairment.

Caffeine. An occasional caffeine-containing beverage is allowed. Our patients are encouraged to limit these to no more than one per day.

Employment. Healthy women with uncomplicated pregnancies are allowed to work during pregnancy. Adequate periods of rest are important.

Travel. In our experience, travel during the third trimester has been associated with many problems. These include, but are not limited to, premature labor, preterm rupture of membranes, development or worsening of pregnancy-induced hypertension, venous thrombosis, and vehicular accidents. When such complications occur, the patient often finds herself remote from appropriate facilities for care. Even if she obtains good-quality care, premature delivery far from home is a real possibility and poses tremendous financial and logistic obstacles. Our patients are strongly urged to avoid any travel beyond a 100-mile radius after 28 weeks.

Sexual Relations. In our experience, patients often ignore the counsel of their physician in this area. In addition to this finding, we also know of no compelling reason to prohibit sexual activity during normal pregnancy. However, patients are advised to avoid vaginal intercourse if they have any of the following conditions: threatened abortion, premature labor, known partial or complete placenta previa, or preterm rupture of membranes.

ULTRASOUND IN OBSTETRICS

The past decade has seen rapid advances in our ability to use ultrasound to evaluate the fetus and placenta. Because of its ability to visualize fetal movement, real-time obstetric ultrasonography has, in most centers, replaced static scanning. A report from the National Institutes for Health recently enumerated indications for diagnostic ultrasound, including verification of dates, exclusion of the possibility of twins, placental localization, amniotic fluid volume assessment, and search for fetal anomalies.

Dating the pregnancy is the most common indication for obstetric sonography. Measurements of fetal biparietal diameter, head circumference, abdominal circumference, and femur length and assessment of placental location and amniotic fluid volume, in addition to fetal presentation and a brief anatomic survey, are essential components of the basic dating examination. Such multiparameter evaluation allows more precise dating than older techniques based on biparietal diameter alone. In using such information clinically, it is important to keep in mind the uncertainty that accompanies any assessment of fetal age. This ranges from plus or minus several days in the first trimester to plus or minus 2 to 3 weeks in the third trimester. If a patient's menstrual dates fall within this range, it is in-

appropriate to change the dates based on the ultrasound examination. This principle is often ignored and may lead to clinical errors. For example, if the sonogram indicates a mean gestational age of 30 plus or minus 2 weeks, and the patient's menstrual age is 29 weeks, it is inappropriate to redate the patient to 30 weeks; rather, this examination is properly interpreted as confirming the patient's menstrual dates. In a similar manner, this uncertainty must be remembered when the patient has unknown menstrual dates and is dated solely on the basis of the ultrasound examination. For example, if a patient with no known date of last menstrual period received ultrasound dating of 28 plus or minus 2 weeks, she could be between 26 and 30 weeks. This has important implications for documenting fetal pulmonary maturity before consideration of elective delivery near term, and for the initiating of antepartum fetal testing for postdates when the patient *could* be in week 41 to 42 of pregnancy.

Patients at increased risk for fetal anomalies or those in whom an anomaly is detected should be referred to a center with experience in the diagnosis of fetal anomalies. In experienced hands, hundreds of conditions can be diagnosed as early as the middle of the second trimester. Knowledge of such conditions or their absence is often of great importance both in counseling parents and in planning proper prenatal care and fetal surveillance.

Should every pregnant patient receive a fetal ultrasound examination? This question remains controversial only in respect to the cost effectiveness of such a policy. It is clear that referring patients for ultrasound only for standard indications results in failure to detect some cases of twins, intrauterine growth retardation, fetal anomalies, amniotic fluid volume disturbances, and other clinically important conditions. Such a realization has led many authorities to recommend routine scanning for all pregnancies. In several European countries, universal scanning has been practiced for many years and has been demonstrated to be a cost-effective way of improving perinatal outcome. Although such a policy is often opposed by third-party payers in the United States and currently is not standard care in this country, there is little question that routine scanning will soon be a part of each woman's prenatal care in the United States. If a patient is to receive a routine ultrasound examination, a scan at 18 to 20 weeks not only will allow precise dating (provided multiple parameters are used) but will also allow the detection of many fetal anomalies that would otherwise be missed in a first trimester scan. Advocates of two screening examinations in every pregnancy recommend a second ultrasound scan at 32 to 34 weeks to detect intrauterine growth retardation.

PRENATAL DIAGNOSIS

High-resolution sonography and sophisticated amniotic fluid analysis have revolutionized our ability to diagnose fetal abnormalities before birth. Several categories of patients are candidates for genetic counseling and prenatal diagnosis. The most common indication for prenatal diagnosis is advanced maternal age because of its association with an increased risk of fetal trisomy. Standard care involves informing any woman who will be 35 years of age or older at the time of the birth of her child of her age-specific risk for trisomy and of the availability of genetic amniocentesis (Table 1). Patients with a family history of certain conditions such as Tay-Sachs disease, various hemoglobinopathies, or inborn errors of metabolism are also candidates for genetic counseling, and, in some circumstances, diagnostic amniocentesis. Parents who

TABLE 1. **Risk of Having a Live-Born Child with Chromosomal Abnormalities***

Maternal Age (yr)	Down's Syndrome	All Abnormalities Except 47,XXX
20	1/1923	1/526
21	1/1695	1/526
22	1/1538	1/500
23	1/1408	1/500
24	1/1299	1/476
25	1/1205	1/476
26	1/1124	1/478
27	1/1053	1/455
28	1/990	1/435
29	1/935	1/417
30	1/885	1/384
31	1/826	1/384
32	1/725	1/322
33	1/592	1/285
34	1/465	1/243
35	1/365	1/178
36	1/287	1/149
37	1/225	1/123
38	1/177	1/105
39	1/139	1/80
40	1/109	1/63
41	1/85	1/48
42	1/67	1/39
43	1/53	1/31
44	1/41	1/24
45	1/32	1/18
46	1/25	1/15
47	1/20	1/11
48	1/16	1/8
49	1/12	1/7

*From Simpson JL, Golbus MS, Martin AO, et al: Genetics in Obstetrics and Gynecology. New York, Grune & Stratton, 1982, p. 5B. Used by permission.

have previously had a child with a neural tube defect are also candidates for prenatal diagnostic evaluation. It has recently been demonstrated that assessment of maternal serum alpha-fetoprotein (MSAFP) between 16 and 20 weeks of gestation allows the detection of 80 to 90 per cent of open neural tube defects (high values) and up to 20 per cent of fetuses with trisomy 21 (low values). Further, abnormal MSAFP values often lead to the detection of twins or incorrect dates after an ultrasound examination. Thus every patient should be offered the option of MSAFP screening in the middle of the second trimester.

ANTEPARTUM ASSESSMENT OF FETAL WELL-BEING

The antepartum assessment of fetal well-being in high-risk patients is an important part of prenatal care. Throughout this decade the NST has become the most widespread technique for antepartum fetal surveillance. Although excellent results have been demonstrated with both the contraction stress test (CST) and the fetal biophysical profile, in most centers these tests are used principally as arbiters of an abnormal NST. Recently, several investigators have suggested improved perinatal outcome when the NST is supplemented with amniotic fluid volume assessment or Doppler umbilical flow measurements. Such modifications of the standard NST are now used in most academic centers in the United States. In interpreting such tests, several pitfalls must be avoided. First, the NST must be interpreted as reactive or nonreactive according to standard criteria. A reactive NST is defined as two accelerations of fetal heart rate lasting at least 15 seconds and peaking at 15 beats per minute above an established baseline, occurring within 10 or 20 minutes. "It looks OK" is not a proper interpretation and may lead to major clinical errors. For the CST, it is important to realize that a *negative* test requires three uterine contractions in 10 minutes without late decelerations. There are, however, no time criteria for a *positive* CST. A fetus subjected to one contraction an hour, and having a late deceleration with each contraction, has a positive CST. Recent definitions of positive have included a late deceleration with 50 per cent or more contractions. Although a reactive NST is always associated with a nonacidotic fetus, a nonreactive NST is usually also associated with fetal well-being. Thus, a nonreactive NST should be followed by a CST or biophysical profile to reduce unnecessary intervention. Recent investigations have focused on the use of fetal sound stimulation to reduce the rate of nonreactive NSTs, and on the significance of variable decelerations and simultaneous amniotic fluid volume assessment in reducing the present 2 or 3 per 1000 rate of antepartum demise that occurs in high-risk patients despite a reactive standard NST. Indications for antepartum fetal surveillance include postdates (beyond 41 weeks of gestation), maternal diabetes, previous stillbirth, decreased fetal movement, maternal hypertension, intrauterine growth retardation, and other conditions associated with an increased risk of antepartum fetal demise. If the NST is elected, it is best performed twice a week in fetuses beyond 41 weeks, in diabetics, and in premature fetuses with significant intrauterine growth retardation. Most other indications require weekly testing. However, specific clinical circumstances may dictate more or less frequent testing.

COMMON PRENATAL PROBLEMS

Anemia. A precise definition of anemia is difficult during pregnancy because a woman's hematocrit normally falls moderately, particularly during the second trimester. This reduction is caused by a relatively greater increase in plasma volume compared with red cell mass. However, a normal pregnant patient can still be expected to maintain a hematocrit above 30 per cent and a hemoglobin level above 10 grams per dl. Values less than these are considered to be evidence of anemia in our practice. The most common form of anemia during the prenatal course is that of iron deficiency. This anemia is somewhat more common in multiparous patients who may experience depletion of iron stores either from repeated fetal growth requirements or from blood loss during previous deliveries. Anemia is customarily presumed to be iron deficiency and is initially treated as such except in the black patient, in whom a sickle cell preparation should first be checked. Traditional microcytic and hypochromic findings on the complete blood count and peripheral smear are less pronounced in the pregnant patient unless anemia is severe. Treatment is with divided doses of oral ferrous sulfate in an amount sufficient to provide 150 mg daily of elemental iron. This amount is in addition to the 60 mg of elemental iron taken daily in the prenatal vitamin. If this treatment does not produce a satisfactory elevation of the hemoglobin or hematocrit value within 4 to 6 weeks, a more complete evaluation of the anemia is undertaken.

Diabetes Mellitus. The diabetic patient is seen earlier than our customary 10 menstrual weeks to begin prenatal care, as are most high-risk patients. In fact, the ideal situation would be to control a diabetic patient's blood sugar level be-

TABLE 2. **Three-Hour Glucose Tolerance Test Values***

Time	Value (mg/dl)
Fasting	105
After a 100-gram glucose challenge	
1 hr	190
2 hr	165
3 hr	145

*Modified from National Diabetes Data Group. Diabetes *28*:1039–1057, 1979. Reproduced with permission of the American Diabetes Association, Inc.

fore conception. If this is not possible, she is brought into the office as soon as pregnancy is diagnosed to begin careful control of blood sugar. In some cases, hospitalization may be required. As mentioned earlier, patients with any risk factor for diabetes are tested with a 50-gram, 1-hour blood sugar screen. We do not usually wait until 28 weeks to perform this screen, but rather do so during the early or middle second trimester (around 16 to 18 weeks). We believe that overtly diabetic patients thus diagnosed benefit from being treated earlier than 28 weeks. If suspicious findings are present or persist later into the pregnancy, we do not hesitate to repeat the screen. Patients with a screening blood sugar level higher than 140 mg per dl are further evaluated by a 100-gram, 3-hour glucose tolerance test. Our laboratory performs tests of plasma glucose levels; our normal limits are found in Table 2. Diabetics are classified according to the traditional White's scheme shown in Table 3. Class A (gestational or chemical) diabetes is diagnosed in women with normal fasting sugar tests who have elevation of two or more other values on the 3-hour oral glucose tolerance test. If repeated fasting sugar values are higher than 105 mg per dl, the gestational diabetic is classified as Class B. Class A patients are followed with routine prenatal care plus weekly fasting blood sugar checks. Studies have indicated no

TABLE 3. **White's Classification of Diabetes in Pregnancy***

Class	Age at Onset (yr)		Duration (yr)	Vascular Involvement
A	Any		Any	None
B	>20		<10	None
C	10–19	*or*	10–19	None
D	<10	*or*	>20	Benign retinopathy
F	Any		Any	Nephropathy
R	Any		Any	Proliferative retinopathy
H	Any		Any	Cardiac disease

*Modified from American College of Obstetricians and Gynecologists: Management of diabetes mellitus in pregnancy. ACOG Technical Bulletin 92. Washington, DC: ACOG, 1986:2.

greater risk of antepartum fetal loss in this group of patients. The only other exception to otherwise normal prenatal care in the Class A patient is that "postdates" fetal testing is begun at 40 weeks by performing weekly NSTs combined with sonographic determination of amniotic fluid volume. Patients with a "ripe" cervix are induced at 40 weeks. No Class A diabetic is allowed to exceed 42 weeks of gestation. Class A patients with preeclampsia or a previous stillbirth receive antepartum fetal heart rate testing beginning no later than 32 weeks. Overtly diabetic patients (Class B and beyond) are seen in the office frequently throughout the entire prenatal course. At each visit, standard prenatal care is conducted and blood sugar levels are reviewed with insulin adjustments as required. Most of our patients do well on a combination of NPH (or Lente Insulin) and regular insulin with the total daily dose divided into morning and evening injections. Occasionally, the continuous infusion insulin pump has been used. Blood sugar levels are monitored at home by the patient using a finger stick monitor system four times daily: morning fasting, before lunch, before dinner, and bedtime, for example, 7:00 a.m., 11:00 a.m., 4:00 p.m., and 9:00 p.m. The patient maintains a log book of blood sugar values that she brings to her weekly office visit. The goal is to keep all four daily blood sugar levels under 100 mg per dl. In a well-controlled patient, twice weekly fetal antepartum testing is begun at 32 weeks. In patients who are not well controlled, antepartum testing is begun as early as 28 weeks. If the fetus remains reactive and the patient's diabetes remains well controlled, amniocentesis for fetal pulmonary maturity is performed at 37 to 38 weeks when the cervix is favorable for induction, and delivery is accomplished if phosphatidylglycerol is present. Usually, fetal pulmonary maturity is achieved somewhat before 40 weeks, and overt insulin-dependent diabetics are not allowed to go beyond their expected date of confinement.

Hypertensive Disorders. Hypertension is defined as a systolic pressure of at least 140 mmHg or a diastolic pressure of at least 90 mmHg or a rise of at least 30 mmHg systolic or 15 mmHg diastolic on two separate occasions at least 6 hours apart. If such findings occur before 20 weeks of gestation in the absence of gestational trophoblastic disease, the patient is considered to have chronic hypertension. Occurrence after 20 weeks is considered to be pregnancy-induced hypertension. If significant proteinuria or generalized edema accompanies the rise in blood pressure, the diagnosis is pre-eclampsia. Eclampsia is the occurrence of convulsions in a patient with pre-eclampsia. A patient with chronic hypertension may develop superimposed pre-eclampsia or eclampsia during pregnancy. Pre-eclampsia is considered to be severe if any one of the following conditions is present: diastolic pressure more than 110 mmHg; proteinuria more than 2 + persistent headache or visual disturbances; raised liver function values; decreased platelet count; decreased renal function (oliguria or abnormally low creatinine clearance); epigastric pain; or fetal growth retardation. Pre-eclampsia is usually more common in the nulliparous patient, particularly those at either end of the reproductive age spectrum. Patients with pre-existing chronic hypertension or renal disease are likewise at higher risk, as are those with any condition that tends to increase the total placental mass such as gestational trophoblastic disease, diabetes, erythroblastosis, or multiple fetuses. Patients with a family history of pre-eclampsia may also be at higher risk. Patients with minor elevations of blood pressure who do not meet the diagnostic criteria of severe pre-eclampsia may be treated conservatively at home. They are placed at bed rest in the left lateral recumbent position for most of the day and are seen in the office two or three times weekly. Such patients must be reliable and their condition must be monitored carefully. If a patient becomes overtly pre-eclamptic, immediate hospitalization is often advisable. Under certain conditions, patients with mild pre-eclampsia before term may be cautiously managed as outpatients. We rely on the guidelines set forth in the American College of Obstetrics and Gynecology's Technical Bulletin No. 91 for such management. However, if signs and symptoms of pre-eclampsia progress, the pregnancy is terminated.

Postdates Pregnancy. The appropriate management of postdates pregnancies depends heavily on the accuracy of each patient's due date. Thus the importance of accurate dating of every pregnancy cannot be overstated. This dating should be accomplished within the first 20 weeks of gestation. Ultrasound dating gradually becomes less accurate as pregnancy advances. If dates are reliable, we begin evaluation of the fetus at 41 completed weeks of gestation with twice weekly NSTs and amniotic fluid volume assessments. However, if the cervix is favorable for induction, the baby is simply delivered at that time. Sonographic evaluation of amniotic fluid is important to detect developing oligohydramnios as well as variable decelerations (often indicative of cord compromise), which may be seen somewhat more frequently in the postdates patient. At 42 completed weeks, most patients have delivery induced. However, with close monitoring (twice weekly fetal surveillance as outlined), an occasional patient may be followed to 43 weeks if the condition of the cervix is hopeless. No patient is allowed to continue beyond that point. We have had good results with the use of prostaglandin gel applied within the cervical canal to "ripen" the unfavorable cervix before actual induction.

ABORTION

method of
WILLIAM D. WALDEN, M.D.
Cornell University Medical College
New York, New York

CLASSIFICATION

Early first trimester—from the first day of the last *normal* menstrual period through the eighth week. Simple suction evacuation is most appropriate. No fetal parts are recognizable yet; the best correlation with duration of gestation is measurement of tissue volume.

Late first trimester—9 through 12 weeks. Small fetal parts are revealed on close inspection. The appropriate procedure is suction evacuation followed by sharp curettage when necessary to check for retained tissue or uterine anomalies.

Early second trimester—13 through 16 weeks. Termination either involves removal of the fetus by the D & E (dilatation and evacuation) method or expulsion of the intact fetus by initiating labor with prostaglandin vaginal suppositories.

Late second trimester—17 through 24 weeks. Pregnancy may be terminated by the D & E method, the intra-amniotic instillation of abortifacient agents, or the use of prostaglandin vaginal suppositories. Methods involving the expulsion of the intact fetus are preferred when autopsy or genetic studies are needed. It should be emphasized that the D & E procedures should be performed only by the most skilled and experienced operator.

DIAGNOSIS

The new urine or serum pregnancy tests can detect human chorionic gonadotropin (hCG) at the time of a missed menstrual period or anytime thereafter. If a test is positive prior to the missed period, evacuation of the uterus should be delayed to ensure removal of adequate volume of tissue for examination. These judgments must be correlated with a careful pelvic examination to ensure that the patient did not miscalculate her last menstrual period. A quantitative beta subunit serum test should be performed to verify an initial negative test, suspected ectopic pregnancy, or missed abortion. Serum hCG levels double approximately every $2\frac{1}{2}$ days in early intact viable pregnancies; therefore, a repeat test a few days later is necessary to verify a rise or fall in hCG levels.

Pelvic ultrasonography has its limitations in very early pregnancy; however, a fetal sac is usually seen 6 weeks after the last period. At this time the serum hCG levels should be above 5000 mIU per ml. Between 8 and 9 weeks fetal heart activity can be detected.

Office pregnancy tests with a sensitivity of less than 50 mIU per ml on *random* urine samples (not morning urine) are now readily available. Two such tests are the Abbott TESTPACK hCG urine (Abbott Laboratories, North Chicago, Il. 60064) and the Access ICON pregnancy test (Access Medical Systems, Inc., Branford, Ct. 06405).

Each patient should receive counseling and detailed information regarding the procedure in a nonjudgmental atmosphere. The patient should be told that the suction method will enhance her fertility and that the rhythm and withdrawal method of contraception will fail and lead to another pregnancy. In my practice information regarding the "morning-after pill" is given to the patient to avoid a similar situation in the future. It is emphasized, however, that this method of pregnancy prevention is *not* a method to be used for routine contraception but only to prevent an inevitable unwanted pregnancy due to contraceptive failure or accident. The medication must be taken *within 36 hours* after unprotected intercourse. Conjugated estrogen (Premarin*), 2.5 mg four times a day for 5 days, is most effective. Prior to prescription of the "morning-after pill" the patient must understand the potential for fetal damage and agree to have an abortion if the medication fails. Once the medication is taken, the next menstrual period should occur at approximately the expected time. It is good practice to tell the patient to inform her doctor when she gets her next period or if she misses her period. In that case, an immediate pregnancy test should be performed and if found to be positive, a termination of that pregnancy should be scheduled.

FIRST TRIMESTER ABORTION

Most patients with proper psychologic support will do well with local paracervical block anesthesia combined with diazepam (Valium), 5 to 10 mg intravenously. Local is preferred to general anesthesia because there is less bleeding and less risk of major anesthetic complications.

After the preliminary pregnancy testing, counseling, pelvic examination, and blood studies (hematocrit and blood type) have been performed, diazepam (Valium) is injected intravenously slowly. The effect of the medication is immediate in relaxing the patient.

The preferred instrument for exposure is the *small* Graves's speculum. The shorter blades on this instrument permit appropriate traction on the uterus, thereby permitting the fundal cavity to be straightened. This in turn provides relatively easy access with dilators and suction cannula and minimizes the possibility of inadvertent perforation. The medium-sized and large specula

---

*This use is not listed by the manufacturer.

should be used only on extremely obese patients in whom visualization of the cervix would be impossible with the smaller instrument.

After the speculum is in place, povidone-iodine (Betadine) solution is poured into the vagina, which is then thoroughly swabbed dry with sterile 4 × 4 inch gauze. A sterile drape under the patient is sufficient for placement of the instruments.

The next step involves injecting a 2-ml dose of 1 per cent lidocaine *without* epinephrine submucosally on the anterior lip of the cervix at the site of attachment of the single-toothed tenaculum. The patient will describe a "pulling feeling" as traction is applied but no pain from the bite of the instrument. Vertical application is preferred to the traditional horizontal position because bleeding will be minimal should the tenaculum tear through the cervix. With a retroverted uterus, application on the posterior lip of the cervix not only serves as a reminder of the position of the cavity but also minimizes the risk of perforation by not tenting the anterior lower uterine segment as the dilators are inserted posteriorly. Off-center application (at 11 o'clock on the anterior lip or 7 o'clock on the posterior lip of the cervix for right-handed operators holding the tenaculum in the left hand) permits easier access through the external os with dilators and curettes.

Completion of the cervical block is accomplished with a 10-ml disposable syringe with a 1½-inch, No. 22 needle. Longer needles are absolutely not necessary and can result in intravascular injection with symptoms of mild systemic toxicity with circumoral paresthesias, voices sounding more distant, and a feeling of fearfulness. With an extremely anxious patient, manipulations during the procedure may cause a vasovagal reaction with momentary loss of consciousness. The treatment is simple—stop the procedure temporarily and elevate the patient's legs 45 degrees. She will regain consciousness almost immediately. This reaction is uncommon, and when it occurs the operator should not overreact by giving unnecessary drugs. Once the patient is awake the procedure may be completed.

Injecting the cervix submucosally at the 2, 5, 7, and 10 o'clock positions should produce a distinct wheal that blanches the cervical mucosa from the original pink to white. Occasionally after completion of the block a patient may still feel excessive pain during dilatation. In such cases an extra 5 ml of lidocaine is injected submucosally within the length of the endocervical canal at 3 and 9 o'clock. This usually eliminates the sensation of instrumentation within the cervix.

Pratt's dilators are the instruments of choice because of their long, tapered, balanced structure. Hegar's dilators should *not* be used in abortion procedures because they are blunt-ended instruments requiring more force during insertion, which can lead to cervical tears and uterine perforation. Pratt's dilator is held with the thumb and third finger, and the little finger is held out and braced against the patient's buttock in order to avoid use of excessive, uncontrolled force. Firm traction on the tenaculum with the operator's opposite hand is essential to perceive the resistance of the internal os. The tenaculum should never be held by a first assistant, since this eliminates all sense of touch for the operator. *Laminaria* is not used in the first trimester.

The use of a metal sound to measure cavity depth is hazardous in a pregnant uterus and can only increase the risk of perforation. The appropriate-sized cannula with centimeter markings etched in the plastic should be gently inserted into the uterine cavity initially without the tubing attached. The cannula used in this way acts as a sound for determining uterine depth, which is far safer than a metal sound. A reliable formula for nulliparous patients is

$$\text{Cavity depth (cm)} - 2 = \text{no. weeks}$$
from last menstrual period

Example: Uterus sounds to 10 cm
minus 2 = 8 weeks

The choice of the flexible Karmen cannula or the rigid cannula of Berkeley design is based on the operator's preference and experience. Many prefer the flexible cannula for early first trimester abortions and choose the rigid cannula for those from 9 through 12 weeks. Once the appropriate-sized cannula is in place, the tubing is connected and the aspirator is turned on. Specifically designed machines for abortions provide suction pressure between 500 and 750 mmHg. The cannula should be rotated 360 degrees within the uterine cavity to cover all surfaces and periodically withdrawn from the cavity to prevent plugging. With the flexible cannula the proximal opening provides the most effective suction and the distal opening acts as a curette. Special attention should be given to ensure that the proximal opening covers all surfaces within the uterus. An occasional complication with the flexible cannula is the breaking off of the suction tip. Tip inspection should be routine, and if it has broken off it can be retrieved with a curette. Once the uterus has contracted a smaller-diameter cannula may be used to complete the procedure. Occasionally one may misjudge the initial size of the cavity and need to step up to a larger size to evacuate the uterus quickly and efficiently. For example, one may start with a No. 6 flexible cannula and find that one needs a No. 7; then, when the contents have been removed, the operator may return to a No. 6 cannula to ensure that all the tissue is out and the fundus is well contracted. The decision whether to use a sharp curette is based on the operator's experience. With increasing experience the use of the sharp curette diminishes. When it is used, the operator should avoid overzealous curetting to prevent postabortal amenorrhea and/or Asherman's syndrome.

The usual duration of applied suction is less than 2 minutes and it is during this time that the patient may experience the most severe cramps. The cervical block does not usually relieve the cramping sensations of the contracting uterus. Patients who have cramps during menstruation will also experience cramps with an abortion procedure.

First trimester terminations with local anesthesia do not require continuous intravenous therapy, or routine use of oxytocin (Pitocin) or ergonovine maleate (Ergotrate). Routine prophylactic antibiotics are not used. In patients with cardiac problems such as mitral valve prolapse or a history of endocarditis, prophylaxis with antibiotics is indicated as recommended by the American Heart Association.

Postoperatively the patient is allowed to rest and is given appropriate analgesic medication either by mouth or by injection to relieve cramping. For mild cramps ibuprofen (Motrin) or its equivalent is adequate. Some patients prefer acetaminophen with codeine phosphate (Tylenol with Codeine No. 3). Patients with severe postabortal cramping need an intramuscular analgesic. My preference is nalbuphine hydrochloride (Nubain), 3 to 4 mg* intramuscularly. An ice bag on the lower abdomen also helps to reduce the discomfort of uterine cramps. Within 10 to 15 minutes all cramps have dramatically subsided. Vital signs are checked, and if the patient is Rh negative and unsensitized, she receives anti-D immune globulin (MiniRhoGAM) intramuscularly. The minidose is used for first trimester terminations only. The usual postoperative recovery time is 40 to 60 minutes.

Prior to discharge the patient's chart should be checked to ensure that written consent for the procedure was obtained.

Written postoperative instructions should include

1. Telephone number to call in case of emergency.
2. Shower only—no baths for at least 5 days.
3. Use ice bag on stomach for 1 hour at a time to control bleeding or to relieve cramping.
4. Avoid sexual activity, douching, tampons, and strenuous exercise like jogging for about 10 days.
5. Next menstrual period should occur in 4 to 6 weeks. If no bleeding occurs by the seventh week, notify your doctor.
6. Use a thermometer to check your temperature if necessary. If there is a temperature over 101° F or heavy bleeding or severe cramping, notify your doctor.
7. No alcoholic beverages today because of Valium injection!

During the patient's recovery period the tissue should be examined after it is removed from the suction bottle. All tissue is sent to the laboratory after inspection. Prior to 9 weeks only tissue volume can provide information regarding duration of gestation. Although volume may fluctuate over a wide range, an easy rule of thumb is

> 5 to 6 weeks—average volume 7 ml
> 7 to 8 weeks—average volume 14 ml
> 9 to 10 weeks—average volume 21 ml

After 9 weeks identification of fetal parts provides information as to length of gestation.

If no tissue is obtained after inspecting the suction bottle, the following six conditions must be considered:

1. False passage created by overzealous dilatation of a stenotic cervix. Avoidance of forceful dilatation reduces the likelihood of this complication. Mechanical devices to dilate the cervix have no place in this procedure.
2. A nonpregnant uterus with a false-positive pregnancy test.
3. Ectopic pregnancy. Scanty decidual tissue with a volume that does not correlate with the history. A quantitative beta subunit serum test is indicated and should be repeated a few days later.
4. Excessive size for dates. In such a case no tissue may be obtained since the suction tip is too small for tissue retrieval. An error in judgment can occur on pelvic examination with a very obese patient, especially when the abdominal hand is below the fundus in a second trimester pregnancy. Obviously the reported date of last menstruation is completely wrong.
5. Uterine perforation, most commonly occurring in the severely anteverted or retroflexed uterus.

---

*This dose is lower than that recommended by the manufacturer (8 to 10 mg).

6. Anomalous uterus (incidence 12 per cent). A septate uterus should be considered after the preceding five conditions have been ruled out. A curette is used to evaluate the anomaly. In rare cases, a uterine didelphys—a double vagina, cervix, and uterus—may be missed since the speculum may compress the septum and hide the second vaginal opening. This is another reason for using the *small* Graves's speculum. Once this condition is discovered, suctioning of each cavity is necessary using separate sterile instruments for each cavity to prevent possible cross-contamination with different cervical bacterial flora.

SECOND TRIMESTER ABORTION

Ten per cent of all women seeking pregnancy termination in the United States fall in the second trimester group. A special category exists with women who have received unfavorable reports from genetic studies obtained by amniocentesis. For this group the methods involving expulsion of the intact fetus are preferred in order to perform genetic studies on the fetus. Dinoprost tromethamine (Prostin F_2 Alpha) is administered intra-amniotically or dinoprostone (Prostin E_2) is administered intravaginally to stimulate the myometrium of the gravid uterus to contract in a manner similar to that seen in the term uterus during labor. The first medication can be used only between the sixteenth and twentieth weeks of gestation as calculated from the first day of the last normal menstrual period. The vaginal suppositories may be administered from the twelfth through the twentieth gestational week. In addition, they may be used to evacuate the uterine contents in the management of missed abortion or intrauterine fetal death up to 28 weeks of gestation. Both medications are potent oxytocic agents and should be administered only in a hospital by trained medical personnel. Intensive care and acute surgical facilities should be available. Contraindications include hypersensitivity to the drug, acute pelvic inflammatory disease, and active cardiac, pulmonary, renal, or hepatic disease. Caution is advised with patients with a history of asthma, hypotension or hypertension, anemia, jaundice, or epilepsy. Vaginal suppositories have a greater tendency to produce a transient pyrexia that may be due to its effect on hypothalamic thermoregulation. The onset is within 15 to 45 minutes of suppository administration. The elevations revert to pretreatment levels within 2 to 6 hours after discontinuation of therapy.

Prior to initiating therapy, diphenoxylate hydrochloride with atropine (Lomotil), four tablets, is given to reduce the tendency to diarrhea. Also prochlorperazine (Compazine), 10 mg intramuscularly, is given to reduce the tendency to vomit. The suppositories are administered intravaginally every 2 hours. Fifty units of oxytocin is added to 1000 ml of lactated Ringer's solution 6 hours after the initial insertion. After a latent period of 6 to 8 hours without uterine contractions the patient begins to experience increasing uterine contractions. Demerol may be used in small doses (25 to 50 mg) intramuscularly to ease the discomfort. Labor must be allowed to continue until expulsion of the fetus occurs into a bedpan. The total time from start to finish can vary from 6 to 27 hours. The average is 12 hours. The placenta is not always expelled with the fetus. It is imperative that the physician be informed immediately that expulsion has occurred, and preferably the physician should be present at the time of expulsion. The patient should be examined without delay and removal of the placenta accomplished by fundal pressure with a medium-sized Graves's speculum in place in the vagina. Sponge forceps may be necessary to assist in the removal of the placental tissue from the external os. Bleeding is minimal when the placenta is removed as soon as possible after expulsion. No benefit is gained by waiting. The patient is then returned to her bed. The oxytocin dosage is reduced to 20 units in 1000 ml of lactated Ringer's solution and kept running at approximately 1 ml per minute until the next morning. The patient is discharged the following day with the same postabortal instructions as listed earlier. A follow-up visit within 10 days is scheduled. RhoGAM if indicated is given prior to discharge.

The D & E procedure is the most common method of midtrimester abortion in the United States, with labor-inducing techniques accounting for most of the remainder. The more advanced the gestation, the greater is the potential for complications such as excessive bleeding and uterine perforation. Only the most experienced physician should perform these procedures.

Since the D & E procedure requires extracting large fetal parts, it is essential that the cervix be adequately dilated by placement of multiple *Laminaria* tents within the cervical canal 12 to 24 hours prior to the procedure. After insertion, the vagina is packed loosely with two 4 × 4 inch Betadine-soaked sponges. With the use of *Laminaria,* prophylactic antibiotics are given orally, usually tetracycline 500 mg four times per day for 7 days. The seaweed in the Japanese Mizutani disposable *Laminaria* is superior to other products. It is thinner, thus permitting easier insertion into a stenotic cervix. It also swells to as much as 10 times its original diameter. Precautions when using *Laminaria* are summarized in Table 1.

TABLE 1. **Precautions for Use of *Laminaria***

Do Not
— force insertion of *Laminaria*
— insert *Laminaria* into a purulent cervix
— leave in place more than 24 hr
Do
— instruct patient *not* to douche or have intercourse with *Laminaria* in place
— reassure patient that slight bleeding and cramping are normal
— allow patient to lie recumbent for 10 to 15 min following insertion; this may prevent vertigo, weakness, or syncope

All second trimester cases should be evaluated as to fetal size by ultrasonography. On the day of surgery, general anesthesia is preferred. Some important points are

1. A pelvic examination should be performed with the patient under anesthesia.

2. A weighted speculum is preferred to a Graves's speculum in those cases that are over 16 weeks.

3. The *Laminaria* tents are removed with a sponge stick and *counted*.

4. Thorough preparation of the vagina with Betadine is necessary.

5. A sponge forceps is attached to the anterior lip of the cervix; a tenaculum should not be used.

6. The cervix should be evaluated as to adequacy of dilatation by the *Laminaria*. Inadequate dilatation is due to placement of the *Laminaria* below the internal os. For early second trimester cases the use of large Pratt's dilators may be sufficient for additional cervical dilatation.

7. The membranes must be ruptured prior to suction. Any instrument may be used to rupture membranes. Once rupture has occurred, suction with a No. 12 or No. 14 Berkeley cannula should be started only to remove the amniotic fluid at this time (to prevent amniotic fluid embolism). Suctioning should be brief at this point, since one wants to *avoid removing the placenta first by suction*. This is to prevent premature contraction of the uterus and trapping of the fetal parts.

8. Once the amniotic fluid has been drained as much as possible by gentle suction, the Bierer forceps or similar instrument should be gently inserted into the uterine cavity to grasp the fetal parts and extract them. Oxytocin and ergonovine maleate should be withheld until the cranium, spine, rib cage, and all four limbs have been identified.

9. The placenta may be removed by use of suction and curettage after all the fetal parts are out. At this point oxytocin may be added to the intravenous solution and ergonovine maleate, 0.2 mg, given intramuscularly. Estimated blood loss may vary from 300 to 1500 ml.

10. The physician should avoid premature removal of the placenta and premature administration of oxytocic medications, which can cause trapping of the fetal parts.

Postoperatively the patient is observed and cared for as with first trimester cases. The recovery from general anesthesia will be prolonged as compared with recovery from local anesthesia.

The saline method utilizing 20 per cent sodium chloride by transabdominal intra-amniotic injection induces fetal death and is preferred in the late second trimester cases beyond 20 weeks. Hypertonic saline generally causes fewer adverse side effects than prostaglandins; however, the induction interval is much longer. In addition, there is a higher risk of serious complications such as tissue necrosis, infection, defibrination, and hypernatremia.

COMPLICATIONS AND THEIR MANAGEMENT

The postabortal syndrome occurs in approximately 1 in 300 cases. The patient begins complaining of severe uterine pain and cramps, usually within an hour or two following an abortion. Examination reveals a tender midline mass extending two to three fingerbreadths above the symphysis that cannot be relieved either by voiding or by catheterization. Rebound tenderness and guarding may lead one to suspect an acute abdomen and to conclude that surgical intervention is necessary. The correct treatment, however, is immediate resuctioning, which results in the removal of 50 to 400 ml of dark blood and clots with no tissue. This procedure brings immediate relief, and ergonovine maleate, 0.2 mg given orally every 4 hours for six doses, should prevent recurrence of the symptoms. A milder form of this syndrome, which may be delayed for as long as 7 days, is frequently associated with a severely retroflexed uterus. Again, resuctioning leads to a dramatic recovery.

Postabortal amenorrhea is more common than the above complication. Cramping occurs at the time of the expected next menses, but there is no sign of blood. The treatment is simple. Probing the cervix either with a No. 5 Karmen cannula or with a plastic disposable uterine sound will open an internal os in which stenosis occurred secondary to trauma of the aspiration. Once the os is open, dark blood will ooze forth, which represents a menstrual period. Cramping subsides almost instantly.

Delayed complications such as retained placental products, postabortal bleeding, fever, and pelvic infection are all managed by re-exploring and emptying the uterine cavity. Ampicillin by mouth

TABLE 2. Clinical Classification and Treatment of Uterine Perforation During Abortion*

Clinical Classification	Treatment
A. *Immediate recognition with cessation of the procedure* (suspected or actual perforation by any instrument including suction cannula *with no suction applied*)	
1. *Completed abortion.* Perforation after contents of uterus completely evacuated.	In-hospital observation of clinical status, serial complete blood counts for at least 48 hr.
2. *Intact sac.* Gestation undisturbed.	As above, then readmit in about 2 wk for repeat surgical evacuation.
	Immediate diagnostic laparoscopy.
3. *Incomplete abortion.* Perforation occurs during evacuation; uterus partially emptied.	Laparotomy and repair if needed. Completion of abortion, either transcervically under laparoscopic observation or, if laparotomy, via uterine rent if transcervical approach inappropriate.
B. *Delayed recognition after operative manipulation* (suction or curettage). No abdominal contents identified. Uterine evacuation may have been attempted before possible perforation was recognized.	All require immediate diagnostic laparoscopy with laparotomy if indicated (bowel trauma, uncontrolled bleeding, etc.).
1. *Completed abortion*	
2. *Intact sac*	
3. *Incomplete abortion*	B.2, B.3: Abortion may be completed as in case A.3.
C. *Perforation with identification of abdominal contents* (bowel, omentum, fat, etc.)	All require immediate laparotomy and surgical repair as needed.
1. *Completed abortion*	
2. *Intact sac*	C.2, C.3: Abortion may be completed as in case A.3.
3. *Incomplete abortion*	

*Adapted from Walden W and Birnbaum S: Contemp Obstet Gynecol 15:47, 1980. Used with permission.

as initial therapy usually is effective. However, failure to respond in 24 hours may require hospitalization and parenteral antibiotics.

Uterine perforation, the most serious complication of either first or second trimester procedures, must be evaluated when one of the following occurs:

1. The stenotic cervix, most commonly seen in very early pregnancy. *Correction:* Firm pressure with a No. 5 Karmen cannula with good countertraction will invariably dilate the cervix, and the flexible cannula will find its way through the cervical canal without the risk of creating a false passage.

2. Physical interference by the weighted posterior vaginal speculum in first trimester cases. *Correction:* Remove and replace with a *small* Graves's speculum. Since it is mobile it cannot interfere with placement of the dilators.

3. The acutely anteverted uterus or retroflexed uterus. *Correction:* Direct the dilators in the correct direction with good traction on the cervix.

4. Inappropriate use of the metal sound. *Correction:* Substitute the cannula as a sound with appropriate centimeter markings.

5. Overzealous suction with the rigid Berkeley cannula. *Correction:* Make allowances for the shortening of the uterine cavity as it empties.

6. Improper selection of the suction tip, using one far too big for the size of the uterus. *Correction:* Re-evaluate using a smaller cannula.

7. Broken tip on the Karmen cannula. *Correction:* Inspect all tips after each withdrawal from the uterine cavity.

8. Unanticipated shortening of the uterine cavity. *Correction:* Avoid forcing the cannula to its original depth on repeated suctioning.

9. Miduterine stenosis. *Correction:* Be gentle and use a smaller cannula to pass through the stenotic area to obtain a true sounding of the cavity. Proceed with caution.

10. Improper use of the sharp curette. *Correction:* Do not force into the uterine cavity.

Table 2 summarizes the management of uterine perforation. The classification is concerned with assessing potential maternal injury and pregnancy status. It can be a useful guide to therapy, particularly in centers where many physicians with varied experience and training perform this operation. It can also help in evaluating patients transferred to hospitals from outpatient facilities.

ECTOPIC PREGNANCY

method of
PHILLIP C. GALLE, M.D.
Southern Illinois University School of Medicine
Springfield, Illinois

An ectopic pregnancy is a pregnancy that has not become implanted in the fundus of the uterus. It can be located in the fallopian tube, abdomen, cervix, or ovary. Most ectopic pregnancies are located in the tube, usually in the ampullary portion. Women with a history of pelvic inflammatory disease are at high risk for ectopic pregnancy. Pregnant women who have had a tubal ligation have a higher incidence of ectopic pregnancy. In a series of women who became pregnant with an intrauterine device in place, the incidence of ectopic pregnancy was 4 to 9 per cent. In women who have had an ectopic pregnancy, the risk of a subsequent ectopic pregnancy is approximately 10 to 15 per cent. There are sufficient data to show that with conservative treatment, the rate of women with subsequent ectopic pregnancy does not differ from the rate of those who undergo salpingectomy. Previous abdominal or tubal surgery, such as tubal anastomosis, fimbriolysis, or neosalpingostomy, is associated with an increased rate of ectopic pregnancy. The rate is approximately 8 to 10 per cent, similar to that in women who have had a previous ectopic pregnancy.

Ectopic pregnancy remains an important obstetric emergency, and its incidence is increasing. The incidence is 1 to 1.5 per cent in a normal population. The treatment of ectopic pregnancies has changed because more of them can be diagnosed before tubal rupture. A high index of clinical suspicion, more sensitive pregnancy tests, and high-resolution ultrasound aid in early diagnosis. Early diagnosis, in turn, can affect the type of treatment and enable more conservative treatment.

PRESENTATION

The clinical presentation depends on whether the tube is ruptured or unruptured. The classic symptoms of an acutely ruptured extrauterine pregnancy are severe abdominal pain, hematoperitoneum, and hemorrhagic shock. The classic triad of clinical symptoms is pain, amenorrhea, and vaginal bleeding. The typical patient presents with unilateral lower abdominal pain with rebound tenderness. On pelvic examination there is a unilateral tender adnexal mass, and the uterus is normal in size or slightly enlarged and soft.

In patients who are followed closely, the diagnosis can often be made before tubal rupture and before the development of typical symptoms. Patients who are at high risk should be counseled before pregnancy so that early diagnosis and close follow-up are possible. They should be advised that during pregnancy certain symptoms must be reported to their physician. These symptoms include vaginal bleeding, abdominal pain, dizziness, or syncope. At the same time, couples need reassurance so that they are not overly concerned. They can be reassured that bleeding is not always associated with a bad outcome, but that when bleeding occurs, it may indicate that additional tests and follow-up are necessary. It is also helpful to inform high-risk patients that they need not be overly alarmed because the incidence of an intrauterine pregnancy after a previous ectopic pregnancy is 85 per cent or greater.

Patients with an ectopic pregnancy commonly fall into one of two categories. In one category, the pregnancy is diagnosed in the office or emergency room, and the patient has clinical signs or symptoms suggestive of an ectopic pregnancy. In the other category are patients who have been followed early in pregnancy and who have remained asymptomatic. In the former category, one must diagnose the pregnancy and then confirm or rule out an ectopic pregnancy; in the latter category, the diagnosis of pregnancy has been established.

DIAGNOSIS

The key to management of the patient with an ectopic pregnancy is early diagnosis. Earlier diagnosis is possible because of more sensitive pregnancy tests, ultrasound scans with better resolution, and laparoscopy. In patients presenting with symptoms, the first step is to confirm or exclude the diagnosis of pregnancy. Greater sensitivity is obtained when using pregnancy tests that are specific for the beta subunit of human chorionic gonadotropin (hCG). The sensitivity of most serum radioimmunoassay pregnancy tests ranges from 3 to 20 mIU per ml. This results in diagnosing 96 to 100 per cent of ectopic pregnancies. For clinical purposes, a negative serum radioimmunoassay pregnancy test excludes the possibility of an ectopic pregnancy.

In women who have a positive pregnancy test, early detection of an ectopic pregnancy presents a clinical challenge. Definitive diagnosis is usually made or confirmed by laparoscopy. Early diagnosis is valuable in prevention of tubal rupture and hemorrhage and in improvement of reproductive potential. However, in women with an intrauterine pregnancy, it is preferable to avoid fetal exposure to the risks of laparoscopy and general anesthesia.

With the use of ultrasound and quantitative values of hCG, one can diagnose ectopic pregnancy earlier: A level of hCG is sought that discriminates ectopic from intrauterine pregnancy. The discriminatory hCG zone is defined as the hCG level that distinguishes patients with intrauterine pregnancy in whom a gestational sac can be seen by gray scale or real-time ultrasound from those in whom it cannot be visualized. A value of 6500 mIU per ml (first International Reference Preparation) is defined as the discriminatory zone. To avoid confusion, two standards have been used for quantitative hCG levels: the First International Reference Preparation and the Second International Standard. The hCG values obtained with the first preparation are double those obtained with the second. The hCG values in the following discussion refer to the First International Reference Preparation. With a serum hCG level of 6500 mIU per ml, most patients with a normal intrauterine pregnancy (96 per cent) have a gestational sac. In the absence of a sac at this hCG level, the incidence of ectopic pregnancy is 86 per cent. The absence of a sac does not completely rule out a normal intrauterine pregnancy when the hCG level is above 6500 mIU per ml.

A frequent clinical problem concerns patients who present with an initial hCG titer below 6500 mIU per ml and are either at high risk and asymptomatic or have minimal symptoms that do not necessitate immediate surgical intervention. In normal pregnancy hCG titers increase with advancing age during the first trimester, with some variability in the doubling time; however, the doubling time is approximately 2 days. In ectopic pregnancy, hCG levels are often lower, and the doubling time is increased slightly. When serial hCG titers are evaluated, the accuracy in diagnosing ectopic pregnancy is increased. If the hCG titer plateaus or decreases on serial measurements, the pregnancy is clearly abnormal. To increase the accuracy of diagnosing ectopic pregnancy, high-risk patients are followed by measuring the rate at which the serum hCG level is increasing rather than by correlating the hCG level with the gestational age. One method of comparing serial changes in hCG level uses the log hCG time curve and the assumption that under normal circumstances hCG titers increase a minimum of 66 per cent every 48 hours. In women with ectopic pregnancy, abnormal increases occur in 76 to 87 per cent, compared with 11 to 15 per cent of those with normal pregnancy.

With the widespread use and availability of ultrasound, an earlier diagnosis of intrauterine pregnancy is possible, thereby increasing the diagnostic accuracy of ectopic pregnancy. The definitive diagnosis of an intrauterine pregnancy is the demonstration of fetal heart activity within the uterus, whereas that of an ectopic pregnancy is fetal heart activity in the adnexa. Because the probability of an intrauterine pregnancy and a coexistent ectopic pregnancy is 1 in 30,000, fetal heart activity within the uterus can, for all practical purposes, rule out an ectopic pregnancy. Endovaginal ultrasound transducers enable visualization of the gestational sac, yolk sac, and fetal heart activity earlier than is possible with abdominal transducers. Often a gestational sac with a yolk sac can be seen before 6 weeks' gestation. The presence of an intrauterine yolk sac provides more reassurance of a pregnancy within the uterus; this often is apparent before the appearance of fetal heart activity.

The data presented on quantitative hCG levels and ultrasound indicate that there is no test or combination of tests that can be used to diagnose an ectopic pregnancy with 100 per cent accuracy. With this information as background, one can provide a method to diagnose ectopic pregnancy. High-risk patients are counseled and encouraged to present early in pregnancy so that close follow-up is possible. The initial evaluation includes the date of the last menstrual period and, if possible, review of other data, such as basal body temperature charts, to determine the date of conception. Blood tests for a quantitative beta hCG level are obtained, and a pelvic examination and an initial transvaginal ultrasound scan are done. Patients are given the symptoms of ectopic pregnancy and are encouraged to notify the physician if any of them occur. They are followed closely, usually weekly, with pelvic examinations, hCG level tests, and ultrasound scans.

In women whose pregnancy is diagnosed in the emergency room, the initial evaluation differs from that of the asymptomatic office patient. If the signs and symptoms strongly suggest an ectopic pregnancy, the patient is admitted for laparoscopy unless the ultrasound scan shows unequivocal evidence of a viable intrauterine pregnancy. However, if the patient has mild or moderate symptoms that suggest an ectopic pregnancy, a quantitative hCG level is obtained, and

the patient is scheduled to return to the office and is followed closely as an outpatient.

If the hCG level is increasing at a rate of approximately 66 per cent every 48 hours, the patient is followed until fetal heart activity is seen. When fetal heart activity is visualized, the patient receives routine obstetric care. If the hCG titer fails to demonstrate an increase of 66 per cent extrapolated for every 48 hours, the patient is followed more frequently. If symptoms such as vaginal bleeding or pain occur, a laparoscopy is scheduled.

If the ultrasound scan fails to demonstrate a gestational sac with a yolk sac but the hCG titer has increased at a normal rate, laparoscopy is deferred until the patient becomes symptomatic, until the hCG level plateaus or falls, or until fetal heart activity is present. If the hCG level plateaus or decreases and the ultrasound scan shows lack of a yolk sac or fetal heart activity, or the sac has decreased in size, the prognosis for a normal intrauterine pregnancy is grave. When this situation occurs, surgery is scheduled. In patients who are not at high risk for ectopic pregnancy, a dilatation and curettage with frozen section analysis is done. If there is no evidence of villi and the patient has been relatively asymptomatic, hCG levels are obtained on an outpatient basis every 3 to 4 days until the hCG level is undetectable. In women who are symptomatic or who are at high risk for ectopic pregnancy, when the frozen section fails to show villi, a laparoscopy is done. Occasionally, the patient must undergo an exploratory laparotomy if one cannot completely visualize both adnexae or cannot completely rule out an ectopic pregnancy at laparoscopy.

TREATMENT

The mainstay in the treatment of ectopic pregnancy is surgery. Other types of therapy include observation and chemotherapy with methotrexate. Until more data are available, treatment with methotrexate, observation, or both should probably be restricted to well-controlled studies and research protocols. In the surgical management of ectopic pregnancy, the least invasive approaches should be selected relative to the patient's condition.

Management of an ectopic pregnancy varies, depending on the patient's age, her desire for future fertility, and other gynecologic data, such as a history of abnormal cervical cytology or pelvic infections. The location and severity of the ectopic pregnancy and the condition of the patient are additional considerations. When an ectopic pregnancy is suspected, the patient or couple should be informed of the range of treatment modalities, including conservative tubal surgery or extirpative surgery, which might consist of salpingectomy, salpingo-oophorectomy, salpingectomy with tubal ligation, and even hysterectomy. Hysterectomy is probably indicated only if there is a major problem in obtaining hemostasis with an interstitial ectopic pregnancy, if there is extensive pelvic inflammatory disease, or if there is a coexisting gynecologic condition. The informed patient can assume a more active role in her own management. She should be cautioned that with conservative surgery the risk of another ectopic pregnancy is increased.

In the patient who desires future fertility, conservative surgery provides the best opportunity to preserve reproductive function. Microsurgical techniques, copious saline heparin irrigation and suction, and meticulous hemostasis are paramount. The type of conservative surgery depends on the location of the ectopic pregnancy and the condition of the tube. The two most common conservative procedures are a linear salpingectomy and a segmental resection. In a linear salpingostomy, the initial incision is made over the portion of the tube containing the ectopic pregnancy and extended so that the products of conception can be removed. The initial incision may be made with cautery, a scalpel, or a laser. After the initial incision along the antimesenteric portion of the tube, the products of conception are gently removed from the tube. Meticulous hemostasis is essential. A controversy exists as to whether it is better to close the linear salpingostomy or leave it open. If the tube is closed, a two-layer closure is provided, with a first layer of interrupted fine sutures and a second layer of fine sutures that reapproximate the serosa. Closure has the advantages of obtaining adequate hemostasis along the margins of the incision and reducing the raw surface of the tube to prevent adhesion formation.

The second technique for conservative tubal surgery is a tubal resection. In this procedure, the tube with the ectopic pregnancy is resected, leaving as much normal tube as possible. This technique is useful when the tube has ruptured or when one cannot obtain adequate hemostasis after an ectopic pregnancy is removed from the tube. Another advantage of this technique concerns ectopic pregnancies located in the isthmic portion of the tube. In these pregnancies, there is a higher incidence of salpingitis isthmica nodosa of the tube. When a tubal resection is done, it is best to perform an anastomosis at a later time. The delay in performing the anastomosis is recommended because the patient's condition and anatomic distortion from edema and tissue engorgement may prevent optimal reconstruction. Because there is a high incidence of salpingitis isthmica nodosa in isthmic ectopic pregnancies, a hysterosalpingogram is recommended to evaluate the contralateral tube. If salpingitis isthmica nodosa exists in the contralateral tube, a resection and reanastomosis of the contralateral tube are planned at the time that the anastomosis is performed on the tube where the ectopic pregnancy was excised.

Laparoscopic treatment of an ectopic pregnancy is being done more often. If this treatment is considered, the patient must be hemodynamically stable. Laparoscopic treatment requires an experienced laparoscopic surgeon with an armamentarium of special instruments and equipment. These include adequate suctioning equipment, lavage, coagulating and cutting cauteries, and/or a laser. The techniques of linear salpingostomy are similar, and the incision along the antimesenteric portion of the tube is not closed.

With a ruptured ectopic pregnancy, the procedures used include linear salpingostomy or tubal resection, depending on the location of the pregnancy. Salpingectomy is indicated when the tube is irreparably damaged or when it is not possible to obtain adequate hemostasis during a conservative procedure.

In the patient who is hemodynamically unstable secondary to blood loss, there is little controversy as to the best management. The main objectives are to obtain prompt hemostasis, fluid and electrolyte replacement, and appropriate blood transfusions. Stabilization of the patient may not be possible until bleeding is controlled. Prompt intervention is essential to control the bleeding. In these cases, removing the ectopic pregnancy and controlling bleeding, salpingectomy, or even salpingo-oophorectomy may be necessary.

POSTOPERATIVE CONSIDERATIONS

If a patient is Rh negative and has not been sensitized, RhoGAM should be given. The dose recommended is 50 micrograms before 13 weeks' gestation and 300 micrograms for gestations of 13 weeks or more. It is often more convenient to give this in the immediate postoperative period while the patient is in the recovery room.

When patients are treated conservatively, it is important that all functioning trophoblastic tissue be removed. There have been cases where residual trophoblastic tissue resulted in hemoperitoneum, additional surgery, or additional treatment. Patients who have undergone conservative treatment must have serial hCG levels determined postoperatively until the levels are undetectable.

VAGINAL BLEEDING IN LATE PREGNANCY

method of
VICTOR R. KLEIN, M.D.
North Shore University Hospital
Manhasset, New York

Vaginal bleeding in the third trimester of pregnancy occurs in approximately 2 to 4 per cent of pregnancies. Although such bleeding may be of minor consequence, in some cases it may be life-threatening to both the mother and the fetus. Pregnancies complicated by late bleeding are associated with an increased rate of premature delivery and perinatal morbidity and mortality. It is important to differentiate the bleeding associated with the "bloody show" occurring at the onset of labor from potentially life-threatening conditions such as placenta previa or abruptio placentae, which may rapidly evolve from minor vaginal bleeding to uncontrollable hemorrhage. Careful evaluation to determine the volume of blood loss, the hemodynamic status of the patient, and the condition of the fetus must occur concomitantly with a search for the etiology of the bleeding.

The causes of late bleeding are summarized in Table 1 and discussed in the next section.

CAUSES OF THIRD TRIMESTER BLEEDING

Labor

Extrusion of the cervical mucus plug (bloody show) occurs when blood vessels rupture as the cervix effaces and dilates. Often heralding the onset of labor, either term or preterm, it is rarely accompanied by significant bleeding. However, the passage of the bloody show is one of the signs of preterm labor and should alert the physician to its possibility.

Trauma and Cervical Lesions

The increased vascularity of the cervix and the fragility of small blood vessels lead to an increased bleeding tendency during pregnancy. Cervical eversions, polyps, and varices may lead to bleeding when a pelvic examination is performed, when a cervical culture or Papanicolaou's smear is obtained, or when sexual intercourse occurs. Invasive carcinoma of the cervix, although rare in pregnancy, may lead to severe blood loss and often requires cesarean delivery to prevent hemorrhage and possible tumor spread, which may occur during vaginal delivery.

Blood Dyscrasias

Bleeding disorders such as idiopathic thrombocytopenic purpura and von Willebrand's disease are associated with bleeding during labor and delivery. Several patients were diagnosed with these disorders only after postpartum hemorrhage occurred.

Disseminated intravascular coagulation, the most serious blood dyscrasia complicating pregnancy, causes a depletion of fibrinogen and clotting factors. Complications of pregnancy associated with the development of disseminated intravascular coagulation include amniotic fluid embolism, pregnancy-induced hypertension, abruptio placentae, and prolonged retention of a dead fetus.

Placenta Previa

Placenta previa occurs when the placenta implants over or close to the internal os rather than in the body of the uterus. The various types of placenta previa are differentiated by the relationship of the placenta to the internal cervical os. Complete placenta previa occurs when the placenta covers the entire cervical os; partial placenta previa when the os is only partially covered; and marginal placenta previa when the placental edge extends to the margin of the cervical os. A low-lying placenta denotes implantation in the lower uterine segment but entirely clear of the internal os.

Risk factors for abnormal placental implantation include multiparity, multiple gestation, advanced maternal age, and previous uterine surgery, particularly cesarean section. The incidence of placenta previa at term is approximately 0.5 per cent. At 20 weeks' gestation, the incidence is 20 per cent. The development of the lower uterine segment leads to the cephalad migration of the placenta as pregnancy progresses. Preterm labor is associated with a higher incidence of placenta previa because of the earlier gestational age.

Bleeding associated with placenta previa is maternal in origin. It is caused by premature separation of the placenta from the implantation site during normal formation of the lower uterine segment or during labor when the cervix effaces and dilates and the placenta becomes separated from the cervix. Classically, bleed-

TABLE 1. Causes of Late Antepartum Bleeding

Blood dyscrasias
  Disseminated intravascular coagulation
  Idiopathic thrombocytopenic purpura
  Leukemia

Cervical causes
  Carcinoma
  Condylomas
  Erosion
  Infection
  Labor
  Polyps

Placental causes
  Abruptio placentae
  Marginal sinus separation
  Placenta previa
  Vasa previa

Uterine rupture

Vaginal causes
  Condylomas
  Varices

ing is painless and the first episode is often not associated with significant blood loss.

Placenta previa can cause significant morbidity and mortality to both the mother and the fetus. Maternal blood loss can be severe, requiring blood transfusion or massive hemorrhage and shock. Severe anemia may lead to decreased placental perfusion and fetal compromise. A review of 30,000 deliveries at Parkland Memorial Hospital in Dallas revealed that perinatal morbidity was caused mainly by complications of premature labor and delivery, such as respiratory distress and pulmonary immaturity, compared with term placenta previas with a good fetal outcome. Placenta previa increases the incidence of premature labor, fetal growth retardation, maternal morbidity during operative delivery, infection, and increased blood loss.

Abruptio Placentae

Abruptio placentae is the premature separation of a normally implanted placenta before delivery of the fetus. This complication of pregnancy is found in 0.3 to 1 per cent of deliveries occurring after 30 weeks' gestation. The incidence of abruptio placentae, although variable, leads to fetal death in approximately 1 in 750 deliveries. Although the cause of placental abruption is unknown, several conditions are associated with it. These include pregnancy-induced hypertension, chronic hypertension, trauma, cocaine abuse, smoking, dietary deficiency, and rapid decompression of the uterus, such as in rupture of the membranes in the patient with polyhydramnios.

Bleeding from abruptio placentae may be either internal or external. Blood usually is situated between the uterus and membranes and is lost through the cervix. When bleeding occurs between the placenta and uterus, the hemorrhage is concealed, leading to delayed diagnosis and an increased chance of disseminated intravascular coagulation.

The risk of recurrence of abruptio placentae is estimated to be 10 per cent after one abruption and 25 per cent after two abruptions.

Signs and symptoms of abruptio placentae include vaginal bleeding, uterine tenderness, labor, fetal distress, and fetal demise. Approximately 80 per cent of patients have heavy vaginal bleeding. When there is maternal tachycardia and hypotension with a normal hematocrit, concealed hemorrhage as a result of an acute event must be considered.

Disseminated intravascular coagulation occurs in 10 to 25 per cent of patients with abruptio placentae. The more severe the coagulopathy, the less likely is the fetus to survive. Abruptio placentae is the most common etiology of disseminated intravascular coagulation in pregnancy.

Abruptio placentae complicating pregnancy may lead to hypovolemia, shock, acute renal failure secondary to delayed or inadequate treatment of hypovolemia, Sheehan's syndrome, and uteroplacental apoplexy (Couvelaire's uterus).

Uterine Rupture

Spontaneous rupture of the uterus is a rare complication of pregnancy, occurring in 0.05 per cent of all deliveries. It may occur before the onset of labor, as in patients with previous vertical cesarean sections, or during labor, in patients with transverse uterine incisions or no previous scars. It can be associated with significant maternal and perinatal morbidity and mortality if diagnosis is delayed. Factors associated with uterine rupture include previous uterine surgery (cesarean section, myomectomy, uterine perforation from a dilatation and curettage), multiparity, uterine anomalies, neglected labor, excessive fundal pressure, and oxytocin use. Uterine rupture in patients undergoing vaginal birth after cesarean section is an uncommon event. The patient with one or even multiple cesarean sections where the uterine incision in the lower uterine segment is transverse is now encouraged to deliver vaginally because of the safety and low frequency of uterine rupture.

Vasa Previa

This uncommon complication occurs when the blood vessels of the umbilical cord separate in the membranes away from the placental margin (velamentous insertion of the cord) and the fetal vessels traverse the internal cervical os. The presenting part on pelvic examination is the cord. Vasa previa occurs more frequently in women with multiple gestations and is associated with severe, rapid fetal blood loss and fetal demise. Occasionally, the physician may palpate the fetal vessels during pelvic examination and note a corresponding change in fetal heart rate on the fetal monitor. Blood that is lost is fetal in origin.

EVALUATION AND MANAGEMENT

The patient with vaginal bleeding late in pregnancy requires a review of the antepartum record, a review of the events antecedent to the bleeding, and an assessment of the hemodynamic status and estimation of blood loss. Although vaginal bleeding is a common complaint early in pregnancy, it is less common as pregnancy progresses. It is often difficult to differentiate between benign causes and those that are potentially life-threatening to both the mother and the fetus. Hemorrhage is the major cause of obstetric death in the United States.

Evaluation

The patient complaining of third trimester bleeding should be evaluated in the labor and delivery unit of a hospital capable of caring for both the compromised mother and the fetus. This is most important when bleeding is heavy and the pregnancy is less than 36 weeks' gestation. Although a careful assessment is usually sufficient when bleeding is not heavy and the fetus is stable, an emergency cesarean section and massive fluid resuscitation are sometimes necessary.

Thus, the time of labor and delivery is usually the best setting to evaluate the mother and fetus.

Initial assessment includes the history and vital signs. The volume of blood lost before arrival at the hospital is usually estimated by the number of pads used or the clothing soiled by blood. The presence or absence of uterine contractions, fetal activity, trauma, rupture of membranes, onset of bleeding, and a history of previous uterine surgery are all ascertained. The patient should be asked whether she is bleeding from sites other than the vagina, which may suggest blood dyscrasias or disseminated intravascular coagulation. Maternal pulse, respiratory rate, and blood pressure with evaluation of orthostasis are assessed. Fetal heart rate monitoring with Doppler examination, followed by external monitoring of the fetal heart rate and uterine activity, should be initiated. Blood volume loss and sites of bleeding, abdominal examination including measurements of fundal height, the presence or absence of uterine tenderness, contractions, and fetal position are assessed. Vaginal examination is deferred until placenta previa has been ruled out and preparations for management of hemorrhage and emergency cesarean delivery have been made.

While members of the team are reviewing the patient's history and obtaining vital signs, others should begin an intravenous line with a large-bore catheter to correct hypovolemia. A baseline hematocrit should be obtained, but this may be falsely reassuring in the face of acute blood loss. Additional laboratory tests include a coagulation profile, prothrombin time, partial thromboplastin time, fibrinogen, complete blood count with platelet count, fibrin degradation products, electrolyte studies, and liver function tests.

A wall clot to assess fibrinogen and clotting capacity usually rapidly alerts the physician to the presence and severity of a coagulopathy. If the blood fails to clot within 6 minutes or a clot forms and then lyses within 30 minutes, a coagulopathy is probably present. Crystalloid solutions should be given until whole blood or packed cells and blood components are available. In the event of massive hemorrhage, non–cross-matched whole blood may prove to be lifesaving. The patient should be given oxygen support during the evaluation period. Continuous external fetal monitoring and uterine contractile activity should be assessed for the number of contractions and hypertonicity. A Foley's catheter should be placed to assess fluid output. Central venous monitoring is rarely required. The "rule of 30"—maintenance of a hematocrit of 30 per cent and urine output of 30 ml per hour—has been found to be associated with fewer sequelae in the face of hypovolemia.

If ultrasound equipment is immediately available, a sonogram is performed to localize the placenta and to determine its relationship to the cervical os. Sonography can identify placenta previa in 95 per cent of cases. It is not as helpful in diagnosing placental abruption, particularly if the placenta is posterior. It is often noted that by the time sonography detects abruptio placentae, the clinical diagnosis has been made. Historically, if the patient had a sonogram earlier in pregnancy, the information that it provides (the absence of placenta previa) may negate the need for emergency sonography and the danger of massive hemorrhage by perforation of a placenta previa during vaginal examination. If sonography is unavailable, palpation of the cervix and the lower uterine segment should be delayed until the double setup is performed. In this situation, the patient is taken to the operating room and two teams are available. The patient's blood is cross-matched, blood is readily available, and the scene is set for an emergency cesarean section. The second team then examines the patient vaginally to assess the placental location even if there is a previous sonogram. If bleeding occurs or if it is determined that vaginal delivery is unsafe, a cesarean section is immediately performed.

Management

The management of late vaginal bleeding depends on the severity of the bleeding, its etiology, and the gestational age. In the face of rapid, heavy bleeding, fetal distress, or coagulopathy, stabilization and fluid resuscitation are followed by emergency delivery. Minor bleeding, such as that associated with benign cervical and vaginal lesions, is treated by local therapy and outpatient management. Often the plan is simple, consisting of either observation or rapid intervention. The most difficult situations occur when the fetus is stable and there is moderate blood loss requiring transfusion therapy. The question of when to deliver the preterm fetus versus the maternal risk is difficult to answer.

Lower Tract Bleeding

Vaginal bleeding caused by vaginal or cervical lesions usually can be controlled locally. Cervical inflammation can be treated with many oral antibiotics and vaginal creams. Carcinoma of the cervix is rarely associated with bleeding when in situ but may be associated with hemorrhage if it is invasive. Condylomas may be treated locally by laser therapy but usually do not create blood loss unless they are part of an episiotomy incision.

Placenta Previa

Classically, the first episode of bleeding associated with placenta previa is both painless and light. Usually the patient presents late in the second trimester or early in the third trimester with bright red vaginal bleeding. After the diagnosis of placenta previa is confirmed, as previously outlined, the patient is admitted to the hospital for labor and delivery for the first 12 to 24 hours. In this setting, where close observation is possible, she is observed for changes in vital signs, assessment of labor, and fetal monitoring. After an accurate estimation of gestational age based on the last menstrual period and sonographic measurements, several options are available. If the patient is at or near term, delivery by cesarean section is indicated if the previa is central. Sometimes a previa partially covering the os may move cephalad during labor as the cervix effaces and dilates, and a vaginal delivery may be possible. The double setup is then performed in labor to view the cervix during gentle speculum examination, and a careful digital examination is done to form the vaginal fornices for placental tissue.

If the patient is preterm, the amount of blood loss must be carefully estimated. Although blood transfusion therapy is indicated to replace lost blood, a decision must be made about how many units of blood will be transfused before cesarean section is performed.

If the vaginal bleeding is light, the patient is admitted to the hospital for expectant arrangements including bed rest, fetal surveillance, a pad count to assess bleeding, sonography, and daily checks of fetal heart tones and maternal vital signs. When the patient has increased bleeding, approaches term, or goes into labor, the management is as described on early admission. If a patient has a confirmed diagnosis of placenta previa and goes into preterm labor, the management is controversial. Some physicians believe that tocolytic therapy is contraindicated in the face of third trimester bleeding. However, it is anticipated that with placenta previa and labor, bleeding will occur. Therefore, tocolytic therapy to abate labor may be used to prevent preterm delivery and stop the bleeding. Although the list of tocolytic agents is small (ritodrine, terbutaline, magnesium sulfate, indomethacin), most proponents of tocolysis prefer to avoid ritodrine and terbutaline, which, as beta agonists, cause a widened pulse pressure and maternal and fetal tachycardia—signs that may indicate anemia and alert the physician to blood loss. The patient with a placenta previa at the time of delivery must have several units of blood cross-matched, and the surgeon must be prepared for possible cesarean hysterectomy if uncontrollable bleeding occurs.

Abruptio Placentae

The management of abruptio placentae includes stabilization and delivery. Although there are rare cases of partial abruption or marginal placental separation with little effect, the majority of cases require delivery after diagnosis. The patient with abruptio placentae faces the possibility of severe perinatal and maternal morbidity and mortality. The patient usually presents with moderate to heavy vaginal bleeding, abdominal tenderness, and uterine irritability. If the fetus is stable with a good heart tracing, vaginal delivery may be possible. However, blood loss often causes decreased placental perfusion and fetal heart rate abnormalities, warranting expedient delivery.

It is important to assess blood loss carefully. Often blood loss is underestimated, and hematocrits after an acute event are normal. An assessment of blood loss and the presence of a coagulopathy is critical before emergency cesarean section. Although prompt delivery is the treatment for abruptio placentae, a stable mother is of the utmost importance. Fluid resuscitation, especially blood transfusion, is important early in the management. If the fetus is not alive, vaginal delivery is preferred, and either spontaneous labor or oxytocin induction of labor is necessary. Volume replacement with either whole blood or packed cells and cryoprecipitate should not be delayed.

Uterine Rupture

Management of uterine rupture includes emergency laparotomy and blood replacement therapy. Uterine rupture poses a great threat to both mother and fetus. Blood loss may be rapid and massive. The fetus may be free-floating in the abdominal cavity or may still be in utero. If the rupture is small or is simply a separation of a previous uterine incision, it may be possible to suture the separated edges if the patient desires future fertility. If there is irreparable damage or if bleeding cannot be controlled, a hysterectomy is indicated.

HYPERTENSIVE DISORDERS OF PREGNANCY

method of
KATHARINE D. WENSTROM, M.D., and
CARL P. WEINER, M.D.
University of Iowa Hospital
Iowa City, Iowa

The various hypertensive disorders of pregnancy affect 6 to 10 per cent of pregnant women. Complications of hypertension result in significant perinatal morbidity and mortality and are associated with 25 per cent of maternal deaths. The American College of Obstetricians and Gynecologists (ACOG) classifies hypertension during pregnancy as (1) pre-eclampsia–eclampsia, (2) chronic hypertension, (3) chronic hypertension with superimposed pre-eclampsia, and (4) late or transient hypertension. This and other classifications are based largely on signs and symptoms because the pathophysiologic mechanism underlying each type is not known and there appears to be considerable overlap among the groups.

NORMAL PREGNANCY

Blood pressure is ordinarily regulated by the interaction of four distinct mechanisms: (1) renal control of fluid volume through the interplay of many complex functions; (2) arterial baroreflex control of vascular tone and heart rate; (3) renin-angiotensin modulation of adrenal function and vasoconstriction; and (4) vascular autoregulation for local control of blood flow and perfusion. Each is affected to some degree by pregnancy. A 50 per cent expansion of plasma volume and a 30 to 40 per cent increase in cardiac output by the twenty-fourth week of pregnancy are accompanied by a large decrease in peripheral vascular resistance (probably the result of baroreflex and vascular autoregulation adjustments). As a result of these changes, the renal blood flow and glomerular filtration rate increase. Consequently, blood urea nitrogen, creatinine levels, plasma osmolality, and plasma sodium concentration all decline during pregnancy. Sodium delivery to the distal tubule increases, and in the nonpregnant subject causes renin secretion to decrease. Paradoxically, renin secretion remains high during normal pregnancy and is associated with an increase in angiotensin II. Blood pressure remains stable in part because of the relative resistance to angiotensin II associated with increased vascular synthesis of prostacyclin. The prostacyclin/thromboxane ratio at the endothelial level increases and protects the microvasculature from platelet aggregation and subsequent vascular damage. Levels of certain blood coagulation factors (specifically, fibrinogen and Factors II, VII, VIII, IX, and X) are increased in pregnancy, but in general, the peripheral maternal vessels are protected from coagulation-related damage. Only the placental vasculature is subject to continuous generation of thrombin, formation of fibrin, and resultant microinfarcts, and these changes are believed to reflect the normal gestational age–related senescence of the placenta.

PRE-ECLAMPSIA–ECLAMPSIA

The term "pre-eclampsia" describes a clinical entity typically occurring late in gestation and characterized by hypertension, proteinuria, and edema. It is a systemic illness that is sometimes difficult to diagnose because of its variable presentation. Central nervous system irritability may be present; if seizure activity occurs, the preferred term is "eclampsia." The underlying mechanism

of pre-eclampsia–eclampsia remains theoretical despite years of research. Several observations concerning differences between pre-eclampsia–eclampsia and the normal pregnant state suggest a primary role for the alteration of prostaglandin synthesis in producing this condition. As previously noted, increased synthesis of prostacyclin during normal pregnancy is associated with resistance to the pressor effects of angiotensin II and protects the vasculature from platelet aggregation and damage. In pre-eclampsia–eclampsia, endothelial damage occurs and, as a result, the ratio of prostacyclin to thromboxane is altered. The pathologic mechanism underlying the endothelial damage is unknown. The result is an increased sensitivity to angiotensin II, norepinephrine, and epinephrine. Vasoconstriction of peripheral blood vessels produces turbulent blood flow, more vascular endothelial damage, and, of necessity, platelet aggregation. The platelets release serotonin and other vasoactive substances that potentiate vasoconstriction, turbulent blood flow, and vascular damage. Platelet activation also initiates the clotting cascade, and certain clotting factors, particularly Factor VIII and antithrombin III, are consumed. Because antithrombin III is the principal inhibitor of thrombin generation, its decrease further increases thrombin formation. Increased fibrin generation results. Because fibrinolytic activity usually decreases after 30 weeks' gestation, soluble fibrin monomer obstructs the microvasculature, producing turbulent blood flow and exacerbating endothelial injury. The hypertension and local ischemic changes that result impair blood flow to the kidneys, liver, and placenta. The pathologic changes just described become self-perpetuating and ultimately destructive to placental function and the fetal-placental unit. Such changes also manifest at the clinical level and account for the characteristic signs and symptoms of the pre-eclamptic–eclamptic state.

In the interests of uniformity, the ACOG has established a standard definition for pre-eclampsia–eclampsia: hypertension (rise in systolic pressure of at least 30 mmHg or a rise in diastolic pressure of at least 15 mmHg, or systolic pressure of at least 140 mmHg, or diastolic pressure of at least 90 mmHg) documented on at least two occasions 6 hours or more apart, plus either proteinuria (300 mg or more protein in a 24-hour urine collection or a concentration of 1 gram per liter or more in at least two random urine collections 6 hours or more apart), or pathologic edema (1+ pitting edema after 12 hours of bed rest or a weight gain of 5 pounds or more in 1 week) occurring after the twentieth week of pregnancy. The criteria for severe pre-eclampsia are a systolic blood pressure of at least 160 mmHg and a diastolic blood pressure of at least 110 mmHg on two occasions 6 hours apart during bed rest; oliguria (24-hour urine output of less than 400 ml); cerebral or visual disturbances (altered consciousness, headache, scotoma, or blurred vision); pulmonary edema or cyanosis; right upper quadrant pain (caused by stretching of the hepatic capsule secondary to hematoma); impairment on liver function tests; and thrombocytopenia. Another criterion is proteinuria (protein level exceeding 5 grams in 24 hours). This criterion may not be reliable because a patient with significant proteinuria without other signs or symptoms of pre-eclampsia may actually have underlying renal disease. In practice, the distinction between mild and moderate pre-eclampsia is probably of limited usefulness because management is dictated by individual patient considerations, and even the mild pre-eclamptic patient may suddenly progress to eclampsia. Eclampsia is defined as the occurence of seizure activity in a pre-eclamptic patient that is not the result of pre-existing neurologic disease.

All the characteristic findings in pre-eclampsia–eclampsia can be related to the pathophysiologic changes already discussed. Vasoconstriction produces hypertension and decreases blood flow to the kidneys and liver. Not only is the urine output decreased, but glomerular damage occurs and correlates with proteinuria. The hematocrit rises, and peripheral edema increases as plasma is forced into subcutaneous tissues through damaged and leaky endothelium. Contracted and damaged microvessels are also associated with pulmonary edema, liver dysfunction, and central nervous system abnormalities. The decreased platelet counts observed are related to the occurrence of a chronic and usually compensated disseminated intravascular coagulopathy, described earlier. Placental damage occurs in the form of multiple infarcts and acute arteriosclerosis. These changes can compromise placental perfusion and may produce signs of uteroplacental insufficiency in the form of intrauterine growth retardation or fetal distress.

Treatment

The treatment for pre-eclampsia after 36 weeks' gestation is delivery. The patient should be protected against convulsions, and blood pressure should be controlled. Magnesium sulfate ($MgSO_4$) is the most common anticonvulsant in use in the United States, although debate continues as to its efficacy and mechanism of action. Some maintain that it exerts a specific anticonvulsant effect on the cerebral cortex. Others insist

that, in therapeutic doses, it does not cross the blood-brain barrier and must therefore act on the motor end plate (if it is effective) to prevent a peripheral response to eclamptic cortical dysfunction. The $MgSO_4$ can be given either intravenously or intramuscularly, although the latter is quite painful. The intravenous method consists of a 6-gram loading dose (30 ml of a 20 per cent solution) followed by a maintenance dose of 1 to 3 grams per hour, depending on the patellar reflex and peripheral blood levels (therapeutic range is 4 to 8 mg per dl). For intramuscular administration, the intravenous loading dose is combined with an intramuscular injection of 10 grams of $MgSO_4$ (5 grams in each buttock) and followed by 5 grams intramuscularly every 4 hours. Patellar reflexes should be tested, and the respiration rate should be monitored closely. $MgSO_4$ is withheld if patellar reflexes are absent. In the event of $MgSO_4$ toxicity, a 10 per cent calcium gluconate solution can be given intravenously with a good response. Respiration may have to be supported until the toxicity is reversed.

$MgSO_4$ is not an effective antihypertensive agent. Diastolic pressures in excess of 110 mmHg are dangerous to both mother and fetus and should be normalized. The degree to which blood pressure can be lowered safely is more dependent on intravascular volume than on any particular diastolic pressure. When intravascular volume is contracted, low pressures may be less well tolerated. Further, in view of this underlying intravascular volume contraction, diuretic use is not logical and should be avoided. Hydralazine, which reduces vascular resistance by directly relaxing arteriolar smooth muscle, is the most widely used drug in this situation and can be given in 5-mg intravenous boluses every 20 to 30 minutes or administered as a constant infusion beginning at 5 mg per hour after the initial 5-mg bolus. It is then increased by 1 mg per hour every half hour to maintain blood pressure in the targeted range. Care must be taken to wait a full 20 to 30 minutes between boluses and to avoid exceeding the optimal therapeutic dose, as sudden hypotension can result from overmedication. Occasionally, this drug produces maternal tachycardia, which, if sustained and uncomfortable, can be treated with intravenous propranolol (asthmatics should not receive propranolol, and diabetics must have glucose levels monitored closely while taking this drug). Labetalol, a mixed alpha and beta blocker, has been used effectively in pre-eclamptics. It can be given in boluses of 20 mg intravenously every 10 minutes until an appropriate response is observed. It has the advantage of not appearing to produce sudden hypotension. Diazoxide, a potent vasodilator with immediate action, has the disadvantage of frequently producing sudden hypotension and uterine relaxation (and thus fetal distress). It is also incompatible with either hydralazine or methyldopa. Although the use of minibolus doses (150 mg) decreases these risks, this drug must be used cautiously as first line therapy. Until the patient is stable, care of the severe hypertensive gravida mandates 1:1 nursing.

Steps toward delivery should be taken, with the ultimate route (vaginal versus abdominal) chosen after consideration of all aspects of maternal and fetal status. Delivery remains the ultimate therapy for pre-eclampsia, as most of the pathologic changes in physiology can be expected to begin resolving after expulsion of the fetus and placenta. As long as blood pressure remains controlled and the fetal and maternal conditions continue to be stable, aggressive induction of labor and vaginal delivery should be attempted. Severe pre-eclampsia in itself is not an indication for cesarean section.

Intravenous oxytocin is administered according to a standard protocol, with careful attention paid to fluid balance, especially pulmonary status and urine output. Membranes should be artificially ruptured as soon as possible, and every attempt should be made to induce active labor rapidly. It is usually not too difficult to induce labor in pre-eclamptic patients, and most can deliver vaginally despite a poor initial Bishop's score. Some patients, because of an unstable fetal or maternal condition, are not candidates for vaginal delivery and must be delivered by cesarean section. Well-controlled lumbar epidural anesthesia, when administered by a skilled anesthesiologist who carefully and slowly raises the anesthetic level, is the preferred anesthetic method for most pre-eclamptic patients. It not only aids blood pressure control but increases placental blood flow as well. Care must be taken to hydrate the patient adequately before its induction to account for the increase in intravascular space that occurs with sympathetic blockade. If emergency delivery is necessary, general anesthesia may be used, with care taken to minimize exacerbation of maternal hypertension on endotreacheal intubation. Intravenous nitroprusside and labetalol have been given in this situation to stabilize blood pressure and have proven efficacy with rapid onset and a short duration of activity.

Pulmonary Edema and Motor Seizures

On occasion, two life-threatening conditions can occur: pulmonary edema and major motor seizures. Pulmonary edema (often, although not always, accompanied by heart failure) causes maternal hypoxia and fetal compromise. Eclampsia increases maternal mortality in direct proportion to the number of seizures, the degree of blood pressure elevation, and the age and parity of the patient. Pulmonary edema must be diagnosed and treated quickly. Oxygen should be delivered by mask and 20 mg of furosemide given intravenously. Intravenous morphine should be considered if the patient is still symptomatic after these measures are taken. If respiratory distress continues, or if uncertainty about the patient's fluid status or cardiac function exists, a Swan-Ganz catheter and an arterial line should be placed and used to guide therapy. A simple central venous pressure measurement may be misleading in such circumstances and should be avoided. If the pulmonary catheter wedge pressure is high, hydralazine or nitroprusside infusion plus furosemide may produce relief of vasospasm and diuresis. If cardiac function is poor, consideration can be given to digoxin therapy. If the pulmonary wedge pressure is low and the edema is noncardiogenic, positive airway pressure and volume expansion may be helpful. Stabilization of the patient should be rapidly followed by delivery and continued postpartum observation in an intensive care unit.

When seizures occur, attention must focus on maintaining an airway and preventing aspiration or other trauma. The patient should be turned to her side and suctioned thoroughly. Oxygen by mask should be instituted. The fetal heart rate monitor may show bradycardia, but this is not the time for an emergency cesarean section, as the fetal heart rate usually recovers after the seizure has resolved. An intravenous line must be placed and an anticonvulsant medication given rapidly. Good choices include a rapidly acting barbiturate such as thiopental, 50 to 100 mg; diazepam, 2.5 to 5 mg; or $MgSO_4$, 2 to 4 grams given by slow intravenous push. The arterial blood gas content should be determined. Endotracheal intubation is useful in the occasional circumstance where aspiration seems likely or ventilation is inadequate. Because eclamptic seizures may be accompanied by pulmonary edema, evaluation should include a thorough examination to detect this entity. Aggressive efforts to control blood pressure and effect delivery should continue, along with anticonvulsive therapy. Continuous fetal monitoring aids fetal assessment and may alter decisions regarding the route and timing of delivery.

The patient should be monitored closely post partum, and intravenous $MgSO_4$ should be continued until diuresis (>150 ml per hour) and blood pressure stabilization have occurred. Although eclamptic seizures can occur up to 7 days post partum, they are extremely unlikely after diuresis has begun. Antihypertensive medications may have to be continued into the postdelivery period, but true pre-eclamptic hypertension usually resolves completely within 2 weeks.

Patient with Premature Fetus

The management of a patient whose fetus weighs less than 1500 grams is less straightforward. The desire to avoid significant fetal morbidity and mortality in the nursery secondary to immaturity must be balanced against maternal well-being and the hostility of the intrauterine environment. If the maternal condition permits, a trial of bed rest is warranted. The goal is to allow time for the fetus to mature and the cervix to ripen while the mother is closely observed for evidence of disease progression. In women whose blood pressure does not exceed 135/85 mmHg and who do not have proteinuria or hematologic alteration, bed rest at home with twice weekly blood pressure checks is indicated. If the blood pressure responds favorably, weekly nonstress tests document continued fetal well-being, and adequate fetal growth continues, further intervention is not necessary. If any of these parameters deteriorates, however, the patient must be admitted to the hospital for thorough evaluation and close supervision. There is no place for the outpatient management of pre-eclampsia. It is impossible to predict who will remain stable and who will develop rapidly progressive disease.

Laboratory evaluation includes a complete blood count with platelet quantification; liver function tests; serum blood urea nitrogen, creatinine, and uric acid determinations; and 24-hour urine collection. The patient should be weighed daily to estimate fluid retention. The fetus should be evaluated for growth (i.e., ultrasound) and continued well-being (i.e., nonstress test or biophysical profile). Decisions about when and how to terminate the pregnancy must be based on both maternal and fetal considerations. If the maternal diagnosis changes from mild to severe pre-eclampsia, clinical judgment must dictate management. For example, isolated severe hypertension, especially in the multipara whose diagnosis is unclear, may respond well to pharmacologic manipulation and allow delay of delivery. Fetal status must be thoughtfully and frequently evaluated. If fetal growth stops, amniotic fluid volume decreases, or tests of fetal well-being indicate stress, the ability of the fetus to survive in the nursery should be weighed against its survival in a hostile intrauterine environment and delivery initiated.

Patients with either a family history of pre-eclampsia or a personal history of severe, early-onset pre-eclampsia in a previous pregnancy are at increased risk of hypertensive complications in a subsequent pregnancy. Such patients may benefit from low-dose aspirin therapy (80 mg per day) during succeeding pregnancies. Aspirin at this dose inhibits thromboxane synthesis and may help to restore a more protective prostacyclin/thromboxane ratio in the peripheral vasculature.

CHRONIC HYPERTENSION

Chronic hypertension is defined as hypertension that antedates the pregnant state, is noted before the twentieth week of gestation, or is diagnosed in a patient with a persistently elevated mean arterial pressure. In most cases, the cause of such arterial hypertension is unknown, but it is often related to undiagnosed renal pathology. Predisposing factors to this condition include obesity, black race, low socioeconomic class, increased age, smoking, elevated cholesterol level, glucose intolerance, high salt intake, and possible altered renin activity. The hypertensive patient may have altered cardiac, renal, and vascular functions as a result of her disease. The young hypertensive gravida develops left ventricular hypertrophy in response to sustained systemic hypertension. The renal glomerular filtration rate may decrease in consequence of arteriosclerotic lesions of afferent and efferent arterioles and glomerular capillary tufts. Damage to vasculature occurs throughout the body and decreases the compliance while increasing the resistance of all vessels. An indication of the extent of such underlying pathology may be gained by performing an ophthalmologic examination and an analysis of urine sediment and by obtaining an echocardiogram. Even if a hypertensive gravida demonstrates no abnormalities in any of these tests, she still enters pregnancy at a disadvantage and faces increased risk of maternal and fetal morbidity and mortality. There is a 10 to 50 per cent chance of superimposed pre-eclampsia, a 0.45 to 10 per cent chance of abruption, and a high associated risk of preterm delivery and intrauterine growth retardation in hypertensive pregnancies.

Some of the normal physiologic alterations of pregnancy are diminished in the chronic hypertensive. The normal decrease in vascular resistance and expansion of blood volume may not occur. The decidual vasculature of the hypertensive gravida may demonstrate pathologic changes and may be responsible for decreased uteroplacental perfusion and an increased incidence of placental abruption. Decreased maternal blood volume and uteroplacental vascular compromise inhibit the delivery of oxygen and nutrients to the fetus and probably account for the increased incidence of intrauterine growth retardation observed in hypertensive women.

Treatment

Management of the chronic hypertensive during pregnancy should focus on control of the underlying maternal disease and improvement of the intrauterine environment. Of primary importance is the normalization of blood pressure. Proper nutrition, limitation of physical activity, and planned periods of rest in the left lateral decubitus position may aid uteroplacental blood flow and the delivery of nutrients to the fetus. The patient should be seen frequently (every 2 weeks in the first half of pregnancy and once a week thereafter) for blood pressure measurement and laboratory evaluation. Fetal well-being should be assessed weekly after 30 to 32 weeks. Serial ultrasound examinations can be used to document adequate fetal growth. The possibility of superimposed pre-eclampsia should be kept constantly in mind, and every effort should be made to diagnose this entity correctly as soon as it appears. Helpful laboratory tests include hematocrit and platelet count, serum creatinine and uric acid levels, creatinine clearance, antithrombin III activity, and quantification of 24-hour urinary protein excretion. Although antihypertensive medications are not usually necessary in the mild to moderate hypertensive patient, the severe hypertensive or the patient already receiving medication may need further pharmacologic intervention.

Control of blood pressure significantly improves the outcome of pregnancy. Many patients begin their pregnancies without antihypertensive medication and may require drug therapy only in the late second or third trimesters or not at all. Some patients, however, are receiving medication before conception. The regimen of these patients should be carefully re-evaluated on the first prenatal visit to determine if it is necessary. Chronic diuretic therapy may prevent the appropriate expansion of intravascular blood volume. Angiotensin-converting enzyme inhibitors (e.g., captopril) should definitely be discontinued during gestation because of their potential toxic effects on the developing fetus. Clonidine (a centrally acting alpha$_2$-adrenergic agonist) may likewise be a suboptimal selection for the pregnant patient because of the risk of hypertensive crisis on withdrawal of the drug. Although some gravidas do well when their antihypertensive medications are discontinued, the severe hypertensive, and especially the patient with diabetes, connective tissue disease, or renal pathology, needs a carefully chosen drug regimen to prevent exacerbation of disease. Whatever drug regimen is ultimately chosen, blood pressure must be carefully monitored so that dosages can be adjusted as the volume of distribution changes and so that other drugs can be added if necessary. The following is a brief discussion of several classes of antihypertensive medication commonly prescribed for the pregnant patient.

Methyldopa

Methyldopa (Aldomet) is a centrally acting alpha$_2$-adrenergic agonist that decreases peripheral resistance without increasing heart rate or cardiac output. Its popularity with obstetricians stems from its minimal side effects on the mother, its safety for the fetus, and the large body of information and experience regarding its use. The usual initial dose is 250 mg three times a day, with steady increases in response to maternal blood pressure until a maximum of 3 grams per day is reached.

Beta-Adrenergic Blockers

Propranolol, atenolol, and metoprolol have all been used successfully in pregnancy. Propranolol decreases beta stimulation of the heart, inhibits renin secretion by the kidneys, and has a direct effect on the central nervous system. It also directly affects the pulmonary tree and therefore should not be given to asthmatics. An initial dose of 80 mg per day can be gradually increased according to the maternal response up to a maximum of 120 to 240 mg. Neonatal hypoglycemia and bradycardia are associated with propranolol, but when it is used carefully, the benefits appear to outweigh the risks. Atenolol and metoprolol have more selective beta-blocking activity than propranolol, but less experience exists with their use in pregnancy.

Alpha- and Beta-Adrenergic Blockers

Labetalol, a drug recently approved for use in the United States, has been used successfully to treat acute severe hypertension. Because of its combined alpha- and beta-blocking properties, it lowers blood pressure without reducing cardiac output or uteroplacental flow and thus seems to avoid the risk of sudden hypotension found with intravenous hydralazine. Its value for treatment of the chronic hypertensive gravida has been less well studied.

Vasodilators

Hydralazine, prazosin, diazoxide, and nitroprusside have all been used for the treatment of hypertension, although diazoxide and nitroprusside are commonly used only for hypertensive emergencies. A great deal of experience with hydralazine, however, has made it the drug of choice for the treatment of chronic hypertension. It causes direct relaxation of the smooth muscle of the arteriolar bed and acts primarily on the precapillary resistance vessels. It is rapidly absorbed after oral administration, quickly reaches peak concentrations, and has a duration of action of 6 to 8 hours. The common dosing regimen is 20 to 50 mg orally every 8 hours. Although it probably crosses the placenta, no adverse fetal effects have been reported. Drawbacks include a compensatory tachycardia and fluid retention.

Calcium Channel Blockers

Calcium channel blocking agents prevent vasospasm and produce vasodilatation of many arterial systems (coronary, vertebral, basilar, gastrosplenic) by a direct effect on vascular smooth muscle. Nifedipine, verapamil, and diltiazem are most commonly used. Nifedipine is the most potent drug and has been used to treat acute severe hypertension with success. The value of these agents for chronic therapy and their effects on the developing fetus are presently under investigation.

CHRONIC HYPERTENSION WITH SUPERIMPOSED PRE-ECLAMPSIA

Chronic hypertensive gravidas are at higher risk for the development of pre-eclampsia than normotensive gravidas. The ACOG defines superimposed pre-eclampsia as an elevation of systolic blood pressure by 30 mmHg and of diastolic blood pressure by 15 mmHg, along with the appearance of proteinuria or generalized edema, in a gravida who already bears the diagnosis of chronic hypertension. Because many hypertensives begin pregnancy with proteinuria secondary to renal disease and have changing requirements for antihypertensive medications as pregnancy advances, this diagnosis may be difficult to make. Attempts to correlate this diagnosis with biopsy-proven underlying renal pathology have confirmed that the diagnosis is incorrect in a majority of cases. If the hypertensive patient's condition deteriorates, however, regardless of the cause, decisions about management and delivery must be made based on the considerations discussed earlier.

LATE OR TRANSIENT HYPERTENSION

Transient hypertension is the development of hypertension unassociated with other signs or symptoms of pre-eclampsia, occurring late in gestation or within the first 24 hours post partum. Because it is unaccompanied by proteinuria or edema, it cannot be considered pre-eclampsia, yet it is clearly related to the pregnant state. The risk it imposes on the mother and fetus is less than the risk of pre-eclampsia. Management decisions should be based on the absolute blood pressure values and the clinical situation. Most patients respond well to delivery, but their blood pressure should be closely monitored and pharmacologic therapy given if warranted.

OBSTETRIC ANESTHESIA
method of
MARSHA L. WAKEFIELD, M.D.
Medical College of Georgia
Augusta, Georgia

In obstetric circles the comment is often made that the ideal anesthetic would be the one that best benefits the patient, the passenger, and the power (to effect delivery). All of these factors must be considered in choosing the most appropriate anesthetic technique for an obstetric procedure.

"Natural" childbirth encompasses many methods (e.g., those of Read, Jacobson, and Lamaze). It is most effective when "prepared" childbirth allows an informed parturient and her partner to participate in a satisfying birth experience. However, it is important to remember that this concept does not mean a denial of regular medical care or an endurance test, and that pain medications or regional anesthesia may be used without the feeling of failure.

SYSTEMIC MEDICATIONS

Systemic medications have long been used for pain relief in childbirth. However, the emphasis has shifted from the era of total oblivion (i.e., twilight sleep) to the current recommendations to use the minimal drug dose that is effective. The primary concerns of excessive systemic medication include (1) maternal respiratory depression, (2) diminished maternal consciousness and cooperativeness, and (3) neonatal depression. The selection, timing, mode of administration, and dose of drug administered to the parturient should be based on knowledge of the effect of the drug on the mother and the fetus.

The dose and site of administration, the maternal distribution and metabolism of the drug, and the physiochemical properties of the drug itself (e.g., pH, lipid solubility, molecular weight) influence the amount of drug transferred to the fetus. Narcotics are the most widely used systemic medications for labor analgesia. Because they are lipid soluble and have molecular weights less than 500, they all cross the placenta easily by diffusion. Incremental intravenous injection is preferred to intramuscular injection because of its more prompt, predictable, and smoother action.

Meperidine (Demerol) is still the most popular narcotic for labor analgesia. Meperidine is usually administered in doses of 50 to 100 mg intramuscularly or 10 to 50 mg intravenously. When the drug is given intramuscularly, the peak analgesic effect occurs 40 to 45 minutes after injection. When the drug is administered intravenously, analgesia begins within 30 seconds and peaks at 5 to 10 minutes. The duration of action is 2 to 4 hours. Because meperidine rapidly crosses the placenta, the maternal and fetal equilibrium occurs within 6 minutes after intravenous administration. The incidence of neonatal respiratory depression is greatest in the second, third, and fourth hours after administration. This corresponds to the time of maximal fetal uptake of meperidine. The half-life of meperidine is 3 hours in the mother but 23 hours in the neonate. Other analgesics that have been used are morphine, pentazocine (Talwin), and fentanyl (Sublimaze). More recently, the narcotic agonist-antagonists butorphanol (Stadol) and nalbuphine (Nubain) have gained some popularity because of potentially less respiratory depression.

Morphine administered in doses of 5 to 10 mg intramuscularly or 2 to 3 mg intravenously has not been as popular as meperidine because it has been shown to cause more neonatal respiratory depression at equipotent doses. Pentazocine, usually administered in doses of 20 to 30 mg intramuscularly or 10 to 20 mg intravenously, never gained widespread use because of its psychomimetic properties. Fentanyl, although widely used in general anesthetic procedures, has not been as useful as an analgesic in obstetrics because of the rapid onset of respiratory depression and its shorter duration of action. The usual dose administered is 50 to 100 micrograms intramuscularly and 25 to 50 micrograms intravenously.

Butorphanol is usually administered in doses of 1 to 2 mg intramuscularly or intravenously during labor. A potential advantage with butorphanol is the mild sedative effect in addition to the narcosis. This effect would otherwise be achieved only by giving a tranquilizer with the other narcotics. Nalbuphine can be administered in doses of 10 to 15 mg intramuscularly. Smaller incremental doses may be given intravenously.

If a narcotic antagonist is needed, the preferred one is naloxone (Narcan). This drug is a pure antagonist and reverses the analgesic effect of narcotics as well as the respiratory depression. If respiratory depression in the neonate is a concern, it is best to administer naloxone directly to the neonate at birth. There is unreliable placental transfer of naloxone when administered to the mother shortly before delivery. Also, administering naloxone just before delivery leads to loss of analgesia in the mother. The maternal dose of naloxone is 0.1 to 0.4 mg intravenously. The neonatal dose is 0.01 mg per kg intravenously or intramuscularly (only with adequate tissue perfusion).

Phenothiazines are also widely used in combination with the narcotics because of their anxiolytic and antiemetic activities. Promethazine (Phenergan) is frequently used in combination with meperidine for labor analgesia and has been noted to reduce the dose requirement of meperidine. If it is given alone, promethazine may have a mild antianalgesic effect. Promethazine crosses the placenta rapidly and reaches equilibrium within 15 minutes. Promethazine and propiomazine (Largon) are the most commonly used phenothiazines in obstetrics. Others such as promazine (Sparine), chlorpromazine (Thorazine), and prochlorperazine (Compazine) are seldom used because of their greater alpha-adrenergic blocking properties and thus the potential for hypotension to occur. Neonates whose mothers had received meperidine (50 mg) plus promethazine (50 mg) intramuscularly or meperidine (50 mg) plus propiomazine (20 mg) intravenously had Apgar scores similar to those whose mothers received only meperidine.

ANESTHESIA FOR VAGINAL DELIVERY

Continuous Lumbar Epidural Analgesia for Labor and Vaginal Delivery

Continuous lumbar epidural analgesia is the most effective means of pain relief for labor. Once continuous epidural anesthesia has been established, it can be used for either spontaneous or operative delivery as the need arises. Epidural analgesia has been shown to decrease the level of circulating maternal catecholamines and, in the absence of hypotension, may actually improve uteroplacental blood flow.

Once the patient has been committed to delivery and the fetus has been evaluated, the epidural block may be administered. To prepare the parturient for the anesthetic, the physician must be able to monitor both the mother and the fetus. It is important to remember that aspiration pneumonitis is still a major cause of maternal morbidity and mortality. Although regional anesthesia has the advantage of maintaining the maternal protective airway reflexes, loss of consciousness is a remote possibility with an unintentional subarachnoid or intravenous placement of an epidural dose of local anesthetics. Therefore, it is important that measures be taken to minimize the hazard of aspiration by administering a non-particulate antacid such as 0.3 M sodium citrate (Bicitra). Because epidural anesthesia causes sympathetic blockade with vasodilation, it is important that the patient be acutely hydrated with 500 to 1000 ml of a non–dextrose-containing intravenous solution. Rapid increases in maternal blood glucose level, as with rapid volume expansion with dextrose-containing intravenous fluids, may put the neonate at increased risk for hypoglycemia. Adequate preloading helps to maintain venous return and, therefore, to prevent maternal hypotension and decreased uteroplacental perfusion. Aortocaval compression or supine hypotensive syndrome occurs in 15 to 20 per cent of parturients at term. This syndrome is a result of compression of the aorta and vena cava by the gravid uterus when the parturient is supine, which impedes venous return to the heart and may cause hypotension, nausea, vomiting, and changes in cerebration. Most women can compensate by vasoconstriction in the lower extremities. The sympathetic blockade of regional anesthesia may exacerbate supine hypotensive syndrome if the mother is not kept in the lateral or semilateral position (left uterine displacement) after the epidural anesthesia is established. In addition to preparing the mother, it is important that proper resuscitation equipment be in good working order and readily available in the area where the block is being placed. This equipment should include an oxygen flow meter, Ambu bag and masks, suction apparatus, and intubation supplies.

After appropriate preparation of the mother and the equipment, the epidural space may be identified from either the caudal or the lumbar approach. The lumbar epidural approach has advantages over the caudal approach for labor, including (1) ability to achieve a segmental block of specific pathways for each stage of labor; (2) finer control of autonomic blockade; (3) higher success rate; (4) smaller drug doses; (5) quicker uterine pain relief because injection is nearer to T_{11}–T_{12}; (6) less maternal discomfort; (7) no risk of puncturing the rectum or fetal head; and (8) less risk of infection. Potential disadvantages of the lumbar or caudal epidural approach compared with spinal anesthesia (for delivery) include (1) delayed onset of anesthesia, usually 10 to 20 minutes; (2) "patchy" or incomplete pain relief; (3) a more difficult technique to master; and (4) larger doses of drug needed.

In the adult the spinal cord usually ends at the L_1 level, occasionally extending as far as the vertebral body of L_2. The dural sac extends as far as the level of S_1–S_2. The epidural space extends from the foramen magnum rostrally to the sacral hiatus caudally. The L_2–L_5 interspaces are usually chosen for obstetric epidural block. The landmarks for epidural anesthesia are the same as those for spinal anesthesia. A line between the left and right iliac crests crosses either the spinous process of the L_4 vertebra or the L_4–L_5 vertebral interspace. The patient may be in either the lateral decubitus position or the sitting position.

After positioning the patient, the lumbar area is prepared and draped in sterile fashion. The interspace is identified and a small-gauge needle is used to make a skin wheal. The epidural needle is then inserted into the intervertebral space 1.2 to 3.7 cm until the needle is anchored in the interspinous ligament. The stylet is then removed and the needle is slowly advanced by using the loss-of-resistance technique (saline or air-filled syringe) or "hanging drop" method to identify the epidural space. After identification of the epidural space has been confirmed by negative aspiration for blood or cerebrospinal fluid, a test dose of local anesthetic may be administered.

The most appropriate test dose in the obstetric setting is controversial. The addition of epinephrine 1:200,000 (15 micrograms in a 3-ml test dose) has been recommended to rule out possible intravascular placement. However, in the patient in active labor, the maternal heart rate and blood pressure may change as much or more with a contraction than may be noted in response to the epinephrine test done. The physician should also usually wait 3 to 5 minutes for evidence of spinal blockade before administering additional drug. The most effective means of preventing the sequelae of unintentional intravenous or subarachnoid placement is to use incremental dosing. Only 3 to 5 ml of drug should be given at a time and verbal contact should be maintained with the patient. Early detection is the key to preventing serious reactions.

For continuous lumbar epidural block, a catheter is usually inserted and the needle carefully removed leaving 3 to 4 cm of catheter in the epidural space. The catheter should then be aspirated to detect the presence of cerebrospinal fluid or blood. If the aspiration is negative, incremental dosing can continue via the catheter until an adequate level of analgesia is obtained. Our initial dose of local anesthetic is usually 8 to 15 ml of 0.25 per cent bupivacaine with an onset of action of 5 to 10 minutes and an expected duration of action of 1.5 to 2 hours. Each repeat dose or "top up" is usually about two-thirds of the initial dose. Other local anesthetics may be used. Lidocaine, 1 to 1.5 per cent, usually is effective for about 60 minutes, but it has been associated with tachyphylaxis when used for prolonged periods. 2-Chloroprocaine (Nesacaine), 2 per cent, may also be used with an expected duration of action of only 45 minutes.

Use of the continuous infusion technique for epidural analgesia has become popular especially in busy obstetric suites. It has been suggested that a continuous infusion would cause fewer episodes of hypotension and more constant analgesia. Continuous infusion has not been found to result in lower total drug requirements or greater maternal satisfaction when compared with regularly administered intermittent top-up doses. The larger volumes and more dilute solutions of local anesthetics may be used to provide suitable analgesia with the least amount of motor blockade. It is important to regularly evaluate the patient being infused because the catheter could potentially migrate into a blood vessel (noted by decreasing analgesia with or without systemic signs from the low doses of local anesthetic) or it could migrate into the subarachnoid space (noted by increasing sensory level and motor block). After epidural anesthesia has been established with the initial loading dose, the infusion is usually begun at a rate of 10 ml per hour. The rate is then adjusted to maintain a T_{10} sensory level. The most commonly used solutions are 0.25 per cent bupivacaine, 0.125 per cent bupivacaine, and 1 per cent lidocaine.

Epidural narcotics are beginning to be widely used, not only for postcesarean pain relief, but also as an adjunct to local anesthetics for labor. The potential advantages include additional analgesia and a decrease in total dose of local anesthetic used. Because of their site of action at opiate receptors in the spinal cord, motor function and sympathetic blockade are not affected by the use of epidural narcotics. Epidural narcotics alone have not been as effective in providing adequate analgesia for labor and delivery as has the combination of local anesthetics and epidural narcotics. Morphine (Duramorph) is the only narcotic for epidural use currently approved. Morphine has the greatest potential for late respiratory depression (8 to 12 hours) and a delayed onset of action (60 minutes). Therefore, it has limited usefulness as an adjunct to labor analgesia. However, fentanyl has been widely studied and used as either an addition to the initial dose (50 micrograms in 10 ml of 0.25 per cent bupivacaine) or an addition to a continuous infusion (2 to 5 micrograms per ml of 0.125 per cent bupivacaine infused). Butorphanol, in doses of 1 to 2 mg (initial bolus), and sufentanil (Sufenta), in doses of 20 to 30 micrograms (initial bolus) or 2 micrograms per ml infusion, have also been used. There has been no noted increase in neonatal effects as reflected in the Apgar scores by the addition of these low-dose epidural narcotics. As for all narcotics, there may occasionally be side effects such as pruritus, nausea, and urinary retention.

During the second stage of labor, pain from the pelvis and perineum is carried by the pudendal nerve (S_2, S_3, and S_4). The most difficult root to block is S_2 because of its large diameter. Therefore, it may be necessary in the second stage to reinforce a block with a "delivery" dose. Usually, 10 to 15 ml is needed with the mother in the semisitting position to ensure good perineal analgesia. Lidocaine, 2 per cent, or 2-chloroprocaine, 3 per cent, may be useful just before delivery because of their more rapid onset of action.

Because epidural analgesia for labor is almost exclusively an elective procedure, it is imperative that the safety of the mother and the fetus be given primary consideration. Proper equipment, monitors, and personnel must be available to ensure the safest and most satisfying birth experience.

Spinal Block for Vaginal Delivery

Spinal anesthesia for vaginal delivery is usually administered just before delivery. It is not a useful technique for prolonged labor analgesia. Spinal anesthesia is less popular now than it was previously. The occurrence of postdural puncture headache, the increased risk of hypotension, and the greater use of continuous epidural anesthesia in obstetrics account for this decline in popularity. However, the ease with which spinal anesthesia may be induced and its rapid onset make this method an attractive option in certain situations.

Spinal anesthesia produces excellent analgesia for spontaneous and instrumental vaginal delivery, for a cerclage operation, for manual removal of the placenta, and for cesarean section. A T_{10} level suffices for vaginal deliveries and cerclage procedures; a T_4 level is required for a cesarean section.

A saddle block or a low spinal block produces adequate anesthesia for vaginal delivery. The saddle block anesthetizes only the sacral roots, but the low spinal block extends also to the T_{10} level. With the patient sitting, a 25-gauge or 26-gauge spinal needle is placed in the subarachnoid space. After return of cerebrospinal fluid, a hyperbaric solution of local anesthetic is injected and the patient is kept in a sitting position for 1 to 2 minutes and is then returned to the lithotomy position. The most commonly used drug is hyperbaric solution with 5 per cent lidocaine. Typically, a dose of 40 mg (range 30 to 60 mg) for an average-size patient is used. Other solutions such as hyperbaric tetracaine (average dose 4 to 5 mg) or hyperbaric bupivacaine (average dose 8 mg) may be used for low spinal anesthesia with longer duration of action. Because of the more rapid onset of sympathetic block, an appropriate fluid preload is necessary to avoid hypotension.

Peripheral Nerve Blocks

For the first stage of labor, the pain is transmitted by afferent fibers, which travel along with sympathetic fibers to T_{10}–L_1. These may be blocked peripherally by either a lumbar sympathetic or a paracervical block. To give effective analgesia for first stage of labor, the lumbar sympathetic block must be bilateral and even with bupivacaine provides only 2 to 3 hours of analgesia. With this block it is important to aspirate the needle before giving local anesthetic to avoid unintentional subarachnoid or intravenous injection. Lumbar sympathetic block may also produce systemic hypotension.

The visceral afferent fibers that transmit labor pain lie in the paracervical area where they are known as Frankenhäuser's plexus. Paracervical block gives good analgesia for first stage of labor, does not impair motor power, and does not cause systemic hypotension. It was very popular in the 1950s and 1960s until the occurrence of fetal bradycardia and fetal hypoxia were reported. There are several mechanisms proposed for the bradycardia. It may result from excessive absorption of local anesthetic into the fetal circulation, which causes fetal myocardial depression. It might also result either from uterine artery vasoconstriction or from an increase in uterine tone, both of which are caused by a high concentration of the local anesthetic. The degree and duration of fetal bradycardia correlate with fetal hypoxia and acidosis.

The pudendal nerve (S_2–S_4) is a branch of the sacral plexus. The pudendal block is performed to relieve pain from the second stage of labor and to provide anesthesia for episiotomy and low forceps delivery. A pudendal block does not provide adequate analgesia for midforceps rotations or extractions. The transvaginal approach is the more widely used and practical route in the obstetric patient. It is performed just before delivery, and although it is a relatively easy and uncomplicated block for the obstetrician, it results in adequate anesthesia only about 50 per cent of the time.

General Anesthesia for Vaginal Delivery

Rarely, general anesthesia may be required for delivery, for example, when the baby is in distress or when uterine relaxation may be needed for a difficult breech delivery or delivery of a second twin. Endotracheal anesthesia is necessary under those circumstances. A nonparticulate antacid should be administered, if possible, and a rapid-sequence induction must be performed using cricoid pressure until the trachea has been secured with a cuffed endotracheal tube. General anesthesia may also occasionally be needed for manual removal of the placenta and may be the technique of choice in the rare event of uterine inversion.

ANESTHESIA FOR CESAREAN SECTION

Regional Anesthesia: Epidural

As previously mentioned in the discussion of epidural anesthesia for labor and delivery, proper preparation is important to prevent potential side effects. The potential for supine hypotension to be exacerbated by sympathetic blockade is even more significant when surgical levels of anesthesia are necessary. Sympathetic blockade has been reported to be from two to six dermatomal levels higher than the level of sensory block. Because of the higher level of sensory block needed for cesarean section (i.e., T_4–T_2), there is limited ability to compensate for the near-complete sympathetic blockade by vasoconstriction in unblocked segments or increased heart rate. Two simple precautions can minimize the cardiovascular effects of high epidural block: the intravenous administration of 1.5 liters of a non–dextrose-containing intravenous fluid just before the block and maintaining left uterine displacement. Likewise, it is important to remember to administer 30 ml of a nonparticulate antacid such as 0.3 M sodium citrate as a prophylaxis against acid aspiration.

The effects of epidural anesthesia on respiratory muscle activity is not clinically significant in the healthy parturient. A sensory level of T_3 is not usually accompanied by a change in vital capacity, and even at a T_1 sensory level there is no blockade of the phrenic nerve. Apnea from a high epidural block is not caused by direct blockade of the phrenic nerve but by the decreased perfusion of the medullary centers related to systemic hypotension. However, a total spinal block affects the respiratory center as well as the respiratory muscles. During an epidural block with a high thoracic sensory level, the patient may complain of dyspnea because of the lack of sensory input from the intercostal muscles. Slow diaphragmatic breathing should be encouraged, and patients should be reassured that such a feeling is to be expected.

Especially when the epidural block is used for an elective cesarean delivery, it is important to use an epinephrine-containing test dose. In this instance the epinephrine is a more reliable marker of intravascular injection, and the toxicity risk is greater because of the higher doses (volume and concentration) needed for surgical anesthesia. After proper placement of the catheter has been confirmed, incremental doses of 2 per cent lidocaine with epinephrine, 0.5 per cent bupivacaine, or 3.0 per cent 2-chloroprocaine may be administered to achieve an adequate sensory level for surgery. Blood pressure and pulse should be checked frequently, and any hypotension (systolic less than 100 torr) should be treated with 5- to 10-mg increments of ephedrine. Proper intravenous fluid preloading helps to offset the potential for a decrease in maternal arterial pressure. Also, the mother should be maintained in the left tilt position to avoid aortocaval compression. It is important to maintain maternal blood pressure (systolic of 100 torr or mean of 70 torr) because of its direct influence on uterine perfusion. During the surgery the mother should receive supplemental oxygen to optimize fetal oxygenation before delivery.

After delivery of the infant, epidural narcotics may be used to provide both intraoperative and postoperative analgesia. It has also been noted that epidural fentanyl (onset of action 5 to 6 minutes) provides additional analgesia during the exteriorization of the uterus. The delayed onset of action of epidural morphine (30 to 60 minutes) makes it less useful for this purpose. The more fat-soluble opiates such as fentanyl have a shorter duration of action and therefore require repeated dosing or a continuous infusion with the catheter left in place for at least 24 hours. A single dose of epidural morphine lasts 12 to 24 hours. The most common side effects of the epidural opioids are respiratory depression, puritus, nausea, and urinary retention. Intraspinal morphine has the highest incidence of respiratory depression. The risk of respiratory depression is greater in patients with underlying lung disease and those receiving additional parenteral narcotics. Because morphine is the least lipid-soluble narcotic, a higher concentration of free drug remains in the cerebrospinal fluid and slowly moves rostrally in the cerebrospinal fluid. This concentration of free drug accounts for the late respiratory depression (6 to 12 hours) as the drug reaches the brain stem. These effects can be treated with small doses (0.1 to 0.4 mg) of naloxone (Narcan). The usual doses of the most commonly used epidural opioids are given in Table 1.

Regional Anesthesia: Spinal

Spinal anesthesia may be used for cesarean section with the advantages of rapid onset of anesthesia, more profound sensory and motor blocks, and the least maternal and fetal drug exposure. Potential disadvantages include a more unpredictable sensory level, greater incidence of significant hypotension, and the risk of postdural puncture headache. It has been noted that even with adequate fluid preload (1.5 to 2 liters) and left uterine displacement, there may be significant hypotensive episodes in up to 40 per cent of parturients with spinal anesthesia. These hypotensive episodes are usually effectively treated by aggressive use of ephedrine. Some physicians have even advocated the use of prophylactic intramuscular ephedrine (25 to 50 mg). There is no untoward effect on the neonate as long as hypotension is avoided. Hyperbaric formulations of the spinal agents are used because they give the most reliable and predictable thoracic levels when compared with isobaric or hypobaric solutions. Lidocaine (5 per cent in 7.5 per cent dextrose), tetracaine (0.5 per cent in 5 per cent dextrose), tetracaine (1 per cent) and procaine (10 per cent) in a 1:1 mixture, and bupivacaine (7.5 per cent in 8.25 per cent dextrose) are the most commonly used spinal preparations. Recent comparisons of hyperbaric bupivacaine, hyperbaric tetracaine, and the mixture of tetracaine and procaine for cesarean section suggest that there may be less hypotension with the hyperbaric bupivacaine. A suggested dosing regimen is shown in Table 2.

More recently, spinal opiates such as morphine or fentanyl in small doses (0.2 mg and 6.25 micrograms, respectively) have been added to the group of spinal local anesthetic agents to provide postoperative analgesia. Respiratory depression is a potential side effect, but the most frequently noted side effect is itching.

General Anesthesia for Cesarean Section

General anesthesia is necessary in cases of fetal distress, in patients who refuse regional anesthesia, or in patients with contraindications for regional anesthesia (i.e., coagulation abnormalities, anatomic spinal anomalies, or hemodynamic instability). All the monitors that are available in the surgical suite should also be available in the area where a cesarean section is performed. Preparation for general anesthesia includes adequate assessment of the airway, prophylactic antacid administration, left uterine displacement, adequate intravenous access for hydration, and

TABLE 1. **Epidural Opioids**

Narcotic	Dose	Onset of Action (min)	Duration of Action (hr)
Morphine	3–5 mg	30–60	16–24
Fentanyl	50–100 μg	6–9	3–5
Sufentanil	15–50 μg	2–8	3–6
Butorphanol	2–4 mg	10–15	6–12
Hydromorphone	1–2 mg	10–13	6–8

preoxygenation. Preoxygenation is important for increasing both the maternal and fetal oxygen stores. Because of a decreased functional residual capacity and increased oxygen consumption, the pregnant patient develops arterial desaturation faster than the nonpregnant patient. Likewise, because of the enlarged breasts and venous engorgement of the airway in the pregnant patient, laryngoscopy may be more difficult. With a potentially longer period of apnea before intubation, it is imperative that all pregnant patients be adequately preoxygenated.

Because of the high risk of aspiration pneumonitis, all pregnant patients receiving general anesthesia must be considered to have a full stomach. Therefore, use of a rapid sequence induction, with cricoid pressure until the airway has been secured with a cuffed endotracheal tube, is preferred. Thiopental (Pentothal) is the most commonly used induction agent in a dose of 3 to 4 mg per kg. Alternatively, ketamine (0.75 to 1 mg per kg) can be used in patients in whom hypovolemia or bronchospasm may be a concern. Succinylcholine is still unsurpassed at offering the best intubating conditions in the shortest time. The usual dose of succinylcholine is 1 to 1.5 mg per kg. Cricoid pressure must be applied correctly to avoid distorting the airway. When pressure is applied correctly, the esophagus is compressed between the back of the cricoid cartilage and the anterior surface of the body of the sixth cervical vertebra. Thus, passive regurgitation is prevented. It is important to maintain the cricoid pressure until the airway has been secured. The surgical incision should not be made until the endotracheal tube has been verified to

be in the trachea. This verification allows the option of awakening the mother and securing the airway in the event of a failed intubation. After the trachea has been successfully intubated, the anesthesia is maintained with nitrous oxide and oxygen (a minimum of 50 per cent oxygen until delivery). Lower doses of a volatile agent (0.5 per cent halothane, 0.75 per cent isoflurane, 1 per cent enflurane) can be added without a significant increase in uterine relaxation or in blood loss. The addition of the volatile agent does decrease the chance of maternal recall, which may be present when nitrous oxide and oxygen are used alone. Muscle relaxation may be maintained with either a succinylcholine drip or the nondepolarizing relaxants. Although all of these agents cross the placenta and can be detected in fetal blood, at the usual clinical doses the amount is not sufficient to cause any neonatal problems. Unnecessary haste to deliver the infant is not warranted just because of the use of general anesthesia. However, an interval from induction to delivery of more than 8 to 10 minutes may have some neonatal effect from the equilibration of the nitrous oxide. This effect is dealt with by oxygen administration and ventilation of the neonate. An interval from uterine incision to delivery of more than 3 minutes has also been shown to be associated with fetal acidosis and lower 1-minute Apgar scores. This interval delay must be limited regardless of whether a regional or general anesthetic is used.

Once the infant has been delivered, Pitocin is added to the intravenous fluids (20 units per liter), and the volatile agent is decreased or discontinued while narcotics are added. If the

TABLE 2. **Spinal Anesthetic Doses in Parturients**

Anesthetic	Dose (mg) for Heights of				
	152 cm	160 cm	168 cm	176 cm	182 cm
Hyperbaric lidocaine 5%*	60	65	70	75	80
Hyperbaric tetracaine 0.5%†	7	8	9	10	11
Hyperbaric bupivacaine 0.75%*	7.5	10	12	14	15
Mixture‡ of tetracaine and procaine, 1% in 10%	6 in 60 mg	7 in 70 mg	8 in 80 mg	9 in 90 mg	10 in 100 mg

*Both lidocaine and bupivacaine are marketed in a premixed formulation with dextrose.
†Tetracaine is available in a 1% solution and in a lyophilized form made hyperbaric by mixing with 10% dextrose.
‡Tetracaine 1% mixed with procaine 10% results in a hyperbaric solution.

oxygen saturation is acceptable, the nitrous oxide may be increased to 70 per cent. Either very-low-dose volatile agents or a small dose of a benzodiazapine (1 to 2 mg of midazolam* [Versed] or 2 to 5 mg of diazepam [Valium]) may be used to supplement amnesia. The addition of narcotics after the delivery allows for decreased use of volatile agents, thus reducing the concern about their potential for uterine relaxation and increased blood loss. Narcotics such as fentanyl (1 to 3 micrograms per kg), morphine (0.1 to 0.2 mg per kg), and meperidine (1 to 2 mg per kg) can be used. The narcotics also provide some analgesia in the postanesthesia care unit and allow for a smoother and potentially more rapid emergence from anesthesia. On emergence from anesthesia, the mother should demonstrate complete reversal of neuromuscular blockade, ability to maintain her airway, and the ability to follow verbal commands. It is important that she be awake and able to cooperate before extubation because of the risk of vomiting and aspiration if protective reflexes are still depressed.

POSTPARTUM CARE

method of
KENNETH J. MOISE, JR., M.D.
Baylor College of Medicine
Houston, Texas

The postpartum period has been arbitrarily divided into the immediate puerperium (first 24 hours after delivery), early puerperium (24 hours to 7 days), and late puerperium (7 days to 6 weeks). Surveillance in the immediate and early postpartum periods is aimed at the detection of infection, bleeding, and complications related to administration of anesthesia.

HOSPITAL CARE

Recovery Room

After vaginal delivery, the patient is usually observed in the recovery room for 1 hour; if epidural anesthesia has been used for labor, the patient should be observed until return of motor function of the lower extremities. After cesarean section (CS), the patient is observed for 2 hours. Vital signs are monitored every 15 minutes for the first hour and every 30 minutes thereafter.

Postpartum Floor

Vital Signs. The patient's temperature, blood pressure, pulse, and respiratory rate are recorded

*Product labeling states that this drug is not recommended for obstetric use.

every 4 to 6 hours. CS patients should have careful monitoring of their fluid status (intravenous fluids, urine output, surgical drain output), with totals noted after each shift. Intake and output records are discontinued when the patient is taking oral fluids.

Laboratory Testing. The hematocrit of all patients should be done 24 hours after delivery. CS patients should have an additional determination on the third postoperative day. This value represents the equilibrated hematocrit related to blood loss after delivery. Any patient whose immunity to rubella is unknown should have this determined before discharge.

Physician's Rounds. The physician should see the patient in the morning and afternoon of each day.

Diet. After vaginal delivery, a regular diet is permitted. After CS, ice chips are allowed until the return of flatus, at which time clear liquids are introduced. A regular diet can be allowed on the following day. The introduction of clear liquids when "bowel sounds are present" often leads to abdominal distention and the need for various enemas and cathartics. The ascultation of bowel sounds represents the return of small bowel function. Postoperative ileus is usually related to decreased motility of the cecum and large intestine. Patients who are breast-feeding should include 500 to 800 additional calories in their diet to promote milk production.

Activity. Ambulation is allowed after vaginal delivery. If an epidural anesthetic was used in labor, the patient should be assisted during her first attempts at walking. CS patients should be placed in a bedside chair in the morning and afternoon the day following surgery. Ambulation with assistance is encouraged by the second postoperative day.

Wound Care. In cases of episiotomy or perineal lacerations, ice packs are applied to the perineum for the first 24 hours, then warm water sitz baths are begun twice a day. Stool softeners are indicated with third- and fourth-degree extensions of the episiotomy. Because the surgical wound is sealed by 24 hours, a CS patient should remove her bandage on the second postoperative day, beginning at the edges of the bandage. The patient should be informed that the *physician* will remove the bandage at evening rounds if it is still in place. The patient should defer showering until skin staples are removed. These staples should be removed on the third postoperative day with a Pfannenstiel's incision or just before discharge with a vertical skin incision. There is no need to remove skin staples over 2 successive days. Benzoin is applied to the skin edges and staples are removed two or three at a time. A reinforced tape strip (Steristrip) is placed before proceeding with removal of additional staples.

Medications

ANALGESIA. Postpartum pain after vaginal delivery is usually related to the episiotomy site or to painful uterine contractions (afterbirth pains). Acetaminophen with codeine is usually sufficient to relieve episiotomy pain. Local anesthetics such as hydrocortisone foam (Epifoam) or benzocaine spray (Dermoplast) may be beneficial. Prostaglandin synthetase inhibitors such as naproxen (Anaprox DS, one tablet every 8 hours) are beneficial for afterbirth pains. CS patients usually require intramuscular medications such as morphine (6 to 8 mg), meperidine (Demerol, 50 to 75 mg), or a synthetic narcotic such as butorphanol (Stadol, 2 mg) every 3 to 4 hours. Patient-controlled analgesia using intravenous bolus therapy of these same medications by sophisticated parenteral pumps is gaining widespread acceptance and has several advantages over standard intramuscular analgesia. The patient can usually be switched to oral analgesics such as acetaminophen with codeine when she is tolerating oral intake.

LACTATION SUPPRESSION. Bromocriptine (Parlodel, 2.5 mg twice daily for 14 days) is usually successful. Occasionally, a patient requires an additional week of therapy. The patient should be cautioned to discontinue the medication if she experiences severe headaches or syncope with standing.

RUBELLA IMMUNIZATION. Any patient who is not immune should be administered intramuscular immunization; breast-feeding is not a contraindication.

RHESUS IMMUNE GLOBULIN. Three hundred micrograms (1 unit) of rhesus immune globulin (RHIG) is given intramuscularly within 72 hours of delivery to Rh-negative women delivering Rh-positive infants. The blood bank may advise the administration of more than 1 unit of RHIG if there is evidence of more than 30 ml of fetal blood in the maternal circulation (this recommendation is based on maternal testing that is routinely performed on all postpartum Rh-negative women in most hospitals).

Breast-Feeding. The infant should be encouraged to suckle soon after birth. Suckling in the delivery room after vaginal delivery stimulates oxytocin release, which aids in preventing uterine atony. Although actual milk production does not begin until the second or third postpartum day, colostrum (with its many important components) is almost always present at birth. The patient should be encouraged to breast-feed at approximately 4-hour intervals. The infant should be allowed to suckle each breast for 5 minutes; the duration of suckling should be increased by 5 minutes every other day until a 20-minute period

of suckling on each breast is achieved. The patient should begin breast-feeding with the opposite breast from the one last used in the previous feeding. Sore nipples are best treated by changing the position of the infant during subsequent feeding. Another patient who has breast-fed a previous child or an experienced nurse is often helpful in demonstrating various feeding positions. Cracked or bleeding nipples can be treated with the contents of a vitamin E capsule. Lanolin cream, although commonly used, does not promote healing of the breast.

Length of Stay in the Hospital. Women who had uncomplicated vaginal deliveries can be discharged within the first 24 hours post partum; CS patients are usually hospitalized for 3 to 5 days.

DISCHARGE PLANNING

Exercise. If an episiotomy or vaginal laceration occurred, the patient should abstain from vigorous physical activity that might stress this area for 2 to 3 weeks. CS patients should not drive or participate in strenuous activities until they are seen at their 4-week postpartum office visit.

Sexual Activity. Coitus should be avoided for 2 to 3 weeks in CS patients and in those patients whose vaginal delivery was complicated by episiotomy or vaginal laceration. Encourage breast-feeding patients to use a lubricating preparation before coitus as the hypoestrogenic state that is secondary to breast-feeding often results in atrophy of the vaginal mucosa. On rare occasions, estrogen vaginal cream (Premarin) can be used two or three times per week to rejuvenate the vaginal mucosa.

Wound Care. Tub soaks should continue twice daily for 1 to 2 weeks to aid in episiotomy healing. CS patients may shower or bathe. Steristrips should be removed 1 week after discharge.

Medications. Discharge medications should include the following:

Analgesics: acetaminophen with codeine or prostaglandin synthetase inhibitors

Bromocriptine (if lactation suppression is desired), 2.5 mg twice daily, to complete a 2-week course

Ferrous sulfate, 325 mg two or three times daily for several weeks if the postpartum hematocrit was less than 30 per cent

Stool softeners: docusate sodium (Colace) twice daily for 2 weeks is effective and should be prescribed especially for a third- or fourth-degree extension of the episiotomy

Prenatal vitamins: continue once daily, especially if the patient is still breast-feeding

Contraception. Breast-feeding patients should be encouraged to use spermicidal foam in conjunction with condoms until they are seen for their postpartum visit because oral contraceptives are contraindicated. Involution of the pelvic organs is usually complete by this time and a diaphragm can be fitted. An intrauterine device can be inserted in the immediate postpartum period; however, the expulsion rate is much higher than if insertion is postponed until the postpartum visit. Most physicians postpone initiation of oral contraceptives until 2 weeks after delivery. This decision is based on the increased incidence of thromboembolism in the postpartum period and the association of oral contraceptives with thromboembolic complications. The patient should begin taking birth control pills after completing the course of bromocriptine.

POSTPARTUM OFFICE VISITS

Cesarean Section Patients. CS patients are examined at 1 week to assess the integrity of the surgical incision. At 4 weeks post partum, a complete physical examination is performed, including Papanicolaou's smear. Contraceptive issues should be addressed.

Vaginal Delivery Patients. A complete physical examination should be performed at 4 weeks post partum, including Papanicolaou's smear. Contraceptive issues should be addressed.

RESUSCITATION AND STABILIZATION OF THE NEWBORN

method of
JAMES M. ADAMS, M.D.
Baylor College of Medicine
Houston, Texas

The depressed infant represents a true medical emergency. The primary physician may encounter such an emergency in a variety of settings, including the delivery room, the nursery, the emergency room, or even an office environment. Resuscitation and stabilization of depressed infants are best accomplished by using a simple but physiologically sound approach applied in a consistent manner and requiring minimal ancillary tools.

The American Academy of Pediatrics has noted the need for specific delivery room arrangements for care of the newborn and has recently made recommendations regarding such care; anticipation of problems is a central theme of these recommendations. The American Heart Association has markedly expanded its emphasis on resuscitation of the newborn, and its most recent guidelines stress a simple, heart rate–oriented resuscitation sequence.

ANTICIPATION OF PERINATAL ASPHYXIA

Most newborns requiring resuscitation have respiratory failure, whether in utero or in the postnatal environment. Many of the conditions leading to such circumstances can be anticipated. Table 1 gives many of the high-risk conditions associated with perinatal or neonatal asphyxia. Placental insufficiency and umbilical cord accidents may be associated with abnormal fetal heart rate patterns on fetal monitoring. When such conditions are known to exist, arrangements must be made for availability of personnel to provide immediate care of the neonate in the delivery room, and the possibility of a critically ill infant should be anticipated. If any of the postnatal conditions noted exist, personnel skilled at resuscitation must be available at all times while the infant is receiving nursery care.

PHYSIOLOGY OF ASPHYXIA

The lung is the organ of respiration for the neonate whereas the placenta is that of the fetus. Both are gas exchange organs that facilitate diffusion of oxygen into blood and the removal of carbon dioxide. The carbon dioxide tension, in turn, acutely determines extracellular pH. Failure of the respiratory organ leads to a

TABLE 1. **Perinatal Conditions Predisposing to Fetal or Neonatal Asphyxia**

Placental Insufficiency
  Maternal diabetes
  Toxemia
  Chronic hypertension
  Postmaturity
  Maternal hyperventilation
  Maternal hypotension
  Cigarette smoking
  Uterine tetany

Fetal bradycardia may occur in such instances and may be of the late deceleration type on the fetal monitor.

Umbilical Cord Accidents
  Cord compression
  True knot in cord
  Cord laceration
  Anomalous insertion with disruption

Fetal bradycardia occurring in these circumstances is often of the variable deceleration type.

Postnatal Asphyxia
  Narcotics, sedatives, anesthetics
  Infection
  Cardiopulmonary disease
  Congenital anomalies

In these circumstances fetal acid-base balance is normal at birth, but derangements occur when lung function is inadequate to replace the detached placenta.

Other Causes of Bradycardia
  Head compression during terminal labor
  Local anesthetic toxicity

stereotyped series of metabolic derangements. There is rapid development of hypoxemia and hypercarbia with acute respiratory acidosis. If such circumstances persist for a more prolonged period, tissue hypoxia occurs with the appearance of superimposed metabolic (lactic) acidosis. During the early course, heart rate and circulatory function are maintained at the expense of vasoconstriction and diversion of blood flow away from noncritical organs. If asphyxia continues, however, the heart rate falls and essential organ perfusion fails. From this sequence of events, it can be readily appreciated that the establishment of adequate alveolar ventilation promptly reverses many of the metabolic consequences of respiratory organ failure. Thus ventilation is the primary tool in the resuscitation process.

Maintenance of adequate circulatory function during asphyxia is critical in determining survival and outcome. Ischemia has a more profound effect on tissue oxygenation than low blood oxygen content alone. Cardiac output and blood flow in the newborn are related to the heart rate; thus, persistent bradycardia in the fetus or neonate may be accompanied by a profound fall in cardiac output. Closed-chest cardiac massage is the most important method of maintaining circulatory function in the face of persistent bradycardia during resuscitation.

Because hypoxia and acidosis may depress myocardial pump function, drugs have historically been used as ancillary means of improving circulatory status during resuscitation. Epinephrine is currently used to increase heart rate, as well as to augment cardiac contractility. The use of buffer agents such as sodium bicarbonate remains controversial. If alveolar ventilation is inadequate, bicarbonate administration exacerbates acidosis and may be accompanied by a fall in cardiac output, as well as increased lactic acid production by the gut. Early animal studies, however, demonstrated improved circulatory function and survival after bicarbonate administration. More recent data have confirmed improvement in arterial and brain intracellular pH after bicarbonate use despite an increase in Pa_{CO_2}. Thus, a role for sodium bicarbonate remains in circumstances of prolonged resuscitation or documented persistent metabolic acidosis.

CLINICAL COURSE OF ASPHYXIA

The classic course of events in perinatal asphyxia has been described in three clinical phases: primary apnea, gasping, and secondary apnea. These represent progressively more severe phases of asphyxia with increasing metabolic derangements. As such, they are clinically useful in attempting to judge the duration and severity of such an episode.

1. Primary apnea
   a. Metabolic derangements mild
   b. Heart rate more than 80 beats per minute
   c. Blood pressure normal or increased (palpable pulses)
   d. Response to tactile stimuli
   e. "Gasp before pink" response
   f. Apgar score usually 4 or higher
2. Gasping respirations

    a. Indicative of serious acidemia and the need for immediate initiation of resuscitation with mask and bag ventilation; without such intervention, the infant will soon enter the phase of secondary apnea
3. Secondary apnea
   a. Metabolic derangements severe
   b. Heart rate less than 80 beats per minute
   c. Blood pressure low (pulses poor or absent)
   d. No response to tactile stimuli
   e. Resuscitation requires positive pressure ventilation
   f. "Pink before gasp" response
   g. Apgar score may be 3 or less

In the clinical setting, however, these phases may progress in utero making primary and secondary apnea indistinguishable at the time of birth. *When faced with an apneic infant, secondary apnea should always be assumed and positive pressure ventilation initiated with a mask and bag without delay for elaborate clinical staging.*

Apgar scoring has likewise been widely used to assess the overall state of reactivity of infants at birth, as well as being an ancillary tool to evaluate the need for intervention. Although it remains useful in the general evaluation of the infant, the Apgar score neither establishes nor rules out the diagnosis of asphyxia. The score frequently correlates poorly with the underlying acid-base status of the infant at birth, particularly in preterm infants. The need for resuscitation can be more accurately assessed by evaluating heart rate, respiratory activity, and color than the Apgar score. These are the key signs guiding the operator in neonatal resuscitation, and they cannot be emphasized too strongly. Resuscitation should be immediately initiated when indicated and never delayed for assessment of the 1-minute Apgar score.

RESUSCITATION-STABILIZATION PROCEDURE

Neonatal resuscitation requires the combined efforts of two trained individuals. The procedure is carried out in two phases, the first of which is performed on every newborn at birth. The need for Phase 2 intervention is determined by the evaluation done during Phase 1. The Phase 1 and 2 sequences are presented in Figure 1 and 2. The keys to the resuscitation sequence are respirations, heart rate, and color.

Phase 1

The following steps should be carried out in all newborns immediately after delivery:

1. Prevent heat loss. Place the infant under a radiant warming device and dry off the amniotic fluid.
2. Open the airway. Position the infant with the neck slightly extended and gently suction first the mouth and then the nose. If mechanical

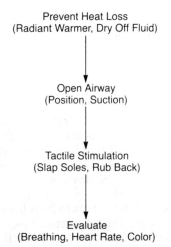

Prevent Heat Loss
(Radiant Warmer, Dry Off Fluid)

↓

Open Airway
(Position, Suction)

↓

Tactile Stimulation
(Slap Soles, Rub Back)

↓

Evaluate
(Breathing, Heart Rate, Color)

Figure 1. Resuscitation-stabilization, Phase 1 (all deliveries).

suction is used, limit negative pressure to 100 mmHg. (Intubation and direct tracheal suctioning should be performed at this point on infants with thick meconium staining. Specific management of the meconium-stained infant is discussed at the end of this chapter.)

3. Provide tactile stimulation. Gently slap the soles of the feet or rub the infant's back. This may be sufficient to stimulate respirations in some apneic infants. Drying off the amniotic fluid also provides tactile stimulation.

4. Evaluate the infant. Is respiratory effort present? Is the heart rate above 100 beats per minute? Is cyanosis present?

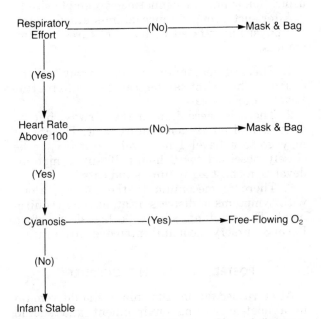

Respiratory Effort ——————(No)————————►Mask & Bag

↓ (Yes)

Heart Rate Above 100 ——————(No)————————►Mask & Bag

↓ (Yes)

Cyanosis——————(Yes)————————►Free-Flowing O₂

↓ (No)

Infant Stable

Figure 2. Resuscitation-stabilization, Phase 2 (intervention).

Phase 2

The following definitive steps should be taken if Phase 1 evaluation reveals apnea or inadequate respirations, a heart rate less than 100 beats per minute, or the presence of cyanosis. The response of each is the key to the next step in the sequence. The basic tools in this sequence are ventilation by mask and bag and closed-chest massage. This type of ventilation is the basic skill for resuscitation of the newborn because it can be mastered and used by all caregivers, both physician and nonphysician. This technique alone adequately resuscitates almost all depressed infants.

1. If the infant is apneic or has inadequate respirations, provide mask-and-bag ventilation with 100 per cent oxygen at a rate of 60 breaths per minute until the heart rate is above 100 beats per minute and spontaneous respirations are established. If the technique is adequate, the heart rate should rise above 100 beats per minute within 30 seconds.

2. If the heart rate is less than 100 beats per minute, provide mask-and-bag ventilation until the heart rate is stable above 100 beats per minute and spontaneous respiratory activity occurs. If the heart rate is less than 80 beats per minute or remains below 100 beats per minute despite adequate ventilation, begin cardiac massage. This can be done at a rate of 120 beats per minute in conjunction with a ventilation rate of 60 beats per minute. Alternatively, both ventilation and massage may be done in a 1:1 ratio at a rate of 100 per minute.

3. If cyanosis is present but the infant is breathing spontaneously with a heart rate above 100 beats per minute, deliver free-flowing oxygen at a rate of 5 liters per minute directly from oxygen tubing held 0.5 inch from the nose.

4. If an infant required mask-and-bag ventilation, with or without cardiac massage, and intubation is indicated for ongoing care, the intubation can be carried out under controlled conditions once the heart rate is stable above 100 beats per minute and the color has been improved using mask-and-bag ventilation.

MEDICATIONS

Medications are rarely needed in resuscitation of the newborn because establishment of adequate ventilation usually reverses the metabolic consequences of respiratory organ failure. Drugs are indicated, however, if the heart rate remains less than 80 beats per minute despite good ventilation with 100 per cent oxygen and chest compressions. The umbilical vein is the preferred route for administration of drugs in the delivery room, but epinephrine can be administered via endotracheal tube if no other route is available. Only the following are currently of proven value in newborn resuscitation:

1. Epinephrine (1:10,000) increases the heart rate, as well as stimulates cardiac contractility and raises peripheral vascular resistance. The dose is 0.1 to 0.2 ml per kg given intravenously or via endotracheal tube (not to exceed 1 ml).

2. Sodium bicarbonate (0.5 mEq per ml) is not indicated for brief resuscitation but may play a role if the course of asphyxia is prolonged or if documented metabolic acidosis is present. The dose is 1 to 2 mEq per kg given intravenously at a rate of 1 mEq per minute.

3. Five per cent albumin in saline is indicated for blood volume expansion if the history suggests acute blood loss. A 20 per cent or greater loss in blood volume may be suspected if there is pallor and poor perfusion despite normal pH and P_{O_2}, if pulses remain weak despite a good heart rate, or if the response to resuscitation is poor. The dose is 10 to 15 ml per kg initially, to be repeated until signs of circulatory insufficiency are improved.

4. Naloxone hydrochloride (Narcan Neonatal) is a narcotic antagonist for reversal of a variety of narcotic analgesics. The drug may be indicated if severe respiratory depression is present with a history of maternal narcotic administration within the past 4 hours. The infant should receive prompt, adequate ventilatory assistance *before* administration of the drug, and such support should be continued until naloxone exerts its effect. The dose is 0.5 ml per kg (0.01 mg per kg) given intravenously, intramuscularly, or via endotracheal tube.

MANAGEMENT OF THE MECONIUM-STAINED INFANT

The passage of meconium into the amniotic fluid may be a sign of fetal distress or asphyxia, but not invariably. The presence of thick or particulate meconium is, however, associated with increased perinatal morbidity and mortality. This includes the risk of meconium aspiration syndrome with severe respiratory distress and complications such as pneumothorax.

The presence of thick, meconium-stained amniotic fluid necessitates a combined obstetric and pediatric approach. When the head of the infant appears on the perineum, the mouth and hypopharynx should be quickly but gently suctioned by the delivering physician. Once delivery has occurred, the trachea should be intubated for removal of any meconium present by direct suc-

tioning. This is best done by applying suction directly to the endotracheal tube, using a regulated suction source limited to 100 mmHg and connected via a commercial adaptor. The suction is applied while withdrawing the tube from the trachea. If no meconium is present, one proceeds with the usual stabilization sequence. If meconium is present, the heart rate should be evaluated. If the heart rate is more than 80 beats per minute, intubation should be repeated if needed to remove any further meconium. Color should be observed and free-flowing oxygen given if needed. One should observe for signs of respiratory distress. If the heart rate falls below 80 beats per minute after initial suctioning, one should ventilate with a mask and bag until the heart rate is stable above 100 beats per minute and then proceed with repeat suctioning if needed.

Suctioning should be done directly via endotracheal tubes. Viscid meconium is not effectively removed by passing a suction catheter into the endotracheal tube. Saline lavage of the trachea should not be done, as this may hasten peripheral deposition of meconium.

It is important that conditions be provided after suctioning to optimize the postnatal fall in pulmonary vascular resistance. Oxygen should be delivered initially and withdrawn progressively rather than abruptly. If cyanosis or respiratory distress is present, oxygen should be continued in amounts adequate to achieve good color; then more definitive studies of the adequacy of oxygenation, such as blood gas analysis or oxymetry, should be done. The dangers of the meconium aspiration syndrome cannot be overemphasized.

After suctioning of a meconium-stained infant, the physician is faced with one of three circumstances:

1. There is meconium in the airway and no distress. The infant can be transferred to routine Level 1 nursery care.

2. There is meconium in the airway, but no distress and no oxygen requirement. The infant may go to a Level 1 or Level 2 nursery, to be closely observed for 6 hours. If any symptoms develop, a chest x-ray film is indicated.

3. There is meconium in the airway, along with symptoms of distress or an oxygen requirement. These infants should be transferred to a Level 3 nursery (neonatal intensive care unit).

POSTRESUSCITATION PROCEDURE

After resuscitation, the infant should remain in a heat-conserving environment and should receive continued positive pressure ventilation or oxygen until an optimal fall in postnatal pulmonary vascular resistance has occurred. The infant should not be moved until ventilation is adequate, the heart rate is stable above 120 beats per minute, the color is pink, and the temperature is in the normal range. Adequate stabilization may require biochemical monitoring of pH and blood gases, hematocrit determination, or a glucose oxidase strip test. Patients requiring intubation should not be extubated until transported to a final nursery where ongoing care and biochemical monitoring demonstrate recovery. Many such infants continue to have respiratory distress. (An exception is the infant intubated for suctioning of meconium who has no meconium in the trachea and no symptoms.) Adequate alveolar ventilation and circulatory support, if needed, must be ensured during transport. After stabilization, infants requiring resuscitation should have a source of intravascular glucose provided to prevent the occurrence of hypoglycemia. The peak period of risk for hypoglycemia in the compromised neonate occurs between 30 and 60 minutes after birth.

CARE OF THE HIGH-RISK NEONATE

method of
LAWRENCE J. FENTON, M.D.
University of South Dakota
Sioux Falls, South Dakota

The care of a high-risk neonate actually begins prior to birth. Therefore, it is important to recognize when such an infant may be born so that steps can be taken to prevent or minimize serious complications. Table 1 summarizes the reasons to anticipate ill health in the neonate and the typical problems associated with each risk category. The scoring system developed by Creasy and colleagues is also helpful in determining the risk of premature labor (Table 2). Most problems arise from either the failure to recognize potential problems or lack of aggressiveness in diagnostic evaluation and treatment.

One can sometimes begin to assume that a baby is well until a crisis is reached, even though signs and symptoms may have been pointing toward a problem for several hours. It is helpful, especially during the first 6 hours after a birth, to maintain an attitude that all newborn babies are in a recovery phase and must *prove* themselves to be well. Of course, infants can become ill after the first 6 hours of life, but in most cases clues to the diagnosis of ill health appear in the first 6 hours, or at least during the first 48 hours.

HISTORY AND PHYSICAL EXAMINATION

Many of the risk factors in Table 1 can be recognized by taking a careful, thorough history. Others can be found in the physical examination performed soon after birth. If there are any questions about the normality of findings on the physical examination, these should be pursued immediately by consultation, appropriate diagnostic tests, or a concrete plan for re-examination in a short time. Close attention should be paid to instability of temperature, poor sucking, or any major change in behavior.

General Appearance. Any unusual aspects of the baby's activity or facial appearance should be noted. The baby's gestational age and physical maturity should be assessed and plotted on a graph to determine percentile rankings (Figures 1 and 2).

Head. The head should be examined for anomalies, including palpation of the hard palate to determine whether there is a submucosal cleft. The ears, eyes, nose, and throat should also be examined.

Respiration. Sounds should be equal bilaterally at the base of the lungs and at the axillae. Abnormalities such as grunting or retraction or a respiratory rate above 60 may also indicate a problem. If there is any reason for doubt about the health of the lungs, transillumination, a chest x-ray, and a complete blood count should be performed to determine whether there is spontaneous pneumothorax, pneumonia, or a congenital pulmonary or cardiac anomaly.

Cardiovascular System. Peripheral perfusion can be tested by pressing on the chest, abdomen, or thigh and timing the return of blood to the skin. If the return of blood takes more than 3 seconds, peripheral perfusion should be considered diminished. Possible causes of this include hypovolemia, infection, hypoplastic left heart syndrome, hypoglycemia, and hypothermia. A chest x-ray, complete blood count, and blood glucose measurement are helpful in pursuing the cause of diminished peripheral perfusion.

The baby should also be examined for signs of congenital heart disease. Bilateral inequality of pulses and blood pressure in the arms or legs may suggest coarctation. Other signs of congenital heart disease include an unusual second heart sound (single, widely split, or loud) and central cyanosis as evidenced by blue coloration of the trunk, face, or lips.

Abdomen. The examiner should palpate the abdomen carefully for the presence of masses and to locate the liver, spleen, and kidneys. If the liver is more than 2 cm below the right costal margin, infection, heart failure, or hemolytic disease may be present. If more than the tip of the spleen is palpable, bacterial or viral infection or hemolysis should be suspected. A complete blood count and a platelet count should be obtained. The examiner should be able to feel both kidneys clearly. If this is not possible despite repeated palpation, renal ultrasonography is indicated.

Genitalia. Careful inspection for genital abnormalities should be performed routinely.

Extremities. In addition to checking the pulses and blood pressure as mentioned earlier, the examiner should look carefully for anomalies of the extremities. A thorough examination of the hips should include both the Barlow's and Ortolani's maneuvers.

Nervous System. Neurologic problems may be indicated by asymmetry of facial movements during crying, or asymmetry of movement or tone of the arms or legs.

TABLE 1. **Major Categories of Risk of Ill Health in the Neonate**

Risk Category	Reasons to Anticipate High-Risk Birth	Typical Problems
Prematurity (less than 38 wk gestation)	Premature labor Premature rupture of membranes Vaginal bleeding after 12 wk gestation History of previous premature delivery or abortion Multiple gestation Maternal infection, e.g., of urinary tract Maternal smoking Low income Uterine anomaly Placenta previa Abdominal surgery History of cesarean section Maternal diabetes	Hyaline membrane disease Apnea and bradycardia Hypoglycemia Hypocalcemia Intraventricular hemorrhage Feeding problems Necrotizing enterocolitis Other fluid and electrolyte disorders Infection Anemia
Postmaturity (more than 42 wk gestation) and intrauterine growth retardation	Poor intrauterine growth Maternal hypertension or other vascular disease Maternal illness during pregnancy possibly compatible with the TORCH group of infections Maternal smoking Oligohydramnios	Birth asphyxia and brain damage Hypoglycemia Polycythemia Clotting disorders, e.g., thrombocytopenia Necrotizing enterocolitis
Birth asphyxia	Postmaturity Intrauterine growth retardation Meconium-stained amniotic fluid Fetal distress, e.g., persistent fetal heart rate greater than 160 beats/min, loss of beat-to-beat variability, persistent abnormal pattern, fetal acidosis	Brain damage Seizures Meconium aspiration Apnea and bradycardia Necrotizing enterocolitis Feeding disorders Persistence of fetal circulation Hypoglycemia Clotting disorders Renal failure (acute tubular necrosis) Poor cardiac output hypotension
Infants of diabetic mothers	Maternal diabetes, either pre-existing or appearing during pregnancy	Hypoglycemia Polycythemia Hypocalcemia Feeding problems Congenital anomalies Respiratory problems Hyaline membrane disease Transient tachypnea
Congenital anomalies	Intrauterine growth retardation Oligohydramnios Polyhydramnios Elevated or depressed alpha-protein Breech presentation	Surgical Life-threatening conditions Major handicaps Need for genetic counseling Parental guilt With elevated alpha-protein: neural tube defect, omphalocele, gastroschisis, congenital nephrosis, upper gastrointestinal obstruction, Turner's syndrome With depressed alpha-fetoprotein: chromosomal anomalies, especially trisomy 21
Infection	Maternal infection, e.g., of urinary tract Chorioamnionitis Birth asphyxia Premature labor Premature rupture of membranes Prematurity Membrane rupture occurring more than 24 hr before delivery	Respiratory failure Hypotension Hypoglycemia Anemia Hyperbilirubinemia Persistent fetal circulation Clotting disorders

TABLE 2. **Scoring System for Risk of Preterm Delivery***

Points†	Socioeconomic Status	Past History	Daily Habits	Current Pregnancy
1	Two children at home Low socioeconomic status	One abortion less than 1 yr since last birth	Work outside home	Unusual fatigue
2	Younger than 20 yr Older than 40 yr Single parent	Two abortions	More than 10 cigarettes per day	Less than 13-lb gain by 32 wk Albuminuria Hypertension Bacteriuria
3	Very low socioeconomic status Shorter than 150 cm Lighter than 45 kg	Three abortions	Heavy work Long, tiring trip	Breech at 32 wk Weight loss of 2 kg Head engaged Febrile illness
4	Younger than 18 yr	Pyelonephritis		Metrorrhagia after 12 wk gestation Effacement Dilatation Uterine irritability
5		Uterine anomaly Second trimester abor- tion Diethylstilbestrol expo- sure		Placenta previa Hydramnios
10		Premature delivery Repeated second trimes- ter abortion		Twins Abdominal surgery

*Adapted with permission from The American College of Obstetricians and Gynecologists (Obstetrics and Gynecology, vol 55, 1980, p 692).

†Score is computed by addition of the number of points given any time. 0–5 = low risk; 6–9 = medium risk; 10 or more = high risk.

The overall vigor of the infant's tone, suck, and cry should also be assessed.

PREMATURE BIRTH

Fluid and Electrolyte Treatment

Intravenous administration of fluids and electrolytes should be started if the baby weighs less than 2500 grams, is less than 36 weeks of gestational age, is unable to suck or swallow, needed resuscitation by intubation or by prolonged bag-and-mask ventilation in the delivery room, or has an Apgar score less than 4 at 1 minute or less than 6 at 5 minutes. If an intravenous line is needed, use of a peripheral vein is preferable if it is possible. A 23- or 25-gauge scalp vein needle may be very useful. In an emergency, an umbilical vein catheter can be used, positioned just above the diaphragm as located on an x-ray or placed in just far enough to allow blood return. No hypertonic solutions should be infused through the umbilical vein catheter unless the tip is known to be above the diaphragm in the inferior vena cava.

In general, 80 ml per kg per 24 hours is a safe amount of fluid to administer when beginning intravenous therapy for premature babies. For babies weighing more than 1200 grams, 10 per cent dextrose in water (D10W) should be used. For infants weighing 1200 grams or less, 5 per cent dextrose in water (D5W) is preferable. Rates of administration can be adjusted on the basis of electrolyte levels, weight changes, urinary output, and specific gravity of urine; however, specific gravity is an unreliable indicator for several weeks or longer in premature babies because of their inability to concentrate urine. If weight increases or fails to decrease, the baby may be overloaded with fluid (unless there was a major loss of volume at delivery). If weight decreases by more than 2 per cent per day, the baby probably needs more fluids.

Usually no electrolytes are needed for the first 6 to 12 hours after birth unless there is reason to suspect electrolyte abnormalities in the mother, as could occur if the mother received a large volume of hypotonic fluid prior to delivery. Serum sodium and potassium levels should be measured at 12 hours of age. Maintenance sodium chloride (3 mEq per kg per day) should be added if the sodium level is below 135 mEq per liter; the desired range for serum sodium is 135 to 145 mEq per liter. Maintenance potassium chloride (2 mEq per kg per day) should be added if the potassium level is less than 4.5 mEq per liter and urine output is established.

Hypocalcemia is common in premature babies. A serum calcium level of less than 7 mg per dl in a premature baby is usually considered a deficiency. The serum calcium level usually reaches its lowest point at about 48 hours of age.

Neuromuscular Maturity

	0	1	2	3	4	5
Posture						
Square Window (wrist)	90°	60°	45°	30°	0°	
Arm Recoil	180°		100°–180°	90°–100°	<90°	
Popliteal Angle	180°	160°	130°	110°	90°	<90°
Scarf Sign						
Heel to Ear						

PHYSICAL MATURITY

Skin	gelatinous red, transparent	smooth pink, visible veins	superficial peeling &/or rash few veins	cracking pale area rare veins	parchment deep cracking no vessels	leathery cracked wrinkled
Lanugo	none	abundant	thinning	bald areas	mostly bald	
Plantar Creases	no crease	faint red marks	anterior transverse crease only	creases ant. 2/3	creases cover entire sole	
Breast	barely percept.	flat areola no bud	stippled areola 1–2 mm bud	raised areola 3–4 mm bud	full areola 5–10 mm bud	
Ear	pinna flat, stays folded	sl. curved pinna; soft with slow recoil	well-curv. pinna; soft but ready recoil	formed & firm with instant recoil	thick cartilage ear stiff	
Genitals ♂	scrotum empty no rugae		testes descending, few rugae	testes down good rugae	testes pendulous deep rugae	
Genitals ♀	prominent clitoris & labia minora		majora & minora equally prominent	majora large minora small	clitoris & minora completely covered	

MATURITY RATING

Score	Wks
5	26
10	28
15	30
20	32
25	34
30	36
35	38
40	40
45	42
50	44

Figure 1. Assessment of gestational age. (Modified from Ballard JL, Novak KK, and Driver M: J Pediatr 95:769, 1979.)

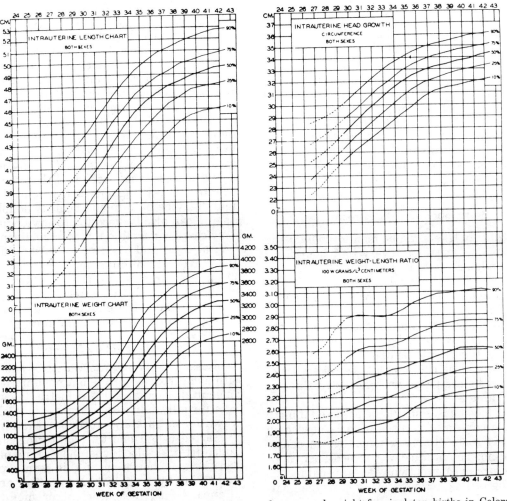

Figure 2. Intrauterine growth curves for length, head circumference, and weight for singleton births in Colorado. (From Lubchenco L, Hansman C, and Boyd, E. Reproduced by permission of Pediatrics *81*:102, 1988.)

I usually begin treatment of hypocalcemia by adding maintenance calcium gluconate to the intravenous fluids at a dose of 1 mEq of elemental calcium per kg per day or 200 mg of calcium gluconate per kg per day. (This is equivalent to 2 ml of 10 per cent calcium gluconate per kg per day.) An alternative to adding the calcium gluconate to the intravenous fluid is to give it as four divided boluses; this should be done very slowly with the infant on a cardiac monitor to allow quick recognition of bradycardia. We prefer this latter method because we occasionally substitute sodium bicarbonate for sodium chloride in the intravenous line when there is significant metabolic acidosis; the sodium bicarbonate and calcium cannot be kept in the same solution, so the calcium in these cases must be administered separately. Another approach is to "drip" the calcium and "push" bicarbonate very slowly if needed. The major risk of rapid pushing of sodium bicarbonate is intraventricular hemorrhage.

The pharmacist should be asked to make up these solutions on a per kilogram basis, rather than giving the electrolytes as a specified measurement per 100 ml. The amount of sodium, potassium, or other electrolyte a baby may need can be quite independent of the baby's need for fluids. Therefore, whenever the rate of infusion of fluid is changed, the electrolyte concentration of the fluid should be adjusted to maintain the desired level of electrolyte administration based on the baby's weight.

A constant weight, typically the birth weight, should be used as the reference weight for determining how much fluid to administer. Otherwise, the normal loss of weight during the first days of life may offset to some extent any increase in fluid administration ordered on a per kilogram basis, or cause an unwanted reduction in total fluid administration in an infant who started out receiving an adequate amount of fluid when infusion was originally based on birth weight.

Fluid intake and output should be carefully monitored and totaled at least every 8 hours. Measurement of urine specific gravity and testing with a urine test-tape should be done frequently, in some cases with every void.

If the baby can tolerate it, weight should be measured once or twice a day. The baby should be kept warm during the weighing process. Emerson lights over the scale are helpful, and adequate staff should be assigned to the procedure to ensure that it is done quickly. Respiratory stability should never be compromised for the sake of monitoring weight.

Basic Laboratory Assessment

Blood glucose levels can be monitored by using Chemstrips or Dextrostix every half hour for 2 hours, then hourly for 2 hours, then 2 hours later, and then at 4-hour intervals until the patient is stable. If the blood sugar reading is 40 mg per dl or lower, a blood sample should be taken for laboratory analysis to confirm the finding. If the laboratory finding is also below 40 mg per dl, an intravenous line should be started.

A complete blood count should be taken. Findings should be compared with normal values as listed in Table 3.

Arterial blood gases should be assessed if birth asphyxia occurs or if resuscitation is needed in the delivery room. If arterial blood gas measurements cannot be obtained, a warmed-heel capillary puncture in conjunction with transcutaneous monitoring of Pa_{O_2} or monitoring of oxygen saturation may be helpful.

A chest radiograph should be obtained if there is respiratory distress or an abnormal blood gas value found on laboratory study. A chest radiograph should also be taken prior to transportation of the infant, especially if air transportation is anticipated.

Routine Care

The infant should be placed on a cardiorespiratory monitor if he or she is less than 36 weeks' gestational age, has any respiratory distress or cyanosis, or needs intravenous therapy, or if there is a historical factor indicating that the baby is at risk for infection. We monitor *all* babies in the newborn intensive care unit from admission to discharge. The monitoring unit should be set to give an alarm if an episode of apnea continues for 15 seconds or if the heart rate rises above 180 or falls below 100 beats per minute. (The lower limit of the heart rate can be adjusted to 80 beats per minute when the baby is fully stabilized or becomes a "grower"; the upper limit may need to

be adjusted to over 200 beats per minute if the baby is active or crying frequently.)

If the infant is less than 35 weeks' gestational age or has an unstable temperature, a neutral thermal environment should be provided (Table 4). An open warmer or an Isolette can be used. If the baby weighs less than 1500 grams and is placed in an open warmer, use of a plastic shield to enclose the baby and addition of warmed humidity (not enough to cause condensation or to form fog) will greatly reduce insensible water loss and preserve the skin. This is especially useful for very small babies. If the baby is in an Isolette that is being opened frequently, Emerson lights may be used to add heat. A double-walled Isolette can also be used to preserve heat, and in some cases a warming mattress is essential.

Vital signs and blood pressure should be monitored every 15 minutes for 2 hours, then every 30 minutes for 2 hours, then 2 hours later, and at 4-hour intervals thereafter. However, if a baby is very unstable, these orders should be modified to keep disturbances to a minimum.

Respiratory Distress

Assessment of respiratory distress should begin with a chest x-ray to rule out pneumothorax and congenital anomalies. If the distress is sustained or is initially fairly significant, blood should be drawn for culture and antibiotic therapy should be started (see Table 6). Monitoring should include arterial blood gas measurements taken every 1 to 4 hours or, if this is not practical, monitoring by warmed heel puncture and transcutaneous Pa_{O_2} measurement or monitoring of oxygen saturation. The Pa_{O_2} should be maintained in the range of 60 to 80 torr. A Pco_2 measurement greater than 50 torr may indicate impending respiratory failure.

If pH is below 7.25 and Pco_2 is above 50 torr, the patient should be intubated and placed on a ventilator or ventilated with a bag. If endotracheal intubation is not feasible, an orogastric tube should be placed and bag-and-mask ventilation should be instituted. A tertiary referral center should be consulted in these cases.

Any sudden adverse change in a premature infant's respiratory status should indicate the need for a repeat physical examination as well as a chest x-ray or transillumination of the chest or both. The endotracheal tube should be checked to ensure that it has not become dislodged or plugged; direct visualization of the tube's position may be needed. If there is doubt, the tube should be pulled and bag-and-mask ventilation begun.

Pneumothorax

If transillumination of the chest unquestionably shows pneumothorax, measures to relieve this

TABLE 3. **Hematologic Values in the Newborn**

NORMAL HEMATOLOGIC VALUES*

Parameter	Gestational Age (wk) 28	Gestational Age (wk) 34	Full-Term Cord Blood	Day 1	Day 3	Day 7	Day 14
Hb (grams/dl)	14.5	15.0	16.8	18.4	17.9	17.0	16.8
Hematocrit (ml/dl)	45	47	53	58	55	54	52
Red cells (mm³)	4.0	4.4	5.25	5.8	5.6	5.2	5.1
MCV (μm³)	120	118	107	108	99	98	96
MCH (pg)	40	38	34	35	33	32.5	31.5
MCHC (%)	31	32	31.7	32.5	33	33	33
Reticulocytes (%)	5–10	5–10	3–7	3–7	1–3	0–1	0–1
Platelets (1000s/mm³)			290	192	213	248	252

WHITE CELL AND DIFFERENTIAL COUNTS IN PREMATURE INFANTS*

	Less Than 150 Grams Birth Weight			1500–2500 Grams Birth Weight		
Age (wk)	1	2	4	1	2	4
Total count (× 10³/mm³)						
Mean	16.8	15.4	12.1	13.0	10.0	8.4
Range	6.1–32.8	10.4–21.3	8.7–17.2	6.7–14.7	7.0–14.1	5.8–12.4
% of total						
Polymorphs	54	45	40	55	43	41
Unsegmented	7	6	5	8	8	6
Eosinophils	2	3	3	2	3	3
Basophils	1	1	1	1	1	1
Monocytes	6	10	10	5	9	11
Lymphocytes	30	35	41	9	36	38

LEUKOCYTE VALUES AND NEUTROPHIL COUNTS IN TERM AND PREMATURE INFANTS†

Age (hr)	Total White Cell Count	Neutrophils	Bands/Metas	Lymphocytes	Monocytes	Eosinophils
Term Infants						
0	10.0–26.0	5.0–13.0	0.4–1.8	3.5–8.5	0.7–1.5	0.2–2.0
12	13.5–31.0	9.0–18.0	0.4–2.0	3.0–7.0	1.0–2.0	0.2–2.0
72	5.0–14.5	2.0–7.0	0.2–0.4	2.0–5.0	0.5–1.0	0.2–1.0
144	6.0–14.5	2.0–6.0	0.2–0.5	3.0–6.0	0.7–1.2	0.2–0.8
Premature Infants						
0	5.9–19.0	2.0–9.0	0.2–2.4	2.5–6.0	0.3–1.0	0.1–0.7
12	5.0–21.0	3.0–11.0	0.2–2.4	1.5–5.0	0.3–1.3	0.1–1.1
72	5.0–14.0	3.0–7.0	0.2–0.6	1.5–4.0	0.3–1.2	0.2–1.1
144	5.5–17.5	2.0–7.0	0.2–0.5	2.5–7.5	0.5–1.5	0.3–1.2

*From Klaus MH and Fanaroff AA: Care of the High-Risk Neonate, 3rd ed. Philadelphia, W. B. Saunders Co., 1986.

†Oski F and Naima J: Hematologic Problems in the Newborn. Philadelphia, W. B. Saunders Co., 1972.

Abbreviations: MCV = mean corpuscular volume; MCH = mean corpuscular hemoglobin; MCHC = mean corpuscular hemoglobin concentration.

condition should be instituted without delay for chest x-rays. This is especially true if the baby is doing poorly. If the baby is unstable, an 18-gauge scalp vein needle can be inserted at the second intercostal space in the midclavicular line. The needle should be connected to a three-way stopcock and a 12- to 35-ml syringe and inserted to a depth of approximately 5 to 10 mm, depending on the thickness of the chest wall. Air should be aspirated, and preparation should be done for placement of a chest tube. If a chest tube cannot be inserted, needle aspiration can be used to maintain control until more definitive treatment can be instituted.

The chest tube can be inserted either in the second intercostal space in the midclavicular line or at the fourth or fifth interspace in the anterior axillary line. The axillary approach avoids anterior scarring, which is more noticeable than axillary scarring. The insertion of a chest tube requires sterile technique, including use of a gown and gloves. A ¼-inch incision should be made over the rib, with care taken to avoid blood vessels that run along the inferior edge. A small, curved hemostat ("mosquito") is used to spread the skin, and pressure by the index finger on top of the curve of the hemostat will "pop" the hemostat through the pleura. The hemostat is then spread gently to allow a No. 10 French (for a small baby) or a No. 12 French (for a baby weighing more than 2000 grams) chest tube to be inserted without use of a stylet. If the axillary approach is used, the tip of the tube should be aimed anteriorly. The tube should be inserted no

TABLE 4. **Neutral Thermal Environmental Temperatures**[*],[†]

Age and Weight	Range of Temperature (° C)	Age and Weight	Range of Temperature (° C)
0–6 hr		72–96 hr	
Under 1200 grams	34.0–35.4	Under 1200 grams	34.0–35.0
1200–1500 grams	33.9–34.4	1200–1500 grams	33.0–34.0
1501–2500 grams	32.8–33.8	1501–2500 grams	31.1–33.2
Over 2500 (and >36 wk)	32.8–33.8	Over 2500 (and >36 wk)	29.8–32.8
6–12 hr		4–12 days	
Under 1200 grams	34.0–35.4	Under 1200 grams	33.0–34.0
1200–1500 grams	33.5–34.4	1501–2500 grams	31.0–33.2
1501–2500 grams	32.2–33.8	Over 2500 (and >36 wk)	
Over 2500 (and >36 wk)	31.4–33.8	4–5 days	29.5–32.6
12–24 hr		5–6 days	29.4–32.3
Under 1200 grams	34.0–35.4	6–8 days	29.0–32.2
1200–1500 grams	33.3–34.3	8–10 days	29.0–31.8
1501–2500 grams	31.8–33.8	10–12 days	29.0–31.4
Over 2500 (and >36 wk)	31.0–33.7	12–14 days	
24–36 hr		Under 1500 grams	32.6–34.0
Under 1200 grams	34.0–35.0	1501–2500 grams	31.0–33.2
1200–1500 grams	33.1–34.2	Over 2500 (and >36 wk)	29.0–30.8
1501–2500 grams	31.6–33.6	2–3 wk	
Over 2500 (and >36 wk)	30.7–33.5	Under 1500 grams	32.2–34.0
36–48 hr		1501–2500 grams	30.5–33.0
Under 1200 grams	34.0–35.0	3–4 wk	
1200–1500 grams	33.0–34.1	Under 1500 grams	31.6–33.6
1501–2500 grams	31.4–33.5	1501–2500 grams	30.0–32.7
Over 2500 (and >36 wk)	30.5–33.3	4–5 wk	
48–72 hr		Under 1500 grams	31.2–33.0
Under 1200 grams	34.0–35.0	1501–2500 grams	29.5–32.2
1200–1500 grams	33.0–34.0	5–6 wk	
1501–2500 grams	31.2–33.4	Under 1500 grams	30.6–32.3
Over 2500 (and >36 wk)	30.1–33.2	1501–2500 grams	29.0–31.8

[*]Adapted from Scopes J and Ahmed I: Arch Dis Child *41*:417, 1966. These investigators had the walls of the incubator 1° to 2° C warmer than the ambient air temperatures.

[†]Generally, the smaller infants in each weight group will require a temperature in the higher portion of the temperature range. Within each time range, the younger the infant, the higher the temperature required.

more than 3 cm but should be placed far enough in so that it "steams up" with each expiration. A purse-string suture should be tied, with use of 4-0 nonabsorbable suture material.

When the chest tube is sutured in place it should be attached to a suction apparatus with a negative pressure of approximately 10 cmH$_2$O. (Heimlich's valve can also work very well for a short time. Excessive drainage can cause rubber to stick together.) Once the tube is in place, its position should be checked radiographically. A lateral view is helpful. Cross-table supine films can often be taken with minimal disturbance to the baby.

Hypoglycemia

Chemstrips can be used to monitor for hypoglycemia. The blood sugar level should be checked at least once every 4 hours until feeding is well established and the baby is stable. If readings on Chemstrips indicate blood sugar less than 40 or more than 150 mg per dl, a blood sample should be drawn for laboratory analysis of blood sugar.

If blood sugar is confirmed as being less than 40 mg per dl and the baby is stable, an increase in the amount of sugar in the intravenous line can be considered. I usually do not exceed D10W in a peripheral vein because the hypertonicity will decrease the time that the intravenous line will remain usable. However, D12.5W can be used on a temporary basis. Unless there is a contraindication, the rate of fluid infusion can be increased by 20 ml per kg per day to increase sugar intake.

If the blood sugar level is below 30 mg per dl or if there are symptoms (seizures, lethargy, excessive tremors) with blood sugar below 40 mg per dl, a bolus of D10W at 2 to 4 ml per kg (or 0.2 to 0.4 gram of glucose per kg) can be given intravenously over a 15-minute period. Chemstrips should be rechecked every 30 to 60 minutes until the patient is stable. No bolus with a sugar concentration greater than D10W should ever be given.

Feeding

Overly aggressive feeding of small babies, babies with respiratory distress, or babies recovering from birth asphyxia may cause aspiration or necrotizing enterocolitis. A lethargic or tachypneic baby may frequently aspirate liquid feedings, and this may greatly complicate any other problems the baby has had. Adequate time for recovery and stabilization should be allowed before feeding is attempted. The first feeding should always be plain sterile water.

The first feeding should be delayed in a number of situations. If the infant is less than 36 weeks' gestational age, or less than 2500 grams of birth weight, the first feeding should be given 24 hours after birth if no problems have developed. If the infant has had respiratory distress, the first feeding should be delayed until the distress is nearly gone—that is, when the respiratory rate is less than 60 and the infant appears comfortable. For infants affected by birth asphyxia, hypotension, acidosis, hypothermia, or severe anemia, the first feeding should not be given until the child is at least 7 days old in order to avoid necrotizing enterocolitis. If the infant has been unstable for any reason, the first feeding should be delayed until the infant has been stable for at least 24 hours; delay of as much as 7 days may be advisable if the instability involved prolonged hypoxia, hypotension, acidosis, or hypothermia.

If the infant is younger than 35 weeks' gestational age, has impaired ability to suck or swallow, or appears to lack vigor, a conservative approach to feeding is advisable. The first feeding, as for all babies, should be sips of sterile water. If aspiration should occur, water will do no damage to the airway. D5W is as harmful to the airway as formula. If there are no problems with the first feeding, the next feeding is with quarter-strength to half-strength sterile formula; smaller or sicker babies should receive the more diluted formula. Babies weighing less than 1500 grams should receive a specially designed formula for the premature that contains 24 kcal per ounce. The first feeding of formula should be approximately 2 to 3 ml per kg. Subsequent feedings can be given every 2 hours for the infant weighing less than 1500 grams or every 3 hours for the infant weighing more than 1500 grams.

The feedings should be adjusted gradually so that full-volume, full-strength feedings are being given at the end of the seventh day of feeding. Table 5 shows a typical 7-day regimen designed for a 2-kg infant who needs gavage feeding and was quite sick for the first 3 to 4 days of life. In this example, the infant's eventual need is 120 kcal per kg per day, which would require 180 ml per kg per day using a formula providing 20 kcal per ounce. The eventual amount of the daily feedings should therefore be 360 ml (180 ml per kg, times 2 kg), divided into eight feedings of 45 ml per feeding. This example assumes that there is no requirement to limit water intake; in some situations, such as bronchopulmonary dysplasia, water intake may need to be limited.

If feeding is not tolerated, as may be indicated by abdominal distention, diarrhea, or vomiting, feeding should be stopped and the baby should be reassessed. If the baby seems well, feeding can be resumed in 24 hours at reduced strength and/ or reduced volume. This schedule is cautious and conservative and rarely is followed by necrotizing enterocolitis.

Oxygen

Oxygen should be used liberally but monitored closely, especially if the baby is less than 35 weeks' gestational age. If the baby is unstable, continual transcutaneous monitoring of Pa_{O_2} or monitoring of oxygen saturation is indicated. If oxygen needs remain greater than 40 per cent for a sustained period, an arterial line is generally indicated. If the baby is unstable, arterial gases should be checked every 1 to 4 hours. Also, when the transcutaneous monitor is changed, arterial gases should be measured so that the values provided by the monitor can be compared for appropriateness and accuracy.

Apnea

Apnea and bradycardia are very common problems that affect most premature babies at some time. Several possible causes of apnea should be considered. A complete blood count, blood culture, and possibly a lumbar puncture should be performed to rule out infection. We have found sepsis due to coagulase-negative staphylococci an important cause of apnea that may be associated with normal results of the blood count. Blood sugar and electrolytes should be measured. A chest x-ray may reveal any of a variety of causes of respiratory disturbances. A careful physical examination should focus on new findings that might change pulmonary dynamics, such as a patent ductus arteriosus, excessive weight gain, or increased fluid in the lungs. An electroencephalogram should be considered to rule out seizures. Computed tomography or ultrasonography of the head may reveal an intracranial malformation or hemorrhage. Conduction abnormalities may be discovered by electrocardiography. A 12-hour pneumogram may be helpful in quantitating and documenting events. The addition of oximetry and nasal thermistry to this technique may

TABLE 5. **Sample Regimen for Increasing Feeding for a Premature Infant***

Day No.	Strength	Initial Volume	Volume (ml) by End of Day
1	¼	5 ml—advance 1 ml/feeding	12
2	¼	12 ml	20
3	½	20 ml (hold volume for 2 feedings after strength change)	26
4	½	26 ml	34
5	¾	34 ml (hold volume after 2 feedings again)	40
6	¾	40 ml	45
7	Full strength	45 ml	45

*See text for details of sample case this regimen applies to.

greatly increase the diagnostic power of the pneumogram recording. Gastroesophageal reflux should be considered as a cause; an esophageal pH study and a barium esophagogram may be required to rule out anomalies.

In practice, the main early work-up should focus on new physical changes, infections, glucose and electrolyte levels, and seizures, because immediate treatment of these problems is necessary, available, and curative.

In most cases apnea in premature infants has no discernible cause. Mild cases of idiopathic apnea are handled merely by stimulation. Low-dose oxygen (22 to 23 per cent) may be helpful, but careful monitoring is required. If apnea is associated with feeding, helpful techniques may include reducing the volume of feeding, adding oxygen, or positioning the baby on the abdomen with the head up. When these methods fail or when spells are significant with associated bradycardia, cyanosis, or pallor, aminophylline is our drug of choice. A loading dose of 5 mg per kg, orally or intravenously, can be followed with 5 to 6 mg per kg per day in four divided doses to achieve a therapeutic level. In our experience, this level usually ranges from 7 to 14 micrograms per ml. Occasionally lower levels are effective, and in some infants higher levels may be needed. After the baby has been stable for several weeks, weaning may be attempted. Some infants will require aminophylline for 2 to 4 months after discharge from the hospital. Levels must be closely followed. Peak levels must be kept below 20 micrograms per ml. Toxic symptoms may appear at levels greater than 10 micrograms per ml. A few infants become extremely irritable at even lower levels.

Home Monitors

Although there is no certain relationship between apnea and sudden infant death syndrome, we tend to use home monitoring if apnea has been a significant problem in the nursery or if a baby requires theophylline after discharge to control apnea. We insist that all babies be free of apnea for at least 1 week prior to discharge. Home monitoring is then frequently carried through for a 6-month period and discontinued if there have been no apneic spells for at least 2 months and the infant has tolerated an infection without having any apneic spells.

POSTMATURITY AND INTRAUTERINE GROWTH RETARDATION

If the fetus is older than 42 weeks' gestation or if there is evidence of intrauterine growth retardation, delivery room personnel and equipment should be prepared for major resuscitation.

Monitoring of blood sugar is mandatory. Chemstrips should be checked every 1 to 2 hours for the first 6 hours and then intermittently until feeding is established. It is especially important to check the sugar level prior to feeding, when blood glucose may be at its lowest value.

A complete blood count should be obtained. Thrombocytopenia may be found in association with intrauterine infection or with toxemia of pregnancy. Polycythemia is frequently seen, and its management is controversial. The presence of polycythemia should be verified by at least two measurements and by use of a central venous or central arterial puncture. If the central hematocrit is 65 to 70 ml per dl and the baby is perfectly well, no treatment is indicated. Higher values may indicate the need for aggressive management. If the central hematocrit is 70 to 75 ml per dl and the baby is symptomatic, for example showing neurologic abnormalities, respiratory distress, or signs compatible with congestive heart failure, such as hepatomegaly, tachypnea, cardiomegaly, or pulmonary edema on x-ray, partial exchange transfusion is indicated. If the central hematocrit is greater than 70 ml per dl, a partial exchange transfusion may be indicated even if the baby shows no symptoms. If the baby is symptomatic or if the hematocrit is above 70 ml per dl, the case should be discussed with a specialist from a tertiary care center.

A postmature baby who is well can be fed ad

libitum as for a normal term infant. If there is extreme growth retardation, cautious feeding as for a premature baby is advisable, because of the risk that chronic hypoxia may have affected the gut.

BIRTH ASPHYXIA

Clinically birth asphyxia should be suspected when there is an Apgar score of less than 3 at 1 minute after birth or an Apgar score of less than 5 at 5 minutes. Severe birth asphyxia, which places the baby at high risk for cerebral palsy, can be recognized when the Apgar score is less than 5 at 10 minutes, when cord blood gases indicate metabolic acidosis, when the baby is hypotonic for more than 30 minutes (hypotonicity for more than 2 hours is an ominous sign), or when seizures develop.

Following birth asphyxia the baby must not be fed. An intravenous line should be started, with fluids restricted to 60 ml per kg per day. Blood sugar levels should be kept fairly high, in the range of 75 to 100 mg per dl. Oxygen levels should be monitored closely. The baby must be kept *well oxygenated*; it is essential to avoid a second episode of hypoxia. If the baby is having apnea or a seizure and begins to become hypoxic, mechanical ventilation may be necessary to maintain good oxygenation until the spell is brought under control. Severely asphyxiated babies should be cared for in a tertiary care center because the chance of deterioration is so great. If further hypoxic events can be avoided and metabolic normality can be maintained, there is a reasonable possibility of a favorable outcome.

Seizures

If the baby is having seizures, a tertiary care center should be contacted. I use phenobarbital to control seizures, with a loading dose of 10 to 20 mg per kg intravenously, followed by a maintenance dose of 3 to 5 mg per kg per day given in two divided doses. The loading dose may be increased to as much as 30 mg per kg, but if a dose this large is given, the physician must be prepared to institute ventilation. The blood level of phenobarbital should be measured in 24 hours. Therapeutic levels are usually achieved between 20 and 30 micrograms per dl, but sometimes higher levels are used in the first several days. Blood levels of sugar, calcium, and sodium must be checked.

Counseling of Parents

In counseling parents of babies with birth asphyxia, I am as honest as I can be. If I have great concern over the prognosis, I say so. However, until the effects of the cerebral edema are gone and the seizures are controlled, the baby cannot be adequately assessed. Prognostic discussions are more valid after about 7 days. Parents should be encouraged to be with their baby and should be given as much emotional support as possible. The health care team should be prepared for the parents' feelings of anger, guilt, and frustration. Parents need to know that no matter what the outcome, the health care team will help them with every step and every difficult decision and will be available to talk with them as frequently as possible. Criticism of the delivering physician, either by direct statements or as implied by attitude, should be avoided.

CONGENITAL ANOMALIES

If surgical anomalies such as omphalocele, gastroschisis, or meningomyelocele are present, the baby must be transported immediately to an appropriate surgical center. The exposed tissues of a meningomyelocele should be covered with moist gauze soaked in sterile saline and then covered with plastic (Saran Wrap, Op-site) and a large, bulky dressing. Exposed bowel can be managed with a commercially available plastic bowel bag. As is done for any major intestinal problem, the stomach should be decompressed with a gastric tube.

Babies with syndromes and malformations that are diagnostic puzzles should also be transferred to a tertiary care center so that a diagnosis can be obtained as soon as possible. A great deal of parental anxiety is frequently relieved when a "name" can be put on something, a definite prognosis given, and genetic counseling obtained. If an infant with multiple anomalies dies, a careful autopsy should be performed that includes blood or tissue sampling for chromosomal analysis as well as x-rays of the chest and skeleton.

INFECTION

The key to successful management of an infection is to begin an appropriate work-up and treatment long before the signs and symptoms have reached a critical point. This requires a prompt and aggressive response to early signs and symptoms or major risk factors.

Signs and Symptoms Requiring Prompt Attention

Diagnostic procedures should be instituted promptly if the baby has respiratory distress of any kind. Disturbances in breathing should not be assumed to be due to transient tachypnea. Grunting should be considered abnormal. A normal appearance on a chest x-ray does not rule out pneumonia, since pneumonia in the newborn is often diffuse and may be difficult to distinguish from hyaline membrane disease or transient tachypnea of the newborn. Cyanosis or an oxygen requirement after 20 minutes of age should *always* be considered abnormal.

Unstable body temperature with axillary temperatures above 37.4° C (99.4° F) or below 36.7° C (98° F) requires prompt diagnosis and adequate treatment. Gastrointestinal signs and symptoms necessitating work-up without delay include poor feeding, vomiting, distention, diarrhea, and bloody stools. Also, lethargy, unexplained metabolic acidosis, unexplained hypoglycemia, pallor, or hypotension demands prompt attention.

A number of findings on blood tests may indicate sepsis. A white blood cell count of less than 5000 per microliter, an absolute neutrophil count of less than 1200 polymorphonuclear leukocytes per microliter, or a ratio of bands to total polymorphonuclear leukocytes (including bands) greater than 0.4 should be considered as evidence of sepsis until proved otherwise.

Risk Factors

Some risk factors require prompt treatment even if the baby is perfectly asymptomatic. Birth trauma, perinatal asphyxia, maternal infection, chorioamnionitis, and prematurity are the major risk factors. Prolonged rupture of membranes becomes of major importance only when the above factors coexist.

The approach to infants with other risk factors depends to some extent on the maturity of the baby. Observation alone is sufficient initially for a term infant with prolonged rupture of membranes, fetal distress, or difficult or traumatic delivery as the sole risk factor. Any one of these accompanying risk factors in a preterm infant is sufficient reason for investigating by obtaining a blood culture, complete blood count, and platelet count. These studies should also be performed in a term infant with prolonged rupture of membranes plus either fetal distress or traumatic delivery, with maternal infection, or with minimal or questionable amnionitis, and in the baby who has required invasive resuscitation.

Work-up for Sepsis

Suspected sepsis is a medical emergency. There may be less than 1 hour between the development of minimal symptoms and respiratory failure with shock. A complete work-up for sepsis should be done for any term infant with any risk factor accompanied by abnormal laboratory data indicating sepsis, with frank (purulent) chorioamnionitis, or with any risk factor in combination with a history of maternal infection. A complete work-up for sepsis is also indicated for any preterm infant with abnormal laboratory data and any risk factor, with two or more risk factors, with early or questionable chorioamnionitis, or with a history including maternal infection or invasive resuscitation.

A blood culture study using a sample of 2 ml of blood and a complete blood count should always be included in the work-up when sepsis is suspected. If the baby is symptomatic, a spinal tap should also be done; however, the spinal tap may have to be delayed if the baby is unstable. In most cases of meningitis, culture will not become negative for 1 to 3 days, and abnormalities of cells, protein, and sugar usually persist for a much longer time. A suprapubic urine collection for culture is indicated if the baby is more than 7 days of age. If the baby is ill but appropriate specimens cannot be obtained, it is advisable to begin treatment; it is better to have a good outcome with an uncertain diagnosis than a poor outcome with a known diagnosis.

Treatment

Initial therapy, especially if the baby is less than 7 days of age, should include both ampicillin and gentamicin (Table 6). Ampicillin covers group B streptococci, which are the most common cause of infection in the newborn, *Listeria,* some gram-negative organisms, and some anaerobes. Gentamicin covers most gram-negative organisms. *Bacteroides* and *Staphylococcus* infections are not covered by this regimen. Staphylococci rarely cause infection in the first week of life. If an anaerobic infection with *Bacteroides* is suspected, cefoxitin can be added to the ampicillin-gentamicin regimen. An older baby has an increased risk for nosocomial infections, which are commonly caused by coagulase-negative staphylococci. Vancomycin and cefotaxime can be used empirically in this situation.

If sepsis is proved or clinically likely, therapy should be continued for 7 to 10 days. If pneumonia is present, with or without positive cultures, treatment for 10 to 14 days is indicated. Meningitis should be treated for a minimum of 14 days if the infecting organism is a group B streptococcus. Meningitis involving *Escherichia coli* or other gram-negative organisms should be treated for at least 21 days.

If cultures are negative, antibiotic treatment can be discontinued if (1) the initial reason for

TABLE 6. **Commonly Used Drugs for Infections in Neonates**

Drug	Usual Dose	Comment
Ampicillin	Less than 7 days of age: 50 mg/kg/dose every 12 hr IV push 7 days of age or more: 70 mg/kg/dose every 8 hr IV push	For babies less than 7 days of age, increase to 100 mg/kg/dose every 12 hr if group B streptococcal infection or meningitis is suspected
Gentamicin	2.5 mg/kg/dose every 12 hr given IV over 20 min	Measure levels to keep peak less than 8 $\mu g/ml$ and trough between 1.5 and 2.5 $\mu g/ml$. Frequency of dose decreased for premature babies or those with decreased creatinine clearance (as with birth asphyxia)
Cefotaxime	50 mg/kg/dose every 8 hr IV push	May be substituted for gentamicin, especially if gentamicin levels cannot be measured. May be used empirically with vancomycin in baby with suspected nosocomial infection
Vancomycin	10 mg/kg/dose every 8–12 hr (less frequent if premature); give IV over 45 min—1 hr	Must monitor drug levels. Keep peak at 20–30 $\mu g/ml$. Keep trough at 5–10 $\mu g/ml$. Watch for flushing, hypothermia, and tachycardia. Indicated for proven or suspected resistant staphylococcal infections
Cefoxitin	40 mg/kg/dose IV every 6 to every 8 hr	Indicated for empiric treatment of anaerobic infection

treatment was a risk factor only, the baby was asymptomatic, and laboratory values were normal, or (2) the baby was symptomatic but review of clinical circumstances indicates that the symptoms were probably due to another cause and laboratory values did not support the diagnosis of infection. Antibiotic treatment should be continued for a full 7-day course despite negative cultures if (1) initial signs and symptoms were clinically convincing, (2) the baby was asymptomatic but laboratory values were highly abnormal, or (3) the baby was asymptomatic but at high risk and the mother received intrapartum antibiotics.

INFANT OF A DIABETIC MOTHER

If the mother is diabetic, the infant's blood sugar level should be monitored by use of Chemstrips. Levels should be checked every 30 minutes for the first 2 hours, then hourly for the next 2 hours, and at 2-hour intervals thereafter. If the level is questionable or is below 40 mg per dl, blood should be obtained for measurement of blood sugar. If blood sugar is less than 40 mg per dl, there are no contraindications to feeding, and the initial feeding with sips of sterile water has been handled without difficulty, 3 to 4 ml of D5W per kg can be offered to the baby. If the sugar level remains above 30 mg per dl and the baby is asymptomatic, D5W or formula can be fed as tolerated.

If the baby will not take feedings or if there are contraindications to feeding, such as prematurity or respiratory distress, an intravenous line should be started with D10W infused at 80 ml per kg per day. Intravenous boluses of sugar should be avoided, as they may exacerbate the problem that was the initial contraindication to feeding. However, if the baby is showing symptoms such as lethargy, seizures, or apnea or seems jittery and the sugar level is remaining below 40 mg per dl and not responding to the intravenous infusion, 4 ml of D10W per kg can be given by intravenous push over 5 to 10 minutes and the intravenous infusion rate can be increased to 100 ml per kg per day. If there is still no response to this therapy, a central line will be needed to increase the blood sugar concentration. The central line can be established with either an umbilical venous catheter with the tip above the diaphragm, or an umbilical artery catheter with the tip between the levels of the sixth and tenth thoracic vertebrae.

TRANSFER TO A TERTIARY CARE CENTER

A baby should be transported to a tertiary care center whenever the baby's current problems exceed the capabilities of either the physician or the hospital to manage them. Similarly, the baby should be transferred if there is a high likelihood that such problems will develop. The goal of transportation is to avoid a crisis rather than being forced to treat one with inadequate resources.

The following items should be considered in the decision of whether to transport the baby to a tertiary care center, even if the physician in charge of the case has the medical skills to care for the baby:

1. Can an intravenous line be maintained 24 hours per day by in-hospital personnel?

2. Is in-house resuscitation available with staff skilled in intubation?

3. If the baby is at high risk for an air leak (for example, due to hyaline membrane disease, meconium aspiration, or any form of mechanical ventilation), is there an in-house team capable of treating acute pneumothorax?

4. Are facilities for x-rays, blood gas testing, and most basic laboratory tests available in the hospital 24 hours per day?

If the answer to any of the above questions is no, transportation to a tertiary care center may be advisable.

NORMAL INFANT FEEDING

method of
RUSSELL J. MERRITT, M.D., PH.D.
University of Southern California
School of Medicine
Los Angeles, California

BREAST-FEEDING

Breast-feeding is the preferred initial method of feeding infants. Almost all term infants thrive on human milk, the advantages of which include optimal nutrient content, lack of microbial contamination, anti-infective properties, possible protection from allergies and obesity, and close mother-infant contact. Exclusive breast-feeding is nutritionally adequate for at least 3 to 4 months.

The lactating mother should consume an adequate amount of fluids, and at least 1800 to 2000 kcal per day from a balanced diet, including four or five servings of dairy products if possible. Consumption of caffeine- and alcohol-containing beverages should be limited, and smoking should be avoided. Contraindications to breast-feeding include debilitating maternal illness, untreated tuberculosis, maternal acquired immunodeficiency syndrome, infections of the breast affecting the nipple area, use of certain antithyroid and antimetabolite medications, medical tests that make the milk radioactive, and the rare inborn errors of galactosemia and homozygous hypercholesterolemia in the infant.

Most breast-fed infants initially nurse eight times or more per day and have frequent (five to eight per day) loose stools. Stool frequency may decrease markedly after 6 to 10 weeks. Adequate intake is confirmed by frequent wet diapers and satisfactory gains in weight and length.

Common problems during early lactation include difficulty with milk let-down, inadequate milk supply, and mastitis (warmth and tenderness over part of a breast with or without fever). These problems are best managed in an anticipatory and supportive fashion. More frequent and longer suckling increases the milk supply. Warm compresses (or warm showers) and continued nursing or manual expression of milk speed resolution of mastitis.

COMMERCIAL FORMULAS

For infants who are not breast-fed, there are safe substitutes for human milk. The most commonly used commercial formulas (Similac, Enfamil, SMA) provide 20 calories per ounce. The formulas are based on use of cow milk, have reduced protein content (and curd tension), contain vegetable oil (which is more easily absorbed than butterfat), and are supplemented with vitamins and minerals. Iron-fortified formulas are adequate as the sole source of infant nutrition. By 1 to 2 weeks of age, most infants take 5 to 6 ounces per kg per day (100 to 120 kcal per kg). After 6 months of age, if the infant is taking at least one-third of the calories from various foods including alternative sources of dietary iron, fresh whole cow milk can be substituted.

Common problems associated with infant feeding include regurgitation, constipation, and colic. Mild to moderate regurgitation (gastroesophageal reflux) generally responds to upright positioning when the infant is held and prone positioning when the infant is in bed. Thickening of formula with rice cereal (1 to 2 tablespoons per 4 ounces) decreases the severity of reflux. Prune juice or dark Karo syrup added to formula can increase stool frequency, but corn syrup adds extra calories and salt. Colic can be related to parental misunderstanding of infant cues for hunger, need for diaper changing, sleep, or holding. In the minority of infants in whom colic is based on allergy, elimination of dairy products from the diet of the breast-feeding mother or use of a protein hydrolysate formula (Nutramigen, Good Start) may help.

Hydrolysate formulas may also be used to prevent allergies in atopic formula-fed infants or to treat infants with signs of allergy to cow milk. Soy formulas also are used in the treatment of this allergy and for suspected lactose intolerance. Some infants develop sensitivity to soy protein as well.

SUPPLEMENTS

A vitamin D supplement is needed by breast-fed infants with limited sunlight exposure. By 4 to 6 months of age, breast-fed infants need additional sources of iron in their diet. All infants in low-fluoride areas need fluoride supplementation. Homemade milk-based formulas need supplementation with vitamin C and a source of iron.

SOLIDS

Weaning to a more varied diet is usually initiated with iron-fortified single-grain cereals and juices. Other single-ingredient foods from the various food groups should then be sequentially added to the diet by using a progression of pureed to finger foods as development and dentition allow. Optimally, by 1 year of age two-thirds of energy intake is derived from nonmilk foods.

DISEASES OF THE BREAST

method of
SHARON GRUNDFEST-
BRONIATOWSKI, M.D., and
ROBERT E. HERMANN, M.D.
Cleveland Clinic Foundation
Cleveland, Ohio

In the newborn, the breast is usually mildly enlarged as a result of the stimulation from the mother's hormones. Occasionally this even causes nipple discharge. The engorgement subsides in a few days, and the breast glands stay in a quiescent state until puberty. At this time, the breast glands differentiate and proliferate under the influence of estrogen, progesterone, and other hormones. Occasionally the mother of an adolescent girl will become concerned that the developing breast bud represents a tumor. The practitioner must not fall into the trap of removing this area, since it contains all the developing cells of the new breast. With the onset of menstruation, the breast will be periodically engorged and tender during the luteal phase of the cycle. These changes are physiologic and should not be a cause for concern.

The normal breast is a mixture of glandular tissue, supporting stroma, and fat. In younger women, the proportion of glandular tissue and stroma to fat is increased, as compared with the breasts of older women, in whom fatty replacement is predominant. Therefore, in premenopausal women one should expect the breast to feel rather granular. After menopause (in the absence of exogenous estrogens) the breast becomes softer and more homogeneous.

CONGENITAL DISORDERS

Rarely, the breast may be completely absent (amastia), or the gland may be present with an absent nipple (athelia). More commonly, the nipple is present, but the breast is hypotrophic (hy-poplasia). Breast hypoplasia may be associated with absence or hypoplasia of the pectoral muscles, deformities of the rib cage, and deformities of the ipsilateral upper extremity (synbrachydactyly). These deformities may all be corrected by reconstructive surgery.

Supernumerary breasts or nipples may appear anywhere along the embryologic milk line. Generally these do not require excision unless they are large or tender.

ACQUIRED DISORDERS

Breast development may sometimes be seen at an early age, along with other signs of early sexual maturation *(precocious puberty)*. Such cases should be referred to an endocrinologist for evaluation to exclude hormone-secreting tumors. *Premature development* may also occur in the absence of any other signs of puberty, such as axillary and pubic hair, clitoral and labial pigmentation, and pigmentation of the areolae. In such cases, only observation and reassurance are required.

Asymmetry in growth may also occur because of chest wall deformities (e.g., pectus excavatum) or because of an abnormal growth spurt in one breast (probably as a result of end-organ hypersensitivity). When *gigantomastia* occurs during puberty it generally requires reduction mammoplasty for correction. Most authorities recommend that this be delayed until the growth spurt has ended. Gigantomastia may also occur during pregnancy or lactation. There have been some case reports of regression after danazol treatment.

In males the breast usually remains undeveloped; however, *benign gynecomastia* may be encountered at puberty, in senescence, or after administration of certain drugs (e.g., digitalis, cimetidine, isoniazid, and spironolactone). It has also been associated with liver disease, testicular tumors, androgen or estrogen excess, thiamine deficiency, and Klinefelter's syndrome. Removal of the enlarged tissue (subcutaneous mastectomy) is indicated for pain or for cosmetic reasons. It may also be performed as a diagnostic measure in older men to exclude carcinoma. For men undergoing estrogen therapy for prostatic carcinoma, prophylactic breast irradiation is useful to prevent subsequent breast engorgement.

Breast pain *(mastodynia)* may occur as a result of hormonal stimulation of the breast, in which case it is usually cyclical. Most women do not require medical treatment, and wish only to be reassured that no damaging pathologic process is involved. In more severe cases, medical therapy may be tried. A wide range of treatments have been advocated, including dietary manipulation (e.g., abstention from caffeine), cold compresses, thiamine, vitamin E, diuretics, iodine, thyroid hormone, and danazol. Caffeine in large doses can cause breast pain in susceptible women, and abstention is sometimes beneficial. Vitamin E has not been shown effective in double-blind trials. Danazol (Danocrine) is helpful (in doses of 100 mg twice a day), but it is expensive and causes virilizing side effects at high doses. Further, its effects on fetal development are not known. The other treatments have not been the subjects of rigorous testing. Noncyclical mastodynia is often associated with stress or depression but may be caused by neuritis, arthritis, or post-traumatic inflammation. When inflammation or arthritis is suspected, an anti-inflammatory medication may be tried. Costochondritis is frequently mistaken for breast pain.

Inflammatory Disorders (Mastitis)

During lactation an area of edema and erythema may develop in the breast as a result of incomplete emptying of milk. This usually responds to emptying the breast by massage or with a breast pump.

The most common inflammatory condition is a *breast abscess*. Abscesses frequently occur as a result of trauma to the nipple during lactation and are usually caused by *Staphylococcus aureus*. Typically the breast is red, swollen, and tender. The patient may be febrile and may have an elevated white blood cell count. Fluctuance is slow to develop owing to the many septations in the breast. An initial trial of antibiotics directed against penicillin-resistant staphylococci and warm compresses should be tried. If the woman is breast-feeding, she should stop using the abscessed breast and empty it with a breast pump. If these measures do not resolve the problem, incision and drainage will be necessary. Skin abscesses and infected sebaceous cysts are also common.

Squamous metaplasia of the lactiferous ducts (Zuska's disease) may cause an inflammation in the subareolar tissues with secondary infection. Anaerobes are found in 20 to 30 per cent. Initially this presents as a tender, erythematous swelling adjacent to the edge of the areola and may be accompanied by a nipple discharge. The infection will sometimes resolve with warm compresses and oral antibiotics. If incision and drainage are performed a *chronic mamillary duct areolar fistula* will frequently be the result. Treatment consists of wide excision of the diseased lactiferous ducts from beneath the nipple. Many authors

have remarked on the high recurrence rates if diseased tissue is left behind.

A variety of other infections have been reported to involve the breast, including tuberculosis, blastomycosis, cryptococcosis, and actinomycosis. Tubercular infection is rare in the United States. It presents as a mass accompanied by multiple draining sinuses and adenopathy. There is almost always a primary lung infection. Antibiotic therapy is indicated, with surgery being reserved for residual masses.

Another common inflammatory process is *duct ectasia* or *plasma cell mastitis*. Its etiology is unknown, and it may occur at any age. Typically it presents as a multicolored, sticky discharge that can be expressed from several ducts in both breasts. It may also be noted incidentally at operation as a grayish-green material within the ducts. Occasionally it produces itching. No therapy is needed for this condition, although if the patient finds it bothersome, or if the physician has some doubt as to the nature of the nipple discharge, an excision of the subareolar ducts will relieve symptoms and establish the diagnosis.

A rare cause of breast pain is *superficial thrombophlebitis (Mondor's disease)* of the thoracoepigastric vein. The condition is self-limited and requires no treatment.

Traumatic Disorders

An injury to the breast may result in *fat necrosis*. Clinically this presents as a firm, irregular mass. There may be overlying erythema. The lesion may be indistinguishable from carcinoma on mammography. The history of trauma may not always be obtained and, even if it is clear that there has been an injury, biopsy is necessary to exclude the presence of cancer. Generally a core-needle biopsy or fine-needle aspiration cytology will be sufficient. However, if excision is not performed, it is imperative that the patient be maintained under observation to be sure that the mass is resolving (which it generally does within a month).

Neoplastic Disorders

Benign Lesions

In teenagers and women in their early twenties the most common breast tumor is a *fibroadenoma*. This lesion may also arise later in life. These tumors are easily recognized; they are firm, rounded, and usually mobile. They are solid on aspiration. Breast cancers are rare in women below the age of 25, and small fibroadenomas in this age group may be safely observed for a period. Usually they are slow growing, and with time some lesions actually involute. They are not generally considered to be premalignant. Fibroadenomas may occasionally grow rapidly under the influence of estrogen during adolescence or pregnancy, or with the use of exogenous hormones. Occasionally, these tumors may achieve a large size accompanied by an exuberant overlying vasculature. Simple excision is sufficient, and mastectomy is never indicated.

As women enter their late twenties and thirties the increased nodularity and thickening that were seen primarily during the luteal phase (physiologic nodularity) may develop into a persistent two-dimensional thickening (mastoplasia). These areas may be distinguished from carcinoma by their tendency to vary in size with the menstrual cycle and the presence of tenderness. In general, carcinomas present as a three-dimensional thickening and are nontender, but this is not invariably the case. Histologically, mastoplasia may include areas of glandular hypertrophy or hyperplasia (adenosis, or epithelial hyperplasia) or of stromal hypertrophy. These diagnoses are often lumped together under the rubric "fibrocystic disease"; however, it is better to attach a more precise diagnosis whenever possible. Adenosis and epithelial hyperplasia do not carry an increased risk of future malignancy unless atypia is present.

As women enter the decade before menopause, cysts become more frequent. These are usually easily diagnosed by aspiration, although mammography and ultrasound may be helpful. Cysts are not associated with an increased risk of malignancy unless there is a strong family history of breast cancer (e.g., in a mother or a sister) and are treated by evacuating the fluid with a syringe. If there is a persistent mass after aspiration or if the cyst recurs, biopsy should be performed to exclude the presence of carcinoma. Although some have advocated abstention from methylxanthines, there has been no double-blind study that unequivocally shows a reduction in cyst formation after such dietary manipulation.

Benign papillary lesions such as an intraductal papilloma may present as palpable masses, but more commonly cause a nipple discharge. They can occur at any age. Unlike the discharge associated with duct ectasia, only one breast and one duct are usually involved, and the discharge is usually spontaneous. The discharge may be clear, serous, or bloody. Because there is no way to distinguish such a discharge from that seen in association with carcinoma, biopsy is mandatory if the nipple fluid cytology does not yield malignant cells. Simple excision is sufficient. Rarely an adenoma of the nipple may be seen. This tumor also presents with a bloody nipple discharge. On inspection of the nipple, a raised area with multiple fissures is seen. The diagnosis is easily made by biopsy, and excision is curative.

A rare tumor usually found in middle-aged women is the phyllodes tumor, also called cystosarcoma phyllodes. These lesions usually present as bulky, multilobulated tumors. They have a strong tendency to invade locally, but only 10 per cent are malignant. Microscopically they bear a resemblance to the fibroadenoma; however, the stroma is more cellular. The malignant potential depends on the number of mitotic figures and the cytologic characteristics of the stromal cells. Wide excision is the treatment of choice. Since this tumor almost never metastasizes to lymph nodes, axillary dissection is unnecessary.

Noninvasive Carcinomas

There is great debate over the management of in situ lesions. Intraductal carcinoma (also called in situ ductal carcinoma, comedocarcinoma, and cribriform carcinoma) may present as a palpable lump or a cluster of microcalcifications. Occasionally, the tumor will attain a very large size (3 cm or more) and axillary involvement will be found despite the diagnosis of "noninvasive" cancer. At other times, no mass will be palpable, but mammography will demonstrate widespread calcifications. Small (less than 2 cm) intraductal lesions not associated with a nipple discharge and not located beneath the nipple areolar complex have been treated by wide excision and radiotherapy with acceptable short-term results. No data are available as to the long-term results of conservative therapy, and mastectomy remains an option. Larger lesions should be treated by mastectomy and axillary sampling (if not a total axillary clearance).

Lobular carcinoma in situ, also called lobular neoplasia, is not considered a malignancy by some authors. Nevertheless, it is associated with an increased risk of carcinoma in both breasts (25 to 30 per cent at 20 years). There is a 30 per cent incidence of multicentricity in this condition. It is interesting to note that the carcinoma that may eventually develop is more likely to be ductal than lobular in origin. Treatment options include careful follow-up with a physical examination of the breast three times a year and a yearly mammography, or bilateral "prophylactic" mastectomy removing all the glandular tissue and the nipple areolar complex. Which choice is taken depends on the age of the patient, the family history, the ease of examination of the breasts, and the preference of the patient.

Invasive Carcinoma

Carcinoma of the breast is the leading cause of cancer mortality among American women. Carcinomas may arise in either the ductal or lobular portions of the breast glands. The most common malignancy (90 per cent) is the *infiltrating ductal cancer*. Well-differentiated forms of this tumor are sometimes called tubular carcinomas. About 10 per cent of tumors are *infiltrating lobular carcinomas*. Other invasive carcinomas include medullary, mucinous, metaplastic, and adenoid cystic carcinomas.

Cancer should be suspected when the patient presents with a three-dimensional, irregular, hard mass; skin retraction or nipple inversion of recent onset; a unilateral nipple discharge coming from one duct; nipple ulceration; or a mammogram showing a spiculated density or a cluster of microcalcifications.

Screening Techniques. Physical examination and mammography remain the principal means of detecting carcinomas of the breast. Breast self-examination is to be encouraged, but unfortunately it has not been shown to improve cancer detection rates.

Palpation of the breast will rarely detect tumors less than 1 cm in size. A number of studies have shown a decrease in mortality when women are regularly screened by mammography (Swedish National Board of Health, the New York Health Insurance Plan trial, the Nijmegen Project, and the Breast Cancer Detection Demonstration Project). The American Cancer Society recommends the following guidelines: (1) women should have a baseline mammogram between the ages of 35 and 40, (2) biannual screening between the ages of 40 and 49, and (3) annual mammography thereafter for life. Women with a history of breast cancer in a first-degree relative should have annual mammography beginning at 40 years of age. Only about 0.5 per cent of asymptomatic women screened will actually have a cancer.

Mammography alone will miss approximately 20 to 30 per cent of palpable tumors. However, mammography when combined with physical examination will detect 95 per cent or more of cancers. Biopsy of a suspicious breast lump should always be performed regardless of the mammographic findings. Mammography helps the surgeon to ascertain the presence of multicentric disease, improves the estimation of tumor size, and may detect unsuspected tumors in the contralateral breast.

Other techniques such as thermography, ultrasound, and diaphanography have not been shown to be sufficiently accurate to be used for cancer screening at this time.

Biopsy Techniques. Histologic samples of vast majority of breast masses may be obtained in the office using either a fine-needle aspiration for cytology or a core-needle biopsy (e.g., Tru-Cut or drill biopsy). Where the diagnosis is equivocal, an open excisional biopsy should be performed. Care should be taken when planning the biopsy incision so as not to interfere with subsequent surgical therapy. Nonpalpable lesions found by mammography are localized first by Kopan's hook-wire technique, and the surgeon follows the wire to the mass.

In past years it was popular to combine biopsy and subsequent mastectomy during one period of general anesthesia because of fears that the tumor would spread if definitive therapy was not immediately carried out. However, it appears that a delay of even 3 weeks does not carry any increased risk. Further, the use of the two-step biopsy procedure allows the surgeon to fully discuss all the options with the patient. A one-anesthesia procedure is still useful when the planned therapy is a partial mastectomy for a small lesion or when a clinically suspicious lesion cannot be diagnosed by needle biopsy and the patient has agreed to undergo mastectomy if the frozen section is positive for carcinoma.

Prognosis of Breast Cancer. The prognosis for an invasive carcinoma of the breast is determined by the size of the tumor, its histologic grade, and the number of axillary nodes involved. Unlike some tumors, breast cancer may appear to be dormant for many years, only to reappear as a systemic or local recurrence. Tumor, nodes, and metastases (TNM) staging is given in Table 1. Five-year survival rates are as follows: Stage I, 80 to 95 per cent; Stage II, 70 to 75 per cent; Stage III, 38 to 42 per cent; and Stage IV, 25 per cent.

Treatment of Operable Breast Cancer. The treatment of invasive carcinoma is a matter of great controversy at present. Treatment options include radical mastectomy; modified radical mas-

TABLE 1. **Clinical TNM Staging for Breast Cancer (UICC–AJC)**

Stage I	T1 —Tumor size 2 cm or less
	N0 —No suspicious lymph nodes
	M0 —No distant metastases
Stage II	T2 —Tumor size 2–5 cm and/or
	N1 —One or more palpable, suspicious nodes
	M0 —No distant metastases
Stage III	T3 —Tumor larger than 5 cm or
	N2 —Ipsilateral nodes fixed to one another or other structures or
	N3 —Ipsilateral supraclavicular or infraclavicular suspicious nodes, or arm edema
	M0 —No distant metastases
Stage IV	T4 —Tumor of any size with fixation to chest wall, edema or ulceration of breast skin, satellite skin nodules, or inflammatory carcinoma, or
	M1 —Any distant metastasis

tectomy (with or without immediate reconstruction); segmental mastectomy and axillary dissection (with or without radiotherapy); and local excision, axillary dissection, and radiotherapy. The vast majority of clinical trials have shown that survival for Stages I and II breast cancer is the same regardless of the local treatment, whether it be radical mastectomy, modified radical mastectomy, segmental mastectomy, or excision and radiotherapy. Dissection of the internal mammary nodes does not appear to confer any benefit. Axillary dissection is usually performed for staging information and to control possible local recurrence in the axilla, but it has not been shown to improve survival. Local recurrence may be higher after local excision and axillary dissection than after local excision, axillary dissection, and radiotherapy (National Surgical Adjuvant Breast Project trial B-06). This, too, is controversial since the local excision in this trial may not have been extensive enough to have eradicated nearby foci of intraductal cancer found in the vicinity of a primary tumor.

Radical mastectomy is rarely performed for Stage I and II lesions in the United States now. Modified radical mastectomy (removal of the breast and axillary nodes with conservation of one or both pectoralis muscles) is usually the treatment of choice for tumors that are centrally located or are larger than 2.5 cm. It is accomplished with little morbidity, with a minimal hospital stay, and at relatively little expense. It also alleviates the concern about multicentric tumors. Breast reconstruction often provides a satisfactory cosmetic result, although the older woman may not wish to be subjected to the added operative time and expense. There are many satisfactory external breast prostheses available. Breast reconstruction can often be accomplished at the time of mastectomy using either a silicone implant or an expandable posthesis. Where skin coverage is a problem, a latissimus dorsi or a rectus muscle myocutaneous flap may be used. Some surgeons prefer to delay reconstruction for several months after mastectomy, but there is no evidence that reconstruction adversely affects local recurrence or survival.

Partial mastectomy with breast conservation is preferred for small (less than 2 cm), peripheral lesions. The addition of radiotherapy to surgery is generally thought to reduce the risk of local recurrence; however, it adds 6 weeks of treatment time and almost doubles the cost of treatment. If a salvage mastectomy is needed after radiotherapy, the skin may be more prone to wound healing problems, making breast reconstruction more difficult. Finally, there is some concern about late morbidity and even mortality as a result of radiation damage to the heart, lungs, and other structures in the radiation field. Ultimately the choice of treatment depends on the size of the tumor, its histology, the stage of the disease, the size of the breast, the location of the tumor in the breast, and the preferences of the patient after a detailed discussion of the options.

Adjuvant Therapy. Adjuvant therapy is given in an effort to improve either local or systemic control of disease. In 1985 the National Institutes of Health convened a Consensus Conference that recommended that adjuvant chemotherapy be reserved for premenopausal women with positive nodes. There is still debate as to whether chemotherapy in this group results in an improvement in survival, but there is a prolongation in disease-free survival.

Premenopausal women with positive nodes are usually given adjuvant cytotoxic chemotherapy utilizing three drugs or more (e.g., cyclophosphamide, 5-fluorouracil, and methotrexate [CMF]; cyclophosphamide, 5-fluorouracil, methotrexate, vincristine, and prednisone [CMFVP]; or 5-fluorouracil, doxorubicin [Adriamycin], and cyclophosphamide [FAC]) for a period of 6 to 12 months. Patients with estrogen receptor–positive tumors may undergo hormonal manipulation in addition. Adjuvant castration alone has not been shown to improve survival over that produced by chemotherapy.

Postmenopausal women with Stage II receptor-positive tumors are treated with tamoxifen (Nolvadex), 10 mg twice a day for at least 2 years. Several trials have demonstrated an improvement in the disease-free interval, and one trial appear to show a small survival advantage in postmenopausal women treated with this estrogen blocker. Toxicity is minimal. No benefit for adjuvant chemotherapy in postmenopausal women with estrogen receptor–negative tumors has been established.

Adjuvant radiotherapy is used to reduce local recurrence in women with poorly differentiated tumors, multiple lymph node involvement, angioinvasion, or neural invasion.

Post-Treatment Follow-up. Patients with Stage I or II breast cancer should probably be seen by a physician every 3 months for the first year, every 6 months for the next 4 years, and yearly thereafter. Mammograms and chest x-rays are obtained once a year, and liver function tests and a complete blood count are usually done twice a year. There is little justification for yearly bone and liver scans unless the patient is in an experimental protocol. These tests are usually reserved for patients with symptoms or an abnormal alkaline phosphatase level, or patients who presented with more advanced disease.

Advanced Breast Cancer. The treatment of advanced breast cancer is dependent on the menopausal status of the patient, the presence or absence of nodal involvement, the presence of systemic disease, and the degree of local involvement.

Patients with bulky chest wall disease but without overt systemic disease are usually treated by modified radical mastectomy followed by chemotherapy and radiation. Alternatively, radiotherapy may be given first to reduce the size of the tumor before resection.

Many different chemotherapy regimens have been advocated. Slightly higher response rates are found for those containing doxorubicin, but no clear survival advantage has been demonstrated for any combination therapy or single agent.

Inflammatory breast cancer is a relatively rare form of breast cancer (1.5 to 4 per cent of all breast carcinomas) characterized by diffuse swelling, erythema, tenderness, warmth, and peau d'orange. Pathologically there is invasion of the dermal lymphatics. Multimodal therapy is recommended. There is a very high rate of local recurrence when surgery alone is used, and 75 per cent of patients develop systemic disease when radiotherapy is used alone. Therefore, the initial treatment is usually a combination of chemotherapy (e.g., FAC) for two or three cycles, followed by mastectomy if the tumor has significantly decreased in size, and postoperative radiotherapy. If no initial response to chemotherapy is seen, radiotherapy is added. Surgery may then be performed at a later time if residual disease is present and appears resectable.

Local Recurrence. Patients presenting with a local recurrence are at significant risk for subsequent systemic disease and should have a complete metastatic evaluation (chest x-ray), bone scan, liver scan, and laboratory studies). Excision and radiotherapy or radiotherapy alone will initially control most local and regional recurrences, but there is a high rate of relapse. The addition of chemotherapy should be considered for patient with widespread or large deposits.

Systemic Recurrence. Radiotherapy provides useful palliation for patients with metastases to bone, brain, spinal cord, orbit, or the brachial plexus. Malignant pleural effusions are treated by chest tube drainage with instillation of tetracycline for pleurodesis. Where possible, biopsy for hormone receptor data should be accomplished in patients with systemic disease. If the tumor is hormone receptor positive, oophorectomy or treatment with tamoxifen, medroxyprogesterone, or aminoglutethimide may be helpful. A significant number of patients will be palliated by combination chemotherapy, although it has not been shown that such treatment improves survival.

ENDOMETRIOSIS
method of
DAVID R. MELDRUM, M.D.
Redondo Beach, California

ETIOLOGY AND SYMPTOMS

Endometriosis generally results from chronic retrograde flow of menses, with implantation of viable endometrial fragments in the cul-de-sac, along the broad ligaments, and on or within the ovaries. If the uterus is anterior, thus creating an anterior cul-de-sac for menstrual debris to accumulate, implantation may also occur on the bladder peritoneum. The fresh or old blood that accumulates in the tissues creates the typical visual appearance, which is sufficient for diagnosis without biopsy confirmation. Yellow papular lesions, hemosiderin, stellate scarring, and peritoneal windows may also signal its presence. In reaction to the blood, scarring may progress to obliterate the cul-de-sac and cause the ovaries to adhere densely to the posterior peritoneum. Visualization of these typical changes at laparoscopy or laparotomy is necessary for the diagnosis, although tender nodularity on rectovaginal examination may be suggestive. Use of a staging system such as the revised classification by the American Fertility Society (1985) is helpful in defining the extent of disease. The locations described readily explain the pain during intercourse, defecation, or urination that commonly occurs. Severe dysmenorrhea, particularly starting a few or several days before menstrual bleeding, is probably due to bleeding and resultant swelling in the pelvic tissues. Premenstrual spotting may occur because of cervical implants. Infertility is a common symptom, apparently mediated by the inflammatory reaction in the pelvic cavity that results in increased macrophage phagocytosis of sperm, embryotoxic leukocyte products, intratubal inflammatory membranes altering ciliary activity, ovulatory dysfunction (luteinized but unruptured follicles), and anatomic disruption of ovum pickup by the fimbria because of scarring.

TREATMENT

Choice of surgical or medical therapy (Table 1) depends on the setting and the patient's goals. Because the diagnosis is usually made at laparoscopy, it has become common to eradicate the disease at that time by using laser vaporization or bipolar coagulation. If infertility is present and there is significant scarring of the tubes or ovaries, laparotomy with lysis of adhesions, tubal repair, and excision, cautery, or vaporization of endometrial tissue is generally preferred if this cannot be done adequately by operative laparos-

TABLE 1. **Medical Therapy of Endometriosis**

1. Acyclic combined oral estrogen/progesterone, using a low estrogen dose with an androgenic progesterone such as ethinyl estradiol and norgestrel (Lo/Ovral, Ovral). Begin with 0.03/0.3 mg and increase to 0.05/0.5 mg if breakthrough bleeding occurs.
2. Continuous progestins using medroxyprogesterone acetate (Provera, Depo-Provera), norethindrone acetate (Aygestin, Norlutate), or megestrol acetate (Megace). Provera should be given in the range of 30–60 mg/day* orally; Depo-Provera,† 150 mg, parenterally every 1–3 mo; Aygestin and Norlutate, 15–30 mg/day*; Megace,† 40–60 mg/day. For Provera, Aygestin, Norlutate, and Megace, the total dose should be achieved in increments, with lower doses being given over several weeks.
3. Methyltestosterone (Metandren)† should be given as 5–10 mg linguets (buccal) daily.
4. Ethinyltestosterone (danazol) should be given orally at a dose of 400–800 mg/day.
5. 19-Nortestosterone derivatives (Gestrinone) should be given orally, 2.5–5 mg 2 or 3 times/wk (not available in the United States).
6. Gonadotropin-releasing hormone agonists: dose varies with potency and route (nasal, subcutaneous, depot injection).

*May exceed manufacturer's recommended dose.
†This use is not listed by the manufacturer.

copy. A collection of endometrial tissue within the ovary (endometrioma) exceeding 1 cm generally does not respond to hormonal therapy and thus requires excision or ablation by laparoscopy or laparotomy. If disease is minimal, use of a cyclic, low-dose, progestin-balanced oral contraceptive may retard progression of the disease. Pregnancy is probably the ideal treatment, and full breast-feeding may add further benefit by continued ovarian suppression.

When pain relief is the treatment goal, a trial of hormonal therapy is commonly used. Danazol is the most extensively used and documented treatment. It acts by suppressing ovarian estrogen secretion (probably mainly at the ovary itself), and it probably also acts directly on the ectopic endometrium. Because of its 4.5-hour half-life, it is best given every 6 or 8 hours. Because its side effects are not clearly lessened by reducing the dose, 600 to 800 mg daily is most effective. Body weight and extent of disease are also variables to consider when deciding about dosage; the lower doses should be used only in thinner women or in those with lesser amounts of disease. About 30 per cent of women have a recurrence in 3 years. If weight gain and androgenic side effects are of concern, a continuous progestin (see Table 1) may be used. Although these drugs have been less thoroughly studied, their effectiveness may be similar to that of danazol. Continuous use of oral contraceptives has been inferior when compared with that of danazol, but newer agents (Table 1) may be more effective; lower cost may be beneficial for some

patients. Methyltestosterone is not generally used because of lesser effectiveness and frequent androgenic side effects. Agonists of gonadotropin-releasing hormone have a similar effectiveness to danazol and are becoming available. Menopausal side effects may be significant and can be relieved by adding small doses of estrogen or norethindrone, probably without affecting efficacy. Calcium supplementation may also help to prevent significant bone loss. With all hormonal agents, a 6- to 9-month treatment course is generally used.

If surgical intervention is required, preoperative or postoperative treatment with danazol has yielded superior results in some studies, particularly in patients with extensive disease. Division or ablation of the uterosacral ligaments or presacral neurectomy may be done if central pelvic pain is a major complaint. If more definitive surgical therapy is chosen, hysterectomy and unilateral oophorectomy may be considered if all disease has been eradicated. If both ovaries are removed, estrogen may be used with a low risk of recurrence if all disease has been excised. With residual endometriosis, a 6-month delay of estrogen replacement may be prudent, during which time medroxyprogesterone acetate may be used for menopausal symptoms. If fertility remains a goal, oophorectomy without hysterectomy should be considered if the patient wishes to consider egg donation.

DYSFUNCTIONAL UTERINE BLEEDING

method of
WILLIAM REVELLE PHIPPS, M.D.
University of Minnesota Medical School
Minneapolis, Minnesota

Dysfunctional uterine bleeding (DUB) is a form of abnormal uterine bleeding that results from abnormal, generally anovulatory, menstrual cycles. The pathophysiology and optimal treatment of DUB are best understood by comparing it with what occurs during the normal menstrual cycle. In the proliferative phase of the normal cycle, estrogen produced by the dominant follicle causes endometrial glands and stroma to proliferate. After ovulation, the corpus luteum produces relatively large amounts of progesterone, in addition to estrogen, which causes secretory changes in the endometrium. Menses occurs because the withdrawal of estrogen and progesterone leads to endometrial desquamation. Menses is an orderly, self-limited event that involves the entire endometrium. In contrast, DUB in general involves exposure of the endometrium to estrogen unopposed by progesterone for relatively long times. This prolonged exposure to estrogen leads to an abnormally thick and structurally unstable endometrium. The tissue is delicate and undergoes essentially spontaneous breakdown with associated bleeding. The process is not an orderly one, may continue more or less indefinitely, and involves different portions of the endometrium at different times.

The clinical picture of DUB is one of irregular episodes of often painless bleeding occurring in an unpredictable fashion, with episodes ranging from a day of spotting to several weeks of continuous, heavy bleeding. Long periods of amenorrhea may or may not be interspersed among bleeding episodes. Both mittelschmerz and premenstrual molimina are absent. Patients particularly at risk for DUB include postmenarchal teenagers, perimenopausal women, and women with polycystic ovarian disease or obesity-related anovulation.

MANAGEMENT

To make the diagnosis of DUB, other entities that may be responsible for abnormal bleeding per vagina must first be excluded with reasonable certainty. The more common of these entities are shown in Table 1. A careful history and physical examination are of course essential. The laboratory testing necessary depends on the details of the individual situation. Patients with any significant degree of bleeding should have a complete blood count. It is particularly important to rule out pregnancy with a blood pregnancy test before endometrial sampling is performed. When

TABLE 1. **Causes of Abnormal Vaginal Bleeding**

Dysfunctional uterine bleeding
Pelvic malignancies
    Endometrial adenocarcinoma
    Uterine sarcoma
    Cervical or vaginal carcinoma
    Gestational trophoblastic neoplasia
Benign anatomic lesions
    Endometrial hyperplasia
    Uterine leiomyoma(s) or adenomyosis
    Endometrial or endocervical polyp(s)
    Cervical or vaginal endometriosis
    Vaginal adenosis
Inflammatory processes
    Endometritis
    Cervicitis
    Vaginitis (infectious, atrophic)
Pregnancy-related bleeding
    Threatened abortion
    Missed or incomplete abortion
    Ectopic pregnancy
    Molar pregnancy
    Third trimester or puerperal bleeding
Bleeding diatheses
Miscellaneous
    Pelvic lacerations or trauma
    Intrauterine device
    Intravaginal foreign body
    Drugs
    Hypothyroidism

a tentative diagnosis of DUB is made, endometrial sampling before medical therapy may be indicated. This is especially true for patients at significant risk for endometrial hyperplasia or adenocarcinoma, two conditions that, similar to DUB, may occur as a result of chronic anovulation. In general, sampling can be accomplished in the office using a Karman cannula or similar device. Occasionally, it is necessary to perform a traditional diagnostic dilatation and curettage.

After initial diagnostic measures, attention is directed to therapeutic intervention. The first goal of DUB therapy is to stop the acute bleeding episode. Either endometrial aspiration with a Karman cannula or dilatation and curettage by itself may provide a substantial therapeutic effect, although in general there is no reason not to start medical therapy immediately after endometrial sampling. In many cases, the bleeding can be stopped with the administration of a progestin. A typical progestin regimen is medroxyprogesterone acetate (Provera), 10 mg orally once daily for 10 days. This treatment usually stops the bleeding during the time it is being administered, followed by more or less orderly withdrawal bleeding starting immediately after the drug is discontinued. This sequence of events is similar to that occurring during the secretory phase of the normal cycle. It is important to advise the patient at risk for pregnancy that occasionally ovulation will occur as a result of progestin administration.

Another therapeutic option useful in stopping acute bleeding involves using oral contraceptive pills (OCPs), for example, having the patient take four low-dose (30 to 35 micrograms each of estrogen) pills daily for 5 days. The bleeding should stop within 1 to 2 days, and again withdrawal bleeding is to be expected within a few days of the last pill. For the patient who has been bleeding heavily for a prolonged time, with little residual endometrial tissue, it may be best to use high-dose estrogen therapy initially, for example, conjugated estrogens (Premarin), 25 mg by intravenous bolus every 4 hours for two or three doses. The immediate improvement with such therapy is due more to a pharmacologic effect of estrogen on small vessel hemostasis than to estrogen's ability to cause proliferation and healing of endometrial tissue. Once the bleeding has stopped in response to the Premarin, an OCP regimen should usually be started immediately.

Patients who are diagnosed as having DUB but who are not responsive to the regimens just outlined require additional evaluation, including endometrial sampling if not previously performed, or possibly hysteroscopy.

Once the acute episode of bleeding has been

treated, attention is directed to the possible need for long-term treatment. For the patient who is usually ovulatory, for whom it is thought that the bleeding episode just treated is unlikely to recur, a period of observation may be all that is necessary. On the other hand, some form of chronic therapy is indicated for patients whose anovulatory state responsible for the DUB is unlikely to abate spontaneously. The goals of this long-term therapy, which must include a progestin component, are to prevent recurrences of the unpredictable bleeding episodes, prevent endometrial hyperplasia, and possibly lower the patient's risk for endometrial or breast cancer. An iron supplement may be started at this time if needed as well.

OCPs given in the usual cyclic fashion are especially useful on a long-term basis for patients with DUB who may occasionally undergo spontaneous ovulation and need birth control. Women with polycystic ovarian disease derive additional benefit from OCP use related to amelioration of the hyperandrogenic state. Patients who are not candidates for OCP use may be treated with cyclic progestin treatment, for example, Provera, 10 mg orally once daily the first 10 to 14 days of each month. Anovulatory patients with DUB who desire pregnancy should of course have an appropriate hormonal evaluation followed by initiation of ovulation induction therapy.

At times, a patient may have a consistently poor response to long-term medical therapy or unacceptable side effects. In that situation, hysterectomy may be considered. Another newly available option for such a patient is endometrial ablation by laser.

AMENORRHEA

method of
EDWARD L. MARUT, M.D.
Michael Reese Hospital and Medical Center
Chicago, Illinois

DEFINITION AND EVALUATION

The common definition of amenorrhea is absence of menses for 3 months or three usual cycle lengths, whichever is shorter. Primary amenorrhea, the failure of menarche to occur by age 16 years, is often associated with delayed puberty, whereas secondary amenorrhea occurs in an individual who has experienced at least one menstrual period. There is significant overlap between the etiologies of amenorrhea and the more general condition of ovulatory dysfunction. The latter encompasses luteal abnormalities, oligo-ovulation, anovulation, and dysfunctional bleeding.

The specific treatment for amenorrhea is linked directly to laboratory tests. Because hormone levels are affected by therapy, they should be measured before initiation of therapy.

Initial endocrine testing should include measurement of follicle-stimulating hormone (FSH), luteinizing hormone (LH), thyroid-stimulating hormone (TSH), and prolactin levels. If the patient is hirsute, levels of androgens, specifically testosterone and dehydroepiandrosterone sulfate (DHEAS), should be measured to rule out ovarian or adrenal tumors. The prevailing endogenous estrogen effect on the endometrium should then be tested with 100 to 200 mg progesterone in oil intramuscularly; the failure to withdraw from progesterone administration suggests either severe dysfunction of the hypothalamic-pituitary-ovarian axis or endometrial disease (Asherman's syndrome). Treatment is determined in part by the results of these endocrine tests and manipulations as well as by the patient's needs and wishes.

ETIOLOGY

The most common cause of secondary amenorrhea, and one that must not be forgotten even in cases of primary amenorrhea, is pregnancy, either normal or pathologic (e.g., tubal or molar). The physician must rule out pregnancy before embarking on a diagnostic or therapeutic course. The availability of rapid sensitive serum pregnancy tests using radioimmunoassay of beta–human chorionic gonadotropin (hCG) makes this task relatively easy, provided that the diagnosis is considered.

Diseases of High Morbidity or Mortality

Ovarian and adrenal tumors, generally manifesting with hyperandrogenism and palpable or radiologically and sonographically detectable masses, require prompt surgical management. Likewise, large pituitary, hypothalamic, pineal, or other intracranial tumors may necessitate surgical attention. Specific endocrine diseases such as Cushing's syndrome, acromegaly, hypothyroidism, and hyperthyroidism must be dealt with specifically and appropriately.

Congenital or Acquired Anatomic Abnormalities

Failure of normal embryologic development of the müllerian system or genital sinus can result in either obstruction of menstrual flow (imperforate hymen, vaginal atresia) or failure of endometrial response (absence of the uterus) in the face of normal ovarian function and thus can require surgical correction, if possible. Included here are intersex disorders, such as androgen insensitivity syndrome (testicular feminization) in XY individuals, as well as a host of chromosomal disorders involving phenotypic females with absence of ovaries as well as müllerian structures; these disorders would manifest as primary amenorrhea. Their acquired counterpart is Asherman's syndrome (amenorrhea traumatica), which features endometrial synechiae or fibrosis after use of instrumentation, manifests as secondary amenorrhea, and requires surgical therapy.

Aberrations of the Hypothalamic-Pituitary-Ovarian Axis

HYPOTHALAMIC DYSFUNCTION. Previously a diagnosis

of exclusion, hypothalamic amenorrhea is generally associated with emotional or physical stress. The extreme examples are anorexia nervosa and marathon running, with a vast middle ground including simple weight loss, change of job, and jogging. It may also be reflected in a delay in resumption of normal menses after suppression by oral contraception or pregnancy. The underlying neuroendocrine abnormality is a derangement in the normal pulsatile secretion of gonadotropin-releasing hormone (GnRH), which results in loss of normal FSH and LH pulsatility. The GnRH abnormality may be modulated by endogenous opioids or by dopaminergic or adrenergic neurotransmission dysfunction. It may be caused by various pharmacologic agents, especially those that elevate prolactin levels via dopamine interference. The severity of the loss of GnRH pulse frequency and amplitude dictates the ultimate treatment, as discussed later. A picture similar to this "functional" amenorrhea may be caused by a hypothalamic tumor. Primary amenorrhea related to the absence of GnRH secretion (Kallmann's syndrome) previously had been thought to be pituitary in origin. LH and FSH are at low or normal levels in hypothalamic amenorrhea but have diminished pulse amplitude or frequency.

PITUITARY DYSFUNCTION. Most pituitary dysfunction is actually due to the aforementioned GnRH abnormalities. Most primary pituitary disease tends to be congenital complete or partial hypopituitarism (including isolated gonadotropin deficiency—not GnRH failure), or pituitary tumors. The most common pituitary tumor involved in amenorrhea is the prolactinoma. Many share the opinion that hyperprolactinemia is actually hypothalamic in origin, because of dopaminergic abnormalities, with or without an identifiable tumor. However, other experts believe that all hyperprolactinemia is tumor related. Interference with gonadotropin secretion may be due to a mass effect, or it may be secondary to the excess prolactin, which suppresses GnRH. Thus, hypothalamic and pituitary origins of the amenorrhea are difficult to separate. The same holds true for other functioning or nonfunctioning tumors (which may raise prolactin levels but not secrete this hormone). Empty-sella syndrome is likely to be due to an infarcted tumor and tends to be associated with hyperprolactinemia. Postpartum ischemic necrosis (Sheehan's syndrome) is another example of acquired pituitary hypofunction, in which LH and FSH levels tend to be low or normal, and includes loss of other trophic and peptide hormones.

OVARIAN DYSFUNCTION. The most common ovarian etiology for secondary amenorrhea is ovarian failure; in a woman in her late forties or older, this event is quite normal. In a woman less than 40 years, it takes the pathologic title "premature ovarian failure." When failure occurs in a karyotypically abnormal individual, treatment is aimed at hormonal replacement alone. Primary amenorrhea may also be the result of prenatal or postnatal follicular depletion. The apparent ovarian failure, with elevated FSH and LH levels, may actually spontaneously resolve in certain individuals, which suggests a resistant ovary syndrome. More likely in a young amenorrheic woman is polycystic ovary syndrome (PCOS), classically manifesting as hyperandro-

genism and obesity from puberty. The primary defect is still unknown, with evidence suggesting several etiologies including a primary ovarian androgen abnormality, adrenal disease (including enzyme defects), hyperprolactinemia, hyperinsulinemia, and dopaminergic dysfunction. The findings on endocrine testing can provide direction to treatment. Classic PCOS demonstrates an LH/FSH ratio higher than 2, but this may not be noted; in addition, prolactin levels may be elevated up to 25 per cent of the time.

OVULATION INDUCTION THERAPY

If the amenorrheic woman desires, immediate fertility ovulation induction is undertaken. In general, unless ovarian failure has been diagnosed or the patient is hyperprolactinemic, clomiphene citrate (Serophene, Clomid) is the first line treatment. For all modes of ovulation induction, basal body temperature (BBT) charting provides an inexpensive, although somewhat gross, presumptive diagnosis of ovulation. Confirmation by luteal phase progesterone levels or endometrial biopsy is helpful, but follicular development is more properly and critically followed by serial ultrasonography and measurement of serum estradiol levels. However, because of the fixed dosage (at least per cycle) of most ovulation induction cycles with clomiphene, ultrasonography and estradiol levels have their greatest importance in difficult inductions and with gonadotropin therapy.

Clomiphene Citrate

Clomiphene is an attenuated nonsteroidal estrogen related to diethylstilbestrol (DES). The action of clomiphene may occur in the hypothalamus, pituitary, or ovary in effecting folliculogenesis and ovulation. By competing with the feedback action of endogenous estrogen, clomiphene causes a rise in FSH and LH levels and thus initiates folliculogenesis. An intact hypothalamic-pituitary axis is necessary because folliculogenesis results in adequate estrogen levels to trigger the LH surge only when appropriate feedback sensitivity is present. An effect on the ovary, which may be beneficial or deleterious, has also been noted.

Clomiphene has an effect in the presence of the estrogenic milieu because its action depends on competition for estrogen receptors. Thus, an endometrial withdrawal in response to a progesterone challenge predicts a potential effect of clomiphene. However, ovulation has been reported in low-estrogen situations on rare occasions, including puberty and hypothalamic amenorrhea, which suggests a direct effect on the pituitary or ovary. Thus, the most likely condition to respond to clomiphene is PCOS, with a normal or elevated estrogen level and a normal prolactin level.

The starting dose of clomiphene is 50 mg per day for 5 days beginning on days 2 to 5 after progesterone withdrawal. By following a BBT chart, the physician may detect presumptive ovulation by noting the temperature rise. If no ovulation occurs and the patient remains amenorrheic, progesterone should again be withdrawn, and the next course of clomiphene should be increased to 100 mg (two tablets) on a similar schedule. Because the failure to cause ovulation is related to either too low or too high a prevailing estrogen level, stepwise increases of clomiphene up to 250 mg per day may be necessary. At doses above 100 mg per day, folliculogenesis without ovulation may occur; although a spontaneous LH surge and ovulation are preferred, it may be necessary to induce ovulation by the addition of hCG (Profasi HP, Pregnyl, A.P.L.), 10,000 units intramuscularly, as an LH surrogate. Thus, at the higher doses of clomiphene, monitoring follicular growth by ultrasonography and measurement of serum estradiol levels may determine whether follicles are developing. If folliculogenesis takes place without ovulation, the hCG may be given with the dominant follicle at a mean diameter of about 20 mm (range, 18 to 24 mm). Clomiphene may result in multifollicular development, so a decision must be made to give hCG or not if several mature follicles are present. This problem becomes greater with gonadotropin therapy (discussed later). Estradiol by rapid assay tends to reflect total estrogen by radioimmunoassay at about 300 pg per ml per mature follicle. This information may be used to detect adequate folliculogenesis and decide whether to increase the dosage or to use hCG.

Even if ovulation occurs with clomiphene, it may be followed by a luteal phase abnormality, which may occur because of inadequate folliculogenesis related to too low or, paradoxically, too high a dose of clomiphene. The luteal phase defect may be diagnosed by an endometrial biopsy or measurement of serum progesterone levels, and the dose of clomiphene may be adjusted empirically in either direction. A short luteal phase (less than 11 days) may be seen on BBT charting. The titration of dosage by 25-mg increments may be necessary to achieve ovulation with adequate luteal function. Overdosage with clomiphene is probably due to antiestrogenic effects on the ovary. Contrariwise, the excessively sensitive patient may develop multiple follicles, ovarian cysts, and even hyperstimulation syndrome. This development is not related to high doses as much as individual sensitivity. A pelvic examination or ultrasonography should precede each treatment cycle.

In patients who fail to ovulate while taking clomiphene alone, the finding of elevated adrenal androgen levels may suggest the addition of low-dose corticosteroids, such as 0.25 to 0.5 mg of dexamethasone nightly. A full replacement of dose of steroids may be necessary, especially if an adult-onset or partial enzyme defect is present; this condition may be diagnosed by stimulation of adrenal androgens by synthetic adrenocorticotropic hormone (ACTH). If this is not the case, alternative regimens of clomiphene may be tried: prolonged treatment at a low dose for 7 to 10 days, or incremental dosage, increasing every 5 days to the next multiple of 50 mg until ultrasonography and estrogen levels demonstrate folliculogenesis. If the initial LH/FSH ratio was higher than 2, addition of bromocriptine at 2.5 mg daily may occasionally result in ovulation when low doses of clomiphene are given. Realistically, the use of gonadotropin therapy as discussed later is indicated if clomiphene therapy fails. In all cases, the cycle length may be shortened by earlier administration of the first clomiphene tablet(s) (e.g., day 3) because the withdrawal bleed is arbitrary in an amenorrheic woman. However, if folliculogenesis is about to occur spontaneously, the earlier administration may over-ride a potentially abnormal cycle.

Human Menopausal Gonadotropins and Human Chorionic Gonadotropin

In the patient with a normal prolactin and low estrogen level (no withdrawal to progesterone), or in one who fails to ovulate even while given an incremental regimen of clomiphene, human menopausal gonadotropin (hMG) (Pergonal) and hCG offer the maximal potential for successful treatment. Unlike other modes of ovulation induction, use of hMG requires no hypothalamic-pituitary function because it has FSH and LH activity extracted from menopausal women's urine. Pergonal is available in ampules for intramuscular administration with an activity of 75 IU of FSH and 75 IU of LH per ampule. (Ampules containing 150 IU of each hormone are also available.) Because of the nonmodulated direct ovarian effect, multifollicular development with ovarian enlargement and hyperstimulation syndrome are potential dangers, which necessitates close monitoring with ultrasonography and measurement of estrogen levels.

Initial treatment with Pergonal begins at one ampule daily; the first estrogen level and ultrasound evaluation can rationally be delayed until the fifth day of therapy because selection of the dominant follicle(s) occurs no earlier than day 5 of a normal cycle. If no follicular development is detected after 5 days of Pergonal, the dosage is increased by one ampule for another 3 to 4 days. The follicular development is followed daily, with incremental increases by one or two ampules every 3 to 4 days, depending on the response. Once folliculogenesis begins, it tends to do so exponentially; thus, no change in dosage should be made in fewer than 3 days. The eventual dosage needed to effect folliculogenesis may require many days to attain in the first cycle. In subsequent cycles, the initial dosage may be selected on the basis of the dosage that led to ovulation.

The immediate dangers of Pergonal therapy are multifollicular development, which is detectable by ultrasonography, and hyperstimulation syndrome, which can often be predicted via estrogen levels. When one or two follicles reach a mean diameter of at least 18 mm as seen on ultrasound scan and estrogen levels are at least 700 pg per ml, Pergonal is not given that day, but hCG, 10,000 IU, is given, and the couple is instructed to have intercourse the next day. If four follicles or more mature or the estrogen level exceeds 1500 pg per ml, multiple pregnancy or hyperstimulation syndrome may result, and the hCG should be withheld. Ovulation is unlikely to occur, and after progesterone withdrawal a new treatment cycle may be begun with a modified, lower dosage. Women with low gonadotropin levels are likely to require an additional dose of hCG (5000 IU 1 week after the ovulating dose) to support the luteal phase.

The experience with Pergonal is critical, and recognition of patterns of folliculogenesis results in more successful and safer induced cycles. The levels of estrogen mentioned earlier are not absolute. The specific assay used sets the minimal and maximal concentrations that determine cessation of Pergonal or withholding of hCG. In addition, the woman with primary amenorrhea or long-standing hypoestrogenism should have endometrial priming for one or two cycles with estrogen and progestin, as outlined later for hormonal replacement.

The discrepancy between ovulation and pregnancy rate as well as the high spontaneous abortion rate may be related to the high levels of estrogen attained. This situation may be due to the nonphysiologic, fixed ratio of FSH and LH. Women with PCOS are typically hypersensitive to Pergonal because they already have an excess LH effect. The advent of the pure FSH preparation Metrodin has provided an alternative to Pergonal in these patients.

Urofollitropin (Metrodin)

The relatively recent introduction of a pure urinary FSH formulation, Metrodin, has added an important agent to the limited armamentarium for ovulation induction. Available in ampules containing 75 IU of FSH and less than 1 IU of LH, Metrodin is approved for use in PCOS, in which amenorrhea results from a relative excess of LH and deficiency of FSH. As mentioned, control of folliculogenesis and hormonogenesis with Pergonal may be difficult in PCOS because of the multiple arrested follicles and sensitivity to the LH component. Metrodin provides the deficient hormone, FSH, without adding LH and can result in a more physiologic response. Unlike the use of Pergonal in a hypoestrogenic state, Metrodin is administered at a lower dose with less dosage adjustment, and often for a longer time. The goal is to allow normal folliculogenesis to occur by exposing the immature follicles to FSH and over-riding the atretogenic effect of LH. Because women with PCOS usually have intact hypothalamic-pituitary function, they can mount a spontaneous LH surge in many cases, as they do with clomiphene therapy. Thus, Metrodin can be administered at one ampule daily for 7 to 10 days before follicular development would be noted. Increases in dosage are more gradual, at one additional ampule daily every 5 to 7 days. Monitoring by ultrasonography and measurement of estrogen levels is necessary to detect the efficiency of the regimen and to avoid hyperstimulation. Estradiol levels at ovulation may approximate those in a spontaneous cycle (300 to 500 pg per ml), as opposed to the supraphysiologic levels attained with Pergonal therapy. If spontaneous ovulation is not possible or not desirable, 10,000 IU of hCG is given when the lead follicle has a mean diameter of 18 mm. Premature increases in dosage may result in multifollicular development, as with Pergonal. This development is common when higher doses of Metrodin are used in an attempt to speed up folliculogenesis; increased recruitment is more often the outcome. Because endogenous LH levels are high, luteal support is unlikely to be necessary. Amenorrhea associated with normal levels of LH and FSH and with a normal estrogen milieu may also be treated by Metrodin therapy instead of Pergonal. Theoretically, the absence of excessive LH makes for more synchrony of follicle maturation. Also, relative resistance of the ovaries in Pergonal cycles may respond to addition of Metrodin to the Pergonal treatment once the dose of three ampules of Pergonal is reached. For both gonadotropin preparations, increased dosages may be required in obese women.

Gonadotropin-Releasing Hormones and Analogues

GnRH (Factrel) is available for diagnostic use in assessing pituitary gonadotrope competence; it can also be used on a clinical protocol for ovulation induction. GnRH must be administered via an automated infusion pump subcutaneously or intravenously at a fixed dose on a 1- to 2-hour pulse frequency schedule to mimic the endogenous pulsatility seen in normal cycles. This fixed dose, fixed frequency regimen results in pulsatile release of FSH and LH, folliculogenesis, and ovulation in the presence of a responsive pituitary-ovarian axis. The dosage and frequency schedule need not be varied through the cycle to duplicate the normally seen changes. Its use is most appropriate in hypothalamic disorders (e.g., Kallmann's syndrome, anorexia nervosa, or stress- or exercise-induced amenorrhea) in which endogenous GnRH pulsatility is negligible. Any disorder with significant GnRH secretion may frustrate the exogenous GnRH action. Because of the technical and clinical limitations of use, GnRH has not been as widely used as originally expected.

It is surprising that the use of a GnRH analogue, leuprolide acetate (Lupron), has become relatively common as an adjunct to hMG therapy despite the fact that Lupron is approved for use only as a gonadal suppressant in men with prostatic cancer. GnRH analogues are synthetic forms of the native GnRH decapeptide molecule with amino acid substitutions or deletions. Depending on the actual amino acid sequence, the molecule has either an exaggerated GnRH effect (agonist) or a blocking effect (antagonist). Paradoxically, the GnRH agonist Lupron is used for its antigonadotropic effect, which occurs via a process called down-regulation. After a stimulatory effect on LH and FSH secretion lasting 7 to 10 days, the secretion of biologically active gonadotropin is suppressed, thus effectively mimicking an antagonist. Lupron has been used to block endogenous LH secretion in individuals with PCOS so that hMG can be used more efficiently. However, FSH is the more logical therapy, as discussed earlier, and avoids the use of two different drugs. The most common use of leuprolide is to prevent LH surges that can prematurely luteinize the follicles.

If Lupron is used to suppress endogenous gonadotropins, 1 mg subcutaneously is administered daily until down-regulation occurs, that is, until the estradiol level reaches menopausal levels. In PCOS, this may take more than 7 to 10 days, as it does in normal women. Pergonal therapy is then initiated as described earlier; often higher doses than usual are required. Once Pergonal is begun, Lupron is reduced to 0.5 mg subcutaneously daily until hCG is given. Luteal phase hCG is necessary because endogenous LH is suppressed.

Bromocriptine (Parlodel)

The treatment of hyperprolactinemia is most successful with bromocriptine. Prolactin levels can be lowered and pregnancy achieved even with microadenomata and macroadenomata. In the latter situations, the risk of tumor expansion during pregnancy must be weighed against the benefits. Bromocriptine is a dopamine agonist that acts on the pituitary dopamine receptors to effect a reduction in prolactin secretion (as well as a reduction in tumor size). Its main drawbacks are the gastrointestinal and orthostatic side effects, which are usually temporary and avoided by night-time administration or split dosing with meals. Vaginal administration has been reported to avoid some of these effects. There are essentially no risks involving multifollicular development or hyperstimulation because the reduction of prolactin permits normal hypothalamic-pituitary-ovarian function to resume. Ultrasonography and monitoring of estrogen levels are rarely needed, although some patients require clomiphene or Pergonal if hypothalamic or pituitary disease also exists. A pituitary magnetic resonance imaging or computed tomography scan should precede therapy.

Parlodel should be initiated at a dose of one 2.5-mg tablet daily for 1 week, with an increase to one tablet twice a day after that. Ovulation should be confirmed by BBT and a normalized prolactin level, which should be checked in a few weeks in case a higher dose is required to reduce the prolactin level to normal. Although ovulatory menses should resume in 1 or 2 months, any accompanying galactorrhea may remain several months longer. If side effects are relentless, a reduction in dosage may relieve them while maintaining the prolactin-inhibiting effect.

Another use for bromocriptine has been occasionally demonstrated in normoprolactinemic women with PCOS in whom the LH level is at least twice the FSH level. There may be dopaminergic deficiency here as well (prolactin may be elevated too), so that an option or addition to clomiphene is provided. For PCOS, a dosage similar to that for hyperprolactinemia may be used. For any use of Parlodel, other agents may be needed if prolactin is suppressed but ovulation does not occur.

Corticosteroids

The amenorrheic patient with elevated adrenal androgen levels may respond to corticosteroid therapy with regular ovulation. Because the level of the androgen marker for adrenal function, DHEAS, may be elevated because of a functional enzyme block (3-β-ol-dehydrogenase), an elevated DHEAS level should not immediately direct the treatment to corticosteroid therapy. Such a patient usually ovulates when given clomiphene, which is safer for long-term use. However, in the patient with adrenal hyperplasia related to an enzyme abnormality, corticosteroid therapy is the treatment of choice. It can initiate menarche in a primary amenorrheic patient as well as result in resumption of menses. Unless the adrenal component is clearly the primary abnormality, or ACTH stimulation demonstrates an enzyme blockade, corticosteroid therapy should be second line, treatment, that is, if clomiphene does not adequately induce ovulation or if ovarian suppression of androgens is incomplete. In the case of frank congenital adrenal hyperplasia, full replacement with corticosteroids may be necessary, with an a.m./p.m. ratio of 2:1, such as cortisol 20 mg/10 mg or prednisone 5 mg/2.5 mg, or dexamethasone 1 mg nightly because of its long action.

In the adult-onset or attenuated enzyme defect, an attempt to give a subreplacement dose of dexamethasone, such as 0.5 mg nightly, is likely to be successful in suppressing androgens without fully suppressing cortisol. This treatment would have the advantage of being safer than a fully suppressive dose. As mentioned earlier, this regimen may need to be added to clomiphene if ovulation does not occur with persistent DHEAS elevation. Proper withdrawal from the steroid is necessary regardless of dosage if the patient wishes to discontinue use.

SEX STEROID REPLACEMENT THERAPY

If fertility is not desired, ovulation induction should not be undertaken for fear of an unwanted pregnancy. Treatment of hyperprolactinemia would be an exception to this rule. Other amenorrheic patients require some type of estrogen or progestin replacement. There are two different types of amenorrheic patients for whom a mode of sex steroid replacement must be decided on: those who have a normal or high estrogenic milieu and withdraw to progesterone injection, and those who are hypoestrogenic and do not bleed.

Progestin

Amenorrheic patients who withdraw to progesterone are at risk for endometrial hyperplasia and adenocarcinoma, especially if they are obese. Thus, periodic withdrawal from a secretory endometrium is necessary to prevent endometrial disease. If ovulation induction is undertaken, the endogenous progesterone provides this sloughing, as in a normal spontaneous cycle. However, if fertility is not desired, conversion of the proliferative (or hyperplastic) endometrium to a secretory one can be achieved by administration of an oral progestin for 12 to 14 consecutive days, after which a withdrawal bleed should occur. If amenorrhea without prior withdrawal exceeds 6 months, especially with a history of dysfunctional bleeding, an endometrial biopsy should be done first to rule out malignancy.

A progestin such as medroxyprogesterone acetate (Provera), 10 mg given daily for 10 days every 6 to 8 weeks, should prevent endometrial hyperplasia as well as permit spontaneous ovulation. Allowing spontaneous return of menses may be important with more reversible types of hypothalamic amenorrhea, such as that related to stress or weight loss. Provera is chosen owing to the absence of androgenic side effects that are seen with other compounds.

The patient must be warned about a continued theoretical risk of pregnancy, albeit small, with intermittent withdrawal. The patient who requires contraception or suppression of ovarian androgens may be given low-dose combination oral contraceptives (30 to 35 micrograms of ethinyl estradiol). The use of spironolactone (Aldactone), 100 to 200 mg daily, in a hirsute amenorrheic woman with polycystic ovaries may cause ovulation by lowering testosterone levels, but the patient also will require contraception because of the potential teratogenicity of the drug. (Oral contraceptive and spironolactone therapy is discussed in the chapter on hirsutism.)

Estrogen-Progestin

The patient who has primary amenorrhea with no progesterone withdrawal and who has failure of secondary sex development and no other treatable entity requires estrogen and progestin replacement. This combination is needed to cause secondary sex characteristics to develop as well as to prevent the morbidity of hypoestrogenism, such as osteoporosis and cardiovascular disease. Conjugated equine estrogens (Premarin), 1.25 to 2.5 mg daily, or the equivalent (estradiol [Estrace], 2 to 4 mg; ethinyl estradiol, 10 to 20 micrograms) or estradiol via transdermal therapeutic system (Estraderm, one or two 0.1-mg patches twice a week) should be sufficient to prime the endometrium, cause breast development and vulvovaginal maintenance, and prevent the morbidity of hypoestrogenism. Higher dosages are probably unnecessary, may have unwanted side effects, and may accelerate development unnaturally. The final 12 to 14 days of the estrogen therapy should be accompanied by medroxyprogesterone acetate, 10 mg, for the previously discussed purpose of preventing endometrial disease. Once development of secondary sexual characteristics is achieved, the estrogen dose is reduced to typical replacement doses for ovarian failure.

The woman who has secondary amenorrhea with low estrogen requires a similar regimen, regardless of etiology: premature ovarian failure, weight loss amenorrhea, exercise-associated amenorrhea, or menopause. The estrogen dosage is lower, however, when full pubertal development has already occurred: 0.625 to 1.25 mg of conjugated estrogens or the equivalent in a woman younger than 40 years, and 0.625 mg in a woman older than 40 years. These dosages provide appropriate maintenance of breasts and genitalia as well as adequate prophylaxis against hypoestrogenic morbidity. Persistent symptoms or side effects dictate adjustments. The 12 to 14 days of medroxyprogesterone acetate should also be given as described. Women with no expectation of return of menses because of pituitary disease and those with premature ovarian failure with abnormal karyotypes should take estrogen and progestin indefinitely. Others should stop the replacement for 1 or 2 months to assess return of hypothalamic-pituitary-ovarian function because even "premature ovarian failure" may resolve spontaneously or because of the estrogen effect on gonadotropins or their receptors. We tend to use estradiol patches at 0.05 mg twice a week because of theoretical benefits of avoiding first-pass effects through the liver.

Asherman's Syndrome (Amenorrhea Traumatica)

The diagnosis of Asherman's syndrome is made by the failure of uterine bleeding to occur in an estrogenic milieu after progestin administration, the lack of bleeding when cyclic estrogen-progestin or oral contraceptives are given, and the findings of intrauterine synechiae on hysterosalpingography or hysteroscopy. This syndrome is the one nonendocrine cause of amenorrhea because the patient will have every other evidence of ovulation save menses. Therapy is therefore surgical: hysteroscopic lysis using scissors or laser.

CONCLUSION

Although the etiologies of amenorrhea vary, the full elucidation of the process is virtually always possible with endocrine testing. Depending on the specific conditions, therapy aimed at fertility or maintenance of quality of life is available.

DYSMENORRHEA

method of
ALVIN F. GOLDFARB, M.D.
Jefferson Medical College of Thomas Jefferson University
Philadelphia, Pennsylvania

Painful menstruation, or dysmenorrhea, is the most common medical disorder occurring in women. The recurrent crampy lower abdominal pain experienced by many young women is usually accompanied by one or more nonspecific complaints, including nausea, vomiting, diarrhea, headaches, and muscle cramps. Although considerable attention has been focused on the psychosocial aspects of this process, work during the last two decades has shifted the emphasis toward physiologic changes. The important role of prostaglandins in the pathophysiology of this condition and the value of the prostaglandin synthetase inhibitors in the treatment of dysmenorrhea have made the management of this problem much more simple.

Primary dysmenorrhea is usually associated with an ovulatory cycle. Most young women who have painful periods do not consult their physicians. They have found that the use of prostaglandin blockers used on an over-the-counter basis controls the symptoms. However, when a young adult complains of dysmenorrhea, it becomes our obligation to find out whether or not it is primary or secondary dysmenorrhea. Once the recognizable causes of secondary dysmenorrhea (painful menses associated with pelvic disease) have been excluded, a diagnosis of primary dysmenorrhea may be entertained. The diagnosis is made on the basis of a history and physical examination. Patients with primary dysmenorrhea have regular cycles and experience pain with the period, which usually develops 1 year after menarche. Thus, most of these cycles are ovulatory.

Our present understanding of dysmenorrhea suggests that prostaglandins, which are synthesized from phospholipids in the plasma membranes of endometrial cells, account for severe uterine contractions. It is well known that primary dysmenorrhea occurs only in ovulatory cycles, and therefore only in the presence of progesterone. It is believed that regression of the corpus luteum and a decrease in progesterone cause disruption of the lyosomes containing enzymes such as phospholipase, thus triggering the onset of menstruation and the conversion of phospholipids in the endometrial cell membranes into prostaglandins.

Prostaglandins have been identified and measured in endometrial tissue, and both prostaglandin E_2 and prostaglandin $F_{2 \, alpha}$ have been found in higher levels in the endometrium during the luteal phase than during the follicular phase of the ovulatory cycle. Moreover, it has been shown that patients with dysmenorrhea have higher endometrial levels of prostaglandins than do women with no complaints of dysmenorrhea. The metabolites of prostaglandins that may be measured in peripheral plasma samples are also elevated in women with dysmenorrhea compared with normal subjects.

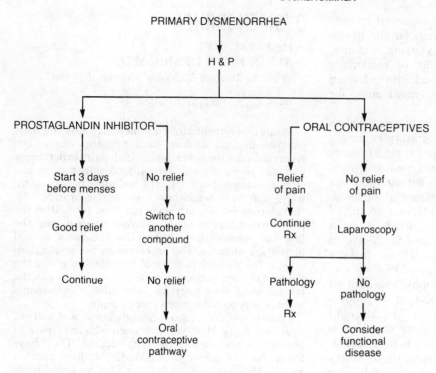

Figure 1. Flow sheet illustrating a simple approach to the management of primary dysmenorrhea.

It is known that intravenous $PGF_{2\ alpha}$ produces menstrual-like cramps and intense uterine contractions with an increase in amplitude and frequency, plus an increased resting tone. It is believed that the resulting pain is essentially ischemic as a result of the release of prostaglandins causing contractions and reduced blood flow. It has also been postulated that the pain may be simply secondary to increased uterine activity, more specifically, to increased sensitization of nerve terminals to pain by prostaglandins.

TREATMENT

Treatment consists of the use of either ovulation suppressors or prostaglandin synthetase inhibitors. Most of these inhibitors act by blocking the enzyme cyclo-oxygenase, thereby preventing the synthesis of prostaglandins, but they do not affect the prostaglandins already in circulation. Ibuprofen, naproxen, and naproxen sodium act by blocking the enzyme. Fenamates interfere with synthesis of prostaglandin but also act as prostaglandin antagonists by blocking the action of prostaglandins at the target organs. The only fenamate approved for use in the United States is mefenamic acid. Table 1 gives the prostaglandin inhibitors that are presently used for the management of primary dysmenorrhea.

All prostaglandin synthetase inhibitors are effective in the treatment of primary dysmenorrhea and may prove to be beneficial in some cases of secondary dysmenorrhea. The side effects of the approved drugs at the recommended dosages are minimal. If a trial of one prostaglandin inhibitor in two consecutive cycles fails to relieve dysmenorrhea, a different agent may be prescribed for the next cycle. In this fashion, most women with primary dysmenorrhea can use one of these inhibitors with great success.

Figure 1 best describes a simple technique for working with the patient who has primary dysmenorrhea.

Secondary dysmenorrhea is best studied by laparoscopic evaluation of the pelvis so that the etiology of the symptom, whether it is endometriosis or pelvic inflammatory disease, can be properly identified. At present, some gynecologists include presacral neurectomy as a procedure done at the time of surgery for endometriosis. This can be performed by laser laparoscopy or at the time of open laparotomy for endometriosis. When the diagnosis of endometriosis is made, medical management may consist of the use of danazol (Danocrine), gonadotropin-releasing hormone agonists, or pseudopregnancy. If the patient has pelvic inflammatory disease, the use of antibiotic therapy and surgery may be in order. If

TABLE 1. **Prostaglandin Inhibitors**

Generic Name	Trade Name	Dose
Ibuprofen	Motrin, Advil	400–600 mg q 6 hr
Naproxen	Naprosyn	250 mg tid
Naproxen sodium	Anaprox	275 mg q 6 hr
Mefanamic acid	Ponstel	250 mg q 6 hr

the individual is wearing an intrauterine device, its removal will decrease the exacerbation of dysmenorrhea.

The evaluation and treatment of the symptom of dysmenorrhea depend on whether the patient is ovulatory, whether there is pelvic pathology, and whether psychosomatic causes for the symptom have been ruled out. Many individuals do not wish to use prostaglandin inhibitors for the relief of dysmenorrhea and would rather use oral contraceptives for this purpose.

MENOPAUSE

method of
DANIEL R. MISHELL, JR., M.D.
University of Southern California School of Medicine
Los Angeles, California

The mean age of menopause is about 51 years, with a normal distribution curve and 95 per cent confidence limits between ages 45 and 55. The average life expectancy for a woman in the United States is about 78 years, and about one-third of a woman's life will be spent postmenopausally. This time of life should be considered an estrogen deficiency state, and improvement in both the quality and the quantity of life can be obtained with the use of estrogen replacement during the postmenopausal years.

GENITOURINARY EFFECTS

Atrophy in the genitourinary tract can produce symptoms of atrophic vaginitis with itching, burning, dyspareunia, and possibly vaginal bleeding. Local estrogen therapy rapidly relieves these symptoms, but because vaginal administration of estrogen results in irregular systemic absorption, estrogen is best administered systematically for long-term prevention of vaginal atrophy as well as osteoporosis. Estrogen deficiency may also cause uterine prolapse as the supporting ligaments lose their tonicity. In addition, cystocele and rectocele may develop as a result of estrogen deficiency. These changes can be prevented or alleviated by administering estrogen. The trigone of the bladder and the urethra are embryologically derived from estrogen-dependent tissue, and postmenopausal estrogen deficiency can cause atrophy of these structures producing symptoms of urinary urgency, incontinence, dysuria, and urinary frequency. Because of atrophy of the vaginal elastic tissue, urinary stress incontinence can also occur. If these symptoms develop postmenopausally, they are best initially treated with estrogen replacement.

CENTRAL NERVOUS SYSTEM CHANGES

The pathognomonic symptom of the menopause is the hot flush or flash, which is caused by a decrease in circulating estrogen levels. The best treatment for the hot flush is estrogen, which has been shown to alleviate symptoms better than placebo. It is best to administer the estrogen at bedtime to alleviate the hot flushes that can interfere with sleep. The usual dosage is 0.625 mg of conjugated estrogen or 1 mg of estradiol, although higher doses may be necessary, especially when the ovaries are removed in a premenopausal individual. For women with contraindications to estrogen therapy, specifically, cancer of the breast or endometrium, other medications that are effective in treating hot flushes include oral medroxyprogesterone acetate (Provera) in a dosage of 10 mg per day. Hot flushes can also be relieved by a single injection of Depo-Provera,* 150 mg given once every 3 months. In addition, clonidine in a dosage of 150 micrograms per day can also reduce the incidence of hot flushes.

Symptoms such as anxiety, depression, irritability, and fatigue increase after the menopause, and it has been shown that estrogen replacement significantly relieves these symptoms even in women who do not have hot flushes that interfere with their sleep.

SKIN CHANGES

Recent studies have shown that postmenopausal estrogen users have a significantly thicker skin and a greater amount of collagen in the dermis than do postmenopausal women who do not use estrogen. Thus systemic estrogen use can retard wrinkling and thinning of the skin that occur postmenopausally.

OSTEOPOROSIS

Postmenopasual osteoporosis affects about 25 per cent of women but is uncommon in black persons and in obese women. In thin caucasian and Oriental women, about 1 to 1.5 per cent of bone mass is lost each year after the menopause. Bone loss is more rapid in trabecular bone, which is found mainly in the thoracic spine, than in cortical bone, which is present in the axial skeleton. Beginning about age 60, fractures occur in the vertebral spine as well as the distal portion of the radius, which is also composed of trabecular bone. Fractures in the neck of the femur, made up mainly of cortical bone, usually start about age 70 to 75 and increase at a logarithmic rate

---

*This use is not listed by the manufacturer.

thereafter. Estrogen replacement therapy will reduce the bone loss associated with postmenopausal osteoporosis and thus reduce the fracture rate in women, prolonging women's productive life span as well as providing a tremendous saving in health care costs. Supplemental calcium therapy and weight-bearing exercise are ancillary measures that by themselves without estrogen will not prevent postmenopausal bone loss. To determine if a patient is at risk for osteoporosis, a careful history and physical examination should be performed. The following factors are known to increase the risk of osteoporosis: (1) caucasian or Oriental race; (2) reduced weight for height, (3) early spontaneous menopause or early surgical menopause, (4) family history of osteoporosis, (5) diet low in calcium, high in caffeine, or high in alcohol, (6) cigarette smoking, and (7) sedentary lifestyle. Routine screening by densitometry or computed tomography scanning is not cost effective and is not recommended.

Osteoporosis is associated with an increased rate of bone resorption, and the administration of estrogen will return the resorption rate to normal. Numerous prospective and retrospective epidemiologic studies have shown that estrogen therapy reduces the amount of postmenopausal bone loss as well as the incidence of fractures. Once estrogen therapy is stopped, bone loss resumes at the same rate as that occurring immediately postmenopausally. Therefore, estrogen replacement therapy should be maintained as long as a woman is ambulatory. The minimum dosage of estrogen needed to prevent osteoporosis is 0.625 mg of conjugated equine estrogen or an equivalent amount of other estrogen formulations. It is recommended that in addition to estrogen, 1.5 grams of calcium should be ingested daily, and weight-bearing exercise such as walking should be encouraged. Supplemental use of vitamin D is of no benefit.

CARDIOVASCULAR EFFECTS

Because estrogen replacement regimens have a minimal effect on liver globulins, postmenopausal estrogen users do not have an increase in mean blood pressure compared with women not ingesting estrogen. It is safe to provide estrogen replacement for postmenopausal women with or without hypertension. Because natural estrogens do not produce a hypercoagulable state, there is no evidence that postmenopausal women with or without a past history of thrombophlebitis have an increased incidence of thrombophlebitis with estrogen replacement therapy. Use of estrogen replacement has been shown in numerous retrospective as well as prospective epidemiologic

studies to reduce the risk of myocardial infarction by about 50 per cent. Estrogen replacement also reduces the risk of stroke by about 50 per cent. Oral estrogen increases levels of the protective high-density lipoprotein cholesterol. Although it has not been determined that this is the mechanism by which estrogen prevents myocardial infarction, the demonstrated reduction of this entity, the major cause of mortality in women, is a major beneficial effect of estrogen. Age-adjusted data indicate that mortality from all causes is significantly lower in estrogen users than nonusers regardless of whether their uteri are intact or have been removed (Table 1).

NEOPLASTIC EFFECTS

Only a few of many epidemiologic studies investigating the relation of estrogen use and breast cancer have shown an increased risk of breast cancer in some subsets of postmenopausal estrogen users, whereas the majority of studies show no effect of estrogen on this cancer. Since estrogen can stimulate the growth of a nonpalpable breast cancer, it is advisable that all women have mammograms performed before initiation of estrogen therapy. If no tumor is found, current evidence indicates that oral estrogen use will not increase the risk of developing breast cancer. Epidemiologic data indicate that there is a significant increased risk of developing endometrial cancer in postmenopausal women who are ingesting estrogen without progestins. This risk increases with increased duration of use of estrogen as well as with increased dosage. The endometrial cancer that develops in estrogen users is usually well differentiated and is usually cured by performing a simple hysterectomy. The risk of developing this endometrial carcinoma in women receiving estrogen replacement can be markedly reduced by also administering progestins. The duration of progestin therapy is more important than the dosage, and it is now recommended that the progestin be administered for at least 12 days per month. The addition of progestin to the estrogen therapy acts synergistically to cause a slight increase in bone density. However, progestins reverse some of the beneficial effects of estrogen on serum lipids and thus should not be given to women without a uterus. There are no well-controlled epidemiologic studies yielding evidence that the use of progestins with estrogen alters the risk of breast cancer.

TREATMENT REGIMENS

The treatment regimen most commonly used in the United States is the sequential regimen of

TABLE 1. **Age-Adjusted All-Cause Mortality Rates (Per 1000 Per Year) by Hysterectomy Status and Estrogen Use**[*][†]

Hysterectomy Status	Estrogen Use		Total
	Nonuser	User	
Intact uterus and ovaries	9.0 (6.5–12.0)	4.9 (1.8–10.7)	8.2 (6.1–10.8)
Hysterectomy	8.2 (3.3–16.8)	2.8 (0.3–10.0)	5.7 (2.6–10.8)
Oophorectomy	11.8 (5.9–21.2)	1.4 (0.0–7.6)	7.2 (3.7–12.6)
Total	9.3 (7.2–11.9)	3.4 (1.5–6.4)	

*From Bush TL, Cowan LD, Barrett-Connor E, et al: JAMA 249:903, 1983.
†Ninety-five per cent confidence limits on rate.

0.625 mg of conjugated estrogen or 1 mg of estradiol orally for the first 25 days each month. Beginning on day 12 to 15 of estrogen (or estradiol) treatment, 5 to 10 mg of medroxyprogesterone acetate is added daily for 10 to 13 days. With this regimen more than half the women have regular withdrawal bleeding, an annoying problem for the postmenopausal woman that decreases patient compliance to continue use. It is not necessary to have withdrawal bleeding to slough the endometrium to reduce the risk of cancer. A continuous regimen in which the estrogen is given daily together with a small dose of oral progestin such as 2.5 to 5 mg of medroxyprogesterone acetate reduces the change of developing uterine bleeding as well as avoiding a week off treatment, in which symptoms may appear. Data from several recent studies indicate that most women do not bleed on this regimen and the endometrium usually remains atrophic. A routine pretreatment endometrial biopsy is unnecessary, as it is not cost effective, and routine annual endometrial biopsies are not necessary unless breakthough bleeding occurs.

Estrogen replacement therapy is indicated for nearly all postmenopausal women because of its numerous beneficial effects. Contraindications to estrogen replacement are uncommon. These include a history of breast cancer, recent history of endometrial cancer, active liver disease, or the presence of thrombophlebitis. A past history of thrombophlebitis is not an absolute contraindication for estrogen replacement.

VULVOVAGINITIS

method of
HUNTER A. HAMMILL, M.D.
Baylor College of Medicine
Houston, Texas

Complaints of irritation in the genital area, both inside the vagina and on the vulva, or skin on the outside, are common among female patients. One-third of all women are affected by vaginitis during their reproductive years. There are various types of vulvovaginal irritations that exhibit different symptoms requiring vastly different therapies.

The most commonly thought-of entities causing vulvovaginal irritation are infectious, including yeast infections with *Candida albicans;* parasitic infections with *Trichomonas vaginalis;* and bacterial vaginitis associated with a mixture of organisms including *Gardnerella vaginalis* and anaerobic bacteria.

The term "normal vaginal flora" may be a misnomer. The only definitive statement about the vaginal flora is that the vagina cannot be sterilized. Since the days of Pasteur and Minchnikoff, there has been a debate about whether the indigenous flora of the human is a sign of health or disease. Vaginal flora and various bacteria composing the flora of an individual patient change with events in the patient's life. These hormonal changes—from the prepubertal state to puberty, and to menopause—are nature's interventions. Additional variables include sexual activity, birth control, antibiotic therapy for distant site infections (e.g., dental), and surgery. These factors are further compounded by pregnancy, which alters the vaginal flora and the symptoms that may result from an overgrowth of different organisms. It should be noted that only certain organisms are clearly pathogens such as *Neisseria gonorrhoeae* and herpes simplex virus, as opposed to potential pathogens, such as *G. vaginalis*. The vagina should have secretions with a pH of 3.2 to 4.0 and no odor. The secretions should be of a quantity so that a pad does not have to be worn. Any disruption of the vaginal environment may result in a heavy discharge with or without itching or odor. It is important to ask patients if their symptoms involve the vulva, vagina, or both. It is also important to ask if the symptoms are itching, odor, or quantity of discharge. Most patients present initially with such minor complaints, or they may have a chronic problem that has been treated with multiple medications prescribed by a physician or one that has been treated with home remedies. It is also important to ask questions about the lifestyle of the patient. Douching is classified by the U.S. Food and Drug Administration (FDA) as cosmetic, and, although it can cause some reduction in bacterial counts, there are no scientific studies showing any therapeutic efficacy for treating vaginitis; the vagina should be self-cleaning. The nature of the patient's sexual activity is also important. Certain patients who practice anal intercourse followed by vaginal relations continually inoculate themselves and cause recurrent bacterial vaginosis. Some patients also may have a modification of vaginal flora because of the use of birth control pills and/or other contraceptive methods. Some patients may use barrier contraceptive methods such as sponges, which, if retained for long periods, enhance bacterial growth. Retained tampons are another source of vaginal irritation.

After these historical questions are considered, examination of the patient and culture are performed. It is important to understand the limitations in interpreting culture data. The normal vaginal flora may be more aptly called "resident flora" of the lower genital tract because endogenous flora are often cultured but may not be the source of the problem. One might ask why a culture should be done because all results are positive.

Specific entities causing vulvovaginal disease will be dealt with in the following sections on an individual basis. It should be noted that before the diagnosis is attempted, any vaginal discharge should be evaluated microscopically. Phenaphthazine paper (Nitrazine), which is used for vaginal pH measurements, costs approximately 5 cents per patient and may give great insight into the bacterial disruption if an infection is present.

FUNGAL INFECTIONS

The primary presenting symptom of a fungal infection in the female genital tract is itching. It should be noted that the sex steroid stimulation of yeast increases during pregnancy. The patient may complain of an irritation with itching in the vagina as well as on the vulva. Classically, the discharge has been described as cottage cheese, although this appearance is not essential. The vaginal pH is in the normal range, not elevated above 4.5. The diagnosis can be made by noting hyphae or germ cells from *C. albicans,* if they are present, on a wet preparation. Additional verification can be provided by use of selective media such as Nickersons or Biggys. In some studies, 30 to 50 per cent of direct microscopic examinations failed to show the organisms.

Treatment

Currently, the drugs for treatment of vaginal fungal infections may be divided into imidazoles, such as clotrimazole (Lotrimin) and miconazole (Monistat), and the polyenes, such as nystatin (Mycostatin). Studies in the past have included therapies ranging from single 500-mg clotrimazole suppositories to intravaginal use twice a day for 7 to 14 days and with efficacies ranging from 86 to 94 per cent. The number of products available for this type of infection has multiplied, and

some of the newer agents are to be applied topically for 5 to 7 days. The newer topical antifungals are probably safe for use in pregnancy; however, many have not received FDA approval because they have not been tested. Systemic therapy for antifungal infections of the vagina includes ketoconazole. Ketoconazole (Nizoral), unfortunately, has shown hepatotoxicity in 1 per 10,000 exposed patients. This effect is usually reversible, although there was one reported death. This agent should be held in reserve, and it is recommended for culture-verified recurrent infections. Additional therapies in the past have included gentian violet, boric acid, and the introduction of lactobacillus (i.e., yogurt) into the vagina. These therapies may not be harmful but are cosmetically discomforting to the patient. Gentian violet dramatically stains the clothes, but it may be ineffective. The problem with yeast infections has been recurrences. It may be helpful for the patient to keep a calendar of when symptoms recur and to have a culture verified. A short course of treatment, from the fifth to eleventh day of a cycle, should be considered if the pattern appears to follow the menstrual cycle.

Special consideration should be given to patients with an underlying disorder, such as diabetes, to control this disorder. It has also been recommended that the patient wear loose-fitting clothing and that the patient use a hairdryer to enhance personal perineal hygiene after bathing.

BACTERIAL VAGINOSIS

Bacterial vaginosis was initially thought to involve a single organism called *Haemophilus vaginalis,* which was later named *Corynebacterium* and finally *Gardnerella.* Patients presenting with bacterial vaginosis complain of an odor, which the physician should elicit in the office. A history of retained tampons or retained vaginal sponge may be related to this condition. The examination by Nitrazine Paper often reveals an pH above 4.5. Clue cells, seen by microscopic examination, are believed to be desquamated vaginal epithelial cells with adherent bacteria. Unfortunately, this finding is not 100 per cent reliable in all patients with bacterial vaginosis. The terminology for this entity has been further changed and is now "bacterial vaginosis" because the vagina does not appear to be inflamed.

If the patient has an elevated vaginal pH, a foul odor from the vagina, and a wet preparation verifying the lack of yeast organisms and lack of *T. vaginalis,* bacterial vaginosis is the probable diagnosis. Past therapies have involved the use of topical sulfa agents, doxycycline, ampicillin, and metronidazole. One study by TA Pheifer and colleagues comparing all of these agents (see New England Journal of Medicine *298*:1429, 1978) showed a 66 to 100 per cent success rate in patients who were diagnosed as having *G. vaginalis* infections. It is significant to note that *G. vaginalis* has been implicated as the etiologic agent—mixed with anaerobic organisms—and may be the cause of the odor.

Treatment

Successful treatment with metronidazole (Flagyl) further illustrates this point because *G. vaginalis* is usually resistant to metronidazole in in vitro laboratory testing. Therapy usually entails metronidazole, 250 mg three times daily for 7 days, although in recurrent infections, 500 mg four times daily may be used. Alternative therapies addressing the anaerobic nature of this entity have entailed the use of Augmentin, 250 mg three times daily for 7 days, although there are no reported studies showing its efficacy. Other agents such as clindamycin may have a therapeutic role with patients allergic to penicillin or metronidazole.

A new organism, *Mobiluncus,* has been implicated in patients with resistant vaginitis. *Mobiluncus* can be resistant to metronidazole, and its presence would explain therapeutic failures in a subgroup of patients.

TRICHOMONAS VAGINALIS INFECTION

It has been estimated that annually more than 180 million women throughout the world suffer from *Trichomonas* infections; 2.5 million women are affected in the United States each year. This problem is further complicated by the incidence of *Trichomonas* infection during pregnancy (ranging in various studies from 4 to 24 per cent). Patients present with complaints of a yellow, copious, frothy discharge, occasionally have inflammation of the vagina, and are classically described as having a strawberry cervix. The pH of the discharge may be higher than 4.5, or the patient may have minimal complaints with a normal vaginal pH. Controversies associated with *Trichomonas* infection involve treatment, particularly during pregnancy. In a series of studies involving more than 2000 patients, there was no association with premature labor, and infection was not thought to be an indication for therapy. *Trichomonas* infection may be associated with other venereal diseases that should be evaluated.

Treatment

Therapy has classically involved the use of metronidazole, 250 mg three times daily for 7

days, or the use of a single 2-gram dose. One important consideration is that if the partner is treated, the successful outcome of therapy will be enhanced. Concerns about the use of metronidazole during pregnancy stem from its category B classification and from reproductive studies in rats with up to five times the human dose. Because of these studies there has been some hesitancy to treat patients during the first trimester. Alternative treatment with clotrimazole may help the patient symptomatically; however, topical clotrimazole does not eradicate the organism. There has also been some concern about resistant *Trichomonas* isolates. This problem has occasionally been addressed by the use of metronidazole suppositories that have been prepared on an individual basis to circumvent possible inactivation of metronidazole to its less active metabolite by the vaginal flora.

Trichomonas organisms are usually passed in a venereal fashion, although there are testimonial reports from the British literature involving splashing in the water closet and from the U.S. literature involving the use of towels in confined populations. Although these are unusual routes of transmission, it should be noted that *Trichomonas* can be dormant, causing no symptoms, and that patients should be appropriately counseled about the venereal, nonvenereal, and dormant nature of *Trichomonas.*

AMEBIC ETIOLOGIES OF VAGINITIS

Entamoeba histolytica, which causes amebiasis, is usually associated with ulcerative lesions of the colon; however, it can also be present in healthy, asymptomatic patients. It has been noted on Papanicolaou's smears and wet preparations, and some patients present with vulvar pruritus related to *E. histolytica.* Therapy for this entity is metronidazole, 250 mg orally three times daily for 10 days, which provides a 90 per cent cure rate.

Enterobiasis, or pinworm infection, is caused by *Enterobius vermicularis* and is not uncommon in children. It is estimated that more than 4 million cases occur in the United States annually. It can be associated with pruritus and vaginal irritation. Vaginal enterobiasis is less common; however, the diagnosis can be established by visual inspection, which reveals a "white thread" appearance. The classic diagnostic method uses clear cellophane tape over the rectum in the morning for 30 seconds, which is then removed and examined for moving pinworms. With repeated examination, this method has a 99 per cent accuracy rate. Current therapy is a single dose of 100 mg of mebendazole (Vermox). *Schis-*

tosoma haematobium infection has been reported with genital irritation, although usually not in the United States but rather in endemic areas of Egypt and Africa. *Phthirus pubis,* which is also referred to as "crabs," is a species of lice that can be involved in the genital area, causing excoriations and irritations. Diagnosis is usually based on finding nits or eggs in the pubic hair. Treatment of this entity involves the use of several agents, most commonly lindane (Kwell) lotion or shampoo.

AGE-RELATED VAGINITIDES

Postmenopausal patients may complain of an atrophic vaginitis. This vaginitis is usually apparent on physical examination and is due to the loss of vaginal mucosa ridges. There may be white coloration instead of pink. The vaginal pH may also rise. Therapy for this condition involves estrogen replacement by a topical, oral, or patch system. Lessening of postmenopausal hot flashes is a side benefit to this therapy.

Prepubertal vaginitis occurs as leukorrhea. The lack of estrogen may result in pediatric vaginitis's being caused by organisms such as coliform bacteria and *Escherichia coli.* In this age group, hyperestrogenic adolescent leukorrhea may also resurface at the time of puberty in the young patient. Evidence of recurrent vaginal irritations and problems in the genital area in a premenarchal female requires further evaluation by a specialist because of the possibility of child abuse.

VULVAR IRRITATIONS

Patients may have exclusively vulvar irritation. The physical examination may direct the practitioner to the problem by the presence of lesions of the vulva. Examination may be enhanced with the application of 5 per cent acetic acid to the vulvar area to look for evidence of human papillomavirus. Colposcopic examination may help in evaluation of the area when indicated. If a suspicious lesion is seen, it is essential to perform a biopsy. In the absence of vulvar lesions, a random biopsy may also be helpful. Biopsies may show evidence of atrophic changes, hypertrophic dystrophies, or lichen sclerosus. Hypertrophic dystrophies can be treated with topical corticosteroid creams such as Hytone in percentages up to 1 per cent twice a day for several weeks. Atrophic dystrophies are treated with estrogen replacement. Lichen sclerosus is treated with testosterone propionate, 2 per cent in a white petrolatum, applied two times daily as needed. It is important that such suspicious areas be followed by doing appropriate biopsies.

The most disturbing finding with current vulvar irritations, aside from cancer, is the presence of human papillomavirus. Evidence of a flat type of this virus, not a classic visible wart, is increasingly being diagnosed by biopsy in vulvodenia. Topical treatment of these viral infections has involved applications of 5-fluorouracil cream or podophyllin to gross warts; laser and other surgical ablations have also been used. It is essential that this disease is recognized as a potentially sexually transmitted disease. It is also essential that its latent nature is explained to the patient. The partner of the patient should also be referred for colposcopy and evaluation by a urologist or dermatologist when human papillomavirus infection is noted.

TOXIC SHOCK SYNDROME

method of
JOHN L. WHITING, M.D., and
ANTHONY W. CHOW, M.D.
University of British Columbia
Vancouver, British Columbia

Toxic shock syndrome (TSS) is an acute multisystemic illness characterized by sudden onset of high fever; diarrhea; hypotension; hyperemia of the conjunctival, oropharyngeal, and urogenital mucous membranes; and a diffuse scarlatiniform rash followed by desquamation from the hands and feet. Other organ systems, including the hepatic, renal, muscular, hematologic, gastrointestinal, cardiopulmonary, and central nervous systems, may also be involved. Since a definitive diagnostic test for TSS currently does not exist, recognition of the syndrome is primarily based on clinical findings (Table 1) and epidemiologic considerations (Table 2). Although TSS was primarily described in menstruating women and was associated with tampon use and vaginal *Staphylococcus aureus* infection, nonmenstrual cases are increasingly recognized. Nonmenstrual TSS has been associated with use of contraceptive diaphragms or sponges and with any of the myriad infections caused by *S. aureus.* Many such infections are acquired in the hospital, particularly infections associated with postoperative wounds, parturition, and nasal packing. The overall mortality of TSS remains high (3 to 7 per cent). Recurrence of disease is frequent in menstrual TSS, but is quite rare in nonmenstrual cases.

ETIOLOGY AND PATHOGENESIS

The precise etiology and pathogenesis of TSS remain unclear. Since bacteremia rarely occurs despite multisystemic involvement, it is widely believed that staphylococcal exotoxins are implicated. Among these

TABLE 1. **Clinical Manifestations of Toxic Shock Syndrome**

Almost Always Present (>80%)	Commonly Present (20–80%)	Rarely Present (<20%)
Temperature ≥ 38.9° C	Headache	Arthritis
Rash and desquamation	Confusion or agitation	Lymphadenopathy
Hypotension	Meningismus	Hepatosplenomegaly
Nausea or vomiting	Pharyngitis	Pulmonary infiltrates
	Vaginitis	Pericarditis
	Conjunctivitis	Photophobia
	Strawberry tongue	Seizure
	Nonpitting edema	
	Myalgia	
	Arthralgia	
	Diarrhea	

staphylococcal products, the toxic shock syndrome toxin-1 (TSST-1), a 24-kilodalton protein that can be demonstrated in over 95 per cent of vaginal *S. aureus* strains associated with menstrual TSS, is a leading candidate as a causative agent of TSS. However, since up to 30 per cent of *S. aureus* strains associated with nonmenstrual TSS may be negative for TSST-1 production, other staphylococcal exotoxins may be responsible in these latter cases. The exact mechanisms for cellular injury by these exotoxins remain unknown, but the most important pathophysiologic effect is extensive capillary leakage of intravascular fluid resulting in rapidly progressive hypovolemia and end-organ dysfunction. Whether staphylococcal exotoxins act directly on target organ sites or indirectly by triggering major biologic mediator systems such as interleukins, cachectin, prostaglandins, kallikrein, complement, and coagulation cascades remains to be determined. Answers to these important questions could provide new therapeutic options.

DIAGNOSTIC APPROACH

TSS should be considered in the differential diagnosis in any patient who is febrile, is in shock, and has a rash. This applies not only to previously healthy, menstruating women, but also to anyone with a suspected *S. aureus* infection. A diligent effort should be made to uncover any occult focus, particularly since infected wounds associated with nonmenstrual TSS often show only minimal signs of local inflammation. Presence of a characteristic sunburn-like rash is particularly helpful in the differential diagnosis; however,

the rash may be evanescent or atypical. Laboratory findings, although striking, are nonspecific, and are useful only for monitoring target organ dysfunction and the severity of complications (Table 3). Blood should be drawn for baseline investigations, and cultures from blood, urine, wounds, or other body sites should be obtained. Although the distinction between TSS and other illness can be quite difficult at times, a careful history and physical examination in combination with a strong index of suspicion and appropriate laboratory tests of exclusion will usually provide the correct diagnosis.

TREATMENT

The major goals of treatment in TSS are (1) resuscitative measures for hypovolemia and shock, (2) eradication of toxin-producing *S. aureus*, (3) removal or neutralization of preformed toxin(s), and (4) treatment of complications.

Resuscitation

Supportive and resuscitative measures should be commenced as soon as the patient has been examined. In patients who have mild hypotension and are otherwise stable, the insertion of a wide-bore intravenous catheter may be all that is necessary. Those with profound hypotension, however, will require rapid infusions of intravenous fluids. As hypotension is largely due to

TABLE 2. **Risk Factors for Toxic Shock Syndrome*†**

High	Moderate	Low
Absence of antibody to TSS toxin-1	Regular absorbency tampons used regularly during menstruation	Contraceptive diaphragm
Infection with TSST-1–positive *S. aureus*	Alternating use of tampons and pads	Intrauterine contraceptive device
Menstruating female less than 35 years of age	Contraceptive sponge	Surgical wound infections
Super absorbency tampon used continuously during menstruation		Early postpartum state
Nasal surgery with packing		

*Modified with permission from Smith CB and Jacobson JA: Toxic shock syndrome. Disease-a-Month *32*(2), 1986. Chicago, Year Book Medical Publishers.

†Oral contraceptives may be protective.

TABLE 3. **Complications of Toxic Shock Syndrome**

Common (>20%)	Rare (<20%)
Acute renal failure	Disseminated intravascular
Adult respiratory distress	coagulation
syndrome	Ataxia
Hypocalcemia	Toxic encephalopathy
Hypomagnesemia	Memory impairment
Menorrhagia	Cardiomyopathy
Alopecia	Protracted malaise
Nail loss	

increased capillary wall permeability and leakage of fluids into extravascular compartments, colloid should be included in the intravenous fluid regimen. Oxygen is administered and a urinary catheter is inserted for monitoring of urine output. Many patients will quickly respond and can then be managed under close observation in a general ward.

If the hypotension persists and the patient is oliguric after 1 or 2 hours of aggressive intravenous fluid management, the patient is best moved to an intensive care facility where hemodynamic parameters can be closely monitored and more effectively controlled. Monitoring devices such as a central venous pressure line, a Swan-Ganz catheter, or an intra-arterial catheter should be inserted if responses remain inadequate after reasonable fluid challenge, or if significant renal impairment or pulmonary edema is present. If the patient remains unresponsive to fluid management, a pressor agent such as dopamine hydrochloride should be considered. It is worth noting that cardiac indices in most patients with TSS usually indicate a state of high cardiac output. If a diminished cardiac output is observed, a toxin-mediated cardiomyopathy causing depressed myocardial contractility should be suspected. In this instance, alternative management, including decreased fluid volume and reduction of cardiac afterload, should be instituted. Dobutamine (Dobutrex) rather than dopamine is preferable when myocardial damage is evident.

High-dose corticosteroids (e.g., methylprednisolone, 10 to 20 mg per kg every 6 to 8 hours), although commonly used, have not been prospectively evaluated in acute TSS. A retrospective study of a limited number of patients did suggest that corticosteroids are of some benefit when administered within the first 2 to 3 days of illness. Such therapy should be considered for the critically ill patient, but is probably unnecessary for most patients. Similarly, there has been only limited experience with the use of naloxone (Narcan) (0.4 mg intravenously followed by an infusion at a rate of 0.05 mg per kg per hour), and such investigational treatment should be reserved for patients with refractory shock.

Antimicrobial Therapy

Although antimicrobial therapy has not been shown to affect the course of the acute illness in menstrual TSS, it definitely reduces the frequency of recurrent episodes. Antimicrobial therapy is clearly important in the management of nonmenstrual TSS. There is no unique susceptibility profile of TSS-associated S. aureus compared with strains not associated with TSS. The choice of specific antistaphylococcal agents is therefore based on other considerations, such as tissue penetrance, bactericidal activity, and known history of hypersensitivity reactions. Beta-lactamase–stable penicillins and cephalosporins such as nafcillin, cloxacillin, and cefazolin* (100 mg per kg per day given every 6 hours), and other agents such as clindamycin (Cleocin) (25 mg per kg per day every 8 hours) or vancomycin (Vancocin) (30 mg per kg per day every 6 hours), are all appropriate choices.

Interestingly, clindamycin, at subinhibitory concentrations for bacterial growth, can "switch off" in vitro production of TSST-1 by toxin-positive strains of S. aureus, presumably by its action at the ribosomal level where protein synthesis takes place. However, the therapeutic implication of this observation is unknown. Antistaphylococcal therapy should be administered intravenously and at maximal doses. In addition, if gram-negative sepsis cannot be ruled out clinically, empiric coverage with an aminoglycoside may be prudent until blood culture results are available. Therapy should be continued until the patient is afebrile and clinically stable. The benefit of additional oral antimicrobial therapy after this time is unproved, but many physicians prefer to complete a 10- to 14-day course of total treatment. Obviously, antibiotics alone may be ineffective in the presence of a loculated infection. Such areas should be adequately drained or débrided as indicated.

Toxin Removal and Neutralization

Apart from antimicrobial therapy to eliminate a continuing reservoir of toxin-producing bacteria, measures to minimize systemic absorption of preformed toxin from infected wounds or vagina may be worthwhile. Surgical wounds, if present, should receive special attention, since most cases of postoperative TSS occur in the absence of obvious local signs of infection. Thus, any surgical wound, even if grossly uninfected, should be closely examined and probably surgically explored. Any foreign body, such as an infected

---

*Usual dose is 500 mg to 1 gram every 8 hours.

prosthesis, intravenous catheter, tampon, diaphragm, or contraceptive sponge, should be removed and cultured. Some clinicians have advocated liberal irrigations of wounds or douching the vagina with saline or povidone-iodine. This is of unproven benefit but unlikely to be harmful.

Since seroprevalence studies in humans and animal protection studies in experimental TSS suggest that antibody to TSST-1 is protective, attempts to rapidly neutralize systemically absorbed TSST-1 by hyperimmune serum appear promising. Human immune globulin has been shown to have high antibody titer to TSST-1, and the protective and therapeutic efficacy of such immune serum has been demonstrated in a rabbit model of TSS. Whether immune globulin will be effective in patients with established disease remains to be ascertained.

Treatment of Complications

While the relative contribution of hypotension versus direct toxin effect to multiple organ dysfunction in TSS is uncertain, it is clear that close attention to the potential for such late complications will be particularly important (see Table 3). Severe electrolyte and acid-base disturbances such as hyponatremia, hypocalcemia, hypomagnesemia, and acidosis should be corrected. Seizures and arrhythmias should be controlled. Patients with acute renal failure may require hemodialysis, whereas those with adult repiratory distress syndrome will need aggressive ventilatory support. Although such complications are rare, patients with late and debilitating sequelae such as persistent neuromyasthenia, severe depression, lack of concentration, and memory loss will require continued support and psychologic counseling.

PREVENTION

Recurrence of TSS is primarily limited to women with menstrual TSS who had received inadequate antimicrobial therapy. With antibiotic treatment and appropriate precautions, fewer than 5 per cent of patients will have a second episode of TSS. Subsequent episodes may be mild or severe, and generally occur under circumstances similar to the initial illness. Recurrence is rare in nonmenstrual TSS. Serologic studies have indicated that women who developed TSS during menses may take many months to acquire a detectable antibody titer to TSST-1, whereas patients with nonmenstrual TSS generally develop a significant antibody response soon after their illness.

Until more is understood about the nature of the disease and its relationship to menstruation and tampon use, patient education remains the mainstay of prevention. Women need to be aware of the symptoms of TSS, and should be instructed to remove tampons and seek medical attention at the first sign of such symptoms. Women who have not developed TSS but wish to reduce future risk should diminish tampon use to a minimum, and wear sanitary pads as an alternative. For those in whom total abstinence from tampon use is impractical, frequent changes and choice of the lowest absorbency compatible with their needs should be recommended.

The value of routine vaginal cultures and screening for serum antibody titers to TSST-1 in the general population is unclear at present. Certainly among women who have had a recent episode of menstrual TSS, surveillance culture of the vagina, nares, oropharynx, and perineum for recurrence of toxin-positive *S. aureus* could be obtained at regular intervals. Colonization by such strains should be eliminated by oral antibiotics until serum antibody to TSST-1 has clearly developed. The ability to detect TSST-1 production by *S. aureus* and serum antibody levels to TSST-1 is now readily available at a number of medical centers.

Since TSS is likely to be a continuing problem and probably occurs more frequently than is currently recognized, there is clearly the need for effective screening methods to identify the susceptible population and for effective vaccines or toxoids for the individuals at risk.

CHLAMYDIAL INFECTIONS

method of
LEWIS H. HAMNER, III, M.D., and
JOHN H. GROSSMAN, III, M.D., PH.D.
George Washington University
Washington, D.C.

Genitourinary infections caused by the bacterial pathogen *Chlamydia trachomatis* are now recognized to be the most common sexually transmitted disease in the United States. It is estimated that 3 to 4 million or more cases occur annually, making chlamydial infections more common in the United States than the estimated new cases of gonorrhea, syphilis, and herpes simplex infection combined. The incidence of cervical colonization in the general population is 3 to 5 per cent. However, among certain high-risk patient populations, cervical carriage rates may approach 15 to 20 per cent.

C. trachomatis is the leading cause of pneumonia in infants less than 6 months of age and has replaced gonococcal infection as the leading cause of neonatal conjunctivitis. Neonatal chlamydial pneumonia is thought to affect 3 to 10 per 1000 live births. However, in populations with a high prevalence of cervical infection this may be as high as 50 to 60 per 1000 live births. In the United States, estimates suggest that in low-prevalence populations (3 to 5 per cent), 26,000 cases of pneumonia and 29,000 cases of conjunctivitis due to *Chlamydia* will occur each year. The number of infections attributed to *Chlamydia* in populations with a higher prevalence of disease will be even greater. The risk to the infant of an infected mother is 60 to 70 per cent for acquiring the disease, with 10 to 20 per cent risk of pneumonia and 25 to 55 per cent risk for conjunctivitis.

MICROBIOLOGY

The genus *Chlamydia* contains two species, *C. psittaci*, found in avian species and some lower mammals, and *C. trachomatis*. *C. trachomatis* is a bacterium; DNA and RNA are present, as is a cell wall. These bacteria lack the enzymes necessary for oxidative phosphorylation, however, and so they are obligate intracellular parasites for at least a portion of their life cycle. During the extracellular portion of their life cycle, infectious particles (called "elementary bodies") are extremely small, approximately 0.3 micrometer in diameter. These elementary bodies attach to columnar epithelium and gain entry to the cell through phagocytosis. During the intracellular portion of their life cycle, chlamydiae utilize the adenosine triphosphate (ATP) and amino acids of the cell to replicate via binary fission and produce new infectious particles that are released with cell lysis.

Fifteen serotypes of *C. trachomatis* have been identified. Serotypes A, B, Ba, and C are associated with blinding trachoma in adults, and serotypes L1, L2, and L3 are the causative agents in lymphogranuloma venereum. Serotypes D to K are most commonly found in genitourinary infections. The remainder of this article will deal specifically with these infectious organisms.

EPIDEMIOLOGY

Chlamydial infections are most prevalent in young, promiscuous, indigent patient populations. As would be expected from this profile of risk factors, they are more likely to occur among unmarried, inner-city women, especially those who are concomitantly infected with or who have a prior history of other sexually transmitted diseases. Women with positive endocervical cultures for gonorrhea, for example, have a 25 to 50 per cent incidence of simultaneous chlamydial infections.

CLINICAL PRESENTATION

Many adult women with genital chlamydial infection are either asymptomatic or minimally symptomatic. Diagnostic testing in the former group may be prompted by discovery of another sexually transmitted disease. Mucopurulent cervicitis has been associated with a 50 per cent incidence of chlamydial infection.

The diagnosis of mucopurulent cervicitis is established by visualization of yellowish mucopurulent endocervical secretions on a white swab and the presence of 10 polymorphonuclear leukocytes or more per field in a gram-stained smear of secretions at ×1000 magnification. Women with symptoms of urethral irritation and pyuria whose urine specimens show no evidence of infection by Gram's stain or conventional bacteriologic culture are at high risk for chlamydial infection as well.

Chlamydial infection has been found to cause 5 to 10 per cent of cases of acute salpingitis in the United States. When compared with women who have gonococcal or mixed aerobic/anaerobic salpingitis, women with chlamydial salpingitis are often less clinically ill, with minimal or even no leukocytosis. Subsequent scarring of the fallopian tubes can lead to infertility and an increased risk for ectopic pregnancy.

The majority of cases of acute epididymitis in men under the age of 35 are caused by *Chlamydia*. Infertility has been described as a long-term complication, as a result of scarring and occlusion of the vas deferens.

Chlamydial infection is the leading cause of conjunctivitis and afebrile interstitial pneumonitis among infants less than 6 months of age. Recent experience suggests that prior or concomitant chlamydial infection may be associated with a significantly higher prevalence of neonatal otitis media and gastroenteritis in the same childhood population.

Follow-up examination of children 7 to 8 years after hospitalization for chlamydial pneumonia during infancy has shown long-term pulmonary changes. Obstructive pulmonary function studies and a significantly greater rate of physician-diagnosed asthma have been reported in these children.

LABORATORY DIAGNOSIS

The isolation of *C. trachomatis* using tissue culture from presumptively infected individuals remains the "gold standard" for definitive laboratory diagnosis. In addition to being somewhat expensive and cumbersome, the tissue culture methodologies that assure reliable recovery are relatively stringent and, consequently, few health care facilities are optimally equipped to perform cultural isolation on a large scale.

Diagnostic methods other than isolation in tissue culture are less sensitive and slightly less specific but are appropriate and may be preferable as cost-effective alternatives in certain patient populations. There are two major rapid direct antigen kits commercially available. One utilizes an enzyme-linked immunosorbent assay (immunoperoxidase) and the other an immunofluorescent indicator system. The sensitivity of either method in testing endocervical specimens ranges from 70 to 90 per cent and the specificity ranges from 94 to 98 per cent. A recent study comparing the immunofluorescent method with tissue culture in a patient population with a 13 per cent prevalence of infection noted a predictive value of a positive (PVP) rapid test of only 65 per cent. Lower-prevalence populations would have even lower PVPs. Of more importance may be the potential 20 to 30 per cent incidence of false-negative results of rapid direct tests of specimens from the cervices of asymptomatic individuals subjected to screening. Nevertheless, the cost and labor of tissue culture isolation make it an impractical albeit scientifically desirable alternative. The rapid direct methods seem most useful for large-scale screening in high-risk, high-prevalence populations.

Papanicolaou's smears are not acceptable substitutes for either screening or diagnosis, since their sensitivity ranges from 40 to 60 per cent among culture-positive individuals. Serologic testing is of little clinical value, since neither seropositives nor seronegatives reliably correlate with infection or absence of infection.

PERINATAL IMPLICATIONS

The extent to which chlamydial infection adversely affects pregnancy and causes perinatal complications remains controversial. Several retrospective studies have demonstrated a significantly higher incidence of stillbirth, premature delivery, and neonatal death among pregnant women with chlamydial infection compared with uninfected, matched controls. However, the most recent prospective information shows no statistical difference between cases and controls for premature rupture of the membranes, preterm delivery, amnionitis, intrapartum fever, delivery of infants that are small for gestational age, postpartum endometritis, and neonatal sepsis. In a subset of women with recent or invasive chlamydial infection, indicated by the presence of IgM antibody against *C. trachomatis,* preterm delivery and premature rupture of the membranes occurred in 19 per cent of patients, which was statistically higher than in controls. Further prospective studies are needed to determine whether there is an association between perinatal chlamydial infection and preterm labor or amniorrhexis.

At present, it seems reasonable to screen certain "high-risk" obstetric populations for chlamydial infection. Adolescents, women with "sterile" pyuria or mucopurulent cervicitis, women with other venereal diseases, and contacts of individuals with chlamydial infections should be included in such testing, either for diagnosis or for follow-up after treatment. Some studies have suggested that obstetric populations with a prevalence of infection greater than 12 per cent are groups in which such screening is likely to be cost effective.

TREATMENT

The treatment of choice for genitourinary chlamydial infections is tetracycline, 500 mg orally

TABLE 1. **Treatment of *Chlamydia trachomatis* Infection**

Tetracycline, 500 mg PO qid for 7 days
or
Doxycycline, 100 mg PO bid for 7 days
Pregnant patients or patients unable to tolerate tetracycline derivatives
    Erythromycin, base 500 qid for 7 days
    or
    Erythromycin ethylsuccinate, 400–800 mg qid for 7 days

four times daily for 7 days, or doxycycline (Vibramycin), 100 mg orally twice daily for 7 days (Table 1). Since treatment with tetracycline derivatives during pregnancy should be avoided, erythromycin is the obstetric treatment of choice. Erythromycin base, 500 mg, or erythromycin ethylsuccinate, 400 to 800 mg, four times daily for 1 week, is the preferred treatment for pregnant women. A recent study has been associated with a cure rate in excess of 90 per cent when the ethylsuccinate regimen was employed in 400-mg dosages. Erythromycin in the ethylsuccinate form seems to be well tolerated and is associated with better patient compliance and less nausea than erythromycin base. Since the neonatal infection rate among offspring of untreated infected women approaches 50 per cent, all women in whom chlamydial infection is diagnosed during pregnancy should receive treatment, follow-up with culture testing, and appropriate testing for other associated sexually transmitted disease.

In the patient hospitalized for parenteral treatment of pelvic inflammatory disease, therapy should include coverage for *Chlamydia.* Penicillin derivatives, cephalosporins, and aminoglycosides are generally not effective against *Chlamydia.* Although some of the broad-spectrum antibiotics such as ticarcillin, mezlocillin, and clindamycin have antichlamydial activity, resolution of clinical symptoms does not correlate with eradication of the chlamydial organism. Recent experience with fluorinated quinolones (e.g., ofloxacin) suggests that these agents may be an effective treatment alternative, although the safety of such agents in pregnancy has not yet been established. Current sexually transmitted disease treatment guidelines suggest the use of cefoxitin (Mefoxin), 2 grams intravenously four times daily, plus doxycycline (Vibramycin), 100 mg intravenously twice daily for at least 4 days and at least 48 hours after the patient improves. Doxycycline, 100 mg by mouth twice a day, is then used to complete 10 to 14 days of total therapy.

PELVIC INFLAMMATORY DISEASE

method of
MICHEL E. RIVLIN, M.D.
University of Mississippi Medical Center
Jackson, Mississippi

Pelvic inflammatory disease (PID) is a broad term that includes a variety of upper genital tract infections unrelated to pregnancy or surgery, such as salpingitis, salpingo-oophoritis, endometritis, peritonitis, and tubo-ovarian inflammatory masses. Usually the patient has had a lower genital tract infection, generally via sexual transmission, which ascends through intermediate stages of cervicitis and endometritis to the fallopian tubes. Recurrence of PID is common but must be differentiated from periodic lower abdominal pain without reinfection, which occurs in nearly 20 per cent of women after an initial episode. Primary infection is due to virulent organisms, such as *Neisseria gonorrhoeae* or *Chlamydia trachomatis* and probably *Mycoplasma hominis* and *Ureaplasma urealyticum*, introduced by sexual contact. Once the cervical barrier has been overcome, secondary colonization by virulent organisms that usually colonize the vagina occurs within a few days. These organisms create a polymicrobial infection including facultative gram-negative bacilli such as *Escherichia coli* and anaerobic bacteria such as *Bacteroides* species and, rarely, *Actinomyces israelii*. Once damaged, the genital tract often does not recover completely, and many women thereafter have recurrent infections with their own endogenous vaginal or rectal organisms. True chronic disease, for instance with tuberculosis, is very rare in the United States.

The important risk factors frequently overlap. These include young age, early coital debut and promiscuity, single status, socioeconomically disadvantaged status, and nonwhite race. The intrauterine device (IUD) increases the relative risk two to nine times, whereas oral contraceptives and barrier methods appear to exert some protective effect. Bacterial vaginosis (nonspecific vaginitis) may predispose to PID, but this is still hypothetical.

CLINICAL PICTURE

Symptoms include abdominal pain and dyspareunia, fever, vaginal discharge and irregular bleeding, urinary and rectal symptoms, nausea, and vomiting. Signs include pyrexia, vaginal discharge, cervical excitation tenderness, and tenderness and adnexal masses evident on bimanual examination. Investigations include endocervical Gram's stain for gonorrhea, complete blood count, urinalysis, serum pregnancy test, erythrocyte sedimentation rate test, serologic tests, and culture for aerobes, anaerobes, *Chlamydia,* and *N. gonorrhoeae* from the cervix, urethra, and rectum. In selected cases, culdocentesis, ultrasound, or laparoscopy should be performed. All these investigations would be extremely expensive if done routinely, and clinical judgment must therefore be used. Differential diagnoses include acute appendicitis, endometriosis, ectopic pregnancy, mesenteric adenitis, and complications of ovarian cysts. Chlamydial infection is probably a more common cause of PID than gonorrhea, and while the older division of PID into gonococcal and nongonococcal variants is no longer emphasized, it is true that gonococcal infections tend to cause a more florid clinical picture, usually within a week of menstruation. By contrast, chlamydial infections are more insidious and as a result the sequelae of infection are greater in nongonococcal PID, probably because of delay in recognition and therapy. Anaerobic infections are clinically the most severe and are relatively more resistant to therapy. They usually occur in patients using an IUD or with a previous history of PID.

DIAGNOSIS AND SEQUELAE

The clinical diagnostic accuracy using classic criteria is low, with the diagnosis being incorrect in 17 to 63 per cent of cases. This is because all the hallmark signs and symptoms are very variable. Standardized criteria have been proposed to improve diagnostic accuracy, but have probably not entered general use as yet. Laparoscopy is thought to be the definitive technique for diagnosis, but routine use of the procedure is impractical in most circumstances. It should probably be reserved for situations in which more information is necessary, for example, if appendicitis or ectopic pregnancy is suspected or for pelvic pain of unknown origin.

The sequelae of PID include involuntary infertility from tubal occlusion, which is related to the number and severity of the infections. Twelve, 35, and 75 per cent of women were found to be infertile after one, two, and three episodes of PID, respectively. Chronic abdominal pain, possibly related to adhesions, occurs in 20 per cent and recurrent infection in approximately 25 per cent of women who have had PID. Tubal damage from previous PID is the most common cause of ectopic pregnancy, increasing the risk six- to tenfold. This risk is also increased with recurrent infections.

TREATMENT

Medical Management

Infertility is probably less frequent when PID therapy is started early. Patients with uncomplicated disease (Grade I, limited to tubes and ovaries) are usually treated as outpatients, although there is a move toward more liberal hospitalization criteria. Patients with cases complicated by inflammatory adnexal masses and/or pelvic peritonitis (Grade II) and patients with suspected ruptured abscess (Grade III) must be hospitalized. Other suggested criteria for inpatient management include temperature greater than 38° C; uncertain diagnosis; pregnancy; inability to follow or tolerate outpatient regimen or lack of response to outpatient management; inability to arrange follow-up within 48 to 72 hours; and disease in a prepubertal or adolescent patient.

As no single antibiotic is active against all possible pathogens, combination regimens directed against *N. gonorrhoeae,* including PPNG (penicillinase-producing *Neisseria gonorrhoeae*), and *C. trachomatis* are recommended by the Centers for Disease Control (CDC) (Table 1). Cefoxitin (Mefoxin), or an equally effective cephalosporin, plus either doxycyline (Vibramycin) or tetracycline provides this activity. If nongonococcal polymicrobial infection is suspected, the patient can be treated with metronidazole (Flagyl), 500 mg orally four times daily, and trimethoprim plus sulfamethoxazole (Bactrim DS or Septra DS), twice daily. Bed rest, sexual abstinence,

TABLE 1. **Centers for Disease Control Recommendations for Outpatient Treatment of Pelvic Inflammatory Disease**

Non–penicillin-allergic patients
  After 1 gram of probenecid PO
    Amoxicillin, 3 grams PO
    Ampicillin, 3.5 grams PO
    Aqueous procaine penicillin G, 4.8 million U IM
    Cefoxitin, 2 grams IM
  Ceftriaxone or equivalently effective cephalosporins
Penicillin-allergic patients
    Spectinomycin, 2 grams IM
  Tetracycline loading dose plus maintenance dose as indicated below
All patients also receive a 7-day course of one of the following:
    Tetracycline, 0.5 gram qid
    Doxycycline, 0.1 gram bid
    Erythromycin base, 0.5 gram qid
    Erythromycin stearate, 0.5 gram qid
    Erythromycin ethylsuccinate, 0.8 gram qid

analgesics, referral of sexual partners, removal of IUD if present, and contraceptive counseling are further important aspects of management. If specific pathogens are cultured, the cultures should be repeated 7 days after therapy is completed.

The CDC recommends two regimens for inpatient PID therapy (Table 2). Intravenous therapy is recommended for at least 4 days and at least 48 hours after the patient improves. In practice, patients who require hospitalization but who do not have an adnexal mass are often treated with single-agent regimens with results equal to those of the CDC recommendations and with lower costs and side effects. Thereafter, outpatient therapy with an agent active against *Chlamydia* (doxycycline, erythromycin) is commonly prescribed. Many of the newer broad-spectrum cephalosporins have proved efficacious against PID; these include ceftizoxime, 1 gram every 8 hours. The expanded-spectrum penicillins (mezlocillin [Mezlin], piperacillin [Pipracil]) are effective in doses of 3 to 4 grams every 6 hours, but probably should be reserved for therapy of *Pseudomonas* infections. Good results are also reported with

TABLE 2. **Centers for Disease Control Recommendations for Inpatient Treatment of Pelvic Inflammatory Disease**

Regimen A
  Cefoxitin, 2 grams IV q 6 hr
  Doxycycline, 0.1 gram IV q 12 hr
  Doxycycline, 0.1 gram PO q 12 hr for 6–10 days
Regimen B
  Clindamycin, 0.6 gram IV q 6 hr
  Gentamicin
    2 mg/kg IV, loading dose
    1.5 mg/kg IV q 8 hr
  Clindamycin, 0.45 gram PO q 6 hr for 6–10 days

other agents, such as ticarcillin-clavulanic acid and imipenem plus cilastatin (Primaxin).

Adnexal abscesses are generally treated with combination regimens including an aminoglycoside or aztreonam (Azactam), and an agent with specific antianaerobic activity (clindamycin, chloramphenicol, metronidazole). Patients with true abscess formation as distinct from inflammatory complexes require surgery for clinical cure in a significant number of cases.

Surgical Management

Indications for surgery include ruptured tubo-ovarian abscess, failure to respond to appropriate antibiotic therapy within 48 to 96 hours, a persistent pelvic mass, or persistent pelvic pain. Surgical cure may be expected with removal of the uterus and adnexa; however, this is a procedure usually reserved for older, parous women. Advances in tubal microsurgery and in vitro fertilization provide some hope of childbearing even in patients with badly damaged tubes, so that conservative surgery, such as unilateral adnexectomy, is recommended for younger patients who have not completed their families.

LEIOMYOMAS OF THE UTERUS

method of
CHARLES H. LIVENGOOD, III, M.D.
Duke University Medical Center
Durham, North Carolina

Leiomyomata uteri are solid, benign, sex hormone–responsive tumors arising from the myometrium. Their prevalence increases with age up to menopause such that 25 per cent or more of women in their forties are affected; they are more common among black women. The tumors are always multiple, and size varies from microscopic to more than 100 pounds. The natural history of leiomyomata uteri is one of slow growth, often intermittent, until menopause when regression occurs. Spontaneous regression before menopause rarely occurs, if ever.

Leiomyomata uteri may become complicated by degeneration, which is characterized by central necrosis of the tumor from hypoperfusion; by extrusion, wherein uterine contractions deliver into the vagina a pedunculated submucosal tumor in a process identical to labor; by pyomyoma, abscess formation within a uterine leiomyoma; and by leiomyosarcoma, which arises in 0.2 per cent of patients.

Symptoms of leiomyomata uteri include dysmenorrhea, dyspareunia, pelvic pressure, pelvic pain, irritative bladder symptoms, and abnormal uterine bleeding; patients may also be asymptomatic. Acute severe pelvic pain accompanies degeneration, extrusion, and pyomyoma. Leiomyosarcoma becomes symptomatic only late in the disease. A history of infertility, early pregnancy loss, or premature labor may be found.

DIAGNOSIS

Diagnosis is generally made on pelvic examination, when the uterus is found to be enlarged, hard, and usually irregular in surface contour. A pelvic sonogram should usually be done to confirm the diagnosis; all too often ovarian cancer treatment has been delayed by expectant management of presumed leiomyomata uteri. Furthermore, abnormal uterine bleeding should never be ascribed to these tumors until sampling of the endometrium has shown no other active process. A plain flat plate radiograph of the pelvis is essentially diagnostic of postmenopausal leiomyomata uteri when calcium deposition in a lamellar pattern is seen. With degenerating tumors, marked uterine tenderness, modest leukocytosis and fever, and peritoneal signs are often encountered; in pyomyoma a progression of these findings, often with evidence of sepsis, is the rule. With extrusion, findings are like those of degenerating tumors, and a hemorrhagic, friable mass presents in the cervix or vagina. The differential diagnosis of leiomyomata uteri includes ovarian tumors, endometriosis externa, intra- or extrauterine pregnancy, tubo-ovarian abscess, colonic diverticular abscess, other bowel tumors, arteriovenous malformation, and malignancies of the uterus and uterine cervix.

TREATMENT

Expectant management is intended for asymptomatic patients who have no abnormal uterine bleeding, a confident diagnosis confirmed by sonogram, and an overall uterine size that does not exceed the size of a pregnant uterus at 12 weeks. These patients may be seen every 6 months to ensure that there has been no rapid growth of the tumors—any more than 10 to 20 per cent growth. After menopause, the tumors should slowly decrease in size, although they may not resolve completely.

Medical Treatment

Medical treatment is of variable efficacy and is generally intended for temporary control of mild symptoms in patients with a confident diagnosis and overall uterine size no more than that of a 12-week gestation; undiagnosed abnormal uterine bleeding is a contraindication to such therapy. Therapy consists of medroxyprogesterone (Provera, others), 10 mg by mouth daily for 10 to 14 days before each expected menses, to be used for a minimum of 3 months. Also, today's low-dose oral contraceptives induce relative hypoestrogenism, so that any effect on leiomyomata uteri will be inhibitory, and in some cases this inhibition is of symptomatic significance. Degeneration of leiomyomata uteri often occurs during pregnancy because of the associated high estrogen levels. These patients are treated with close inpatient observation—because of the possibility of misdiagnosis of placental abruption, appendicitis, and other major complications of pregnancy—and analgesia; improvement usually occurs within a few days. In the nonpregnant woman, nonsteroidal anti-inflammatory agents (Motrin, Anaprox, others) and medroxyprogesterone (Provera, others), 10 mg by mouth three times daily* for 7 to 10 days, are added to the treatment regimen for the pregnant woman.

Surgical Treatment

Conservative surgical treatment refers first to myomectomy, an abdominal operation in which as many leiomyomata are removed from the uterus as allowed by blood loss, which is usually brisk, and by the need to retain an adequate volume of normal uterine tissue to permit reconstruction of a potentially functional organ. The procedure is appropriate only for women strongly desiring retention of reproductive function and those in whom pregnancy loss has been attributed to the tumors. More than 50 per cent of these women develop recurrent tumors. The second conservative surgical procedure is that for an extruding tumor, wherein the tumor is pulled downward into the vagina, its pedicle is ligated, and the tumor is removed. Postoperatively, the patient is watched closely for evolution of uterine infection, which is common.

Curative surgical therapy consists of hysterectomy, using a vaginal approach for small tumors and an abdominal approach for larger ones. The ovaries may be left in place unless there is another indication for their removal. Curative surgery is indicated for patients who have rapid growth of the uterus, intractable pain that is believed to be the result of the tumors, and abnormal bleeding of a severity to induce anemia despite no other active abnormality within the uterus as shown by dilatation and curettage. Hysterectomy early in the process is always indicated in pyomyoma, along with broad-spectrum parenteral antibiotic therapy.

Estrogen replacement therapy is not contraindicated for the postmenopausal woman with leiomyomata uteri. Low-dose treatment should be given with cyclic estrogen and progestin. Any abnormal bleeding or uterine enlargement should be investigated immediately.

---

*The usual dose is 5 to 10 mg daily.

CANCER OF THE ENDOMETRIUM

method of
JOHN H. MALFETANO, M.D.
The Albany Medical College
Albany, New York

Carcinoma of the body of the uterus is the most common gynecologic malignancy and has remained so for the past decade. Throughout the 1970s, there was a 1.5-fold increase in the number of endometrial cancer patients. In 1975, 27,000 new cases were reported, reaching a high of 40,000 cases in 1986; the estimated number of new cases annually now appears to be stable at 36,000. Endometrial carcinoma is the sixth leading cause of death in females after breast, colorectal, lung, ovarian, and cervical carcinomas.

EPIDEMIOLOGY

Uterine cancer is a disease of the postmenopausal female (75 per cent of cases), with a peak incidence at 58 years of age. Some 25 per cent of the patients are premenopausal, 5 per cent of whom are under the age of 40 at the time of diagnosis. Endometrial carcinoma is more common in caucasian women than in black or Asian persons. The apparent rise in the incidence of carcinoma of the corpus is attributed primarily to two factors: obesity and the use of unopposed exogenous estrogens for menopausal symptoms. Other associated risk factors include living in a highly industrialized Western country, familial history, upper socioeconomic class, history of anovulation, nulliparity, estrogen-producing ovarian neoplasms, and the coincident disorders of adult-onset diabetes mellitus and hypertension. The high-risk woman characterized by obesity, failure of ovulation, or prolonged estrogen administration produces continuous, unopposed estrogen stimulation to the endometrium and appears to be causally subject to subsequent development of endometrial carcinoma. This continuous endometrial stimulation in susceptible individuals leads to hyperplastic states within the endometrium and thereafter to frank carcinoma.

DIAGNOSIS AND DETECTION

The first symptom in virtually all women with carcinoma of the endometrium is abnormal bleeding, spotting, or discharge. The frequency, amount, and duration of bleeding are of no consequence, and all forms of bleeding demand investigation, especially in the postmenopausal female. Nearly 30 to 50 per cent of postmenopausal bleeding is caused by carcinoma. Papanicolaou's smear, which has been so successful in detecting early cervical carcinoma, is not reliable for detection of endometrial carcinoma. The false-negative rate of cervical and vaginal smears in endometrial carcinoma ranges from 50 to 80 per cent.

A variety of sampling techniques, both cytologic and histologic, are available for the detection of endometrial carcinoma. It is axiomatic that any woman with postmenopausal bleeding must have the endometrial cavity sampled, either by an office endometrial biopsy or by formal curettage of the endometrium. Only with an office biopsy that is positive for carcinoma can the physician be certain about the etiology of the abnormal bleeding. Any other pathologic result from the office sampling necessitates a formal dilatation and curettage of the uterus. A small carcinoma within atypical adenomatous hyperplasia may be missed by office biopsy alone. Repeat sampling is also necessary if symptoms persist without any etiology, and in rare circumstances, hysterectomy is indicated for diagnosis.

Carcinoma of the uterine corpus is clinically staged according to the International Federation of Gynecology and Obstetrics staging classification (Table 1). This process depends on the physical examination, chest and x-ray roentenograms, and blood chemistry. The stage is not influenced by subsequent surgical pathologic findings. Evaluation of the uterine size and extension of the disease to the cervix differentiate Stage I and Stage II disease. A high false-positive rate remains with endocervical curettage, especially with

TABLE 1. **FIGO Classification of Carcinoma of the Corpus Uteri***

Stage	Characteristics
0	Carcinoma in situ exists. Histologic findings are suspicious of malignancy; cases of Stage 0 should not be included in any therapeutic statistics.
I	The carcinoma is confined to the corpus.
IA	The length of the uterine cavity is 8 cm or less.
IB	The length of the uterine cavity is more than 8 cm.
Stage I cases should be subgrouped with regard to the histologic type of the adenocarcinoma as follows:	
G1	Highly differentiated adenomatous carcinoma exists.
G2	Differentiated adenomatous carcinoma with partly solid areas exists.
G3	Predominantly solid or entirely undifferentiated carcinoma exists.
II	The carcinoma has involved the corpus and the cervix but has not extended outside the uterus.
III	The carcinoma has extended outside the uterus but not outside the true pelvis.
IV	The carcinoma has extended outside the true pelvis or has obviously involved the mucosa of the bladder or rectum. A bullous edema as such does not permit a case to be allotted to Stage IV.
IVA	The growth has spread to adjacent organs.
IVB	The growth has spread to distant organs.

*From Beahrs OH and Myers MH (eds): Manual for Staging of Cancer. Philadelphia, J. B. Lippincott, 1983, pp. 139–141. Used by permission.

TABLE 2. **Five-Year Survival in Carcinoma of the Uterine Corpus**

Stage	5-Year Survival (%)
I	63–94
II	50–65
III	25–35
IV	5–10

lower uterine segment carcinomas. Disease should be classified as Stage II only when there is carcinoma involving the cervical stroma.

TREATMENT

Adenocarcinoma of the endometrium remains one of the most treatable gynecologic malignancies despite a previous lack of unanimity concerning the best treatment. Nearly 70 per cent of patients with endometrial cancer present with Stage I disease, which portends a favorable prognosis. Survival ranges from 63 to 94 per cent for patients with Stage I cancer; however, extrauterine disease is more difficult to control (Table 2).

Although endometrial carcinoma is clinically staged, its treatment is based on the surgical pathologic findings at operation. Treatment, planning, and prognosis are related to the risk factors of tumor grade, myometrial invasion, extension to the cervix or adnexa, and possibly positive peritoneal cytology. These virulence factors are helpful in selecting women who are at risk for pelvic and para-aortic nodal metastasis and, therefore, who are to be candidates for postoperative radiation therapy. As the tumor becomes more undifferentiated, with deeper invasion into the myometrium, the incidence of nodal disease increases (Tables 3 and 4).

The approach to Stage I carcinoma of the uterine corpus is surgical. In opening the abdominal cavity, pelvic and paracolic washings are obtained by instilling 100 to 150 ml of saline and sending the specimens for cytologic evaluation and cell block. The entire abdomen is then explored. An extrafascial hysterectomy and bilateral salpingo-oophorectomy are performed. Bilateral pelvic lymph nodes, as well as aortic lymph nodes, are sampled and sent for histologic evaluation, followed by resection or biopsy of any other sites that may harbor metastatic disease.

TABLE 3. **Endometrial Cancer Grade versus Positive Pelvic and Para-Aortic Nodal Disease**

Grade	Pelvic Nodes (%)	Para-Aortic Nodes (%)
1	3	0–2
2	10	4.0–13.6
3	36	28–37.5

TABLE 4. **Depth of Myometrial Invasion and Pelvic and Para-Aortic Nodal Disease**

Myometrial Invasion	Pelvic Nodes (%)	Para-Aortic Nodes (%)
Endometrium only	1–3.6	1–1.8
Inner one-third	5–11.5	3–9.8
Middle one-third	6–10	0–1
Outer one-third	25–43	17–21

POSTOPERATIVE MANAGEMENT

The radiation fields are tailored to the surgical and pathologic findings at surgery. Standard pelvic fields should deliver midplane doses of 4500 to 5000 cGy and cover the upper one-third of the vagina. The upper extent of the radiation field should cover the L_4–L_5 vertebral interspace. Extended para-aortic fields to cover T10 and deliver 4500 to 5000 cGy are necessary if there is para-aortic nodal disease. Patients with Grade 3 lesions, positive pelvic nodes, extension to the cervix, or tumor of any grade with myometrial invasion of 50 per cent or more are candidates for postoperative therapy.

Endometrial cancer patients with no risk factors can be considered for postoperative vaginal treatment. Vaginal cylinders produce a surface dose to the vaginal apex of 6000 cGy and reduce vaginal cuff recurrences to approximately 1 per cent.

Patients with para-aortic nodal disease represent a difficult problem because they probably have systemic disease. To date, there is no known effective therapy for this group; however, extended-field radiation therapy to the para-aortic chain, with or without chemotherapy, has been quite promising.

Patients with occult clinical Stage II endometrial carcinoma should be treated in the same manner as other Stage I patients. Postoperative pelvic radiation is indicated if there is stromal involvement of the cervix. Patieents with gross Stage II carcinoma of the uterus are treated like patients with Stage IB carcinoma of the cervix. This includes radical hysterectomy and bilateral salpingo-oophorectomy, pelvic and para-aortic lymphadenectomy, or pelvic radiation therapy plus an interstitial implant combined with extrafascial hysterectomy and bilateral salpingo-oophorectomy. The experienced pathologist may have difficulty distinguishing Stage II carcinoma of the endometrium from adenocarcinoma of the endocervix, and the final diagnosis may be discovered only postoperatively.

GROUP II PATIENTS (MEDICALLY INOPERABLE)

Some patients, because of advanced stage or a poor medical condition that prevents surgery, fall into the Group II category. This relatively rare group of patients can be treated with external pelvic radiation and intracavitary therapy. The overall survival rate with radiation therapy alone in Stage I disease ranges from 28 to 78 per cent at 5 years.

STAGE III AND STAGE IV ENDOMETRIAL CANCER

Adequate treatment of advanced endometrial cancer is not available and must be individualized. Depending on the sites of metastatic disease, surgery, radiation therapy, and chemotherapy may be used.

RECURRENT DISEASE

Cytotoxic chemotherapy for endometrial cancer has been slow to evolve because of high cure rates with surgery and radiation therapy. Hormonal therapy had been the mainstay of treatment of recurrent disease. Estrogen and progesterone receptors are contained in endometrial cancers, and tumors should be sent for determination of these receptors at the time of initial operation. Tumors can be hormonally manipulated if the receptor status is known. Progestational agents alone or with tamoxifen, which may increase progesterone receptors, can be used.

Recent studies have shown that progestational agents are not nearly as effective as earlier studies had suggested and that pulmonary lesions may be the only ones to respond. Ongoing present clinical trials using systemic agents, cisplatin (Platinol), doxorubicin (Adriamycin), and cyclophosphamide (Cytoxan) are encouraging.

CARCINOMA OF THE UTERINE CERVIX

method of
MAUREEN A. JARRELL, M.D.
University of Vermont
Burlington, Vermont

Carcinoma of the cervix is the third most common gynecologic malignancy, with approximately 13,000 new cases reported each year. Squamous carcinoma of the cervix, which comprises more than 95 per cent of these cases, is a sexually transmissible disease. The association between this cancer and the sexual promiscuity of the patient and her male partners is clear. Early age at first coitus, multiple sexual contacts, and male partners who have had multiple contacts contribute to the risk. The search for a sexually transmissible agent has led to the recent implication of the human papillomavirus. Both clinically overt and subclinical infections with this virus are important in the development of preinvasive and invasive cancers of the cervix. Women who smoke also increase their risk of developing cervical cancer. This factor is independent of other risk factors.

DIAGNOSIS

The squamocolumnar junction of the cervix is the site where neoplastic cervical changes begin. This area is sampled by Papanicolaou's (Pap) smear. When taken correctly, the Pap smear includes a sampling of the exocervix and endocervix. A smear in which endocervical cells are absent indicates that the zone at highest risk was not sampled. This smear should be repeated. If a smear shows evidence of persistent atypia, dysplasia, carcinoma in situ, or invasive cancer, the patient should be referred for colposcopic examination of the cervix. If a gross cervical lesion is present, a biopsy should be obtained regardless of the results of the Pap smear. Cervical infection with human papillomavirus is often recognized by the presence of koilocytes on a Pap smear. This constitutes an additional reason for referral for colposcopic examination. This examination should include a search for the squamocolumnar junction, directed biopsies of the exocervix, and endocervical curettage.

Colposcopic examination helps to select those preinvasive lesions that can be treated by conservative methods. These methods include the use of cryotherapy, the carbon dioxide laser, and 5-fluorouracil cream. Lesions that require cone biopsy are those for which colposcopy has failed to explain the cytologic lesion and those that involve the endocervical canal. For these patients, the cone biopsy not only is therapeutic but also helps to rule out the possibility of invasive disease.

The most common symptom of cervical carcinoma is abnormal vaginal bleeding. Bleeding may be associated with sexual intercourse. Adenocarcinoma of the cervix is increasing in frequency, representing 10 to 15 per cent of the reported cases in many series. This increase in adenocarcinoma reinforces the need for endocervical sampling during the Pap smear and the need to perform an adequate endocervical curettage at the time of colposcopic evaluation.

A patient who has been treated for a preinvasive cervical carcinoma should be followed with repeated Pap smears every 3 months for 1 year after treatment and at 6-month intervals for 5 years. If there is no evidence of recurrent disease, the Pap smear may then be taken on a yearly shedule. It is extremely important to sample the endocervix at the time of the Pap smear in the follow-up of these patients.

TREATMENT

Staging

Staging of cervical carcinoma is primarily based on pelvic examination. The stage may be modified by the findings of the physical examination, chest x-ray film, skeletal survey, intravenous pyelogram, and cystoscopy or sigmoidoscopy. The stage is not modified by body imaging scans or by operative findings. Table 1 shows the current international staging for invasive carcinoma of the cervix. When available, information gathered from computed tomography and magnetic resonance imaging scans may alter the choice of treatment regardless of the assigned clinical stage. Often a barium enema may be added to the work-up of patients who are likely to receive pelvic radiation therapy. In these patients, knowledge of diverticular disease or other colon pathology before pelvic irradiation may help in the assessment of rectal bleeding or other problems on follow-up.

Stage IA

The diagnosis of Stage IA carcinoma of the cervix is most often made by cone biopsy. The diagnosis of microinvasive disease identifies those patients who have invasive disease but a negligible risk of metastases. For the patient who desires future childbearing, treatment may be limited to cone biopsy. In these patients, the cone biopsy margins must be negative and the endo-

TABLE 1. FIGO Classification of Cancer of the Cervix

Stage	Characteristics
I	Carcinoma is confined to the cervix.
IA	Preclinical carcinomas; visible only with a microscope.
IA1	Minimal microscopically evident stromal invasion.
IA2	Measurable lesions not exceeding 5 mm in depth from the base of the epithelium, either surface or glandular. The horizontal spread must not exceed 7 mm.
IB	Lesions larger than those of Stage IA2 or clinically evident lesions.
II	The carcinoma extends beyond the cervix but has not extended onto the pelvic wall, or the carcinoma involves the vagina but not the lower third.
IIA	No obvious parametrial involvement.
IIB	Obvious parametrial involvement.
III	The carcinoma has extended onto the pelvic wall. On rectal examination there is no cancer-free space between the tumor and the pelvic wall, or the tumor involves the lower third of the vagina.
IIIA	No extension onto the pelvic wall.
IIIB	Extension onto the pelvic wall and/or hydronephrosis or a nonfunctioning kidney.
IV	The carcinoma has extended beyond the true pelvis or has clinically involved the mucosa of the bladder or rectum.
IVA	Spread of the growth to adjacent organs.
IVB	Spread of the growth to distant organs.

Abbreviation: FIGO = International Federation of Gynecology and Obstetrics.

cervical curettage above the level of the cone must show no disease. The patient who has completed childbearing should be treated by simple hysterectomy, with or without preservation of the ovaries. Patients who are in poor physical condition may be treated with radiation therapy in the form of implants (brachytherapy).

Stages IB and IIA

Carcinomas of the cervix that are confined to the cervix or upper vagina can be treated with radical hysterectomy and pelvic lymphadenectomy, radiation therapy, or a combination of the two. Radiation therapy and radical surgery are equally effective treatments for these stages. Surgical therapy allows preservation of ovarian and vaginal function and avoids the long-term side effects of radiation therapy. The operation is best performed on young women with small, exophytic tumors. The operative procedure begins with a thorough abdominal exploration and para-aortic lymph node biopsies to determine the extent of disease. If exploration and biopsies show that the extent of disease is still appropriate for radical hysterectomy, the operation is performed. Patients with negative pelvic lymph nodes and clear surgical margins need not receive any supplemental radiation therapy. When metastatic disease to the pelvic lymph nodes is found by the pathologist, the patient may receive adjuvant external pelvic radiation therapy of approximately 4500 to 5000 rad.

Radiation therapy is widely used as a treatment for Stages IB and IIA disease. It is always the treatment of choice when the patient is elderly or medically compromised or when the initial surgical exploration shows that the tumor has spread beyond the cervix. In these cases, external megavoltage radiation therapy is combined with brachytherapy. In young patients, when radiation treatment is anticipated, one or both ovaries may be moved out of the pelvis to avoid radiation castration.

Large, bulky Stage IB cervical tumors may fail treatment with either surgery or radiation therapy. Ongoing clinical trials are testing the role of combinations of surgery, radiation therapy, and chemotherapy in these tumors.

Stages IIB, III, and IV

Patients with advanced cervical carcinoma are treated with radiation therapy. Body imaging scans are extremely valuable in treatment planning for these patients. A large, necrotic cervical carcinoma may give rise to reactive lymph nodes in the absence of metastatic spread. Guided fine-needle aspiration of suspicious findings should be used to confirm the presence or absence of metastatic disease. When disease has spread to the para-aortic region, radiation treatment fields may be extended to include these areas.

External radiation therapy delivers uniform doses to the entire pelvis, including the pelvic lymph nodes, and is often administered first in the treatment sequence to shrink the tumor volume. Radiation implants deliver high-energy doses to the cervix and surrounding areas and usually follow the external therapy.

High failure rates in the treatment of advanced cervical carcinomas are caused by the bulk of the tumor and the spread of disease outside the treatment field. Radiation therapists and gynecologic oncologists are currently studying both hyperthermia and radiation-sensitizing agents as potentiators of radiation in the treatment of this disease. It is still unknown whether single-agent or combination chemotherapy given in association with radiation therapy can alter the course of systemic spread of disease.

Pregnancy

Patients in whom invasive cervical carcinoma is diagnosed at the time of pregnancy present difficult management problems. Within each stage of disease, survival is similar to that of nonpregnant women. Disease management is generally the same during pregnancy, with the added consideration of the fetus. Decisions that may require interrupting the pregnancy before treatment or delaying the treatment for a number of weeks until the pregnancy is viable are highly stressful for the patient and staff. It is important that this diagnosis be made as early as possible during the pregnancy; therefore, visualization of the cervix and a Pap smear are recommended at the first antepartum visit. Abnormal Pap smears are evaluated by colposcopy and, when necessary, by cervical biopsy. The examination is aided by the natural eversion of the endocervix during pregnancy.

Recurrent Disease

Patients treated for carcinoma of the cervix are examined every 3 months for the first year, every 4 months for the second year, and every 6 months in years 3 to 5. Some high-risk patients are followed more closely during the first year. Most recurrent disease appears within the first 2 years of follow-up. Fifty per cent of all recurrences occur in the pelvis. These are generally found by Pap smear, transvaginal and transrectal fine-needle aspiration of suspicious nodules, or body imaging techniques.

Patients who were initially treated by surgery and have a pelvic recurrence are treated with radiation therapy. Patients who were initially treated with radiation therapy and have central pelvic recurrences are candidates for pelvic exenteration when there is no evidence of extrapelvic disease.

Solitary recurrences outside of the pelvis can be treated with surgical excision or radiation therapy. Patients with unresectable pelvic disease or widespread distant disease may be treated with chemotherapy. Often this modality of treatment is severely compromised by bone marrow suppression caused by previous radiation therapy or decreased renal function resulting from ureteral compromise.

Pain management can be a most difficult problem in the patient with recurrent cervical cancer. Invasion of bone and nerve trunks is not uncommon. Some success has been obtained with permanently implanted epidural catheters, which allow the benefit of pain relief without central nervous system suppression.

NEOPLASMS OF THE VULVA

method of
ALAN N. GORDON, M.D.
Vanderbilt Medical Center
Nashville, Tennessee

Cancer of the vulva is a relatively uncommon lesion. Invasive cancer arising on the vulva probably accounts for 5 per cent or less of female genital cancers. Squamous cell carcinomas probably account for 90 to 95 per cent of all cancers arising in the vulva.

During the last two decades, the number and percentage of preinvasive squamous cell lesions have increased. These lesions are occurring in younger patients and are often multifocal. This has often led to the use of therapies designed for better preservation of function. The concern with preservation of function has also led to the introduction of less radical therapies in the treatment of invasive diseases.

VULVAR DYSTROPHIES

The vulvar dystrophies were previously believed to be premalignant on the basis of guilt by association. However, although many cases of invasive cancer have associated areas of dystrophy, only a rare patient has cancer arising within a focus of dystrophy.

Classification

Studies of dystrophy in the past were hampered by the use of clinically descriptive terms that were often confusing. Terms such as "leuko-plakia" and "kraurosis vulvae" actually describe clinical entities and not the underlying disease process. The International Society for the Study of Vulvar Diseases has recommended a classifi-cation based on the histology of the lesion (Table 1). This allows prediction of the possible malig-nant potential and proper selection of therapy.

The hyperplastic lesions often develop in re-sponse to irritants and may or may not be as-sociated with atypia. These lesions are often pruritic. They are usually associated with hyper-keratosis, and atypical maturation of the epithe-lium may or may not be present. The degree of atypia is graded mild, moderate, or severe, de-pending on the percentage of epithelium in-volved.

Atrophic dystrophy is characterized by thin-ning of the vulvar epithelium. In atrophic dystro-phy, or lichen sclerosus, there is thinning of the dermal papillae, along with infiltration of the dermis by a collagenous matrix. This is usually accompanied by a leukocytic infiltration. Clini-cally, the skin is pale and thin, and the labial folds are lost. Ecchymoses may be seen as a result of bruising.

Mixed dystrophies are those in which both types of dystrophies are seen within the epithe-lium. Only if there is a mixed dystrophy can preinvasive or invasive disease occur with lichen sclerosus.

Treatment

In all types of dystrophy, good perineal hygiene is essential to help avoid the irritation that causes further itching and then sets up a vicious cycle. The use of synthetic undergarments should be avoided because these help to retain moisture rather than absorb it, as cotton undergarments do. Liberal use of cornstarch helps to keep the perineum and vulvar tissues dry. In general, tight-fitting clothes should also be avoided be-cause these help to retain moisture in affected areas.

In all types of dystrophy, topical corticosteroids

TABLE 1. **ISSVD Classification
of Vulvar Dystrophy**

Hypertrophic dystrophy
    Without atypia
    With atypia

Atrophic dystrophy (lichen sclerosus)
Mixed dystrophy
    Without atypia
    With atypia

Abbreviation: ISSVD = International Society for the Study of Vulvar Disease.

usually help to decrease the itching. The halo-genated steroids have a longer half-life, providing more prolonged relief than hydrocortisone. These must be well rubbed into the skin to provide relief. If the topical route is not effective, steroids may be given in the subcutaneous tissue. A small amount is injected subcutaneously and then mas-saged in. In intractable cases, absolute alcohol has been given by injection into the subcutaneous tissue. However, this should be reserved for the most severe cases, as it may cause sloughing of the tissues.

In cases of hyperplastic dystrophy, local estro-gens may help to thin the skin. In cases of lichen sclerosus, however, it is necessary to thicken the epithelium. Two per cent testosterone in petro-latum base can be applied daily to provide some thickening and can then be used twice weekly. If patients are reluctant to use male hormones, progesterone 5 per cent can be used instead in a petrolatum base.

Before therapy, the liberal use of punch biop-sies is encouraged to ensure that there is no evidence of pre-existing carcinoma. Repeat biop-sies are warranted in any area that fails to respond to medical therapy. For the hyperplastic and mixed dystrophies, areas that fail to respond are suitable for either laser ablation or wide local excision. If ablative therapy is chosen, multiple biopsies must be performed before therapy. There is limited experience with the laser in lichen sclerosus and atrophic dystrophies. In these le-sions, wide local excision is preferred.

PREINVASIVE DISEASE

Squamous Cell Carcinoma in Situ

The last few decades have seen a marked in-crease in the incidence of squamous cell carci-noma in situ of the vulva. There has also been an increased understanding of the natural history of this disease. This has slowly led to the use of less destructive procedures with preservation of vulvar function.

In approximately one-half of the cases, carci-noma in situ is completely asymptomatic and is diagnosed only after close inspection. One-fourth to one-third of patients have a history of cancer, usually a squamous cancer involving the genital canal. The remainder of the patients usually present with itching as their main complaint. However, in some cases, a lesion may be noted by the patient.

The lesions have different appearances, de-pending on the histopathology. They may be white because of hyperkeratosis. If parakeratosis is the predominant pattern, they are red. They may be pigmented because of increased deposition of melanocytes in the epithelium. Ulceration may be present, usually when there is associated pruritus. Careful inspection is necessary because lesions may be multifocal, especially in younger patients. Toluidine blue can be applied to the vulva and then washed with acetic acid. However, this procedure may give false-positive results in areas of ulceration and may be negative because of areas of hyperkeratosis. Application of 5 per cent acetic acid, which is then allowed to dry, often aids in defining abnormal areas on the vulva. Colposcopy may be helpful, but it is of limited value in areas with hyperkeratosis.

Definitive diagnosis is made through the use of key punch biopsies. In large areas or multifocal lesions, multiple biopsies should be obtained. Previously, multiple terms were used to describe the different histologic appearances of carcinoma in situ. Because these terms have no bearing on the diagnosis or prognosis, their use should be avoided.

Treatment

In the past, treatment for carcinoma in situ of the vulva usually involved a simple vulvectomy. As it became clear that this was an intraepithelial process, a skinning vulvectomy, whereby the epithelium alone was removed and replaced with a skin graft, was often used. This treatment allowed preservation of the labial folds. In most cases, however, unless there is widespread multifocal involvement, even this is no longer indicated.

Lesions in the hair-bearing regions are best treated by wide local excision. An adequate margin of 1.5 to 2.0 cm of normal tissue should be obtained around the lesion. Almost all excisions can be closed primarily through mobilization of lateral skin flaps. If the defect is too large to allow simple closure, a flap of skin can usually be rotated inward for closure. The laser can be used to ablate these lesions. However, if there is extension into appendages that are then ablated, scarring usually occurs during healing.

Lesions in the non–hair-bearing area (e.g., the vestibule, frenulum) or involving the clitoris are well suited to ablative therapy after biopsy. In these areas, excision usually results in some distortion or scarring, which can lead to dyspareunia. The carbon dioxide laser is excellent for treating the epithelium in these areas. Ablation can be carried down to just below the epidermal-dermal junction, and rapid healing ensues from the periphery. There is no need to worry about skin appendages, which do not occur in this part of the vulva. Multiple biopsies are necessary to rule out invasion before any form of ablative therapy.

Topical therapies have been used. 5-Fluorouracil has been reported to have some success. This is applied until a "burn" develops that results in loss of the epithelium; re-epithelialization then occurs from the edges. However, the accompanying discomfort often causes patients to fail to complete the therapy. Sensitization with dinitrochlorobenzene and other immunogens has also met with limited success.

Recurrence rates tend to be 15 to 20 per cent, regardless of the method used. When a lesion recurs, it is imperative to perform another biopsy before instituting therapy.

Paget's Disease

This lesion on the vulva is similar to Paget's disease of the breast. It typically appears as a velvety to fiery red lesion with raised edges. Clinically, it is associated with an intense pruritus.

Histologically, the lesion has a classic appearance, with Paget's cells infiltrating the base of the epithelium, often in the parabasal layers. It has often been stated that this disease is associated with an underlying carcinoma. However, although an underlying invasive carcinoma is often seen in Paget's disease of the breast, it is only rarely seen in Paget's disease of the vulva. Also rare is an invasive form of Paget's disease. However, there does appear to be increased frequency of subsequent cancer in these patients, especially of the colon or breast, and patients should therefore be followed closely.

Therapy

The therapy for Paget's disease of the vulva typically involves wide local excision. At least 2 cm of normal tissue should be taken around the visible lesion to prevent recurrence. The underlying tissue should be carefully examined to rule out a coexisting apocrine cell carcinoma or an invasive form of Paget's disease. Where no evidence of invasion is found, close follow-up is all that is indicated. However, because these patients often have isolated nests of Paget's cells some distance from the main lesion, recurrence is seen in 20 to 30 per cent of cases. Repeat wide local excisions are indicated for cases of symptomatic recurrence. Where there is no evidence of invasion, consideration can be given to following recurrences if they are asymptomatic. Recently, the carbon dioxide laser has been used to vaporize areas of recurrence with limited success; recurrence remains a problem.

Basal Cell Carcinoma

These lesions are usually asymptomatic. Classically, they are ulcerative lesions with rolled edges. Histologically, they have a rather monotonous appearance, consisting of small cells with indistinct features. The hallmark is a palisading of the cells along the edges of the tumor.

Because these lesions are not invasive, wide local excision is again the treatment of choice. The recurrence rate is approximately 10 to 15 per cent. However, repeat excision is all that is indicated.

INVASIVE SQUAMOUS CELL CARCINOMA

Several factors place patients at high risk for squamous cell carcinoma of the vulva. This is still predominantly a disease of older women. Many patients also have a history of carcinoma involving the genital tract, usually a squamous cancer. Many patients have a history of vulvar irritation or dystrophy. However, it is important to remember that few patients who have dystrophy develop carcinoma. Pruritus may be the chief complaint. Pain or bleeding is usually seen only in more advanced lesions. In early cases, the lesions may present as a superficial ulceration or nodule. It is necessary to confirm the diagnosis of invasion by biopsy. In many early cases, the diagnosis may be made only after wide local excision of what was thought to be a carcinoma in situ.

Squamous cell carcinoma of the vulva tends to spread by direct extension or via lymphatic metastases; hematogenous dissemination is unusual except in advanced cases. As the tumors advance, they may involve adjacent genital organs: the vagina, urethra, or rectum. Review of results in patients treated by radical vulvectomy, bilateral inguinal lymphadenectomy, and pelvic lymphadenectomy has shown that spread via the lymph nodes proceeds in an orderly fashion. The tumors first metastasize to the superficial inguinal nodes (above the cribriform fascia), then to the deep inguinal nodes (femoral nodes), then through the inguinal ligament to involve the pelvic nodes, and then finally to the para-aortic nodes and above. Direct spread to the pelvic nodes, although feasible for midline lesions, is exceedingly uncommon. It has also been found that lateralized lesions rarely involve the contralateral lymph node groups unless the ipsilateral lymph node groups are involved first. The incidence of spread to the primary node groups (the superficial and deep inguinal nodes) depends on the size of the lesion, the depth of invasion, and the clinical stage. The best predictor of overall survival is whether or not the primary lymph nodes are involved with disease.

Staging

The International Federation of Obstetrics and Gynecology has a staging system similar to that used for other genital cancers. However, in cases of vulvar cancer, this system often fails to give specific information about the tumor. Although the tumor, node, and metastases (TNM) classification (Table 2) proposed by the International Union Against Cancer is somewhat more cumbersome, it does provide more valuable information in comparing tumors of various stages (Table 3). In vulvar cancer, the stage is based on the clinical examination. The biopsy specimen is used to confirm the presence of invasion, and the physical examination and chest x-ray film are the most pertinent studies. Although the clinical examination can be misleading in classifying the inguinal nodes, there is currently no accurate

TABLE 2. **TNM Classification for Vulvar Carcinoma**

T	Primary tumor	
	T1	Confined to the vulva, diameter ≤ 2 cm
	T2	Confined to the vulva, diameter > 2 cm
	T3	Adjacent spread to the urethra, vagina, perineum, or anus (any size)
	T4	Infiltration of the upper urethral mucosa, bladder mucosa, or rectal mucosa, or fixed to bone
N	Regional lymph nodes	
	N0	Nodes not palpable
	N1	Nodes palpable but not clinically suspicious
	N2	Clinically suspicious nodes
	N3	Fixed or ulcerated nodes
M	Distant metastases	
	M0	No clinical metastases (disregarding inguinal lymph nodes)
	M1a	Palpable deep pelvic lymph nodes
	M1b	Other distant metastases

Abbreviation: TNM = tumor, node, and metastases.

TABLE 3. **FIGO Classification and Corresponding TNM Classification**

FIGO Stage	TNM		
I	T1	N0	M0
	T1	N1	M0
II	T2	N0	M0
	T2	N1	M0
III	T3	N0	M0
	T3	N1	M0
	T3	N2	M0
	T1	N2	M0
	T2	N2	M0
IV	T1	N3	M0
	T2	N3	M0
	T3	N3	M0
	T4	N0	M0
	T4	N1	M0
	T4	N2	M0
	T4	M3	M0
	All M1 lesions		

Abbreviations: FIGO = International Federation of Gynecology and Obstetrics; TNM = tumor, mode, and metastases.

test to diagnose preoperatively the presence of tumor within the nodes.

Treatment

The most significant complication associated with radical vulvectomy is wound breakdown caused by the large bulk of tissue removed and the subsequent tension on the flaps used for closure. Musculocutaneous flaps can be used to help fill the defects. However, this only results in larger procedures. The trend over the last few decades has been toward smaller, more conservative procedures that result in less disfigurement. In addition, pelvic lymphadenectomy has been abandoned. Patients with negative inguinal nodes do not benefit from its addition to radical vulvectomy. Patients with positive pelvic nodes have poor survival. In patients who are at risk for spread to the pelvic nodes (patients with positive inguinal nodes), adjuvant pelvic radiation therapy postoperatively provides survival equal to that obtained with pelvic lymphadenectomy, with lower morbidity.

Early Lesions

Currently, there is no accepted definition of "microinvasion," and this term should be avoided in discussing carcinoma of the vulva. Its use is misleading because there is a low, but still present, risk of lymph node metastases even with the earliest invasive lesions (Table 4). Only cases with the very earliest invasion are not at risk for lymph node metastases. Most T1 lesions seen in recent series have less than 5 mm of invasion.

The inguinal lymph nodes can be approached through separate skin incisions without excising the skin bridge from the lesion. Midline lesions and those approaching the midline require bilateral lymphadenectomy. Lateralized lesions can be treated with an ipsilateral lymphadenectomy. In favorable lesions (those with 3 mm or less of invasion), only the superficial nodes need be removed. If they demonstrate metastases, the deeper nodes and contralateral nodes can either be excised or be treated with adjuvant radiation therapy.

Virtually all early lesions can be handled with

TABLE 4. Incidence of Regional Node Metastases by Depth of Tumor Invasion

Depth of Invasion (mm)	% of Positive Inguinal Nodes
<1	1–5
1–3	10–15
3–5	15–30
5–10	30–45
>10	≥40

radical local excision. At least a 2-cm margin of tissue is obtained, and all deep tissue is excised to the inferior fascia of the urogenital diaphragm. This approach has a recurrence rate equal to that obtained with radical vulvectomy.

Advanced Lesions

Larger lesions or those with clinically involved nodes present a greater challenge. These often require a radical excision and en bloc resection of the inguinal nodes, which may or may not be involved. If the defect is large, a musculocutaneous flap may be needed from either the gracilis or the tensor fascia lata to close the defect. Adjuvant external radiation therapy can be given to the inguinal or pelvic nodes if the inguinal nodes contain metastasis. Implantation of radioactive sources can be used for compromised margins.

Lesions that extend to involve other organs have been traditionally treated with pelvic exenteration combined with vulvectomy. However, preoperative radiation therapy may shrink these tumors away from the other organs, allowing excisional therapy for the lesion with preservation of function of other organs. Often these excisions require the use of musculocutaneous flaps to fill in the defect and bring in the new blood supply to allow adequate healing.

Survival

Survival varies according to the stage of the primary tumor and is proportional to the status of the inguinal nodes (Table 5). The inguinal nodes are a better predictor of survival than the stage.

Recurrent Tumor

Local recurrence is seen more often with larger lesions or where a margin may have been com-

TABLE 5. Survival Rate by FIGO Stage and Nodal Status for Patients with Invasive Squamous Cell Vulvar Carcinoma

FIGO Stage and Nodal Status	% Surviving for 5 Years
Stage	
I	70–90
II	50–80
III	30–50
IV	10–15
Nodal Status	
0 positive	97
1 positive	94
2 positive	80
≥3 positive	12

Abbreviation: FIGO = International Federation of Gynecology and Obstetrics.

promised rather than cut across adjacent organs. Wherever feasible, resection of the recurrence is the treatment of choice. This may be curative in many cases, and if the patient has not had previous irradiation, adjuvant radiation therapy can be given postoperatively.

Groin recurrences carry a worse prognosis. Usually by the time these are clinically manifest, tumor has spread to secondary node groups and often beyond. Excision followed by adjuvant radiation therapy may be curative in some cases.

Disease that has spread to the para-aortic nodes, or systemic disease, is exceedingly difficult to treat. Local irradiation may provide palliation for symptomatic metastases. Platinum-based combination chemotherapy has produced responses but has not prolonged survival.

OTHER VULVAR NEOPLASMS

Verrucous Carcinoma

Clinically, these lesions appear to be large, fungating cancers. Histologically, they are a well-differentiated form of squamous cancer and can even resemble a condylomatous tumor. They are characterized by local invasion but do not metastasize. They are best treated by wide local excision with at least a 2- to 3-cm margin around the tumor. Radiation therapy should be avoided because it has been reported to cause these tumors to develop a more malignant growth pattern.

Bartholin's Gland Carcinoma

The duct of Bartholin's gland can give rise to either squamous or transitional cell cancers. These behave like other squamous cancers of the vulva and are treated similarly. The gland itself can give rise to either an adenocardinoma or an adenoid cystic carcinoma. Clinically, these cancers appear as local swellings. Because they occur in an older age group, they should not be mistaken for a Bartholin's abscess. In the older patient, a suspected abscess requires biopsy. Adenocarcinomas are best treated by radical local excision with an ipsilateral inguinal lymphadenectomy. It is often difficult to obtain adequate margins because of the location of the gland. Adjuvant postoperative irradiation of the involved hemipelvis appears to improve survival.

Melanoma

Malignant melanoma accounts for approximately 5 per cent of vulvar cancers. Typically it is a pigmented, raised lesion within the epidermis. If it reaches a significant size, it may ulcerate and cause bleeding. The best predictors of survival are the size and thickness of the lesion.

Malignant melanomas are best treated by wide local excision of the primary lesion. There are no data showing significant improvement in survival with more radical procedures. In lesions that measure less than 0.75 mm in thickness, the risk of nodal metastasis is quite small. There is controversy regarding the effectiveness of lymphadenectomy in lesions more than 0.75 mm and up to 3 mm in thickness. Patients who already have metastatic disease in the lymph nodes have low survival rates, and patients with negative nodes tend to do well. To date, no form of systemic therapy has produced significant improvement in survival when used as adjuvant therapy.

Sarcoma

Sarcomas rarely arise on the vulva but may consist of virtually any histologic type. The prognosis depends on the grade of the lesion rather than the histologic type. Wide local excision is the treatment of choice because more radical therapy does not increase survival. As with sarcomas in other areas, adjuvant chemotherapy has not produced significant improvement in survival. Local radiation therapy may decrease the risk of recurrence in some cases.

THROMBOPHLEBITIS IN OBSTETRICS AND GYNECOLOGY

method of
RIAD CACHECHO, M.D., and
SUZANNE K. WEDEL, M.D.
Boston University School of Medicine
Boston, Massachusetts

Deep venous thrombosis (DVT) is a serious disorder that can be life-threatening, especially if untreated. Its incidence in the general population is more than 200,000 cases per year. The incidence in pregnant women is estimated at 1 per 250 deliveries; compared with other women of the same age, pregnant women have a fivefold increase in the incidence of DVT. This risk increases further with cesarean section. The risk of DVT in the gynecologic population is comparable to that of general surgical patients. Table 1 presents risk factors in surgery and the associated incidence of DVT; Table 2 gives risk factors for DVT.

ETIOLOGY AND PATHOPHYSIOLOGY

More than a century ago, Virchow described the classic pathologic changes that predispose to DVT

TABLE 1. **Risk of DVT in Surgical Patients**

Group	Age	Surgical Procedure	Incidence of DVT (%)
Low risk	<40 yr	Minor surgery (<30 min)	<3
Moderate risk	40–70 yr	Major surgery (>30 min)	10–40
High risk—Patients with risk factors listed in Table 2			50

development: venous stasis, endothelial injury, and hypercoagulability. Today these remain the inciting factors. All of them may be implicated in DVT formation in the obstetric and gynecologic populations.

Venous stasis occurs during pregnancy as the enlarged uterus compresses the iliac veins. A large pelvic tumor may also compress the iliac veins, producing a low-flow state. Prolonged bed rest in both groups exacerbates this problem.

Endothelial injury occurs during labor and surgical procedures. This injury triggers a cascade of events, including initiation of platelet aggregation, activation of coagulation pathways, and release of vasoactive mediators, resulting in clot formation.

Estrogens inhibit antithrombin III and Factor X inhibitor, both of which are naturally occurring anticoagulants. This inhibition produces a hypercoagulable state that is especially pronounced during the third trimester of pregnancy. Congenital deficiencies of antithrombin III, protein-C, or protein-S increase this predisposition to venous thrombosis.

DIAGNOSIS

Calf pain and tenderness, ankle edema, a palpable venous cord, or pain on ankle dorsiflexion (Homan's sign) are the classic signs of thrombophlebitis. However, these signs are present in only approximately 50 per cent of patients who have DVT. Thus, the clinical examination is insensitive, and a careful medical history becomes vital in determining which patients are at risk for developing deep venous thrombosis.

NONINVASIVE METHODS OF DETECTING DEEP VENOUS THROMBOSIS

Doppler Ultrasound. This method uses sound waves to evaluate venous blood flow and its alteration with the

TABLE 2. **Risk Factors for DVT**

Previous DVT
Oral contraceptives and estrogen
Pregnancy
Immobilization
Obesity
Cancer
Trauma
Long bone or pelvic fracture
Age > 60 yr
Hypercoagulability
Pelvic or abdominal surgery
Congestive heart failure
Dehydration

respiratory cycle. When DVT develops, there is loss of blood flow with absence of respiratory fluctuations in the involved vein. Although Doppler ultrasound is an accurate method of detection, marked variation in examiners makes interpretation of scans inconsistent.

Impedance Plethysmography. Impedance plethysmography (IPG) uses a high-frequency electrical current and records variations in electrical resistance, or impedance to blood flow. Because blood is an excellent conductor, test results depend on the blood volume in the extremity and its fluctuation in response to temporary occlusion with a pressure cuff. IPG is especially sensitive in popliteal, femoral, and iliac veins. It is of little value, however, in calf vein thrombosis, and it cannot distinguish between old and fresh blood clots. External compression of venous outflow by a gravid uterus or a pelvic tumor produces false-positive test results. Hence, IPG has limited value in such circumstances.

Phleborrheography. Phleborrheography (PRG) evaluates changes in blood flow recorded with special cuffs in relation to a respiratory pattern. PRG has many of the same advantages and limitations as IPG. In addition, PRG does not localize the site of venous thrombosis.

IPG and PRG are useful as serial monitoring studies in patients who are at high risk for DVT. These tests are also helpful in follow-up assessment of patients who are recovering from DVT and those who are undergoing treatment with anticoagulants.

Duplex Venous Imaging. This recently popularized technique uses simultaneous ultrasound imaging and Doppler signals to evaluate anatomic and functional changes in the venous system. Its sensitivity in detecting clots in the major veins of the calf, thigh, and groin approaches 100 per cent. Differentiation between old and new thrombi is also possible.

INVASIVE METHODS OF DETECTING DEEP VENOUS THROMBOSIS

Radioactive Fibrinogen Imaging. This method uses radiolabeled fibrinogen (with ^{125}I) and follows its incorporation into an actively forming thrombus. This study is extremely sensitive and can detect clots that may be clinically insignificant. The radioactive isotope crosses the placenta and is excreted in breast milk. Thus, this method is contraindicated in pregnant women and nursing mothers.

Contrast Venography. This method is the "gold standard" of DVT diagnosis; all other methods of detection are compared with it when assessing efficacy. Venography requires injection of intravenous contrast medium to look for filling defects in the involved vein. It is highly sensitive and can differentiate between both old and new clots and between thrombosis and external compression. If this test is performed during pregnancy, appropriate protection (lead apron on the lower abdomen) for the fetus is required.

An algorithm for DVT diagnosis is illustrated in Figure 1.

TREATMENT

General Treatment

Patients with DVT are initially treated with rest with leg elevation. This treatment continues for several days, usually until a therapeutic level of anticoagulation is achieved. Warm soaks and wraps with Ace bandages are used to alleviate local inflammatory symptoms.

Anticoagulation Therapy

The purposes of anticoagulation therapy are to stop formation and propagation of the thrombus and to prevent embolization to the lungs. Pulmonary embolism (PE) may be fatal and may be prevented with proper anticoagulation.

The acute phase of anticoagulation extends for 3 to 7 days from the time of DVT diagnosis. The recommended therapy during this initial period is intravenous heparin, beginning with a loading dose of 5000 to 10,000 IU. This bolus is followed by a maintenance dose of 1000 IU per hour as a continuous intravenous infusion. The subsequent dosage is adjusted to maintain the activated par-

tial thromboplastin time (APTT) at one and one-half to two times the control level. The half-life of heparin is 90 minutes and its effect can be reversed with protamine sulfate (1 mg per 100 IU of heparin).

Once the patient is adequately heparinized, we recommend initiation of oral therapy with warfarin (Coumadin). A daily dose of 10 mg is administered for the first 2 to 3 days, followed by 2.5 to 7.5 mg daily to maintain the prothrombin time at one and one-half times the control level. Once the prothrombin time is adequate, heparin is discontinued and the patient is discharged with warfarin. Warfarin's half-life is approximately 48 hours, and its action on the coagulation system is detected 36 to 72 hours after the initial dose. The effect of warfarin is reversed with vitamin K in 6 to 8 hours or is reversed promptly with fresh-frozen plasma. Fresh-frozen plasma is used to treat bleeding complications or to prepare patients for urgent surgery.

Warfarin crosses the placenta and may cause fetal or neonatal hemorrhage, as well as central nervous system deformities. It is contraindicated in pregnancy. Therefore, we recommend using heparin for the chronic phase of anticoagulation in pregnant women. One may administer 5000 IU of heparin every 8 to 12 hours subcutaneously or continuously infuse heparin intravenously to maintain the APTT at one and one-half times the control level. Continuous infusion requires a pump and a tunneled central line. Either treatment option is suitable for outpatients.

Bleeding into the central nervous system, gas-

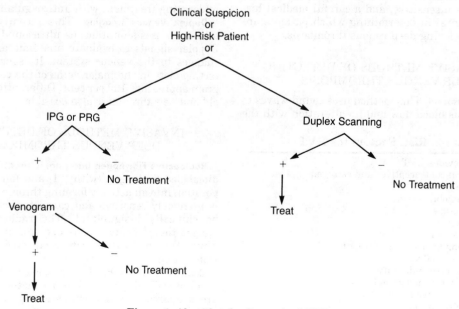

Figure 1. Algorithm for diagnosis of DVT.

trointestinal system, genitourinary tract, or retroperitoneum is a complication of both heparin and warfarin therapy. This complication is most likely to occur in patients with platelet disorders, especially those concomitantly taking aspirin or nonsteroidal anti-inflammatory agents.

Skin necrosis is a rare complication of warfarin therapy. This necrosis presents as an erythematous rash evolving into a full-thickness skin necrosis. Treatment consists of stopping the drug, resuscitating the patient with intravenous fluids, and using topical antibiotics.

Specific complications of heparin therapy include thrombocytopenia and arterial thromboembolism. These complications occur during the first 2 weeks of therapy and may require heparin discontinuation. Osteopenia caused by inhibition of renal vitamin D metabolism is also a complication of heparin therapy. This inhibition is observed especially if high doses of heparin are used for more than 4 months. Patients with osteopenia often complain of back pain.

Table 3 lists the absolute and relative contraindications to anticoagulation therapy.

The length of maintenance anticoagulation therapy is individualized. If DVT occurred during pregnancy, treatment is stopped during delivery and reinstated for 3 months post partum. If DVT extended to the femoral or iliac veins or resulted in PE, therapy is continued for at least 6 months. Warfarin is used after delivery in non–breast-feeding mothers and in gynecologic patients. Follow-up is accomplished by IPG testing, which is an easy, cost-effective method of detecting resolutions or propagation of the clot and, therefore, of determining the duration of anticoagulation therapy.

Fibrinolytic Therapy

Streptokinase and urokinase activate the plasminogen system, resulting in clot dissolution. This activation prevents both the acute and chronic complications of DVT. Fibrinolytic therapy is generally contraindicated in pregnant or postoperative women because of the severe bleeding complications that may occur.

Thrombectomy

Surgical removal of the venous blood clot may be indicated in rare clinical situations. For example, an ileofemoral DVT allowed to propagate may produce total venous occlusion, leading to extensive edema in the affected limb. This edema may impede arterial inflow. Failure to treat this condition adequately, called phlegmasia cerulea dolens, or blue phlebitis, leads to gangrene.

PROPHYLAXIS

Early postpartum or postoperative ambulation is the key to prevention of DVT in all risk groups. The perioperative use of pneumatic compression devices is also warranted in moderate- and high-risk patients. These devices prevent venous stasis and may enhance fibrinolytic activity. Subcutaneous heparin (5000 IU every 8 to 12 hours) therapy, beginning 2 hours preoperatively and continuing until full ambulation occurs, is an alternative method of prevention in moderate- and high-risk patients. Adjusted-dose subcutaneous heparin (maintaining the APTT at one and one-half times the control level 6 hours after heparin injection) increases the efficacy of subcutaneous heparin without increasing the risk of bleeding. Perioperative use of warfarin is an alternative, effective method of prevention in high-risk groups. However, bleeding complications are greater with warfarin than with the other methods previously discussed.

Discontinuation of contraceptive pills and estrogen before elective surgery is recommended. Pregnant women with a history of DVT and PE are given subcutaneous heparin antenatally, and the initiation of this anticoagulation therapy is individualized. Low-dose heparin is used post partum until full ambulation occurs.

COMPLICATIONS

Pulmonary Embolism

PE is a life-threatening complication of DVT. It may present with shortness of breath, tachycardia, tachypnea, chest pain, and hypoxia, all of which are nonspecific signs or symptoms. PE may also be asymptomatic. Chest x-ray films and electrocardiograms are usually nonspecific and nonsensitive.

The pulmonary arteriogram is the "gold standard" diagnostic test. Because of its invasiveness, it is usually preceded by an isotope lung scan. If

TABLE 3. **Contraindications to Anticoagulation Therapy**

Absolute
Central nervous system surgery
Eye surgery
Bleeding gastrointestinal ulcer
Drug allergy
Active bleeding after trauma
Relative
Recent major surgery
Recent major trauma
Gastrointestinal ulcer
Necrotic tumor

the isotope scan is completely normal, no further work-up is needed. If the scan indicates a low or moderate probability of PE, a positive pulmonary arteriogram is needed to confirm the diagnosis. A highly suspicious lung scan does not require a confirmatory pulmonary arteriogram before proceeding to anticoagulation therapy.

The treatment of PE is similar to that of DVT, except that it is continued for at least 6 months. Patients who have a contraindication to or a complication of anticoagulation, or who develop PE while receiving full anticoagulation, require inferior vena cava disruption. This disruption is achieved by either surgical application of a venocaval clip or percutaneous insertion of a venocaval filter.

Postphlebetic Syndrome

Occlusion of the deep veins of the lower extremities or destruction of the venous valves by local inflammatory reactions to venous thrombosis results in venous pooling in the affected limb. This pooling leads to chronic swelling, hyperpigmentation, and ulceration, which may be a debilitating, crippling process. If simple leg elevation and properly fitted stockings fail to alleviate the edema, surgical removal of dilated varicose veins, repair of the incompetent valves, or ligation of the perforating veins is indicated.

CONTRACEPTION

method of
CYNDA ANN JOHNSON, M.D.
University of Kansas
Kansas City, Kansas

Contraceptive technology affects the lives of 327 million couples, the number worldwide estimated to use some form of birth control. Physicians caring for these couples must be knowledgeable in the variety of birth control methods available and the advantages and disadvantages of each. The final decision and responsibility for use of the method belong to the patients, but the concerned physician can assist patients in choosing the method best suited to their age, lifestyle, medical profile, and stage of reproductive life.

Safety and efficacy are the critical factors in the choice of contraceptive method. It is incumbent on the physician to identify those issues for their patients and to present them with optimal alternatives. Table 1 lists failure rates for birth control methods commonly used in the United States. A woman who has unprotected intercourse has a 90 per cent chance of becoming pregnant within a year. The safety of the various methods is discussed as each method is reviewed.

TABLE 1. **First-Year Failure Rates for Common Contraceptive Methods***

Method	Lowest Observed Failure Rate (%)	Failure Rate in Typical Users (%)
Tubal sterilization	0.4	0.4
Vasectomy	0.4	0.4
Injectable progestin	0.25	0.25
Combined oral contraceptives	0.5	2
Progestin-only pill	1	2.5
Intrauterine device	1.5	5
Condom	2	10
Diaphragm (with spermicide)	2	19
Sponge (with spermicide)	9–11	10–20
Foams, creams, jellies, and vaginal suppositories	3–5	18
Coitus interruptus	16	23
Fertility awareness techniques (basal body temperature, mucous method, calendar, and rhythm)	2–20	24
Douche		40

*Adapted from Hatcher RA, et al (eds): Contraceptive Technology 1986–1987, 13th rev ed. New York, Irvington Publishers, 1986, p 102.

PERMANENT STERILIZATION

Permanent sterilization is the most prevalent method of birth control worldwide. It is both safe and effective. Choice of procedure and its permanence are the two most important issues in counseling patients before sterilization. Factors influencing whether the man undergoes a vasectomy or the woman a tubal ligation are risk, cost of procedure, lifestyle, and future considerations. Overall, a vasectomy is the simpler, safer, and less expensive alternative. In many cases the woman wishes to protect herself as completely as possible from future pregnancies and prefers to have a tubal ligation. In either case the patient must understand that the procedure should be considered to be permanent. Sterilization reversal procedures have become popularized so that the patient may naively expect a reversal operation to be routine if the social situation changes. The fact is that the overall success rate for tubal reconstruction is less than 30 per cent; clinical success is achieved in only 18 to 60 per cent of vasectomy reversals, depending on the initial surgical procedure, type of ligation material used, and time elapsed between the vasectomy and the reversal procedure.

COMBINED ORAL CONTRACEPTIVES

The combined oral contraceptive is the most popular reversible form of contraception used in the United States. Probably for that reason, physicians frequently offer and patients often ask for birth control pills when patients first seek contraceptive advice. Although the choice may be a good one, the physician should review other alternatives with the patient before automatically prescribing oral contraceptives.

A complete history and physical examination including pelvic examination with Papanicolaou's smear and appropriate tests for sexually transmitted diseases should be carried out on any woman before oral contraceptives are prescribed. The necessity for routine laboratory tests before starting oral contraceptives is controversial. If the cost is not prohibitive to the patient, fasting glucose and serum lipid assays should be done within the first 6 months of use. Patients who continue to take oral contraceptives after the age of 35 years and those at high risk for diabetes or cardiovascular disease should be tested yearly.

Use of birth control pills is absolutely contraindicated by a history of thromboembolic disorder, cerebrovascular accident, coronary artery disease, known or suspected carcinoma of the breast or other estrogen-dependent neoplasm, pregnancy or undiagnosed abnormal vaginal bleeding, and liver tumor or impaired liver function.

There are many other relative contraindications to use of the combined oral contraceptive. There is little justification to prescribing them for any patient older than 40 years and for patients older than 35 years who smoke cigarettes. They generally should not be used by patients with severe recurrent headaches or hypertension, lactating women, patients requiring long-term immobilization, and those with active gallbladder disease.

More than 30 different formulations of oral contraceptives are available in the United States. A few simple guidelines will help avoid confusion in initial prescribing and pill changes. To minimize estrogenic side effects, women should begin taking a pill with less than 50 micrograms of estrogen. These pills all contain ethinyl estradiol as their estrogenic compound.

Pills with less than 30 micrograms of ethinyl estradiol, however, are associated with a higher risk of intermenstrual spotting and a slightly higher pregnancy rate. These pills may be tried by women who wish to continue to take a combined oral contraceptive despite the presence of nausea, breast tenderness, or water retention when taking 30 micrograms of ethinyl estradiol.

The triphasic birth control pills, in which the hormonal content varies every 7 days during the pill pack, are an excellent first choice. They all contain between 30 and 40 micrograms of ethinyl estradiol and a variable progestin content during the first 21 days. (The last seven pills of a 28-day pack are inert, as in all types of combined oral contraceptive.) The total amount of progestin in the triphasic pills is less than that in the monophasic varieties, which minimizes progestin-related complications and side effects. Potential problems related to progestin excess that may be avoided include hypertension, decreased levels of high-density lipoproteins, dilated leg veins, pelvic congestion syndrome, acne and oily skin, depression, tiredness, decreased libido, and cholestatic jaundice. The clinical importance of decreasing levels of high-density lipoprotein, which are associated with the progestin norgestrel, is unclear at this time.

Women taking oral contraceptives for the first time should be re-evaluated in 3 to 6 months. Rarely should the pill type one be changed sooner. As with all low-dose pills, the patient may expect some intermenstrual spotting during the first 3 months of use of the triphasic pills. If abnormal bleeding continues, the pill type is often changed to one with higher estrogenic content. However, changing to another triphasic pill with a different ratio of estrogen to progestin or to a monophasic pill with a higher total progestin content may be adequate, and estrogenic side effects will be minimized.

Women taking low-dose pills may also have episodes of amenorrhea. Although the amenorrhea is not harmful, pregnancy is often a concern. With the ease of pregnancy testing, patients should generally be investigated if amenorrhea occurs, rather than pill exchange advice being carried out by the telephone. If the patient is not pregnant, there is no urgency to make a pill change. Often a course of conjugated estrogens given along with the oral contraceptive during the subsequent cycle will replenish the endometrial lining, and withdrawal bleeding will be re-established.

Patients who forget to take a pill for 1 or 2 days during a cycle should catch up on the missed pill and finish the pill pack while optimally using a back-up method of birth control. Patients who routinely skip pills should be re-evaluated. These women should probably be offered another form of birth control instead of high-dose pills. Certain medications, particularly antibiotics, may interfere with the effectiveness of the birth control pill. During a short course of antibiotics, a back-up birth control method should be used, but a higher-dose pill may have to be selected for women who are given long-term antibiotic therapy. Women who are taking birth control pills should be instructed to talk to the doctor before simply stopping the pills for any reason. These patients may unintentionally become pregnant before further contraceptive advice is sought.

PROGESTIN-ONLY CONTRACEPTION

Progestin-only contraception, which may be administered orally or by injection, is underused in this country. The progestin-only birth control pill, or minipill, is indicated in situations where estrogen administration is undesirable. Patients with headaches, leg pain, chloasma, nausea, weight gain, or hypertension (suspected to be secondary to the estrogen content of the combined oral contraceptive) may be given progestin-only pills. Lactating women and women older than age 35 years are also good candidates for the minipill.

Progestin-only pills are taken daily without a pill break or placebo pill. Patients must be warned that their periods will usually be light, irregular, and unpredictable. This pattern is unacceptable to many patients. If they are not counseled carefully on the advantages of the minipill, its use will continue to be limited.

Injectable, long-acting progestins, most commonly medroxyprogesterone acetate, are used in more than 80 countries for routine contraception. They are not approved for this indication by the U.S. Food and Drug Administration but are an excellent second line choice for certain individuals. They are useful in patients with endometriosis; women with dysfunctional uterine bleeding related to estrogen excess or with ovulatory dysfunctional bleeding that is hard to control; and unreliable patients in whom reliable contraception is critical. This last group grew greatly when the intrauterine device (IUD) fell into disfavor.

INTRAUTERINE DEVICES

Although the IUD is the second most common form of contraception worldwide, its use in the United States dropped precipitously after January 1986 when costly litigation led to the withdrawal of all types of IUDs but the Progestasert. Among IUD users there is a higher incidence of abnormal uterine bleeding and cramping and an increase in ectopic pregnancies, infertility, sexually transmitted diseases (STDs), and pelvic inflammatory disease. Many IUD users, however, experience no undesirable side effects over many years of continued reliance on the method. Patients who have completed their families but do not wish permanent sterilization are good candidates for an IUD.

Recently the Copper T has been placed back on the market with specific patient selection guidelines. In all cases, written informed consent from the patient should be obtained and pregnancy and infection ruled out before IUD placement. Patients should be multiparous and without a history of STDs. Patients with multiple sexual partners are at increased risk of infection. Patients becoming pregnant with an IUD in place or contracting an STD or other pelvic infection should have the IUD removed promptly. IUDs should also be replaced after the time period specified by the product information brochure.

BARRIER METHODS

Barrier methods of contraception, known to have existed for at least 600 years, are those in which a physical and/or chemical barrier blocks the entrance of sperm into the uterus. Commonly available products include the condom (rubber), diaphragm, and vaginal sponges, foams, creams, jellies, and suppositories. These methods are not costly, and all except the diaphragm are available to the patient without a prescription. The major disadvantage is that they must be used at every episode of intercourse for maximum efficacy. A potential side effect is allergy to the spermicide, rubber, or polyurethane, which necessitates a change to a different substance or device. The lambskin condom is the least allergenic of that group.

The condom is certainly the most important barrier method. It is the best prophylactic against STDs and when used with a vaginal spermicide is a superb contraceptive, the failure rate being 2 per cent per year or less. A spermicidal condom is also available. For couples at risk for STDs, the physician should encourage the use of a condom in addition to any other chosen birth control method.

The diaphragm (with spermicidal agent placed in the cup and around its rim) and vaginal sponge both provide physical and chemical barriers to the sperm. The diaphragm is somewhat more difficult to insert and must be fitted by a health care provider, but with repeated use it is cheaper than the vaginal sponge and somewhat more effective as a contraceptive. It should fit snugly but comfortably behind the pubic bone and over the cervix. Its position should be checked on every insertion by the patient or partner. Although the diaphragm provides some protection against cervicitis, pelvic inflammatory disease, and cervical intraepithelial neoplasia, it is responsible for an increased incidence of cystitis in some users. Both diaphragm and vaginal sponge may rarely be associated with toxic shock syndrome and should always be removed within 24 hours of insertion.

The vaginal spermicides consist of an inert base and one of two spermicidal compounds, nonoxynol 9 and octoxynol 9. Previously there had been some concern that spermicides were associated with an increased incidence of birth defects. Subsequent research has not supported that claim. These compounds have modest activity against STDs, particularly the gonococcus. Vaginal spermicides should not be the contraceptive of choice in patients who require an extremely high degree of protection from pregnancy. Women who have stopped birth control pills and who do not wish to become pregnant for a few months and mothers who are breast-feeding their babies full-time may be acceptable candidates for vaginal spermicide only. Foam and suppositories are superior to creams and jellies when used alone, but the latter are the better choice for use with the diaphragm.

FERTILITY AWARENESS METHODS

These methods of contraception, often termed "natural family planning," include rhythm (or calendar), basal body temperature, and cervical mucous methods, or a combination thereof. All are based on determination of the fertile period of the menstrual cycle and avoidance of intercourse during that time. The advantages of these methods include cost, safety, and acceptability to groups that oppose other contraceptive methods. The failure rate of these methods is highly variable and depends on correct interpretation of the fertile period and the care with which intercourse is avoided for an adequate interval. Failure in couples who follow the methods strictly is often secondary to the unusual and unpredictable long-lived sperm, which may survive in the female genital tract for 5 days or more.

Psychiatric Disorders

ALCOHOLISM

method of
A. WODAK, M.D.
St. Vincent's Hospital
Darlinghurst, New South Wales, Australia

Although patients labeled "alcoholics" are familiar to all medical practitioners, few physicians are confident about the diagnosis and management of this important condition. In the United States alone, 18 million persons 18 years of age and older are estimated to have problems associated with the use of alcohol. The difficulties that both society and the medical profession have in responding to alcoholism may be partly explained by the protean nature of alcohol-related disabilities, uncertainty regarding the etiology and definition, and the acceptance of alcohol as a social beverage. In recent decades, much progress has been made in defining concepts and expanding knowledge of the biologic and psychosocial consequences of alcohol consumption.

THE NATURE OF ALCOHOLISM

In the traditional view, alcoholism has been regarded as a unitary phenomenon with overtones of moral turpitude and irreversibility. Alcoholism has been considered to be a disease of unknown etiology with an assumed physical cause, in addition to psychologic and spiritual elements. The concept of "loss of control" has been regarded as a central and absolute component of alcoholism, with total and permanent abstinence therefore regarded as indispensable for salvation. In recent years, the term "alcoholism" has fallen somewhat into disfavor, both because of the association with this somewhat subjective conceptualization and because of its pejorative overtones. The term "problem drinker," referring to any person with any problem consequent on alcohol consumption, is being increasingly adopted. A fundamental component of the contemporary approach is the delineation of an alcohol dependence syndrome, which can be crudely summarized as a scientific description of alcohol addiction, and alcohol-related problems, which include any harmful consequences regarded as resulting from alcohol use.

Alcohol-related disabilities are now increasingly regarded as biopsychosocial phenomena with both etiology and consequences involving biologic, physiologic, and social domains. Problem drinkers are characterized by

1. A heavy pattern of drinking that may be either persistent or sporadic
2. A pattern of abnormal drinking behavior, such as secrecy or a preoccupation with drinking
3. Harmful consequences of drinking, which may be psychologic (such as tolerance or dependence), physical (such as liver cirrhosis), or social (such as marital or employment problems).

THE ALCOHOL DEPENDENCE SYNDROME

The term "syndrome" emphasizes the clustering of phenomena with no assumption that all elements are invariably present. The alcohol dependence syndrome is regarded as a graded continuum from mild to severe. As with many other sequelae of alcohol abuse, there is a poor correlation between the quantity and duration of hazardous alcohol consumption and the risk of development of alcohol dependence. The assessment of the alcohol dependence syndrome is based on the recognition and summation of its composite parts. The components of this syndrome are now discussed and are summarized in Table 1.

Narrowing of the Drinking Repertoire

As alcohol dependence becomes more firmly established, the ability to choose from among a range of alcoholic beverages and to vary the quantity consumed according to the social occasion lessens. Instead of a few dry sherries in genteel surroundings or a couple of cans of beer after sport, the alcohol-dependent drinker insists on an excessively generous consumption of a preferred beverage on all occasions.

Salience of Drink-Seeking Behavior

With increasing alcohol dependence, alcohol consumption gains priority over all other competing

TABLE 1. Components of the Alcohol Dependence Syndrome

Narrowing of the drinking repertoire
Salience of drink-seeking behavior
Increased tolerance of alcohol
Repeated withdrawal symptoms
    Tremor
    Nausea
    Sweating
    Mood disorders
Relief or avoidance of withdrawal symptoms by further drinking
Subjective awareness of a compulsion to drink
Reinstatement after abstinence

claims for attention. Even when faced with potentially catastrophic consequences if discovered drinking, such as divorce or dismissal from employment, the alcohol-dependent drinker increasingly ignores all warnings and continues to imbibe.

Increased Tolerance of Alcohol

This is demonstrated by the need for ever-increasing quantities of alcohol to achieve the same desired effect. The development of tolerance has a predominantly neurologic basis, with only a trivial contribution from increased metabolism. Tolerance is often described by alcohol-dependent patients in terms of the curious observation that no quantity of alcohol produces intoxication, with the convenient assumption that this represents greater resistance to the baleful consequences of alcohol abuse. Cross-tolerance extends to some other sedative drugs.

Repeated Withdrawal Symptoms

At first, withdrawal symptoms are mild and intermittent. With increasing dependence, the frequency and severity of symptoms increase, as does the likelihood of their occurrence after a decrease or cessation of alcohol consumption. The symptoms are often first apparent in the early morning soon after waking (when the blood alcohol level is at its nadir), but with increasing dependence, withdrawal symptoms may develop at any time of day and may even wake the patient at night.

The common symptoms of alcohol withdrawal consist of

1. Tremor of the hands. This symptom may be a minor inconvenience but in severe cases can be incapacitating.

2. Nausea. In mild cases, morning anorexia may be the only manifestation. Later, nausea may develop, followed by the onset of retching or vomiting. Many patients pay little attention to the fact that breakfast has been lost from the daily routine. Later, they may notice that an attempt to brush their teeth in the morning results in dry retching.

3. Sweating. This may consist merely of clamminess on waking in patients with mild dependence. More severely dependent patients may complain of drenching sweats.

4. Mood disturbance. Initially, patients may complain of being "frightened" or "edgy." When dependence is severe, agitation or depression, or a combination of the two, may be vividly described.

Relief or Avoidance of Withdrawal Symptoms by Further Drinking

As alcohol dependence increases in severity, the first drink of the day is taken earlier and earlier. In severe alcohol dependence, alcoholic beverages may be kept in the bedroom to relieve withdrawal symptoms that interrupt sleep. Often the daily routine is planned in advance to allow access to alcohol to prevent the onset of distressing withdrawal symptoms.

Subjective Awareness of a Compulsion to Drink

This is a subjective preoccupation with the consumption of alcohol and is often referred to by patients as a "craving" for a drink. Although it is often thought that control is lost entirely, it is probably more accurate to consider that control is intermittently impaired and to a variable degree.

Reinstatement After Abstinence

Individuals who have developed dependence may notice that if alcohol consumption begins after a prolonged period of abstinence, the development of alcohol dependence for the second time is telescoped into a brief period.

ALCOHOL-RELATED PROBLEMS

The consequences of alcohol abuse are as diverse as the range of professionals and organizations from which help is subsequently requested. Alcohol-related problems in an individual may exist singly or in combination. One person who has consumed alcohol steadily for many years may have developed only mild alcohol dependence, whereas a neighbor with an identical pattern of alcohol consumption may have suffered irreversible organ damage, unemployment, and social disgrace. Much of the harm related to alcohol abuse in a community is associated with alcoholic intoxication. Impaired psychomotor function and judgment resulting from acute ingestion of alcohol are associated with high morbidity and mortality from automobile crashes and often violent deaths, including suicide. Acute intoxication is also associated with behavioral manifestations that may result in marital and family disharmony or loss of employment. Recent consumption of alcohol is also linked to a wide variety of crimes, especially crimes of violence such as assault, rape, and homicide. The records of patients presenting with alcohol-related problems in middle age often show a history of several "driving while intoxicated" offenses one or two decades earlier.

The range of organic conditions associated with excessive chronic alcohol consumption covers all of the major systems of the body, with the gastrointestinal system bearing the brunt of the damage. Chronic excessive alcohol ingestion often results in financial hardship and sometimes homelessness.

EPIDEMIOLOGY

Approximately two-thirds of adults in Western countries consume alcohol; one-half of the alcohol is consumed by the heaviest-drinking 10 per cent of the society. For the entire U.S. population 14 years of age or older, the estimated per capita consumption in 1984 was the equivalent of 2.65 gallons of pure alcohol per person, which is the eighteenth highest per capita consumption in the world. Per capita consumption has been declining in recent years in the United States and a number of other Western countries. It is generally recognized that the extent of alcohol-related harm in a community varies with the per capita alcohol consumption. Seven per cent of adult U. S. drinkers surveyed in 1984 experienced moderate dependence symptoms; 10 per cent (14 per cent male, 6 per cent female) experienced moderate social or personal consequences associated with alcohol abuse. Women generally have fewer drinking-related problems and fewer dependence symptoms than men, but when allowance is made for the fact that they consume far less alcohol and weigh considerably less, women may be more susceptible to the harmful consequences of alcohol than men.

High alcohol consumption tends to be found in a number of occupations, including all sections of the alcohol beverage industry, business and administration, the armed forces and police, occupations associated with lengthy separations from home, and the medical profession. Alcohol consumption generally declines with age. It is far higher in men than in women and in persons who live alone.

DIAGNOSIS

The diagnosis of problem drinking is now discussed and is summarized in Table 2.

The Drinking History

A small minority of patients with a drinking problem spontaneously volunteer this information to their physician. Usually a constellation of nonspecific symptoms forms the presenting complaint, and the diagnosis is missed without a high index of suspicion on the part of the clinician. The experienced diagnostician may be alerted by the combination of seemingly unrelated, vague findings, such as diarrhea, Monday absenteeism, and hypertension in a divorced person known to be experiencing difficulties at work.

A drinking history should be obtained from all adult patients and can usually be ascertained with surprising ease in a few minutes. The supposed unreliability of the information gained generally reflects a poor interview technique, which uses leading questions and carries judgmental overtones. Questions should be framed in a neutral fashion, beginning with "On how many days a week do you usually drink alcohol?" rather than "Do you drink?" It is helpful to prompt

TABLE 2. Diagnosis of Problem Drinking

History of persistent consumption of six or more standard drinks a day (males) or four or more standard drinks a day (females)
History of injury caused by driving a car or operating equipment while intoxicated
History of abnormal drinking behavior (e.g., secrecy)
Harmful consequences of alcohol abuse
  Alcohol dependence syndrome
  Alcohol-related problems
    Medical
    Social
    Family
    Employment
    Criminal
    Legal
    Financial

answers, beginning with the top of the range (e.g., "Seven days a week?") and then prompting with the bottom of the range (e.g., "Less than once a week?"). The beverage of preference is ascertained and then the number of drinks consumed per day is established, again providing high and then low prompts to give the patient "permission" to reveal high levels of consumption. This information can be extended by ascertaining the drinking history over several years or even decades. Depending on the information obtained, further questioning regarding symptoms of alcohol dependence or specific alcohol-related problems may be required. The primary care physician is often well informed about the patient's family and background and thus is often well placed to draw on various sources of information for the diagnosis. This is significant because in many countries almost 80 per cent of the population see their primary care physician at least once a year.

A number of questionnaires have been devised in recent years to assist in the diagnosis of alcohol-related disabilities in different medical settings. One of the best-known of these questionnaires is the Michigan Alcoholism Screening Test, which was devised for an inpatient psychiatric population. General health questionnaires have also been devised with disguised alcohol-related content and adapted for personal computers with simplified controls operated by patients. The use of pen-and-paper and computer-assisted questionnaires is still largely confined to research.

The history obtained should also include an attempt to establish precipitating or related factors such as the presence of psychiatric conditions or factors causing undue stress.

The Physical Examination

Once again, the remarkable feature is the diversity of physical abnormalities and the paucity of pathognomonic anomalies associated with hazardous alcohol consumption. The combination of physical findings is usually of more assistance than any individual findings. The detection of alcohol on the breath during the day, especially if alcohol consumption has been categorically denied, clearly supports a suspicion based on the history alone. Normal cognitive function in the presence of strong alcoholic fetor is evidence of tolerance to alcohol reflecting dependence.

Laboratory Investigations

Estimation of blood (or urinary) alcohol levels is a simple test that can often assist the clinician. A high blood alcohol level in the presence of either denial of drinking or normal cognitive function must be regarded as strong evidence supporting the physician's suspicions. The results of a number of standard hematologic and biochemical tests are elevated in the presence of sustained, excessive alcohol consumption, but lack of sensitivity and specificity when used individually remains a problem. These tests include alanine transaminase, aspartate transaminase, alkaline phosphatase, gamma-glutamyltransferase, erythrocyte mean corpuscular volume, uric acid, and high-density-lipoprotein cholesterol. A low platelet count that returns to normal over several days is often found in heavy drinkers admitted to the hospital. The likelihood of abnormality in any of these tests increases with the quantity of alcohol consumed and the duration of heavy drinking. Combinations of tests improve the sensitivity and specificity of single tests, and composite indices based on discriminant function analysis show promise but are still mainly confined to research.

MANAGEMENT

The first step in management is to assemble the evidence compiled covering the drinking history, alcohol dependence, and alcohol-related problems. Judgments can then be made about whether the patient is at risk because of a persistent or sporadic pattern of heavy drinking or has already developed alcohol-related disabilities. The severity of the problems and the existence of any primary disorders should be considered. Questionnaires are available to facilitate assessment of some of these aspects, but they are not yet in widespread use.

The next step in management is to give the patient a succinct summary of the assessment so that an informed and responsible choice for the future can be made by the patient. Some patients may be ambivalent about their objectives or may even strive for contradictory aims. However, many patients are clear about their intentions. Some wish to abstain permanently, whereas others desire a period of abstinence followed by a review of the situation. Still others do not wish to abstain for any period but seek to control their alcohol consumption by reducing it to a safe level. The task for the physician in this instance is to attempt to reconcile the patient's aims with the medical reality. There is little to be gained by encouraging a severely jaundiced patient with cirrhosis in the belief that a mere reduction in alcohol consumption is sufficient. However, a patient who has had many unsuccessful attempts to achieve total abstinence may be best advised to seek a middle alternative and attempt a meaningful reduction in alcohol consumption. The consumption of six or more standard drinks a day for men or four or more standard drinks a day for women should be regarded as harmful.

Patients who wish to achieve total abstinence generally experience great difficulty in attempting to stop while carrying out their normal routine and should be encouraged to seek admission to a detoxification center. Detoxification is the process of providing a safe, caring environment for the duration of the body's metabolism of a drug of dependence and the associated withdrawal symptoms in order to facilitate subsequent rehabilitation. The patient should be nursed in a quiet, nonthreatening environment with subdued, even lighting. The staff should have a sympathetic and sensitive manner. In many cases, detoxification is conducted in a psychiatric clinic or general hospital. Outpatient detoxification should be reserved for carefully selected patients.

Sedative medication to which the patient is cross-tolerant prevents the development of withdrawal symptoms. A variety of oral agents with long half-lives have proved to be satisfactory, including the benzodiazepines diazepam (Valium) and chlordiazepoxide (Librium). Diazepam has the advantage of having additional anticonvulsant properties and can be conveniently administered in 20-mg doses hourly while the patient is agitated until a state of sedation has been achieved. Usually the end point occurs with three or fewer doses. No further doses are then required. Alternatively, diazepam can be administered in 10- to 20-mg doses every 4 to 6 hours, tapering down to zero over several days. Another agent used is chlormethiazole (Hemineurin), which itself is associated with the development of dependence. The intravenous administration of chlormethiazole is effective but also dangerous, as it can result in respiratory depression. The major tranquilizer haloperidol (Haldol) lowers the seizure threshold and may cause hypotension. Therefore, it should be reserved for patients with delirium tremens who have not responded to benzodiazepines.

However, detoxification can also be achieved satisfactorily without any medication and without undue discomfort, using a tranquil environment and a carefully selected and trained staff (who need not be health professionals). The experience of overcoming a major life problem without recourse to a psychoactive substance may even be an important experience.

Detoxification should be accompanied by a plan for future management that includes follow-up by a family physician, referral to a psychiatrist or other specialist, or referral to Alcoholics Anonymous.

The family must not be neglected at this time of crisis, and medical support is an important ingredient in management. The spouse may be advised to attend Alanon, a community-based organization established for the close relatives of alcoholics and based on a philosophy similiar to that of Alcoholics Anonymous. Another organization resembling Alcoholics Anonymous, Alateen, has been established for the benefit of teenage children of alcoholics.

Alcoholics Anonymous is a remarkable organization that exists in many countries and was established more than 50 years ago. It is a self-help organization, but many patients are unable to accept its quasi-religious nature. Every encouragement should be provided for attendance at the meetings of Alcoholics Anonymous, although it must be acknowledged that the organization does not suit everybody. Alcoholics Anonymous is free, has no waiting list or bookings, and keeps no records. Many large towns and cities have several meetings a week that follow a standard format. Identification with the central tenets of the organization is an important ingredient in its success. There are, without question, many people today who owe their lives and sobriety to Alcoholics Anonymous. However, it has not been possible to devise satisfactory research methods to assess the efficacy of Alcoholics Anonymous scientifically.

The role of pharmacologic agents in the management of patients with problems resulting from alcohol abuse is surprisingly limited. Multivitamins, especially vitamin B, should be used generously and may reduce the incidence of the Wernicke-Korsakoff syndrome. Intravenous rehydration with aqueous solutions containing dextrose can precipitate Wernicke's encephalopathy in thiamine-deficient patients and should therefore be initiated only after administration of adequate doses of parenteral thiamine. Hypokalemia is common in severe alcohol withdrawal and should be managed by administration of oral potassium. Anticonvulsants are frequently prescribed for alcohol withdrawal, but because of hepatic enzyme induction, therapeutic levels of phenytoin (Dilantin) are difficult to maintain after cessation of drinking. In the long-term management of patients with epilepsy who also have fluctuating alcohol consumption, the administration of anticonvulsants often causes more problems than it solves because of erratic compliance. Antidepressant medication is also frequently prescribed, but the evidence of its efficacy in the depressed alcohol-dependent patient is doubtful. Although depression is common in persons who consume excessive quantities of alcohol, it is often limited to the period of alcohol withdrawal or may be secondary to the social sequelae of drinking. It is difficult to achieve therapeutic plasma levels with tricyclic antidepressants because of hepatic enzyme induction. The monoamine oxidase inhibitors are not recommended because of the risk of precipitating a hypertensive crisis, as many alcoholic beverages contain tyramine.

Alcohol-sensitizing drugs have been available for almost 40 years. More experience has been gained with disulfiram (Antabuse) than any other similar agent, although the mode of action of all of them is identical. The inhibition of aldehyde dehydrogenase results in the buildup of the primary alcohol metabolite acetaldehyde, which is a toxic substance that causes a flushing reaction consisting of extreme dizziness, hypotension, nausea, vomiting, and sweating. The sensitizing reaction after administration of disulfiram can even occur several days after the last dose and can result from minimal quantities of alcohol. This agent should be used only after the patient has been fully informed about its interaction with alcohol. It is probably best reserved for situations where administration of the drug can be supervised. It may be considered for patients who need to get through a difficult period of festivities or anniversaries of personal loss or bereavement. In general, disulfiram should be prescribed for at least several months only in carefully selected patients who are medically fit. Only in recent years has the efficacy of this drug been scientifically evaluated. Some studies indicate a small to modest effect when disulfiram is included in a comprehensive treatment program. A new form of pharmacotherapy involving serotonin uptake blockers appears encouraging in animal research and limited clinical studies, but these agents are still restricted to research.

INPATIENT ALCOHOLISM TREATMENT PROGRAMS

Until recently, programs involving 3 to 4 weeks of hospital admission were the major form of treatment. However, they have not been demonstrated to be more effective than far cheaper and simpler outpatient treatment. The high relapse rates after both intensive inpatient and outpatient treatment appear similar. The inpatient programs typically include education regarding the effects of alcohol, individual and group therapy, stress management and assertiveness training, an introduction to Alcoholics Anonymous, and special sessions with health professionals. The goal of treatment is generally abstinence, with admission contingent on a satisfactory assessment of motivation. Despite high relapse rates after completion of treatment, a number of studies have found a positive outcome in terms of cost/benefit analysis.

EARLY INTERVENTION AND CONTROLLED DRINKING

Discouraging evaluations of the effectiveness of prolonged inpatient programs for severely alcohol-dependent patients have been followed by an interest in early intervention for less severely dependent patients for whom goals other than abstinence may be more appropriate. The choice between controlled drinking (i.e., a reduction from previous high levels) and abstinence should be made jointly by the patient and the physician. It is generally considered that younger patients who are only mildly dependent on alcohol do better with controlled drinking, whereas older, more dependent patients achieve more satisfactory results when they aim for abstinence. However, these guidelines are not universally accepted and lack precision. Moreover, many patients agree to reduce their alcohol consumption, but not to the degree suggested by their physician. The culmination of the negotiation between patient and physician may be written into the patient's notes, suggesting a form of a contract.

The results of several early intervention studies with a controlled drinking approach are promising, but the area remains extremely controversial. The techniques used in controlled drinking begin with setting goals agreed to by the patient and clinician. The next step is to monitor alcohol consumption, often using a daily diary to record drinking and its context. A set of rewards and punishments is often established for success or failure in complying with the targets. Simple principles to be followed include never drinking alcohol to quench thirst; alternating alcoholic and nonalcoholic beverages; not gulping alcoholic drinks; and setting a minimum time for consuming each alcoholic drink. Textbooks and self-help manuals with various degrees of sophistication, length, and expense are available.

A variety of psychologically based techniques for outpatient management have been developed in the last decade. In recognition of the fact that abstinence is usually relatively easy to achieve, even in severely dependent patients, with failure attributed almost always to relapse, new techniques have been devised. These techniques anticipate situations likely to lead to relapse by developing successful coping strategies to prevent a return to drinking. These cognitive techniques emphasize the distinctions among cognition, feeling, and action to provide patients with power to change their behavior. These forms of therapy can include the spouse and the entire family. At present, cognitive-behavioral techniques with controlled drinking objectives are still developing and expanding. Impressive evidence is accumulating regarding the effectiveness of these approaches. The remaining unresolved question is, For whom are these techniques most suitable?

PREVENTION

The first element of any intervention should be an attempt to prevent, if possible, the occurrence of the condition. In the case of alcohol abuse, the relationship between per capita alcohol consumption and alcohol-related disabilities has already been noted. Although a number of factors influence per capita alcohol consumption, the increasing price and decreasing availability of alcohol are generally regarded as the most important measures. The development of national health policies on alcohol has been encouraged by the World Health Organization as part of the movement for Health for All in the Year 2000. Medical practitioners who would like to see the incidence of alcohol-related disabilities decline should support the implementation of national alcohol strategies designed to reduce either per capita alcohol consumption or alcohol-related harm without reducing consumption (e.g., safety belt legislation). Improving the quantity and quality of treatment services provides additional benefits. Noting that members of the medical profession have a high risk of developing alcohol-related disabilities, physicians should consider supporting efforts to assist their impaired colleagues.

The renewed interest in preventing alcohol-related problems follows partly from the failure of treatments to deliver expected results. However, it also follows from the evolving view of alcohol dependence and alcohol-related problems that emphasizes a public health application more than previously. Support for prevention has also followed from the recognition that a treatment system adequate to manage all persons with alcohol-related problems would bankrupt the health system.

It is generally assumed that most alcohol-related problems in the community are caused by the few individuals who have the highest consumption of alcohol. However, from a community perspective, it is the drinker who consumes far more than average but less than the maximum who is responsible for more problems simply because there are so many "heavy social drinkers" and so few "alcoholics." Lowering the per capita alcohol consumption can reduce the number of heavy social drinkers at risk, to the benefit of the whole community. The provision of earlier intervention with goals more specifically developed for less dependent populations can also be of benefit.

In 1983, alcohol cost the United States almost $117 billion, of which $71 billion was attributed to lost employment and reduced productivity. In an era of increasing concern about economic growth, the development of improved treatment and more effective prevention strategies has a new and urgent meaning.

NARCOTIC POISONING

method of
FRANK J. BAKER, II, M.D.
MacNeal Hospital
Berwyn, Illinois

Narcotic overdose is a common occurrence and remains a frequent cause of death in young and middle-aged adults. If it is treated early before irreversible hypoxic damage occurs, the response can be rapid and dramatic and the patient may have no long-term sequelae.

"Narcotic" is a nonspecific term that originally referred to any drugs that could cause sleep or narcosis. Legally, the term has come to refer to any drugs or medicines that are addictive. Medically, the term generally refers to opiates or compounds related to opium. This article deals with overdoses caused by opiates and their analogues, and the term "narcotic" refers specifically to these compounds.

The various generally available narcotic preparations are presented in Table 1. They are generally divided into three groups: the pure agonists, such as morphine and heroin; the mixed agonist-antagonists, such as pentazocine and butorphenol; and the pure antagonists, such as naloxone and naltrexone.

CLINICAL SETTING

Narcotic overdose occurs in a relatively small number of clinical settings. Accidental overdoses occur when agents such as heroin or pentazocine are used recreationally. In children they can occur when medicines that have not been secured out of reach are accidentally ingested. One specific circumstance of note is the child who drinks methadone (Dolophine)-laced orange juice that is part of an adult family member's methadone maintenance program and that has been casually left in the refrigerator. Intentional overdoses also occur, usually in patients who are being treated with opiates for intractable pain and who have become suicidal. Finally, overdoses can occur in the therapeutic setting because of overzealous use for analgesia.

The narcotic overdose frequently is the result of injection or ingestion of multiple compounds. The concomitant presence of other agents such as alcohol, barbiturates, sedatives, hypnotics, and stimulants, especially cocaine, can significantly alter the clinical presentation, and this should always be kept in mind. Also, street drugs are frequently adulterated with diluents before their final use. These diluents may produce pharmacologic effects of their own such as pulmonary edema.

PRESENTATION

The triad of coma, depressed respirations, and pinpoint pupils is pathognomonic for narcotic overdose. Opiates produce analgesia and respiratory depression before suppressing the level of consciousness. Indeed, most patients with narcotic overdose respond to irritating verbal or physical stimuli, and a search for other causes should be made in patients who are deeply comatose. On occasion, dilated pupils are seen; this reaction may be due to hypoxia, the anticholinergic effects of meperidine (Demerol), or other drugs.

LABORATORY TESTS

In the comatose patient with suspected narcotic overdose, baseline tests should include a complete blood count, glucose, electrolytes, blood urea nitrogen, creatinine, arterial blood gases, urinalysis, urine toxicology screen, chest x-ray film, and electrocardiogram.

TREATMENT OF ACUTE NARCOTIC OVERDOSE

Death is almost universally due to respiratory depression and resultant hypoxia. Thus the priority of care in all settings and locations is the maintenance of an adequate airway and assisted ventilation. In comatose patients this should consist of endotracheal intubation and mechanical ventilation with high concentrations of oxygen delivered by a bag-valve-tube device (Ambu bag) or ventilator.

An intravenous infusion of D5W should be established at a keep-open rate. Blood should be taken for baseline values. Glucose should be given in a dose of 50 ml of a 50 per cent solution. Naloxone should be given intravenously in a dose of 0.4 mg. If there has been some response, additional incremental intravenous doses of naloxone (Narcan), 0.4 mg, should be given every 2 to 3 minutes until the patient is aroused and respiratory depression has beeen relieved. Under no circumstances should therapeutic doses be reduced or withheld for fear of producing an acute withdrawal syndrome.

If the initial dose of naloxone, 0.4 mg, failed to give a clinical response, additional doses of 2 mg should be given intravenously every 2 to 3 minutes until the patient responds or until a total dose of 10 mg has been given. If the patient has not responded to a total dose of 10 mg, a narcotic overdose is unlikely and other causes should be considered and investigated.

Narcotics delay gastric emptying, which slows absorption and prolongs the clinical syndromes of orally ingested opiates. Patients with oral overdoses who are conscious and alert should have emesis induced with 30 ml of syrup of ipecac followed by 250 ml of water. After emesis has occurred, they should be given 50 grams of activated charcoal in 500 ml of water. Emesis may be difficult to provoke with ipecac because of narcotic suppression of the chemoreceptor trigger zone. If the patient's level of consciousness is suppressed, the airway should be secured with endotracheal intubation before gastric lavage.

TABLE 1. **Generally Available Narcotics**

Generic Name	Trade Name	Street Name	Toxic Dose (mg) (Equivalent to 10 mg Morphine)	Plasma Half-Life (hr)	Comments
Agonists					
Codeine	Codeine	Cough medicine	120	2.5–3	May require large doses of naloxone for reversal
Diphenoxylate	Lomotil		300	14	Long duration of action, concomitant atropine poisoning
Fentanyl	Sublimaze, Innovar	China White	0.1	3.5	May produce muscular rigidity
Heroin		Smack, H, Horse, Speedball	3	2.5–3	Frequently adulterated before injected; may be taken with cocaine (Speedball)
Hydrocodone	Hycodan	Hyke	10	2–4	Common in cough syrup
Hydromorphone	Dilaudid	Little D	1.5	3	Potent therapeutic substitute for morphine
Meperidine	Demerol	Big D	75	3	May cause seizures and mydriasis
Methadone	Dolophine	Meth	10	24–48	Long duration of action requires special measures
Morphine		Dreamer, Miss Emma	10	2.5–3	
Opium	Pantopon	Big O, Black Stuff	12	2.5–3	
Oxycodone	Percodan	Perks	15	3	
Propoxyphene	Darvon	Dummies	120	4–12	May cause seizures; clinical course prolonged and unpredictable
Sufentanil	Sufenta	China White	0.01	2.5	May cause muscular rigidity
Agonist-Antagonists					
Buprenorphine	Buprenex		0.3	1–7	Not easily reversed by naloxone
Butorphanol	Stadol		2.0	3	Not easily reversed by naloxone
Nalbuphine	Nubain		10	5	May require large doses of naloxone
Pentazocine	Talwin	Ts (and Blues with pyrabenzamine)	30	2–3	Tablets for oral use now contain 0.5 mg of naloxone
Antagonists					
Naloxone	Narcan			1–1.5	Pure agonist with no known antagonist actions
Naltrexone	Trexan			4–10	Not approved for use in narcotic poisoning

Gastric lavage should be followed by administration of activated charcoal, as noted previously.

Codeine, propoxyphene (Darvon), and pentazocine (Talwin) are generally resistant to naloxone, and doses in the range of 10 to 20 mg may be required. Most narcotics have a longer duration of action than naloxone, and repeat doses may be necessary every 20 to 60 minutes. If symptoms recur, a continuous intravenous infusion of naloxone, 0.4 to 0.8 mg per hour, may be helpful. This method is particularly useful in cases of methadone poisoning because methadone has a particularly long duration of action.

In the out-of-hospital setting, when an intravenous line cannot be started, appropriate airway management and mechanical ventilation should suffice until the patient reaches the hospital. However, naloxone, 0.4 mg, can be given by sublingual injection.

Although opiates initially stimulate the nervous system, only a few, such as meperidine and propoxyphene, cause convulsions in adults. Should convulsions occur, they can be treated with standard doses of intravenous diazepam (Valium).

Noncardiogenic pulmonary edema is common, is sometimes delayed as much as 12 hours in onset, and is most likely caused by hypoxia. Pulmonary edema, although transient and usually lasting for less than 24 to 36 hours, exacerbates pre-existing hypoxia and should be treated aggressively. Endotracheal intubation, followed by positive-pressure ventilation with oxygen at a high fractional inspired flow rate, is frequently required to maintain adequate oxygenation. Positive end-expiratory pressure is occasionally required. Because the pulmonary edema is noncardiogenic, digitalis and diuretics are not indicated and indeed may predispose to dysrhythmias.

Narcotics are metabolized principally by conjugation in the liver, and hepatic metabolism determines their duration of action. Hepatic disease prolongs the metabolic half-life of opiates. The long duration of action of methadone and diphenoxylate (Lomotil) is caused by their slow hepatic metabolism.

The kidney excretes the conjugated metabolites of opiates. The rate of hepatic metabolism is not affected by the rate of urinary excretion of these metabolites. Thus forced diuresis is of no value in narcotic overdose.

In normal adults, opiates cause slight hypertension. The occurrence of hypotension in narcotic overdose suggests involvement of other drugs, pre-existent hypovolemia, or preterminal hypoxia.

A small percentage of patients are febrile; in these patients, aspiration pneumonia should be investigated. Hypothermia should be looked for and may be due to prolonged environmental exposure in select cases involving long-acting agents. In such cases, the possibility of rhabdomyolysis should be considered.

Hypoglycemia is occasionally seen and has been thought to be secondary to other associated agents, such as alcohol.

In children the initial intravenous dose of naloxone is 0.01 mg per kg. If a total dose of naloxone of 0.20 mg per kg has been administered without clinical improvement, other causes of coma and respiratory depression should be considered and investigated. In contrast to adults, convulsions can be produced by most of the opiates in children. They can be treated with diazepam, 0.25 mg per kg, up to a total dose of 10 mg, and at a rate not to exceed 1 mg per minute.

Naloxone is the most frequently used narcotic antagonist. Unlike its predecessor nalorphine (Nalline), which was a mixed agonist-antagonist, naloxone is a pure antagonist and has no agonist activity. Naloxone acts within 1 to 2 minutes when given intravenously and has a half-life of 12 to 20 minutes. It must be given parenterally.

Naloxone is exceedingly safe, although a few complications have been reported. These have been almost exclusively confined to patients who have receved general anesthesia and in whom opiates have been used as adjuncts for analgesia and sedation. In such patients, when naloxone is used to lighten sedation, cardiac dysrhythmias and pulmonary edema have occasionally occurred.

Naltrexone (Trexan) is a newer agent similar to naloxone, except that it is given orally and has a prolonged duration of action. Currently, naltrexone is approved only as an adjunct for the maintenance of an opiate-free state in a patient who is not under the influence of opiates at the time that therapy is started. It is not approved for use in opiate poisoning.

SPECIAL CONSIDERATIONS

Some narcotics are atypical and deserve special mention. Propoxyphene, unlike other narcotics that are not stored in the body, is fat soluble and is therefore stored in various tissue compartments from which it is later released. This explains the unpredictable and prolonged course that can be seen in propoxyphene overdose. Butorphanol, like propoxyphene, is fat soluble and has a prolonged duration of action. Methadone and diphenoxylate have prolonged durations of action because of their slow metabolism by the liver. Overdose or poisoning by these agents produces protracted symptoms that require repeated intravenous doses of naloxone or a continuous intravenous drip of naloxone, as mentioned previously.

Agonist-antagonist drugs such as pentazocine, butorphanol, and nalbuphine (Nubain) usually require higher doses of naloxone (on the order of 10 to 20 mg) to reverse the symptoms of overdose completely.

DISPOSITION

The initial response to therapy with naloxone is so dramatic that one can be fooled into thinking that the patient has recovered and can be discharged. Such is not the case. Because all narcotics have plasma half-lives exceeding that of naloxone, it should be assumed that these patients will relapse and will require additional treatment. All patients with narcotic overdoses should be observed for a minimum of 24 hours and possibly longer, depending on the agents involved. Finally, patients with intentional overdoses require psychiatric evaluation when they are medically clear and when they are no longer under the influence of narcotics.

ANXIETY DISORDERS

method of
WILLIAM E. FANN, M.D.
Baylor College of Medicine and VA Medical Center
Houston, Texas

All humans experience anxiety, and not all anxiety is pathologic, even when it is severe. Nevertheless, some individuals suffer from anxiety persistently, severely, and in a manner that effectively disables them.

Severe, chronic anxiety is probably induced or learned, but there may be a primary neurophysiologic (perhaps familial or genetic) component to the condition. It is often mixed with moderate depression and as such is the most frequent psychiatric diagnostic category with which the primary physician is confronted.

Anxiety is an unpleasant affect manifesting in its free-floating form as fear, apprehension, or even terror, with physical concomitants of tremor, sweating, tachycardia, dry mouth, urgency to micturate, diarrhea, paresthesias, inability to concentrate, insomnia, and easy fatigue. The revised third edition of the American Psychiatric Association's *Diagnostic and Statistical Manual of Mental Disorders* (DSM-III-R) can be consulted for extensive categorizations and manifestations.

Anxiety, like syphilis, is one of medicine's great imitators and can manifest itself in the guise of many physical diseases. Thus, the anxious patient may present with weakness, easy fatigue, or multiple aches and pains. Symptoms may be referable to one or more organ systems.

APPROACH TO THE PATIENT

A complete evaluation of the patient's physical complaints is necessary to establish the diagnosis of generalized anxiety disorder. Diminishing the severity of the patient's experience of discomfort as "nerves" or "all in your mind" will neither resolve the problem nor strengthen the therapeutic alliance necessary for its resolution. If the patient has (or believes that he or she has) a significant physical illness, the anxiety may be a response to the disease and may be associated with fears of pain, disability, or death. The patient may suffer from one of the many physical diseases in which anxiety is a prominent symptom or may have an anxiety disorder that looks like a physical disease. It is usually helpful to explain to the patient that anxiety exists in everyone, that for reasons we do not always understand it may become severe enough to affect functioning, that it may have an underlying neurophysiologic cause, and that it can be treated.

Generalized anxiety disorder is typically experienced at a persistent relatively low but nevertheless uncomfortable level, as opposed to the periodic intense highly uncomfortable attack, with physiologic components of tachycardia, diaphoresis, and flushing that are characteristic of panic disorder. Although reassurance that the unpleasant feelings of anxiety will not result in death can be helpful, medication is indicated as a therapeutic adjunct when anxiety is chronic and appears to exceed the limits of normal response to environmental threats. Panic disorder, with associated phobia, was once believed to represent an extreme manifestation of generalized anxiety. It is now better understood as a complex neurophysiologic disease that does not respond to the treatment regimens usually prescribed for relief of other anxiety disorders.

TREATMENT

There are several types of medications that are effective in relieving symptoms of generalized anxiety disorder and associated anxiety conditions such as post-traumatic stress disorder. These are benzodiazepines, tricyclic antidepressants, buspirone, and beta-adrenergic blockers. Each of these medications has limitations as well as advantages and should be used only after careful evaluation of the patient's mental and physical status.

The benzodiazepines are highly effective and safe but can produce euphoria and are therefore susceptible to abuse. They have the potential for physiologic dependency when used at high doses for protracted periods. When dependency does develop, drug withdrawal symptoms can include seizures, insomnia, irritability, and increased anxiety. Patients with a history of drug abuse should not be given benzodiazepines if other therapeutic modes are available. For the patient with generalized anxiety disorder, a longer-acting benzodiazepine such as diazepam (Valium) may be preferable, providing symptomatic relief for up to 6 hours. Compounds with shorter half-lives, such as alprazolam (Xanax), may quickly quell a period of acute anxiety but may lose effectiveness between scheduled doses. It is often useful to advise the patient to take one 5-mg diazepam tablet when anxiety symptoms are first felt and a second if symptoms remain intolerable after 30 minutes. Usually, 10 mg of diazepam is sufficient to control the symptoms of even intense anxiety; if this dosage is ineffective, the patient may be suffering from a physical disease such as hyperthyroidism, which manifests with anxious symptoms that do not respond to anxiolytics. Subsequent dosages should be administered in response to symptoms rather than on a fixed schedule. This dosing schedule puts the patient in control of the condition and avoids a constant condition of medication intoxication. On return office visits the patient should bring the bottle for a pill count as an index of the frequency and severity of the anxiety.

Tricyclic antidepressants are the medication of choice for patients who may be at risk for dependency on benzodiazepines. Imipramine (Tofranil-PM), doxepin (Sinequan), or amitriptyline (Elavil) should be administered on a regular basis (usually 25 mg three times daily), rather than on an as needed basis. Tricyclics are potent sedatives that can interfere with daytime functioning until the patient becomes accustomed to their effects. Doses at supper and bedtime will minimize interference with regular activities and will help the anxious patient to sleep. A steady-state blood level will usually be achieved in about 2 weeks, with anxiolytic effect evenly distributed around the clock. In some cases tricyclic antidepressants can paradoxically worsen the symptoms of anxiety, and the physician should be alert to this possibility.

Buspirone (BuSpar) is a new compound differing in most respects from other antianxiety agents now on the market. Its principal advantage is that it does not appear to produce euphoria or dependency; its chief disadvantage is that it may require 1 week to 10 days to achieve therapeutic effect. It is neither cross-tolerant nor cross-sensitive to sedative medication and therefore cannot be used to treat the effects of withdrawal from alcohol, sedatives, or benzodiazepines. The usual prescribing pattern is 5 mg four times daily.

Beta-adrenergic blocking agents have some antianxiety efficacy, primarily in patients with a strong cardiovascular component to their symptoms. It is helpful in reducing tachycardia and tremor, especially in situations such as public speaking, where there may be a powerful anticipatory anxiety element. Propranolol (Inderal), 20 mg, can be given three or four times daily beginning 2 to 3 days before the anticipated triggering event. Beta blockers can cause hypotension, bradycardia, and impairment of short-term memory and are specifically contraindicated in asthmatics.

BULIMIA NERVOSA

method of
JAMES E. MITCHELL, M.D.
University of Minnesota
Minneapolis, Minnesota

Bulimia nervosa is an eating disorder that is characterized by episodic binge-eating and other abnormal eating-related behaviors designed to promote weight loss or prevent weight gain. The diagnostic criteria for bulimia nervosa from the American Psychiatric Association's *Diagnostic and Statistical Manual of Mental Disorders,* third revised edition, are shown in Table 1.

TABLE 1. **Diagnostic Criteria for 307.51 Bulimia Nervosa***

A. Recurrent episodes of binge-eating (rapid consumption of large amount of food in a discrete period of time)
B. A feeling of lack of control over eating behavior during the eating binges
C. Regular self-induced vomiting, use of laxatives or diuretics, strict dieting or fasting, or vigorous exercise to prevent weight gain
D. A minimum average of two binge-eating episodes a week for at least 3 months
E. Persistent overconcern with body shape and weight

*From Diagnostic and Statistical Manual of Mental Disorders DSM-III-R, 3rd rev. ed. Washington, D.C., American Psychiatric Association, 1987. Used by permission.

Although isolated case reports of this disorder have appeared for at least 100 years, it was recognized as a common, distinct syndrome only in 1979. Therefore, research on this condition has been limited, and long-term data are not yet available.

The term "bulimia" implies a voracious appetite and, indeed, as reflected in the criteria, most individuals with bulimia nervosa report a strong appetitive drive and a feeling of lack of control while eating. Binge-eating episodes generally last about an hour or less. The amount of food ingested during eating binges varies dramatically, with some patients consuming approximately 1000 kcal and others as much as 10,000 to 15,000 kcal, with a typical intake of about 3500 to 4000 kcal. Most individuals isolate themselves while binge-eating, the most common locations being one's house or apartment; binge-eating also occurs while driving around in a car. Individuals tend to have a set pattern of binge-eating, and they tend to binge-eat in the same place at the same time of day and to ingest the same sorts of foods. Binge-eating episodes typically begin in the late afternoon or early evening. High-fat, low-protein foods, such as ice cream and doughnuts or cookies, are preferred. It is not uncommon for women with bulimia nervosa to spend $50 or more a week on binge foods. Over time, bulimic behaviors tend to crowd out normal eating behavior, and most patients with bulimia nervosa rarely eat regular, nutritionally balanced meals.

The most common weight control techniques used are self-induced vomiting, present in about 90 per cent of patients who present for treatment with bulimia nervosa, and laxative abuse, present in about 30 per cent of those who present for treatment but used intermittently by about 60 per cent of patients with this disorder. Early in the course of the illness, vomiting is usually induced by mechanical stimulation of the gag reflex; however, most patients learn to vomit reflexively when they have been symptomatic for several years. Laxative abuse usually involves the ingestion of a large number of over-the-counter stimulant-type laxatives. The goal of the laxative use is to stimulate an abrupt watery diarrhea, which results in a sense of thinness and weight loss but which in reality induces a loss of fluid and electrolytes rather than ingested food. The individual feels thinner, and thus the behavior is reinforced. Smaller percentages of patients misuse several other classes of agents, including diuretics (15 per cent), diet pills (25 per cent), and ipecac (5 per cent), which is ingested by some patients to help them vomit.

EPIDEMIOLOGY

A large cross-sectional population-based survey of this disorder has not been completed. Available epidemiologic studies of target populations suggest that 50 to 60 per cent of college-age women will experiment with bulimic behaviors. However, only 1 to 3 per cent develop an ongoing pattern of binge-eating coupled with self-induced vomiting or laxative abuse, a pattern likely to result in adverse medical consequences or psychosocial sequelae. The few data available would suggest that bulimia nervosa is seen most commonly in industrialized societies where there is an abundance of food and where there is a strong cultural emphasis on thinness, particularly for young women. In Third World countries, where food availability is more limited and the model of attractiveness for women is somewhat heavier, this disorder appears to be quite rare.

The typical age of onset is around 18 years. About 5 to 8 per cent of cases occur in males. Most patients are symptomatic for approximately 6 years before seeking treatment, and most are of normal weight when they seek treatment.

ASSOCIATED PROBLEMS

Several other forms of psychiatric problems have been associated with bulimia nervosa. The most common are affective disorders, particularly unipolar depression. This association has led to some speculation that bulimia nervosa might actually be a variant of affective disorder, although the data in this regard are far from clear.

There is also an enhanced co-morbidity for problems with alcohol and drug abuse. The rate of such problems among patients with bulimia nervosa appears to be four to five times the rate of these problems in age-matched controls. The results of some studies suggest an association between bulimia nervosa and certain types of personality disorders, in particular borderline personality disorder, but again the data here are not clear, and further research is necessary to determine what personality problems result from the illness rather than being present premorbidly.

COMPLICATIONS

Although bulimia nervosa is more medically benign than anorexia nervosa, in which many of the medical complications can be attributed to starvation, there are some significant physical hazards associated with this disorder. It is important to remember that the medical complications result from the specific behaviors involved. For example, erosion of dental enamel, a common complication, is directly attributable to the vomiting behavior. The fluid and electrolyte abnormalities are directly attributable to vomiting and laxative abuse and the resulting depletion of fluids.

Three physical symptoms are useful in diagnosing bulimia nervosa. The first is erosion of dental enamel. This change was originally observed in patients with anorexia nervosa but has more recently been shown to be present in patients with bulimia nervosa who vomit. What is observed clinically is decalcification of the lingual, palatal, and posterior occlusal surfaces of the teeth, where the acid hits as it is projected from the throat. A second sign is hypertrophy of the salivary glands, particularly the parotid glands. The exact prevalence of this among bulimic women is unknown, and the pathophysiology is unclear. The third sign of diagnostic utility is scar and callous formation on the back of the hand, caused by using the hand to self-induce vomiting and thereby macerating the surface of the skin against the teeth.

There are several possible cardiovascular complica-tions in this disorder. Dehydration secondary to vomiting or laxative or diuretic abuse can be associated with intravascular fluid contraction, hypotension, light-headedness, dizziness, or fainting. Electrolyte abnormalities are present in at least 50 per cent of patients with bulimia nervosa, the most common being metabolic alkalosis, hypochloremia, and hypokalemia. Abuse of ipecac is of particular concern because of the propensity of this agent to induce myopathies, including cardiomyopathies, when used repeatedly.

There appears to be an association between bulimia nervosa and diabetes mellitus. Several reports of individuals with diabetes mellitus who developed bulimia nervosa have been published, and some of these patients withheld insulin as a way of purging to rid themselves of the excess calories and promote weight loss.

Patients with bulimia nervosa frequently evidence changes suggestive of starvation despite a normal body weight, including elevated serum beta-hydroxybutyric acid and reduced fasting blood glucose levels.

It is common to discover elevated serum amylase levels among these patients. Although these are usually assumed to be salivary in origin, recent research suggests that at times the elevation may be pancreatic, and pancreatic abnormalities have been reported by computed tomography (CT) scanning in some patients with bulimia nervosa.

Two rare but dangerous complications associated with binge-eating and vomiting are esophageal or gastric perforation. Most of the fatalities associated with bulimia nervosa probably have resulted from gastric rupture. There is also some evidence that patients with bulimia nervosa develop delayed gastric emptying, which may help to explain the postprandial bloating that many of them report.

A recent study suggests that there is evidence of atrophic changes on CT scan of the head in a subgroup of these patients, which again suggests a state of relative starvation despite a normal body weight.

EVALUATION

Assessment of patients with bulimia nervosa should include a careful history, physical examination, and screening laboratory tests. The history should include, in addition to the standard medical history, information on the following factors:

1. Weight history including current weight, desired weight, highest and lowest weights, and concerns about body shape and weight issues
2. Dieting behavior
3. Binge-eating behavior (characterize binge-eating episodes; what foods are consumed, in what amounts, how often)
4. Purging behavior (laxative abuse, diuretic abuse, self-induced vomiting)
5. Other weight control techniques (exercise, fasting, rumination, chewing and spitting out food)
6. Evidence of alcohol or drug abuse
7. Evidence of concomitant affective disorder
8. On family history, evidence of familial loading for affective disorder or alcohol/drug abuse problems

The physical examination should focus on evidence of abnormalities attributable to the behavior. Particular attention should be paid to hydration status, cardiovascular functioning, and any evidence of gastrointestinal bleeding.

Screening laboratory tests should include, at minimum, serum electrolyte determination and stool examination for blood. Strongly recommended are complete blood count, blood urea nitrogen, screening liver tests, electrocardiogram, a dental examination, and levels of creatinine, glucose, calcium, phosphorous, triiodothyronine, thyroxine, and serum amylase. In atypical cases, consideration should be given to obtaining a CT scan of the head to rule out a central nervous system lesion. Electromyography should also be considered in individuals who have been abusing ipecac, and gastrointestinal radiographic/scoping procedures if there is evidence of gastrointestinal blood loss.

TREATMENT

The initial treatment must be geared to medical stabilization. Fortunately, most patients with bulimia nervosa are not critically ill when they appear for evaluation; however, 10 to 15 per cent may need overnight rehydration in the emergency room or a brief hospital stay for stabilization.

Treatment beyond this point depends on the individual symptoms and the age of the patient. Most patients with bulimia nervosa are adults living independently of their families. Most of this discussion will focus on this group. Younger patients who are living at home may need referral to a family therapist in addition to other treatment interventions. Rarely, placement outside the home is indicated.

For adult patients with bulimia nervosa, there are two major types of treatment that have been advocated, which can be used in combination. One type of treatment is antidepressant therapy. These drugs were originally used in the treatment of bulimia nervosa in the hope that they would alleviate some of the depressive symptoms and allow patients to better control their eating behavior. However, it has been determined subsequently that antidepressant therapy works in patients with bulimia nervosa whether or not they are depressed at baseline. The mechanism of action of these drugs in bulimia nervosa may be different from their mechanism of action in depression.

In general, antidepressants need to be used in regular antidepressant dosages to be effective. The onset of action is frequently delayed, as in the treatment of depression. The antidepressants that have been shown to be effective in suppressing bulimic behaviors in double-blind placebo-controlled trials include imipramine (Tofranil), desipramine (Norpramin), the monoamine oxidase (MAO) inhibitor phenelzine (Nardil), and the nontricyclic fluoxetine hydrochloride (Prozac). Many patients with bulimia nervosa do not tolerate the side effects of the more highly anticholinergic tricyclics such as amitriptyline (Elavil) and imipramine. Therefore, if tricyclics are to be used, I would recommend low anticholinergic agents such as desipramine or nortriptyline (Aventyl). The MAO inhibitors may also be used successfully but require patients to follow the usual tyramine-free diet, which is difficult for some of these patients. The new antidepressant fluoxetine appears to be particularly useful in the treatment of this condition, given its favorable side effects profile, lack of sedation, and lack of anticholinergic effects.

In most controlled trials there has been a highly statistically significant reduction in the frequency of target eating behaviors among patients taking antidepressants, generally in the range of 60 to 75 per cent. However, in most studies the majority of patients are still actively bulimic, although they are much improved. Therefore, there are significant questions that could be raised about whether or not antidepressant treatment should constitute the sole intervention for these patients.

There have been 11 studies of psychotherapy of this disorder with adequate controls, one of which compared a form of cognitive behavioral psychotherapy to antidepressant treatment. Most of these studies have relied heavily on cognitive behavioral techniques, often coupled with nutritional counseling. I have given some of the techniques commonly used in these programs in Table 2. Again, these studies suggest that these interventions tend to be quite useful for patients and quite effective in suppressing binge-eating behavior, but again in many studies an unfortunately large number of patients are still symptomatic at the end of treatment. A recent comparison study of psychotherapy and drug therapy demonstrated that an intensive outpatient cognitive behavioral group therapy, wherein patients are seen multiple times during the week and strong emphasis is placed on interrupting bulimic symptoms, will result in an outcome that is superior to that achieved with antidepressants alone, and indeed the majority of patients can achieve remission using such an approach. Therefore, some general treatment guidelines can be offered, as follows:

1. Antidepressant treatment appears to be quite helpful in suppressing target eating behaviors in patients with bulimia nervosa. However, few patients are cured with drug therapy. I think it is preferable to offer a psychotherapy approach when a highly structured program is available, adding antidepressant therapy for individuals

TABLE 2. **Elements of Treatment Programs for Bulimia Nervosa**

Type of Program	Components
Nutritional counseling	Teach meal planning. Have patient eat regular, balanced meals.
Self-monitoring	Monitor and record patterns of binge-eating, vomiting, and other significant behaviors. Monitor other eating behavior.
Alternative behaviors	Have patient develop a repertoire of behaviors to engage in as alternatives to bulimic behavior.
Cue restriction	Early in treatment have patient avoid foods and situations associated with bulimic behavior.
Exposure/response prevention	Have patient eat with others ("exposure" to food) in situations where the patient cannot vomit ("response prevention").
Cognitive restructuring	Examine thoughts/assumptions/beliefs underlying the behavior such as, "I need to lose weight," "I am too fat," "If I eat regular meals, I'll become obese."

who are quite depressed or for those who make only limited progress.

2. Psychotherapy approaches that include cognitive behavioral techniques similar to those used in the treatment of depression are quite helpful. There appears to be an advantage in using an intensive approach, particularly early in treatment, and in placing a strong emphasis on eating regular, balanced meals as part of the intervention.

DELIRIUM

method of
BARRY S. FOGEL, M.D.
Brown University
Providence, Rhode Island

Delirium, or the acute confusional state, is an abnormal mental state associated with physical illness and characterized by impaired attention and orientation, impaired memory, a disturbed sleep-wake cycle, lethargy or agitation, and an assortment of additional psychologic and behavioral symptoms. Delirious patients always have impaired attention, usually are disoriented, always have memory problems, usually show other intellectual defects, and frequently display hallucinations, paranoid thinking, or labile mood and affect. The more severe forms of agitated delirium may resemble mania; severe retarded delirium resembles stupor or impending coma. Mild agitated delirium may present as anxiety; mild retarded delirium may mimic depression. Currently accepted criteria for the diagnosis of delirium are given in Table 1.

DETECTION

The syndrome of delirium is best diagnosed by combining historical information with a mental status examination. The relevant history is of an acute or subacute change in mental status, with a waxing and waning level of consciousness or fluctuating attention, accompanied by disorientation, agitation or lethargy, and confusion. Mental status examination invariably reveals deficits in attention, orientation, and memory if sufficiently sensitive tests are used.

ASSESSMENT

Although virtually any visceral, toxic-metabolic, or primary central nervous sysem (CNS) disorder can provoke delirium, particularly in a very elderly or mildly demented patient, assessment must first address the most likely possibilities given the patient's age, medical problems, and epidemiologic setting. For example, delirium in a patient with chronic lung disease always indicates a blood gas determination; delirium in a diabetic always requires a blood glucose assessment. Computed tomography (CT) scans are indicated for patients at high risk for stroke, such as those with atrial fibrillation; lumbar puncture to rule out infection should be done promptly in the presence of unexplained fever, meningeal signs, or immune compromise.

All patients require basic laboratory screening, with sodium, calcium, blood urea nitrogen and creatinine, liver enzymes, and thyroid-stimulating hormone most likely to identify metabolic factors. A careful review of the drug list, including drugs recently discontinued, is essential. Although hundreds of drugs are occasionally associated with delirium, a relatively small number are most often implicated in causing delirium. These are given in Table 2. Withdrawal deliria are most often seen with alcohol and sedative-hypnotic drugs. Tachycardia, hypertension, agitation, and tremor are also commonly encountered in withdrawal deliria.

Drug levels should be obtained, if available and meaningful, for all prescription drugs the patient is taking. However, drugs may cause delirium even at levels within the conventional therapeutic range. Toxic screens may be indicated if drug abuse is suspected but not confirmed; false-negative results may occur, however, with cocaine and stimulants because of their short half-lives.

The electroencephalogram (EEG) in delirium usually shows diffuse slow activity. It is most helpful when the diagnosis of delirium is in doubt or when the patient has a known metabolic problem, such as liver failure, and one wants to estimate its effect on the brain. Brain imaging by CT or magnetic resonance imaging is indicated when the patient is at risk for primary brain disease or shows unexplained neurologic signs of CNS dysfunction.

TABLE 1. **Diagnostic Criteria for Delirium***

A. Reduced ability to maintain attention to external stimuli (e.g., questions must be repeated because attention wanders) and to appropriately shift attention to new external stimuli (e.g., perseverates answer to a previous question).
B. Disorganized thinking, as indicated by rambling, irrelevant, or incoherent speech.
C. At least two of the following:
    1. Reduced level of consciousness, (e.g., difficulty keeping awake during examination).
    2. Perceptual disturbances: misinterpretations, illusions, or hallucinations.
    3. Disturbance of sleep-wake cycle with insomnia or daytime sleepiness.
    4. Increased or decreased psychomotor activity.
    5. Disorientation to time, place, or person.
    6. Memory impairment, e.g., inability to learn new material, such as the names of several unrelated objects after five minutes, or to remember past events, such as history of current episode of illness.
D. Clinical features develop over a short period of time (usually hours to days) and tend to fluctuate over the course of a day.
E. Either (1) or (2):
    1. Evidence from the history, physical examination, or laboratory tests of a specific organic factor (or factors) judged to be etiologically related to the disturbance.
    2. In the absence of such evidence, an etiologic organic factor can be presumed if the disturbance cannot be accounted for by any nonorganic mental disorder, e.g., manic episode accounting for agitation and sleep disturbance.

*From Diagnostic and Statistical Manual of Mental Disorders DSM-III-R, 3rd rev. ed. Washington, D.C., American Psychiatric Association, 1987. Used by permission.

TREATMENT

Treatment begins with rapidly identifying the likely cause of the delirium and treating it whenever possible. However, the delirious state may persist for hours or even days after correction of measurable metabolic disturbance or obvious visceral disease. The EEG, if initially abnormal, can be used to follow the return of brain function to normal.

Safety issues must be addressed. Harmful substances, sharp objects, and other instruments of self-injury should be put out of the patient's reach. The patient who is agitated should be under continual observation. Having a concerned family member with the patient continuously is the ideal.

TABLE 2. **Drugs Commonly Implicated in Delirium**

Anticholinergic drugs (including over-the-counter cold remedies and sedatives)
Corticosteroids
Digoxin*
Cimetidine (Tagamet)
Antiparkinsonian drugs (includes carbidopa-levodopa, bromocriptine, and amantadine)
Lidocaine*
Narcotic analgesics (especially meperidine [Demerol] and pentazocine [Talwin])
Nonsteroidal anti-inflammatory drugs (especially indomethacin [Indocin])
Salicylates*
Theophylline*
Methyldopa (Aldomet)
Anticonvulsants*
Tricyclic antidepressants* (especially amitriptyline [Elavil] and imipramine [Tofranil])
Antiarrhythmics* (especially procainamide [Pronestyl] and quinidine)

*Drug levels for these agents are widely available, meaningful, and usually helpful diagnostically.

If psychotic features such as hallucinations or paranoid thinking are present, a low-dose, high-potency neuroleptic drug such as haloperidol or fluphenazine may be prescribed. A dose of 0.5 mg two to four times per day is adequate for most frail or elderly patients; younger patients occasionally may require substantially higher doses.

Agitation also responds to low-dose neuroleptics. However, benzodiazepines, such as lorazepam (Ativan) are preferable for three types of patients: (1) the patient who is withdrawing from alcohol, sedative-hypnotics, or anxiolytic drugs; (2) the patient who has an agitated delirium because of anticholinergic drug toxicity but who must receive medication for severe agitation; and (3) the patient with past or present intolerance of neuroleptics, particularly with muscle rigidity or an elevated creatine phosphokinase level thought to be due to neuroleptic drug treatment. Typical initial doses of lorazepam are 0.5 to 1 mg orally or intramuscularly for an elderly or frail person and 1 to 2 mg for other patients. The drug is repeated every 1 to 2 hours until the patient is calm; the total dose needed for sedation is then repeated every 8 to 12 hours and tapered as the delirium resolves. Quiet deliria that verge on lethargy usually do not require drug treatment.

An appropriate environment comforts the patient and reduces agitation while the delirium resolves. The ideal environment (1) provides orienting cues such as an easily readable clock, a calendar, and pictures of family members; (2) provides a different lighting level during the daytime and at night, with enough low-level light at night to comfort the patient who awakens at that time; (3) provides freedom from dangerous objects and substances; and (4) provides an optimal level of stimulation. Some patients do better in rooms with other patients; others find them too stimulating. Likewise, some patients are comforted by a constant attendant, whereas others are irritated. The proper level of stimulation should be determined by a systematic trial and should then be continued until the delirium resolves. Overstimulation usually produces agitation and disorientation; understimulation may lead to hallucinations, sensory illusions, or yelling for attention.

FOLLOW-UP

After the resolution of an acute delirium, reexamination of the patient is warranted for residual neurologic signs or cognitive impairment suggestive of mild dementia. If these are encouragered, further neurologic assessment may be indicated.

The patient, who is usually totally or partially amnesic for the episode of delirium, should be educated about what happened, and the basis of the delirium should be explained. Likewise, family members, who may be frightened by the patient's bizarre behavior during the delirium, should be offered information about the cause of the delirium and the self-limited nature of the process.

If neuroleptic drugs were begun during the delirium, they should definitely be tapered and discontinued over the next several days. A recurrence of psychotic symptoms after resolution of the delirium is an occasion for psychiatric consultation.

AFFECTIVE DISORDERS

method of
DAVID L. DUNNER, M.D.
University of Washington
Seattle, Washington

"Affective disorders" is a term denoting disorders of mood with particular reference to depression. Although the prevalence of the depressive disorders is unknown, several estimates suggest that depression is perhaps the most frequent psychiatric condition and that 15 to 20 per cent of the population will experience a significant depression at some time. Most depressions are extremely responsive to treatment. However, inaccurate clinical diagnosis results in many depressed patients being inadequately treated. In this article, I will review classifications of depression that are useful in delineating specific treatments for depressed patients, with emphasis on the recently revised nomenclature of the revised third edition of the American Psychiatric Association's *Diagnostic and Statistical Manual of Mental Disorders* (DSM-III-R).

Depression is a word that has both psychiatric and commonplace meanings. Thus, people will use the word depression to mean that they are upset about a particular life event. Depressed mood in the absence of specific symptoms of depression is essentially not of sufficient significance to be clinically treatable. Depression as a psychiatric disorder consists of depressed mood plus depressive symptoms. Other terms for depressed mood include feeling sad, blue, hopeless, low, down in the dumps, and irritable. Typical depressive symptoms include change in appetite and weight, with either poor appetite and weight loss or increased appetite and weight gain; change in sleeping habits, with either insomnia or hypersomnia; change in motor activity, with either agitation or motor retardation; loss of interest in usual activities and in sexual relations; loss of energy; feelings of worthlessness, self-reproach, or guilt; decreased ability to think or concentrate; and recurrent thoughts of death or suicide or suicide attempts. In this article, I will use depressed mood plus symptoms to define psychiatric depression in contrast to depression without symptoms.

SUBCLASSIFICATION

It is generally recognized that there is affective response to the death of a close friend or relative. This depression, which is termed "uncomplicated bereavement," is associated with depressed mood and depressive symptoms. Bereavement tends to be prompt in onset and relatively short-lived. Feelings of worthlessness and psychomotor retardation are uncommon with this disorder. In general, bereavement is not treated by psychiatrists but is usually treated by internists or family physicians. Bereavement is often not treated except with supportive care. Brief courses of small doses of antianxiety agents may be of benefit. It is unusual for psychiatrists to treat bereaved persons. However, when the syndrome fails to respond to brief therapy or the symptoms persist for several months, one should consider a major depression as a diagnostic possibility.

Depression occurring shortly after a traumatic life event is termed "adjustment disorder with depressed mood." Such depressions are usually time limited and often respond to supportive measures. By definition in DSM-III-R, adjustment disorder with depressed mood lasts less than 6 months. If the mood disorder persists, rediagnosis to major depression should be considered.

Depression (or elated mood) occurring with evidence of a specific organic factor that is judged to be etiologically related to the mood disturbance is termed "organic mood syndrome." Such etiologic factors may include stroke, endocrine disturbance, medication or drug use or abuse, or cancer. Treatment of the etiologic factor is the main therapeutic approach.

The primary mood disorders can be divided into those with mania or hypomania (bipolar disorder) and those with depression only (unipolar disorder or depressive disorders).

Mania is defined as a change in mood state (euphoria or irritability) and presents with symptoms such as increase in activity, increase in talkativeness, flight of ideas or racing thoughts, grandiosity, decreased need for sleep, distractability, and impulsive behavior. The severe form of this disorder, which is often accompanied by delusions of grandeur or frank psychosis, usually results in the patient's being hospitalized specifically for the manic condition. Such patients have been termed "bipolar I." In DSM-III-R these patients would be termed as "having a bipolar disorder." Patients who have manic symptoms but not to the degree resulting in hospitalization (i.e., hypomanic symptoms) are termed "bipolar II." Bipolar II patients typically have recurrent depressions and hypomania. Their hypomanic symptoms are rarely incapacitating and may be productive or beneficial to their life status. In DSM-III-R, bipolar II patients are classified as "bipolar disorder, not otherwise specified." Patients with less severe forms of bipolar and unipolar depression, cyclothymic personality and depressive personality, respectively, were defined as those who had mood disorder but not of sufficient severity to require treatment. The DSM-III-R terms "cyclothymic" and "dysthymic" would probably correspond well to the older terms cyclothymic and depressive personality, respectively.

One other point of diagnostic clarification concerns the presence of Schneiderian first rank symptoms in affective disorders. These symptoms, such as bizarre delusions, somatic delusions, auditory hallucinations such as a voice commenting on the patient's behavior or two or more voices conversing with one another, and delusions such as audible thoughts and thought broadcasting, represent psychotic symptoms, which in the past have been used synonymously with schizophrenia. However, in the past few years schizophrenia has been narrowly defined to include patients who have the above psychotic symptoms associated with a chronic course and absence of affective symptoms. Research studies clearly demonstrate a high prevalence of Schneiderian first rank symptoms during manic episodes.

The term "schizoaffective disorder" is defined in DSM-III-R in such a way that psychotic symptoms occur in the absence of symptoms of mood disorder in patients who also have prolonged periods of mood disorder. Such patients clearly are complicated to treat and require symptomatic treatment for both mood and psychotic symptoms.

In contrast to the rather clearly defined bipolar and unipolar disorders, there are other disorders in which the illness is presumably affective, although the data to support this assumption may be scant. An example is "masked depression," in which a patient will present clinically with somatic complaints rather than depressive symptoms. Masked depressions may be more frequently seen among older patients. The recognition of this problem is important, since it is believed that masked depression represents a significant portion of patients with depression and that most frequently such patients do not have their psychiatric problems adequately recognized or treated. Another less well-defined illness is depression occurring in a patient whose psychiatric disorder becomes complicated by a second psychiatric illness, for example, alcoholism or polydrug abuse. An underlying depression is often suspected in such patients, particularly if they have positive family histories of depression and if there are atypical features to the course of their secondary illness.

BIPOLAR-UNIPOLAR DIFFERENTIATION

Recent data support the separation of bipolar from unipolar primary affective disorders. In general, bipolar I illness is a well-characterized clinical condition in comparison to other primary affective disorder subtypes. Patients with bipolar I illness tend to have extreme psychomotor retardation and often have hypersomnia when depressed, whereas patients with unipolar depression may either be agitated or have psychomotor retardation. Furthermore, the age of onset of illness tends to be earlier in life in bipolar disorders than in unipolar disorders, with the former occurring at a mean age of approximately 30 years and the latter occurring at a mean age of 40 years. Of some interest is the fact that bipolar disorders may have a more frequent postpartum onset than unipolar disorders. There is considerable evidence relating genetic and biologic factors to the etiology of bipolar depression, although these factors have not been elucidated to the point at which a clear biologic-genetic etiology has been determined. Recent studies have pointed toward a possible genetic defect on chromosome 11 or the X chromosome in certain selected families with bipolar illness. Bipolar depression tends to be familial, and approximately 25 per cent of the first-degree relatives of a patient with bipolar disorder will experience either bipolar or unipolar depression. In contrast, unipolar depression probably represents a very heterogeneous group of patients, with various causes for their disorders. For example, the genetic and biologic factors associated with bipolar disorder are not nearly as well delineated among families of patients with unipolar disorders, and the relationship of unipolar disorders to other psychiatric illnesses such as alcoholism is often striking.

CLINICAL COURSE

The course of affective disorders can be recurrent attacks or single episodes. The bipolar disorders tend to be marked by recurrent episodes, sometimes on a regular cyclic basis in such a way that the timing of subsequent attacks is quite predictable. Unipolar disorders tend not to be recurrent, and the frequency of attacks tends to be much reduced in unipolar depression as compared with bipolar depression. Rapid cycling (four or more episodes per year) occurs in about 10 per cent of bipolar disorders, and such patients present particular treatment problems. Mania usually begins early in bipolar illness, with about 80 per cent of patients having experienced a manic attack at the onset of their disorder. About one-third of patients have a significant premanic depression, and almost 100 per cent of patients have a significant postmanic depressive episode. Indeed, the concept of "unipolar mania" (defined as patients who have only recurrent manic episodes) was studied and found not to be useful in that most patients who have recurrent manic episodes also have some depressive features. Between episodes of illness, patients with bipolar and unipolar illness tend to be free of affective symptoms.

TREATMENT

Treatment considerations should relate to diagnosis, current mood state, and the clinical history. For example, one could be treating a patient with bipolar disorder who is manic or who is depressed or who is euthymic but prone to recurrent cycles. Similarly, one could be treating a patient with unipolar disorder who is depressed or who is prone to recurrent attacks.

Finally, it should be noted that the suicide risk in depressive illness is considerable. About 15 to 20 per cent of patients with depression die from suicide, and approximately 30 to 50 per cent of primary affective disorder patients have a history of suicide attempts. Suicide generally occurs during the depressed phase of illness. Although it has been stated that suicide is unusual early in the course of depression and more common later in the course of depression, we suggest that the clinician should be carefully aware of suicidal behavior during any phase of the depressive illness. Suicide during mania and during the interim euthymic phases between depressions is unusual. Suicidal behavior tends to occur more frequently among men, among older patients, and among patients who are single, widowed, or divorced. It should be noted that there has been a considerable increase in the reported suicides among adolescents in the past few years.

Most patients who have committed suicide have indicated their intent to commit suicide to other people, and such communication of suicidal intent should be taken quite seriously in the depressed patient. In terms of assessing suicidal risk in an individual patient, it is important to have an underlying assumption that all patients with depression are suicidal but that their tendency to commit suicide at any given point in time may be contingent upon a number of factors. For example, very few patients with depression will have active plans for suicide. A higher percentage of patients will have thoughts of death or suicide, and a majority of patients with depression will wish they would not wake up in the morning or will wish they were dead. The recognition of this hierarchy of suicidal behavior is important in order to establish rapport with the patient and to apply appropriate treatment. It should be stressed that hospitalization should be advocated for any patient in whom the suicidal risk is thought to be high at that period of time. Depression is a highly treatable disorder, and the suicide of a patient during the course of a severe depression might have been prevented with appropriate treatment.

In the following section I will discuss modes of treatment for various types of depression. In general, these modes include electroconvulsive therapy (ECT), pharmacotherapy, and various forms of psychotherapy. The decision about which mode or combination of modes to use is often based upon the severity of the depressive symptoms as well as diagnostic considerations. It should be emphasized that the best guide to treatment is the past response to treatment.

Modes of Treatment

Electroconvulsive Therapy. ECT was widely used in the 1940s, but the beneficial effects of other forms of treatment as well as some attempts to regulate its use legally have resulted in decreased use of ECT. However, it should be noted that ECT is the most effective of all the forms of antidepressant treatment.

ECT is usually administered to hospitalized patients, although patients who have family members to take care of them can receive this treatment on an outpatient basis. A course of therapy usually consists of a series of 8 to 12 treatments, with a frequency of approximately one every other day. Before the treatment is administered, the physician should have good knowledge of the patient's medical condition, including cardiovascular and pulmonary status. The only absolute contraindication to ECT is a space-occupying brain lesion. During ECT, there is a temporary increase of intracranial pressure, which could result in brain stem herniation if a space-occupying lesion is present.

The patient is prepared for ECT by maintaining an empty stomach for at least 8 hours prior to ECT. Approximately half an hour before ECT a small dose of atropine is administered in order to reduce bronchial secretions. Prior to ECT, the patient should void, and dentures should be removed. Furthermore, hairpins should be removed, and any constricting garments around the chest should be removed or loosened. Immediately before administering ECT, the patient should receive an anesthetic intravenously, usually a short-acting barbiturate. The patient is then given succinylcholine in a dose sufficient to cause relaxation of all muscles but not so excessive as to reduce spontaneous respiration for too prolonged a period after ECT. The usual dose of succinylcholine is about 20 to 40 mg intravenously. It is important to maintain the airway and respirate the patient during the succinylcholine-induced paralysis. With bilateral ECT the electrodes are placed on both temples; with unilateral ECT both electrodes are placed over the nondominant hemisphere. In either case a short period of electrical current is applied to the electrodes, usually at the point of maximal muscle depolarization from the succinylcholine. This current application induces a grand mal convulsion characterized by a tonic phase, followed by a brief clonic phase. It is important to respirate the patient with oxygen until the effects of succinyl-choline wear off and the patient begins to breathe spontaneously. At this point the patient will be drowsy and somewhat confused. The patient's airway should be protected, and the patient should be observed for approximately half an hour after ECT or until such time as confusion has cleared sufficiently for the patient to resume usual functioning. There is a considerable amount of confusion that occurs just after each treatment; as the number of treatments increases, the patient may become confused for longer periods of time between treatments. Usually, a course of eight treatments suffices to treat a severe depression, at which time a few days are necessary to enable the confusion to clear up sufficiently so that the patient can return home. Although much has been made recently of permanent brain damage resulting from ECT, ECT remains the safest and most effective treatment for severe depression. ECT is useful in the treatment of acute depression. There is no reliable evidence that chronic ECT prevents occurrence of future attacks of depression.

ECT has also been used successfully to treat acute manic episodes. Lithium carbonate therapy should be discontinued about 1 week prior to ECT in order to reduce the risk of neurotoxicity.

Antidepressant Medication. Antidepressant medication can be divided into three types: the tricyclic antidepressants, newer antidepressants, and monoamine oxidase inhibitors (MAOIs). The tricyclic antidepressants (Table 1) have become the most widely used treatment of depression and are efficacious in approximately 80 per cent of depressed patients. Recently, measurement of these compounds in the blood has become available, and for most compounds there seems to be some relationship with either a threshold or a range of blood levels and therapeutic response. Thus, if a patient is not responding to a tricyclic antidepressant and is believed to have an adequate dose, it may be useful to obtain a plasma

TABLE 1. Tricyclic Antidepressant Medication

Generic Name	Trade Names	Dose Range* (mg/day)
Amitriptyline	Amitid, Amitril, Elavil, Endep	150–300
Imipramine	Imavate, Janimine, Presamine, SK-Pramine, Tofranil	150–300
Nortriptyline	Aventyl, Pamelor	50–150
Trimipramine	Surmontil	75–300
Desipramine	Norpramin, Pertofrane	150–200
Protriptyline	Vivactil	10–60
Doxepin	Adapin, Sinequan	150–300

*Some doses may be higher than those listed in the manufacturers' official directive.

TABLE 2. Newer Antidepressant Medication

Generic Name	Trade Names	Dose Range* (mg/day)
Amoxapine	Asendin	150–300
Maprotiline	Ludiomil	150–225
Trazodone	Desyrel	300–600
Fluoxetine	Prozac	20–80
Bupropion†	Wellbutrin	Up to 450

*Some doses may be higher than those listed in the manufacturers' official directive.
†This drug has been taken off the market in the United States.

tricyclic level approximately 12 hours after the last dose of tricyclic medication to determine whether the blood level is in the adequate range.

The tricyclic antidepressants can be generally divided into two types: sedating (such as amitriptyline [Elavil], imipramine [Tofranil], trimipramine [Surmontil], and doxepin [Adapin]) and alerting (such as nortriptyline [Pamelor], desipramine [Norpramin], and protriptyline [Vivactil]).

"Newer" antidepressants (Table 2) include amoxapine (Asendin), maprotiline (Ludiomil), trazodone (Desyrel), and fluoxetine (Prozac). All of these agents have advantages and disadvantages as compared with the standard tricyclic compounds. Amoxapine is sedating, but this compound has a major metabolite that has dopamine-blocking effects. Concern for the development of tardive dyskinesia might limit its use to patients who are refractory to other agents. Maprotiline is similar to imipramine; however, an increased risk for seizures has been associated with this compound. Trazodone is among the most frequently prescribed antidepressants. It seems safer than the tricyclic antidepressants, in that the effects of overdose are less severe with trazodone. A small percentage of males will develop priapism with trazodone, and we have therefore not recommended this drug for initial treatment of male patients. Fluoxetine has been recently released, and this compound lacks the anticholinergic side effects and weight gain associated with the tricyclic compounds. The suggested dose of fluoxetine is 20 mg in the morning, and the drug is activating. Side effects include nausea, tremulousness, and insomnia. In addition, there are reports of increased tricyclic compound blood levels when these agents are used with fluoxetine. Bupropion has at this time not been rereleased by the U.S. Food and Drug Administration for prescription use. The compound is activating and seems not to cause cycling among bipolar depressives. Cardiovascular and anticholinergic side effects are lacking, but seizures are reported with bupropion if administered at too high a dose, if the dose is increased too rapidly, or if certain patients (e.g., bulimics) are treated with bupropion.

MAOIs (Table 3) were introduced to psychiatry before the tricyclic antidepressants and in the early years of their use were noted to be quite effective. A potentially serious side effect of these drugs results from inhibition of MAO in the liver. Tyramine, which is present in many food substances, is ordinarily metabolized by liver MAO. If tyramine-containing foods are ingested while the patient is treated with an MAOI, tyramine enters the blood stream, and sudden increases in blood pressure may occur. Because of these potentially serious side effects (headache, strokes), MAOIs were little used for many years. They have been reintroduced recently and are gaining considerable popularity for the treatment of refractory depressions, "atypical" depressions, anxious patients, and postmanic depressive episodes in bipolar patients.

There are two general types of MAOIs. Tranylcypromine (Parnate) has a structure very similar to that of amphetamine and is stimulating, whereas phenelzine (Nardil) is somewhat less stimulating. MAOI drugs have the usual side effects of tricyclic antidepressants, and orthostatic hypotension is the most frequent serious side effect. Hypertensive crisis can be avoided completely if patients follow a low-tyramine diet and avoid medication that affects biogenic amines. The appropriate dose of the medication can be determined by the dose required to inhibit MAO in platelets. In general, a dose of 45 mg per day of phenelzine inhibits this enzyme in about 50 per cent of patients, and thus a somewhat higher dose is required of this medication.

Approaches to Treatment

General Principles. As a general principle of psychopharmacology, it is inadvisable to use fixed-dose regimens. Thus, patients who are outpatients should be encouraged to alter the dose frequently, within certain guidelines, depending on symptoms or side effects, and for hospitalized patients the physician should carefully assess the dose on a daily basis, balancing therapeutic effect with side effects. Fluoxetine has become a frequently used antidepressant because of its ease of administration and lack of severe side effects.

TABLE 3. **Monoamine Oxidase Inhibitors**

Generic Name	Trade Names	Dose Range (mg/day)
Isocarboxazid	Marplan	10–30
Phenelzine	Nardil	15–75
Tranylcypromine	Parnate	10–60

In treating unipolar depression one should be cognizant of two general types of depression: those patients with agitation and insomnia and those patients with psychomotor retardation and hypersomnia. For the former patients, who also may experience anxiety as a prominent feature of the depression, a sedating antidepressant often given at bedtime seems to be most effective. For the latter patients, a more alerting antidepressant, often given toward morning hours in divided doses, seems to be the most logical choice of medication. The target dose for hospitalized patients should be approximately 3.5 mg per kg (imipramine or amitriptyline). It should be noted that protriptyline is given in approximately one-fifth the dose of the other tricyclic antidepressants.

In considering the starting dose, one should take into account previous responses to antidepressants, the general medical state of the patient, and the patient's age. Patients who are older should be started on lower doses of antidepressants than younger patients, and older patients have a lower target dose. The initial dose should be increased progressively toward the target dose with an attempt to achieve the target dose within the first 2 weeks of treatment. During the first week of treatment, there is usually no apparent improvement in depression. Toward the end of this period, the patient, when questioned carefully, may experience very brief periods of feeling well, followed by a feeling of sinking back into the depressive condition. The patient should be encouraged to see this as a beneficial sign that the antidepressant will be working, and the dose should be increased appropriately. For outpatients the general starting dose of amitriptyline or imipramine is approximately 25 to 100 mg per day, and the dose should be increased by the patient every 3 to 4 days as tolerated.

It is advisable, considering the suicidal potential of such patients, to have the patient seen or phone in during the first week of treatment so that the dose can be adjusted upward or downward, depending on therapeutic response or side effects. In general, outpatient depressives have less severe depression than hospitalized patients and often require less antidepressant total dosage, although many depressed outpatients will require doses in the range of 3.5 mg per kg.

At times, inpatients or outpatients will not respond to antidepressants at the target dose, and the dose will have to be increased, perhaps even above the therapeutic levels recommended in the *Physicians' Desk Reference.* For example, it is not uncommon to have patients respond to 350 mg of amitriptyline, whereas they had not responded to a daily dose of 300 mg. Special attention should be paid to the patient's cardiovascular status when doses are increased, and in general outpatients should be told that they should reduce the dose and increase their salt and food intake if they feel dizzy. The typical side effects of tricyclic antidepressants are dry mouth, constipation, blurring of vision, and orthostatic hypotension (experienced as dizziness when one changes position). Later in the course of treatment patients may experience a craving for sweets and weight gain.

Patients tend to respond within 2 to 4 weeks of instituting treatment, although on close questioning they may not feel 100 per cent back to normal. At this point the patient should be maintained on the antidepressant for 2 to 6 months. Frequently, toward the end of this interval the dose can be gradually reduced with approximately 10 per cent reduction in dose every week or every other week. Having the patient reduce the dose and then waiting 1 or 2 weeks to see if symptoms recur is a satisfactory way of determining whether the patient still requires that dose of medication. The patient should be advised not to stop the dose suddenly, as a brief confusional episode may ensue.

The acute depressions of bipolar patients are often somewhat refractory to treatment with tricyclic antidepressants. In general, such patients have retarded depression, and imipramine-like drugs seem to be more indicated than amitriptyline-type drugs. The patient often will improve somewhat but not completely, and the depression in general will take several months to improve in spite of using maximal doses. For this reason, it may be preferable to treat the acute postmanic depressive phase of a bipolar patient with an MAOI rather than with a tricyclic antidepressant. The premanic depressive phase of bipolar patients often spontaneously ends in manic or hypomanic episodes. Thus, the patient should be alerted to the possibility of a manic occurrence during the course of tricyclic treatment, and it may be advisable to treat the patient simultaneously with lithium carbonate. In general, tricyclic antidepressants seem to accentuate mania and are contraindicated during manic or hypomanic episodes. Lithium carbonate has an antidepressant effect, but treatment of the acute depressed phase of bipolar or unipolar depression with lithium carbonate alone is not recommended, although some favor lithium for bipolar depressions because of the tendency for tricyclic antidepressants to cause rapid cycling.

It has been claimed that low doses of antipsychotic agents may be useful in treating some depressive episodes. Furthermore, it has been suggested that patients with psychotic depression often are nonresponders to antidepressant therapy and that antipsychotic drugs should be added to the tricyclic antidepressant. In general, antipsychotic drugs are not the treatment of choice for depression. The addition of an antipsychotic drug to antidepressant therapy in psychotic depressives is of clinical benefit at times. However, ECT should also be considered in these patients.

Prophylaxis of Depression. Recently, tricyclic antidepressants such as amitriptyline and imipramine have been administered on a long-term basis to patients with recurrent unipolar depression to effect a reduction in the frequency of future attacks of this disorder. Such reduction in frequency and/or severity of future episodes with long-term treatment is termed prophylaxis or maintenance therapy, and several studies support the efficacy of chronic tricyclic antidepressants in unipolar recurrent depression. However, it should be noted that some of these studies report a high incidence of manic or hypomanic failures while supposedly unipolar patients are being treated with tricyclic antidepressants. The bipolar II category includes patients who have brief hypomanic episodes before or after their depression, and such patients probably were included as unipolar in those studies mentioned earlier, resulting in the reported hypomanic failures with chronic tricyclic treatment. Lithium carbonate has also been shown to have a prophylactic effect for recurrent unipolar and bipolar depression, and lithium carbonate is preferred over tricyclic antidepressants for such treatment.

The appropriate dose of tricyclic antidepressants in prophylactic treatment has not been established, although most physicians seem to prefer a maintenance dose of approximately 100 to 150 mg daily of amitriptyline or imipramine. Other antidepressants have not been systematically studied for their long-term prophylactic effect. Lithium carbonate maintenance will be discussed later in this article. Maintenance efficacy for recurrent depression may not become clinically apparent until the patient has been in treatment for about 2 years.

Patients with the rapid cycling form of bipolar illness will experience recurrent depressions and hypomanic episodes. Their depressions are seen as illness, whereas the hypomanic episodes are not viewed by the patient as being clinically significant. However, treating such patients with tricyclic antidepressants alone or in combination with lithium carbonate seems to result in a perpetuation of the cyclic process, whereas treating rapid cyclers with lithium carbonate alone or perhaps with a small dose of antipsychotic agent (such as thioridazine) may be of benefit.

Special Uses in Depression. The use of tricyclic

antidepressants in the secondary depressions and in bereavement has not been systematically studied. In my experience if such patients require an antidepressant based on the presence of depressive symptoms, they usually respond at relatively low doses of the antidepressant, such as 50 mg daily of amitriptyline. One should be cautious in treating depression associated with alcoholism, since the antidepressants are sedating, as is alcohol, and the sedative effects of alcohol may be potentiated. Also, particular attention should be paid to treating depression in the elderly, as such patients are particularly prone to the hypotensive and cardiovascular effects of tricyclic antidepressants. The beginning dose for elderly patients is low, on the order of 10 to 25 mg of amitriptyline daily, and very slow increments of the dose are advised, along with careful assessment of blood pressure and cardiovascular status. New antidepressants lacking the cardiovascular side effects of the tricyclic compounds may be of particular benefit in the treatment of the elderly depressed patient.

An important drug-drug interaction of the tricyclic antidepressants occurs with guanethidine, an antihypertensive agent. The antihypertensive effects of guanethidine can be blocked with the administration of tricyclic antidepressants. Thus, if patients are hypertensive and prone to depression, it is advised that they be treated with an antihypertensive agent other than guanethidine. In addition, antidepressants are not advocated during the first trimester of pregnancy.

Acute Mania. Acute manic disturbances may present particular problems because the patient may not be willing to be hospitalized for treatment. Treating manic patients on an outpatient basis is difficult because of the lack of control regarding medication that can be exercised in such circumstances. Thus, the optimal plan is to hospitalize the patient for treatment of an acute manic disorder. ECT is effective in the treatment of acute manic disturbances. Lithium should be discontinued about 1 week before administering ECT because neurotoxicity has been noted with combined treatment. The usual method of treating acute mania is with lithium carbonate, antipsychotics, or a combination of lithium carbonate and antipsychotics. In general, treatment of acute mania consists of beginning either a benzodiazepine or an antipsychotic drug and instituting lithium carbonate as soon as the patient is willing to take medication orally. The severity of the acute manic disorder and cooperation of the patient are the critical factors in the choice of the antipsychotic drug. For example, patients who are uncooperative in taking oral medication will require intramuscular medication, such as haloperidol or chlorpromazine. Chlorpromazine (Thorazine) can be given in 25 to 50 mg doses intramuscularly every 1 to 3 hours, with careful attention being paid to blood pressure, since orthostatic hypotension often accompanies this route of administration. Haloperidol (Haldol) has been used more recently as an acute antimanic drug and is often given as 5 to 10 mg intramuscularly every 1 to 2 hours. Haloperidol has a great propensity for causing parkinsonian symptoms, which should be treated with antiparkinsonian drugs. Haloperidol has very little effect on blood pressure, and although it is not as sedating as chlorpromazine, manic patients can be successfully sedated with haloperidol. For patients who are more cooperative or whose manic episodes are less severe, thioridazine is an excellent drug in that it has very few blood pressure effects or parkinsonian side effects. The thioridazine dose should not exceed 800 mg per day. Starting doses on the order of 200 to 400 mg per day can be used in combination with lithium carbonate to treat the acute manic episode. Two serious side effects can occur with antipsychotic medication—tardive dyskinesia and neuroleptic malignant syndrome. Therefore, sedating benzodiazepines may be useful to reduce the doses of antipsychotic drugs.

Lithium carbonate is perhaps more effective in treating acute manic episodes than are the antipsychotic agents. However, lithium carbonate cannot be given in an intramuscular form, and thus the patient must be cooperative to be treated with lithium carbonate. Prior to treatment with lithium carbonate it is advisable to have a medical work-up, which would include physical examination, electrocardiogram, thyroid studies, white blood count, urinalysis, blood urea nitrogen, and creatinine. There have been several regimens described for determining the dose of lithium carbonate. These involve giving a "test dose" of 600 to 900 mg of lithium carbonate and determining a blood lithium level at a fixed time thereafter. This blood level is used to select a "therapeutic" dose. In our experience these projected doses often result in a high daily dose being administered to the patient with resulting lithium toxicity. We prefer to start lithium carbonate at 300 to 600 mg the first day and increase the dose daily until therapeutic blood concentrations of lithium result. This method requires frequent measurement of blood levels but is safe for the patient and produces fewer acute side effects, such as nausea and vomiting. The therapeutic blood lithium concentration for acute mania is about 1.0 to 1.5 mEq per liter. Blood levels should be measured frequently for hospitalized patients who are receiving increasing doses of lithium, particularly older patients or patients with borderline renal function. Patients should be examined daily for the presence of lithium side effects, such as nausea, vomiting, diarrhea, or tremor. Signs of neurotoxicity for lithium should also be observed; these would include confusion, gross tremor, ataxia, slurring of speech, and sedation. These neurotoxic symptoms may occur in some patients at doses within the therapeutic range, particularly if the patient is receiving high doses of antipsychotic drugs concomitantly. It is vital that the patient have an adequate fluid and salt intake during lithium treatment because lithium urinary excretion is dependent on sodium metabolism. In many but not all cases, manic symptoms will improve at about 10 to 14 days, at which time the dose of the antipsychotic drug can be tapered. The dose of lithium may also have to be reduced somewhat, as while manic, the patient may be drinking copious amounts of fluid, and this phenomenon will decrease as the mania abates. The physician should be cautioned about premature discharge of the manic patient from the hospital, as insight and judgment seem to be the last manic symptoms to improve in contrast to sleep and activity. Patients who are discharged from the hospital prematurely may stop their medication and have a relapse of manic symptoms. As a general guide, the manic episode has not been completed until the patient enters into a postmanic depressive phase.

Patients who are refractory to lithium treatment may respond to treatment with anticonvulsants such as carbamazepine, valproic acid, or benzodiazepines. These compounds, although effective in the treatment of acute mania, have been less studied than lithium or antipsychotic medication.

Lithium Carbonate Maintenance. Prophylaxis of manic episodes is the most striking reason why lithium carbonate became the accepted drug of the 1970s. It was found that the administration of this simple salt on a long-term basis reduced the frequency and intensity of subsequent manic episodes in patients who are prone to bipolar cyclic manic-depressive illness. The maintenance dose is that dose sufficient to produce a blood level of 0.7 to 1.0 mEq per liter. During proper administration of chronic lithium treatment, there are minimal side effects, mainly occasional diarrhea or occasional tremor. A slight polyuria is frequently found, but this is usually not of clinical significance.

There are several medical concerns about long-term administration of lithium. An antithyroid effect is often noted early in the course of administration and can be corrected by giving thyroid

supplements if clinical manifestations of hypothyroidism persist. Cardiac effects, especially in older patients, have been noted during lithium treatment. Sinus node dysfunction may be accentuated during lithium therapy. A third effect has been related to severe polyuria and the possibility of renal disease in patients undergoing chronic lithium treatment or who have experienced lithium toxicity. For this reason, patients should have monitoring of medical status, including thyroid tests, blood urea nitrogen, creatinine, and electrocardiogram at least yearly while undergoing lithium treatment. If symptoms develop referable to a primary medical illness, appropriate consultations should be obtained. It should not be too lightly stressed that patients must be carefully monitored during long-term lithium treatment and that it is important to obtain blood lithium levels at least several times a year. Blood for lithium concentrations should be obtained 8 to 12 hours after a lithium dose. It is best to keep the interval between the patient's taking the medication and the blood level being determined constant from visit to visit. During steady-state lithium treatment, the blood level generally does not vary more than 0.1 mEq per liter, and variations greater than this are probably due to irregularities in the patient's taking the medication. The most likely time for a relapse during lithium treatment is in the initial 6 months of treatment, based on actuarial life table statistics. Patients have a risk of developing an affective episode when starting lithium treatment of about 5 per cent per month through the initial 6 months of treatment, and subsequent to that the risk is about 1 per cent per month. Maintenance lithium treatment for outpatients (who are generally euthymic) is usually initiated with low doses, that is, one capsule per day. The dose is increased on a weekly basis until the therapeutic blood level is achieved. Patients are generally seen every 1 to 2 weeks initially, and when they are stable, the interval visits can be lengthened to once per month.

While it is clear that lithium has an effect on reducing manic and hypomanic episodes very dramatically in the first year of treatment, its effect against depression in both bipolar and unipolar recurrent depression takes longer to achieve. Recent data suggest that it takes approximately 1½ to 2 years of treatment before the prophylactic effect of lithium against recurrent depression can be statistically demonstrated. However, the data also suggest that there may be subclinical beneficial effects on mild mood states during this initial period. Thus, in starting patients on lithium one should carefully explain that it is likely that they will have recurrent depressions at least for 1 to 2 years in spite of treatment and that these depressions initially may seem as severe as their prior depressions before they began taking lithium. Second, patients should notice a decrease in the frequency and severity of manic and hypomanic attacks, although manic episodes may not be completely obliterated during lithium treatment. Those patients who have had a recurrence of severe manic episodes at least once every 7 years or at least two recurrent depressive episodes in 5 years are candidates for lithium prophylactic treatment. It should also be noted that the prophylactic efficacy of lithium carbonate in unipolar recurrent depression is controversial, although its use has been supported by several research studies. Patients frequently feel well for long intervals during lithium treatment, and some may wish to stop their medication. This should not be advised, since on stopping medication patients tend to return to their previous rate of episodes, and the failure rate on stopping lithium treatment seems to be the same as if the patient never was on lithium treatment.

Although there are few drug-drug interactions with lithium, diuretics should be avoided. Lithium excretion requires sodium, and concomitant diuretic administration often results in lithium retention and can provoke episodes of lithium toxicity. Thus, patients should be cautioned not to change their sodium intake or their sodium metabolism in any way while taking lithium carbonate. Lithium toxicity, in contrast to lithium side effects, tends to be a fairly acute-onset illness. Usually, the symptoms occur over a week or so, and these symptoms are characterized by polyuria, confusion, agitation, and tremor and may eventually progress to coma and death. As the patients continue to take lithium they become progressively dehydrated because of polyuria resulting from lithium toxicity. The treatment of lithium toxicity is to stop lithium and to rehydrate the patient, particularly with water, sodium, and potassium.

Rapid-cycling patients who continue to cycle in spite of lithium maintenance therapy may benefit from long-term treatment with carbamazepine or valproic acid. Laboratory tests for blood counts and liver function should be obtained regularly if these compounds are prescribed. Neurotoxicity from the combination of lithium carbonate and carbamazepine has been reported.

Barbiturates and Stimulants. Barbiturates should be avoided as sleeping medications for patients with depression. Barbiturates are totally un-needed for treatment of depressed patients with insomnia because such patients can be treated with a sedating antidepressant such as amitriptyline. In addition, barbiturates tend to activate liver enzymes that metabolize tricyclic antidepressants. Thus, the effect of a barbiturate in combination with a tricyclic antidepressant would be to lower the dose of the antidepressant. Stimulants such as methylphenidate or amphetamine are of only temporary benefit in depression and should be avoided.

Psychotherapy. Although psychotherapy is generally believed to be of importance in the treatment of depression, there has been a considerable change in the emphasis on psychotherapy for depressed patients over the past several years. In the late 1960s in some centers, analytically oriented psychotherapy was considered the treatment of choice for both bipolar and unipolar affective disorders. The efficacy of psychopharmacologic agents resulted in the need for greater specificity and efficacy in the psychotherapies employed for affective disorders.

Educational and supportive psychotherapies are helpful for the depressed patient. It is very important to have the patient understand the illness as thoroughly as possible and to understand the need for and the role of medication and therapy. The patient should be taught to recognize early symptoms and to adjust medication according to agreed-upon guidelines. Decisions that could alter life situations, such as job changes, marital changes, moves, and the like, should be avoided if at all possible until the depression is over. It is important to have the patient try to get out of the house as much as possible, even if only for an hour a day. Physical exercise, such as jogging, may be of benefit to some patients. However, patients should be cautioned that physical exercise is usually of only brief benefit in depression. More specific psychotherapies, such as cognitive-behavioral psychotherapy and interpersonal psychotherapy, have been used successfully with some depressives.

Psychotherapy of a manic patient during such episodes is extremely difficult, as the patient attempts to maintain control of the therapy situation. Family and/or marital therapy may be indicated in some manic patients after remission of the manic episode. A flexible approach to psychotherapy is probably best. Some patients may benefit from certain types of therapy but not other types, and some patients may need little psychotherapy.

SCHIZOPHRENIC DISORDERS

method of
WILLIAM T. CARPENTER, Jr., M.D., and
ALAN BREIER, M.D.

*Maryland Psychiatric Research Center and
    University of Maryland School of Medicine
Baltimore, Maryland*

Schizophrenia is a clinical syndrome comprising an unknown number of disease entities. Each entity within the syndrome may have multiple factors that contribute to etiology and pathogenesis, and specific etiologic factors probably vary among patients. Clinical manifestations of these disorders include hallucinations, delusions, many forms of disordered cognition and attention, and impairment in core attributes of personality functioning. Examples of the latter, which are sometimes referred to as negative or deficit symptoms, are diminished drive, diminished volition, diminished capacity for emotional arousal, inability to experience gratification and pleasure, and impoverished content of mental activity. These deficit manifestations often account for the severe and long-lasting impairments associated with schizophrenia, whereas the so-called positive symptoms (e.g., hallucinations, delusions, thought disturbance) often have an exacerbating and remitting course, account for many of the large number of admissions to hospitals, and are the target symptoms for most therapeutic approaches.

Schizophrenia is a common disorder with a lifetime prevalence of between 0.5 and 1 per cent in the United States and most other countries where population surveys are reported. These figures double when schizophrenia-like psychoses are included. These illnesses usually occur early in life, with the peak age of onset of psychosis occurring in adolescence and early adulthood. The course of illness varies; some patients have chronic, unremitting symptoms, whereas others have a series of symptom exacerbations with few or no symptoms between active episodes. The long-term outcome of schizophrenia is also variable; some patients recover completely and others have severe symptoms throughout life. Negative symptoms often precede psychosis and last indefinitely.

The etiology and pathogenesis of schizophrenia remain an enigma, but it is now clear that there is an important genetic contribution to vulnerability to this illness. Less robust contributions to vulnerability may come from complications related to gestation and birth and from birth during the winter, which are modest risk factors for schizophrenia. There may be many other contributors to vulnerability, and there is also considerable interest in environmental factors that may increase or decrease the likelihood of a vulnerable individual's developing manifest illness.

The clinician needs a broad biopsychosocial-medical model to define the range of treatment interventions and the integration of therapeutics necessary for comprehensive care of the schizophrenic patient.

Treatments may be characterized as somatic and psychosocial (the mode of intervention initiated is biologic, psychologic, or social). Regardless of the type of therapeutic intervention, it is anticipated that treatment effects on the patient will encompass changes in brain physiology, subjective experience, and behavior and will have an impact on social interaction.

SOMATIC TREATMENTS

For all practical purposes, somatic treatments are limited to pharmacotherapy. Many treatments espoused in the past, such as insulin coma therapy and use of megavitamins, have not developed an accepted empiric basis for therapeutic efficacy, and the risks associated with insulin treatment make it an entirely unwarranted therapeutic approach in schizophrenia. Psychosurgery is sometimes performed, but there is no adequate definition of benefits to justify risks, and consideration of such an experimental procedure for schizophrenia would be warranted only under extraordinary circumstances. A few years ago, positive reports from an uncontrolled study of hemodialysis prompted intense interest in the therapeutic potential of this procedure. However, subsequent controlled clinical trials have failed to demonstrate any therapeutic advantage associated with hemodialysis. Electroconvulsive therapy (ECT) is not often used in the treatment of schizophrenia today. However, moderate courses of ECT may have applicability in certain circumstances. Patients in catatonic stupor or catatonic excitement not responsive to antipsychotic drugs may respond to ECT. Although there have been few controlled studies, available data suggest that a brief course of ECT (6 to 12 treatments) may be effective to treat acute psychoses. Such treatment might be justified in patients for whom pharmacotherapy is contraindicated or in patients who prove to be chronically unresponsive to antipsychotic drugs. A key limiting factor in the use of ECT is the absence of long-lasting effects and the failure to develop an acceptable long-term continued therapy or prophylactic approach.

Pharmacotherapy

The use of neuroleptic antipsychotic medication is ubiquitous in the treatment of schizophrenia and is considered to be the mainstay for pharmacotherapy of this illness. These medications have many different physiologic effects but share in common an affinity for postsynaptic dopamine receptors. This effect is believed to be important for initiating a poorly understood chain of actions that provide the mode of therapeutic efficacy for neuroleptic drugs. These neuroleptic medications are called antipsychotic because they are effective on symptoms of psychosis regardless of etiology or diagnostic group. The principal effects of neuroleptics in schizophrenia are reduction of the severity of a broad range of symptoms and behavioral manifestations of the illness, and reduction of the rate of psychotic exacerbation by about 50 per cent in the context of long-term outpatient treatment. These effects contribute to higher levels of functioning of patients and less reliance on inpatient care. The limitations of antipsychotic drug therapy are (1) many patients do not derive sufficient reduction of the severity of symptoms, (2) these drugs are not decisively effective for long-standing deficit manifestations of the illness, (3) there are significant adverse side effects, and (4) because of the dysphoric side effects, patients are often noncompliant in their use of the drugs.

The clinician must consider a number of factors before instituting neuroleptic antipsychotic drug therapy. First, an accurate diagnosis is critical. There are many causes of psychosis, and in some forms of psychosis the use of neuroleptic drugs may be contraindicated (e.g., anticholinergic properties of neuroleptics may exacerbate anticholinergic-induced psychosis). Ascertaining a detailed history of past illness and previous pharmacotherapeutics is crucial. Past history can guide the selection of drug administration strategy, and the prior history of clinical response to and side effects of various neuroleptic medications may guide the selection of the specific compound. The prescribing doctor should be knowledgeable about at least one neuroleptic drug from each major group (i.e., piperidine, piperazine, phenothiazines, thioxanthenes, butyrophenones, dihydroindolones, dibenzoxazepines). Because all of the neuroleptics are thought to have equal therapeutic efficacy, the selection of a specific agent is often guided by its side effect profile. In general, high-potency neuroleptics (e.g., haloperidol) are associated with less sedation and more extrapyramidal effects than low-potency neuroleptics (e.g., chlorpromazine). Baseline evaluation includes measures of vital signs, blood pressure with the patient in standing and reclining positions, complete blood count, liver profile, and electrocardiogram. The specific range of side effects and monitoring requirements are detailed for each drug in the *Physicians' Desk Reference* and are not given here.

It is crucial that the clinician identify target symptoms and goals of pharmacotherapy and reevaluate these periodically. For example, substantially lower doses are associated with prophylactic maintenance and higher doses are used for exacerbations. Long-term prophylactic therapeutics should be restricted to patients who are known to have recurrent forms of illness, and maintenance therapy should be restricted to patients who are known to have continuous manifestation of symptoms responsive to the drug.

It is important to use the lowest dose necessary to achieve control of symptoms and to avoid the temptation of maintaining patients on high-dose regimens. This issue has become important because the incidence of tardive dyskinesia is about 3 per cent of the cohort of patients per year cumulative over time, and data from recent studies demonstrate diminished dyskinesia associated with low-dose strategies. Another consideration is empiric data demonstrating that standard doses are as effective as high doses in treating hospitalized patients. Long-term treatment of outpatients has usually been continuous medication at doses approximating daily doses of 300 mg of chlorpromazine (Thorazine), 25 mg of haloperidol (Haldol), or biweekly injections of 0.5 to 1 ml of fluphenazine (Prolixin). For high-potency neuroleptics, an 80 to 90 per cent reduction of this medication level effectively controls symptoms for most outpatients and is associated with fewer side effects and better compliance. When exacerbation of symptoms occurs in outpatients treated with low-dose neuroleptics, brief increases in the level of medication at the time of the exacerbation are often sufficient to prevent a full relapse. A targeted drug strategy using neuroleptic drugs only at time of exacerbations in selected outpatients has also proved to be an effective therapeutic strategy to reduce dosage. The choice of a neuroleptic dosage reduction strategy is guided by the risk/benefit ratio for the individual patient.

Contraindications. Severe cardiovascular disease may be a contraindication to the use of antipsychotic medication. Serious liver damage requires special precautions in using these medications. Data are not available demonstrating the safety of neuroleptic drugs during pregnancy, and the clinician and pregnant patient must make informed judgments about potential risks and benefits of these drugs. The *Physicians' Desk Reference* should be consulted for specific contraindications and precautions for each compound.

Side Effects. Side effects of neuroleptic medications include drowsiness, contact dermatitis, photosensitivity, weight gain, anticholinergic effects, gynecomastia, galactorrhea, amenorrhea, ocular changes in pigmentation of lens and cornea, retinitis pigmentosa, electrocardiographic changes, jaundice, hematologic changes, extrapyramidal signs, and dysphoric subjective experience. Many of these effects are frequent, and the clinician must be thoroughly familiar with them. A particularly problematic side effect is akathisia. This common extrapyramidal symptom causes considerable patient discomfort. It involves restless legs, constant movement, and intense inner feelings of tension. These manifestations are often mistaken for increased schizophrenic symptoms or agitation, which may erroneously lead to an increase in medication. A reduction of the dosage, switch to a different neuroleptic, and use of antiparkinsonian drugs are indicated for patients with akathisia.

Acute dystonic reactions to neuroleptic drugs can be extremely uncomfortable and frightening to patients. These reactions include torticollis and oculogyric crisis. Diagnosis needs to be rapid, and patients can be effectively treated with anticholinergic drugs. Tardive dyskinesia is a syndrome of abnormal involuntary movements that is a frequent complication of longer-term neuroleptic treatment. It is sometimes persistent and severe. Tardive dyskinesia is most often observed in buccolingual movements or involuntary jerks in distal extremities. The syndrome sometimes progresses to whole-body jerks or diaphragmatic dyskinesia, which can be frightening and dangerous. There is no effective treatment for tardive dyskinesia. It is thought that the best approach is to diminish the incidence with strategies to reduce the dosage of medication. Once dyskinesia is manifest, efforts at reduction of dosage or periodic discontinuation of use of the drug may afford the best opportunity to delay progression or prevent irreversibility of the syndrome.

The neuroleptic malignant syndrome involving fever, muscle rigidity, autonomic instability, and alterations in consciousness is a rare but potentially fatal adverse effect of neuroleptic treatment.

Conclusions About Neuroleptic Pharmacotherapy. The following guidelines will prove to be useful to the physician treating patients with antipsychotic medication.

1. Differential diagnosis is critical. Therapeutics of nonschizophrenic psychoses usually do not depend on a neuroleptic as the primary drug. Parenthetically, patients without schizophrenia may be more vulnerable to the risk of adverse effects of neuroleptics.

2. Restrict the use of neuroleptic drugs to acute management therapeutics in the psychosis, except in patients who have longer-lasting or recurrent forms of schizophrenia or related disorders.

3. At times of exacerbation of symptoms, rapid intervention with medication is desirable, but the loading strategies leading to high doses are not more effective than rapid intervention with standard therapeutic doses.

4. In longer-term maintenance and prophylactic therapy, the physician should avoid high doses when possible. Doses that are substantially lower than standard guidelines (e.g., 300 mg of chlorpromazine equivalence) can be safely administered to most patients and can accomplish a diminution in the frequency of side effects, better compliance, and effective therapeutics. Such dose reduction strategies, whether continuous low dose or targeted intermittent, should be accompanied by overall clinical care, which facilitates rapid increase of the level of medication at the warning sign of an exacerbation. Patients with frequent, abrupt, or severe relapses or patients who are uncooperative may not be good candidates for reduction strategies.

5. It is crucial that physicians integrate antipsychotic drug therapy with psychosocial treatment.

Other Medications

A number of other compounds merit consideration as special treatment of schizophrenia. Empiric evidence is scant, but patients with severe and long-lasting illness merit consideration for use of experimental therapeutics when a reasonable basis for anticipating therapeutic efficacy exists. It should be a high priority in the field of psychiatry to provide more adequate scientific evaluation of the following supplemental drug therapies.

Lithium. Lithium has proved to be an effective drug in the acute forms of schizophrenia-like illnesses, but it has not been established as an alternative drug for the treatment of florid psychosis or in the treatment of chronic forms of schizophrenia. Preliminary evidence suggests that lithium supplementation of neuroleptic drug therapy may enhance the antipsychotic effect in drug-resistant patients. Schizophrenic patients who have affective symptoms may be good candidates for the addition of lithium to existing neuroleptic treatment. In circumstances where careful monitoring of the side effects of lithium therapy can be assured, patients who have chronic illness and unsatisfactory responses to neuroleptic drugs should be considered for a trial of lithium supplementation lasting a few weeks.

Antiseizure Medication. There are interesting hypothetical considerations and a number of anecdotal reports with regard to patients with schizophrenia and schizophrenia-like illnesses who responded to antiseizure medication. Here, the empiric data are scant and fail to document a treatment-responsive subgroup. Because carbamazepine (Tegretol) has been effective in atypical affective disorders with psychosis, and because there is preliminary evidence that carbamazepine may be effective as a neuroleptic supplement, physicians may wish to test short-term carbamazepine treatment in a highly selected subpopulation of schizophrenia patients. Evidence of sudden inexplicable violence, amnesia for episodes of violence, alcohol-induced psychotic exacerbation, and abnormal electroencephalography are factors that provide a hypothetical basis for selecting occasional patients for therapeutic trial. This approach should be limited to patients who are inadequately responsive to neuroleptic drugs and should be considered as an addition to the use of neuroleptic therapeutics.

Antianxiety Drugs. Antianxiety drugs, including the benzodiazepines, have not proved to be effective antipsychotic agents, although high doses in selected inpatients reduce symptoms and behavioral manifestations. During remission, patients may manifest symptoms of anxiety that will prove to be responsive to periodic administration of antianxiety drugs. In an effort to accomplish long-term neuroleptic dose reduction, the physician should consider targeted treatment of anxiety symptoms with antianxiety drugs in stable outpatients rather than increases in neuroleptic medication. A small number of recent reports have indicated that high-potency benzodiazepines (e.g., alprazolam, clonazepam) used in conjunction with neuroleptics may be effective in some schizophrenic patients, but additional data are needed to confirm these preliminary findings.

Antidepressant Medication. Antidepressant medication is not an effective treatment for the schizophrenia-like psychoses. However, depression is a common finding in patients with schizophrenia, and in selected cases where the depression constitutes a major depressive episode during periods of remission of psychosis, the physician may consider treatment with antidepressant medication. In this circumstance a special alertness for signs of exacerbation of psychosis is required, and if the patient is not receiving neuroleptic drugs, the rapid initiation of this therapy may be warranted. Differential diagnosis of depression is critical because demoralization is a concomitant of chronic severe illness, anxiety and depression are concomitants of acute psychosis, and some negative symptoms mimic depression. These features are common in schizophrenia and do not respond to antidepressant medication.

Atypical Neuroleptics. An exciting development in the treatment of schizophrenia has been the introduction of antipsychotic drugs with an atypical pharmacologic profile. Clozapine is an atypical neuroleptic that has been used extensively in Europe and, at the time of this writing, is anticipated to be available for general use in the American market soon. This drug may differ from other neuroleptics in a differential ratio of affinity for D_1 and D_2 dopamine receptors, heightened activity in serotoninergic systems, heightened anticholinergic properties, preferential affinity for neuronal systems in limbic brain regions with less affinity for basal ganglia systems, and failure to increase serum prolactin levels. A large-scale, well-designed study has demonstrated substantial therapeutic effects in patients with well-established treatment resistance to ordinary neuroleptics. Clozapine is associated with a diminished or absent effect in extrapyramidal systems, which gives promise that this compound will be far more benign than standard neuroleptics in causing extrapyramidal side effects including tardive dyskinesia. The most worrisome side effect of clozapine is agranulocytosis, which occurs in approximately 1 to 2 per cent of patients who receive this agent. The risk of agranulocytosis will lead to the selection of clozapine for treatment-resistant patients, but subsequent development of safer atypical neuroleptics may provide substantially enhanced pharmacotherapeutics of schizophrenia.

PSYCHOSOCIAL TREATMENTS

Continuity of clinical care is indispensable in the long-term treatment of schizophrenia. The clinician must establish an effective working relationship, offer support and guidance to the patient, be in a position to detect subtle changes in the patient's clinical condition, and use longitudinal observation of phenomenology as a basis for all therapeutic decision-making.

The general context for psychosocial care is the continuity of the clinical relationship. The clinician must develop a broad treatment context to include the family or other household members, the staff from supervised apartment or psychosocial rehabilitation centers, and other members of the treatment team. It is important to include those close to the patient in the treatment process to enable a shared understanding of the illness and to develop an alliance to facilitate the management of relapses. The patient and family also need the clinician's help and advice regarding issues such as seeking an occupation, living arrangements, social functioning, and a legion of issues of daily life that are vexing to patients, their families, and caretakers. Schizophrenia is often a chronic illness with impairments in many areas of social and occupational functioning. Treatment strategies must be nested in this overall clinical context.

With regard to some specifics about interpersonal therapy, the labor-intensive insight-oriented psychotherapies derived from psychoanalytic theory and psychodynamic tradition have not proved to be superior to more practical day-to-day supportive clinical care. Furthermore, these intensive strategies have often precluded the careful integration of other therapeutic procedures and have had the unfortunate and unnecessary adverse effect of suggesting to many patients and families that they can find the cause and cure of their illness by understanding and modifying their interpersonal and intrapsychic spheres. Currently recommended interpersonal therapies contrast with the intensive, insight-oriented psychotherapy or family therapy. For example, training in social skills targets certain impairments, enhances the patient's performance, and may play an important role in improving overall functioning. Teaching patients and families stress reduction and coping procedures has been proved to decrease the rate of relapses in outpatients. Along these lines, psychoeducational approaches that include family members aimed at reducing the intensity and negativity sometimes encountered in the homes of schizophrenic patients may reduce relapse rates. All of these interpersonal therapeutic strategies have defined and understandable aims and are closely integrated with pharmacotherapeutic strategies.

Another important focus for psychosocial treatment is rehabilitation. Rehabilitation is an important and underdeveloped area in the treatment of patients with schizophrenia. Available rehabilitation resources vary considerably across communities. It is vital that clinicians appreciate the importance of rehabilitation and integrate these opportunities into the overall, long-term treatment plan.

Clinical care of patients with schizophrenia is one of the great challenges in modern medicine. The range of skills and knowledge required is exceptional, and the task of integrating widely divergent therapies is ever present. Present-day advances in the relevant basic and clinical sciences provide a continuous flow of scientific data germane to therapeutics. As new knowledge is gained about etiology and pathophysiology, we can anticipate new approaches to prevention and therapeutics for one of today's most important perplexing diseases.

PANIC DISORDER AND AGORAPHOBIA

method of
LASZLO A. PAPP, M.D., and
JACK M. GORMAN, M.D.
College of Physicians and Surgeons,
Columbia University, New York

Anxiety is a ubiquitous human experience. The popular usage of the term refers to various conditions ranging from appropriate and normal everyday worries to severe, debilitating fears. The psychiatric terminology defines anxiety as the experience of fear, tension, worry, and autonomic nervous system hyperactivity out of proportion to the circumstances. The term does not include the experience of fear during truly life-threatening situations.

For a long time, anxiety had been considered a homogeneous condition varying only in severity. Because the differential diagnosis had little practical consequence, physicians in general tended to dismiss the anxious patient. During the past 15 years, a substantial body of new knowledge has challenged this idea. It is now widely recognized that anxiety disorders differ from each other qualitatively and respond specifically to different therapeutic interventions, including both medications and psychotherapy.

The single most important new development in anxiety research was the finding that spontaneous panic attacks are qualitatively dissimilar from, rather than more intense versions of, chronic unremitting anxiety. Patients with panic attacks represent a biologically and psychologically distinct subgroup of anxiety disorder patients. Their repeated panic attacks often lead to severe, debilitating secondary complications like avoidance (agoraphobia), anticipatory anxiety (fear of the fear), and depression. Attempts at self-medication may result in secondary alcohol or other substance abuse. The appropriate diagnosis of panic disorder and specific treatment result in recovery in up to 90 per cent of patients.

PANIC DISORDER

The hallmark of panic disorder is the spontaneous panic attack. Essential to the definition of this syndrome is that the attacks are initially unprovoked by environmental stimuli. The first attacks may occur in the context of a major life event (e.g., illness, accident, birth, and death in the family) or after the use of psychoactive substances, especially marijuana, cocaine, or amphetamine.

Typically, during a panic attack, a patient is engaged in a routine activity—perhaps driving a car, eating in a restaurant, or reading a book—when suddenly overwhelmed by fear, apprehension, and a sense of impending doom. Some of the associated physical symptoms, representing a massive overstimulation of the autonomic nervous system accompanied by hyperventilation, include the experience of chest pain or discomfort, palpitations, choking or smothering sensations, dizziness, faintness or unsteady feelings, paresthesias, hot and cold flushes, sweating, trembling or shaking, and feelings that things and self appear unreal. The patient is afraid of dying, going crazy, or doing something uncontrolled. A typical attack lasts from 5 to 20 minutes, rarely as long as an hour. Patients who complain of longer attacks may misperceive the exhaustion and tension that frequently follow the actual panic attack or may suffer from other types of pathologic anxiety.

The patient experiencing the first panic attack generally fears that a heart attack or a stroke is occurring. Extensive medical work-ups usually find no abnormalities, and the patient is told that the cause of the problem is psychologic. Experiences like these eventually discourage the patient from seeking medical attention. The natural course of the illness is characterized by brief active periods lasting weeks to months during which there are frequent panic attacks alternating with years of complete or partial remissions. The condition may affect up to 30 million Americans and together with agoraphobia may be the most prevalent psychiatric illness. Women are approximately twice as likely to have panic disorder as men. The mean age of onset is the late twenties.

Many people experience occasional spontaneous panic attacks; however, the diagnosis of panic disorder is made only when the attacks occur in a specific manner. Current diagnostic criteria of the American Psychiatric Association from the *Diagnostic and Statistical Manual of Mental Disorders* (DSM-III-R) require at least four attacks in a 4-week period or one or more attacks followed by "a period of at least a month of persistent fear of having another attack." Panic attacks with 4 symptoms or more from a list of 13 are arbitrarily called full-blown attacks; episodes with fewer than 4 symptoms are defined as limited attacks.

AGORAPHOBIA

The most serious outcome of panic disorder is the development of phobic avoidance, which can progress to the full agoraphobic syndrome. The term "agoraphobia" is a misnomer. Instead of fearing the marketplace (agora) or open spaces, these patients experience anxiety in all situations in which they feel that escape may be difficult or embarrassing in case an attack occurs. The severity of agoraphobia ranges from distress with only mild or occasional avoidance of phobic situations to being completely housebound for decades. At this point there is no reliable way of predicting which patient will develop agoraphobia and to what degree. Although cases of agoraphobia without a prior history of panic attacks have been described, a careful history almost always reveals at least one spontaneous panic attack preceding the development of agoraphobia.

DIFFERENTIAL DIAGNOSIS

Many medical and psychiatric conditions present with the signs and symptoms of acute anxiety attacks.

These conditions must be systematically ruled out before the diagnosis of panic disorder can be made.

Thyroid Conditions. Both hypo- and hyperthyroidism may present in the early clinical stages as panic attacks without any of the typical symptoms of thyroid dysfunction. Thus, any patient with panic attacks should be screened with thyroid function tests.

Cardiovascular Disorders. Panic patients frequently complain of palpitations, skipped beats, and even chest pain. Mitral valve prolapse (MVP) may be more common in panic patients than in controls. Because chest pain and cardiac dysrhythmias can accompany some cases of MVP, panic disorder patients may have a higher rate of cardiac complaints than the general population. Significant cardiac pathology, however, is almost never found.

Certain arrhythmias can cause acute anxiety. An electrocardiogram is recommended in all patients over 40 years of age complaining of an anxiety attack to rule out acute myocardial ischemia. Paroxysmal atrial tachycardia has been found to cause panic-like symptoms. Twenty-four-hour cardiac monitoring, however, is almost invariably normal in panic patients.

Pheochromocytoma. The symptoms of this rare adrenal medullary tumor might be difficult to differentiate from those of an acute panic attack. Contrary to common belief, pheochromocytoma cannot be differentiated from anxiety on the basis of hypertension. The workup for pheochromocytoma requires determination of the total amount of catecholamine metabolites in the 24-hour urine sample. However, screening for pheochromocytoma is not recommended in all patients with anxiety attacks.

Hypoglycemia. During the 1950s, reactive or idiopathic hypoglycemia was thought to be responsible for almost all emotional disturbance. The elimination of carbohydrates from the American diet was seen as a solution to depression, hyperactivity, and anxiety. Today, few studies support the belief that low blood glucose level is the cause of any psychiatric illness.

Vertigo. Panic patients frequently experience lightheadedness, dizziness, and unsteady feeling but almost never true vertigo. If patients feel that the room or their body is spinning in the same direction with each attack, the differential diagnosis should include lesions of the cerebellum, brain stem, or eighth cranial nerve; acute labyrinthitis; benign positional vertigo; or Meniere's disease.

Substance Abuse. Patients in the midst of acute withdrawal may show symptoms that simulate acute panic attacks. Alcohol, barbiturate, or opiate withdrawal should be suspected and ruled out carefully. A number of patients experience their first panic attack during or immediately after cocaine or marijuana use, and some develop full-blown panic disorder.

Complex Partial Seizures. There is some overlap between the symptoms of panic and seizure disorders. Some seizure patients will become agoraphobic. Transient amnesia or incontinence during a panic attack should prompt a complete work-up for seizures.

TREATMENT

Essential to the successful treatment of panic disorder is blocking spontaneous panic attacks.

Once the attacks are blocked, the phobic avoidance may diminish automatically. Some patients with extensive agoraphobia require additional, primarily behavioral, therapy. Although the mechanism of panic blockade remains largely obscure, several classes of medications have well-established, specific properties of blocking spontaneous panic attacks. More recently, of the numerous psychotherapies claiming success, certain types of cognitive or behavioral treatments seem to emerge as potential alternatives to pharmacotherapy.

Medications

Tricyclic Antidepressants*

Although almost all antidepressants possess antipanic properties, the most systematically studied antipanic drug remains imipramine (Tofranil). After organic causes of anxiety have been ruled out and the patient has been educated to distinguish between spontaneous and situational panic, imipramine should be started in the patient with panic disorder. Approximately 20 per cent of panic patients are unusually sensitive to imipramine. This "hypersensitivity" response manifests as jitteriness, insomnia, and a "speeded up" feeling. For this reason patients should be started with 10 mg of imipramine and the dose raised by 10 mg every other day until a dose of 50 mg is reached. This regimen usually obviates the hypersensitivity reaction. If not, the dose can be lowered by 10 mg temporarily or benzodiazepines can be added. Because of its long half-life, the entire dose of imipramine can be administered once a day, usually at night. The average dose required is about 200 mg per day with a range from 10 to 400 mg per day.

If attacks are still occurring after 1 week of 50 mg of imipramine, the dose is raised more rapidly (by 25 mg every 2 to 3 days up to 150 mg daily). Patients who continue to panic have the dose raised by 50 mg every 3 to 4 days up to 300 mg. The exact rate of increase depends on the tolerance of the patient.

This treatment leads to complete elimination of panic attacks in more than 80 per cent of cases. Over subsequent weeks, anticipatory anxiety and phobic avoidance decline. Patients should be maintained with the highest dose of imipramine tolerable for 6 to 9 months after clinical remission. Most patients tolerate 200 to 300 mg of imipramine well, and there is little reason to reduce the dose. However, anticholinergic symptoms—constipation, dry mouth, difficulty with

erection—may require dosage reduction or switching to desipramine (Norpramin, Pertofrane). Desipramine appears to be an effective antipanic drug with fewer anticholinergic side effects than imipramine.

Approximately 15 per cent of patients with panic disorder are refractory to this regimen. We know of no associated clinical features that predict which patients will be affected. Several steps need to be taken with the refractory patient.

The most common reason for "failure" with the medication is that the patient is confusing anticipatory anxiety with panic attacks. Analysis of daily diaries and discussion with informed spouses, relatives, and friends can be helpful. Next, increasing the dose of imipramine above 300 mg should be considered. Before this is done, however, an electrocardiogram should be obtained and the imipramine level in the blood determined.

All tricyclic drugs lengthen the conduction intervals on the electrocardiogram, which is generally not a matter of concern. PR intervals over 0.20 and even incomplete right bundle branch block are not uncommon in patients taking therapeutic doses of imipramine. Increasing the dose of imipramine above 300 mg, however, may increase the chances of inducing more serious heart block. Hence, patients who already have increased PR or QRS intervals at 300 mg of imipramine should probably not take a higher dose. If conduction intervals are normal, the dose can safely be raised to 350 mg and a repeat electrocardiogram obtained.

In terms of toxicity, it appears that a QRS interval higher than 0.10 is a far better indicator of toxicity than the blood level of imipramine. Hence, obtaining the imipramine level in the blood is intended only to identify those patients who have unusually low blood levels, which probably indicates an idiosyncratically rapid hepatic metabolism of the drug. We have seen patients who continue to panic while taking 300 mg but respond to 350 or even 400 mg. There is no good evidence that doses above 400 mg are clinically useful.

A "novel" antidepressant fluoxetine (Prozac), acting primarily on the serotonergic system, appears to be a good alternative for patients who cannot tolerate the anticholinergic side effects of the tricyclics. After the initial hypersensitivity reaction, the drug is well tolerated at a dose ranging from 20 to 80 mg per day.

Monoamine oxidase inhibitors (MAOIs)*

MAOI drugs are now making a comeback in clinical practice. Many patients who are refrac-

---

*This use is not listed by the manufacturer.

*This use is not listed by the manufacturer.

tory to imipramine respond to MAOIs. Because of the absolute need to place the patient on a special MAO diet, however, these drugs are not the first choice for treating panic disorder. Although some authors assert that adding MAOIs to a tricyclic antidepressant is a safe procedure, we recommend discontinuing imipramine over a 2-week period before starting phenelzine (Nardil) at 30 mg daily. The dose can be divided initially to reduce side effects, but ultimately the total amount can be taken at once, usually in the morning. The dose is increased to between 45 and 90 mg in a manner similar to that for imipramine until the attacks are completely blocked. The usual effective dose of another MAOI, tranylcypromine (Parnate), is between 30 and 60 mg* daily.

In starting an MAOI, the clinician must warn the patient about the serious risk of toxicity if the special monoamine oxidase diet is not maintained, must review the diet list in detail, and must explain how the enzyme monoamine oxidase works and what tyramine is. Certain medications, including sympathomimetics and meperidine, must be avoided. For unclear reasons, the clinican must never switch a patient from one MAOI to another without at least a 2-week drug-free hiatus. MAOIs are safe if the patient is compliant.

Common side effects include insomnia, restlessness, euphoria, weight gain, various sexual dysfunctions, muscle aches or twitching, and orthostatic hypotension. Proper management techniques include switching the timing of the drug, reducing the dose, adding pyridoxine, and increasing fluid or salt intake.

Benzodiazepines

Recently, it has been shown that alprazolam (Xanax)† is an effective antipanic medication. Patients often begin to respond to alprazolam within the first week, whereas response is rare to the other drugs in fewer than 3 to 4 weeks. Alprazolam has no cardiovascular or anticholinergic effects, little potential for causing suicide, no special dietary requirements, and appears to effectively reduce anticipatory anxiety as well as the actual panic attack.

Alprazolam has some disadvantages compared with tricyclic antidepressants. First, it has been shown to be disinhibiting in some patients, leading to unexpected and sometimes dangerous behavior. Second, it has a relatively short half-life (5 to 10 hours) so that it must be taken at least three or four times daily to be effective. Finally,

and most troublesome, patients frequently have difficulty during tapering of alprazolam. In our experience, panic attacks recur during the tapering phase of alprazolam more frequently than with either imipramine or phenelzine. In addition, many patients complain of severe withdrawal symptoms, including agitation, insomnia, derealization, and tremulousness.

Alprazolam should be used in situations in which there are medical contraindications to taking either imipramine or desipramine. This might apply to patients with significant cardiovascular disease or with medical problems that make administering anticholinergic drugs dangerous. Doses up to 6 mg,* or even more, are often necessary to block panic completely.

In the occasional patient in whom panic attacks are so severe that the clinician believes that a rapidly acting drug is necessary, a low dose of alprazolam might be given for 1 or 2 weeks while imipramine is concomitantly started. These doses usually do not exceed 0.5 mg four times a day. This therapy usually does not completely block the attacks but attenuates their severity. Then, when the patient is stabilized with therapeutic doses of imipramine, the alprazolam is slowly discontinued by reducing it 0.5 mg every 4 days.

Although dosage schedules are not yet well established, clonazepam (Klonopin†), a long-acting (half-life 20 to 40 hours) benzodiazepine, has also been reported to block panic attacks.

Psychotherapy

Most psychotherapies are unsuccessful in blocking panic attacks. Traditional behavioral techniques, such as desensitization, flooding, or exposure both individually or in groups, can be helpful for patients with extensive and/or refractory phobic avoidance. More recently, a specific cognitive or behavioral treatment has been shown to block panic attacks. The treatment is based on the theory that panic patients are vulnerable to perceived internal and external events as uncontrollable, unpredictable, and dangerous. To correct this the clinician uses breathing retraining, interoceptive exposure, and cognitive restructuring within the framework of time-limited (10 to 15 sessions), structured, individual treatment sessions. If its comparative efficacy with pharmacotherapy is established, cognitive or behavioral treatment would become a viable and preferrable nonpharmacologic alternative in the treatment of panic disorder.

---

*This dose may exceed manufacturer's recommended dose.
†This use is not listed by the manufacturer.

*This dose may exceed manufacturer's recommended dose.
†This use is not listed by the manufacturer.

Physical and Chemical Injuries

BURNS

method of
JOHN L. HUNT, M.D., and
GARY F. PURDUE, M.D.
Southwestern Medical School
Dallas, Texas

More than 2.5 million people in the United States sustain a thermal injury each year of sufficient magnitude to require medical attention. More than 100,000 people are hospitalized and in excess of 12,000 die as a direct result of this injury. Time away from work, lost revenue, rehabilitation time, and the psychologic impact are major problems the victim must overcome after discharge.

The severity of the thermal injury depends on the amount of heat and the time of exposure of the skin surface. It is often difficult to assess burn depth accurately in the first 24 hours after the injury. Although burns are often divided into first, second, and third degree, more recent nomenclature identifies two classes. (1) *Partial-thickness* burns involve only the epidermis and the dermis. Skin regeneration will occur, and, depending on the depth, the burn may be treated either conservatively or with surgical excision and skin grafting. The latter is often done because of the time it takes to heal and the severe scarring associated with spontaneous healing of deep partial-thickness burns. (2) *Full-thickness*, or third-degree, burns involve the entire thickness of the skin. All skin appendages are destroyed. Ultimately, skin grafting must be done to close the wound.

EMERGENCY CARE

The burn victim must be considered to be a trauma victim. A primary survey including the ABC's (airway, breathing, and circulation) must be carried out initially to identify and treat any life-threatening conditions. Approximately 5 per cent of victims of high-speed motor vehicle accidents have an associated thermal injury. Therefore, immobilization of the cervical spine may be indicated at the scene of the accident.

A severe inhalation injury or carbon monoxide intoxication may be the cause of respiratory arrest requiring that cardiopulmonary resuscitation and even emergency airway intubation be instituted in the field. If possible, expeditious insertion of a large-bore intravenous catheter is advisable to begin resuscitation, but if the patient is within 20 to 30 minutes of a hospital, it is best to transport the patient immediately to that facility and eliminate the delay associated with initiation of intravenous therapy. All patients should be administered either nasal or mask oxygen during transportation. Wound coverage need be with only a sterile or clean sheet. The patient must be kept warm.

The American Burn Association has established the following criteria for referral of a patient to a burn center:

1. Partial- and full-thickness burns
   a. > 10 per cent total body surface area
      i. < 10 years and > 50 years
   b. > 20 per cent
      i. All other age groups
         Face, eyes, ears, hands, feet, genitalia, perineum, and major joints
2. Full-thickness burn > 5 per cent in any location
3. Electric burns, including lightning
4. Chemical burns
5. Burns with associated significant fractures or other organ injury
6. Inhalation injury
7. Burns plus significant pre-existing disease

TREATMENT

Patients with all other types of burns can be treated adequately as outpatients. The burn wound should initially be débrided of all loose skin and blisters everywhere except on the hand where they are left intact for the patient's comfort. The wound is cleaned with a mild soap and washed with isotonic saline solution or tap water. It is then covered with a topical antimicrobial agent, such as silver sulfadiazine, and a bulky dressing. Burned extremities should be kept elevated. All burns should be followed up within 24 to 48 hours of injury to assess the condition of the burn wound and burn depth and to evaluate for possible infection. Prophylactic antibiotics are not used for routine outpatient burn care.

Burns of the face and the ears are not wrapped with an occlusive dressing but are treated by an open method with an antibiotic ointment such as a polymyxin or bacitracin. A tetanus booster is administered to all burn patients if they have not had one in the last 5 years. If there has been no previous immunization, both hyperimmune tetanus globulin, 250 units, and a booster dose of 0.5 ml of tetanus toxoid are administered intramuscularly, followed by a booster dose at 1 and 2 months after the injury.

Burn wound cellulitis is an infrequent complication of outpatient treatment of burns. Clinically, it is associated with a low-grade temperature, wound edema, erythema, and pain. When cellulitis occurs, the topical antimicrobial agent, if it is not silver sulfadiazine, is removed and replaced with this cream and an appropriate broad-spectrum antibiotic is administered (usually a first-generation cephalosporin).

EMERGENCY ROOM MANAGEMENT

The patient must be completely undressed to evaluate the extent of burn injury. The estimation of burn size is based on the total amount of both partial- and full-thickness injury and excludes first-degree burns. Figure 1 shows the "rule of nines" for estimating percentage of total body surface area burn (TBSA). Because of the disproportion of the surface area–to–weight ratio in a child, the Lund and Browder chart is used for ages up to 15 years (Figure 2).

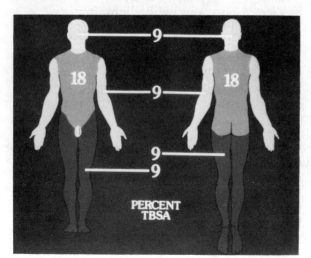

Figure 1. Rule of nines for estimation of percentage of total body surface area burn.

The average burn patient presents in an agitated, generally alert, hyperventilating state. Obtundation, disorientation, or confusion may be caused by hypoxia or carbon monoxide intoxication. Therefore, arterial blood gas analysis must be performed. One or two large-bore (16 gauge) intravenous lines are inserted through either burned or unburned skin. The subclavian intravenous route is discouraged because a pneumothorax would be devastating in a patient with an inhalation injury. Central lines are for *monitoring,* not resuscitation. Otherwise, central sites are saved for intravenous hyperalimentation. All intravenous lines are changed every 3 days to minimize the risk of suppurative thrombophlebitis. A Foley's catheter and nasogastric tube are inserted. Analgesia is given intravenously, not intramuscularly. The intramuscular route may be associated with erratic and unpredictable absorption of medication because of peripheral vasoconstriction and hypovolemia.

FLUID RESUSCITATION

Most burn patients can be adequately resuscitated. Only a minority, those with burns less than 5 per cent and more than 85 per cent TBSA, do not respond to resuscitation regardless of how much fluid is administered. Burn injury, particularly if more than 30 per cent TBSA, is associated with a generalized disruption of capillary integrity resulting in increased vascular permeability and loss of electrolyte and protein-rich fluid. A generalized capillary leak, which is greatest in the area of the burn injury, occurs almost immediately after the injury. Red blood cells remain within the intravascular space resulting in hemoconcentration, increased blood viscosity, and capillary thrombosis, unless the patient is promptly and adequately resuscitated. The capillary leak is greatest in the first 8 hours after the burn. Because of this leak, colloid does not remain within the intravascular space, and therefore Ringer's lactate is the recommended resuscitation fluid. Crystaloid, 2 to 4 ml per kg per percentage of TBSA burn, is administered in the first 24 hours. One-half of the calculated amount is given during the first 8 hours, and the remaining amount is given over the next 16 hours. In general, any adult with a burn of 15 per cent TBSA or greater or child with a burn greater than 10 per cent TBSA requires intravenous fluid resuscitation.

Close patient monitoring, usually hourly, is necessary to evaluate the adequacy of resuscitation. This assessment is best done by maintaining an hourly urine output of 0.5 ml per kg per hour in an adult and 1 ml per kg per hour in a child. Despite adequate resuscitation, hemoconcentra-

AREA	AGE-YEARS					% 2°	% 3°	% TOTAL
	0–1	1–4	5–9	10–15	ADULT			
Head	19	17	13	10	7			
Neck	2	2	2	2	2			
Ant. Trunk	13	17	13	13	13			
Post. Trunk	13	13	13	13	13			
R. Buttock	2½	2½	2½	2½	2½			
L. Buttock	2½	2½	2½	2½	2½			
Genitalia	1	1	1	1	1			
R.U. Arm	4	4	4	4	4			
L.U. Arm	4	4	4	4	4			
R.L. Arm	3	3	3	3	3			
L.L. Arm	3	3	3	3	3			
R. Hand	2½	2½	2½	2½	2½			
L. Hand	2½	2½	2½	2½	2½			
R. Thigh	5½	6½	8½	8½	9½			
L. Thigh	5½	6½	8½	8½	9½			
R. Leg	5	5	5½	6	7			
L. Leg	5	5	5½	6	7			
R. Foot	3½	3½	3½	3½	3½			
L. Foot	3½	3½	3½	3½	3½			
					Total			

Figure 2. Lund and Browder Chart (From Lund CC and Browder NC: Surg Gynecol Obstet 79:352, 1944. By permission of Surgery, Gynecology & Obstetrics.)

tion, which is reflected by a rising hematocrit, will occur. Therefore, serial hematocrit determinations are not adequate to evaluate the patient's response to resuscitation. Other parameters to follow include mentation, blood pressure, and pulse.

By 24 hours after the burn, the capillary leak has sealed and colloid remains within the intravascular space. At this time the plasma volume deficit, which was not corrected with the administration of crystalloid, can be corrected by the use of fresh-frozen plasma, 0.5 ml per kg per TBSA. The plasma furnishes clotting factors, which are decreased in the early postburn period. Plasma is administered over a 2- to 4-hour period. Potassium is not administered in the first 24 hours postburn. At the end of the first 24 hours postburn, salt infusion is no longer necessary in the adult; 5 per cent dextrose in water is given to replace evaporative losses (a rule of thumb is 1.0 ml per kg per per cent TBSA). The serum sodium level should be maintained at about 135 mEq per liter.

In the child younger than 3 years of age, the resuscitation requirements are unique because of the discrepancy between surface area and weight, which is different from that of the adult. Fluid requirements are based on the formula 3 to 4 ml per kg per per cent TBSA for the first 24 hours. *Fluid for maintenance must be added* to this calculated amount. The physician should give 100 ml of Ringer's lactate per kg for the first 10 kg, 50 ml of Ringer's lactate per kg for the second 10 kg, and then 20 ml for each additional kilogram. After the first 24 hours, the pediatric patient is given a small amount of salt in the maintenance fluid with 5 per cent dextrose in 0.25 N saline.

In a child younger than 1 year of age, especially one younger than 6 months, hypoglycemia can be a lethal complication within the first few hours of a burn. Children of this age have a limited amount of glycogen stored in the liver, and after several hours of burn stress, glucogen is depleted. Consequently, hourly monitoring of serum glucose by dipstick is mandatory. Alterations in the clinical status of the patient, such as lethargy, obtundation, or increased irritability, may indicate hypoglycemia.

Common clinical circumstances associated with fluid requirements in excess of the calculated amounts are (1) delayed resuscitation, (2) inadequate initial volume replacement, (3) inhalation injury, (4) extremely deep (fourth-degree) burns, (5) electrical injuries, and (6) burn with associated trauma.

CIRCUMFERENTIAL BURNS

A circumferential full-thickness eschar may cause vascular ischemia of both underlying and distal tissues, which may be manifested within 4 to 6 hours of burn injury. The earliest signs of impending ischemia are numbness and tingling. Absence of pulse is a late sign of tissue ischemia. Because of overlying eschar or edema, pulses may not be palpable, and a Doppler ultrasonic flow meter is used to assess tissue perfusion. This assessment is done every 30 minutes to 1 hour during the first 24 hours postburn. In the upper extremity, the superficial palmer arch of the hand is monitored to determine the need for escharotomy. In the feet, both the dorsalis pedes and posterior tibial pulses are monitored. When an escharotomy is necessary, both medial and lateral incisions on the extremity are carried out from the most proximal to the most distal portion of the burn. The incisions are carried down through the superficial fascia and across the wrist if the hand is burned or across the ankle if the foot is burned. Electrocautery is used to minimize bleeding.

INHALATION INJURY

The incidence of an inhalation injury may be more than 15 per cent in large TBSA burns. Mortality in patients with a significant inhalation injury is uniformly between 50 and 85 per cent. There are two types of inhalation injury: (1) upper airway obstruction secondary to edema from the injury, which is accentuated by the fluid administered during resuscitation, and (2) small airway damage, which is manifested 48 to 72 hours after the injury and which causes progressive pulmonary insufficiency associated with deteriorating Pa_{O_2} and a worsening of findings on chest x-ray film. Acute upper airway obstruction can occur as early as 2 to 4 hours postburn. If airway patency is not maintained, acute upper airway obstruction and asphyxia occur. An inhalation injury can be suspected with the following: (1) a history of injury in a closed space; (2) singed nasal and eyebrow hair; (3) facial edema, oral erythema, edema, or hoarseness; (4) carbonaceous sputum; and (5) bronchorrhea and/or wheezing. If the arterial carbon monoxide level is higher than 15 per cent or if Po_2 in room air is less than 65 mmHg, inhalation injury should be suspected. All patients should be treated with 100 per cent oxygen, which reduces the carboxyhemoglobin level by one-half in approximately 40 minutes. If significant upper airway injury is suspected, "prophylactic" intubation should be performed to prevent acute upper airway occlusion from rapid formation of edema. Fiberoptic bronchoscopy is ideal to both diagnose the injury and aid in intubation of the patient. Bronchoscopic criteria of an inhalation injury include

mucosal ulceration, edema, erythema, bronchorrhea, and carbonaceous sputum. The chest x-ray film is usually normal on admission and will remain so for the first 24 to 48 hours postburn. Bronchodilators are used if wheezing is present. Prophylactic antibiotics and steroids are contraindicated in the burn patient with an inhalation injury because they promote the emergence of resistant microbes and increase the incidence of sepsis.

ELECTRICAL BURNS

Electrical burns are arbitrarily classed as either high-voltage (more than 1000 volts) injury or low-voltage injury. Generally, low voltage involves household-type exposure and causes minimal deep tissue injury. A common low-voltage injury occurs when a child bites on an electric cord and sustains burns of the mouth. These injuries are generally treated conservatively on an outpatient basis, with late reconstruction if necessary. The cardiac abnormalities associated with electrical burns are usually manifested either at the scene of the accident or soon thereafter. Cardiac evaluation should consist of a 12-lead electrocardiogram and continuous monitoring in the emergency room. If no cardiac abnormalities are present during this evaluation, 24-hour cardiac monitoring is not necessary. If cardiac abnormalities are noted during this period and they are treated appropriately, the patient is monitored for 24 hours. There is a poor correlation between myocardial enzymes and electrocardiogram abnormalities. A low incidence of myocardial damage is associated with electrical burns.

The high-voltage electrical burn is similar to a crush injury. Although the cutaneous manifestations may be minimal, soft tissue damage is often devastating. The presence of pigment (either hemoglobin or myoglobin) in the urine indicates underlying muscle damage. The extent of cutaneous burn injury is a poor indicator of the total amount of resuscitation fluid required for the patient with an electrical injury. In the electrically burned patient with underlying muscle damage, an unknown quantity of additional fluid is required. Ringer's lactate is the resuscitation fluid of choice. Mannitol, 25 grams, is given as an intravenous bolus to establish an immediate osmotic diuresis. This treatment is immediately followed by two ampules (88 mEq) of sodium bicarbonate, which is in turn followed by Ringer's lactate at a rate sufficient to maintain a urine output of approximately 100 ml per hour. This initial alkalinization of the urine minimizes precipitation of pigment in the renal tubules. Once the urine is grossly clear, intravenous rates may be adjusted to maintain a urine output of 50 ml per hour. The presence of myoglobinuria or hemoglobinuria indicates nonviable muscle, and fasciotomy of all compartments of affected extremities may be needed. This procedure should be performed in the operating room with the patient under general anesthesia to minimize ischemic damage in adjacent areas of viable muscle caused by compartment syndromes. The topical agent of choice for electrical injuries is mafenide acetate (Sulfamylon). This agent diffuses into deep tissues and provides adequate antimicrobial levels. Systemic antibiotic coverage of both anaerobic and aerobic bacteria is given intravenously until all nonviable tissue is removed. A technetium-99m stannous pyrophosphate muscle scan accurately identifies the extent of muscle damage within the first 48 hours after injury and provides a guide for surgical exploration. Serial neurologic examinations should be performed on all high-voltage electrical injury patients for up to 2 years. There is a significant risk both early and late (up to 2 years) after injury of neuromuscular dysfunction, spasticity, paresis, and paralysis. For medicolegal reasons, spinal and regional anesthesia should be avoided in these patients. Ocular cataracts may occur in both the early and late postburn periods and are usually associated with burns of the head and upper torso.

CHEMICAL BURNS

The severity of the chemical burn is related directly to length of time that a given agent is exposed to the skin. Patients sustaining chemical burns must have all clothing removed and copious tap water lavage begun on affected areas. Medical personnel must wear protective gloves. After transport to an emergency facility, lavage should be continued in a shower. As a general rule, almost all chemical burns can be treated with water. Exact identification of the burning chemical may suggest appropriate specific measures, but an acid should not be neutralized with a base or vice versa. If there is any suspicion that the chemical entered the eyes, irrigation of the eyes should be continued for a minimum of 20 to 30 minutes. After irrigation with tap water, treatment of chemical burns is identical to that of a thermal injury. The exact depth of the chemical burn is difficult to determine by its initial gross clinical appearance; it is often 5 to 7 days before the depth of the burn becomes apparent. The depth is often greater than thought initially, with alkali injuries generally being worse than acid injuries.

BURN MANAGEMENT

Significant bacterial colonization of the burn wound does not generally occur before the fifth postburn day, if appropriate wound débridement and coverage with a topical antimicrobial agent are instituted promptly. Topical antimicrobial agents are the mainstay of burn care. Although no topical agent sterilizes the burn wound, bacterial growth is minimized. Silver sulfadiazine (Silvadene) is the initial topical agent of choice because of its broad antibacterial spectrum and lack of significant complications. Eschar penetration is moderate. A thin (1.5 to 3 mm), even layer is applied with a sterile, gloved hand every 8 to 12 hours. Leukopenia, which is unrelated to either burn size or burn depth, has been rarely noted. Occasionally, allergy may require use of an alternative form of therapy.

Mafenide acetate has excellent penetration of eschar, thereby achieving effective concentration at the interface between viable and nonviable tissue. It is the agent of choice to treat *Pseudomonas aeruginosa* infections. Mafenide acetate inhibits carbonic anhydrase, which decreases urinary bicarbonate reabsorption and may result in a metabolic acidosis. The patient usually hyperventilates to compensate for this, but pulmonary complications such as bronchopneumonia may cause insufficient pulmonary compensation. Mafenide acetate causes pain when applied on partial-thickness wounds and has an allergy rate of about 10 per cent. It is the agent of choice for electrical burns with underlying damaged muscle and for fourth-degree burns.

Continual surveillance of the burn wound for bacterial infection is mandatory (done three times a week) to identify infection at the earliest possible time. Quantitative wound biopsies are performed on full-thickness injuries; contact plate cultures are done on partial-thickness burns. Quantitative bacterial counts of 10^5 organisms or more per gram of tissue represent burn wound sepsis, the harbinger of septicemia. Lower quantitative counts in patients with large surface area burns may also represent a significant overall bacterial wound inoculum, with subsequent risk of sepsis. Cellulitis adjacent to a burn wound is often the earliest sign of burn wound infection. Cellulitis characteristically appears on the fifth to seventh postburn day and is often associated with minimal systemic symptoms. A wound culture should be obtained. In the absence of clinical illness, an antimicrobial agent that is effective against gram-positive organisms (usually a first-generation cephalosporin) is administered until specific organisms are cultured. An increase of two logarithm counts in bacterial concentration between two successive biopsies warrants close re-evaluation of both topical and systemic antimicrobial therapy.

The hypermetabolic burn patient often metabolizes aminoglycoside antibiotics extremely rapidly and requires two to two and one-half times the recommended dose to achieve adequate peak and trough serum levels. Any burn patient receiving a nephrotoxic drug must have frequent determinations of serum drug levels, serum creatinine levels, and creatinine clearance.

Burn Wound Closure

The goal of burn therapy is early wound closure. In general, the longer the burn wound remains open and unhealed, the greater the risk of infection and of rehabilitative and cosmetic complications.

Partial-Thickness (Second-Degree) Burns. Partial-thickness burns may take 2 to 6 weeks to heal spontaneously. Many of these wounds can be closed immediately by application of a biologic dressing directly to the burn wound after initial débridement. Porcine xenograft or Biobrane is especially effective for these burns and results in significant improvement in patient comfort. Pain is diminished, as are evaporative water loss and protein losses. As re-epithelialization occurs, the overlying biologic dressing lifts off from the healed wound and can be trimmed. If this dressing is adherent 24 hours later, re-epithelialization will generally occur within 2 weeks and surgical intervention is unwarranted. Conservative management includes twice daily applications of an antimicrobial cream and whirlpool therapy for wounds of indeterminate depth.

Full-Thickness (Third-Degree) Burns. Full-thickness burns, unless extremely small (smaller than 2 to 3 cm), must ultimately be autografted. Conservative treatment allowing natural separation of the eschar by underlying bacterial autolysis may require weeks because of effective topical antimicrobial therapy. Consequently, nearly all third-degree burns are treated by early surgical excision and grafting.

Burn Wound Excision

Early burn wound excision is performed on all deep partial-thickness and full-thickness burns. Deep partial-thickness burns are difficult to identify in the early postburn period. These wounds are tangentially excised with a Humby's or Goullian-Weck knife. This technique involves sequential excision of eschar in thin layers until the underlying viable dermal bed is reached, as evidenced by uniform, diffuse, punctate bleeding. Hemostasis is obtained by the application of top-ical thrombin, hot laparotomy packs, and compression. Autograft, 0.010 to 0.012 inches thick, is obtained from selected donor sites and immediately applied either unmeshed or meshed at a ratio of 1.5:1 to the excised wound. Meshed graft has the advantages of wider coverage and minimal subgraft accumulation of serum or blood at the expense of worse scar appearance. Blood loss is minimized when excising burns on extremities by the proximal application of a blood pressure cuff tourniquet. Full-thickness burns are excised tangentially as just described to viable deeper tissues or are excised to viable fascia with a scalpel or electrocautery. Sheet or meshed autograft is then applied depending on the availability of donor sites. Excision to fascia results in significant cosmetic and functional deformity. Large burns (more than 30 per cent body surface area) usually require staged excision. Burns of between 10 and 15 per cent body surface area are excised and autografted at one time. All third-degree eschar is excised first. With limited available donor sites, either cadaver allograft or Biobrane is applied as temporary coverage to the wound bed. Autografting is usually begun at the first procedure rather than waiting until all eschar has been excised. Autograft is meshed at a ratio of 2:1 to 4:1 depending on donor site availability. Autograft meshed more than 3:1 is then overlaid with either Biobrane or allograft. The graft is then covered with an antibiotic-impregnated gauze and a bulky compressive dressing. This overlay technique permits coverage of the exposed wound interstices in the meshed graft until complete re-epithelialization occurs.

Excision of large burns requires a specialized team to achieve optimal results. Operative time is limited to approximately 2 hours because blood loss may be massive and intraoperative hypothermia can occur rapidly. Raising operating room temperature to above 80° F lessens the risk of hypothermia. In pediatric patients, both the percentage of burn excised and the operative time are reduced. Excision of large burns should be undertaken only in a hospital offering good blood bank support and ready availability of homograft.

NUTRITIONAL SUPPORT

Post-traumatic metabolic response of the patient with a major burn consists of a severe catabolic state characterized by hypermetabolism, weight loss, and protein wasting. Aggressive nutritional support must be provided to all burned patients, especially those with a burn larger than 35 per cent TBSA. The hypermetabolic response is even greater in the patient who is stressed with surgery or associated sepsis. An approximation of the caloric requirements is obtained by multiplying the Harris-Benedict equation by 1.5. A nitrogen/calorie ratio of 1:150 is maintained. Indirect calorimetry at the bedside provides a method of realistically evaluating these needs. Use of a metabolic cart to measure oxygen consumption and carbon dioxide production allows exact determination of caloric needs.

When possible, nutritional support is always begun by the oral route. If this method supplies insufficient calories, enteral tube feedings are added. If this treatment still is inadequate, intravenous hyperalimentation is begun. Ideally, nutrition is begun within the first 24 hours of the burn and maintained throughout the postburn course with minimal disruption. Twice weekly nutritional assessment, including caloric counts and patient weight, is imperative in all patients with large burns.

REHABILITATION

Patient rehabilitation is begun soon after admission to the hospital. Initial evaluation and assessment by the physical and occupational therapy team evaluate the need for splints, appropriate positioning, and institution of both active and passive range-of-motion exercises. An overall treatment plan is developed and carried out through the patient's hospital course. This program should be continually re-evaluated to ensure maximal potential recovery and return to the best possible functional status.

DISTURBANCES CAUSED BY COLD

method of
FAITH T. FITZGERALD, M.D.
University of California, Davis
Sacramento, California

HYPOTHERMIA

Human hypothermia has been arbitrarily defined as a rectal temperature less than 95° F. Although hypothermia is seen principally in winter and in cold climates, even physicians practicing in temperate climates encounter this often puzzling condition. Advances in the understanding and therapy of hypothermia have led to a decrease in mortality. Compared with an 80 per cent mortality in 1960, mortality currently ranges between about 6 and 75 per cent, depending on the severity of the underlying disease predisposing to the hypothermia.

Fundamental pathophysiology of hypothermia

involves exposure (although it need not be to severe cold, but only to an ambient temperature of less than 98.6° F), caloric restriction (because calories are the major source of heat in endotherms), or, most commonly, abnormalities in thermoregulation caused by drugs or disease. Maintenance of body heat in mammals is mediated by hypothalamic thermoregulators and sensory receptors in the skin. Retention of body heat depends on the integrity of the dermal covering, layers of insulation (fat), and restriction of blood flow to the skin. Body heat is generated by conversion of mechanical to caloric energy by muscle movement, as well as by intrinsic metabolic processes. Loss of heat occurs by conduction, convection, and evaporation. Exposure, central nervous system disease, thermoregulatory dysfunction through vasodilation of the skin, excess sweating, and muscle immobility, as well as mixed causes, are the underlying pathogeneses of human hypothermia. The causes of hypothermia are given in Table 1.

Acute hypothermia, such as may occur with immersion in cold water, may protect the organism, because metabolic consumption of oxygen declines rapidly as body temperature falls. The physician must, therefore, remember that even patients who appear to be dead because of prolonged anoxia (as in 45 minutes of immersion at the bottom of a cold lake) may be able to be resuscitated. It is well to keep in mind, in both acute and chronic hypothermia, the clinical ax-

TABLE 1. **Causes of Hypothermia**

Exposure (need not be to marked cold) plus:

Central nervous system disease
  Brain tumor, injury, seizure
  Cord transection
  Hypoglycemia
  Thiamine deficiency
  Hepatic failure
  Drugs

Interference with vasoconstriction
  Drugs (alcohol, bethanechol, phenothiazines)
  Sepsis
  Erythroderma
  Burns

Interference with muscle movement
  Paresis, paralysis
  Extremes of age
  Drugs (alcohol, phenothiazines, narcotics, barbiturates)
  Hypothyroidism

Mixed causes
  Starvation, cachexia
  Adrenal insufficiency
  Acute myocardial infarction
  Hypothyroidism
  Hypopituitarism

iom "Not dead until warm and dead," because many of the physical manifestations of hypothermia are similar to those of death.

Stages

Animal studies and experience with human hypothermia have led to a clinical categorization of chronic hypothermic patients into three major phases based on body temperature.

1. *Responsive phase (95° to 90° F).* In this range, characteristic of mild exposure in the elderly, for example, the intact organism makes physiologic adjustments to retain and generate heat. Shivering occurs, blood pressure and pulse increase, and cutaneous vasoconstriction forces volume into the central circulation, precipitating diuresis. Early volume loss may become important therapeutically if hypothermia progresses.

2. *Slowing phase (89° to 75° F).* In this range, enzyme kinetics slow, decreasing the patient's ability to generate heat. Muscles grow stiffer, gross shivering decreases to a fine tremor, and blood pressure, pulse, and respirations may all fall. The majority of chronically hypothermic patients tend to be in this range.

3. *Poikilothermic phase (below 75° F).* In this range, patients are very cold. They now lose heat as would an inanimate object. In this range the differential diagnosis is death.

Hypothermic Review of Systems

Systemic effects that occur in the hypothermic patient are given in Table 2. In general, the hypothermia victim can look like a corpse—immobile, cold, and stiff to the touch. It may be

TABLE 2. **Pathophysiologic Changes That May Occur in the Temperature Range 90°–75° F**

Decreased respiration, pulse
Cold, dry, pale skin
Tissue edema
Depressed hearing, pupillary reflexes
Generalized muscle rigidity
Aspiration, bronchorrhea, pulmonary edema
Arrhythmias
Hemoconcentration, microvascular sludging and infarcts
Increased creatine kinase level (with myocardial bands)
Coagulopathy
Increased amylase level and pancreatitis
Gastrointestinal bleeding
Decreased bowel sounds
Decreased glomerular filtration rate
Decreased urine-concentrating capacity
Renal glycosuria
Prerenal azotemia
Acute tubular necrosis
Depressed consciousness
Depressed deep tendon reflexes
Decreased drug metabolism

necessary to use a thermocouple rectal probe or a specially designed low-reading thermometer for proper diagnosis because many clinical thermometers in use in emergency rooms do not record temperatures below 94° F. Rectal temperatures as low as 50° F have been recorded in patients who have subsequently survived. Respiratory rates may be depressed or increased. Blood pressure tends to fall with a progressive drop in temperature, or blood pressure obtained by sphygmomanometer may be factitiously low because of intensive peripheral vasoconstriction induced by the cold state. The pulse rate tends to slow below 90° F, with atrial fibrillation and a slow ventricular response occurring as one approaches 80° F and ventricular fibrillation or asystole occurring below 80° F. There is no direct, predictable correlation between depth of hypothermia and pulse rate, however. Atrial fibrillation is the most common hypothermic arrhythmia in humans, but the risk of ventricular fibrillation increases as the temperature drops below 86° F and is probably greatest between 70 and 75° F.

The skin gives clues to the disorder predisposing to hypothermia, such as uremia, starvation, hepatic failure, alcoholism, or erythroderma. Although the skin of the hyothermic person is cold, dry, and pale, there may also be a generalized edema, perhaps caused by cold-induced loss of cell membrane integrity and the shift of intravascular fluid into skin. Tissue edema in the hypothermic patient, therefore, cannot be used to testify to total volume status.

A careful search for head trauma should be made in all stuporous patients, whether hypothermic or not. Neurologic examination is made more difficult in the hypothermic patient, however, by the cold-induced decrease in or blockage of pupillary reflexes, decreased response to hearing, and neck muscle rigidity, which may mimic meningismus. Examination of the neck should obviously include a search for a palpable goiter or a thyroidectomy scar.

Respiratory infection is common in hypothermia because of cold-induced depression of the cough reflex, reduction in vital capacity, diminished consciousness, and thickening of bronchial secretions from dehydration. Cold bronchorrhea is the response of the tracheal bronchial tree to cold and involves the production of thick, copious secretions. This can further predispose to atelectasis and aspiration. A noncardiogenic pulmonary edema may occur in hypothermia.

Assessment of pulmonary status on admission depends on the physician's awareness of the proper interpretation of arterial blood gas measurements in the hypothermic patient. There is considerable controversy about whether or not the blood gases should be corrected for the hypothermic state because the laboratory automatically warms the blood sample to normal body temperature as the measurements are made. This warming tends to decrease the pH and increase the P_{CO_2} and P_{O_2} above the warmed solution. The patient is, therefore, less acidemic, less hypercarbic, and less well oxygenated than appears from the uncorrected gas measurements. Others have argued that corrected values cannot be properly interpreted without knowing the normal values at the patient's reported temperature, and that the pH, P_{CO_2}, and bicarbonate are true values, regardless of the temperature of the patient. Moreover, because different temperatures may exist in the hypothermic human (blood, rectal, bladder, and esophageal temperatures often vary by several degrees), there is no "true" temperature to use in correction. For this reason, it is recommended that blood gas values be reported in uncorrected form and that principal attention be paid to the pH, trying to maintain it at 7.4 in the uncorrected state. It is well to remember that even if the gases show significant hypoxemia, cold protects the victim by decreasing tissue oxygen requirements.

Cardiovascular volume is depleted in most chronically hypothermic patients. This volume depletion may lead to hemoconcentration, which, along with the increased viscosity of cold plasma and circulatory slowing, can result in intravascular sludging and microvascular occlusion.

Both skeletal and cardiac creatine phosphokinase and lactate dehydrogenase levels may be elevated in the hypothermic patient in consequence of a tissue leak of intramuscular enzymes because of the cold-induced loss of cell membrane integrity. These elevations may also be caused by vaso-occlusive myocardial damage; histopathologic studies of the hypothermic heart at autopsy have shown microinfarcts, fatty change, and subendocardial hemorrhage. Electrocardiographic changes in hypothermic humans include increases in the PR and QT intervals, nodal rhythm, and the classic (although not pathognomonic) "camel hump" sign of Osborn, also called the "J wave."

The bowel becomes hypomotile in the cold, with a decrease in bowel sounds. This condition, associated with the rigid musculature of the abdominal wall, may make clinical assessment of the abdomen difficult. Gastric submucosal hemorrhage and erosion may be present at autopsy, although significant gastrointestinal bleeding from hypothermia alone is rare. Platelet levels may be low in hypothermia as a result of sequestration in the liver and spleen, and volume constriction in the hypothermic patient may falsely elevate the hematocrit. Hypothermia blunts both exocrine and endocrine pancreatic functions, and hemorrhagic pancreatitis has been attributed to microvascular sludging in hypothermia. Of most pertinence to the therapist is the progressive slowing of blood flow through the liver, with alteration in conjugation and detoxification of drugs.

In the hypothermic patient, azotemia may result from decreased glomerular filtration, cardiac slowing, or hypovolemia. If severe and prolonged, azotemia may lead to acute tubular necrosis with renal shutdown, and the rhabdomyolysis of marked hypothermia and immobility may contribute to renal failure. A cold-induced renal tubular concentrating defect leads to the production of urine with low specific gravity, even in the face of decreased glomerular filtration. Hypothermia may also induce renal tubular glycosuria and makes it impossible to rule out hypoglycemia on the basis of glucose in the urine alone.

There is a rough correlation in the literature between depression of consciousness and reduction of body temperature. Cerebral oxygen consumption and blood flow are reduced in hypothermia, and the electroencephalogram may be flat below 68° F. For this reason, hypothermia is one of the exclusionary states defying the use of the electroencephalogram in the definition of brain death. Deep tendon reflexes, peripheral nerve conduction, and pain sensitivity may all be profoundly depressed in the hypothermic patient.

Hypothermia is, paradoxically, an emergency in suspended animation. Although hypothermia induces pathophysiologic change and suggests profound underlying disease in many patients, it is an error to persist in two common assumptions: (1) that one must normalize all values in the hypothermic patient as rapidly as possible and (2) that rapid restoration of normal body temperature is necessarily lifesaving. It is clear from accumulated data that the major cause of death in hypothermia is, in fact, the underlying disease that predisposed the individual to become hypothermic, and that the rate of rewarming is more dependent on the severity of that disease than on any other single factor. Other causes of death in hypothermia may be distressingly iatrogenic, including rewarming arrhythmias, cardiovascular collapse, pulmonary infection, pulmonary edema, and drug toxicity.

Diagnosis

Initial assessment of the hypothermic patient, therefore, should attend to both the causes and the consequences of hypothermia. A meticulous history and careful physical examination should be relentlessly repeated as the patient rewarms.

The diagnosis of hypothermia should be established with careful thermometry and the temperature monitored throughout the recovery phase. In our hospital, we admit patients with temperatures of 90° F or below to an intensive care unit. Because the patient's status changes rapidly as rewarming occurs, continuous monitoring is required. Because alcoholism, hypoglycemia, and narcotic overdosage are common causes of hypothermia in many populations, we administer intravenously 100 mg of thiamine, 50 grams of glucose, and 1 to 2 mg of naloxone hydrochloride (Narcan) in the emergency room to all significantly hypothermic patients. Because the pharmacology of all drugs is poorly understood at variable body temperatures, we try to avoid using other drugs, particularly antiarrhythmics, cardiotropics, and pressors, unless absolutely necessary to save life. Because infection is fairly common in the hypothermic patient, broad-spectrum or specific antibiotics may be indicated, with due regard to the nephrotoxic potential of many antibacterials. Studies suggest that patients with an elevated cardiac index and decreased systemic vascular resistance with right-sided heart catheterization (which should not be done routinely in patients with hypothermia but may be required in the most seriously ill) tend to be infected. Because infection is frequently masked in hypothermia, careful, repeated evaluation should be carried out and empiric therapy begun at the first suspicion of infection. More arguable is the use of stress-level steroids (300 mg of hydrocortisone or its equivalent per day). There is little evidence for cold-induced adrenal insufficiency, but adrenally insufficient patients may become hypothermic. Again, clinical judgment is needed.

Arterial blood gases should be measured and periodically re-examined, with careful reassessment of physical and chest x-ray evaluations of pulmonary status. Attempts to correct an acidemic pH (corrected or uncorrected) too vigorously with bicarbonate should be avoided because acidemia often clears with either hyperventilation or rewarming. Rebound alkalosis, which may occur if bicarbonate is administered too vigorously to the hypothermic patient, may predispose to arrhythmia.

Cardiac monitoring and titration of volume status are essential in the arrhythmic hypothermic patient.

Therapy

The most vigorous debate concerns the therapy of the hypothermia itself. Three major methods are reported in the literature. *External active rewarming* involves such drastic measures as dipping the patient in hot water or surrounding him or her with hot blankets. Although this method may occasionally be necessary in the profoundly cold patient in whom other methods of rewarming (see later) have failed, it is almost never required and may be dangerous. Most of the deaths reported in the literature have occurred with this type of active rewarming. *Central active rewarming* involves the use of warmed peritoneal lavage fluid, warmed intragastric lavage, or a specialized dialysis system. Complications of aspiration and peritonitis with the first two types of therapy and the enormous investment in personnel and equipment needed to maintain dialysis make these techniques useful only in exceptional circumstances.

Passive rewarming is preferred in the majority of patients who are not in cardiopulmonary arrest and who require less than immediate rewarming. Passive rewarming uses warm (not hot) blankets, warm intravenous fluids, and incremental warm supplemental oxygen heated and delivered as mist (keeping the inspired oxygen at a temperature of 104° F or less to avoid pulmonary burns). Except for the patient in cardiopulmonary arrest who may need active, invasive rewarming to 80° to 90° F, in whom defibrillation may be successful, most patients rewarm if they are simply removed from the exposed environment, covered with a blanket, warmed with intravenous fluids to 98.6° F, and allowed to rewarm at their own pace (Table 3). Data suggest that failure to rewarm by this method indicates serious underlying disease, and the rate of active rewarming in this population may have no influence on mortality.

TABLE 3. **Recommended Therapy for Hypothermia**

1. Check all temperatures of 94° F or less with thermistor or long thermometer.
2. Administer
   Thiamine, 100 mg IV
   Glucose, 50 grams IV   } in the emergency room
   Naloxone hydrochloride,
      1–2 mg IV.
3. Avoid other drugs except for:
   Antibiotics if indicated
   Stress-level (300 mg/day) steroids if indicated.
4. Admit patients with a temperature of 90° F or less to the intensive care unit.
5. Reassess the patient continually.
6. Follow arterial blood gases, both corrected and uncorrected.
7. Assess the patient's cardiac status using the cardiac monitor.
8. Use careful titration to assess volume status.
9. Use central passive rewarming:
   Warm (not hot) blankets
   IV fluids warmed to 98.6° F
   Inhalant warmed mist, if available, to 104° F.

FROSTBITE

Frostbite is the freezing of tissue, generally caused by exposure to temperatures or a wind-chill factor less than 0° F. It is most common in persons who are exposed to moist, cold environments or who have prolonged exposure and immobility of the affected parts. It affects unacclimatized individuals with clothing that is inadequate for the degree of external cold, those who use peripheral vasoconstrictors (such as nicotine), or those who have an intrinsic disease (such as Raynaud's phenomenon or atherosclerotic disease) that involves reduced perfusion to fingers and toes. It appears to be more common in the black races and in people born in tropical areas and with increased age, and it may occur as a result of the contiguous application of ice or cold, as with the prolonged use of ice packs on poorly perfused tissue (Table 4).

The pathogenesis of frostbite involves the formation within the frozen tissue of tiny particles of ice in the extracellular space, which leads to the drawing of water out of surrounding cells and into the extracellular space. This water accretionally joins the ice crystals and mechanically compresses the surrounding cells, possibly rupturing membranes either during freezing or during later thawing. This process, associated with the intracellular dehydration that occurs by the loss of intracellular water, may result in extensive tissue death and necrosis.

Diagnosis

The diagnosis of frostbite can be easily made. The affected part (generally fingers, toes, or ears and occasionally the nose) becomes white and cold and hard to the touch; later, the color may change to a bluish gray. Mobility is decreased, and the patient's sensation of cold discomfort gradually changes to one of warmth and then to total anesthesia as freezing occurs. Clinical distinction between superficial and deep frostbite (i.e., frostbite affecting only the skin and upper subcutaneous tissue versus that affecting those areas and underlying muscle) may be impossible in the field.

TABLE 4. **Factors Predisposing to Frostbite**

Ambient temperature or wind chill less than 0° to −5° F
Moisture, prolonged exposure, immobility
Inadequate clothing
Use of peripheral vasoconstrictors (e.g., nicotine) or intrinsic disease (Raynaud's phenomenon)
Black race
Increased age
Contiguous ice or cold (e.g., ice pack application)

Therapy

Therapy of frostbite can be divided into three phases: prethaw, thaw, and post-thaw (Table 5). Because many physicians believe that thawing and refreezing compound tissue damage, it is important to keep the frostbitten part frozen until the patient can be transported to a proper facility for care. If transport within several hours is impossible, thawing can be undertaken in the field. Caution must be taken to avoid refreezing the part. As transport is being arranged, the frozen part must be protected from trauma with padding or splints.

Thawing of the part is best done by immersing it in a whirlpool or tub of warm water at a temperature of 100° to 108° F. Rubbing the tissue with snow or ice, towels, or fingers should be avoided because it may compound tissue trauma. As the tissues thaw, severe pain may occur, and sedatives and analgesics may be required for comfort. Rapid rewarming of the part appears to preserve the greatest amount of tissue, but the use of excessive heat (water temperature higher than 115° F) may exacerbate the injury. As thawing occurs, a pink flush progresses distally down the extremity. Immersion should continue until the distal tip of the thawed part flushes, remains flushed when removed from the bath, and is warm to the touch. The actual color of the thawed part—pink or blue—does not immediately indicate whether the frostbitten part is recoverable. Persistent cyanosis, however, may suggest compartment syndrome and may require fasciotomy. Blebs or blisters on the affected part commonly develop over the several hours after thawing and should be kept intact. Because tissue may be débrided, the affected areas should be treated in the same sterile manner as one would a burn. In

TABLE 5. **Therapy of Frostbite**

Prethaw
Keep the frostbitten part frozen until the patient arrives at a proper facility for care if rapid transport can be arranged.
Protect the frozen part from trauma (with padding, splints).
If thawing has occurred (or if transport to a definitive facility is unavailable), avoid refreezing the affected part.

Thaw
Use whirlpool or tub immersion at a temperature of 100°–108° F.
Avoid tissue trauma.
Give sedatives and/or analgesics.

Post-Thaw
Watch for compartment syndrome.
Elevate the affected extremity.
Use whirlpool immersion and débridement.
Give antibiotics as required and a tetanus booster.
Provide physical therapy.

the post-thaw period, the affected part should be elevated to avoid dependent edema, and continuing treatment with a whirlpool bath at least twice a day for 20 minutes at a temperature of 90° to 95° F provides gentle cleansing and physiologic débridement. Antibiotics are seldom useful, but evidence of infection requires their use. Tetanus toxoid should be given if the patient's tetanus immune status is uncertain. Physical therapy is an indispensable part of treatment, and gentle movement by the patient of the fingers or toes, particularly in the whirlpool bath, prevents flexion contracture of the digits. If the blebs that form develop into dry, hard eschars, and if these prevent motion of the digits, careful splitting of the eschars along the dorsal or lateral borders may be necessary for mobilization of the joint. One should not try to remove the eschars, however; they will slough in the whirlpool by the second or third week.

Only after about 3 weeks will it be known, in many cases, whether the soft tissue is irrevocably injured. If the distal parts of an extremity become cold and black, they often undergo spontaneous amputation over the next several weeks to months, but they may require surgical attention.

DISTURBANCES CAUSED BY HEAT

method of
T. MICHAEL HARRINGTON, M.D.
The University of Alabama
Birmingham, Alabama

In the United States, heat-related fatalities occur more commonly than deaths related to any other natural phenomenon. From 1962 through 1986, 1000 to 2000 excess deaths per year were attributable to heat. By comparison, during the same 25-year period, the annualized death rate from flooding was 151 deaths per year; from lightning, 94 per year; from tornados, 87 per year; and from hurricanes, 31 per year. The 1980 heat wave in the southwestern United States claimed more than 1265 lives. In July 1987, in Greece, 878 people died during a 6-day heat wave when daily temperatures approached 115° F.

PHYSIOLOGY

An understanding of heat physiology is essential for the adequate treatment of the heat-related disorders. Homeostatic mechanisms limit the human temperature range to 96.5° to 99° F. This narrow range is essential for proper bodily functions and enzymatic processes. There is a constant interchange between heat production and heat loss maintained through complex hormonal, cardiovascular, renal, and neural influences. The largest producers of heat in the human

body are the muscles. Muscles produce heat through exercise or shivering. However, the body remains only 25 per cent efficient in fuel consumption, with 75 per cent of metabolic energy converted into heat. Without *any* ability to lose heat the human body would increase core temperature by 1° C (1.8° F) every 5 minutes.

Heat loss is largely accomplished by four separate mechanisms: radiation, convection, conduction, and evaporation. Radiation is the photon emission of electromagnetic energy from the skin and accounts for approximately 50 per cent of heat loss. Convection is heat transfer to an air current, and conduction is heat loss by direct contact. These mechanisms account for about 15 per cent of the body's heat loss. Evaporation (conversion of a liquid to a vapor) is responsible for around 25 per cent of heat loss. Several other factors account for the remaining 10 per cent, such as heat loss in stool and urine. When ambient temperature exceeds skin temperature (92° F), radiation, convection, and conduction are largely nonoperative. In addition, when relative humidity exceeds 60 per cent, heat loss by evaporation is reduced, and there is very little heat loss when the relative humidity exceeds 75 per cent.

It becomes clear then that in a hot, humid environment, the body's heat loss mechanisms are largely impaired. Any cardiovascular, renal, neural, or endocrine abnormality that hinders the body's capacity to dissipate heat compounds the situation.

HEAT CRAMPS

Heat cramps, also known as miner's, stoker's, logger's, or fireman's cramps, are incapacitating but *not* life-threatening. They generally occur in an acclimatized individual during or after heavy labor. The diagnosis is suspected when the large muscle groups of the abdomen or legs sustain severe cramps occurring during or after exercise. The patient's temperature and vital signs are normal, the skin is moist, and there are no central nervous system (CNS) symptoms (Table 1). Pathophysiologically, there is sodium loss in excess of water loss.

The treatment of choice is oral hydration with salt water. This can be easily made with a teaspoon of salt added to 500 to 1000 ml of water. This is a simple, safe, and effective treatment. Alternatively, normal saline via an intravenous route can be used, but generally is not necessary. It is important to have the patient liberally salt his or her food for the next 2 to 3 days and recognize that residual soreness may be present for 24 to 48 hours.

Current recommendations do *not* include use of salt tablets. Adverse effects of salt tablets include gastric pooling of oral fluid, vomiting, and potassium depletion. At times salt tablets remain undigested and pass through the gastrointestinal tract with little or no therapeutic benefit.

TABLE 1. Signs, Symptoms, and Treatment of Heat Disorders

Disorder	Vital Signs	Central Nervous System Symptoms	Skin Signs	Treatment
Heat cramps	Temperature: usually normal Blood pressure: normal Pulse: usually normal	None	Sweaty	Oral salt replacement, outpatient
Heat exhaustion	Temperature: less than 104°F Blood pressure: normal to low Pulse: elevated	Headache Nausea Dizziness Confusion	Sweaty or cool and clammy	Oral or IV salt and water replacement, outpatient or inpatient
Heat stroke	Temperature: greater than 104°F (often 106°–108°F) Blood pressure: low, normal, or high Pulse: elevated	Seizure Delirium Coma	Hot and dry (classic) Sweaty (exertional)	Rapid cooling Admission to intensive care unit

HEAT EXHAUSTION

Heat exhaustion is also known as heat prostration and heat collapse. This is the most common heat disorder. The diagnosis is suspected when the patient develops nausea, vomiting, dizziness, or a headache. The patient may also be confused or disoriented. Occasionally muscle cramps may intervene. Vital signs can vary from a normal to an elevated pulse and a normal or low blood pressure. Body temperature may be elevated, but is less than 104° F.

Pathophysiologically, both salt and water are depleted in the patient. At times salt depletion is in excess of water depletion, and at other times the reverse is true. There are some clinical differences between heat exhaustion with salt depletion (hypotonic) and heat exhaustion with water depletion (hypertonic), yet these distinctions have minimal significance for treatment.

Treatment includes moving the patient to the shade, removing any constricting garments, and keeping him or her recumbent. Oral hydration with salt and water is adequate if the patient is conscious and the airway is maintained. If this is not achievable, then intravenous hydration with either hypotonic or isotonic solution can be used. The patient should be hospitalized if he or she is elderly, has a chronic disease, or has a severe case of heat exhaustion. If there is *any* concern whatsoever about heat stroke, that would constitute a clear-cut need for hospitalization.

HEAT STROKE

Heat stroke is also known as heat pyrexia, sun stroke, or siriasis. Heat stroke is a true medical emergency. It is generally accepted that therapy must be instituted within 30 minutes to make an impact on the disease. Mortality ranges from 10 to 80 per cent depending on other factors, most notably the patient's age, general health, and other chronic diseases.

The diagnosis is entertained when a patient has significant CNS dysfunction coupled with extreme hyperthermia. The CNS disturbance may present as seizures, delirium, or coma. The skin can be hot and dry (classic heat stroke) or moist (exertional heat stroke). Blood pressure can be normal, elevated, or decreased, and the pulse is generally normal or elevated. Temperature is greater than 104° F, and the 106° to 108° F range is not unusual. (The highest recorded temperature in a surviving patient was 115.7° F.)

There are important differences in presentation between classic and exertional heat stroke that are worthy of discussion. Classic heat stroke is typically found in an older patient after a 3- to 5-day prodrome of headache, nausea, lassitude, and confusion. It is often found during a heat wave in the summer months. The differential diagnosis would include other CNS disorders, stroke, sepsis, and other causes of shock, but the key feature is the extremely elevated core temperature.

Exertional heat stroke is more commonly found in the young, active patient and with no prodrome. It is more typically found in the military recruit or the athlete. Pathophysiologically there is total hypothalamic and/or sweat gland failure. There is a complete inability to lose body heat.

Primary Treatment

The fundamental treatment for acute heat stroke is rapid cooling. The patient should be moved to a cool, shady area and his or her clothing should be removed. Ice packs, ice bags, or iced sheets or towels can be placed on the patient if available. Fans will promote evapora-

tion and aid cooling. The airway should be secured, oxygen supplied, and intravenous access
established. A Foley catheter and nasogastric
tube may be used; however, they can be inserted
later in the hospital. En route to the hospital,
the patient should be splashed or cooled with cold
water and either the windows of the vehicle left
open or the air conditioning turned on to provide
the coldest environment for transportation.

The optimal and recommended method of cooling is total immersion in an ice bath with active
muscle massage. This is the most reliable, time-
honored, and effective method. The patient is
placed in a tub of ice and water and a minimum
of four people actively and vigorously massage
the skeletal muscles and extremities. Muscle
massage is critical to prevent vasoconstriction
and paradoxical temperature rise. It will also
promote effective heat exchange.

In many larger hospitals, the physical therapy
department has a whirlpool tank that is quite
adequate. Ice can be delivered from the cafeteria.
In the smaller community hospital, an emergency
facility should have the availability of a large
tub (a small rubber boat or children's wading
pool works nicely) and a planned means of securing ice for the tub. Body cooling units are being
developed that deliver a cool mist and a fan for
rapid cooling by evaporation, yet these should be
considered investigational and are not universally available. Ice bath massage remains the
only specific treatment for heat stroke.

The core temperature should be monitored with
a rectal probe and the patient removed from the
tub when the temperature reaches 101° F. This
will prevent overcooling of the patient with subsequent hypothermia. If shivering due to the ice
bath presents a major problem (and thus increases heat production) small doses of chlorpromazine, 25 to 50 mg intravenously, can be
used.

Hospital Care

Once the temperature is reduced, attention is
directed toward the complications of heat stroke.
Organ systems that may sustain damage include
the CNS, cardiac, respiratory, renal, hepatic, pancreatic, and musculoskeletal systems. Several
laboratory tests should be ordered on admission
to assess for organ damage (Table 2).

CNS problems include seizures and cerebral
edema. Seizures can be controlled in the acute
setting with small doses (5 to 10 mg) of intravenous diazepam (Valium). Cerebral edema can be
managed with mannitol (12.5 to 25 grams intravenously) and careful fluid management.

Cardiac manifestations include hypotension

TABLE 2. **Initial Laboratory Assessment
for Heat Stroke**

Complete blood count (CBC) with platelet count
Blood urea nitrogen (BUN), creatinine
Creatine phosphokinase (CPK), serum glutamic-oxaloacetic
    transaminase (SGOT), serum glutamic-pyruvic transami-
    nase (SGPT), bilirubin
Electrolytes, glucose
Prothrombin time (PT), partial thromboplastin time (PTT)
Amylase, arterial blood gases, serum lactate
Chest x-ray, electrocardiogram
Urinalysis

and myocardial damage. While not all patients
with heat stroke are hypotensive and volume
depleted, many are. The volume-depleted patients usually respond well to volume replacement guided by monitoring of urine output and
central venous pressure. If fluid resuscitation is
not completely successful, an intravenous drip of
dopamine or isoproterenol drips may be used.

Respiratory complications include pulmonary
edema. This can result from myocardial damage
or fluid overload from overhydration. Monitoring
is done with physical examination and central
venous pressure readings. Management includes
careful fluid resuscitation, diuretics, and digitalis
as for classic pulmonary edema.

Renal complications include acute tubular necrosis and myoglobinuria. Extensive rhabdomyolysis can occur secondary to heat stroke. The
resulting colored urine is related to the myoglobin pigment from the muscle destruction. Myoglobin is thought to be nephrotoxic, at least in
part resulting from a direct toxic affect on the
renal tubule. Therefore, adequate renal blood
flow should be maintained. Furosemide (Lasix)
and mannitol are used to minimize renal damage.
Early dialysis might be carried out in some situations.

Hepatic, pancreatic, and skeletal muscle damage is monitored with liver function tests and
measurements of amylase levels and total creatine phosphokinase. Damage to these systems is
managed supportively. Disseminated intravascular coagulopathy (DIC) may appear within the
first 48 to 72 hours. Prothrombin time, partial
thromboplastin time and platelet counts are used
to monitor for DIC. Treatment is supportive.

Steroids or antibiotics are not indicated for the
general care of the heat stroke patient. Their use
would be predicated upon a specific indication
only.

PREVENTION

It is apparent from this discussion that an "at
risk" population can be defined and preventive
measures should be employed prior to the onset

of one of the heat disorders. Athletes, laborers, and military personnel are at risk when working in a hot environment. Obese and nonacclimatized people are at risk. The elderly patient is at risk owing to reduced cardiovascular ability to respond to a heat challenge. A large group of medications impair an individual's ability to respond to heat. Anticholinergics, phenothiazines, tricyclics, and antihistamines can all promote hypohidrosis. Dehydration is aggravated by diuretics. Alcohol and drug withdrawal promote increased muscular activity (and thus increased heat). Vasoconstrictors decrease cutaneous blood flow, and myocardial reserve is reduced by beta blockers. Finally, hot, humid, and windless days add to everyone's risk.

Anyone working or exercising in a warm environment should have adequate acclimatization. This is generally achieved after 10 to 14 days of gradually acclimatizing to the heat. There are definite renal and hormonal adaptations made to the heat. Salt and water conservation mechanisms are enhanced, and the sweating apparatus is modified so that there is more extracellular fluid volume for sweating. Sweating can increase up to two and one-half times. Under aldosterone influence salt and water are conserved at the kidney and sweat gland level. After acclimatization it is still necessary to maintain hydration. The best solution for this is cool or cold water. Cold water is more rapidly absorbed from the gastrointestinal tract, and solutions with high concentrations of electrolytes and sugar are generally not needed (one exception to this might be the endurance athlete, such as the marathon runner or bicycle racer). In addition, hypotonic solutions empty more rapidly from the stomach than isotonic or hypertonic solutions. Other common sense approaches would be to wear light-colored and loose-fitting clothing, to avoid the mid-day heat, and to pay attention to the temperature-humidity index provided by the National Weather Service. Temperature-humidity indexes, wet-bulb thermometers, and wet-bulb globe thermometer indexes all provide useful information for predicting and avoiding heat disorders.

SPIDER BITES AND SCORPION STINGS

method of
RONALD W. SWINFARD, M.D.
East Tennessee State University
Johnson City, Tennessee

For all that is written about arthropod envenomations, nearly all are trivial and require only conserv-

ative management. This therapy consists principally of rest and symptomatic treatment (Table 1), but with an expectant approach to detect the rare systemic reaction that requires aggressive intervention. A patient may also have a hypersensitivity reaction (immediate or delayed) to the venom, which is unrelated to its usual toxicity. Certain categories of patients should be considered at higher risk, including the very young (pre–school-age children), the elderly, the physically debilitated, and those with a prior history of adverse reaction. These patients, as well as those in whom a significant systemic reaction is documented or suspected, should be hospitalized for close monitoring and treatment. Even persons at low risk or without apparent systemic toxicity should be re-evaluated 6 to 24 hours after the initial visit to reassess local and systemic reactions.

Prophylactic antibiotics are seldom indicated because secondary bacterial infection of arthropod bites is uncommon and occurs days after envenomation. There is thus ample time for the initiation of therapy that is directed by culture and sensitivity test results. Because of the significant morbidity from use of horse serum antivenins, these should also not be used prophylactically but should be reserved for persons who have demonstrated complications or who are in the high-risk group.

BROWN RECLUSE SPIDER BITES (LOXOSCELISM)

Several species of *Loxosceles* are found in the New World, with *L. reclusa* having received the most intensive study and worst reputation. Also known as the "fiddleback" spider, this species may be recognized by the dark, violin-shaped marking on the dorsal thorax. As the name implies, the brown recluse spider prefers a reclusive environment, usually indoors in closets or storage boxes. It tends to be nocturnal, and patients are frequently bitten while putting on clothes that have been left overnight in the spider's territory. Although this species was originally found mostly in the central and southern United States, al-

TABLE 1. **General Management of Arthropod Bites and Stings**

1. General rest, with immobilization of bite site and elevation of an affected extremity
2. Cold packs to the site of the bite to provide topical anesthesia and to reduce enzymatic activity of venom
3. Tetanus toxoid, as indicated
4. Symptomatic control of pain and itching, including narcotics, if indicated (except for scorpion stings), and antihistamines
5. Systemic steroids, if hypersensitivity is suspected (prednisone, 1–2 mg/kg/day, tapered over 10–20 days)
6. Identification of the biting arthropod
   a. Recovery of organism preferred, with identification by reputable entomologist
   b. Analysis of geographic likelihood of organisms in region
   c. As a minimum, reaction matched to likely organism
7. Attentive follow-up

leged bites have now been described widely, possibly the result of spider transport during household moves.

As a rule, pain at the bite site is absent or, at worst, mild and transient. In the vast majority of patients (90 to 95 per cent) there will be mild erythema and discomfort at the site in 3 to 6 hours, with subsequent uncomplicated healing without morbidity. This sequence is particularly true for individuals raised in the spider's habitat who seem to have acquired some immunity to the venom. Those with a significant reaction have considerable pain and erythema, which prompt them to seek medical treatment several hours after the bite. The erythema then progresses to dusky cyanosis surrounded by vasoconstrictive blanching, with this surrounded by reactive erythema. Noticeable edema to the entire region is common. Other spiders, notably *Chiracanthium,* may produce a similar necrotic reaction easily mistaken for loxoscelism.

Twenty-four to 36 hours later, the central cyanotic area frequently develops a serohemorrhagic or hemorrhagic blister, eccentrically shaped as determined by the gravitational spread of venom. Some lymphangitis is common, with a generalized morbilliform, nearly petechial, eruption occasionally developing a few days after the bite. By about 1 week, the central area has become necrotic with purple to black eschar showing separation from the surrounding tissue. This area is usually relatively small (2 to 5 cm in diameter), with areas greater than 10 cm in diameter suggesting alternative diagnoses such as a necrotizing bacterial process or pyoderma gangrenosum. The largest areas of necrosis are usually seen over prominent subcutaneous fat, no doubt because a major component of the venom is the enzyme sphingomyelin phosphodiesterase. The necrotic ulcer should be permitted to heal completely; only conservative therapy is needed. Surgery has been demonstrated to have no role acutely, and, in fact, may be contraindicated. Repair by plastic surgery of resultant defects or deformities may be undertaken in 6 to 12 months, if necessary or desired. Most ulcerations heal in 6 to 12 weeks without appreciable deformity.

Rarely, a patient develops systemic loxoscelism manifested by lassitude, fever, chills, arthralgias, and nausea, which is probably due to hypersensitivity to the venom. Even more uncommon, intravascular hemolysis may develop and progress to full-blown disseminated intravascular coagulation with its attendant complications, including renal injury with anuria, coma, or both. Serial urinalyses and hematologic evaluations (including complete cell count with platelet count, prothrombin time, and partial thrombo-plastin time) are appropriate for the patient in whom a systemic reaction is suspected. These patients are usually from the aforementioned high-risk groups, especially the young. Early intervention wiith peritoneal dialysis in children with loss of renal function has resulted in rapid and complete recovery. With careful monitoring and appropriate treatment of complications, death is exceedingly rare.

Treatment

For the overwhelming majority of brown recluse spider bites, management as given in Table 1 is all that is required. For this reason, many therapeutic regimens have been touted as successful because of favorable outcomes. Currently popular is dapsone (50 to 100 mg every 12 hours for 2 to 3 weeks), instituted as soon as possible after the bite.* Caution is encouraged because dapsone itself may also produce hemolysis and methemoglobinemia. Serial complete blood counts are required to monitor this therapy, and a glucose-6-phosphate dehydrogenase level should be obtained before initiating therapy. No studies comparing dapsone with vigilant conservative management have yet been published, although they are anticipated in the near future. For patients with systemic toxicity, corticosteroids (prednisone, 1 to 2 mg per kg per day) have traditionally been used, also without rigorous scientific validation. A *Loxosceles* antivenin derived from rabbit serum has been developed at Vanderbilt University and appears to be promising, although it is not yet available.

BLACK WIDOW SPIDER BITES (LATRODECTISM)

Several species of the *Latrodectus* genus of widow spiders are found in the United States, the black species (*L. mactans*) having the greatest notoriety. The popularly described hourglass on the ventral abdomen is inconstant, which emphasizes the importance of expert entomologic identification of arachnids for accurate reporting of cases. The venom and hence toxicity are similar among all members of the genus. Widow spiders are generally found outdoors, spinning a web with a characteristic geometric pattern. Contact with humans is accidental, often when the spider is found in outbuildings.

After envenomation, there is usually, although not always, local pain with mild erythema. If the patient is seen shortly after the bite, two puncta may be visible at the bite site. Local reaction with ecchymosis, edema, and necrosis is *not* char-

---

*This use is not listed by the manufacturer.

acteristic of latrodectism. Within the hour, systemic symptoms begin, the most notorious of which is abdominal cramping. When accompanied by similar muscle cramping in adjacent areas (proximal extremities, pelvis, chest) this may simulate the classic "board-like" rigidity of an acute abdomen. Generalized muscle tightness, aches, pain, and occasional tremors, along with hyperesthesia, are predictably seen with this neurotoxic venom. Other variably described features include headache, tachypnea, restlessness, hypertension, and cardiac arrhythmias. Obviously, sympathetic discharge related to feelings of anxiety about the incident complicates the overall clinical picture. The most severe findings are seen in young children, including near-paralysis with altered consciousness, convulsions, or both. In addition to the previously described high-risk groups, patients with hypertensive cardiovascular disease have traditionally been singled out for increased likelihood of complication. Rarely, life-threatening hypersensitivity reactions may occur, which are manifested by paralysis, intravascular hemolysis, renal failure, and/or coma.

Treatment

Aside from the general measures outlined in Table 1, specific therapy is aimed at treating the neuromuscular symptoms and assessing the need for *Latrodectus* antivenin. For the former treatment, calcium gluconate (10 ml of 10 per cent solution, given intravenously) or muscle relaxants (diazepam [Valium] or methocarbamol [Robaxin]), or both are most frequently used. It is frequently necessary to repeat these drugs, as indicated, during the first 24 hours. *Latrodectus* antivenin is seldom required except in the most threatened or high-risk cases. Its use is further discouraged because it is derived from horse serum, which necessitates skin testing for sensitivity, and a small percentage of patients still have adverse reactions despite negative skin tests. As the product insert from the manufacturer describes, only a single 2.5-ml intramuscular injection is required, but severe cases may need a subsequent dose diluted in normal saline and given slowly, by the intravenous route, 60 to 90 minutes after the first dose. Those with life-threatening complications should, of course, be in an intensive care setting, with current protocols for specific complications (e.g., hemolysis) used.

SCORPION STINGS

In the United States, scorpion stings are medically important only in the desert Southwest, principally from *Centruroides sculpturatus* and its relatives. These scorpions tend not to be aggressive, and stings result when the scorpions are inadvertently disturbed or threatened. Their normal habitant is above ground under logs and stones. They exhibit greatest activity at night.

Envenomation is typically painful and produces local paresthesias and occasional numbness of the envenomized extremity, which is characteristic of injected neurotoxins. Any systemic toxicity usually occurs within a few hours of the sting, mostly as an extension of the neurotoxicity: facial pruritus, excessive salivation, muscle twitching and spasm (especially of jaw muscles, rarely progressing to bowel or bladder incontinence), and occasional nausea with vomiting. Severe reactions, seen especially in the young, may include convulsions. Life-threatening reactions such as respiratory and circulatory collapse are rare and may be due as much to an allergic reaction as to the direct effects of the venom.

Treatment

Initial treatment is as described in Table 1, except that morphine and its derivatives are contraindicated. Reports from several decades suggest that the opiates have a synergistic effect with scorpion venom. Treatment of systemic toxicity, if present, is based on the mechanisms of venom toxicity:

1. Calcium gluconate, 10 ml of 10 per cent solution, intravenously, for muscle symptoms
2. Phenobarbital sodium, slowly by the intravenous route, for convulsions
3. Atropine sulfate, for excessive salivation
4. Antivenin, rarely necessary, especially in adults (available from the Antivenom Production Laboratory, Department of Microbiology at Arizona State University; derived from goat serum and, for regulatory reasons, available only to licensed physicians in Arizona)
5. Standard protocols for cardiopulmonary collapse

SNAKEBITE

method of
WILLIS A. WINGERT, M.D.
University of Southern California
Los Angeles, California

Approximately 10,000 victims are bitten by venomous snakes annually, which results in 8 to 12 deaths. The venomous snakes in the United States belong to two families: the Crotalidae, or pit vipers, including

17 species of rattlesnakes (genera *Crotalus* and *Sistrurus*) and the copperheads and moccasins, or cottonmouths (*Agkistrodon*); and *Elapidae,* or coral snakes, including two species that are limited to the southern and southwestern states. However, bites by legally or illegally imported foreign venomous snakes are not uncommon.

Snake species are limited geographically. The major offenders in each region are

Northeast

Copperheads	*Agkistrodon contortrix*
Timber rattlesnake	*Crotalus horridus*
Massasauga	*Sistrurus catenatus*

South

Eastern diamondback	*Crotalus adamanteus*
Water moccasin	*Agkistrodon piscivorus*
Copperhead	*Agkistrodon contortrix*
Eastern coral snake	*Micrurus fulvius*

Midwest

Prairie rattlesnake	*Crotalus viridis viridis*
Timber rattlesnake	*Crotalus horridus*

Southwest, including deserts

Western diamondback	*Crotalus atrox*
Sidewinder	*Crotalus cerastes*
Mojave Rattkesnake	*Crotalus scutulatus*

West Coast

Pacific rattlesnake	*Crotalus viridis helleri* and *viridis oreganus*

The diamondback rattlesnakes are large, irritable, and aggressive and are able to deliver a large quantity of venom during a strike. The venom of the Pacific rattlesnake is highly toxic, and the venom of the Mojave rattlesnake contains potent neurotoxins.

The severity of envenomation depends on two factors: the quantity of venom injected and the relative toxicity of the venom. Snakes do not inject all of their venom in a single bite. Twenty to 25 per cent of all bites result in minimal or no envenomation. Factors that determine the quantity of venom injected include the species of snake, the number of bites, the length of time that the fangs remained embedded, the irritability of the snake, and the size of the snake. Venom toxicity varies, especially according to species. Bites by copperheads usually do not require treatment, whereas envenomation by the highly toxic Mojave rattlesnake is a medical emergency.

Pit viper venoms are complex poisons that contain two major components: small lethal proteins (molecular weight 4800 to 100,000) that are designed to kill the prey, and 5 to 15 digestive enzymes. The pharmacologic actions of these components include

1. Local tissue necrosis
2. Capillary endothelial cell injury resulting in increased permeability with transudation of plasma and erythrocytes into tissues and pulmonary alveoli
3. Local progressive swelling
4. Hypovolemic shock
5. Pulmonary edema
6. Hemolysis of erythrocytes
7. Renal shutdown secondary to hypovolemia or to tubular deposition of hemoglobin
8. Coagulation defects caused by disseminated intravascular coagulation, with consumption of fibrinogen and platelets
9. Disturbance of neuromuscular transmission leading to curare-like muscular paralysis (venoms of coral snakes and the Mojave rattlesnake)
10. Probable liberation of histamine, bradykinin, and prostaglandins with specific autopharmacologic actions

Venom poisoning therefore causes complex reactions involving almost all organ systems except the central nervous system, either primarily or secondarily. Signs and symptoms of pit viper envenomation are

1. Moderately severe stinging or a brief burning pain at the bite site, but occasionally no pain
2. Swelling at the site of the bite, which may progress rapidly and involve the entire extremity within 1 to 2 hours
3. Ecchymosis at the bite site, extending proximally
4. With progressive edema, bullae and hemorrhagic blebs, also occurring at the bite site and progressing proximally
5. Paresthesias (tingling, numbness) of the scalp, face, and lips and a metallic taste in the mouth, particularly in bites by the Pacific, timber, and eastern diamondback rattlesnakes
6. Cranial nerve palsies (hoarseness, diplopia, dysphagia) progressing to respiratory paralysis, after Mojave rattlesnake envenomation
7. Muscular fasciculations
8. General symptoms of weakness, faintness, nausea, and vomiting
9. In untreated patients with severe envenomation, hypovolemic shock, pulmonary edema, and renal failure

MANAGEMENT

First Aid in the Field

Avoid panic. Toxic effects of the venom are increased by muscular activity.

Move the victim immediately out of the snake's striking range, put at rest, and keep warm.

Remove rings and constrictive items.

Locate and observe the offending snake, if possible. Especially, estimate the snake's length because more severe envenomations usually are inflicted by large snakes. If only one species inhabits a geographic area, species identification is not necessary. If identification is required, kill the snake by a blow on the neck and transport in a closed bag or sealed box to the closest trained person.

Immobilize the injured extremity by splinting. Application of an elastic bandage at less than venous pressure (50 mmHg) may be of value if transport time is prolonged.

Mark, preferably with ink, the proximal level of the swelling and record the time.

Transport the patient to a medical facility as quickly as possible.

Do not apply ice or tourniquet. Do not incise and suction the bite site.

Hospital Management

Step 1 Establish a Physiologic Baseline

If the snake *is* available, verify the species as venomous. Pit vipers have a triangular head, vertical elliptic pupils, maxillary fangs, indentation ("pit") between eye and nostril, and one or more rattles. Coral snakes have round pupils, small fixed maxillary fangs, black snout, and a sequential pattern of color bands (red-yellow-black) completely encircling the body.

If the snake *is not* available, diagnose envenomation by presenting signs and symptoms: fang marks (one or more distinctive puncture wounds with ragged edges, often with slight bleeding); local edema; local subcutaneous hemorrhage; and paresthesias of the face, mouth, and tongue.

Obtain a history of the bite and of any known allergies to drugs or horse serum.

Record vital signs.

Obtain blood for the following determinations: complete blood count and erythrocyte morphology (spherocytosis, pyknocytosis); platelet count (decreased in severe envenomation); coagulation screen, especially fibrinogen level and split products, partial thromboplastin time, bleeding time (template); and levels of electrolytes, serum protein, and creatine kinase, a reliable marker for tissue necrosis.

Perform urinalysis for hematuria, proteinuria, and specific gravity.

Obtain electrocardiogram for patients older than 40 years or for patients with a history of cardiac disease.

Measure and record the circumference of the injured extremity at the proximal point of edema and approximately 10 cm proximal to this level. Record the time of the observations.

Step 2: Determine the Severity of Envenomation.
Grade the reaction according to Table 1.

Step 3: Perform a Skin Test for Sensitivity to Horse Serum.
Inject 0.02 ml of a 1:10 dilution of horse serum (included in antivenin package) intradermally. Inject 0.02 N saline at another site as a control. Note: This test is neither highly reliable nor sensitive.

Step 4: Start Intravenous Infusions in Two Extremities.
Use one line to administer antivenin; use the second line for life support if needed, such as administration of blood, plasma expanders, or epinephrine or measurement of central venous pressure.

Step 5: Administer Adequate Amount of Specific

TABLE 1. **Grade of Severity of Pit Viper Envenomation**

Severity	Characteristics
No envenomation	Fang marks but no local or systemic reaction.
Minimal	Fang marks with local edema, but no systemic reaction.
Moderate	Fang marks. Edema progressing rapidly beyond the bite site, together with a systemic reaction. Paresthesias. Laboratory changes including decrease in platelet count, fibrinogen, or hematocrit; increase in split products and creatine kinase; hematuria, proteinuria. History of bite by large snake; provoked bite.
Severe	Fang marks, very rapidly progressing swelling, subcutaneous ecchymoses, severe general symptoms, especially hypotension, laboratory changes noted above. History of multiple bites, large snake, highly toxic species (Mojave, diamondback, and Pacific rattlesnakes), prolonged embedding of fangs (snake "hung on").

Antidote (Antivenin). Administer neutralizing antibodies supplied in Wyeth Laboratory Antivenin (Crotalidae) Polyvalent according to Table 2. Dilute the antivenin 1:5 with 0.5 N saline and administer slowly over a period of 2 hours. In children, administer at a rate of 20 ml per kg of body weight per hour.

Step 6: Monitor Progress of Poisoning and Repeat Antivenin Dose If Required.
Measure the circumference of the affected extremity every 20 minutes and compare with the initial determinations. Mark the progress of the edema with a timed line. Note the development of any systemic reactions, such as falling blood pressure or hemorrhages. Repeat the initial dose of antivenin every 2 hours until no further progression of swelling occurs and general symptoms, such as paresthesias, are controlled.

If the skin test is highly positive or if anaphylactic symptoms (pruritus, urticaria, hypotension, bradycardia) occur when antivenin is administered, consultation with a poison control center is strongly recommended before proceeding.

TABLE 2. **Initial Dose of Wyeth Polyvalent (Crotalidae) Antivenin**

Severity of Envenomation	Dose
No envenomation	No antivenin and no skin test
Minimal	5 vials (50 ml)
Moderate	10 vials (100 ml)
Severe	15 vials (150 ml)
Known Mojave (*C. scutulatus*) bites	10 vials (100 ml)

Step 7: Monitor and Support Physiologic Status of Circulatory, Respiratory, and Renal Systems.
Monitor vital signs, especially blood pressure. Insert a central venous catheter in severely envenomated patients. Treat hypovolemic shock by administering 10 to 20 ml per kg of a plasma expander (*not* a crystalloid solution).

Repeat assays for hemoglobin, hematocrit, and platelet levels every hour until the patient is stable. Correct decreased hematocrit with packed red blood cells, 10 ml per kg, or whole blood if indicated.

Monitor intake and output of fluids. Perform periodic urinalyses for evidence of hematuria, proteinuria, or both.

Obtain serial electrolyte determinations and correct abnormalities in fluid and electrolyte balance as required.

Administer oxygen by mask if the patient becomes hypoxemic. In coral snake or Mojave rattlesnake envenomation, prepare to ventilate the patient mechanically if cranial nerve palsies, dysphagia, diplopia, ptosis, or hoarseness appears.

Step 8: If envenomation is severe, or if wound was incised, suctioned, or both, use broad-spectrum antibiotic. Administer the antibiotic (ampicillin, amoxicillin, or a second-generation cephalosporin) prophylactically for at least 7 days.

Step 9: Prevent Tetanus. Use tetanus toxoid booster for previously immunized patients or 250 units of human immune tetanus globulin for unimmunized patients.

Step 10: Local Tissue Care. Lightly immobilize the extremity in position of function on a well-padded splint. Cleanse the fang wounds daily with an antiseptic solution and cover with dry, sterile dressing. Débride blebs, vesicles, and superficial necrotic tissue aseptically on the fourth or fifth day if coagulation values are normal.

Begin active and passive rehabilitation therapy within 5 days to prevent contractures. Swelling usually subsides completely within 10 days if antivenin therapy has been adequate.

Step 11: Observe for Serum Sickness. Type III IG-g immune complex allergic reaction may develop after 7 to 14 days. Administer prednisone, 10 mg every 6 hours, at the onset of pruritus and urticaria (2 mg per kg per day in children). Continue treatment until all signs and symptoms have subsided for 24 hours. Antihistamines are of value only for sedation or for alleviation of pruritus.

Step 12: Avoid Medicolegal Liability. Notify the police or the state's Department of Fish and Game if the patient has been bitten by a captive venomous snake. Most states require a license to collect or maintain wild or venomous animals.

Coral Snake (Micrurus fulvius) Envenomation

Obtain a history with the salient factors: size of the snake, sequence of the color bands, length of time the fangs remained embedded (most coral snakes tend to hold on and chew), length of time from accident to evaluation, and allergies, especially to drugs or horse serum.

Observe the patient for signs and symptoms of poisoning: one or more fang marks, usually on a finger, often slightly oozing blood; local swelling; paresthesia; cranial nerve palsies, as manifested by dyspnea, diplopia, dysphagia, or slurred speech.

Perform a skin test for horse serum sensitivity. A negative test does *not* guarantee an anaphylactic reaction.

If the test is negative, administer Antivenin (*Micrurus fulvius*) Wyeth intravenously, diluted 1:5 with 0.5 N saline, over a period of 2 hours. The initial dose depends on the circumstances of the bite: for large snakes, plus difficulty in disengaging the snake, delay of over 2 hours in treatment, and small size of patient: 10 vials. All others: 6 vials.

Monitor the patient especially for neurologic (bulbar paralytic) symptoms for at least 72 hours. Additional doses of 5 vials of antivenin may be required.

If the skin test or the history of allergy is positive, obtain consultation from a poison control center before proceeding.

Bites of Exotic Foreign Snakes

Consult an expert at a poison control center. Antivenin usually may be obtained only from the herpetology department of major zoos. The *Antivenin Index* in Oklahoma City (405–271–5454) or the Poison Control Center in Tucson (602–626–6016 or 602–626–6200) may suggest the closest source of antivenin. Dosage varies according to the species of offending snake.

ACUTE POISONINGS

method of
HOWARD C. MOFENSON, M.D.
THOMAS R. CARACCIO, PHARM.D., and
JOSEPH GREENSHER, M.D.
Long Island Regional Poison Control Center
East Meadow, New York

BASIC MANAGEMENT OF POISONINGS

The severity of the manifestations of acute poisoning exposures varies greatly with the age and intent of the

The assistance of Lauren Leader and Helene Jacobs in the preparation of this manuscript is gratefully acknowledged.

victims. Accidental poisoning exposures make up 80 to 85 per cent of all poisoning episodes and are most frequent in children under 5 years of age. Many of these episodes are actually ingestions of relatively nontoxic substances that require minimal medical care. Intentional poisonings constitute 10 to 15 per cent of poisonings, and often these patients require the highest standards of medical and nursing care and the occasional use of sophisticated equipment for recovery. Suicide attempts are a significant number, and the use of toxic substances is often involved. The majority of the drug-related suicide attempts involve a central nervous system depressant, and "coma management" is vital to the treatment.

Sixty per cent of patients who take a drug overdose do so with their own prescribed medication and 15 per cent with drugs prescribed for relatives. The top poisoning categories for all ages are over-the-counter analgesics, sedative-hypnotics, benzodiazepines, cleaning agents and petroleum products, alcohol and substance abuse, pesticides, tricyclic antidepressants, plants, carbon monoxide, and opioids.

ASSESSMENT AND MAINTENANCE OF VITAL FUNCTIONS

Upper airway obstruction is the most common cause of death in intoxicated patients outside the hospital. Any patient who is comatose and has absent protective airway reflexes is able to tolerate an endotracheal tube (cuffed for those over ages 7 to 9 years) and should have it inserted as soon as possible.

Ventilation is required if the respiratory rate and depth are inadequate.

The circulatory status is best assessed by the blood pressure and heart rate and rhythm. The circulatory clinical status and tissue perfusion may be inferred from the skin temperature, the return of color after pressure blanching (capillary filling), and the urine output. Intra-arterial blood pressure measurements are essential for adequate monitoring.

If the circulation fails to improve after adequate ventilation and oxygenation, then a 15- to 20-cm elevation of the foot of the bed may aid by increasing the venous return to the heart. A fluid challenge also may improve the circulatory status if hypovolemia is the cause. If these measures fail, plasma expanders and similar products may be required. As a last resort vasopressors may be needed. If these measures fail to produce a response, a central venous pressure or a pulmonary artery wedge pressure (PAWP) line should be inserted to monitor for heart failure and fluid overload.

The level of consciousness of all intoxicated patients should be assessed and the time of assessment recorded. The Glasgow Coma Score used in head trauma is not useful in intoxications, as alcohol, depressant drugs, and hypotension may give falsely lowered scores. The Reed Coma Scale is preferred (Table 1).

PREVENTION OF ABSORPTION AND REDUCTION OF LOCAL DAMAGE

Ocular exposure should be immediately treated with water or saline irrigation for 20 minutes with eyelids fully retracted. Do not use neutralizing chemicals. All caustic and corrosive injuries should be evaluated by an ophthalmologist.

Dermal exposure is treated immediately with rinsing, not a forceful flushing in a shower, which might result in deeper penetration of the toxic substance. The skin should be rinsed with copious amounts of water for at least 30 minutes. Hair shampoo, cleansing of fingernails and navel, and irrigation of the eyes are necessary in an extensive exposure. The clothes may have to be discarded. Leather goods are often irreversibly contaminated and must be abandoned. Caustics (alkali) often require hours of irrigation until the "soapy" feeling of the burn is gone. Dermal absorption may occur with pesticides, hydrocarbons, and cyanide.

Injected exposures to drugs and toxins or those introduced by envenomation may require a proximal tourniquet and early incision and suction. (See Antidotes 4 through 6 in Table 4.)

Inhalation exposures to toxic substances are treated by immediately removing the victim from the contaminated environment.

Gastrointestinal exposure is the most common route of poisoning, and an estimate of what, when, and how much of the toxic substance was ingested must be made. If there is a possibility of potential intoxication, gastrointestinal decontamination is performed rather than waiting for symptoms to develop.

Gastrointestinal Decontamination

To decrease gastrointestinal absorption, emesis should be induced or gastric aspiration and lavage performed. Neither of these methods is completely effective; each removes only 30 to 50 per cent of the ingested substance. They are recommended up to 3 to 4 hours postingestion; however, to elect *not* to remove a potential toxin after 4 hours requires reliance on an often unreliable history of the substance and the time of ingestion. Therefore, it is safer to evacuate the stomach up to 12 hours after an ingestion in most significant intoxications.

Emesis

Relative contraindications to the induction of emesis are (1) petroleum distillate ingestion of

TABLE 1. **Level of Consciousness (Reed Coma Scale)**

Stage	Conscious Level	Pain Response	Reflexes	Respiration	Circulation
0	Asleep	Normal	Normal	Normal	Normal
1	Coma	Decreased	Normal	Normal	Normal
2	Coma	None	Normal	Normal	Normal
3*	Coma	None	None	Normal	Normal
4†	Coma	None	None	Abnormal	Abnormal

*Patients in Stages 3 and 4 require intubation and placement in an intensive care unit.
†Patients in Stage 4 need intervention to sustain life.

high-viscosity agents; (2) agents that are likely to rapidly produce coma (short-acting barbiturates) or convulsions (propoxyphene, camphor, isoniazid, strychnine) in less than 30 minutes and therefore may predispose to aspiration during emesis; and (3) prior significant vomiting.

Absolute contraindications to the induction of emesis are (1) caustic (alkali) or corrosive (acid) ingestions; (2) convulsions because of the danger of aspiration and possible induction of laryngospasm; (3) coma because of the possibility of aspiration with the loss of protective airway reflexes; (4) absence of a cough reflex—absence of the gag reflex is not a reliable indication of lack of airway protection, since a number of healthy people lack gag reflexes; (5) hematemesis, in which vomiting may produce additional damage; (6) an infant under 6 months of age, because of immature protective airway reflexes; and (7) foreign bodies—emesis is ineffective and risks obstruction or aspiration.

Inducing Emesis. *Syrup of ipecac* is the preferred agent, but never fluid extract of ipecac, which is too potent, or salt water, which has produced fatal hypernatremia. Emesis is not recommended to be induced at home in children under 1 year of age but can be performed in a medical facility under supervision when indicated. The dose of syrup of ipecac in the 6- to 9-month-old infant is 5 ml; in the 9- to 12-month-old, 10 ml; and in the 1- to 12-year-old, 15 ml. In children over 12 years and in adults, the dose is 30 ml. The dose may be repeated *once* if the child does not vomit in 15 to 20 minutes. The vomitus should be inspected for remnants of pills or toxic substances and the appearance and odor noted.

Apomorphine is a parenteral emetic that must be freshly prepared. Its use is fraught with complications, although it produces more rapid onset of emesis than syrup of ipecac. We do not recommend its use in the cooperative patient. Naloxone should be available to reverse central nervous system (CNS) depression.

Gastric aspiration and lavage may be preferable to the induction of emesis in cooperative adolescents or adults because a large tube can be introduced through the oral cavity. *Contraindi-*

cations to gastric aspiration and lavage in intoxicated patients are (1) caustic (alkali) and corrosive (acid) ingestions, because of the risk of esophageal perforation, (2) uncontrolled convulsions, because of the danger of aspiration and injury during the procedure, (3) petroleum distillate products, (4) coma or absent protective airway reflexes, which require the insertion of an endotracheal tube to protect against aspiration, (5) significant cardiac dysrhythmias, which should be controlled first, and (6) hematemesis, which may be a relative contraindication.

The best results with gastric aspiration and lavage are obtained with the largest possible orogastric tube that can be reasonably passed (nasogastric tubes are not large enough for this purpose). In adults, use a large-bore orogastric Lavacuator hose or a No. 36 French Ewald tube; in children, use a No. 22–28 French orogastric-type tube.

The amount of fluid used will vary with the patient's age and size, but in general 300 ml per lavage is used in an adult and 100 ml in a child.

Continuous gastric suction has been used for substances that have an enterohepatic recirculation or are actively secreted into the gastrointestinal tract, such as tricyclic antidepressants (imipramine [Tofranil]) and local anesthetics such as mepivacaine (Carbocaine) (Table 2).

Activated charcoal is produced by combustion of organic material in the absence of air until the carbon particle is formed. There are few *relative contraindications* to the use of activated charcoal: (1) it should not be administered prior to, concom-

TABLE 2. **Substances with Enterohepatic Recirculation**

Chloral hydrate
Colchicine
Digitalis preparations (digoxin, digitoxin)
Glutethimide
Halogenated hydrocarbons (DDT derivatives)
Isoniazid
Methaqualone
Phenothiazines
Phenytoin
Salicylates
Tricyclic antidepressants

itantly with, or shortly after syrup of ipecac since it may adsorb the ipecac and interfere with its emetic properties; (2) it should not be given prior to, concomitantly with, or shortly after oral antidotes unless proved not to interfere significantly with their absorption; (3) it does not effectively adsorb caustics and corrosives and may produce vomiting or cling to the esophageal or gastric mucosa and falsely appear as a burn on endoscopy; and it should not be given if there are no bowel sounds. Activated charcoal has no *absolute contraindications*, but it does not effectively adsorb alcohols, boric acid, caustics, corrosives, cyanide, metals, and drugs insoluble in aqueous acid solution (Table 3). Activated charcoal is a stool marker, indicating that the toxin has passed through the gastrointestinal tract and that no further significant absorption from the original ingestion will occur.

The dose of activated charcoal is 1 gram per kg per dose orally with a minimum of 15 grams. The usual adolescent and adult dose is 60 to 100 grams. It is administered as a slurry mixed with water or by orogastric tube. It is too thick to get down by nasogastric tube. It should not be mixed with milk, marmalade, or starch because these interfere with charcoal's adsorptive action. Charcoal should be mixed with sorbitol, which acts as a cathartic, enhances palatability, and does not interfere with charcoal's adsorptive capacity.

Activated charcoal may be administered orally every 4 hours as long as bowel sounds are present, and it may be especially beneficial in intoxications that have an enterohepatic recirculation (see Table 2). Repeated dosing with oral activated charcoal has been shown to increase the clearance of many drugs without enterohepatic recirculation (see individual poisonings).

Catharsis is used to hasten the elimination of any remaining toxin in the gastrointestinal tract. Cathartics are *relatively contraindicated* (1) when ileus is indicated by absence of bowel sounds, (2) in intestinal obstruction or evidence of intestinal perforation, and (3) in cases with a pre-existing electrolyte disturbance. Magnesium sulfate (Epsom salts) is contraindicated in renal failure;

TABLE 3. **Toxic Substances Not Effectively Adsorbed by Activated Charcoal**

Alcohols
Aliphatic hydrocarbons
Boric acid
Caustic alkali
Corrosive acids
Cyanide
Glycols
Metals—iron, lead, lithium, mercury
Mineral acids
Saline cathartics—sodium, magnesium

sodium sulfate (Glauber's salts), in heart failure or diseases requiring sodium restriction. Magnesium sulfate or sodium sulfate is administered in doses of 250 mg per kg per dose as 20 per cent solutions. The adolescent and adult doses are 30 grams. Sorbitol is given at 2.8 ml per kg to a maximum of 214 ml of a 70 per cent solution, for adults. The cathartic should be given with the initial dose of activated charcoal. *Note:* Super Char with sorbitol (Gulf Biosystems, Inc.) has been shown to be a more efficacious charcoal preparation because it has three times the surface area as compared with standard activated charcoal preparations.

Dilutional treatment is indicated for the immediate management of caustic and corrosive poisonings but is otherwise not useful. *Contraindications* to dilution are (1) inability of the patient to swallow, resulting in aspiration of the diluting fluid, and (2) signs of upper airway obstruction, esophageal perforation, and shock. The administration of large quantities of diluting fluid—above 30 ml in children and 250 ml in adults—may produce vomiting, re-exposing the vital tissues to the effects of local damage and possible aspiration.

Neutralization has not been proved to be scientifically effective.

THE USE OF ANTIDOTES

Antidotes are available for only a relatively small number of poisons. An available antidote should be administered only after the vital functions are established. Table 4 summarizes the commonly used antidotes and their indications and methods of administration. Most informational, so-called first aid measures and antidotes on commercial product labels are notorious for their inaccuracy; it is preferable to contact the regional poison control center rather than follow recommendations on these labels.

ENHANCEMENT OF ELIMINATION

The medical methods for elimination of the absorbed toxic substances are diuresis, dialysis, hemoperfusion, exchange transfusion, plasmapheresis, enzyme induction, and inhibition. The methods to increase urinary excretion of toxic chemicals and drugs are being studied extensively, but the other modalities have not been well evaluated.

In general, these methods are needed in only a minority of instances and should be reserved for life-threatening circumstances or when a definite benefit is anticipated.

Diuresis. Diuresis increases the renal clearance

Text continued on page 1062

TABLE 4. **Antidotes***

Medications	Indications	Comments
1. *N*-Acetylcysteine (NAC, Mucomyst), Mead Johnson. Glutathione precursor that prevents accumulation and helps detoxify acetaminophen metabolites. **Dose:** *Adult,* 140 mg/kg PO of 5% solution as loading dose, then 70 mg/kg PO q 4 hr for 17 doses as maintenance dose. *Child,* same as adult. **Packaged:** 10 and 20% solution in 5-, 10-, and 30-ml vials.	Acetaminophen toxicity. Most effective within first 8 hr (to make more palatable, administer through a straw inserted into closed container of citrus juice). **AR:** Stomatitis, nausea, vomiting. See Acetaminophen in text. The full course of therapy is required in any patient whose level falls in the toxic range.	IV preparation experimental. The dose of NAC should be repeated if the patient vomits within 1 hr after administration. Methods to stop vomiting of the NAC are (1) placement of a tube in the duodenum, (2) slow administration over 1 hr, (3) ½ hour before NAC dose use metoclopramide (Reglan), 1 mg/kg IV over 1–2 min (max dose 10 mg) every 6 hr or droperidol (Inapsine), 1.25 mg IV; for extrapyramidal reactions use diphenhydramine (see 18. Diphenhydramine).
2. **Ammonium chloride**, USP, usually given via nasogastric tube. **Dose:** *Adult,* 2 grams q 6 hr in 60-ml dose to maximum of 12 grams/day or 1.5 grams as 1–2% IV q 6 hr up to 6 grams/day. *Child,* 75 mg/kg (2.75 mEq/kg) 4 times/day to maximum of 2–6 grams IV or PO. **Packaged:** 325-, 500-, and 1000-mg tablets: 2.14% in 500 ml, 21.4% in 30 ml, 26.75% in 20 ml.	Acidification of urine may enhance the elimination of phencyclidine and other weak bases (amphetamines and strychnine), but the danger of rhabdomyolysis and precipitation of myoglobin in the renal tubules in an acid milieu indicates that this therapy is too dangerous to recommend routinely.	Goal in acid diuresis is to keep urine pH 4.5–5.5 and output 3–6 ml/kg/hr. Monitor blood pH, keep at 7.2–7.3. A diurectic may be used to enhance acid diuresis. Contraindications: weak acid drugs, rhabdomyolysis and myoglobinuria, liver dysfunction, renal dysfunction, closed-head injury.
3. **Amyl nitrite.**	See 14. Cyanide antidote kit	
4. **Antivenin Black Widow Spider** (*Latrodectus mactans*) **Dose:** 1–2 vials infused over 1 hr. **Packaged:** 6000 U/vial with 2.5 ml sterile water and 1 ml horse serum 1:10 dilution.	Black widow spider; all *Latrodectus* species with severe symptoms. Most healthy adults will survive with supportive care. Used in elderly or infants or if underlying medical condition causing hemodynamic instability. **AR:** Same as antivenin polyvalent because derived from horse serum.	Preliminary sensitivity test. Supportive care alone is standard management.
5. **Antivenin Polyvalent** for Crotalidae (pit vipers), Wyeth. IV only. **Dose:** depends on degree of envenomation: minimal: 5–8 vials, moderate: 8–12 vials, severe: 13–30 vials. Dilute in 500–2000 ml of crystalloid solution and start IV at a slow rate, increasing after the first 10 min, if no reaction occurs. **Packaged:** 1 vial (10 ml) lyophilized serum, 1 vial (10 ml) bacteriostatic water for injection, 1 vial (1 ml) normal horse serum.	Venoms of crotalids (pit vipers) of North and South America. **AR:** (Shock anaphylaxis) reaction occurs within 30 min. Serum sickness usually occurs 5–44 days after administration. It may occur less than 5 days, especially in those who have received horse serum products in the past. Symptoms include fever, edema, arthralgia, nausea, and vomiting, as well as pain and muscle weakness.	Consider consulting with Regional Poison Control Center and herpetologist. Administer IV. Preliminary sensitivity test. Never inject in fingers, toes, or bite site.
6. **Antivenin**, North American coral snake. Wyeth. IV only. **Dose:** 3–5 vials (30–50 ml) by slow IV injection. First 1–2 ml should be injected over 3–5 min. **Packaged:** 1 vial antivenin, 10 ml. 1 vial bacteriostatic water 10 ml for injection.	*Micrurus fulvius* (Eastern coral snake); *Micrurus tenere* (Texas coral snake) **AR:** Anaphylaxis (sensitivity reaction). Usually 30 min after administration. Signs/symptoms: Flushing, itching, edema of face, cough, dyspnea, cyanosis. Neurologic manifestations: Usually involve the shoulders and arms. Pain and muscle weakness are frequently present, and permanent atrophy may develop.	Same as for Antivenin polyvalent for Crotalidae. Will not neutralize the venom of *Micrurus euryxanthus* (Arizona or Sonoran coral snake).

*This is for informational purposes and is not intended to substitute for independent judgment. It is always advisable to review the package insert for the most up-to-date information. Contact Regional Poison Control Center for additional details on use.

Abbreviations: AR = adverse reactions to antidotes; MP = monitor parameters; FDA = U.S. Food and Drug Administration; ECG = electrocardiogram; CNS = central nervous system; GI = gastrointestinal.

TABLE 4. **Antidotes*** *Continued*

Medications	Indications	Comments
7. **Atropine** (various manufacturers). Antagonizes cholinergic stimuli at muscarinic receptors. **Dose:** *Adult,* Initial dose 2–4 mg IV. Dose every 10–15 min as necessary until cessation of secretions. Severe poisoning may require doses up to 2000 mg. *Child,* Initial dose of 0.02 mg/kg to a maximum of 2 mg every 10–15 min as necessary until cessation of secretions. Use preservative-free atropine for infusion. **Packaged:** 0.3 mg/ml in 30 ml; 0.4 mg/ml in 0.5-, 1-, 20-, and 30-ml vials; 1 mg/ml in 1- and 10-ml vials.	Therapy in carbamate and organophosphate insecticide poisonings. Rarely needed in cholinergic mushroom intoxication (*Amanita muscaria, Clitocybe, Inocybe* spp.). Lack of signs of atropinization confirms diagnosis of cholinesterase inhibition. **Diagnostic Test:** *Child,* 0.01 mg/kg/ IV. *Adult,* 1 mg total. **AR:** Flushing and dryness of skin, blurred vision, rapid and irregular pulse, fever, and loss of neuromuscular coordination.	If cyanosis, establish respiration first because atropine in cyanotic patients may cause ventricular fibrillation. If severe signs of atropinization, may correct with physostigmine in doses equal to one-half dose of atropine. If symptomatic, administer until the end point of drying secretions and clearing of lungs. Hallucinations, flushing of the skin, dilated pupils, tachycardia, and elevation of body temperature are not end points and do not preclude atropine administration. Atropinization should be maintained for 12 to 24 hours; then taper dose and observe for relapse. Atropine has been administered successfully by IV infusion, although this method has not received FDA approval. **Dose:** Place 8 mg of atropine in 100 ml D5W or saline. Conc. = 0.08 mg/ml. Dose range = 0.02–0.08 mg/kg/hr or 0.25–1 ml/kg/hr. Severe poisoning may require supplemental doses of IV atropine intermittently in doses of 2–4 mg until drying of secretion occurs.
8. **BAL**	See 17. Dimercaprol	
9. **Bicarbonate**	See 35. Sodium bicarbonate	
10. **Botulism antitoxin**, Connaught Medical Research Laboratories. **Dose:** *Adult,* 1 vial IV stat then 1 vial IM repeat in 2–4 hr if symptoms appear in 12–24 hr. *Child,* Check with state health department.	Prevention or treatment of botulism.	Contact local or state health department for full management guidelines.
11. **Calcium disodium edetate** (EDTA), Disodium Versenate, Riker. **Dose:** *Adult,* Maximum 4 grams. *Child,* 1 gram. Moderate toxicity, IM or IV, 50 mg/kg day for 3–5 days. Severe toxicity, IV or IM, 75 mg/kg day for 4–5 days, divided into 3–6 doses daily. Dilute 1 gram in 250–500 ml saline or D5W, infuse over 4 hr twice daily for 5–7 days. *Child,* Maximum 1 gram. For lead levels over 69 µg/dl or if symptoms of lead poisoning or encephalopathy: Add BAL alone initially, 4 mg/kg, then combination BAL and EDTA at different sites. EDTA dose: 12.5 mg/kg IM.	For chelation of cadmium, chromium, cobalt, copper, lead, magnesium, nickel, selenium, tellurium, tungsten, uranium, vanadium, and zinc. **AR:** 1. Thrombophlebitis. 2. Nausea, vomiting. 3. Hypotension. 4. Transient bone marrow suppression. 5. Nephrotoxicity, reversible tubular necrosis (particularly in acid urine). 6. Fever 4–8 hr after infusion. 7. Increased prothrombin time.	Hydrate first and establish renal flow. Avoid plain sodium EDTA since hypocalcemia may result. Procaine 0.25–1 ml of 0.5% for each ml of IM EDTA to reduce pain. Do not use EDTA orally. Limit use to 7 days (otherwise loss of other ions and cardiac dysrhythmias may occur). **MP:** Calcium levels, urinalysis, renal profile, erythrocyte protoporphyrin, blood lead, and liver profile. Contraindicated in iron intoxication, hepatic impairment, and renal failure.

*This is for informational purposes and is not intended to substitute for independent judgment. It is always advisable to review the package insert for the most up-to-date information. Contact Regional Poison Control Center for additional details on use.

Abbreviations: AR = adverse reactions to antidotes; MP = monitor parameters; FDA = U.S. Food and Drug Administration; ECG = electrocardiogram; CNS = central nervous system; GI = gastrointestinal.

Table continued on following page

TABLE 4. **Antidotes*** *Continued*

Medications	Indications	Comments
(See Lead in text for latest recommendations.) Modify dose in renal failure. **Packaged:** 200 mg/ml, 5-ml ampules.		
12. (A) **Calcium gluconate**, various manufacturers. **Dose:** *Adult,* 10 grams in 250 ml of water PO or by nasogastric tube; 30 grams maximum daily dose. **Packaged:** 500-, 650-mg, 1-gram tablets.	To precipitate fluorides, magnesium, salts, and oxalates after oral ingestion.	
(B) **Calcium gluconate** 10%. **Dose:** IV 0.2–0.5 ml/kg of elemental calcium up to maximum 10 ml (1 gram) over 5–10 min with continuous ECG monitoring. Titrate to adequate response. **Packaged:** 10% in 10 ml vial.	Calcium channel blocker poisoning, e.g., nifedipine (Procardia), verapamil (Calan), diltiazem (Cardizem). It improves the blood pressure but does not affect the dysrhythmias. Hypocalcemia as result of poisonings. Black widow spider envenomation.	Repeat dose as needed. Monitor calcium levels. Contraindicated with digitalis poisoning.
(C) **Calcium chloride.** **Dose:** IV 0.2 ml/kg up to maximum 10 ml (1 gram) with continuous IV monitoring. Titrate to adequate response.	Hydrofluoric acid (if irrigation with cool water fails to control the pain). **AR:** IV bradycardia, asystole, necrosis with extravasation.	Infiltration with calcium gluconate should be considered if hydrofluoric acid exposure results in immediate tissue damage and erythema and pain persist following adequate irrigation.
(D) **Infiltration of calcium gluconate.** **Dose:** Infiltrate each square cm of the affected dermis and subcutaneous tissue with about 0.5 ml of 10% calcium gluconate using a 30-gauge needle. Repeat as needed to control pain. **Packaged:** 10% in 10-ml vial.		
(E) **Calcium gel** 3.5 grams USP, calcium gluconate powder added to 5 oz of water-soluble lubricating jelly.	Dermal exposures of hydrofluoric acid less than 20%.	Gel must have direct access to burn area. If pain persists, a calcium gluconate injection may be needed.
13. **Chlorpromazine,** various manufacturers. Phenothiazine derivative. **Dose:** *Adult,* 1 mg/kg dose† IV/IM or 0.5 mg/kg dose if taken with barbiturate or if exhausted. **Packaged:** 25 mg/ml in 1-, 2-, and 10-ml vials.	Only in *pure* amphetamine overdose, with life-threatening manifestations. (Diazepam [Valium] is preferred.) Toxicity: CNS depression, coma, hypotension, extrapyramidal syndrome, agitation, fever, convulsions, dry mouth, cardiac arrhythmias, ECG changes.	Do not use if any signs of atropinization or "street drug" amphetamines are present. Watch for hypotension. In general it is safer to use diazepam (Valium) or haloperidol (Haldol).
14. **Cyanide antidote kit,** Lilly. Nitrite-induced methemoglobinemia attracts cyanide off cytochrome oxidase and thiosulfate forms nontoxic thiocyanate. **Doses:** *Adult,* amyl nitrite.‡ Inhale for 30 sec of every min. Use a new ampule every 3 min. Reapply until sodium nitrite can be	Cyanide poisoning. **AR:** Hypotension, methemoglobinemia.	*Note:* If a child is given the adult dose of sodium nitrite, a fatal methemoglobinemia may result. *Do not use methylene blue* for methemoglobinemia in cyanide therapy. Observe for hypotension and have epinephrine available. Cyanide kits should have amyl nitrite changed annually.

*This is for informational purposes and is not intended to substitute for independent judgment. It is always advisable to review the package insert for the most up-to-date information. Contact Regional Poison Control Center for additional details on use.

†This dose may exceed the manufacturer's recommended dose.

‡This use is not listed by the manufacturer.

Abbreviations: AR = adverse reactions to antidotes; MP = monitor parameters; FDA = U.S. Food and Drug Administration; ECG = electrocardiogram; CNS = central nervous system; GI = gastrointestinal.

TABLE 4. **Antidotes*** *Continued*

Medications	Indications	Comments
given. Then inject IV 300 mg (10 ml of 3% solution) of sodium nitrite at a rate of 2.5 to 5 ml/min. Then inject 12.5 grams (50 ml of 25% solution) of sodium thiosulfate. *Child*, Use the following chart for children's dosage. **Packaged:** 2- to 10-ml ampules sodium nitrite injection: 2- to 50-ml ampules sodium thiosulfate injection; 0.3-ml amyl nitrite inhalant.		Administer 100% oxygen between inhalations of amyl nitrite. Monitor hemoglobin, arterial blood gases, methemoglobin concentration (nitrite given to obtain a methemoglobin of 25%). Some add nitrite ampule to resuscitation bag.

Hemoglobin	*Initial Child Dose of Sodium Nitrite 3% (do not exceed 10 ml)*	*Initial Child Dose of Sodium Thiosulfate (do not exceed 12.5 grams)*
8 gram	0.22 ml/kg (6.6 mg/kg)	1.10 ml/kg
10 gram	0.27 ml/kg (8.7 mg/kg)	1.35 ml/kg
12 gram	0.33 ml/kg (10 mg/kg)	1.65 ml/kg
14 grams	0.39 ml/kg (11.6 mg/kg)	1.95 ml/kg

If signs of poisoning reappear, repeat above procedure at one-half the above doses.

Medications	Indications	Comments
15. **Deferoxamine mesylate** (DFOM, Desferal), Ciba. Has a remarkable affinity for ferric iron and chelates it. **Therapeutic Dose:** *Adult*, 90 mg/kg† IM or IV q 8 hr to a maximum of 1 gram per injection; may repeat to maximum of 6 grams in 24 hr. *Child*, Same as adult. IV administration can be given by slow infusion at rate not exceeding 15 mg/kg/hr. **Packaged:** 500 mg/ampule (powder).	DFOM is useful in the treatment of symptomatic iron poisoning or cases where the serum iron level > 350 μg/dl. A positive result of a DFOM challenge test is not a definite indication that therapy is necessary in the asymptomatic patient. Oral DFOM is not recommended. Iron intoxication. Therapeutic: See dose in left column. *Diagnostic trial*: Give deferoxamine, 50 mg/kg IM (up to 1 gram). If serum iron exceeds total iron-binding capacity, unbound iron is excreted in urine, producing a "vin rose" color of chelated iron complex in the urine (pink orange). However, may be negative with high serum iron exceeding total iron-binding capacity. **AR:** Flushing of the skin, generalized erythema, urticaria, hypotension, and shock may occur. Blindness has occurred rarely in patients receiving long-term, high-dose DFOM therapy. Contraindicated in patients with renal disease or anuria.	Therapy is usually continued until urine color and/or iron levels are normal. Therapy is rarely required over 24 hr. Establish a good renal flow. To be effective DFOM should be administered in first 12–16 hr. In mild to moderate iron intoxication, IM or IV route. In severe intoxication or shock, IV route only. Monitor serum iron levels, urine output, and urine color.
16. **Diazepam** (Valium), Roche. **Dose:** *Adult*, 5–10 mg IV (maximum 20 mg) at a rate of 5 mg/min until seizure is controlled. May be repeated 2 or 3 times. *Child*, 0.1–0.3 mg/kg up to 10 mg IV slowly over 2 min. **Packaged:** 5 mg/ml, 2- to 10-ml vials.	Any intoxication that provokes seizures when specific therapy is *not* available, e.g., amphetamines, PCP, barbiturate and alcohol withdrawal. Chloroquine poisoning. **AR:** Confusion, somnolence, coma, hypotension.	IM absorption is erratic. Establish airway and administer 100% oxygen and glucose.

*This is for informational purposes and is not intended to substitute for independent judgment. It is always advisable to review the package insert for the most up-to-date information. Contact Regional Poison Control Center for additional details on use.

†This dose may exceed the manufacturer's recommended dose.

Abbreviations: AR = adverse reactions to antidotes; MP = monitor parameters; FDA = U.S. Food and Drug Administration; ECG = electrocardiogram; CNS = central nervous system; GI = gastrointestinal.

Table continued on following page

TABLE 4. **Antidotes*** *Continued*

Medications	Indications	Comments
17. **Dimercaprol** (BAL), Hynson, Westcott, and Dunning. **Dose:** Recommendations vary, contact Regional Poison Control Center. Prevents inhibition of sulfhydryl enzymes. Given deep IM only. For *severe lead poisoning:* see 11. EDTA. For *mild arsenic or gold:* 2.5 mg/kg q 6 hr for 2 days, then q 12 hr on the third day, and once daily thereafter for 10 days. For *severe arsenic or gold:* 3–5 mg/kg q 6 hr for 3 days, then q 12 hr thereafter for 10 days.† For *mercury:* 5 mg/kg initially, followed by 2.5 mg/kg 1 or 2 times daily for 10 days. **Packaged:** 100 mg/ml 10% in oil in 3-ml ampules.	For chelation of antimony, arsenic, bismuth, chromates, copper, gold, lead, and mercury nickel. **AR:** 30% of patients have reactions: fever (30% of children), hypertension, tachycardia; may cause hemolysis in glucose-6-phosphate dehydrogenase deficiency patients. Doses greater than recommended may cause various adverse effects: nausea, vomiting, headache, chest pain, tachycardia, and hypertension.	Contraindicated in instances of hepatic insufficiency, with the exception of postarsenic jaundice. Should be discontinued or used only with extreme caution if acute renal insufficiency is present. Monitor blood pressure and heart rate (both may increase), urinalysis, qualitative urine excretion of heavy metal. Contraindicated in iron, silver, uranium, selenium, and cadmium poisoning.
18. **Diphenhydramine** (Benadryl), Parke-Davis. Antiparkinsonian action. **Dose:** *Adult,* 10–50 mg IV over 2 min. *Child,* 1–2 mg/kg IV up to 50 mg over 2 min. Maximum in 24 hr 400 mg. **Packaged:** 10 mg/ml in 10- and 30-ml vials. 50 mg/ml in 1-, 5-, 10-, and 30-ml vials. Capsules, tablets 25 mg. Elixir, syrup 12.5 mg/5 ml.	Used to treat extrapyramidal symptoms and dystonia induced by phenothiazines and related drugs. **AR:** Fatal dose, 20–40 mg/kg. Dry mouth, drowsiness.	Continue with oral diphenhydramine 5 mg/kg/day to 25 mg 3 times a day for 72 hr to avoid recurrence.
19. **EDTA**	See 11. Calcium disodium edetate	
20. **Ethanol** (ETOH). Competitively inhibits alcohol dehydrogenase. **Loading Dose:** Administer 7.6–10.0 ml/kg of 10% ETOH in D5W over 30 min IV or 0.8–1.0 ml/kg 95% ETOH PO in 6 oz of orange juice over 30 min. While administering loading dose start maintenance. **Maintenance Dose:** Volume of 10% ETOH needed IV or 95% oral solution (not in dialysis). (See table of maintenance dose below.) If patient is on dialysis, add 91 ml/hr in addition to regular maintenance dose. See comments to prepare 10% solution if not commercially available. **Packaged:** 10% ethanol in D5W 1000 ml; 95% ethanol. May be given as 50% solution orally.	Methanol, ethylene glycol. Ethanol infusion therapy may be started in cases of suspected methanol and ethylene glycol poisoning presenting with increased anion gap and osmolal gap, or if the urine shows the crystalluria of ethylene glycol poisoning or the hyperemia of the optic disk of methanol intoxication. **AR:** CNS depression, hypoglycemia.	Monitor blood ethanol 1 hr after starting infusion and every 4–6 hr. Maintain a blood ethanol concentration of 100–200 mg/dl. Monitor blood glucose, electrolytes, blood gases, urinalysis, and renal profile at least daily. Continue infusion until safe concentration of ethylene glycol or methanol is reached. Ethanol-induced hypoglycemia may occur. Dialysis, preferably hemodialysis, should be considered in severe intoxication not controlled by ethanol alone. To prepare 10% ethanol for infusion for infusion therapy: Remove 100 ml from 1 liter of D5W and replace with 100 ml of tax-free bulk absolute alcohol after passing through 0.22 μm filter. 50-ml vials of pyrogen-free absolute ethanol for injection are available from Pharm-Serve, 218–20 96th Avenue, Queen's Village, NY 11429. Telephone 718-475-1601.

*This is for informational purposes and is not intended to substitute for independent judgment. It is always advisable to review the package insert for the most up-to-date information. Contact Regional Poison Control Center for additional details on use.

†This dose may exceed the manufacturer's recommended dose.

Abbreviations: AR = adverse reactions to antidotes; MP = monitor parameters; FDA = U.S. Food and Drug Administration; ECG = electrocardiogram; CNS = central nervous system; GI = gastrointestinal.

TABLE 4. **Antidotes*** *Continued*

Medications	Indications	Comments

Maintenance Dose:

Patient Category	ml/kg/hr using 10% IV	ml/kg/hr using 50% oral
Nondrinker	0.83	0.17
Occasional drinker	1.40	0.28
Alcoholic	1.96	0.39

Medications	Indications	Comments
21. **Fab** (antibody fragment) (Digibind). **Dose:** The average dose used during clinical testing was 10 vials. Dosage details are specified by the manufacturer. It should be administered IV over 30 min. Calculate on basis of body burden either by known amount ingested or by serum digoxin concentration. *Calculation of dose of Fab:* 1. Known amount ingested multiplied by bioavailability (0.8) = body burden. Body burden divided by 0.6 = number of vials. 2. Known serum digoxin (obtained 6 hr postingestion) multiplied by volume distribution (5.6 liters/kg) and weight in kg divided by 1000 = body burden. Body burden divided by 0.6 = number of vials.	Digoxin, digitoxin, oleander tea with life-threatening intoxications, refractory dysrhythmias, hyperkalemia. 40 mg binds 0.6 mg digoxin.	Contact Regional Poison Control Center. Preliminary sensitivity test. Administer through a 0.22-μm filter. It causes a rise in measured bound digoxin but a fall in free digoxin.
22. **Glucagon.** Works by stimulating production of cyclic adenyl monophosphate. **Dose:** 50–150 μg/kg over 1 min IV followed by a continuous infusion of 1–15 mg/hr in dextrose and then taper over 5–12 hr. 2 mg of phenol is in 1 mg of glucagon; 50 mg is the maximum amount of phenol recommended and therefore toxicity may result when high doses of glucagon are used. **Packaged:** 1-mg (1-unit) vial with 1-ml diluent with glycerin and phenol; also in 10-ml size.	Propranolol and other beta blocker intoxication. **AR:** Generally well tolerated—most frequent are nausea, vomiting.	Do not dissolve the lyophilized glucagon in the solvent packaged with it when administering IV infusion because of possible phenol toxicity. Use 0.9% saline or D5W. Effects of single dose observed in 5–10 min and last for 15–30 min. A constant infusion may be necessary to sustain desired effects.
23. **Labetalol hydrochloride** (Normodyne) Schering; (Trandate) Glaxo. Nonselective beta and mild alpha blocker. **Dose:** IV 20 mg over 2 min. Additional injections of 40 or 80 mg can be given at 10-min intervals until desired supine blood pressure achieved. Maximum dose 300 mg. Alternative: Slow IV infusion: 200 mg (40 ml) is added to 160 or 250 ml of D5W and given at 2 mg/min. Titrate infusion according to response. **Packaged:** Solution 5 mg/ml in 20 ml.	Hypertensive crises secondary to cocaine. **AD:** GI disturbances, orthostatic hypotension, bronchospasm, congestive heart failure, atrioventricular conduction disturbances, and peripheral vascular reactions.	Concomitant diuretic enhances therapeutic response. Patient should be kept in a supine position during infusion. **MP:** Monitor blood pressure during and after administration.

*This is for informational purposes and is not intended to substitute for independent judgment. It is always advisable to review the package insert for the most up-to-date information. Contact Regional Poison Control Center for additional details on use.

Abbreviations: AR = adverse reactions to antidotes; MP = monitor parameters; FDA = U.S. Food and Drug Administration; ECG = electrocardiogram; CNS = central nervous system; GI = gastrointestinal.

Table continued on following page

TABLE 4. **Antidotes*** *Continued*

Medications	Indications	Comments
24. **Methylene blue**, Harvey and others. Physiologically transformed to reduced form, leukomethylene blue, which is then oxidized to methylene blue in the presence of methemoglobin. The methemoglobin is converted to hemoglobin. **Dose:** *Adult,* 0.1–0.2 ml/kg of 1% solution (1–2 mg/kg over 5 min IV). *Child,* Same as adult. **Packaged:** 1% 10-ml ampules. May repeat in 1 hr if necessary, only once.	Methemoglobinemia. **AR:** GI (nausea, vomiting), headache, hypertension, dizziness, mental confusion, restlessness, dyspnea when IV dose exceeds 7 mg/kg. Also, hemolysis, dysuria, blue skin or urine, burning sensation in vein. Treatment is unnecessary unless methemoglobin is over 30% or respiratory distress.	Saliva, urine, and other body fluids may turn blue. *Contraindications:* Renal insufficiency; cyanide poisonings when sodium nitrite is used to induce methemoglobinemia; in glucose-6-phosphate dehydrogenase deficiency patients. Monitor hemolysis, methemoglobin level, and arterial blood gases. Avoid extravasation because of local necrosis.
25. **Naloxone** (Narcan). Pure opioid antagonist. **Dose:** *Adult,* 0.4–2.0 mg IV and repeat at 3-min intervals until respiratory function is stable. Before excluding opioid intoxication on the basis of a lack of naloxone response, a minimum of 2 mg in a child or 10 mg in an adult should be administered. *Child,* Initial dose is 0.01 mg/kg. If no response, a subsequent dose of 0.1 mg/kg may be administered. **Packaged:** 0.02 and 0.4 mg/ml ampules, and 10-ml multidose vial.	Narcotic, opiate, CNS depression. This drug is relatively free of adverse reactions. Rare report of pulmonary edema. Should be administered with caution in pregnancy. It is used only to reverse depression and hypoxia.	Naloxone infusion therapy should be used if a large initial dose was required, repeated boluses are necessary, or a long-acting opiate is involved. In infusion therapy the initial response dose is administered every hour and may need to be boostered in ½ after starting. The infusion may be tapered after 12 hr of therapy. Naloxone infusion: Calculate daily fluid requirements, add initial response dose of naloxone multiplied by 24 to the solution. Divide fluid by 24 to determine ml/hr of naloxone infusion. Does not cause CNS depression. Routes: IV or endotracheal are preferred routes. Pentazocine (Talwin), dextromethorphan, propoxyphene (Darvon), and codeine may require larger doses.
26. **Nicotinamide** (various manufacturers). **Dose:** *Adult,* 500 mg IM or IV slowly, then 200–400 mg q 4 hr. If symptoms develop, the frequency of injections should be increased to every 2 hr (maximum 3 grams/day). *Child,* One-half suggested adult dose. **Packaged:** 100 mg/ml: 2-, 5-, 10-, 30-ml vials; 25- and 50-mg tablets.	Vacor poisoning: phenylurea pesticide intoxication. *Note:* Vacor 2% is now available only to professional exterminators. 0.5% Vacor is available to the general public and can be toxic to children if swallowed. **AR:** Large doses: flushing, pruritus, sensation of burning, nausea, vomiting, anaphylactic shock.	Nicotinamide is most effective when given within 1 hr of ingestion. Do not use niacin or nicotinic acid in place of nicotinamide. Monitor liver profile.
27. **Oxygen** 100%. **Dose:** *Adult,* 100% oxygen by inhalation or 100% oxygen in hyperbaric chamber at 2–3 atm. *Child,* Same as adult.	Carbon monoxide, cyanide, methemoglobinemia. Any inhalation intoxication.	Half-life of carboxyhemoglobin is 240 min in room air 21% oxygen; if a patient is hyperventilated with 100% oxygen, half-life of carboxyhemoglobin is 90 min; in chamber at 2 atm, half-life is 25–30 min.
28. **Pancuronium bromide** (Pavulon). Nondepolarizing (competitive) blocking agent. **Dose:** *Adults and children,* Initially, 0.1 mg/kg IV; for intubation, 0.1 mg/kg IV, repeated as required (generally every 40 to 60 min).†	Neuromuscular blocking agent. Used for intubation and seizure control, acts in 2 min, lasts 40–60 min. **AR:** Main hazard is inadequate postoperative ventilation. Tachycardia and slight increase in arterial pressure may occur owing to vagolytic action.	The required dose varies greatly and a peripheral nerve stimulator aids in determining appropriate amount. Should monitor electroencephalogram, since motor effect may be abolished without decreasing electrical discharge from brain.

*This is for informational purposes and is not intended to substitute for independent judgment. It is always advisable to review the package insert for the most up-to-date information. Contact Regional Poison Control Center for additional details on use.

†This dose may exceed the manufacturer's recommended dose.

Abbreviations: AR = adverse reactions to antidotes; MP = monitor parameters; FDA = U.S. Food and Drug Administration; ECG = electrocardiogram; CNS = central nervous system; GI = gastrointestinal.

TABLE 4. **Antidotes*** *Continued*

Medications	Indications	Comments
Packaged: Solution 1 mg/ml in 10 ml; 2 mg/ml in 2- and 5-ml containers.		
29. D-**Penicillamine** (Cuprimine) Merck; (Depen) Wallace. Effective chelator and promotes excretion in urine. **Dose:** 250 mg 4 times daily PO for up to 5 days for long-term (20–40 days) therapy; 30–40 mg/kg/day in children. Maximum 1 gram/day. For chronic therapy, 25 mg/kg/day in 4 doses. **Packaged:** 125- and 250-mg capsules.	Heavy metals, arsenic, cadmium, chromates, cobalt, copper, lead, mercury, nickel, and zinc. **AR:** Leukopenia (2%); thrombocytopenia (4%); GI: nausea, vomiting, diarrhea (17%); fever, rash, lupus syndrome, renal and hepatic injury; anaphylactic shock.	This is not considered standard therapy for lead poisoning after chelation therapy. May produce ampicillin-like rash, allergic reactions, neutropenia, and nephropathy. Contraindication: hypersensitivity to penicillin. **MP:** Routine urinalysis, white differential blood count, hemoglobin determination, direct platelet count, renal and hepatic profiles. Collect 24-hr urine; quantify for heavy metal.
30. **Physostigmine salicylate** (Antilirium), Forest. Cholinesterase inhibitor. A diagnostic trial is not recommended. **Dose:** *Adult,* 1–2 mg IV over 2 min: may repeat every 5 min to maximum dose of 6 mg. *Child,* IV, 0.02 mg/kg over 2 min to a maximum dose of 2 mg.† Once effect accomplished give lowest effective dose every 30–60 min if symptoms recur. **Packaged:** 1 mg/ml in 2 ml/ampule.	Used if conventional therapy fails for coma, convulsions, severe cardiac dysrhythmias, severe hypertension, hallucinations secondary to anticholinergics, antihistamines, and anticholinergic plants. **AR:** Death may result from respiratory paralysis, hypertension/hypotension, bradycardia/tachycardia/asystole, hypersalivation, respiratory difficulties/convulsions (cholinergic crisis).	Do not consider for the following: antidepressants, amoxapine, maprotiline, nomifensine, bupropion, trazodone, imipramine. IV administration should be at a slow controlled rate, not more than 1 mg/min. Rapid administration can cause adverse reactions. Can be reversed by atropine. Lasts only 30 min. Contraindicated in asthma, cardiovascular disease, intestinal obstruction.
31. **Pralidoxime chloride** (2-PAM, Protopam) Ayerst.Cholinesterase reactivator by removing-phosphate. **Dose:** *Adult,* 1–2 grams in 100–250 ml saline IV over 5–30 min. May repeat every 8–12 hr. In severe cases may repeat in 1 hr. May also be given as 5% solution in not less than 5 min. *Child,* 25–50 mg/kg IV over 15–30 min, no faster than 10 mg/kg/min. Maximal dose 12 grams/day. **Packaged:** 1 gram/20 ml vials.	Organophosphate insecticide poisoning. Not usually needed in carbamate insecticide poisoning. Most effective if stated in first 24 hr before bonding of phosphate. **AR:** Rapid IV injection has produced tachycardia, muscle rigidity, transient neuromuscul→ blockade. IM: cxonjunctival hyperemia, subconjunctival hemorrhage, especially if concentrations exceed 5%–. Oral: nausea, vomiting, diarrhea, malaise.	Should be used only after initial treatment with atropine. Draw blood for erythrocyte cholinesterase level prior to giving 2-PAM. The use of 2-PAM may require a reduction in the dose of atropine. **MP:** Monitor renal profile and reduce dose accordingly.
32. **Propranolol** (Inderal). Nonselective beta blocker. **Dose:** *Adult,* 0.1–0.15 mg/kg IV, administered in increments of 0.5 to 0.75 mg every 1–2 min with continuous ECG and blood pressure monitoring up to 10 mg. *Child,* 0.01–0.15 mg/kg per dose slow IV with repeat dose q 6–8 hr as needed. **Packaged:** 1 mg/ml; tablets: 10, 20, 40, 60, 80, 90 mg; capsules: 20, 80, 160 mg.	Cocaine intoxication. Has not been scientifically proved to be safe and effective. Anecdotal reports only. Labetalol is theoretically preferred agent for cocaine intoxication. **AR:** Bradycardia, hypotension, pallor; neurologic effects include hallucinations, coma, and seizures.	Not a specific antidote; used for catecholamine storm and dysrhythmias. Increased mortality has been reported in animals that received propranolol for cocaine poisoning, and hypertension has occurred in humans following its use in cocaine intoxication.

*This is for informational purposes and is not intended to substitute for independent judgment. It is always advisable to review the package insert for the most up-to-date information. Contact Regional Poison Control Center for additional details on use.

†This dose may exceed the manufacturer's recommended dose.

Abbreviations: AR = adverse reactions to antidotes; MP = monitor parameters; FDA = U.S. Food and Drug Administration; ECG = electrocardiogram; CNS = central nervous system; GI = gastrointestinal.

Table continued on following page

TABLE 4. **Antidotes*** Continued

Medications	Indications	Comments
33. **Protamine sulfate.** **Dose:** 1 mg neutralizes 90–115 U of heparin. Maximum dose 50 mg IV over 5 min at 10 mg/ml. **Packaged:** 5 ml = 50 mg; 25 ml = 250 mg.	Heparin overdose. **AR:** Rapid administration causes anaphylactoid reactions.	**MP:** Monitor thromboplastin times. Doses of up to 200 mg have been tolerated over 2 hr in an adult.
34. **Pyridoxine (Vitamin B₆).** Gamma-aminobutyric acid agonist. **Dose:** *Unknown amount ingested:* 5 grams over 5 min IV. *Known amount:* Add 1 gram of pyridoxine for each gram of INH ingested IV over 5 min. **Packaged:** 50 and 100 mg/ml; 10 and 30 ml.	Isoniazid (INH), hydrazine. **AR:** Unlikely owing to the fact that vitamin B_2 is water soluble. However, nausea, vomiting, somnolence, and paresthesia have been reported from chronic high doses.	Pyridoxine is given as 5–10% solution IV mixed with water. It may be repeated every 5–20 min until seizures cease. Some administer pyridoxine over 30–60 min. **MP:** Correct acidosis, monitor liver profile, acid-base parameters. Lethal dose of pyridoxine is 1 gram/kg.
35. **Sodium bicarbonate.** **Dose:** IV 1–3 mEq/kg as needed to keep pH 7.5 (generally 2 mEq/kg q 6 hr). When alkalinization is desired to correct acidosis to a pH of 7.3, use 2 mEq/kg to raise pH 0.1 unit. **Packaged:** 50 ml, 44.6 mEq, 50 mEq ampule.	To promote urinary alkalinization for salicylates, phenobarbital (weak acids with low volume of distribution excreted in urine unchanged). To correct severe acidosis. To promote protein-binding and supply sodium ions into Purkinje cells in cyclic antidepressant intoxication. **AR:** Large doses in patients with renal insufficiency may cause metabolic alkalosis. In patients with ketoacidosis, rapid alkalinization with sodium bicarbonate may result in clouding of consciousness, cerebral dysfunction, seizures, hypoxia, and lactic acidosis.	Alkaline diuresis. The assessment of the need for bicarbonate should be based on both the blood and urine pH. Maintain the blood pH at 7.5. Keep the urinary output at 3–6 ml/kg/hr. May use a diuretic to enhance diuresis. Potassium is necessary to produce alkaline diuresis. Monitor electrolytes, calcium, pH of both urine and blood, arterial blood gases.
36. **Sodium nitrite.**	See 14. Cyanide antidote kit.	
37. **Sodium thiosulfate.**	See 14. Cyanide antidote kit.	
38. **Vitamin K** (AquaMEPHYTON) Merck. Promotes hepatic biosynthesis of prothrombin and other coagulation factors. Competitive antagonist of warfarin. It may be administered orally in the absence of vomiting. **Dose:** *Adult,* 2.5–10 mg IV, depending on potential for hemorrhage. Oral dose is 15–25 mg/day. Severe bleeding, 5–25 mg slow IV push. Rate 1 mg/min. Repeat q 4–8 hr depending on prothrombin time. *Child,* 1–5 mg IV may be given orally when vomiting ceases at a dose of 5–10 mg/day. **Packaged:** 2 mg/ml in 0.5-ml ampules. 2.5- or 5-ml vials.	Warfarin (coumarin), salicylate intoxication.	Fatalities from anaphylactic reaction have been reported following IV route. It takes 24 hr for vitamin K to be effective. The need for further vitamin K is determined by the prothrombin time test. If severe bleeding, fresh blood or plasma transfusion may be needed.

*This is for informational purposes and is not intended to substitute for independent judgment. It is always advisable to review the package insert for the most up-to-date information. Contact Regional Poison Control Center for additional details on use.

Abbreviations: AR = adverse reactions to antidotes; MP = monitored parameters; FDA = U.S. Food and Drug Administration; ECG = electrocardiogram; CNS = central nervous system; GI = gastrointestinal.

of compounds that are partially reabsorbed in the renal tubules. *Forced-fluid diuresis* is based on the principle that it will shorten exposure for reabsorption at the *distal* renal tubules. The risks of diuresis are fluid overload, with cerebral and pulmonary edema, and disturbances in acid-base and electrolyte balance. Failure to produce a diuresis may imply prerenal or renal failure. If renal failure is present, dialysis should be considered.

Osmotic diuresis is meant to increase the osmotic gradient and prevent reabsorption from the *proximal* loop and *distal* tubules. Mannitol is used to initiate this type of diuresis, and then fluids are added in sufficient amounts to produce a diuresis similar to forced-fluid diuresis.

Acid and alkaline diuresis is based on the principle that to inhibit reabsorption of certain toxic agents the urinary pH can be adjusted so that the substance is maintained in its ionized form, which interferes with its passage back into the blood. Electrolyte and acid-base monitoring is necessary. Hypokalemia and hypocalcemia are frequent complications. *Acid diuresis* is accomplished by using ammonium chloride (Antidote 2, Table 4). Ascorbic acid may be used as an adjunct. It enhances the elimination of weak bases such as amphetamines and fenfluramine (Pondimin). Ammonium chloride is contraindicated if rhabdomyolysis is present. *Alkaline diuresis* with sodium bicarbonate can be utilized in the therapy of weak acids, such as salicylates, and long-acting barbiturates, such as phenobarbital (Antidote 35, Table 4).

Dialysis. Dialysis is the extrarenal means of removing certain toxins from the body or can substitute for the kidney when renal failure occurs. Dialysis is never the first measure instituted; however, it may be lifesaving later in the course of the severe intoxication. It is needed only in a small minority of intoxications (Table 5). *Peritoneal dialysis* is only one-twentieth as effective as hemodialysis. It is easier to use and less hazardous to the patient but also less reliable in removing the toxin. *Hemodialysis* is the most effective means of dialysis but requires experience with sophisticated equipment. *The patient-related criteria for dialysis* are anticipated prolonged coma and the likelihood of complications, renal impairment, and deterioration despite careful medical management.

Hemoperfusion. Hemoperfusion is the extracorporeal exposure of the patient's blood to an adsorbing surface (charcoal or resin). This procedure has extended extracorporeal removal to a large range of substances that were either poorly dialyzable or nondialyzable. Hemoperfusion may be used for agents that have high protein binding, low aqueous solubility, and poor distribution in the plasma water. In these cases hemodialysis is relatively ineffective. Hemoperfusion has proved useful in glutethimide (Doriden) intoxication, barbiturate overdose even with short-acting barbiturates, theophylline, cyclic antidepressants, and chlorophenothane (DDT). The commonly used types are activated charcoal and resin cartridges. In general, supportive care is all that is required. Analysis of studies with hemodialysis

and hemoperfusion does not indicate that they reduce morbidity or mortality substantially except in certain cases (Table 6).

TABLE 5. Indications and Contraindications for Dialysis

Immediate Consideration of Dialysis
Ethylene glycol with refractory acidosis
Methanol with refractory acidosis and levels consistently over 50 mg/dl
Lithium levels consistently elevated over 4 mEq/liter
Amanita phalloides

Indications on Basis of Patient's Condition (coma greater than Stage 3 of Reed Coma Scale)

Alcohol*	Iodides
Ammonia	Isoniazid*
Amphetamines	Meprobamate
Anilines	Paraldehyde
Antibiotics	Potassium*
Barbiturates* (long-acting)	Quinidine
Boric acid	Quinine
Bromides*	Salicylates*
Calcium	Strychnine
Chloral hydrate*	Thiocyanates
Fluorides	(Certain other drugs also dialyzable)

Indicated for General Supportive Therapy
Uncontrollable metabolic acidosis or alkalosis
Uncontrollable electrolyte disturbance, particularly sodium or potassium
Overhydration
Renal failure
Hyperosmolality not responding to conservative therapy
Marked hypothermia
Nonresponsive Stage 3 or greater coma (Reed Coma Scale)

Contraindicated on Pharmacologic Basis Except for Supportive Care
Antidepressants (tricyclic and monoamine oxidase inhibitors)
Antihistamines
Barbiturates (short-acting)
Belladonna alkaloids
Benzodiazepines (Valium, Librium)
Digitalis and derivatives
Hallucinogens
Meprobamate (Equanil, Miltown)
Methyprylon (Noludar)
Opioids (heroin, Lomotil)
Phenothiazines (Thorazine, Compazine)
Phenytoin (Dilantin)

*Most useful.

SUPPORTIVE CARE, OBSERVATION, AND THERAPY OF COMPLICATIONS

The comatose patient is on the threshold of death and must be stabilized initially by establishing an airway. Intubation should be attempted in any comatose patient. This is the best means to check for the presence of the protective airway reflexes.

An intravenous line should be inserted in all comatose patients and blood collected for appro-

TABLE 6. **Plasma Concentrations Above Which Removal by Extracorporeal Means May Be Indicated***

Drug	Plasma Concentration (mg/dl)	Method of Choice
Phenobarbital	10	HP>HD
Other barbiturates	5	HP
Glutethimide	4	HP
Methaqualone	4	HP
Salicylates	80	HD>HP
Ethchlorvynol	15	HP
Meprobamate	10	HP
Trichloroethanol	5	HP
Paraquat	0.1	HP>HD
Theophylline	6 (chronic), 10 (acute)	HP
Methanol	50	HD
Ethylene glycol	Unknown	HD
Lithium	4 mEq/liter	HD
Ethanol	500	HD

*Modified from Haddad L and Winchester JF (eds): Clinical Management of Poisoning and Drug Overdose. Philadelphia, W. B. Saunders Co., 1983, p 162.

Abbreviations: HP = hemoperfusion; HD = hemodialysis.

priate tests, including toxicologic analysis (10 ml of clotted blood, initial gastric aspirate, 100 ml of urine). The initial management of the comatose patient should include the administration of 100 per cent oxygen, 100 mg of thiamine intravenously, 50 per cent glucose as an intravenous bolus, and 2 to 10 mg of naloxone (Narcan) intravenously. Other causes associated with coma and mimicking intoxications should be eliminated by examination and laboratory tests (trauma, infection, cerebrovascular accident, hypoxia, and endocrine-metabolic causes).

Pulmonary edema complicating poisoning may be cardiac or noncardiac in origin. Fluid overload during forced diuresis may cause the cardiac variety, particularly if the drugs have an antidiuretic effect (opioids, barbiturates, and salicylates). Some toxic agents produce increased pulmonary capillary permeability, and other agents may cause a massive sympathetic discharge resulting in neurogenic pulmonary edema (opioids and salicylates). Management consists of minimizing the fluid administration, diuretics, and oxygen. If renal failure is present, dialysis may be necessary. The noncardiac type of pulmonary edema occurs with inhaled toxins such as ammonia, chlorine, and oxides of nitrogen or with drugs such as salicylates, opioids, paraquat, and intravenous ethchlorvynol (Placidyl). This type does not respond to cardiac measures, and oxygen with intensive respiratory management using mechanical ventilation with positive end-expiratory pressure (PEEP) is necessary.

Hypotension and circulatory shock may be caused by heart failure due to myocardial depression, hypovolemia (fluid loss or venous pooling), decrease in peripheral vasculature resistance (adrenergic blockage), or loss of vasomotor tone caused by central nervous system depression.

Renal failure may be due to tubular necrosis as a result of hypotension, hypoxia, or a direct effect of the poison on the tubular cells (salicylate, paraquat, acetaminophen, carbon tetrachloride). Hemoglobinuria or myoglobinuria may precipitate in the renal tubules and produce renal failure.

Cerebral edema in intoxications is produced by hypoxia, hypercapnia, hypotension, hypoglycemia, and drug-impaired capillary integrity. Computed tomography may aid in diagnosis. Therapy consists of correction of the arterial blood gas and metabolic abnormalities and the hypotension. Reduction of the increased intracranial pressure may be accomplished by 20 per cent mannitol, 0.5 gram per kg, run in over a 30-minute period, and hyperventilation to reduce the Pa_{CO_2} to 25 mmHg. The head should be elevated, and intracranial pressure monitoring should be considered. Fluid administration should be minimized.

Seizures are caused by many substances, such as amphetamines, camphor, chlorinated hydrocarbon insecticides, cocaine, isoniazid, lithium, phencyclidine, phenothiazines, propoxyphene, strychnine, tricyclic antidepressants, and drug withdrawal from ethanol and sedative-hypnotics. Isolated brief convulsions require no therapy, but recurring or protracted seizures require intravenous diazepam (Valium) and phenytoin.

Cardiac dysrhythmias occur with poisoning. A wide QT interval occurs with phenothiazines and a wide QRS interval occurs with tricyclic antidepressants, quinine, or quinidine overdose. Digitalis, cocaine, cyanide, propranolol, theophylline, and amphetamines are among the more frequent toxic causes of dysrhythmias. Correction of metabolic disturbances and adequate oxygenation will correct some of the dysrhythmias; others may require antidysrhythmic drugs or a cardiac pacemaker or cardioversion.

Metabolic acidosis with an increased anion gap is seen with many agents in overdose. Assessment of the arterial blood gases, electrolytes, and osmolality may be a clue to the etiologic agent. Intravenous sodium bicarbonate may be needed when the pH is below 7.1.

Hematemesis can be produced by caustics and corrosives, iron, lithium, mercury, phosphorus, arsenic, mushrooms, plant poisons, fluoride, and organophosphates. Therapy consists of fluid and blood replacement and iced saline lavage if there is no esophageal damage.

TOXICOKINETICS FOR THE PRACTICING PHYSICIAN

Toxicokinetics is clinical pharmacokinetics from the viewpoint of the toxicologist. Pharmacokinetics is a mathematical description of what the body does to a drug. Knowledge of the toxicokinetics of a specific toxic agent will allow the physician to plan a rational approach to the definitive management of the intoxicated patient after the vital functions have been stabilized.

The *LD*$_{50}$ (the lethal dose for 50 per cent of experimental animals) and the *MLD* (the minimum lethal dose) are seldom relevant in human intoxications but indicate potential toxicity of the substance. *Protein binding* of toxic agents influences the volume distribution, elimination, and action of the drug. Diuresis and dialysis are usually reserved for drugs with less than 50 per cent protein binding. The *therapeutic blood range* is the concentration of any drug at which the majority of the treated population can be expected to receive therapeutic benefit. The *toxic blood range* is the concentration at which this majority would be expected to have toxic manifestations. The range is not an absolute value. *Blood concentrations* are a quantitative aid in determining whether more specific measures need to be instituted in correlation with the clinical manifestations. The *apparent volume distribution (Vd)* is the percentage of body mass in which the drug is distributed. It is determined by dividing the amount absorbed by the blood concentration. When a substance has a large volume distribution, as in most lipid-soluble chemicals (above 1 liter per kg), and is concentrated in the body fat, it will not be available for diuresis, dialysis, or exchange transfusion. *Elimination routes* of detoxification will allow the physician to make therapeutic decisions, such as using ethanol to interfere with the metabolism of methanol and ethylene glycol into more toxic metabolites. *Urine identification* is qualitative and allows only the identification of an agent.

Never manage a poisoned patient solely by laboratory tests, and always treat according to the manifestations of poisoning, not the laboratory test results. The laboratory toxicology analyst should be given whatever historical information is available so that the agent can be sought and identified as rapidly as possible. Toxicologic analysis is like a miniresearch project, unlike most other laboratory tests. *Specimens* for toxicologic analysis require the patient's name, date, time of ingestion, time specimen was drawn, therapeutic drugs administered, patient's manifestations, and other relevant data. The toxicologic specimens that should be obtained for analysis are (1) vomitus or initial gastric aspiration, (2) blood, 10 ml (ask the analyst about the type of container and anticoagulant), and (3) urine, 100 ml.

COMMON POISONS AND THERAPY

Abbreviations Used in Following List of Common Poisons

t½ = half-life (time required for blood level to drop by 50 per cent of the original value)
Vd = volume of distribution (liter per kg)
TLV = threshold limit value in air
TWA = time-weighted average
PPM = parts per million in air and water

Conversion Factors

1 gram	= 1000 milligrams (mg)
1 milligram (mg)	= 1000 micrograms (μg)
1 microgram (μg)	= 1000 nanograms (ng)

Standard International Units:

1 mole	= mol wt in grams per liter
1 millimole	= mol wt in milligrams per liter
1 micromole	= mol wt in micrograms per liter

Blood levels:

1 microgram per ml	= 100 micrograms per dl
	= 1 milligram per liter
	= 1000 nanograms per ml
100 mg per dl	= 0.1 gram per dl
	= 1000 mg (1 gram) per liter
	= 1 mg per ml

Acetaminophen, APAP (Tylenol). *Toxic dose:* Child, 3 grams or more; adult, 7.5 grams or more. Liver toxicity, 140 mg per kg. *Toxicokinetics:* Absorption time, 0.5 to 1 hour. Vd, 0.9 liter per kg. Route of elimination by liver. Draw peak blood level after 4 hours in overdose. *Manifestations:* First 24 hours: malaise, nausea, vomiting, and drowsiness, followed by a latent period of 24 hours to 5 days; then hepatic symptoms, disturbances in clotting mechanism, and renal damage. *Management:* (1) Activated charcoal has been contraindicated when *N*-acetylcysteine is contemplated; use gastric lavage. However, recently activated charcoal may be given in the first few hours or alternated 2 hours after the *N*-acetylcysteine. (2) *N*-Acetylcysteine for toxic overdose (Antidote 1, Table 4). Start and give a full course if a toxic dose has been ingested or if blood concentrations are above the toxic line on the nomogram shown in Figure 1. (3) In this instance, a saline sulfate cathartic is preferred to sorbitol. *Laboratory aids:* APAP level, optimally at 4 to 6 hours. Plot levels on nomogram in Figure 1 as a guide for treatment. Monitor liver and renal profiles daily.

Acids. See Caustics and Corrosives.

Alcohols

1. ***Ethanol*** (grain alcohol). *Manifestations:* Blood ethanol levels over 30 mg per dl produce euphoria; over 50, incoordination and intoxication; over 100, ataxia; over 300, stupor; and over 500, coma. Levels of 500 to 700 mg per dl may be fatal. Chronic alcoholic patients tolerate higher levels, and the correlation may not be valid. *Management:* (1) Gastrointestinal decontamination up to 1 hour postingestion. Activated charcoal and cathartics are not indicated. (2) Give 0.25 gram per kg of dextrose, 25 to 50 per cent, intravenously if the blood glucose level is less than 60 mg per dl. (3) Thiamine, 100 mg intravenously, if chronic

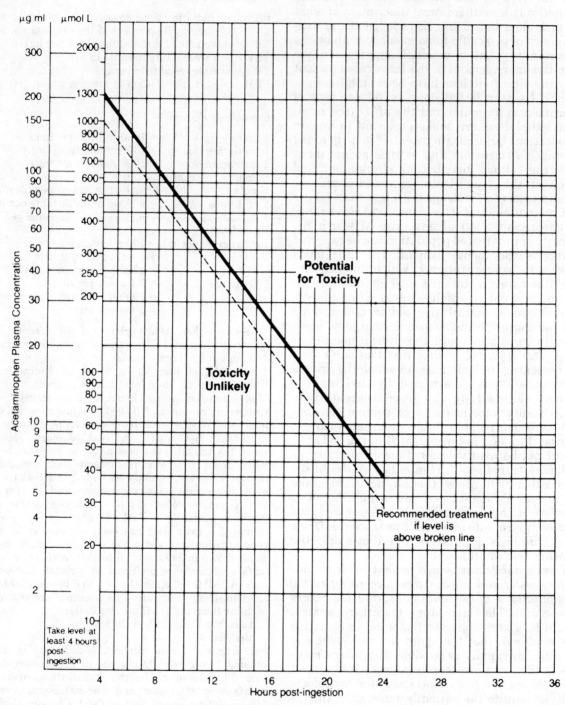

Figure 1. Nomogram for acetaminophen intoxication. Start *N*-acetylcysteine therapy if levels and time coordinates are above the lower line on the nomogram. Continue and complete therapy even if subsequent values fall below the toxic zone. The nomogram is useful only in acute, single ingestions. Serum levels drawn before 4 hours may not represent peak levels. (From Rumack BH and Matthew H: Acetaminophen poisoning and toxicity. Reproduced by permission of Pediatrics 55:871, 1975.)

alcoholism is suspected, to prevent Wernicke-Korsakoff syndrome. (4) Hemodialysis is indicated in severe cases when conventional therapy is ineffective (rarely needed). (5) Treat seizures with diazepam (Valium) followed by phenytoin (Dilantin) if unresponsive. (6) Treat withdrawal with hydration and chlordiazepoxide (Librium) or diazepam. Large doses of sedatives may be required for delirium tremens. *Laboratory aids:* Arterial blood gases, electrolytes, blood ethanol levels, glucose, determine anion and osmolar gap, and check for ketosis. Chest radiograph to determine whether aspiration pneumonia is present. Liver function tests and bilirubin levels.

2. ***Isopropanol*** (rubbing alcohol). Normal propyl alcohol is related to isopropanol but is more toxic. *Manifestations:* Ethanol-like intoxication with acetone odor to breath, acetonuria, acetonemia without systemic acidosis, gastritis. *Management:* (1) Gastrointestinal decontamination. Activated charcoal and cathartics not indicated. (2) Hemodialysis in life-threatening overdose (rarely needed). *Laboratory aids:* Isopropyl alcohol levels, acetone, glucose, and arterial blood gases.

3. ***Methanol*** (wood alcohol). *Toxic dose:* One teaspoonful is potentially lethal for a 2-year-old child and can cause blindness in an adult. The toxic blood level of methanol is above 20 mg per dl, the potentially fatal level over 50 mg per dl. *Manifestations:* Hyperemia of optic disk, violent abdominal colic, blindness, and shock. *Management:* (1) Gastrointestinal decontamination. Activated charcoal and cathartics are not indicated. (2) Treat acidosis vigorously with sodium bicarbonate intravenously. (3) If clinically suspect methanol because of metabolic acidosis, with an anion gap and/or osmolar gap methanol concentration above 20 mg per dl, immediately initiate ethanol IV or PO to produce a blood ethanol concentration of 100 to 150 mg per dl (Antidote 20, Table 4). (4) Folinic acid and folic acid have been used successfully in animal investigations. Administer leucovorin, 1 mg per kg up to 50 mg IV every 4 hours for six doses. (5) Consider hemodialysis if the blood methanol level is greater than 50 mg per dl or if significant metabolic acidosis or visual or mental symptoms are present. *Note:* The ethanol dose has to be increased during dialysis therapy. (6) Continue therapy (ethanol and hemodialysis) until blood methanol level is below 20 mg per dl and preferably undetectable and there are no acidosis and no mental or visual disturbances. This will often require 2 to 5 days. (7) Ophthalmology consultation. *Laboratory aids:* Methanol and ethanol levels, electrolytes, glucose, and arterial blood gases.

Alkali. See Caustics and Corrosives.

Amitriptyline (Elavil). See Tricyclic Antidepressants.

Amphetamines (diet pills, various trade names). *Toxicity:* Child, 5 mg per kg; adult, 12 mg per kg has been reported as lethal. *Toxicokinetics:* Peak time of action is 2 to 4 hours. $t^{1/2}$, 8 to 10 hours in acid urine (pH less than 6.0) and 16 to 31 hours in alkaline urine (pH, 7.5). *Route of elimination:* Liver, 60 per cent; kidney, 30 to 40 per cent at alkaline urine pH; at acid urine pH, 50 to 70 per cent. *Manifestations:* Dysrhythmias, hyperpyrexia, convulsions, hypertension, paranoia, violence. *Management:* (1) Gastrointestinal decontamination. Avoid induced emesis because of rapid onset of action. (2) Control extreme agitation or convulsions with diazepam. Chlorpromazine (Thorazine) may be dangerous if ingestion is not pure amphetamine. (3) Treat hypertensive crisis with diazoxide. (4) Acidification diuresis is not recommended. (5) Treat hyperpyrexia symptomatically. (6) If focal neurologic symptoms, consider cerebrovascular accident. Obtain computed axial tomography scan. (7) Observe for suicidal depression that may follow intoxication. (8) In life-threatening agitation use haloperidol (Haldol). (9) Significant life-threatening tachydysrhythmia may respond to the alpha and beta blocker labetalol (Normodyne; Antidote 23, Table 4) or other appropriate antidysrhythmic agents. In a severely hemodynamically compromised patient, use immediate synchronized cardioversion. *Laboratory aids:* Monitor for rhabdomyolysis (creatine phosphokinase [CPK]), myoglobinuria, hyperkalemia, and disseminated intravascular coagulation. Toxic blood level, 10 micrograms per dl.

Aniline. See Nitrites and Nitrates.

Anticholinergic Agents. Examples are antihistamines—hydroxyline (Atarax), diphenhydramine (Benadryl); antipsychotics (neuroleptics)—phenothiazines (Thorazine); antidepressant drugs (tricyclic antidepressants)—imipramine (Tofranil); antiparkinsonian drugs—trihexyphenidyl (Artane), benztropine (Cogentin); over-the-counter sleep, cold, and hayfever medicine (methapyrilene); ophthalmic products (atropine); plants—jimsonweed *(Datura stramonium),* deadly nightshade *(Atropa belladonna),* henbane *(Hyoscyamus niger);* and antispasmodic agents for the bowel (atropine). *Toxicokinetics:* See Table 7. *Manifestations:* Anticholinergic signs—hyperpyrexia, dilated pupils, flushing of skin, dry mucosa, tachycardia, delirium, hallucinations, coma, and convulsions. *Management:* (1) Gastrointestinal decontamination up to 12 hours postingestion. (2) Control seizures with diazepam. (3) Control ventricular dysrhythmias with lidocaine. (4) Physostigmine (Antidote 30, Table 4) for life-threatening anticholinergic effects refractory to conventional

TABLE 7. **Toxicokinetics of Anticholinergic Agents**

Drug	Potential Fatal Dose	Peak Effect	Vd (Liters/kg)	$t^{1/2}$ (hr)	Excretion Route (%)
Atropine	Child: 10–20 mg; adult: 100 mg	1–2 hr, may be prolonged in overdose	2.3	2–3	Renal (30–50) hepatic (50–70)
Diphenhydramine	20–40 mg/kg; 2 oz has been fatal in 2-year-old child	3–4 hr, may be prolonged in overdose	3–4	5–8	Renal (some hepatic)

TABLE 8. **Anticonvulsants**

Drug	Peak Time of Action/Hr (Steady State)	Vd (Liters/kg)	t½ (hr)	Route of Elimination (%)	Protein Binding (%)	Blood Level (μg/ml)	Comment*
Carbamazepine (Tegretol)	8–24 (2–4 days)	1.0	18–54	Liver (98)	70	Therapeutic, 5–12	Related to tricyclic antidepressants, can cause dysrhythmias
Ethosuximide (Zarontin)	24–48 (5–8 days)	0.8	36–56	Liver (80–90) Renal (10–20)	0	Therapeutic, 40–100	
Phenytoin (Dilantin)	PO, 6–12 IV, 1 (5–10 days)	0.6–1.0	20–30; varies in toxic doses: zero-order kinetics	Liver (95)	87–93	Therapeutic, 10–20; toxic, 20–30; nystagmus only, 30–40; ataxia, 40+; coma, convulsions	Dysrhythmias with parenteral use only
Primidone (Mysoline)	3–4? (4–7 days)	0.6	Parent, 3–12; metabolites, 30–36	Liver	60	Therapeutic, 6–12 primidone and 15–40 phenobarbital (PB); toxic, over 50 primidone and over 40 PB (see Barbiturates)	Metabolized to active metabolites phenyl-ethylmalonamide and PB; overdose gives white crystals in urine†
Valproic acid (Depakene)	? (1–2 days)	0.4	5–15	Liver (80–100)	20	Therapeutic, 60–100	Produces nausea and vomiting, changes in liver function
Clonazepam (Clonopin)	? (4–12 days)		20–60	Liver (98)	90	Therapeutic, 20–70 ng/ml	

*Manifestations: The major manifestations of these agents are depression of consciousness and respiratory depression. Other significant manifestations are mentioned in this column.

†Primidone produces whorls of shimmering white crystals in the urine from precipitation of intact primidone in massive overdose.

treatments. (5) Treat urinary retention. (6) Treat cardiac dysrhythmias only if tissue perfusion is not adequate or if the patient is hypotensive.

Anticonvulsants. See Table 8. *Toxic dose:* Specific anticonvulsant blood levels and the clinical manifestations will indicate toxicity. In general, the ingestion of five times the therapeutic dose is expected to have the potential for toxicity. *Management:* (1) Gastrointestinal decontamination up to 12 hours postingestion. Repeated doses of activated charcoal will shorten t½ of carbamazepine, phenobarbital, primidone, phenytoin, and possibly others. (2) Monitor specific anticonvulsant blood levels. (3) The effectiveness of hemoperfusion and dialysis has not been established.

Antidepressants. See Tricyclic Antidepressants.

Antifreeze. See Alcohols (Methanol) and Ethylene Glycol.

Antihistamines (H₁ Receptor Antagonists). See Anticholinergic Agents.

Arsenic and Arsine Gas. *Toxic dose:* In humans, the inorganic arsenic trioxide toxic dose is 5 to 50 mg; the potential fatal dose is 120 mg or 1 to 2 mg per kg. Sodium arsenite is nine times more toxic than arsenic trioxide. Organic arsenic is less toxic. The maximum allowable concentration for prolonged exposure is 0.05 PPM. See Table 9. Humans are more sensitive than rodents to arsenic. Acute poisoning results from accidental ingestion of arsenic-containing pesticides. (Ant traps sold in some states contain arsenic.) *Toxicokinetics:* Rapidly absorbed by inhalation and ingestion. Crosses placenta and can cause fetal damage. Distributes into spleen, liver, kidneys. *Excretion:* In urine, 90 per cent. Following acute ingestion, it takes 10 days to clear a single dose; chronic ingestion takes up to 70 days. *Arsine gas:* Forms when active hydrogen comes in contact with arsenic. This may occur when zinc, antimony, lead, or iron is contaminated with arsenic and comes in contact with acid. This causes arsine

inhalation intoxication characterized by a latent period of 2 to 48 hours and a triad of abdominal pain, jaundice (due to hemolysis), and hematuria. *Manifestations:* Gastroenteritis, neurologic and cardiac abnormalities, subsequent renal involvement. A garlic odor to the breath may be a clue. Smaller doses and prolonged low-level exposure produce subacute (stomatitis) and chronic (peripheral neuropathy) symptoms.

Management: (1) Gastrointestinal decontamination. Follow with abdominal radiographs, as arsenic is radiopaque. Consider whole-bowel washout if usual methods fail to remove arsenic. (2) Intravenous fluids to correct dehydration and electrolyte deficiencies. (3) Treat shock with oxygen, blood, and fluids as needed. (4) In severe cases, administer BAL (dimercaprol) (Antidote 17, Table 4). (5) In chronic poisoning, D-penicillamine (Antidote 29, Table 4) may be used to chelate arsenic. Therapy should be continued in 5-day cycles until the urine arsenic is less than 50 micrograms per

TABLE 9. **Comparative Acute Toxicities of Some Common Arsenicals***

Arsenical	Oral LD₅₀ in Rats (mg/kg)	Estimated Mortality in Human Poisoning (%)
Arsenic trioxide	385	12
Sodium arsenite	42	65
Calcium arsenite	ca. 275	?
Lead arsenite	1500+	5
Ortho Crabgrass Killer†	3719	None known

*From Done AK: . . . And old lace. Emerg Med 5:246, 1973. Used by permission.

†Product containing 8 per cent each of only mildly toxic octyl NH₄ and dodecyl NH₄ methanearsonate.

TABLE 10. **Barbiturates: Examples and Elimination***

	Long Acting		Intermediate	Short Acting	
Generic name	Barbital	Phenobarbital	Amobarbital	Pentobarbital	Secobarbital
Trade name	Veronal	Luminal	Amytal	Nembutal	Seconal
Slang name	—	Purple hearts	Blue heaven	Yellow jackets	Red devils
pKa	7.74	7.24	7.25	7.96	7.9
Detoxification	Renal	Renal 30%, hepatic 70%	Hepatic 98%	Hepatic 90–100%	Hepatic 90–100%
Onset: IV	22 min	12 min	—	0.1 min	0.1 min
PO	Over 6 hr	6–18 hr (peak 6–18 hr)	Less than 3 hr (peak 3–4 hr)	10–15 min (peak 2–4 hr)	10–15 min (peak 2–4 hr)
Protein binding (%)	5	20–40	—	35	44
Hypnotic dose (mg)	300–500	100–200	50–200	50–100	50–100
Fatal dose (grams)	10	8	5	3	3
Toxic dose (mg/kg)	8	15–35	Over 6	3–5	3–5
Therapeutic level (μg/ml)	5–8	15–40	5–6	1–4	3–5
Toxic level (μg/ml)	Over 30	Over 40	10–30	Over 10	Over 10
Lethal level† (μg/ml)	Over 100	Over 100	Over 50	Over 35	Over 35
Duration of action (hr)	Over 16	Over 6	6 hr	6 hr	6 hr
Half-life (hr)	58–96	50–120	8–42	15–48	19–34
Rate of metabolism (hr)	—	0.7	2.5	—	—
Volume distribution (liters/kg)	—	0.75	0.5–1.1	0.65–1.5	0.65–1.5

Manifestations

Low dose: Euphoria, ataxia, incoordination, nystagmus on lateral gaze

High dose: Flaccid coma, hypotension, respiratory depression, pulmonary edema (particularly with the short-acting barbiturates), subcutaneous bullae (6%), dermatographia

*Classification into long acting, intermediate, and short acting has no relationship to the duration of coma.

†These levels are not absolute, and tolerance occurs.

liter. (6) Hemodialysis is effective in acute poisoning and can be used concurrently with chelation therapy in severe cases, especially if renal failure develops. (7) Arsine intoxication is treated by exchange transfusion and hemodialysis if renal failure occurs. BAL is ineffective. *Laboratory aids:* Blood arsenic and 24-hour urine arsenic levels. Excessive exposure is indicated by a level of 50 micrograms per liter of arsenic in urine, but persons whose diets are rich in seafood may excrete 200 micrograms per day. View values over 100 micrograms per day with suspicion. Monitor electrocardiogram (ECG) and renal function. A blood arsenic level above 1.0 mg per liter is toxic and one of 9 to 15 mg per liter is potentially fatal (false values occur in inexperienced laboratories).

Aspirin. See Salicylates.

Atropine. See Anticholinergic Agents.

Barbiturates. See Table 10. *Management:* (1) Gastrointestinal decontamination up to 8 to 12 hours. Avoid emesis in short-acting barbiturates. Activated charcoal and a cathartic in repeated doses have been shown to reduce the serum half-life and increase the nonrenal clearance over 50 per cent. Give every 4 hours while the patient is comatose. (2) Supportive and symptomatic care is all that is necessary in the majority of cases. (3) Alkalinization with sodium bicarbonate, 2 mEq per kg IV during the first hour, followed by sufficient sodium bicarbonate (Antidote 35, Table 4) to keep the urinary pH at 7.5 to 8.0, enhances excretion of long-acting barbiturates. Forced diuresis should be used with caution because of fluid overload. At present, alkalinization without diuresis is advocated. (4) In severe cases that do not respond to conservative measures, consider hemodialysis and hemoperfusion. (5) Treat any bullae as a local second-degree

skin burn. (6) Give intensive care monitoring to comatose patient. *Treatment of withdrawal: In an emergency,* use pentothal or diazepam intravenously. If the patient is stable, a pentobarbital tolerance test may be given; 200 mg of pentobarbital is given orally and the patient examined after 1 hour for signs of intoxication (nystagmus, slurred speech, and ataxia). If none are present, the dose is repeated every 3 hours until these signs develop. This is the stabilizing dose; the patient is maintained on this dose for 72 hours and then changed to phenobarbital, 30 mg substituted for each 100 mg of pentobarbital. The phenobarbital is tapered, decreasing by 10 per cent or 30 mg every 3 to 5 days. *Laboratory aids:* Emergency plasma barbiturate concentrations rarely alter management.

Benzene. See Hydrocarbons.

Benzodiazepines (BZP). See Table 11. *Toxicity:* Low toxic potential. More than 500 mg has been ingested without respiratory depression. Benzodiazepines have an additive effect with sedatives such as alcohol and barbiturates. Most patients intoxicated with benzodiazepines alone recover within 24 hours. Many of these agents have active metabolites with a long plasma $t\frac{1}{2}$, so performance in skilled tasks such as driving may be impaired. Withdrawal may be delayed. *Manifestations:* CNS depression. Deep coma leading to respiratory depression suggests presence of other drugs. *Management:* (1) Gastrointestinal decontamination. (2) Supportive and symptomatic care. (3) Withdrawal, if it occurs, is treated with a long-acting benzodiazepine on a tapering schedule. *Laboratory aids:* Document benzodiazepines in urine. Quantitative blood levels are not useful.

Bleach. Household bleaches are 4 to 6 per cent sodium hypochlorite. Commercial types are 10 to 20 per cent.

TABLE 11. **Benzodiazepines (BZP)**

Drug	Oral Dosage Range	Peak Oral Plasma Levels (hr)	Half-Life (hr)	Major Active Metabolites (Half-life in hr)	Elimination Rate
ANXIOLYTICS					
Diazepam (Valium)	6–40 mg/day	1–2	20–50	Desmethyldiazepam (30–60)	Slow
Chlordiazepoxide (Librium, Libritabs, various others)	15–100 mg/day	2–4	5–30	Desmethylchlordiazepoxide, demoxepam, desmethyldiazepam	Slow
Clorazepate (Tranxene)	15–60 mg/day	1–2.5	30–60	Desmethyldiazepam	Slow
Prazepam (Centrax)	20–60 mg/day	6	78	3-Hydroxyprazepam, desmethyldiazepam	Slow
Halazepam (Paxipam)	60–160 mg/day	1–3	7	N-3-Hydroxyhalazepam, desmethyldiazepam	Slow
Oxazepam (Serax)	30–120 mg/day	1–2	3–10	None	Rapid to intermediate
Lorazepam (Ativan)	2–6 mg/day	2	10–20	None	Intermediate
Alprazolam (Xanax)	0.75–4 mg/day	0.7–1.6	12–19	α-Hydroxyalprazolam	Intermediate
HYPNOTICS					
Flurazepam (Dalmane)	15–60 mg	3–6	50–100	Desalkylflurazepam (50–100)	Slow
Midazolam (Versed)	5–30 mg/day IV	0.3–0.8	3–5	None	—
Flunitrazepam (Rohypnol— investigational, Roche)	1–2 mg	<1	—	7-Aminoflunitrazepam (23), N-desmethylflunitrazepam (31)	—
Temazepam (Restoril)	15–30 mg	2–3	9–12	None	Intermediate
Triazolam (Halcion)	0.125–0.5 mg	0.5–1.5	2–3	α-Hydroxytriazolam	Rapid
ANTICONVULSANT					
Clonazepam (Klonopin)	1.5–20 mg/day	1–4	24–48	None	—

Manifestations: Difficulty in swallowing; pain in mouth, throat, chest, or abdomen. General household strength bleach does not produce burns; commercial strength bleach may. Inhalation of gases produced by mixing chlorine bleach with acids (toilet bowl cleaner and rust removers—chlorine gas) or with household ammonia (chloramine gas) is irritating to mucous membranes, eyes, and upper respiratory tract. *Management:* (1) Ingestion—Avoid GI decontamination procedures. Dilute with small amounts of water or milk. Avoid acids. (2) Esophagoscopy only if unusually large amounts have been ingested, the patient is symptomatic, or the product was stronger than the average household bleach. (3) Inhalation—Remove from contaminated area. Observe for pulmonary edema. (4) Ocular exposure requires immediate gentle irrigation with water for at least 15 minutes, followed by fluorescein dye stain for damage.

Botulism. See article on Foodborne Illnesses in Section 2.

Brake Fluid. See Ethylene Glycol.

Calcium Channel Blockers. Used in treatment of effort angina and supraventricular tachycardia. See Table 12. *Manifestations:* Hypotension, bradycardia within 1 to 5 hours, CNS depression, and gastric distress. *Management:* (1) Gastrointestinal decontamination. (2) Treat hypotension and bradycardia with positioning, fluids, and calcium gluconate or chloride (see Antidote 12B, Table 4). Dopamine or norepinephrine may be used if necessary. (3) Heart block—may respond to intravenous calcium (Antidote 12B, Table 4) or atropine sulfate, 0.5 to 1 mg, if no response. (4) Ventricular pacing may be required in the severely intoxicated patient. (5) Patients receiving digitalis run the risk of toxicity and should be carefully monitored. *Laboratory aids:* Specific drug levels, blood sugar and calcium, ECG.

Camphor (External analgesic rubs, Vicks Vaporub 4.8 per cent, Campho-Phenique 11 per cent). Many camphorated oil products were removed from the marketplace in September, 1982. Five milliliters of camphorated oil (20 per cent camphor) equals 1 gram of camphor. *Toxicity:* Adult, 5 grams; child, 1 gram has been fatal. *Toxicokinetics:* Onset of manifestations, 5 to 90 minutes. Readily and rapidly absorbed through the skin, mucous membranes, and gastrointestinal tract and crosses the placenta. Route of elimination: Rapidly metabolized in liver to the glucuronide form, which is excreted in urine. Pulmonary excretion causes a distinctive odor on the breath. *Manifestations:* Nausea, vomiting, and burning epigastric pain. Seizures may occur suddenly and without warning within 5 minutes of ingestion. Apnea and vision disturbances may occur. *Management:* (1) Induction of emesis is

TABLE 12. **Kinetics and Other Actions of Calcium Channel Blockers**

Parameter	Nifedipine (Procardia)	Verapamil (Calan, Isoptin)	Diltiazem (Cardiazem)
Bioavailability (%)	65	20	<40
Dose			
Adult, PO (mg/day)	30	240	90
Maximum mg/day	120–180	480–720	240–360
IV (mg/kg)	0.1	—	
Preparations	10- and 20-mg tablets	80- and 120-mg tablets	30-, 60-, 90-, and 120-mg tablets
Slow release	480-mg capsules		
Onset of action (min)			
PO	<20	<30	<15
IV	<1	<1	—
Sublingual	3	—	—
Peak effect			
PO	1–2 hr	5 hr	1–2 hr
IV		5–15 min	
Sublingual	20 min		
Peak blood concentration (min)	30–60	90–120	120–180
t½ (hr)	3–5	3–7	4–9
Protein binding (%)	90	90	90
Vd (liters/kg)	3	4.5–7	4–5
Elimination	Hepatic	Hepatic	Hepatic
Toxic blood concentration (ng/ml)	>100	>300	>200
Coronary vasodilation	+ + +	+ + +	+ + +
Peripheral vasodilation	+ + +	+ +	+
Negative inotropy	−	+	+
Slow atrioventricular conduction	−	+ +	+
Preload	Decrease	—	Decrease
Heart rate	Increase	Decrease	Decrease

contraindicated because of early seizures. (2) Remove residual drug by gastric lavage. (3) Administer activated charcoal and a saline cathartic. Avoid giving oils or alcohol. (4) Treat seizures with intravenous diazepam. (5) Treat apnea with respiratory support.

Carbon Monoxide (CO). This is an odorless gas produced from incomplete combustion; it is found also as an in vivo metabolic breakdown product of methylene chloride (paint removers). Observe for the symptoms described in Table 13. Contrary to popular belief, the skin rarely shows a cherry-red color in the live patient.

Toxicokinetics: CO is rapidly absorbed through the lungs. The rate of absorption is directly related to alveolar ventilation. Elimination occurs through the lungs. The t½ in room air equals 5 to 6 hours; in 100 per cent oxygen, 90 minutes; in hyperbaric oxygen, 20 minutes. The nomogram pictured in Figure 2 can be used to decide quickly whether serious CO intoxication is likely to have occurred and to select patients at high risk or who need early management in the intensive care unit or hyperbaric oxygen.

Management: (1) Remove the patient from contami-

TABLE 13. **Carbon Monoxide (CO)**

CO in Atmosphere (PPM)	Duration of Exposure	Saturation of Blood (%)	Symptoms
Up to 0.01	Indefinite	1–10	None
0.01–0.02	Indefinite	10–20	Tightness across forehead, slight headache, dilation of cutaneous vessels
0.02–0.03	5–6 hr	20–30	Headache, throbbing temples
0.04–0.06	4–5 hr	30–40	Severe headache, weakness and dizziness, nausea and vomiting, collapse, leukocytosis
0.07–0.10	3–4 hr	40–50	Above, plus increased tendency to collapse and syncope, increased pulse and respiratory rate
0.11–0.15	1.5–3 hr	50–60	Increased pulse and respiratory rate, syncope, Cheyne-Stokes respiration, coma with intermittent convulsions
0.16–0.30	1–1.5 hr	60–70	Coma with intermittent convulsions, depressed heart action and respirations, death possible
0.50–1.00	1–2 hr	70–80	Weak pulse, depressed respirations, respiratory failure, and death

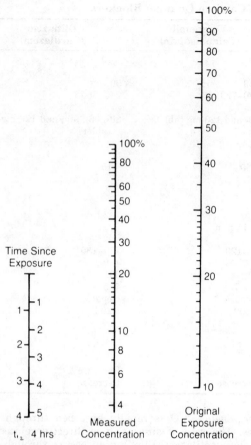

Figure 2. Nomogram for calculating carboxyhemoglobin concentration at time of exposure. The time since exposure is given on two scales to allow for the effects of previous oxygen administration on the half-life of carboxyhemoglobin (left-hand scale assumes a half-life of 3 hours). *Note:* The nomogram assumes a half-life of carboxyhemoglobin of 4 hours in a subject breathing room air. Most patients will not have received supplementary oxygen before admission, and at best this will have been administered via a face mask, giving a maximum fractional inspired oxygen concentration of 50 to 60 per cent with little effect on carboxyhemoglobin elimination. The scale on the left side of the time column makes allowances for prior oxygen supplements by assuming a short half-life of 3 hours. The nomogram may help decide quickly whether serious carbon monoxide intoxication is likely to have occurred and may help select patients at high risk for early management in the intensive care unit. The nomogram may be an oversimplification because patients usually are not resuscitated with constant concentrations of oxygen, and many patients may hyperventilate, thus changing elimination characteristics. (Redrawn from Clark CJ, et al: Blood carboxyhaemoglobin and cyanide levels in fire survivors. Lancet *1*:1332, 1981.)

nated area and expose to fresh air. Establish vital functions. (2) Give 100 per cent oxygen to all patients until the carboxyhemoglobin level falls to 5 per cent or less. Assisted ventilation may be necessary. The exposed pregnant woman should be kept in 100 per cent oxygen for several hours after the carboxyhemoglobin level is zero because carboxyhemoglobin concentrates in the fetus and oxygen are needed five times

longer to ensure elimination of CO from fetal circulation. CO or hypoxia may be teratogenic. (3) Monitor arterial blood gases and carboxyhemoglobin levels. Determine carboxyhemoglobin level at time of exposure by using nomogram. *Note:* A near-normal carboxyhemoglobin level does not rule out significant CO poisoning. (4) Only if pH is below 7.1 after correction of hypoxia and adequate ventilation, give sodium bicarbonate to correct acidosis. (5) Indications for 100 per cent oxygen and possible therapy with hyperbaric oxygen (controversial): (a) carboxyhemoglobin level higher than 25 per cent; (b) carboxyhemoglobin level higher than 15 per cent in a child or in a patient with cardiovascular disease; (c) carboxyhemoglobin level higher than 10 per cent in a pregnant woman (and monitor fetus); (d) abnormal or ischemic chest pain or ECG abnormality; (e) abnormal chest x-ray; (f) presence of hypoxia, myoglobinuria, or abnormal renal function; (g) history of unconsciousness, syncope, or neuropsychiatric symptoms. A list of hyperbaric oxygen chambers can be obtained by contacting a regional poison control center. (6) Treat seizures with intravenous diazepam. (7) Monitor ECG, chest radiograph, and serum CPK and lactate dehydrogenase levels. (8) Treat cerebral edema with elevation of the patient's head, minimizing intravenous fluid, hyperventilation, and, if needed, mannitol and intracranial pressure monitor. (9) Re-evaluate after recovery for neuropsychiatric sequelae. *Laboratory aids:* Arterial blood gases show metabolic acidosis and normal oxygen tension but reduced oxygen saturation.

Carbon Tetrachloride. See Hydrocarbons.

Caustics and Corrosives. Common acid substances are hydrochloric acid, sulfuric acid (battery acid), carbolic acid (phenol), nitric acid, oxalic acid, hydrofluoric acid, and aqua regia (mixture of hydrochloric and nitric acids). These are used as cleaning agents. Common alkali substances are sodium or potassium hydroxide (lye), sodium hypochlorite (Clorox) (bleach), sodium carbonate (nonphosphate detergents), potassium permanganate, ammonia, electric dishwashing agents, cement, and flat disk batteries. *Toxicity:* Acids produce mucosal coagulation necrosis. They usually do not penetrate deeply (exception: hydrofluoric acid). The gastric mucosa is the primary site of injury. Alkalis produce liquefaction necrosis and saponification and penetrate deeply. Oropharyngeal and esophageal damage by solids is more frequent than by liquids. Liquids are more likely to produce gastric damage. *Toxic dose:* Adult potential fatal dose of concentrated acid/alkali is 5 ml. The absence of oral burns does not exclude the possibility of esophageal burns (10 to 15 per cent).

Management: (1) Dilute with milk or water immediately up to 30 ml in children or 250 ml in adults. Neutralization with acidic or alkalinic agents is contraindicated. Dilute only if patient can swallow. (2) Gastrointestinal decontamination is contraindicated. However, in acid ingestions some authorities advocate nasogastric intubation and aspiration in the early postingestion phase. Patient should receive only intravenous fluids following dilution until surgical consultation is obtained. Dermal and ocular decontamination should be carried out. (3) Endoscopy at 12 to 48 hours may be indicated postingestion to assess severity of burn. (4) Steroids are controversial. Some recommend administration of steroids if burns are found or esophagoscopy is not performed. (5) Antibiotics are not useful prophylactically. (6) Barium swallow may be necessary at 10 days to 3 weeks to assess severity of damage. (7) Esophageal dilation may need to be performed at 2- to 4-week intervals if evidence of stricture is found. (8) Intraposition of the colon may be necessary if dilation fails to provide an adequate-sized esophagus. (9) Inhalation management requires immediate removal from the environment, and clinical, x-ray, and arterial blood gas evaluation when appropriate. Oxygen and respiratory support may be required.

Chloral Hydrate. See Sedative Hypnotics.

Chlordane. See Organochlorine Insecticides.

Chlordiazepoxide (Librium). See Benzodiazepines.

Chlorine Gas. Chlorine gas is a yellow-greenish gas with an irritating odor used in bleach, in manufacture of plastics, and for water purification. Exposure usually results from transportation mishaps, industrial accidents, chemistry experiments, the mixing of household cleaners with bleach containing hypochlorite, and accidental release around swimming pools. Its density is greater than that of air, and an odor is detected at concentrations of less than 0.5 PPM. Chlorine acts as an oxidizing agent and also acts with tissue water to form hypochlorite and hydrochloric acid and generate free oxygen radicals. *Toxic dose:* The threshold limit value is less than 1 PPM; 4 PPM is tolerated for 0.5 hour; 15 PPM immediately irritates mucous membranes of eyes, ears, nose, and throat; 30 PPM produces choking and chest pain; 60 PPM produces pulmonary edema; 400 PPM for 30 minutes is lethal; and 1000 PPM is fatal in a few minutes.

Management: (1) Remove the patient from contaminated environment and stabilize vital functions. Decontamination procedures for dermal and ocular contamination as indicated. Protect rescue personnel with breathing apparatus. Classification—If symptomless or with a cough that clears up in less than 1 hour, rest for 12 hours and report if symptoms occur; no vigorous exercise for 24 hours. If symptoms persist beyond period of exposure, admit to hospital and treat with bronchodilators (use theophylline, not epinephrine) and humidified oxygen. Noncardiac pulmonary edema is treated with PEEP; corticosteroids are controversial; furosemide (Lasix) may be used. For conjunctival irritation, copious water irrigation and fluorescein stain for corneal damage. For dermal burns, copious water irrigation and conventional treatment of burns. *Laboratory aids:* Chest radiograph (may not reflect damage for 24 hours), arterial blood gases, cardiac monitor for dysrhythmias.

Chlorpromazine (Thorazine). See Phenothiazines and Other Major Neuroleptics.

Clinitest Tablets. See Caustics and Corrosives.

Cocaine (Benzoylmethylecgonine). Toxic dose: The potential fatal dose is 1200 mg, but death has occurred with 20 mg parenterally. *Toxicokinetics:* See Table 14. *Manifestations:* Hypertension, convulsions, hyperthermia, and cardiac dysrhythmias. *Management:* (1) Supportive care. Avoid induction of emesis or gastric lavage because of rapid onset of action of cocaine. Blood pressure and thermal monitoring. Phenytoin

may be effective for ventricular dysrhythmias, whereas lidocaine may be ineffective and enhance toxicity. Nitroprusside infusion, 0.5 to 10 micrograms per kg per minute, may be used for severe hypertension. Avoid propranolol. Control anxiety and convulsions with diazepam. Labetalol intravenously (Antidote 23, Table 4) has been used to control life-threatening hypertension and tachycardia. A nonthreatening environment to reduce all sensory stimuli and protect patient from injury is required. Apply precautions against suicide attempts and monitor the fetus if a pregnant woman. The management of the "body packer" and "body stuffer" is to administer repeated doses of activated charcoal (except plastic vials), secure venous access, and have drugs readily available for treating life-threatening manifestations until contraband is passed in the stool. Surgical removal may be indicated if material does not pass the pylorus. Endoscopy may be used to remove hard plastic vials, but not the bags, containing crack.

Codeine. See Opioids.

Corrosives. See Caustics and Corrosives.

Cyanide. See Table 15. Hydrocyanic acid and sodium and potassium salts act rapidly and are extremely poisonous. The acid is extremely volatile, producing cyanide, which has a distinctive odor of bitter almonds and can produce death within minutes after inhalation. Cyanide interferes with the cytochrome oxidase system. *Classes of cyanides and derivatives:* (1) Hydrogen cyanide and simple salts in large doses act to produce death in 15 minutes. (2) Halogenated cyanides such as cyanogen chloride produce irritant and vesicant gases that may cause pulmonary edema. (3) Nitriles such as acrylonitrile and acetonitrile. Cyanides are used as fumigants (hydrogen cyanide), in synthetic rubber (acrylonitrile), in fertilizers (cyanamide), in metal refining (salts), and in the home in some silver and furniture polishes. Cyanide in the seeds of fruit stones is harmful only if the capsule is broken. *Manifestations:* Seizures, stupor, cardiac dysrhythmias, pulmonary edema, lactic acidemia, decreased arterial venous oxygen difference. Bright red venous blood.

Management: Attendants should not administer mouth to mouth resuscitation. (1) Immediately, 100 per cent oxygen. If inhaled, remove patient from contaminated atmosphere. (2) Cyanide antidote kit (Antidote 14, Table 4). Use antidote only if certain of diagnosis and (a) significant toxicity (impairment of consciousness); (b) manifestations not corrected by oxygen and out of proportion to carboxyhemoglobin level; and (c) lactic acidosis and bright red venous blood with high or normal Pa_{O_2}. (3) Gastrointestinal decontamination by gastric lavage. *No* syrup of ipecac. Activated charcoal not very effective (1 gram binds only 35 mg of cyanide). (4) Treat seizures with intravenous diazepam. (5) Correct acidosis. (6) Other antidotes: In Europe, dicobalt edetate, 600 mg, is used intravenously, followed by 300 mg if the response is not satisfactory. Hydroxycobalamin (vitamin B_{12}) is a useful antidote but must be given immediately after exposure in very large doses. Dose: 1800 mg of vitamin B_{12} per dl of KCN is usually required (forms cyanocobalamin).

DDT and Derivatives. See Organochlorine Insecticides.

Desipramine (Norpramin, Pertofrane). See Tricyclic Antidepressants.

TABLE 14. **Pharmacotoxicokinetics of Cocaine**

Type	Route	Onset	Peak	Duration t½ (min)	Possible Fatal Dose (Adult)
Hydrochloride	Insufflation	1–5 min	30–60 min	60–75	750–800 mg
	Ingested	Delayed	50–90 min	Sustained	1.4 grams
	IV	2–3 min	15–30 min	60–90	20–800 mg
Coca paste	Smoked			Not known	
Crack and free base	Smoked	(Fastest) 4–6 sec	8–16 sec	Up to 20 min	Not known

Diazepam (Valium). See Benzodiazepines.

Digitalis Preparations. See Table 16. *Manifestations*: Abdominal pain, nausea, vomiting, diarrhea, dysrhythmias, heart block, CNS depression, colored-halo vision. *Management*: (1) Gastrointestinal decontamination. Avoid ipecac syrup; it may increase the vagal effect if patient is symptomatic. Repeated doses of activated charcoal may interrupt enterohepatic recirculation. (2) Treat ventricular premature contractions, including bigeminy, trigeminy, quadrigeminy, ventricular tachycardia, and atrial tachycardia, with phenytoin. Lidocaine also may be administered for ventricular dysrhythmias. (3) Treat bradycardia and second- and third-degree atrioventricular block with atropine or isoproterenol. External pacing may be needed. (4) Treat hyperkalemia (above 6 mEq per liter) with intravenous glucose 5 to 10 per cent, intravenous sodium bicarbonate, intravenous insulin (insulin is not used in children), and Kayexalate retention enema (25 per cent in sorbitol 25 per cent) in severe cases. If hyperkalemia is present (ominous sign), insertion of a pacemaker should be seriously considered. Hemodialysis is treatment of choice for severe or refractory hyperkalemia. (5) Direct current countershock may cause life-threatening dysrhythmias. (6) Specific Fab antibody fragments (Digibind) (Antidote 21, Table 4) have been used for life-threatening cardiac dysrhythmias, hyperkalemia, and cases refractory to conventional measures. *Laboratory aids*: Monitor ECG and potassium and digitalis levels. Draw digoxin levels 6 to 8 hours postingestion. An endogenous digoxin-like substance that cross-reacts with most common immunoassay antibodies, with values as high as 4.1 ng per ml, has been reported in newborns, patients with chronic renal failure, and patients with abnormal immunoglobulin levels. The bound digoxin blood concentrations rise after use of Fab, but the free (usually unmeasured) digoxin level falls.

Diphenhydramine (Benadryl). See Anticholinergic Agents.

Doxepin (Sinequan, Adapin). See Tricyclic Antidepressants.

Ethchlorvynol (Placidyl). See Sedative Hypnotics.

Ethyl Alcohol. See Alcohols.

Ethylene Glycol (solvent, antifreeze). *Toxic dose*: Death has occurred after a 60-ml ingestion; fatal dose = 1.4 ml per kg of 100 per cent solution. The TLV is 50 PPM. *Toxicokinetics*: Time of onset, 30 minutes to 12 hours for CNS and metabolic abnormalities to occur (Phase I). Twelve to 36 hours postingestion, cardiopulmonary depression (Phase II). In Phase III (2 to 3 days

postingestion), renal failure occurs. The t½ is 3 hours (during ethanol therapy this is prolonged to 17 hours). *Management*: (1) Gastrointestinal decontamination up to 2 to 4 hours postingestion. Activated charcoal and cathartics are not indicated. (2) Treat seizures with intravenous diazepam. Exclude hypocalcemia. (3) Correct acidosis with intravenous sodium bicarbonate. (4) Initiate ethanol therapy to block metabolism (Antidote 20, Table 4) if the blood ethylene glycol level is higher than 20 mg per dl, or if the patient is symptomatic or acidotic with increased anion gap or osmolar gap. Ethanol should be administered intravenously or orally to produce a blood ethanol concentration of 100 to 150 mg per dl. (5) Early hemodialysis is indicated if the ingestion was large; if the blood ethylene glycol level is greater than 50 mg per dl; if severe acid-base or electrolyte abnormalities occur despite conventional therapy; or if renal failure occurs. (6) Thiamine and pyridoxine have been recommended for 48 hours but have not been extensively studied. *Laboratory aids*: Complete blood count, electrolytes, urinalysis (look for oxalate crystals), and arterial blood gases. Obtain ethylene glycol and ethanol levels, plasma osmolarity (use freezing point depression method). Calcium, creatinine, and blood urea nitrogen studies. An ethylene glycol level of 20 mg per dl is usually toxic (levels are very difficult to obtain).

Flurazepam (Dalmane). See Benzodiazepines.

Glutethimide (Doriden). See Sedative Hypnotics.

Hallucinogens

1. **LSD** (lysergic acid diethylamide). *Toxic dose*: ≥ 35 micrograms. Street doses are typically 50 to 300 micrograms. *Toxicokinetics*: Peak effect, 1 to 2 hours. Duration, 12 to 24 hours. t½, 3 hours. Route of elimination, hepatic.

2. **Morning-Glory Seeds** (*Rivea corymbosa* or *Ipomoea*). These have one-tenth the potency of LSD.

3. **Mescaline/Peyote** (trimethoxyphenylethylamine or *Lophophora williamsii*). *Toxic dose*: ≥ 5 mg per kg. Each button of mescaline contains 45 mg (4 to 12 produce symptoms). *Toxicokinetics*: Peak effect, 4 to 6 hours. Duration, 14 hours.

4. **Psilocybin.** Similar in effect to LSD but short acting. Peak effect, 90 minutes. Duration, 5 to 6 hours.

5. **Nutmeg** (*Myristica*). *Toxic dose*: 5 to 15 grams (1 to 3 nutmegs). Peak effect, 3 to 6 hours. Duration, up to 60 hours.

6. **Marijuana** (*Cannabis sativa*) (Δ⁹-tetrahydrocannabinol, THC). One joint equals 500 mg of marijuana; when smoked, 50 per cent is destroyed. *Toxicokinetics*: Time of onset, 2 to 3 minutes (smoked).

TABLE 15. Sources of Cyanide and Their Toxicity

PLANTS CONTAINING CYANIDE GLYCOSIDES

Common Name	Part of Plant	Botanical Name
Apple	Seeds	*Malus* spp.
Appricot		*Prunus armeniaca*
Arrow grass		*Triglochin* spp.
Bamboo	Sprouts, stems	Tribe Bambuseae
Bermuda grass		*Cynodon dactylon*
Bird's-foot trefoil		*Lotus corniculatus*
Bitter almond		*Prunus amygdalus amara*
Blackthorn, sloe		*Prunus spinosa*
Calabash tree		*Crescentia cujete*
Cassava	Beans and roots	*Manihot esculenta*
Catclaw		*Acacia greggi*
Cherry laurel		*Prunus laurocerasus*
Chokecherry		*Prunus virginiana*
Cotonester		*Cotoneaster* spp.
Cycad nut		*Zamia pumila*
Elderberry	Leaves and shoots	*Sambucus* spp.
Eucalyptus		*Eucalyptus cladocalyx*
False sago palm		*Cycas circinalis*
Flax		*Linum usitatissimum*
Hyacinth bean	Bean	*Dolichos lablab*
Hydrangea	Leaves and bulb	*Hydrangea* spp.
Jetbead		*Rhodotypos tetrapetala*
Johnson grass		*Sorghum halepense*
Lima bean		*Phaseolus lunatus* (not in United States)
Mountain mahogany		*Cercocarpus montanus*
Passionflower (African)		*Adenia volkensii*
Peach		*Prunus persica*
Pear	Seeds	*Pyrus communis*
Plains bahia		*Bahia oppositifolia*
Plum		*Prunus domestica*
Poison suckleya		*Suckleya suckleyana*
Queen's delight		*Stillingia sylvatica*
Sudan grass		*Sorghum* spp.
Velvet grass		*Holcus lanatus*
Vetch	Seed	*Vicia sativa*

HYDROGEN CYANIDE LIBERATED FROM SAMPLES OF CARCINOGENIC GLYCOSIDES

Sample	HCN (mg/gram or ml)
Laetrile (amygdalin)	
Sigma	55.9
Tablet yellow	400
Kemdalin	14.1
Apricot seeds	2.92
Peach seeds	2.60
Apple seeds	0.61

Laetrile is 500-mg tablet for oral use, which is 6% cyanide by weight.

FORMS OF CYANIDE AND THEIR TOXICITY

Product	Toxicity (Potential Lethal Dose)
Hydrocyanic acid	50 mg (1.0 mg/kg)
Potassium/sodium cyanide	150–300 mg (2 mg/kg)
Ferriferrocyanide (Prussian Blue)	50 grams
Sodium nitroprusside	5 mg/kg causes toxicity
Bitter almonds	
Oil	2 oz
Almonds	50–60 (each contains 0.001 grams of cyanide)
Pulp	240 grams
Apricot	
Wild	100 grams of moist seed = 217 mg of cyanide
Cultivated	100 grams = 8.7 mg of cyanide

TABLE 16. Digitalis Preparations

	Digoxin	Digitoxin
Trade name	Lanoxin	Crystodigin
Onset time PO, min	15–30	25–120
Peak, hr	1.5–6	4–12
Half-life	31–40 hr	4–6 days
Protein bound (%)	25	90
Vd, liters/kg	7–8	0.6
Route of elimination	Renal, 75%	Liver, 80%
Toxic blood levels, ng/ml	2.4	>30
Enterohepatic route	Small	Large

Duration, 2 to 3 hours. t½, 28 to 47 hours (shorter for chronic user). *Note:* 1 per cent of the metabolite can be detected in urine up to 2 weeks after use. *Manifestations:* Visual illusions, sensory perceptual distortions, depersonalization, and derealization. *Management:* "Talk-down" technique.

7. **Inhalants.** Nitrites (amyl and isobutyl nitrite)—act immediately; aromatic hydrocarbon in airplane model glues, plastic cements (benzene, toluene, xylene)—see Hydrocarbons; *nitrous oxide* and *halogenated hydrocarbons.*

8. **Tryptamine Derivatives** (DMT, *N*-dimethyltryptamine; DET, diethyltryptamine; DPT, dipropyltryptamine). Rapid onset of action, but duration is only 1 to 2 hours.

9. **STP** or **DOM** (2,5-dimethoxy-4-methylamphetamine). Acts like LSD but lasts 72 hours or longer.

10. **MDA** (3-methoxy-4,5-ethylenedioxyamphetamine). Related to amphetamine, produces a mild LSD-like reaction lasting 6 to 10 hours ("love pill").

See also Alcohols, Amphetamines, Anticholinergic Agents, Barbiturates, Cocaine, Opioids, Phencyclidine, Phenothiazines and Other Major Neuroleptics, and Tricyclic Antidepressants.

Haloperidol (Haldol). See Phenothiazines and Other Major Neuroleptics.

Heroin. See Opioids.

Hydrocarbons

1. **Petroleum Distillates.** Gasoline (petroleum spirit), 2 to 5 per cent benzene; kerosene (coal oil, kerosene, jet aviation fuel No. 1, charcoal lighter fluid); petroleum naphtha (cigarette lighter fluid, ligroin, racing fuel); petroleum ether (benzine); turpentine (pine oil, oil of turpentine); and mineral spirits (Stoddard solvent, white spirits, varasol, mineral turpentine, petroleum spirit). *Manifestations:* Materials aspirated during the process of ingestion may produce pneumonitis. Hypoxia associated with aspiration is the cause of CNS depression, not absorption. It is *unlikely* that a child accidentally or an adult during siphoning would ingest a sufficient quantity to warrant the induction of emesis.

2. **Aromatic Hydrocarbons.** *Benzene*, a solvent used in manufacturing dyes, phenol, and nitrobenzene, has a TLV of 10 PPM by inhalation according to the Occupational Safety and Health Administration

TABLE 17. **Common Examples of Aliphatic Halogenated Hydrocarbons**

Hydrocarbon	Estimated Fatal Dose (Ingested)	TLV-TWA (PPM)	Synonyms
1,1,1-Trichloroethane	15.7 grams/kg	50	Methyl chloroform, Triethane, chlor-ethane, Glamorene Spot Remover, Scotchgard
1,1,2-Trichloroethane	580 mg/kg	10	Vinyl trichloride
Trichloroethylene	Controversial, 3–5 ml/kg	50	—
Tetrachloroethanene	Not known	5	Acetylene tetrachloride
Dichloromethane	25 ml	100	Methylene chloride
Tetrachloroethylene	5 ml	50	Tetrachloroethene Perchloroethylene
Dichloroethane	0.5 ml/kg	200	—
Carbon tetrachloride	3–5 ml	5	—

(OSHA). The National Institute for Occupational Safety and Health (NIOSH) value is 1 PPM. The adult ingested toxic dose is 15 ml. Chronic exposure may cause leukemia. Two hundred PPM is fatal in 5 minutes. *Toluene,* used in manufacturing TNT, has an OSHA TLV of 200 PPM by inhalation; the NIOSH figure is 100. The adult ingested toxic dose is 50 ml. *Styrene* has an OSHA TLV of 100 PPM by inhalation. *Xylene,* used in the manufacture of perfumes, has an OSHA TLV of 100 PPM by inhalation. The adult ingested toxic dose is 50 ml. *Manifestations*: Asphyxiation, CNS depression, defatting dermatitis, and aspiration pneumonitis. A bite into a tube of household plastic cement by a young child does not warrant the induction of emesis. Ingestion of hydrocarbon with a benzene fraction over 5 per cent may warrant induction of emesis.

3. **Aliphatic Halogenated Hydrocarbons.** See Table 17 for common examples. *Manifestations*: Myocardial sensitization and irritability, hepatorenal toxicity, and CNS depression. Dichloromethane may be converted into carbon monoxide in the body. Trichloroethylene concentrates in the fetus (pregnant women should not be exposed) and causes a disulfiram (Antabuse) reaction ("degreaser's flush") when associated with ingestion of ethanol. The decision to induce emesis must be based on the toxicity of the agent.

4. **Dangerous Additives.** Dangerous additives to the hydrocarbons, such as heavy metals, nitrobenzene, aniline dyes, insecticides and demothing agents, may warrant the induction of emesis.

5. **Heavy Hydrocarbons.** These have high viscosity, low volatility, and minimal absorption, so emesis is unwarranted. Examples are asphalt (tar), machine oil, motor oil (lubricating oil, engine oil), diesel oil (engine fuel, home heating oil), petrolatum liquid (mineral oil, suntan oils), petrolatum jelly (Vaseline), paraffin wax, transmission oil, cutting oil, and greases and glues.

6. **Products Treated as Petroleum Distillates.** Essential oils (e.g., turpentine, pine oil) are treated as petroleum distillates. Mineral seal oil (signal oil), found in some furniture polishes, is a heavy, viscous oil that *never* warrants emesis; it can produce severe pneumonia if aspirated. It has minimal absorption. *Management*: Dermal decontamination. Removal from the environment in inhalation.

First Aid Treatment. See Table 18. *The use of activated charcoal, oils, and cathartics is not advised in petroleum distillate ingestions. General management*: (1) In the asymptomatic patient: observe several hours for development of respiratory distress. (2) In the symptomatic patient: supportive respiratory care for respiratory distress. Bronchospasm may be treated with intravenous aminophylline. Avoid epinephrine. Monitor ECG; arterial blood gases; liver, pulmonary, and renal function; serum electrolytes; serial radiographs. Observe for intravascular hemolysis and disseminated intravascular coagulation. If cyanosis is present that does not respond to oxygen or the arterial Pa_{O_2} is normal, suspect methemoglobinemia that may require therapy with methylene blue. Steroids have not been shown to be beneficial. Antimicrobial agents are not useful in prophylaxis. (Fever or leukocytosis may be produced by the chemical pneumonitis itself.) It is not necessary to treat pneumatoceles. Most infiltrations resolve spontaneously in 1 week except for lipoid pneumonia, which may last up to 6 weeks.

Imipramine (Tofranil). See Tricyclic Antidepressants.

Iron. The iron content of some preparations appears in Table 19. *Toxic dose*: Range, 20 to 60 mg per kg or greater of elemental iron. Dose to induce emesis, ≥ 20 mg per kg. The potential fatal dose is 180 mg per kg (600 mg of elemental iron). *Toxicokinetics*: Absorption occurs chiefly in the small intestine. For excretion there is no normal route except blood loss or gastrointestinal desquamation. *Manifestations*: Phase I—Mucosal injury possibly with hematemesis (1 to 6 hours postingestion). Phase II—patient appears improved (6 to 48 hours). Phase III—cardiovascular collapse and severe metabolic acidosis. Phase IV—sequelae of intestinal stricture and obstruction or anemia (weeks to months). Patients asymptomatic for 6 hours rarely develop serious intoxication manifestations.

Management: (1) Gastrointestinal decontamination. Emesis should be induced in ingestions of elemental iron of over 20 mg per kg. Emesis should be followed by gastric lavage if large amounts have been ingested (over 60 mg per kg). The solution to be used for lavage is 1 to 1.5 per cent sodium bicarbonate to form ferrous carbonate salts, which are poorly absorbed. One hundred milliliters of this solution should be left in the stomach (prepared by dilution of a sodium bicarbonate ampule with saline). The use of deferoxamine

TABLE 18. **Initial Management of Hydrocarbon Ingestions**

Symptoms	Contents	Amount	Initial Management
None	Petroleum distillate only	<5 ml/kg	None
None	Heavy hydrocarbon Mineral seal oil Petroleum distillate	Any amount >60 ml	None* None ? Emesis
None	Petroleum distillate with dangerous additive (heavy metals, pesticide)	Depends on toxicity of additives	Emesis
	Aromatic	>1 ml/kg	Emesis
	Halogenated hydrocarbons Trichlor compound Tetrachlor compound	 >1 ml/kg Any amount ingested	 Emesis Emesis
Loss of protective airway reflex, seizures	Petroleum distillate with dangerous additive, aromatic or halogenated hydrocarbon	Depends on toxicity	Use endotracheal tube before gastric lavage

*Emesis may be necessary if machine oil contains triorthocresyl phosphate (TOCP), which causes weakness, sensory impairment, and "partially reversible damage to the spinal cord."

(Desferal) in the gastrointestinal tract is controversial. The use of diluted Fleet's enema solution risks severe hypertonic phosphate poisoning. (2) Postlavage abdominal radiograph—if significant amounts of residual radiopaque material are present, consider removal by endoscopy or surgery since coalesced tablets have produced hemorrhagic infarction and perforation peritonitis. (3) Protect the mucosal surfaces with demulcents if damage is evident. (4) Diagnostic chelation test—deferoxamine not reliable. (5) Indications for chelation therapy with deferoxamine are serum iron level greater than total iron binding capacity, or positive diagnostic chelation test; serum iron level over 350 mg per dl; and systemic signs of intoxication independent of serum iron level. Chelation should be performed within 12 to 18 hours to be effective.

Laboratory aids: Serum iron levels correlate with the clinical course. Iron levels taken at 2 to 6 hours that are below 350 mg per dl predict an asymptomatic course; levels of 350 to 500 are associated with mild gastrointestinal symptoms (rarely serious); and levels greater than 500 suggest the possibility of serious Phase III manifestations. White blood cell counts greater than 15,000 per microliter, blood glucose levels over 150 mg per dl, radiopaque material present on abdominal radiograph, vomiting, and diarrhea predict iron levels greater than 300 mg per dl. Monitor complete blood counts, blood glucose, serum iron, stools,

TABLE 19. **Iron Content of Some Preparations**

Salt	Elemental Iron Content (%)	Average Tablet Strength (mg)	Iron Content Per Tablet (mg)
Ferrous sulfate	20	300	60
Ferrous sulfate (dried)	29.7	200	65
Ferrous gluconate	11.6	320	36
Ferrous fumarate	33	200	67

and vomitus for occult blood; electrolytes; acid-base balance; urinalysis and urinary output; liver function tests; blood urea nitrogen; and creatinine. Obtain type and match of blood in severe cases. Abdominal radiographs. Follow-up is necessary for sequelae in significant intoxications—gastrointestinal series for intestinal strictures and anemia secondary to blood loss. Patients who develop fever or toxic symptoms following iron overdose should have blood and stool cultures checked for *Yersinia enterocolitica*.

Isoniazid (INH, Nydrazid). This is an antituberculosis drug frequently used in suicides by American Indians and Eskimos. *Mechanism of toxicity:* It produces pyridoxine deficiency (doubles excretion of pyridoxine). *Toxic dose:* 1.5 grams, 35 to 40 mg per kg, produces convulsions; severe toxicity is seen at 6 to 10 grams; 200 mg per kg is an obligatory convulsant. *Toxicokinetics:* Absorption is rapid, with a peak in 1 to 2 hours (clinical symptoms may start in 30 minutes). Volume distribution is 0.6 liter per kg. It passes the placenta and into breast milk at 50 per cent of the maternal serum level. Not protein bound. Elimination is by the liver, which produces a hepatotoxic metabolite, acetylisoniazid. The t½: Slow acetylators (2 to 4 hours) may develop peripheral neuropathy (50 per cent of blacks and whites). Fast acetylators (0.7 to 2 hours) may develop hepatitis (90 per cent of Orientals and a majority of patients with diabetes). Excreted unchanged, 10 to 40 per cent. *Major toxic manifestations:* Visual disturbances, convulsions (90 per cent or more with one or more seizures), coma, resistant severe acidosis (due to lactate secondary to hypoxia, convulsions, and metabolic blocks).

Management: (1) Control seizures with large doses of pyridoxine, 1 gram for each gram of isoniazid ingested (Antidote 34, Table 4). If the dose ingested is unknown, give at least 5 grams of pyridoxine intravenously. (2) Correct acidosis with fluids and sodium bicarbonate (pyridoxine may spontaneously correct the acidosis). (3) Diazepam may be used as a supplement to control the seizures. (4) After patient is stabilized, or if asymptomatic, gastrointestinal decontamination procedures may be carried out, keeping in mind the rapid onset of convulsions. Asymptomatic patients should be observed for 4 hours. (5) Hemodialysis is rarely needed but may be used as an adjunct for uncontrollable acidosis and seizures. Hemoperfusion has not been adequately evaluated. Diuresis is ineffective. *Laboratory aids:* Isoniazid toxic levels are above 10 to 20 micrograms per ml. Monitor the blood glucose (often hyperglycemia), electrolytes (often hyperkalemia), bicarbonate, and arterial blood gases. Monitor the temperature closely (often hyperpyrexia).

Isopropyl Alcohol. See Alcohols.

Kerosene. See Hydrocarbons.

Lead. *Acute* lead poisoning is rare. *Acute toxic dose:* 0.5 gram. *Management:* (1) Gastrointestinal decontamination. (2) Supportive care, including measures to deal with the hepatic and renal failure and intravascular hemolysis. (3) Ethylenediaminetetraacetic acid (EDTA) in all severe cases if lead levels confirm absorption. *Chronic* lead poisoning occurs most often in children 1 to 6 years of age who are exposed in their environment and in adults in certain occupations or from illicit whiskey. *Chronic toxic dose:* Determined by blood lead level and clinical findings. Over 25 micrograms per dl indicates excess body burden. A chronic dose of 0.6 mg a day will increase the body burden, 2.5 mg a day will result in toxicity in 4 years, and 3.5 mg a day will cause toxicity in a few months.

Toxicokinetics: Absorption—10 to 15 per cent of the ingested dose is absorbed in adults; in children up to 40 per cent is absorbed with iron deficiency anemia. Inhalation absorption is rapid and complete. Vd—95 per cent present in bone. In blood, 95 per cent is in red blood cells. t½, 35 days; in bone, 10 years. The major elimination route for inorganic lead is renal. Organic lead is metabolized in the liver to inorganic lead; 9 per cent is excreted in the urine per day. *Manifestations of acute symptoms of chronic lead poisoning* (ABCDE): Anorexia, apathy, anemia; behavior disturbances; clumsiness; developmental deterioration; and emesis. Manifestations of encephalopathy are "PAINT": *P,* persistent forceful vomiting; *A,* ataxia; *I,* intermittent stupor and lucidity; *N,* neurologic coma and convulsions; *T,* tired and lethargic. In adults one may see peripheral neuropathies and "lead gum lines."

Management: (1) Gastrointestinal decontamination with enemas if radiopaque foreign bodies are noted. Do not delay therapy until clear. (2) Remove from exposure. For children, see Table 20. *Laboratory aids:* (1) Provocation mobilization test—500 mg per M² of EDTA for one dose given deeply intramuscularly with 0.5 per cent procaine diluted 1:1 and collect the urine for 6 to 8 hours. A ratio of micrograms excreted in the urine to milligrams of Ca-EDTA administered greater than 0.6 represents an increased lead body burden, and chelation should be administered. (2) Evaluate complete blood count, levels of serum iron, or ferritin; repeat blood lead levels and erythrocyte protoporphyrin. (3) Flat plate of the abdomen and long bone radiographs (knees usually). (4) Renal function tests. (5) Monitor electrolytes, serum calcium, phosphorus, blood glucose.

Lindane. See Organochlorine Insecticides.

Lithium (Eskalith, Lithane). Most cases of intoxica-

tion have occurred as therapeutic overdoses. The toxic dose is determined by serum levels, although intoxication has occurred with levels in the therapeutic range.

Toxicokinetics: Absorption is rapid, with complete peaking in 1 to 4 hours. Vd is 0.5 to 0.9 liter per kg. It is not protein bound. The t½ therapeutically is 18 to 24 hours. Eighty-nine to 98 per cent is excreted by the kidney unchanged, one-third to two-thirds in 6 to 12 hours. Excretion is decreased in the presence of hyponatremia and dehydration. The cerebrospinal fluid concentration is one-half the plasma concentration. The breast milk level is 50 per cent of the maternal serum level—toxic to the nursling. *Manifestations:* The first sign of toxicity may be diarrhea. Fine tremor of hands, lethargy, weakness, polyuria and polydipsia, goiter and hypothyroidism, and fasciculations are side effects. Severe toxicity is manifested by ataxia, impaired mental state, coma, and seizures (limbs held in hyperextension with eyes open in "coma vigil"). Cardiovascular manifestations are dysrhythmias, hypotension, flat T waves, and increased QT interval.

Management: (1) Gastrointestinal decontamination may not be useful after 2 hours because of rapid absorption. In slow-release preparations, decontamination may be useful up to 24 hours postingestion. Activated charcoal is not indicated. (2) Hospitalize if intoxication is suspected because seizures may occur unexpectedly. (3) Restore normothermia and fluid and electrolyte balance, particularly sodium. If diabetes insipidus is present, an infusion of sodium may cause hypernatremia. Current evidence supports saline infusion as enhancing excretion of lithium. (4) Forced diuresis has no role, unless the glomerular filtration rate is low. Consider only when the lithium level is not above 2.5 mEq per liter and fails to fall below 1 mEq per liter within 30 hours. (5) Hemodialysis is the treatment of choice for severe intoxication. Lithium is the most dialyzable toxin known. Long runs of 12 hours or longer should be used until the lithium level is less than 1 mEq per liter because of extensive reequilibration rebound. Follow levels every 4 hours after dialysis. Dialysis may have to be repeated. Expect a time lag in neurologic recovery. If hemodialysis is not available or delayed, peritoneal dialysis can be used but is less effective. (6) Monitor ECG. Refractory dysrhythmias may be treated with magnesium sulfate and sodium bicarbonate. (7) Aminophylline may increase lithium excretion and decrease lithium reabsorption but has not been extensively studied. (8) Avoid thiazides and spironolactone diuretics, which increase lithium levels.

Laboratory aids: Lithium level determinations should be performed every 4 hours. Although they do not always correlate with the manifestations at low levels, they are predictive in severe intoxications. Levels of 0.6 to 1.2 mEq per liter are usually therapeutic. Levels over 4.0 mEq per liter are severely toxic. Other tests to be monitored are complete blood count (lithium causes leukocytosis), renal function, thyroid, ECG, and electrolytes. Factors that predispose to lithium toxicity are febrile illness, sodium depletion, concomitant drugs (thiazide and spironolactone diuretics), impaired renal function, advanced age, and fluid loss in vomiting and diarrheal illness.

TABLE 20. **Choice of Chelation Therapy Based on Symptoms and Blood Lead Concentration***

Clinical Presentation	Treatment	Comments
Symptomatic children		
Acute encephalopathy	BAL, 450 mg/M²/day CaNa₂-EDTA, 1500 mg/M²/day (EDTA not used alone if blood Pb > 72 μg/dl or symptoms present)	Start with BAL, 75 mg/M² IM q 4 hr After 4 hr start continuous infusion of CaNa₂-EDTA, 1500 mg/M²/day Therapy with BAL and CaNa₂-EDTA should be continued for 5 days Interrupt therapy for 2 days Treat for 5 additional days, including BAL if blood Pb remains high Other cycles may be needed depending on blood Pb rebound
Other symptoms	BAL, 300 mg/M²/day CaNa₂-EDTA, 1000 mg/M²/day Monitor BUN, creatinine, AST, ALT, urine	Start with BAL, 90 mg/M² IM q 4 hr After 4 hr start CaNa₂-EDTA, 1000 mg/M²/day, preferably by continuous infusion, or in divided doses IV (through a heparin lock) Therapy with CaNa₂-EDTA should be continued for 5 days BAL may be discontinued after 3 days if blood Pb < 50 μg/dl Interrupt therapy for 2 days Treat for 5 additional days, including BAL if blood Pb remains high (>50 μg/dl) Other cycles may be needed depending on blood Pb rebound
Asymptomatic children BEFORE TREATMENT, MEASURE VENOUS BLOOD LEAD		
Blood Pb > 70 μg/dl	BAL, 300 mg/M²/day CaNa₂-EDTA, 1000 mg/M²/day	Start with BAL, 50 mg/M² IM q 4 hr After 4 hr start CaNa₂-EDTA, 1000 mg/M²/day, preferably by continuous infusion, or in divided doses IV (through a heparin lock) Treatment with CaNa₂-EDTA should be continued for 5 days BAL may be discontinued after 3 days if blood Pb < 50 μg/dl Other cycles may be needed depending on blood Pb rebound
Blood Pb 56–69 μg/dl	CaNa₂-EDTA, 1000 mg/M²/day	CaNa₂-EDTA for 5 days, preferably by continuous infusion, or in divided doses (through a heparin lock) Alternatively, if lead exposure is controlled, CaNa₂-EDTA may be given as a single daily outpatient dose IM or IV Other cycles may be needed depending on blood Pb rebound
Blood Pb 25–55 μg/dl PERFORM CaNa₂-EDTA PROVOCATION TEST TO ASSESS LEAD EXCRETION RATIO		
If ratio > 0.70	CaNa₂-EDTA, 1000 mg/M²/day	Treat for 5 days IV or IM, as above
If ratio 0.60–0.69 Age < 3 yr	CaNa₂-EDTA, 1000 mg/M²/day	Treat for 3 days IV or IM, as above
Age > 3 yr	No treatment	Repeat blood Pb and CaNa₂-EDTA provocation test periodically
If ratio < 0.60	No treatment	Repeat blood Pb and CaNa₂-EDTA provocation test periodically

*From Piomelli S., et al.: Management of childhood lead poisoning. J. Pediatr. *105*:523–532, 1984. Used by permission.

Lomotil (Diphenoxylate and Atropine). See Opioids and Anticholinergic Agents.

LSD (Lysergic Acid Diethylamide). See Hallucinogens.

Marijuana. See Hallucinogens.

Meperidine (Demerol). See Opioids.

Meprobamate (Equanil, Miltown). See Sedative Hypnotics.

Mercury. *Management:* (1) Inhalation of elemental mercury—remove from exposure. (2) Ingestion of mercuric salt—gastrointestinal decontamination. A protein solution such as egg white or 5 per cent salt-poor albumin can be given to reduce salt to mercurous ion (less toxic). Give activated charcoal and cathartic. (3) Chelating agents (do not use Ca-EDTA because of nephrotoxicity): Dimercaprol (BAL) enhances mercury excretion through the bile as well as the urine and would be the choice if there were renal impairment from the mercury (Antidote 17, Table 4). Penicillamine (Antidote 29, Table 4) or *N*-acetyl-DL-penicillamine (investigational use). Use of BAL in methyl mercury intoxication increases the brain mercury and appears to be contraindicated; penicillamine and its analogue should be used (decreases mercury in brain). A new chelator, 2,3-dimercaptosuccinic acid, holds promise of less toxicity and more specific therapy and is now available under the Orphan Drug Program.* (4) Monitor fluid and electrolyte levels, renal function, hemoglobin levels. Obtain blood and urine mercury levels (consult the laboratory for proper collection technique and containers). (5) Hemodialysis early in the symptomatic patient is useful. (6) New but not established

---

*Inquiries can be made to the National Information Center for Orphan Drugs and Rare Diseases, 800–336–4797.

approaches are Polythiol resin to bind the methyl mercury excreted in the bile; heat and sauna treatment to increase mercury excretion through perspiration; and a regional dialyzer system using L-cysteine. (7) Surgical excision of *local injection sites*.

Laboratory aids: (1) Blood levels are below 2 to 4 micrograms per dl and urine levels below 10 to 20 micrograms per liter in 90 per cent of adult population. Levels above 4 micrograms per dl in blood and 20 micrograms per liter in urine probably should be considered abnormal. Blood levels are not always reliable. Exposed industrial workers' urine levels are 150 to 200 micrograms. (2) In asymptomatic patients with urine levels under 300 micrograms per liter, a chelating challenge with BAL or penicillamine may bring a significant increase that may aid in establishing the diagnosis. (3) Approximately 150 micrograms per liter of mercury in urine is equivalent to 3.5 micrograms per dl in blood. (4) Methyl mercury is excreted mainly through the feces, so urine mercury would not be a reliable measurement. (5) Mercury is also excreted in the sweat and saliva. The parotid fluid level is approximately two-thirds that of the blood. Since the hair is porous, it may absorb mercury from the atmosphere; however, hair concentrations of 400 to 500 micrograms are likely to be associated with neurologic symptoms.

Methadone. See Opioids.

Methanol. See Alcohols.

Methaqualone. See Sedative Hypnotics.

Methyprylon (Noludar). See Sedative Hypnotics.

Narcotic Analgesics. See Opioids.

Neuroleptics. See Phenothiazines and Other Major Neuroleptics.

Nitrites (NO₂) and Nitrates (NO₃). These are readily available in both inorganic and organic forms. Organic nitrates used for angina pectoris are listed in Table 21. Inorganic nitrates have more toxicologic importance in natural foods and contaminated well water. *Potential fatal doses:* Nitrite, 1 gram; nitrate, 10 grams; nitrobenzene, 2 ml; nitroglycerin, 0.2 gram; and aniline dye (pure), 5 to 30 grams. *Toxicokinetics:* Onset of action of nitroglycerin sublingually is 1 to 3 minutes,

with a peak action of 3 to 15 minutes and a duration of 20 to 30 minutes. Other routes have a slower onset (2 to 5 minutes) and longer duration of action (1.5 to 6 hours). Nitrites are potent oxidizing agents converting ferrous to ferric iron, which cannot carry oxygen. Normally, humans have 0.7 per cent of methemoglobin, which is converted by methemoglobin reductase into oxygen-carrying hemoglobin. Liver detoxification by dinitration is the route of elimination. *Toxic manifestations* depend on the level of methemoglobinemia. At 10 per cent, "chocolate cyanosis" occurs; at 10 to 20 per cent, headache, dizziness, and tachypnea occur; and at 50 per cent, mental alterations are present and coma and convulsions may occur. Headache, flushing, and sweating are due to the vasodilatory effect; hypotension, tachycardia, and syncope may also occur. Severe hypoxia may produce pulmonary edema and encephalopathy. Levels above 50 per cent produce metabolic acidosis and ECG changes; cardiovascular collapse occurs at levels of 70 per cent.

Management: (1) Dermal decontamination, if indicated. Aniline dyes may be removed with 5 per cent acetic acid (vinegar). (2) Gastrointestinal decontamination if ingested. (3) Hypotension can be treated by the Trendelenburg position and fluid challenge. Vasoconstrictors (dopamine or norepinephrine) are rarely needed. (4) Methylene blue (Antidote 24, Table 4) is indicated for methemoglobin levels above 30 per cent, dyspnea, metabolic acidosis (lactic acidosis), or an altered mental state. (5) Oxygen, 100 per cent, or a hyperbaric chamber should be used in symptomatic patients if methylene blue fails or is not effective, e.g., chlorate intoxication or glucose-6-phosphate dehydrogenase deficiency. *Laboratory aids:* Methemoglobin levels, arterial blood gases. Blood has a chocolate-brown appearance and fails to turn red on exposure to oxygen.

Nortriptyline (Aventyl, Pamelor). See Tricyclic Antidepressants.

Opioids (Narcotic Opiates). See Table 22. The major metabolic pathway differs for each opioid but they are 90 per cent metabolized in the liver. Patients should be observed for CNS and respiratory depression and hypotension. Pulmonary edema is a potentially lethal complication of mainlining (intravenous use). *Manifestations:* All opiate agonists produce miotic pupils (except meperidine and Lomotil early), respiratory and CNS depression, physical dependence, and withdrawal.

Management: (1) Supportive care, particularly an endotracheal tube and assisted ventilation. (2) Gastrointestinal decontamination up to 12 hours postingestion, as opiates delay gastric emptying time, but this is of no benefit if overdose is by injection. Convulsions occur rapidly with propoxyphene (Darvon) and codeine overdose, and this may be an indication not to use an emetic for gastrointestinal decontamination in this drug overdose. (3) Naloxone (Narcan) (Antidote 25, Table 4) may be given in bolus intravenous doses and by continuous drip. Naloxone must be titrated against the clinical response and precipitation of withdrawal in narcotic addicts. It should be repeated as often as necessary, since many opioids in overdose can last 24 hours to 48 hours, whereas the action of naloxone lasts only 2 to 3 hours. *Larger doses are*

TABLE 21. **Organic Nitrates for Angina Pectoris**

Drug and Route	Trade Name	Onset (min)	Duration (hr)
Nitroglycerin			
Oral	Many	Varies	4–6
Sublingual	Many	1–3	¼–½
2% ointment	Nitrobid Nitrol	Varies	3–6
Isosorbide dinitrate	Isordil		
Sublingual		1–3	1.3–3
Oral		2–5	4–6
Chewable		2–5	2–3
Timed release		Varies	—
Pentaerythritol tetranitrate, oral	Peritrate	2–5	3–5
Erythrityl tetranitrate, oral	Cardilate	2–5	4–6

TABLE 22. **Opioids (Narcotic Opiates)***

Drugs		Equivalent IM Dose† (mg)	Oral† (mg)	Peak Action (hr)	Half-Life (hr)	Duration of Action (hr)	Potential Toxic Dose (mg)
Generic	Trade						
Alphaprodine	Nisentil	45	—	0.5	—	1–2	—
Butorphanol	Stadol	2	12	0.5–1.0	3	3–4	—
Camphorated tincture of opium	Paregoric	2–4 ml	25 ml	—	—	4–5	—
Codeine	Various	120	200	—	3	3–6	800
Diacetylmorphine	Heroin	3.0	60	—	0.5	3–4	100
Dihydrocodeine	Hycodan	5–10	—	—	—	—	100
Diphenoxylate	Lomotil	40–60	—	Delayed by atropine	—	—	—
Fentanyl	Sublimaze	0.2	—	0.5	1.5	1–2	—
Hydromorphone	Dilaudid	1.5	6.5	0.5–0.75	2–3	4–5	100
Meperidine	Demerol	75–100	300	0.5–1	0.5–5	4–6	1000
Methadone	Dolophine	10.0	20	4	22–97	4–6	120
Morphine	Various	10.0	60	0.75–1.5	2–3	4–6	200
Nalbuphine	Nubain	10.0	60	—	5	3–6	—
Oxycodone	Percodan	15	30	—	—	3–4	—
Oxymorphone	Numorphan	1.0	6.5	1	2–3	4–5	—
Pentazocine	Talwin	60	180	0.75	2	4–7	—
Propoxyphene	Darvon	240	—	2–4	8–24	2–4	500

*"Ts and blues" are a combination of pentazocine (Talwin) and tripelennamine (Pyribenzamine) used intravenously. Pentazocine now has naloxone added to it to counter this abuse. Innovar is fentanyl plus droperidol, used as an IV anesthetic.
†Dose equivalent to 10 mg of morphine.

needed for codeine, pentazocine, and propoxyphene. (4) Pulmonary edema does not respond to naloxone and needs respiratory supportive care. Fluids should be given cautiously in opioid overdose, because these agents stimulate antidiuretic hormone effect and pulmonary edema is frequent. (5) *If the patient is comatose, give 50 per cent glucose* (3 to 4 per cent of comatose narcotic overdose patients have hypoglycemia). (6) *If the patient is agitated,* consider hypoxia rather than withdrawal and treat as such. (7) *Observe for withdrawal* (nausea, vomiting, cramps, diarrhea, dilated pupils, rhinorrhea, piloerection). If these occur, stop naloxone.

OPIOID ADDICT WITHDRAWAL SCORE. Symptoms of withdrawal are diarrhea, dilated pupils, gooseflesh, hyperactive bowel sounds, hypertension, insomnia, lacrimation, muscle cramps, restlessness, tachycardia, and yawning. Each sign or symptom is given 0, 1, or 2 points, depending on the severity. A score of 1 to 5 is mild; 6 to 10, moderate; and 11 to 15, severe. Seizures are very unusual with withdrawal. They indicate severity regardless of the rest of the score. *Management:* Mild withdrawal is treated with diazepam orally, 10 mg every 6 hours; moderate withdrawal, with intramuscular diazepam; and severe withdrawal, with diazepam and diphenoxylate (Lomotil) for the diarrhea. Methadone orally may be used, 20 to 40 mg every 12 hours, decreased by 5 mg every 12 hours. When 10 mg is reached, add Lomotil. Clonidine (Catapres), 6 micrograms per kg every 6 hours, can be used with informed consent. (This is an unlisted use of clonidine; the manufacturer states that relief from withdrawal symptoms has been reported with 0.8 mg per day.)

Laboratory aids: For acute overdose obtain levels of blood gases, blood glucose, and electrolytes; chest x-ray; and ECG. Blood opioid levels confirm diagnosis but are not useful for making a therapeutic decision. For drug abusers, consider testing for hepatitis B,

syphilis, and HIV antibody (HIV testing usually requires consent).

PROPOXYPHENE (Darvon). *Manifestations:* Onset may be as early as 30 minutes after ingestion. Convulsions occur early. Patients may develop diabetes insipidus, pulmonary edema, and hypoglycemia. *Elimination:* Metabolism is 90 per cent by demethylation in the liver. Peak plasma level of 1 to 2 hours after oral dose. Half-life is 1 to 5 hours. As little as 10 mg per kg has caused symptoms, and 35 mg per kg has caused cardiopulmonary arrest. Therapeutic blood level is less than 200 micrograms per ml. *Treatment* (in addition to the general management): (1) Emesis can be dangerous because of the rapid onset of seizures. (2) Indications for naloxone are respiratory depression, seizure activity, coma, and miotic pupils. Signs of naloxone effect are dilation of pupils, increased rate and depth of respirations, reversal of hypotension, and improvement of obtunded or comatose state. Larger doses of naloxone are often required and can be continued as an infusion of the initial response dose every hour. (3) Naloxone and intravenous glucose should be tried first to control seizures. If these fail, diazepam may be tried.

Organochlorine Insecticides (DDT Derivatives). See Table 23 for a listing of these agents. The *toxic dose* varies greatly. Chlorophenothane (DDT), 200 to 250 mg per kg, is fatal; 16 mg per kg causes seizures. Methoxychlor, 500 to 600 mg per kg, is fatal. Chlordane, 200 mg per kg, is fatal (chlordane house air guidelines are below 5 micrograms per m³; the occupational TLV is 500 micrograms per m³). These insecticides interfere with axon transmission of nerve impulses. Metabolism varies; they resist degradation in human tissue and the environment. They accumulate in adipose tissue; the elimination route is via the liver. *Manifestations:* CNS stimulation, convulsions, late respiratory depression, increased myocardial irritability. Endrin produces liver toxicity with guarded prognosis.

TABLE 23. **Organochlorine Pesticides (DDT Derivatives)**

Chemical Name	Trade Name	Toxicity Rating	Elimination Time	Comment
Endrin	Hexadrin	Highest	hr–days	Banned
Lindane	1% in Kwell; Benesan; Isotox; Gamene	Moderate to high	hr–days	Scabicide; general garden insecticide
Endosulfan	Thiodan	Moderate	hr–days	
Benzene hexachloride	BHC, HCH	Moderate	wk–mo	Banned, produces porphyria (cutanea tarda)
Dieldrin	Dieldrite	High	wk–mo	
Aldrin	Aldrite	High	wk–mo	
Chlordane (10% is heptachlor)	Chlordan	High	wk–mo	Restricted; termiticide
Toxophene	Toxakil Strobane-T	High	hrs–days	
Heptachlor	—	Moderate	wk–mo	Malignancy in rats
Chlorophenothane	DDT	Moderate	mo–yr	Banned in 1972
Mirex	—	Moderate	mo–yr	Banned; red anticide
Chlordecone	Kepone	Moderate	mo–yr	Tidewater, Virginia, contamination
Methoxychlor	Marlate	Low	hr–days	
Perthane	—	Low	hr–days	
Dicofol	Kelthane	Low	hr–days	
Chlorobenzilate	Acaraben	Low	hr–days	Banned

Chronic exposure causes liver and kidney damage. *Management:* (1) Dermal decontamination, discard contaminated leather goods. Protect personnel. Gastrointestinal decontamination, no oils. Emesis can be dangerous owing to rapid seizures. Many are dissolved in petroleum distillates, presenting an aspiration hazard. (2) No adrenergic stimulants (epinephrine) should be used because of myocardial irritability. (3) Cholestyramine, 4 grams every 8 hours, has been reported to increase the fecal excretion. (4) Anticonvulsants, if needed.

Organophosphate and Carbamate Insecticides (OPI). These may cause (1) irreversible inhibition of cholinesterase, either direct (TEPP) or delayed (parathion or malathion), or (2) reversible inhibition of cholinesterase (carbamates). Examples of OPI are listed in Table 24. Absorption is by all routes. The onset of acute toxicity is usually before 12 hours and always before 24 hours. *Toxic manifestations:* Early, cholinergic crisis—cramps, diarrhea, excess secretion, bronchospasms, bradycardia. Later, sympathetic and nicotine effects occur—twitching, fasciculations, weakness, tachycardia and hypertension, and convulsions. CNS effects are anxiety, confusion, emotional lability, and coma. Delayed respiratory paralysis and neurologic disorders have been described.

Management: (1) Basic life support and decontamination with careful protection of personnel. (2) Atropine (Antidote 7, Table 4), if symptomatic, every 10 to 30 minutes until drying of secretions and clear lungs occur. Maintain for 12 to 24 hours, then taper the dose and observe for relapse. (3) Intravenous pralidoxime (2-PAM) may be required after atropinization (Antidote 31, Table 4). It should be given in the first 24 hours. It is used in the presence of weakness, respiratory depression, or muscle twitching. Its use may require reduction in the dose of atropine. (4) Careful dermal and gastrointestinal decontamination when stable. (5) Suction secretions until atropinization

drying is achieved. Intubation and assisted ventilation may be needed. (6) *Do not* use morphine, aminophylline, phenothiazine, or reserpine-like drugs or succinylcholine. *Laboratory aids:* Draw blood for red blood cell cholinesterase determination before giving pralidoxime. Levels are usually more than 50 per cent depressed for severe symptoms. Monitor chest radiograph, blood glucose, arterial blood gases, ECG, blood coagulation status, liver function, and the urine for the metabolite alkyl phosphate p-nitrophenol. *Note:* If the diagnosis is probable, do not delay therapy until it is confirmed by laboratory tests. Atropine is both a diagnostic and a therapeutic agent. A test dose of 1 mg in adults and 0.01 mg per kg in children may be administered parenterally. In the presence of severe cholinesterase inhibition, the patient fails to develop signs of atropinization.

It is not medically advisable to administer atropine or pralidoxime prophylactically to workers exposed to organophosphate pesticides.

CARBAMATES (esters of carbonic acid). Carbamates cause reversible carbamylation of acetylcholinesterase. Pralidoxime is usually not indicated in the management but atropine may be required. The major differences from OPI are (1) toxicity is less and of shorter duration; (2) they rarely produce overt CNS effects because of poor penetration; and (3) cholinesterase returns to normal rapidly so that blood values are not useful in confirming the diagnosis. Some common examples of carbamates are Ziram, Temik (alkicarb) (taken up by plants and fruit), Matacil (aminocarb, carazol), Vydate (oxamyl), Isolan, furadan (Carbofuran), Lannate (methomyl, Nudrin), Zectran (mexacarbate), and Mesural (methiocarb). These agents are all highly toxic. Moderately toxic are Baygon (propoxur) and Sevin (carbaryl). Some of these agents may be formulated in wood alcohol and have the added toxicity of methyl alcohol.

Paradichlorobenzene. See Hydrocarbons.

TABLE 24. **Examples of Organophosphate Insecticides (OPI)**

Common Name	Synonym	EFD*
Agricultural Products (highly toxic; LD_{50} is 1–40 mg/kg)		
Tetraethyl pyrophosphate	TEPP, Tetron	0.05
Phorate	Thimet	
Disulfoton†	Di-Syston	0.2
Demeton†	Systox	
Terbufos	Counter	
Chlortriphos	Calathion	
Mevinphos	Phosdrin	0.15
Parathion	Thiophos	0.10
Methamidophos	Monitor	Delayed neuropathy
Monocrotophos	Azodrin	
Octamethyl-diphosphoramide	OMPA, Schradan	
Azinphosmethyl	Guthion	0.2
Ethyl–nitrophenyl thiobenzene PO₄	EPN	
Animal Insecticides (moderately toxic; LD_{50} is 40–200 mg/kg)		
DEF	DeGreen	
Dichlorvos	DDVP, Vapona	
Coumaphos	Co-ral	
Trichlorfon	Dylox	
Ronnel	Korlan	10.0
Dimethoate	Cygon, De-Fend	
Fenthion	Baytex	Long acting
Leptophos	Phosvel	
Chlorfenvinophos (tick dip)	Supona, Dermaton	
Household and Garden Pest Control (low toxicity; LD_{50} is 200–1400 mg/kg)		
Malathion	Cython	60.0
Diazinon‡	Spectracide, Dimpylate	25.0
Chlorpyrifos‡	Lorsban, Dursban	
Temephos	Abate	

*Estimated fatal dose (grams/70 kg).
†Most OPI degrade in the environment in a few days to nontoxic radicals. These are taken up by the plants and fruits.
‡Some classify these as moderately toxic.

Paraquat and Diquat. Paraquat is a quaternary ammonia herbicide rapidly inactivated in the soil by clay particles. Nonindustrial preparations of 0.2 per cent are unlikely to cause serious intoxications. *Toxic dose:* Commercial preparations such as Gramoxone 20 per cent are very toxic; one mouthful has produced death. Systemic absorption in the course of occupational use is apparently minimal. Paraquat on marijuana leaves is pyrolyzed to nontoxic dipyridyl. *Toxicokinetics:* "Hit and run" toxin. Less than 20 per cent is absorbed. The peak is 1 hour postingestion. The route of elimination is the kidney. Most of the dose is eliminated in the first 40 hours; it is detected in urine for 15 days. Volume distribution is over 500 liters per kg. *Manifestations:* Local corrosive effect on skin and mucous membranes. Acute renal failure in 48 hours (often reversible). Pulmonary effects in 72 hours are progressive, and oxygen aggravates the pulmonary fibrosis. Diquat does not produce effects on the lungs but

produces convulsions and gastrointestinal distention. Long-term exposure may cause cataracts. Chlormequat's target organ is the kidney.

Management: (1) Gastrointestinal decontamination despite corrosive effects should be done cautiously with a nasogastric tube; administer local adsorbent. Repeated doses of activated charcoal are recommended. Dermal and ocular decontamination as needed. (2) Hemodialysis and hemoperfusion may be carried out in tandem. Hemoperfusion with charcoal alone is the present choice; however, the results are still poor. Continue hemoperfusion until blood paraquat levels cannot be detected. (3) Diuresis may be of value but consider the risk of fluid overload. (4) Niacin and vitamin E have not been effective. (5) Avoid oxygen unless absolutely necessary (Pa_{O_2} below 60 mmHg) because this aggravates fibrosis. Some use hypoxic air, FI_{O_2} 10 to 20 per cent. (6) Corticosteroids may help prevent adrenocortical necrosis. *Laboratory aids:* Blood levels above 2 micrograms per ml at 4 hours or above 0.10 micrograms per ml at 24 hours are usually fatal. Blood level testing and advice may be obtained from ICI American, 800–327–8633. Monitor renal, liver, and pulmonary functions and chest radiographs. Urine test for paraquat exposure: alkalinization and sodium dithionite give an intense blue-green color in exposure.

Parathion. See Organophosphate Insecticides.

Pentazocine (Talwin). See Opioids.

Perphenazine. See Phenothiazines and Other Major Neuroleptics.

Petroleum Products. See Hydrocarbons.

Phencyclidine (Angel Dust, PCP, Peace Pill, Hog). This is the "drug of deceit" because it is substituted for many other drugs, such as THC and mescaline. There are now at least 38 analogues. Smoking may give cyanide poisoning. Improper mixing has caused explosions. *Toxic dose:* Two to 5 mg smoked or "snorted" produces drunken behavior, agitation, and excitement. Five to 10 mg produces stupor, coma, and myoclonus convulsions. Ten to 25 mg smoked, snorted, or taken orally results in prolonged coma and respiratory failure. It is usually fatal over 25 mg (250 ng per ml blood concentration). *Toxicokinetics:* Weak base. Rapidly absorbed when smoked, snorted, or ingested and secreted into stomach gastric juice. Absorbed in alkaline intestine, but ion trapping takes place in acid gastric media. Half-life is 30 to 60 minutes. Lipophilic drug with extensive Vd. The onset of action if smoked is 2 to 5 minutes (peak in 15 to 30 minutes); orally, 30 to 60 minutes. The duration at low doses is 4 to 6 hours and normality returns in 24 hours. At large overdoses coma may last 6 to 10 days (waxes and wanes). An adverse reaction in overdose occurs in 1 to 2 hours. *Route of elimination:* By liver metabolism (50 per cent). Urinary excretion of conjugates and free PCP. *Manifestations:* Sympathomimetic, cholinergic, cerebellar. Observe for violent behavior, paranoid schizophrenia, self-destructive behavior. Clues to diagnosis are bursts of horizontal, vertical, and rotary nystagmus, coma with eyes open.

Management (avoid overtreatment of mild intoxications): (1) Gastrointestinal decontamination up to 4 hours postingestion, but this may not be effective because PCP is rapidly absorbed. Insert nasogastric tube into stomach for administration of activated charcoal every 6 hours, because PCP is secreted into the stomach even if it is smoked or snorted. (2) Protect patient and others from harm. "Talk down" is usually ineffective. Low sensory environment. Diazepam (Valium) may be used orally or intramuscularly in the uncooperative patient. (3) For behavioral disorders and toxic psychosis—haloperidol (Haldol), 2 to 5 mg, or diazepam or both. (4) Seizures and muscle spasm—control with diazepam, 2.5 mg, up to 10 mg (Antidote 16, Table 4). (5) Dystonia reaction—diphenhydramine (Benadryl) intravenously (Antidote 18, Table 4). (6) Hyperthermia—external cooling. (7) Hypertensive crisis (dopaminergic)—diazoxide, 3 to 5 mg per kg intravenously up to 300 mg bolus, or nitroprusside. (8) Acid diuresis ion trapping (controversial). Ammonium chloride use is not routinely recommended. If rhabdomyolysis occurs, myoglobin may precipitate in the renal tubules (Antidote 2, Table 4). (9) No phenothiazines in the acute phase of intoxication because they lower the convulsive threshold. May be needed later for psychosis.

Laboratory aids: (1) CPK level will be clue to the amount of rhabdomyolysis occurring and the chance of myoglobinuria developing. Values up to 20,000 units have been reported. (2) Test urine for myoglobin and pigmented casts. Test urine with ortho-toluidine; a positive test without red blood cells on microscopic examination suggests myoglobinuria. (3) Monitor urine and blood pH and urinary output if acidifying patient. (4) Measure PCP level. (5) Evaluate blood urea nitrogen, ammonia, electrolytes, blood glucose (20 per cent of patients have hypoglycemia) levels. (6) Test for PCP in gastric juice; levels are 40 to 50 times higher than in blood. *Complications:* Rhabdomyolysis, myoglobinuria, and renal failure. Dopaminogenic—hypertensive crisis, cerebrovascular accident, encephalopathy, and malignant hyperthermia. Schizophrenic paranoid psychosis (induced in chronic users or precipitated in acute users). Loss of memory for months. Teratogenic cases have been reported. Children have been intoxicated from inhalation in a room where adults were smoking PCP. PCP-induced depression and suicide.

Phenobarbital. See Barbiturates.

Phenothiazines and Other Major Neuroleptics. Phenothiazines are represented by aliphatic compounds: chlorpromazine (Thorazine), promethazine (Phenergan), promazine (Sparine), triflupromazine (Vesprin), methoxypromazine (Tentone); piperazine compounds (dimethylamine series); acetophenazine (Tindal), fluphenazine (Prolixin), prochlorperazine (Compazine), perphenazine (Trilafon), trifluoperazine (Stelazine); and piperidine compounds: mepazine (Pacatal), mesoridazine (Serentil), thioridazine (Mellaril), pipamazine (Mornidine). Nonphenothiazines are the thioxanthines: chlorprothixene (Taractan), thiothixene (Navane); butyrophenones: haloperidol (Haldol), droperidol (Inapsine); dibenzoxazepines: loxapine (Loxitane, Daxolin); and dihydroindolones: molindone (Moban, Lidone). These have pharmacologic properties similar to those of the phenothiazines. *Manifestations:* Clues to phenothiazine overdose are miosis, tremor, hypotension, hypothermia, respiratory depression, radiopaque pills

on radiograph of abdomen, and increased QT waves in the ECG. Anticholinergic actions are also present. Major problems are respiratory depression, myocardial toxicity (quinidine-like), neurogenic hypotension (antidopaminogenic), and idiosyncratic reaction, which may occur at therapeutic levels. Idiosyncratic reaction consists of opisthotonos, torticollis, orolingual dyskinesis, and oculogyric crisis (painful upward gaze) and can be mistaken for a psychotic episode. Extrapyramidal crisis is frequent in children and women. Death is usually due to cardiac effects. Phenothiazines are metabolized by the liver into many metabolites. Some remain in the body longer than 6 months.

Management: (1) Gastrointestinal decontamination. Emesis induction may be useful if symptoms have not occurred. If symptoms are already present, many of these agents have antiemetic action, so lavage may be required. Always provide gastric lavage to comatose patients after the airway is protected regardless of the time of ingestion because of inhibition of gastric motility. (2) Extrapyramidal signs (idiosyncratic reaction) can be treated with diphenhydramine (Benadryl) (Antidote 18, Table 4), or benztropine (Cogentin), 1 to 2 mg intravenously slowly. Symptoms recur, and these drugs should be continued orally for 2 to 3 days. *This is not the treatment of overdose,* only of the idiosyncratic reaction. (3) Monitor ECG for dysrhythmias and treat with antidysrhythmic agents. (4) Hypotension is treated with the Trendelenburg position or fluid challenge or both. Vasopressors are used only if these fail. Dopamine (Intropin) should not be used to treat the hypotension because these drugs are antidopaminogenic. If a pressor agent is needed, use norepinephrine (Levarterenol, Levophed). (5) Treat neuroleptic malignant syndrome by discontinuing the offending agent, reducing temperature with external cooling, and correcting any metabolic imbalance. Dantrolene, bromocriptine, and amantadine are agents that have been shown to be useful pharmacologic adjuncts for the management of this syndrome. (6) Treat hypo- or hyperthermia with external physical measures (not drugs).

Laboratory aids: A ferric chloride test of urine can confirm exposure to phenothiazines if there is a sufficient blood level. Blood levels are *not* useful in management. A radiograph of the abdomen is useful to detect undissolved tablets, which may be radiopaque. Monitor arterial blood gases, renal and hepatic function, and levels of elecrolytes and blood glucose for creatinine kinase and myoglobinemia in neuroleptic malignant syndrome.

Phenylpropanolamine (PPA). See Amphetamines.

Primidone. See Anticonvulsants.

Propoxyphene. See Opioids.

Propranolol and Beta Blockers. Some of these agents available in the United States at this time are listed in Table 25. *Toxic dose:* Varies considerably. *Toxicokinetics:* Peak action is 1 to 2 hours orally and lasts 24 to 48 hours. In drugs with long half-lives, e.g., nadolol, it may take many days to recover from overdose toxicity (Table 25). *Manifestations:* Observe for bradycardia and hypotension. Fat-soluble drugs have more CNS effects. Partial agonists may produce tachycardia and hypertension (oxprenolol, pindolol).

TABLE 25. **Pharmacokinetic Properties of Beta Blockers**

Drug Name	Solubility and Absorption (%)	Plasma t½ (hr)	Elimination Route	Peak Concentration (hr)	Protein Bound (%)	Vd (Liters/kg)	Beta₁ Cardiac Selective
Acebutolol* (Sectral) Dose: 400–800 mg MDD: 800 mg TPC: 200–2000 ng/ml	Moderate, lipid (90)	3–4, metabolite diacetolol	Hepatic, active metabolite	—	26	1.2	+
Alprenolol* (Aptin, Betapin; Betacard) Dose: 200–800 mg MDD: 800 mg TPC: 50–200 ng/ml	Lipid (10)	3.1	Hepatic	1–3	85	3.4	−
Atenolol (Tenormin) Dose: 50–100 mg MDD: 100 mg TPC: 200–500 ng/ml	Water (46–62)	6–9	Renal, 95%	2–4	3–10	0.7	+
Betaxolol (Betoptic) Dose: 1 drop in eye twice daily MDD: not available	Water (70–90)	12–22	Hepatic, 3–12%	—	50–60	4.9–13	+
Esmolol (Brevibloc) Dose: IV 50–500 µg/kg/min (loading dose) MDD: 300 µg/kg/min	Water	9 min	Hepatic, plasma esterases	—	55	3.4	+
Labetalol (Normodyne, Trandate) Dose: 400–800 mg MDD: 1–2 grams	Water (50)	6–8	Hepatic, 95% Blocks alpha (weakly) and beta activity	—	50	11	−
Levobunolol (Betagan) Dose: Ophthalmologic: 1 drop twice daily, 0.5%, 1%	Water (100)	6.1	Hepatic	—	—	—	−
Metoprolol (Lopressor) Dose: 50–100 mg MDD: 450 mg TPC: 50–100 ng/ml	Lipid (>95)	3–4	Hepatic	1–2	10	5.6	+
Nadolol (Corgard) Dose: 40–320 mg MDD: 320 mg TPC: 20–400 ng/ml	Water (15–25)	14–23	Renal, 70%	3–4	25	2.1	−
Oxyprenolol (Trasicor) Dose: 80–320 mg MDD: 480 mg TPC: 80–100 ng/ml	Lipid (70–95)	1.5–3	Hepatic	1–2	80	1.5	−
Pindolol* (Visken) Dose: 20–60 mg MDD: 60 mg TPC: 50–150 ng/ml	Lipid (>90)	3–4	Hepatic, 60%; renal, 40%	1.25	57	2.0	−
Practolol* (Eraldin) Dose: 25–600 mg MDD: 800 mg TPC: 1500–5000 ng/ml	Water (100)	6–8	Renal No longer available in United States because of adverse reactions	3	40		+

Table continued on following page

TABLE 25. **Pharmacokinetic Properties of Beta Blockers** *Continued*

Drug Name	Solubility and Absorption (%)	Plasma t½ (hr)	Elimination Route	Peak Concentration (hr)	Protein Bound (%)	Vd (Liters/kg)	Beta₁ Cardiac Selective
Propranolol (Inderal) Dose: 40–160 mg MDD: 480 mg TPC: 50–100 ng/ml	Lipid (100) (70% first pass)	2–3	Hepatic; renal (<1%), active hydroxy metabolite.	1.5	90–95	3.6	–
Sotalol (Beta-cardone, Sotacor) Dose: 80–320 mg MDD: 480 mg TPC: 500–4000 ng/ml	Water (70)	5–13	Renal — Prolongs QT and may produce torsades de pointes	2–3	54	0.7	–
Timolol†‡ (Blocadren) Dose: 20 mg; ophthalmologic (Timoptic, 0.25%, 0.5%), 1 drop twice daily MDD: 60 mg TPC: 5–10 ng/ml	Lipid (>90)	3–5	Hepatic, 80%; renal, 20%	4–5	<10	5.5	–

*Partial agonists.
†Substantial first pass.
‡Mitochondrial calcium protection during ischemia.
Abbreviations: MMD = maximum daily dose; TPC = therapeutic plasma concentration.

Management: (1) Gastrointestinal decontamination with gastric lavage and activated charcoal/cathartic. Before gastric lavage, treatment with atropine, 0.01 mg per kg for a child and 0.5 mg for an adult, has been suggested to decrease the vagal effect in patients with bradycardia or significant intoxications. Avoid induced emesis because of early onset of seizures and vagal stimulation. Asymptomatic patients may be discharged after 12 to 24 hours of observation. (2) Treat hypoglycemia (frequent in children) and hyperkalemia. (3) Control convulsions. (4) Cardiovascular manifestations: Bradycardia—if hemodynamically stable and asymptomatic, no therapy. If unstable (hypotension or atriovenous block), use atropine, isoproterenol, glucagon, and pacemaker. Ventricular tachycardia or premature beats—use lidocaine, phenytoin, or overdrive pacing. Myocardial depression and hypotension—correct dysrhythmias, institute Trendelenburg positioning, and fluids. Monitor with PAWP catheter. If low cardiac output with low PAWP, give more fluids. If low cardiac output with normal PAWP, use glucagon (Antidote 22, Table 4). Avoid quinidine, procainamide, and disopyramide (Norpace). Glucagon is probably the drug of choice since it works through adenyl cyclase mechanism not affected by the beta blockers. It is given as a bolus and may be continued as an infusion (Antidote 22, Table 4). If bronchospasm, give aminophylline. Hemodialysis or hemoperfusion for low volume distribution drugs that are low protein binding and water soluble (nadolol and atenolol), particularly with evidence of renal failure. If hypoglycemia, give intravenous glucose. *Laboratory aids*: Monitor blood glucose, potassium, ECG, PAWP. Fatal blood level of propranolol is 0.8 to 1.2 mg per dl (8 to 12 micrograms per ml).

Quinidine and Quinine (Antidysrhythmic and Antimalarial Agents). *Toxic dose* in child is 60 mg per kg; in adult, 2 to 8 grams. There is 95 to 100 per cent absorption, peak action in 2 to 4 hours. Half-life is 3 to 4 hours (quinidine gluconate, 8 to 12 hours). Large Vd. Metabolized predominantly by the liver. *Manifestations*: Cinchonism (headache, nausea, vomiting, tinnitus, deafness, diplopia, dilated pupils). Myocardial depression, dysrhythmias, ECG changes—prolongation of PR, QRS, and QT intervals. Rashes and flushing. Hemolysis in glucose-6-phosphate dehydrogenase deficiency. Dementia reported. *Management*: (1) Gastrointestinal decontamination. (2) Monitor ECG and liver function. (3) May need antidysrhythmic drugs and pacemaker and alkalinization.

Salicylates. *Toxic dose*: See Table 26. Methyl salicylate (oil of wintergreen): 1 ml equals 1.4 grams of salicylate. One teaspoonful equals 21 adult aspirins. *Toxicokinetics*: Plasma concentration is significant in 30 minutes and peaks in 1 to 2 hours. Half-life is 3 to 6 hours (therapeutic) to 12 to 36 hours (toxic). Urine pH influences urine salicylate elimination. *Manifestations of acute ingestion* (see Table 26): The metabolic disturbance in adults and older children is usually respiratory alkalosis; in children under 5 years of age the initial respiratory alkalosis will usually change to metabolic or mixed metabolic acidosis and respiratory alkalosis with acidosis predominating within a few hours.

Management: (1) Gastrointestinal decontamination is useful up to 12 hours postingestion, as some factors

TABLE 26. **Quantities of Aspirin Ingested: Deposition and Manifestations***

Category	Amount Ingested (mg/kg)	Toxicity Expected	Gastrointestinal Decontamination	Manifestations Anticipated
Nontoxic	<150	No	No	None
Usually nontoxic	>150	No	Yes (home)	None
Mild intoxication	150–200	Yes	Yes (ECF)	Vomiting, tinnitus, mild hyperventilation
Moderate intoxication	200–300	Yes	Yes (ECF)	Hyperpnea lethargy or excitability
Severe intoxication	300–500	Yes	Yes (ECF)	Coma, convulsions, severe hyperpnea
Very severe intoxication	>500	Yes	Yes (ECF)	Potentially fatal

*See toxic dose indications for gastrointestinal decontamination.
Abbreviation: ECF = emergency care facility.

delay absorption (food, enteric-coated tablets, other drugs); pylorospasm may delay emptying; and concretions may form. Activated charcoal should be administered every 4 hours until stools are black. Concretions may be removed by lavage, whole-body irrigation, endoscopy, or gastrostomy. (2) Intravenous fluid should be given as recommended in Table 27. Alkalinization enhances salicylate excretion. Potassium is essential to produce adequate alkalinization. Monitor *both* the urine and blood pH. Do not use the urine pH alone to assess the need for alkalinization (Antidote 35, Table 4). (3) Fluid retention can be treated with mannitol (20 per cent), 0.5 gram per kg over 30 minutes, or furosemide, 1 mg per kg intravenously. (4) Hyperpyrexia should be treated with external cooling. (5) Abnormal bleeding or hypoprothrombinemia will need vitamin K, 10 to 50 mg intravenously, and, if bleeding continues, fresh blood or platelet transfusion (Antidote 38, Table 4). (6) Dialysis (hemodialysis) or hemoperfusion is indicated if there is persistent acidosis (pH < 7.1) and lack of response to fluid or alkali in 6 hours; if serum salicylate levels are initially greater than 160 mg per dl or greater than 130 mg per dl at 6 hours postingestion (do *not* use the salicylate level as the sole criterion for dialysis); or if there are coma and uncontrollable seizures, congestive heart failure, acute renal failure, and progressive deterioration despite good management. (7) Chronic toxicity is usually a more severe intoxication because of the cumulative pharmocokinetics of salicylates. Management needs are outlined in Table 28.

Laboratory aids: The metabolic acidosis of salicylism has a moderately elevated anion gap. Hyper- or hypoglycemia may exist. Serum salicylate levels used in conjunction with the Done nomogram (Figure 3) are useful predictors of expected severity following *acute single ingestions.* The Done nomogram is *not* useful in chronic intoxications, methyl salicylate, phenyl salicylate, or homomethyl salicylate ingestions. The salicylate level for use in the Done nomogram should be obtained 6 hours postingestion. Before 6 hours, levels in the toxic range should be treated, and patients with levels below the toxic range should be retested if a potentially toxic dose is ingested. Monitor urine output, urine pH, electrolytes, arterial blood gases, blood glucose, prothrombin time, renal function, serum salicylate level, and urine salicylate with the ferric chloride test. Arterial blood pH should be kept at 7.5. *Prognosis:*

TABLE 27. **Recommendations for Fluid Management for Moderate or Severe Salicylism***

Purpose	Rate (ml/kg/hr)	Duration (hr)	Na	K	Cl	HCO₃	Glucose (%)
			mEq/Liter				
Volume expansion	20	0.5–1.0	100	0	77	23	5–10
Administered as 0.45% saline with 23 mEq/liter NaHCO₃							
Hydration Ongoing losses Alkalinization	4–8	Until therapeutic blood serum concentration 30 mg/dl	56	40	56	1–2 mEq/kg child; 50–100 mEq adult	5–10
Administered as 0.33% saline and NaHCO₃ to obtain urine pH 7.5–8.0, blood pH 7.5							
			mEq/kg/day				
Maintenance	2–6	—	3	2	4		

*For severe acidosis pH < 7.15, may require 1–2 mEq/kg every 1–2 hr. Usual fluid loss is 200–300 ml/kg, but carefully monitor for fluid overload. Potassium may be needed in excess of 40 mEq/liter when alkalinizing.

TABLE 28. **Management of Chronic Salicylate Intoxication**

Classification	Urine pH	Blood pH	Hydration	NaHCO₃ (mEq/liter)	Potassium (mEq/liter)
Mild	Alkaline	Alkaline	Yes	Yes	20
Moderate	Acid*	Alkaline	Yes	pH 7.5†	40
Severe	Acid	Acid	Yes	pH 7.5	40‡ 80§

*Paradoxical acid urine and alkaline blood indicate potassium depletion.
†Bicarbonate administered to keep blood pH 7.5 and urine pH 7.5–8.0.
‡Normal serum potassium and ECG.
§Low serum potassium and/or abnormal ECG indicating potassium deficiency.

Persistent vigorous treatment of salicylate ingestion is essential, as recovery has occurred despite decerebrate rigidity.

Sedative Hypnotics, Nonbarbiturate. See Table 29. *Management* is primarily supportive (especially intubation and ventilator therapy with continuous positive airway pressure for adult respiratory distress syndrome) and with the use of hemoperfusion or hemodialysis in patients who are severely intoxicated and fail to respond to good supportive care and whose intoxication is life-threatening. Avoid emesis because of rapid onset of convulsions, apnea, and coma. (1) *Chloral hydrate* management includes cautious gastrointestinal decontamination. Avoid the use of epinephrine

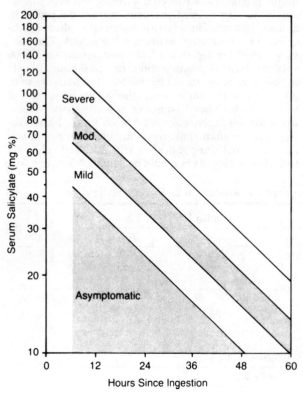

Figure 3. The Done nomogram for salicylate intoxication. For limitations of use, see *Laboratory aids*. (Redrawn from Done A: Salicylate intoxication: significance of measurements of salicylate in blood in cases of acute ingestion. Reproduced by permission of Pediatrics *26*:800, 1960.)

and catecholamines that may produce dysrhythmias. Propranolol, 0.1 mg per kg in 1-mg increments, appears to be more effective than lidocaine for ventricular dysrhythmias. (2) *Ethchlorvynol* management includes gastrointestinal decontamination up to 12 hours postingestion. Resin hemoperfusion (Amberlite XAD-4) is the best method of extracorporeal removal when other measures fail in a life-threatening situation (ingestion of over 10 grams or 100 mg per kg, with serum levels of over 100 micrograms per ml in the first 12 hours or 70 micrograms per ml after 12 hours in patients with prolonged life-threatening coma). External rewarming if temperature is below 32° C. (3) *Glutethimide* management includes gastrointestinal decontamination up to 24 hours postingestion. Concretions may form. Resin hemoperfusion appears to be the best method of extracorporeal removal in life-threatening protracted coma when the patient has ingested over 10 grams and has a serum level of over 30 micrograms per ml. Treat hyperthermia with external cooling. (4) *Meprobamate* management includes gastrointestinal decontamination up to 12 hours postingestion, with charcoal hemoperfusion in prolonged coma with life-threatening complications. Concretions may form in the stomach and may require breaking up or surgical removal. (5) *Methaqualone* management includes gastrointestinal decontamination. Forced diuresis, dialysis, and hemoperfusion are not indicated. Fatalities are rare. (6) *Methyprylon* management includes gastrointestinal decontamination and may require treatment of the hypotension with vasopressors of the alpha adrenergic variety—levarterenol (Levophed). The hypotension usually does not respond to position or fluids alone. This is a dialyzable drug, but dialysis usually is not necessary. Fatalities are rare.

Strychnine. Primarily available as a rodenticide and component of cathartics and "tonics." Adulterant of "street drugs," particularly marijuana and cocaine. *Toxic dose*: 5 to 10 mg; fatal in doses of 15 to 30 mg. *Toxicokinetics*: Rapid absorption. Manifestations may occur within 15 to 30 minutes. Low protein binding. Hepatic metabolism, which appears to be saturable. Twenty per cent is excreted in urine. Has been found in the urine up to 48 hours after a 700-mg dose. *Manifestations*: Interferes with postsynaptic neurotransmitter inhibition by glycine. Hyperacusis is often the first sign. Mild cases—face stiffness (trismus and risus sardonicus). Moderate cases—extensor muscle thrusts. Severe cases—tetanic convulsions with opisthotonos. Death occurs within 1 to 3 hours after inges-

TABLE 29. **Nonbarbiturate Sedative Hypnotic Drugs**

Drug	Absorption and Toxic Dose	Peak (hr)	Vd (Liter/kg)	Protein Bound (%)	Elimination Route	Serum Half-life (hr)	Toxic Level (μg/ml)	Manifestations and Comment*
Chloral hydrate (Noctec)	Rapid TD, 2 grams FD, 4–10 grams	1–2	0.75–0.9	40	Hepatic 90% to active metabolite trichloroethanol (TCE)	4–8	100 (80 TCE—very toxic)	Pear-like odor; dysrhythmias (especially ventricular), hepatotoxicity, irritant to mucosa of GI tract; ARDS; radiopaque capsules
Ethchlorvynol (Placidyl)	Rapid TD, 2.5 grams FD, 5 grams	1–2	3–4	35–50	Hepatic 90%	10–25 in OD over 100	20–80	Prolonged coma up to 200 hr, apnea, hypothermia, pulmonary edema, pink gastric aspirate, pungent odor
Glutethimide (Doriden) (highest mortality of all sedative hypnotics, 14%)	Slow, erratic TD, 5 grams FD, 10 grams	6	Large, 2–2.7	50	Hepatic 98% to toxic metabolite 4-hydroxyglutarimide	10 in OD over 100	20–80	Prolonged, cyclic coma up to 120 hr, anticholinergic signs, convulsions, recurrent apnea, hyperthermia
Meprobamate (Equanil, Miltown)	Rapid TD, 10 grams	4–8	10	20	Hepatic 90%	6–16	30–100	Coma, convulsions, pulmonary edema, apnea, concretions in stomach
Methaqualone (Quaaludes, "love drugs")	Rapid TD, 800 mg FD, 125 mg/kg	1–3	2–6	80	Hepatic 90%	10–40	8–10	Hypertonia, hyper-reflexia, convulsions, apnea, acts "drunk," bleeding tendencies
Methyprylon (Noludar)	Rapid TD, 3 grams	2–4	1–2	97	Hepatic 97%	3–6; over 8 in OD over 50	30	Hyperactive coma lasts 30 hr, miosis, persistent hypotension, pulmonary edema; mortality rare

*Comment includes other features besides the typical manifestations of all these agents—coma, respiratory depression, psychologic and physiologic withdrawal, hypotension, hypothermia (except glutethimide hyperthermia).

Abbreviations: TD = toxic dose; FD = fatal dose; OD = overdose; ARDS = adult respiratory distress syndrome; GI = gastrointestinal.

tion. The prognosis for survival improves if the patient survives beyond 5 hours. The complications of intoxication are lactic acidosis, hyperthermia, rhabdomyolysis and renal damage from precipitation of myoglobin in the renal tubules, and death from hypoxia. *Management*: (1) Emesis is contraindicated because of rapid absorption and the early onset of seizures. Gastric aspiration and lavage may be used after the seizures are controlled. Activated charcoal should be given and repeated. (2) Control convulsions with diazepam or phenobarbital. (3) Supportive care for respiratory depression. (4) Acid diuresis and dialysis do not appear to be justified on the basis of available studies. (5) Paralysis with assisted ventilation is useful.

Tear Gas (Lacrimators). CS (chlorobenzylidine), "riot control"; CN powder (chloroacetophenone, 1 per cent); Mace (chloroacetophenone). *Management:* Dermal and ocular decontamination. Protect attendants from contamination. Ophthalmologic evaluation. Oxygen ther-

apy may be needed for dyspnea and respiratory distress.

Theophylline. *Toxic dose*: Acute, single dose greater than 10 mg per kg yields mild toxicity. Greater than 20 mg per kg, moderate manifestations. *Toxicokinetics*: Absorption is complete. Peak levels occur within 60 to 90 minutes after ingestion of liquid preparations; 1 to 3 hours after regular tablets; and 3 to 10 hours after slow-release preparations. Vd, 0.3 to 0.7 liter per kg. Protein binding, 15 to 40 per cent. Half-life varies: 3.5 hours average in a child and 4.5 hours in an adult (range from 3 to 9 hours). In neonates and young infants the drug's half-life is much longer. Overdose increases the half-life. *Elimination*: Hepatic metabolism, 90 per cent (demethylation and oxidation); 8 to 10 per cent is excreted unchanged in the urine. *Manifestations*: Acute toxicity generally correlates with blood levels; chronic toxicity does not. Ten to 20 micrograms per ml is the therapeutic range, but some mild gastrointestinal toxicity may occur. Twenty to 40 micrograms per ml is moderate toxicity, with gastrointestinal and CNS stimulation. Over 50 micrograms per ml—seizures and dysrhythmias may occur, but they may also occur at lower levels and without gastrointestinal symptoms. Children tolerate higher serum levels. Chronic intoxication is more serious and difficult to treat. Many factors increase theophylline concentration.

Management: (1) Gastrointestinal decontamination in acute overdose, up to 4 hours with regular preparations and up to 8 to 12 hours with slow-release preparations. Test aspirate or vomitus for blood. Give activated charcoal every 4 hours. Do not induce emesis if hematemesis exists. (2) Monitor ECG, obtain theophylline levels every 4 hours until in the therapeutic range of 10 to 20 micrograms per ml. (3) Control seizures with diazepam. If coma, convulsions, or vomiting exists, intubate immediately. (4) Hypotension is treated with fluid challenge and if this fails, vasopressors. (5) Hematemesis is managed with iced saline lavage and blood replacement if needed. (6) Charcoal hemoperfusion is the management of choice in life-threatening convulsions, dysrhythmias, hematemesis, or intractable vomiting refractory to conventional measures. Differences in slow-release preparations from regular preparations: few or no gastrointestinal symptoms with high levels; peak concentration times may be 10 to 24 hours postingestion; and onset of seizures may occur 10 to 12 hours postingestion. *Laboratory aids*: Monitor theophylline levels, check for occult blood in vomitus and stools, monitor vital signs and hemoglobin and hematocrit (for hemorrhage). Monitor cardiac, renal, and hepatic function, electrolytes, blood glucose, arterial blood gases, and acid-base balance.

Toluene. See Hydrocarbons.

Tranquilizers. See Sedative Hypnotics.

Trichloroethylene. See Hydrocarbons.

Tricyclic Antidepressants (TCAD). These agents are generally rapidly absorbed from the gastrointestinal tract, but absorption may be prolonged in overdose owing to anticholinergic action. Their bioavailability has considerable variation among patients, and they are highly bound to plasma and tissue proteins. Protein binding decreases with decreasing pH. The Vd is large, usually 10 to 20 liters per kg. The TCAD are metabolized primarily in the liver. *N*-Demethylation of the tertiary amines yields the active secondary amine metabolites; hydroxylation gives rise to inactive metabolites. Forty per cent is excreted in the feces and only 3 per cent in the urine unchanged. The t½ varies from 9 to 198 hours. In an overdose, the half-life may be much longer. Tricyclic tertiary amines (metabolized to active metabolites) are amitriptyline (Elavil), imipramine (Tofranil), and doxepin (Sinequan). Tricyclic secondary amines (metabolized to nonactive metabolites) are desipramine (Norpramin, Pertofrane), protriptyline (Vivactil), and nortriptyline (Aventyl). Tricyclic dibenzoxazepine (metabolized to a major metabolite) is amoxapine (Asendin).

Manifestations: The onset of action varies from less than 1 hour to 12 hours after ingestion. The phases of intoxication are (1) consciousness with dry mouth, mydriasis, ataxia, increased deep tendon reflexes, and changes in the ST segment; (2) Stages I and II coma with hypertension, tachycardia above 160, mydriasis, and supraventricular tachycardia; and (3) Stages III and IV coma with hypotension, heart rate under 120, respiratory depression, tonic-clonic seizures, and ventricular dysrhythmias. The CNS effects occur early, and seizures are common. *Cardiovascular toxicity* is frequent in the serious poisonings and results from anticholinergic effects, sympathomimetic activity (by blocking reuptake of catecholamines), quinidine activity, catecholamine depletion, and alpha-adrenergic blockage. Cardiotoxic effects include cardiac dysrhythmias, hypertension, hypotension, and pulmonary edema.

Toxic dose: The TCAD have a narrow margin of safety. In a child, a 375-mg dose and in adults, as little as 500 to 750 mg has been fatal. The following dosages may serve as a guide to the degree of toxicity: Less than 10 mg per kg produces light coma, mydriasis, and tachycardia and has a good prognosis. At 20 mg per kg, Stage III manifestations are produced. At 30 mg per kg, fatalities may result. At 50 mg per kg, the mortality rate is increased. Over 70 mg per kg is rarely survived. Therapeutic blood levels are in the range of 50 to 170 ng per ml. If the QRS interval is less than 0.10 second for 6 hours, the prognosis is good. If it is greater than 0.10 second, seizures may occur, and if it is over 0.16 second, serious dysrhythmia may occur.

Newer Antidepressants. Amoxapine (Asendin) allegedly has less cardiotoxicity. Patients with amoxapine overdose may develop the syndrome of seizures, rhabdomyolysis, and acute renal tubular necrosis. Recent reports indicate more fatalities with amoxapine than with TCAD. Maprotiline (Ludiomil) is a tetracyclic compound with cardiac toxicity similar to the existing tricyclic antidepressant drugs. Trazodone hydrochloric acid (Desyrel) is an antidepressant chemically unrelated to the other antidepressants. It produces less serious toxicity, although orthostatic hypotension, vertigo, and priapism have been reported. Bupropion (Wellbutrin) is a phenylaminoketone antidepressant that produces dose-related seizures. Nomifensine (Merital) was withdrawn in 1986 because of reports of hemolytic anemia associated with it.

Management: (1) Maintenance of vital functions. Intensive care unit care until there are no abnormalities in the ECG for 24 to 48 hours. (2) Gastrointestinal decontamination (omit emesis) if the patient is alert. Intact pills have been recovered by lavage up to 18 hours after ingestion. Suspected cases should have ECG monitoring. (3) Activated charcoal cathartic every 4 to 6 hours and continuous nasogastric suction for the first 48 hours may interrupt enterohepatic recycling of tricyclic antidepressants. (4) Control seizures with intravenous diazepam. Intravenous phenytoin (Dilantin) may be added for seizures not responding to diazepam alone. For refractory seizures, physostigmine may be used (Antidote 30, Table 4). (5) Life-threatening delirium and hallucinations can be treated with physostigmine. Physostigmine was the drug of choice, but recently its use has been advocated only when conventional therapy has failed. (6) All cardiovascular complications of TCAD should *first* be treated by alkalinization of blood with sodium bicarbonate to a pH of 7.5 to 7.55 (Antidote 35, Table 4). Serum potassium levels should be followed, as a sudden increase in blood pH can aggravate or precipitate hypokalemia. Specific cardiovascular complications should be treated as follows: *Hypotension*— norepinephrine (Levophed), a predominantly alpha-adrenergic drug, is preferred over dopamine. (Hypertension that occurs early rarely requires treatment.) *Serious conduction defects* are best managed with phenytoin, and patients may need a temporary transvenous pacemaker. *Sinus tachycardia* usually does not require treatment. *Supraventricular tachycardia* that does not respond to alkalinization alone may be treated with phenytoin, physostigmine, or synchronized car-dioversion. *Ventricular tachycardia*—after alkalinization and phenytoin, intravenous lidocaine (for one dose only) may be required for persistent ventricular tachycardia. Synchronized cardioversion may be needed if lidocaine fails. *Ventricular fibrillation* should be treated with direct current countershock. *Torsades de pointes* is treated with isoproterenol, lidocaine, phenytoin, and atrial or ventricular overdrive pacing to shorten the QT interval. *Laboratory aids*: Arterial blood gases with blood pH, ECG, serum electrolytes, blood urea nitrogen and creatinine, serum phenytoin level, urine output, and, in severe cases, central venous pressure and/or PAWP should be monitored.

Turpentine. See Hydrocarbons.

Xylene. See Hydrocarbons.

Appendices and Index

LABORATORY VALUES OF CLINICAL IMPORTANCE

method of
REX B. CONN, M.D.
Thomas Jefferson University
Philadelphia, Pennsylvania

INTRODUCTION

The quantitative procedures carried out in a clinical laboratory represent measurements of substances normally present within rather narrow ranges of concentration. In order to use such data, we must know the values to be expected in a normal individual and what is considered a significant deviation from normal. Actually, there can be no sharp dividing line between abnormal and normal values, since there is a gradual transition during any pathologic process from what is clearly normal to what is clearly a pathologic condition.

In medicine, it is a logical impossibility to define normality, and the term "reference values" has replaced the earlier term "normal values." Reference values are derived from statistical studies on subjects believed to have no condition that might affect the measurements under consideration. The traditional and most widely used statistical approach is to carry out the measurement on a large group of subjects and to set the reference limits at the mean value plus or minus two standard deviations. Since values obtained for many measurements are not Gaussian in distribution, additional steps are frequently used in calculation of the reference ranges. The important consideration is that the reference ranges derived by these statistical methods contain only 95 per cent of the reference population. Thus, a value slightly outside the reference range might be due either to chance distribution or to an underlying pathologic process.

A single reference range for all individuals may be inadequate for some clinical measurements. Values obtained on presumably normal persons may vary because of age, sex, body build, race, environment, and state of gastrointestinal absorption. A universal caveat in the use of reference values is that for many procedures the reference range will vary with the method used. This is particularly true for enzyme measurements and measurements based upon immunochemical principles.

THE INTERNATIONAL SYSTEM OF UNITS FOR LABORATORY MEASUREMENTS (LE SYSTÈME INTERNATIONAL D'UNITÉS)

An extensive modification of the metric system has been adopted by clinical laboratories in many countries. This adaptation is the International System of Units (Le Système International d'Unités), usually abbreviated S.I. units. Whereas the metric system utilizes the centimeter, the gram, and the second as basic units, the International System uses the meter, the kilogram, and the second as well as four other basic units.

The International System is a coherent approach to all types of measurement that utilizes seven dimensionally independent basic quantities: mass, length, time, thermodynamic temperature, electric current, luminous intensity, and amount of substance. Each of these quantities is expressed in a clearly defined *base unit* (Table 1).

Two or more base units may be combined to provide *derived units* (Table 2) for expressing other measurements such as mass concentration (kilograms per cubic meter) and velocity (meters per second). Standardized prefixes (Table 3) for base and derived units are used to express fractions or multiples of the base units so that any measurement can be expressed in a value between 0.001 and 1000.

TABLE 1. **Base Units**

Property	Base Unit	Symbol
Length	metre	m
Mass	kilogram	kg
Amount of substance	mole	mol
Time	second	s
Thermodynamic temperature	kelvin	K
Electric current	ampere	A
Luminous intensity	candela	cd

TABLE 2. **Derived Units**

Derived Property	Derived Unit	Symbol
Area	square metre	m^2
Volume	cubic metre	m^3
	litre	l
Mass concentration	kilogram/cubic metre	kg/m^3
	gram/litre	g/l
Substance concentration	mole/cubic metre	mol/m^3
	mole/litre	mol/l
Temperature	degree Celsius	C = K − 273.15

TABLE 3. **Standard Prefixes**

Prefix	Multiplication Factor	Symbol
atto	10^{-18}	a
femto	10^{-15}	f
pico	10^{-12}	p
nano	10^{-9}	n
micro	10^{-6}	μ
milli	10^{-3}	m
centi	10^{-2}	c
deci	10^{-1}	d
deca	10^1	da
hecto	10^2	h
kilo	10^3	k
mega	10^6	M
giga	10^9	G
tera	10^{12}	T

Medical Applications

The most profound change in laboratory reports will result from expressing concentration as amount per volume (moles per liter) rather than mass per volume (milligrams per 100 milliliters). The advantages of the former expression can be seen in the following:

Conventional Units

1.0 gram of hemoglobin
Combines with 1.37 ml of oxygen
Contains 3.4 mg of iron
Forms 34.9 mg of bilirubin

S.I. Units

1.0 mmol of hemoglobin
Combines with 4.0 mmol of oxygen
Contains 4.0 mmol of iron
Forms 4.0 mmol of bilirubin

Chemical relationships between lactic acid and pyruvic acid and the glucose from which both are derived, as well as the relationship between bilirubin and the binding capacity of albumin, are other examples of chemical relationships that will be clarified by using the new system.

There are a number of laboratory and other medical measurements for which the S.I. units appear to offer little advantage, and some that are disadvantageous because the change would require replacement or revision of instruments such as the sphygmomanometer. The cubic meter is the derived unit for volume; however, it is inappropriately large for medical measurements, and the liter has been retained. Thermodynamic temperature expressed in kelvins is not more informative for medical measurements. Since the Celsius degree is the same as the kelvin degree, the Celsius scale is used. Celsius rather than centigrade is the preferred term.

Selection of units for expressing enzyme activity presents certain difficulties. Literally dozens of different units have been used in expressing enzyme activity, and interlaboratory comparison of enzyme results is impossible unless the assay system is precisely defined. In 1964, the International Union of Biochemistry attempted to remedy the situation by proposing the International Unit for enzymes. This unit was defined as the amount of enzyme that will catalyze the conversion of 1 micromole of substrate per minute under standard conditions. Difficulties remain, however, as enzyme activity is affected by temperature, pH, the type and amount of substrate, the presence of inhibitors, and other factors. Enzyme activity can be expressed in S.I. units, and the katal has been proposed to express activities of all catalysts, including enzymes. The katal is that amount of enzyme that catalyzes a reaction rate of 1 mole per second. Thus, adoption of the katal as the unit of enzyme activity would provide no more information than is obtained when results are expressed in International Units.

Hydrogen ion concentration in blood is customarily expressed as pH, but in S.I. units it would be expressed in nanomoles per liter. It appears unlikely that the very useful pH scale will be discarded.

Pressure measures, such as blood pressure and partial pressures of blood gases, would be expressed in S.I. units using the pascal, a unit that can be derived from the base units for mass, length, and time. This change probably will not be adopted in the early phases of the conversion to S.I. units. Similarly, a proposed change in expressing osmolality in terms of the depression of freezing point is inappropriate, because osmolality may be calculated from vapor pressure as well as freezing point measurement.

Conventions

A number of conventions have been adopted to standardize usage of S.I. units:

1. No periods are used after the symbol for a

unit (kg not kg.), and it remains unchanged when used in the plural (70 kg not 70 kgs).

2. A half space rather than a comma is used to divide large numbers into groups of three (e.g., 5 400 000 not 5,400,000).

3. Compound prefixes should be avoided (nanometer not millimicrometer).

4. Multiples and submultiples are used in steps of 10^3 or 10^{-3}.

5. The degree sign for the temperature scales is omitted (38 C not 38°C).

6. The preferred spelling is metre not meter, litre not liter.

7. Report of a measurement should include information on the system, the component, the kind of quantity, the numerical value, and the unit. For example: *System,* serum. *Component,* glucose. *Kind of quantity,* substance concentration. *Value,* 5.10. *Unit,* mmol/l.

8. The name of the component should be unambiguous; for example, "serum bilirubin" might refer to unconjugated bilirubin or to total bilirubin. For acids and bases, the maximally ionized form is used in naming the component; for example, lactate or urate rather than lactic acid or uric acid.

Tables of Reference Values

Tables accompanying this article indicate "normal values" for most of the commonly performed laboratory tests. The title of the tables has been changed from the "normal values" of previous years to "reference values" to conform to current usage. The reference value is given in conventional units, and the value in S.I. units is calculated from these figures. Notes (page 1077) provide additional information.

Reference Values in Hematology

	Conventional Units		S.I. Units		Notes
Acid hemolysis test (Ham)	No hemolysis		No hemolysis		
Alkaline phosphatase, leukocyte	Total score 14–100		Total score 14–100		
Carboxyhemoglobin	Up to 5% of total		0.05 of total		a
Cell counts					
Erythrocytes					
Males	4.6–6.2 million/cu mm		$4.6–6.2 \times 10^{12}/l$		
Females	4.2–5.4 million/cu mm		$4.2–5.4 \times 10^{12}/l$		
Children (varies with age)	4.5–5.1 million/cu mm		$4.5–5.1 \times 10^{12}/l$		
Leukocytes					
Total	4500–11,000/cu mm		$4.5–11.0 \times 10^9/l$		
Differential	*Percentage*	*Absolute*			
Myelocytes	0	0/cu mm	0/1		b
Band neutrophils	3–5	150–400/cu mm	$150–400 \times 10^6/l$		
Segmented neutrophils	54–62	3000–5800/cu mm	$3000–5800 \times 10^6/l$		
Lymphocytes	25–33	1500–3000/cu mm	$1500–3000 \times 10^6/l$		
Monocytes	3–7	300–500/cu mm	$300–500 \times 10^6/l$		
Eosinophils	1–3	50–250/cu mm	$50–250 \times 10^6/l$		
Basophils	0–0.75	15–50/cu mm	$15–50 \times 10^6/l$		
Platelets	150,000–350,000/cu mm		$150–350 \times 10^9/l$		
Reticulocytes	25,000–75,000/cu mm		$25–75 \times 10^9/l$		b
	0.5–1.5% of erythrocytes				

Bone marrow, differential cell count

	Range	*Average*	*Range*	*Average*	
Myeloblasts	0.3–5.0%	2.0%	0.003–0.05	0.02	a
Promyelocytes	1.0–8.0%	5.0%	0.01–0.08	0.05	
Myelocytes: Neutrophilic	5.0–19.0%	12.0%	0.05–0.19	0.12	
Eosinophilic	0.5–3.0%	1.5%	0.005–0.03	0.015	
Basophilic	0.0–0.5%	0.3%	0.00–0.005	0.003	
Metamyelocytes	13.0–32.0%	22.0%	0.13–0.32	0.22	
Polymorphonuclear neutrophils	7.0–30.0%	20.0%	0.07–0.30	0.20	
Polymorphonuclear eosinophils	0.5–4.0%	2.0%	0.005–0.04	0.02	
Polymorphonuclear basophils	0.0–0.7%	0.2%	0.00–0.007	0.002	
Lymphocytes	3.0–17.0%	10.0%	0.03–0.17	0.10	
Plasma cells	0.0–2.0%	0.4%	0.00–0.02	0.004	
Monocytes	0.5–5.0%	2.0%	0.005–0.05	0.02	
Reticulum cells	0.1–2.0%	0.2%	0.001–0.02	0.002	
Megakaryocytes	0.3–3.0%	0.4%	0.003–0.03	0.004	
Pronormoblasts	1.0–8.0%	4.0%	0.01–0.08	0.04	
Normoblasts	7.0–32.0%	18.0%	0.07–0.32	0.18	

Table continued on following page

Reference Values in Hematology *Continued*

	Conventional Units	S.I. Units	Notes
Coagulation tests			
Antithrombin III (synthetic substrate)	80–120% of normal	0.8–1.2 of normal	
Bleeding time (Duke)	1–5 min	1–5 min	
Bleeding time (Ivy)	Less than 5 min	Less than 5 min	
Bleeding time (template)	2.5–9.5 min	2.5–9.5 min	
Clot retraction, qualitative	Begins in 30–60 min / Complete in 24 hrs	Begins in 30–60 min / Complete in 24 h	
Coagulation time (Lee-White)	5–15 min (glass tubes) / 19–60 min (siliconized tubes)	5–15 min (glass tubes) / 19–60 min (siliconized tubes)	
Euglobulin lysis time	2–6 hrs at 37°	2–6 h at 37 C	
Factor VIII and other coagulation factors	50–150% of normal	0.50–1.5 of normal	a
Fibrin split products (Thrombo-Wellco test)	Less than 10 mcg/ml	Less than 10 mg/l	
Fibrinogen	200–400 mg/dl	5.9–11.7 µmol/l	c
Fibrinolysins	0	0	
Partial thromboplastin time, activated (APTT)	20–35 sec	20–35 sec	
Prothrombin consumption	Over 80% consumed in 1 hr	Over 0.80 consumed in 1 h	a
Prothrombin content	100% (calculated from prothrombin time)	1.0 (calculated from prothrombin time)	a
Prothrombin time (one stage)	12.0–14.0 sec	12.0–14.0 sec	
Tourniquet test	Ten or fewer petechiae in a 2.5 cm circle after 5 min	Ten or fewer petechiae in a 2.5 cm circle after 5 min	
Cold hemolysin test (Donath-Landsteiner)	No hemolysis	No hemolysis	
Coombs' test			
Direct	Negative	Negative	
Indirect	Negative	Negative	
Corpuscular values of erythrocytes (values are for adults; in children, values vary with age)			
MCH (mean corpuscular hemoglobin)	27–31 picogm	0.42–0.48 fmol	d
MCV (mean corpuscular volume)	80–96 cu micra	80–96 fl	
MCHC (mean corpuscular hemoglobin concentration)	32–36%	0.32–0.36	a
Haptoglobin (as hemoglobin binding capacity)	100–200 mg/dl	16–31 µmol/l	d
Hematocrit			
Males	40–54 ml/dl	0.40–0.54	a
Females	37–47 ml/dl	0.37–0.47	
Newborn	49–54 ml/dl	0.49–0.54	
Children (varies with age)	35–49 ml/dl	0.35–0.49	
Hemoglobin			
Males	14.0–18.0 grams/dl	2.17–2.79 mmol/l	d
Females	12.0–16.0 grams/dl	1.86–2.48 mmol/l	
Newborn	16.5–19.5 grams/dl	2.56–3.02 mmol/l	
Children (varies with age)	11.2–16.5 grams/dl	1.74–2.56 mmol/l	
Hemoglobin, fetal	Less than 1% of total	Less than 0.01 of total	a
Hemoglobin A_{1c}	3–5% of total	0.03–0.05 of total	a
Hemoglobin A_2	1.5–3.0% of total	0.015–0.03 of total	a
Hemoglobin, plasma	0–5.0 mg/dl	0–0.8 µmol/l	d
Methemoglobin	0–130 mg/dl	4.7–20 µmol/l	e
Osmotic fragility of erythrocytes	Begins in 0.45–0.39% NaCl / Complete in 0.33–0.30% NaCl	Begins in 77–67 mmol/NaCl / Complete in 56–51 mmol/l NaCl	
Sedimentation rate			
Wintrobe: Males	0–5 mm in 1 hr	0–5 mm/h	
Females	0–15 mm in 1 hr	0–15 mm/h	
Westergren: Male	0–15 mm in 1 hr	0–15 mm/h	
Females	0–20 mm in 1 hr	0–20 mm/h	
(May be slightly higher in children and during pregnancy)			

Reference Values for Blood, Plasma, and Serum
(For some procedures the reference values may vary depending upon the method used)

	Conventional Units	S.I. Units	Notes
Acetoacetate plus acetone, serum			
Qualitative	Negative	Negative	
Quantitative	0.3–2.0 mg/dl	3–20 mg/l	
Adrenocorticotropin (ACTH), plasma			
6 AM	10–80 picogm/ml	10–80 ng/l	
6 PM	Less than 50 picogm/ml	Less than 50 ng/l	
Alanine aminotransferase, *see* Transaminase			
Aldolase, serum	0–11 milliunits/ml (30°)	0–11 units/l (30 C)	f
Aldosterone			
Adult, supine	3–10 nanogm/dl	0.08–0.3 nmol/l	
standing			
male	6–22 nanogm/dl	0.17–0.61 nmol/l	
female	5–30 nanogm/dl	0.14–0.8 nmol/l	
Alpha amino nitrogen, serum	3.0–5.5 mg/dl	2.1–3.9 mmol/l	
Ammonia (nitrogen), plasma	15–49 mcg/dl	11–35 μmol/l	
Amylase, serum	25–125 milliunits/ml	25–125 units/l	
Anion gap	8–16 mEq/liter	8–16 mmol/l	
Ascorbic acid, blood	0.4–1.5 mg/dl	23–85 μmol/l	
Aspartate aminotransferase, *see* Transaminase			
Base excess, blood	0 ± 2 mEq/liter	0 ± 2 mmol/l	
Bicarbonate, serum	23–29 mEq/liter	23–29 mmol/l	
Bile acids, serum	0.3–3.0 mg/dl	3.0–30.0 mg/l	
Bilirubin, serum			
Direct	0.1–0.4 mg/dl	1.7–6.8 μmol/l	
Indirect	0.2–0.7 mg/dl (Total minus direct)	3.4–12 μmol/l (Total minus direct)	
Total	0.3–1.1 mg/dl	5.1–19 μmol/l	a
Calcium, serum	4.5–5.5 mEq/liter	2.25–2.75 mmol/l	
	9.0–11.0 mg/dl		
	(Slightly higher in children)	(Slightly higher in children)	
	(Varies with protein concentration)	(Varies with protein concentration)	
Calcium, ionized, serum	2.1–2.6 mEq/liter	1.05–1.30 mmol/l	
	4.25–5.25 mg/dl		
Carbon dioxide content, serum			
Adults	24–30 mEq/liter	24–30 mmol/l	
Infants	20–28 mEq/liter	20–28 mmol/l	
Carbon dioxide tension (Pco₂), blood	35–45 mm Hg	35–45 mm Hg	g
Carotene, serum	40–200 mcg/dl	0.74–3.72 μmol/l	
Ceruloplasmin, serum	23–44 mg/dl	230–440 mg/l	h
Chloride, serum	96–106 mEq/liter	96–106 mmol/l	
Cholesterol, serum			
Total	150–250 mg/dl	3.9–6.5 mmol/l	
Esters	68–76% of total cholesterol	0.68–0.76 of total cholesterol	a
Cholinesterase			
Serum	0.5–1.3 pH units	0.5–1.3 pH units	f
Erythrocytes	0.5–1.0 pH unit	0.5–1.0 pH unit	f
Copper, serum			
Males	70–140 mcg/dl	11–22 μmol/l	
Females	85–155 mcg/dl	13–24 μmol/l	
Cortisol, plasma			
8 AM	6–23 mcg/dl	170–635 nmol/l	
4 PM	3–15 mcg/dl	82–413 nmol/l	
10 PM	Less than 50% of 8 AM value	Less than 0.5 of 8 AM value	
Creatine, serum	0.2–0.8 mg/dl	15–61 μmol/l	
Creatine kinase, serum (CK, CPK)			
Males	12–80 milliunits/ml (30°)	12–80 units/l (30 C)	f
	55–170 milliunits/ml (37°)	55–170 units/l (37 C)	f
Females	10–55 milliunits/ml (30°)	10–55 units/l (30 C)	f
	30–135 milliunits/ml (37°)	30–135 units/l (37 C)	f
Creatine kinase isoenzymes, serum			
CK-MM	Present	Present	
CK-MB	Absent	Absent	
CK-BB	Absent	Absent	
Creatinine, serum	0.6–1.2 mg/dl	53–106 μmol/l	
Cryoglobulins, serum	0	0	
Fatty acids, total, serum	190–420 mg/dl	7–15 mmol/l	i
nonesterified, serum	8–25 mg/dl	0.30–0.90 mmol/l	
Ferritin, serum	20–200 nanogm/ml	20–200 μg/l	

Table continued on following page

Reference Values for Blood, Plasma, and Serum *Continued*
(For some procedures the reference values may vary depending upon the method used)

	Conventional Units	S.I. Units	Notes
Fibrinogen, plasma	200–400 mg/100 ml	5.9–11.7 µmol/l	c
Folate, serum	1.8–9.0 nanogm/ml	4.1–20.4 nmol/l	
Erythrocytes	150–450 nanogm/ml	340–1020 nmol/l	
Follicle-stimulating hormone (FSH), plasma			
Males	4–25 milliunits/ml (I.U.)	4–25 IU/l	
Females	4–30 milliunits/ml (I.U.)	4–30 IU/l	
Postmenopausal	40–250 milliunits/ml (I.U.)	40–250 IU/l	
Gamma glutamyltransferase			
Males	6–32 milliunits/ml (30°)	6–32 units/l (30 C)	f
Females	4–18 milliunits/ml (30°)	4–18 units/l (30 C)	f
Gastrin, serum	0–200 picogm/ml	0–200 ng/l	
Glucose (fasting)			
Blood	60–100 mg/dl	3.33–5.55 mmol/l	
Plasma or serum	70–115 mg/dl	3.89–6.38 mmol/l	
Growth hormone, serum	0–10 nanogm/ml	0–10 µg/l	
Haptoglobin, serum	100–200 mg/dl	16–31 µmol/l	d
	(As hemoglobin binding capacity)	(As hemoglobin binding capacity)	
Hydroxybutyric dehydrogenase, serum (HBD)	0–180 milliunits/ml (30°)	0–180 units/l (30 C)	f
17-Hydroxycorticosteroids, plasma	8–18 mcg/dl	0.22–0.50 µmol/l	j
Immunoglobulins, serum			
IgG	550–1900 mg/dl	5.5–19.0 g/l	
IgA	60–333 mg/dl	0.60–3.3 g/l	
IgM	45–145 mg/dl	0.45–1.5 g/l	
IgD	0.5–3.0 mg/dl	5–30 mg/l	
IgE	<500 nanogm/ml	<500 µg/l	
	(Varies with age in children)	(Varies with age in children)	
Insulin, plasma (fasting)	5–25 microunits/ml	36–179 pmol/l	
Iodine, protein bound, serum	3.5–8.0 mcg/dl	0.28–0.63 µmol/l	k
Iron, serum	75–175 mcg/dl	13–31 µmol/l	
Iron binding capacity, serum			
Total	250–410 mcg/dl	45–73 µmol/l	
Saturation	20–55%	0.20–0.55	a
Lactate, blood, venous	4.5–19.8 mg/dl	0.5–2.2 mmol/l	
arterial	4.5–14.4 mg/dl	0.5–1.6 mmol/l	
Lactate dehydrogenase, serum (LD, LDH)	45–90 milliunits/ml (I.U.) (30°)	45–90 units/l (30 C)	f
	100–190 milliunits/ml (37°)	100–190 units/l (37 C)	
LDH$_1$	22–37% of total	0.22–0.37 of total	
LDH$_2$	30–46% of total	0.30–0.46 of total	a
LDH$_3$	14–29% of total	0.14–0.29 of total	
LDH$_4$	5–11% of total	0.05–0.11 of total	
LDH$_5$	2–11% of total	0.02–0.11 of total	
Leucine aminopeptidase, serum	14–40 milliunits/ml (30°)	14–40 units/l (30 C)	f
Lipase, serum	0–1.5 units (Cherry-Crandall)	0–1.5 units (Cherry-Crandall)	f
Lipids, total, serum	450–850 mg/dl	4.5–8.5 g/l	m
Lipoprotein cholesterol, serum			
LDL cholesterol	60–180 mg/dl	600–1800 mg/l	
HDL cholesterol	30–80 mg/dl	300–800 mg/l	
Luteinizing hormone (LH), serum			
Males	6–18 milliunits/ml (I.U.)	6–18 IU/l	
Females, premenopausal	5–22 milliunits/ml (I.U.)	5–22 IU/l	
midcycle	3 times baseline	3 times baseline	
postmenopausal	Greater than 30 milliunits/ml (I.U.)	Greater than 30 IU/l	
Magnesium, serum	1.5–2.5 mEq/liter	0.75–1.25 mmol/l	
	1.8–3.0 mg/dl		
5'-Nucleotidase, serum	3.5–12.7 milliunits/ml (37°)	3.5–12.5 units/l (37 C)	f
Nitrogen, nonprotein, serum	15–35 mg/dl	10.7–25.0 mmol/l	
Osmolality, serum	285–295 mOsm/kg serum water	285–295 mmol/kg serum water	n
Oxygen, blood			
Capacity	16–24 vol % (varies with hemoglobin)	7.14–10.7 mmol/l (varies with hemoglobin)	o
Content Arterial	15–23 vol %	6.69–10.3 mmol/l	o
Venous	10–16 vol %	4.46–7.14 mmol/l	o
Saturation Arterial	94–100% of capacity	0.94–1.00 of capacity	a
Venous	60–85% of capacity	0.60–0.85 of capacity	a
Tension, PO_2 Arterial	75–100 mm Hg	75–100 mm Hg	g
P$_{50}$, blood	26–27 mm Hg	26–27 mm Hg	g

Reference Values for Blood, Plasma, and Serum *Continued*
(For some procedures the reference values may vary depending upon the method used)

	Conventional Units	S.I. Units	Notes
pH, arterial, blood	7.35–7.45	7.35–7.45	p
Phenylalanine, serum	Less than 3 mg/dl	Less than 0.18 mmol/l	
Phosphatase, acid serum	0.11–0.60 milliunit/ml (37°)	0.11–0.60 units/l	f
	(Roy, Brower, Hayden)		
Phosphatase, alkaline, serum (ALP)	20–90 milliunits/ml (30°)	20–90 units/l (30 C)	f
	(Values are higher in children)	(Values are higher in children)	
Phosphate, inorganic, serum			
Adults	3.0–4.5 mg/dl	1.0–1.5 mmol/l	
Children	4.0–7.0 mg/dl	1.3–2.3 mmol/l	
Phospholipids, serum	6–12 mg/dl	1.9–3.9 mmol/l	
	(As lipid phosphorus)	(As lipid phosphorus)	
Potassium, serum	3.5–5.0 mEq/liter	3.5–5.0 mmol/l	
Prolactin, serum			
Males	1–20 nanogm/ml	1–20 μg/l	
Females	1–25 nanogm/ml	1–25 μg/l	
Protein, serum			
Total	6.0–8.0 grams/dl	60–80 g/l	m
Albumin	3.5–5.5 grams/dl	35–55 g/l	q
	52–68% of total	0.52–0.68 of total	a
Globulin			
Alpha$_1$	0.2–0.4 gram/dl	2–4 g/l	m
	2–5% of total	0.02–0.05 of total	a
Alpha$_2$	0.5–0.9 gram/dl	5–9 g/l	m
	7–14% of total	0.07–0.14 of total	a
Beta	0.6–1.1 grams/dl	6–11 g/l	m
	9–15% of total	0.09–0.15 of total	a
Gamma	0.7–1.7 grams/dl	7–17 g/l	m
	11–21% of total	0.11–0.21 of total	a
Protoporphyrin, erythrocyte	27–61 mcg/dl packed RBC	0.48–1.09 μmol/l packed RBC	
Pyruvate, blood	0.3–0.9 mg/dl	0.03–0.10 mmol/l	
Sodium, serum	136–145 mEq/liter	136–145 mmol/l	
Sulfates, inorganic, serum	0.8–1.2 mg/dl	83–125 μmol/l	
Testosterone, plasma			
Males	275–875 nanogm/dl	9.5–30 nmol/l	
Females	23–75 nanogm/dl	0.8–2.6 nmol/l	
Pregnant	38–190 nanogm/dl	1.3–6.6 nmol/l	
Thyroid-stimulating hormone (TSH), serum	0–7 microunits/ml	0–7 milliunits/l	
Thyroxine, free, serum	1.0–2.1 nanogm/dl	13–27 pmol/l	
Thyroxine (T$_4$), serum	4.4–9.9 mcg/dl	57–128 nmol/l	
Thyroxine binding globulin (TBG), serum (as thyroxine)	10–26 mcg/dl	129–335 nmol/l	
Thyroxine iodine, serum	2.9–6.4 mcg/dl	229–504 nmol/l	k
Triiodothyronine (T$_3$), serum	150–250 nanogm/dl	2.3–3.9 nmol/l	
Triiodothyronine (T$_3$) uptake, resin (T$_3$RU)	25–38% uptake	0.25–0.38 uptake	a
Transaminase, serum			
SGOT (aspartate aminotransferase, AST)	8–20 milliunits/ml (30°)	8–20 units/l (30 C)	
	7–40 milliunits/ml (37°)	7–40 units/l (37 C)	
SGPT (alanine aminotransferase, ALT)	8–20 milliunits/ml (30°)	8–20 units/l (30 C)	f
	5–35 milliunits/ml (37°)	5–35 units/l (37 C)	f
Triglycerides, serum	40–150 mg/dl	0.4–1.5 g/l	r
		0.45–1.71 mmol/l	
Urate, serum			
Males	2.5–8.0 mg/dl	0.15–0.48 mmol/l	
Females	1.5–7.0 mg/dl	0.09–0.42 mmol/l	
Urea			
Blood	21–43 mg/dl	3.5–7.3 mmol/l	
Plasma or serum	24–49 mg/dl	4.0–8.3 mmol/l	
Urea nitrogen			
Blood	10–20 mg/dl	7.1–14.3 mmol/l	k
Plasma or serum	11–23 mg/dl	7.9–16.4 mmol/l	
Viscosity, serum	1.4–1.8 times water	1.4–1.8 times water	
Vitamin A, serum	20–80 mcg/dl	0.70–2.8 μmol/l	
Vitamin B$_{12}$, serum	180–900 picogm/ml	133–664 pmol/l	

Reference Values for Urine
(For some procedures the reference values may vary depending upon the method used)

	Conventional Units	S.I. Units	Notes
Acetone and acetoacetate, qualitative	Negative	Negative	
Albumin			
Qualitative	Negative	Negative	
Quantitative	10–100 mg/24 hrs	10–100 mg/24 h	q
		0.15–1.5 μmol/24 h	
Aldosterone	3–20 mcg/24 hrs	8.3–55 nmol/24 h	
Alpha amino nitrogen	50–200 mg/24 hrs	3.6–14.3 mmol/24 h	
Ammonia nitrogen	20–70 mEq/24 hrs	20–70 mmol/24 h	
Amylase	1–17 units/hr	1–17 units/h	f
Amylase/creatinine clearance ratio	1–4%	0.01–0.04	
Bilirubin, qualitative	Negative	Negative	
Calcium			
Low Ca diet	Less than 150 mg/24 hrs	Less than 3.8 mmol/24 h	
Usual diet	Less than 250 mg/24 hrs	Less than 6.3 mmol/24 h	
Catecholamines			
Epinephrine	Less than 10 mcg/24 hrs	Less than 55 nmol/24 h	
Norepinephrine	Less than 100 mcg/24 hrs	Less than 590 nmol/24 h	
Total free catecholamines	4–126 mcg/24 hrs	24–745 nmol/24 h	s
Total metanephrines	0.1–1.6 mg/24 hrs	0.5–8.1 μmol/24 h	t
Chloride	110–250 mEq/24 hrs	110–250 mmol/24 h	
	(Varies with intake)	(Varies with intake)	
Chorionic gonadotropin	0	0	
Copper	0–50 mcg/24 hrs	0–0.80 μmol/24 h	
Cortisol, free	10–100 mcg/24 hrs	27.6–276 mmol/24 h	
Creatine			
Males	0–40 mg/24 hrs	0–0.30 mmol/24 h	
Females	0–100 mg/24 hrs	0–0.76 mmol/24 h	
	(Higher in children and during pregnancy)	(Higher in children and during pregnancy)	
Creatinine	15–25 mg/kg body weight/24 hrs	0.13–0.22 mmol·kg⁻¹body weight/24 h	
Creatinine clearance			
Males	110–150 ml/min	110–150 ml/min	
Females	105–132 ml/min	105–132 ml/min	
	(1.73 sq meter surface area)	(1.73 m² surface area)	
Cystine or cysteine, qualitative	Negative	Negative	
Dehydroepiandrosterone	Less than 15% of total 17-ketosteroids	Less than 0.15 of total 17-ketosteroids	a
Males	0.2–2.0 mg/24 hrs	0.7–6.9 μmol/24 h	
Females	0.2–1.8 mg/24 hrs	0.7–6.2 μmol/24 h	
Delta aminolevulinic acid	1.3–7.0 mg/24 hrs	10–53 μmol/24 h	
Estrogens			
Males			
Estrone	3–8 μg/24 hrs	11–30 nmol/24 h	
Estradiol	0–6 μg/24 hrs	0–22 nmol/24 h	
Estriol	1–11 μg/24 hrs	3–38 nmol/24 h	
Total	4–25 μg/24 hrs	14–90 nmol/24 h	u
Females			
Estrone	4–31 μg/24 hrs	15–115 nmol/24 h	
Estradiol	0–14 μg/24 hrs	0–51 nmol/24 h	
Estriol	0–72 μg/24 hrs	0–250 nmol/24 h	
Total	5–100 μg/24 hrs	18–360 nmol/24 h	u
	(Markedly increased during pregnancy)	(Markedly increased during pregnancy)	
Glucose (as reducing substance)	Less than 250 mg/24 hrs	Less than 250 mg/24 h	
Hemoglobin and myoglobin, qualitative	Negative	Negative	

Reference Values for Urine *Continued*
(For some procedures the reference values may vary depending upon the method used)

	Conventional Units	S.I. Units	Notes
Homogentisic acid, qualitative	Negative	Negative	
17-Hydroxycorticosteroids			
Males	3–9 mg/24 hrs	8.3–25 μmol/24 h	j
Females	2–8 mg/24 hrs	5.5–22 μmol/24 h	
5-Hydroxyindoleacetic acid			
Qualitative	Negative	Negative	
Quantitative	Less than 9 mg/24 hrs	Less than 47 μmol/24 h	
17-Ketosteroids			
Males	6–18 mg/24 hrs	21–62 μmol/24 h	l
Females	4–13 mg/24 hrs	14–45 μmol/24 h	
	(Varies with age)	(Varies with age)	
Magnesium	6.0–8.5 mEq/24 hrs	3.0–4.3 mmol/24 h	
Metanephrines (see Catecholamines)			
Osmolality	38–1400 mOsm/kg water	38–1400 mmol/kg water	n
pH	4.6–8.0, average 6.0	4.6–8.0, average 6.0	p
	(Depends on diet)	(Depends on diet)	
Phenolsulfonphthalein excretion (PSP)	25% or more in 15 min	0.25 or more in 15 min	a
	40% or more in 30 min	0.40 or more in 30 min	
	55% or more in 2 hrs	0.55 or more in 2 h	
	(After injection of 1 ml PSP intravenously)	(After injection of 1 ml PSP intravenously)	
Phenylpyruvic acid, qualitative	Negative	Negative	
Phosphorus	0.9–1.3 gram/24 hrs	29–42 mmol/24 h	
Porphobilinogen			
Qualitative	Negative	Negative	
Quantitative	0–0.2 mg/dl	0–0.9 μmol/l	
	Less than 2.0 mg/24 hrs	Less than 9 μmol/24 h	
Porphyrins			
Coproporphyrin	50–250 mcg/24 hrs	77–380 nmol/24 h	
Uroporphyrin	10–30 mcg/24 hrs	12–36 nmol/24 h	
Potassium	25–100 mEq/24 hrs	25–100 mmol/24 h	
	(Varies with intake)	(Varies with intake)	
Pregnanediol			
Males	0.4–1.4 mg/24 hrs	1.2–4.4 μmol/24 h	
Females			
Proliferative phase	0.5–1.5 mg/24 hrs	1.6–4.7 μmol/24 h	
Luteal phase	2.0–7.0 mg/24 hrs	6.2–22 μmol/24 h	
Postmenopausal phase	0.2–1.0 mg/24 hrs	0.6–3.1 μmol/24 h	
Pregnanetriol	Less than 2.5 mg/24 hrs in adults	Less than 7.4 μmol/24 h in adults	
Protein			
Qualitative	Negative	Negative	
Quantitative	10–150 mg/24 hrs	10–150 mg/24 h	m
Sodium	130–260 mEq/24 hrs	130–260 mmol/24 h	
	(Varies with intake)	(Varies with intake)	
Specific gravity	1.003–1.030	1.003–1.030	
Titratable acidity	20–40 mEq/24 hrs	20–40 mmol/24 h	
Urate	200–500 mg/24 hrs	1.2–3.0 mmol/24 h	
	(With normal diet)	(With normal diet)	
Urobilinogen	Up to 1.0 Ehrlich unit/2 hrs	Up to 1.0 Ehrlich unit/2 h	
	(1–3 PM)	(1–3 PM)	
	0–4.0 mg/24 hrs	0–6.8 μmol/24 h	
Vanillylmandelic acid (VMA) (4-hydroxy-3-methoxymandelic acid)	1–8 mg/24 hrs	5–40 μmol/24 h	

Reference Values for Therapeutic Drug Monitoring

Drug	Therapeutic Range	Toxic Levels	Proprietary Names
Antibiotics			
Amikacin, serum	15–25 mcg/ml	Peak: >35 mcg/ml	Amikin
		Trough: >5–8 mcg/ml	
Chloramphenicol, serum	10–20 mcg/ml	>25 mcg/ml	Chloromycetin
Gentamicin, serum	5–10 mcg/ml	Peak: >12 mcg/ml	Garamycin
		Trough: >2 mcg/ml	
Tobramycin, serum	5–10 mcg/ml	Peak: >12 mcg/ml	Nebcin
		Trough: >2 mcg/ml	
Anticonvulsants			
Carbamazepine, serum	5–12 mcg/ml	>12 mcg/ml	Tegretol
Ethosuximide, serum	40–100 mcg/ml	>100 mcg/ml	Zarontin
Phenobarbital, serum	10–30 mcg/ml	Vary widely because of developed tolerance	
Phenytoin, serum (diphenylhydantoin)	10–20 mcg/ml	>20 mcg/ml	Dilantin
Primidone, serum	5–12 mcg/ml	>15 mcg/ml	Mysoline
Valproic acid, serum	50–100 mcg/ml	>100 mcg/ml	Depakene
Analgesics			
Acetaminophen, serum	10–20 mcg/ml	>250 mcg/ml	Tylenol
			Datril
Salicylate, serum	100–250 mcg/ml	>300 mcg/ml	
Bronchodilator			
Theophylline (aminophylline)	10–20 mcg/ml	>20 mcg/ml	
Cardiovascular drugs			
Digitoxin, serum	15–25 nanogm/ml (Specimen obtained 12–24 hrs after last dose)	>25 nanogm/ml	Crystodigin
Digoxin, serum	0.8–2 nanogm/ml (Specimen obtained 12–24 hrs after last dose)	>2.4 nanogm/ml	Lanoxin
Disopyramide, serum	2–5 mcg/ml	>5 mcg/ml	Norpace
Lidocaine, serum	1.5–5 mcg/ml	>5 nanogm/ml	Anestacon
			Xylocaine
Procainamide, serum	4–10 mcg/ml	>16 mcg/ml	Pronestyl
	*10–30 mcg/ml (*Procainamide + N-Acetyl Procainamide)	*>30 mcg/ml	
Propranolol, serum	50–100 nanogm/ml	Variable	Inderal
Quinidine, serum	2–5 mcg/ml	>10 mcg/ml	Cardioquin
			Quinaglute
			Quinidex
			Quinora
Psychopharmacologic drugs			
Amitriptyline, serum	*120–150 nanogm/ml (*Amitriptyline + Nortriptyline)	*>500 nanogm/ml	Amitril
			Elavil
			Endep
			Etrafon
			Limbitrol
			Triavil
Desipramine, serum	*150–300 nanogm/ml (*Desipramine + Imipramine)	*>500 nanogm/ml	Norpramin
			Pertofrane
Imipramine, serum	*150–300 nanogm/ml (*Imipramine + Desipramine)	*>500 nanogm/ml	Antipress
			Imavate
			Janimine
			Presamine
			Tofranil
Lithium, serum	0.8–1.2 mEq/liter (Specimen obtained 12 hrs after last dose)	>2.0 mEq/liter	Lithobid
			Lithotabs
Nortriptyline, serum	50–150 nanogm/ml	>500 nanogm/ml	Aventyl
			Pamelor

Reference Values in Toxicology

	Conventional Units	S.I. Units	Notes
Arsenic, blood	3.5–7.2 mcg/dl	0.47–0.96 μmol/l	
Arsenic, urine	Less than 100 mcg/24 hrs	Less than 1.3 μmol/24 h	
Bromides, serum	0	0	
	Toxic levels: Above 17 mmol/l	Toxic levels: Above 17 mmol/l	
Carbon monoxide, blood	Up to 5% saturation	Up to 0.5 saturation	
	Symptoms occur with 20% saturation	Symptoms occur with 0.20 saturation	a
Ethanol, blood	Less than 0.005%	Less than 1 mmol/l	
Marked intoxication	0.3–0.4%	65–87 mmol/l	
Alcoholic stupor	0.4–0.5% mcg/dl	87–109 mmol/l	
Coma	Above 0.5%	Above 109 mmol/l	
Lead, blood	0–40 mcg/dl	0–2 μmol/l	
Lead, urine	Less than 100 mcg/24 hrs	Less than 0.48 μmol/24 h	
Mercury, urine	Less than 100 mcg/24 hrs	Less than 50 nmol/24 h	

Reference Values for Cerebrospinal Fluid

	Conventional Units	S.I. Units	Notes
Cells	Fewer than 5/cu mm; all mononuclear	Fewer than 5/μl; all mononuclear	
Chloride	120–130 mEq/liter	120–130 mmol/l	
	(20 mEq/liter higher than serum)	(20 mmol/l higher than serum)	
Electrophoresis	Predominantly albumin	Predominantly albumin	
Glucose	50–75 mg/dl	2.8–4.2 mmol/l	
	(20 mg/dl less than serum)	(1.1 mmol/less than serum)	
IgG			
Children under 14	Less than 8% of total protein	Less than 0.08 of total protein	a,m
Adults	Less than 14% of total protein	Less than 0.14 of total protein	
Pressure	70–180 mm water	70–180 mm water	g
Protein, total	15–45 mg/dl	0.150–0.450 g/l	m
	(Higher, up to 70 mg/dl, in elderly adults and children)	(Higher, up to 0.70 g/l, in elderly adults and children)	

Reference Values for Gastric Analysis

	Conventional Units	S.I. Units	Notes
Basal gastric secretion (1 hour)			
Concentration	(Mean ± 1 S.D.)	(Mean ± 1 S.D.)	
Males	25.8 ± 1.8 mEq/liter	25.8 ± 1.8 mmol/l	
Females	20.3 ± 3.0 mEq/liter	20.3 ± 3.0 mmol/l	
Output	(Mean ± 1 S.D.)	(Mean ± 1 S.D.)	
Males	2.57 ± 0.16 mEq/hr	2.57 ± 0.16 mmol/h	
Females	1.61 ± 0.18 mEq/hr	1.61 ± 0.18 mmol/h	
After histamine stimulation			
Normal	Mean output 11.8 mEq/hr	Mean output 11.8 mmol/h	
Duodenal ulcer	Mean output 15.2 mEq/hr	Mean output 15.2 mmol/h	
After maximal histamine stimulation			
Normal	Mean output 22.6 mEq/hr	Mean output 22.6 mmol/h	
Duodenal ulcer	Mean output 44.6 mEq/hr	Mean output 44.6 mmol/h	
Volume, fasting stomach content	50–100 ml	50–100 ml	
Emptying time	3–6 hrs	3–6 h	
Color	Opalescent or colorless	Opalescent or colorless	
Specific gravity	1.006–1.009	1.006–1.009	
pH (adults)	0.9–1.5	0.9–1.5	p

Gastrointestinal Absorption Tests

	Conventional Units	S.I. Units
D-Xylose absorption test	After an 8 hour fast, 10 ml/kg body weight of a 0.05 solution of D-xylose is given by mouth. Nothing further by mouth is given until the test has been completed. All urine voided during the following 5 hours is pooled, and blood samples are taken at 0, 60, and 120 minutes. Normally 0.26 (range 0.16–0.33) of ingested xylose is excreted within 5 hours, and the serum xylose reaches a level between 25 and 40 mg/100 dl after 1 hour and is maintained at this level for another 60 minutes.	No change
Vitamin A absorption	A fasting blood specimen is obtained and 200,000 units of vitamin A in oil is given by mouth. Serum vitamin A level should rise to twice fasting level in 3 to 5 hours.	No change

Reference Values for Feces

	Conventional Units	S.I. Units	Notes
Bulk	100–200 grams/24 hrs	100–200 g/24 h	
Dry matter	23–32 grams/24 hrs	23–32 g/24 h	
Fat, total	Less than 6.0 grams/24 hrs	Less than 6.0 g/24 h	
Nitrogen, total	Less than 2.0 grams/24 hrs	Less than 2.0 g/24 h	
Urobilinogen	40–280 mg/24 hrs	40–280 mg/24 h	
Water	Approximately 65%	Approximately 0.65	a

Reference Values for Immunologic Procedures

	Conventional Units
Lymphocyte subsets	
T cells	60–85%
B cells	1–20%
T-helper cells	35–60%
T-suppressor cells	15–30%
T-H/S ratio	1.5–2.5
Complement	
C3	85–175 mg/dl
C4	15–45 mg/dl
CH_{50}	25–55 H_{50} units/ml
Tumor markers	
Carcinoembryonic antigen (CEA)	
(Roche)	Less than 5 nanogm/ml
(Abbott)	Less than 4.1 nanogm/ml
Alpha-fetoprotein (AFP)	Less than 10–30 nanogm/ml (depends on method)

Reference Values for Semen Analysis

	Conventional Units	S.I. Units	Notes
Volume	2–5 ml; usually 3–4 ml	2–5 ml; usually 3–4 ml	
Liquefaction	Complete in 15 min	Complete in 15 min	
pH	7.2–8.0; average 7.8	7.2–8.0; average 7.8	p
Leukocytes	Occasional or absent	Occasional or absent	
Count	60–150 million/ml	60–150 million/ml	
	Below 60 million/ml is abnormal	Below 60 million/ml is abnormal	
Motility	80% or more motile	0.80 or more motile	a
Morphology	80–90% normal forms	0.80–0.90 normal forms	a

Oral Glucose Tolerance Test

The oral glucose tolerance test (OGTT) may be unnecessary if the fasting plasma glucose concentration is elevated (venous plasma ≥140 mg/dl or 7.8 mmol/l) on two occasions. The OGTT should be carried out only on patients who are ambulatory and otherwise healthy and who are known not to be taking agents that elevate the plasma glucose (see reference 10). The test should be conducted in the morning after at least 3 days of unrestricted diet (≥150 grams of carbohydrate) and physical activity. The subject should have fasted for at least 10 hours but no more than 16 hours. Water is permitted during the test period; however, the subject should remain seated and should not smoke throughout the test.

The dose of glucose administered should be 75 grams (1.75 grams per kg of ideal body weight, up to a maximum of 75 grams for children). Commercial preparations containing a suitable carbohydrate load are acceptable. If criteria for gestational diabetes are used, a dose of 100 grams of glucose is required.

A fasting blood sample should be collected, after which the glucose dose is taken within 5 minutes. Blood samples should be collected at 30 minute intervals for 2 hours (for gestational diabetes, fasting 1, 2, and 3 hours). The following diagnostic criteria have been recommended by the National Diabetes Data Group:

Normal OGTT in Nonpregnant Adults	Fasting venous plasma glucose <115 mg/dl (6.4 mmol/l); ½ h, 1 h, and 1½ h OGTT venous plasma glucose <200 mg/dl (11.1 mmol/l); 2 h OGTT venous plasma glucose <140 mg/dl (7.8 mmol/l)
Diabetes Mellitus in Nonpregnant Adults	Both the 2 hour sample *and* some other sample taken between administration of the 75 gram glucose dose and 2 hours later must show a venous plasma glucose ≥200 mg/dl (11.1 mmol/l)
Impaired Glucose Tolerance in Nonpregnant Adults	Three criteria must be met: Fasting venous plasma glucose <140 mg/dl (7.8 mmol/l); ½ h, 1 h, or 1½ h OGTT value ≥200 mg/dl (11.1 mmol/l); 2 h OGTT venous plasma glucose between 140 and 200 mg/dl (7.8 and 11.1 mmol/l)
Gestational Diabetes	Two or more of the following values after a 100 gram oral glucose challenge must be met or exceeded: (values are for venous plasma glucose)

Fasting	105 mg/dl	5.8 mmol/l
1h	190 mg/dl	10.6 mmol/l
2h	165 mg/dl	9.2 mmol/l
3h	145 mg/dl	8.1 mmol/l

NOTES

a. Percentage is expressed as a decimal fraction.

b. Percentage may be expressed as a decimal fraction; however, when the result expressed is itself a variable fraction of another variable, the absolute value is more meaningful. There is no reason, other than custom, for expressing reticulocyte counts and differential leukocyte counts in percentages or decimal fractions rather than in absolute numbers.

c. Molecular weight of fibrinogen = 341,000 daltons.

d. Molecular weight of hemoglobin = 64,500 daltons. Because of disagreement as to whether the monomer or tetramer of hemoglobin should be used in the conversion, it has been recommended that the conventional grams per deciliter be retained. The tetramer is used in the table; values given should be multiplied by 4 to obtain concentration of the monomer.

e. Molecular weight of methemoglobin = 64,500 daltons. See note d above.

f. Enzyme units have not been changed in these tables because the proposed enzyme unit, the katal, has not been universally adopted (1 International Unit = 16.7 nkat).

g. It has been proposed that pressure be expressed in the pascal (1 mm Hg = 0.133 kPa); however, this convention has not been universally accepted.

h. Molecular weight of ceruloplasmin = 151,000 daltons.

i. "Fatty acids" includes a mixture of different aliphatic acids of varying molecular weight. A mean molecular weight of 284 daltons has been assumed in calculating the conversion factor.

j. Based upon molecular weight of cortisol 362.47 daltons.

k. The practice of expressing concentration of an organic molecule in terms of one of its constituent elements originated when measurements included a heterogeneous class of compounds (nonprotein nitrogenous compounds, iodine-containing compounds bound to serum proteins). It was carried over to expressing measurements of specific substances (urea, thyroxine), but the practice should be discarded. For iodine and nitrogen 1 mole is taken as the monoatomic form, although they occur as diatomic molecules.

l. Based upon molecular weight of dehydroepiandrosterone 288.41 daltons.

m. Weight per volume is retained as the unit because of the heterogeneous nature of the material measured.

n. The proposal that osmolality be reported as freezing point depression using the millikelvin as the unit has not been received with universal enthusiasm. The milliosmole is not an S.I. unit, and the unit used here is the millimole.

o. Volumes per cent might be converted to a decimal fraction; however, this would not permit direct correlation with hemoglobin content, which is possible when oxygen content and capacity are expressed in molar quantities. One millimole of hemoglobin combines with 4 millimoles of oxygen.

p. Hydrogen ion concentration in S.I. units would be expressed in nanomoles per liter; however, this change has not received general approval. Conversion can be calculated as antilog ($-$pH).

q. Albumin is expressed in grams per liter to be consistent with units used for other proteins. Concentration of albumin may be expressed in mmol/l also, an expression that permits assessment of binding capacity of albumin for substances such as bilirubin. Molecular weight of albumin is 65,000 daltons.

r. Most techniques for quantitating triglycerides measure the glycerol moiety, and the total mass is calculated using an average molecular weight. The factor given assumes a mean molecular weight of 875 daltons for triglycerides.

s. Calculated as norepinephrine, molecular weight 169.18 daltons.

t. Calculated as metanephrine, molecular weight 197.23 daltons.

u. Conversion factor calculated from molecular weights of estrone, estradiol, and estriol in proportions of 2:1:2 daltons.

REFERENCES

1. AMA Drug Evaluations, 6th ed. Chicago, American Medical Association, 1986.
2. AMA Council on Scientific Affairs: J.A.M.A. *253*:2552, 1985.
3. Goodman, A. G., Gilman, L. S., Rall, T. W., and Murad, F.: Goodman and Gilman's The Pharmacological Basis of Therapeutics, 7th ed. New York, Macmillan, 1985.
4. Henry, J. B.: Clinical Diagnosis and Management by Laboratory Methods, 17th ed. Philadelphia, W. B. Saunders Company, 1984.
5. Henry, R. J., Cannon, D. C., and Winkleman, J. W.: Clinical Chemistry—Principles and Techniques, 2nd ed. New York, Harper & Row, 1974.
6. International Committee for Standardization in Hematology, International Federation of Clinical Chemistry and World Association of Pathology Societies: Clin. Chem. *19*:135, 1973.
7. Lundberg, G. D., Iverson, C., and Radulescu, G.: J.A.M.A. *255*:2247, 1986.
8. Miale, J. B.: Laboratory Medicine—Hematology, 6th ed. St. Louis, C. V. Mosby, 1982.
9. National Diabetes Data Group: Diabetes *28*:1039, 1979.
10. Page, C. H., and Vigourex, P.: The International System of Units (S.I.). U.S. Department of Commerce, National Bureau of Standards, Special Publication 330, 1974.
11. Physicians' Desk Reference, 43rd ed. Oradell, N.J., Medical Economics Company, 1989.
12. Scully, R. E., McNeely, B. U., and Mark, E. J.: N. Engl. J. Med. *314*:39, 1986.
13. Tietz, N. W.: Clinical Guide to Laboratory Tests. Philadelphia, W. B. Saunders Company, 1983.
14. Tietz, N. W.: Textbook of Clinical Chemistry. Philadelphia, W. B. Saunders Company, 1986.
15. Williams, W. J., Beutler, E., Erslev, A. J., and Lichtman, M. A.: Hematology, 3rd ed. New York, McGraw-Hill Book Company, 1983.

Some of the values have been established by the Clinical Pathology Laboratories, Emory University Hospital, Atlanta, Georgia, or by the Clinical Laboratories, Thomas Jefferson University Hospital, Philadelphia, Pennsylvania, and have not been published elsewhere.

NOMOGRAM FOR THE DETERMINATION OF BODY SURFACE AREA OF CHILDREN AND ADULTS*

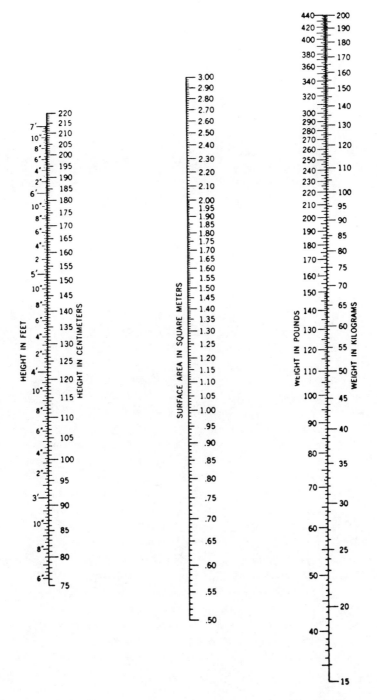

*From Boothby, W. M., and Sandiford, R. B.: Boston Med. Surg. J. *185*:337, 1921.

Index

Note: Page numbers in *italics* refer to illustrations; page numbers followed by (t) refer to tables.

Skin *(Continued)*
T cell lymphoma involving, 383, 390
tumors of, malignant, 708–709
premalignant, 731–734
ulcers of, 751–755
vasculitic lesions of, 718–721
lupus erythematosus and, 714
viral infection of, 737(t), 737–740
Skin care, for decubitus ulcers, 753–754
Skin graft, for burns, 1036
Skull fracture, 859–860. See also *Head, trauma to.*
Small cell lung cancer, 151
treatment of, 154–155
Small intestine, bacterial overgrowth in, 464–465
due to diverticula, 438
diverticula of, 437–438
ischemia of, 466
malabsorption due to primary disorders of, 465
resection of, diet after, 466
Small noncleaved cell lymphoma, 388–389
Smoking cessation, in management of COPD, 145, 146(t)
Snake bite, 1047–1050, 1049(t)
antivenin for, 1049, 1049(t), 1050, 1054(t)
Social worker, role of, in rehabilitation of stroke patient, 789
Sodium, diminished serum levels of, 550, 551(t)
as complication of prostate surgery, 632
treatment of, 552
elevated serum levels of, treatment of, 552
Sodium nitroprusside, for heart failure, 284(t), 286
in patient presenting with acute pulmonary edema, 242, 243, 243(t)
for hypertension, 262(t)
in advanced cardiac life support, 214(t)
Sodium restriction, in management of hypertension, 252
in management of renal failure, 638, 643
Sodium stibogluconate, for leishmaniasis, 80
Sodium tetradecyl sulfate, for mucoid cyst involving nail, 725
Soft tissue bleeding, in hemophilia, 343
Solar cheilitis, 746
Solar lentigines, 769
Solar urticaria, 775
Solitary plasmacytoma, osseous, 395
Solvents, poisoning by, 1074
Sotalol, 1086(t)
Spacers (reservoir devices), for administration of beta-adrenergic agonists, 146, 147(t)
Spasm, diffuse esophageal, 435
infantile, 806
Spasticity, in multiple sclerosis, 824
Spectinomycin, for gonorrhea, 666
Speech pathology, after stroke, 789
Spermicides, 996–997

Spider bites, 1045(t), 1045–1047
antivenin for, 1047, 1054(t)
Spine, osteoarthritis of, 886–887
Spiramycin, for toxoplasmosis, 127, 128
Spirillum minus infection, 106, 106(t)
Spironolactone, for Cushing's syndrome, 566
for hypertension, 254(t)
Splenectomy, and infection, 326
for autoimmune hemolytic anemia, 314
for hemolytic anemia, 319
for leukemia, 378, 381, 382
for thalassemia, 326
Splenic sequestration, 350
in sickle cell disease, 331
Splenorenal shunt, for bleeding esophageal varices, 421, 422
Spondylitis, ankylosing, 878–880
in Crohn's disease, 450
Spontaneous bacterial peritonitis, in patients with cirrhotic ascites, 427
Sporotrichosis, 746
Sports injuries, 893–895
Sprains, 895(t)
Sprue, 465–466
Sputum, abnormal, 25
Squamous cell carcinoma, of oral cavity, 749
of skin, 708
of vulva, 986–990, 988(t), 989(t)
Squaric acid dibutyl ester, induction of dermatitis with, to promote hair growth, in alopecia areata, 707
Staging, of acquired immunodeficiency syndrome, 37, 38(t)
of cancer, of adrenals, 649(t)
of breast, 954(t)
of cervix, 984(t)
of lung, 151–152, 152(t)
of penis, 659(t)
of testis, 658(t)
of uterus, 981(t)
of vulva, 988, 988(t)
of chronic lymphocytic leukemia, 379–380, 380(t)
of Hodgkin's disease, 359(t)
of mycosis fungoides, 390, 390(t)
of myeloma, 393
of non-Hodgkin's lymphoma, 384, 385(t)
Stanford protocol, for non-Hodgkin's lymphoma, 387(t)
Staphylococcal endocarditis, antimicrobials for, 247(t), 247–248, 248(t)
Staphylococcal enterotoxins, 69
Staphylococcal scalded skin syndrome, 735
Staphylococcal skin infection, 734, 735
in atopic dermatitis, 756, 758
Status asthmaticus, treatment of, 689–690
Status epilepticus, drugs for, 800–801, 804(t), 807
Stenosis, aortic valve, 234–235
carotid, surgery for, 786
pulmonary valve, 234
Sterilization, 994
Steroid(s). See also specific drugs, e.g., *Prednisone.*
for acne, 704

Steroid(s) *(Continued)*
for acne rosacea, 705
for allergic rhinitis, 694
for asthma, 680, 680(t), 682, 683, 687, 689, 690
for atopic dermatitis, 757
for bullous pemphigoid, 760–761
for carditis, in rheumatic fever, 110
for cerebral edema, due to brain tumor, 866
due to surgery for brain abscess, 778
for chronic obstructive pulmonary disease, 142, 148(t), 148–149, 149(t)
for contact dermatitis, 762, 763
for Crohn's disease, 449
for dermatitis, 724
for dermatomyositis, 716
for epidermolysis bullosa acquisita, 762
for erythema multiforme, 758
for gouty arthritis, 515
for hepatitis, 460
for herpes gestationis, 764
for hyperpigmentation, 769
for hypersenstivity pneumonitis, 186
for hypoadrenocorticism, 561, 562, 577
for hypogonadotropic hypogonadism, 576
for increased intracranial pressure, due to brain tumor, 866
for keloids, 725
for leukemia, 380
for multiple sclerosis, 827
for myasthenia gravis, 832–833
for nail psoriasis, 724
for osteoarthritis, 885
for pemphigoid, 751, 760–761
for pemphigus, 751, 760–761
for pruritic urticarial papules and plaques, in pregnant patient, 764
for pruritus, 33, 34, 764, 765
in lichen planus, 712, 713
in pityriasis rosea, 712
for psoriasis, 710
for renal disease, in lupus erythematosus, 715
for rheumatoid arthritis, 872
in children, 876
for rosacea, 705
for sarcoidosis, 181
for seborrheic dermatitis, 709–710
for tendinitis, 884
for tetanus, 125
for ulcerative colitis, 444, 445, 446
for vasculitis, 720, 721
for vitiligo, 770–771
replacement therapy with, after surgery for Cushing's disease, 566
use of, in patients with AIDS, 50
Stevens-Johnson syndrome, 750, 758
Stings, allergic reactions to, 698–700, 700(t)
Stomach, adenocarcinoma of, 483
adenoma of, 482
atrophy of mucosa of, 657
bleeding from, due to stress ulcers, 656